DISEASES AND ICD-9CM CODES

Acne   706.1
Adrenal Insufficient   255.4
Alcoholism   303.9
Alopecia   704.00
Altered Mental State   780.9
Altitude Sickness   993.2
Alzheimer's Disease   331.0
Amebiasis   006.9
Amenorrhea   626.0
Anaphylaxis   995.0
Anemia, Megaloblastic   281.9
Anemia, Sickle Cell   282.60
Angina   413.9
Angioedema   995.1
Animal Bites   879.8
Ankle Fractures   824.8
Anorexia Nervosa   307.1
Anuria   788.5
Aortic Dissection   441.00
Appendicitis   541
Arrhythmias   427.9
Arthritis, Rheumatoid   714.0
Ascaris Infection   127.0
Ascites   789.5
Asthma   493.9
Atelectasis   518.0
Atrial Fibrillation   427.31
Bacteremia   790.7
Basal Cell Carcinoma   173.9
Bell's Palsy   351.0
Bladder Cancer   188.9
Blastomycosis   116.0
Bleeding Disorders   287.9
Blood Transfusion, Adverse Reaction to   999.8
Bowel Obstruction (small and large bowel)   560.9
Brain Tumor   239.6
Breast Cancer   174.9
Bronchiectasis   494
Bronchiolitis   466.19
Bronchitis   490
Bulimia Nervosa   307.51
Burns   949.0
Bursitis   727.3
Calluses   700
Cancer Screening   V76.9
Cardiac Arrest   427.5
Cardiomyopathy   425.4
Carpal Tunnel Syndrome   354.0
Cellulitis   682.9
Cellulitis, Orbital   376.01
Cervical Cancer   180.9
Cervicitis   616.0
Cheilitis   528.5
Cheilitis, Angular   528.5
Cholecystitis   575.1
Chronic Fatigue Syndrome   780.71
Chronic Obstructive Pulmonary Disease   496

Cirrhosis   571.5
Claudication   443.9
Coccidiodomycosis
Colorectal Cancer   1
Condyloma Acumina
Congestive Heart Fail
Conjunctivitis   372.3(
Constipation   564.0
Contraception   V25.9
Corneal Ulceration   370.00
Corns   700
Costochondritis   733.6
Crohn's Disease   555.9
Croup   464.4
Cushing's Syndrome/Disease   255.0
Decubitus Ulcer   707.0
Deep Venous Thrombosis   453.8
Dementia   294.8
Depression   311
Dermatitis, Atopic   691.8
Dermatitis, Contact   692.9
Dermatitis, Seborrheic   690.1
Diabetes Mellitus, Type I   250.01
Diabetes Mellitus, Type II   250.02
Diarrhea, Acute   787.91
Diarrhea, Chronic   787.91
Diarrhea, Infectious   009.2
Disseminated Intravascular Coagulation   286.6
Diverticulitis   562.11
Domestic Violence   995.81
Drug Allergy   995.2
Dysfunctional Uterine Bleeding   626.8
Dyslexia   784.61
Dysmenorrhea   625.3
Dysuria   788.1
Earache   388.70
Ectopic Pregnancy   633.9
Edema, Leg   782.3
Elbow Dislocations   832.0
Endocarditis   424.90
Endometrial Cancer   182.0
Endometriosis   617.9
Endometritis   615.9
Enuresis   788.30
Epicondylitis   726.32
Epidymitis   604.90
Epistaxis   784.7
Erysipelas   035
Erythroplasia   233.5
Fecal Impaction   560.30
Fetal Alcohol Syndrome   760.71
Fetal Lung Immaturity   770.4
Fever and Chills   780.6
Fever of Unknown Origin (FUO)   780.6
Fibrocystic Disease of the Breast   610.1
Finger Dislocations   834
Finger Fractures   816

Listing continues on the back end paper.

Saunders
Manual
of Medical
Practice

Saunders Manual of Medical Practice

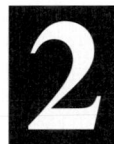

Edition **2**

ROBERT E. RAKEL, MD

Professor
Department of Family and Community Medicine
Baylor College of Medicine
Houston, Texas

Illustrations by Jan Redden

W.B. SAUNDERS COMPANY
A Harcourt Health Sciences Company
Philadelphia   London   New York   St. Louis   Sydney   Toronto

W.B. SAUNDERS COMPANY
A Harcourt Health Sciences Company

The Curtis Center
Independence Square West
Philadelphia, Pennsylvania 19106

Library of Congress Cataloging-in-Publication Data

Saunders manual of medical practice / [edited by] Robert E. Rakel ;
  illustrations by Jan Redden and foreword by Roger C. Bone. — 2nd ed.
     p.   cm.
  Includes bibliographical references and index.
  ISBN 0-7216-8002-X
  1. Internal medicine Handbooks, manuals, etc. I. Rakel, Robert E.
II. Title: Manual of medical practice.
  [DNLM: 1. Clinical Medicine Handbooks. WB 39 S257 2000]
RC55.S325   2000
616—dc21
DNLM/DLC   99-29018

CPT five digit codes, nomenclature and other data are copyright 1998 American Medical Association. All Rights Reserved. No fee schedules, basic units, relative values or related listings are included in CPT. The AMA assumes no liability for the data contained herein.

Acquisitions Editor: Raymond R. Kersey
Developmental Editor: Lynne Gery

SAUNDERS MANUAL OF MEDICAL PRACTICE   ISBN 0-7216-8002-X

Printed in the United States of America.

Last digit is the print number: 9   8   7   6   5   4   3   2   1

Contributors

ALLAN V. ABBOTT, M.D.
Professor of Family Medicine and Associate Dean for Curriculum, University of Southern California School of Medicine, Los Angeles, California
Ankle Fractures

LOUISE S. ACHESON, M.D.
Associate Professor of Family Medicine and Assistant Professor of Reproductive Biology, Case Western Reserve University and University Hospitals of Cleveland, Cleveland, Ohio
Office Endometrial Biopsy

BOBBI B. ADCOCK, M.D.
Assistant Professor of Family Medicine, University of Alabama School of Medicine; Active Teaching Staff, DCH Regional Medical Center, Tuscaloosa, Alabama
Rhabdomyolysis

DAVID M. ADELSON, M.D.
Clinical Assistant Professor, University of Oklahoma Health Care Center, Oklahoma City, Oklahoma
Fungus Infections of the Skin

DAVID C. AGERTER, M.D.
Assistant Professor of Family Medicine, Mayo Medical School and Mayo Graduate School of Medicine, Mayo Family Medicine Residency Program, Mayo Clinic; Chair, Department of Family Medicine, Mayo Clinic, Rochester, Minnesota
Whiplash

SYED M. AHMED, M.D., M.P.H., Dr.P.H.
Associate Professor, Department of Family Medicine, and Director, Alliance for Research in Community Health (ARCH), Wright State University, Dayton, Ohio
Dysuria; Acute Urinary Tract Infection in Children; Insomnia

JAMES D. ALEXANDER, M.D.
Assistant Professor, Department of Family Practice, University of Texas Health Sciences Center-San Antonio; Medical Director, Family Health Center-Downtown, University Health System, San Antonio, Texas
Palpitations

EZRA A. AMSTERDAM, M.D.
Professor, Internal Medicine, and Director, CCU, University of California, Davis, School of Medicine, Davis, California; Fellow, American College of Cardiology; Fellow, American Heart Association; Editor-in-Chief, *Preventive Cardiology*
Ventricular Tachyarrhythmias; Atrioventricular Block and Sick Sinus Syndrome

LINDA B. ANDREWS, M.D.
Director of Residency Education, Department of Psychiatry and Behavioral Sciences and Assistant Dean, Office of Student Affairs, Baylor College of Medicine, Houston, Texas
Schizophrenia

JOHN A. ANDRILLI, M.D.
Assistant Professor of Medicine, New York Medical College, Valhalla; Attending Physician, Saint Vincent's Hospital and Medical Center, New York, New York
Penile Discharge

DAVID ARAUJO, M.D.
Clinical Assistant Professor, Department of Family Practice, University of California at Davis, Sacramento; Program Director, Sutter Merced Family Practice Residency, Sutter Merced Medical Center, Merced, California
Vasectomy: Traditional Method

THURAYYA ARAYSSI, M.D.
Assistant Professor, American University of Beirut, Beirut, Lebanon
Hip Pain

SUSAN B. ARJMAND, M.D.
Instructor, Department of Family Medicine, Rush Medical College; Physician, Department of Family Medicine, Rush Presbyterian St. Luke's Medical Center, Chicago, Illinois
Fibrocystic Breast Disease

JAMES M. ATKINS, M.D.
Professor of Internal Medicine, University of Texas Southwestern Medical School; Senior Active Attending, Parkland Memorial Hospital, Dallas, Texas
Cardiopulmonary Resuscitation

GLEN F. AUKERMAN, M.D.
Professor, Department of Family Medicine, The Ohio State University; Associate Medical Director, Nationwide Insurance, Columbus, Ohio
Transient Ischemic Attack

CAROL A. BAASE, M.D.
Assistant Professor, Pennsylvania State University/The Good Samaritan Hospital, Family Practice Residency Program, Lebanon, Pennsylvania
Amenorrhea

GREGORY BAHTIARIAN, D.O.
Family Practice Physician, Bayside Health Association, Chtd, Lewes, Delaware
Seborrheic Dermatitis

VINCENT M. BALESTRINO, M.D.
Clinical Associate Professor, Department of Family Medicine, University of Pittsburgh School of Medicine; Associate Director, Family Residency Program, University of Pittsburgh Medical Center-St. Margaret Hospital, Pittsburgh, Pennsylvania
Otitis Externa

KENNETH A. BALLEW, M.D., M.S.
Assistant Professor, Division of General Internal Medicine, Department of Medicine, University of Virginia School of Medicine, Charlottesville, Virginia
Cardiac Arrest

DAVID M. BARCLAY, III, M.D., M.P.H.
Assistant Professor, Temple University School of Medicine; Chair, Fundamentals of Clinical Care Curriculum Committee, Philadelphia, Pennsylvania
Runner's Injuries

JAMES R. BARRETT, M.D.
Associate Professor, Department of Family Medicine, University of Oklahoma Health Sciences Center; Director, Primary Care Sports Medicine Fellowship, Oklahoma City, Oklahoma
Ankle and Foot Pain

KATHLEEN C. BARRY, M.D.
Private Practice, St. Petersburg, Florida
Chest Tube Insertion

ROBERT L. BASS, M.D.
Associate Professor Emeritus, Department of Family and Community Medicine, University of Nebraska College of Medicine, Omaha, Nebraska
Ingrown Toenail

DENNIS J. BAUMGARDNER, M.D.
Associate Professor of Family Medicine, University of Wisconsin Medical School, Madison; Director, Family Practice Residency, St. Luke's Medical Center, Aurora Health Care, Milwaukee, Wisconsin
Blastomycosis

DIANE K. BEEBE, M.D.
Professor, Residency Director, and Vice Chairman for Academic Programs, Department of Family Medicine, University of Mississippi Medical Center, Jackson, Mississippi
Abnormal Vaginal Bleeding

MARK H. BELFER, D.O.
Program Director, Family Practice Residency, Trinity Lutheran Hospital, Kansas City, Missouri
Hemorrhoids

JOSHUA O. BENDITT, M.D.
Associate Professor of Medicine, University of Washington School of Medicine; Medical Director, Respiratory Care Services, University of Washington Medical Center, Seattle, Washington
Pneumothorax

ROBERT L. BENZ, M.D.
Clinical Professor of Medicine, Thomas Jefferson University Medical College; Chief, Division of Nephrology, and Director, Haverford Dialysis Unit, Jefferson Health System-Main Line Health Hospitals, Philadelphia, Pennsylvania
Chronic Renal Failure

DAN BENZIE, M.D., M.S.P.H.
Associate Professor, University of Minnesota School of Medicine, Duluth; Medical Director/President, Gateway Family Health Clinic, Moose Lake, Sandstone, Minnesota
Diagnostic Upper Gastrointestinal Endoscopy

MICHAEL DAVID BERNSTEIN, M.D.
Assistant Clinical Professor of Medicine, Health Science Center at Brooklyn; Attending Gastroenterologist, Department of Gastroenterology, Coney Island Hospital, Brooklyn, New York
Hyperbilirubinemia

SHAUN BERRY, M.D.
Assistant Professor, Department of Family Medicine, John A. Burns School of Medicine, University of Hawaii, Honolulu; Director of Long Term Care Unit, Residency Faculty, Wahiawa General Hospital, Wahiawa, Hawaii
Swimmer's Injuries

KENNETH M. BIELAK, M.D.
Assistant Professor, Department of Family Medicine, University of Tennessee Graduate School of Medicine, Knoxville, Tennessee
Wrist and Hand Pain

JAMES R. BLACKMAN, M.D.
Assistant Dean and Clinical Professor of Family Medicine, WWAMI Center for Clinical Medical Education, Boise, Idaho; University of Washington School of Medicine, Seattle, Washington
Animal Bites

REID B. BLACKWELDER, M.D.
Associate Professor, Family Medicine, and Program Director, Kingsport Family Practice Residency, East Tennessee State University, Kingsport, Tennessee
Alternative Medicine; Wrist Fractures

GREGORY H. BLAKE, M.D., M.P.H.
Professor and Chairman, Department of Family Medicine, Graduate School of Medicine, University of Tennessee Medical Center, Knoxille, Tennessee
Aphthous Stomatitis

MARK BLUMENTHAL, M.D., M.P.H.
Assistant Professor, Department of Family Medicine, University of Tennessee; Attending Physician, University of Tennessee Medical Center, Knoxville, Tennessee
Iron Deficiency Anemia

WILLIAM Z. BORER, M.D.
Professor of Pathology, Thomas Jefferson University, Philadelphia, Pennsylvania
Reference Intervals for the Interpretation of Laboratory Tests

WAYNE A. BOTTNER, M.D.
Section Chief, Hematology, Gundersen Lutheran, La Crosse, Wisconsin
Megaloblastic Anemia

DANIEL E. BREWER, M.D.
Assistant Professor, Department of Family Medicine, University of Tennessee; Medical Staff, University of Tennessee Medical Center, Knoxville, Tennessee
Endometrial Cancer

MICHAEL S. BRONZE, M.D.
Professor, Internal Medicine and Infectious Diseases, and Vice Chairman, Department of Internal Medicine, University of Tennessee, Memphis, Memphis, Tennessee
Endocarditis

MICHAEL JON BROOKS, M.D.
Staff Gastroenterologist and Instructor, Delaware County Memorial Hospital, Lansdowne; Mercy Community Hospital, Havertown, and Mercy Fitzgerald Hospital, Darby, Pennsylvania
Diverticulitis

MARY T. BROPHY, M.D.
Assistant Professor of Medicine, Boston University School of Medicine; Staff Physician, Boston Veterans Affairs Medical Center, Boston, Massachusetts
Bleeding Disorders

LEE K. BROWN, M.D.
Clinical Professor of Medicine, University of New Mexico School of Medicine; Medical Director, New Mexico Center for Sleep Medicine, and Chairman, Department of Sleep Medicine, Lovelace Health Systems, Inc., Albuquerque, New Mexico
Sleep Apnea

WARD M. BROWN, M.D.
Associate Professor of Clinical Science, University of Wisconsin, La Crosse; Assistant Clinical Professor of Medicine, University of Wisconsin, La Crosse, La Crosse, and University of Wisconsin School of Medicine, Madison; Chairman, Gundersen Lutheran Heart Institute, Gundersen Lutheran Medical Center, La Crosse, Wisconsin
Syncope

ELIZABETH E. BROWNELL, M.D.
Private Practice, Family Practice and Obstetrics, Waukesha Health Care, Waukesha Memorial Hospital, Waukesha, Wisconsin
Rosacea

STEPHEN A. BRUNTON, M.D.
Director of Faculty Development, The Stamford Hospital/Columbia University Family Practice Residency Program, Stamford, Connecticut
Gastroesophageal Reflux Disease

JAMES K. BUCK II, M.D.*
Allergist, Indian Path Medical Group, Kingsport, Tennessee
Anaphylaxis

DAVID M. BURKHART, M.D.
Assistant Professor, Department of Family Medicine, Wright State University School of Medicine; Associate Director, Dayton Community Family Practice Residency Program, Dayton, Ohio
Bladder Tap

FRANK C. BURWICK, M.D.
Private Practice, Pediatrics and Internal Medicine, Aloha, Oregon
Sore Throat

MARK BYLER, M.D.
Assistant Professor, Department of Community and Family Medicine, University of Missouri, Kansas City, School of Medicine, Kansas City, Missouri
Local and Regional Anesthesia of the Lower Extremity; Ascaris and Hookworm Infection

ROBERT J. CARR, M.D.
Associate Professor and Program Director, Georgetown University/Providence Hospital Family Practice Residency Program, Washington, D.C.
Ectopic Pregnancy

LEE M. CARTER, M.D.
Clinical Assistant Professor, Department of Family Medicine, College of Medicine, University of Tennessee, Memphis, Memphis; Private Practice, Baptist of Physicians, R.B. Wilson Medical Center, Huntingdon, Tennessee
Dilatation and Curettage of the Uterus

ANNE CAWLEY, M.D.
Assistant Clinical Professor, Department of Family and Community Medicine, University of California, San Francisco, San Francisco, California
Dry Skin

FRANK S. CELESTINO, M.D.
Associate Professor, Department of Family and Community Medicine, Wake Forest University School of Medicine; Attending Staff, North Carolina Baptist Hospital, Winston-Salem, North Carolina
Frostbite

---

*Deceased.

ASHISH CHABRA, M.D.
Clinical Faculty, Midwestern University, Glendale; Medical Director, Foothills Family Medicine, Phoenix, Arizona
Corneal Ulceration

BENJAMIN H. CHADI, M.D.
Instructor, Medicine, Mount Sinai School of Medicine; Attending Physician, Beth Israel Hospital, New York, New York
Shock; Cardiomyopathy

S. SHEKAR CHAKRAVARTHI, M.B.
Associate Clinical Professor, Department of Family Medicine, East Carolina University School of Medicine, Greenville, North Carolina
Hyperparathyroidism

JASON CHAO, M.D.
Associate Professor, Department of Family Medicine, Case Western Reserve University School of Medicine; Department of Family Practice, University Hospitals of Cleveland, Cleveland, Ohio
Abnormal Liver Function Tests

MILTON C. CHAVEZ, M.D.
Assistant Professor of Family Medicine, Rush Presbyterian St. Luke's Medical Center, Chicago, Illinois
Seizure Disorder

ANTHONY L.-T. CHEN, M.D.
Clinical Assistant Professor, Department of Family Medicine, University of Washington; Provisional Staff, Providence Hospital; Consulting Staff, Swedish Medical Center, Seattle, Washington
Fatigue

EUGENE Y. CHENG, M.D.
Professor of Anesthesiology and Medicine, Medical College of Wisconsin; Co-Director Medical and Surgical ICU, Froedtert Memorial Lutheran Hospital, Milwaukee, Wisconsin
Local and Regional Anesthesia: Head and Neck

MARC J. CHERNOFF, D.O.
Hematology Oncology, Abington Memorial Hospital, Abington, and Holy Redeemer Hospital, Meadowbrook, Pennsylvania
Leukemia

SUBRAMANYAM CHITTIVELU, M.D.
Assistant Professor, Texas Tech University Health Sciences Center, Amarillo, Texas
Arterial Puncture

ROBERT TAO-PING CHOW, M.D.
Assistant Professor of Medicine, Johns Hopkins University School of Medicine; Director, Division of General Internal Medicine, and Associate Program Director, Sinai Hospital of Baltimore, Baltimore, Maryland
International Travel Disease Prevention

LILI CHURCH, M.D.
Assistant Professor, Department of Family Medicine, University of Washington School of Medicine; University of Washington Medical Center, Seattle, Washington
Dysfunctional Uterine Bleeding

JUDITH Z. CLARK, Ph.D.
Private Practice, Avalon, Catalina Island, California
Marital Discord

TODD J. COHEN, M.D.
Associate Professor of Medicine, State University of New York at Stonybrook, Stonybrook; Director of Electrophysiology and Director of Pacemaker-Arrhythmia Center, Winthrop-University Hospital, Mineola, New York
Defibrillation

MARILEE C. S. COLE, M.D.
Clinical Assistant Professor, Georgetown University and Georgetown University Medical Center, Washington, D.C.
Acute Diarrhea; Chronic Diarrhea

JOSEPH V. CONNELLY, M.D.
Adjunct Assistant Clinical Professor of Medicine, Columbia University College of Physicians and Surgeons, New York, New York; Director, Family Practice Residency Program, The Stamford Hospital/Columbia University Family Practice Residency Program, Stamford, Connecticut
Rubella

BRIAN CONNOLLY, M.D.
Assistant Professor and Program Director, Department of Family Medicine, State University of New York at Buffalo, Buffalo, New York
Nasal Fracture Reduction

JOHN B. COOMBS, M.D., M.N.S.
T.J. Phillips Professor of Family Medicine, and Adjunct Professor, Department of Pediatrics, University of Washington School of Medicine; Associate Dean, Regional Affairs and Rural Health, and Associate Vice President of Medical Affairs, Clinical Systems and Networks, University of Washington Academic Medical Center, Seattle, Washington
Loss of Appetite

JOHN J. COON, M.D.
Clinical Associate Professor of Family Medicine, and Vice Chair, Department of Family and Community Medicine, University of Illinois College of Medicine; Senior Associate Director, Family Practice Residency, Methodist Medical Center, Peoria, Illinois
Purpura

DAVID J. COOPER, M.D.
Assistant Professor of Medicine, New York University School of Medicine, New York; Attending, ProHEALTH Care Associates, North Shore University Hospital, Manhasset, New York
Parenteral Nutrition

JANE E. CORBOY, M.D.
Assistant Professor and Residency Program Director, Baylor College of Medicine, Houston, Texas
Exercise Prescribing

LOUISA COUTTS-van DIJK, M.D.
Assistant Professor, Baylor College of Medicine, Houston, Texas
Otitis Media with Effusion

JACK L. COX, M.D.
Clinical Associate Professor, Department of Family and Preventive Medicine, University of Utah School of Medicine, Salt Lake City; Regional Medical Director, USR, Intermountain Health Care, Provo, Utah
Nicotine Dependence

PAUL T. CULLEN, M.D.
Clinical Associate Professor, University of Pittsburgh, Pittsburgh; Director, Washington Hospital Family Practice Residency Program, Washington Hospital, Washington, Pennsylvania
Tinnitus

T. K. CUMARASAMY, M.D., M.S.
Director, Family Practice, Virtua Health: Hospital Affiliations; West Jersey Hospital System, Cooper University Hospital, and Our Lady of Lourdes Medical Center, Camden, New Jersey
Temporomandibular Joint Syndrome

ANNE CATHER CUTLIP, M.D.
Associate Professor, Family Medicine, and Vice Chair, Department of Family Medicine, West Virginia University School of Medicine; Staff Physician, Burby Memorial Hospital, Morgantown, West Virginia
Cervical Biopsy/LEEP; Condyloma Acuminata

TONI M. CUTSON, M.D., M.H.S.
Clinical Assistant Professor, Department of Family and Community Medicine and Department of Medicine, Duke University Medical Center; GRECC, Durham Veterans Affairs Medical Center, Durham, North Carolina
Thoracic Outlet Syndrome

TIMOTHY P. DAALEMAN, D.O.
Assistant Professor, Department of Family Medicine, University of Kansas School of Medicine, University of Kansas Medical Center; Attending Physician, University of Kansas Hospital, Kansas City, Kansas
Undescended Testicle; Disseminated Intravascular Coagulation

DIANA S. DARK, M.D.
Associate Professor of Medicine, Division of Pulmonary Disease and Critical Care Medicine, University of Missouri, Kansas City, School of Medicine; Staff Physician, St. Luke's Hospital, Kansas City, Missouri
Coccidioidomycosis; Malnutrition

MARC A. DARR, M.D.
Clinical Assistant Professor, University of Arizona College of Medicine, Tucson; Associate Director, St. Joseph's Hospital Family Practice Residency Program, Phoenix, Arizona
Vitiligo

TERRY F. DAVIES, M.D., M.B.
Professor of Medicine, and Director, Division of Endocrinology and Metabolism, Mount Sinai School of Medicine; Attending Physician, The Mount Sinai Hospital, New York, New York
Thyroiditis

DANIEL T. DAVISON, D.O.
Clinical Associate Professor of Family Medicine, Chicago College of Osteopathic Medicine, Downers Grove, and Midwestern University, Chicago; Staff Physician, SportsMed-Wheaton Orthopaedics, Carol Stream, Illinois
Tendinitis and Tendinosis

O. DAVID DELLINGER, III, M.D.
Assistant Professor, University of Alabama at Birmingham, Birmingham, Alabama; Physician, Gainesville Internal Medicine Group, Gainesville, Georgia
Diabetes Mellitus, Type I

ALICIA DERMER, M.D.
Clinical Associate Professor, Department of Family Medicine, University of Medicine and Dentistry of New Jersey-Robert Wood Johnson Medical School, New Brunswick, New Jersey
Neonatal Jaundice

D. TODD DETAR, D.O.
Clinical Assistant Professor and Medical Director, Medical University of South Carolina; Medical Staff, Trident Medical Center, Charleston, South Carolina
Scrotal Pain Or Mass

MILIND R. DHOND, M.B.B.S.
Assistant Clinical Professor of Medicine and Cardiovascular Diseases, University of California, Davis, School of Medicine, Davis; Consultant Cardiologist, University of California, Davis, Medical Center, Sacramento, California
Sinus Rhythms and Ectopic Beats; Supraventricular Tachyarrhythmias

SHIRLEY L. DICKINSON, M.D.
Faculty Physician, Natividad Family Medicine Residency, Natividad Medical Center, Salinas, California
Menopause

MARIANNE DIETERICH, M.D.
Professor of Neurology, Department of Neurology, Klinikum Grosshadern, Ludwig Maximilians University, Munich, Germany
Dizziness and Vertigo

ROBERT A. Di TOMASSO, Ph.D.
Professor, Vice Chair, and Director of Clinical Research, Department of Psychology, Doctoral Program in Clinical Psychology, Philadelphia College of Osteopathic Medicine, Philadelphia, Pennsylvania
Deep Muscle Relaxation Exercises

JON DIVINE, M.D., M.S.
Assistant Professor, and Director, Sports Medicine Program, Department of Family and Community Medicine, Baylor College of Medicine, Houston; Private Practice, Baylor and Methodist Primary Care Associates, Sugar Land, Texas
Joint Aspiration and Injection

MICHAEL N. DOUPÉ, M.D.
Clinical Instructor, Boston University School of Medicine, Boston; Faculty Member, Tufts University Family Practice Residency, Malden, Massachusetts
Hypernatremia

DAVID DOVNARSKY, M.D.
Clinical Instructor, Department of Family Medicine, University of Medicine and Dentistry of New Jersey-Robert Wood Johnson Medical School, New Brunswick; Faculty, West Jersey Family Practice Residency-Virtua Health, Voorhees, New Jersey
Hyperlipidemia

MARSHA DuPREE, M.D.
Assistant Professor, Albany Medical College, Albany, New York
Basal and Squamous Cell Carcinoma

CHARLES B. EATON, M.D., M.S.
Associate Professor, Department of Family Medicine, Brown University School of Medicine, Providence; Predoctoral Director, Department of Family Medicine, Memorial Hospital of Rhode Island, Pawtucket, Rhode Island
Bell's Palsy

GERRY EDWARDS, M.D.
Assistant Professor, Department of Family Medicine, State University of New York, Health Science Center at Syracuse, Syracuse; Faculty, St. Joseph's Hospital Family Practice Residency, East Syracuse, New York
Swallowing Difficulty

WILLIAM G. ELDER, Jr., Ph.D.
Associate Professor of Family Practice, University of Kentucky Chandler Medical Center, Lexington, Kentucky
Reading Disabilities, Including Dyslexia

C. GREGORY ELLIOTT, M.D.
Professor of Medicine, University of Utah School of Medicine; Chief, Pulmonary Division, LDS Hospital, Salt Lake City, Utah
Pulmonary Embolism

CAROL L. ELLIS, M.D.
Associate Professor, Residency Program Director, University of Tennessee Medical Center, Knoxville, Tennessee
Cellulitis

JOHN W. ELY, M.D., M.S.P.H.
Associate Professor, Department of Family Medicine, University of Iowa College of Medicine, Iowa City, Iowa
Excision of a Sebaceous (Epidermal) Cyst

ESTHER ENTIN, M.D.
Clinical Associate Professor, Department of Family Medicine, Brown University School of Medicine, Providence, Rhode Island
Attention-Deficit Hyperactivity Disorder; Fetal Alcohol Syndrome

RANDOLPH W. EVANS, M.D.
Clinical Associate Professor, Department of Neurology, University of Texas at Houston Medical School; Clinical Associate Professor, Department of Family and Community Medicine, Baylor College of Medicine; Chief of Neurology, Park Plaza Hospital, Houston, Texas
Postconcussion Syndrome; Hyperventilation Syndrome

A.E. EYLER, M.D., M.P.H.
Clinical Associate Professor, Department of Family Medicine, University of Michigan Medical School, Ann Arbor, Michigan
Sexual Function and Dysfunction in Women

GEORGE T. FANTRY, M.D.
Associate Professor of Medicine, University of Maryland School of Medicine; Director, Clinical Gastroenterology, University of Maryland Medical Systems, Baltimore, Maryland
Peptic Ulcer Disease

RAYMOND H. FEIERABEND, Jr., M.D.
Professor, Department of Family Medicine, James H. Quillen College of Medicine, East Tennessee State University, Johnson City; Residency Program Director, Bristol Family Practice Residency, Bristol, Tennessee
Rheumatoid Arthritis

JOEL FEIGIN, M.D.
Clinical Associate Professor of Family Medicine, University of Medicine and Dentistry of New Jersey-Robert Wood Johnson Medical School, New Brunswick; Coordinator of Procedural Medicine, Warren Hospital Family Practice Residency Program, Phillipsburg, New Jersey
Vasectomy: No-Scalpel Technique

EUGENE A. FELMAR, M.D.
Clinical Professor of Family Medicine, University of California, Los Angeles, School of Medicine, Los Angeles; Director Emeritus, Family Practice Residency Program, Santa Monica-University of California, Los Angeles, Medical Center, Santa Monica, California
Hemorrhoid Sclerotherapy, Infrared Coagulation, and Banding

BRADLEY W. FENTON, M.D.
Clinical Associate Professor of Medicine, Thomas Jefferson University, Philadelphia, Pennsylvania
Infectious Diarrhea

MITCHELL F. FINNIE, M.D.
Assistant Director, Santa Rosa Family Practice Residency Program, San Antonio, Texas
Atopic Dermatitis

BRUCE FLAREAU, M.D.
Clinical Associate Professor, University of South Florida, Tampa; Director of Medical Education and Clinical Research, and Program Director, Morton Plant Mease Family Practice Residency of University of South Florida, Morton Plant Mease Health Care, Clearwater, Florida
Aquatic Injuries

JEAN FORMAN, M.D.
Assistant Professor of Clinical Medicine, Keck School of Medicine at University of Southern California; Staff Physician, University Hospital at University of Southern California, Los Angeles, California
Pediculosis (Body and Head Lice)

GRANT C. FOWLER, M.D.
Associate Professor and Vice Chair, Department of Family Practice and Community Medicine, University of Texas at Houston Health Science Center-Medical School, Houston, Texas
Hydrocele/Spermatocele

KEITH A. FREY, M.D., M.B.A.
Chair, Department of Family Medicine, Mayo Clinic Scottsdale, Scottsdale, Arizona
Infertility

JOSIAH FRIEDLANDER, M.D.
Assistant Professor of Family Medicine, University of Southern California, Los Angeles, California
Psoriasis

ERNEST FRUGÉ, Ph.D.
Assistant Professor, Department of Pediatrics, and Department of Family and Community Medicine, Baylor College of Medicine; Director, Psychosocial Programs, Texas Children's Cancer Center, Texas Children's Hospital, Houston, Texas
Substance Abuse

YANGHENG FU, M.D., Ph.D.
Assistant Clinical Professor, Department of Internal Medicine, University Medical Center, University of California, San Francisco, at Fresno, Fresno, California
Toxic Shock Syndrome

WILLIAM FULCHER, M.D.
Associate Professor, Family Medicine, University of Alabama at Birmingham School of Medicine, Birmingham, Alabama
Chronic Fatigue Syndrome

NICHOLAS J. GALIOTO, M.D.
Associate, Department of Family Practice, University of Iowa College of Medicine, Iowa City; Director, Transitional Residency Program, and Associate Director, Family Practice Residency Program, Broadlawns Medical Center, Des Moines, Iowa
Croup

JOSEPH P. GARRY, M.D.
Assistant Professor, Department of Family Medicine, East Carolina University School of Medicine; Chief Physician, L.T. Walker International Human Performance Center, Greenville, North Carolina
Thoracentesis

DAVID L. GASPAR, M.D.
Associate Professor, Department of Family Medicine, University of Colorado Health Sciences Center, Denver, Colorado
Upper Respiratory Infections

ELLEN T. GEMINIANI, M.D.
Assistant Professor of Family Medicine, Pennsylvania State University College of Medicine; Clinical Faculty, Pennsylvania State Geisinger Health System, Hershey, Pennsylvania
Finger Dislocations

ROBERT M. GERBO, M.D.
Assistant Professor of Family Medicine, West Virginia University School of Medicine, Charleston Division, Charleston, West Virginia
Small and Large Bowel Obstruction

ERIK O. GILBERTSON, M.D.
Clinical Instructor, Voluntary, University of California, San Diego, La Jolla; Clinical Dermatologist, Scripps Clinic, Division of Dermatology and Cutaneous Surgery, San Diego, California
Hyperhidrosis

BEN L. GLASPEY, D.O.
Family Practitioner, Martin Memorial Hospital/Medical Group, Stuart, Florida
Ankle Sprain

RICHARD A. GLECKMAN, M.D.
Chairman of Medicine, and Chief, Infectious Disease Division, St. Joseph's Hospital and Medical Center, Paterson, New Jersey
Bronchitis

LYNNE J. GOEBEL, M.D.
Associate Professor of Internal Medicine, Marshall University School of Medicine, Huntington, West Virginia
Eye Pain

CHRIS GOERDT, M.D., M.P.H.
Assistant Professor, University of Iowa, Iowa City, Iowa
Peripheral Arterial Disease

GARY A. GOFORTH, M.D., M.T.M.H.
Associate Professor of Family Medicine, Medical University of South Carolina, Charleston; Director of Medical Education and Residency Program Director, Self Memorial Hospital Family Practice Residency Program, Greenwood, South Carolina
Malaria

ARNOLD GOLDBERG, M.D.
Clinical Assistant Professor, Brown University, Providence; Medical Director of Family Care Center, Memorial Hospital of Rhode Island, Pawtucket, Rhode Island
Alopecia

AVRA GOLDMAN, M.D.
Clinical Instructor, Department of Family Medicine, Boston University School of Medicine; Family Physician, Boston Medical Center, Boston, Massachusetts
Kaposi's Sarcoma

THOMAS B. GOLEMON, M.D.
Clinical Associate Professor, Department of Family and Community Medicine, University of Illinois College of Medicine at Peoria; Director, Family Practice Residency, Methodist Medical Center of Illinois, Peoria, Illinois
Osteomyelitis; Hair Disorders

RUSSELL P. GOLLARD, M.A., M.D.
Adjunct Professor of English, University of Nevada at Las Vegas, Las Vegas, Nevada
Neutropenia

SUSANA GONZALEZ, M.D.
Assistant Professor of Obstetrics/Gynecology and Family Medicine, University of Southern California School of Medicine, Los Angeles, California
Intrauterine Device Insertion and Removal

MARK A. GRABER, M.D.
Associate Professor of Clinical Family Medicine and Surgery, University of Iowa College of Medicine, Iowas City, Iowa
Recurrent Infections

MARGARET GRADISON, M.D.
Assistant Clinical Professor, Department of Community and Family Medicine, Duke University Medical School, Durham, North Carolina
Diaphragm Fitting

ALISON GRANN, M.D.
Clinical Assistant, Memorial-Sloan-Kettering Cancer Center, New York, New York
Oncologic Emergencies

JOSEPH W. GRAVEL, Jr., M.D.
Assistant Clinical Professor, Department of Family Medicine, Tufts University School of Medicine, Boston; Program Director, Tufts University Family Practice Residency, Malden; Vice Chairman, Department of Family Medicine, New England Medical Center Hospitals, Boston; Chief, Department of Family Medicine, Malden Medical Center, Hallmark Health System, Malden, Massachusetts
Lipoma

LELAND GRAVES, III, M.D.
Assistant Professor of Medicine, University of Missouri, Kansas City, School of Medicine, Kansas City, Missouri
Hypocalcemia

GARY R. GRAY, D.O.
Assistant Professor, Department of Family Medicine, Georgetown University School of Medicine, Washington, D.C.
Conjunctivitis

MARTHA S. GRAYSON, M.D.
Senior Associate Dean for Primary Care and Associate Professor of Clinical Medicine, New York Medical College, Valhalla; Chief, Section of General Internal Medicine, Saint Vincent's Hospital and Medical Center of New York, New York, New York
Breast Cancer

BRUCE D. GREENWALD, M.D.
Associate Professor of Medicine, University of Maryland School of Medicine, Baltimore, Maryland
Ulcerative Colitis

DAWN M. GRINENKO, M.D.
Clinical Assistant Professor and Director, Adolescent/Young Adult Program, University of Florida School of Medicine, Gainesville, Florida
Bulimia and Anorexia Nervosa

DAVID E. GUTSTEIN, M.D.
Cardiology Fellow, Mount Sinai School of Medicine and Mount Sinai Medical Center, New York, New York
Acute Pulmonary Edema (Heart Failure); Chronic Heart Failure

DAVID L. HALL, M.D.
Associate Physician, Baylor-Methodist Primary Care Associates, Houston, Texas
Bladder Cancer

NEIL K. HALL, M.D., M.B.A.
Clinical Associate Professor, Department of Family Practice, State University of New York Health Science Center at Syracuse, Syracuse; Chief of Geriatrics, United Health Services, Binghamton, New York
Benign Prostatic Hyperplasia

ECKART HANEKE, M.D., Ph.D.
Lecturer, University of Witten/Herdecke, Witten; Professor and Chairman, Department of Dermatology, Wuppertal Hospitals Ltd., Wuppertal, Germany
Diseases of the Nails

JIMMY H. HARA, M.D.
Associate Clinical Professor, Department of Family Medicine, University of California, Los Angeles, School of Medicine; Residency Program Director and Assistant Chief of Service, Department of Family Practice, Kaiser Los Angeles Medical Center, Los Angeles, California
Myofascial Syndromes (Fibromyalgia and Myofascial Trigger Points)

THOMAS P. HARDER, M.D.
Rheumatology Fellow, University of California, Los Angeles, San Fernando Valley Program, Veterans Affairs Medical Center, Sepulveda, California
Gout

MICHAEL B. HARPER, M.D.
Professor of Clinical Family Medicine and Residency Program Director, Louisiana State University School of Medicine in Shreveport, Shreveport, Louisiana
Nasogastric Intubation

JOHN J. HART, M.D.
Associate Clinical Instructor, University of Kansas School of Medicine, Wichita, Kansas
Myasthenia Gravis

SUSAN HART-HESTER, M.A., Ph.D.
Associate Professor, Department of Family Medicine, University of Mississippi Medical Center, Jackson, Mississippi
Autism

ROBERT B. HASH, M.D.
Associate Professor of Family Medicine, Mercer University School of Medicine, Macon, Georgia
Ketoacidosis

ROBERT L. HATCH, M.D., M.P.H.
Associate Professor, Department of Community Health and Family Medicine, University of Florida School of Medicine, Gainesville, Florida
Foot Fractures

VALERIE L. HEARNS, M.D.
Assistant Professor, Department of Family Medicine, and Predoctoral Director, University of South Dakota School of Medicine, Sioux Falls, South Dakota
Pinworms

JOHN M. HEATH, M.D.
Associate Professor of Family Medicine, University of Medicine and Dentistry of New Jersey-Robert Wood Johnson Medical School, New Brunswick, New Jersey; Fellow, American Geriatric Society
Chronic Obstructive Pulmonary Disease

ROBERT M. HEILIGMAN, M.D., M.P.H.
Associate Professor of Clinical Medicine, University of Arizona College of Medicine, Tucson; Associate Program Director for Curricular Affairs, Internal Medicine Residency Program, St. Joseph's Hospital and Medical Center, Phoenix, Arizona
Bone Marrow Aspiration and Biopsy

JEFFREY W. HEMP, M.D.
Clinical Assistant Professor, University of Illinois College of Medicine; Associate Director, Methodist Family Practice Residency, Peoria, Illinois
Cheilitis and Angular Cheilitis

SCOTT T. HENDERSON, M.D.
Associate Professor of Family Practice, and Program Director, University of Wyoming Family Practice Residency Program at Cheyenne; Active Staff, United Medical Center, Cheyenne, Wyoming
First Trimester Bleeding

ARTHUR H. HEROLD, M.D.
Associate Professor of Family Medicine, University of South Florida College of Medicine; Associate Professor of Public Health, University of South Florida College of Public Health, Tampa, Florida
Rectal Bleeding

CARLOS R. HERRERA, M.D., M.P.H.
Associate Professor, University of Texas at Houston Medical School; Memorial Hermann Hospital, Houston, Texas
Hypertension

HILARY I. HERTAN, M.D.
Assistant Professor of Medicine, New York Medical College, Valhalla; Associate Program Director, Division of Gastroenterology and Clinical Nutrition, and Chief of Gastrointestinal Endoscopy, Our Lady of Mercy Medical Center, Bronx, New York
Nutritional Assessment in Clinical Practice

THOMAS F. HESTON, M.D.
Editor, The Internet Medical Journal, *http://www.Medjournal.com*
Lead Poisoning

JOE E. HIMES, M.D.
Family Practitioner, Table Rock Family Practice, Shell Knob, Missouri
Shoulder Dislocations

RENEE A. HOFFMANN, M.B.B.C.H.
Clinical Instructor in Ambulatory Care, Boston University, Harvard University, and Tufts University, Boston, Massachusetts
Endotracheal Intubation

HOWARD A. HOLTZ, M.D.
Clinical Associate Professor of Medicine, Mount Sinai School of Medicine, New York, New York; Associate Chairman of Medicine, Saint Barnabas Medical Center, Livingston, New Jersey
Domestic Violence

DIANE D. HOMAN, M.D.
Assistant Professor of Family Medicine, Rush-Presbyterian-St. Luke's Medical Center, Chicago, Illinois
Pregnancy

MARK E. HRONCICH, M.D.
Clinical Assistant Professor of Medicine, Loyola University Medical School, Maywood; Attending Physician, MacNeal Hospital, Berwyn, Illinois
Paget's Disease of Bone

WILLIAM Y. HUANG, M.D.
Assistant Professor, Department of Family and Community Medicine, Baylor College of Medicine, Houston, Texas
Abdominal Pain

WILLIAM J. HUESTON, M.D.
Professor and Chair, Department of Family Medicine, Medical University of South Carolina, Charleston, South Carolina
Chronic Cough

PAUL J. HUGHES, M.D.
Medical Director, Durable Medical Equipment Regional Carrier, United Healthcare, Nanticoke, Pennsylvania
Altitude Sickness

THOMAS K. HUNT, M.D.
Affiliate Assistant Professor and Biomedical Professor, University of Alaska; Active Staff, Providence Hospital and Humane Hospital, Anchorage Alaska
Stomatitis

CHARLEEN ISÉ, M.D.
Associate Director, Bayfront Family Practice Residency, St. Petersburg; Assistant Clinical Professor, University of South Florida College of Medicine, Tampa; Attending Physician, Bayfront Medical Center, and All Children's Hospital, St. Petersburg, Florida
Percutaneous Incision and Drainage of Abscess

NICOLA J. JACOBUCCI, M.D.
Community Preceptor, University of North Carolina Medical School, Chapel Hill, and Wake Forest University Medical School, Winston-Salem; Secretary, Family Practice Section, High Point Regional Hospital, High Point, North Carolina
Fine-Needle Aspiration of the Breast

STEPHEN P. JAMES, M.D.
Professor of Medicine, University of Maryland, Baltimore; Head, Division of Gastroenterology and Hepatology, University of Maryland Medical Center, Baltimore, Maryland
Crohn's Disease

ARMANDO JOSE JARQUIN, M.D.
Clinical Assistant Professor, Department of Family and Community Medicine, Baylor College of Medicine (Voluntary Faculty); Staff Physician, Kelsey-Seybold Clinic, Houston, Texas
Lyme Disease

P. GEORGE JOHN, M.D.
Associate Professor of Family Medicine, Wright State University School of Medicine; Associate Director, Family Practice Residency, Franciscan Medical Center, Dayton, Ohio
Hypercalciuria and Renal Calculi

MARK S. JOHNSON, M.D., M.P.H.
Chairman, Department of Family Medicine, University of Medicine and Dentistry-New Jersey Medical School; Chief of Service, Family Practice, University Hospital, Newark, New Jersey
Sickle Cell Disease

PHILIP C. JOHNSON, M.D.
Professor and Director, Division of General Medicine, Department of Internal Medicine, University of Texas at Houston Medical School, Houston, Texas
Late Symptomatic HIV Infection

TANYA Y. JONES, M.D.
Clinical Associate Professor, Department of Family Medicine, Morehouse School of Medicine, Atlanta, Georgia
Sjögren's Syndrome

JAI H. JOSHI, M.D.
Assistant Professor of Medicine, The Johns Hopkins University School of Medicine, Baltimore, Maryland
Metastatic Cancer of Unknown Origin

GREGORY JUCKETT, M.D.
Associate Professor of Family Medicine, West Virginia University; Staff Physician, Ruby Memorial Hospital, Morgantown, West Virginia
Advance Directives; Tapeworm Infections; Snakebite

VICTORIA S. KAPRIELIAN, M.D.
Associate Clinical Professor, Department of Community and Family Medicine, Duke University School of Medicine; Staff Physician, Duke University Medical Center, Durham, North Carolina
Osgood-Schlatter Disease

RAJANI KATTA, M.D.
Assistant Professor of Dermatology, Baylor College of Medicine, Houston, Texas
Lichen Planus

MICHAEL D. KAUFMAN, M.D.
Director, Multiple Sclerosis Center, Carolinas Medical Center, Charlotte, North Carolina
Multiple Sclerosis

RICK KELLERMAN, M.D.
Professor and Chair, Department of Family and Community Medicine, University of Kansas School of Medicine at Wichita, Wichita, Kansas
Immunization Schedules

STEPHEN F. KEMP, M.D.
Assistant Professor of Medicine and Pediatrics, and Co-Director, Division of Allergy and Immunology, Department of Medicine, The University of Mississippi Medical Center, Jackson, Mississippi
Drug Allergy

JOHN I. KENNEDY, Jr., M.D.
Associate Professor of Medicine, Division of Pulmonary, Allergy, and Critical Care Medicine, Department of Medicine, University of Alabama at Birmingham, Birmingham, Alabama
Ventilator Support

JENNIFER R. KESSMANN, M.D.
Assistant Professor, Department of Family and Community Medicine, University of Texas Southwestern Medical Center, Dallas, Texas
Vaginal Discharge

EDWARD D. KIM, M.D.
Assistant Professor of Urology, Baylor College of Medicine, Houston, Texas
Sexual Dysfunction in Men

LISA G. KING, M.D.
Private Practice, Utica Park Clinic, Tulsa, Oklahoma
Salmonellosis

JUDITH D. KINZY, M.D.
Assistant Professor of Medicine, University of Tennessee; University of Tennessee Medical Center, Knoxville, Tennessee
Gonorrhea; Chlamydia; Lymphogranuloma Venereum; Granuloma Inguinale (Donovanosis); Chancroid; Syphilis

DONALD F. KIRBY, M.D.
Professor of Medicine, Psychiatry, Biochemistry, and Molecular Physics, and Chief, Section of Nutrition and Wellness, Division of Gastroenterology, Virginia Commonwealth University, Medical College of Virginia Campus, Richmond, Virginia
Obesity

JEFFREY T. KIRCHNER, D.O.
Associate Director, Family Practice Residency Program, Lancaster General Hospital, Lancaster, Pennsylvania
Lymphadenopathy

MICHAEL O. KIRKPATRICK, M.D.
Assistant Professor, Department of Family and Community Medicine, Texas A&M University College of Medicine; Senior Staff, Department of Family Medicine, Scott and White Clinic, Temple, Texas
Prostatitis

ISAAC KLEINMAN, M.D.
Associate Professor, Department of Family and Community Medicine, Baylor College of Medicine; Active Staff, St. Luke's Episcopal Hospital, Houston, Texas
Corneal Foreign Body Removal; Goiter; Common Symptoms of Protozoan/Helminthic Diseases

MICHAEL H. KLEINMAN, M.D.
Clinical Assistant Professor of General Surgery, Baylor College of Medicine; Clinical Assistant Professor of Surgery, University of Texas; Physician Liaison, Memorial Hermann Hospital System, Houston, Texas
Gallstones and Cholecystitis

AUBREY L. KNIGHT, M.D.
Associate Professor of Clinical Family Medicine, University of Virginia School of Medicine, Charlottesville; Director, Family Practice Education, Carilion Health System, Roanoke, Virginia
Fecal Impaction

SARAH S. KRAMER, M.D.
Clinical Associate Professor of Family Medicine, University of Washington; Clinic Chief, Federal Way Clinic, University of Washington Physicians, Seattle, Washington
Back Pain

ELANA NUDEL KRIPKE, M.D.
Assistant Professor of Medicine, Medical College of Pennsylvania, Philadelphia, Pennsylvania
Nipple Discharge

LINDA L. KRISHNA, M.D.
Member, AAFP and TAFP; Staff Physician, St. Luke's Episcopal Hospital, Houston, Texas
Early Symptomatic HIV Infection

LINDA L. KURIBAYASHI, M.D.
Associate Clinical Professor of Medicine, University of California, San Francisco, Fresno Medical Education Program, Fresno, California
Pleural Effusions

KURT KUROWSKI, M.D.
Associate Professor, Department of Family Medicine, F.U.H.S./The Chicago Medical School, North Chicago; Staff Physician, Department of Family Practice, Highland Park Hospital, Highland Park, Illinois
Hypercalcemia

MARK A. LANDIS, M.D.
Private Practice, Bluff City, Tennessee
Giardiasis

PETE LANE, D.O.
Associate Professor, Department of Family and Community Medicine, University of Alabama at Birmingham, Birmingham; Staff Physician, Bessmer Carraway Medical Center, Bessmer, Alabama
Oliguria/Anuria

LARS C. LARSEN, M.D.
Professor of Family Medicine, East Carolina University School of Medicine, Greenville, North Carolina
Poisonings

VICTOR R. LAVIS, M.D.
Professor of Internal Medicine, University of Texas at Houston Medical School, Houston, Texas
Pheochromocytoma

THOMAS L. LEAMAN, M.D.
Professor Emeritus, Department of Family and Community Medicine, Pennsylvania State University College of Medicine, The Milton S. Hershey Medical Center, Hershey, Pennsylvania
Generalized Anxiety Disorder

KIM EDWARD LeBLANC, M.D., Ph.D.
Associate Professor of Family Medicine, Louisiana State University Medical Center, New Orleans; Family Practice Residency Program Director, and Family Practice Department Head, University Medical Center, Lafayette, Louisiana
Elbow Dislocations

PETER S. P. LEE, M.D.
Chief Resident, Department of Family and Community Medicine, Baylor College of Medicine, Houston, Texas
Scabies

JEANNE PARR LEMKAU, Ph.D.
Departments of Family Medicine and Community Health, Wright State University School of Medicine, Dayton, Ohio
Phobias

GARY I. LEVINE, M.D.
Associate Professor, Department of Family Medicine, East Carolina University School of Medicine, Greenville, North Carolina
Acne (Vulgaris)

RUTH LEVINE, M.D.
Associate Professor of Clinical Psychiatry and Internal Medicine, and Director of Undergraduate Education, Department of Psychiatry and Behavioral Sciences, University of Texas Medical Branch, Galveston, Texas
Personality Disorders

MICHAEL P. LEWKO, M.D.
Clinical Assistant Professor of Family Practice, University of Medicine and Dentistry of New Jersey-Robert Wood Johnson Medical School, New Brunswick, New Jersey; Clinical Instructor of Internal Medicine, Mount Sinai School of Medicine, New York, New York; Clinical Assistant Professor of Medicine, St. George's University School of Medicine, Grenada; Chief of Geriatrics, St. Joseph's Hospital and Medical Center, Paterson, New Jersey
Temporal Arteritis

EDGAR LICHSTEIN, M.D.
Professor of Medicine, State University of New York Health Science Center at Brooklyn; Chairman, Department of Medicine, Maimonides Medical Center, Brooklyn, New York
Myocardial Infarction

JOSEPH J. LIEBER, M.D.
Clinical Associate Professor of Medicine, Mount Sinai School of Medicine, New York; Chief, Medical Consult Service, and Associate Attending in Medicine, Elmhurst Medical Center, Elmhurst, New York
Proteinuria

JANET C. LINDEMANN, M.D.
Associate Professor, Department of Family Medicine, University of South Dakota School of Medicine, Sioux Falls, South Dakota
Premenstrual Syndrome

DAVID R. LITTLE, M.D., M.S.
Associate Professor, Department of Family Medicine, Wright State University School of Medicine, Dayton, Ohio
Hemochromatosis

ANNE R. LOCKETT, M.D.
Associate Professor of Family and Community Medicine, Eastern Virginia Medical School, Norfolk; Residency Director, Portsmouth Family Medicine, Portsmouth, Virginia
Contact Dermatitis

DAVID P. LOSH, M.D.
Associate Professor and Residency Program Director, Department of Family Medicine, University of Washington School of Medicine, Seattle, Washington
Decubitus Ulcer

REGGIE LYELL, M.D.
Private Practice, Harrison Family Medicine, Corydon, Indiana
Exercise Stress Testing

PAUL LYONS, M.D.
Assistant Chair for Clinical Education, Department of Family and Community Medicine, Temple University School of Medicine, Philadelphia, Pennsylvania
Abnormal Pap Smear

BONNIE P. MALVEA, M.D., M.P.H.
Associate Professor, Department of Family Medicine, Morehouse School of Medicine, Atlanta, Georgia
Appendicitis

VIPUL N. MANKAD, M.D.
Professor and Chairman, Department of Pediatrics, University of Kentucky and University of Kentucky Children's Hospital, Lexington, Kentucky
Thalassemia Syndromes

JON V. MARTELL, M.D.
Associate Professor of Family Practice and Internal Medicine, John A. Burns School of Medicine, University of Hawaii, Honolulu, Hawaii
Hyponatremia

F. ALLAN MARTIN, M.D.
Residency Director, Northwest Arkansas Family Practice Residency Program, University of Arkansas for Medical Sciences; Assistant Professor of Family and Community Medicine, Area Health Education Center-Northwest; Medical Director, Generations Geropsychiatry Unit, Washington Regional Medical Center, Fayetteville, Arkansas
Delirium

HENRY MARTIN-del-CAMPO, M.D.
Clinical Assistant Professor of Family and Community Medicine, University of Illinois College of Medicine at Peoria; Associate Medical Director, OSF Health Plans, Peoria, Illinois
Epididymitis

JOSEPH R. MASCI, M.D.
Associate Professor of Medicine, Mount Sinai School of Medicine, New York; Associate Director of Medicine, Elmhurst Hospital Center, Elmhurst, New York
Erysipelas

THOMAS MASCIANGELO, M.D.
Assistant Professor, Department of Family and Community Medicine, Baylor College of Medicine, Houston, Texas
Nausea and Vomiting

CHRISTI A. MATTEONI, M.D.
Senior Fellow, Department of Gastroenterology, The Cleveland Clinic Foundation, Cleveland, Ohio
Viral Hepatitis

DALE A. MATTHEWS, M.D.
Associate Professor of Medicine, Georgetown University School of Medicine, Washington, D.C.
Somatoform Disorders

HAROLD J. MAY, Ph.D.
Head, Behavioral Medicine, and Professor of Family Medicine, Department of Family Medicine, East Carolina University School of Medicine, Greenville, North Carolina
Sexual Assault

TODD A. MAY, M.D.
Assistant Clinical Professor, University of California, San Francisco; Co-Director, Family Practice Inpatient Service, San Francisco General Hospital, San Francisco, California
Ascites

ELIZABETH C. McCORD, M.D., M.S.
Assistant Professor, East Tennessee State University, Johnson City, Tennessee
Health Promotion Protocols

DOUGLAS C. McCRORY, M.D., M.H.Sc.
Assistant Professor of Medicine, Division of General Internal Medicine, Department of Medicine, Duke University Medical Center; Staff Physician, Ambulatory Care, Durham Veterans Affairs Medical Center, Durham, North Carolina
Stroke

JOHN C. McKECHNIE, M.D.
Clinical Professor, Baylor Medical School, Houston, Texas
Flexible Sigmoidoscopy/Colonoscopy

JAMES P. McKENNA, M.D.
Adjunct Assistant Professor of Family Medicine and Clinical Epidemiology, and Director, Family Practice Residency, The Medical Center, Beaver, Pennsylvania
Paresthesias

KEVIN M. McKOWN, M.D.
Associate Professor, Department of Internal Medicine, University of Tennessee, Memphis, Memphis, Tennessee
Neck Pain

BARRY R. MEISENBERG, M.D.
Head, Division of Hematology/Oncology, and Deputy Director, Greenebaum Cancer Center, University of Maryland School of Medicine, Baltimore, Maryland
Lymphoma

DOMINICK MEMOLI, M.D.
Medical Director, Glen Burnie Veterans Affairs Clinic, Baltimore Veterans Affairs Medical Center, Baltimore, Maryland
Anemia Work-up

GARY R. MENNIE, M.D.
Assistant Professor, Department of Family Medicine, and Assistant Clinical Professor, Department of Obstetrics and Gynecology, University of Texas Medical Branch, Galveston; Attending Physician, Family Medicine Residency, St. Elizabeth Hospital Family Medicine Residency, Beaumont, and St. Mary Hospital Family Medicine Residency, Port Arthur, Texas
Pregnancy-Induced Hypertension

LINDA N. MEURER, M.D., M.P.H.
Assistant Professor of Family and Community Medicine, Medical College of Wisconsin, Milwaukee, Wisconsin
Developmental Surveillance

JOHN MEYERHOFF, M.D.
Assistant Professor of Medicine, Johns Hopkins University School of Medicine; Clinical Scholar in Rheumatology, Sinai Hospital of Baltimore, Baltimore, Maryland
Polymyositis and Dermatomyositis; Polymyalgia Rheumatica

GIULIA MICHELINI, M.D.
Assistant Professor of Medicine, University of California, Los Angeles, Los Angeles; Staff Internist, Veterans Affairs Greater Los Angeles Healthcare System-Sepulveda, Sepulveda, California
Allergic Rhinitis

THOMAS C. MICHELS, M.D., M.P.H.
Clinical Instructor in Family Medicine, University of Washington School of Medicine, Seattle; Chief, Department of Family Practice, Madigan Army Medical Center, Tacoma, Washington
Insects and Spiders

JOHN MIDTLING, M.D., M.S.
Professor and Head, Department of Family and Community Medicine, and Associate Dean, University of Illinois College of Medicine at Rockford, Rockford, Illinois
Knee Injuries

ETAN C. MILGROM, M.D., M.S.
Associate Clinical Professor of Family Medicine, and Associate Pre-doctoral Director, University of California, Los Angeles, School of Medicine, Los Angeles, California
Rhinolaryngoscopy

KARL E. MILLER, M.D.
Associate Professor, Department of Family Medicine, University of Tennessee College of Medicine, Chattanooga Unit, Chattanooga, Tennessee
Bone Pain and Swelling

JEFFREY F. MINTEER, M.D.
Assistant Professor of Family and Community Medicine, Pennsylvania State University, Philadelphia, and University of Pittsburgh, Pittsburgh; Associate Director of Family Practice Residency, Washington Hospital, Washington, Pennsylvania
Raynaud's Phenomenon

ALIASGHAR MOHYUDDIN, M.D.
Assistant Professor of Medicine, University of Kansas School of Medicine at Wichita; Staff Physician, Via Christi Regional Medical Center, and Wesley Medical Center, Wichita, Kansas
Hemolytic Anemia

MYRTHO MONTES, M.D.
Assistant Professor of Medicine, New York Medical College, Valhalla; Associate Section Chief of General Internal Medicine, Saint Vincent's Hospital and Medical Center, New York, New York
Amebiasis

CYNTHIA M. MOORE-SLEDGE, M.D.
Assistant Professor, Department of Family Medicine, University of Alabama at Birmingham, Birmingham, Alabama
Fever of Unknown Origin

KIMBERLY L. MORRIS, M.D.
Associate Professor, Department of Internal Medicine, University of Tennessee, Knoxville, College of Medicine; Assistant Program Director, Internal Medicine Residency Program, University of Tennessee Medical Center, Knoxville, Tennessee
Orbital and Periorbital Cellulitis; Pelvic Pain

MARY HELEN MORROW, M.D.
Assistant Professor, Texas A&M College of Medicine, College Station; Director of Orientation and Recruitment, Family Practice Residency of the Brazos Valley, Texas
Postpartum Depression

R. MICHAEL MORSE, M.D.
B. Lewis Barnett, Jr., M.D., Professor of Family Medicine, University of Virginia School of Medicine, Charlottesville, Virginia
Rib Fractures

ROBERT J. MOSS, M.D.
Clinical Instructor, University of Illinois, Chicago; Director of Geriatric Medicine, Department of Family Practice, Lutheran General Hospital: Advocate Health Care System, Park Ridge, Illinois
Alzheimer's Disease

JULIE GRAVES MOY, M.D., M.P.H.
Assistant Professor, Texas A&M University School of Medicine, College Station; Medical Director, Mother's Milk Bank at Austin, Austin, Texas
Induction of Labor

VASKAR MUKERJI, M.D.
Professor of Medicine, and Chief, Division of Cardiology, Southern Illinois University School of Medicine, Springfield, Illinois
Chest Pain

J. DENNIS MULL, M.D., M.P.H.
Professor of Clinical Family Medicine, Department of Family Medicine, University of Southern California School of Medicine, Los Angeles, California
Bronchiolitis

BRIAN S. MURPHY, M.D., M.P.H., M.S.
Assistant Professor of Medicine, New York Medical College, Valhalla; Director, Clinical Strategies Program, Saint Vincent's Hospital and Medical Center, New York, New York
Paracentesis and Abdominal Diagnostic Tap; Urinary Incontinence; Restless Legs Syndrome

DAVE G. MUTHALI, M.D.
Assistant Professor, Department of Internal Medicine, and Director of Residency Training, Texas Tech University Health Sciences Center; Consultant Pulmonologist, Veterans Affairs Medical Center, Amarillo, Texas
Histoplasmosis

VISHWANATHA S. NADIG, M.D.
Fellow, Cardiovascular Medicine, Medical College of Wisconsin, Milwaukee, Wisconsin
Pericarditis

SHERIF F. NAGUEH, M.D.
Assistant Professor of Medicine, Baylor College of Medicine; The Methodist Hospital, Houston, Texas
Mitral Valve Disease

LAETH S. NASIR, M.D.
Associate Professor, Department of Family Medicine, University of Nebraska College of Medicine, Omaha, Nebraska
Impetigo; Childhood Behavioral Problems

NANCY E. NEFF, M.D.
Assistant Professor, Department of Family and Community Medicine, Baylor College of Medicine; Attending Physician, Harris County Hospital District; Member, American College of Physicians, Houston, Texas
Tuberculin Skin Testing

HOLLI K. NEIMAN, M.D., B.S.N.
Assistant Professor, Department of Family Medicine, Wright State University School of Medicine; Associate Director, St. Elizabeth Family Practice Residency Program, Franciscan Medical Center, Dayton, Ohio
Heartburn and Indigestion

KEVIN R. NELSON, M.D.
Associate Professor of Neurology and Assistant Chief of Staff, University of Kentucky Medical Center, Lexington, Kentucky
Carpal Tunnel Syndrome and Other Nerve Entrapments

DAVID H. NEUSTADT, M.D.
Clinical Professor of Medicine, University of Louisville School of Medicine, Louisville, Kentucky
Osteoarthritis

MARK W. NIEDFELDT, M.D.
Assistant Professor and Associate Director, Sports Medicine Fellowship; Departments of Family and Community Medicine, Orthopaedic Surgery, and Cell Biology, Neurobiology, and Anatomy, Medical College of Wisconsin, Milwaukee, Wisconsin
Patellofemoral Pain Syndrome

J. MICHAEL NIEHOFF, M.D.
Associate Director, Department of Family Practice, Franklin Square Hospital Center, Baltimore, Maryland
Casting Techniques

W. ANDERSON NISH, M.D.
Private Practice, Allergy-Immunology, Allergy and Asthma Care Center, Gainesville, Georgia
Food Allergy

ANDREW J. NORTON, M.D.
Associate Professor of Medicine, Medical College of Wisconsin; Senior Vice President of Medical Affairs, Froedtert Memorial Lutheran Hospital, Milwaukee, Wisconsin
Cushing's Syndrome/Disease

TRACEY LEE NORTON, D.O.
Associate Professor of Clinical Family Medicine, and Family Medicine Residency Director, University of Southern California School of Medicine, Los Angeles, California
Preterm Labor

LAURA NOVAK, M.D.
Assistant Professor of Clinical Family Medicine, Northeastern Ohio University College of Medicine, Rootstown; Assistant Director, Barberton Area Family Practice Center, Barberton, Ohio
Hirsutism

JIM NUOVO, M.D.
Associate Professor, Department of Family and Community Medicine, University of California, Davis, Sacramento, California
Cervical Cancer

MARY E. O'BRIEN, M.D.
Associate Professor of Medicine, University of North Carolina, Chapel Hill; Director of Geriatrics, Coastal AHEC, Wilmington, North Carolina
Pneumonia

FRANCIS G. O'CONNOR, M.D.
Assistant Professor of Family Medicine, and Director, Primary Care Sports Medicine Fellowship Program, Uniformed Services University of the Health Sciences, Bethesda, Maryland
Elbow Pain

MICHAEL L. O'DELL, M.D.
Associate Professor, Division Director of Family Medicine, University of Alabama School of Medicine-Huntsville Campus, Huntsville, Alabama
Heat-Related Illness

KEVIN C. OEFFINGER, M.D.
Associate Professor, Department of Family Practice and Community Medicine, University of Texas Southwestern Medical Center, Dallas, Texas
Hypokalemia

JOHN G. O'HANDLEY, M.D.
Clinical Associate Professor, Department of Family Medicine, The Ohio State University College of Medicine; Program Director, Family Practice Residency, Mount Carmel Medical Center, Columbus, Ohio
Acute Otitis Media; Excision of Thrombosed Hemorrhoid

NORMANDI OMAR, M.D.
Assistant Professor, and Associate Director of Family Practice Residency Program, Rush Medical College; Associate Director of Family Practice Residency Program, Rush-Illinois Masonic Family Practice Residency, Chicago, Illinois
Ménière's Disease

SIDNEY C. ONTAI, M.D., M.B.A.
Associate Clinical Professor of Family Medicine, University of Southern California School of Medicine, Los Angeles, California, and Texas Tech University School of Medicine, Lubbock, Texas
Preferred Imaging Modalities in Common Specific Conditions

LARS OSTERBERG, M.D.
Clinical Assistant Professor of Medicine, Stanford University School of Medicine; Staff Physician, Veterans Affairs Palo Alto Health Care System, Palo Alto, California
Swan-Ganz Catheter Monitoring

TOMÁS P. OWENS, Jr., M.D.
Associate Clinical Professor, Department of Family and Preventive Medicine, Department of Internal Medicine, Adjunct, and Department of Geriatric Medicine, Adjunct, University of Oklahoma Health Sciences Center, University of Oklahoma College of Medicine; Chair, Department of Family Practice, Integris Baptist Medical Center; Associate Director, Great Plains Family Practice Residency Program; Board of Directors, Oklahoma Academy of Family Physicians (OAFP) Integris Mental Health Board, Oklahoma City, Oklahoma
Removal of Impacted Cerumen

WILLIAM O. OWINGS, M.D.
Clinical Professor of Family and Community Medicine, University of Alabama School of Medicine Tuscaloosa Program-College of Community Health Sciences; Department of Surgery, DCH Regional Medical Center, Tuscaloosa, Alabama
Wound Management; Wound Revision

JAMES T. PACALA, M.D., M.S.
Associate Professor, Program in Geriatrics, and Director, Program in Medical Student Education, Department of Family Practice and Community Health, University of Minnesota, Minneapolis, Minnesota
Falls in the Elderly

KRISHNAN PADMANABHAN, M.B.B.S.
Associate Professor of Clinical Medicine, State University of New York Health Science Center at Brooklyn; Associate Director, Department of Pulmonary Medicine, Coney Island Hospital, Brooklyn, New York
Atelectasis

JON S. PARHAM, D.O., M.P.H.
Assistant Professor and Pre-doctoral Director, Department of Family Medicine, University of Tennessee Graduate School of Medicine, Knoxville, Tennessee
Parotid Gland Enlargement

STEPHEN PAUL, M.D.
Assistant Clinical Professor, Department of Family and Community Medicine, and Staff, Campus Health, University of Arizona, Tucson, Arizona
Dysmenorrhea

THOMAS R. PELLEGRINO, M.D.
Professor of Neurology, Eastern Virginia Medical School; Staff Physician, Sentara Hospitals, Norfolk, Virginia
Tremor

LINDA F. PESSAR, M.D.
Associate Professor of Clinical Psychiatry and Family Medicine; Director of Medical Student Education in Psychiatry, State University of New York at Buffalo, School of Medicine and Biomedical Sciences, Buffalo, New York
Irritability

JOHN L. PFENNINGER, M.D.
Clinical Professor of Family Medicine, Michigan State University College of Human Medicine, East Lansing; President and Medical Director, The National Procedures Institute, Midland, Michigan
Laceration Repair

ANDY G. PINSON, M.D.
Assistant Professor of Medicine, Medical College of Virginia at Virginia Commonwealth University; Assistant Professor of Medicine, Medical College of Virginia Hospital, Richmond, Virginia
Pyelonephritis

C. S. PITCHUMONI, M.D.
Professor of Medicine and Professor of Preventive Medicine, New York Medical College, Valhalla; Director of Medicine and Chief of Gastroenterology, Our Lady of Mercy Medical University Hospital, Bronx, New York
Pancreatitis

J. STEVEN POCETA, M.D.
Staff Physician, Department of Neuropharmacology, Scripps Research Institute and Green Hospital/Scripps Clinic, La Jolla, California
Sleep Disorders

MARTIN H. POLESKI, M.D.C.M.
Clinical Professor of Medicine, University of California, San Diego, San Diego; Consultant, Scripps Clinic Medical Group, La Jolla, California
Pancreatic Carcinoma

JOHN B. POPE, M.D.
Associate Professor of Clinical Family Medicine, Louisiana State University Medical Center-Shreveport, Shreveport, Louisiana
Nausea and Vomiting; Gastritis

LAWRENCE D. POWELL, M.D.
Assistant Professor, and Primary Care Sports Medicine Director, Department of Family Medicine, Morehouse School of Medicine, Atlanta, Georgia
Bursitis

THOMAS P. POWER, M.B.
Assistant Professor of Medicine, MCP/Hahnemann Allegheny General Hospital; Senior Attending, Division of Cardiology, Department of Medicine, Allegheny General Hospital, Pittsburgh, Pennsylvania
Aortic Dissection

JANET L. PURKEY, M.D.
Associate Professor, Department of Medicine, University of Tennessee Graduate School of Medicine; Director, Medicine Resident Practice, University of Tennessee Memorial Hospital, Knoxville, Tennessee
Calluses and Corns

RONALD E. PUST, M.D.
Professor of Family and Community Medicine, and Professor of Public Health, University of Arizona College of Medicine, Tucson; Family Practice Physician, Carondelet-St. Mary's Hospital, Tucson, Arizona, and Wapenamanda Hospital, Enga Province, Papua New Guinea
Leprosy

DAVID P. RAKEL, M.D.
Affiliate Faculty, Family Practice Residency Program, Idaho State University, Pocatello; Active Staff, Teton Valley Hospital, Driggs, Idaho
Controlling Epistaxis; Hiccups

ROBERT E. RAKEL, M.D.
Professor, Department of Family and Community Medicine, Baylor College of Medicine, Houston, Texas
Circumcision: Plastibell; Depression

TIMOTHY J. J. RAMER, M.D.
Assistant Professor, University of Minnesota School of Medicine; Faculty, Smiley's Clinic, Minneapolis, Minnesota
Circumcision: Gomco

GOUTHAM RAO, M.D., C.M.
Clinical Assistant Professor, University of Pittsburgh; Director, Predoctoral Education, University of Pittsburgh Medical Center-St. Margaret Hospital, Pittsburgh, Pennsylvania
Cirrhosis

NORMAN H. RASMUSSEN, Ed.D.
Consultant, Department of Psychiatry and Psychology, Consultant, Department of Family Medicine, and Assistant Professor, Mayo Medical School, Mayo Clinic, Rochester, Minnesota
Obsessive Compulsive Disorder

ROSE A. RECCO, M.D.
Assistant Professor of Medicine, State University of New York Downstate Medical Center; Director of Infectious Diseases, Coney Island Hospital, Brooklyn, New York
Nongonococcal Urethritis

BARBARA D. REED, M.D., M.S.P.H.
Associate Professor, Department of Family Medicine, University of Michigan, Ann Arbor, Michigan
Vaginitis

EILEEN M. REICKERT, M.D.
Clinical Instructor, Department of Family Medicine, University of Michigan; Physician, University of Michigan Medical Center, Ann Arbor, Michigan
Intussusception

KATHRYN REILLY, M.D., M.P.H.
Associate Professor, Department of Family and Preventive Medicine, University of Oklahoma Health Sciences Center, Oklahoma City, Oklahoma
Hodgkin's Disease

PETER M. REISER, M.D.
Associate Professor of Clinical Medicine, New York University School of Medicine, New York; Chief, Division of Critical Care Medicine, North Shore University Hospital, Manhasset, New York
Bacteremia/Sepsis

RONALD D. REYNOLDS, M.D.
Associate Professor of Family Medicine, University of Cincinnati College of Medicine, Cincinnati; Private Practice, New Richmond Family Practice, New Richmond, Ohio
Circumcision: Mogen Technique

J. RANDALL RICHARD, M.D.
Professor of Clinical Family Medicine, Northeast Ohio Universities College of Medicine, Rootstown; Associate Program Director, Family Practice Residency, Barberton Citizens Hospital, Barberton, Ohio
Punch and Shave Biopsy

MARC RINGEL, M.D.
Northeast Colorado Family Health Center, Brush, Colorado
Enuresis

SHERRY L. ROBBINS, M.D.
Assistant Professor, James H. Quillen College of Medicine, East Tennessee State University, Johnson City; Active Medical Staff, Wellmont-Holston Valley Hospital and Medical Center, Kingsport, Tennessee
Suicide Assessment

VIRGINIA E. ROBERTSON, M.D.
Clinical Assistant Professor, State University of New York Downstate Medical Center; Vice Chair, Department of Family Practice, Long Island College Hospital, Brooklyn, New York
Varicella Infections; Warts and Nevi

JAMES K. RONE, M.D.
Chief of Endocrinology, Murfreesboro Medical Clinic, Murfreesboro, Tennessee
Adrenal Insufficiency

JO ANN ROSENFELD, M.D.
Director of Women's Health, Franklin Square Family Practice, Baltimore, Maryland
Epistomy and Vaginal Laceration Repair

HEATHER ROSSI, M.D.
Rush Medical College; Resident, Department of General Surgery, Rush-Presbyterian-St. Luke's Medical Center, Chicago, Illinois
Colorectal Cancer

STEVEN K. ROTHSCHILD, M.D.
Associate Professor, Department of Family Medicine, Rush Medical College; Chairman, Department of Family Medicine, Illinois Masonic Medical Center; Associate Chair for Clinical Programs, Department of Family Medicine, Rush-Presbyterian-St. Luke's Medical Center, Chicago, Illinois
Peripheral Neuropathy

MICHAEL P. ROWANE, D.O., M.S.
Assistant Professor of Family Medicine, Department of Family Medicine, Case Western Reserve University School of Medicine; Residency Director, University Hospitals of Cleveland Family Practice Residency Program, Cleveland, Ohio
Endometritis

AARON RUBIN, M.D.
Team Physician, University of California, Riverside, Riverside; Program Director, Kaiser Permanente/S.P.O.R.T. Fellowship Program, Kaiser Permanente Family Medicine Residency Program, Fontana, California
Epicondylitis; Head Injuries in Sports

TERRY S. RUHL, M.D.
Associate Director, Allegheny Family Physicians Family Practice Residency Program, Altoona, Pennsylvania
Itching

GEORGE RUST, M.D., M.P.H.
Associate Professor of Family Medicine, and Director, National Center for Primary Care at Morehouse School of Medicine, Morehouse School of Medicine, Atlanta, Georgia
Peritonsillar Abscess Drainage

JERRY RYAN, M.D.
Associate Professor, Department of Family Medicine, and Medical Director, Physician Assistant Program, University of Wisconsin, Madison; Director, Family Medicine Impatient Service, University of Wisconsin Hospital and Clinics, Madison, Wisconsin
Shoulder Pain

CONSTANTINE SAADEH, M.D.
Clinical Professor, Internal Medicine and Pediatrics, Texas Tech University Health Sciences Center; Private Practice, Allergy Asthma Rheumatology Treatment Specialist; President, Amarillo Allergy, Asthma, and Arthritis Research Foundation, Amarillo, Texas
Urticaria and Angioedema

AKRAM SADAKA, M.D., M.P.H.
Assistant Clinical Professor of Family Medicine and Preventive Medicine, The Ohio State University, Columbus, Ohio
Preoperative Evaluation

REBECCA B. SAENZ, M.D.
Assistant Professor of Family Medicine, University of Mississippi Medical Center, Jackson, Mississippi
Colposcopy

STEPHEN D. SAGLIO, M.D.
Assistant Clinical Professor, Department of Family and Community Medicine, University of California, San Francisco, School of Medicine, San Francisco; Faculty Physician, Natividad Medical Center, Salinas, California
Pityriasis Rosea

SAMUEL J. SALIBA, M.D.
Clinical Professor of Family Medicine, University of Alabama at Birmingham School of Medicine, Birmingham; Program Director, Montgomery Family Medicine Residency, Baptist Health Medical Center, Montgomery, Alabama
Gynecomastia

WILLIAM R. SCHEIBEL, M.D.
Professor of Family Medicine, Department of Family Medicine, University of Wisconsin, Madison, Wisconsin
Infectious Mononucleosis

DAWN SCHISSEL, M.D.
Associate Professor, University of Iowa, Iowa City; Faculty Physician, Broadlawns Medical Center, Des Moines, Iowa
Meningitis

KATHERINE R. SCHLAERTH, M.D.
Associate Clinical Professor of Family Medicine and Pediatrics, University of Southern California School of Medicine; Attending Physician, LAC-University of Southern California Medical Center, Los Angeles, California
Food Poisoning

E. ROBERT SCHWARTZ, M.D.
Professor and Chair, Department of Family Medicine and Community Health, University of Miami School of Medicine; Chief of Service, Department of Family Medicine, Jackson Memorial Hospital, Miami, Florida
Varicocele

ROBERT J. SCHWARTZMAN, M.D.
Professor and Chairman, Department of Neurology, MCP Hahnemann University School of Medicine, Philadelphia, Pennsylvania
Reflex Sympathetic Dystrophy

WILLIAM A. SCHWER, M.D.
Professor and Chairman, Rush Medical College, Chicago, Illinois
Hoarseness

PATRICIA A. SERENO, M.D., M.P.H.
Clinical Instructor, Department of Family Medicine, Boston University School of Medicine; Lecturer, Department of Family Medicine and Community Health, Tufts University School of Medicine; Faculty Member, Tufts University Family Practice Residency, Boston, Massachusetts
Endometriosis

ANIL SHAH, M.D.
Chief, Division of Internal Medicine, Samaritan Medical Center, Watertown, New York
Aortic Valve Disease

GYANENDRA K. SHARMA, M.D.
Assistant Professor, Department of Internal Medicine, University of Kansas School of Medicine; St. Francis Regional Medical Center, Wichita, Kansas
Central Venous Catheter Insertion

ANGELA J. SHEPHERD, M.D.
Assistant Professor, and Director, Residency Program, University of Texas Medical Branch, Galveston, Texas
Adult Jaundice

HAL S. SHIMAZU, M.D.
Associate Clinical Professor, Department of Family Medicine, University of California, Irvine, College of Medicine, Orange, California
Thrombocytopenia

CYNTHIA L. SHORT, M.D.
Clinical Assistant Professor, Albany Medical College; Capital District Renal Physicians, Albany, New York
Acute Renal Failure

PESACH SHVARTZMAN, M.D.
Chair, Division of Community Health, and Chair, Department of Family Medicine, Ben Gurion University; Director, Department of Family Medicine, and Consultant, Home Palliative Care Unit, Kupat Holim Chalit, Beer-Sheva, Israel
Pain Management

MOHAMAD A. SIDANI, M.D., M.S.
Assistant Professor, Department of Family Practice, Associate Program Director, and Family Practice Center Clinic Director, Louisiana State University School of Medicine Family Practice Residency Program, Kenner, Louisiana
Tympanocentesis

RICHARD T. SILVER, M.D.
Clinical Professor of Medicine, Weill Medical College, Cornell University; Attending Physician, Department of Medicine, Division of Hematology and Medical Oncology, New York Presbyterian Hospital, New York, New York
Polycythemia

WILLIAM M. SIMPSON, Jr., M.D.
Professor of Family Medicine, Medical University of South Carolina, Charleston, South Carolina
Varicose Veins

MARION H. SIMS, M.D.
Residency Director, Family Practice Residency Program, Medical Center East, Birmingham, Alabama
Use of Blood Products

DANIELLE SINK, M.D.
Assistant Professor of Clinical Medicine, University of Arizona College of Medicine, Tucson; Director of House Staff Affairs, Department of Internal Medicine, St. Joseph's Hospital and Medical Center, Phoenix, Arizona
Sclerotherapy for Varicose Veins

W. MICHAEL SKEENS, M.D.
Associate Professor of Medicine, Department of Medicine, Marshall University School of Medicine, Huntington, West Virginia
Flashing Lights and Floaters; Optic Neuritis

ARTHUR R. SLAUGHTER, M.D.
Associate Professor of Clinical Family Medicine, University of Virginia, Charlottesville; Associate Director of Family Medical Education, Carilion Health System, Roanoke, Virginia
Herpes Simplex Infection; Herpes Zoster Infection

JOHN T. SLEVIN, M.D.
Professor, Departments of Neurology and Pharmacology, University of Kentucky Medical School; Staff Neurologist, Veterans Administration Medical Center, Lexington, Kentucky
Parkinson's Disease

LAWRENCE G. SMITH, M.D.
Professor of Medicine, Mount Sinai School of Medicine; Attending Physician, Mount Sinai Hospital, New York, New York
Weight Loss

RICHARD H. SNYDER, M.D., M.B.A.
Associate Professor of Clinical Medicine, The Milton S. Hershey Medical Center, Pennsylvania State University College of Medicine, Hershey; Vice Chairman, Department of Medicine, Internal Medicine and Transitional Residency Program Director, and Medical Director of Critical Care, Lehigh Valley Hospital, Allentown, Pennsylvania
Acute Respiratory Distress Syndrome

BECK B. SODERBERG, M.D.
Private Practice, Lancaster General Hospital, Lancaster, Pennsylvania
Cat-Scratch Disease

AUGUSTINE J. SOHN, M.D., M.P.H.
Assistant Professor, Department of Family Medicine, University of Illinois at Chicago College of Medicine; Attending Physician, University of Illinois Medical Center, Chicago, Illinois
Burns

GLEN D. SOLOMON, M.D.
Associate Professor of Medicine, The Ohio State University, Columbus; Consultant, Section of Headache, Department of Neurology, The Cleveland Clinic Foundation, Cleveland, Ohio
Headache

GREGORY T. SOLTNER, D.O.
Family Practice Physician, Family Practice Association Upper Dublin, Fort Washington, and Abington Memorial Hospital, Abington, Pennsylvania
Miliaria

JOHN G. SPANGLER, M.D., M.P.H.
Assistant Professor, Department of Family and Community Medicine, Wake Forest University School of Medicine; Attending Physician, Wake Forest University Baptist Medical Center, Winston-Salem, North Carolina
Influenza; Leukoplakia and Erythroplasia

JOHN P. SPECK, M.D.
Medical Director, CAPD Program, South East Michigan Kidney Center, Berkley, Michigan
Hyperkalemia

FERNANDO F. STANCAMPIANO, M.D.
Staff Physician, Department of Internal Medicine, Cleveland Clinic Florida, Fort Lauderdale, Florida
Claudication

JOHN B. STANDRIDGE, M.D.
Assistant Professor, Department of Family Medicine, University of Tennessee College of Medicine, Chattanooga Unit; Baroness Erlanger Medical Center, Chattanooga, Tennessee
Growth and Development Guidelines

J. STEPHAN STAPCZYNSKI, M.D.
Chair and Associate Professor, University of Kentucky College of Medicine, Lexington, Kentucky
Fever and Chills

KENNETH K. STEINWEG, M.D.
Associate Professor, Geriatric Division, Department of Family Medicine, East Carolina University School of Medicine, Greenville, North Carolina
Osteoporosis

MICHAEL B. STEVENS, M.D.
Clinical Associate Professor, Division of Family and Community Medicine, Department of Medicine, Stanford University School of Medicine, Palo Alto; Associate Director, San Jose Medical Center Family Practice Residency Program, San Jose, California
Migraine Headache

M. DAVID STOCKTON, M.D., M.P.H.
Associate Professor, Department of Family Medicine, University of Tennessee Graduate School of Medicine; Active Staff, University of Tennessee Medical Center, Knoxville, Tennessee
Pulmonary Function Testing

ERIC B. STONE, M.D.
Family Practice Residency Teaching Staff, David Grant Medical Center, Travis Air Force Base, California
Starting an Intravenous Infusion: Adult and Infant

FREDERICK C. STONE, Jr., M.D., M.P.H.
Assistant Professor of Family Medicine, James H. Quillen College of Medicine, East Tennessee State University, Johnson City, Tennessee
Hyperprolactinemia

MARIAN R. STUART, Ph.D.
Clinical Professor, Department of Family Medicine, University of Medicine and Dentistry of New Jersey-Robert Wood Johnson Medical School, New Brunswick, New Jersey
The BATHE Technique

FRED M. SUTTON, Jr., M.D.
Associate Professor of Medicine, Baylor College of Medicine; Chief, Gastroenterology, Ben Taub General Hospital, Houston, Texas
Irritable Bowel Syndrome

S. ANTHONY SWALDI, M.D.
Clinical Faculty, University of Texas Southwestern Medical School, Dallas, Texas
Fungal Infections

CARLOS M. SWANGER, M.D.
Part-time Faculty, Department of Medicine, University of Rochester School of Medicine and Dentistry; General Internist, Unity Health System, Park Ridge Hospital, Unity Medical Group-Park Ridge Internal Medicine, Rochester, New York
Scleroderma (Systemic Sclerosis)

STEVEN K. SWEDLUND, M.D.
Associate Director, Miami Valley Hospital Family Practice Residency; Associate Clinical Professor, Department of Family Medicine, Wright State University School of Medicine, Dayton, Ohio
Acute Urinary Tract Infection in Adults

DAVID J. TANAKA, M.D.
Associate Professor of Medicine, Division of Internal Medicine, Department of Medicine, University of Colorado Health Sciences Center, Denver, Colorado
Deep Venous Thrombosis

HOWARD B. TANDETER, M.D.
Lecturer and Coordinator of Family Development Program, Department of Family Medicine, Faculty of Health Sciences, Ben-Gurion University, Beer-Sheva; Chairman, Israeli Society of Teachers of Family Medicine, Israel
Earache/Ear Pain

EROL TAŞDEMIROĞLU, M.D.
Attending Neurosurgeon, İncirli Hospital, Neurosurgery Service, Istanbul, Turkey
Subdural Hematoma

NANCY O. TATUM, M.D.*
Associate Professor, Department of Family Medicine, University of Mississippi Medical Center, Jackson, Mississippi
Asymptomatic HIV Infection

NADER TAVAKOLI, M.D.
Clinical Assistant Professor of Family Medicine, Georgetown University School of Medicine, Washington, D.C.; Co-Chairman, Department of Family Medicine, Ross University School of Medicine, Dominica, West Indies
Pap Smear

HARRIS C. TAYLOR, M.D.
Associate Clinical Professor of Medicine (Endocrinology), Case Western Reserve University School of Medicine; Director of Resident Research, Fairview Health System Internal Medicine Residency, Cleveland, Ohio
Hypoglycemia

ROSLYN D. TAYLOR, M.D.
Associate Director, Memorial Health Family Practice Residency, Savannah; Associate Professor, Department of Family Medicine, Mercer University School of Medicine, Macon; Clinical Associate Professor, Department of Family Medicine, Medical College of Georgia, Augusta; Memorial Health University Medical Center, Savannah, Georgia
Low Back Pain Exercises

---

*Deceased.

KENNETH L. TAYLOR-BUTLER, M.D.
Faculty Physician, Trinity Lutheran Hospital, Kansas City, Missouri
Finger Fractures

JONATHAN L. TEMTE, M.D., M.S., Ph.D.
Assistant Professor of Family Medicine, Department of Family Medicine, University of Wisconsin, Madison, Wisconsin
Abdominal Pain

LINDA E. TEPPER, M.D.
Clinical Instructor of Medicine, Albert Einstein College of Medicine of the Yeshiva University of New York; Voluntary Faculty, Long Island Jewish Medical Center, New Hyde Park, and North Shore University Hospital, Manhasset, New York
Hematuria

JOANNA M. THOMAS, M.B., Ch.B.
Assistant Professor, Department of Family and Community Medicine, University of Arkansas Medical School, Area Health Education Center, North West Arkansas Residency Program, Fayetteville; Chief of Family Practice, Washington Regional Medical Center, Fayetteville; Staff Member, North West Medical Center, Springdale, Arkansas
Norplant Insertion and Removal

WARREN G. THOMPSON, M.D.
Associate Professor of Medicine, University of Tennessee Graduate School of Medicine; Chairman, Department of Medicine, University of Tennessee Medical Center, Knoxville, Tennessee
Alcoholism

GEORGE ALLEN TINDOL, Jr., M.D.
Assistant Professor of Internal Medicine, Mercer University School of Medicine, Macon; Assistant Clinical Professor of Internal Medicine, Medical College of Georgia, Augusta; Associate Director of Internal Medicine Education, Memorial Health University Medical Center, Savannah, Georgia
Sarcoidosis

PETER P. TOTH, M.D., Ph.D.
Clinical Assistant Professor, Department of Family Medicine, University of Illinois College of Medicine at Rockford, Rockford; Attending Physician, Sullivan Clinic/Sarah Bush Lincoln Health System, Sullivan, Illinois
Management of Bartholin's Gland Duct Cysts and Abscesses

DAVID E. TRACHTENBARG, M.D.
Clinical Professor of Family Practice, University of Illinois College of Medicine at Peoria; Medical Director, Family Medical Center, Methodist Medical Center, Peoria, Illinois
Venous Stasis Ulcer

HOWARD TUNG, M.D.
Assistant Professor of Neurological Surgery, Division of Neurological Surgery, University of California, San Diego, San Diego, California
Trigeminal Neuralgia

JOSEPH VALENTINO, M.D.
Assistant Professor, Department of Surgery, University of Kentucky Chandler Medical Center, Lexington, Kentucky
Epistaxis; Cricothyrotomy/Tracheostomy

DEEPA VASUDEVAN, M.D., M.B.B.S.
Assistant Professor, Department of Family and Community Medicine, University of Texas at Houston School of Medicine; Faculty, Herman Hospital, Houston, Texas
Glaucoma

MIRIAM T. VINCENT, M.D., M.S., Ph.D.(c)
Associate Professor of Family Practice, State University of New York Health Science Center at Brooklyn; Associate Professor, and Interim Chair, Department of Family Practice, University Hospital of Brooklyn, Kings County Hospital Medical Center, Brooklyn, New York
Typhoid Fever

CAREY VINSON, M.D., M.P.M.
Clinical Assistant Professor of Clinical Epidemiology and Family Medicine, University of Pittsburgh School of Medicine; Medical Director, Quality Improvement, Highmark Blue Cross Blue Shield, Pittsburgh, Pennsylvania
Cervicitis

H. BRUCE VOGT, M.D.
Professor and Chair, Department of Family Medicine, and Medical Director, University of South Dakota Physician Assistant Studies Program, University of South Dakota School of Medicine, Sioux Falls, South Dakota
Nasal Polyps

KIMBERLE J. VORE, M.D.
Clinical Assistant Professor of Family Medicine, Department of Family Medicine and Clinical Epidemiology, University of Pittsburgh School of Medicine, Pittsburgh; Clinical Instructor, Washington Hospital, Washington, Pennsylvania
Gestational Hyperglycemia/Diabetes

DIANE S. VOSS, M.D.
Clinical Instructor of Medicine, University of Missouri School of Medicine and University of Missouri School of Nursing, Kansas City, Missouri
Fluid Balance

CYNTHIA M. WAICKUS, M.D., Ph.D.
Assistant Professor and Director of Predoctoral Education, Department of Family Medicine, Rush Medical College, Chicago, Illinois
Hemoptysis

MARGARET WALSH, M.S.
Assistant Professor, Albert Einstein College of Medicine; Family Nurse Practitioner, and Faculty, Bronx Lebanon Family Practice Residency Program, Bronx Lebanon Hospital, Bronx, New York
Pelvic Inflammatory Disease

BENNET M. WANG, M.D., M.P.H.
Assistant Chief, North Region Pulmonary and Critical Care Medicine, Group Health Cooperative of Puget Sound, Seattle, Washington
Laryngitis; Bronchiectasis

RANDY K. WARD, M.D.
Clinical Assistant Professor, Department of Family Medicine, University of Michigan, Ann Arbor, Michigan
Wernicke-Korsakoff Syndrome

BENJAMIN C. WARF, M.D.
Associate Professor of Surgery and Pediatrics, Chief of Pediatric Neurosurgery, and Director of Surgical Education, University of Kentucky Medical School, Lexington, Kentucky
Brain Tumor

PETER R. WARRINGTON, D.O.
Teaching Faculty-Obstetrics/Gynecology Coordinator, Wyoming Valley Family Practice Residency, Kingston, Pennsylvania
Third Trimester Bleeding

MICHAEL L. WATERS, M.D.
Active Staff at Baptist Medical Center-Downtown and Wolfson Children's Hospital; Team Physician Jacksonville University Football Team, Jacksonville, Florida
Red Eye

DEANNA J. WATHINGTON, M.D., M.P.H.
Assistant Professor, Department of Family Medicine, University of South Florida College of Medicine; Active Staff, Tampa General Hospital, Tampa, Florida
Kidney Cancer

MONICA O. WATTS, M.D.
Assistant Professor, Morehouse School of Medicine, Atlanta, Georgia
Systemic Lupus Erythematosus

RONALD S. WATTS, M.D.
Endocrinology Staff, St. Joseph's Hospital, Atlanta, Northside Hospital, Atlanta, and North Fulton Regional Medical Center, Roswell, Georgia
Hypothyroidism; Hyperthyroidism

RALPH WEBER, M.D.
Instructor, Cardiovascular Medicine, Johns Hopkins University School of Medicine; Attending Physician, Johns Hopkins Hospital, Sinai Hospital of Baltimore, and Union Memorial Hospital, Baltimore, Maryland
Leg Edema

DAVID G. WEISMILLER, M.D., Sc.M.
Assistant Professor of Family Medicine, and Director, Program in Women's Health, Department of Family Medicine, East Carolina University School of Medicine; Attending Physician, Pitt County Memorial Hospital, Greenville, North Carolina
Fetal Lung Immaturity

KENNETH A. WELLER, M.D.
Clinical Assistant Professor, University of Colorado Health Sciences Center, Denver; Assistant Residency Director, Swedish Family Medicine Residency, Littleton, Colorado
Impaired Hearing

MARK D. WELLS, M.D.
Associate Professor of Surgery, Case Western Reserve University, Cleveland, Ohio
Tattoo Removal

HAROLD V. WERNER, M.D.
Professor, Internal Medicine, Texas Tech University School of Medicine, Amarillo, Texas
Thyroid Nodule; Thyroid Carcinoma

RUSSELL D. WHITE, M.D.
Clinical Associate Professor, Department of Family Medicine, University of South Florida College of Medicine, Tampa; Associate Director, Family Practice Residency, and Director, Sports Medicine Fellowship Program, Bayfront Medical Center, St. Petersburg, Florida
Asthma; Costochondritis

LORI A. WHITTAKER, M.D., Ph.D.
Member of Medical Staff, Steven's Hospital, and Birth and Family Clinic, Edmonds, Washington
Cancer Screening; Ovarian Cancer

JOHN W. WILLIAMS, Jr., M.D., M.H.S.
Associate Professor, University of Texas Health Science Center-San Antonio; Staff Physician, South Texas Veterans Health Care System, San Antonio, Texas
Sinusitis

REBECCA WILLIAMS, M.D.
Assistant Professor of Clinical Family Medicine, University of Illinois at Chicago, Chicago, Illinois
Breast-Feeding

SEYMOUR G. WILLIAMS, M.D.
Epidemiologist/Medical Officer, Air Pollution and Respiratory Health Branch, National Center for Environmental Health, and Centers for Disease Control and Prevention, Atlanta, Georgia
Vulvar Pruritus

SANDRA K. WILLSIE, D.O.
Interim Chair of Medicine and Professor of Medicine, University of Missouri, Kansas City, School of Medicine, and Truman Medical Center, Kansas City, Missouri
Pulse Oximetry; Cancers of the Larynx and Lung

BRUCE E. WILSON, M.D.
Director, Smohalla Metabolism, Richland, Washington
Diabetes Mellitus, Type II

TIMOTHY J. WILT, M.D., M.P.H.
Associate Professor of Medicine, University of Minnesota; Staff Physician, Section of General Medicine, Minneapolis Veterans Affairs Center for Chronic Diseases Outcomes Research, Minneapolis, Minnesota
Prostate Cancer

CARL WINFIELD, M.D.
Clinical Assistant Professor of Family Medicine, and Team Physician, Athletic Department, The Ohio State University; Medical Director, The Ohio State University Center for Wellness and Prevention-Downtown, The Ohio State University Hospitals, Columbus, Ohio
Patellar Dislocations

WILLIAM H. WINKLER, M.D.
Assistant Professor, Department of Family Medicine, University of Texas Medical Branch, Galveston; Associate Director, Conroe Family Practice Residency, Conroe, Texas
Coronary Artery Disease

KELLEY WITHY, M.D.
Assistant Professor of Family Medicine, Department of Family Practice and Community Health, John A. Burns School of Medicine, University of Hawaii, Honolulu; Staff Physician, Residency Faculty, Wahiawa General Hospital, Wahiawa, Hawaii
Plantar Fasciitis

ANDREW M. D. WOLF, M.D.
Associate Professor of Medicine, University of Virginia School of Medicine and University of Virginia Health System, Charlottesville, Virginia
Constipation

IRVING D. WOLFE, M.D.
Associate Clinical Professor of Dermatology, University of Maryland School of Medicine; Instructor in Dermatology, Johns Hopkins University School of Medicine, Baltimore, Maryland
Cyrosurgery and Electrocautery of Skin Lesions

MICHAEL S. WOLKOMIR, M.D., M.A., D.E.C.H.
Associate Professor of Family and Community Medicine, Medical College of Wisconsin; Obstetrics/Gynecology Education Director, St. Michael Hospital Family Practice Residency, Milwaukee, Wisconsin
Postpartum Hemorrhage

LAURIE J. WOODARD, M.D.
Associate Professor of Family Medicine, University of South Florida, Tampa, Florida
Lumbar Puncture

JACK R. WOODSIDE, Jr., M.D.
Assistant Professor, Department of Family Medicine, East Tennessee State University College of Medicine, Johnson City, Tennessee
Intercostal Nerve Block; Local and Regional Anesthesia of the Upper Extremity

ROBERT J. WOOLLEY, M.D.
Staff, Boynton Health Service, University of Minnesota, Minneapolis, Minnesota
Contraception

SEIJI YAMADA, M.D., M.P.H.
Associate Professor of Family Medicine, Department of Family Practice and Community Health, John A. Burns School of Medicine, University of Hawaii, Mililani, Hawaii
Tuberculosis

DAVID H. YAWN, M.D.
Professor of Pathology, Baylor College of Medicine; Medical Director of Transfusion Service, The Methodist Hospital, Houston, Texas
Adverse Reactions to Blood Transfusions

RAM YOGEV, M.D.
Professor of Pediatrics, Northwestern University Medical School; Associate Division Head, Division of Infectious Diseases, and Director, Section of Pediatric and Maternal HIV Infection, Children's Memorial Hospital, Chicago, Illinois
Measles (Rubeola)

CRAIG C. YOUNG, M.D.
Associate Professor and Medical Director of Sports Medicine, Medical College of Wisconsin, Milwaukee, Wisconsin
Knee Pain

ZOBAIR M. YOUNOSSI, M.D., M.P.H.
Staff, Department of Gastroenterology, The Cleveland Clinic Foundation, Cleveland, Ohio
Acute Upper Gastrointestinal Bleeding

KHALID ZAFAR, M.D.
Teaching Staff and Consultant Nephrologist, William Beaumont Hospital, Royal Oak; Consultant Nephrologist, Grace Hospital, Affiliate of Wayne State University, Detroit, Michigan
Glomerulonephritis

ANDREW H. ZALSKI, M.D.
Assistant Professor, Rush Medical College; Director, Rush Illinois Masonic Family Practice Center, Illinois Masonic Medical Center, Chicago, Illinois
Guillain-Barré Syndrome

MUHAMMAD K. ZAMAN, M.D.
Associate Professor of Medicine, University of Tennessee, Memphis, College of Medicine, Memphis; Chief of Pulmonary Section and Director of Respiratory Therapy Service, Veterans Affairs Medical Center, Memphis, Tennessee
Interstitial Lung Disease; Technique of Sputum Induction

MARK A. ZAMORSKI, M.D., M.H.S.A.
Clinical Assistant Professor of Family Medicine, University of Michigan Medical School, Ann Arbor, Michigan
Panic Disorder

THERESE ZINK, M.D., M.P.H.
Assistant Professor of Clinical Family Medicine, Department of Family Medicine, University of Cincinnati Medical Center, Cincinnati, Ohio
Herbal Medicine

ROGER J. ZOOROB, M.D., M.P.H.
Associate Department Chair and Program Director, Department of Family Practice, Louisiana State University School of Medicine Family Practice Residency Program, Kenner, Louisiana
Melanoma

Foreword to the First Edition

> Knowledge is of two kinds. We know a subject ourselves, or we know where we can find information upon it.
>
> *Samuel Johnson, 1775*

James Boswell's quote from the *Life of Johnson* is appropriate for the world's first great lexicographer. Samuel Johnson was the first person to use illustrative historical quotations and his *Dictionary*, published in 1755, is a milestone of the English language. In the creation of his *Dictionary*, Johnson knew that the educated 18th century man or woman needed a dependable reference source.

Today, the educated physician also needs a dependable reference source. *Saunders Manual of Medical Practice* offers that source with a thoroughness and clarity that is admirable.

Dr. Johnson's method of organizing his *Dictionary* was preordained—he simply depended on the English alphabet. However, the *Saunders Manual* editors were faced with a more daunting task. They had to develop a system of organizing medical knowledge so that it became readily accessible to the diligent primary care physician as well as the overwhelmed medical student. The organization had to be as easy to use—and as dependable—as looking up the word "lung" under "L."

The editors chose to organize *Saunders Manual of Medical Practice* into 20 organ system sections. The outline format within each organ system allows for instant recognition of symptoms, laboratory tests needed, treatment, and other basic relevant medical information. While allowing for a quick look-see when appropriate, each section also contains more than enough information for extensive study, including reference follow-ups for additional information.

Dr. Johnson's *Dictionary* became famous because the author took the extra step in explaining the English language. Similarly, *Saunders Manual of Medical Practice* also takes an extra step to distinguish it from other manuals. There are 58 procedures interspersed in the text. They are highly illustrated to give physicians the opportunity to quickly review procedures which they may not have the need to do every day yet are necessarily part of the lexicon of the primary care physician.

Samuel Johnson's *Dictionary of the English Language* was not the first dictionary, the only dictionary, or even the largest dictionary of his day. Yet, it survives as one of the most famous dictionaries of all time because of its energy and illustrative language and ambition to explain words in the most precise way possible.

Similarly, *Saunders Manual of Medical Practice* is not the only medical manual available to the primary care physician or medical student. However, I believe that its ambition, scope, and organization make it an outstanding volume that will soon be the standard text in every physician's office. With *Saunders Manual*, today's physician or medical student can be comfortable with Dr. Johnson's quote— "If you don't know the answer, you'll know where to find it."

ROGER C. BONE, M.D.

Preface

This is an expanded and revised version of the first edition, designed to help the busy primary care physician and allied health professional. The goal is to provide concise information regarding the diagnosis and treatment of problems frequently encountered in practice. Material is presented in outline format to facilitate ease of retrieval. Key points are highlighted and boxed to assist in identifying essential information rapidly.

Twenty-four new topics and five new procedures have been added. Among the new topics are herbal medicine, PPD testing, polymyositis, Sjögren's syndrome, autism, cat scratch disease, and attention deficit disorder. New procedures include pulse oximetry, Mogen circumcision, and treatment of a Bartholin cyst infection.

There are 18 new illustrations drawn by Jan Redden, and four from the first edition were modified.

There are 486 chapters consisting of 343 diseases, 79 symptoms, 64 procedures, and an appendix of normal laboratory values. Each chapter has recent or classic references for those who desire additional information. Tables are frequently used to provide a maximum of information in a concise and rapidly retrievable format.

Many topics are included that are not found in most traditional texts. Examples are deep muscle relaxation exercises, costochondritis, removal of impacted cerumen, reflex sympathetic dystrophy, techniques for sputum induction, chronic fatigue syndrome, aphthous stomatitis, restless legs syndrome, and the use of glue in laceration repair.

Every attempt has been made to keep the material current up to the date of publication. One example is the lead information on immunization schedules, which continue to change as new and better vaccines become available.

Special credit for the quality of this edition goes to Ray Kersey and the excellent editorial staff at W.B. Saunders, and to Caroline Kosnik, my editorial assistant, whose excellent attention to detail ensures that manuscripts and galley proof are managed in a timely manner and the book published on schedule.

ROBERT E. RAKEL, M.D.

Contents

Detailed table of contents begins on following right hand page

Part IV Cardiovascular Diseases

Part XVIII Neurology

Appendix

1 Immunization Schedules

Rick Kellerman

Diphtheria-Tetanus-Pertussis (DTaP, DTwP, DT, dT, DTaP-HbCV, DTwP-HbCV)

General Information
1. DTaP (diphtheria-tetanus–acellular pertussis)
   a. Combination vaccine with diphtheria and tetanus toxoids and acellular pertussis component
   b. Lower incidence of fever, local reactions, and systemic symptoms than with DTwP
   c. Administer at 2, 4, 6, and 15 to 18 months and 4 to 6 years (see Table 1–1).
   d. Allow 6 months between doses 3 and 4; allow 6 months between doses 4 and 5.
   e. Dose 5 is unnecessary if dose 4 is administered after age 4.
   f. Antipyretics are indicated before administration.
   g. When possible, use the same DTaP product for first three doses; if not available, may use interchangeably.
   h. DTaP preferred over DTwP for all primary series doses in children.
   i. Future immunization schedules may recommend DTaP booster after age 6.
2. DTwP (diphtheria-tetanus–whole-cell pertusis)
   a. Pertussis component is whole cell.
   b. Acceptable alternative to DTaP using same schedule; higher rate of fever, local reactions, and systemic symptoms than with DTaP
   c. Antipyretics indicated before and after administration.
   d. Do not use after age 6 years.
3. DT (pediatric diphtheria-tetanus): Substitute for DTaP and DTwP if pertussis component is contraindicated in child under age 7 years.
4. dT (booster diphtheria-tetanus)
   a. Adolescent booster is given at age 11 to 16 years.
   b. Adult booster is given every 10 years after the adolescent booster.
   c. Use for primary series in unimmunized adults and children older than age 6 years: 0, 4 to 8 weeks, 6 to 12 months.
   d. All primary series doses after age 6 years should be dT.
5. DTaP–*Haemophilus influenzae* type b conjugate vaccine (HbCV)
   a. TriHIBiT is the only licensed DTaP-HbCV combination vaccine.
   b. Licensed only for the fourth dose at age 15 to 18 months
   c. Must administer within 30 minutes of reconstitution.
   d. Local and systemic reaction profile no different than separately injected vaccines.
6. DTwP-HbCV
   a. Tetramune and ActHIB/DTP allow simultaneous immunization of DTP and HbCV at 2, 4, 6, and 15 to 18 months.
   b. Of limited usefulness because DTaP is now the preferred vaccination against diphtheria, tetanus, and pertussis.

Precautions
1. Diphtheria and tetanus toxoid components
   a. Rarely cause systemic reactions.
   b. May cause local reactions.
   c. Reactions more common with too-frequent immunization.
   d. Although rare, available evidence favors causal relationship between tetanus toxoid and both brachial neuritis and Guillain-Barré syndrome in adult vaccinees.
   e. Exaggerated local Arthus-type reactions may occur 2 to 8 hours after immunization, probably as a result of very high serum tetanus antitoxin levels.
   f. Bleeding disorders
2. Pertussis component
   a. Precautions apply equally to DTaP and DTwP.
   b. DTaP preferred over DTwP for all vaccinations in children less than 7 years.
   c. DTaP preferred over DTwP if previous vaccination resulted in pertussis-associated "Precaution" and risk/benefit ratio favors further immunization.

TABLE 1–1.   RECOMMENDED CHILDHOOD IMMUNIZATION SCHEDULE, UNITED STATES—JANUARY 1999 TO DECEMBER 1999[1]

Vaccine	Birth	1 mo	2 mo	4 mo	6 mo	12 mo	15 mo	18 mo	4–6 yr	11–12 yr	14–16 yr
Hepatitis B[2]	Hep B										
		Hep B			Hep B					Hep B	
Diphtheria, tetanus, pertussis[3]			DTaP	DTaP	DTaP		DTaP[3]		DTaP	Td	
Haemophilus influenzae type b[4]			Hib	Hib	Hib	Hib					
Poliovirus[5]			IPV	IPV	IPV				IPV		
Measles-mumps-rubella[6]						MMR			MMR[6]	MMR[6]	
Varicella[7]						Var				Var[7]	

[1]This schedule has been approved by the Advisory Committee on Immunization Practices (ACIP), the American Academy of Pediatrics and the American Academy of Family Physicians (AAFP). It indicates the recommended ages for routine administration of currently licensed childhood vaccines. Clear bars indicate range of recommended ages for immunization. Any dose not given at the recommended age should be given as a "catch-up" immunization at any subsequent visit when indicated and feasible. Shaded bars indicate vaccines to be given if previously recommended doses were missed or given earlier than the recommended minimum age. Combination vaccines may be used whenever any components of the combination are indicated and its other components are not contraindicated. Providers should consult the manufacturers' package inserts for detailed recommendations.

[2]Infants born to hepatitis B surface antigen (HBsAg)-negative mothers should receive the second dose of hepatitis B (Hep B) vaccine at least one month after the first dose. The third dose should be administered at least four months after the first dose and at least two months after the second dose, but not before six months of age for infants. Infants born to HBsAg-positive mothers should receive Hep B vaccine and 0.5 mL hepatitis B immune globulin (HBIG) within 12 hours of birth at separate sites. The second dose is recommended at one to two months of age and the third dose at six months of age. Infants born to mothers whose HBsAg status is unknown should receive Hep B vaccine within 12 hours of birth. Maternal blood should be drawn at the time of delivery to determine the mother's HBsAg status; if the HBsAg test is positive, the infant should receive HBIG as soon as possible (no later than one week of age). All children and adolescents (through 18 years of age) who have not been immunized against Hep B may begin the series during any visit. Special efforts should be made to immunize children who were born in or whose parents were born in areas of the world with moderate or high endemicity of Hep B virus infection.

[3]Diphtheria and tetanus toxoids and acellular pertussis vaccine (DTaP) is the preferred vaccine for all doses in the immunization series, including completion of the series in children who have received one or more doses of whole-cell diphtheria, tetanus, pertussis (DTP) vaccine. Whole-cell DTP is an acceptable alternative to DTaP. The fourth dose (DTP or DTaP) may be administered as early as 12 months of age, provided six months have elapsed since the third dose and if the child is unlikely to return at age 15 to 18 months. Tetanus and diphtheria toxoids (Td) is recommended at 11 to 12 years of age if at least five years has elapsed since the last dose of DTP, DTaP or DT. Subsequent routine Td boosters are recommended every 10 years.

[4]Three *H. influenzae* type B (Hib) conjugate vaccines are licensed for infant use. If PRP-OMP (PedvaxHIB and COMVAX) is administered at two and four months of age, a dose at six months is not required. Because clinical studies in infants have demonstrated that using some combination products may induce a lower immune response to the Hib vaccine component, DTaP/Hib combination products should not be used for primary immunization in infants at two, four or six months of age, unless it is approved by the U.S. Food and Drug Administration for these ages.

[5]An all-IPV immunization schedule is recommended as of January 2000. Oral poliovirus vaccine is no longer recommended for routine immunization.

[6]The second dose of measles, mumps-rubella (MMR) vaccine is recommended routinely at four to six years of age but may be administered during any visit, provided at least four weeks has elapsed since receipt of the first dose and that both doses are administered beginning at or after 12 months of age. Those who have not previously received the second dose should complete the schedule by the 11- to 12-year-old visit.

[7]Varicella (Var) is recommended at any visit on or after the first birthday for susceptible children, i.e., those who lack a reliable history of chickenpox (as judged by a health care provider) and who have not been immunized. Susceptible persons 13 years of age or older should receive two doses, given at least four weeks apart.

Adapted from Centers for Disease Control Advisory Committee on Immunization Practices: Notice to readers recommended childhood immunization schedule—United States, 1999. MMWR Morbid Mortal Wkly Rep 1999;48(1):8–16.

d. May induce febrile seizures.

e. No increased risk of permanent brain damage in neurologically normal child

f. Not a cause of sudden infant death syndrome

g. Consider risk/benefit ratio of administration if previous immunization was followed by:

   (1) Fever 105° F (40.5° C) or greater within 48 hours

   (2) Hypotonic-hyporesponsive episode within 48 hours

   (3) Persistent, inconsolable crying lasting 3 hours or longer within 48 hours

   (4) Seizures, with or without fever, within 3 days

h. Bleeding disorder

Contraindications

1. Immediate anaphylactic reaction

2. Moderate or severe acute illness, with or without fever

3. Pertussis component–specific contraindications

   a. Encephalopathy, not due to other identifiable cause, within 7 days of previous immunization

   b. Neurologic disorder with progressive developmental delay or changing neurologic status

   c. Whole-cell pertussis component over age 6 years

Special Considerations

1. Persons who develop allergic or unusual adverse effects or who require medical attention after immunization: Report through the Vaccine Adverse Event Reporting System (VAERS) at 1-800-822-7967.

2. Suspected allergy but in need of further tetanus immunizations: Consider referral to allergist for desensitization; may check serum tetanus titer to determine need for additional vaccination; have resuscitation equipment and medication available if reimmunized.

3. When immunization with pertussis vaccine is contraindicated: Use DT after child's neurologic status is clarified; do not use DTaP, DTwP, or pertussis combination vaccine.

4. Child with family history or personal history of seizures without other neurologic disorder: May receive the pertussis component, but risk for seizure exists; DTaP preferred.

5. Child with stable cerebral palsy or nonprogressive developmental delay without seizure dis-

position: The child is not at increased risk for seizures.

6. Prolonged interval between doses: Reinitiation of primary series is not required.

7. Patient who tests positive for human immunodeficiency virus (HIV): May receive vaccination.

8. Immunosuppressed: Expected antibody response may not be obtained. If immunosuppressive medication will soon be discontinued, defer immunization until 3 months after therapy.

9. Preterm infants: Vaccinate according to chronologic age from birth; do not give fractional or reduced doses.

Polio (IPV, OPV)

General Information

1. IPV (inactivated poliovirus vaccine)

   a. All-IPV immunization schedule recommended as of January 2000

   b. Enhanced, inactivated virus; administered subcutaneously; no viral shedding

   c. Administer IPV at 2, 4, 6 to 18 months, and 4 to 6 years.

   d. Primary series in unimmunized non-infant under age 18 years: administer 3 doses of IPV with second dose 4 weeks after the first dose and the third dose 6 months after the second dose.

2. OPV (oral poliovirus vaccine)

   a. As of January 2000, no longer recommended for routine immunization.

   b. Live virus; administered orally

   c. Excreted in stool; nonimmune contacts have risk of vaccine-associated paralysis; risk of paralysis is 1 per 2.4 million doses distributed

   d. May be recommended in rare situations: wild-type polio virus outbreak or unimmunized child traveling to polio-endemic country within four weeks.

Precautions

1. Pregnancy: theoretical; no known adverse effects on fetus

2. Bleeding disorders

Contraindications

1. Anaphylaxis

2. Moderate to severe acute systemic illness, with or without fever

3. IPV-specific contraindications

a. Anaphylactic reaction to neomycin, polymyxin B, or streptomycin
4. OPV-specific contraindications
   a. HIV infection, immunocompromise, household member who is known HIV positive or immunocompromised

Special Considerations

1. Incompletely immunized infants and children who have received previous OPV vaccination: transition to IPV for next recommended dose; no need to repeat any doses.
2. Incompletely immunized adults in the United States: Primary vaccination and booster doses unnecessary unless there is risk because of foreign travel or occupation. If primary vaccination necessary, use IPV.
3. Low-to-moderate steroid use: not a contraindication
4. If third dose is administered after age 4: the fourth dose is not needed.
5. Patient inadvertently received OPV and family member is immunodeficient: avoid or minimize contact for 4 to 8 weeks.

Measles, Mumps, Rubella (MMR)

General Information

1. Combination live virus vaccine administered subcutaneously; also available as single-antigen vaccines
2. Primary dose: age 12 to 15 months; booster dose: age 4 to 6 years
3. Physicians should scrutinize immunization record of adolescents for completion of two doses.
4. Arthralgias may develop 1 to 3 months after immunization, especially in women, because of rubella component.
5. Five per cent have transient rash.
6. May temporarily suppress TB skin test reactivity; administer the TB skin test on the same day or 4 to 6 weeks after the MMR vaccine.

Precautions

1. Immune globulin administered within previous 3 months
2. Anaphylaxis to gelatin-containing products
3. History of seizure disorder
4. Bleeding disorders

Contraindications

1. Anaphylaxis to vaccine component, egg ingestion, or neomycin
2. Moderate to severe acute illness with or without fever

3. Pregnancy
4. Immunodeficiency (cancer, lymphoma, leukemia, chemotherapy, radiation therapy, high-dose steroids)
5. Symptomatic, severely immunocompromised HIV positive

Special Considerations

1. Women of childbearing age: Screen for rubella immunity and vaccinate unless the patient is pregnant or there is some other contraindication. Avoid pregnancy for 3 months after vaccination.
2. Pregnant woman with child in need of vaccination: The child may be immunized; the vaccine is not transmitted from the vaccinee to susceptible contacts.
3. Adults born before 1957 are considered immune.
4. Health care workers, college students, and international travelers born after 1956: Give special attention to vaccination and immunity status.
5. Community epidemic: The vaccine may be administered to a child under age 12 months, but it does not count as the first dose. The child must be revaccinated at age 15 months and receive a booster dose at 4 to 6 years.
6. Low- to moderate-dose steroid use: not a contraindication
7. Asymptomatic HIV positive: not a contraindication
8. Symptomatic HIV positive: May vaccinate unless severely immunocompromised.
9. Infants less than 6 months: usually protected by maternal-derived antibodies
10. Breastfeeding: not a contraindication
11. Leukemia in remission with chemotherapy terminated or previous high-dose steroids: Administer after 3-month waiting period.

HbCV and Combination Vaccines

General Information

1. Most important in children under age 15 months to prevent *H. influenzae* meningitis
2. Three vaccines approved for children under age 15 months.
   a. PedvaxHIB: The primary series is administered at ages 2 and 4 months; the booster at age 12 to 15 months.
   b. HibTITER: The primary series is administered at ages 2, 4, and 6 months; the booster at age 12 to 15 months.

c. ActHIB or OmniHIB: The primary series is administered at ages 2, 4, and 6 months; the booster at age 12 to 15 months.

d. Interchangeable for primary and booster vaccines. If different vaccines must be used for primary vaccination of a child under 15 months, a total of three doses, regardless of manufacturer, should be administered.

3. Combination vaccines

a. DTaP-HbCV (TriHIBiT): ActHIB or OmniHIB reconstituted with Pasteur Merieux Connaught DTaP; licensed only for fourth dose of vaccination series (see "Diphtheria, Tetanus, Pertussis"). Should not be used for primary vaccination of infants.

b. DTwP-HbCV (see "Diphtheria, Tetanus, Pertussis")

   (1) Tetramune: Contains HibTITER and DTwP.
   (2) ActHIB or OmniHIB reconstituted with Pasteur Merieux Connaught DTwP

c. HBV-HbCV: (Comvax); contains Recombivax HB and PedvaxHIB (see "Hepatitis B Virus").

d. Other combination vaccines expected in future.

e. Combination vaccines may decrease number of injections but complicate the number of vaccines stocked in office.

f. No increase in side effects if combination vaccine is used compared to two separate injections.

4. Children under 15 months, incompletely immunized: Consult package insert for dosing schedule.

5. ProHIBiT: licensed only for primary dose at ages 15 to 59 months

Precautions
1. Bleeding disorders
2. Combination vaccines: Refer to DTaP, DTwP, and hepatitis B virus (HBV) contraindications as appropriate.

Contraindications
1. Anaphylaxis
2. Moderate to severe systemic acute illness with or without fever
3. Combination vaccines: Refer to DTaP, DTwP, and HBV contraindications as appropriate.

Special Considerations
1. Previously unvaccinated child, 15 to 59 months: Give a single dose of any HbCV vaccine.

2. After age 5 years: HbCV vaccination is unnecessary unless a special circumstance, sickle cell disease, asplenia, HIV, certain immune deficiency syndromes, chemotherapy for malignancy.

3. Day care centers: Special attention should be given to vaccinating all children.

4. Children under 24 months with history of invasive *H. influenzae* disease do not develop immunity to natural disease; ensure vaccination.

Hepatitis B Virus (HBV)

General Information
1. Two licensed hepatitis B vaccines: Recombivax HB and Engerix-B; equally immunogenic
2. May be used interchangeably in their respective recommended dosages.
3. Consult package insert for dosage administration because of differing formulations and schedules.
4. Administered intramuscularly.
5. Recommended for all infants and adolescents. May administer at any time during childhood.
6. Combination vaccine (Comvax) contains Recombivax HB and PedvaxHIB (HbCV); should not be used before 6 weeks of age.
7. Physicians should scrutinize immunization records of adolescents for completion of series.

Indications
1. Infants born to hepatitis B surface antigen (HBsAg)-negative mothers: Administer a thimerosal-free hepatitis B vaccine at 0, 2, and 6 to 18 months.

   a. If thimerosal-containing hepatitis B vaccine is used, administer the first dose at 2 months, not at birth. Administer subsequent doses at 4 and 6 to 18 months.

   b. Premature infants should not receive thimerosal-containing hepatitis B vaccine until they weight 2.5 kg and are of term gestational age. They may receive thimerosal-free hepatitis B vaccine at birth.

2. All infants born to HBsAg-positive mothers: Administer hepatitis B vaccine (with or without thimerosal) within 12 hours of birth in combination with hepatitis B immune globulin (HBIG). Administer additional doses of hepatitis B vaccine at 1 to 2 months and 6 months.

3. All adolescents

4. Health care and public safety workers

5. Clients and staff of institutions for the developmentally disabled; inmates of correctional facilities

6. Hemodialysis patients; recipients of certain blood products; hemophiliacs

7. Injection drug users

8. Multiple sex partners; sexually active homosexual and bisexual men; high-risk adults (sexually transmitted diseases are "red flags"); prostitutes

9. Household contacts, sex partners of HBV carriers

10. International travelers, especially if they are staying for more than 6 months in an area with a high rate of HBV.

11. Adoptees from countries where HBV is endemic

12. Children in households of Pacific Islanders or first-generation immigrants from countries where hepatitis is endemic

13. Therapy after HBV exposure in combination with HBIG

14. Persons who test positive for hepatitis C virus

Precautions
Bleeding disorders

Contraindications
1. Anaphylaxis to previous vaccination, common baker's yeast, or thimerosal

2. Moderate or severe acute illness, with or without fever

Special Considerations
1. Periodic serologic testing: no consensus

2. Periodic revaccination: no consensus

3. Health care workers, dialysis patients, regular sexual contactants of HBV carriers, infants born to HBsAg-positive mothers, anticipated suboptimal response (HIV, immunosuppressed): Consider serologic testing after immunization.

4. Patient does not respond to the initial three-dose regimen: Revaccinate with one or more doses.

5. Elderly, smokers, chronic illness, obese: less likely to develop immunity. Consider serologic testing after immunization.

6. Subcutaneous, intradermal, or buttock administration of vaccine: less likely to develop immunity. Consider serologic testing after immunization.

7. Pregnancy: not a contraindication to vaccination. Routinely screen for HbsAg.

8. Prolonged interval between doses: not problematic. Continue series regardless of intervals between doses.

Hepatitis A Virus (HAV)

General Information
1. Inactivated virus; administered intramuscularly (IM); not derived from blood products

2. Two licensed vaccines: Havrix (720 and 1440 ELISA units) and Vaqta. Both available in two-dose schedule at 0 and 6 to 12 months. Can use interchangeably.

3. Three-dose schedule 360-ELISA-unit Havrix is being phased out.

4. Not approved for children under age 2

5. Side-effects are mild and transient; most frequent are injection site soreness and headache.

6. Duration of long-term immunity under study; may be at least 20 years.

7. Administer at least 2 weeks prior to expected exposure.

8. Pre-exposure vaccination recommendations

   a. International travelers to intermediate- and high-risk areas for hepatitis A, especially if extended or frequent short-term travel

   b. Children living in communities with high rates or periodic outbreaks of hepatitis A (Alaskan Native villages, Native American reservations, selected Hispanic communities)

   c. Men who have sex with men

   d. Illegal-drug users

   e. Persons with chronic liver disease or who test positive for hepatitis C

   f. Occupational risk (hepatitis A research settings or infected primate handlers)

   g. Persons with bleeding disorders receiving clotting factor concentrates

9. Consider vaccination for these groups:

   a. Occupational risk: health care workers, day care workers, military personnel, food handlers, staff of institutions for developmentally disabled, sewage workers

   b. Children at day care centers and parents, siblings, and other close contacts

   c. Persons with repeated sexually transmitted diseases

   d. Consumers of high-risk foods such as raw shellfish

Precautions
1. Moderate or severe acute illness with or without fever

2. Bleeding disorders

3. Pregnancy

Contraindications

Anaphylactic reactions to previous dose, aluminum or aluminum hydroxide

Special Considerations

1. Immunocompromised: May not develop immune response.
2. Postexposure prophylaxis: not recommended
3. Postvaccination testing for anti-HAV: not recommended; high rate of response. Detectable antibody may not be present but individual may still be protected.
4. Vaccination of immune person: Does not increase risk of adverse reaction.
5. Prevaccination testing for anti-HAV: indicated only if testing costs less than vaccination and a high likelihood of previous infection.
6. For travelers leaving for high-risk area within 4 weeks and who need both immediate and long-term protection: May administer simultaneously with immune globulin.
7. Future vaccine schedules may include routine use for children.

Varicella Vaccine

General Information

1. Live attenuated vaccine; administer subcutaneously; deltoid site preferred; store frozen at $-15°$ C; use within 30 minutes of reconstitution.
2. Most common side effect: injection site pain, redness, swelling
3. Fifteen per cent report fever; febrile seizures not clearly associated.
4. Some vaccinees report upper respiratory illness, cough, irritability, joint pain, diarrhea.
5. Five per cent or less develop generalized chickenpox rash with a median of five lesions or injection site rash within 3 weeks.
6. Cost-benefit analysis shows $5.40 of societal savings for every dollar invested in varicella vaccine, based on medical and parental work-loss costs.
7. Within 3 years, 1 per cent of children immunized will develop chickenpox, a 93 per cent decrease compared to expected attack rates; most cases are milder.
8. Mild herpes zoster rarely follows vaccination.
9. May interfere with TB skin test; administer TB skin test on the same day or 4 to 6 weeks after varicella vaccine.
10. Postmarketing studies on duration of immunity are ongoing.
11. No evidence that vaccination will prevent disease if administered immediately after exposure to natural virus.
12. Probably decreases long-term risk of herpes zoster.

Indications

1. Age 12 months and older if without history of natural chickenpox
   a. Age 12 months to 12 years: one dose
   b. Adults and adolescents age 13 years or older: two doses, administered 4 to 8 weeks apart
2. Susceptible adults and adolescents at high risk of exposure targeted: teachers of young children and day care workers, college students, military personnel, residents/staff of institutional settings, inmates/staff of correctional institutions, international travelers to endemic areas, health care workers, and family contacts of immunocompromised.

Precautions

1. Avoid aspirin for 6 weeks after immunizations.
2. Immunoglobulin administered within previous 5 months may decrease immunogenic response.
3. Breast-feeding

Contraindications

1. Hypersensitivity to any component of the vaccine, including gelatin and neomycin
2. Moderate or severe acute illness, with or without fever
3. History of blood dyscrasias, lymphoma, leukemia, or other malignant neoplasms of the bone marrow or lymphatic system (may not apply to children with acute lymphoblastic leukemia in remission)
4. Use of high-dose steroids and immunosuppressants; may administer vaccine after 3-month waiting period.
5. Primary or acquired immune deficiencies, including symptomatic or asymptomatic HIV
6. Family history of congenital or hereditary immunodeficiency unless immune competence is clear
7. Active untreated tuberculosis
8. Pregnancy: Avoid for 3 months postvaccination. May vaccinate household contacts.
9. Children or adolescents on chronic aspirin therapy (because of risk of Reye's syndrome)

Special Considerations

1. Children and adolescents age 12 months to 17 years with acute lymphoblastic leukemia in re-

mission: May receive Varivax under investigational protocol.

2. Low- to moderate-dose steroid therapy: not a contraindication

3. Vaccinees may transmit virus to susceptible contacts; avoid contact with known nonimmune pregnant women, immunocompromised, and other high-risk persons, especially if postvaccination chickenpox rash.

4. In some cases, benefits of vaccinating susceptible household contact of immunocompromised contact may outweigh risk of transmission of vaccine virus to immunocompromised contact.

Pneumococcal Vaccine

General Information
1. Contains capsular polysaccharides of the 23 most prevalent pneumococcal types.
2. Administered only once in a lifetime, unless indication for booster (see below)

Indications
1. Age over 65 years
2. Ages 2 to 64 with
   a. Chronic disease—cardiovascular, respiratory, hepatic, renal; diabetes; immunosuppression; cancer; lymphoma; multiple myeloma; leukemia; organ transplantation
   b. HIV positive
   c. Native Americans
   d. Asplenia (anatomic or sickle cell disease)
   e. Chronic alcohol abuse
   f. Closed groups: nursing home and institutional
   g. Chronic cerebrospinal fluid leakage
3. Booster recommended for
   a. Age 65 or older, if vaccine received 5 or more years previously and patient was 65 years old or younger when first vaccinated
   b. Age 10 to 64 years and immunocompromised or with anatomic or functional asplenia and 5 or more years since first dose
   c. Age 2 to 10: Revaccinate after 3 to 5 years if asplenic, sickle cell disease, or nephrotic syndrome, or have other high risk for severe infection.
   d. Immunocompromised or highest risk at any age and 5 or more years since first dose

Precautions
1. Febrile illness or active infection
2. Pregnancy

3. Bleeding disorders

Contraindications
Anaphylaxis to vaccine or hypersensitivity to any vaccine component, including thimerosal

Special Considerations
1. Under age 2 years: Vaccination is not effective.
2. Administer 2 weeks before elective splenectomy.
3. Most patients who are candidates for pneumococcal vaccine are candidates for influenza vaccine.

Influenza Vaccine

General Information
1. Killed virus; cannot cause influenza.
2. Needed yearly because of antigenic variation
3. Split-virus vaccine preferred over whole-virus vaccine (fewer reactions); only use split-virus if under age 13.
4. Intranasal vaccine may be available in the future.

Indications
1. Over age 50
2. Ages 6 months to 50 years with chronic heart disease, lung disease (including asthma), diabetes and other metabolic disorders, renal dysfunction, hemoglobinopathy, sickle cell disease, immunosuppression, HIV positive
3. Women who will be in the second or third trimester of pregnancy during influenza season
4. Residents of nursing homes and other chronic care facilities
5. Ages 6 months to 18 years receiving long-term aspirin therapy; at risk for Reye's syndrome after influenza
6. Those capable of transmitting influenza to high-risk patients: health care workers, home care volunteers, household members
7. Liberally administer to any person wishing to minimize illness from influenza, college students in dormitories, people in institutional settings, essential community service providers.
8. The American Academy of Family Physicians (AAFP) recommends routine immunization for all patients over age 50.

Precautions
1. Immunosuppression: May decrease immunogenic response.
2. Bleeding disorders
3. Moderate or severe acute illness, with or without fever

Contraindications

1. Anaphylaxis to previous vaccination, chicken eggs, aminoglycosides, neomycin, polymyxin, or sulfites
2. Past history of Guillain-Barré syndrome

Special Considerations

1. Children under age 6 months: Vaccine is not approved for use.
2. Children ages 6 months to 9 years not previously vaccinated: Give two doses of split-virus vaccine 4 weeks apart.
3. Northern hemisphere: Vaccinate in the fall.
4. Except for the 1976–1977 swine influenza vaccine, subsequent vaccines have not been clearly associated with Guillain-Barré syndrome.
5. If vaccine cannot be given to a high-risk patient, amantadine or rimantadine may be used for prophylaxis. In the future, oseltamavir and zanamivir may prove useful for prophylaxis.
6. Vaccination considered safe at all stages of pregnancy.
7. Do not unnecessarily delay vaccination in children with asthma on steroid therapy.

Meningococcal Polysaccharide Vaccine

General Information

1. Contains serotypes A, C, Y, W135.
2. Does not include serotype B and is not effective against serotype C in children under age 2 years. These serotypes are those most likely to cause disease in U.S. children.

Indications

1. Functional or anatomic asplenia
2. Sickle cell anemia
3. Terminal complement component deficiencies
4. Travelers to endemic areas
5. Outbreaks of serotypes included in vaccine

Precautions

1. Pregnancy
2. Moderate or severe acute illness, with or without fever

Contraindications

Anaphylaxis

Special Considerations

1. Not routinely recommended for U.S. children
2. Due to increasing incidence of meningococcal disease on college campuses, consider immunizing college students, especially those who live on campus.
3. For short-term protection against serogroup A, may vaccinate as young as 3 months.

Rabies

General Information

1. Inactivated virus vaccine
2. Three vaccines are available: human diploid cell vaccine (HDCV) (Imovax), rabies virus adsorbed (RVA), and chick embryo culture vaccine (PCEC [Rabavert]).
3. HDCV is available as IM and intradermal (ID) formulations
4. Pre-exposure prophylaxis indications
   a. Veterinarians, animal handlers, animal control and wildlife workers, park rangers
   b. Cave explorers
   c. Certain rabies laboratory workers
   d. People visiting or living in countries where rabies risk is high
5. Postexposure treatment of previously unvaccinated
   a. Thoroughly clean wound.
   b. Administer five-dose series (1.0 ml IM) of HDCV, RVA, or PCEC on days 1, 3, 7, 14, and 28; deltoid muscle preferred.
   c. Administer human rabies immune globulin (HRIG), 20 IU/kg. Infiltrate full dose around the wound; if not anatomically feasible, administer remainder IM at site distant from HDCV/RVA/PCEC injection site.
6. Postexposure treatment of previously vaccinated
   a. Thoroughly clean wound.
   b. Administer a two-dose series IM of HDCV, RVA, or PCEC on days 0 and 3; deltoid muscle preferred.
   c. Do not administer HRIG.
7. HRIG often not available abroad and locally available vaccines may pose risks.

Precautions

1. Immunosuppression may interfere with immunity; give IM only; monitor rabies antibody response.
2. Pre-exposure: pregnancy, moderate or severe illness
3. Postexposure treatment: hypersensitivity
4. Bleeding disorders: Consider ID administration of HDCV if pre-exposure prophylaxis.

Contraindications

Pre-exposure prophylaxis: anaphylaxis

Special Considerations

1. Bite, scratch, or mucous membrane exposure by bat: Regard as rabid and give HRIG and vaccination even if evidence is not visible but exposure occurred.
2. Bite by wild skunk, fox, coyote, raccoon, bobcat, other carnivores: Regard the animal as rabid unless lab test results are negative.
3. Bite by squirrel, hamster, guinea pig, gerbil, chipmunk, rat, mouse, other rodent, livestock, rabbit, hare: Consider individually; consult public health officials; such bites seldom require rabies treatment.
4. Bite by dog or cat
   a. Rabid or suspected rabid: postexposure treatment
   b. Healthy and available for 10 days of observation: Observe the animal. No treatment is required unless the animal is rabid. Destroy the animal for lab testing if any doubt.
   c. Unknown or escaped: Consult public health officials; postexposure treatment may be required.
5. Chloroquine phosphate and mefloquine: May weaken antibody response to HDCV. Do not use HDCV ID. Check antibody response.
6. If revaccination of person with hypersensitivity is required: Pretreat with antihistamines; use alternate vaccine; have epinephrine available; observe closely.

Tetanus Prophylaxis in Wound Management

General Information

1. Thoroughly clean wound; débride if necessary.
2. If the patient is over age 6 years, dT is preferred.
3. If the patient is under age 7 years, review the immunization record; use the incident as an opportunity to update immunizations.
4. For passive immunization, tetanus immune globulin (TIG) is indicated; adult dose is 250 units IM.
5. In the United States, tetanus is a disease of the elderly; pay attention to their immunization status; ensure completion of primary immunizations.

Indications for TIG

1. Patients who require immediate immunity against tetanus toxoid, especially those with little or no active immunity

2. Treatment for active case of tetanus

Precautions

1. TIG: Do not use for skin testing; reaction is easily misinterpreted.
2. Bleeding disorders
3. See "Diphtheria, Tetanus, Pertussis."

Contraindications

1. TIG: anaphylaxis to previous gamma globulin or thimerosal
2. See "Diphtheria, Tetanus, Pertussis."

Special Considerations

1. Clean minor wound; three or more dT immunizations: Immunization is not necessary if the last dT injection was given within the past 10 years; if it was not given within the past 10 years, update the immunization status with dT.
2. Clean minor wound; unknown status or fewer than three dT immunizations: Update the immunization status with dT and schedule the patient for the remaining primary series; TIG is unnecessary.
3. Contaminated dirty wound, puncture, avulsion, crush, burn, frostbite; three or more dT immunizations: Administer dT if 5 years have passed since last dose; TIG is unnecessary.
4. Contaminated dirty wound, puncture, avulsion, crush, burn, frostbite; unknown status or fewer than three dT immunizations: Update the immunization status with dT and schedule the patient for the remaining primary series; administer TIG.
5. Persons recovering from tetanus should be immunized; disease does not confer immunity.

Rotavirus

The RotaShield rotavirus vaccine was removed from the market in 1999 due to increased risk of intussusception within two weeks of receiving the vaccine. Several other rotavirus vaccines are being developed. These are bovine based rather than rhesus based, which some predict will be less likely to cause intussusception.

Lyme Disease Vaccine

General Information

1. Inactivated recombinant OspA (bacterial outer surface lipoprotein A) vaccine
2. Administer at 0, 1, and 12 months IM, deltoid muscle
3. Not approved for ages less than 15 years or more than 70 years

4. Time vaccine so that second and third doses precede *Borrelia burgdorferi* transmission seasons (April and May) by several weeks.

5. Immunization efforts should be targeted to high risk populations based on geographic location, residental characteristics, occupation, and leisure activities.

6. High risk vaccination targets: those with frequent or prolonged exposure to deer tick-infested habitats of the northeast United States, Michigan, Wisconsin such as outdoor workers or frequent recreators in wooded areas or who live in periresidential areas that are heavily wooded or unkempt.

7. Moderate risk vaccination targets: consider vaccinating those who live in high risk geographic areas but have neither frequent nor prolonged exposure to wooded areas.

8. Vaccination not recommended for low risk groups regardless of where they live in the United States if there is minimal or no contact with wooded, grassy areas.

9. Vaccination does not prevent all cases of Lyme disease.

10. Vaccination does not substitute for standard preventive measures such as long pants tucked into socks, long sleeves, hats, and tick repellent.

Contraindications

1. Severe allergic reactions to vaccine components
2. Febrile illness or active infection
3. Safety not yet established in children less than age 15

Precautions

1. Thrombocytopenia or bleeding disorder
2. Treatment resistant (antibiotic refractory) Lyme arthritis

3. Immunodeficiency (diminished antibody response)
4. Pregnant and lactating women
5. Age over 70 years (studies not yet conducted)

Special Considerations

1. Adverse effects include injection site soreness, influenza-like illness, myalgias.

2. Most cases of Lyme disease are thought to be acquired during routine activities of property maintenance, exercise of pets and recreation in periresidential areas

3. Those with a past history of Lyme disease may benefit from vaccination

4. Further study may result in a proven need for booster doses, alternative rapid dosing schedules, and recommendations for children and elderly

5. Effect on laboratory tests for Lyme disease diagnosis are uncertain

6. Studies on vaccine safety have not shown link with inflammatory arthritis, though follow-up was limited to two years

Bibliography

Centers for Disease Control and Prevention: Recommended Childhood Immunization Schedule–United States, 1999. MMWR Morb Mortal Wkly Rep 1999; 48(1).

Centers for Disease Control and Prevention: Human Rabies Prevention–United States, 1999. Recommendations of the ACIP. MMWR Morb Mortal Wkly Rep 1999;48(RR-1).

Centers for Disease Control and Prevention: Prevention and Control of Influenza. Recommedendations of the ACIP. MMWR Morb Mortal Wkly Rep 1999;48(RR-4).

Thompson RF: Travel and Routine Immunizations: A Practical Guide for the Medical Office. Milwaukee, WI, Shoreland Inc, 1998.

Zimmerman RK: Lowering the age for routine influenza vaccination to 50 years: AAFP leads the nation in influenza vaccine policy. Am Fam Physician 1999;60: 2061–2066.

2 Health Promotion Protocols

Elizabeth C. McCord

Current Health Status (Table 2–1)

Assess risk factors utilizing interval history, including past medical history, family history, and social history.

Nutritional Status

1. Address developmentally appropriate foods, patterns, changes.
2. Address adequacy/excess of calories, nutrients: vitamins, minerals (e.g., calcium, iron), vegetables and fruits, soluble/nonsoluble fiber, fats, concentrated sweets, carbohydrates, amount and type of protein; pattern of intake.
3. Address dietary adjustments suggested by weight and/or growth changes, family risks, lab results, physiologic changes (e.g., toddler, adolescent, anticipated pregnancy/childbearing years, breast-feeding, menopause).
4. Supplement as needed: fluoride, specific vitamins, antioxidants, folate, calcium, iron.

Activity

1. Physical
   a. Utilize developmental screens for motor milestones, gains and losses.
   b. Assess play/exercise for aerobic exercise, flexibility, weight bearing, strength-enhancing activities, endurance, balance, and gait training.
   c. Address adequacy and developmental appropriateness of weight recommendations and make adjustments/adaptations as necessitated by weight changes, family risks, lab results, physiologic changes, and/or anatomic changes.
   d. Target adult aerobic exercise at (220 − age) × 0.7 for at least 20 minutes five times a week.
2. Mental/intellectual: verbal, math, spatial, memory, judgment, abstraction. Utilize developmental screens; assess speech, reading, academic performance, learning difficulties, work performance, intellectual stimulation (e.g., reading, discussion), memory, judgment difficulties; Mini-Mental Status Exam (MMSE).
3. Emotional
   a. Assess developmentally appropriate emo-

tional milestones throughout the lifespan for positive mental health strategies, behaviors, strengths, and coping mechanisms.
   b. Be alert for attention-deficit disorder with or without hyperactivity, autism, depression, grief, anxiety, stress, thought disorders, and substance use and abuse throughout the lifespan.
   c. Consider specific counseling regarding adequate daylight exposure, physical activity, stress reduction and management strategies, coping strengths and strategies.
4. Spiritual
   a. Gauge moral development.
   b. Note activity, development, practices, preferences, and plans.
5. Social
   a. Utilize developmental screens for adjustments to home, school, peers, work, and community.
   b. Be alert for family dysfunction, violence.
6. Sexual: Assess sexual development; provide contraceptive and preconception counseling.

Developmentally Appropriate Accident and Injury Prevention

1. Motor vehicle accident and boating injury prevention
   a. Recommend age-appropriate vehicle restraints and placement in vehicles.
   b. Recommend avoiding speeding 5 mph over speed limit.
   c. Advise to avoid impaired driving or riding with impaired driver (alcohol and/or drug use, sleep deprived, emotional state, or poor peer judgment).
   d. Encourage selection of vehicle safety equipment for cars/vehicles, boats, jet skis, and farm equipment (tractor roll bars, PTO shields, auger and combine cutoffs, etc.).
2. Fall prevention
   a. Utilize developmentally appropriate guidance for infants and toddlers (infant rolling, stairs, window guards, childproofing the home) and for elders (ladders, loose rugs, hand rails).

TABLE 2–1. HEALTH PROMOTION PROTOCOLS BY AGE GROUP

PROTOCOL ▼ / AGE GROUP ▶	Infants	2–6 Years	7–12 Years	13–18 Years	19–39 Years	40–64 Years	65+ Years
Assess Current Health Status, Risk Factors, Interval History, Past Medical, Family, and Social Histories	■	■	■	■	■	■	■
Nutritional Status and Counseling	■	■	■	■	■	■	■
Activity							
1. Physical							
a. Motor milestones/gains and losses	■	■				■	■
b. Play/exercise recommendations		■	■	■	■	■	■
2. Mental							
a. Developmental screenings, speech, reading	■	■	■				
b. Memory, judgment, MMSE							■
3. Emotional							
a. Developmentally appropriate milestones	■	■	■	■	■	■	■
b. ADD, ADHD, autism, behavioral development	■	■	■				
c. Depression, grief, anxiety, stress, suicide, thought disorders			■	■	■	■	■
d. Substance abuse			■	■	■	■	■
4. Spiritual							
a. Moral development, activity, practices & preferences		■	■	■	■	■	■
5. Social							
a. Adjustment		■	■	■	■	■	■
b. Family dysfunction		■	■	■	■	■	■
c. Family violence	■	■	■	■	■	■	■
6. Occupational							
a. Risks				■	■	■	■
b. Injury				■	■	■	■
c. Toxins/poisoning/chemicals				■	■	■	■
d. Sun exposure				■	■	■	■
e. Stress				■	■	■	■
f. Infections				■	■	■	■
7. Functional assessment	■						■

(Table continued on following page)

TABLE 2–1.   HEALTH PROMOTION PROTOCOLS BY AGE GROUP (*Continued*)

Protocol ▼ / Age Group ▶	Infants	2–6 Years	7–12 Years	13–18 Years	19–39 Years	40–64 Years	65+ Years
Accident/Injury Prevention							
1. Motorized vehicle and watercraft	███	███	███	███	███	███	███
2. Fall prevention	███	███					███
3. Sports/helmets		███	███	███			
4. Burns/smoke detectors	███	███	███	███	███	███	███
5. Drowning/pools	███	███	███	███	███	███	
6. Farm & home poisoning	███	███					
7. Mower safety			███	███	███	███	
8. Firearm safety		███	███	███	███	███	███
9. Violence							
a. Sibling rivalry	███	███	███				
b. Violent behavior				███	███		
c. Family violence	███	███	███	███	███	███	███
10. Miscellaneous							
a. CO & radon detectors					███	███	███
b. Suffocation/SIDS	███						
11. Skin & eye protection	███	███	███	███	███	███	███
Infection Prevention							
1. Immunizations	███	███	███	███	███	███	███
2. Kitchen food habits						███	███
3. Hand washing		███	███				
4. Sexual practices				███	███	███	
5. Travel	███	███	███	███	███	███	███
Dental Health	███	███	███	███	███	███	███

Abbreviations: ADD, attention-deficit disorder; ADHD, attention-deficit hyperactivity disorder; CO, carbon monoxide; MMSE, Mini-Mental Status Exam; SIDS, sudden infant death syndrome.

    b. Assess medications that increase fall risk in elderly.
3. Sports/exercise injury prevention
    a. Recommend helmets/protective gear for bicycles, motorcycles, roller skates/blades, ice skates/hockey, and football; advise about street safety and pedestrian accidents.
    b. Suggest back conditioning exercises.
4. Burn prevention
    a. Lower hot water heater to less than 120° F for infants and elders.
    b. Advise about placement and installation of smoke detectors and alarms.
    c. Inform parents about school-age children playing with matches.
5. Drowning/pool accident prevention
    a. Avoid the use of alcohol and/or drugs when around water.
    b. Review boating/jet ski safety and required flotation devices.
    c. Discuss pool safety; fences with locks, pool alarms, and covers that lock.
    d. Discuss safe diving practices and to avoid swimming alone.
6. Farm and home poisoning prevention
    a. Discuss importance of ipecac and provide the local Poison Control Center hot line number.
    b. Review safe storage of medications, household chemicals, farm chemicals and poisons.
7. Mower safety: Discuss use of protective eye shields and appropriate footwear.
8. Violence prevention
    a. Screen for violent behavior.
    b. Utilize family violence screens for partners, children, teens, and elders.
    c. Discuss sibling rivalry.
9. Firearm safety
    a. Recommend that, for home storage, unloaded guns and ammunition be locked and in separate locations, inaccessible to children.
    b. Discuss practicing safe firearm procedures while hunting, supervision of novices, and avoiding alcohol.
10. Miscellaneous
    a. Discuss importance of smoke, carbon monoxide, and radon detectors.
    b. Suffocation/sudden infant death syndrome (SIDS): Inform parents about bedding, crib, bassinet, cradle, and playpen recommendations, infant and car seat safety, and proper positioning of infant on back or side.
    c. Discuss safety of infants and children when pets are present in the home.
    d. Discuss proper skin and eye protection from ultraviolet light.

Infection Prevention
1. Immunizations (see Ch. 1, Immunization Schedules)
2. Avoid unnecessary exposures to contagious persons.
3. Review proper hand-washing technique.
4. Discuss appropriate kitchen and food habits.
5. Discuss sexual habits.
6. Review need for chemoprophylaxis in specific situations.

Dental Health
1. Discuss baby bottle teeth.
2. Assess need for brushing and flossing.
3. Assess need for fluoride supplementation.
4. Urge periodic dental visits.

Chemoprophylaxis
1. Ophthalmic ointment for all newborns
2. Assess need for fluoride supplementation.
3. Discuss daily aspirin over age 40.
4. Discuss estrogen replacement therapy perimenopause.
5. Consider folate supplementation for childbearing, older adults.

Community
Be aware of the following for frequency, patterns, and trends in the community:
1. Environmental concerns
2. Violence/crime
3. Trauma/accidents
4. Infectious diseases
5. Toxins
6. Epidemiologic concerns

Screening for Early Detection (Table 2–2)
1. Congenital diseases
2. Obesity and growth disorders
3. Cardiovascular diseases
4. Hyperlipidemia/diabetes
5. Sensory loss
6. Anemia
7. Orthopedic diseases

TABLE 2–2. SUGGESTED SCREENINGS BY AGE GROUP*

	First Week	Birth–18 Months	2–6 Years	7–12 Years	13–18 Years	19–39 Years	40–64 Years	65+ Years	Pregnancy
Suggested frequency of patient visits	Once	5 times or more	Yearly	None recommended	Once	Once every 1–3 yr	Once every 1–3 yr	Yearly	
Physical screening examination									
Abuse/neglect		✓	✓	✓	✓	✓	✓	✓	✓
Blood pressure			✓	✓	✓	✓	✓	✓	✓
Breast examination						✓	✓	✓	✓
Carotid bruit							✓✓	✓✓	
Complete functional status assessment		✓	✓					✓	
Dental/oral cavity		✓	✓	✓	✓	✓✓	✓✓	✓✓	
Digital rectal examination							✓	✓	
Hearing	✓✓	✓✓	✓✓		✓✓	✓✓	✓✓	✓	
Height and weight	✓	✓	✓	✓	✓	✓	✓	✓	✓
Peripheral artery disease							✓✓	✓✓	
Sexual development/ contraception/practices					✓	✓	✓		
Scoliosis					✓				
Skin examination/ protection					✓✓	✓✓	✓✓	✓✓	
Testicular examination					✓✓	✓✓			
Thyroid nodules						✓✓	✓✓	✓✓	
TIA symptoms								✓	
Vision/eye examination		✓	✓	✓				✓✓	
Screening Tests & Procedures									
Amniocentesis for karyotyping									✓✓
Bone densitometry							✓✓		
Cholesterol—nonfasting						✓	✓	✓	
Colonoscopy						✓✓	✓✓	✓✓	
ECG						✓✓	✓✓	✓✓	
Flex. sig. (q5–7yr)							✓	✓	
Fecal occult blood (q1yr)							✓	✓	
Glucose—fasting						✓✓	✓✓	✓✓	
Hepatitis B antibody					✓✓	✓✓	✓✓		✓
Hgb	✓✓	✓			✓✓	✓✓	✓✓	✓✓	✓

(Table continued on opposite page)

TABLE 2–2. SUGGESTED SCREENINGS BY AGE GROUP* (*Continued*)

	FIRST WEEK	BIRTH–18 MONTHS	2–6 YEARS	7–12 YEARS	13–18 YEARS	19–39 YEARS	40–64 YEARS	65+ YEARS	PREGNANCY
Hgb electrophoresis	✓✓				✓✓				✓✓
Lead		✓✓	✓✓						
Mammogram (q1–2yr)						✓✓	✓	✓	
MSAFP									✓
OGTT									✓
PAP (q1–2yr)					✓✓	✓	✓	✓✓	
PKU (once)	✓								
PPD			✓✓	✓✓	✓✓	✓✓	✓✓	✓✓	
PSA							✓✓		
Rh factor typing & testing									✓
Rubella antibodies									✓
STDs/HIV counseling & testing; needle sharing counseling					✓✓	✓✓	✓✓		✓
Thyroid function (q5yr for women)	✓							✓	
Urinalysis			✓			✓✓	✓✓	✓	✓
Ultrasound for growth									✓✓

Abbreviations: ECG, electrocardiogram; Flex. sig., flexible sigmoidoscopy; Hgb, hemoglobin; MSAFP, maternal serum α-fetoprotein; OGTT, oral glucose tolerance test; PAP, Papanicolaou smear; PKU, phenylketonuria; PPD, purified protein derivative (tuberculin test); PSA, prostate-specific antigen; STDs/HIV, sexually transmitted diseases/human immunodeficiency virus; TIA, transient ischemic attack.

*✓✓ = to be checked in high-risk patients only.

8. Infections
9. Cancer
10. Dental diseases

Bibliography

Abraham CL, Seremetis S: Breast health at midlife: guidelines for screening and patient evaluation. Geriatrics 1997;52:58–65.

Littrup PJ: Future benefits and cost-effectiveness of prostate carcinoma screening. Cancer 1997;80:1864–1870.

Public Health Service: Put Prevention into Practice: Clinician's Handbook of Preventive Services, 2nd ed. Washington, DC, U.S. Department of Health and Human Services, 1998.

U.S. Preventive Services Task Force: Guide to Clinical Preventive Services: An Assessment of the Effectiveness of 169 Interventions, 2nd ed. Washington, DC, U.S. Preventive Services Task Force, 1996.

Woolf SH, Jonas S, Lawrence RS: Health Promotion and Disease Prevention in Clinical Practice. Baltimore, Williams & Wilkins, 1996.

3 Growth and Development Guidelines

John B. Standridge

Natural History

1. Normal growth is a dynamic process that requires adequate genetic, hormonal, nutritional, and psychosocial components.
2. Normal growth occurs in three distinct phases:
   a. In utero and in infancy: very fast and then decelerates
   b. Ages 2 through 10: steady but slower growth rate with linear growth gradually slowing and growth in weight gradually increasing
   c. Pubertal phase: rapid, up to 4 inches a year. Menarche, around age 13, signals the slowing of linear growth for females. Males reach peak growth velocity around age 14 and plateau around age 18.

Detecting Abnormal Growth

1. Height and weight measurements are a fundamental and necessary part of every office visit.
2. Abnormal growth patterns are recognizable only through sequential plotting of growth data and analysis of the growth curve trajectory (see "Growth and Development Charts" at end of chapter).
3. Regardless of cause, the best treatment occurs when early recognition leads to timely mobilization of resources.

Interpreting Abnormal Growth

1. Remeasure and reweigh the child, and rechart the data to confirm abnormal trajectory.
2. Inquire about recent illness, caloric intake, stature and weight of siblings, and stature and weight of parents.
3. Typical growth patterns stay within channels (canalization) as a result of genetic influences. Two normal exceptions are small-for-gestational-age infants who shift percentiles upward toward their parents' mean percentile, and large neonates who shift downward toward their smaller parents' mean.
4. Compensate for prematurity by subtracting the weeks of prematurity from the postnatal age.
5. Acute undernutrition causes decreases on the weight-for-age and weight-for-height curves (wasting), whereas months of caloric deprivation decrease the height-for-age curve (stunt-ing). Chronic severe undernutrition depresses head circumference growth, a predictor of later cognitive disability.
6. Analyze the trajectory patterns:
   a. In endocrine etiologies, the length declines before or with the weight; weight-for-height is normal or elevated.
   b. In nutritional insufficiency, the weight declines before the length and weight-for-height is low.
   c. In congenital pathologic short stature (e.g., chromosomal, infectious, teratogenic, or extreme prematurity etiologies), the infant is born small and growth gradually tapers off throughout infancy.
   d. In constitutional growth delay, weight and height decrease near the end of infancy, then parallel the norm before accelerating toward the end of adolescence.
   e. In familial short stature, growth runs parallel to and just below the normal curves (see Fig. 3–7 at end of chapter).

Differentiating Abnormal Growth Patterns

1. Short, looks normal; low growth velocity
   a. Organic failure to thrive
      (1) Neurologic: mental retardation, cerebral palsy, diencephalic syndrome, swallowing dysfunction
      (2) Endocrine: hypothyroidism, diabetes, panhypopituitarism, adrenogenital syndrome
      (3) Gastrointestinal: pyloric stenosis, esophageal stricture, inflammatory bowel disease, celiac disease (growth delay may precede diarrhea and abdominal distention) (see Figs. 3–11 and 3–12 at end of chapter)
      (4) Renal: pyelonephritis, uremia, renal tubular acidosis
      (5) Cardiac: patent ductus arteriosus, coarctation of the aorta, septal defects (see Figs. 3–9 and 3–10 at end of chapter)
      (6) Pulmonary: recurrent pneumonia, asthma, tracheomalacia, cystic fibrosis

(7) Chronic infection: tuberculosis, human immunodeficiency virus (HIV) infection

(8) Miscellaneous: immune disorders (connective tissue disease, juvenile rheumatoid arthritis), tumors, hematologic disease (sickle cell disease, thalassemia), multiple congenital abnormalities

b. Malnutrition

(1) Kwashiorkor, marasmus: listlessness, apathetic, decreased lean body mass and adiposity, pallor, hair thin or sparse, hypotonia, protuberant abdomen

(2) Iron deficiency

(3) Zinc deficiency

c. Nonorganic failure to thrive (psychosocial)

(1) Inadequate nutritional information (maternal)

(2) Disturbance in attachment (deficiency in care), parental inadequacy, drug and alcohol abuse, marital or family discord, neglect, mental illness, depression, or mental retardation

(3) Disturbance in separation-individualization (food refusal on the part of the child)

2. Short, looks normal; growth velocity normal

a. Intrauterine growth retardation: term birth weight less than 2000 gm or preterm size small for gestational age

(1) Fetal factors: chromosomal, congenital infections, metabolic disorders, numerous syndromes

(2) Placental factors: implantation or vascular abnormalities (twins, single umbilical artery)

(3) Maternal factors: malnutrition, toxemia, drugs (cigarettes, cocaine, ethanol, phenytoin, propranolol, steroids, warfarin), uterine malformations, chronic disease (severe diabetes mellitus, hypertension, nephritis, sickle cell anemia, HIV infection)

b. Genetic short stature: family history, normal bone age. Exclude genetic growth disorder in parents.

c. Constitutional delay: family history; slowing of the growth rate between ages 1 and 3, delay in physical maturation and bone age. Growth normalizes but remains 2 to 3 years behind chronologic age, then accelerates toward the end of adolescence.

3. Short, looks abnormal; proportionate growth

a. Noonan's syndrome: features similar to Turner's syndrome (mental retardation, webbed neck, cryptorchidism, pulmonary stenosis) but more often male; normal karyotype

b. Russell-Silver syndrome: intrauterine growth retardation, café au lait spots, asymmetry, craniofacial dysostosis, short limbs, small triangular face, variable features

c. Fetal alcohol syndrome: hypertelorism, microcephaly, small palpebral fissures, midface hypoplasia, flat philtrum

4. Short, looks abnormal; disproportionate growth

a. Skeletal disorders

(1) Achondroplastic dwarfism: short upper arms and thighs, large head and forehead, small nose, normal intelligence

(2) Hypochondroplasia: milder form, short limbs, normal face

(3) Other skeletal dysplasias: number more than 50; consult *Smith's Recognizable Patterns of Human Malformation* (Jones, 1997).

b. Chromosomal abnormalities

(1) Trisomy 21 (Down's syndrome): mental retardation, delayed bone maturation, characteristic physical features

(2) Turner's syndrome: female, variable stigmata, short limbs, no adolescent growth spurt. Confirm with karyotype.

(3) Trisomy 18: micrognathia, overlapping fingers, horseshoe kidney, rocker-bottom feet, cardiac defects, diaphragmatic hernia, omphalocele

(4) Trisomy 13: microcephaly, cleft lips and/or palate, polydactyly, cardiac defects

5. Short, obese

a. Laurence-Moon-Biedl syndrome: mental deficiency, poly/syndactyly, retinitis pigmentosa, hypogonadism

b. Prader-Willi syndrome: hypotonia, mental retardation, hypogonadism, small hands and feet

6. Tall, looks normal; increased growth velocity

a. Precocious puberty: secondary sex characteristics before age 8 in girls and before age 9 in boys

b. Excess growth hormone: coarse facial features, organ enlargement, abnormal glucose tolerance test, abnormal hand and skull radiographs

c. Hyperthyroidism: goiter, staring, lid lag, dermopathy; abnormal thyroid function studies

7. Tall, looks normal; normal growth velocity— genetic tall stature: family history, tall parents

8. Tall, looks abnormal; proportionate growth—cerebral giantism: birth weight and height above the 90th percentile, mental retardation, advanced bone age

9. Tall, looks abnormal; disproportionate growth
   a. Marfan's syndrome: long limbs, narrow hands, arachnodactyly; arm span exceeds height; dissecting aortic aneurysm common.
   b. Klinefelter's syndrome (XXY): hypergonadotropic hypogonadism

Failure to Thrive Syndrome

1. Hallmark is failure to gain weight at an expected rate for the age of the child, as represented by a weight below the 5th percentile or a decline of greater than two major percentile lines (see Fig. 3–8 at end of chapter).

2. Etiology (see "Differentiating Abnormal Growth Patterns")
   a. The immediate cause is inadequate nutrition.
   b. The ultimate cause may be a consequence of physical problems, psychosocial problems, or both.
   c. Mixed etiology is common. The child in a stressed family may also have a physical problem; the child with a medical disorder resulting in poor growth may have a stressed family situation compounding the feeding and nutritional problems.

3. Evaluation
   a. A thorough and focused history, physical, and neurologic assessment
   b. Developmental evaluation: Denver Developmental Screening Test II (DDST II)
   c. Calorie count, intake and output, frequent weight measurement
   d. Laboratory tests: as appropriate, obtain complete blood count; multiple chemistry profile; glucose tolerance test; urinalysis; Venereal Disease Research Laboratory (VDRL) test; thyroxine, thyroid-stimulating hormone, somatomedin C (insulin-like growth factor I), immunoglobulin levels; erythrocyte sedimentation rate; stool for pH, reducing substances, and fat; jejunal biopsy; cultures of urine, blood, and stool; tuberculosis and HIV testing; sweat chloride test; arterial blood gases; chromosomal studies
   e. Radiologic: left wrist for bone age, chest film, intravenous pyelogram, trauma survey, upper and lower gastrointestinal series, various scans
   f. Electrocardiogram and echocardiogram
   g. Electroencephalography and neuroimaging should be considered if there is suspicion of seizure, encephalopathy, microcephaly, or rapidly expanding head circumference.

4. Indications for hospitalization
   a. Strong suspicion of organic cause
   b. Signs of physical abuse
   c. Suspected neglect: poor infant hygiene (e.g., severe cradle cap, diaper rash, long dirty fingernails), parental unconcern, no previous medical attention
   d. History of frequent vomiting or diarrhea
   e. Infant over age 2 months and still near birth weight
   f. Infant between ages 3 and 6 months with minimal weight gain over previous 2 months
   g. Potentially life-threatening malnutrition
   h. Mother overtly depressed or rejecting baby
   i. History of bizarre diet
   j. Insignificant weight gain after 1 month of outpatient management

5. Management
   a. Get involved. Earn and sustain trust. Advocate for the child without becoming an adversary of the parents.
   b. Approach the parents or caregivers with a sense of urgency to determine whether they are willing to make the required changes. If not, change the caregiving situation.
   c. Identify, then eliminate or reduce environmental stresses.
   d. Find supportive, empathetic relatives and neighbors.
   e. Find parenting classes, self-help groups, lactation consultant, professional counseling, drug or alcohol treatment programs, and so on, when indicated, for parents.
   f. Find age-appropriate day care programs, respite centers, and so on for the child.
   g. Find social worker, psychologist, nurse, or other human services providers who can become intensely involved with the family for 1 to 2 years; but know when and when not to enlist protective service agents and visiting nurses.

Assessing Abnormal Development

1. In the first months, abnormal development manifests as poor suck, floppy or spastic tone, and a lack of auditory response.

2. In the first year, motor delay in sitting and crawling suggests a developmental delay.

3. In the second and third year, language and behavioral abnormalities are manifest.

4. By school age, evidence of learning disabilities and attention-deficit hyperactivity disorder may be present.

5. Medical evaluation for mental retardation and autism should include chromosomal and molecular biologic testing for fragile X syndrome, the most common inherited cause for mental retardation. Classic findings for fragile X (long facies, large ears, and large testes) may be absent in infancy.

6. Testing for mental retardation includes phenylketonuria, thyroid, galactosemia, biotinidase deficiency, and maple syrup urine disease, usually done in the newborn period. Additional metabolic investigation might include plasma amino acids, urine organic acids, and blood lactate.

Developmental Screening Instruments

1. DDST II is a general screening tool that assesses personal-social, fine motor–adaptive, language, and gross motor skills in children ages 0 to 6 years (see Ch. 4, Developmental Surveillance).

2. CLAMS (Clinical Linguistic Auditory Milestones Scale) and ELM (Early Language Milestones) scale are language screening tools that assess receptive and expressive language by observation and interview for ages less than 36 months.

3. The Brazelton Neonatal Behavioral Assessment Scale (NBAS) assesses neurologic intactness, adaptation to extrauterine life, primitive reflexes, state organization, self-regulatory ability, and interactive capacities in infants from birth to 1 month.

4. No child is too young for formal audiologic testing.

Anticipatory Guidance to Promote Normal Growth and Development

1. Diet and exercise
2. Injury prevention measures
3. Reassurance of safety and self-worth
4. Parental advice, counseling, and moral support

Bibliography

Behrman RE, Kliegman RM, Arvin AM (eds): Nelson Textbook of Pediatrics, 15th ed. Philadelphia, WB Saunders Company, 1996.

Gahagan S, Holmes R: A stepwise approach to evaluation of undernutrition and failure to thrive. Pediatr Clin North Am 1998;48:169–186.

Jones KL: Smith's Recognizable Patterns of Human Malformation. Philadelphia, WB Saunders Company, 1997.

Kliegman RM, Nieder ML, Super DM (eds): Practical Strategies in Pediatric Diagnosis and Therapy. Philadelphia, WB Saunders Company, 1996.

Levy SE, Hyman SL: Pediatric assessment of the child with developmental delay. Pediatr Clin North Am 1993;40:465–473.

Sturtz GS: Common Sense Guide to Growth and Nutrition. Watertown, NY, Hojack Publishing, 1991.

Growth and Development Charts

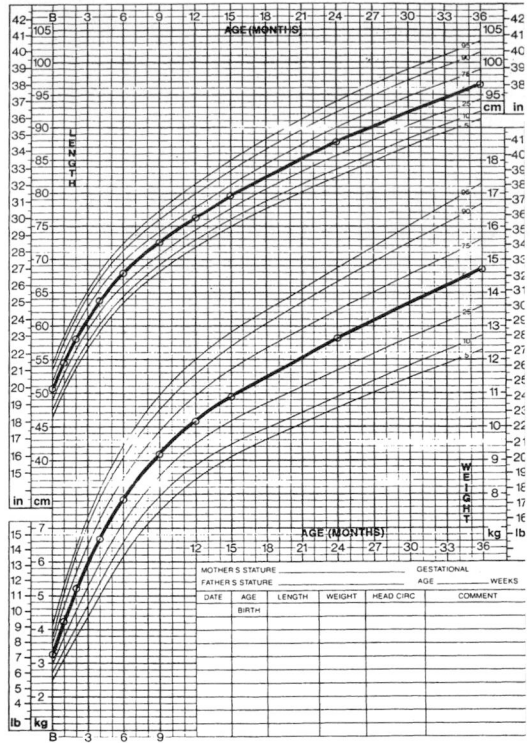

Figure 3–1 Growth at the 50th percentile. Average United States boy. (From Sturtz GS: Common Sense Guide to Growth and Nutrition, p 37. Watertown, NY, Hojack Publishing Company, 1991, with permission.)

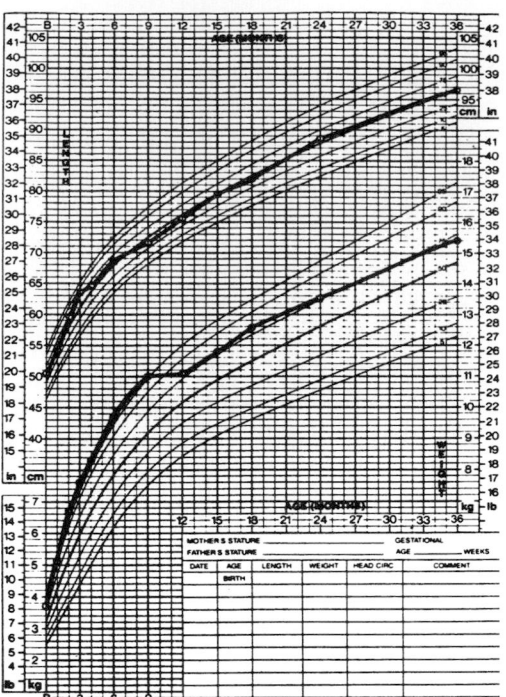

Figure 3–3 Breast-fed male infant with rapid weight gain that regressed toward the 50th percentile. (From Sturtz GS: Common Sense Guide to Growth and Nutrition, p 87. Watertown, NY, Hojack Publishing Company, 1991, with permission.)

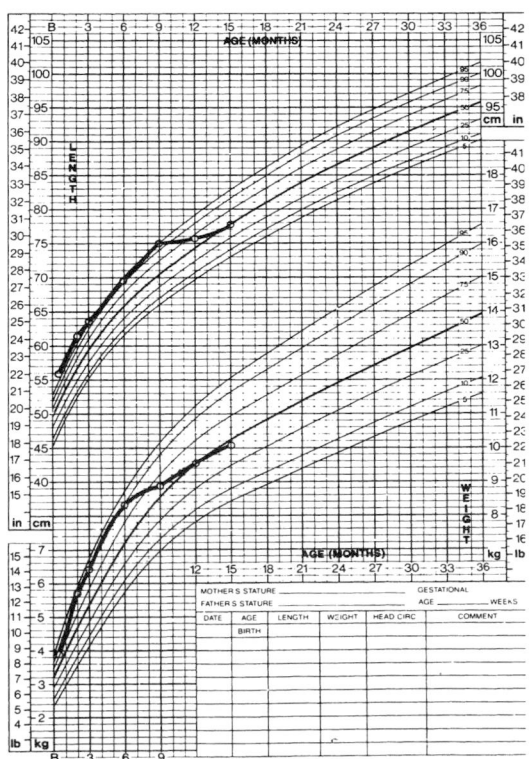

Figure 3–2 Neonatal growth near the 95th percentile regressing to the 50th percentile by age 15 months. (From Sturtz GS: Common Sense Guide to Growth and Nutrition, p 81. Watertown, NY, Hojack Publishing Company, 1991, with permission.)

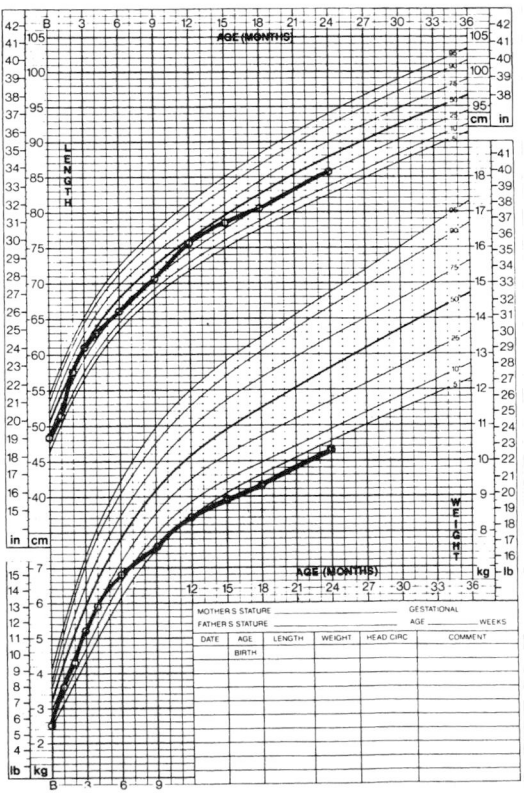

Figure 3–4 Length is at the 25th percentile. Weight is below the 5th percentile. The small, thin son of small, thin parents. (From Sturtz GS: Common Sense Guide to Growth and Nutrition, p 52. Watertown, NY, Hojack Publishing Company, 1991, with permission.)

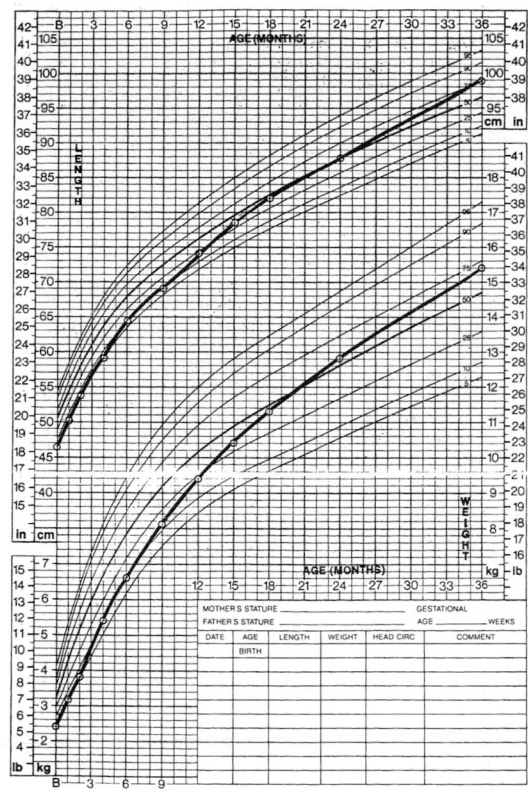

Figure 3–5 Catch-up growth in an infant at the 5th percentile at birth. (From Sturtz GS: Common Sense Guide to Growth and Nutrition, p 42. Watertown, NY, Hojack Publishing Company, 1991, with permission.)

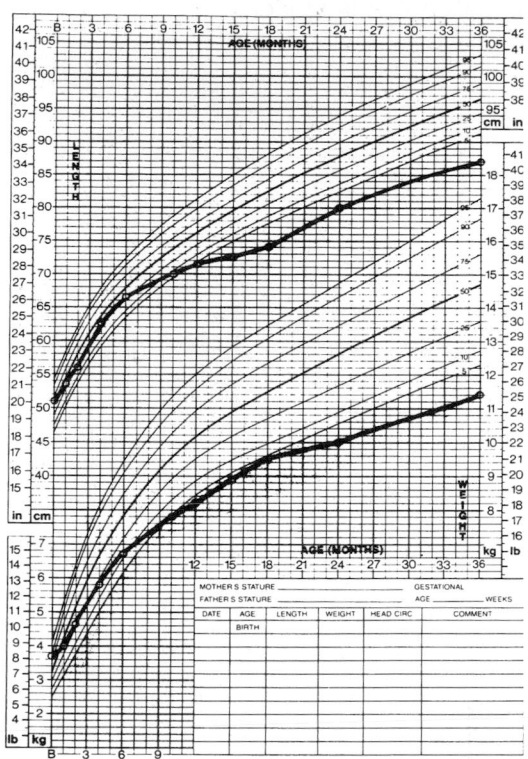

Figure 3–7 Length and weight fell below the 5th percentile in this boy with familial short stature. (From Sturtz GS: Common Sense Guide to Growth and Nutrition, p 91. Watertown, NY, Hojack Publishing Company, 1991, with permission.)

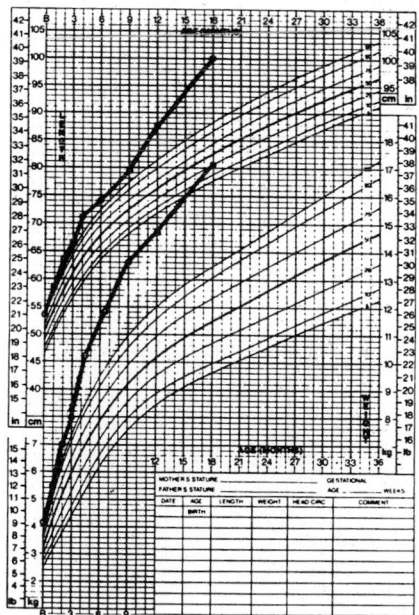

Figure 3–6 Enormous child who was fed enormous amounts of food despite dietary counseling. (From Sturtz GS: Common Sense Guide to Growth and Nutrition, p 54. Watertown, NY, Hojack Publishing Company, 1991, with permission.)

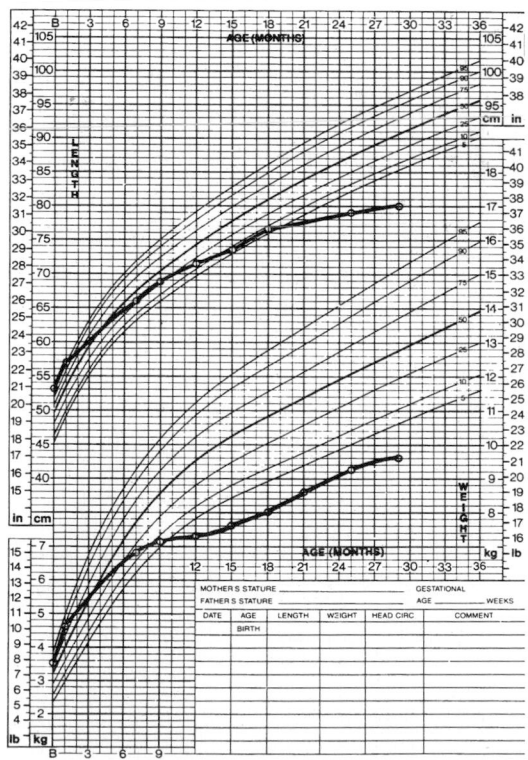

Figure 3–8 Classic case of failure to thrive. (From Sturtz GS: Common Sense Guide to Growth and Nutrition, p 66. Watertown, NY, Hojack Publishing Company, 1991, with permission.)

3 Growth and Development Guidelines • 23

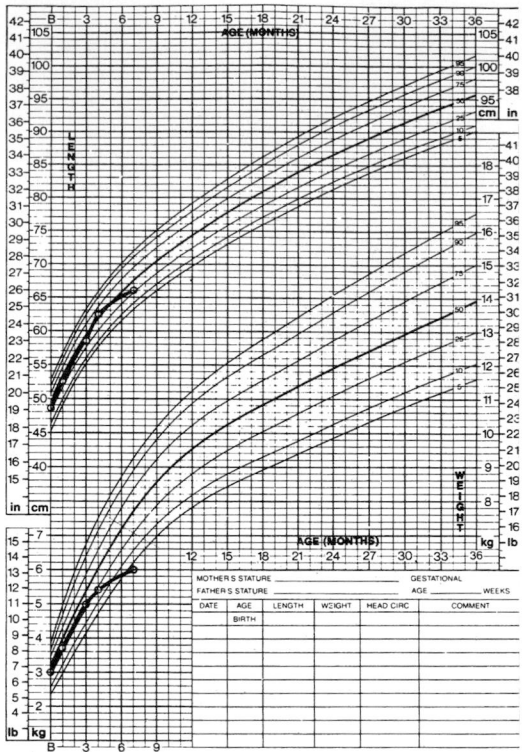

Figure 3–9 Example of heart failure secondary to patent ductus arteriosus. Closed surgically at age 7 months. (From Sturtz GS: Common Sense Guide to Growth and Nutrition, p 65. Watertown, NY, Hojack Publishing Company, 1991, with permission.)

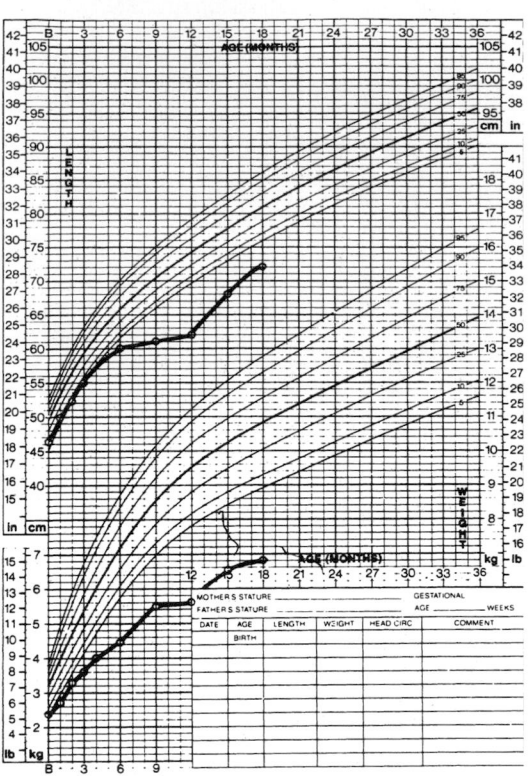

Figure 3–11 Example of giardiasis (contaminated family water supply) treated at age 12 months. (From Sturtz GS: Common Sense Guide to Growth and Nutrition, p 61. Watertown, NY, Hojack Publishing Company, 1991, with permission.)

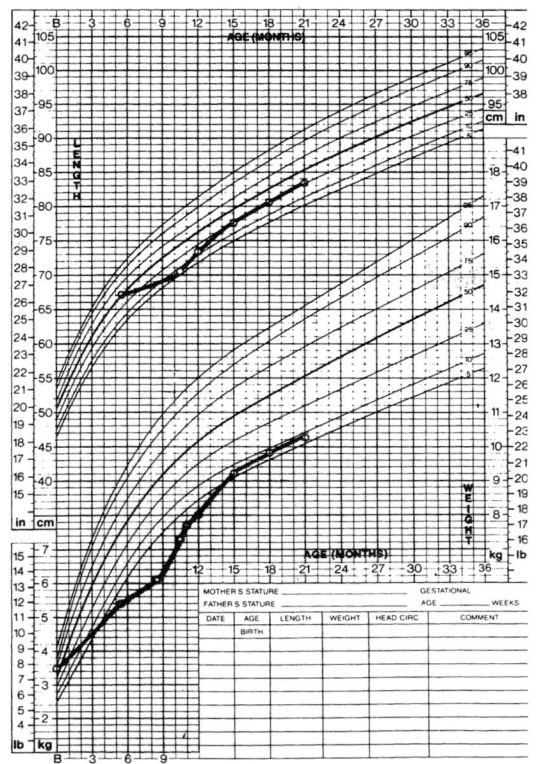

Figure 3–10 Example of heart failure secondary to ventricular septal defect. Repaired surgically at 6 months. (From Sturtz GS: Common Sense Guide to Growth and Nutrition, p 76. Watertown, NY, Hojack Publishing Company, 1991, with permission.)

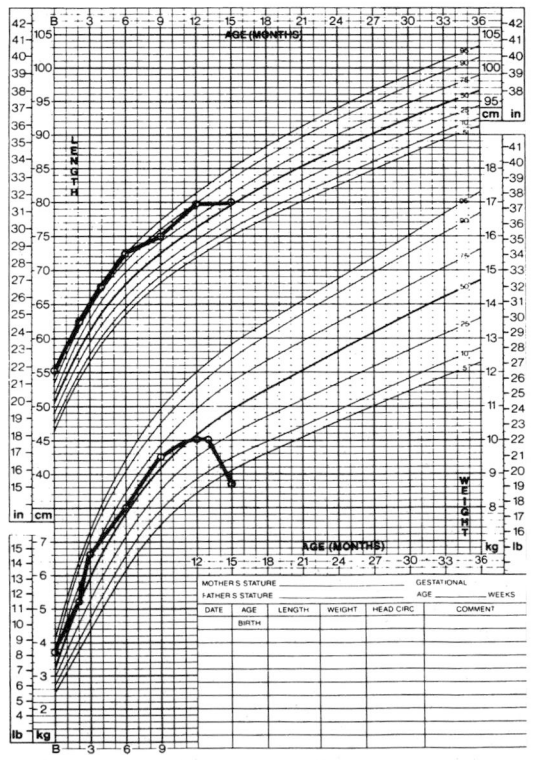

Figure 3–12 Example of celiac disease, beginning at 12 months and diagnosed at 15 months. Gluten-free diet led to appropriate weight gain. (From Sturtz GS: Common Sense Guide to Growth and Nutrition, p 93. Watertown, NY, Hojack Publishing Company, 1991, with permission.)

4 Developmental Surveillance

Linda N. Meurer

Etiology

1. Definitions
   a. Developmental screening: assessment of whole populations of children to identify those at high risk for developmental delay for whom more intensive investigation may be warranted; may involve the administration of brief tests.
   b. Developmental surveillance: longitudinal and collaborative process whereby parents and knowledgeable professionals assess the developmental progress of a child in the context of his or her environmental and medical risk factors. Providers elicit and attend to parental concerns, review relevant developmental milestones, and make clinical judgments based on careful, skilled observation of age-appropriate tasks. Formal screening tests are sometimes used as adjuncts to clinical evaluation.
   c. Developmental assessment: detailed multidisciplinary investigation of demonstrated or suspected developmental delay, designed to be diagnostic and provide prognoses
   d. Developmental delay: broad term referring to a failure to reach developmental milestones appropriately. Children develop at different rates but acquire their developmental skills in a strikingly similar and predictable sequence. Delay may occur in any or all of several domains, including fine or gross motor (e.g., cerebral palsy), language, social (e.g., infantile autism), and cognitive (e.g., mental retardation) skills.
2. Epidemiology of developmental delay
   a. Two to 5 per cent of children suffer from potentially reversible visual deficits.
   b. One to 2 per cent of infants and children have hearing deficits that may interfere with the development of language, social, and cognitive skills if not identified early.
   c. Gross motor delays are the easiest to identify very early and may be associated with other developmental delays. The level of motor delay, however, does not predict future cognitive abilities.
   d. An estimated 8.5 per cent of children under age 3 years have significant language delays. Disorders of communication are the most sensitive early predictors for cognitive and school difficulties.
   e. Although advocated for all, less than 15 per cent of children under age 5 receive regular screening for vision, hearing, language, and other developmental milestones. Providers fail to identify up to 95 per cent of preschool children with speech and language disorders.
3. Risk factors
   a. Medical
      (1) Hereditary disorders: gene and chromosomal aberrations, such as fragile X and Down's syndromes, inborn errors of metabolism
      (2) Perinatal morbidity: fetal alcohol syndrome, fetal malnutrition, prematurity, hypoxic encephalopathy, low birth weight, intrauterine growth retardation
      (3) Acquired childhood diseases: infection, brain trauma, lead poisoning, iron deficiency, malnutrition
   b. Environmental
      (1) Social deprivation
      (2) Parents with emotional disturbances, mental retardation, substance abuse
      (3) Low socioeconomic status—associated with many other risk factors

Presentation and History

1. Developmental delay may be suspected by health professionals because of parental concerns, a history of risk factors, medical conditions, or physical findings likely to be associated with delays or demonstrated delays at the time of observation.
2. History for every child elicits potential risk factors and includes the following:
   a. Family history
   b. Pregnancy, labor, delivery
   c. Neonatal problems
   d. Illnesses and accidents
   e. Diet and growth
   f. Developmental milestones
   g. Family and home environment

3. Parental description of a child's development may be inaccurate and must be supplemented by the direct, skilled observation of professionals.

4. Developmental history can serve as an educational intervention by introducing developmental stages and stimulatory methods to parents.

Clinical Findings

Physical examination includes the following:

1. General examination with observation for malformations or dysmorphology

2. Growth pattern

3. Neurologic examination

4. Hearing and vision tests (see below)

5. Direct observation of developmental milestones in the various domains

Key Components of Screening Process

- Sensitive attention to parental concerns

- Thoughtful inquiry about parental observations

- Observations of a wide variety of child's behaviors

- Examination of specific developmental attainments

- Use of all encounters for observing and recording developmental status

- Screening of vision and hearing to rule out sensory impairment as cause

- Observation of parent-child interaction

Adapted from American Academy of Pediatrics Committee on Children with Disabilities: Screening infants and young children for developmental disabilities. Pediatrics 1994;93: 863–865. Copyright 1994 American Academy of Pediatrics, with permission.

Screening Tests

1. All infants should be examined by 6 months of age to evaluate fixation preference, ocular alignment, and the presence of eye disease. Vision testing is recommended for all children starting at 3 years of age.

2. The National Institutes of Health recommends universal screening for hearing deficits within the first 3 months of life, and screening of all high-risk infants before hospital discharge. Hearing loss during early childhood should be

identified early through the eliciting of parental concerns and surveillance of speech and language development.

3. Developmental screening tests should be viewed as one of many sources of information obtained over multiple points in time to monitor child development.

   a. They are meant to identify children at high risk or with suspected delay who may benefit from further developmental assessment.

   b. They are not diagnostic or designed to predict function or IQ.

   c. Major pediatric organizations in the United States and Great Britain do not advocate routine administration of formal screening tests to all children but recommend their use to reinforce suspicions of delay and to monitor children at risk for developmental problems.

4. The Denver Developmental Screening Test, revised as the Denver II, is the best known instrument and is used worldwide (Fig. 4–1). Features of the Denver II are as follows:

   a. Designed to be used with apparently well children between birth and age 6 years

   b. Administered by assessing a child's performance on age-appropriate tasks in four areas:

      (1) Personal-social: getting along with people and caring for personal needs

      (2) Fine motor–adaptive: eye-hand coordination, manipulation of small objects, problem solving

      (3) Language: hearing, understanding, using language

      (4) Gross motor: sitting, walking, jumping, overall large muscle movement

   c. The Denver II also serves as a valuable aid to provider memory and helps to communicate interest in the child's development and encourage parents to raise questions.

5. Other useful screening instruments include the following:

   a. Minnesota Child Development Inventory: for screening general development and conceptual, number, fine motor, and language skills

   b. Early Language Milestones (ELM) scale: for

Figure 4–1 Denver Developmental Screening Test II. (From Frankenburg WK, Dodds J, Archer P, et al: Denver II Training Manual, 2nd ed, pp 1–4. Denver, Denver Developmental Materials, 1992, with permission.) *Illustration on opposite page*

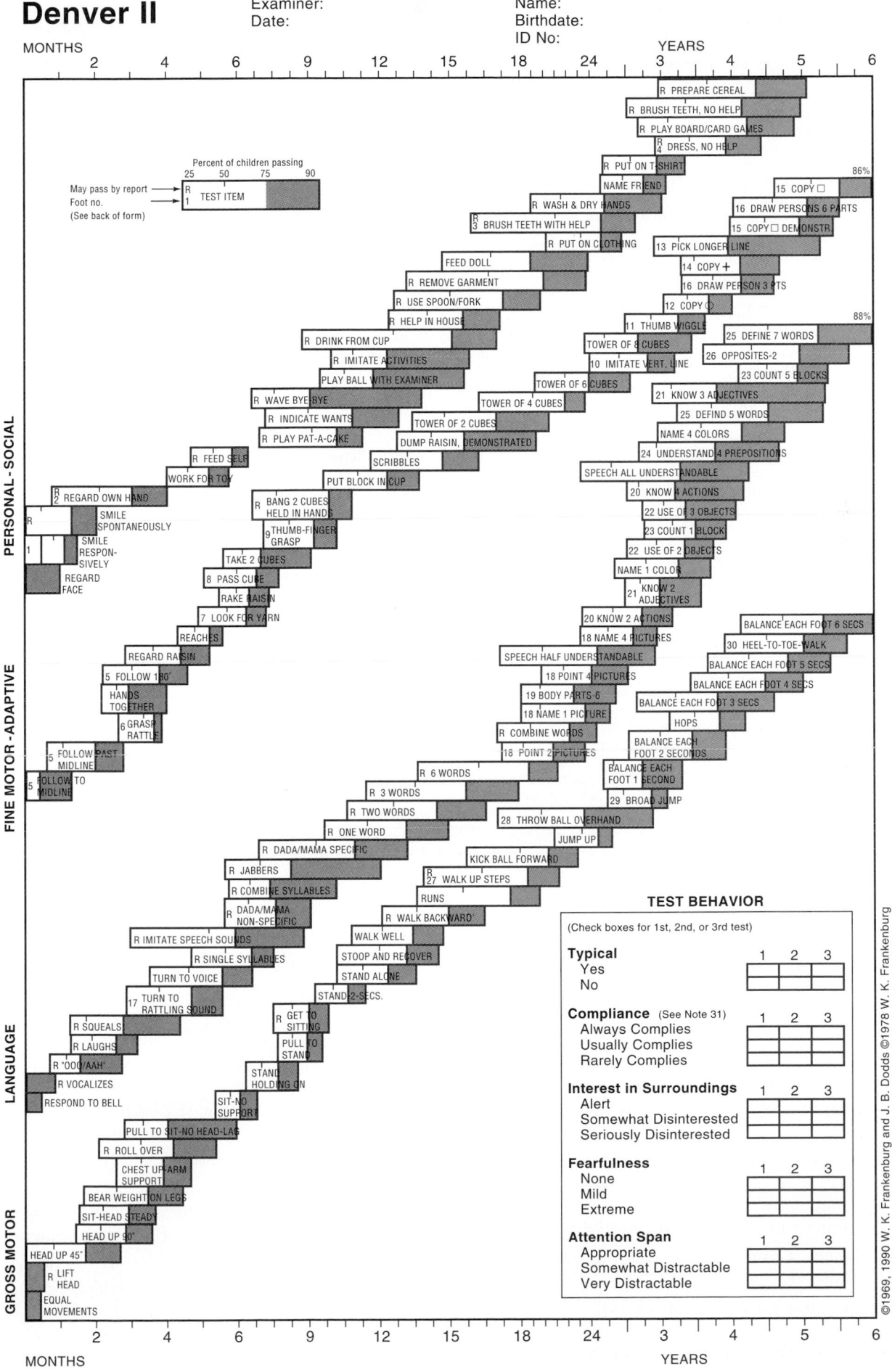

DIRECTIONS FOR ADMINISTRATION

1. Try to get child to smile by smiling, talking or waving. Do not touch him/her.
2. Child must stare at hand several seconds.
3. Parent may help guide toothbrush and put toothpaste on brush.
4. Child does not have to be able to tie shoes or button/zip in the back.
5. Move yarn slowly in an arc from one side to the other, about 8" above child's face.
6. Pass if child grasps rattle when it is touched to the backs or tips of fingers.
7. Pass if child tries to see where yarn went. Yarn should be dropped quickly from sight from tester's hand without arm movement.
8. Child must transfer cube from hand to hand without help of body, mouth, or table.
9. Pass if child picks up raisin with any part of thumb and finger.
10. Line can vary only 30 degrees or less from tester's line.
11. Make a fist with thumb pointing upward and wiggle only the thumb. Pass if child imitates and does move any fingers other than the thumb.

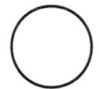   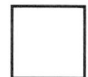

12. Pass any enclosed form. Fail continuous round motions.

13. Which line is longer? (Not bigger.) Turn paper upside down and repeat. (pass 3 of 3 or 5 of 6)

14. Pass any lines crossing near midpoint.

15. Have child copy first. If failed, demonstrate.

When giving items 12, 14, and 15, do not name the forms. Do not demonstrate 12 and 14.

16. When scoring, each pair (2 arms, 2 legs. etc.) counts as one part.
17. Place one cube in cup and shake gently near child's ear, but out of sight. Repeat for other ear.
18. Point to picture and have child name it. (No credit is given for sounds only.)
    If less than 4 pictures are named correctly, have child point to picture as each is named by tester.

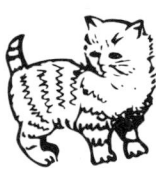   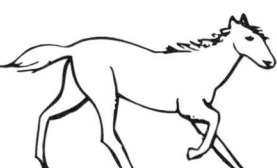   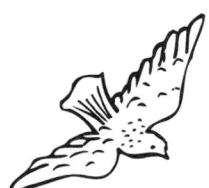   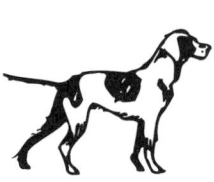   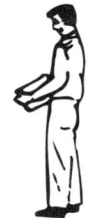

19. Using doll, tell child: Show me the nose, eyes, mouth, hands, feet, tummy, hair. Pass 6 of 8.
20. Using pictures, ask child: Which one flies?... says meow?... talks?... gallops? Pass 2 of 5, 4 of 5.
21. Ask child: What do you do when you are cold?... tired?...hungry? Pass 2 of 3, 3 of 3.
22. Ask child: What do you do with a cup? What is a chair used for? What is a pencil used for?
    Action words must be included in answers.
23. Pass if child correctly places <u>and</u> says how many blocks are on paper. (1, 5).
24. Tell child: Put block **on** table; **under** table; **in front of** me, **behind** me. Pass 4 of 4.
    (Do not help child by pointing, moving head or eyes.)
25. Ask child: What is a ball?... lake?... desk?... house?... banana?... curtain?... fence?... ceiling?... Pass if defined in terms of use, shape, what it is made of, or general category (such as banana is fruit, not just yellow). Pass 5 of 8, 7 of 8.
26. Ask child: If a horse is big, a mouse is___? If fire is hot, ice is___? If the sun shines during the day, the moon shines during the___? Pass 2 of 3.
27. Child may use wall or rail only, not person. May not crawl.
28. Child must throw ball overhand 3 feet to within arm's reach of tester.
29. Child must perform standing broad jump over width of test sheet (8 1/2 inches).
30. Tell child to walk forward, ∞∞∞∞→ heel within 1 inch of toe. Tester may demonstrate.
    Child must walk 4 consecutive steps.
31. In the second year, half of normal children are non-compliant.

OBSERVATIONS:

Figure 4–1 (*Continued*)

testing language skills in children under age 3

  c. Clinical Linguistic and Auditory Milestones Scale (CLAMS): for testing language development in all children and cognitive development in children with motor delays

  d. Milani-Comparetti scale: for assessing motor skills

  e. Simultaneous Technique for Acuity and Readiness Testing (START): for testing vision and general development

  f. Stanford-Binet test: for estimating intelligence

  g. Home Screening Questionnaire (HSQ): for identifying high-risk home environments

6. Additional tests may be necessary to determine the cause of an identified developmental delay and might include chromosomal and DNA

testing, metabolic screening, thyroid studies, imaging studies such as computerized tomography and magnetic resonance imaging, and others.

Interventions

1. Primary prevention
   a. Educate pregnant women as to the importance of good nutrition and avoidance of alcohol and drugs.
   b. Improve parental understanding of normal child development and developmental expectations, assist understanding of the individual developmental characteristics and temperament of their child, and encourage parental feelings of confidence and competence to affect their child's development.
2. Secondary prevention
   a. Perform developmental surveillance in all children, using all encounters as opportunities to observe developmental progress.
   b. Recognize high-risk medical and environmental situations and early delay.
   c. Obtain a complete developmental assessment of children with suspected delay.
   d. Rescreen periodically as expectations change.
3. Tertiary prevention
   a. Maintain updated information on community resources for children and families at risk for or with developmental delay.
   b. Maintain linkages with these resources and coordinate patient care with them.

Bibliography

American Academy of Pediatrics Committee on Children with Disabilities: Screening infants and young children for developmental disabilities. Pediatrics 1994;93:863–865.

American Academy of Pediatrics Committee on Practice and Ambulatory Medicine, Section on Ophthalmology: Eye examination and vision screening in infants, children, and young adults. Pediatrics 1996;98:153–157.

Frankenburg WK, Dodds J, Archer P, et al: Denver II Training Manual, 2nd ed, pp 1–4. Denver, Denver Developmental Materials, 1992.

Green M (ed): Bright Futures: Guidelines for Health Supervision of Infants, Children, and Adolescents. Arlington, VA: National Center for Education in Maternal and Child Health, 1994.

National Institutes of Health Consensus Development Conference on Early Identification of Hearing Impairment. NIH Consensus Statement. 1993;11:1–24.

5 Preoperative Evaluation

Akram Sadaka

General Rules

All patients need to be evaluated as follows:

1. Complete history and physical examination
2. Complete blood count (CBC), prothrombin time, partial thromboplastin time, SMA 7, and urinalysis.
3. Electrocardiogram (ECG) in all males over 40, females over 50, patients at high risk for coronary heart disease (CHD), heavy smokers, or patients known to have a history of CHD.
4. Posteroanterior and lateral chest film in all patients over 40, smokers, and patients with chronic obstructive pulmonary disease (COPD).
5. Liver function tests, Mg^{2+}, and Ca^{2+} in all alcoholics, heavy drinkers, and those who are known to have liver disease.
6. Room air arterial blood gases (ABGs) in all COPD cases.
7. Pregnancy test in all female patients of childbearing age who still have even one ovary.

Diabetes

1. Make sure there is no underlying coronary or peripheral vascular disease. If so, work up as indicated.
2. All diabetics must have 12-lead ECG, SMA 7, glycosylated hemoglobin A_{1c} (Hb A_{1c}), and urinalysis. The higher the Hb A_{1c}, the greater the potential for postoperative complications in terms of wound healing, cardiovascular function, and infections.
3. Because diabetics are prone to skin and systemic infections, their skin must be carefully and thoroughly inspected.

Management

1. Type II diabetes that is controlled by diet, oral hypoglycemics, or small doses of insulin (<25 units/day): Simply withhold medications the day of surgery. Metformin must be held for at least 48 hours postoperatively.
2. Type I diabetes or type II diabetes that is controlled with high doses of insulin (>25 units/day)
   a. Give one third to one half (depending on the time of surgery and how brittle the diabetes

is) of the morning dose of insulin in the morning of the day of surgery.
   b. Dextrose 5 per cent must be included in the IV solution until full recovery is achieved. This is along with immediate pre- and postoperative glucose determinations.

Coronary Heart Disease

1. After myocardial infarction (MI), there is a decrease in reinfarction risk over time. It is advisable to postpone elective procedures as long as possible to lower reinfarction potential.
   a. Less than 3 months post-MI, the operative risk of reinfarction is about 33 per cent.
   b. From 3 to 6 months post-MI, the operative risk of reinfarction is about 15 per cent.
   c. Over 6 months post-MI, the operative risk of reinfarction is about 5 per cent.
2. All patients who are known to have CHD must have 12-lead ECG, CBC, SMA 7, and chest radiograph.
3. The administration of perioperative nitroglycerin must be individualized. Generally speaking, for those patients who are asymptomatic or had remote or non–Q-wave MI, perioperative nitropaste is best.
4. Those who have stable angina or a history of MI less than 6 months must receive complete cardiac evaluation, including two-dimensional echocardiogram, multiple gated acquisition blood pool scan, and cardiology consult. After cardiology clearance, it is advisable that this group of patients receive perioperative intensive care unit monitoring along with sampling of the MB isoenzyme of creatine kinase, nitroglycerin drip, and serial ECGs.

Chronic Obstructive Pulmonary Disease

1. All patients must have preoperative posteroanterior and lateral chest radiographs, room air ABGs, and determination of forced expiratory volume in 1 second and forced vital capacity. If pulmonary function testing equipment is not readily accessible, a simple test can be done in the office by asking the patient to blow a lit candle from a distance of 8 inches. If the patient

fails the lit candle test, then the likely postoperative pulmonary complications are great and possibly grave ones.

2. In moderate to severe cases of COPD, it is advisable to refer patients to preoperative respiratory training programs.

3. Smoking cessation is a must at least 2 weeks preoperatively in all cases of COPD and otherwise.

Central Nervous System

1. Head injury or intracranial blood can increase intracranial pressure (ICP). Therefore, the fundi need to be carefully checked.

2. Anesthesia should avoid all drugs known to increase cerebral blood flow, such as halothane and narcotics.

3. Perioperative hyperventilation is a crucial step in the prevention of grave outcome of increased ICP.

Psychiatric Disorders

With the exception of monoamine oxidase (MAO) inhibitors, most psychotropic drugs do not require special management. MAOs must be discontinued and substituted at least 2 weeks before surgery.

Endocrine Disorders

Patients who received adrenal steroids in the 6 to 12 months prior to surgery will need supplemental steroids perioperatively. This can be accomplished by giving the patient 300 mg of hydrocortisone on the day of surgery and tapering over the subsequent few days.

Renal Failure

Renal failure is handled best by scheduling the dialysis as close as possible to the day of surgery. Check CBC, SMA 7, and acid-base balance. Conservative correction of abnormalities is advisable.

Bibliography

Goldman L, Caldera DL, Nassbaum SR, et al: Multifactorial index of cardiac risk in noncardiac surgical procedures. N Engl J Med 1977;297:845.

Kennedy SK, Longneck DE: History and principles of anesthesiology. In Hardman JG and Limbird LE (eds): Goodman and Gilman's The Pharmacological Basis of Therapeutics, pp 295–306. New York, McGraw Hill, 1996.

Marsh ML, Marshall LF, Shapiro HM: Neurosurgical intensive care. Anesthesiology 1977;47:149.

Riggs JRA, Jones NL: Clinical assessment of respiratory function. Br J Anaesthesiol 1978;50:3.

Stein M, Cassara EL: Preoperative pulmonary evaluation and therapy for surgery patients. JAMA 1970;211:787.

Symposium on the postoperative period. Br J Anaesthesiol 1975;47:91.

6 Advance Directives

Gregory Juckett

Advance Directive Types

An advance directive is a legal document that permits adults with decision-making capacity (DMC) to express their intentions regarding future medical intervention in the event they lose that capacity. Two main types of advance directives exist:

1. The living will (instruction or treatment directive)
2. The durable power of attorney for health care (DPAHC) or proxy directive.

Living Will

A living will is a written legal document stating the patient's preference for future interventions (and commonly requesting they be withheld) in the event of terminal illness or persistent vegetative state (Fig. 6–1).

1. Increasingly, these interventions are specified (cardiopulmonary resuscitation, artificial hydration/nutrition, intravenous medications, antibiotics, blood products, dialysis and mechanical ventilation), although until recently the vaguer phrases "heroic measures" or "artificial life support" were used. The intention is usually for a more natural death with comfort care rather than aggressive life support.
2. Living wills are designed to provide care instructions at the end of life, so they are only activated by a terminal illness (or, in most states, a persistent vegetative state) when the patient's DMC is lost.
3. Living wills pertain primarily to forgoing end-of-life treatment and usually make no provision for a surrogate decision maker.
4. One serious drawback is that no legal penalties exist in the event the living will is ignored or overridden.

Durable Power of Attorney for Health Care

1. A DPAHC, or medical power of attorney, is a legal document in which an individual (principal) designates a representative (surrogate or proxy) to make medical decisions whenever the individual loses DMC.
2. It is called durable because, unlike a regular power of attorney, it continues to be in effect after the principal becomes incompetent. It also may designate specific limitations or instructions to the degree these can be anticipated.
3. Many people elect to have a living will in addition to the DPAHC or else incorporate the living will's instructions into the same document. A DPAHC is more versatile than the living will in that it is activated whenever DMC is lost and not just in a terminal illness or persistent vegetative state.

Health Care Surrogate Selection and Decision Making

Choosing a Surrogate Without an Advance Directive

1. Although advance directives of both types are increasingly popular, relatively few patients (10 to 20 per cent) ever complete them. Therefore, a process is needed to ensure that patients who lack advance directives and have lost DMC are able to have health care decisions made on their behalf.
2. Most states now have adopted legislation that permits physicians or others to appoint a health care surrogate decision maker for the patient in this setting. Surrogate selection legislation minimizes judicial involvement and provides legal protection to the parties involved.
3. The surrogate should have certain qualifications (competence, emotional stability, demonstrated care and concern, regular contact with the patient, and availability to make decisions).
   a. Granted these qualifications are present, surrogates are usually chosen in rank order according to their relationship to the patient (e.g., guardian, spouse, adult child, either parent, adult sibling, adult grandchild, close friend, sheriff, or adult protective services).
   b. The exact order and who is included varies slightly from state to state.
   c. Surrogates do not always need to be a blood relative, and, for patients who are estranged from their families, often a close friend can be the best choice.

Types of Surrogate Decision Making

Surrogate decisions may be based on three different standards:

LIVING WILL

I, _____, being of sound mind, willfully and voluntarily make this declaration to be followed if I become incompetent. This declaration reflects my firm and settled commitment to refuse life-sustaining treatment under the circumstances indicated below.

I direct my attending physician to withhold or withdraw life-sustaining treatment that serves only to prolong the process of my dying, if I should be in a terminal condition or in a state of permanent unconsciousness.

I direct that treatment be limited to measures to keep me comfortable and to relieve pain, including any pain that might occur by withholding or withdrawing life-sustaining treatment.

In addition, if I am in the condition described above, I feel especially strong about the following forms of treatment:

I ( ) do ( ) do not want cardiac resuscitation.
I ( ) do ( ) do not want mechanical respiration.
I ( ) do ( ) do not want tube feeding or any other artificial or invasive form of nutrition (food) or hydration (water).
I ( ) do ( ) do not want blood or blood products.
I ( ) do ( ) do not want any form of surgery or invasive diagnostic tests.
I ( ) do ( ) do not want kidney dialysis.
I ( ) do ( ) do not want antibiotics.

I realize that if I do not specifically indicate my preference regarding any of the forms of treatment listed above, I may receive that form of treatment.

OTHER INSTRUCTIONS:

I ( ) do ( ) do not want to designate another person as my surrogate to make medical treatment decisions for me if I should be incompetent and in a terminal condition or in a state of permanent unconsciousness. Name and address of surrogate (if applicable):

Name of Surrogate: _____

Address of Surrogate: _____
_____
_____
_____

Name and address of substitute surrogate (if surrogate designated above is unable to serve):

Substitute Surrogate: _____

Address of Substitute: _____
_____
_____
_____

I made this declaration on the _____ day of _____ (mo)_____ (yr)

Declarant's signature: _____

Declarant's address: _____
_____
_____
_____

The declarant or the person on behalf of and at the direction of the declarant knowingly and voluntarily signed this writing by signature or mark in my presence.

Witness's signature: _____

Witness's address: _____
_____
_____
_____

Witness's signature: _____

Witness's address: _____
_____
_____
_____

Figure 6–1 Example of a living will.

1. The *autonomy standard* refers to respecting known verbal (unwritten) directives given by a previously competent person that now help answer the question of what he or she would have desired.

2. The *substituted judgment standard* refers to choosing the decision the incompetent person would have made if competent, whether or not this decision is in his or her best interest. Of course, the surrogate must know what the patient would have wanted in the present circumstances.

3. The *best interest standard* is based on the surrogate weighing the benefits versus burdens of

various courses of action to find which option provides the maximal benefit or best quality of life ("what a reasonable person in the same or similar situation would want"). For patients who have never been competent, the best interest standard is the most appropriate.

Decision-Making Capacity

1. Unlike incompetency as determined by a court, DMC is a clinical judgment about whether a patient can make his or her own health care decisions.
2. Once DMC is deemed absent, an advance directive should be followed or a surrogate decision maker should be appointed. Patients with mental retardation, mild dementia, and depression may still possess DMC.
3. Key elements of DMC
   a. Possession of a set of values and goals
   b. The ability to understand and communicate information
   c. The ability to reason and deliberate about the available choices
4. Questions to ask when determining DMC
   a. Does the patient have the ability to understand his or her condition?
   b. Can the patient appreciate the benefits and risks of the various treatment options, including the withholding of treatment?
   c. Does the patient have the ability to judge how treatment options affect his or her values and goals?
   d. Can the patient reason and deliberate about the available options?
   e. Can the patient communicate his or her decisions meaningfully?
5. DMC is not absolute (all or none) or static. Some patients can only make simple decisions by themselves. Some patients have fluctuating levels of consciousness so DMC may be present only during lucid intervals.

Patient Self Determination Act of 1991

1. This act mandates that all health care facilities receiving Medicare or Medicaid funds (hospitals, nursing homes, health maintenance organizations, hospices, and home care agencies) inform patients of their right to accept or refuse medical treatment and provide information on advance directives according to the specific state laws.
2. Although patients are not required to possess advance directives, this act has promoted their use. Many patients now appoint a surrogate decision maker as part of the hospital admission process in the event they lose DMC later.

Potential Problems with Advance Directives

1. Lack of advance planning
   a. Most patients are understandably reluctant to plan for or even discuss a terminal illness, and so they postpone legal documentation of their wishes.
   b. Physicians are in an excellent position to address patient concerns and to document their decisions during a routine office visit. A good way to open the discussion is to ask: Would you like to discuss with us what you would want us to do in case you become too sick to tell us yourself? Other windows of opportunity are prior to surgery or on admission to the hospital.
   c. Once the patient knows what he or she wants, an advance directive can often be completed in minimal time using standardized forms. Advance directives for the various states may be obtained through "Choice in Dying" at 1-800-989-WILL or on the Internet at *www.choices.org*. Having this form witnessed and notarized in a hospital or larger clinic setting is seldom difficult.
2. Objections of conscience
   a. Health care providers may, at times, find themselves unable to comply with an advance directive as a matter of conscience. In such a situation, the best course of action is to notify the surrogate or family about the provider's objection and, if no compromise can be reached, to attempt to transfer the patient to another provider who will be able to comply with the directive.
   b. If these measures are undertaken "in good faith," the noncomplying physician is usually immune from prosecution or charges of abandonment.
3. Unacceptable conflicts of interest
   a. Surrogate decision makers may be confronted by mounting health care debts, the prospect of a large inheritance, or the possibility that pension checks may be terminated upon the death of their loved one. All of these conflicts of interest could potentially interfere with decisions by the surrogate solely according to the patient's previously stated desires or best interests.
   b. Social workers should be consulted when a surrogate is selected because they are more

likely to be aware of potential problems than the physician.

   c. Surrogate decisions that are clearly against the patient's best interests or wishes should be challenged. More often, it is a spouse's intense emotional involvement rather than a financial factor that impairs judgment enough to warrant further discussion or selection of an alternative surrogate.

4. Limited foresight

   a. Situations may arise in patient care that were not and indeed could not have been reasonably anticipated. Clearly there are even greater limitations to the average patient's foresight stemming from a lack of medical expertise. Sometimes, a patient's fear of medical technology results in a directive that encourages premature withdrawal of care. Instructions can be overexplicit (too many treatment options denied) or underexplicit and vague, leaving the physician with many questions. Proper advance counseling by the patient's own physician may correct some of these shortcomings.

   b. Patients should also be instructed to change their advance directives if and when their preferences change.

   c. If several advance directives exist for a given patient, the most recent document supersedes the others.

5. Failure to discuss advance directives with family or surrogate

   a. Unfortunately, DPAHCs are sometimes completed without adequate communication between the principal and the surrogate about his or her wishes.

   b. There should also be an alternate surrogate named in the event that the patient's first choice is unavailable or unable to serve. This person, as well, needs to be kept updated regarding the patient's desires.

   c. Likewise, living wills are more likely to be disputed and even overturned by surviving family members if the patient never discussed them when competent.

Bibliography

Arenson CA, Novielli KD, Chambers CV, et al: The importance of advance directives in primary care. Primary Care 1996;23:67–82.

Beauchamp TL, Childress JF: Nonmaleficence. In Principles of Biomedical Ethics, 4th ed, pp 189–258. New York, Oxford University Press, 1994.

Beauchamp TL, Childress JF: Respect for autonomy. In Principles of Biomedical Ethics, 4th ed, pp 120–188. New York, Oxford University Press, 1994.

King NMC: In Making Sense of Advance Directives (Clinical Medical Ethics), rev ed. Washington, DC, Georgetown University Press, 1996.

Moss AH: Assessing Decision-Making Capacity: Ethical Principles and Practical Application [brochure]. Morgantown, WV, Center for Health Ethics and Law, West Virginia University, 1998.

Rich BA: Advance directives, the next generation. J Legal Med 1998;19:63–97.

7 Cancer Screening

Lori A. Whittaker

Mortality and morbidity from cancer can be reduced by early detection of disease through regular cancer screening. Unfortunately, there is no consensus on uniform screening guidelines among various medical organizations. Listed here are the recommendations of two primary groups, the U.S. Preventive Services Task Force (USPSTF) and the American Cancer Society (ACS), as well as those of several subspecialty groups such as the American Gastroenterology Association (AGA), the American College of Obstetrics and Gynecology (ACOG), and the American Urology Association (AUA). Clinical judgment should be used when applying these guidelines to individual patients.

When considering cancer screening guidelines, it is important to identify individuals at particularly high risk for disease, because they may require more intensive screening strategies than the general population. High-risk groups include those with a strong family history of cancer (two or more first-degree relatives, one first-degree and two-second degree relatives, or one first-degree relative with onset of cancer at an early age), or other specific high-risk conditions. Risk factors that place an individual in a high-risk category are identified in boldface type.

Cancer screening strategies will continue to evolve as new insight into the pathogenesis of cancer is gained, and improved techniques for early detection are identified.

Breast Cancer

Risk Factors
1. Age >50
2. **Family history of breast cancer or cancer family syndrome**
3. **Personal history of breast, colon, endometrial, or ovarian cancer**
4. **Cellular atypia or lobular carcinoma in situ on breast biopsy**
5. Hormonal factors: nulliparity or low parity, age over 30 years at first live birth, early menarche or late menopause
6. Use of hormone replacement therapy after menopause

General Screening
1. USPSTF: mammogram every 1 to 2 years at ages 50 to 69. There is insufficient evidence to recommend for or against mammograms in women younger than 40 or older than 70. Screening in these age groups should be individualized.
2. ACS: monthly breast self-examination beginning at age 20; clinical breast examination every 3 years at ages 20 to 39 and annually beginning at age 40; and annual mammograms beginning at age 40
3. ACOG: monthly breast self-examination beginning at age 20; annual clinical breast examination beginning age 40; and mammograms every 1 to 2 years at ages 40 to 49 and annually beginning at age 50

High-Risk Screening
1. ACS and ACOG: Physicians may elect to begin mammography at age 35 in women at high risk, especially those with a family history of early-onset breast cancer.
2. Future recommendations may include screening for the breast cancer genes *BRCA1* and *BRCA2* in individuals with a strong family history of breast and/or ovarian cancer.

Cervical Cancer

Risk Factors
1. **Infection with human papillomavirus (HPV)**
2. **Early age at first intercourse**
3. **Multiple sexual partners**
4. **Previous history of cervical dysplasia**
5. **Male partner in a high-risk group**
6. **Human immunodeficiency virus (HIV) infection**
7. Smoking

General Screening
1. USPSTF: Papanicolaou (Pap) smears at least every 3 years in all women with a cervix who are sexually active and by age 18 in adolescents whose sexual history is considered unreliable. Testing more frequently may be indicated by the presence of risk factors. Pap smears may be discontinued at age 65 in women who have had consistently normal smears.
   a. There is insufficient evidence to recommend

routine screening by other methods such as cervicography, colposcopy, or HPV testing.

b. There is no evidence to indicate the need for Pap smears in women who have had a hysterectomy unless the hysterectomy was performed for cervical cancer or its precursors.

2. ACS and ACOG: annual Pap smears in all women who are sexually active or age 18 or over, with testing less frequently after three consecutive normal smears at the discretion of the physician

High-Risk Screening

1. ACS and ACOG: annual Pap smears in high-risk women
2. USPSTF: See above. HIV-infected women require more frequent screening.

Colorectal Cancer

Risk Factors

1. Age >50
2. **Family history of colorectal cancer, cancer family syndrome, or familial polyposis syndrome**
3. **Previous history of colorectal cancer; colorectal adenomas; inflammatory bowel disease; familial polyposis syndrome; or breast, ovarian, endometrial, or prostate cancer**
4. High-fat and/or low-fiber diet

General Screening

1. USPSTF: beginning at age 50, annual fecal occult blood testing and/or flexible sigmoidoscopy at an unspecified interval (although it is suggested that every 10 years may be adequate)
2. ACS: beginning at age 50, annual fecal occult blood testing with flexible sigmoidoscopy every 5 years; or total colon screening with either colonoscopy every 10 years or double-contrast barium enema every 5 to 10 years; digital rectal examination at time of endoscopy or barium enema (i.e., every 5 to 10 years)
3. AGA and ACOG: flexible sigmoidoscopy every 3 to 5 years after age 50 and annual digital rectal examination age 40 and over

High-Risk Screening

1. USPSTF: periodic screening with colonoscopy
2. ACS: careful colonoscopic surveillance with timing and intervals dependent on the degree of risk; consideration of genetic testing in individuals with strong family history of colon cancer or known hereditary colorectal cancer syndrome

Endometrial Cancer

Risk Factors

1. Age over 40
2. Obesity
3. Diabetes
4. Late menopause
5. **History of infertility or anovulatory cycles**
6. **History of unopposed estrogen replacement**
7. **Tamoxifen therapy**
8. **Personal or family history of breast, ovarian, or colon cancer**
9. **History of irregular vaginal bleeding after age 40**
10. *Lower risk associated with use of oral contraceptives.*

General Screening

ACS: annual pelvic exam age 40 and over

High-Risk Screening

ACS: Endometrial biopsy may be performed at menopause and periodically thereafter at the discretion of the physician in symptomatic or high-risk women.

Lung Cancer

Risk Factors

1. Exposure to tobacco smoke (direct or secondhand)
2. Exposure to asbestos, radon gas, polyhydrocarbons

General and High-Risk Screening

No current recommendations for routine screening

Ovarian Cancer

Risk Factors

1. **Family history of ovarian, breast, endometrial, or colon cancer**
2. Personal history of breast, endometrial, or colon cancer
3. History of infertility or use of infertility drugs
4. Nulliparity
5. *Lower risk associated with oral contraceptive use, breast-feeding, and tubal ligation.*

General Screening

No current recommendations for routine screening for ovarian cancer

High-Risk Screening

1. USPSTF: no current recommendations. There is no evidence to support aggressive screening strategies in high-risk women.
2. ACS: Transvaginal ultrasound and CA-125 levels may assist in diagnosis but are not recommended for routine screening.

Prostate Cancer

Risk Factors

1. Age >50
2. **African American race**
3. **Family history of prostate,** breast, endometrial, or colon **cancer**
4. Personal history of colon cancer
5. High-fat diet
6. Occupational exposure to cadmium or rubber

General Screening

1. USPSTF: Routine screening for prostate cancer is not recommended.
2. ACS and AUA: annual digital rectal examination and prostate-specific antigen (PSA) determination beginning at age 50 in men who have a life expectancy of at least 10 years

High-Risk Screening

ACS and AUA: PSA determination beginning at age 40 to 45.

Skin Cancer (Melanomatous and Nonmelanomatous)

Risk Factors

1. Cumulative sun exposure
2. Fair skin that burns easily; red or blond hair; freckles
3. History of blistering sunburns in childhood
4. **Giant congenital nevi**
5. **Dysplastic nevi (especially with family history of melanoma)**
6. **Family history of skin cancer**
7. **Previous history of skin cancer or preneoplastic lesions (e.g., actinic keratoses)**
8. **Xeroderma pigmentosum, albinism, basal cell nevus syndrome**
9. **Exposure to hydrocarbons, arsenic, ionizing radiation**

General Screening

ACS: regular skin self-examination, and clinical skin examination every 3 years at ages 20 to 39 and annually after age 40

High-Risk Screening

USPSTF: Clinical skin examinations recommended only for those at high risk of skin cancer (frequency not specified).

Testicular Cancer

Risk Factors

1. Age 15 to 40 and >60
2. Caucasian race
3. **Cryptorchidism, gonadal dysgenesis, Kleinfelter's syndrome, orchiopexy, testicular atrophy**

General Screening

1. ACS: clinical testicular examination every 3 years at ages 20 to 39 and annually after age 40
2. AUA: annual testicular examinations beginning at age 15
3. No recommendations regarding testicular self-examination

High-Risk Screening

USPSTF: discussion with patients with cryptorchidism or testicular atrophy of increased risk and option for screening with testicular self-examination.

Bibliography

American Cancer Society Guidelines
Byers T, Levin B, Rothenberger D, et al: ACS guidelines for screening and surveillance for early detection of colorectal polyps and cancer: update 1997. CA Cancer J Clin 1997;47:154–160.
Leitch AM, Dodd GD, Costanza M, et al: ACS guidelines for the early detection of breast cancer: update 1997. CA Cancer J Clin 1997;47:150–153.
von Eshenbach A, Ho H, Cunningham M, et al: ACS guideline for the early detection of prostate cancer: update 1997. CA Cancer J Clin 1997;47:261–264.

For more information on cancer screening, see
Branch WT Jr, Crouch M: Periodic health exams: what really matters? Patient Care 1998;January 15:21–41.
Office of Disease Prevention, U.S. Department of Health and Human Services: The Clinician's Handbook of Preventive Services. Alexandria, VA, International Medical Publishing, Inc, 1994.
U.S. Preventive Services Task Force: Guide to Clinical Preventive Services: Report of the U.S. Preventive Services Task Force, 2nd ed. Alexandria, VA, International Medical Publishing, Inc, 1996.

8 International Travel Disease Prevention

Robert Tao-Ping Chow

Each year, an estimated 8 million U.S. citizens travel to countries where tropical diseases are endemic. Most of these diseases are preventable through limiting exposure to infectious agents, obtaining appropriate vaccinations, and anticipating potential health hazards. When asked to provide advice to international travelers, physicians should consider both the travel itinerary and the pre-existing medical history of the traveler. Chronic obstructive lung disease, for example, may exacerbate at high altitudes, and achlorhydria increases susceptibility to enteric pathogens. After assessing the traveler's medical condition and the rigors of the proposed itinerary, the physician should provide counsel regarding the following:

1. Vaccinations (required and suggested)
2. Prevention of traveler's diarrhea
3. Malaria prophylaxis, if appropriate
4. Environmental illnesses

Vaccinations

Routine Vaccinations

1. Regardless of their destinations, travelers should be current with routine immunizations. These include the influenza, pneumococcal, measles, mumps, rubella, diphtheria, tetanus, and polio vaccinations. The recommended dosages and schedules appear in Ch. 1 (Immunization Schedules).
2. Tetanus and polio vaccinations warrant further comment. Certain high-risk travelers should receive tetanus booster immunization every 5 years rather than every 10 years because patients with possible tetanus infection require either tetanus immune globulin or booster if they were vaccinated more than 5 years previously. In addition, adult travelers who anticipate being in close contact with citizens of developing countries where polio may be endemic should consider reimmunization against polio. For those who received the primary series during childhood, one dose of the oral (OPV) or inactivated (IPV) polio vaccine conveys immunity. IPV is recommended over OPV because of the rare but real risk of vaccine-related paralytic polio.

3. The dosage schedule of required and recommended vaccines for adult travelers is provided in Table 8–1. Patients may receive multiple immunizations on the same day without apparent loss of efficacy. However, it is recommended that patients receive at most three live vaccines at one sitting, and live vaccines should be given at least 2 weeks before or 6 weeks after hepatitis A immune globulin.

Required Vaccinations

Certain countries may require incoming travelers to provide proof of vaccination against yellow fever, as regulated by the World Health Organization. This vaccine is provided at state-designated vaccination centers and is charted on a valid passport-sized document entitled "International Certificate of Health."

1. Those who travel to equatorial Africa or the jungle regions of South America should receive the yellow fever vaccine, irrespective of whether it is required. The vaccine is effective and confers immunity for 10 years.
2. Cholera vaccination should no longer be required of any traveler, because the cholera vaccine has an estimated efficacy of only about 30 to 50 per cent. However, some countries may require documentation of immunization if the traveler is arriving from a cholera-infected country. The primary cholera series requires two injections given at least 1 week apart. Two oral cholera vaccines against *Vibrio cholerae* O1 have recently become available, but they offer no protection against *V. cholerae* O139. Cholera can be largely prevented by following hygienic precautions regarding proper use of food and water.

Recommended Vaccinations

1. Typhoid fever vaccination should be considered for travelers who will be exposed to potentially contaminated food or drink. Three forms of the vaccine exist: a parenterally administered inactivated form that requires two injections at least 4 weeks apart and has a high incidence of side effects; an oral live, attenuated form taken over 1 week (Ty21a); and an improved inactivated injectable vaccine. The latter two forms appear to confer a longer lasting immunity than the

TABLE 8-1. VACCINE SCHEDULES FOR ADULT TRAVELERS

VACCINE	DOSE	BOOSTERS	COMMENTS
Cholera	0.2 ml ID on days 0 and 7	Every 6 months; give concurrently with yellow fever vaccine or separate by 3 weeks	Rarely indicated; efficacy <30–50 per cent; not recommended unless required by law at destination country
Hepatitis A	1.0 ml IM on day 0 and in 6 months	Every 10 years	Preferred over immune globulin
Hepatitis B	1.0 ml IM on day 0, 1 month, and 6 months	Every 5–7 years as needed based on titers	High prevalence in Asia and sub-Saharan Africa
Immune globulin	0.02 ml/kg (2.0 ml) IM 0.06 ml/kg (5.0 ml) IM	Every 3 months Every 5 months; give with or 2 weeks after live vaccines	Recommended for all travelers visiting developing countries, unless they have had hepatitis A
Japanese encephalitis	1.0 ml SC on days 0, 7, and 30	Every 2 years	Local irritation at injection site and generalized flu-like symptoms occur in 10–20 per cent of patients
Measles-mumps-rubella	0.5 ml IM	Once if no booster given since 1980 and birth date after 1957	Worldwide risk; live vaccine
Meningococcal	0.5 ml SC	Every 3 years; polysaccharide vaccine	Risk in sub-Saharan Africa, the Himalayas, and for travelers to Mecca
Poliovirus, inactivated	0.5 ml SC	In adults (>12 years of age), one booster lasts for life	High risk in Asia and Africa; minimal risk in Americas
Poliovirus, oral/live	Single-dose unit	One adult booster; live vaccine	See above; potential for mutation of live virus to a paralytic strain
Rabies pre-exposure	1.0 ml IM on days 0, 7, and 21 or 28 0.1 ml ID on days 0, 7, and 28	Every 2 years or based on titers; if exposure occurs, two additional doses are needed	For occupational risk or children, especially long-term overseas residents
Tetanus-diphtheria	0.5 ml IM	Every 10 years or at 5 years with exposure	Recommended for all travelers
Typhoid injectable	0.5 ml SC on day 0 and 1 month later	Every 3 years with 0.1 ml ID	High risk for most travelers
Typhoid live/oral Ty21a	One capsule every other day for 4 doses	Every 5 years; live bacteria vaccine	Fewer side effects and better efficacy than injectable
Yellow fever	0.5 ml SC	Every 10 years; live vaccine; give with or 3 weeks apart from cholera vaccine	Required by some countries; risk in sub-Saharan Africa and Amazon basin

Abbreviations: ID, intradermally; IM, intramuscularly; SC, subcutaneously.
Adapted from Mathews DS, Pust RE, Cordes DH: Prevention and treatment of travel-related illness. Am Fam Physician 1991;44: 1343.

original form and have a lower incidence of side effects.

2. Epidemics of meningococcal meningitis have occurred in sub-Saharan Africa and Nepal. Travelers to these areas who anticipate significant contact with the local populace should receive meningococcal vaccine, including all pilgrims on the hajj.

3. Rabies and plague vaccinations are recommended only for travelers who may have contact with potentially rabid animals or with wild rodents or rabbits. Plague occurs during warm, humid weather and is found in rural areas throughout the world. Candidates for vaccination include farm workers, veterinarians, and hunters.

4. Japenese B encephalitis is transmitted by mosquitoes and has caused epidemics in the Far East, especially during the summer months. A killed vaccine should be administered in three injections with at least 1 week between each. The vaccine is available in the United States, but there are significant local and systemic side effects.

5. Hepatitis B vaccination is recommended for travelers who may contact the blood or secretions of infected people. Southeast Asia and sub-Saharan Africa have a high prevalence of hepatitis B.

6. Hepatitis A is prevalent throughout the developing world and is spread through contaminated water or food. Active immunization with the recently developed hepatitis A vaccine (Havrix) is recommended for most travelers to these regions. A 1.0-ml intramuscular dose 2 weeks prior to travel achieves 80 to 90 per cent immunity. A 1.0-ml booster dose in 6 months provides immunity for up to 10 years. Travelers departing in less than 2 weeks can receive both the new vaccine and immune gamma globulin.

Traveler's Diarrhea Prevention

About 25 to 50 per cent of travelers to developing countries contract traveler's diarrhea. Because it is transmitted by way of the fecal-oral route, most cases can be prevented through careful hygienic measures. The clinical syndrome is described in more detail in Ch. 250 (Infectious Diarrhea).

1. Travelers should be counseled to avoid tap water, ice made from tap water, unpeeled fruits, raw vegetables, unpasteurized milk, dairy products, raw meat, and raw seafood. Tap water can be purified by boiling or by using iodine or chlorine additives (available at camping supply stores and pharmacies).

2. Foods should be cooked thoroughly and recently and served steaming hot.

3. Bottled carbonated beverages, canned fruit juices, and beer and wine are usually safe.

4. Pharmacologic prophylaxis against traveler's diarrhea is controversial. Travelers at high risk may benefit from doxycycline, 100 mg once daily; ciprofloxacin (Cipro), 500 mg once daily; trimethoprim-sulfamethoxazole (Bactrim, Septra), one double-strength tablet once a day; or bismuth subsalicylate (Pepto-Bismol), two tablets four times a day. It is generally recommended that antibiotics be reserved for use if diarrhea occurs.

Malaria Prevention

1. Transmitted by the bites of infected female anopheline mosquitoes, malaria is caused by four species of the genus *Plasmodium*. It is endemic to many developing tropical countries, including Central America, South America, sub-Saharan Africa, India, Southeast Asia, and Oceanic Asia. Travelers to these areas should be instructed to use mosquito repellent that contains no more than 35 per cent N,N-diethyl-*m*-toluamide (DEET), daily and liberally; minimize exposed skin surfaces; sleep in screened or netted areas; and be especially vigilant during the evening or nighttime hours, when anopheline mosquitoes usually feed.

2. Pharmacologic prophylaxis is recommended in addition to these preventive measures. For travelers to Central America, the Caribbean, or the Middle East and Egypt, chloroquine (for adults, 300 mg of the base or 500 mg of the phosphate salt) should be taken weekly, starting the week before entering and continuing until 6 weeks after leaving the endemic area. *Plasmodium falciparum* in the remainder of the world has become chloroquine resistant. Adult travelers to those areas should take mefloquine (Lariam), 250 mg, once a week for 4 weeks and every other week thereafter. Mefloquine should be started 1 week before entering and continued for 4 weeks after leaving the endemic area. Travelers who have experienced heavy mosquito exposure should be considered candidates for a 2-week course of primaquine after finishing chloroquine or mefloquine, to prevent relapse caused by the exoerythrocytic hepatic phase of *P. vivax* or *P. ovale*. The clinician should be familiar with the potentially serious side effects and drug interactions of these agents before administration.

3. Multidrug-resistant strains of *P. falciparum* have been documented in eastern Thailand; the traveler to those remote regions should be advised to take doxycycline 100 mg daily. Mefloquine resistance has also been found in West Africa as well, but prophylactic recommendations have yet to be revised to reflect what may be an increasingly prevalent health concern.

4. Physicians with specific questions regarding malaria prophylaxis and other travel-related infections should consult the Centers for Disease Control and Prevention hot line at 1-404-332-4555, or its comprehensive travel information Internet site.

Other Travel-Related Conditions

1. Travelers should be aware of the high prevalence of *sexually transmitted diseases* in developing countries and be counseled to take appropriate preventive measures. These diseases include gonorrhea (especially penicillinase-producing *Neisseria gonorrhoeae*), syphilis, chancroid, granuloma inguinale, and human immunodeficiency virus infection.

2. Sudden disruption of the body's sleep-awake cycle may cause fatigue, insomnia, anorexia, constipation, headache, and mild incoordination. A short-acting benzodiazepine or a feast-fast–feast-fast dietary schedule may alleviate the symptoms of *jet lag*. Although the evidence for melatonin is too limited to recommend its widespread use, many travelers have found it beneficial.

3. Rapid ascent to high altitudes (>10,000 ft) may cause a syndrome of headache, nausea, anorexia, dyspepsia, insomnia, and fatigue. *Acute mountain sickness* (AMS) is usually self-limiting, but rare patients can develop altitude-related pulmonary or cerebral edema. The immediate treatment is descent to a lower altitude, followed by symptomatic supportive care. Those who have previously experienced AMS or anticipate rapid ascents have benefited from

acetazolamide (Diamox), 500 mg two times daily, to be initiated before ascent.

4. Despite the plethora of potential infectious agents, the most common cause of death among international travelers is *trauma*, usually sustained in motor vehicle accidents. Unfamiliar with local road conditions and traffic patterns, travelers must also cope with the unavailability of safety devices, such as seat belts, motorcycle helmets, and traffic signals. Travelers should proceed cautiously and select safe and reliable means of transportation.

Emergency Medical Care

If medical care is needed abroad, the American embassy or consulate can usually provide names of hospitals and physicians. The quality of health care varies in developing countries, and travelers should be cautioned against consenting to blood transfusion, injection with a previously used needle, and placement of an intravenous catheter. Once stabilized, the patient should consider transportation to a modern medical facility or to the United States.

 ## Bibliography

Centers for Disease Control and Prevention: Health Information for International Travel, 1996–1997. Atlanta, Centers for Disease Control and Prevention, 1997. (Published annually).

DuPont HL, Ericsson CD: Prevention and treatment of traveler's diarrhea. N Engl J Med 1993;328:1821–1827.

Rose SR: International Travel Health Guide, 7th ed. Northhampton, MA, Travel Medicine Inc, 1996.

World Health Organization: International Travel and Health Vaccination Requirements and Health Advice 1997. Geneva, World Health Organization, 1997. (Published annually).

Wyler DJ: Malaria chemoprophylaxis for the traveler. N Engl J Med 1993;329:31–37.

The most up-to-date and accessible sources of information on travel medicine appear on the Internet

Centers for Disease Control and Prevention: *www.cdc.gov/travel*

Travel Health on Line: *www.tripprep.com*

World Health Organization: *www.who.ch/programmes/ctd*

9 Pain Management

Pesach Shvartzman

Pain is one of the most common symptoms people complain to the doctor about. It is of critical importance to address pain properly and prevent suffering. The International Association for the Study of Pain defined pain as an unpleasant emotional experience associated with physical damage, or damage perceived so by the brain. It is a complex, multidimensional concept that includes physical, emotional (anger, anxiety, depression), spiritual, and social components.

Pain is a prevalent symptom among cancer patients and in the general population, increasing with age and progression of disease. In all, 70 to 90 per cent of cancer patients will suffer from pain in the latter stages of their disease. Arthritic pains are also common and observed in more than one third of those 65 years of age or older. Often, patients report on more than one source for their pain (80 per cent), and approximately one third report pain in four or more places. Each pain source must be evaluated and diagnosed in order to choose the appropriate approach.

Types of Pain

1. Pain can be characterized as chronic or acute.
   a. Acute pain is often characterized by subjective complaints and by well-observed physical symptoms, which in most cases are a result of an overactive sympathetic system (facial expressions of pain, sweating, palpitations, irritability, anxiety).
   b. In chronic pain, the physical manifestations of pain are not apparent, although it may lead to changes in lifestyle and general functioning and to depression.
2. Pain can be categorized as somatic, visceral, or neuropathic.
   a. *Somatic pain*: the most common pain, caused by the activation of the nociceptive or sensory receptors in the skin or in deeper layers (e.g., bone pain)
   b. *Visceral pain*: Originates from the extension or stretching of the hollow organs in the chest or abdomen. The pain is most often deep and colic-like in nature (e.g., pancreatic, gallbladder, or liver pain).
   c. *Neuropathic pain*: Caused by damage to the peripheral or central nervous system. The pain can be described as paresthesia, electricity, or burning sensation.

History and Clinical Findings

1. Accurate diagnosis is vital because specific conditions will respond to specific strategies. For example, metastasis in the bone may respond to radiation treatment, neuropathic pain may respond to tricyclic antidepressants, and headache caused by intracranial pressure will respond to steroid treatment.
2. Pain is defined by what the patient relates and not what seems or appears to be. Unfortunately, there are no tests that can indicate the severity of the pain. To evaluate the intensity of the pain, the use of a visual analogue scale (VAS) is an acceptable method. The VAS is a scale on which the patient marks the intensity of the pain (0 indicating no pain and 10 the worst possible pain) (Fig. 9–1).
3. There are many situations that influence the sensation of pain: insecurity, fear, loneliness, lack of sleep, boredom, anxiety, and depression.

Evaluation of Pain

Pain evaluation includes

- Detailed history of the pain complaint (since when, where, pain characteristics, severity, factors that increase or relieve the pain)
- Background diseases
- Evaluation of the sociopsychological status
- Detailed physical examination and use of tests as needed

Management

General Principles

The aim of pain treatment is to relieve the patient while maintaining the patient's consciousness level and minimizing the side effects. The essence of the pain approach must be explained to each patient. The treatment of pain includes pharmacologic and nonpharmacologic methods, or a combination of both, while complying with the following general principles:

On a scale of 0 to 10, what is the worst pain you suffered during the last 24 hours?

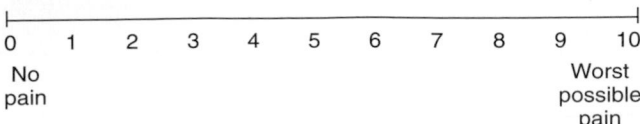

| 0 | 1 | 2 | 3 | 4 | 5 | 6 | 7 | 8 | 9 | 10 |

No pain

Worst possible pain

Figure 9–1 Visual analogue pain scale.

1. Leave the patient and his or her family in control—use oral, transdermal, or rectal medications as much as possible.
2. Use a variety of methods:
   a. Approaches that influence the disease directly: radiation, hormonal treatment, palliative chemotherapy, palliative surgery
   b. Methods that affect the pain: education, mental support, medications, relaxation, neural blocks, transcutaneous electrical nerve stimulation (TENS)
   c. Changes in lifestyle
3. Use the most effective and simple method: minimize medications and dosages as much as possible.
4. Respond to the accompanying complaints of pain and treat them: nausea, vomiting, constipation, hiccups.
5. Avoid the use of placebo.
6. Define the expectations of the patient and his or her family, such as activity without pain, rest without pain.
7. Evaluate the different factors that affect pain: anxiety, depression, relationship with the patient's family and caregivers.

Principles of Pain Management

- Determine the cause.
- Explain symptoms and treatment.
- Treat simply.
- Give medications regularly—around the clock.
- Plan "breakthrough" pain-relieving doses.
- Provide complementary therapy (e.g., massage, physiotherapy, diet, relaxation).
- Provide psychosocial support.
- Review.

Nonpharmacologic

The nonpharmaceutical treatments include radiation (very effective against bone metastases), neural blocks, and alternative methods such as relaxation, physiotherapy, TENS, and acupuncture.

Pharmacologic

1. The main treatment course is pharmacologic treatment: the appropriate analgesic, the pertinent administrative route, the correct dosage, and the appropriate timing must be chosen (Table 9–1).
2. Oral, transdermal, or rectal administration is preferred. If the patient cannot swallow, it is also possible to administer medications subcutaneously or intravenously especially in those cases where there is a coma status, dysphagia, or intractable vomiting. The analgesic treatment must be given *continually* so that the next dose is administered before the effect of the previous dose expires. Some of the patients taking opioids will need "supplements" between regular dosages; these are called *rescue dosages*—between 50 and 100 per cent of the daily dose divided by 6.
3. The analgesic treatment should be given in accord with the three-steps ladder of the World Health Organization. For mild pain, step 1 medications (nonopioid analgesic drugs) are prescribed; for moderate pain, step 2 drugs (weak opioids) are added; and for severe pain, step 3 drugs (strong opioids) are approved. If the pain does not respond to drugs from a certain step, then there is a need to proceed to the next step. At each step on the ladder adjuvant drugs can be added for specific conditions (for treatment of side effects of the analgesic treatment). Studies examining the effectiveness and reliability of the three-step ladder found effectiveness to be 70 to 100 per cent in a total of 2649 patients who were examined and treated.
4. The *mild analgesic drugs* include the weak opioids (codeine, dihydrocodeine, hydrocodone, propoxyphene), nonsteroidal anti-inflammatory drugs, and acetaminophen. With these drugs there is no dependency or addiction development but there is a maximal analgesic dosage (ceiling effect).
5. The *strong analgesic drugs* include the strong opioids. With these drugs there is no ceiling effect, and the correct dosage is the one achieving the best analgesic effect without side effects.
6. Within the opioid products, there are short-term opioids (need to be administered every 4 hours) and long-term products (can be administered every 8, 12, 24, or 72 hours).
7. The most common side effects of opioid treatment include constipation, nausea, vomiting, sleepiness, dizziness, and sweatiness. All pa-

TABLE 9–1. PAIN MEDICATIONS

GENERIC NAME	ROA*	INITIAL DOSE (mg)	USUAL DOSE (mg)	MAXIMUM DOSE (mg)
Nonopioid Analgesics				
Paracetamol/acetaminophen	PO, PR	500	500–1000 q4h	1000 q4h
Acetylsalicylic acid/aspirin	PO	500–650	500–650 q4h	900–1000 q4h
Diclofenac (Voltaren)	PO, PR	25 q8h	50 q6–8h	50 q4h
	SR		100 q24h	100 q12h
Diflunisal (Dolobid)	PO	500	250 q12h	500 q12h
Ibuprofen	PO	400	400–600 q6h	800 q6h
Indomethacin	PO, PR	25	25 q12h–50 q8h	50 q6h
	SR	75	75 q24h	75 q12h
	SR	100	100 q24h	100 q12h
Naproxen	PO, PR	250	250 q8h	500 q8h
Picroxicam (Feldene)	PO	10	10–20 q24h	20 q24h
Nimesulide†	PO	100 q12h	100 q12h	400
Nabumetone (Relafen)	PO	500 q12h	500 q12h	2000
Tramadol (Ultram)	PO	100 q12h		
Dipyron†	PO, PR	500	500 q4h–1000 q6h	1000 q6h
Opioid Analgesics				
Codeine phosphate (methylomorphine)	PO	30	30 q4–6h	60 q4h
Propoxyphene	PO	32.5	50–100 q4h	100 q4h
Oxycodone 5 mg	PO	5 q4h	q4h	None
	SR	5 q12h		
Morphine sulfate	PO, PR	2.5	q4h	None
	SR	10	q12h	None
Morphine HCl	SC, IV	2.5; 5–10	q4h	None
Methadone‡	PO	10		None
Buprenorphine	SL	0.2	0.8 q8h	3–5
Fentanyl	TC	25 μg		None
Adjuvant Drugs				
Dexamethasone	PO, IV		16–96	
Prednisone	PO		40–100	
Carbamazepine	PO	200	200–1600	1600
Phenytoin	PO	200 q24h	300–500 q24h	500 q24h
Amitriptyline	PO	25 q24h	25–150 q24 h	300

*Route of administration: IV, intravenous; PO, oral; PR, rectal; SC, subcutaneous; SL, sublingual; SR, slow release; TC, transcutaneous.

†Not available in the United States.

‡Methadone can be prepared by a pharmacist in different concentrations. Maximal analgesia and side effects are not achieved until 4 to 14 days of use. Methadone should not be used in elderly or demented patients. It should be given every 6 hours for the first 2 days, and then every 8 to 12 hours.

tients who receive opioids are also prescribed on a regular basis a laxative treatment that promotes bowel movement and softening of stools. Because only one third of the patients will develop vomiting, there is no need to prescribe an antiemetic as a precaution/prevention treatment. The vomiting usually subsides after 2 to 3 weeks.

Treatment Steps

In order to maximize the benefit from the treatment, the following steps should be followed:

1. Choose the correct method and dosage.

2. Start with the lowest possible dosage.

3. Tiltrate according to the response and the side effects.

4. Use increased dosage as needed.

5. Use a logical combination.

6. Avoid side effects.

Bibliography

Agency for Health Care Policy and Research: Management of Cancer Pain: Clinical Practice Guideline No 9 (AHCPR Publication no 94-0592). Washington, DC, Agency for Health Care Policy and Research, 1994.

Doyle D, Hanks G, MacDonald N: Oxford Textbook of Palliative Medicine, 2nd ed, pp 299–390. Bath, Oxford University Press, 1998.

Fields HL, Liebeskind JC: Pharmacological Approaches to the Treatment of Chronic Pain. Seattle, IASP Press, 1994.

International Association for the Study of Pain: Rheumatic pain. Newsletter IASP Special Interest Group Rheum Pain 1998;July:1.

World Health Organization: Cancer Pain Relief. Geneva, World Health Organization, 1996.

10 Alternative Medicine

Reid B. Blackwelder

One of the more debated topics in medicine today is variously called alternative, complementary, traditional, and integrative medicine, among others. This particular topic is extremely difficult to define clearly and, therefore, many different healing systems have been classified in different ways. The original definition as proposed by Eisenberg in his landmark article, stated that alternative medicine was what was not routinely taught in U.S. medical schools or regularly available in U.S. hospitals. However, this definition is no longer particularly useful because over 50 per cent of U.S. medical schools now provide some training in alternative medicine; more and more hospitals are broadening their formularies to include botanicals and their treatment options to include massage, aromatherapy, and so on; and insurance companies are even regulating required repayments for alternative treatments.

Many studies are in existence that review why patients might use complementary and alternative medicine. Moreover, many conjectures are being made as to why the prevalence of this use exists. Regardless, anywhere from 30 to 70 per cent of patients are using treatments that have not been prescribed by their physician. In 1997, over $21 billion was spent on alternative treatments, of which over $12 billion was out of pocket and not reimbursed. Although the alternative medicine movement has been thought to be due to a backlash against western allopathic medicine, studies have suggested that many patients who utilize these treatments are not necessarily dissatisfied with their regular medical care. It seems that a large number of patients believe alternative therapies are more congruent with their own philosophical views of health and healing. This is an important concept because it allows easier integration of art and style into patient therapy as opposed to learning a new field.

One of the most important results of the investigations into alternative medicine has been the realization that physicians generally do not allow their patients to tell much of a story. One study documented that physicians take control of an interview within 18 seconds. Moreover, the total time spent with patients has been on the decline as managed care and time pressures have taken precedence. Well over 70 per cent of patients will not discuss their use of alternative treatments with their physician and, in most of these cases, the physician has not asked. It

has been documented that a patient-centered interview that is open ended in nature is beneficial to outcome. More and more medical schools are beginning to stress patient-centered interviewing, in which an open and tolerant style is utilized to explore the patient's perspective in great detail. This includes more awareness of the biopsychosocial-spiritual aspects of the patient's life as a whole rather than viewing the patient as someone carrying a disease into the doctor's office. This change in approach to the medical interview could be considered an aspect of alternative medicine.

The Office of Complementary and Alternative Medicine (OCAM) was established by the National Institutes of Health in 1992. In 1998 it became the National Center for Complementary and Alternative Medicine (NCCAM). This organization is designed to research different alternative techniques and to fund controlled studies in these different areas. The NCCAM has utilized seven broad categories to help categorize all manner of techniques. This is one of the easier ways to approach alternative medicine and is utilized in this chapter. By no means is this brief listing all inclusive; it is merely an introduction to this broad area. The format for description of each category is structured as follows:

 a. Types of practices included
 b. Defining characteristics
 c. Potential for interaction for western physician
 d. Scientific support

Categories of Alternative Medicine

 1. Alternative systems of medical practice
    a. Include traditional Chinese medicine, ayurveda, homeopathy, tribal systems (such as curanderismo and Native American practices).
    b. The interview allows long sessions with patients and often intense interaction with the practitioner one on one. Treatments are often individualized and address many aspects of both patients' health and interaction with disease.
    c. Over 80 per cent of the world uses some form of tribal or traditional medicine. Because this country is made up of people from all over the world, this creates the potential

for interaction in any patient encounter. The most likely systems to be encountered by western physicians include traditional Chinese medicine, or more specifically acupuncture; ayurvedic herbs, available in health food stores; homeopathic general remedies, available similarly; and, depending upon region of practice, some specific tribal practices. Although many different disease processes may be impacted by an alternate system of medical practice, the potential for cross-cultural interaction is probably most important.

d. A great deal of research exists supporting at least aspects of some of these systems, such as acupuncture. Other areas, such as homeopathy, are hotly debated. Regardless, many years of experiential use exist for all these systems.

2. Botanical/herbal medicine/phytopharmaceuticals

   a. Even today, 25 to 50 per cent of the U.S. pharmacopeia is comprised of plants or plant-based products. Many current synthetic products originally began as botanical medicines.

   b. The use of botanicals varies in different parts of the world, and even in different regions of this country. Different systems believe in the use of single herbs versus combinations. The issue of whether dried plant material, fresh teas, capsules, or alcohol-based extractions should be used is beyond the scope of this chapter.

   c. Western physicians are likely to see patients using botanicals. These are some of the more prevalent alternative medicines that are readily available. These are also the most easily assimilated by western physicians because botanicals are often used according to a "prescription" that involves dosing patterns physicians are familiar with.

   d. Examples of some of the more prevalent uses of herbs to treat diseases that are supported by strong research include St. Johns wort for depression, feverfew for migraine headaches, gingko for vascular dementia, and echinacea for immune support and infections.

3. Bioelectromagnetic applications

   a. Various systems are based on the premise that bioelectromagnetic fields influence health.

   b. Bioelectromagnetic methods are already integrated into medical practice in many ways with items such as transcutaneous electrical nerve stimulation units, electrostimulation for bone healing, and various diagnostic testing dependent upon the generation of electromagnetic fields.

   c. As with botanicals, western physicians are likely to see or utilize some of these techniques.

   d. Good studies and experience exist for treating problems such as fractures and muscle spasm. Other areas, such as the use of magnets, await well-designed study support.

4. Mind-body interactions that explore the mind's capacity to affect the body

   a. Include biofeedback, guided imagery, relaxation techniques, meditative techniques, hypnotherapy, and prayer.

   b. Distinguishing characteristics include very individualized treatment approaches, as well as more time spent with the patient.

   c. Western physicians are likely to see or recommend such techniques. Many physicians are trained in some aspects of biofeedback during their medical education. Many individuals, including physicians, have utilized some form of meditation in their personal lives and recommend it to their patients. This can also include such things as yoga breathing exercises and prayer. Hypnotherapy is becoming more and more popular and possible for physicians to train in.

   d. Diseases that would benefit from such approaches include mood disorders such as depression and anxiety, general stress, and chronic illnesses. Supportive studies exist.

5. Manipulative/manual healing

   a. Includes acupressure, osteopathy (although this is considered mainstream medicine now, it is still included in the NCCAM listing), chiropractic, Alexander and Feldenkreis techniques, and healing touch.

   b. These techniques are often utilized by other health professionals, including nurses and physical therapists, often without the order or awareness of physicians.

   c. Because chiropractic is recognized in all 50 states, osteopaths are our peers, and nurses are gaining training in touch therapy, it is highly likely that such therapies are used by patients.

   d. Studies have suggested that movement therapies in particular have been quite beneficial in decreasing symptoms and slowing the progression of osteoarthritis. Moreover, the initial management of acute back pain should be manipulative therapy. Conversely, one study suggested that the human energy field cannot be sensed, although other studies have demonstrated decreased pain in children and increased wound healing by touch therapy.

6. Pharmacologic and biologic treatments

    a. These are treatments that are "silver bullet" approaches not yet accepted by mainstream medicine and include such things as shark cartilage therapy, chelation therapy, and hydrogen peroxide therapy.

    b. Often seem to offer rapid benefits or "cures" to chronic, serious problems.

    c. Western physicians are likely to have patients ask questions about these techniques because clinics utilizing chelation and hydrogen peroxide therapy are becoming very prevalent. Moreover, substances such as shark cartilage and other agents are readily available to patients over the counter.

    d. The scientific basis of many of these products is either unknown or controversial. Some studies may have suggested positive effects on peripheral vascular disease with the use of chelation therapy; however, other studies have not supported these findings. Although shark cartilage may not pan out in formal study, substances isolated during this research may have ultimate utility in treatment of cancers, for example.

7. Diet, nutrition, and lifestyle changes

    a. Include the Ornish lifestyle modification trial, the Gerson diet, macrobiotics, megavitamins, and supplements.

    b. It is ironic and disappointing that this is indeed a recognized area at the NCCAM. This suggests that use of diet, nutrition, and behavioral changes is not fully taught to physicians or incorporated into the care of patients, and is essentially an "alternative" approach.

    c. This is an area that must be addressed by all physicians for every patient. Current medical training is still basically insufficient to obtain the knowledge needed to make some of these recommendations. Even so, more and more information is available to physicians. As noted above, every patient should have these issues addressed in every encounter for any disease.

    d. The scientific basis of such approaches has been well established, particularly with the lifestyle modification trial demonstrating reversal of coronary arthrosclerosis with the combination of intense diet, meditation, and exercise. Moreover, many vitamins and supplements, when used in doses other than RDA recommendations, are useful in treating or preventing illnesses. For example, since folic acid has been noted to prevent neural tube defects it has been added to fortify all cereals.

Using Alternative Techniques in Western Medical Practice

The bottom line in addressing alternative medicine is to recognize that patients utilize these techniques. We should be aware that asking patients what they use for health and to fight disease is critically important in designing individualized treatment plans. The open communication style that involves patient perspective and some patient control over the interview is critical in identifying patient needs, as well as avenues for integrative therapy. Although it may well be impossible for a western physician to be able to learn enough to feel comfortable incorporating many of the techniques described above, the appreciation of the role of diet, nutrition, and lifestyle changes should be one that is addressed.

Information exists in multiple resources to assist in obtaining these important skills. The following list of resources is not exhaustive but reflects some of the availability.

1. Offices and associations

    a. The National Center for Complementary and Alternative Medicine

    b. The American Medical Association and Society of Teachers of Family Medicine special sections on alternative medicine

    c. The American Holistic Medical Association

2. Books in the lay press

    a. Weil A: Health and Healing. Boston, Houghton, Mifflin, 1995

    b. Micozzi MS (ed): Fundamentals of Complementary and Alternative Medicine. New York, Churchill Livingstone, 1996.

    c. Fugh-Berman A: Alternative Medicine: What Works. Tucson, AZ, Odonian Press, 1996. (a comprehensive, easy-to-read review of the scientific evidence, pro and con)

    d. Time-Life: The Medical Advisor: The Complete Guide to Alternative and Conventional Treatments. New York, Time-Life Books, 1996.

3. Magazines, both lay and professional: Many of these are now peer reviewed and can be accessed through Medline.

4. Newsletters, including those put out by Dr. Andrew Weil, and the University of Berkeley Wellness Letter.

5. Regularly updated reviews
   a. *The Review of Natural Products*, published by Facts and Comparisons (1-314-878-2515)
   b. *Quarterly Review of Natural Medicine*, which includes a great deal on nutrition and diet, accessed at 1-206-623-2520.
6. Internet
   a. The NCCAM e-mail address at the National Institutes of Health is nccam/info@altmed.od.nih.gov; their web site is at http://nccam.nih.gov
   b. The alternative medicine home page is located at http://www.pitt.edu/~cbw/altm.html
7. Additional training
   a. A fellowship in integrative medicine exists at the University of Arizona.
   b. Numerous continuing medical education opportunities exist statewide, nationally, and internationally for training in acupuncture, hypnosis, and botanical medicine.

11 Herbal Medicine

Therese Zink

One third of the adult U.S. population are self-medicating with herbs for preventive or therapeutic use, spending several billion dollars annually. Patients perceive that herbal products are safe because they are "natural." This may or may not be true. Herbs contain hundreds of constituents. Some are responsible for adverse effects and others have the potential to interact with pharmaceuticals. Because the United States lacks a regulatory system, these concerns are not addressed. Herbal products are marketed as "foods" or "dietary supplements." They are not regulated under federal drug laws; safety and effectiveness do not need to be demonstrated before they are marketed. There are no legal standards for their processing, harvesting, or packaging, and the possibility of poor quality, adulteration, contamination, and varying strengths must be kept in mind when evaluating them.

Herbs are available in a variety of forms (teas, tinctures, tablets, and bulk), with the standardized extract becoming more prevalent. An herbal extract is considered standardized when a guaranteed level of a certain constituent or group of constituents from the herb is present in the final product. Usually it is expressed as a percentage of the weight of the extract. For example, standardized extracts of St. John's wort use one of the plant's constituents, hypericin, as the reference, and the per cent composition ranges from 0.13 to 0.3.

Table 11–1 summarizes some of the popular herbs that patients are taking, including what is currently known in the literature about their effectiveness, dosage, side effects, toxicities, and possible drug interactions. All doses are adult doses.

Safety

There are many safety issues for herbal products.
1. There have been reports in the literature of herbal remedies containing lead, arsenic, and other heavy metals, as well as pharmaceuticals such as steroids and benzodiazepines.
2. Currently, only substances legally considered drugs must have labeling on the product package that includes approved uses, doses, possible side effects, toxicity, and contraindications. Under current law, herbs are not classified as drugs, so packaging gives little guidance to the consumer. A federal Commission on Dietary Supplement Labels is examining this issue.

3. Postmarketing surveillance for adverse reactions to herbal supplements has been limited. The Commission on Dietary Supplement Labels has recommended that the herb industry and the Food and Drug Administration (FDA) work together to improve the adverse effects tracking system. Physicians are encouraged to report individual cases of potential drug and herb interactions or suspected herb side effects to FDA MED WATCH: 1-800-FDA-1088 or www.fda.gov/medwatch/index.html. Physicians may request reports of adverse reactions to herbs.
4. Herbs can enhance or block the effects of conventional drugs; for example, ginkgo potentiates aspirin, and licorice counteracts antihypertensive medications.

How to Talk With Patients

Talking with patients about their use of herbs does not require new skills. Physicians talk with patients about controversial subjects all the time.
1. After asking about medications being taken, inquire about the use of herbs, vitamins, or other remedies. This discussion also fits into the social history when cigarette, exercise, alcohol, and other health prevention discussion occurs.
2. The information a physician obtains may be vexing. Patients may have made some choices on their own and the physician may be unfamiliar with such remedies. Physicians may want to consider not judging a remedy they are unfamiliar with.
3. Physicians should educate patients about the potential for drug and herbal interactions that are known. Simply telling a patient to stop using a specific product if there is no clear indication of risk can be harmful to the doctor-patient relationship. Continuing the relationship and monitoring the patient's success or failure with an herbal product provides a mutual learning opportunity.

Comments

Patients use alternative modalities for a variety of reasons, often when conventional modalities are not working. In chronic illness there is the possibility that herbs that have been shown to be safe and nontoxic

Text continued on page 55

TABLE 11–1. PHARMACOLOGY OF MEDICINAL HERBS

HERB	USE	DOSE	MECHANISM; PRECAUTIONS; POSSIBLE INTERACTIONS
ALOE *Aloe vera* *Aloe barbadensis*	Two commercial products: gel and latex GEL: used *topically*, promotes wound healing and treatment of burns and frostbite. Used *orally*, a component of the gel or juice, Acemannan, may enhance the immune system. LATEX: used orally as cathartic	*Topical gel:* prn *Oral gel or juice:* dose not well defined *Oral latex:* 0.05–0.2 gm powdered aloe or dry extract	*Topical gel:* Two FDA advisory panels found insufficient evidence to show *A. vera* is useful in the treatment of minor burns and cuts; however, several human trials indicate potential benefit. No side effects reported. Best to use fresh products. *Oral gel or juice:* Not shown to exert any consistent therapeutic benefit. No known side effects. *Oral latex:* Can cause abdominal cramping and diarrhea, resulting in electrolyte imbalance and hypokalemia. May potentiate toxicity of cardiac glycosides and thiazide diuretics. May turn urine red. *A. perryi, A. vera, A. ferox* have FDA approval as natural food flavorings. Oral latex contraindicated in children and pregnancy, causes stimulation of the uterine muscle.
BLACK COHOSH *Cimicifuga racemosa* (NOT Blue cohosh)	PMS, dysmenorrhea, menopausal problems	40–80 mg daily for maximum of 6 mo duration Can take 4 wk for effect	Estrogen-like action is controversial; no effect on LH, FSH, and prolactin. Causes menopausal symptoms to subside. Seems to be safe when hormone replacement therapy is contraindicated. Do not know if cardiac- or bone-protective properties exist. May cause GI disturbances. May potentiate antihypertensive drugs. Be careful about combining with other hormonal therapies. Contraindicated in pregnancy and lactation. BEWARE: blue cohosh is entirely different and more toxic.
DONG QUAI *Angelica sinensis*	Stimulates normal menstrual flow and prevents cramping	Benefit not worth the risk; not recommended	Used successfully in China for centuries, but mixed with other herbs. Scientific evidence in studies of don quai alone is lacking. Essential oil contains safrole, a carcinogen. Causes photodermatitis. Slight laxative effect. Can cause hypertension. Contains coumarins; should not be used in patients on anticoagulants. Contraindicated in pregnancy.
ECHINACEA *Echinacea purpurea* *Echinacea angustifolia*	Immune stimulation	No well-controlled studies define dosing Traditional dosing: maximum daily dose in adults: 6–9 ml of expressed fresh juice, or 1.5–7.5 ml of tincture, or 2–5 gm of dried root	Human and animal studies: Increases phagocytosis, lymphocytic activity, cellular respiration, and activity against tumor cells. No bactericidal and bacteriostatic properties. Limit treatment period to 8 successive weeks. No known side effects, drug interactions, or toxicity. Do not use in patients with AIDS, HIV infection, TB, collagen vascular disease, multiple sclerosis, and autoimmune diseases.
FEVERFEW *Tanacetum parthenium*	Migraine headache prophylaxis ? Antiarthritic	50–200 mg of dried leaves equivalent to 0.2–0.6 mg of parthenolide	Inhibits prostaglandin production and acts as serotonin antagonist. No long-term studies, no documented problems. Stopping abruptly may cause rebound headache. Used OTC in Canada. Caution with anticoagulants. Has short shelf life. Not recommended in pregnancy; induces menstruation.
GARLIC *Allium sativum*	Slows atherosclerosis ? Antihypertensive properties	No well-controlled studies define dosing Traditional dosing: 4 gm of fresh garlic or 1 clove or 8 mg of alliin daily Must either chew or use enteric-coated capsule because alliin/allinase are unstable in gastric acid	Effectiveness in reducing cholesterol is controversial, but a number of double-blind, placebo-controlled, or crossover studies (with design problems) show a reduction in total cholesterol, decrease in LDL and rise in HDL. Studies also show promise for lowering blood pressure. Antimicrobial and anticancer properties under investigation. Increases serum insulin and improves glycogen storage. Because of effect on platelet aggregation, use cautiously with patients on anticoagulants. Concerns of increased bleeding postoperatively. No adverse effects.

(Table continued on following page)

TABLE 11–1. PHARMACOLOGY OF MEDICINAL HERBS (Continued)

Herb	Use	Dose	Mechanism; Precautions; Possible Interactions
GINGER *Zingiber officinale*	Used for treatment of motion sickness and nausea Anti-inflammatory properties for treatment of arthritis	1 gm 30 minutes prior to travel, then 0.5–1 gm q4h (max daily dose 2–4 gm)	Inhibits thromboxane synthetase (platelet aggregation inducer) and is a prostacyclin agonist (inhibitor of platelet aggregation). May result in prolonged bleeding time. Good evidence to support use for motion sickness. Effective for treating morning sickness, but safety is controversial in pregnancy. May be useful in rheumatoid arthritis at 5 gm of fresh ginger, 50 gm of lightly cooked ginger, or 0.1–1 gm of powdered ginger. No reports of toxicity in humans.
GINKGO *Ginkgo biloba*	Mild to moderate cerebral insufficiency Dementia ? Favorable for PMS and vertigo ? Use for antioxidant and lowering cholesterol	120–240 mg daily of standardized extract (standardized to 24 per cent flavone glycosides and 5 per cent terpene lactones), divided in 2–3 doses 120–160 mg daily of standardized extract, as above	Numerous European clinical trials show efficacy for cerebrovascular insufficiency. U.S.-based trial in 1997 corroborates efficacy for mild to moderate dementia (mild Alzheimer's or multi-infarct). European studies suggest improvement of claudication symptoms. Complaints of transient headache, GI upset, skin rash. No known severe side effects. One case report of spontaneous subdural hematoma in a healthy adult. Caution with concurrent use of aspirin and NSAIDs. No known restrictions in pregnancy or breast-feeding.
GINSENG *Panax ginseng* *Panax quinquefolius* (Siberian ginseng is NOT true ginseng)	Increases endurance and stamina, enhances performance Used as an "adaptogen," helps the body adapt to internal and external stressors	Contents of commercial products vary Frequently mislabeled or adulterated Roots must be at least 3 yr old to be effective; 1–2 gm root daily or 100–300 mg of extract (standardized to 7 per cent gingenosides) tid taken for 3–4 wk	Human studies lacking. Nervousness the first few days of intake. Overuse can cause headache, insomnia, palpitations. May cause hypertension. May lower blood cholesterol and improve LDL and HDL ratios. Estrogenic effects may cause vaginal bleeding and breast nodules. Ginseng may affect platelet adhesiveness and blood coagulation. Caution in patients using anticoagulants. Ginseng can cause hypoglycemia; monitor use in diabetics cautiously. Do not use in patients on MAOIs. In Asia used commonly by pregnant women and newborns, but due to lack of clinical trials do not recommend use in pregnancy, lactation, or children.
GOLDEN SEAL *Hydrastis canadensis*	Used to treat mucous membrane infections (mouth, respiratory, GI or GU system) Used to treat inflammation of the gallbladder and to treat metabolic abnormalities in cirrhosis	0.5–1 gm of dried root or 2–4 ml of tincture tid A tea from 6 gm in 240 ml of water is used for mouth sores	Poor studies to assess antiseptic and astringent properties. Often combined with *Echinacea* to stimulate the immune system. Nontoxic at recommended therapeutic doses. High-dose symptoms include nausea, vomiting, diarrhea, and CNS stimulation. Contraindicated in pregnancy because of uterine stimulation activity. Avoid if breast-feeding. Used in attempt to mask positive urine tests for illicit drugs, although it does not. An isolated constituent of golden seal, berberine has been shown to be effective for treating bacterial diarrhea.
GRAPESEED EXTRACT *Vitis vinifera* Also Pinebark extract, which contains the same constituents, trademarked Pycnogenol	Used as an antioxidant to treat hypoxia from atherosclerosis, inflammation, and cardiac or cerebral infarction	75–300 mg daily for 3 wk, then 40–80 mg daily maintenance dose	Potent antioxidants, free-radical scavengers, and inhibitors of lipid peroxidation. Also active inhibitors of collegenase, elastase, etc., which are involved in the degradation of the main structural components of the extravascular matrix, but prevention of connective tissue breakdown is not clinically proven. Small double-blind clinical trials suggest effectiveness for symptoms of chronic venous insufficiency. No adverse reactions reported.

Herb	Uses	Dosage/Recommendation	Comments
HORSECHESTNUT *Aesculus hippocastanum* (buckeye) NOT the same as sweet chestnut (*Castanea sativa*) used for cooking	Used to treat the leg swelling of varicose veins, hemorrhoids, and other venous insufficiencies	High risk/benefit ratio. Not recommended for self-preparation because whole chestnuts are toxic. Distinguish between whole horse chestnut seeds and horse chestnut seed extract; however, Venastat, a commercially prepared seed extract, does NOT include the principal toxin aesculin or esculin and may be safe. 1 capsule bid	Active ingredient in seed extract, aescin, reduces edema by increasing the permeability of capillary membranes. Antioxidant properties. The seed extract with the aesculin/esculin removed appears well tolerated other than reports of GI irritation, nausea, pruritis, and giddiness. Renal and hepatic toxicity and anaphylaxis have been reported rarely with intravenous administration. Eight double-blind, placebo-controlled studies (some with questionable study designs) using a standardized horse chestnut extract with 100 mg/day of aescin suggested good evidence that horse chestnut extract is efficacious in reducing the leg edema and improving typical subjective complaints associated with chronic venous insufficiency. Used extensively in Germany with and without elastic compression stockings.
KAVA KAVA *Piper methysticum*	Relieves anxiety, relaxes muscles, induces sleep, and counteracts fatigue	60–300 mg daily kava pyrones. Do not exceed 3 mo of therapy	Uncertain about use in pregnancy. Naloxone does not block kava, so it works via a nonopiate pathway. Potentiates alcohol and other CNS depressants (benzodiazepines). Six controlled, double-blind studies on patients (some with design problems) suggested good evidence that kava is an alternative to synthetic anxiolytics and tranquilizers. Side effects include GI complaints, allergic skin reactions, eye disturbances, and skin discoloration. Heavy use leads to poor health, including dermopathy and visual effects.
LICORICE *Glycyrrhiza glabra*	Used for stomach ulcers and mouth sores and a variety of other conditions, including cough, skin problems, liver function in patients with hepatitis B, antibacterial and antiviral activity, anti-inflammatory and hormonal effects (weak estrogenic activity)	Potent drug, but can be toxic. Better used in low doses (<10 gm/day) and for less than 6 wk for acute, not chronic conditions	Contraindicated in pregnancy, lactation, and endogenous depression. Primary active ingredient is glycyrrhizin and its derivative, glycyrrhetinic acid, which bind to glucocorticoid and mineralocorticoid receptors. This affects renal cortisol levels, which blocks the renin-aldosterone axis, causing low-renin hypertension. The elevated blood pressure can last up to 4 mo after discontinuing the licorice. Can also cause hyperaldosteronism (sodium retention, potassium loss). At high doses has antiestrogenic activities, causing amenorrhea and hyperprolactemia. Avoid in pregnancy. Interacts with Lasix and potentiates potassium depletion. Potentiates hydrocortisone. Affects insulin activity. Do not combine with laxatives. Increases nitrofurantoin absorption by 50 per cent. Licorice is used to flavor smokeless tobacco, gum, soft drinks, and candy.
MA HUANG *Ephedra*—over 40 species whose contents vary; some contain ephedrine and pseudoephedrine	Respiratory conditions such as asthma. Used for weight loss, but not shown to be effective or safe	Not recommended	Because of deaths in several states, a total ban of ephedrine has been initiated except for sale by pharmacists. Sold OTC for treatment of asthma (Primatene). Promoted for years as a natural herbal stimulant and weight loss remedy. St. John's wort and ephedrine marketed as herbal Phen-Fen. A component of the currently popular Metabolife weight loss remedy. Side effects: insomnia, motor disturbances, high BP, glaucoma, elevated glucose, urinary problems, impaired cerebral circulation. Do not use if diabetic, have benign prostatic hypertrophy, pregnant, or less than 18 years of age.

(Table continued on following page)

TABLE 11–1. PHARMACOLOGY OF MEDICINAL HERBS (Continued)

HERB	USE	DOSE	MECHANISM; PRECAUTIONS; POSSIBLE INTERACTIONS
ST. JOHN'S WORT *Hypericum perforatum*	Mild to moderate depression	300 mg tid for 450 mg bid standardized extract (standardized to 0.13–0.3 per cent hypericin) Maximum in studies 1000 mg daily	Inhibits uptake of neurotransmitters (serotonin, norepinephrine, dopamine) and binds to GABA receptors in vitro. MAOI activity in vitro, not in vivo. No major side effects; minor complaints of dry mouth, dizziness, constipation, and confusion. Photosensitivity with high doses (600 mg tid of 0.24–0.32 per cent hypericin). No known drug interactions, but because of neurotransmitter activity should exercise caution in taking with other antidepressants. Uterotonic in animals in pregnancy.
SAW PALMETTO *Serenoa repens*	Treats urinary difficulties of BPH: frequency, dysuria, nocturia	320 mg daily of standardized lipoidal extract (85–90% fatty acids and sterols) or 1–2 gm of ground, dried fruit daily	Well studied. No known adverse effects. Need long-term effectiveness studies. Action similar to finasteride (Proscar), with similar improvement in urinary symptoms and flow measures, with fewer adverse treatment events and cheaper. Use in combination cautiously. Does not reduce the size of the prostate gland. Acts via antiandrogenic and anti-inflammatory actions. Do not use in pregnancy, lactation, or children.
VALERIAN *Valeriana officinalis* and other species	Restlessness and sleep disturbance	1–3 gm of extract qd–tid and qhs 1–3 ml tincture	Improves latency to sleep, but does not reduce night awakenings. Controversy about use as a short term sleep aid. Takes 2–4 weeks to achieve improvements, including daily mood. Risk of dependence uncertain. No adverse health effects known. Ten controlled clinical trials, with study design issues, suggested efficacy for sleep problems. Animal studies show inhibition of reuptake of GABA. Case report of interaction with alprazolam (Xanax). Avoid concomitant use with benzodiazepines and other sedative-hypnotics. Chronic use can cause headache, excitability, uneasiness, cardiac disturbance. Case report of overdose (20× recommended) with fatigue, abdominal pain, and tremor. Not synergistic with alcohol.

Abbreviations: AIDS, acquired immunodeficiency syndrome; BP, blood pressure; BPH, benign prostatic hypertrophy; CNS, central nervous system; FDA, Food and Drug Administration; FSH, follicle-stimulating hormone; GABA, γ-aminobutyric acid; GT, gastrointestinal; GU, genitourinary; HDL, high-density lipoprotein; HIV, human immunodeficiency virus; LDL, low-density lipoprotein; LH, luteinizing hormone; MAOI, monoamine oxidase inhibitor; NSAIDs, nonsteroidal anti-inflammatory drugs; OTC, over-the-counter; PMS, premenstrual syndrome; TB, tuberculosis.

may enhance the patient's sense of control and self-care.

Herbs are complex. Scientific clarity and sorting through the marketing hype will be a slow and arduous process.

Bibliography

McGuffin M (ed): Botanical Safety Handbook. Boca Raton, FL, American Herbal Products Association, 1997.

Newall CA, Anderson LA, Phillipson JD: Herbal Medicine: A Guide for Health-Care Professionals. London, The Pharmaceutical Press, 1996.

Schulz V, Hansel R, Tyler VE: Rational Phytotherapy: A Physician's Guide To Herbal Medicine, 3rd ed. New York, Springer-Verlag, 1998.

Additional resources

German Commission E Monographs, available from the American Botanical Council, PO Box 144345, Austin, Texas 78714-4345; 1-512-926-4900 or *www.herbalgram.org*

Prescriber's Letter: Therapeutic Uses of Herbs, Parts 1 and 2, 2 booklets on most popular herbs, 1998; 1-209-472-2240, Fax 1-209-472-2249.

The Review of Natural Products, published by Facts and Comparisons (A Wolters Kluwer Company), 111 West Port Plaza, Suite 400, St. Louis, MO 63146-3098; 1-314-216-2100.

12 Common EENT Symptoms

SYMPTOM **RED EYE**   *Michael L. Waters*

Scleral injection, or the "red eye," can be a sign and symptom of a variety of underlying abnormalities of the eye. Infection, allergy, drugs, chemical exposure, trauma, and systemic disease may cause scleral injection as well as many other ocular manifestations.

Differential Diagnosis

1. Conjunctivitis
   a. Bacterial (most common: *Staphylococcus aureus*, pneumococcus, *Haemophilus influenzae*): purulent conjunctival discharge with a gritty foreign body sensation and matting of the lids and lashes
   b. Viral (most common: adenovirus): serous conjunctival discharge with erythematous, edematous eyelids and palpable preauricular lymphadenopathy. Fever and other upper respiratory symptoms may be present.
   c. Allergic: watery conjunctival discharge with pruritus
2. Drug induced (marijuana, alcohol, benzodiazepines): decreased or absent pupillary light reaction, corneal glaze, nystagmus, nonconvergence
3. Chemical exposure: eye pain; burning with lid edema and possible burn of periocular skin
4. Blepharitis: erythematous, edematous lid margins with crusting
5. Subconjunctival hemorrhage: asymptomatic blood underneath conjunctiva
6. Ophthalmia neonatorum/inclusion conjunctivitis: mucopurulent/purulent conjunctival discharge with preauricular adenopathy
7. Corneal abrasion: eye pain, photophobia, and history of injuring eye
8. Corneal foreign body: foreign body sensation with blurred vision
9. Canaliculitis: tearing with tenderness over nasal aspect of lower or upper eyelid
10. Acute angle-closure glaucoma: halos around lights with nausea, vomiting, and frontal headache; increased intraocular pressure (IOP)
11. Scleritis/episcleritis: bluish hue of sclera(e) with severe pain radiating to forehead and/or jaw
12. Anterior uveitis: eye pain, photophobia with diminished vision. Light to uninvolved eye is painful to involved eye.

> Refer to Ch. 15, Glaucoma; Ch. 17, Conjunctivitis; Ch. 18, Corneal Ulceration; Procedure on Corneal Foreign Body Removal (after Ch. 18); Ch. 23, Allergic Rhinitis; Ch. 321, Meningitis; and Ch. 346, Substance Abuse.

History: Key Questions to Ask

When a patient presents complaining of a red eye, a thorough history alone can often lead to the diagnosis.

1. When did the redness appear?
2. Is there pain, burning, visual changes, foreign body sensation, photophobia, discharge, pruritus, excessive or diminished tearing?
3. Are there systemic symptoms such as fever, upper respiratory involvement, nausea, vomiting, joint pain, rash, urethral or vaginal discharge?
4. Was there precipitating injury, drug use, or chemical exposure?
5. Do any family members or contacts have similar symptoms?
6. Have you had any previous eye disease?
7. Do you have any other medical problems?

These questions pertain to the most common etiologies for scleral infection and can help the primary care physician arrive at a differential diagnosis.

Clinical Findings

For any eye complaint, a thorough examination of both eyes should be performed to evaluate

1. Visual acuity: should be tested with glasses or contacts if possible. Also, testing should be performed prior to treatment except in chemical burns, when emergent irrigation is essential.

2. Extraocular eye movements
3. Pupil size/reaction: various street drugs cause concomitant scleral infection and pupillary size/reactivity changes.

In addition to the gross eye examination outlined above, microscopic evaluation with a slit-lamp is sometimes indicated. Chemical burn, corneal abrasion, foreign body, acute angle-closure glaucoma, scleritis, episcleritis, and anterior uveitis are all causes of scleral infection requiring slit-lamp examination for accurate diagnosis and therapy. For this reason, patients in whom these possible diagnoses are considered should be referred for ophthalmologic evaluation after gross eye examination and initial treatment have been instituted.

Management

Conjunctivitis

1. Bacterial
   a. Cultures usually are not required in patients with mild conjunctivitis of suspected bacterial origin. However, culture should be obtained with hyperacute purulent conjunctivitis, chronic/recurrent conjunctivitis, or in patients who do not respond to treatment.
   b. Conjunctiva(e) should be swabbed for Gram's stain, culture, and sensitivity. Topical ciprofloxacin (Cipro), erythromycin, or bacitracin should be instituted for 5 to 7 days.
   c. *Haemophilus influenzae* conjunctivitis should be treated with oral amoxicillin-clavulanate (Augmentin), 20 to 40 mg/kg/day tid, because of occasional concomitant otitis media, pneumonia, or meningitis.
   d. In hyperacute (onset within 12 hours) bacterial conjunctivitis possibly from *Neisseria gonorrhoeae*, single-dose ceftriaxone (Rocephin), 1 gm intramuscularly; oral tetracycline, erythromycin, or doxycycline for 2 to 3 weeks (for associated chlamydia); and topical ciprofloxacin, erythromycin, or bacitracin are all indicated. If corneal involvement is present, ophthalmologic consultation is indicated for hospitalization and intravenous ceftriaxone. The patient needs to be reevaluated every 1 to 2 days until definite improvement is seen and then every 3 to 5 days until completely resolved.
   e. Antibiotic therapy may need to be altered depending on culture results and patient response.
2. Viral
   a. Treatment consists of artificial tears and cool compresses several times per day for 1 to 3 weeks. If itching is severe, use naphazoline-pheniramine (Naphcon-A), levocabastine (Livostin), ketorolac tromethamine (Acular), or diclofenac sodium (Voltaren).
   b. Patients should be advised that symptoms may worsen for the first 4 to 7 days and may not resolve for 3 weeks.
   c. Patients should be educated on contagiousness of conjunctival secretions, which may last 2 weeks after onset. Follow up if symptoms worsen.
3. Allergic
   a. If possible, remove the precipitating allergen.
   b. Artificial tears and cool compresses several times per day are adequate in mild cases. More severe cases may require Naphcon-A, Livostin, Voltaren, Acular, or oral antihistamines.
   c. If patient response is inadequate, ophthalmology referral is indicated for topical steroid therapy. Follow up if symptoms worsen.

Chemical Exposure

1. With any chemical exposure, vigorous irrigation should be instituted immediately. If possible, anesthetize the eye with any topical agent (e.g., proparacaine [Ophthaine]). Evert the upper lid and pull down the lower lid to expose the fornices. Irrigate quickly with 1 L of Ringer's lactate, normal saline, or even unsterile water. Check conjunctival pH by placing litmus paper in inferior cul-de-sac and irrigate until pH is 7.
2. Make sure fornices are clean and then apply a cycloplegic (cyclopentolate 1% [Cyclogyl]), a topical antibiotic ointment (erythromycin or bacitracin), and a pressure patch for 24 hours.
3. Ophthalmologic consultation should be sought to measure IOP and further evaluate.

Blepharitis

Treatment consists of scrubbing the eyelid margins with mild shampoo (e.g., Johnson's Baby Shampoo) twice a day and applying warm compresses several times a day. If severe, apply antibiotic ointment (erythromycin or bacitracin) to the eyelid(s) at night. Oral tetracycline may be necessary as well. Follow up if symptoms worsen.

Subconjunctival Hemorrhage

No treatment is required. If eye irritation is present, artificial tears four times a day is adequate. However, hypertension, bleeding diathesis, and eye trauma must be ruled out. The hemorrhage usually resolves spontaneously within 2 weeks. Return for follow-up if bleeding does not resolve or with recurrence.

Ophthalmia Neonatorum

1. Ocular *Chlamydia trachomatis* in the newborn (ophthalmia neonatorum) manifests in the first 5 to 12 days of life and ophthalmologic consultation is essential. Adult inclusion conjunctivitis typically presents in sexually active individuals 18 to 30 years of age.

2. Initial therapy is based upon results of Gram's and Giemsa stains.

   a. Gram-positive bacteria without suspicion of gonorrhea and no corneal involvement require erythromycin ointment for 2 weeks. Gram-negative bacteria without suspicion of gonorrhea and no corneal involvement require gentamicin ointment for 2 weeks.

   b. If bacteria are present on Gram's stain and the cornea is involved, obtain ophthalmologic consultation for hospitalization and treatment.

   c. If no information can be obtained from Gram's or Giemsa stains, then treat with erythromycin ointment and erythromycin syrup, 50 mg/kg/day in divided doses for 2 to 3 weeks, and modify according to culture results.

   d. If chlamydia is suspected, treat with erythromycin ointment and erythromycin syrup, 50 mg/kg/day for 2 to 3 weeks. If chlamydia is confirmed by immunofluorescent stain or culture, remember to treat mother and sexual partner(s).

   e. If *Neisseria gonorrhoeae* is suspected, then hospitalize for evaluation and possible treatment of disseminated gonococcal infection as well as ophthalmologic consultation.

3. All of the remaining causes of the red eye require ophthalmologic consultation for slit-lamp evaluation.

   a. The size of a corneal abrasion must be measured and its location diagrammed for a baseline necessary in evaluating a therapeutic response. In addition, an anterior-chamber reaction must be ruled out.

   b. A corneal foreign body must be removed under slit-lamp with a foreign body spud or rust-ring drill.

   c. The punctal concretions present in canaliculitis must be removed under slit-lamp and possibly via surgical canaliculotomy for complete success.

   d. Acute angle-closure glaucoma requires continuous IOP monitoring as well as gonioscopy of anterior chamber angles.

   e. Scleritis and episcleritis require slit-lamp examination for diagnosis and may need steroid therapy and/or surgery for resolution.

   f. Anterior uveitis has a multitude of causes; therefore, accurate diagnosis is essential before extensive work-up is indicated.

PEARLS

- Urine drug screening for possible drug-induced (marijuana, alcohol, benzodiazepine) redness. Scleral injection may not detect drugs taken and usually takes 1 to 2 hours to become positive after exposure. However, eye signs are evident within 15 minutes.

- *Neisseria* meningitis is a cause of hyperacute conjunctivitis.

- Ocular epithelial defects take up fluorescein slowly; repeating of dye applications is occasionally necessary.

- A pressure patch is generally not applied when an abrasion is at significant risk of infection.

- Inadequately treated chlamydial conjunctivitis in a neonate can lead to chlamydial pneumonia.

Bibliography

Cullom RD Jr, Chang B: The Wills Eye Manual: Office and Emergency Room Diagnosis and Treatment of Eye Disease, 2nd ed. Philadelphia, JB Lippincott Company, 1994.

Morrow GL, Abbott RL: Conjunctivitis. Am Fam Physician 1998;57:735–746.

Potts AM: Diagnostic eye instruments for the general physician. J Florida Med Assoc 1994;81:234.

Tennant F: The rapid eye test to detect drug abuse. Postgrad Med 1988;84:108–114.

Zimmerman TJ: Topical ophthalmic beta blockers: a comparative review. J Ocular Pharmacol 1993;9:373–384.

Differential Diagnosis

The first step in evaluation of eye pain is to decide whether the pain is coming from the eye itself or is referred from surrounding structures.

Intrinsic Eye Pain

The lid, conjunctiva, cornea, and uveal tract are richly innervated by the ophthalmic nerve. The retina, the vitreous, and the optic nerve, in contrast, are less well innervated and thus seldom are a source of pain.

1. Pain with swelling around the eye
   a. Stye or hordeolum: on lid margin, inflammation of glands of Zeis or Moll
   b. Chalazion: Points away from lid margin; usually chronically inflamed meibomian gland.
   c. Dacryocystitis and dacryoadenitis: inflammation of lacrimal system
   d. Orbital and preseptal cellulitis: May need computerized tomographic scan to differentiate the two; orbital cellulitis requires parenteral antibiotics.
2. Pain with foreign body sensation, usually referred to outer portion of upper eyelid regardless of location of lesion
   a. Conjunctivitis: red eye, bright red vessels located peripherally
   b. Corneal abrasion: ingrown lashes, contact lens overuse, trauma
   c. Corneal ulcer: requires referral
   d. Foreign matter on lid or surface of eye
   e. Ultraviolet overexposure (sun, sun lamp, welding)
   f. Trauma

PEARL

A drop of local anesthetic in the conjunctival sac alleviates the pain from superficial abrasion and foreign body but not that from deeper structures.

---

3. Pain with burning or itching
   a. Conjunctivitis
   b. Allergy
   c. Dry eyes: May be secondary to collagen-vascular disease (sicca syndrome).
   d. Overuse or fatigue: seen in people who work with video display terminals because of infrequent blinking

   e. Chemical injury: history of exposure
4. Deep pain
   a. Anterior uveitis: purplish red vessels around the limbus of the cornea, miotic pupils, blurred vision, cell and flare in anterior chamber with slit-lamp
   b. Glaucoma: purplish red vessels around the limbus of the cornea; midposition fixed pupils; decreased vision; steamy cornea
   c. Scleritis and episcleritis: Scleritis causes more severe pain and may perforate; episcleritis is easily confused with conjunctivitis, but dilated vessels are more purple and do not disappear with topical decongestants.
5. Pain on movement of eyes
   a. Retrobulbar optic neuritis: some loss of central vision; swollen disk; positive swinging-flashlight test (afferent pupillary defect)
   b. Orbital pseudotumor: idiopathic orbital inflammatory syndrome; pain, lid edema, chemosis, proptosis; no fever or leukocytosis
   c. Posterior scleritis: decreased vision, disk edema
   d. Myositis: diplopia
6. Pain with no or subtle signs
   a. Eye strain
   b. Astigmatism
   c. Tonic pupil

Referred Pain

Referred pain can be either from contiguous structures or from structures innervated by the recurrent meningeal branches of the ophthalmic nerve.

1. Headaches: migraine, sinus, cluster, tension; subarachnoid hemorrhage; pseudotumor cerebri
2. Sinusitis
3. Temporal arteritis
4. Pituitary apoplexy
5. Herpes zoster ophthalmicus prodrome or postherpetic neuralgia
6. Trigeminal neuralgia
7. Occipital neuralgia
8. Cavernous sinus thrombosis: idiopathic, inflammatory, tumor; causes cranial nerve palsies and sensory loss in V1 and V2.
9. Orbital tumors: proptosis, decreased vision, diplopia; severe pain suggests cancer.
   a. Lymphoid tumors
   b. Dermoid cysts: Can rupture spontaneously or with trauma and cause intense pain.

c. Metastatic tumors: lung and breast in adults

d. Locally invasive paranasal tumors: nasopharyngeal carcinoma, squamous cell carcinoma of sinuses

10. Dissecting aneurysm of extracranial internal carotid

11. Carotid cavernous fistula

12. Aneurysm of posterior communicating artery

13. Dissection of vertebral artery

14. Stroke: parieto-occipital or thalamic infarct

15. Pontine tumors and other brain stem lesions such as Wallenberg's syndrome and multiple sclerosis

16. Increased intracranial pressure: boring pain worse with Valsalva maneuver, associated vomiting, papilledema

17. Temporomandibular joint pain

Refer to Ch. 15, Glaucoma; Ch. 17, Conjunctivitis; Ch. 18, Corneal Ulceration; Procedure on Corneal Foreign Body Removal (after Ch. 18); Ch. 19, Optic Neuritis; Ch. 23, Allergic Rhinitis; Ch. 25, Sinusitis; Ch. 26, Orbital and Periorbital Cellulitis; Ch. 227, Polymyalgia Rheumatica; Ch. 228, Temporal Arteritis; and procedure on Removal of Ocular Foreign Body following Ch. 18.

History: Key Questions to Ask

1. Quality, timing, progression, onset, and duration of pain?

2. Relieving or exacerbating factors?

3. Associated symptoms, such as nausea or vomiting?

4. Loss of vision, diplopia, photophobia, discharge, history of trauma, exposure to ultraviolet light, possible foreign bodies, use of contact lenses?

5. History of headache, sinus problems, cancer, joint problems, rash?

Clinical Findings

1. Decreased visual acuity

2. Erythema or swelling of eyelids or conjunctiva

3. Extraocular muscle palsy or pain with movement

4. Decreased pupillary response or positive swinging-flashlight test

5. Papilledema on funduscopic examination

6. Steamy cornea or defect in cornea

7. Narrow anterior chamber or cell and flare present on slit-lamp examination

8. Visual field defect

9. Temporal artery tenderness or swelling

10. Sinus tenderness

11. Proptosis

12. Sensory deficits

13. Unequal carotid pulses

PEARLS

Refer to ophthalmologist if any of the following is present:

- Decreased vision

- Trauma

- Corneal ulcer

- Herpes zoster ophthalmicus

- Metallic foreign body with rust ring

- Any condition that requires topical steroid treatment

- Patient not improved with conservative management

Tests

Diagnostic tests should be carried out based on clinical suspicion. Common office tests include the following:

1. Fluorescein dye: to detect corneal defects

2. Tonometry: to measure intraocular pressure

3. Slit-lamp examination: to detect cell and flare in the anterior chamber

4. Computerized tomographic scan and magnetic resonance imaging, if indicated

Management

Depends on specific diagnosis.

 ## Bibliography

Kohrman B, Warfield C: Eye pain: ocular and nonocular causes. Hosp Pract 1987;22:33–50.

Newell FM: Ophthalmology Principles and Concepts, 8th ed. St. Louis, Mosby, 1996.

Rosenblatt M, Sakol P: Ocular and periocular pain. Otolaryngol Clin North Am 1989;22:1173–1203.

Vaughan D, Asbury T, Riordan-Eva P: General Ophthalmology, 15th ed. Stamford, CT, Appleton & Lange, 1998.

The subjective complaints of flashes of light and floaters are usually of different origins. Light perception by the occipital cortex is commonly due to stimulation of the retina and less frequently due to cerebral causes. Photopsia is the subjective sensation of sparks or flashes of light induced by mechanical or electrical retinal stimulation. The visualization of floaters is primarily due to changes in the vitreous and seldom due to foreign bodies in the anterior aspect of the eye.

Differential Diagnosis

Flashes

1. Bilateral photopsia (unformed visual hallucinations) is of cerebral origin.
   a. Static light and stars arise from the occipital cortex and association areas.
   b. Luminous colored flashes and rings arise from the parastriate area 18.
   c. Other cerebral areas may produce formed images.
2. Monocular
   a. Simple traction of the vitreous on the sensory retina (Moore's lighting streak)
   b. Vitreous detachment causing a fluid-filled optically empty space between the vitreous and the retina, seen especially in women ages 55 through 65
   c. Retinal hole, possibly with hemorrhage from a small vessel tear
   d. Detachment of the retina: May be due to diabetic proliferative retinopathy causing surface wrinkling of the retina.
   e. Cataracts
   f. Migraine headache
   g. Epilepsy
   h. Oculodigital phenomenon
   i. Flick phosphene of quick eye motion
   j. Retinal microembolization
   k. Retinitis (e.g., cytomegalovirus infection)
   l. Vertebral basilar insufficiency
   m. Multiple medications, including clomiphene citrate (Clomid) and many antibiotics
   n. Poisonings: mushroom, cannabis, mescaline, mullet fish, gasoline, *Myristica* (nutmeg), ololiuqui (morning glory seed)

Floaters

1. Tear film debris
2. Material in the vitreous: principally remnants of the embryonic hyaloid vascular system (muscae volitantes)

3. Degenerative vitreous changes: syneresis (fluid replacement in part or whole of the vitreous)
   a. Myopic
   b. Aging
   c. Post-traumatic
4. Hemorrhages
   a. Peripheral: floater
   b. Central: red haze and decreased visual acuity
   c. Caused by neovascularization from diabetes, tumor, or inflammation or rupture of a subhyaloid retinal hemorrhage secondary to a subarachnoid hemorrhage (Tenson's)
5. Corneal foreign body
6. Carbon tetrachloride poisoning

Refer to Ch. 174, Diabetes Mellitus, Type I; Ch. 175, Diabetes Mellitus, Type II; Ch. 309, Migraine Headache; and Ch. 310, Seizure Disorder.

History

A rapid onset of flashing lights (especially a shower of them) is more suspicious of retinal detachment. The rapid onset of floating opacities is more indicative of vitreous or retinal hemorrhages and, possibly, formation of a retinal hole.

Key Questions to Ask

1. Unilateral versus bilateral: Do the symptoms change or go away if one or the other eye is closed?
   a. If the symptoms change with closure of one eye, this suggests that the abnormality is relative to one eye only.
   b. If the symptoms do not change with closure of one eye, the problem is central (cerebral) in origin or, less likely, due to bilateral involvement (in this case, it should generally be asymmetric).
2. If lights are reported, are they colored rings or halos, or are they flashes or streaks?
3. Has there been any change in overall visual acuity aside from the lights or floaters?
4. For floaters, does blinking clear or change the appearance of the opacity? If so, the opacity would be in the rear film layer.
5. For floaters, do the dots dart away when the patient tries to fixate on them? If so, this probably represents hyaloid vascular system remnants (muscae volitantes).

6. If diabetes is present, there is increased risk of hemorrhage from proliferative vessels.

Clinical Findings/Tests

1. A dilated examination, including indirect ophthalmoscopy, is required for any sudden onset of flashing lights or floaters to rule out retinal detachment or hemorrhages.
2. The presence of hyaloid artery remnants on the posterior aspect of the lens capsule (Mittendorf's dot) or on the center of the optic nerve head (Bergmeister's papilla) is not symptomatic.
3. Multiple shiny calcium-lipid deposits in the vitreous on ophthalmoscopy (asteroid hyalosis), usually unilaterally, is also a normal variant that does not cause symptoms.
4. The presence of pus in the conjunctiva and tear film or a foreign body in the cornea can be the cause of floating or fixed densities, respectively.
5. The presence of densities seen while focusing through the vitreous during ophthalmoscopy usually is indicative of benign floaters, which may shift out of the visual axis with further degenerative changes within the vitreous.
6. Myopic patients are at increased risk for spontaneous retinal detachment because of increased traction of the attachment points of the vitreous on the retina.

Management

1. For benign floaters, no treatment is necessary or effective. With further changes and shifts in the vitreous, the densities may shift out of the visual axis, although in time they frequently return.
2. Rapid diagnosis of retinal holes or detachments is necessary for stabilization of holes or reattachment of the retina because the sensory retina cannot survive long without its vascular supply. Therapies include scleral buckling, laser therapy, cryotherapy, diathermy, encircling rod, and silicon or air injection into the vitreous.
3. The responsible drug or medication should be withdrawn.
4. For hemorrhages, vitrectomy may be required to clear the visual axis.
5. For diabetic patients, routine screening ophthalmologic examinations and good glycemic control are paramount in minimizing the risk of hemorrhages and detachments.

Bibliography

Fauci A, Braunwald E, Isselbacher KJ, et al (eds): Harrison's Principles of Internal Medicine, 14th ed. New York, McGraw-Hill, 1998.

Newell FW: Ophthalmology Principles and Concepts, 8th ed. St. Louis, Mosby, 1996.

Roy FH: Ocular Differential Diagnosis, 6th ed. Baltimore, Williams & Wilkins, 1996.

Spalton DJ, Hitchings RA, Hunter PA, et al: Atlas of Clinical Ophthalmology, 2nd ed. London, Mosby–Year Book Europe, 1994.

Vaughan D, Asbury T, Riordan-Eva P: General Ophthalmology, 15th ed. Stamford, CT, Appleton & Lange, 1998.

SYMPTOM EARACHE/EAR PAIN

Howard B. Tandeter

Etiology

Earache (otalgia) is a common symptom with many causes. It can be classified as primary or secondary according to the site in which the pain originates. In primary otalgia, the pain results from pathologic conditions of the ear. In referred otalgia, the pain originates in nonotologic structures (adjacent or distal) that share a common nerve supply (cranial nerves V, VII, IX, and X, and the cervical plexus C2 and C3). Acute otitis media is probably the most common cause of otalgia, especially in the pediatric age group. In adults, up to 50 per cent of all complaints of earache are referred, and about half of these may be due to dental pathology.

Differential Diagnosis

Local Causes

1. External ear

a. Pathologies of the auricle
   (1) Perichondritis
   (2) Furunculosis
   (3) Abscess
   (4) Hematoma
   (5) Preauricular cyst or sinus
   (6) Frostbite
   (7) Malignancies
b. Pathologies of the external ear canal
   (1) External otitis
      (a) Bacterial
      (b) Fungal
      (c) Viral
      (d) "Malignant" otitis externa
   (2) Myringitis and myringitis bullosa
   (3) Impacted cerumen
   (4) Foreign bodies

    (5) Eczema of the meatus

    (6) Seborrheic dermatitis

    (7) Trauma

    (8) Necrotizing osteitis

    (9) Neurodermatitis

    (10) Tumors (malignant and benign)

2. Middle ear and mastoid
  a. Acute otitis media
  b. Chronic otitis media
  c. Cholesteatoma
  d. Barotrauma
  e. Acute mastoiditis
  f. Tumors (malignant and benign) of middle ears and mastoid process

Referred Causes

1. Mouth and jaws
  a. Pain originating in teeth (caries, inflamed pulp, exposed dentine, dying nerves, impacted molars and wisdom teeth, traumatic occlusion of teeth, improperly fitting denture)
  b. Glossitis and stomatitis
  c. Aphthous ulcers
  d. Temporomandibular joint (TMJ) dysfunction
  e. Carcinoma of the buccal cavity
  f. Carcinoma of the tongue

2. Pharynx, nose, and sinuses
  a. Tonsillitis
  b. Pharyngitis
  c. Peritonsillar abscess
  d. Retropharyngeal abscess
  e. Postadenoidectomy or tonsillectomy
  f. Elongation of the styloid process
  g. Pharyngeal candidiasis
  h. Nasopharyngeal fibroma
  i. Nasal infections
  j. Malignancies

3. Larynx
  a. Laryngitis
  b. Chondritis/perichondritis
  c. Cricoarytenoid arthritis
  d. Malignancies

4. Esophagus
  a. Hiatus hernia
  b. Esophagitis
  c. Foreign body
  d. Benign tumors
  e. Malignancies

5. Cervical area
  a. Radiculopathy
  b. Osteoarthritis
  c. Spondylosis
  d. Trauma of cervical spine
  e. Tabes dorsalis
  f. Lymphadenitis (postauricular)
  g. Carotidynia

6. Other
  a. Thyroiditis (acute)
  b. Salivary glands (sialoadenitis, mumps)
  c. Neuralgia (glossopharyngeal, trigeminal, sphenopalatine)
  d. Herpes oticus (Ramsay Hunt's syndrome)
  e. Cardiovascular (angina pectoris, thoracic aneurysm)
  f. Lung and bronchial infections
  g. Myofascial pain syndromes

History

1. Duration and onset of pain
  a. Acute
  b. Persistent
  c. Chronic

2. Excessive or unusual crying (children)

3. Accompanying signs and symptoms
  a. Fever
  b. Discharge
  c. Hearing loss
  d. Fullness of ears
  e. Itching

4. When referred pain is suspected: signs of distal pathologies responsible for the pain

Because there are so many different causes of earache, originating from such diverse anatomic sites, there are no key questions that will be able to distinguish between all the causes of this symptom. Physical examination is the tool that will ultimately help us define whether the cause of pain is primary or referred.

Clinical Findings

1. Redness, swelling, tenderness, and fluctuation over the mastoid process (signs of mastoiditis)

2. Macroscopic findings on the auricle
  a. Swollen, red, warm, and tender auricle (perichondritis)
  b. Furuncles, abscesses
  c. Hematomas
  d. Macroscopic malignancies: basal cell carcinoma, squamous cell carcinoma

3. Signs of external auditory canal pathologies
    a. Tenderness on traction of the pinna and on pressure over the tragus: distinguish external otitis from other causes of otalgia
    b. Swollen, red skin of the external auditory canal with moist, purulent debris: sign of external otitis
    c. Foul-smelling, purulent otorrhea and granulation tissue almost occluding the external auditory canal: signs of malignant external otitis
    d. Impacted cerumen
4. Otoscopic signs of middle ear pathologies: Tympanic membrane
    a. Perforation
    b. Retraction
    c. Bulging
    d. Redness
    e. Displacement of light reflex
    f. Vesicles (bullous myringitis)

In patients presenting with earache, physicians should define if the problem is primary or referred. History and physical examination easily diagnose primary causes. If a cause for pain is not found in the ear area, the first sites one should examine for the presence of pathologies are teeth, tonsils, TMJ, tongue, and thyroid. If the cause is not found in these sites, one should perform a thorough investigation based on the knowledge of the causes of this symptom.

Diagnostic Tests
Otoscopy (pneumatic recommended)

Management
1. *External otitis*: solution of neomycin sulfate 0.5%, polymyxin B sulfate 10,000 U/ml, and 1% hydrocortisone (Cortisporin Otic). An analgesic might be necessary for the first 24 to 48 hours. If cellulitis is present and extends beyond the ear canal, systemic antibiotic treatment should be given.
2. *Malignant external otitis*: Control of the diabetes and prolonged IV therapy with an aminoglycoside antibiotic and a semisynthetic penicillin.

3. *Furuncles*: They should be allowed to drain spontaneously, because incision may lead to a spreading perichondritis of the pinna. Analgesics may be used to relieve the pain. In some cases, antibiotics are recommended. Dry heat also helps relieve pain and hastens resolution.
4. *Perichondritis*: Systemic antibiotics are required.
5. *Hematoma*: The clot must be evacuated through an incision.
6. *Bullous myringitis*: Pain may be relieved by rupture of the vesicles with a myringotomy knife. Analgesics are recommended.
7. *Acute otitis media*: Antibiotic therapy is generally indicated for acute otitis media (in the United States) to relieve the symptoms and reduce the chance of complications. Data from the Netherlands suggest that most of the patients with otitis media can be effectively managed without antibiotics (with no differences in outcomes).

PEARLS

Five Ts for Referred Otalgia

- Teeth
- Tonsils
- TMJ
- Tongue
- Thyroiditis

Bibliography

Harvey H: Diagnosing referred otalgia: the ten Ts. Cranio 1992;10:333–334.
Holborow C: Earache. In French H (ed): French's Index of Differential Diagnosis, 12th ed, pp 229–232. Bristol, John Wright & Sons Ltd, 1985.
Paparella MM, Jung TTK: Otalgia. In Paparella MM, Shumrick DA (eds): Otolaryngology, 3rd ed, pp 1237–1242. Philadelphia, WB Saunders Company, 1991.
STAT!-Ref Medical Library [computer software], Windows version. Jackson, WY, Teton Data Systems, 1997.
Yanagisawa K, Kveton JF: Referred otalgia. Am J Otolaryngol 1992;13:323–327.

Unless abnormal, the parotid gland goes unnoticed by patients and is unpalpable by clinicians. From the Greek word meaning "near the ear," the parotid gland is the largest major salivary gland and fills the irregular subcutaneous space between the external auditory canal, the masseter muscle, the zygomatic arch, and the sternocleidomastoid muscle. The parotid gland's contribution of only 25% of all saliva is channeled through Stensen's duct, which forms a punctum adjacent to the second maxillary molar. The facial nerve also is intimately associated with the parotid gland, dividing it into deep and superficial portions. Significant parotid enlargement involving the deep portion can invade the lateral pharyngeal space. The superficial and deep cervical nodes provide lymphatic drainage for the parotid gland.

Because few physicians are called upon to evaluate parotid gland enlargement (PGE) with any frequency, it is challenging to discern true PGE and its etiology. Inherent in this challenge is the fact that development of the parotid gland occurs simultaneously and intimately with that of lymphoid tissue in the same area of the mandible. Generally, the etiology of PGE can be classified as either inflammatory, metabolic/endocrine, or neoplastic, plus some miscellaneous causes.

Differential Diagnosis

1. Inflammatory conditions
   a. Viral infections
      (1) Mumps parotitis
      (2) Epstein-Barr virus
      (3) Cytomegalovirus
      (4) Human immunodeficiency virus (HIV) associated
         (a) Adenovirus
         (b) Malignant salivary gland tumors (lymphoma, Kaposi's sarcoma)
         (c) Diffuse infiltrative lymphocytosis syndrome (DILS)
   b. Benign lymphoepithelial lesion (Mikulicz's disease)
   c. Wegener's granulomatosis
   d. Sarcoidosis
      (1) Uveoparotid fever (Heerfordt's disease)
      (2) Generalized sarcoidosis, including parotid gland
   e. Sjögren's syndrome
   f. Amyloidosis
   g. Granulomatous diseases
      (1) Cat-scratch disease/Parinaud's oculoglandular syndrome
      (2) Syphilis
      (3) Toxoplasmosis
      (4) Actinomycosis
      (5) *Mycobacterium*
   h. Sialadenitis (inflammation of a salivary gland)
      (1) Acute suppurative (bacterial)
      (2) Chronic, nonspecific: painful swelling without exudate; initially nonbacterial
   i. Recurrent parotitis of childhood: usually nonbacterial; some associated with stones
   j. Dental apical abscess

Metabolic/Endocrine Conditions

   a. Alcoholic cirrhosis: parotid gland cellular hypertrophy initially, fatty infiltration late
   b. Cystic fibrosis: usually no significant pathologic affects in or from PGE
   c. Gross obesity: fatty infiltration of parotid gland
   d. Bulimia: protein malnutrition and chronic emesis
   e. Gout (rare)
   f. Toxic exposure: lead, mercury, copper, iodine
   g. Diabetes mellitus: the most common endocrine-associated abnormality
   h. Hypothyroidism (rare)
   i. Cushing's disease (rare)
3. Neoplasm
   a. Benign: 75 to 80 per cent of all parotid tumors
      (1) Pleomorphic adenoma: 60 to 70 per cent of all benign salivary tumors, but no risk factors
      (2) Hemangioma (the most common childhood parotid tumor) and lymphangioma
      (3) Warthin's tumor: adenolymphoma; peak incidence is seventh decade and in males
      (4) Other benign cysts (relatively rare)
         (a) Traumatic
         (b) Congenital: brachial cleft cysts
         (c) Polycystic (dysgenic) disease of parotids: usually females and bilateral
      (5) Lymphoepithelial lesion (rare)
      (6) Oncocytoma (rare)
      (7) Monomorphic adenoma (very rare)
   b. Primary, low-grade malignant (in order of occurrence in adults)

    (1) Mucoepidermoid carcinoma: in children, a relatively frequent parotid malignancy

    (2) Acinar cell carcinoma

    (3) Malignant oncocytoma

  c. Primary, high-grade malignant (in order of occurrence in adults)

    (1) Mucoepidermoid carcinoma

    (2) Adenoid cystic carcinoma

    (3) Adenocarcinoma

    (4) Carcinoma ex pleomorphic adenoma

    (5) Malignant mixed tumor

  d. Metastatic tumor: squamous cell carcinoma, malignant melanoma

4. Miscellaneous

  a. Medications: amitriptyline, clonidine, clozapine, contrast media (iodine), cyclobenzapine, cytarabine, doxycycline, guanethidine, insulin, interferon-α, isoproterenol, methimazole, methyldopa, mirtazapine, nicardipine, nitrofurantoin, phenylbutazone, procyclidine, ritodrine, saquinivar, sulfisoxazole, terbinafine, thioridazine, trimipramine, vinblastine, vincristine

  b. Mechanical

    (1) Sialolithiasis: Only 10 per cent of stones occur in parotid gland or Stensen's duct

    (2) Ductal stricture: caused by punctum trauma

    (3) Pneumoparotitis/oropharyngeal manipulation: with endoscopy or during inhalational anesthesia

  c. Food allergies: strawberries, seafood

  d. Radiation sialadenitis

Unique among the salivary glands, the parotid contains lymphoid tissue within its capsule, making it vulnerable to a variety of inflammatory conditions and neoplastic tumors. PGE in children is most commonly due to either viral parotitis or vascular neoplasm. Because of the mumps vaccine, nonparamyxovirus viral agents (coxsackievirus A, parainfluenza, influenza, echovirus) are the most common cause of individual attacks of parotitis in children and cause a similar clinical picture. Headache, fever, and malaise often precede the unilateral parotid swelling by 2 to 3 days, which becomes bilateral in about 70 per cent of cases. PGE is also usually bilateral (at least eventually) in patients with associated HIV, bulimia, various medications, food allergies, sarcoid, Sjögren's syndrome, and non-Hodgkin's lymphoma. Sialolithiasis, most neoplasms (except Warthin's tumor), parotid gland–associated cat-scratch disease, and tuberculosis usually cause unilateral enlargement. Suppurative parotitis is often seen in debilitated patients with poor oral hygiene, the elderly with dehydration, and patients undergoing courses of chemotherapy or radiation therapy. *Staphylococcus aureus* predominates all cases of suppurative parotitis, but *Streptococcus pneumoniae*, *Haemophilus influenzae*, enteric gram-negative bacilli, and some anaerobes are also possible pathogens.

> **Note**
> Malignancy must be ruled out in any slow-growing, unilateral parotid mass.

Finding a benign lymphoepithelial lesion (Mikulicz's disease) should prompt a search for Sjögren's syndrome and lymphoma. Salivary gland enlargement occurs in 50 per cent of patients with Sjögren's syndrome. PGE in Sjögren's syndrome is usually bilateral, pain-free, firm, and perhaps episodic. Lymphoma should be suspected with asymmetric PGE in Sjögren's syndrome. Pleomorphic adenomas are painless, slow-growing, well-circumscribed, firm, mobile masses usually in the posteroinferior parotid area. Firm, unilateral PGE with fixation, ipsilateral facial nerve dysfunction and/or cervical lymphadenopathy, or trismus is very suspicious for malignancy. Metastatic disease to the parotid gland is very rare.

> Refer to Ch. 16, Sjögren's Syndrome.

History

1. PGE

  a. Duration, rate and symmetry of growth: Rapid suggests inflammatory cause; slow, unilateral suggests neoplasm.

  b. Size variation: Associated with eating?

  c. Unilateral (most common) versus bilateral

  d. Diffuse (most common) versus nodular (suggests neoplasm)

2. Pain associated with eating: If so, how soon afterward; rapid onset suggests sialothiasis.

3. Pet exposure (cats)

4. Recent or concurrent acute illness? If so, what symptoms?

5. Other concurrent symptoms: xerostomia, xerophthalmia, arthritis, constitutional symptoms (weight change, fever, chills), diarrhea, vomiting, bruxism, ipsilateral toothache or gum swelling, ipsilateral facial weakness or numbness

6. Co-morbid medical conditions: autoimmune disease, tuberculosis or other granulomatous disease, HIV-positive or high risk, hypothyroidism, Cushing's disease, diabetes, food allergies/sensitivities, toxic exposure (lead, copper, mer-

cury, iodine), alcohol intake, pancreatitis, gout, malignancy, immunosuppressed (chemical or radiotherapy), ipsilateral scalp infections or skin cancers.

Clinical Findings
1. Parotid gland
   a. Unilateral versus bilateral PGE: Is enlargement truly in parotid gland?
   b. Gland consistency: nodular, compressible
   c. Tenderness?
   d. Fixed (very suspicious for malignancy) or mobile?
   e. Well circumscribed?
2. Skin: induration, ulceration, erythema, abnormal warmth, sinus or fistula tract? (infection)
3. Stensen's duct appearance
   a. Inflamed, erythematous: infection, dental-related trauma, stone
   b. Spontaneous saliva/expressible saliva
      (1) Volume
      (2) Appearance: purulent or clear
   c. Palpable stone or mass
4. Trismus
5. Facial nerve abnormality: weakness of facial muscles, decreased sensation
6. Cervical ipsilateral lymphadenopathy: suggests malignancy
7. Bimanual oral examination; head/neck examination and pertinent other systems: rheumatic/lymphatic/ophthalmic

> **Note**
> Facial nerve dysfunction associated with ipsilateral parotid swelling is highly suspicious for malignant neoplasm of the parotid gland.

Tests
1. Complete blood count with differential: if infection suspected
2. Serum amylase: if acute pancreatitis suspected
3. Blood glucose: if diabetes mellitus suspected or glycosylated hemoglobin to monitor control
4. Uric acid: if gout suspected
5. Microscopic studies of parotid saliva from Stensen's duct
   a. Eosinophils: allergy related
   b. Uric acid crystals: gout
   c. White blood cell count, Gram's stain, culture/sensitivity
6. Serum toxin levels: lead, mercury, iron
7. HIV antibody test

8. Pregnancy test: if bilateral, cystic, and persistent PGE
9. Fine-needle aspiration: usually only used in pre-excisional diagnosis and treatment planning
10. Ultrasound and sialography are usually inferior to computerized tomography (CT) and magnetic resonance imaging (MRI), except
    a. Doppler duplex scanning for children with suspected vascular tumors
    b. Sialography may be diagnostic/therapeutic in chronic parotitis.
11. CT scan: Usually discerns tumor from non-neoplastic lesion.
12. MRI: most definitive diagnostically, especially if neoplasm suspected

> **Note**
> When cervical lymphadenopathy and multicystic parotid enlargement are found on CT scan, HIV must be ruled out.

Management
1. In any suspected neoplasm, get definitive imaging study (CT or MRI scan) and head/neck or ear-nose-throat (ENT) surgical consult.
2. Most non-HIV viral conditions are usually self-limiting, requiring only supportive care.
3. Treatment of chronic sialadenitis is frustrating, but local heat, sialagogues, and antibiotics (if suppurative) may help. Strongly consider ENT referral.
4. Acute suppurative sialadenitis is usually treated with antistaphylococcal antibiotics, initially intravenously in systemically ill patients. Adequate hydration, local intermittent heat, gentle parotid gland massage, and sialagogues (lemon juice and candies) are useful adjunct therapies. Surgical drainage is rarely needed. However, poor response to usual measures warrants CT scanning for abscess formation.
5. Sialolithiasis usually requires gentle probing of the punctum or ENT referral and lithotripsy.
6. In most other secondary PGE (diabetes, granulomatous disease, HIV), treatment centers around the primary diagnosis and local, symptomatic measures for the PGE.

> **Note**
> Suppurative parotitis requires β-lactamase–resistant antibiotics, such as nafcillin (Nafcil, Unipen) or ampicillin-sulbactam (Unasyn).

Follow-Up

With rare exception, parotid tumors should never be merely followed clinically.

Bibliography

Carroll WR, Wolf GT: Salivary glands. In Ballenger JJ, Snow JB Jr (eds): Otorhinolaryngology: Head and Neck Surgery, 15th ed, pp 390–400. Baltimore, Williams & Wilkins, 1996.

Krause GE, Meyers AD: Management of parotid swelling. Compr Ther 1996;22:256–261.

Manifold DK, Thomas JM: Examination and differential diagnosis of parotid swellings. Br J Hosp Med 1993; 50:60–65.

Seibert RW: Disease of the salivary glands. In Bluestone CD, Stool SE, Kenna MA (eds): Pediatric Otolaryngology, 3rd ed, vol 2, pp 1093–1107. Philadelphia, WB Saunders Company, 1996.

Wolf JS, Goldberg AN, Bigelow DC: Pleomorphic adenoma of the parotid. Am Fam Physician 1997;56:185–192.

SYMPTOM IMPAIRED HEARING

Kenneth A. Weller

Hearing loss is a common problem that affects about 10 per cent of the population and as many as 35 per cent of people over age 65. The prevalence increases significantly with age. Subtle hearing loss may be unrecognized, but, with proper diagnosis, patients may benefit substantially. Impaired hearing should be classified as either a conductive hearing loss (usually implying a reversible cause) or a sensorineural hearing loss.

Differential Diagnosis

1. Conductive hearing loss
   a. Otitis media with effusion: common cause of acquired hearing loss, especially in children
   b. Impacted cerumen (or foreign body): common cause in all ages
   c. Chronic or serous otitis media: Typically causes immobility of the tympanic membrane.
   d. External otitis: Inflammation and exudate in the external auditory canal can lead to temporary loss of air conduction.
   e. Perforation of tympanic membrane: Prevents normal sound translation to mechanical impulses.
   f. Otosclerosis: Produces fixation of the stapes over the oval window, preventing transmission of sound to the inner ear. This finding is present at autopsy in 1 out of every 10 adults but clinically significant in only 1 out of 100.
   g. Exostoses: bony outgrowths in the external auditory canal; may be associated with repetitive exposure to cold water, such as with ocean swimming; needs correction (surgical) only if the condition produces significant narrowing of the canal.
   h. Developmental defects: canal atresia (such as Treacher Collins syndrome) and malformation of the ossicles. These defects may or may not be present with abnormalities of the pinna.
   i. Glomus tumors: rare, benign, highly vascular tumors that produce a middle ear mass effect, leading to hearing loss
2. Sensorineural hearing loss
   a. Presbycusis: most common cause of hearing loss; also called age-related hearing loss; multifactorial etiology; produces a typical high-frequency loss that is bilaterally symmetric and irreversible.
   b. Noise induced: produced by chronic exposure to high levels of sound, usually at a specific frequency (typically around 4000 Hz); irreversible cause of hearing loss but preventable with the use of earplugs or other protective devices
   c. Drug induced: most common ototoxic drugs —aminoglycosides, quinidine, furosemide, and salicylates. Salicylate toxicity is reversible.
   d. Ménière's disease: causes fluctuating hearing loss (usually unilateral) associated with vertigo and tinnitus. Hearing loss begins as a low-frequency loss and commonly develops after the vertigo and tinnitus.
   e. Acoustic neuroma: rare but important tumor of cranial nerve VIII that causes unilateral constant or progressive hearing loss, possibly associated with headache; requires surgical removal.
   f. Congenital sensorineural loss: May occur from hereditary defects (e.g., Waardenburg's syndrome), prenatal maternal infections (e.g., rubella, syphilis), or perinatal causes (e.g., erythroblastosis fetalis, anoxia)
   g. Acquired infections: syphilis or viral illnesses

History

1. Hearing loss: Some patients present with a complaint of impaired hearing. Others are unaware

of a problem, although those close to the patient (family members or coworkers) may have noticed it and raise their concern with the physician or to the patient.

2. Associated symptoms

  a. Tinnitus, earache, or vertigo may be present.

  b. Impaired ability to hear normal conversation

    (1) Sensorineural loss: Patients may say that they think they hear fine, but they have difficulty understanding speech (or state that other people do not speak clearly). Noisy environments make hearing more difficult.

    (2) Conductive loss: Patients complain of muffled hearing and may actually hear better than expected in a noisy room.

3. Developmental history: especially important for children. Speech development, perinatal infections or problems, and school difficulties are important.

Clinical Findings

1. Ear

  a. External auditory canal: look for obstruction, deformities, trauma

  b. Tympanic membrane: intact, retracted, middle ear fluid?

2. Cranial nerves

3. Office testing

  a. Weber's test: vibrating 512-Hz (or higher) tuning fork placed in midline of the skull. Normally, the sound should be equal in both ears.

    (1) Sensorineural loss: louder in the *unaffected* (or less affected) ear

    (2) Conductive loss: louder in the *affected* ear

  b. Rinne's test: vibrating tuning fork placed on the mastoid process. When the sound dies away, the fork is promptly placed (without restriking it) over the external auditory meatus. Normally, by way of air conduction, the sound can be heard for twice as long as in bone conduction.

    (1) Sensorineural loss: Ratio of air conduction to bone conduction remains normal (2 to 1).

    (2) Conductive loss: Ratio becomes closer to 1 to 1, or even reversed.

  c. Schwabach's test: Bone conduction of the patient (using a vibrating tuning fork over the mastoid process) is compared with that of the examiner.

    (1) Sensorineural loss: Patient's bone conduction is present for a *shorter* time than the examiner's.

    (2) Conductive loss: Patient's bone conduction is present for a *longer* time than the examiner's.

  d. Whispering: qualitative attempt to test impaired hearing. A whisper heard from about 2 ft away is a good screen for intact hearing. Patients with a sensorineural loss have great difficulty hearing a whisper because of the high-frequency loss.

Tests

1. Office screening audiometry: Sound-generating otoscopes are available and produce sounds at 20, 25, and/or 40 decibels at frequencies of 500, 1000, 2000, and 4000 Hz. This test helps to screen for hearing loss or determine if impaired hearing is present. A loss greater than 20 decibels is considered significant.

2. Audiometry: This is the best test for determining the extent and nature of a hearing loss. It is available for all ages, but is most useful when used with older children and adults. It can be performed in hospital speech and hearing departments as well as in physicians' offices.

3. Brain stem auditory evoked response: This study is used to detect sensorineural loss caused by retrocochlear pathology (e.g., acoustic neuroma). It is also used for neonatal screening.

4. Computerized tomographic scans and magnetic resonance imaging help to detect tumors, such as acoustic neuroma and glomus tumor, and traumatic injuries.

Management

1. Sensorineural loss: Most types of sensorineural loss are not correctable, but some steps can be taken to improve hearing and avoid further damage.

  a. Noise induced: Avoid occupational exposure and wear earplugs or other protective equipment around noisy machinery.

  b. Loss secondary to medication: Stop all ototoxic drugs.

  c. Acoustic neuroma: surgical removal of the tumor

2. Conductive loss: Treatment of the underlying disorder (e.g., removal of cerumen or foreign bodies, treatment of otitis media or externa, surgery for otosclerosis or tympanic membrane perforation) usually results in resolution of the hearing loss.

3. Hearing aids: These devices are useful for patients with irreversible sensorineural loss or with conductive loss when surgical correction is not chosen. Patients with a flat threshold and good speech discrimination usually respond most favorably to hearing amplification, although almost all patients benefit to some degree.

PEARLS

- Determine whether loss is conductive or sensorineural.

- Use audiometry to test hearing.

- Treat if cause is reversible.

- Prescribe a hearing aid if indicated (and loss is irreversible).

Bibliography

For overview of impaired hearing, see
Brechtelsbauer DA: Adult hearing loss. Prim Care 1990; 17:249–265.

For more information on impaired hearing, see
Hughes GB, Nodar RH, Kay PP: Clinical evaluation of hearing loss. In Hughes GB (ed): Textbook of Clinical Otology, pp 91–96. New York, Thieme-Stratton, 1985.

For more information on detailed differential diagnosis, see
Nadol JB Jr: Hearing loss. N Engl J Med 1993;329: 1092–1102.

For more information on pediatric hearing problems, see
Rapin I: Hearing disorders. Pediatr Rev 1993;14:43–49.

Removal of impacted cerumen and foreign bodies is common at primary care and otolaryngology/audiology offices. Approximately 150,000 ears are irrigated each week in the United States, yet this is still an underutilized intervention. Although a minor procedure, severe otologic injury (with subsequent litigation) is possible.

Indications

1. Local discomfort or pain from impaction of cerumen
2. Foreign body
3. Otitis externa associated with cerumen/foreign body
4. Hearing impairment from obstruction or poor transmission of sound as a result of cerumen behind a hearing aid
5. Removal of otitis externa debris to allow wick application of antimicrobic/anti-inflammatory agent
6. Packed scaly desquamation accompanying seborrheic dermatitis or psoriasis
7. Cleansing of post-traumatic debris/blood/clots in the ear canal after thorough evaluation reveals no ongoing bony or tympanic trauma
8. Tinnitus or equilibrium disorders potentially associated with impaction/foreign body
9. Inability to visualize the tympanic membrane

The elderly, hearing aid users, cotton-tipped applicator users, and those who are institutionalized (particularly in a nursing home), mentally and physically disabled, or in custodial care are at the highest risk of impaction; *screening* them regularly is a sensible approach. Hearing loss in mentally disabled individuals can make them become withdrawn, depressed, and socially isolated and generate other behavioral problems; hence, evaluation of the ear canal is indicated in such patients showing these changes.

Contraindications

1. Tympanic membrane perforation
2. Severe ear canal and/or temporal bone trauma with neurosensory loss
3. Irregular, sharp foreign body or very hard wax
4. Protracted unsuccessful efforts
5. Inability to fully immobilize the patient
6. Mimics: cholesteatoma, exostosis of the ear canal, tumors (polyps, chondroma, basal and squamous cell carcinoma, melanoma)

Preparation

1. Obtain informed consent from all patients, emphasizing the risk of perforation, middle and inner ear trauma, and ear canal trauma.
2. Alert the patient about
   a. The possibility of dizziness or vertigo with the irrigation
   b. The bubbling sound and mild heat of peroxide in the canal, which could be distressing
   c. The sensation of the irrigating solution against the canal and the loosening of a bolus of cerumen may produce a small amount of discomfort.
3. Discuss the need to remain still. Ask the patient to tell you if pain occurs at any time.
4. Thorough history is essential to assess the possibility of trauma, perforated tympanic membrane, or tumor cholesteatoma, which would be contraindications to irrigation.
5. Perform careful otoscopy to assess pathologic variations that may appear to be cerumen or foreign bodies and to examine the shape and situation of the cerumen.
6. If removal is not urgent (and it seldom if ever is), the physician can have the patient instill 3 to 6 drops of a softening agent in the affected ear canal(s) for 2 to 5 days before attempting removal. If this is not possible, applying the agent 30 to 45 minutes before the procedure, or at least filling one ear while working on the other, will prove very helpful. If the wax is very hard and dry, this is mandatory to prevent the cutting effect of the borders of the wax on the canal. Several substances have been recommended:
   a. A 10% solution of sodium bicarbonate—approximately 1 teaspoon of baking soda in one quart of water (this has the best wax-dissolving characteristics)
   b. A 50% solution of water and peroxide or plain 3% peroxide (may heat up the canal temporarily)
   c. Liquid docusate sodium (Colace), a detergent
   d. Mineral oil, virgin olive oil, or maize oil
   e. "Baby oil"
   f. Cerumenolytics such as Cerumenex (triethanolamine polypeptide oleate-condensate 10%, which can occasionally be irritating and is sold by prescription only), Debrox, Bausch&Lomb, Auro Ear Drops, Audiolo-

gist's Choice, Murine Ear Drops (carbamide peroxide 65% and glycerine)

g. White vinegar (diluted solution of acetic acid) or commercially available diluted solutions of acetic acid with or without low-potency corticosteroids, such as VôSol or VôSol HC (acetic acid 2% in propylene glycol diacetate 3%, benzethonium chloride 0.22%, and sodium acetate 0.015%), Otic Domeboro HC (acetic acid 2% in modified Burow's solution–water, aluminum acetate, and sodium acetate, with boric acid as stabilizer), if there is evidence of otitis externa and/or inflammation (they may dry up wax in other instances)

h. If infection is present, Cortisporin TC (colistin sulfate, neomycin sulfate, thonzonium bromide, and hydrocortisone acetate), Cipro HC (ciprofloxacin, hydrocortisone), Floxin Otic (ofloxacin), or Cortane-B Otic may be used for 7 days or longer, sometimes averting the need for other removal procedures altogether. The products containing hydrocortisone are preferred if inflammation is significant.

Positioning the Patient

1. Have a good light source, such as
   a. Lamp (may generate too much heat)
   b. "Otolaryngologist's" head mirror and lamp
   c. "Surgical" headlamp
   d. Glasses-mounted lamp
2. It is preferred to have the patient sitting at a slightly lower level than the sitting examiner. In most examination rooms, a standing practitioner can work on a patient seated on the examination table with the back in the upright position.
   a. Prior sedation is seldom necessary in adults but is warranted in small children and the mentally disabled. Chloral hydrate at adequate doses could help.
   b. Restraining small children with a Papoose-type board and having an assistant or parent immobilize the head is important to prevent injury (children are hence treated in the dorsal decubitus position).

Equipment

All methods require a good lighting source and a halogen-light magnifying operating otoscope. Commonly, but not always, direct instrumental removal of some or (rarely) all of the cerumen is necessary.

1. Irrigation: All irrigation methods require the use of a Goldnamer ear basin or a kidney-shaped emesis basin and tap water warmed to 37° C in a clean container. A plastic drape and/or towels are needed to protect the neck and shoulder of the patient.
   a. Chrome-plated tapered (preferred) or short bulbous Reiner-Alexander ear irrigation syringe with or without shield. It comes in 100-, 150-, and 200-ml sizes.
   b. Luer Lock–type 20- to 50-ml syringe with a C-loop irrigation set or butterfly tubing with the needle and butterfly removed.
   c. The Water Pik *with* the Hydro Med Ear Irrigator Tip uses lower pressure settings, making it safe and expeditious. (The Water Pik Oral Jet irrigator with a *dental* tip is *NOT* recommended because it causes significant trauma to the stapes and cochlea; the manufacturer does not endorse its use for ear lavage.)

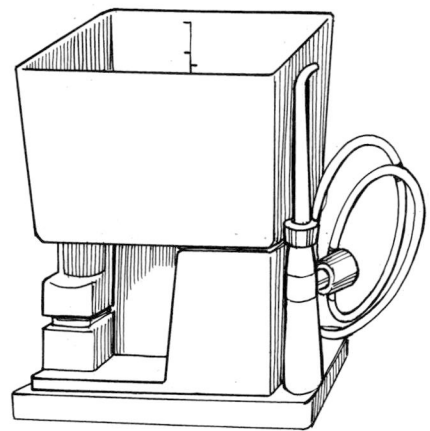

   d. The DeVilbiss Model 177 ear irrigator with 7-ounce bottle requires a pressure generator and connectors.
   e. The Elephant Ear Washer is a very inexpensive, simple, ingenious, and easy-to-use device with a shorter track record.
2. Mechanical removal
   a. Suction
      (1) A small 60-cycle suction machine, as used for endoscopic procedures
      (2) C-loop angulated suction tip catheter set (Coleman, Frazier or Baron), sizes 3 and 5 French
      (3) Magnifying glasses (either operative-telescopic or visor type) are extremely helpful in many instances.
   b. Direct instrumental removal
      (1) Otoscope, Hartman (round) or Farrior (oval) ear speculum, and light source
      (2) Multiple sizes of flexible Billeau wire ear loops

(3) Multiple sizes of Buck, Yankauer, or Shapleigh (preferred because they are less sharp) rigid metallic ear curettes or plastic ear curettes (Flex-loop or Infant Ear Scoop)

(4) Noyes alligator 4- or 5⅛-inch serrated jaw ear forceps

(5) Alternatively, Hartman or Littauer forceps or bayonet-type ear forceps such as Wilde, Blake, Lucae, or Jansen (Gruenwald)

3. Ear candles: This age-old method has somehow regained popularity in the United States over the last few years. Patients should be admonished to avoid it because it has been meticulously studied and found to be totally ineffective (many times worsening the problem significantly by depositing bee's wax in the innermost canal) and potentially very dangerous.

Anesthesia

Sedation of the noncooperative small child or confused mentally disabled adult is recommended. Anesthesia is only necessary in extreme cases.

Technique

1. Irrigation
   a. Fill the irrigator with 37° C water.
   b. With the patient in the recommended position and safely immobilized and draped, direct the tip of the selected irrigator to the most superior gap between the wax plug and the wall, making sure that the stream is aimed at the wall-plug interface itself and not directly at the tympanum.

   c. The pinna can be pulled laterally, posteriorly, and superiorly in adults to make the canal wider and straighter, facilitating the process.
   d. Be sure that the tip does not fully block the ear canal at any time, because it may generate very high pressures and damage the canal and/or perforate the tympanic membrane.
   e. If the plug is totally obstructive, direct the tip to the margin between the superior or posterosuperior aspect of the debris and the wall of the ear canal.

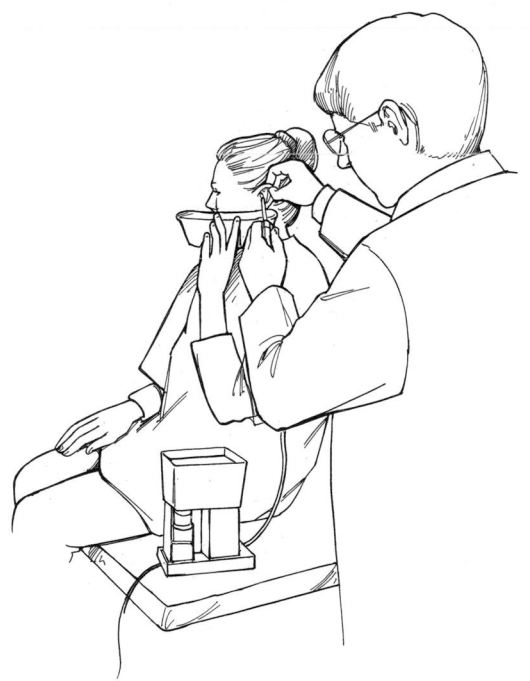

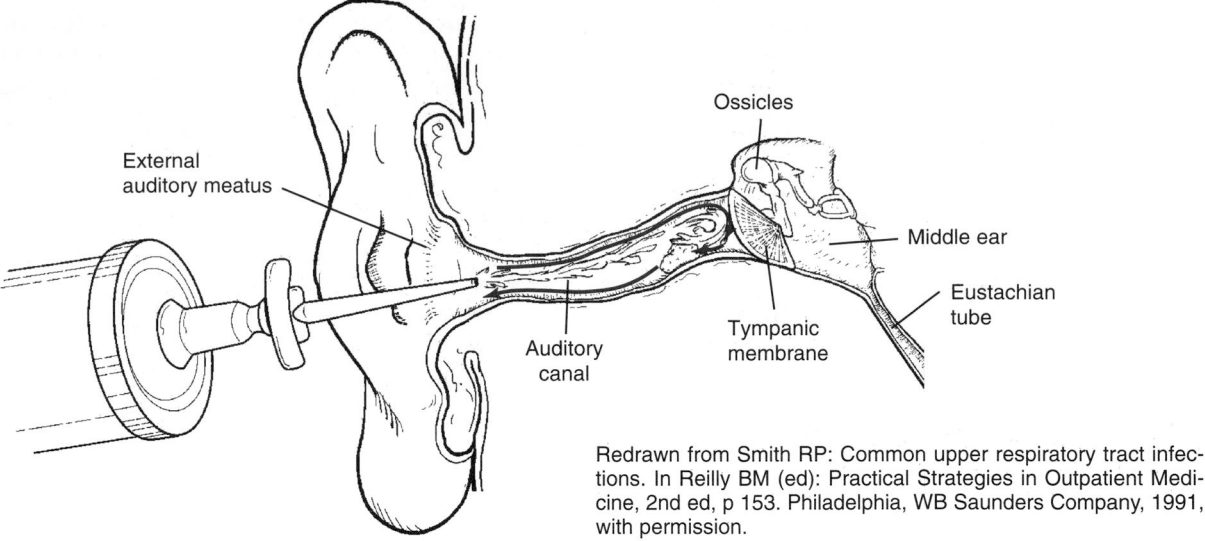

Redrawn from Smith RP: Common upper respiratory tract infections. In Reilly BM (ed): Practical Strategies in Outpatient Medicine, 2nd ed, p 153. Philadelphia, WB Saunders Company, 1991, with permission.

f. Take care not to touch the canal. Stimulation of the posterior ear canal can produce cough in some elderly and the practitioner should be prepared for the potential of sudden movement. It is critical that the operator be in a comfortable position that allows stability and control of the irrigator tip to avoid trauma.

g. Adult patients can hold the ear or emesis basin under the pinna. They should be close to the upright back of the table so as not to fall if dizziness occurs.

h. If true pain occurs, re-evaluate and consider changing the approach.

i. Otoscopic re-assessment should be done each time after material is flushed or after one or two flushes if no material is obtained so the stream can be redirected or to stop the procedure.

j. Following irrigation, swab and dry the ear canal with a cotton-tipped applicator to reduce the risk of infection.

k. The use of 2 to 5 drops of a hygroscopic/drying agent (e.g., alcoholic/acetic acid solution or acetic acid 3%) is sometimes recommended to avoid bacterial and/or fungal overgrowth. In the presence of significant maceration, a brief course of antibiotic/hydrocortisone drops is warranted.

2. Mechanical removal

a. Place the patient in the recommended position and visualize the cerumen with the operating otoscope or speculum.

b. Apply *suction* directly to the plug and, using magnification, remove the fragments in an atraumatic fashion. This method requires experience, occasionally is unsuccessful if the wax is embedded or the suction is too low, and can produce trauma if the wax is hard and sharp.

c. *Direct instrumental removal* is performed in the same fashion.

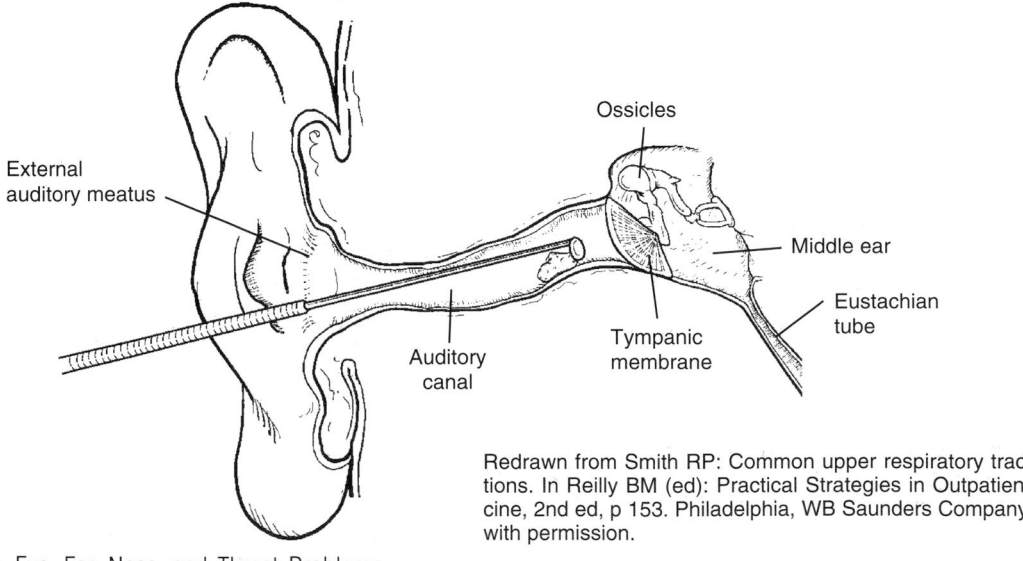

Redrawn from Smith RP: Common upper respiratory tract infections. In Reilly BM (ed): Practical Strategies in Outpatient Medicine, 2nd ed, p 153. Philadelphia, WB Saunders Company, 1991, with permission.

If very hard wax is encountered, cerumenolytics can be used for 5 to 20 minutes and the extraction re-attempted if wax has softened; otherwise, bring the patient back in a few days or attempt irrigation and/or suction.

Follow-Up

1. In the absence of significant trauma or pain, no immediate follow-up is required.

2. Re-evaluation of the canal in 3 months is sensible to assess reoccurrence of impaction.

3. Regular use of cerumenolytics is indicated in recurrent cases. Three to 5 drops should be used each month or more often, depending on pattern.

4. Instruct the patient to contact the physician's office if there is decreased hearing, vertigo, dizziness, drainage, or any pain.

5. Instruct the patient to avoid any instrumentation of the ear canal with cotton-tipped applicators.

Bibliography

Coleman JH: Cerumen and foreign body removal from the ear. In Mayhew HE, Rodgers LA (eds): Basic Procedures in Family Practice, pp 213–220. New York, John Wiley & Sons, 1984.

Forzley GJ, Newkirk GR: Cerumen impaction removal. In Pfenninger JL, Fowler GC (eds): Procedures for Primary Care Physicians, pp 192–196. St. Louis, Mosby, 1994.

Freeman RB: Impacted cerumen: how to safely remove earwax in an office visit. Geriatrics 1995;50:52–53.

Grossan M: Cerumen removal—current challenges. ENT Ear Nose Throat J 1998;77:541–548.

Wilson PL, Ross RJ: Cerumen management: professional issues and techniques. J Am Acad Audiol 1997;8:421–430.

SYMPTOM TINNITUS

Paul T. Cullen

Tinnitus is an abnormal sound that is perceived in the ear or the head area and is unrelated to an external source. Almost 40 million Americans suffer from sustained tinnitus, and 20 per cent of this group report a significant decrease in their quality of life as a result of the symptom. The sound is usually described as a hissing, ringing, or buzzing. It is most commonly a benign disorder associated with high-frequency sensorineural hearing loss. It can be seen in more serious disorders, including acoustic neuroma. Sound transmitted from turbulent blood flow in nearby abnormal or narrowed blood vessels may cause "pulsatile" tinnitus. Neuromuscular spasms of the palate, nasopharynx, and middle ear result in vibratory tinnitus. Anxiety and depressive disorders are frequently found in patients with intractable tinnitus.

Differential Diagnosis

1. Sensorineural hearing loss of aging (presbycusis)
2. Noise-induced hearing loss
3. Ménière's disease (low-pitched, associated with vertigo)
4. Drugs: aspirin, nonsteroidal anti-inflammatory drugs, quinine, tricyclic antidepressants, aminoglycoside antibiotics
5. Muscle spasms of palate and middle ear
6. Uncontrolled hypertension
7. Carotid occlusive disease (pulsatile)
8. Traumatic head injury
9. Acoustic neuroma

About 90 per cent of tinnitus is due to otologic causes. High-frequency hearing loss with deficits at 3000 to 8000 Hz is most common. Ménière's disease is an exception, with low-frequency tinnitus. Other otologic causes include otosclerosis and chronic suppurative otitis. Medical problems, including uncontrolled hypertension, have been associated with tinnitus that resolves when the blood pressure is lowered. Less frequent medical causes include hypothyroidism and hyperlipidemia.

Refer to Ch. 58, Hypertension, and Ch. 323, Ménière's disease.

History

1. Define the duration of symptoms; *acute-onset, short-duration* tinnitus is probably due to an acute process, such as otitis media, traumatic head injury, labyrinthitis, and noise exposure.

2. Define the nature of the sound. A pulsatile noise synchronous with the pulse results from turbulent flow in abnormal blood vessels (e.g., arteriovenous malformation, internal carotid stenosis). A vibratory intermittent noise with a beating or clicking quality is often due to spasm of the tensor tympani, stapedius, or palatine musculature.

3. Determine whether the tinnitus is unilateral. Although 50 per cent of patients with high-frequency sensorineural loss report symptoms in one ear, it should raise concern about a retrocochlear lesion—typically, acoustic neuroma.

4. Determine whether the tinnitus is continuous or fluctuating. Fluctuating tinnitus with fluctuating hearing loss and vertigo is typical of Ménière's disease.

5. Inquire about symptoms of depression. Sleep disorder, loss of interest, feelings of hopelessness and sadness, and trouble concentrating are often found in patients with intractable tinnitus.

6. Determine the medications, both prescription and over-the-counter, that the patient is taking. The most common drug that provokes tinnitus is aspirin.

7. Screen for associated neurologic symptoms that might suggest a more serious cause. Vertigo, abnormalities of facial nerve function, and symptoms of a transient ischemic attack should prompt a more detailed evaluation.

Clinical Findings

1. In the majority of cases resulting from cochlear disease, there are no specific abnormal findings.

2. If symptoms of pulsatile tinnitus are elicited, careful auscultation of the neck, mastoid, and skull for bruits is indicated.

3. In all cases, perform a careful examination of the tympanic membrane.

4. A directed examination of the cranial nerves and cerebellum is indicated, especially if symptoms suggest a neurologic cause.

Tests

1. Complete audiometric testing, including air and bone conduction, is mandatory in the evaluation of all patients with tinnitus. The most common abnormality is bilateral high-frequency (3000 to 8000 Hz) sensorineural loss. Some patients have significant loss into the range of normal speech (500 to 2000 Hz). A unilateral significant abnormality on audiography should be investigated for the possibility of a retrocochlear lesion (i.e., acoustic neuroma).

2. Blood pressure should be measured and treated if elevated.

3. Consider measurement of hemoglobin, blood glucose, and serum lipid levels as well as a serologic test for syphilis and thyroid function tests in selected circumstances. Only a small number of patients with tinnitus have one of these disorders as the primary cause of tinnitus.

4. In pulsatile tinnitus, computerized tomography of the brain and temporal bone, duplex ultrasound examination of the carotid bifurcation, and, possibly, cerebral angiography should be performed.

Management

1. Eliminate all medications that may be contributing to the tinnitus.

2. Avoid the use of stimulants—especially nicotine and caffeine—which may worsen the symptom.

3. If a bilateral high-frequency loss is detected and the patient's primary complaints occur at bedtime, suggest a radio at low volume to mask the tinnitus.

4. If significant hearing loss and tinnitus coexist, referral to an audiologist and evaluation for a hearing aid and masking device are indicated.

5. If depression or an anxiety disorder exists, vigorously treat with appropriate antidepressants, antianxiety drugs, and psychotherapy.

6. In patients without confirmed anxiety or depression, alprazolam, nortriptyline, biofeedback, and relaxation therapy have been used with varying degrees of success.

Patient Education

1. Although the symptom can be quite disturbing, in most cases, tinnitus is a symptom of a benign disorder. The patient should be reassured after evaluation that the symptom is not caused by a life-threatening problem.

2. Tinnitus often decreases with time.

3. Avoid noise exposure.

4. In addition to the therapies above, some patients find relief in support groups. Information can be obtained from the American Tinnitus Association, P.O. Box 5, Portland, OR 97207.

Follow-Up

Depends on the degree of the patient's dysfunction and the results of initial diagnostic tests

Bibliography

Clocon J, Amede F, Lechtenberg C, Astor F: Tinnitus: a stepwise workup to quiet the noise within. Geriatrics 1995;50:18–25.

Meyerhoff W, Ridenour B: Tinnitus. In Meyerhoff W, Rice D (eds): Otolaryngology Head and Neck Surgery, pp 435–446. Philadelphia, WB Saunders Company, 1992.

Schleuning A: Management of the patient with tinnitus. Med Clin North Am 1991;75:1225–1237.

Sismanis A, Smoker W: Pulsatile tinnitus: recent advances in diagnosis. Laryngoscope 1994;104:681–687.

Sullivan M, Katon W, Dobie R, et al: A randomized trial of nortriptyline for severe chronic tinnitus. Arch Intern Med 1993;153:2251–2259.

SYMPTOM EPISTAXIS

Joseph Valentino

Most people have at least one bout of epistaxis in their lifetime. The vast majority of nose bleeds never come to medical attention. The cause is usually local trauma to the anterior portions of the nasal septum; however, epistaxis may be an early sign of a more significant systemic illness. Epistaxis often is intermittent, making it frustrating for both the patient and the physician, because one is never quite certain the bleeding has ceased. Significant bleeding, although unusual, is possible and can be fatal. Primary care physicians must be familiar with epistaxis and should be able to institute basic treatment and temporize severe bleeding until the otolaryngologist arrives.

Differential Diagnosis

Trauma

- Intranasal trauma
- External nasal trauma
- Chemical irritation

Inflammation

- Rhinosinusitis
- Allergic and vasomotor rhinitis
- Rhinitis of pregnancy
- Unusual rhinosinusitis: typhoid, nasal diphtheria, pertussis, ozena, malaria, other parasitic infections
- Wegener's granulomatosis

Vasculopathy

- Hypertensive vasculopathy
- Hereditary hemorrhagic telangiectasias

Hematologic Pathology

- Iatrogenic (e.g., warfarin, aspirin, heparin, nonsteroidal anti-inflammatory drugs [NSAIDs])
- Factor deficiencies (e.g., hemophilia, hepatic failure, vitamin K deficiency)
- Blood dyscrasias (idiopathic thrombocytopenia purpura, leukemia, polycythemia vera, etc.)
- Disseminated intravascular coagulation

Neoplasms of the Nose, Paranasal Sinuses, and Nasopharynx

- Benign: hemangioma, juvenile nasopharyngeal angiofibroma, meningioma, etc.
- Malignant: squamous cell carcinoma, adenocarcinoma, lymphoma, olfactory neuroblastoma, etc.

Other

- Atrophic rhinitis
- Vicarious menstruation

1. Trauma
   a. Intranasal trauma
      (1) The most common cause is self-inflicted trauma to Kiesselbach's area, such as with digital manipulation, blowing, and wiping of the nose, which can mechanically traumatize this area.
      (2) Decreased environmental humidity is associated with mucosal drying and cracking. This explains the increased incidence in colder climates during the winter months.
      (3) Septal deformity or septal perforations can cause turbulent airflow, leading to excessive drying and irritation of the nasal mucosa.
   b. External nasal trauma can cause tearing of intranasal mucous membranes. Fractures of the facial skeleton can disrupt major facial vessels.
   c. Chemical irritation can result from caustic agents or inhaled drugs.

2. Inflammation induces vascular engorgement of the nose, producing an increased friability of the mucous membranes. These patients are also traumatizing their noses with more frequent blowing and wiping.

3. Vascular disorders may produce increased vascular fragility that results in epistaxis. Some may produce granular formations in the nose with resultant epistaxis. The most common vascular disorder producing epistaxis is a loss of adventitial and muscularis integrity of the larger posterior nasal arterial vessels produced by longstanding hypertension in the adult. These patients suffer from more significant posterior nasal hemorrhage that can be very challenging to control.

History: Key Questions to Ask

1. Can you estimate the volume of blood lost?
2. Which side of the nose began to bleed first?
3. Are you swallowing blood?
4. Seek signs of hypovolemia (dizziness, loss of consciousness, last void)
5. Medications? Do not forget over-the-counter medicines such as aspirin and NSAIDs.
6. History of nasal or facial trauma? Surgery of the nose or sinuses?
7. Past medical history: previous epistaxis (which side?), coagulopathy, easy bruising, bleeding, bleeding complications of trauma or surgery, hypertension, liver disease
8. History of rhinosinusitis or allergic rhinitis?

Clinical Findings

1. Vital signs
2. Examine face for evidence of trauma.
3. Intranasal exam: Before treatment or packing, the physician should always attempt to examine the nose to determine the cause and site of bleeding.
   a. Clear the nose of blood and clot with gentle suctioning. Application of topical vasoconstricting agent as well as a topical anesthetic agent for 5 to 10 minutes if possible may greatly facilitate examination. This can be applied by spraying, or using cotton or cottonoid material soaked in the solution and placed into the nose with bayonet forceps under direct visualization.
   b. Inspect for the origin of bleeding, especially if the nose is to be packed. Packing macerates the nasal mucosa, frequently making it difficult to identify the source of bleeding. If the patient's bleeding has stopped, the site is often a prominent erythematous vessel read-

ily visible through the mucosa. If the bleeding is brisk, noting where the blood appears to be originating may be helpful.
   c. Identify predisposing conditions such as septal deformity, tumor, or evidence of sinusitis (mucopurulence).
4. Oral: Examine the lips for telangiectasias, the oropharynx for blood streaming from the nasopharynx.
5. General physical examination: Look for signs of hypovolemia, cutaneous hemangiomata, petechiae, or neck masses.

Tests

If the bleeding is minor and not a recurring problem, no testing is indicated. For more substantial bleeding, or recurrent bleeding, the following may be useful:

1. Complete blood count, including platelet count: The hematocrit does not truly reflect the degree of acute blood loss until the patient has had sufficient volume replacement. It can show anemia from more chronic blood loss and serve as a baseline to compare future laboratory values. The complete blood count reveals blood dyscrasias.
2. Bleeding time: Aspirin use, von Willebrand's disease, and many platelet-based bleeding disorders elevate the bleeding time.
3. Prothrombin time and partial thromboplastin time: Coagulation times are elevated in hemophilia, but more often they detect liver disease and vitamin K deficiency.
4. Invasive angiography: In cases of uncontrollable epistaxis where surgical packing has failed, invasive angiography may be able to identify the blood vessel producing the bleeding. In some cases selective vascular occlusion techniques can be employed.

Management

Refer to Procedure: Controlling Epistaxis, p 80

PEARLS

- Before examining the patient, gather all needed equipment, including head light or head mirror, nasal speculum, Frazier-tipped suction cannula, bayonet forceps, cotton strips or $1/2 \times 3$-inch cottonoids, and 4% cocaine or lidocaine with phenylephrine solution to provide anesthesia and vasoconstriction of the nose.

- Hypertension will exacerbate bleeding, making control more difficult. Control with antihypertensive agents; mild anxiolytics are useful.

- Patients with coagulopathies need to have this corrected. Packing and other significant nasal manipulations can exacerbate bleeding in these patients. Diffuse oozing from multiple areas is common. Expandable foam nasal tampons are useful in these patients.

- Do not cauterize both sides of the nasal septum because this may lead to septal perforation.

- Provide discharge instructions where appropriate, after controlling the bleeding:
  - **Do not blow, wipe or pick the nose.**
  - No heavy lifting, straining, or exertion
  - Vasoconstricting sprays (oxymetazoline or phenylephrine for 2 to 3 days)
  - Humidify the environment.
  - Apply a water-in-oil cream (e.g., Vaseline) to the nose twice daily.
  - Provide treatment for underlying or exacerbating conditions (hypertension, allergy, sinusitis, etc.).

Bibliography

LePore ML: Epistaxis. In Bailey BJ (ed): Head and Neck Surgery—Otolaryngology, pp 428–460. Philadelphia, JB Lippincott Company, 1993.

McGarry G, Moulton C: The first aid management of epistaxis by accident and emergency department staff. Arch Emerg Med 1993;4:298–300.

Pollice PA, Yoder MG: Epistaxis: a retrospective review of hospitalized patients. Otolaryngol Head Neck Surg 1997;117:49–53.

Rubin J, Rood SR, Myers EN, et al: The Management of Epistaxis: A Self-Instructional Package. Alexandria, VA, American Academy of Otolaryngology–Head and Neck Surgery Foundation, 1990.

Strachan D, England J: First-aid treatment of epistaxis—confirmation of widespread ignorance. Postgrad Med J 1998;74:113–114.

The most important aspect of managing epistaxis is localizing the site of bleeding. Ninety per cent of bleeds are anterior and arise from Kiesselbach's plexus (or Little's area) on the nasal septum. Anterior bleeding usually responds to local therapy, but sometimes an anterior pack is required. If the bleeding is posterior, both an anterior and a posterior pack are often needed. Posterior bleeding is usually arterial, is more severe, and arises from the sphenopalatine and the ethmoid arteries. Posterior bleeding can be associated with hypertension, atherosclerosis, and conditions that decrease platelet and clotting functions. Such bleeding is much more common in elderly people. One would suspect that the site is posterior if there is extensive bleeding into the oropharynx while pinching the anterior nose or when bleeding is from both nostrils.

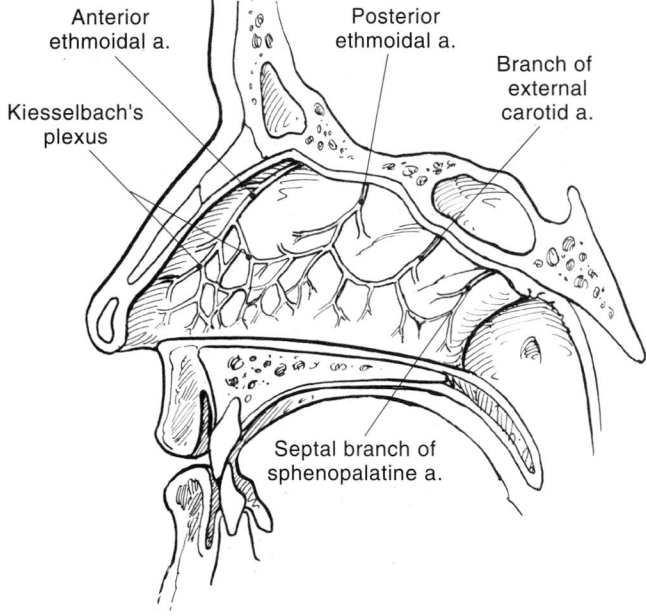

Indications
1. Local therapy: anterior bleeding
2. Anterior packing
   a. Anterior bleeding unresponsive to local therapy
   b. Posterior bleeding
3. Posterior packing: posterior bleeding. *Note:* The posterior packing acts as a buttress against which the anterior packing is placed to tamponade the bleeding site.

Contraindications
1. A history of a coagulopathy is a contraindication to cautery; thus, an anterior pack should be used.

2. Obstruction of the oral airway and a history of tumor in the nasopharynx are contraindications for posterior packing.

Preparation
1. Reassure the patient.
2. Wear a protective gown. The patient should also wear a gown.
3. Position the patient upright with the head forward in a sniffing position.
4. Have the patient blow his or her nose to clear it of all clots so that it is easier to localize the bleeding site.

Equipment
1. Local therapy
   a. Head light
   b. Suction with a No. 8 to No. 10 French tip
   c. Nasal speculum
   d. Cotton balls soaked in topical anesthetic and vasoconstrictor (see "Anesthesia")
   e. Cautery tools
      (1) Silver nitrate sticks
      (2) Electrocautery
   f. Lidocaine 1% (Xylocaine) with 1:100,000 epinephrine if local injection will be attempted
2. Anterior pack
   a. Bayonet forceps
   b. Petrolatum (Vaseline) gauze or Nu-Gauze packing (½ × 72 inch). An expanding nasal tampon such as Merocel Epistaxis packing, can also be used (available in 4-, 8-, and 10-cm lengths).
   c. Antibiotic ointment (bacitracin or neomycin)
3. Posterior pack
   a. Foley catheter, No. 12 or No. 13 French, with 30-ml balloon
   b. A 20-ml syringe
   c. Umbilical clamp
   d. Padding (4 × 4) to place between umbilical clamp and nose
   e. Tape to secure catheter
   f. Tongue blade

Anesthesia
1. Local therapy and anterior packing: Cotton balls soaked in phenylephrine 1% (Neo-Synephrine) and lidocaine 2% with epinephrine. When placed in the nasal cavity for about

5 minutes, good anesthesia and vasoconstriction are produced.

2. Posterior packing: If sedation is required, use morphine sulfate, 5 to 12 mg intramuscularly or intravenously, with or without midazolam (Versed), 1 to 2 mg intravenously. Watch for respiratory depression.

Precautions

1. Patients with nasal packing are at increased risk for infection, such as otitis media, sinusitis, and toxic shock syndrome. They should be placed on prophylactic antibiotics (e.g., amoxicillin–clavulanate potassium [Augmentin]). The packing materials should also be covered with an antibiotic ointment.

2. Patients who require posterior packing should be admitted to the hospital and watched closely for evidence of cardiac arrhythmia and for respiratory failure.

3. Hypoxia is common in patients with posterior packs. Low-flow humidified oxygen may be given by face mask.

Technique

1. Local therapy
   a. Ask the patient to blow his or her nose free of clots.
   b. Determine the site of the bleeding.
   c. Place medicated cotton pledgets in the bleeding nostril, and ask the patient to sit forward, pinching the nostril for about 5 minutes.
   d. Remove the cotton pledgets and see if site is still bleeding.
   e. If the bleeding continues, apply cautery either with silver nitrate sticks or electrocautery. *Note*: Excessive electrocautery can lead to nasal septal perforation.
   f. If the nose is still bleeding, some may choose to inject lidocaine 1% with epinephrine using a 27-gauge needle around the bleeding site.
   g. If the bleeding persists, insert an anterior pack.

2. Anterior packing
   a. Open the nose with a nasal speculum.
   b. With the bayonet forceps, grasp the packing 2 to 3 cm from its end, placing it in the nose in an "accordion" manner so that part of each layer is near the front of the nose.

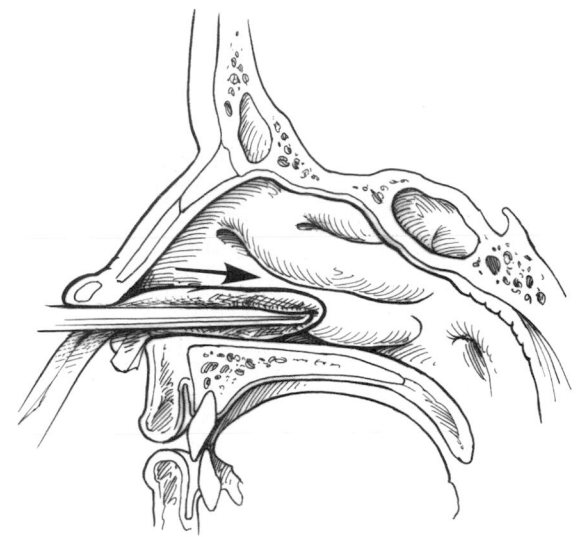

Note: The free ends of packing near the back of the nose can fall into the posterior nasopharynx, which can cause gagging.

   c. After several layers have been placed, push the packing down with the bayonet forceps, making it tighter and more secure. Six feet of packing may be required for an adequate pack on the side that is bleeding.

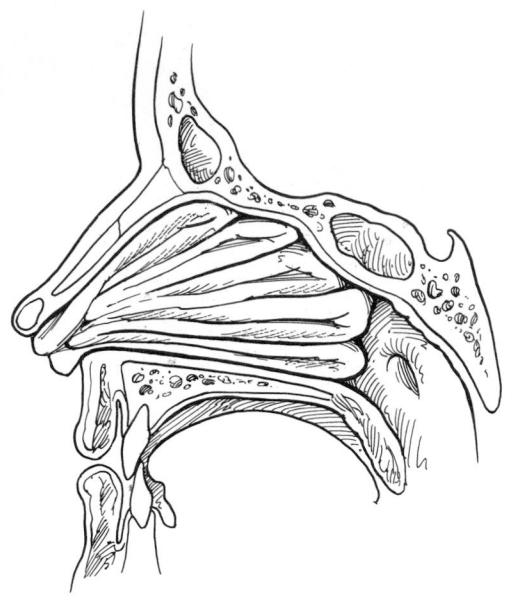

3. Posterior packing
   a. Sedate the patient if necessary.
   b. Take a No. 12 or No. 13 French Foley catheter, and cut off the tip distal to the balloon.
   c. Advance the catheter along the floor of the nostril with the heaviest bleeding until you see the tip in the pharynx.
   d. Inflate the balloon with 5 to 10 ml of water. Then apply gentle traction until the balloon lodges in the choana.

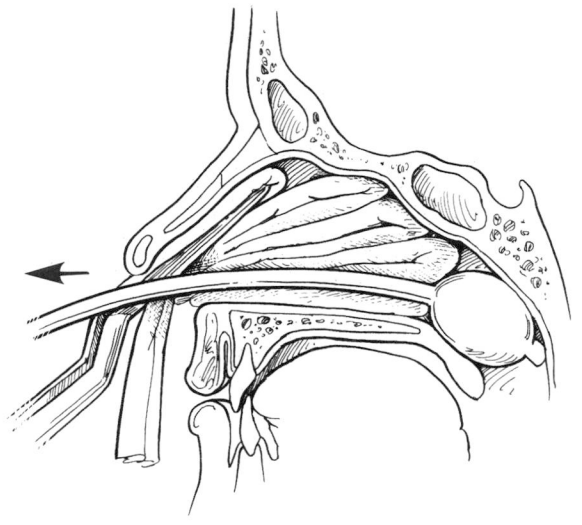

d. An expanding nasal tampon can also be inserted. If needed, trim the compressed tampon with scissors to fit into the nose. Insert as quickly and as far back into the nose as possible. If placed too slowly, the tampon will begin to expand, making insertion more difficult. Then allow for bleeding to expand the tampon, compressing the bleeding site. The end should be just inside the naris.

e. Add an additional 10 to 15 ml of water to the balloon. If the soft palate is grossly displaced inferiorly or there is significant pain, the balloon should be slightly deflated.

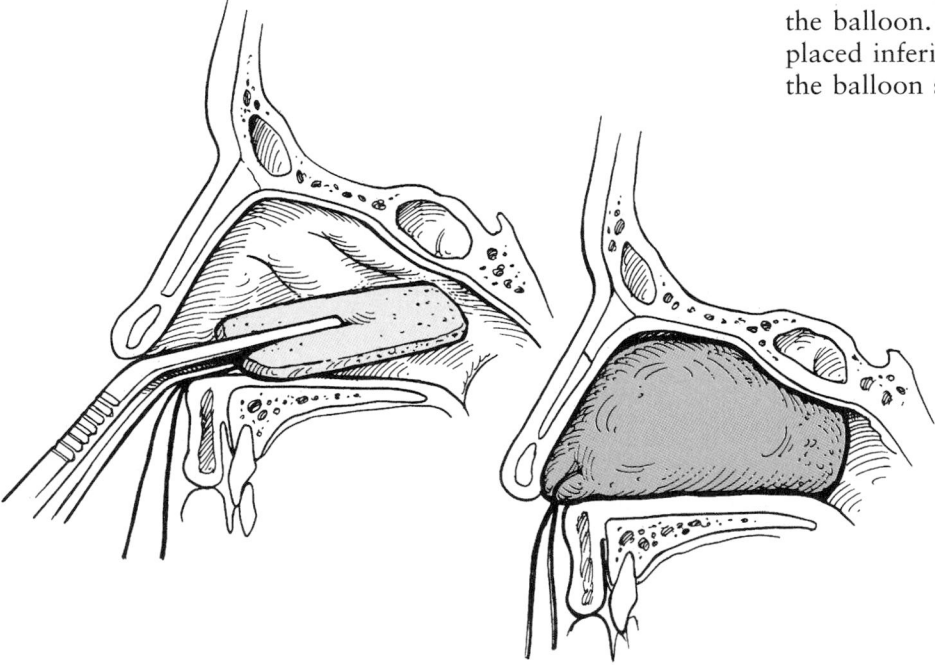

f. Have an assistant apply gentle traction on the catheter while you insert an anterior pack.

g. Fix the catheter in placed using the umbilical clamp. Apply adequate padding (4 × 4) between the clamp and the nose to prevent pressure necrosis.

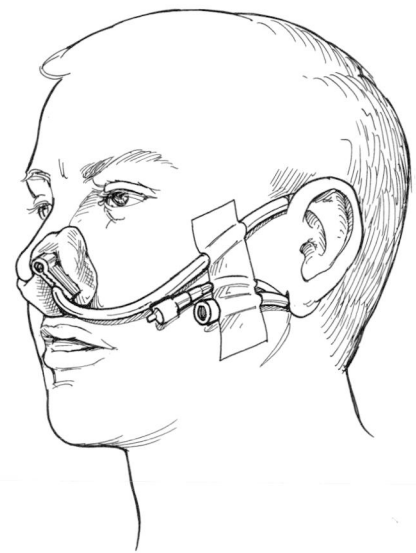

h. Secure the catheter around the ear, as shown. *Note*: If bleeding continues, refer the patient to an otolaryngologist for possible arterial ligation.

Follow-Up

1. Instruct the patient to apply Vaseline to the nasal mucosa three times per day to prevent drying and cracking.

2. Recommend air humidification.

3. Tell the patient not to take aspirin.

4. Remove anterior packing in 1 to 3 days, depending on the severity of the bleeding.

5. For posterior packing, once the bleeding has stopped, deflate the balloon and leave the catheter in place for 2 to 3 hours. Reinflate the balloon if the bleeding starts again.

Bibliography

Pollice PA, Yoder MG: Epistaxis: a retrospective review of hospitalized patients. Otolaryngol Head Neck Surg 1997;117:49–53.

Randall DA, Freeman SB: Management of anterior and posterior epistaxis. Am Fam Physician 1991;43:2007–2014.

Rosen P, Barkin RM: Emergency Medicine: Concepts and Clinical Practice, 3rd ed, pp 2465–2468. St. Louis, Mosby–Year Book, 1992.

Schlesselman LR, Iriarte RI: Controlling posterior epistaxis. In Driscoll CE, Rakel RE (eds): Procedures for Your Practice, 2nd ed, pp 373–377. Los Angeles, Practice Management Information Co, 1991.

Simmen D, Heinz B: Epistaxis strategy—experiences with the last 360 hospitalizations. Laryngorhinootologie 1998;77:100–106.

SYMPTOM HOARSENESS

William A. Schwer

Hoarseness is defined as a change in normal voice quality or abnormal production of sound by the larynx. It may be described by patients as raspiness, harshness, breathiness, roughness, or change in the pitch of the voice. *Dysphonia* is the term used by laryngologists to describe abnormal voice quality.

Differential Diagnosis

Acute hoarseness is defined as the presence of symptoms for less than 2 weeks. The majority of the causes of acute hoarseness are benign. Chronic hoarseness is defined as symptoms persisting for greater than 2 weeks and denote more serious conditions. Patients with chronic hoarseness should generally be referred to an ear-nose-throat (ENT) specialist.

Etiology

Acute Hoarseness

1. Hemorrhage into a vocal fold secondary to voice trauma (i.e., yelling).

2. Viral laryngitis: Usually associated with a sore throat. Coxsackie, Epstein-Barr, influenza A, variola, measles, mumps, varicilla, echo, parainfluenza, and herpes simplex viruses all can be causative agents.

3. Bacterial laryngitis: *Moraxella catarrhalis, Haemophilus influenzae*, streptococcus, staphylococcus, mycoplasma, and pneumococcus all can be causative agents.

4. Other infectious agents: Blastomycosis, mycobacterium, candidiasis, histoplasmosis, coccidioidomycosis, and rhinosporidiosis are all unusual causes of hoarseness.

5. Chemical and environmental irritants: Exposure to certain allergens or irritating agents can cause edema and erythema similar to that seen with infectious agents. Cigarette smoking is a common irritant.

6. Vocal overuse and abuse: This is a very common cause of edema and erythema of the vocal cords. It is seen with patients who need to use their voice frequently (i.e., singers, speakers).

7. Stress: Hoarseness results from a misuse of laryngeal musculature.

Chronic Hoarseness

1. Local disease—benign: Nodules, callus formation, polyps, and papillomas are all causes. Nodules can resolve with proper therapy; all others will require surgery.

2. Local disease—malignant: Most cancers are of squamous cell origin and mainly are located on the vocal cords. Causative agents include smoking and alcohol use.

Other Etiologies

1. Gastroesophageal reflux causes hoarseness as a result of direct irritation. Chronic cough and wheezing can be associated symptoms.

2. Immobility of one or more vocal cords: Paralysis of a vocal cord/cords can result from injury to the recurrent laryngeal nerves during neck surgery. Central neurologic lesions can cause bilateral paralysis. Endotracheal intubation can also cause injury to the recurrent laryngeal nerve. A thoracic process such as a lung carcinoma or left atrial enlargement can cause unilateral left vocal cord paralysis.

3. Systemic diseases: Hypothyroidism causes edema of the vocal cords. Wegener's granulomatosis, amyloidosis, lupus, rheumatoid arthritis, and sarcoidosis can affect the larynx, producing hoarseness.

4. Pregnancy: Hoarseness can result from increased blood volume and resultant swelling of the vocal cords.

5. Presbylaryngeus: This is the most common cause of hoarseness in the elderly. Muscle tone is decreased and therefore the vocal cords bow.

6. Neurologic diseases: Diabetes mellitus can cause a neuropathy leading to vocal cord weakness or paralysis. Parkinson's disease, amyotrophic lateral sclerosis, and Guillain-Barré syndrome all can lead to abnormal voice production or hoarseness.

History

A careful history should include the following:

1. Is hoarseness present for less than or greater than 2 weeks?

2. Are there times the voice is normal? Fixed lesions do not allow the voice to have periods of normality.

3. Does the hoarseness fluctuate during the day? Gastroesophageal reflux causes hoarseness more in the morning.

4. Is there associated ear pain (otalgia)?

5. Is there a history of allergies?

6. Has there been any surgery to the neck region or a history of intubation?

7. Does the patient use tobacco or alcohol?

8. Are there any other systemic diseases that the patient suffers from?

9. What is the occupation of the patient?

10. Any other associated symptoms?

Clinical Findings

1. A complete head and neck examination should be performed on all patients complaining of hoarseness. The oral cavity and oropharynx are examined to look for signs of infection or postnasal drainage. A normal ear examination will rule out ear diseases as a cause of otalgia. The neck should be examined for lymphadenopathy and thyroid enlargement.

2. A more complete general examination may be necessary dependent on the patient's past medical history or associated symptoms.

Diagnostic Tests

Hoarseness lasting longer than 2 weeks requires a complete laryngoscopic examination. Indirect laryngoscopy in the hands of an experienced physician can be adequate. Transnasal fiberoptic laryngoscopy has the advantage of being able to observe motion of the larynx during voice production and can lead to more underlying pathology.

Management

1. The cornerstone of management of hoarseness is good vocal hygiene. The larynx must have a watery, thin lubrication for proper functioning. Therefore, decongestants can actually worsen hoarseness. Six glasses of water per day are recommended for good hydration.

2. If hoarseness is due to vocal overuse or trauma, vocal rest but not total disuse is recommended in most situations.

Medication

1. If bacterial or fungal infections are the causative agent, then appropriate antibiotics need to be employed. Decongestants should not be used.

2. Histamine$_2$ blockers or proton pump inhibitors should be used for gastroesophageal reflux.

3. Nasal steroids are appropriate for allergy-based phenomena.

Diet

1. Excellent hydration is important. Alcohol and caffeine should be avoided as they cause diuresis and therefore mild dehydration.

2. Foods that contribute to gastroesophageal reflux, if that is the causative agent for hoarseness, should be avoided.

Activity

Voice rest is imperative for most benign causes of hoarseness. Avoidance of airborne irritants or allergens may be necessary.

Patient Education

This depends on the underlying cause of hoarseness. Reassurance is key for most benign conditions.

Follow-Up

If a treatment(s) for an acute condition does not result in resolution of hoarseness, or if the symptom has now lasted for more than 2 weeks, a referral to an ENT specialist is advised.

PEARLS

- Acute hoarseness is generally benign. Chronic hoarseness suggests a more serious condition.

- Sporadic hoarseness connotes sporadic irritation. Constant hoarseness connotes a fixed lesion.

- Morning hoarseness suggests gastroesophageal reflux.

Bibliography

Garrett CG, Gossoff RH: Hoarseness: contemporary diagnosis and management. Compr Ther 1995;21:705–710.

Hanson DG, Kamel PL, Kahrilas PJ: Outcomes of antireflux therapy for the treatment of chronic laryngitis. Ann Otol Rhinol Laryngol 1995;104:550–555.

Moragos NE: Hoarseness. Primary Care 1990;17:347–363.

Rosen CA, Anderson D, Murry T: Evaluating hoarseness: keeping your patient's voice healthy. Am Fam Physician 1998;57:2775–2782.

Flexible fiberoptic rhinolaryngoscopy is a safe, convenient, and effective procedure for examining the upper airway. By using rhinolaryngoscopy, physicians can easily examine areas in the nose and pharynx that were previously inaccessible. The vocal cords, larynx, pharynx, and surrounding structures can be more readily and comfortably visualized than with indirect mirrors or rigid telescopes.

Indications

1. Eustachian tube dysfunction
   a. Ear fullness
   b. Ear plugging
   c. Chronic or recurrent otitis media
2. Pharyngeal complaints
   a. Chronic sore throat
   b. Chronic postnasal drip
   c. Dysphagia
   d. Odynophagia
   e. Persistent cough
   f. Suspected laryngeal foreign body
   g. Stridor
3. Nasal complaints
   a. Chronic stuffiness
   b. Chronic rhinitis
   c. Epistaxis (not active)
   d. Suspected nasal foreign body
   e. Halitosis
   f. Evaluation of snoring
4. Sinusitis
   a. Recurrent headache
   b. Chronic sinusitis
5. Hoarseness or voice changes: phonation disturbances
6. Cancer screening (i.e., history of smoking)
7. Post-traumatic evaluation
8. Postsurgery evaluation
9. Caustic ingestion
10. Regional radiation therapy
11. Psychogenic disorders (globus hystericus)

Contraindications

1. Acute epiglottitis
2. Impending airway obstruction
3. Blood dyscrasias
4. Hypersensitivity to topical anesthetics
5. Severe hypertension

Complications

1. Gagging
2. Bleeding
3. Sneezing
4. Coughing
5. Laryngospasm
6. Anesthesia reaction

Equipment

1. Nasal speculum
2. Ephedrine 1%, oxymetazoline (Afrin), phenylephrine 0.05% (Neo-Synephrine), or cocaine 0.5% in spray dispenser
3. Lidocaine 4% (mixed in cromolyn sodium [Nasalcrom] or any nasal steroid spray, 1:1 dilution; end up with a 2% mixture); benzodiazepines and narcotics not necessary.
4. Viscous lidocaine to apply to scope for lubrication (optional)
5. Fiberoptic rhinolaryngoscope with appropriate light source

Structures and Abnormalities To Look For

1. Inferior larynx, hypopharynx, pharynx
   a. Vocal cords (true cords)
      (1) Appearance
      (2) Mobility (paralysis?)
         (a) Quiet breathing
         (b) Deep inspiration
         (c) Panting
         (d) Phonation ("eeee")
      (3) Glottic aperture
         (a) Mucus bridging
         (b) Midline
      (4) Vocal cord trauma, hyperkeratosis, malignancies, inflammatory granulomata, polyps, nodules, ulcerations, granulomatous extensions, papillomas
      (5) Vocal cord dysfunction syndrome
   b. False cords
   c. Arytenoids
   d. Aryepiglottic folds
   e. Epiglottis
   f. Vallecula
   g. Posterior tongue; lingual tonsils: Hypertrophy may result in a sensation of globus.
2. Nasopharynx, superior pharynx
   a. Pharyngeal wall

(1) Spasm of constrictor muscles

(2) Osteophytes from vertebral bodies may cause obstruction

(3) Hypertrophy of lymphoid tissue from chronic inflammation produces a "cobblestoned" appearance

b. Palate

c. Adenoid

(1) Primary lymph node, first line of defense for inflammation involving the nasal airway

(2) May impinge on torus tubarius (opening of Eustachian tube).

(3) Adenoidectomy may damage torus tubarius.

(4) Hypertrophy may partially or totally block nasal airway.

d. Rosenmüller's fossa

(1) Vertical cleft between posterior lip of torus tubarius and adenoidal pad

(2) Many pharyngeal malignancies originate here.

e. Torus tubarius (eustachian orifice)

(1) Obstruction, dysfunction

(2) Cysts

3. Nose

a. Septum

(1) Septal deviation; evaluation of repair

(2) Bony spurs, protrusion, ridging

(3) Perforation

b. Mucosa

(1) Color

(2) Exudate

c. Nasal turbinates (conchae)

(1) Clefting

(a) Both horizontal and sagittal clefting can occur.

(b) Horizontal or sagittal clefting of the middle turbinate can look like a polyp.

(2) Postoperative evaluation of turbinectomy

(3) Polypoid changes

d. Inferior meatus

(1) Nasolacrimal duct

(2) Surgically created antral windows

e. Middle meatus

(1) Frontal sinus ostium

(2) Maxillary sinus ostium

(3) Anterior ethmoid ostia

f. Superior meatus, sphenoethmoidal recess

(1) Sphenoid ostia

(2) Posterior ethmoid ostia

(3) Ethmoidectomy

g. Polyps

(1) Manipulation necessary to distinguish polypoidal degeneration of a turbinate from polyps that are entering the nose from the sinuses.

(2) Most polyps originate from the ethmoids, but they can come from any of the sinuses.

Technique

1. Carefully explain indications and technical procedure to the patient.

2. Discuss patient consent form, and then witness it being signed.

3. Address drug hypersensitivity.

4. Perform routine speculum examination to identify most accessible and patent nasal passage.

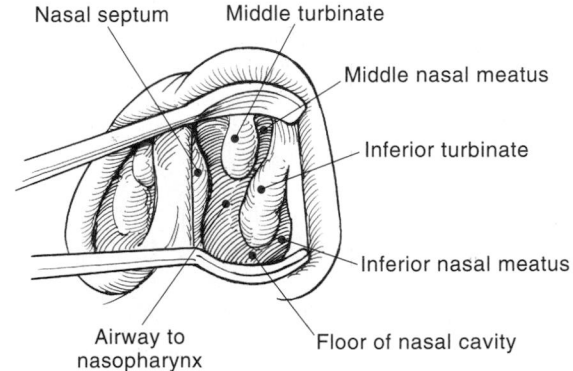

Nasal septum — Middle turbinate — Middle nasal meatus — Inferior turbinate — Inferior nasal meatus — Floor of nasal cavity — Airway to nasopharynx

5. Apply two sprays of ephedrine 1% to the viewed nostril to induce vasoconstriction. This should be followed by lidocaine 2% to 4% spray to each nostril (mix in Nasalcrom or steroid nasal spray [see "Equipment"]).

6. Apply viscous lidocaine 2% to scope for lubrication.

7. Place the patient in a sitting position with the head leaning against the head rest or wall (to avoid sudden jolting away from rhinolaryngoscope). The scope should rest in the clinician's hand on the angle between the first finger and thumb, so that that first finger or thumb is free to manipulate the angulation tip on the scope. The other hand should gently rest against the patient's face and help guide the scope through the nasal passage. The latter hand actually controls the movement of the scope through the nasal passage. Therefore, contact between the patient's face, the clinician's hand, and the scope should be maintained throughout the procedure.

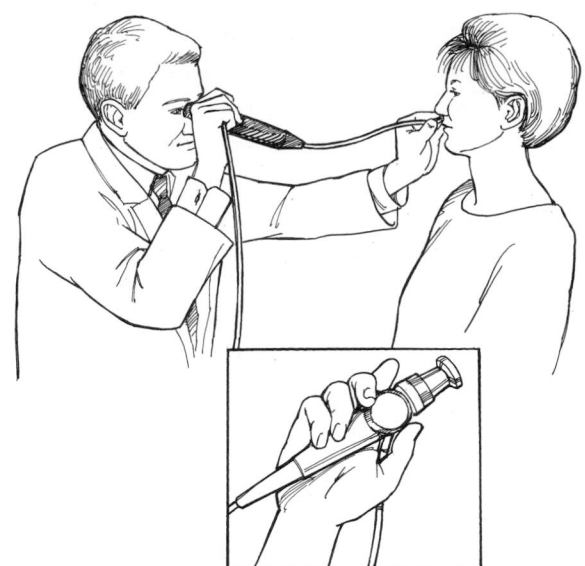

8. It is recommended to advance the scope to the end point and to observe the anatomy and structures in a methodical manner as the scope is withdrawn. Be sure to advance the scope along the floor of the cavity below the turbinates. Avoid making contact with the scope against the nasal septum because this causes discomfort to the patient. Also try to avoid touching the scope against the pharynx because this induces the gag reflex, making the examination more difficult for both the patient and the physician. Advance the scope along the posterior pharyngeal wall (without touching it) and over the uvula until the larynx is in full view. The angulation tip should be pushed forward to move the scope tip inferiorly. This is the end point of the scope insertion and where careful examination should begin.

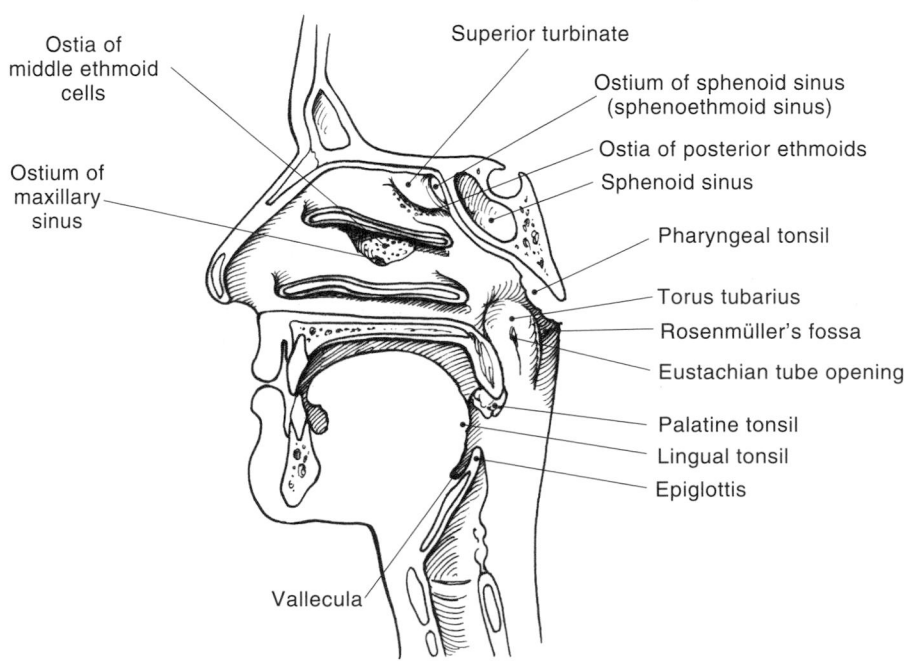

Ostia of middle ethmoid cells

Ostium of maxillary sinus

Superior turbinate

Ostium of sphenoid sinus (sphenoethmoid sinus)

Ostia of posterior ethmoids

Sphenoid sinus

Pharyngeal tonsil

Torus tubarius

Rosenmüller's fossa

Eustachian tube opening

Palatine tonsil

Lingual tonsil

Epiglottis

Vallecula

9. Suggested examination sequence
   a. Withdraw the scope once the end point has been reached.
   b. Larynx
      (1) Piriform sinuses
      (2) Arytenoids
      (3) False vocal cords
      (4) True vocal cords: Ask the patient to say "eeee" to observe vocal cord movement.

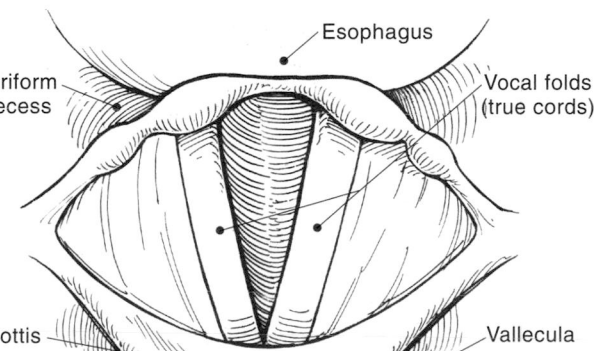

POSTERIOR

Esophagus

Piriform recess

Vocal folds (true cords)

Epiglottis

Vallecula

Lingual tonsil   ANTERIOR

Ask the patient to try not to swallow during the procedure. However, reassure the patient that, if he or she swallows, it will not interfere with the procedure and will not cause harm. It is better to have the patient breathe through the mouth during the procedure because nasal breathing is more likely to fog the scope.

   c. Oropharynx
      (1) Glossal, epiglottic, lateral glottic folds
      (2) Epiglottis
      (3) Vallecula
      (4) Posterior tongue, lingual tonsils
      (5) Posterior pharyngeal wall
      (6) Soft palate
      (7) Lateral pharyngeal walls
   d. Nasopharynx
      (1) Rosenmüller's fossa (most common area for pharyngeal cancer)
      (2) Torus tubarius—both sides ("eeee" for

function of veli palatini). The scope tip should be maintained in the flexed position, and the hand holding the eyepiece portion of the scope should be turned to force the flexed scope tip to view the contralateral torus tubarius.
      (3) Adenoidal pad (palatine tonsil)
   e. Choana (opening to pharynx): Flex tip upward, view
      (1) Introitus, ostea of sphenoid sinus, ostea of posterior ethmoids
      (2) Superior (supreme) turbinate
      (3) Sphenoethmoidal recess
   f. Nasal floor: Move anteriorly, view choana.
   g. Nasal roof: Go over middle turbinate, flex tip upward—cribriform plate
   h. Middle turbinate: Flex tip upward underneath turbinate, if possible; usually this is not possible.
      (1) Maxillary sinus ostium
      (2) Polyps
   i. Superior portion of anterior nose
   j. Nasal vestibule, septum, nasal floor, inferior turbinate (viewed from vestibule)
10. The procedure itself is not hard to perform. The difficult part is developing the skill and experience to differentiate normal anatomy from abnormal pathology. Aside from identifying abnormal structures, pay special attention to color, appearance, mobility, and function of each pertinent structure (e.g., vocal cords). Also take note of abnormal exudates that may help identify pathology (i.e., sinusitis, gastroesophageal reflux).

Bibliography

Curry RW Jr: Flexible fiberoptic nasolaryngoscopy. Fam Pract Recertification 1990;12:21–36.
DeWitt DE: Fiberoptic rhinolaryngoscopy in primary care. Postgrad Med 1988;84:85.
Draf WF, Weber R, Keerl R: Nasal endoscopy. In Schaefer SD (ed): Rhinology and Sinus Disease: A Problem-Oriented Approach, pp 29–39. St. Louis, CV Mosby, 1998.
Netter FH: Atlas of Human Anatomy, plates 32, 75. West Caldwell, NJ, Ciba-Geigy, 1989.
Selner JC: Concepts and clinical application of fiberoptic examination of the upper airway. Clin Rev Allergy 1988;6:303–320.

Hiccups (*singultus*, meaning speech broken by sobs) is the repeated involuntary, spasmodic contraction of the diaphragm associated with sudden closure of the glottis. Hiccups are generally self-limiting and do not require medical attention. The therapeutic challenge is the case of hiccups that is persistent or intractable, lasting weeks or longer, which can lead to fatigue or insomnia. This can cause significant morbidity in the elderly population.

Three categories have seen suggested for defining the duration and severity of hiccups:

1. Hiccup bouts: intermittent episodes comprising several hiccups and persisting as long as 48 hours
2. Persistent hiccups: episodes lasting longer than 48 hours but less than 1 month
3. Intractable hiccups: episodes lasting longer than a month

The anatomy of the hiccup reflex arc is still being defined. The afferent portion arises from the phrenic and vagus nerves along with the sympathetic chain arising from the segments T6 to T12. The central connection has been attributed to a nonspecific anatomic location in the spinal cord between segments C3 and C5. The primary efferent branch is the phrenic nerve, which completes the arc.

Differential Diagnosis (Table 12–1)

1. Hiccup bouts or transient hiccups are often caused by gastric distention and can have many causes. Some include excessive food ingestion, aerophagia, and gastric inflation with upper endoscopy. Other causes include alcohol ingestion, smoking, sudden temperature changes, and emotional stress and excitement.
2. Persistent or intractable hiccups can be a sign of a more serious condition. One must look for a cause localized to the central nervous system, neck, thorax, and abdomen, especially areas that are located along the hiccup reflex arc, specifically the pathways of the vagus and phrenic nerves. This can include more than 100 causes that can be classified into three categories: organic, psychogenic, and idiopathic. Hiccups should be classified as psychogenic or idiopathic only after an organic cause has been ruled out.

Clinical Evaluation

1. A complete history should be performed, covering
   a. Severity, duration, and characteristics of the hiccups
   b. Aggravating and relieving factors
   c. Underlying medical diseases
   d. Ask about alcohol or tobacco use as well as medications such as corticosteroids or benzodiazepines.
   e. Include a psychiatric history.
2. A complete physical should address the head

TABLE 12–1. CAUSES OF HICCUPS

Irritation of Vagus Nerve
Pharyngeal branches
  Pharyngitis
Auricular branches
  Hair or foreign body in ear canal
Thoracic branches
  Pneumonia
  Pleuritis
  Aortic aneurysm
  Pericarditis
  Chest tumors
  Myocardial infarction
Abdominal branches
  Gastric distention
  Gastritis/peptic ulcer disease
  Abdominal abscess
  Gallbladder disease
  Tumors

Diaphragmatic Irritation
Gastric distention
Hiatal hernia
Splenomegaly/hepatomegaly
Subphrenic abscess

Central Nervous System
Structural lesions
Neoplasms
Multiple sclerosis
Brain stem tumors
Syringomyelia
Trauma
Infection (encephalitis, meningitis)
Vascular disease

Postoperative Causes
General anesthesia
Suppression of normal inhibition
Stimulation of oropharynx or glottis
Traction of viscera
Gastric distention
Neck extension

Toxic-Metabolic
Alcohol
Tobacco
Drugs (corticosteroids, benzodiazepines, α-methyldopa)
Uremia
Diabetes mellitus
Electrolyte imbalance (sodium, potassium, carbon dioxide)

Psychogenic
Stress
Excitement
Conversion reaction
Hysterical neurosis
Malingering

Modified from Loft LM, Ward RF: Hiccups: a case presentation and etiologic review. Arch Otolaryngol Head Neck Surg 1992; 118:1115–1119. Copyright 1992 American Medical Association, with permission.

and neck, chest, heart, abdomen, and neurologic systems. Think of potential irritants along the central nervous system and phrenic and vagus nerves. These can be in the form of tumor, trauma, demyelinating disease, arteriovenous malformations, stroke, inflammation, or metabolic compromises. Do not forget to look in the ears for a foreign body.

Tests

1. Complete blood count
2. Renal and electrolyte measurements
3. Further tests depending on the clinical findings
4. If no cause can be found after thorough evaluation, imaging studies with magnetic resonance imaging or computerized tomography scanning of the head and chest may be warranted.

Management

The best therapy for hiccups is to find and treat the underlying cause. If this is unsuccessful, there are numerous therapeutic approaches, emphasizing the ineffectiveness of any one treatment. There is probably no disease that has had more forms of therapy with poor results than intractable hiccups. Made more than 65 years ago, Charles W. Mayo's statement on persistent hiccups remains true today: "The amount of knowledge on any subject such as this can be considered as being in inverse proportion to the number of different treatments suggested and tried for it."

Nonpharmacologic Treatment

1. Physical maneuvers are directed at stimulation or interruption of the reflex arc. Irritation of the nasopharynx may interrupt the vagal afferent limb. Methods to stimulate the phrenic nerve pathway are directed at interruptions of respiration. Many of the methods listed in Table 12–2 have limited scientific basis but occasionally may be helpful.

2. Acupuncture
   a. This modality, if successful, can prevent the sedation common with pharmacologic therapy. The goal is to stimulate the sympathetic chain of the afferent reflex arc arising from the thoracic segments of T6 to T12. Stimulation can be performed by inserting a needle or by injecting dextrose or lidocaine.
   b. Using normal sterile technique, move 1½ inches lateral (either right or left) to the spinous process of T8 on the mid-back and insert a sterile needle ½ to ¾ inch, being careful not to enter the chest cavity. Acupuncture needles are preferred, but if not available a 27- or 25-gauge pediatric spinal needle with

TABLE 12–2. NONPHARMACOLOGIC TREATMENT OF HICCUPS

Stimulation of the Nasopharynx
Forcible traction of the tongue
Lifting the uvula with a spoon
Cotton-tipped swab or catheter stimulation of the nasopharynx
Gargling with water
Sipping ice water
Sucking on hard candy
Swallowing granulated sugar
Swallowing hard bread
Drinking water from the far side of a glass
Biting on a lemon
Inhalation of noxious irritants (nebulized saline or lidocaine)

Counterirritation of the Vagus Nerve
Carotid massage
Supraorbital pressure
Irritation of the tympanic membrane
Valsalva's maneuver
Digital rectal massage

Phrenic Nerve Disruption
Vapocoolant sprays
Ice packs
Electrical stimulation
Alcohol or bupivacaine injection
Phrenic nerve crushing, avulsing, or transection

Counterirritation of the Diaphragm
Pulling knees to chest
Leaning forward to compress chest
Applying pressure at points of diaphragmatic insertion

Interruption of Respiratory Function
Sneezing or coughing
Valsalva's maneuver
Hyperventilation
Use of continuous positive airway pressure
Breath holding
Gasping induced by noxious odors or fright
Rebreathing into a paper bag

Relief of Gastric Distention
Induced vomiting
Nasogastric aspiration
Gastric lavage
Reduction of rate of flow of tube feedings

Miscellaneous
Hypnosis
Behavior modification
Diaphragmatic pacing electrodes
Acupuncture
Prayer

stylet in place can be used to decrease the chance of infection. Leave the needle in for 20 to 30 minutes. If no relief is obtained, spin the needle in the fingers as if winding a watch to further stimulate the sympathetic chain.

Pharmacologic Treatment

1. Baclofen (Lioresal) is currently the most promising drug and has overtaken chlorpromazine (Thorazine) as the drug of choice for intractable hiccups. It is an antispastic drug that exerts its therapeutic effect on suppression of both mono- and polysynaptic reflexes.
   a. Start with 5 mg tid and increase by 5 mg

three times daily every 3 days until the hiccups are suppressed or a maximum dose of 80 mg/day is given. Baclofen comes in 10- and 20-mg scored tablets. If discontinuing, taper this drug slowly over 1 to 2 weeks.

b. If baclofen alone is not effective, add carbamazepine (Tegratol). Baclofen has a strong synergistic effect with this drug. Start carbamazepine at 200 mg bid and increase by a 200-mg additional daily dose (tid and then qid) weekly if needed for therapeutic response. Carbamazepine is particularly helpful in patients with multiple sclerosis as their cause of hiccups.

2. Chlorpromazine (Thorazine) is the most commonly used antipsychotic for the treatment of hiccups. Its success ranges from 0 to 80%. It is more effective if given IV. Watch for postural hypotension, which can be severe. Give 25 to 50 mg IV diluted in 500 ml of saline q6h prn; if effective, can change to oral formulation at the same dose. Continue for 7 days.

3. Haloperidol (Haldol), 2 to 5 mg IM once, than 1 to 4 mg PO tid, can also be tried and may cause less hypotension than chlorpromazine. As will all neuroleptics, watch for sedation, dry mouth, constipation, and extrapyramidal side effects.

4. Metoclopramide (Reglan) has been successful in abating hiccups of many causes, but particularly when they are secondary to gastroparesis, because of its prokinetic effect on the stomach. Give 5 to 10 mg three to four times a day IV, PO, or IM.

5. A study in Germany obtained 60% substantial relief in idiopathic chronic hiccups with the combination of cisapride (Propulsid), omeprazole (Prilosec), and baclofen (Lioresal). Cisapride and omeprazole facilitate gastric emptying and reduce gastric acid, while baclofen suppresses the excitability of the hiccup reflex arc.

6 Other medications

a. Amitriptyline (Elavil) 10 to 25 mg one to three times/day

b. Nifedapine (Procardia), 10 mg three times/day

c. Phenytoin (Dilantin), 200 mg IV once, then 300 mg/day with titration for clinical effect and blood levels

d. Valproic acid (Depakene), 15 mg/kg/day PO with increases of 250 mg/day every 2 weeks as needed

7. Do not use benzodiazepines such as diazepam (Valium) or chlordiazepoxide (Librium) for the treatment of hiccups. These can exacerbate the condition.

Other Methods

1. If hiccups persist despite the above measures, referral to a surgeon for phrenic nerve crushing or ligation can be considered as a last resort.

2. Referral to an anesthesiologist for phrenic nerve blocks, paravertebral block of C3 through C5, or epidural block below C5 can be tried.

3. Electrostimulation of the phrenic nerve as well as continuous positive airway pressure have also had some success.

Bibliography

Friedman NL: Hiccups: a treatment review. Pharmacotherapy 1996;16:986–995.

Lu R, Liu M: Clinical application of single acupoint for treatment. J Tradit Chin Med 1991;11:284–285.

Perez Del Molino A: Treatment of "intractable" hiccup with baclofen. Rev Clin Esp 1996;196:831–833.

Petroianu G, Hein G: Idiopathic chronic hiccup: combination therapy with cisapride, omeprazole, and baclofen. Clin Ther 1997;19:1031–1038.

Rousseau P: Hiccups. In Rakel RE (ed): Conn's Current Therapy, pp 11–13. Philadelphia, WB Saunders Company, 1998.

Wong SK: Treatment of hiccough by acupuncture. Med J Malaysia 1983;38:80–81.

13 Aphthous Stomatitis

Gregory H. Blake

Etiology

1. Stomatitis represents a spectrum of inflammatory changes of the oropharynx, most typically ulcerative or vesicular.

2. Causes are multiple and may be *primary*, such as local infections or trauma in the oral cavity, or *secondary*, such as oral manifestations of systemic diseases. Often, no cause can be identified.

    a. The etiologic agent in the most common ulcerative oral lesion, aphthous stomatitis ("aphtha" means "ulcer"), is unknown and may be multiple. Proposed infectious causes include streptococci and various herpes viruses, including varicella-zoster and cytomegalovirus. Gastrointestinal and nutritional factors may include gluten-sensitive enteropathy and iron, folic acid, zinc, or vitamin B_1, B_2, B_6, and B_{12} deficiencies. Other factors implicated include minor dental trauma, stress, fluctuations in immune status, and genetic predisposition. None of these factors have withstood rigorous analysis.

    b. Viral-induced oral infections are common. Herpes simplex virus type 1 causes several distinct oral diseases, among them acute herpetic gingivostomatitis and herpes simplex labialis ("cold sores"). Coxsackie A viruses cause at least two clinical entities: (1) herpangina and (2) hand-foot-and-mouth disease. Many of the childhood viral exanthems (rubella, rubeola, varicella) present with oral lesions.

    c. Other infectious causes include syphilis, tuberculosis, deep fungal infections, *Mycoplasma pneumoniae*, cytomegalovirus, and anaerobic bacteria.

    d. Stomatitis may reflect systemic disease, particularly inflammatory bowel disease, collagen vascular disease, Behçet's syndrome, Kawasaki's disease, erythema multiforme, cyclic neutropenia, mouth and genital ulcers with inflamed cartilage syndrome, FAPA syndrome (fever, aphthosis, pharyngitis, and adenitis), and immunosuppressive conditions such as human immunodeficiency virus (HIV) infections.

    e. Other etiologies include trauma (from biting or ill-fitting dentures), irritants (aspirin, sharp foods), chemotherapy, and carcinoma.

Symptoms

1. Aphthous ulcers, or "canker sores," are painful and can recur four or more times a year.

2. Stomatitis caused by viral infections have classic prodromal phases of fever, chills, myalgias, and arthralgias.

3. Any stomatitis can be disabling and cause anorexia.

Key Symptoms

- Oral pain
- May have systemic symptoms: fever, chills, malaise, anorexia, arthralgias

Clinical Findings

1. Aphthous stomatitis is characterized by its painful and recurring nature. Aphthous ulcers are rarely found on oral mucosa that is bound to periosteum, such as the attached gingiva and hard palate; this provides an important distinction from herpetic ulcers. Lesions usually are noted in childhood or adolescence and decrease in frequency of recurrence and severity with age. There are three variants:

    a. The *minor* form (80 per cent) is usually a solitary oval ulcer measuring less than 1 cm in diameter and lasting 7 to 10 days. Most patients are young. Disease prevalence is 20 to 50 per cent in the general population.

    b. *Major* ulcers (10 per cent) are multifocal and ragged and may be up to 2 cm in diameter; these frequently last up to 60 weeks, may scar, and are often immediately followed by a recurrent ulcer.

    c. *Herpetic* ulcers (10 per cent) are so named because the papulovesicular lesions occurring in the posterior part of the mouth are grouped, simulating herpes simplex infections.

2. In *acute primary herpetic gingivostomatitis*, the patient is usually young and toxic-appearing with the classic viral prodrome, followed in 24 to 48 hours by mucosal vesicles that quickly rupture and coalesce into large, painful ulcers associated with gingivitis, a white coating on the tongue, and regional lymphadenopathy. The acute phase rarely lasts more than a week. Recurrent episodes, commonly known as *herpes labialis*, or "cold sores," are characterized by single or multiple 2- to 4-mm vesicles around the vermilion border of the lip, frequently following prodromal "itchiness" or "tingling," and rupturing in 36 to 48 hours to form crusts. Frequency of recurrences varies and may be influenced by sunlight, cold, and stress.

3. In HIV-positive patients, discrete ulcers often larger than 1 cm in size and numbering five or less may persist from weeks to months. Ulcers typically occur when CD4+ counts are below 100 cells/ml. Infection and malignancy must be ruled out as causes.

Key Signs

- Oral vesicles or ulcers
- Fever
- Lymphadenopathy
- Toxic appearance (in herpetic infections)

Laboratory Tests

1. Diagnosis of aphthous stomatitis is clinical. Patients with complex aphthosis, troublesome signs and symptoms, or symptoms of malabsorption may be screened with a complete blood count; serum levels of zinc, iron, vitamin B_{12}, and folate; and anti-endomysial or anti-gliadin antibody studies.

2. Herpes infection can be confirmed by titers in acute and convalescent sera and by cytology showing giant cells with viral inclusion bodies.

3. Suspected syphilitic lesions can be sampled by smear for darkfield microscopy.

4. Biopsy may be required where tuberculous, fungal, or carcinomatous etiologies are considered.

Differential Diagnosis

Aphthous ulcers must be differentiated from acute herpetic gingivitis, traumatic ulcers, allergy, and ulcerations caused by systemic disease.

1. Ulcerations caused by herpes simplex virus infections usually follow constitutional symptoms and rupture of vesicles.

2. Traumatic and aphthous ulcers are clinically and histologically identical and are distinguished by anatomic relation to irritating structures.

3. Allergic lesions tend to be diffuse and do not ulcerate.

4. Ulcers of systemic disease are slow to heal but rarely recur.

Treatment

1. Therapy for aphthous stomatitis is palliative and should include avoidance of hot or acidic foods, gently rinsing with saline solution, and topical medications.

   a. Amlexanox (Aphthasol) (5 per cent) oral paste applied to the ulcers four times daily accelerates the resolution of pain and healing.

   b. Hyaluronan with 3 per cent diclofenac relieves pain by coating the ulcer.

   c. Benzocaine (Americaine), dyclonine HCl (Dyclone), benzydamine HCl, and a viscous lidocaine (Alphacaine), pectin/Kaolin, and diphenhydramine (Benadryl) combination may be applied to the ulcer three to four times a day. Topical viscous lidocaine (3 ml of 2% solution) held in the mouth for 1 to 2 minutes before meals is effective.

   d. Tetracycline-cyanoacrylate (Actisite), or doxycycline-cyanoacrylate (Atridox), applied to the ulcer provides 6 days of pain relief after 1 latency day. This treatment is more effective in pain relief than triamcinolone-acetonide or chlorhexidine combined with cyanolate.

   e. Cauterizing the central portion of the ulcer with caustic agents, such as silver nitrate, relieves pain.

   f. Topical steroids provide relief for aphthous but not viral stomatitis.

      (1) Beclomethasone dipropionate (Beclovent) spray reduces the severity and frequency of ulcer pain but not the recurrence rate.

      (2) Dexamethasone (Decadron) elixir is beneficial when ulcers are on the soft palate.

      (3) Triamcinolone suspension (needs to be mixed by pharmacist) 5 ml oral rinse applied after meals and at bedtime produces prompt healing. Kenalog in Orabase when applied to lesions is equally effective.

   g. Moistened sucralfate (Carafate), dabbed onto ulcers several times a day, allows eating on the first day and ulcer healing on day 2.

2. Use systemic or locally injected medications in severe cases of aphthous stomatitis.

   a. Oral prednisone may be needed for persistent ulcers.

   b. Colchicine, administered as 0.6 mg orally three or four times daily, or dapsone during the prodromal stage may terminate ulcer formation, but the lesions may recur within days of drug discontinuance.

   c. Pentoxifylline (Trental), administered as 400 mg orally three times a day, decreases pain, the number of lesions, and their duration.

3. Antibacterial washes (tetracycline mouthwash or chlorhexidine gluconate oral rinse [Peridex]) may diminish secondary bacterial infection.

4. Topical acyclovir (Zovirax) (5 per cent) may help herpes labialis. Consider oral acyclovir during the prodrome.

5. Provide symptomatic relief for viral syndrome.

6. Treat other infections accordingly (e.g., syphilis, tuberculosis).

7. For HIV-positive patients, 100 to 200 mg thalidomide each day for 4 weeks may benefit. Thalidomide is contraindicated in HIV-associated polyneuropathy, polyradiculopathy, and encephalopathy.

Diet

1. Avoid hot, acidic, irritating foods. Encourage fluid intake.

2. Role of iron, B_{12}, and folate supplementation is not clear.

Patient Education

1. Probably a role in aphthous stomatitis for stress reduction.

2. Patients with herpesvirus infection need to understand they are infectious.

Key Treatment

- Saline rinses
- Steroid cream applied locally

Follow-Up

Perform biopsy on any ulcer that fails to heal spontaneously in 10 to 14 days.

Bibliography

Eversole LR: Inflammatory diseases of the mucous membranes. Part 1: Viral and fungal infections; Part 2: Immunopathologic ulcerative desquamative diseases. CDA (Calif Dent Assoc) J 1994;22:52–66.

Greenspan D, Greenspan JS: Oral lesions of HIV infection: features and therapy. AIDS Clin Rev 1992;4:225–239.

Rogers RS III: Common lesions of the oral mucosa: a guide to diseases of the lips, cheeks, tongue, gingivae. Postgrad Med 1992;91:141–148, 151–153.

Ship JA: Recurrent aphthous stomatitis: an update. Oral Surg Oral Med Oral Pathol Oral Radiol Endod 1996; 81:141–147.

Woo SB, Sonis ST: Recurrent aphthous ulcer: a review of diagnosis and treatment. J Am Dent Assoc 1996;127: 1202–1213.

14 Cheilitis and Angular Cheilitis

Jeffrey W. Hemp

Etiology

Cheilitis

1. Contact cheilitis
   a. Irritant; contributing factors include
      (1) Dryness, windburn, and sunburn
      (2) Citrus fruits, mangos, artichokes, and others
   b. Allergic
      (1) Tartar-control toothpastes, lipsticks, sunscreens, lip balms, and cane reed instruments
      (2) Foods and flavorings
2. Plasma cell cheilitis
   a. Rare, benign inflammatory disorder but underlying myeloma occasionally present
   b. Idiopathic but contact hypersensitivity may play a role.
3. Exfoliative cheilitis
   a. Chronic, inflammatory disorder with persistent, recurrent scaling
   b. Factitious activity: repetitive biting, licking, or picking at lips
   c. May be associated with actinic cheilitis, glandular cheilitis, lupus, *Candida*, and human immunodeficiency virus (HIV).
4. Cheilitis glandularis
   a. Rare, chronic inflammatory disorder of labial sweat glands
   b. May be associated with squamous cell carcinoma, actinic exposure, emotional problems, atopy, and familial macrocheilia.
5. Cheilitis granulomatosa
   a. Rare, idiopathic inflammatory disorder
   b. Recurrent lymphedema in young adult years; becomes permanent
6. Actinic cheilitis
   a. Chronic, premalignant condition, usually of lower lip; affects mostly fair-skinned males ages 40 to 80.
   b. Associated with prolonged sun exposure
   c. May evolve into squamous cell carcinoma; may metastasize in 10 per cent of cases.

7. Infectious cheilitis
   a. Herpes simplex, *Candida*, and bacterial forms (especially staphylococcus)
   b. Causative agents similar to those of angular cheilitis.

Angular Cheilitis

1. Synonyms: angular stomatitis, angular cheilosis, rhagades, and perleche
2. Most often seen in elderly
   a. Loss of vertical dimension in denture wearers or edentulous persons
   b. Denture stomatitis, overhanging skinfolds, moisture retention, and drooling
   c. May be associated with xerostomia, Sjögren's syndrome, perioral dermatitis, and orofacial granulomatosis.
3. Infectious
   a. *Candida*, especially in immunocompromised states (HIV, diabetes, cancer) and associated with oral candidiasis
   b. Bacterial, especially *Staphylococcus* and *Streptococcus* species.
   c. Viral, primarily herpes simplex I
4. Nutritional deficiencies
   a. Iron deficiency states, associated with glossitis, anemia, splenomegaly, and spooning of nails
   b. Folate deficiency, associated with glossitis, keratitis, and dermatitis
   c. Ariboflavinosis, associated with glossitis
   d. Vitamin B_{12} deficiency, associated with glossitis
5. Other: mechanical irritation, trauma, activity changes, and chronic irritation from smoking

Symptoms
1. Sensation of dryness
2. Irritation, burning, or discomfort of lips or corners of mouth
3. Intermittent bleeding, intermittent or chronic swelling

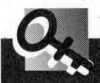

- Burning
- Discomfort
- Swelling
- Irritation
- Bleeding

Clinical Findings

1. Contact cheilitis
   a. Crusts, scales, and/or fissures
   b. Erythema, edema, vesicles
2. Plasma cell cheilitis
   a. Glistening, red lower lip; may involve oral mucosa
   b. Fissures, ulcerations, pain and food sensitivity
3. Exfoliative cheilitis: scaling and desquamation of vermilion epithelium
4. Cheilitis glandularis: swollen, enlarged, and everted lips with crusting and nodularity
5. Cheilitis granulomatosa
   a. Nontender, nodular swelling of one or both lips
   b. May have facial distortion.
   c. Associated findings: sarcoidosis, Crohn's disease, Melkersson-Rosenthal syndrome (facial nerve paralysis, fissured tongue)
6. Actinic cheilitis
   a. Erythema, crusting, erosions, bleeding or painful fissures
   b. Leukoplakia, atrophy, or friable patch
7. Infectious cheilitis
   a. Pustules: staphylococcus; vesicles: herpes
   b. Erythema/scaling: *Candida*
   c. May involve lips or corners of mouth.
8. Angular cheilitis
   a. Atrophy, erythema, ulcerations or fissures confined to corners of mouth
   b. Crusting, scaling
   c. Suppuration and granulation tissue in chronic cases

- Erythema
- Scaling
- Fissures
- Pain
- Swelling
- Ulcers

Laboratory Tests

1. Complete blood count (CBC), glucose, serum albumin, and vitamin B levels in suspected nutritional deficiencies and to rule out diabetes mellitus
2. Smear or culture in suspected infectious etiologies
3. HIV testing, tests for immunodeficiency if indicated
4. Patch testing in atopic or allergic cases
5. Biopsy for diagnosis or to rule out cancer or precancerous conditions

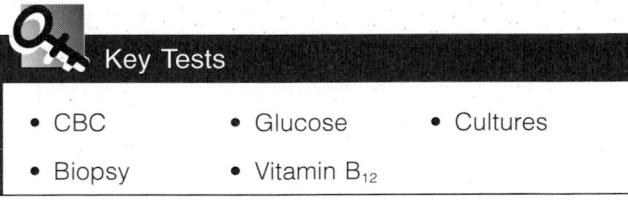

- CBC
- Glucose
- Cultures
- Biopsy
- Vitamin B_{12}

Differential Diagnosis

1. Dysplasia, carcinoma in situ and squamous cell carcinoma
   a. Occurs more often on lower lip
   b. Clinically may appear as leukoplakia or erythroplakia
   c. Risk factors: fair-skinned, low socioeconomic status, sun exposure, tobacco use, male sex, poor dentition, chronic irritation or infection
2. Basal cell carcinoma
   a. Occurs more often on upper lip
   b. Raised, nodular lesions with pearly borders and telangiectasias
   c. Risk factors: sun exposure, fair-skinned, male sex
3. Lichen planus
   a. Inflammatory dermatosis occasionally affecting lips
   b. Lesions are reticular with whitish streaks; papules, plaques, or ulcerations may be present
   c. Diagnose with biopsy.
4. Lichenoid drug eruptions: associated with nonsteroidal anti-inflammatory drugs, thiazides, methyldopa, phenothiazines, and gold
5. Pemphigus and pemphigoid
   a. Blisters and erosions are characteristic.
   b. More often involves oral cavity and not lips.
6. Systemic diseases: Crohn's disease, sarcoidosis, Melkersson-Rosenthal syndrome, Ascher's syndrome, angioedema, urticaria, amyloidosis, and CREST (calcinosis, Raynaud's phenomenon, esophageal involvement, sclerodactyly, telangiectasia) syndrome.

Treatment

1. Surgical
   a. Dysplastic conditions and carcinoma in situ: cryosurgery, CO_2 laser vaporization, or vermilionectomy
   b. Cheilitis glandularis: vermilionectomy or surgical reduction (severe cases)
   c. Basal cell carcinoma: wedge excision
   d. Invasive squamous cell cancer: vermilionectomy or more radical procedures

2. Medication
   a. Infectious etiologies
      (1) Viral: topical/systemic acyclovir (Zovirax) or similar antiviral agents
      (2) Bacterial: mupirocin ointment, systemic antibiotics
      (3) Fungal: topical (clotrimazole [Mycelex, Lotrimin]) or systemic (fluconazole [Diflucan]) agents
   b. Emollients: useful for dryness and crusting in contact cheilitis
   c. B vitamins and iron: in documented cases of deficiency, some use empirically.
   d. Corticosteroids
      (1) Topical
         (a) Contact cheilitis
         (b) Fluorinated forms (e.g., fluocinonide [Lidex]) best; watch out for atrophy.
         (c) May worsen exfoliative cheilitis.
      (2) Systemic: cheilitis glandularis and granulomatosa
      (3) Intralesional or topical useful for plasma cell cheilitis.
   e. Antidepressants and antianxiety agents may be useful in exfoliative cheilitis.

3. Other
   a. Good oral hygiene to prevent infection
   b. Properly fitted dentures should be cleaned and removed at night (angular cheilitis).

Diet

Unless dietary deficiencies exist, there are no specific dietary measures.

Patient Education

Patient understanding of disease and contributing factors is essential to control all forms of these diseases.

Key Treatment

- Directed at specific cause

Follow-Up

1. Every 1 to 2 weeks to assess response in acute or severe cases
2. In stabilized cases, less frequent evaluations indicated.
3. In suspected precancerous lesions, a biopsy is indicated and long-term follow-up recommended.

Bibliography

Archad H: Biology and pathology of the oral mucosa. In Fitzpatrick T, Eisen A, Wolft K, et al (eds): Dermatology in General Medicine, 3rd ed, vol 1, pp 1202–1204. New York, McGraw-Hill, 1987.

Ophaswongsse S, Maibach H: Allergic contact cheilitis. Contact Dermatitis 1995;33:365–370.

Rogers R, Bekic M: Diseases of the lips. Semin Cutan Med Surg 1997;16:328–336.

Samaranayake LP, Wilkieson CA, Lamey PJ, MacFarlane TW: Oral disease in the elderly in long-term hospital care. Oral Dis 1995;1:147–151.

Tanigvchi S, Kono T: Exfoliative cheilitis. Dermatology 1998;196:253–255.

15 Glaucoma

Deepa Vasudevan

1. Glaucoma is defined as a condition in which there is an increase in the intraocular pressure (IOP) of the eyeball (normal pressure being 10 to 23 mm Hg). This condition results in visual deficits and optic disc changes. It may occasionally present in the presence of a normal IOP, which is currently a hot research topic.

2. Glaucoma is among the most common causes of blindness in the United States, with a prevalence of 0.5 per cent of the total population. This condition demonstrates an increasing trend after the age of 60. Glaucoma is thought to occur more frequently in the African American population, the cause of which is still unknown at this time.

3. Aqueous humor produced by the ciliary epithelium flows from the posterior chamber to the anterior chamber, into the chamber angle, and through the trabecular network into the canal of Schlemm. The fluid finally flows into the episcleral veins.

Etiology

1. Increase in the volume of the intraocular contents, which could be secondary to
   a. Increase in the aqueous humor production
   b. Decrease in the drainage of the aqueous humor secondary to obstruction
   c. Increase in the blood volume as a result of capillary and arterial dilatation
   d. Decrease in the venous outflow
   e. Increase in the volume of the lens and the vitreous humor
2. External pressure upon the eyeball

Classification

1. Congenital glaucoma or buphthalmos
   a. Usually inherited as an autosomal recessive trait (80 per cent) with incomplete penetrance
   b. Usually manifests itself by 6 months to 3 years of age and is bilateral
   c. Occurrence is secondary to a defective iridocorneal angle
   d. This condition leads to an enlargement of the eyeball and is also associated with photophobia and defective vision
2. Acquired glaucoma (see Fig. 15–1)

Open-Angle Glaucoma

This constitutes about 90 per cent of all cases of glaucoma. The clinical presentation usually occurs insidiously over a period of months to years. Identification of the problem by the patient may not happen until there is substantial increase in the IOP and development of visual deficits. Ocular risk factors are

1. Genetically prone persons
2. Persons with a positive family history
3. African Americans
4. Myopic prescriptions over −5 diopters
5. Other population groups with a clinical history or examination suggestive for probable development of glaucoma

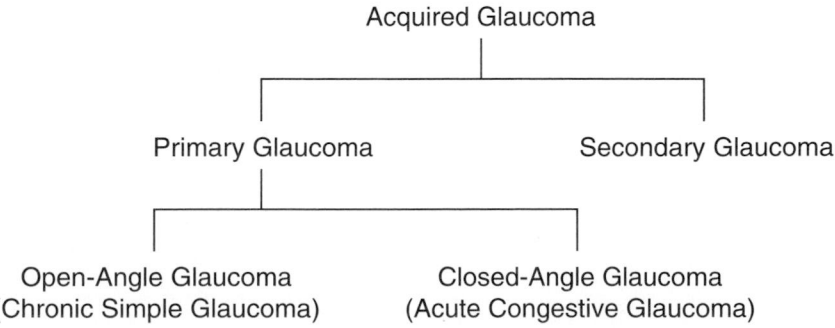

Figure 15–1 Different types of acquired glaucoma. Absolute glaucoma is a stage of glaucoma wherein the sense of perception and projection of light is lost. This can occur as an end stage of both acquired and congenital glaucoma.

Epidemiology and Etiology

1. Incidence is most common in the middle-age to elderly population groups. There is a slight male preponderance and the occurrence is usually bilateral.
2. The cause for the development of this type of glaucoma is thought to be multifactorial, with one of the components most probably being genetically determined, the inheritance pattern of which has not been clearly determined to date.
3. This condition is probably due to a decrease in the outflow of aqueous humor as result of changes in the trabecular pattern of Schlemm's canals or in the exit channels from Schlemm's canal. Over time this leads to an increase in the volume of aqueous humor, which eventually results in an increase in the IOP, which results in atrophy of the retinal nerve fibers and ganglion cells. This condition finally leads to optic disk cupping and optic nerve atrophy, which, if left untreated, can lead to atrophy of the entire uveal tract. It is important to understand that all these changes occur with an open angle.

Symptoms

1. Slow onset with no to minimal symptoms in the early stages is the most common presentation in this type of glaucoma.
2. Mild headaches and eye ache with very minimal loss of peripheral vision can occur initially, which can progress over time to tunnel vision (i.e., persistence of central vision only).
3. Presbyopic prescriptions may need to be changed frequently secondary to accommodative weakness resulting from pressure on the ciliary muscle.
4. Night blindness can also occur as a late change.
5. Untreated cases can lead to complete blindness.

Key Symptoms

- Minimal eye ache/ headache
- Blurred vision/loss of peripheral vision (may be perceived by the patient only in the later stages of the disease)

Clinical Findings

Patients may initially have a normal looking eye but in the later stages usually develop corneal haziness with increase in IOP. Optic disk cupping with an increase in the cup/disk ratio to greater than 0.6 is usually diagnostic. The progressive visual field deficits associated with this type of glaucoma are

1. Baring of the blind spot
2. Development of small wing-shaped scotoma, which appear above and below the blind spot and later coalesce with the blind spot to lead to the development of a sickle-shaped scotoma (positive Seidel's sign). On further progression of the disease, extension of the scotoma occurs and an arcuate or Bjerrum's scotoma is formed. Two arcuate scotoma join around the fixation point to form an annular scotoma.

Key Signs

- Visual field deficits
- Increase in IOP
- Optic disk cupping

Tests

1. Tonometry
2. Perimetry
3. Ophthalmoscopic examination
4. Gonioscopy to measure the angle of the anterior chamber

Differential Diagnosis

1. Immature cataract
2. Optic atrophy

Treatment

1. Medical
   a. Miotic eyedrops (e.g., pilocarpine) help in the absorption of aqueous humor by dilating the blood vessels.
   b. Topical β-adrenergic antagonists act by decreasing the aqueous humor production and helping outflow.
   c. Carbonic anhydrase inhibitors may be used in the oral/parenteral form to tide over the crisis.
2. Surgical: usually undertaken if the medical management fails
   a. Trabeculectomy with subscleral filtration and drainage through opened canals of Schlemm.
   b. Iridencleisis
   c. Elliot's sclerocorneal trephine
   d. Laser trabeculoplasty

Closed-Angle Glaucoma

This is a condition wherein there is an increase in IOP secondary to obstruction of the outflow of aqueous humor caused by an extremely narrow/closed anterior chamber angle. The onset is usually acute and can lead to complete blindness if the condition is not promptly treated. This condition is considered a true ophthalmic emergency.

Epidemiology and Etiology

1. The condition occurs most commonly in the 45- to 60-year-old age group. There is a slight female preponderance. Usually one eye is affected first, followed by the other eye. Ocular risk factors are

    a. Positive family history

    b. Hypermetropia

    c. Shallow anterior chamber

    d. Congenital narrow angle secondary to small eyeball, big ciliary body, or an increase in the size of the lens

2. About 1.5 per cent of the general population have narrow anterior chamber angles, but not all develop glaucoma, and hence this condition is uncommon.

3. The episode occurs suddenly or can be precipitated by pupillary dilatation (which could be secondary to going into a dark room, due to pharmacologic mydriasis for an ophthalmoscopic examination, or due to dilatation in times of stress). In the elderly it is common secondary to the physiologic enlargement of the lens.

Pathology

1. The dilatation of the pupil leads to a narrow angle, as a result of which there is an increase in IOP that further leads to capillary stasis, causing an increase in the capillary permeability. This leads to congestive edema of the corneal epithelium and anterior ciliary veins of the conjunctiva.

2. After 72 hours of an acute episode there is mild papilledema and hydropic degeneration of the nerve fibers anterior to the lamina cribrosa.

3. If untreated, severe papilledema with disintegration of the nerve fibers occurs, which results in optic disk cupping and cavernous atrophy of the optic nerve, similar to the changes that occur in chronic simple glaucoma.

Symptoms

1. Sudden onset of intense pain in the affected eye with headache

2. The local symptoms can be associated with abdominal pain, prostration, nausea, and vomiting.

3. Marked visual deficits that in some cases could be reduced to only projection and perception of light can occur.

4. Other symptoms associated with this condition are photophobia, lacrimation, and visualization of color halos around a light source.

Key Symptoms

- Sudden onset of pain in the affected eye
- Marked visual loss

Clinical Findings

1. Edema of the eyelid with congestion/chemosis of the conjunctiva

2. Steamy and hazy cornea with ciliary injection

3. Anterior chamber is shallow.

4. Pupil is mid-dilated with loss of light and accommodative reflex.

5. Increase in IOP

6. Visual deficits

Key Signs

- Narrow angle
- Increase in IOP
- Marked visual deficits

Tests

1. Tonometry

2. Gonioscopy, which is used to measure the angle of the anterior chamber. A grading system determines the severity of the problem based on the chamber angle.

Differential Diagnosis

1. Mucopurulent conjunctivitis

2. Iridocyclitis

3. Corneal trauma or infection

Treatment

1. Medical

    a. The initial treatment is a combination of oral and topical agents to lower IOP.

    b. Acetazolamide is used orally/parenterally to control IOP initially. Miotic eyedrops (e.g., pilocarpine) can be used, 1 drop in the affected eye every 15 minutes for 1 hour, to drop IOP in the acute setting.

    c. Topical β-blockers, 1 to 2 drops in the affected eye every 30 minutes for 1 hour; can be used about 5 minutes after using the miotic eyedrops.

    d. One or both of these agents may need to be used on a continual basis after the treatment of an acute episode.

2. Surgical

    a. Laser peripheral iridectomy/iridotomy will usually result in permanent cure and is recommended after the initial control of IOP of an acute attack.

    b. The contralateral eye needs to be treated with prophylactic iridectomy/iridotomy.

Prognosis

Untreated acute glaucoma results in severe and permanent visual loss within 2 to 5 days after the onset of clinical symptoms.

Secondary Glaucoma

This is a condition associated with an increase in IOP secondary to a pre-existing condition.

Etiology

Some causes of secondary glaucoma are

1. Postiridocyclitis
2. Scleritis
3. Panophthalmitis
4. Lens-induced glaucoma secondary to cataract
5. Steroid-induced glaucoma
6. Aphakic glaucoma

Treatment

1. The acute phase is treated with carbonic anhydrase inhibitors and, if needed, osmotic diuresis.
2. Once the acute episode is resolved, the underlying pathogenesis is determined and treated.

Bibliography

Chatterjee BM: Handbook of Ophthalmology, 6th ed, pp 162–200. New Delhi, India, CBS Publishers, 1997.

Kanski J: Clinical Ophthalmology, 3rd ed, pp 233–279. London, Butterworth Heinemann, 1994.

Palay D, Krachmir J: Glaucoma. In Beck A (ed): Ophthalmology for the Primary Care Physician, pp 135–142. New York, Mosby–Year Book, 1997.

Pau H: Differential Diagnosis of Eye Diseases, 3rd ed, pp 268–275. New York, Thieme Medical Publishers, 1988.

Tiernay L, McPhee S, Papadakis M: Eye. In Riordan P, Vaughan D (eds): Current Medical Diagnosis and Treatment, 33rd ed, pp 158–161. East Norwalk, CT, Prentice-Hall International, 1994.

Tolbert S: Glaucoma. In Rakel R (ed): Saunders Manual of Medical Practice, pp 66–68. Philadelphia, WB Saunders Company, 1996.

16 Sjögren's Syndrome

Tanya Y. Jones

Sjögren's syndrome is an autoimmune disorder. Patients have a genetic sensitivity that seems triggered by an environmental exposure. It is characterized by dry eyes, dry mouth, endocrine and exocrine dysfunction, peripheral and/or central vasculitis, and other systemic manifestations. Although frequently mild in expression with a waxing and waning course of symptoms, it can be a serious disease.

Etiology

1. Genetic factors
   a. Nonmonozygotic twin concordance
   b. Increased frequency in relatives of patients with Sjögren's syndrome or other autoimmune disorder
   c. *Primary Sjögren's syndrome*: association with human leukocyte antigen (HLA)-D3 in African Americans, most Caucasian Americans, and northern Europeans; HLA-DR5 and DRw-53 in Japanese and Greeks; HLA-D8 in Chinese
   d. *Secondary Sjögren's syndrome* (predominant form): association with HLA-DR4 along with another autoimmune disorder, especially rheumatoid arthritis, mixed connective tissue disease, systemic lupus erythematosus (SLE), scleroderma, or polymyositis
   e. Frequent presence of HLA anti-SS A and anti-SS B
2. Environmental factors
   a. Viral stimulus may trigger expression of Sjögren's sydrome.
   b. Associated viruses include hepatitis C and B, Epstein-Barr, cytomegalovirus, herpesvirus 6, and various retroviruses.
2. Gender and age factors
   a. Can be expressed in either gender and at any age, including children.
   b. Female predominence of 90 per cent suggests a hormonally related neuroendocrine abberation in the autoregulation of the immune system is probably involved.
   c. Average age of expression is 45 to 55 years; coincides with perimenopause.
4. Risk factors
   a. Positive family history of Sjögren's syndrome

b. History of silicone breast implants
c. History of radiation therapy

> **Note**
> Lymphoma, human immunodeficiency virus (HIV), and sarcoidosis must be excluded prior to making a diagnosis of Sjögren's syndrome.

Symptoms

1. Inability to tear properly, with resultant dry eyes and thick mucous discharge and insults to cornea and conjunctiva (keratoconjunctivitis sicca); waking mucous film or excess "rope-like" mucus in the eyes
2. Eye fatigue, burning, itching, foreign body sensation (gritty, sandy)
3. Inability to produce sufficient saliva resulting in dysphagia, especially with dry foods
4. Increased dental caries, oral and upper airway infections
5. Unexplained abdominal pain or dyspareunia
6. Confusion with menopausal symptoms, including stress, arthralgias, gynecologic infections, skin and hair changes, mood, sleep and urination pattern alterations with "normal" aging process
7. Stiff and aching muscles or joints
8. Unexplained rashes
9. Redness, blanching, or swelling of the fingers or hands
10. Stress/depression
11. Nocturnal leg cramps
12. Photosensitive lesions similar to SLE

Key Symptoms

- Dry mouth
- Dry irritated eyes
- Difficulty swallowing
- Difficulty speaking
- Alterations in taste

Clinical Findings

1. Deeply fissured, beefy red tongue
2. Rope-like mucus in the eyes
3. Chapped lips and angular cheilosis
4. Decreased tear formation
5. Decreased saliva formation
6. Corneal or conjunctival abnormalities
7. Decreased papillae of tongue
8. Mutiple dental cavities
9. Oral *Candida* infection
10. Splenomegaly or hepatomegaly
11. Parotid or submandibular gland swelling or enlargement
12. Soft tissue nodules under the skin

Clinical Findings in Sjögren's Syndrome

Ocular

- Dry, "gritty" eyes
- "Rope-like" or filmy mucous eye discharge
- Inability to tear adequately
- Photosensitivity
- Corneal/conjunctival opacities or lesions
- Eye fatigue

Systemic Vasculitis

- Unexplained dyspareunia/abdominal pain
- Skin lesions/reddening, rashes, purpura, urticaria
- Glomerular nephritis/renal tubular acidosis
- Cranial neuropathy, especially trigeminal
- Aseptic meningitis/seizure activity
- Peripheral neuropathy
- Interstitial pneumonia
- Subclinical hypothyroidism

Oral

- Dry "cotton" mouth
- Difficulty swallowing dry foods
- Chapped lips/angular cheilosis
- Yeast or bacterial oral/upper airway infections
- Accelerated dental caries formation
- Loss of sense of taste

Immune Mediated

- Myalgias/arthralgias/myosities
- Fatigue
- Subcutaneous nodules
- Alopecia areata
- Raynaud's phenomenon/reddening or swelling
- Hashimoto's thyroiditis
- Pleuropericarditis
- Diabetes insipidus

Key Signs

- "Click sign": clicking while speaking (tongue sticks to mouth while speaking)
- "Cotton mouth sign": severe dryness of oral mucosa
- "Rope-like" mucus in eyes

WARNING

There is a 44-fold increase in the incidence of malignant lymphoma in Sjögren's syndrome patients.

Tests

1. Schirmer tear formation test: 2 mm or less in 5 minutes (15 mm in 5 minutes is normal)
2. Rose bengal stain test
3. Complete blood count (CBC) for anemia, leukopenia, eosinophilia
4. Salivary gland biopsy
5. Salivary scintigraphy
6. Parotid sialography
7. Erythrocyte sedimentation rate
8. Rheumatoid factor greater than 1:320
9. Antinuclear antibodies greater than 1:320
10. Whole saliva anti-Ro and La antibodies (anti-SS-A and -SS-B; polyclonal B lymphocytes)
11. Homocysteine levels
12. Thyroid function, saliva viscosity, pooling or spin tests

Key Tests

- Schirmer tear formation test
- Rose bengal stain test
- CBC for anemia, leukopenia, eosinophilia
- Erythrocyte sedimentation rate
- Rheumatoid factor test
- Antinuclear antibodies test

Diagnosis

1. History consistent with Sjögren's syndrome
2. Confirmation with salivary or lacrimal gland biopsy demonstrating focal accumulation of mononuclear cells around ducts and acini
3. Fifty or more primarily CD4 lymphocytes, T-helper cells, and B lymphocytes, which produce circulating autoantibodies leading to delayed apoptosis with resultant compromise of glandular function

Differential Diagnosis

1. Primary fibromylagia
2. Multiple sclerosis
3. Chronic fatigue syndrome

4. Hepatitis C– or B–related sicca
5. Autoimmune neuropathy
6. Salivary gland dysfunction
7. Blepharitis or meibomitis
8. Silicone breast implant symptoms
9. HIV-related diffuse lymphocytic syndrome
10. Lymphoma
11. Sarcoidosis
12. SLE, scleroderma, polymyositis, mixed connective tissue disorder
13. Rheumatoid arthritis
14. Drug side effects, especially tricyclics and clonidine
15. Depression or post-traumatic stress syndrome

Treatment

1. Artificial tears and ophthalmologic lubricants without preservatives
2. Frequent water intake and/or artificial saliva, Xylitol chewing gum, or Xyli-Fresh to promote salivation
3. Fluoride dentifrice; frequent flossing; periodic fluoride treatments
4. Frequent mouth rinse with solution of 1/4 tsp. salt, 1/4 tsp. baking soda, and 8 oz water
5. Topical antifungal agents to prevent oral candidiasis
6. Humidifiers in the sleeping area: nasal lavage when necessary to discourage mouth breathing
7. Colloidal oatmeal moisturizing products such as Aveeno and lubricants such as Eucerin after warm baths
8. Nonsteroidal anti-inflammatory medications for mild vasculitis and myalgias
9. Thorough gynecologic care to prevent and treat infections as well as dyspareunia
10. Quinine or alternatively clonazepam (0.5 to 1 mg qhs) for nocturnal myoclonus
11. Steroids, pilocarpine, methotrexate, antimalarials for severe symptoms and vasculitis
12. Appropriate support for organ compromise of kidneys, thyroid, pancreas, lungs

Key Treatment

- Artificial tears
- Frequent water intake and/or artificial saliva

- Fluoride dentifrice; frequent flossing; periodic fluoride treatments
- Frequent mouth rinse with solution of 1/4 tsp. salt, 1/4 tsp. baking soda, and 8 oz water

Diet

1. Low refined sugar, avoidance of alcohol and other gastritis-precipitating foods
2. Herbal teas such as chamomile for mild anti-inflammatory action
3. Increased water intake for skin hydration, salivation, tearing, and maximizing kidney function
4. Multivitamin supplement that includes folic acid, B$_{12}$, and antioxidants
5. Possible dehydroepiandrosterone supplementation in women suspected of androgen-estrogen imbalance

Activity

1. Low-impact exercise such as water aerobics, massage
2. Meditation or reflection time

Patient Education

1. Sjögren's syndrome support group
   a. Sjögren's Syndrome Foundation, 333 North Broadway, Jericho, NY 11753 (1-516-933-6365)
   b. National Sjögren's Syndrome Association, 3201 West Evans Drive, Phoenix, AZ 85023
2. Newsletter such as "The Moisture Seekers," published by the Sjögren's Syndrome Foundation

Bibliography

Fox RI: Sjögren's syndrome: controversies and progress. Clin Lab Med 1997;17:431–444.
Fox RI: Vth International Symposium on Sjögren's Syndrome: Clinical Aspects and Therapy. Clin Rheumatol 1995;14(Suppl 1).
Gobetti JP, Froeschle ML: Sjögren's syndrome: a challenge for dentistry. Gen Dentistry 1997;45:268–272.
Oxholm P, Asmussen K: Primary Sjögren's syndrome: the challenge for classification of disease manifestations. J Intern Med 1996;239:467–474.
Price EJ, Venables PJW: The etiopathogenesis of Sjögren's syndrome. Semin Arthritis Rheum 1995;225:117–133.

17 Conjunctivitis

Gary R. Gray

Conjunctivitis refers to inflammation of the conjunctiva, a thin mucous membrane that lines the inner surface of the eyelid and anterior sclera.

Etiology
Etiologic agents include viral and bacterial infections, as well as allergic disorders. Chemical exposure and impaired lacrimation are less common causes of conjunctival inflammation.

1. Infectious causes
   a. Viral
      (1) Adenoviruses have three clinically distinct presentations: follicular conjunctivitis; pharyngoconjunctival fever types 3, 4, and 7; and epidemic keratoconjunctivitis types 18 and 19.
      (2) Other causes: herpes simplex, coxsackie, varicella, measles, *Enterovirus*
   b. Bacterial: *Haemophilus* species, *Staphylococcus* species, *Streptococcus pneumoniae*, *Chlamydia trachomatis*, *Neisseria gonorrhoeae*, *Neisseria meningitidis*
2. Allergic disorders
3. Impaired tear production: dry eye syndrome, Sjögren's syndrome
4. Chemical exposure: industrial chemicals, household cleaners, cosmetics, topical medications

Symptoms
Patients with conjunctivitis report ocular irritation, itching, and accompanying discharge. Clinical presentation varies depending on etiologic agent.

Key Symptoms

- Eye irritation, itching, burning
- Discharge, tearing

Clinical Findings
Conjunctival hyperemia and discharge are universal findings in patients with conjunctivitis. Specific clinical findings provide clues of underlying cause (Table 17–1).

1. Viral conjunctivitis
   a. Watery discharge
   b. Often bilateral
   c. Preauricular adenopathy
   d. Lymphoid follicles on undersurface of lid
   e. Symptoms of concurrent viral upper respiratory tract infection
2. Bacterial conjunctivitis
   a. Purulent discharge
   b. Marked conjunctival injection
   c. Usually unilateral
   d. History of sexual contact in chlamydial and gonococcal infections
3. Allergic conjunctivitis
   a. Watery discharge
   b. Bilateral involvement
   c. Itching
   d. Associated allergic disorders (asthma, atopic dermatitis, allergic rhinitis)
4. Chemical conjunctivitis
   a. Watery or mucoid discharge
   b. History of chemical exposure
   c. Lack of associated upper respiratory and allergic symptoms
5. Keratoconjunctivitis sicca
   a. Common in older patients with impaired lacrimation
   b. Associated immune disorders (Sjögren's syndrome, rheumatoid arthritis)
   c. Patients complain of dryness and redness

Key Signs

- Hyperemia
- Tearing
- Discharge

Laboratory Tests
The diagnosis of conjunctivitis is often made on clinical findings alone. Evaluation includes a detailed history, physical examination, and appropriate lab-

TABLE 17–1. COMMON CAUSES AND DIAGNOSTIC FEATURES OF CONJUNCTIVITIS

	VIRAL	BACTERIAL	ALLERGIC	CHEMICAL

Etiology	Adenoviruses
	  types 3, 4, 7
	  (pharyngoconjunctival
	  fever)
	  Types 18, 19 (epidemic
	  keratoconjunctivitis)
	Other Causes: herpes
	  simplex, varicella-zoster,
	  measles, coxsackie,
	  Enterovirus
		Haemophilus influenzae,
		Staphylococcus aureus,
		Streptococcus pneumoniae,
		Neisseria gonorrhoeae,
		Neisseria meningitidis,
		Chlamydia trachomatis
			Pollens, molds, animal
			  dander, etc.
				Industrial/household
				  chemicals
				Topical medications

Physical findings				

Conjunctiva	Lymphoid follicles
	Diffuse hyperemia
	Subconjunctival
	  hemorrhage with
	  Enterovirus type 70
		Marked hyperemia	Diffuse hyperemia	Variable hyperemia

Discharge	Watery discharge	Purulent discharge	Watery discharge	Watery or mucoid discharge
Adenopathy	Preauricular adenopathy	Uncommon except in chlamydial infections	Absent	Absent

oratory tests to identify underlying etiology. A systemic evaluation should include

1. History
   a. Duration and progression of symptoms
   b. Precipitating events
   c. Associated symptoms (pharyngitis, nasal congestion, cough)
   d. Allergic disorders
2. Documentation of visual acuity
3. Examination of
   a. Eyelids and lashes
   b. Cornea
   c. Pupil
   d. Bulbar and palpebral conjunctiva
   e. Fluorescein staining will help identify corneal involvement.
   f. Slit-lamp examination if available
4. Gram's stain and culture of conjunctival scrapings if discharge is purulent

Key Tests

- Visual acuity
- Fluorescein staining/slit-lamp exam if available
- Gram's stain and culture

Differential Diagnosis

The primary concern when evaluating the patient with conjunctivitis is to rule out any vision-threatening conditions.

1. Corneal ulceration and abrasions can be diagnosed with fluorescein staining and generally present with pain, foreign body sensation, and photophobia.
2. Keratitis refers to inflammation of the cornea and is characterized by pain, photophobia, tearing, and injection.
3. Iritis presents with photophobia, marked injection, and sluggish pupillary reflex.
4. Acute glaucoma presents with severe globe pain, injection, corneal clouding, and sluggish, dilated pupil.

WARNING

Globe pain, marked photophobia, and decreased visual acuity suggest disease of other eye structures. Prompt referral should be considered.

Treatment

Treatment should be guided by identification of the underlying etiology. Treatment may be primarily supportive or require the use of topical or systemic antimicrobial therapy. Contact lenses should not be worn until infection resolves.

Viral Conjunctivitis

1. Adenoviral conjunctivitis (usually self-limited, lasting 1 to 3 weeks)
   a. Supportive treatment (warm compresses, antipyretics)
   b. Steroids have no effect on outcome, al-

though they may be used to relieve symptoms in severe cases.

c. Topical antibiotics are commonly used to prevent secondary infection.

d. Careful attention to hand washing to avoid spreading infection

2. Herpes simplex/varicella-zoster conjunctivitis

a. Prompt consultation with an ophthalmologist for confirmation of diagnosis and institution of antiviral therapy

b. Steroids are contraindicated.

Bacterial Conjunctivitis

1. Acute bacterial conjunctivitis

a. Topical antimicrobial drops every 3 to 4 hours while awake for 5 to 7 days (Table 17–2)

b. Sulfonamide solutions cause mild transient stinging.

c. Neomycin solutions may cause conjunctival and cutaneous sensitization.

d. Antimicrobial ointments may be easier for young children.

2. Gonococcal infections

a. Systemic antibiotics necessary per Centers for Disease Control and Prevention guidelines.

b. May rapidly progress to corneal perforation; prompt consultation with an ophthalmologist is required.

3. Chlamydial infections

a. Tetracycline 500 mg qid for 3 to 4 weeks

b. Doxycycline 100 mg bid for 3 weeks

c. Erythromycin 500 mg qid for 3 to 4 weeks

d. Refer to ophthalmologist if corneal involvement.

Allergic Conjunctivitis

1. Allergen avoidance

2. Cool compresses

3. Topical antihistamines, nonsteroidal anti-inflammatory drugs, vasoconstrictors, mast cell stabilizers (Table 17–3)

4. Topical steroids should typically be used only under the direction of an ophthalmologist.

Keratoconjunctivitis Sicca

1. Treat underlying cause.

2. Artificial tears and lubricating ointments

Chemical Conjunctivitis

1. Avoidance of offending agent

2. Cool compresses

3. Lubricating eyedrops

4. Consultation with ophthalmologist if persistent or severe symptoms

Key Treatment

- Comfort measures
- Topical antibiotics
- Ocular allergy medications

TABLE 17–2.　COMMONLY USED OPHTHALMIC ANTIBIOTICS

Antibiotic	Recommended Dose*
Sulfonamide	
Sulfacetamide sodium 10% solution† (Sodium Sulamyd)	1–2 drops every 3–4 hr (not recommended under 1 yr)
Quinolones	
Norfloxacin 0.3% solution (Chibroxin)	1–2 drops 4 times daily (not recommended under 1 yr)
Ciprofloxacin HCl 0.3% solution (Ciloxan)	1–2 drops every 4 hr (not recommended under 1 yr)
Ofloxacin 0.3% solution (Ocuflox)	1–2 drops every 4 hr (not recommended under 1 yr)
Aminoglycosides	
Gentamicin 3-mg/ml solution† (Garamycin)	1–2 drops every 4 hr
Tobramycin 0.3% solution† (Tobrex)	1–2 drops every 4 hr
Neomycin-Polymyxin B	
Multiple preparations	1–2 drops 4–6 times daily (neomycin may cause sensitization)
Macrolide	
Erythromycin 5-mg/gm ointment (Ilotycin)	0.5-in ribbon 2–3 times daily

*Dosing frequency may be increased for first 24 to 48 hours and in severe infections.
†Available in ointments.

TABLE 17–3. COMMONLY USED OCULAR ALLERGY MEDICATIONS

ALLERGY MEDICATION	RECOMMENDED DOSE
Antihistamine Levocabastine HCl 0.05% (Livostin)	1 drop 4 times daily Contraindicated with soft contacts
Vasoconstrictor-antihistamine Naphazoline HCl 0.025% with pheniramine maleate 0.3% (Naphcon-A, Naphoptic-A)	1–2 drops 4 times daily Contraindicated with narrow-angle glaucoma, monoamine oxidase inhibitors, contact lenses
Nonsteroidal anti-inflammatory drug Ketorolac tromethamine 0.5% solution (Acular)	1 drop 4 times daily Contraindicated in aspirin sensitivity, pregnancy
Mast cell stabilizers Lodoxamine 0.1% solution (Alomide) Cromolyn sodium 4% solution (Crolom)	1–2 drops 4 times daily 1–2 drops 4–6 times daily Contraindicated with soft contact lenses
Antihistamine-mast cell stabilizer Olopatadine HCl 0.1% (Patanol)	1–2 drops twice daily

---

> **WARNING**
>
> Ophthalmologic consultation should be considered before using ocular steroid preparations.

Follow-Up

Most cases of conjunctivitis are self-limited and respond promptly to therapy. Some authorities recommend routine re-evaluation within 48 to 72 hours. All patients should be re-examined if symptoms persist or worsen despite treatment. Patients who fail to improve after 5 to 7 days of therapy or who develop progressive corneal infiltrates should be referred to an ophthalmologist.

 Bibliography

Cullom RD, Chang B: The Wills Eye Manual: Office and Emergency Room Treatment of Eye Disease, 2nd ed, pp 109–118. Philadelphia, JB Lippincott Company, 1994.

Friedlaender MH: A review of the causes and treatment of bacterial and allergic conjunctivitis. Clin Ther 1995; 17:800–810.

Hara JH: The red eye: diagnosis and treatment. Am Fam Physician 1996;54:2423–2430.

Ruppert SD: Differential diagnosis of pediatric conjunctivitis. Nurse Pract 1996;21:12–26.

Weber CM, Eichenbaum JW: Acute red eye: differentiating viral conjunctivitis from other, less common causes. Postgrad Med 1997;101:189–192, 195–196.

18 Corneal Ulceration

Ashish Chabra

Etiology

1. Infection of the cornea by bacteria, virus, or fungi as a result of breakdown in the protective epithelial barrier
2. Dry eyes, contact lenses, burns, abrasions, or foreign body entry to the eye (i.e., trauma); severe allergic eye disease
3. Inappropriate use of topical anesthetics or antiviral or antibiotic medications
4. Diabetes, thyroid disease (fifth-nerve palsy, exophthalmos)
5. Chronic blepharitis, conjunctivitis, or herpes simplex keratitis
6. Immunosuppression or immunosuppressive drugs resulting in opportunistic infections
7. Vitamin A or protein malnutrition
8. Defective closure of the eyelids (lagophthalmos)
9. Infectious agents include the following:
   a. Gram-positive organisms (e.g., staphylococci, streptococci, bacilli)
   b. Gram-negative organisms (e.g., rods, diplococci)
   c. Anaerobes
   d. Viruses (e.g., herpes)
   e. *Pseudomonas*
   f. Sexually transmitted diseases (trachoma, gonorrhea)
   g. Fungi
   h. Amebas (*Acanthamoeba*)
   i. Various inflammatory disorders (either ocular or part of a systemic vasculitis [e.g., Sjögren's syndrome])

Symptoms

1. Red eyes
2. Sensation of foreign body in affected eye
3. Blurred vision
4. Discharge from affected eye (i.e., mucopurulent or serous if viral)
5. Pain in the eye, especially with movement
6. Photophobia
7. Blepharospasm
8. Tearing

Key Symptoms

- Foreign-body sensation
- Eye discharge
- Blurred vision
- Pain

Clinical Findings

1. Inflammation and edema of eyelid
2. Conjunctival injection or inflammation; circumcorneal injection
3. Discharge from affected eye (i.e., mucopurulent versus serous)
4. Dull, grayish, circumscribed superficial infiltration that may progress to necrosis and ulcer formation (hypopyon)

Key Signs

- Edema and inflammation
- Mucopurulent discharge
- Ciliary injection
- Blepharospasm

Tests

1. Fluorescein stain to confirm ulcer
2. Culture
3. Scrapings for Gram's and Giemsa stains to identify bacteria, yeast, or intranuclear inclusions

Key Tests

- Fluorescein stain
- Culture

Differential Diagnosis

1. Identify infecting organism to determine if viral, bacterial, or fungal
2. Corneal abrasion
3. Corneal foreign body
4. Conjunctivitis

5. Keratitis
6. Blepharitis
7. Dacrocystitis

Treatment

1. Immediate institution of aggressive topical antibiotic treatment
2. Prompt referral to an ophthalmologist
3. Topical cycloplegics to help reduce inflammation and pain
4. Daily evaluation

WARNING

- **Topical steroids should never be used.**
- **Do not bandage the eye.**

Medication

1. Topical gentamicin (Garamycin) and tobramycin (Tobrex) for aerobic gram-negative organisms, *Enterobacter*, *Klebsiella*, and *Pseudomonas*
2. Topical cephalosporins (cefazolin [Kefzol]) for gram-positive organisms
3. Sulfacetamide 10% (Cetamide Ophthalmic) only for low-grade infections
4. Ciprofloxacin (Cipro) for *Pseudomonas* infections
5. Fungal infections need to be treated with parenteral amphotericin B (Fungizone); may also require ketoconazole (Nizoral), clotrimazole (Lotrimin), or miconazole (Monistat).
6. Vidarabine (Vira-A Ophthalmic) or trifluridine (Viroptic Ophthalmic Solution 1%) for herpes simplex infection; oral antivirals (e.g., acyclovir)

7. Propamidine isethionate 0.1% ophthalmic solution (Brolene) and fortified neomycin drops for *Acanthamoeba* infections

Diet

If the patient is vitamin A–deficient or protein-malnourished, increase supplements of these in the diet; otherwise, no special dietary requirements.

Activity

Limit sports or heavy physical activities until healing is complete and vision returns to normal.

Patient Education

1. Proper handling of contact lenses
2. Prevention of abrasions or injury

Key Treatment

- Ophthalmologic referral
- Aggressive use of topical antibiotics
- Combination aminoglycosides and cephalosporins as initial therapy

Follow-Up

Daily follow-up with physician

 Bibliography

Bacon AS, Lewis G, Richards B, et al: *Acanthamoeba* keratitis: the value of early diagnosis. Ophthalmology 1993;100:1238–1239.

Newell FW: Ophthalmic Pathology: Principles and Concepts, 7th ed. St Louis, CV Mosby, 1991.

Tahija SG, Chandler JW: Corneal ulceration: have we advanced in the last 20 years? [review]. Int Ophthalmol Clin 1990;30:33–35.

Whitcher JP: Corneal ulceration [review]. Int Ophthalmol Clin 1990;30:30–32.

Epidemiology

1. Foreign bodies were involved in 57 per cent of all eye injuries and accounted for 3.6 per cent of all emergency department visits to one hospital; 31 per cent were due to wind and dust, 30 per cent due to grinding, 8.5 per cent due to drilling, 6.4 per cent to wood cutting, and 4.3 per cent to welding.

2. Occupational exposure is the major risk factor, along with contact lenses and failure to wear protective goggles.

Symptoms

The principal symptoms of corneal foreign body or abrasion are pain, scratchy sensation, and burning. Any time the patient presents with such symptoms, foreign body should be suspected and searched for regardless of whether the patient complains of a foreign body.

Evaluation

1. Examine both eyes with magnification (binocular loupe, ophthalmoscope, slit-lamp). This is essential to determine whether a foreign body is superficial or deep. The use of a slit-lamp is highly desirable.

2. Evert the tarsal plate of the affected eye to look for foreign material.

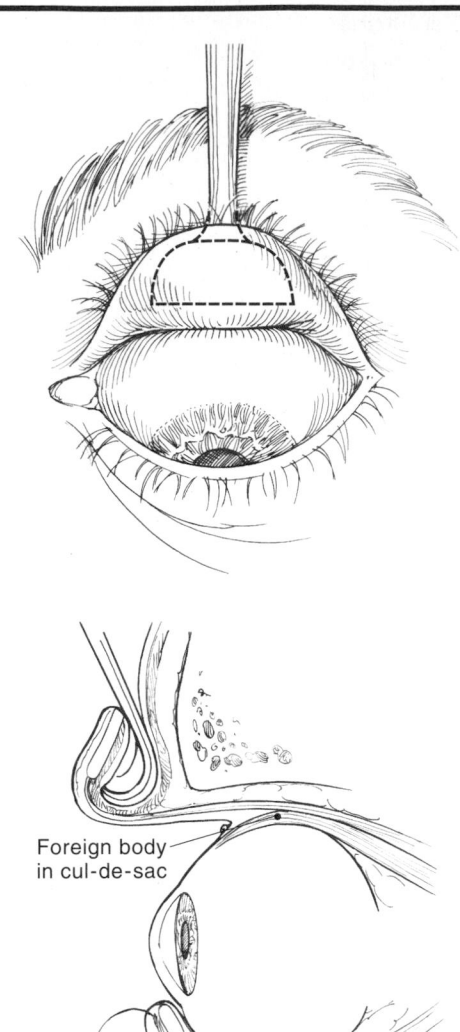

Foreign body in cul-de-sac

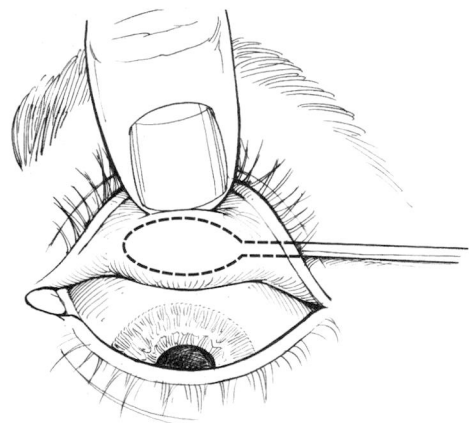

Double eversion of the tarsal plate may be necessary to look high into the cul-de-sac. If a Desmarres retractor is not available, a bent large paper clip will suffice. Pull down on the upper lid, "hook" the superior edge of the tarsal plate, and evert lid upward and outward.

Vertical scratches on the cornea suggest a foreign body in the superior palpebral conjunctiva. Keep in mind that injury from wind and blast (explosion) may result in the presence of more than one foreign body in the eye.

3. Most foreign bodies are superficial and lie on or within the epithelium. If they are beneath the epithelium and if Bowman's membrane has been injured, foreign body removal is usually

best done under an operating microscope by an ophthalmologist.

4. Signs of globe perforation include decreased tone on tactile examination, shallowing of the anterior chamber, altered pupil size, and a positive percolation test (i.e., continuous washing of fluorescein from the site of injury by a stream of aqueous humor leaking through the cornea [Seidel's sign]). If perforation is found, avoid manipulation, protect the eye with a shield, and refer to an ophthalmic surgeon.

5. Note any signs of anterior uveitis (cells or clouding within the anterior chamber).

6. Always test and record visual acuity before performing any procedure or manipulation.

7. If no foreign body is found, search for an inturned eyelash or eyelid (entropion). Be sure to evert the tarsal plate and look under it. If nothing is seen, anesthetize the eye surface with a drop of fluorescein from an impregnated fluorescein strip that has been moistened with a few drops of a topical anesthetic, such as proparacaine 0.5%. Wait a few minutes, and then irrigate the eye obliquely with saline solution.

8. Examine again under magnification. If no ulceration, abrasion, or foreign body can be found, examine the eye by means of a slit-lamp or refer for slit-lamp examination. If a lesion is not acute, there may be signs of infection, such as hypopion, edema and corneal clouding, purulent discharge, or ulceration exceeding the size of the foreign body. Such signs indicated the need for urgent hospitalization.

WARNING

- **When a foreign object, especially a metallic foreign body, is found on the cornea, always obtain orbit radiographs to rule out an unsuspected foreign body within the orbit. This is especially true if the particle has come from a high-velocity source, such as a grinding wheel or a hammer strike.**
- **Wood, plastic, and pencil lead produce intraocular foreign bodies that may not show up on radiography of the orbit; use magnetic resonance imaging or ultrasound.**
- *Avoid magnetic resonance imaging if there is any possibility of a metallic foreign body within the eye.*
- **Document all findings (e.g., visual acuity in both eyes, location of the foreign body [peripheral or central] or abrasion, signs of infection, presence of rust rings).**
- **Avoid use of steroids because they retard healing and can be disastrous in the circumstance of infection.**
- **Never dispense take-home topical anesthesia for pain relief because it delays corneal healing and masks symptoms.**
- **Use sterile single-dose anesthesia and fluorescein.**

Technique

1. If a foreign body is seen on the cornea, it is best removed with the patient lying supine with eyes fixed on the ceiling at a point that makes the foreign body become the uppermost point of the globe.

2. Caution the patient about the need to remain still. Children may require restraint.

3. First try to blot the foreign body from the cornea with a sterile cotton-tipped applicator moistened with normal saline solution. Be careful not to use force or abrasion. Most foreign bodies come away in this manner.

4. If this fails, gently scrape the foreign body from the cornea with an eye spud or a hypodermic needle using a *tangential* approach. Select a needle size appropriate for the size of the foreign body. Having the needle attached to the barrel of a plastic syringe may help achieve hand stability. Resting the hand on the patient's cheek keeps any movements of face and hand in tandem and reduces the risk of injury. Use magnification (binocular loupe).

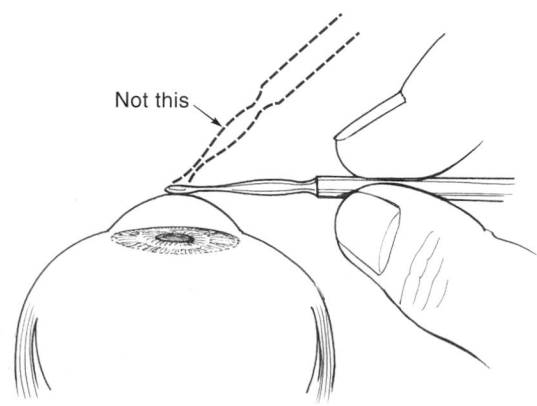

Not this

5. If the foreign body is ferrous, check carefully for a rust ring. If found, it must be removed. This can be done by gently scraping with the spud or by gentle rotation of a dental burr of appropriate size. (This method is not suitable for rust that is in the center of the cornea or for deep rust.) If an ophthalmic magnet is available, it may be used to lift off ferrous foreign bodies.

6. Instill an ophthalmic antibiotic ointment (tobramycin or gentamicin). Patch an anesthetized eye for 2 hours postexamination or have the patient wear protective lenses. Patching per se has not been shown to speed healing of corneal ulcers, but it provides protection against unrecognized foreign body entry while the eye is insensitive. Schedule follow-up in 24 hours and restain the cornea. Do not omit the 24-hour follow-up examination. Failure to show prompt healing requires referral. Give special attention to cases of vegetable foreign body or contaminated substances because they are prone to infection. Use of ketorolac tromethamine 0.5% ophthalmic solution (Acular) postexamination may reduce pain and reduce the time to resumption of normal activities.

7. Cases in which multiple foreign bodies are driven into the cornea, such as blasts or explosions, are best referred. Tropicamide (Mydriacyl) or cyclopentolate hydrochloride (Cyclogyl), one drop in the affected eye, reduces the effects of secondary iridocyclitis and makes the eye more comfortable.

Bibliography

Ban DH, Hedge JR: Corneal foreign body removal and treatment. Optom Clin 1991;1:59–70.

Kaiser PK, Pineda R 2nd: A study of topical nonsteroidal anti-inflammatory drops and no pressure patching in the treatment of corneal abrasions: Corneal Abrasion Patching Study Group. Ophthalmology 1997;104: 1353–1359.

Kruger RA, et al: Emergency eye injuries. Austral Fam Physician 1990;19:934–936.

Patterson J, Fetzer K, Krell J: Eye patch treatment for pain of corneal abrasion. South Med J 1996;89:227–229.

Reich JA: Removal of corneal foreign bodies. Austral Fam Physician 1990;19:719–721.

Santen SA, Scott JL: Ophthalmolgic procedures. Emerg Med Clin North Am 1995;13:681–701.

19 Optic Neuritis

W. Michael Skeens

Optic neuritis is due to inflammation, demyelination, or infection that affects the optic nerve at or anterior to the optic chiasm. This disorder is subdivided into papillitis and retrobulbar neuritis. The division is made based on whether the intraocular portion of the optic nerve is involved, causing papillitis. If the adjacent retina is also involved, it is referred to as optic neuroretinitis. The primary group of entities that optic neuritis must be differentiated from are the disorders that cause optic neuropathy. As well, the papillitis may be confused with papilledema. Optic neuropathy may result from ischemia, compression, or toxic effects. These problems include arteritis, systemic lupus erythematosus, syphilis, accelerated hypertension, diabetes, collagen-vascular diseases, sickle cell disease, migraine headaches, carotid artery disease, acute hypotension (as in sudden gastrointestinal hemorrhage), polycythemia vera, radiation, compression, and atherosclerosis. This also includes entities such as tobacco-alcohol amblyopia.

Etiology

1. Demyelination
   a. Multiple sclerosis
      (1) Fifteen per cent of patients with multiple sclerosis present with optic neuritis.
      (2) Among all patients with multiple sclerosis, 33 per cent develop optic neuritis during some stage of their disease process.
   b. Felty's syndrome (rheumatoid arthritis and hypersplenism)
   c. Behr's disease (hereditary optic atrophy)
   d. Schilder's disease (diffuse periaxial encephalitis)
   e. Diffuse cerebral sclerosis (e.g., metachromatic leukodystrophy)
   f. Brown-Marie syndrome (hereditary ataxia)
   g. Acute disseminated encephalomyelitis
   h. Neuromyelitis (Devic), bilateral, with transverse spinal cord myelitis optica
2. Inflammation (including secondary to infection)
   a. Systemic lupus erythematosus
   b. Autoimmune encephalitis
   c. Meningitis
   d. Syphilis
   e. Tuberculosis
   f. Mumps
   g. Chickenpox
   h. Infectious mononucleosis
   i. Herpes zoster
   j. Vasculitis, including Stevens-Johnson syndrome, Henoch-Schönlein purpura, multiple myeloma (Kahler disease), temporal arteritis, Raynaud's disease, and periarteritis nodosa
   k. Lyme disease: May also present as papilledema with increased cerebrospinal fluid pressure, appearing similiar to pseudotumor cerebri.
3. Infection
   a. Intraocular keratitis, endophthalmitis, and chronic uveitis
   b. Orbital region infections
      (1) Orbital cellulitis
      (2) Orbital abscess (Rollet's syndrome)
      (3) Spread from spheroid and ethmoid sinuses
      (4) Wegener's granulomatosis
      (5) Tolosa-Hunt syndrome (painful ophthalmoplegia)
   c. Systemic infections, including bacterial, fungal, protozoal, helminthic, rickettsial, and viral (e.g., Guillain-Barré syndrome, hepatitis, influenza, polio)
4. Systemic diseases
   a. Diabetes (Willis' disease)
   b. Acquired immunodeficiency syndrome
   c. Alcohol ingestion
   d. Amyloidosis
   e. Sarcoidosis
   f. Behçet's disease
   g. Pregnancy
   h. Chronic glomerulonephritis
   i. Multiple medications
   j. Multiple other disease processes and tobacco use
5. Etiology unknown: frequent

Symptoms

1. Acute monocular vision loss ranging from mild decreased visual acuity to monocular blindness;

abrupt onset, usually over hours, seldom over weeks.

2. Color vision is affected more severely than the overall visual acuity, which is not true in optic neuropathies.

3. Primary vision loss is central in nature. It occurs primarily in the 20- to 50-year age group and equally in both sexes.

4. Pain on motion of the affected eye (especially in the lateral direction) is found with retrobulbar optic neuritis.

5. Elderly patients may present with acute papilledema and monocular vision loss. Anterior ischemic optic neuropathy secondary to arteritis is more common.

Key Symptoms

- Acute monocular vision loss
- Primary vision loss
- Pain on motion of affected eye
- Loss of some color vision

Clinical Findings

1. Retrobulbar optic neuritis
   a. Pain on eye movement
   b. Tenderness on palpation of the globe with the eyelid closed
   c. Diffuse swelling and enhancement of the optic nerve on computerized tomographic (CT) scan
   d. Normal ophthalmoscopy
2. Papillitis (anterior optic neuropathy)
   a. Swollen optic disk with blurred margins giving the appearance of a smaller disk, dilated retinal veins, and, possibly, flame hemorrhages
   b. If severe, an oval pattern of yellow exudates may be seen around the fovea centralis and inflammatory cells may be present in the adjacent vitreous.
   c. May advance to optic atrophy with gliosis over the disk, causing a pale nerve head, permanent visual dysfunction, and distortion of vessels
3. Papillitis and retrobulbar optic neuritis
   a. Causes are the same.
   b. Color vision is more severely affected than overall visual acuity.
   c. Afferent pupillary defect (APD; Marcus Gunn pupil)

d. Central or paracentral scotoma
e. Acute-onset monocular vision loss

Key Signs

Retrobulbar Optic Neuritis

- Pain on eye movement
- Tenderness on palpation of globe with eyelid closed
- Diffuse swelling of optic nerve

Papillitis

- Swollen optic disk
- Oval pattern of yellow exudate seen around fovea centralis
- Inflammatory cells present in adjacent vitreous

Tests

1. Color testing
2. Visual acuity (including pinhole to rule out refractive component) before and after shining a penlight in the affected eye. This further decreases visual acuity in patients with retinal diseases but does not affect the vision of a patient with optic neuritis.
3. CT scan of the orbit when retrobulbar optic neuritis is suspected.
4. Visual fields to demonstrate the central or paracentral scotoma
5. Swinging light test to detect APD
6. Visual evoked potentials are abnormal.

Key Tests

- Color testing
- Visual acuity
- CT scan of orbit when retrobulbar optic neuritis suspected

Differential Diagnosis

1. Optic neuropathy: does not have the early loss of visual acuity seen in optic neuropathy
2. Amaurosis fugax: should resolve quickly over a short period.
3. Cystoid macular edema: central serous choroidopathy also present with painless loss of vision with central scotoma, but there is no APD and color vision is not as severely affected.

4. Papilledema must be differentiated from papillitis. Papilledema does not have the early loss of visual acuity and tends to be bilateral.

Treatment

1. Remove or treat the inciting cause, if known.
2. If optic neuritis is retrobulbar and caused by demyelinating disease, recovery usually is spontaneous within 2 to 6 weeks. Some residual optic atrophy that affects the papillomacular bundle may occur.
3. Extremely high-dose steroids may benefit some patients.

Key Treatment

- Remove or treat inciting cause.
- High-dose steroids may benefit some patients.

Bibliography

Fauci AS, Braunwald E, Isselbacher KJ, et al (eds): Harrison's Principles of Internal Medicine, 14th ed. New York, McGraw-Hill, 1998.

Gorbach SL, Bartlett JG, Blacklow NR: Infectious Diseases, 2nd ed. Philadelphia, WB Saunders Company, 1998.

Roy FH: Ocular Differential Diagnosis, 6th ed. Baltimore, Williams & Wilkins, 1996.

Spalton DJ, Hitchings RA, Hunter RA: Atlas of Clinical Ophthalmology, 2nd ed. London, Wolfe, 1994.

Vaughan D, Asbury T, Riordan-Eva P: General Ophthalmology, 13th ed. East Norwalk, CT, Appleton & Lange, 1992.

20 Acute Otitis Media

John G. O'Handley

Etiology

1. Eustachian tube dysfunction
   a. The peak incidence of acute otitis media is between ages 6 and 24 months because of developmental changes that surround the eustachian tube. They include persistent collapse as a result of abnormal tubal compliance, as well as delayed innervation of the tensor veli palatini muscle, which opens and closes the eustachian tube.
   b. Infection ascends through the eustachian tube.
   c. Normal eustachian tube function
      (1) Maintains atmospheric pressure in the middle ear.
      (2) Protects the middle ear from reflux of secretions from the nasopharynx.
      (3) Clears the middle ear secretions into the nasopharynx by ciliary activity.
   d. When these functions are altered, middle ear infection can result.
2. Infective organisms
   a. The typical occurrence of acute otitis media comes 5 to 7 days after an upper respiratory tract infection. Viruses are believed to play a role in the pathogenesis of this common condition, the principal one being respiratory syncytial virus. However, bacterial cultures are positive in 75 per cent of middle ear aspirates from children with acute otitis media.
   b. Bacterial pathogens
      (1) *Streptococcus pneumoniae* and *Haemophilus influenzae* make up about 60 per cent of isolates from the middle ear.
      (2) *Moraxella catarrhalis*, *Streptococcus pyogenes*, *Staphylococcus aureus*, and anaerobic organisms, either alone or in combination, make up the rest of the 90 per cent of organisms recovered from middle ear fluid in acute otitis media.
      (3) In adults, similar organisms are found, although the incidence of *H. influenzae* in some studies is higher than that of *S. pneumoniae*.
3. Risk factors
   a. Male sex
   b. Bottle feeding, especially in the supine position
   c. Exposure to upper respiratory tract infections (e.g., day care setting, winter season)
   d. Genetic factors
   e. Ethnic factors (e.g., Inuit and Native Americans)
   f. Parental smoking
   g. Allergy
   h. Craniofacial abnormalities (e.g., cleft palate)
   i. Previous episode of acute otitis media, particularly during the preceding 3 months

Signs and Symptoms

These are due to inflammation and fluid in the middle ear.

1. Otalgia
2. Ear-pulling
3. Diminished hearing
4. Fever
5. Loss of appetite
6. Irritability
7. Vomiting
8. Vertigo
9. Tinnitus
10. Otorrhea

Key Symptoms

- Otalgia
- Fever
- Hearing loss

Clinical Findings

Appearance of tympanic membrane
1. Lack of landmarks
2. Limited mobility or complete immobility
3. Erythematous
4. Bulging

Tests

1. Pneumatic otoscopy
2. Complete blood count and blood culture only when patient is considered toxic.

Differential Diagnosis

1. Myringitis: red tympanic membrane without middle ear exudate
2. Pharyngitis or tonsillitis: Can cause referred pain to the ear.
3. Teething
4. Referred pain from temporomandibular joint syndrome

Treatment

Medication

1. Drug of choice: amoxicillin, 40 mg/kg/day in three divided doses for 5 to 10 days (adult dose is 250 mg q8h) in uncomplicated cases. For high risk patients (those with recent antimicrobial exposure, age less than 2 years, and day care attendance) use amoxicillin at 80 to 90 mg/kg/day in three divided doses.
2. Alternative drugs
   a. Amoxicillin/clavulanate (Augmentin), 40 mg/kg/day in three divided doses for 10 days (adult dose is 250 mg q8h)
   b. Cefaclor (Ceclor), 40 mg/kg/day in three divided doses for 10 days (adult dose is 250 mg q8h)
   c. Cefuroxime axetil (Ceftin), children under 2 years, 125 mg twice daily; children 2 years or over, 250 mg twice daily for 10 days
   d. Trimethoprim-sulfamethoxazole (Bactrim, Septra), 8 mg/kg trimethoprim and 40 mg/kg sulfamethoxazole per 24 hours given in divided doses every 12 hours for 10 days
   e. Erythromycin and sulfisoxazole (Pediazole), 50 mg/kg/day erythromycin and 150 mg/kg/day sulfisoxazole in four divided doses for 10 days
   f. Azithromycin (Zithromax), 10 mg/kg on day 1 followed by 5 mg/kg on days 2 to 5 (adult dose is 500 mg on day 1 followed by 250 mg on days 2 to 5)
   g. Clarithromycin (Biaxin), 7.5 mg/kg q12h for 10 days (adult dose is 250 mg q12h for 10 days)
   h. Cefpodoxime proxetil (Vantin), 10 mg/kg q24h for 10 days (maximum 400 mg/dose) or 5 mg/kg q12h for 10 days (maximum 200 mg/dose)
   i. Cefprozil (Cefzil), 30 mg/kg/day in two divided doses for 10 days
   j. Cefixime (Suprax), 8 mg/kg/day as a single daily dose for 10 days
   k. Ceftriaxone (Rocephin), 50 mg/kg IM as a single dose
3. Anhydrous glycerol eardrops or similar eardrops provide symptomatic relief. Acetaminophen may also be used for pain.
4. Systemic decongestants and expectorants for symptoms only

Alternative drugs should be used

- When resistant organisms have been identified on culture of middle ear fluid
- In previous treatment failure with amoxicillin
- If patient is hypersensitive to penicillin

There is increasing evidence that short-course treatment (5 to 7 days) for community-acquired bacterial upper respiratory infections such as uncomplicated acute otitis media may be as or more effective than traditional 10-day therapies. Besides being more cost-effective, short-course treatment reduces the development of bacterial resistance.

Note

Antihistamines are not recommended for the resolution of acute otitis media because they lead to decreased ciliary motility.

Surgical Treatment

1. Tympanocentesis can be used if antibiotics are not effective.

WARNING

Determine compliance with medication before performing tympanocentesis.

2. Myringotomy with polyethylene tube placement if antibiotics and tympanocentesis fail to resolve an effusion lasting 3 months and there is concern over hearing or speech delay

Diet

As tolerated

Activity

1. Pain and fever preclude going to school or work.
2. There are no restrictions after pain and fever are gone.
3. Avoid barotrauma (e.g., flying, scuba diving).

Patient Education

1. Parents should avoid bottle feeding of infants in the supine position. This practice can cause reflux of oral contents into the eustachian tube.
2. Parents should be informed that tobacco smoke increases the risk of middle ear infections in children.
3. Allergens in the home, such as pets, house dust, and mold, should be eliminated as much as possible for people who have an allergic diathesis.

Follow-Up

1. Patients require follow-up in 4 to 6 weeks. Ninety per cent of middle ear effusions have resolved by that time, and pneumatic otoscopy can determine if fluid is still present.
2. Tympanometry is another method of follow-up but increases cost. It is useful in those patients who are unable to cooperate for pneumatic otoscopy and provides an objective measurement of the status of the middle ear.

3. For patients who have had three episodes of acute otitis media in the past 6 months or four episodes in the past 12 months, prophylaxis with amoxicillin (20 mg/kg in a single dose or two divided doses) or sulfisoxazole (50 mg/kg/day at bedtime) is recommended during the winter season.
4. The use of antibiotic prophylaxis to prevent recurrent otitis media is now being questioned because prolonged antibiotic use may increase nasopharyngeal colonization with penicillin-resistant *Streptococcus pneumoniae*, and recent studies suggest no difference between amoxicillin prophylaxis and placebo.

Bibliography

Dowell SF, Butler JC, Giebink GS, et al: Acute otitis media: management and surveillance in an era of pneumococcal resistance—a report from the Drug-Resistant Streptococcus Pneumoniae Therapeutic Working Group. Pediatr Infect Dis J 1999;18:1–9.

Kozyrskyj AL, Hildes-Ripstein GE, et al: Treatment of acute otitis media with a shortened course of antibiotics. JAMA 1998;279:1736–1742.

Roark R, Berman S: Continuous twice daily or once daily amoxicillin prophylaxis compared with placebo for children with recurrent acute otitis media. Pediatr Infect Dis J 1997;16:376–381.

Rosenfeld RM: An evidence-based approach to treating otitis media. Pediatr Clin North Am 1996;43:1165–1181.

Williams RL, Chalmers TC, Stange KC, et al: Use of antibiotics in preventing recurrent acute otitis media and in treating otitis media with effusion. JAMA 1993;270:1344–1351.

21 Otitis Media with Effusion

Louisa Coutts–van Dijk

The current correct terminology for what was called chronic serous otitis media, or "glue ear," is otitis media with effusion. Effusions can be both serous and mucoid.

1. Definition: persistence of serous or mucoid fluid in the middle ear without signs or symptoms of acute infection
2. Central role of eustachian tube (ET) dysfunction with insufficient clearing of fluid from the middle ear. Inflammation and infection also play a role.

Epidemiology and Etiology

1. Otitis media with effusion (OME) is extremely common. Around the age of 2 years it occurs in approximately 20 per cent of children. Another incidence peak occurs around age 5. Annual costs in the United States are estimated at over $2 billion.
2. Middle ear effusions are extremely common after upper respiratory tract infections, acute otitis media, and episodes of allergic rhinitis.
3. Less common contributing factors are enlarged adenoids, hypothyroidism, radiotherapy, and congenital structural abnormality (Down's syndrome).
4. Without intervention, more than two thirds of effusions clear spontaneously within 3 months. Of the remaining cases, another two thirds resolve spontaneously within another 3 months.
5. Chronic middle ear effusion is the most common cause of hearing loss in children.
6. Environmental factors
   a. Exposure to tobacco smoke
   b. Attendance at group child-care facilities
   c. Bottle feeding rather than breast-feeding
7. Infective organisms
   a. Bacteria
      (1) *Streptococcus pneumoniae* (resistant strains are emerging more commonly).
      (2) *Haemophilus influenzae*
      (3) *Moraxella catarrhalis*
      (4) *Streptococcus pyogenes*
   b. Viral
      (1) Respiratory syncytial virus
      (2) Adenovirus

Symptoms

OME is often asymptomatic
1. Pressure in the ear
2. Fullness or "plugged up" sensation
3. Infants and toddlers may present with
   a. Pulling at ear
   b. Fussiness
   c. Nocturnal wakening

Key Symptoms

- Ear fullness or pressure
- Mild to moderate conductive hearing loss that may fluctuate

---

Note
Fever, severe ear pain (otalgia), and vomiting suggest ACUTE otitis media. Refer to Ch. 20, Acute Otitis Media.

Clinical Findings

1. Otoscopy findings
   a. May be normal.
   b. Retraction of tympanic membrane, malleus pulled into horizontal position
   c. Dull or opaque tympanic membrane
   d. Fluid level or bubbles visible behind tympanic membrane
   e. Immobility of tympanic membrane
   f. Two thirds of OME cases are bilateral.
2. Hearing loss in OME, if present, is
   a. Conductive
   b. Mild to moderate and rarely exceeds 40 dB.
3. Possible language or speech developmental delay in children as a result of bilateral hearing loss. Increased concerns about developmental delay if OME occurs during first 3 years of life.

Refer to Ch. 4, Developmental Surveillance.

4. Decreased school performance or behavior problems in older children

Key Signs

- OME is bilateral in two thirds of cases
- Dull and poorly mobile tympanic membranes
- Absent or diminished compliance peak on tympanogram

Note
A red, bulging, and immobile tympanic membrane suggests ACUTE otitis media.

Tests

1. Pneumatic otoscopy
   a. Pneumatic otoscopy is insufflation of a small amount of air into the sealed external ear canal via a small balloon. This is attached to the otoscope, through which the mobility of the tympanic membrane is visualized.
   b. If a middle ear effusion is present, decreased or absent mobility of the tympanic membrane is present.
   c. This test has high false-positive and high false-negative rates for the diagnosis of middle ear effusions. A tympanogram is therefore recommended.

2. Tympanogram (Fig. 21–1)
   a. For ages 6 months and older
   b. A small probe is inserted into the patient's external ear canal until a seal is obtained. A transducer delivers a controlled tone. A microscope picks this up while the air pressure in the ear canal is varied. Compliance of the middle ear is measured as milliliters of displaced air and is displayed on the vertical axis of the resulting graph. The range of negative, atmospheric, and positive pressures is displayed on the horizontal axis in millimeters of water.
   c. Interpretation is based on both the shape of the compliance peak and the pressure at which this peak occurs (Fig. 21–1).

3. Hearing evaluation
   a. Indicated when effusions are present for more than 3 months

Refer to Ch. 12, Symptom: Impaired Hearing.

   b. Auditory brain stem response (ABR) testing, for children under 3 years of age
   c. Pure tone audiometry, for children over 3 years of age

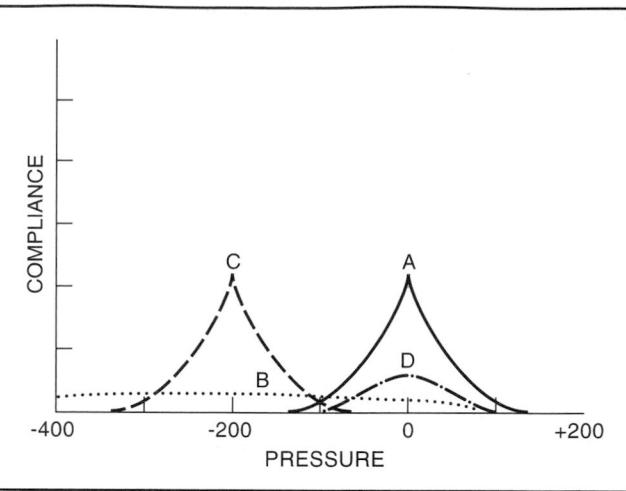

Figure 21–1 System of tympanographic classification. A normal result (*curve A*) is a tall compliance peak (0.2 to 2.0 ml) with maximum compliance located at or near 0 mm H_2O. A flat tympanogram (*curve B*) has no peak and indicates lack of compliance usually as a result of a middle ear effusion. A compliance peak of normal shape that occurs below the normal limit of −150 mm H_2O (*curve C*) indicates eustachian tube dysfunction with or without an effusion. A low peak at or near 0 mm H_2O (*curve D*) indicates an effusion, ossicular stiffening, or thickening of the tympanic membrane. A very high peak (not shown) located at or near 0 mm H_2O indicates ossicular disruption or a flaccid tympanic membrane. (Redrawn from Adams GL, Boies LR Jr, Hilger PA [eds]: Boies Fundamentals of Otolaryngology, 6th ed, p 58. Philadelphia, WB Saunders Company, 1989, with permission.)

Note
Less than one half of children with abnormal tympanograms will have a hearing loss.

   d. Screening tests for hearing loss
      (1) Startle reflex to loud sound, ages 0 to 4 months, evoked otoacoustic emission (EOE) screening
      (2) Distraction test with noisemaker for children ages 4 months to 3 years. A noisemaker is sounded softly at waist level outside of field of vision; depending on age, responses are widening of eyes, interruption of activity, turning of head toward sound, location of sound.
      (3) Pure tone audiometry, useful for children 3 years of age and older; earphones at 1000, 2000, and 4000 Hz; soundproof room noise level at 20 dB, otherwise 25 dB.

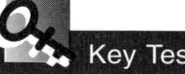

Key Tests

- Pneumatic otoscopy
- Tympanogram
- Hearing evaluation after 3 months and again immediately prior to decision on surgery

Differential Diagnosis

1. Recurrent acute otitis media (three episodes in the past 6 months or four per year)
2. Flat tympanograms caused by
   a. Cerumen impaction
   b. Perforation of the tympanic membrane
   c. Functioning pressure-equalizing (PE) tubes
   d. Thickening of the tympanic membrane
   e. Stenosis of the ear canal
3. These should be evident on otoscopic examination with direct visualization of the tympanic membrane.
4. Increased canal volume (over 2.0 ml) may help differentiate perforation or functioning PE tube. Decreased canal volume (below 0.2 ml) may indicate obstruction or debris (foreign body or cerumen).

Treatment

1. The majority of cases will resolve spontaneously.
2. Watchful waiting is indicated during the first 3 months. This consists of monthly evaluations, follow-up tympanograms, and a hearing evaluation at 3 months if OME (confirmed by tympanogram) persists.
3. Treatment is aimed at preventing long-term hearing loss and developmental delay.

Patient Education

1. Avoidance of tobacco smoke, passive smoking. Smoke enhances attachment of pathogens, prolongs inflammatory response, and impedes ET drainage. Each packet of cigarettes is estimated to increase time with effusion by 11 per cent.
2. If hearing impairment is present, advise
   a. Turning off background noise (television, radio) when communicating
   b. Facing child and obtaining attention before speaking
   c. Placing child in front of classroom
   d. Avoiding exposure to loud noise (fireworks, shots, and loud music)
3. Autoinflation: inflating a balloon device by Vasalva maneuver through one nostril with the other nostril closed. Short-term effects are encouraging but further trials are needed. Only for children ages 3 and older.

Diet

1. Avoid bottle feeding in recumbent position.
2. Encourage breast-feeding. Breast-feeding reduces the incidence of upper respiratory tract infections. Sucking mechanism improves ET drainage.

> Refer to Ch. 129, Breast-Feeding.

3. Avoid known allergens causing allergic rhinitis.

Medication

1. Approximately one of every six children treated with antibiotics will benefit. The effects are transient (1 month), and a long-term benefit of antibiotics for OME has not been shown.
2. After 3 months' duration of OME, a 14- to 28-day course of antibiotics at full therapeutic dose may be tried.
   a. First-line ($): amoxicillin, 40 mg/kg/day; safe and inexpensive, not active against β-lactamase–producing organisms
   b. Second-line ($–$$): trimethoprim-sulfamethoxazole, 8/40 mg/kg/day (Bactrim, Septra), erythromycin-sulfisoxazole (Pediazole)
   c. Third-line ($$$–$$$$$): amoxicillin-clavulanate (Augmentin), cefuroxime (Ceftin), Cefpodoxime (Vantin)
3. In view of concerns about overuse of antibiotics and resulting antibiotic resistance (25 per cent of otitis media organisms), a more conservative approach with longer watchful waiting without medical treatment may be prudent. Consider a nonmedical approach when OME is unilateral or not accompanied by hearing loss or is present in older asymptomatic children.
4. Addition of prednisone 1 mg/kg/day for 7 days may increase the likelihood of resolution. The use of intranasal steroids (beclomethasone) is experimental.
5. Most studies fail to show effectiveness of antihistamines or decongestants.
6. Vaccination: pneumococcal vaccine to prevent acute otitis media for children and adults over 2 years of age (children younger than 2 years of age have poor immune response).
7. Antibiotic prophylaxis may be considered for recurrent acute otitis media. This is defined as three or more episodes per 6 months or four episodes per year.
8. A possible therapeutic effect of the herbal medicine Sairei-to deserves further study.

> **Note**
> The use of prednisone without an antibiotic is not recommended, and steroids are contraindicated when there has been recent exposure to varicella in a previously unexposed patient.

Surgery

1. Surgical treatment may be considered if OME has been present for at least 4 months *and* there is documented *bilateral* hearing loss of at least 20 dB. Because hearing loss may fluctuate or improve over time, it is advisable to repeat hearing evaluation immediately before making decisions about surgery.

2. Children with significant morbidity from recurrent acute otitis media may also benefit from surgery.

3. Surgical treatment consists of myringotomy with placement of PE tubes. These usually come out spontaneously after staying in place for an average of 10 to 12 months.

4. Complications of PE tube placement include tympanosclerosis (10 to 50 per cent), otorrhea (13 per cent), and permanent perforation (1 per cent). PE tubes themselves may result in a long-term 5-dB hearing loss.

5. Adenoidectomy may be indicated in addition to PE tube placement in children with enlarged adenoids who are over 4 years of age.

Key Treatment

- Watchful waiting for first 3 months; avoidance of passive smoke

- Consider antibiotics ± steroids after 3 months.

- PE tube placement after 4 to 6 months if bilateral hearing loss is present.

- More conservative management if OME is unilateral, unaccompanied by hearing loss, or present in older asymptomatic children

Follow-Up

1. Watchful waiting

   a. Indicated during the first 3 months

   b. Consists of monthly evaluations, repeat tympanograms, and hearing evaluation at 3 months.

   c. Longer watchful waiting without medical/surgical treatment may be prudent when OME is unilateral, not accompanied by hearing loss, or present in older asymptomatic children.

2. Referral

   a. If indicated, after 3 months refer infants for hearing evaluation.

   b. OME for more than 4 to 6 months with confirmed bilateral hearing loss: Refer to otolaryngologist.

   c. Language, speech developmental delay: Refer to speech therapist, home language enrichment program

   d. Behavioral problems: Refer to school nurse, psychologist.

 ## Bibliography

Agency for Health Care Policy and Research: Clinical Practice Guideline No 12: Otitis Media with Effusion in Young Children (AHCPR Publication no 94-0623). Washington, DC, Agency for Health Care Policy and Research, 1994.

Culpepper L, Froom J: Otitis media with effusion in young children: treatment in search of a problem? J Am Board Fam Pract 1995;8:305–316.

DeMelker R: Treating persistent glue ear in children, more patience, less surgery. BMJ 1993;306:5–6.

Paap CM: Management of otitis media with effusion in young children. Ann Pharmacother 1996;30:1291–1297.

Williams RL, Chalmers TC, Stange KC, et al: Use of antibiotics in preventing recurrent acute otitis media and in treating otitis media with effusion: a meta-analytic attempt to resolve the brouhaha. JAMA 1993;270:1344–1351.

Tympanocentesis is the puncturing of the tympanic membrane to aspirate fluid from the middle ear. It is used most often to obtain specimens for culture. *Myringotomy* is the incision of the tympanic membrane for drainage of middle ear fluid. Tympanocentesis can be easily performed by a primary care physician in the office setting.

Indications

1. Otitis media in seriously ill or toxic-appearing patients
2. Presence of suppurative complications, such as acute mastoiditis, labyrinthitis, facial paralysis, or meningitis. Under these circumstances, tympanocentesis is performed first to identify causative organisms. Myringotomy is performed afterward for drainage purposes.
3. Otitis media in immunocompromised persons
4. Otitis media in the neonatal period
5. Failure of otitis media to respond to appropriate antimicrobial therapy
6. Onset of otitis media in a patient who is receiving antimicrobial agents

Contraindications

1. Uncooperative patient
2. Improper visualization of the tympanic membrane
3. Known anomalous positioning of the jugular bulb

Preparation

1. Explain the procedure—all indications, risks, and alternative treatments—to the patient, parent, or legal guardian.
2. Obtain signed informed consent.

Equipment

1. Otoscope with a surgical head or an otomicroscope
2. Phenol solution, or midazolam injectable solution
3. 70% alcohol
4. Small sterile cotton-tipped applicator
5. 18-gauge spinal needle
6. Tuberculin syringe or Alden-Senturia trap
7. Goggles

Anesthesia

1. Infants can be adequately restrained by a sheet or board especially designed for this purpose.

2. Intranasal midazolam (Versed), 0.1 to 0.5 ml/kg of the injectable formulation, can be used for sedation in young children, especially preschoolers. The solution is instilled into the nasal cavity by a tuberculin syringe without the needle. (This route is not approved yet.) This drug produces a calm, compliant patient with retrograde and anterograde amnesia. Midazolam has a half-life of 106 ± 29 minutes and a rapid onset of action of 10 to 15 minutes when administered intranasally.
3. A topical solution of phenol (using a small cotton-tipped applicator) applied to the exact spot on the tympanic membrane for tympanocentesis may be enough in older children (school-age) or teenagers.

Precautions

1. Identify the puncture site in the inferior posterior quadrant to avoid injury to the chorda tympani and the ossicles.

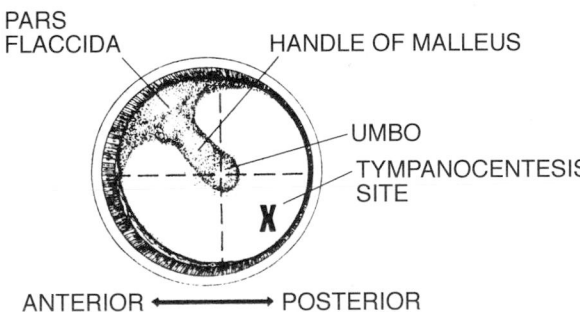

From Hughes WT, Buescher ES (eds): Pediatric Procedures, 2nd ed, p 196. Philadelphia, WB Saunders Company, 1980, with permission.

2. Excessive penetration should be avoided. This can cause fracture of the crura of the stapes.
3. Pulse oximeter should be used on all patients who are sedated for a procedure.
4. Make sure the patient's head is securely immobilized before puncturing the tympanic membrane. This will prevent quick jerks by the patient and trauma to the middle ear.
5. Never perform the procedure blindly. Many vital structures could be damaged, including the ossicles, chorda tympani, facial nerve, jugular bulb, and internal carotid artery.
6. Avoid the contact of phenol with tissues other than the tympanic membrane.
7. Take universal precaution measures and wear goggles.

Technique

1. Position the patient in the sitting or supine position.

2. Choose the largest speculum that fills the ear canal.

3. Use an otoscope with a surgical head or an otomicroscope.

4. Obtain a culture of the external canal; fill the ear canal with 70 per cent alcohol for 1 minute, then aspirate the alcohol if the middle ear fluid will be cultured.

5. Apply phenol at the puncture site if it is to be used.

6. Bend the spinal needle 30 to 45 degrees at its mid-length and mount it on the tuberculin syringe or the Alden-Senturia trap.

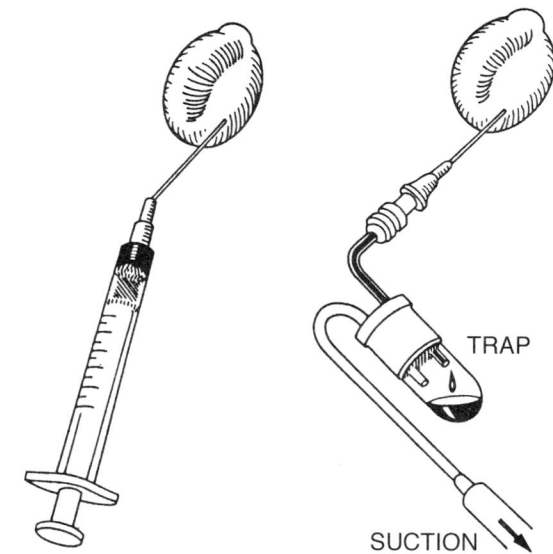

TRAP

SUCTION

From Hughes WT, Buescher ES (eds): Pediatric Procedures, 2nd ed, p 107. Philadelphia, WB Saunders Company, 1980, with permission.

7. Advance the needle slowly into the external canal and toward the inferior posterior quadrant.

8. Puncture the tympanic membrane at the white spot produced by the phenol to a depth of no more than 2 mm. The plunger of the tuberculin syringe can now be pulled to aspirate the middle ear fluid.

9. Remove the needle and clean the external canal of any drainage or blood.

10. Send the aspirated fluid for culture. Check culture results from both the ear canal and the middle ear fluid. If the same organisms grow in both cultures, they are contaminants from the middle ear.

11. Use the following CPT codes for the procedure:

a. 69420—Myringotomy including aspiration and/or eustachian tube inflation

b. 69421—Myringotomy including aspiration and/or eustachian tube inflation requiring general anesthesia

c. 69420 and 69421 services include surgical procedures only.

Follow-Up

1. Observe patients sedated with midazolam for 1 hour.

2. Instruct patients to call back if drainage persists.

3. Instruct patients to call back if otalgia develops or becomes worse.

Complications

1. Persistent otorrhea

2. Dislocation of incudostapedial joint

3. Severing of the facial nerve with facial nerve paralysis

4. Severe hemorrhage can occur following myringotomy. The internal carotid artery may extend as far as the middle of the promontory and can be punctured during the procedure. Also the jugular bulb vein located at the floor of the middle ear with no intervening bone in infants can be punctured during the procedure.

5. Injury to the chorda tympani with impairment of the sense of taste on the same side of the tongue

6. Persistent perforation

7. Atrophic scar

ACKNOWLEDGMENTS: Illustrations reprinted from Hughes WT, Buescher ES: Ear, eye, and nose. In Pediatric Procedures, pp 191–206. Philadelphia, WB Saunders Company, 1980, with permission.

Bibliography

Bluestone CD, Klein JO: Otitis media, atelectasis, and eustachian tube dysfunction. In Bluestone CD, Stool SE, Kenna MA (ed): Pediatric Otolaryngology, 3rd ed, vol 1, pp 388–582. Philadelphia, WB Saunders Company, 1996.

Bluestone CD, Klein JO: Diagnosis. In Bluestone CD, Klein JO: Otitis Media in Infants and Children, pp 69–120. Philadelphia, WB Saunders Company, 1988.

Coté CJ: Sedation for the pediatric patient: a review. Pediatr Clin North Am 1994;41:31–58.

Forzley GJ: Myringotomy. In Pfenninger JL, Fowler GC (eds): Procedures for the Primary Care Physician, pp 188–191. St. Louis, Mosby–Year Book, 1994.

Hughes WT, Buescher ES: Ear, eye, and nose. In Pediatric Procedures, pp 191–206. Philadelphia, WB Saunders Company, 1980.

22 Otitis Externa

Vincent M. Balestrino

Etiology

1. Otitis externa is an infection or inflammation of the auricle and external auditory canal (EAC).
2. Predisposing factors
   a. Moisture
   b. Absence of or impacted cerumen
   c. Hearing aids
   d. Trauma
   e. Dermatoses
   f. Immunocompromised state
3. Classification
   a. Acute diffuse otitis externa (swimmer's ear): most common type. Bacterial infection caused by
      (1) *Pseudomonas aeruginosa* (most common isolate, >60 per cent)
      (2) *Staphylococcus aureus* (20 per cent)
      (3) Anaerobes: *Peptostreptococcus/Proprionibacterium* (8 per cent)
      (4) Gram-negative organisms
   b. Acute localized otitis externa: Begins as a folliculitis and forms a furuncle of the canal. Caused by staphylococcus (occasional streptococcus) species
   c. Chronic otitis externa: persistent low-grade infection and inflammation
   d. Eczematoid otitis externa: secondary to underlying dermatitis
      (1) Atopic dermatitis
      (2) Contact dermatitis
      (3) Seborrheic dermatitis
      (4) Psoriasis
      (5) Allergic/hypersensitivity
      (6) Neurodermatitis
   e. Otomycosis
      (1) Ten per cent of otitis externa in the United States
      (2) Increased incidence in tropics
      (3) Fungal infection: *Aspergillus* (80 to 90 per cent); *Candida* (10 to 20 per cent)
   f. Necrotizing otitis externa: Invasive bacterial (pseudomonal) infection with osteomyelitis of the temporal bone in a diabetic or immunocompromised patient.

Symptoms

1. Acute infectious (bacterial)
   a. Itching
   b. Pain
   c. Discharge
   d. Decreased hearing
2. Chronic
   a. Itching
   b. Decreased hearing
3. Eczematoid
   a. Itching
   b. Crusting
   c. Weeping

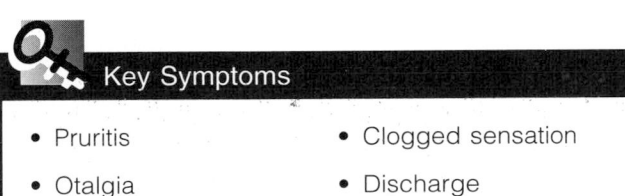

Key Symptoms	
• Pruritis	• Clogged sensation
• Otalgia	• Discharge

Clinical Findings

1. Infectious
   a. Pain caused by manipulation of the auricle or with mastication
   b. Erythema and edema of the EAC
   c. Localized furuncle or abscess
   d. Stenosis of canal secondary to debris and secretions
   e. In necrotizing otitis externa, granulation tissue is seen in the canal, with bony tenderness and regional adenopathy as well as systemic signs of infection with or without cranial neuropathies.
2. Chronic and/or mycotic
   a. Thickening of the EAC
   b. Dry, hypertrophied skin of the EAC
   c. Presence of fungal elements (i.e., conidiophores—small black dots seen with *Aspergillus*)
3. Eczematoid: involvement of the entire ear canal and auricle is common.

a. Seborrhea (dandruff) of the scalp may be present.

b. Hyperemia, edema, and fissuring of the auricle

c. Crusting, weeping, and scaling of the auricle and canal

Key Signs

- Auricular tenderness
- Debris and secretions in canal
- Erythema and stenosis of canal
- Periauricular adenitis—granulation tissue

Complications

1. Stenosis of canal
2. Myringitis
3. Perforation of TM
4. Cellulitis
5. Parotitis
6. Cranial neuropathies
7. Chondritis

Laboratory Tests

For most cases of otitis externa, no routine laboratory tests are needed.

1. Gram's stain with culture and sensitivity may be helpful in recalcitrant cases or immunocompromised host.
2. KOH stain and fungal cultures helpful in chronic infection or history of travel to tropics.
3. Complete blood count, cultures, erythrocyte sedimentation rate, and computerized tomography scan of temporal bone indicated in necrotizing otitis externa.
4. May need a skin biopsy to establish a diagnosis of an underlying dermatitis.

> ### WARNING
>
> **Antibiotic pretreatment will alter laboratory results.**

Key Test

None in uncomplicated otitis externa; cultures (bacterial and fungal)

Differential Diagnosis

1. Otitis media with perforation of the tympanic membrane
2. Foreign body of the EAC
3. Ramsay Hunt syndrome: herpes zoster of VIIth cranial nerve
4. Relapsing polychondritis
5. Facial cellulitis with extension to the auricle
6. Allergic reaction and/or chemical irritation secondary to topical agents used in treatment
7. Insect bite of auricle
8. Tumor

Treatment

The mainstay of treatment is atraumatic cleansing, suctioning, and drying of the EAC, coupled with adequate analgesia.

1. Repeated careful suctioning and débridement is often necessary.
2. Topical hydrogen peroxide is helpful in loosening and removing crusting and debris.
3. A wick may be necessary for a severely stenotic canal. This helps deliver topical treatment deeper into the canal and enlarges the lumen of the canal. It may be left in place for 2 to 5 days.
4. Hypersensitivity reaction: Eliminate the offending agent.

> ### WARNING
>
> **Neomycin sensitivity occurs in 10 per cent of the population, and neomycin is a frequent component of topical agents.**

5. Furunculosis requires incision and drainage (I&D).
6. Necrotizing otitis externa requires systemic antipseudomonal antibiotics and may require surgical débridement and hospitalization.

Topical Therapies

1. Infectious otitis externa
   a. Acute localized otitis externa requires I&D plus an oral antistaphylococcal agent.
   b. Acute diffuse otitis externa
      (1) Topical polymyxin, colistimethate (Coly-Mycin), ofloxacin (Floxin Otic), and ciprofloxacin (Cipro HC Otic) are the most effective antipseudomonal agents and some are available in several different preparations with and without hydrocortisone (i.e., Cortisporin Otic, Coly-Mycin S). These are applied tid for 5 to 7 days.

(2) 2% Acetic acid with or without hydrocortisone (Vo-Sol or Domeboro Otic) tid for 5 to 7 days

(3) 2% Gentian violet or 5% aqueous-silver nitrate applied directly to the canal are bactericidal and fungicidal.

2. Eczematoid variant: Treat the underlying dermatitis.

   a. Seborrhea may respond to ketoconazole (Nizoral) or selenium sulfide shampoo and a midpotency steroid preparation.

   b. Atopic or contact dermatitis: Apply low- to midpotency steroid ointment twice daily.

3. Chronic diffuse otitis externa: 2% acetic acid or gentian violet

4. Otomycosis

   a. 2% Acidic acid, thimerasol drops, gentian violet, topical antifungal agents such as clotrimazole (Lotrimin) or ketoconazole

   b. Occasional recalcitrant cases require the addition of an oral antifungal agent such as itraconozole (Sporonox).

WARNING

Necrotizing otitis externa does not respond to topical therapy and requires institution of systemic antipseudomonal antibiotics and possibly surgical débridement and hospitalization.

Antibiotic Treatment

Antibiotic therapy includes an oral fluoroquinolone (i.e., Cipro, Floxin, Trovan) or a parenteral aminoglycoside and a semisynthetic penicillin or cephalosporin for 4 to 6 weeks.

Key Treatment

- Cleaning and drying canal
- 2% acetic acid
- Topical antimicrobials

Patient Education

Prevention is the key to avoiding recurrence.

1. Swimmer's ear

   a. Use water-impermeable earplugs or Vaseline-impregnated cotton.

   b. 70% alcohol or peroxide after swimming

   c. Blow-drying the canal

2. Avoid manipulation of the canal (i.e., cotton swabs, bobby pins, etc.).

3. Frequent removal and cleansing of hearing aids with alcohol

4. Control of underlying dermatitis

Follow-Up

1. For uncomplicated acute otitis externa that responds to conventional therapy in 3 to 5 days, no follow-up is necessary.

2. Patients requiring oral antibiotic or antifungal therapy should be re-evaluated within 2 weeks.

3. Recalcitrant cases require frequent follow-up (i.e., weekly with repeat cleansing, suctioning, drying, etc.).

4. All patients with acute necrotizing otitis externa or any complications of otitis externa (see under "Clinical Findings") require close follow-up and often referral to an otolaryngologist.

Bibliography

Ballenger JJ: Diseases of the external ear. In Austin DF (ed): Diseases of the Nose, Throat, Ear, Head and Neck, 14th ed, pp 1069–1080. Philadelphia, Lea & Febiger, 1991.

Bojrab D: Otitis externa. Otolaryngol Clin North Am 1996;29:761–782.

Clark WB, Brook I, Bianki D, et al: Microbiology of otitis externa. Head Neck Surg 1997;116:23–25.

Mirza N: Otitis externa—management in the primary care office. Postgrad Med 1996;99:153–158.

Selesnick S: Otitis externa: management of the recalcitrant case. Am J Otol 1994;15:408–412.

23 Allergic Rhinitis

Giulia Michelini

Etiology

1. In genetically susceptible individuals, nasally inhaled allergens cause an immunoglobulin E (IgE)–mediated hypersensitivity response.
2. Symptoms may be seasonal, depending on the allergen and the geographical area.
   a. Ragweed: mid-August to the first frost
   b. Tree pollen: March to May
   c. Grass pollen: May to early July
3. In perennial allergic rhinitis, allergens are present year round.
   a. Dust mites
   b. Molds
   c. Animal dander or saliva
   d. Cockroach antigen
4. Irritants and other stimuli may also trigger symptoms.
   a. Smoke, air pollutants
   b. Perfumes, detergents, or soaps
   c. Solvents or fumes
   d. Changes in air temperature, light, or atmospheric pressure
   e. Emotion

Symptoms

1. Paroxysmal sneezing often occurs in the morning.
2. Nasal itching may result in frequent nose rubbing (allergic salute).
3. Nasal congestion may lead to loss of taste or smell.
4. Acute or chronic sinusitis may complicate nasal obstruction.
5. Rhinorrhea is usually watery (may be profuse and continuous).
6. Chronic postnasal drip may cause cough and/or sore throat.
7. Palatal itching, dry mouth, and halitosis also occur.
8. Conjunctivitis causes ocular itching, redness, and tearing.
9. General symptoms include fatigue and disrupted sleep.

Key Symptoms

- Sneezing
- Nasal discharge
- Postnasal drip
- Nasal congestion
- Conjunctivitis
- Itchy nose

Clinical Findings

Clinical signs cannot be relied on for diagnosis.

1. Pale or bluish, swollen nasal mucosa (in 50 to 60 per cent of patients)
2. Clear, thin nasal discharge
3. Edematous turbinates
4. Allergic salute
5. Lymphoid hyperplasia in posterior oropharynx (cobblestoning)
6. Erythematous throat
7. Conjunctival and scleral injection
8. Chemosis of conjunctivae
9. Dark circles under the eyes (allergic shiners)

Key Signs

- Pale, swollen nasal mucosa
- Allergic shiners
- Nasal discharge
- Turbinate edema
- Conjunctival injection
- Allergic salute

Tests

Diagnosis is usually based on clinical evaluation.

1. Nasal smears: Cytology is examined using a Wright or Hansel stain.
   a. The presence of nasal eosinophils suggests allergy.
   b. Predominance of neutrophils suggests an infectious cause.
2. Allergy testing
   a. Skin testing is useful if the diagnosis is uncertain.
      (1) An allergen is applied with a prick or intradermal injection.

(2) A wheal-and-flare reaction can confirm the allergen that is triggering the symptoms.

(3) Skin tests may be positive in 10 to 15 per cent of asymptomatic patients.

b. Radioallergosorbent testing (RAST) is an in vitro test to measure a person's level of IgE in response to an allergen. It is more expensive and less sensitive than skin testing.

Key Tests

- Nasal smears
- Radioallergosorbent testing
- Skin testing

Differential Diagnosis

1. Infectious causes
   a. Rhinitis
      (1) Viral
      (2) Bacterial
      (3) Fungal
      (4) Atypical organisms (*Mycobacterium tuberculosis*, leprosy)
   b. Sinusitis
2. Noninfectious nonallergic causes
   a. Idiopathic rhinitis is a perennial rhinitis in response to nonspecific irritants and other stimuli (e.g., smoke, air pollutants).
   b. Drug-induced rhinitis is caused by the local or systemic effect of drugs on the nasal mucosa.
      (1) Sympathomimetic nasal drops or sprays
      (2) Cocaine
      (3) Antihypertensives (reserpine, guanethidine, hydralazine, angiotensin-converting enzyme inhibitors, β-blockers)
   c. Mechanical nasal obstruction can cause a secondary rhinitis.
      (1) Nasal polyps
      (2) Deviated septum
      (3) Nasal neoplasms
   d. Systemic conditions can result in nasal symptoms.
      (1) Rhinitis of pregnancy
      (2) Hypothyroidism
      (3) Granulomatous disease (Wegener's, sarcoid)
      (4) Ciliary dysfunction (cystic fibrosis, Kartagener's syndrome)

Treatment

Medication

1. Antihistamines relieve sneezing, rhinorrhea, and pruritus.
   a. The five classes of the first-generation antihistamines differ in sedative and anticholinergic side effects.
   b. For better effect, use before allergen exposure: alkylamine class—chlorpheniramine, 4 mg orally three or four time per day
   c. Newer agents have longer action and reduced side effects.

> **WARNING**
>
> Rare QT prolongation and arrhythmias have occurred with the use of terfenadine or astemizole with erythromycin, clarithromycin, ketoconazole, itraconazole, troleandomycin, and mibefradil dihydrochloride, and in patients with significant hepatic dysfunction.

   (1) Loratadine (Claritin), 10 mg orally daily
   (2) Cetirizine (Zyrtec), 10 mg orally daily
   (3) Fexofenadine (Allegra), 60 mg orally twice per day
   (4) Astemizole (Hismanal), 10 mg orally daily
2. Decongestants are useful for obstructive symptoms (congestion): pseudoephedrine hydrochloride (Sudafed), 30 to 60 mg orally qid
3. Intranasal steroids are the most effective drugs available.
   a. Beclomethasone (Beconase, Vancenase), one spray (42 μg) per nostril bid to qid
   b. Flunisolide (Nasalide), two sprays (50 μg) per nostril bid
   c. Triamcinolone (Nasacort), two sprays (110 μg) per nostril daily

> **Note**
> Side effects of all intranasal steroids include irritation and, rarely, nasal ulceration.

4. Cromolyn sodium (Nasalcrom) (a mast cell stabilizer), one spray (5.2 mg) per nostril three or four times per day. This drug has a less predictable response and should be used with regular (prophylactic) dosing.

Immunotherapy

1. Specific allergens (identified by skin tests or RAST) are injected weekly or monthly.

2. Reserved for patients with severe rhinitis who do not respond to or who cannot or will not take medications and who have symptoms for more than two seasons or six months.

3. The best response is seen with seasonal allergies to pollens.

Patient Education

Avoidance of precipitating allergens is vital.

1. Dust mites
   a. Keep humidity below 50 per cent.
   b. Wash sheets in very hot water at least once a week.
   c. Encase mattress, boxspring, and pillows in plastic.
   d. Dust floors (remove carpets) and surfaces frequently.
2. Mold
   a. Lower the humidity (as above).
   b. Vent and clean bathrooms with fungicides.
   c. Remove books and plants from the bedroom.
   d. Install air filter units.
3. Animal allergens: Remove pets from the house or at least from the bedroom.
4. Pollen
   a. Avoid outdoor exposure.
   b. Keep the bedroom windows closed (use air conditioning).
   c. Install air filter units.

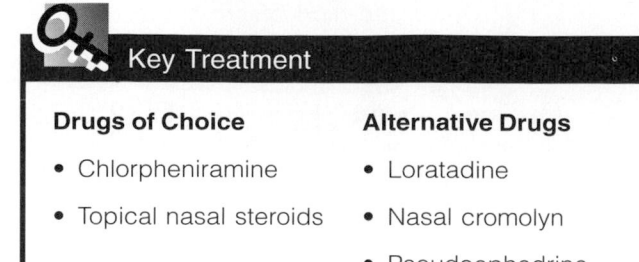

Key Treatment

Drugs of Choice	Alternative Drugs
• Chlorpheniramine	• Loratadine
• Topical nasal steroids	• Nasal cromolyn
	• Pseudoephedrine

Follow-Up

1. If response to treatment is poor, and an anatomic or a secondary disorder is a consideration, refer to a head and neck specialist.

2. If the diagnosis seems correct but the response to treatment is poor, refer to an allergist.

Bibliography

Fornadley JA, Corey JP, Osguthorpe JD, et al: Allergic rhinitis: clinical practice guideline. Otolaryngol Head Neck Surg 1996;115:115–122.

Guarderas JC: Rhinitis and sinusitis: office management. Mayo Clin Proc 1996;71:882–888.

Lund VJ, Aaronson D, Bousquet J, et al: International consensus report on the diagnosis and management of rhinitis: International Rhinitis Management Working Group. Allergy 1994;49(Suppl 19):1–34.

Noble SL, Forbes RC: Allergic rhinitis. Am Fam Physician 1995;51:834–846.

Prenner BM, Scharf M: Prescribing antihistamines: what you need to know. Int Med 1997;18:57–66.

24 Nasal Polyps

H. Bruce Vogt

Etiology and Epidemiology

1. Nasal polyps are non-neoplastic outgrowths of nasal and sinus mucosa. They usually arise from the middle meatus, middle turbinates, and ethmoid (particularly anterior) sinuses, although they may also arise from the superior turbinates and maxillary and sphenoid sinuses. They are rarely found on inferior turbinates or the nasal septum. Nasal polyps are associated with several diseases. Although inflammation appears to be a key factor, their specific etiology remains controversial and is likely multifactorial. The most frequently proposed hypotheses are

   a. Infection: despite a dramatic decrease in chronic (infective) sinusitis, however, the incidence of nasal polyps has not changed.

   b. Allergy: long believed to be an important factor, although several studies contradict its role. An immunoglobulin E–mediated mechanism may be one mechanism for the inflammatory changes in the mucosa that initiate polyp formation.

2. A hereditary factor may exist for nasal polyps; however, the mode of transmission is unknown. The estimated incidence of nasal polyps in the "normal" population is approximately 1 per cent, and men outnumber women 2:1 to 3:1. The prevalence increases with age, peaking at age 50 or older. Predisposing diseases and the incidence of polyps in these diseases are

   a. Nonallergic (intrinsic) asthma (13 per cent)

   b. Allergic asthma (5 per cent)

   c. Aspirin intolerance (36 per cent)

   d. Nonallergic rhinitis (5 per cent)

   e. Allergic rhinitis (1.5 per cent)

   f. Allergic fungal sinusitis (80 to 85 per cent)

   g. Cystic fibrosis (10 to 20 per cent)

   h. Dental sinusitis (16 per cent)

   i. Kartagener's syndrome (27 per cent)

   j. Churg-Strauss syndrome (36 to 50 per cent)

   k. Young's syndrome (?)

3. The triad of nasal polyps, aspirin sensitivity, and asthma is well documented. Polyps are rare in children less than 10 years of age and, when present in any child 16 years of age or younger, suggest the possibility of cystic fibrosis until proven otherwise.

Symptoms

1. Nasal obstruction
2. Hyposmia or anosmia
3. Loss of taste (secondary to hyposmia/anosmia)
4. Nasal voice
5. Snoring
6. Sneezing
7. Rhinorrhea
8. Postnasal draining

Symptoms may be aggravated by temperature changes or environmental exposure to dusts, chemicals, fumes, and odors.

Key Symptoms

- Nasal obstruction
- Hyposmia or anosmia
- Loss of taste
- Nasal voice

Clinical Findings

1. Soft, smooth, pale, round or pear-shaped gelatinous lesions
2. Mobile, insensitive to pain, and typically do not bleed
3. Usually located on the lateral wall of the nose, most often in the middle meatus, and prolapse into the nasal cavity
4. The diagnosis is usually made by anterior rhinoscopy; however, endoscopic (fiberoptic or rigid) examination provides the best visualization.

Key Signs

- Soft, smooth, pale, gelatinous lesions
- Mobile
- Pain insensitive

Laboratory Tests

1. Objective testing to quantify the severity of nasal airway obstruction (nasal inspiratory peak flow, anterior rhinomanometry, acoustic rhinometry) and tests of smell to assess response to treatment are available but not used routinely.
2. Radiology
   a. Sinus films are of limited value.
   b. Computerized tomography with coronal sections is indicated to determine the extent of disease when surgery is to be performed.
3. Allergy testing may be considered when associated allergies are suspected.
   a. Skin tests
   b. Radioallergosorbent testing (RAST)
4. Pulmonary function tests may be considered because some patients have subclinical asthma.
5. Children with nasal polyps should be evaluated for cystic fibrosis (sweat test).

Key Tests

- Sweat test in children
- Allergy testing if indicated
- Computerized tomography prior to surgery

Differential Diagnosis

1. The following conditions may be confused with nasal polyps:
   a. Nasal turbinate congestion (most common)
   b. Hypertrophied or polypoid nasal turbinates
   c. Benign tumors (e.g., squamous papilloma, inverting papilloma, angiofibroma)
   d. Malignant tumors (e.g., mucinous adenocarcinoma, squamous cell carcinoma, sarcoma)
   e. Encephalocele (in infants)
2. An important distinguishing feature of nasal polyps is their insensitivity to pain on manipulation, unlike the well-innervated nasal turbinates. Congested turbinates generally decrease in size upon application of a topical decongestant, whereas nasal polyps do not.
3. Additional characteristics that suggest a diagnosis other than nasal polyps include unilaterality, firmness, friability, and spontaneous bleeding.

Treatment

Effective treatment requires a combination of medications and surgery.

Medical Treatment

1. Intranasal corticosteroids are the mainstay of medical treatment. They have been proven to reduce polyp size and associated nasal symptomatology, and to significantly reduce recurrences following polypectomy. Corticosteroid sprays and inhalers include
   a. Beclomethasone diproprionate (Beconase, Vancenase)—age 6 or older
      (1) Beconase Inhalation Aerosol, 1 inhalation each nostril two to four times daily
      (2) Beconase AQ Nasal Spray, 1 to 2 inhalations each nostril twice daily
      (3) Vancenase Pockethaler, 1 inhalation each nostril two to four times daily
      (4) Vancenase AQ Nasal Spray, 1 to 2 inhalations each nostril twice daily
   b. Funisolide—ages 6 or older: Nasalide or Nasarel Nasal Solution, 2 inhalations each nostril twice daily
   c. Budesnoside—age 6 or older: Rhinocort Nasal Inhaler, 2 inhalations each nostril twice daily, or 4 inhalations each nostril once daily in the morning
   d. Fluticasone proprionate—age 4 or older: Flonase Nasal Spray, 1 inhalation each nostril twice daily, or 2 inhalations each nostril once daily in the morning
   e. Triamcinolone acetonide—age 12 or older: Nasacort Nasal Inhaler or Nasacort AQ Nasal Spray, 2 inhalations each nostril once daily in the morning

   With all of these agents, once control is achieved reduce the effective dose.
2. Systemic steroids are very effective in reducing the size of polyps and rhinitis symptoms, and have been reported to be as effective as surgery. When used preoperatively, they facilitate surgery by reducing polyp size and also delay recurrences. They are often used in patients with intractable disease. They usually relieve anosmia, as opposed to topical steroids. *Contraindications* to their use include advanced osteoporosis, severe hypertension, diabetes mellitus, gastric ulcer, and herpetic keratitis. Intranasal steroids must be used concurrently to retard recurrences. Regimens include
   a. Prednisone, 60 mg/day with 10- to 14-day taper
   b. Prednisolone, 30 mg for 7 days with 10- to 20-day taper
   c. Dexamethasone, 12 mg for 3 days, 8 mg for 3 days, 4 mg for 3 days
3. When allergy is concurrent, environmental con-

trol measures should be instituted, along with antihistamines or decongestant-antihistamine preparations and cromolyn sodium if indicated. Desensitization may also be employed. In patients with aspirin hypersensitivity, elimination of natural salicylates and tartrazine dyes (link with aspirin) is worth a trial. Because wheat-flour hypersensitivity may produce rhinitis symptomatology, dietary exclusion of it may be tried.

4. Antibiotics must be used for associated bacterial sinusitis.

Surgery

1. Referral to an otolaryngologist for possible surgery should be considered when intranasal steroids have been ineffective. Surgery may be the only option in patients who have failed topical steroid therapy and in whom systemic steroids are contraindicated. Intranasal and external approaches are used. Procedures include

   a. Simple snare polypectomy

   b. Powered nasal polypectomy

   c. Laser polypectomy

   d. Functional endoscopic sinus surgery (FESS)

   e. Intranasal ethmoidectomy

   f. Transantral ethmoidectomy

   g. Radical ethmofrontosphenoidectomy

2. Despite meticulous surgery, recurrence is common. Postoperative topical steroids delay recurrences.

Key Treatment	
Medical	Surgical
• Intranasal steroids	• Polypectomy
• Short course of oral steroids	• FESS
	• Ethmoidectomy

Follow-Up

1. Nasal polyposis tends to be a recurrent disease. Although some patients may be able to control their disease with periodic use of intranasal steroids, ongoing therapy is required for many.

2. Periodic office visits are important to determine patient compliance, provide patient education, identify complications, and modify treatment.

Bibliography

Drake-Lee AB: Medical treatment of nasal polyps. Rhinology 1994;32:1–2.

Holmberg K, Karlsson G: Nasal polyps: medical or surgical management. Clin Exp Allergy 1996;26(Suppl 3): 23–30.

Lund VK: Diagnosis and treatment of nasal polyps. BMJ 1995;311:1411–1414.

Mygind MD, Lildholdt T: Nasal polyps treatment: medical management. Allergy Asthma Proc 1996;17:275–282.

Slavin RG: Nasal polyps and sinusitis. JAMA 1997;278: 1849–1854.

A nasal fracture, the most frequent facial bone fracture, should be suspected when any significant facial trauma occurs. Isolated nasal fractures are common. It is important to bear in mind that only displaced fractures require reduction; simple undisplaced fractures require only local application of ice to reduce swelling, and analgesia. In addition, there is often poor correlation between the radiologic findings and the presence of external deformity, the latter determining the need for reduction. In delayed presentations where significant swelling is present, it is wiser to defer attempts at reduction and refer the patient within 5 to 7 days.

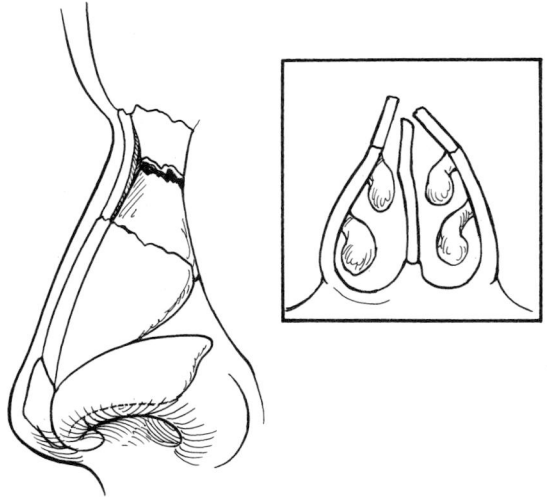

Indications

1. History of recent nasal trauma (within approximately 24 hours)
2. Clinical or radiologic confirmation with visible deformity (verify with patient that deformity is new)
3. Unilateral compromise of the bony pyramid
4. Bilateral fractures with demonstrable integrity of the septum

Contraindications

1. Open nasal fracture
2. Suspected cribriform plate fracture with or without cerebrospinal fluid (CSF) leak
3. Bilateral or complex fractures of the nasal pyramid involving the septum with or without hematoma
4. Nasal fractures with suspected associated midface fractures
5. Blood dyscrasias

Diagnosis

1. History: Review details of the injury, any past history of nasal trauma or deformity, epistaxis, nasal breathing, or blood dyscrasias.
2. Clinical examination
   a. External: Inspect for deformities, swelling, ecchymosis, epistaxis, and rhinorrhea and check ocular movements. Gently palpate the nose and face for tenderness, crepitus, and instability.
   b. Internal: Gentle suctioning is frequently required for adequate evaluation of the nasal cavity and septum. Refer patient if there is CSF leakage, septal hematoma (must be drained urgently), or septal dislocation or fracture.
   c. Examine the oropharynx and look for posterior nasal bleeding; if present, refer.
3. Radiographic evaluation
   a. Review nasal radiographs for nasal fracture
   b. If more extensive injury is suspected, rule out fractures involving the cervical spine, facial bones, and sinuses.

Equipment

1. Headlamp or other good light source
2. Suction equipment with nasal cannulas
3. Nasal speculum
4. Walsham or Asch forceps or other suitable blunt surgical instrument (e.g., a scalpel handle or a large hemostat wrapped in gauze at the tip to protect the nasal mucosa)
5. Bayonet forceps

Anesthesia

1. Intranasal (wait 15 minutes after application before attempting reduction)—Use one of the following:
   a. Cocaine 4%; Soak 3-in rolled cotton pledgets in the solution and squeeze excess out. Under direct visualization, place one pack along the floor of the nose, another along the roof, and the third along the middle turbinate.
   b. Cocaine 10%; Spray the nasal mucosa with 2 ml of 10% cocaine solution.
   c. Benzocaine or lidocaine spray with a topical vasoconstrictor (e.g., 0.5% phenylephrine hydrochloride [Neo-Synephrine] or oxymetazoline [Afrin])
2. Extranasal—Use one of the following:
   a. EMLA cream (eutectic mixture of local anesthetics; lidocaine 2.5%, prilocaine 2.5%):

Apply a thick layer on the nasal pyramid skin and cover with an occlusive plastic dressing. A major disadvantage of this cream is that it must be applied 1 hour prior to reduction.

   b. External infiltration of the nose with 1% lidocaine with 1:100,000 epinephrine: bilateral percutaneous infiltration of the whole bony dorsum with the needle inserted on each side at the anterior (caudal) edge of the nasal bone midway between the nasal bridge and the maxilla.

3. Optional: sedation with a short-acting benzodiazepine such as midazolam (Versed). Monitor patient's oxygenation status when using sedation.

Precautions

1. Absence of contraindications

2. Patient awareness and understanding of the procedure for compliance and cooperation

3. Warn patient that even a perfect nasal fracture reduction at the time of the procedure may develop some deviation a few weeks later (mostly because of a deflection of the septum), and subsequent elective revision may be necessary.

4. Signed consent form prior to procedure

Technique

1. The patient should be sitting in a chair with posterior head support.

2. Perform an external and internal examination as previously described.

3. Anesthetize as previously described.

4. WAIT 15 MINUTES TO ALLOW FOR PROPER ANESTHESIA AND VASOCONSTRICTION before reduction.

5. Digital pressure alone may be sufficient to manipulate the nasal fracture into the midline position (thus avoiding internal nasal instrumentation and reducing the risk of epistaxis).

6. Otherwise insert the instrument chosen into the nostril of the affected side under the nasal bone with the dominant hand.

7. Reduce the fracture by pushing anteriorly and superiorly with the instrument while the nondominant hand verifies the proper position of the nasal bone.

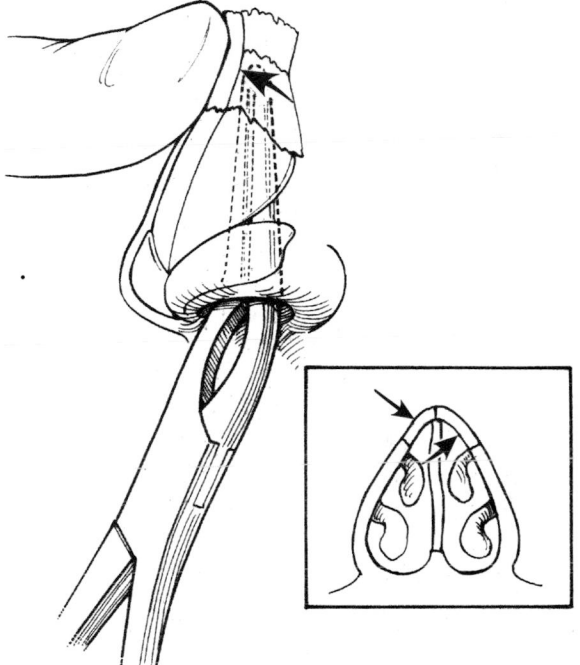

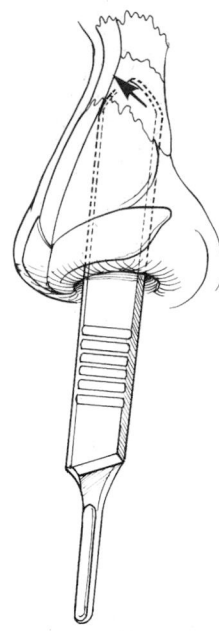

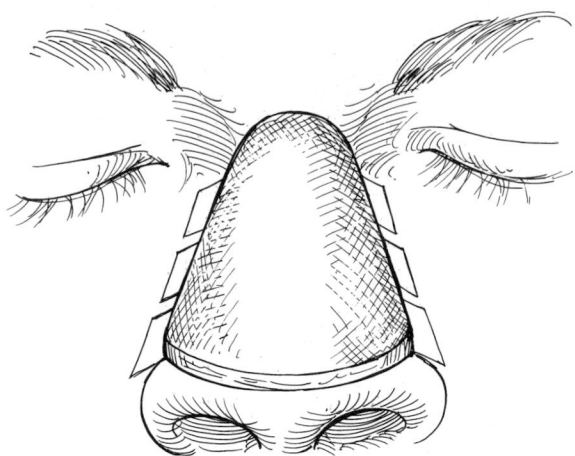

8. In bilateral fractures, insert both blades in the side of the greatest deformity and use the non-dominant hand to apply pressure on the contralateral nasal bone.

9. Inspect and gently palpate the nasal pyramid. It should appear aesthetically adequate for both the physician and the patient. Then perform anterior rhinoscopy to be sure both nasal passages look symmetric, allowing good air flow, that the septum is midline without hematoma; and that there is no epistaxis.

10. Intranasal packing is usually unnecessary. Light packing of the nose should only be utilized to control epistaxis.

11. Routine use of an external nasal splint is unnecessary but may serve to remind the patient of the injury. If one is to be applied, the skin should be cleaned and degreased and two to three layers of paper tape or ½-in Steri-strips applied; a prepackaged nasal splint is placed over this. Alternatively, one can be made from five layers of plaster cast material cut to the shape of the nose.

12. Observe for 15 minutes, and verify the absence of anterior or posterior nasal bleeding.

13. Contrary to previous practice, there is no need to prescribe a broad-spectrum oral antibiotic.

Follow-Up

1. Instruct the patient to watch for and report posterior nasal bleeding, hematemesis, fever, persistent headache, difficulty tasting food, visual disturbances, or dizziness.

2. Re-evaluate in 48 hours (and remove packing if any was placed).

3. Remove the external splint, if used, in 7 days.

4. Recheck the patient in 1 month, and consider referral if results are unsatisfactory.

 Bibliography

Bowerman JE: Fractures of the middle third of the facial skeleton. In Williams JL (ed): Rowe and Williams' Maxillofacial Injuries, vol 2, pp 591–603. New York, Churchill Livingstone, 1994.

Cook JA, Murrant NJ, Evans K, et al: Manipulation of the fractured nose under local anesthesia. Clin Otolaryngol 1992;17:337–340.

Houghton DJ, Hanafi Z, Papakostas K, et al: Efficacy of external fixation following nasal manipulation under local anaesthesia. Clin Otolaryngol 1998;23:169–171.

Nigam A, Goni A, Benjamin A, et al: The value of radiographs in the management of the fractured nose. Arch Emerg Med 1993;10:293–297.

Renner GJ: Management of nasal fractures. Otolaryngol Clin North Am 1991;24:195–213.

25 Sinusitis

John W. Williams, Jr.

Etiology

1. Sinusitis is defined as inflammation of one or more paranasal sinuses but usually refers to infection of the sinuses. The maxillary sinuses are the most frequently infected, either alone or in combination with the ethmoid or frontal sinuses. Isolated sphenoid sinusitis is rare and constitutes a medical emergency. The maxillary sinus drains through a narrow channel, the ostiomeatal complex, that is easily obstructed by inflammation or edema. Obstruction is followed by decreased ciliary action, increased mucus production, and bacterial proliferation. In 5 to 10 per cent of cases, maxillary sinusitis is associated with dental abscess and is thought to result from contiguous spread of bacteria.

2. Factors that predispose to ostial obstruction include viral upper respiratory tract infection, allergic rhinitis, overuse of topical decongestants, deviated nasal septum, nasopharyngeal intubation, nasal polyps, and tumors. Immunodeficiency and bronchiectasis may also predispose to sinusitis.

3. The microbiology of sinusitis is best considered in relation to the duration of symptoms. In adults with acute sinusitis, the most common organisms are *Streptococcus pneumoniae* (35 per cent) and *Haemophilus influenzae* (35 per cent). β-Lactamase–producing strains of *H. influenzae* and *Moraxella catarrhalis* are amoxicillin-resistant but are not prevalent in acute sinusitis. In chronic sinusitis, anaerobic organisms are much more common (more than 50 per cent), and infections are more likely to be polymicrobic.

Symptoms

1. There may be a high degree of overlap between symptoms of acute or chronic sinusitis and other causes of nasal congestion, such as allergic or viral rhinitis. No single symptom or sign is pathognomonic. Despite diagnostic difficulties, the overall accuracy of the clinical evaluation is about 78 per cent and is based on the recognition of a pattern of symptoms and signs.

2. Acute sinusitis should be high on the differential when a patient has a prolonged "cold" (>7 to 10 days) or an unusually severe "cold." Colored rhinorrhea, cough, and pain in the upper teeth are characteristic symptoms. Unilateral facial pain and failure to improve with over-the-counter decongestants or antihistamines increase the likelihood of sinusitis.

3. Chronic sinusitis presents as a protracted course of respiratory symptoms, including nasal congestion and cough. Facial fullness, headache, and nasal drainage may be prominent, but fever is uncommon.

Key Symptoms

- Maxillary toothache
- Colored rhinorrhea
- Poor response to over-the-counter nasal decongestants and antihistamines

Clinical Findings

1. A focused examination is useful diagnostically and to evaluate for predisposing causes. Most commonly the patient is afebrile or has a low-grade fever and does not appear very ill.

2. The focused examination consists of the following:

   a. Examine the nasal mucosa for color, edema, and character of nasal secretions; polyps; and structure of the nasal septum. Purulent secretion, particularly when seen coming from the middle meatus, is predictive of sinusitis.

   b. In a completely darkened room, transilluminate the maxillary sinuses by placing a Welch-Allyn Finnoff transilluminator or Mini Mag-Lite over the infraorbital rim, and judge light transmission through the hard palate. Normal and equal light transmission from side to side makes sinusitis much less likely. Decreased light transmission on either side makes sinusitis more likely but also may be due to polyps or a hypoplastic sinus.

   c. Percuss the maxillary teeth with a tongue blade to check for a dental source of sinusitis.

   d. Facial tenderness elicited by palpation is an

unreliable sign for maxillary sinusitis but may be useful for frontal sinus infection.

When none of the key symptoms or signs is present, the probability of sinusitis is less than 10 per cent; when all are present, the probability of sinusitis exceeds 90 per cent.

Tests

1. Sinusitis is usually diagnosed clinically, but, when considerable uncertainty persists after the clinical evaluation or the patient fails an initial course of therapy, diagnostic testing may be useful.
2. Radiographic evaluation is the most useful diagnostic test for nonspecialists.
   a. Compared with sinus aspiration and culture, conventional radiographs are about 85 per cent sensitive and 75 per cent specific for maxillary sinusitis. A single Waters view is less expensive and correlates highly with the standard four-view sinus series. However, conventional radiographs visualize the ethmoid sinuses poorly.
   b. Sinus computerized tomography is more sensitive (90 to 100 per cent) and images the ethmoid sinuses well but may have poor specificity (60 per cent; therefore, many false positives). It is best used for evaluating the ostiomeatal complex in chronic sinusitis as well as complications of sinusitis, such as orbital cellulitis and cerebral abscess.
3. Nasal cytology may be useful for evaluating chronic nasal symptoms. A sample can be obtained by having the patient blow his nose into wax paper or by using a cotton-tipped applicator to swab the nasal mucosa. The specimen should be stained with a modified Wright-Giemsa or Hansel stain and examined at high power. Five or more neutrophils per high-power field (HPF) has 86 per cent sensitivity and 40 per cent specificity for radiographic evidence of sinusitis. Five or more eosinophils per HPF makes allergic rhinitis or nasal polyposis more likely than sinusitis.
4. Cultures of nasal secretions do not correlate with cultures from sinus antral aspirates and should not be done. Sinus aspiration and culture is the "gold standard" for establishing sinusitis but is most useful for draining the sinus and guiding antibiotic coverage in patients with complicated or refractory sinusitis.
5. Flexible rhinopharyngoscopy allows a detailed inspection of the nasal cavity and posterior nasopharynx. It is most useful for establishing the diagnosis of chronic sinusitis and for identifying anatomic abnormalities that may predispose to recurrent sinusitis.

Differential Diagnosis

1. The differential diagnosis for nasal symptoms is long but can be grouped into three broad categories: inflammatory, noninflammatory, and mechanical causes.
   a. Inflammatory: allergic rhinitis (seasonal or perennial), acute viral infection, acute or chronic bacterial sinusitis, nasal polyps, Wegener's granulomatosis, sarcoidosis
   b. Noninflammatory: idiopathic vasomotor rhinitis, drug-induced vasomotor rhinitis (reserpine, guanethidine, prazosin, angiotensin-converting enzyme inhibitors, cocaine abuse), rhinitis medicamentosa, hormonal (pregnancy, hypothyroidism)
   c. Mechanical: deviated septum, nasal polyps, tumor, foreign body
2. In the primary care setting, the most common causes of nasal symptoms are allergic rhinitis, acute viral infection, acute or chronic sinusitis, idiopathic vasomotor rhinitis, rhinitis medicamentosa, and deviated nasal septum.

Treatment

The management of acute sinusitis is aimed at improving drainage of the sinuses and eradicating bacterial infection.

Medication

1. Antibiotic choice is based on the duration of symptoms, cost, and evidence of efficacy from randomized controlled trials. A recent meta-analysis showed therapeutic equivalency for multiple classes of antibiotics. For acute sinusitis (symptoms present <30 days), 7 to 10 days of trimethoprim-sulfamethoxazole (Bactrim,

Septra), 160/800 mg bid, or amoxicillin, 500 mg tid, leads to 80 to 90 per cent clinical response rates; these are the drugs of choice. In geographic areas with a high prevalence of β-lactamase–producing *H. influenzae* or *M. catarrhalis*, an agent with a broader spectrum, such as amoxicillin-clavulanate (Augmentin), cefaclor (Ceclor), cefuroxime axetil (Ceftin), or azithromycin (Zithromax), is appropriate. For patients with protracted symptoms, a longer course (2 to 3 weeks) of antibiotics is probably indicated.

2. Topical and systemic decongestants promote sinus drainage and ventilation and may be used safely in patients with mild to moderate hypertension. Prolonged use of topical decongestants may lead to rebound vasodilation and rhinitis medicamentosa. For adults, prescribe oxymetazoline (Afrin) nasal spray 0.05%, two sprays bid for 3 to 5 days; pseudoephedrine (Sudafed) extended release, 120 mg bid; or phenylpropanolamine extended release, 75 mg bid.

3. Mucolytics and ciliator activators may thin secretions and promote sinus drainage. Evidence from one clinical trial suggests that guaifenesin, 30 mg qid, speeds recovery.

4. Nasal corticosteroids have a limited role in acute sinusitis but may be useful for selected patients with underlying allergic rhinitis. Nasal steroids inhibit inflammatory responses without inducing adrenal suppression and act to decrease edema of the ostiomeatal complex.

5. Nasal saline or steam may decrease nasal crusting and liquefy secretions, thus facilitating sinus drainage.

6. Antihistamines may thicken nasal secretions, and, therefore, they are not routinely indicated in the initial treatment of acute sinusitis. For patients with underlying allergic rhinitis, the nonsedating antihistamines are less likely to thicken secretions and may be useful ancillary treatment when topical corticosteroids have failed.

Patient Education

1. Most patients feel substantially improved or cured after 5 to 6 days of effective therapy.

2. Emphasize that prolonged use of topical decongestants may cause rebound vasodilation and worsening symptoms.

3. For patients with underlying allergic conditions, avoidance of environmental allergens may be helpful.

4. When prescribing nasal steroids, instruct the patient that it may take 1 to 2 weeks to achieve maximal effect.

Key Treatment

- Drugs of choice: trimethoprim-sulfamethoxazole or amoxicillin; oxymetazoline nasal spray

- Alternative drugs: amoxicillin-clavulanate, cefaclor, cefuroxime axetil, azithromycin, clarithromycin

Follow-Up

1. For most patients, the initial course of therapy leads to clinical cure, and no specific follow-up is needed. For patients who do not improve with initial treatment or have recurrent disease, further evaluation and therapy are indicated.

2. Patients who do not respond to an initial course of treatment should be re-evaluated. If not previously done, sinus radiographs should be taken to confirm the diagnosis. Once confirmed, a longer course of a broad-spectrum antibiotic that is effective against β-lactamase–producing organisms should be prescribed.

3. In patients with sinusitis that recurs three or more times a year, further evaluation by an otolaryngologist is indicated. This evaluation should include a search for anatomic factors that may predispose to sinusitis.

Bibliography

For more information on the bacteriology of acute sinusitis, see
Gwaltney JM Jr, Schel W, Sande MA, et al: The microbial etiology and antimicrobial therapy of adults with acute sinusitis: a fifteen-year experience at the University of Virginia and review of other selected studies. J Allergy Clin Immunol 1992;90:457–462.

For more information on the diagnosis of sinusitis, see
Gwaltney JM, Phillips CD, Miller RD, et al: Computed tomographic study of the common cold. N Engl J Med 1994;330:25–30.
Williams JW Jr, Simel DL: Does this patient have sinusitis? Diagnosing acute sinusitis by history and physical examination. JAMA 1992;270:1242–1246.

For more information on the treatment of sinusitis, see
Coates ML, Rembold CM, Farr BM: Does pseudoephedrine increase blood pressure in patients with controlled hypertension? J Fam Pract 1995;40:22–26.
deBock GH, Dekker FW, Stolk J, et al: Antimicrobial treatment in acute maxillary sinusitis: a meta-analysis. J Clin Epidemiol 1997;50:881–890.
de Ferranti SD, Ioannidis JPA, Lau J, Anninger WV, Barza M: Are amoxicillin and folate inhibitors as effective as other antibiotics for acute sinusitis? A meta-analysis. BMJ 1998;317:632–637.

26 Orbital and Periorbital Cellulitis

Kimberly L. Morris

Etiology

1. Sinusitis is the most common predisposing condition in patients with orbital cellulitis. The ethmoid sinuses are most frequently involved, followed by the maxillary sinuses.

   a. Children under age 4 years

      (1) *Haemophilus influenzae* type b (HIB): less common pathogen in post-HIB vaccination era; if suspected, consider concomitant, life-threatening infections such as meningitis, epiglottitis, and pneumonia.

      (2) Streptococcal species: most common pathogens; *S. pneumoniae* most likely with young children; group A streptococcus common with older children.

   b. Older children and adults

      (1) Acute sinusitis: *H. influenzae, S. pneumoniae, Moraxella (Branhamella) catarrhalis, Staphylococcus aureus, Streptococcus pyogenes,* and *viridans* streptococci

      (2) Chronic sinusitis is often caused by polymicrobial infection with both aerobic and anaerobic bacteria, including *Bacteroides* species, *Peptostreptococcus,* and *Fusobacterium* species.

2. Orbital cellulitis may also occur as a result of contiguous spread from adjacent structures by way of the valveless facial veins.

   a. Dental infection—anaerobes

   b. Facial infection

   c. Infection of the globe or eyelids

   d. Lacrimal system

3. Less common causes of orbital cellulitis include direct trauma to the eye, often with implantation of a foreign body, and, rarely, postsurgical infection. *Staphylococcus aureus* is the most common pathogen in both situations.

4. Hematogenous spread from distal infection may occur and should be considered in patients with serious underlying diseases, such as diabetes, cirrhosis, and immunosuppression.

5. Tumor resulting in sinus obstruction must also be considered in the older patient, particularly in smokers.

6. Nasal cocaine abuse may cause septal and orbital bone destruction and predispose to sinusitis.

Symptoms

1. Pain, erythema, eyelid edema

2. Symptoms of sinusitis, such as facial tenderness, purulent nasal secretions, fever, headache, halitosis

Key Symptoms

- Erythema
- Pain
- Fever
- Purulent secretions
- Eyelid edema
- Facial tenderness
- Headache

Clinical Findings

1. Specific signs of orbital involvement include proptosis, limited extraocular movement, and vision loss.

2. Conjunctival edema (chemosis) and injection are seen frequently. Eyelid edema is a nonspecific finding.

3. A bluish skin discoloration is often seen in children with *H. influenzae* infection.

4. Ominous signs of cavernous sinus and meningeal involvement include sensory loss in the ophthalmic branch of the trigeminal nerve, cranial neuropathy, afferent pupillary defect, and mental status changes.

Key Signs

- Proptosis
- Vision loss
- Pupil abnormality
- Ophthalmoplegia
- Chemosis
- Cranial neuropathy

Tests

1. Laboratory tests
   a. White blood cell count with differential
      (1) In adults, a range of 10,000 to 15,000/mm^3 is common.
      (2) In children, the white blood cell count may exceed 20,000/mm^3.
   b. Blood cultures
   c. Drainage from all wounds should be cultured.
   d. In general, cultures from the conjunctivae, eyelids, and nasal passages are not helpful.
   e. Aspiration of orbital contents is not recommended because of the low yield of cultures and the risk of the procedure.
2. Other tests
   a. Computerized tomography with axial and coronal cuts through the orbit is indicated and may provide additional information that can aid in selecting treatment.
   b. Plain radiographs may assist in ruling out dental abscess in patients with maxillary sinus opacification on computerized tomography.

Key Tests

- Computerized tomography must be performed if signs of orbital infection are present.
- Blood cultures must be obtained.
- Consider cerebrospinal fluid analysis in children who have not received the HIB vaccine.

Differential Diagnosis

1. Preseptal cellulitis may cause pain, redness, eyelid edema, chemosis, and conjunctival injection. Structures anterior to the orbit are involved. A patient with these findings in the absence of orbital signs can be managed more conservatively. However, complications such as meningitis may occur in young children, and therefore hospitalization is warranted.
2. Subperiosteal abscess may involve the medial wall of the orbit. Displacement of the medial rectus muscle by the periosteum may be seen by computerized tomography.
3. Blunt trauma to the eyelid with orbital foreign body or local infection
4. Orbital pseudotumor may present with eyelid edema, proptosis, and ophthalmoplegia, but the characteristic signs of infection are absent.

5. Dacryocystitis can be seen with acute mumps infection or chronic sarcoidosis.
6. Allergic reactions are usually accompanied by pruritus and are nontender and recurrent.
7. Orbital tumors such as rhabdomyosarcoma may be seen in children.

WARNING

Mycotic orbital infection must be suspected in diabetic patients or in those with metabolic acidosis. Necrosis of the palate or nasal mucosa is presumptive evidence.

Treatment

1. The patient should be hospitalized and given empiric intravenous antibiotic treatment. Antibiotic selection should be made on the basis of the most likely cause.
   a. In children, a second-generation cephalosporin with gram-positive coverage and *H. influenzae* coverage would be reasonable.
   b. In adults, ceftriaxone (Rocephin), cefuroxime (Kefurox, Zinacef), or ampicillin-sulbactam (Unasyn) is suggested. In patients with immediate-type hypersensitivity reactions to β-lactam antibiotics, clindamycin (Cleocin) combined with ciprofloxacin (Cipro) or aztreonam (Azactam) would be reasonable.
   c. Amphotericin B is the drug of choice if mucormycosis (*Rhizopus* species) is suspected.
2. A multispecialty approach is optimal and should include a physician who is knowledgeable in antibiotic use, an otolaryngologist, and an ophthalmologist. Surgical intervention may be necessary if clinical response is inadequate or abscess is present.

Key Treatment

Antibiotic selection must be based on the likely cause in view of specific patient characteristics.

Follow-Up

1. Close clinical follow-up is mandatory. Signs of orbital involvement should be assessed twice daily. Repeat computerized tomographic scanning may be indicated if the clinical course is suboptimal.
2. Surgical drainage of the sinuses and orbital exploration may be necessary.

Bibliography

Davis JP, Stearns MP: Orbital complications of sinusitis. Postgrad Med J 1994;70:108–110.

Lessner A, Stern GA: Preseptal and orbital cellulitis. Infect Dis Clin North Am 1992;6:933–952.

Martin-Hirsch DP, Habashi S, Hampton AH, et al: Orbital cellulitis. Arch Emerg Med 1992;9:143–148.

Schwartz GR, Wright SW: Changing bacteriology of periorbital cellulitis. Ann Emerg Med 1996;28:617–620.

Steinkuller PG, Jones DB: Preseptal and orbital cellulitis and orbital abscess. In Linberg JV (ed): Oculoplastic and Orbital Emergencies, pp 51–66. East Norwalk, CT, Appleton & Lange, 1992.

Indications

1. Surgical or dental procedures
2. Pain control: postoperative; terminal cancer
3. Facilitation of orotracheal or nasotracheal intubation
4. Diagnosis and treatment of tic douloureux and trigeminal neuralgia

Contraindications

1. Practitioner's lack of knowledge of anatomic landmarks and local anesthetic characteristics
2. Allergies to all local anesthetics
3. Poor patient cooperation
4. Infection of injection site, severe coagulopathy, lack of clearly identifiable landmarks

Preparation

1. Educate patient about pain on injection and limits of pain control.
2. Premedicate using parenteral sedatives, hypnotics, and/or opioids.
3. Have airway management and cardiopulmonary resuscitative equipment and resuscitation drugs available.

Equipment

1. Syringes (5 to 10 ml) and needles (22 to 27 gauge)
2. Skin preparation materials (sponges, iodine solution, alcohol)
3. Field sterility materials (mask, cap, drapes, gloves)

Anesthesia

1. Lidocaine (Xylocaine)
   a. Standard local anesthetic used for skin infiltration and most peripheral nerve blocks
   b. Lidocaine 1% to 2% solutions are usually used; solutions stronger than 2% may cause motor block.
   c. Duration of action is approximately 2 to 4 hours. Adding epinephrine (1:200,000 concentration) will slow the rate of absorption and prolong the block.
2. Bupivacaine (Marcaine)
   a. Duration of action is two to three times longer than that of lidocaine.
   b. More toxic (dose limit 2 to 3 mg/kg) than lidocaine

   c. For peripheral nerve blocks or skin infiltration, 0.25% to 0.50% solutions are typically used.
3. Ropivacaine (Naropin)
   a. Duration of action is similar to that of bupivacaine.
   b. Cardiac toxicity is greater than that of lidocaine but less than that of bupivacaine. Upper limit of drug dose is approximately 3 mg/kg.
   c. For peripheral nerve blocks or skin infiltration, 0.5% to 1.0% solutions can be used.
4. Lidocaine and Prilocaine (EMLA [eutectic mixture of local anesthetics] cream)
   a. A topical oil-in-water emulsion of lidocaine and prilocaine that permits larger quantities of anesthetic to penetrate to the nerve ending in deeper skin layers
   b. A thick application covered by an occlusive dressing will provide a 3-, 4-, and 5-mm depth of anesthesia after a 60-, 90-, and 120-minute application, respectively. Anesthesia will persist for 1 to 2 hours after wiping off the medication.
   c. Helps minimize the pain of injection of nerve blocks or allows for surgical excision of superficial skin lesions without additional injection of local anesthetic.
5. Cocaine
   a. Topical anesthetic primarily for the nose and throat; vasoconstrictive effect decreases swelling and bleeding.
   b. Total dose should not exceed 200 mg (e.g., 5 ml of 4% solution), regardless of application method.

Precautions

1. Central nervous system toxicity of local anesthetics
   a. Manifested by dysequilibrium, obtundation, confusion, seizures, or respiratory arrest
   b. Symptoms can occur with rapid absorption of perineural-injected local anesthetic or direct injection into the cerebrovascular circulation.
   c. Diazepam (Valium), 5 to 10 mg; midazolam (Versed), 2 to 6 mg; or thiopental (Pentothal Sodium), 2 to 4 mg/kg, is effective in treating local anesthetic-induced seizures.

2. Cardiotoxicity
   a. Cocaine can cause intense vasospasm leading to cardiac ischemia and infarction.
   b. Bupivacaine can cause cardiac arrest if upper dosage limits are exceeded.

WARNING

- Severe pain with needle advancement or injection of local anesthetic could mean intraneural needle placement. Withdraw the needle and reinsert.

- Aspirate before local anesthetic injection. Withdraw the needle and reinsert if blood or cerebrospinal fluid is aspirated.

Techniques

1. Brow and forehead block
   a. Blocking the supraorbital and supratrochlear nerves (terminal branches of the first division [ophthalmic nerve] of the trigeminal nerve) anesthetizes the ipsilateral forehead from eyebrow to vertex and from the midline to the temporal region (A in figure).

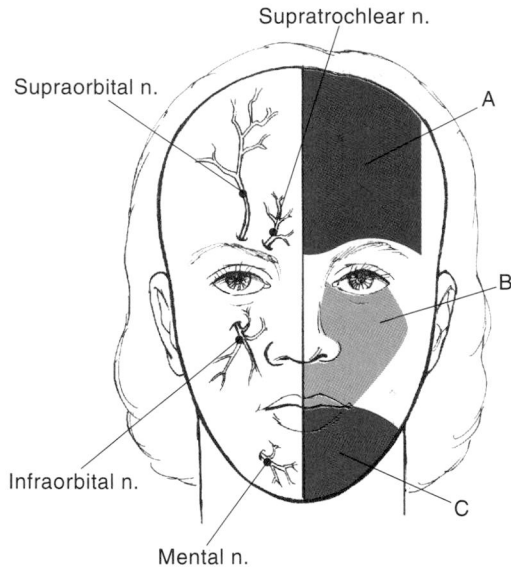

   b. Procedure
      (1) Prepare the block site in a sterile manner.
      (2) Above the eyebrow over the medial aspect, raise a skin wheal with a local anesthetic.
      (3) Insert a small-gauge needle through the skin wheal, and infiltrate 2 to 3 ml of local anesthetic over the medial half of the eyebrow.

2. Upper lip block
   a. Blocking the infraorbital nerve (peripheral nerve of the second [maxillary] division of the trigeminal nerve) anesthetizes the lower eyelid, cheek, lateral aspect of the nose, upper lip, and part of the temple (B).
   b. Procedure
      (1) Prepare the block site in a sterile manner.
      (2) The infraorbital nerve is located one fingerbreadth below the orbital rim in the same vertical plane as the pupil with the eye looking forward. Raise a skin wheal over this site.
      (3) Insert the needle through the wheal slightly cephalad and laterally toward the infraorbital foramen. Infiltrate 2 to 3 ml of local anesthetic in the general area.

3. Lower lip block
   a. Blocking the mental nerve (peripheral branch of the mandibular nerve [third division of the trigeminal nerve]) anesthetizes the ipsilateral lower lip and chin (C).
   b. Procedure
      (1) Prepare the injection site in a sterile manner.
      (2) The foramen through which the mental nerve emerges is found in the same vertical plane as the pupil and slightly above or on the superior aspect of the mandibular ramus. Raise a skin wheal over the mental foramen.
      (3) Insert the needle medially through the wheal, and inject 2 to 3 ml of local anesthetic.

4. External nose block
   a. The external nose is primarily innervated by the infratrochlear and external nasal nerves (terminal branches of the ophthalmic nerve; the lateral portion of the nose is innervated by the infraorbital nerve).
   b. Procedure
      (1) Prepare the injection site in a sterile manner.

(2) The infratrochlear and external nasal nerves are found about 1 cm above the inner canthus and just lateral to the medial wall of the orbit. Place a skin wheal over this site.

(3) Direct the needle posteriorly and slightly medially to a depth of about 2.5 cm. Inject 2 to 3 ml of local anesthetic.

(4) If anesthesia is also required over the lateral part of the nose, the infraorbital nerve should be blocked, as in upper lip block.

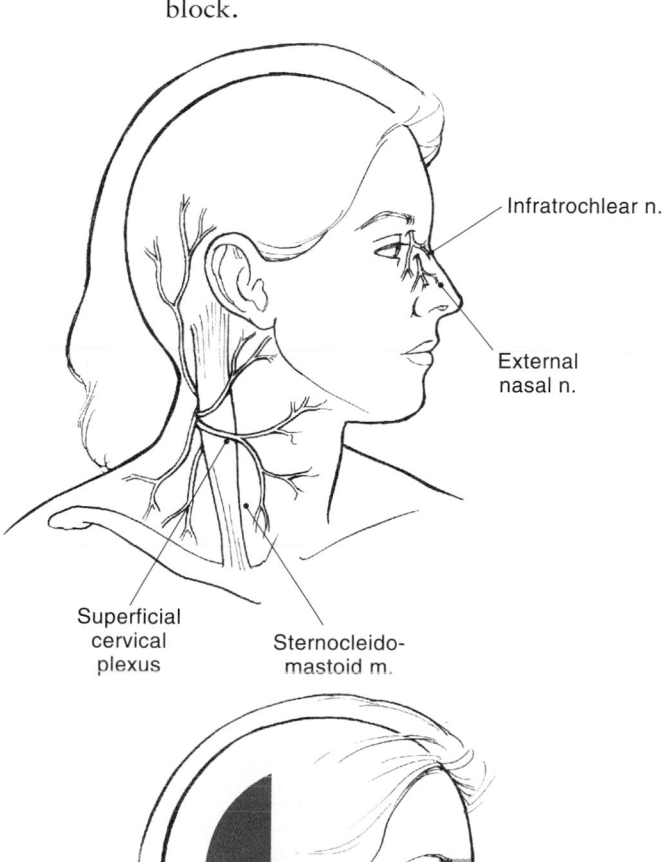

Infratrochlear n.

External nasal n.

Superficial cervical plexus

Sternocleido-mastoid m.

C-2

C-3

C-4

5. Neck block

a. The superficial cervical plexus is derived from the anterior rami of cervical nerves 2 through 4 (C-2 through C-4). Blocking the superficial cervical plexus anesthetizes the skin of the neck from midline to posterior.

b. Procedure

(1) Prepare the block site in a sterile manner.

(2) The superficial cervical plexus is found in the posterior triangle of the neck, emerging at the midpoint of the posterior border of the sternocleidomastoid muscle.

(3) Locate the posterior aspect of the sternocleidomastoid muscle and superficially infiltrate 3 to 4 ml of local anesthetic over the middle third.

Follow-Up

1. Obtain a neurology consult if sensation or motor function does not return within the expected time period (2 to 4 hours with lidocaine; 6 to 10 hours with bupivacaine or ropivacaine).

2. Instruct the patient to return immediately for evaluation if redness or exudation occurs at the injection site.

3. Hospitalize patients for adverse systemic reactions, such as seizures, respiratory arrest, or severe allergic reactions.

4. If peripheral nerve blocks are only partially effective, nerve root or first-division nerve blocks will provide better analgesia.

Bibliography

Carron H, Korbon GA: Common nerve blocks in anesthetic practice. Semin Anesth 1983;2:30–49.

de Jong RH: Local anesthetics. In Raj PP (ed): Practical Management of Pain with Special Emphasis on Physiology of Pain Syndromes and Techniques of Pain Management, pp 539–556. Chicago, Year Book Medical Publishers, 1986.

Ehlert TK, Arnold DE: Local anesthesia for soft-tissue surgery. Otolaryngol Clin North Am 1990;23:831–844.

Kretzschmar JL, Peters JE: Nerve blocks for regional anesthesia of the face. Am Fam Physician 1997;55:1701–1704.

Murphy TM: Somatic blockade of head and neck. In Cousins MJ, Bridenbaugh PO (eds): Neural Blockade in Clinical Anesthesia and Management of Pain, 2nd ed, pp 533–560. Philadelphia, JB Lippincott Company, 1988.

27 Common Respiratory Symptoms

| SYMPTOM | CHRONIC COUGH | *William J. Hueston* |

Etiology

1. Underlying cause for cough: Cough is a common condition that arises from four underlying mechanisms: inflammation, mechanical trauma, chemical irritation, or thermal stimulation. Not all coughing is pathologic in nature. Studies of children have shown that healthy children cough an average of 11 times every day. Even when pathologic, the cause may be a self-limited condition such as acute bronchitis or upper respiratory viral infection, which needs no further evaluation or treatment. The challenge for the primary care physician is to discern when a cough is caused by a benign condition and when it is a manifestation of more severe pathology.

2. Duration of cough: Most benign causes of cough resolve within 14 days. However, it should noted that up to 25 per cent of individuals with acute bronchitis will continue to cough for a month or longer. A cough lasting between 14 and 28 days should begin to raise concern; a cough persisting for over a month is an indication for further evaluation.

Differential Diagnosis

Conditions that should be considered when evaluating a patient with a chronic cough are listed in Table 27–1. Most cases of chronic cough are associated with pulmonary pathology, but clinicians should also be alert that abnormalities in the cardiac, gastrointestinal, and other systems also can result in unremitting cough.

History

1. Characteristic and timing of cough
   a. Cough that is predominantly at night is usually seen with reflux esophagitis or congestive heart failure.
   b. Angiotensin-converting enzyme (ACE) inhibitor–associated cough usually is a nagging, tickling cough that occurs throughout the day; sometimes patients may not even be aware that they are coughing.
   c. Psychogenic cough is often dramatic, featuring a bizarre or honking sound.
   d. Patients with asthma will report a cough with changes in temperature or exercise.

2. Sputum production
   a. Pulmonary infections often, but do not always, produce a cough with sputum. If hemoptysis is present, this is often an indication of bronchial inflammation seen with neoplasms, infection, or autoimmune disorders. In many conditions, such as chronic bronchitis, bronchiectasis, and pneumonia, the amount of sputum produced is large. In particular, bronchiectasis results in very large amounts of sputum that is foul-smelling and is increased when the patient bends over, as when tying shoe laces.

TABLE 27–1. DIFFERENTIAL DIAGNOSIS FOR CHRONIC COUGH

Pulmonary Causes
Infectious
  Postobstructive pneumonia
  Pneumocystis carinii
  Bronchiectasis
  Lung abscess
  Tuberculosis
Noninfectious
  Asthma
  Chronic bronchitis
  Allergic aspergillosis
  Bronchogenic neoplasms
  Sarcoidosis
  Pulmonary fibrosis
  Chemical or smoke inhalation
Cardiovascular Causes
Congestive heart failure/pulmonary edema
Enlargement of left atrium
Gastrointestinal Tract Causes
Reflux esophagitis
Other Causes
Medications, especially ACE inhibitors
Psychogenic cough
Foreign body aspiration

b. Asthma, bronchogenic carcinomas, sarcoidosis, pulmonary fibrosis, and infection with *Pneumocystis carinii* generally result in dry, hacking coughs.

3. Other symptoms: Associated symptoms such as dyspnea on exertion, heartburn or acid-tasting material in the back of the throat after eating, and constitutional symptoms such as weight loss, appetite suppression, and fatigue are also helpful in uncovering the etiology of the cough.

Clinical Findings

1. Pulmonary: A thorough pulmonary examination is essential for evaluating the respiratory tract:
   a. Bilateral wheezing can be a sign of bronchial inflammation present in asthma, sarcoidosis, or autoimmune problems.
   b. Unilateral wheezing should raise suspicion for foreign body aspiration, tumor, or chronic reflux with aspiration into the right lung.
   c. Localized rales suggest a focal pneumonia, which should raise suspicion for bronchial obstruction from a tumor or foreign body.
   d. Dry crackles bilaterally throughout the lung fields are suggestive of fibrotic lung disease.
   e. Dependent rales suggest congestive heart failure.

2. Head, eye, ear, nose, and throat
   a. Signs of chronic sinusitis or allergic rhinitis (posterior pharyngeal drainage or boggy, edematous nasal turbinates) can often help localize the cause of a cough. In some series, chronic postnasal drip is responsible for up to 40 per cent of all cases of chronic cough.
   b. The neck area should be examined carefully to note diffuse or focal thyroid enlargement that could compress the trachea, or enlarged lymph nodes that could arise from lung neoplasms.

3. Cardiac
   a. An S_3 heart sound, lateral displacement of the point of maximal impulse, and resting tachycardia should all raise suspicion for a dilated cardiomyopathy and congestive heart failure.
   b. Murmurs associated with the mitral valve (either regurgitation or stenosis) or irregular rhythms associated with atrial fibrillation suggest possible enlargement of the left atrium, which can result in a cough.

Diagnostic Tests

1. Chest radiograph: If the history and physical examination suggest that a respiratory condition is responsible for the cough, a chest radiograph should be obtained.
   a. Radiographs should be carefully inspected for hilar densities seen with enlarged lymph nodes or tumors and for wedge-shaped infiltrates suggesting postobstructive pneumonia.
   b. Interstitial changes may be noted that suggest sarcoidosis or fibrosis.
   c. Aeration of the lungs may suggest either asthma (bilateral hyperinflation) or a foreign body (which can produce either hypoinflation if complete obstruction is present, but more often hyperinflation from a ball-valve effect).
   d. The size of the heart and left atrium can be determined as a risk factor for congestive heart failure.

2. Laboratory evaluation
   a. If suspicion is high for an infectious source of the cough, a complete blood count may lend further support to an infectious etiology.
   b. Electrolytes or other routine laboratory tests are of little use.

3. Pulmonary function testing
   a. When the etiology of the cough is unclear, often spirometry is useful at determining if an obstructive or restrictive abnormality is present. This is often useful if underlying asthma is suspected.
   b. Diffusing capacity of carbon monoxide can also be useful in detecting interstitial lung disease.

4. Bronchoscopy
   a. If the chest radiograph is normal, but a high likelihood for a bronchogenic problem exists, bronchoscopy may be necessary to make the diagnosis.
   b. Bronchogenic tumors, inflammatory changes associated with infectious agents or gastrointestinal reflux, and foreign bodies may be detected under direct visualization, washings, and biopsies.

5. Echocardiography: If signs and symptoms point to a cardiac condition causing the cough, echocardiogram may be useful to evaluate left atrial size, ejection fraction, and mitral valve function.

Management

Management depends upon the etiology.

1. For young patients with signs of a recent upper respiratory tract infection of acute bronchitis,

an empiric trial of a macrolide antibiotic may be a cost-effective alternative to launching an extensive evaluation for other respiratory, cardiac, or gastrointestinal conditions.

2. For patients at high risk for malignancy, such as older patients with significant smoking history or other exposures, rapid progression to bronchoscopy is warranted.

Follow-Up

1. Follow-up is usually not a problem for patients with chronic cough. For many, the cough is so disruptive to their usual activities (e.g., keeping them awake at night, irritating their co-workers or spouse, or embarrassing them at church) that they will continue to seek care until the underlying condition is discovered and treated.

2. In many cases, consultation with a pulmonologist is indicated when initial studies are negative or if bronchoscopy is advisable.

3. Because a large proportion of chronic cough problems stem from nonpulmonary conditions, it is important that the patient continue to receive support and evaluation from the primary care physician until the problem is resolved.

PEARLS

- Postnasal drip is the cause of chronic cough in 40 per cent of patients.

- Cough associated with viral acute bronchitis can persist up to a month in 25 per cent of patients.

- Asthma and bronchitis (acute or chronic) are the most common primary pulmonary problems causing chronic cough.

- Allergic rhinitis and reflux esophagitis are the most common nonpulmonary problems causing chronic cough.

- The vast majority of causes of chronic cough can be diagnosed by history, physical examination, and chest radiograph. Laboratory studies are rarely useful. Bronchoscopy should be reserved for patients with high risk for malignancy, those with hemoptysis, or those with unrelenting symptoms that cannot be diagnosed by noninvasive means.

Bibliography

Celli BR: Current thoughts regarding the treatment of chronic obstructive pulmonary disease. Med Clin North Am 1996;80:589–609.

Cao WM: Chronic persistent cough: diagnosis and treatment update. Pediatr Ann 1996;25:162–168.

Mello CJ, Irwin RS, Curley FJ: Predictive values of the character, timing, and complications of chronic cough in diagnosing its cause. Arch Intern Med 1996;156:997–1003.

Munyard P, Bush A: How much coughing is normal? Arch Dis Child 1996;74:531–534.

Woolcock AJ: Epidemiology of chronic airways disease. Chest 1989;96(Suppl 3):302S–306S.

SYMPTOM SORE THROAT

Frank C. Burwick

Sore throat is, in its most common form, more or less a nuisance that afflicts humans throughout life. More common in childhood, adolescence, and young adulthood, sore throat can occur at any age. Although it most commonly is a benign disease that need not—and cannot—be treated except with some soothing over-the-counter medications or home remedies of questionable value, sore throat can be a prelude to severe debilitating disease and, on rare occasions, can be a fatal disease if not recognized and treated correctly. The throat, with its lymphoglandular tissue (Waldeyer's tonsillar ring), is the first line of defense against an onslaught of external factors, be they of physical, chemical, or microbial origin.

Differential Diagnosis

1. Infectious

a. Viral: most common; all ages, all seasons, but more prevalent during winter

b. Bacterial: most important, group A β-hemolytic streptococci; most common from ages 5 to 15 years

c. Fungal: *Candida*

2. Environmental: tobacco smoke, smog, dust allergens

3. Drainage from "above" or "below"

a. Postnasal drip

b. Gastroesophageal reflux

4. Rare causes

a. Hypothyroidism or hyperthyroidism

b. Thyroiditis

c. Foreign body

d. Leukemia, agranulocytosis

e. Diphtheria

f. Gonorrhea in 10 per cent of patients with anogenital gonorrhea

5. Sore throat with pharyngeal ulcers

a. Canker sores (aphthous stomatitis)

b. Herpangina

c. Herpes simplex

d. Fusospirochetal infection

e. Candidiasis

f. Herpes zoster

g. Chickenpox

h. Primary or secondary syphilitic ulcerations (usually not painful)

One can argue whether environmental factors or infections are the most common causes of sore throat. For the physician, the infectious reasons and their correct recognition are of greater importance. However, to stress the importance of environmental factors is an important part of patient awareness and education. Among infectious agents that cause sore throat, viruses far outnumber bacteria. Fungal causes are rare but on the rise as the acquired immunodeficiency syndrome epidemic continues unchecked.

Bacterial pharyngitis is often caused by group A β-hemolytic streptococci. Sudden onset of sore throat, general malaise, a temperature that is usually high (104°F [40°C] in adults and even higher in children), and suppurative and nonsuppurative sequelae make recognition of this pathogen extremely important, especially since acute rheumatic fever has become more common.

PEARLS

• Exudate is not specific for streptococcal tonsillitis; viral tonsillitis can look the same.

• Strep throat is extremely rare in children under age 3 years, and, if it occurs, it is associated with purulent rhinitis.

• *Arcanobacterium haemolyticus* (formerly *Corynebacterium haemolyticum*) causes pharyngitis and tonsillitis quite similar to group A β-hemolytic streptococci infection, with anterior neck lymphadenitis as well as scarlatiniform rash that often, as in strep throat, proceeds to desquamate.

• Sore throat becomes worse on swallowing, but throat examination is normal. Palpate the thyroid (thyroiditis?).

Infectious mononucleosis causes about 5 per cent of sore throats. Most often it is caused by Epstein-Barr virus and rarely by cytomegalovirus. Usually a disease of adolescents and young adults, it can, on inspection, mimic strep throat, but the history is different: gradual onset, low-grade temperature, mild pharyngeal symptoms, more pronounced systemic symptoms. Enanthema and petechiae on the palate are almost diagnostic for infectious mononucleosis. Posterior cervical lymphadenitis points strongly toward infectious mononucleosis or other viral cause.

PEARLS

• For the Monospot test, there are essentially no false-negative results except in children under age 6 years. However, false-positive results are found in 10 per cent of children in this age group. Complete blood count with at least 50 per cent lymphocytes and at least 10 per cent atypical lymphocytes also confirms the diagnosis.

• Throat culture, the gold standard for the diagnosis of strep pharyngitis, should be performed in patients at high risk for complications even when the probability of strep throat is low (i.e., patients with diabetes mellitus or a history of rheumatic fever and during outbreak of a nephrogenic strain).

• Pharyngeal exudate is not diagnostic for strep tonsillitis; only 50 per cent of patients with strep throat have exudate, and, of all patients with exudate, only 50 per cent have strep throat.

Refer to Ch. 13, Aphthous Stomatitis; Ch. 23, Allergic Rhinitis; Ch. 180, Thyroiditis; and Ch. 256, Infectious Mononucleosis.

History

In addition to inquiry about onset of symptoms, exposure to other cases with similar symptoms, and so on, it is important to take note of the time of year and age of the patient. Certain diagnoses are common in certain seasons and age groups. The questions to ask are a logical consequence of the patient's signs and symptoms, which might include the following:

1. Fever: high and sudden onset, low-grade and insidious onset

2. Pain: Where? Referred pain?

3. Dysphagia?

4. Drooling?

5. Preferred position?

6. Pain on extension of the neck?

Clinical Findings

1. Inspection
   a. Pharyngeal erythema
   b. Enlargement of tonsils
   c. Asymmetry, position of uvula
   d. Exudate—does it wipe off?
   e. Pseudomembrane
   f. Enanthema
   g. Postnasal drip
   h. Posterior or lateral swelling
   i. Ulcers

2. Palpation
   a. Enlarged and tender anterior cervical nodes suggest a bacterial infection.
   b. Enlarged and tender posterior cervical nodes suggest a viral infection.
   c. Check the thyroid gland if throat inspection is normal.

Tests

1. In patients whose clinical picture is consistent with influenza, common cold, or irritants, no further laboratory tests are needed.

2. A rapid strep test should be done in patients with an intermediate likelihood of strep throat and in patients at high risk for complications, even when the likelihood is small.

3. Obtain a Monospot test or complete blood count if infectious mononucleosis is suspected. If mononucleosis is confirmed, perform liver function tests and antiglobulin (Coombs') test.

4. Obtain a lateral neck radiograph if drooling is present. Look for epiglottitis.

5. Order a computerized tomographic scan of the neck or a magnetic resonance imaging scan if there is retropharyngeal or peritonsillar abscess.

Management

1. Viral: symptomatic only, with aspirin (acetaminophen in children), lozenges, saltwater gargling, and plenty of fluids. Avoid giving antibiotics; they are ineffective for viral sore throat and expensive, and they carry the risks of adverse effects and induction of allergy.

2. Bacterial (e.g., strep throat): if typical presentation (rapid onset, high fever, exudate on tonsils, tender swollen anterior cervical lymph nodes), treat with penicillin (or erythromycin in penicillin allergy). The presence of cough and coryza makes viral infection much more likely.

3. Candidiasis (oral thrush): nystatin solution or ketoconazole

4. Diphtheria: rare but possible even in societies with high immunization rates. Give diphtheria antitoxin within 48 hours of disease onset.

5. Retropharyngeal or peritonsillar abscess: requires surgery and intravenous clindamycin (Cleocin) or nafcillin (Unipen).

Follow-Up

Usually not necessary. Recurrences are common. Penicillin for strep throat prevents nonsuppurative sequelae if treatment is started within 48 hours.

Bibliography

Del Mar C: Managing sore throat: a literature review. Making the diagnosis. Med J Aust 1992;156:5672–5675.

Dippel DW, Touw-Otten F, Habbema JD: Management of children with acute pharyngitis. J Fam Pract 1992; 32:149–159.

Goldstein MN: Office evaluation and management of the sore throat. Otolaryngol Clin North Am 1992;25:837–842.

Little P, Gould C, Williamson I, et al: Reattendance and complications in a randomized trial of prescribing strategies for sore throat: the medicalising effect of prescribing antibiotics. BMJ 1997;315:350–352.

Pichichero ME: Group A beta hemolytic streptococcal infections. Pediatr Rev 1998;19:291–302.

Wald ER, Green MD, Schwartz B, et al: A streptococcal score card revisited. Pediatr Emerg Care 1998;14:109–111.

Indications
Peritonsillar abscess

Contraindications
1. Bleeding disorders or anticoagulant therapy
2. Neck swelling or other signs of abscess extension to deeper fascial planes
3. Impaired mental status (patient unable to protect airway)

Preparation
1. Informed consent
2. Careful examination of oropharynx and neck to rule out retropharyngeal abscess and/or extension of abscess into cervical fascia

Equipment
1. 20-ml syringe (standard or three-finger control)
2. 1.5-inch, 16- or 18-gauge needle
3. Scalpel with No. 11 or No. 15 blade (tape over base of blade to allow only 1 cm depth of incision)
4. Small curved hemostat
5. Head lamp or other light source
6. Suction equipment

Anesthesia
1. Topical anesthesia with 20% benzocaine gel (Hurricane), Cetacaine spray, or 4% topical lidocaine
2. If incision and drainage (I&D) is planned after needle aspiration, follow topical anesthesia with local injection of 1% lidocaine with epinephrine

Precautions
1. Position patient in the upright sitting position with head supported and suction equipment ready to avoid aspiration of blood or pus.
2. Avoid delays in drainage of an established abscess to prevent complications such as necrotizing fasciitis, sepsis, mediastinitis, or even spontaneous hemorrhage from erosion into major vessels.

Technique

1. Place the alert patient in a sitting position with head supported.
2. Use head mirror or lamp for adequate visualization.
3. Apply topical anesthesia gel or spray.
4. Wrap gauze around tongue and gently retract with one hand.
5. Needle aspiration
   a. Using the other hand to hold the needle and syringe, insert the needle 1 to 2 cm into the abscess cavity through the posterior soft palate at a shallow upward and lateral angle, aiming from near the midline toward the superior tonsillar pillar.

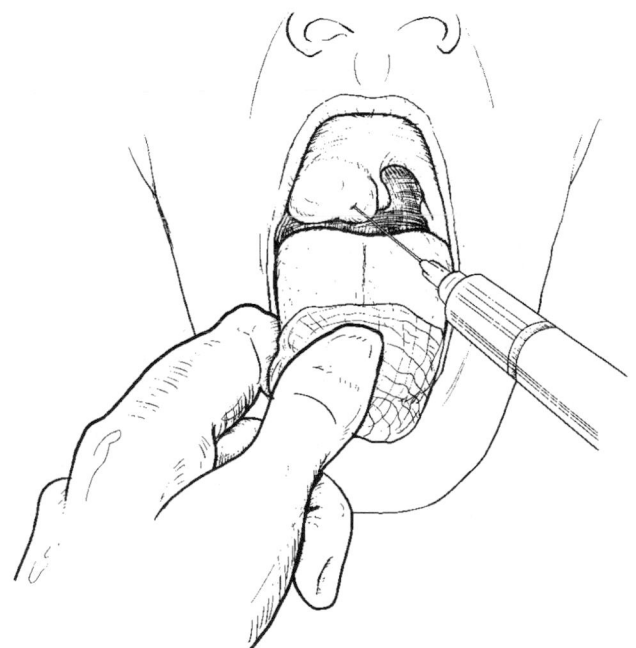

   b. Aspirate with a 20-ml syringe until no more pus is obtained (average case yields 2 to 4 ml of pus, but may range up to 20 ml).
6. If no pus is obtained and the needle has entered the apparent abscess cavity, efforts to drain the lesion should be aborted (the diagnosis may be peritonsillar cellulitis with edema; treat with antibiotics and hydration, obtain imaging studies, and re-evaluate).

Figures redrawn from Dunmire SM, Paris PM: Atlas of Emergency Procedures, p 93. Philadelphia, WB Saunders Company, 1994, with permission.

7. Needle aspiration is the only procedure necessary in uncomplicated cases. Traditional I&D offers no advantages for initial treatment, but may be needed for cases of early recurrence.

8. Incision and drainage: Use a No. 11 scalpel blade with adhesive tape guarding all but 1.0 cm of the tip. With suction ready, make a 0.5- to 1.0-cm mucosal incision. Incise in the supratonsillar region to avoid scarring of the tonsillar pillar.

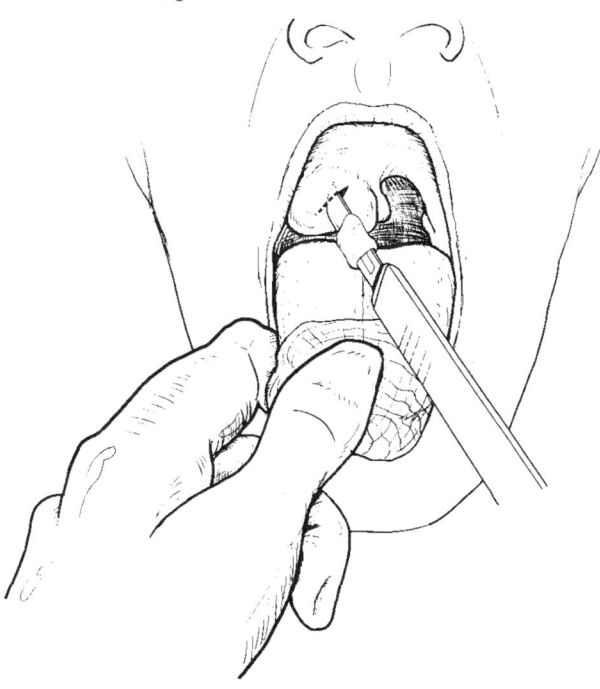

9. Slip a small curved hemostat (closed) into the abscess cavity and open it gently to create a drainage tract.

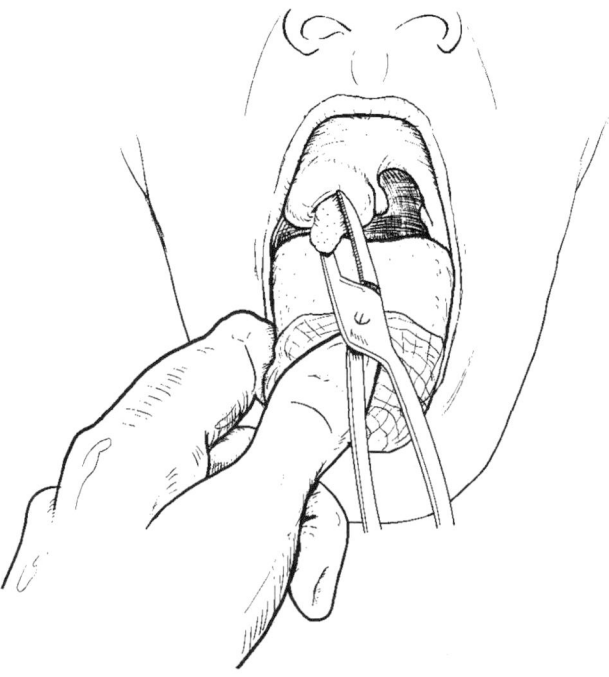

Use suction to clear pus and blood from oropharynx.

10. Consider sending swabs for aerobic and anaerobic culture, although many studies show that this should have no effect on treatment decisions or outcome.

> **Note**
> Needle aspiration is the initial procedure of choice and will result in cure rates of over 90 per cent with appropriate antibiotic therapy; reaspiration may be required in 24 to 48 hours. Incision and drainage is appropriate for treatment failures after two needle aspirations, or perhaps for early recurrences (within 30 days of previous episode).

Follow-Up

1. Prescribe penicillin orally for 10 days. Clindamycin may be used for penicillin-allergic patients.

> **Note**
> Patients treated with penicillin are cured at the same rate as those treated with broader spectrum antibiotics, even when cultures grow penicillin-resistant organisms.

2. Re-evaluate in 24 to 36 hours. Repeat aspiration may be required in 10 to 20 per cent of cases.

3. Ten to 15 per cent of patients may require hospitalization for dehydration, sepsis, or threat of airway obstruction.

4. Patients not responding to antibiotics plus several aspirations or I&D may require more definitive surgery (abscess tonsillectomy). Recurrent episodes may also be an indication for tonsillectomy; a single uncomplicated episode probably is not.

Bibliography

Friedman NR, Mitchell RB, Pereira KD, et al: Peritonsillar abscess in early childhood: presentation and management. Arch Otolaryngol Head Neck Surg 1997;123: 630–632.

Herzon FS: Peritonsillar abscess: incidence, current management practices, and a proposal for treatment guidelines. Laryngoscope 1995;105(8 Pt 3, Suppl 74):1–17.

Kornblut AD: Non-neoplastic diseases of the tonsils and adenoids. In Paparella MM, Shumrick DA (eds): Otolaryngology, 3rd ed, vol 3, pp 2137–2138. Philadelphia, WB Saunders Company, 1991.

Schlossberg D: Infections of the Head and Neck, pp 178–179. New York, Springer-Verlag, 1987.

Stringer SP: Peritonsillar abscess. In Johnson JT, Yu VL (eds): Infectious Diseases and Antimicrobial Therapy of the Ears, Nose, and Throat, pp 435–443. Philadelphia, WB Saunders Company, 1997.

1. Hemoptysis is defined as the coughing up or spitting up of blood (*hemo* = blood; *ptysis* = spitting) that originates from the respiratory tract below the pharynx.
   a. The hemoptysis may consist of pure blood or it may be mixed with sputum, causing a blood-tinged or blood-streaked expectoration.
   b. In true hemoptysis, the sputum is usually bright red and frothy with air bubbles.
   c. Hemoptysis is often characterized by the quantity of blood
      (1) Massive hemoptysis is defined as coughing up of 400 to 600 ml of blood within a 24-hour period
      (2) Moderate hemoptysis is described by volumes greater than 5 ml but less than 400 ml in 24 hours
      (3) Mild hemoptysis is blood-tinged or blood-streaked sputum, with a blood loss of less than 5 ml in 24 hours.
2. There are numerous causes of hemoptysis, and each may be related to sources intrinsic to the pulmonary system or may have its origins in diseases that secondarily affect the lungs. It is very important for the clinician to clearly distinguish true hemoptysis from the expectoration of blood from sites other than the bronchial or pulmonary systems (pseudohemoptysis). Patients are typically frightened and anxious, and may have difficulty distinguishing between blood that is expectorated from pulmonary and nonpulmonary sources, especially because the descriptions may be quite similar.

Differential Diagnosis

Hemoptysis is an occasional complication of adult pulmonary disease and is rare in children. It is, however, an alarming presenting symptom. The etiology varies and typically depends on the criteria used for patient selection, the patient population, and the techniques used for diagnosis. From a practical point of view, it is appropriate to differentiate between hemoptysis that is of small volume and intermittent and that which is massive and potentially life threatening. Most patients cough up small volumes of blood but are nevertheless alarmed and usually regard the symptom as an indication of a serious underlying disease.

There are multiple causes, and almost any pulmonary lesion may result in hemoptysis. The most common causes in adults are infection, bronchiectasis, pulmonary neoplasm, cystic fibrosis, pulmonary

infarction, and trauma. In children the most common causes are infection, congenital abnormalities of the cardiopulmonary vasculature, and foreign body aspiration. The origin of hemoptysis often proves elusive, with nearly 50 per cent of cases remaining undiagnosed despite extensive work-ups. About 50 per cent of patients with lung cancer will have some expectoration of blood (or blood-tinged sputum) during the course of their disease. Hemoptysis can be broken down into four categories:

1. Infectious/inflammatory
   a. Bronchitis
   b. Pneumonia
   c. Bronchiectasis
   d. Tuberculosis
   e. Lung abscess
   f. Fungal infection
   g. Parasitic lung disease (especially in endemic areas)
   h. Connective tissue diseases
   i. Cystic fibrosis
2. Tumors
   a. Carcinoma of the lung (primarily bronchogenic carcinoma)
   b. Benign endobronchial tumors (bronchial adenoma)
3. Cardiovascular disease
   a. Pulmonary embolism
   b. Heart failure
   c. Mitral valve stenosis
   d. Vascular malformations of the lung
4. Other
   a. Hematologic disorders
   b. Foreign body aspiration
   c. Trauma (including iatrogenic causes)

History

The first step in evaluating hemoptysis is to establish that the blood or blood-tinged material has actually originated from the chest, and not the mouth, nose, upper respiratory tract, or gastrointestinal tract. Frequently, patients are unable to distinguish true hemoptysis from hematemesis or expectoration of aspirated blood. It is important to determine the duration and possibly quantify the amount of hemoptysis, and to note whether there is gross blood, clots, or blood-tinged/streaked sputum. As in most other significant medical problems, a careful history is necessary to identify the presence of hemoptysis and localize the source.

1. Duration of hemoptysis
2. Is it gross blood or blood-tinged/streaked?
3. Determine amount of blood produced (if possible).
4. Is there any history of respiratory difficulty preceding or coincident with the hemoptysis?
5. Is there any history of chronic illness?
6. Is there any history of naso/oropharyngeal disorders?
7. Is there any history of bleeding dyscrasias?
8. Fever, chills, sweats, weight loss
9. Presence or absence of cough
10. Sputum production, including quality and quantity
11. Is there any history of cardiovascular disease or chest pain?
12. Smoking, alcohol, recent travel

Clinical Findings

An organized, systematic approach to examining the patient is imperative. The directed physical examination should complement the history taking. In general, the physical examination will correspond to the degree of blood loss and the patient's hemodynamic stability, and will ascertain that the blood is truly originating from the respiratory tract.

1. Note the following about the patient:
   a. General condition and appearance
   b. Skin color
   c. Signs of bruising
   d. Body habitus
   e. Evidence of chronic illness
   f. State of nutrition
   g. Weight loss or debilitation
   h. Psychological attitude, awareness of/anxiety from events
2. Note acute respiratory distress, pain, or mental confusion
3. Vital signs
   a. Respiratory rate
   b. Temperature
   c. Heart rate
   d. Blood pressure
4. Head, eye, ear, nose, and throat examination (especially for evidence of nasopharyngeal or oropharyngeal disease or trauma)
5. Neck
   a. Adenopathy
   b. Jugular venous distention

6. Cardiac examination
   a. Murmurs
   b. Signs of heart failure
7. Careful respiratory examination
8. Edema, cyanosis, varicosities

Diagnostic Tests

There is no clearly defined, optimal diagnostic assessment of hemoptysis. Each case should be handled individually, and be based on the clinical assessment obtained from the history and physical examination.

1. Blood work
   a. Chemistry panel: electrolytes, renal function, nutritional status
   b. Complete blood count: signs of infection, anemia, thrombocytopenia
   c. Coagulation profile
   d. Arterial blood gas: acid-base status, oxygenation
   e. Type and cross match (if transfusion is necessary)
2. Sputum analysis: identification of infection, acid-fast bacilli, cytology
3. Radiologic studies
   a. Chest radiograph (comparison of old films if available)
   b. Computerized tomography
4. Bronchoscopy: with or without biopsy, as both a diagnostic and therapeutic intervention
5. Radioisotopic studies or angiography: to identify vascular abnormalities
6. Ventilation-perfusion scan (if pulmonary embolism is suspected)

Management

Management will clearly be defined by the degree of hemoptysis, the cause, and the patient's prognosis. Immediate management should be directed toward ensuring hemodynamic stability and maintaining a patent airway. Massive hemoptysis should be regarded as an emergency whether or not resuscitation is necessary. Palliative management should be aimed at reducing patient anxiety.

1. Supportive
   a. Maintain a patent airway
   b. Oxygenation (mask vs. intubation)
   c. Fluid support or transfusion if necessary
2. Sedation if necessary: bedrest, reassurance, close observation, and sedation
3. Appropriate antibiotics for infection
4. Antitussives (if appropriate): to minimize further small bleeds

5. Treat coagulation disorder if present.
6. Oral hemostatic drugs: for minor bleeds
7. Anticoagulation: for pulmonary embolism
8. Control of massive bleeding
   a. Cauterization or tamponade of visible site
   b. Bronchial artery embolization
   c. Surgery: for resection of affected vessel or pulmonary site
   d. Radiotherapy: for palliative treatment of lung cancers sites

Bibliography

DiLeo M, Amedee R, Butcher R: Hemoptysis and pseudohemoptysis: the patient expectorating blood. ENT Ear, Nose Throat J 1995;74:822–828.

Hirshberg B, Biran I, Glazer M, et al: Hemoptysis: etiology, evaluation, and outcome in a tertiary referral hospital. Chest 1997;112:440–444.

Marshall T, Flower C, Jackson J: The role of radiology in the investigation and management of patients with haemoptysis. Clin Radiol 1996;51:391–400.

Marshall T, Jackson J: Vascular intervention in the thorax: bronchial artery embolization for haemoptysis. Eur Radiol 1997;7:1221–1227.

Thompson J, Nguyen C, Lazar R, et al: Evaluation and management of hemoptysis in infants and children. Ann Otol Rhinol Laryngol 1996;105:516–520.

28 Upper Respiratory Infections

David L. Gaspar

The common cold is the most frequent upper respiratory tract infection (URTI). In addition, other respiratory structures above the level of the larynx may also be infected, leading to otitis media, sinusitis, pharyngitis, and, more rarely, epiglottitis. Adults experience an average of two to four URTIs per year, while children get on average six to eight per year. The majority of URTIs occur from early autumn to late spring.

Etiology
1. Causes of the common cold
   a. Most often caused by rhinoviruses and coronaviruses
   b. Less frequently caused by parainfluenza or influenza viruses, respiratory syncytial virus (RSV), adenoviruses, and others
2. The bacterial syndromes of the upper respiratory tract are most often caused by *Haemophilus influenzae, Moraxella catarrhalis, Streptococcus pneumoniae,* and *Streptococcus pyogenes.*
3. Transmission is usually self-inoculation via secretions from contaminated fomites and skin or, less commonly, person-to-person directly via droplets.

Symptoms
1. Symptoms begin 1 to 5 days after exposure and usually resolve in 7 to 10 days.
2. Most common complaints are cough, nasal congestion and discharge, and throat irritation.
3. Less commonly seen are mild fever, tender cervical adenopathy, uncomfortable or plugged ears, watery eyes, and sometimes headache and muscle aches.

Key Symptoms
- Nasal discharge or congestion
- Cough
- Throat irritation

Clinical Findings
1. Most times minimal findings
2. Watery to purulent nasal discharge; nasal crusting; red, swollen nasal mucosa
3. Mild conjunctivitis, cervical adenopathy, erythema of the pharynx, or redness and immobility of the eardrums

Key Signs
- Usually minimal
- Watery nasal discharge with crusting
- Swollen, red nasal mucosa

Laboratory Tests
1. None usually are done.
2. Viral cultures possible but almost never used.
3. Throat culture and/or rapid antigen screen for streptococcal infection
4. Sinus radiograph or computerized tomography scan; chest radiograph if concerned about bacterial complications

Differential Diagnosis
1. *Allergic rhinoconjunctivitis*: The seasonal nature or more prolonged course of allergic conditions may be helpful to differentiate them from URTIs. Prominent itching of the nose, palate, or eyes and sneezing are more likely to suggest allergies. The complete blood count may show eosinophilia, and a personal or family history of atopy may be present.
2. *Sinusitis*: Criteria that can help predict those who have sinusitis are poor sinus transillumination, purulent nasal discharge, dental pain, and a poor response to decongestants.
3. *Otitis media*: In children, this can present as ear pain, fever, and fussiness a few days after a common cold. The physical exam may reveal red, bulging, or immobile tympanic membranes.
4. *Influenza*: Many symptoms are similar, but they are usually more intense with influenza and progress more rapidly. Fever and lower respiratory symptoms are more pronounced, as are sys-

temic symptoms such as headache, malaise, and myalgias.

5. *Asthma*: Rhinovirus infections increase lower airway reactivity and may result in a cough that persists following a viral URTI. Prolonged cough, especially if exertional or nocturnal, may be due to reactive airways disease or a flare of a patient's asthma. A past history of asthma or atopic conditions is helpful.

6. *Epiglottitis*: Usually caused by *H. influenzae*, this syndrome may lead to severe respiratory distress or even death. It usually affects young children between ages 2 and 7 with a rapid onset of fever, severe sore throat, and, classically, stridor and drooling. This is an emergency that must be managed in an emergency room setting with airway support.

7. *Croup (laryngotracheobronchitis)*: Children develop a prominent "barking," nonproductive cough. They do not appear particularly ill and classically improve in a cooler or more humid environment (either in a steamy shower or in the car on the way to the Emergency Department!).

8. *Streptococcal pharyngitis*: Fever, anterior cervical adenopathy, pharyngeal exudate, and the absence of cough are more common in streptococcal sore throat.

9. *Bronchiolitis*: This is a disease of children 6 months to 2 years old caused primarily by RSV. After what appears to be a common cold, the infant develops tachypnea, wheezing, and intercostal and subcostal indrawing.

Treatment

Medication

1. Common "cold"
   a. In many cases no treatment is needed.
   b. Antibiotics are not indicated, and studies show that physicians are not very good at predicting which patients expect an antibiotic.
   c. Little evidence supports the use of cough and cold medication in children.
   d. For cough in adolescents and adults
      (1) Dextromethorphan, 10 to 30 mg q4–6h
      (2) If more severe, codeine, 10 to 20 mg q4–6h
   e. For aches and pains: acetaminophen, 325 to 650 mg q6h; ibuprofen, 200 to 400 mg q6h; or naproxen sodium, 225 to 450 mg q12h. Aspirin should not be used in children because of its association with Reye's syndrome.

   f. For nasal symptoms: Pseudoephedrine, 60 mg q6h, or phenylpropanolamine, 25 mg q4h orally, can be helpful.
   g. There is some evidence that zinc lozenges may shorten the symptoms of a URTI in adults. Vitamin C (2 to 4 gm daily) may do the same.
   h. Investigational treatments include alfa-interferon and intranasal ipratropium bromide (Atrovent) and nedocromil sodium (Tilade).

2. If a bacterial syndrome is present, such as sinusitis or otitis media, antibiotic therapy aimed at the most likely pathogens is indicated.

3. Antihistamines, nasal steroids, and in some cases immunotherapy may be used for allergic conditions, whereas inhaled steroids and β-agonists may be used for lower airway reactivity and asthma.

Diet

No specific diet therapy is needed, but general recommendations to drink plenty of fluids may be reasonable, especially if fever is present.

Activity

1. Febrile children should probably be kept home from school.
2. Rest is usually recommended, but activities that the patient can tolerate are acceptable.

Patient Education

The aim is to help patients understand their illness and educate them in issues related to preventing other respiratory diseases and decreasing the frequency of URTIs in the future. At the same time the patients' fears and concerns must be acknowledged. Telling patients that they "just have a virus" can sometimes be misinterpreted as trivializing their problem.

1. Hand washing appears to be the single most important means of infection control.
2. Smoking cessation should be encouraged in patients and the parents of ill children.
3. Influenza immunization will not prevent the common cold, but a visit for an URTI may be the window of opportunity to introduce this measure to susceptible individuals.

Key Treatment

- For cough: dextromethorphan or codeine
- For nasal congestion: oral pseudoephedrine or phenylpropanolamine
- For aches and pains: acetaminophen, ibuprofen, or naproxen sodium

Follow-Up

1. Patients usually need not be seen for a follow-up visit.

2. It is important to make them aware they should return if symptoms persist or if fever or pain worsens.

 ## Bibliography

Glezen WP: The common cold. In Gorbach SL, Bartlett JG, Blacklow NR (eds): Infectious Diseases, pp 548–553. Philadelphia, WB Saunders Company, 1998.

Kirkpatrick GL: The common cold. In Irons TG, Newton DA (eds): Primary Care Clinics in Office Practice, pp 657–675. Philadelphia, WB Saunders Company, 1996.

Low DE, Desrosiers M, McSherry J, et al: A practical guide for the diagnosis and treatment of acute sinusitis. Can Med Assoc J 1997;156(Suppl 6):1S–14S.

Smith MB, Feldman W: Over the counter cold medications: a critical review of clinical trials between 1950 and 1991. JAMA 1993;269:2258–2263.

Zinc for the common cold. Med Lett Drugs Ther 1997; 39(993):9–10.

29 Laryngitis

Bennet M. Wang

Etiology

The history is key to determining the cause of laryngitis and should include any specific inciting events (e.g., vocal abuse, upper respiratory tract infection, intubation); any infectious or toxic exposures (see below); and any associated gastrointestinal or respiratory complaints. A wide variety of infectious and inflammatory (noninfectious) processes can cause laryngitis.

Infectious

1. Acute infection (symptoms less than 2 to 3 weeks)
   a. Viral
      (1) Influenza A and B, parainfluenza
      (2) Adenovirus, rhinovirus, coronavirus
      (3) Epstein-Barr virus (usually in association with pharyngitis)
   b. Bacterial
      (1) *Haemophilus influenzae* (can cause epiglottitis; decreasing incidence in children as a result of vaccination but can still occur in adults [see Bibliography])
      (2) *Mycoplasma pneumoniae* and *Chlamydia* species
      (3) Streptococcal and staphylococcal species (usually secondary to primary pharyngitis, sinusitis, or tonsillitis)
      (4) *Corynebacterium diphtheriae* (usually in association with pharyngitis)
2. Chronic infection (symptoms extending over weeks to months)
   a. Bacterial
      (1) Tuberculosis (see Bibliography)
      (2) Actinomycosis
   b. Fungal
      (1) Histoplasmosis or blastomycosis
      (2) Candidiasis (usually in association with esophageal or disseminated disease)

Inflammatory (Noninfectious)

1. Gastroesophageal reflux (see Bibliography)
2. Postnasal drip
3. Exposure to irritating agents such as tobacco smoke, chemicals, radiation, or excessive heat (smoke inhalation or steam injury)
4. Excessive use of the voice (can lead to vocal cord inflammation ["singer's nodules"])
5. Intubation granuloma (after endotracheal intubation)

Symptoms

1. Hoarseness or a change in vocal quality (dysphonia) are usually the primary symptoms.
2. Nocturnal or early morning cough, throat-clearing, and heartburn can be clues to gastro-esophageal reflux.
3. Nasal stuffiness, frontal headaches, and a history of allergies or hay fever can suggest postnasal drip and/or sinusitis.
4. Pain may be localized to the larynx and throat but can be referred to the ear.
5. Dyspnea, stridor, dysphagia, and odynophagia are late symptoms and suggest more serious disease.

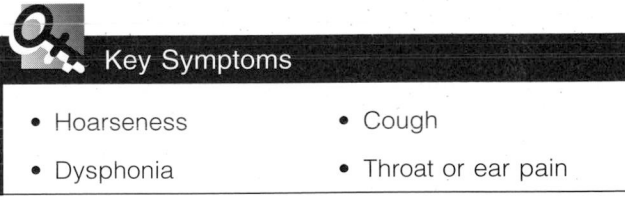

Key Symptoms

• Hoarseness	• Cough
• Dysphonia	• Throat or ear pain

Clinical Findings

1. Fever is present at times in laryngitis, particularly when caused by infection.
2. A thorough head and neck examination, including gag and swallowing reflexes, is essential and may reveal lymphadenopathy and signs of inflammation in the pharynx, sinuses, and lungs.
3. Extreme tenderness or pain on gentle palpation of the larynx area raises the possibility of epiglottitis (see Bibliography).
4. Indirect (mirror) or fiberoptic laryngoscopy is the key to visualization to assess for laryngeal edema, erythema, ulcers, or nodules and to assess vocal cord function.

- Fever

- Tenderness in area of larynx

- Laryngeal edema, erythema, ulcers, or nodules

Tests

1. A white blood cell count with differential may be useful if infection is suspected.

2. Cultures from the throat, larynx, or blood, and other specific tests, such as rheumatoid factor or C1 esterase inhibitor level, may be indicated in selected cases.

3. Laryngeal tissue biopsy by means of direct laryngoscopy may be useful when noninvasive studies are not diagnostic.

- White blood cell count (if infection suspected)

- Cultures (if infection suspected)

- Laryngoscopy (with possible biopsy)

Differential Diagnosis

1. Vocal cord dysfunction, in particular secondary to recurrent and/or superior laryngeal nerve dysfunction, can also present as hoarseness.

2. Neoplasms of the larynx
   a. Papilloma (benign; juvenile and adult forms)
   b. Squamous cell carcinoma (typically presents between ages 50 and 70; increased risk associated with tobacco and alcohol use)

3. Systemic disorders that affect the larynx
   a. Sarcoidosis
   b. Rheumatoid arthritis of cricoarytenoid joint
   c. Systemic lupus erythematosus
   d. Angioedema (*Note*: can be secondary to angiotensin-converting enzyme inhibitor medications, even after prolonged use).

4. Functional disorders
   a. Vocal weakness (lack of usual vigor or tone to voice; typically seen in older patients as a result of vocal cord bowing and muscle atrophy, part of the normal aging process).
   b. Psychogenic aphonia (history of emotional disturbance often present).

Treatment

1. The central goal is to treat the underlying cause if identified and to eliminate or diminish any contributing factors.

2. For most cases of acute laryngitis, the voice eventually returns to baseline spontaneously. Careful management can speed recovery and lessen the risk of permanent damage.
   a. *Voice rest*: Shouting, long telephone conversations, throat clearing, and prolonged whispering are prohibited. The goal is to use as few words as possible.
   b. *Humidification and hydration*: The goal is to increase the lubrication of the laryngeal mucosa. One suggestion for adequate fluid is at least eight glasses of water a day.
   c. *Cough suppression*: For irritative coughs, an over-the-counter preparation of dextromethorphan can be useful.
   d. *Relief of nasal obstruction*: Because the nose functions to help humidify inhaled air, nasal decongestants can be beneficial. In addition, use of nasal steroid sprays can help diminish postnasal drip if present.
   e. Treatment of gastroesophageal reflux if present. Use high-dose histamine$_2$ blockers or proton pump inhibitors such as omeprazole (Prilosec) or lansoprazole (Prevacid).
   f. Antibiotics in selected patients. Use when fever, pain, productive cough, or purulent sputum suggests primary or secondary bacterial infection.

- Voice rest
- Humidification and hydration
- Cough suppression
- Relief of nasal obstruction
- Treatment of gastroesophageal reflux if present
- Antibiotics in selected patients

Follow-Up

With appropriate conservative management, most patients with acute laryngitis recover their voice within 2 to 3 weeks. (*Note*: It may take up to 8 weeks for gastroesophageal reflux laryngitis to resolve completely.) For patients with acute laryngitis who do not improve or for those with chronic laryngitis of unknown cause, referral to an otolaryngologist is indicated.

 ## Bibliography

For more information on laryngitis, see
Fried M, Shapiro J: Acute and chronic laryngeal infections. In Paperella MM, Shumrick (eds): Otolaryngology, 3rd ed, vol 3, pp 2245–2256. Philadelphia, WB Saunders Company, 1991.

For more information on epiglottitis in adults, see
Carey MJ: Epiglottitis in adults. Am J Emerg Med 1996; 14:421–424.

For more information on laryngeal tuberculosis, see
Riley EC, Amundson DE: Laryngeal tuberculosis revisited. Am Fam Physician 1992;46:759–762.

For more information on reflux laryngitis, see
Siegel PD, Katz J: Respiratory complications of gastroesophageal reflux disease. Prim Care 1996;23:433–441.

For more information on the treatment of laryngitis, see
Woodson GE: Hoarseness and laryngitis. In Rakel RE (ed): Conn's Current Therapy 1994, pp 21–26. Philadelphia, WB Saunders Company, 1994.

30 Croup

Nicholas J. Galioto

Etiology

1. Predominantly disease of viral etiology
   a. Parainfluenza 1 virus is the most common type and accounts for about 75 per cent of cases.
   b. Parainfluenza 2 and 3 virus
   c. Influenza serotype A virus
   d. Respiratory syncytial virus
   e. Rhinovirus
2. Mycoplasmal pneumonia is implicated in 3 to 4 per cent of cases.
3. Most commonly occurs in the fall and early winter

Symptoms

1. Occurs primarily in children ages 6 months to 3 years but may be seen in children up to age 6 years
2. Several-day history of progressive upper respiratory tract infection
3. "Barking" or "seal-like" cough developing on the second to third day of illness, especially at night
4. Hoarseness
5. Low-grade fever, generally less than 102.2° F (39° C)

Key Symptoms

- Age: 6 months to 3 years
- Upper respiratory tract infection prodrome
- Barking cough
- Hoarseness
- Low-grade fever

Clinical Findings

1. Inspiratory and expiratory stridor
2. Barking cough
3. Mild wheezing may be present on auscultation in 5 per cent of cases.
4. Position has no effect on airway obstruction.
5. Evaluate for respiratory distress
   a. Color: normal, dusky, or cyanotic
   b. Increased respiratory rate
   c. Stridor: mild or severe
   d. Retractions: supracostal, substernal, or intercostal
   e. Nasal flaring
   f. Air entry on auscultation: normal or decreased
   g. Decreased level of consciousness

If two or more signs of respiratory distress are present, the patient may require further observation and/or hospitalization.

Key Signs

- Stridor
- Barking cough
- Presence or absence of respiratory distress
- Position has no effect on obstruction

Tests

1. Diagnosis is generally made on the basis of clinical findings.
2. White blood cell count is usually normal or only mildly elevated. It is greater than 15,000/mm^3 in about 20 per cent of patients.
3. Lateral and anteroposterior radiographs of the neck
   a. An anteroposterior view may demonstrate a narrowed subglottic region or the "steeple" sign in 40 to 50 per cent of cases.
   b. A lateral view may show widening of the hypopharynx and may be helpful in making the diagnosis of epiglottitis, bacterial tracheitis, or retropharyngeal abscess.
4. Arterial blood gases will help assess the adequacy of ventilation and oxygenation, especially in the setting of severe respiratory compromise.
5. Pulse oximetry may be helpful in determining oxygen saturation but needs to be interpreted in conjunction with clinical presentation. Oxygen saturations greater than 90% may be noted even in the presence of marked hypercapnia.

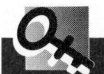

Key Test

Diagnosis usually is made on the basis of clinical findings.

Differential Diagnosis

1. Epiglottitis—must always be considered because it can rapidly lead to complete airway obstruction.
2. Spasmodic croup
3. Bacterial tracheitis
4. Peritonsillar abscess
5. Retropharyngeal abscess
6. Foreign-body aspiration
7. Diphtheria
8. Caustic ingestion
9. Laryngeal web
10. Laryngomalacia

WARNING

The child who presents with rapid onset of disease, absence of cough, and drooling and is leaning forward should alert the physician to the possibility of epiglottitis.

Treatment

1. Hospitalization is based on the degree of stridor, severity of retractions, pulse rate, respiratory rate, and evidence of cyanosis.
2. Frequent reassessments
3. Oxygen if necessary
4. Humidified air
   a. Mist tent in hospital if not overly traumatic to patient
   b. Cool-mist vaporizer, humidifier, or bathroom steam at home
5. Hydration
   a. Intravenous fluids in hospitalized patient (intravenous flow should be based on maintenance plus ongoing losses secondary to decreased oral intake, increased respiratory rate, and fever)
   b. Encourage increased oral fluid intake at home.

Medication

1. Racemic epinephrine, 0.25 to 0.50 ml in 2 to 3 ml normal saline solution given by aerosol.
   a. Onset of action is rapid and clinically detectable within 10 minutes of treatment.
   b. Mechanism of action is through its α-adrenergic effects, causing mucosal vasoconstriction and decreased tracheal edema.
   c. Medication may be repeated as necessary and is limited by the development of tachycardia (greater than 180 beats/min).
   d. Overuse may result in rebound swelling and increased stridor.
   e. Patients who receive racemic epinephrine should be considered for hospitalization. If outpatient management is still contemplated, then patients need to be observed for at least 2 hours for signs of rebound and/or worsening symptoms.
2. Corticosteroids: single dose of dexamethasone, 0.6 mg/kg, given orally, intramuscularly, or intravenously. May be repeated in 24 to 48 hours.
3. Antibiotics: generally not indicated in the treatment of viral croup except for superimposed bacterial infections, such as otitis media

Diet

1. If hospitalized with respiratory distress, patients should receive nothing by mouth and intravenous fluids should be provided.
2. For outpatient treatment or once respiratory distress has resolved, start clear liquids and advance diet as tolerated.

Activity

Level of activity limited by patient's clinical condition.

Patient Education

1. Review signs and symptoms of worsening distress.
2. Provide humidified air either through cool-mist vaporizer or bathroom steam.
3. Walking outside in the cool air may also decrease acute stridor.
4. Giving extra oral fluids is important.
5. Order acetaminophen for fever at a dose of 10 to 15 mg/kg every 4 hours as needed.
6. Avoid preparations that increase tenacity of tracheal secretions or have a drying effect (i.e., antihistamines, cold and cough preparations).

Key Treatment

- Humidified air
- Oxygen if necessary
- Racemic epinephrine
- Corticosteroids
- Hydration

Follow-Up

1. Close follow-up is often indicated by telephone or office visit within 24 hours.
2. Parents should be encouraged to report any change in the child's condition.

Bibliography

Cressman WR, Myer CM III: Diagnosis and management of croup and epiglottitis. Pediatr Clin North Am 1994; 41:265–276.

Custer JR: Croup and related disorders. Pediatr Rev 1993;14:19–29.

Geelhoed GC: Croup. Pediatr Pulmonol 1997;23:370–374.

Orenstein DM: Acute inflammatory upper airway obstruction. In Behrman RE, Vaughan VC, Nelson WE (eds): Nelson Textbook of Pediatrics, 15th ed, pp 1201–1205. Philadelphia, WB Saunders Company, 1996.

Quan L: Diagnosis and treatment of croup. Am Fam Physician 1992;46:747–755.

31 Bronchiolitis

J. Dennis Mull

Etiology

The pathophysiology of bronchiolitis results from the fact that children under age 2 have small airways. When they get a lower respiratory viral infection, swelling may close off those airways and lead to dyspnea. After age 2, children's anatomy changes and the airways do not close off in this way. Respiratory syncytial virus (RSV) accounts for 50% of bronchiolitis cases and other viruses, such as adenovirus, account for the rest.

Symptoms

One should always think of bronchiolitis when a young child presents with dyspnea and the child or a family member has had a recent respiratory infection. Often there is fussiness and poor feeding as a result of difficult or fast breathing.

Key Symptoms

- Dyspnea
- Fussiness

Clinical Findings

1. Clinical findings to look for are a rapid respiratory rate (see Table 31–1 for guidelines), nasal flaring, and retractions of the intercostal or subcostal spaces.
2. Wheezing may or may not be present.
3. The child's temperature is only minimally or not at all elevated.

TABLE 31–1. WORLD HEALTH ORGANIZATION GUIDELINES FOR WHEN TO CONSIDER CHEST RADIOGRAPH OR HOSPITALIZATION FOR FAST BREATHING

AGE OF CHILD	RESPIRATORY RATE
Birth to 1 month	>60 times/minute
1 month to 12 months	>50 times/minute
1 year to 5 years	>40 times/minute

From World Health Organization: Acute Respiratory Infections (ARI) Case Management Charts. Geneva, World Health Organization, 1990, with permission.

Key Signs

- Fast breathing
- Nasal flaring
- Chest retractions
- In severe cases, cyanosis

Laboratory Tests

1. Pulse oximetry is the most important test in bronchiolitis and should be performed on all children with this condition.
2. In severe cases with hypoxemia, arterial blood gases are necessary to rule out CO_2 retention and respiratory acidosis.
3. Chest radiograph may reveal hyperinflation or small local patchy areas of pneumonia.
4. In high-risk cases, other tests may include complete blood count (CBC) and immunoassay of nasal secretions for RSV.

Key Tests

- Pulse oximetry
- Chest radiograph
- Arterial blood gases in severe hypoxia
- CBC

Treatment

1. Hospitalization is mandatory for bronchiolitis in very young or chronically ill children or those with severe hypoxemia.
2. It is customary to give a trial of albuterol because it may help in occasional cases that have a component of bronchospasm. The usual mainstay of treatment is supportive therapy, which consists of placing the child in an oxygen tent with moisture and providing intravenous feeding if necessary. Usually the course of the disease is short, and after 2 or 3 days the child is able to return home, with gradual resumption of normal diet and activity.

3. Antibiotic use is controversial. One school of thought holds that, because bronchiolitis is a viral infection characterized by normal white count and minimal fever, antibiotics are not needed. Others contend that all cases should be treated with a fairly benign antibiotic such as amoxicillin because more than half of children with RSV-caused bronchiolitis go on to develop bacterially caused acute otitis media. Ribavirin (Virazole) is active against RSV and may be used in the most severe cases, but its effectiveness is controversial. Steroids are never indicated.

Patient Education

Although bronchiolitis rarely occurs in children more than 2 years old, it can and does recur up to that age. Therefore mothers should be encouraged to avoid exposing infants and young children to people with respiratory infections.

Prospects for preventing RSV infection in high risk infants have improved since the recent introduction of monoclonol antibody against RSV. Monthly injections of palivizumab (Synagis) during winter months are said to reduce hospitalizations by more than half. At a dosage of 15 mg/kg the cost of this agent in its 100-mg vial will limit its availability: $1,216 wholesale cost to the pharmacist per vial.

Key Treatment

- *Emergency care*: A trial of nebulized albuterol (0.15 mg/kg/dose) is customary. Up to three doses at 20-minute intervals may be given.

- *Supportive treatment*: humidified oxygen tent at a fractional oxygen concentration of 28 to 40 per cent. When feeding is impaired, intravenous fluids (5% dextrose with 0.25 normal saline with potassium) are indicated.

- Antibiotics are controversial, as is antiviral therapy with ribavirin (Virazole).

- Steroids are not appropriate.

- Palivizumab (Synagis) useful for prevention in high risk babies. Expensive.

Follow-Up

Whether hospitalized or not, children need to be followed up carefully in the office every day or so until their respiratory rates have returned to normal and they appear to be thoroughly recovered.

 Bibliography

Adcock PM, Sanders CC, Marshall GS: Standardizing the care of bronchiolitis. Arch Pediat Adolesc Med 1998; 152:739–744.

Andrade MA, Hoberman A, Glustein J, et al: Acute otitis media in children with bronchiolitis. Pediatrics 1998; 101:617–619.

Inkelis SH: Bronchiolitis. In Tintinalli JE, Ruiz E, Krome RL (eds): Emergency Medicine: A Comprehensive Study Guide, pp 642–644. New York, McGraw-Hill, 1996.

Klassen TP: Recent advances in the treatment of bronchiolitis and laryngitis. Pediatr Clin North Am 1997; 44:249–261.

Orenstein DM: Bronchiolitis. In Behrman RE, Kliegman RM, Arvin AM (eds): Nelson Textbook of Pediatrics, 15th ed, pp 1211–1213. Philadelphia, WB Saunders Company, 1996.

The Medical Letter, Vol 41, pp 3–4, January 1, 1999.

32 Fetal Lung Immaturity

David G. Weismiller

Fetal lung immaturity is the result of birth prior to the biochemical maturation of lungs (surfactant production by type II alveolar cells) and may also result from an alteration in extracellular matrix that inhibits lung expandability. The major function of surfactant is to decrease alveolar surface tension and increase lung compliance. Surfactant prevents alveolar collapse at the end of expiration and allows for opening of the alveoli at low intrathoracic pressure. Respiratory distress syndrome (RDS), a consequence of endogenous pulmonary surfactant deficiency, is the primary factor in neonatal morbidity and mortality among infants with immature lungs.

Etiology
1. Preterm infant
2. Maternal diabetes (combined fetal hyperglycemia and hyperinsulinemia)

Clinical Findings
Affected infants characteristically present with tachypnea, grunting, nasal flaring, chest retraction, and cyanosis in the first 3 hours of life.
1. Decreased air entry on auscultation of the chest
2. Hypoxemia
3. Complications associated with fetal lung immaturity that are associated with asphyxia and mechanical ventilation
   a. Pneumothorax
   b. Patent ductus arteriosus
   c. Intraventricular hemorrhage
   d. Necrotizing enterocolitis
   e. Bronchopulmonary dysplasia
   f. Retinopathy of prematurity

Key Signs

- Tachypnea
- Grunting
- Nasal flaring
- Chest retractions
- Cyanosis

Laboratory Tests
1. Pulse oximetry
2. Blood gas determination
3. Complete blood count with differential
4. Cultures: blood, urine, cerebrospinal fluid
5. Blood glucose and electrolytes
6. The diagnosis is confirmed by a chest radiograph that reveals a uniform ground-glass pattern and an air bronchogram that is consistent with diffuse atelectasis.

Key Tests

- Pulse oximetry
- Blood gases
- Chest radiograph

Differential Diagnosis
1. Developmental disorders
   a. Transient tachypnea of the newborn
   b. Persistence of the fetal circulation
   c. Esophageal atresia with tracheoesophageal fistula
   d. Pulmonary hypoplasia
   e. Diaphragmatic hernia
   f. Congenital lobar emphysema
   g. Apnea
2. Acquired disorders
   a. Pneumonia
   b. Bacterial or viral infection/sepsis
   c. Pneumothorax
   d. Hypoglycemia
   e. Meconium aspiration syndrome
   f. Anemia
   g. Polycythemia

Treatment

Medication
1. Antenatal corticosteroids
   a. Reduce mortality, RDS, and intraventricular hemorrhage.
   b. Benefit a broad range of gestational ages, not limited by gender or race.
   c. Although the greatest benefit occurs with

treatment at more than 24 hours, treatment of less than 24 hours may improve outcome.

d. Administering corticosteroids (24 mg betamethasone or 24 mg dexamethasone) to women who are expected to deliver preterm can substantially reduce neonatal morbidity and mortality.

e. No adverse consequences of this treatment have been identified.

f. Recommended for preterm premature rupture of membranes at less than 30 to 32 weeks of gestation in the absence of clinical chorioamnionitis. More data are needed to identify risks and benefits of this treatment.

g. No evidence is available on repeated doses of corticosteroids in women at continued risk of preterm birth 1 week after an initial course of therapy.

h. The decision to use antenatal corticosteroids should not be altered by the availability of surfactant replacement therapy.

i. Treatment substantially decreases neonatal morbidity and mortality and health care costs.

2. Surfactant

a. Intratracheal pulmonary surfactant for infants at risk (prophylactic) or diagnosed with RDS (treatment) ameliorates RDS, decreases the need for supplemental oxygen, and decreases the duration of ventilatory support.

b. Mortality rate and long-term complications of severe RDS decrease.

c. The combined treatment of antenatal corticosteroids and postnatal surfactant reduces mortality, RDS, and intraventricular hemorrhage. Surfactant replacement has little or no impact on the incidence of intraventricular hemorrhage.

d. Current recommendations

(1) Should be directed by physicians trained in respiratory management of low-birth-weight infants and who have experience in mechanical ventilation.

(2) Experienced nursing and respiratory therapy personnel should be available when therapy is administered.

(3) Equipment to manage and monitor low-birth-weight infants, including that needed for mechanical ventilation, should be available.

(4) Radiology and laboratory support for managing very-low-birth-weight infants should be available.

(5) An institutionally approved protocol for administering surfactant therapy should be a mandatory component of a quality assessment program.

(6) In an emergency in which recommended staff and equipment are not available, only a physician skilled in endotracheal intubation should give surfactant. Transfer infants as soon as feasible to a center with appropriate facilities and staff trained to care for multisystem morbidity in low-birth-weight infants.

3. Postnatal corticosteroid therapy

a. The combined use of antenatal corticosteroids and postnatal surfactant has significantly decreased overall morbidity and mortality caused by RDS relative to either treatment alone; however, even the combined use has not demonstrated a reduction in the incidence of bronchopulmonary dysplasia.

b. Although many physicians prescribe corticosteroid therapy for prevention and treatment of chronic lung disease, treatment efficacy is controversial.

4. Thyrotropin-releasing hormone, triiodothyronine, and thyroxine

a. On the basis of currently available evidence, antenatal thyrotropin-releasing hormone cannot be recommended for clinical practice.

b. Thyroid hormones have been found to accelerate fetal lung maturation in various studies. The value of antenatal administration is limited because the hormones are metabolized by the placenta and membranes.

c. There is no conclusive evidence that administering thyrotropin-releasing hormone prior to very preterm delivery reduces the risk of RDS or chronic oxygen dependence. Also, there is no clear effect on neonatal mortality.

Patient Education

1. The benefits vastly outweigh the risks of antenatal administration of corticosteroids to fetuses at risk of preterm delivery.

2. Antenatal corticosteroid use slightly increases the risk of neonatal infection. Because of the effectiveness of antenatal corticosteroids in reducing mortality in fetuses, treatment is appropriate in the absence of chorioamnionitis.

3. The risk of problems during pregnancy is greatest when diabetes is not well controlled. Good control of glucose levels, before and during pregnancy, can lower the risk of fetal lung

immaturity and subsequent respiratory distress syndrome.

a. Goal: fasting blood sugar less than 100 mg/dl

b. Goal: 2-hour postprandial blood sugar less than 120 mg/dl

Key Treatment

Mother (Predelivery)	Infant
• Betamethasone, 12 mg IM q 24h × 2	• Surfactant
	• Oxygen
• Dexamethasone, 6 mg IM q12h × 4	• Mechanical ventilation

Follow-Up

1. Data from trials with follow-up of children up to 12 years indicate that antenatal corticosteroid therapy does not adversely affect physical growth or psychomotor development. No long-term maternal adverse effects have been reported.

2. Both short- and long-term benefits have been associated with the use of surfactant for treatment of RDS as the result of fetal lung immaturity. No long-term adverse effects have been reported.

Bibliography

ACOG Committee on Obstetric Practice: Antenatal Corticosteroid Therapy for Fetal Maturation. (No 210). New York, American College of Obstetricians and Gynecologists, 1998.

American Academy of Pediatrics and The American College of Obstetrics and Gynecology: Guidelines for Perinatal Care, 4th ed, pp 183–206. Elk Grove Village, IL, American Academy of Pediatrics, 1997.

Crowther CA, Alfirevic Z, Haslam RR: Antenatal thyrotropin-releasing hormone (TRH) prior to preterm delivery (Cochrane Review). In: The Cochrane Library, Issue 3. Oxford, Update Software, 1998.

National Institutes of Health: Report of the Consensus Development Conference on the Effect of Corticosteroids for Fetal Maturation on Perinatal Outcomes (NIH Pulication no 95-3784). Bethesda, MD, National Institutes of Health, 1994.

Rastogi A, Akintorin SM, Bez ML, et al: A controlled trial of dexamethasone to prevent bronchopulmonary dysplasia in surfactant-treated infants. Pediatrics 1996; 98:204–210.

33 Asthma

Russell D. White

Definition

1. Asthma is a chronic inflammatory disease of the airways.
2. Asthma is characterized by
   a. Episodic, reversible airway obstruction
   b. Episodic wheezing, cough, and dyspnea secondary to inflammation
   c. Increased bronchial hyperresponsiveness to various stimuli

Epidemiology

1. Asthma affects 5 per cent of U.S. population (14 to 15 million persons).
2. Asthma is the most common chronic disease of childhood.
3. Male/female ratio = 2:1 in childhood; 1:1 ratio in adulthood
4. Worldwide prevalence is increasing!

Etiology

1. Accepted theory is an inflammatory process that is activated by an allergen, chemical irritant, or some other inflammatory factor.
2. An allergic component is identified in 80 to 85 per cent of patients.
3. Asthma is classified as
   a. Allergic asthma: onset in childhood; characterized by history of allergy, increased immunoglobulin E (IgE) levels, and positive response to specific allergens
   b. Idiosyncratic asthma: onset in adulthood; characterized by no allergy history and normal IgE levels. Patients often develop asthma in response to upper respiratory infections.
   c. Mixed asthma: onset in adulthood; characterized by features of both types
4. Common inciting factors include dust mite feces, plant pollens, cigarette smoke, and viral upper respiratory infections

Pathophysiology

1. Hallmark is narrowing of bronchial airway diameter secondary to:
   a. Smooth muscle contraction
   b. Airway edema
   c. Respiratory vascular congestion
   d. Increase in airway secretions
   e. Hypertrophy of basement membrane, remodeling, and fibrosis (chronic). This chronic change may produce *irreversible* obstruction
2. Other respiratory changes include:
   a. Decrease in expiratory flow rates
   b. Increased respiratory workload and muscle fatigue
   c. Ventilation-perfusion mismatch
   d. Arterial blood gas abnormalities
   e. Pulmonary hypertension

Symptoms (Table 33–1)

1. Triad of cough, dyspnea, and wheezing
2. Poor or variable exercise tolerance
3. Abdominal pain (children)
4. Majority of patients experience nocturnal symptoms.

Key Symptoms

- Cough
- Dyspnea
- Wheezing

Clinical Findings (Table 33–1)

1. Increased respiratory and heart rate
2. Wheezing (may be absent with severe bronchospasm)
3. Prolonged expiratory phase of respiration
4. Hyperresonant chest percussion
5. Late, severe signs
   a. Use of accessory muscles for breathing
   b. Increased negative intrathoracic pressure
   c. Cyanosis/diaphoresis with severe respiratory compromise

Key Sign

Wheezing

TABLE 33-1. SEVERITY OF ASTHMA EXACERBATION

	MILD	MODERATE	SEVERE
Symptoms			
Dyspnea	Speaks in sentences	Speaks in phrases	Speaks in single words
Position, preferred	Can lie down	Sitting	Sits upright
Alertness	Normal/agitated	Agitated	Agitated or drowsy
Signs			
Respiratory rate	Normal to 30% above mean	30–50% above mean	>50% above mean
Heart rate	<100 bpm	100–120 bpm	>120 bpm
Color	Normal	Pale	Cyanotic
Accessory muscle use	None/mild intercostal retractions	Moderate intercostal retractions, chest hyperinflation, use of sternocleidomastoid muscles	Moderate intercostal retractions; chest hyperinflation; tracheosternal retraction during inspiration
Auscultation	End-expiratory wheezing	Inspiratory and expiratory wheezing	Inaudible breath sounds (no wheezing)
Pulsus paradoxus	<10 mm Hg	10–25 mm Hg	>25 mm Hg
Tests*			
PEF	80% of predicted or baseline	50–80% of predicted or baseline	<50% of predicted or baseline
O_2 saturation	>95%	91–95%	<91%
PCO_2	<43 mm Hg	<42 mm Hg	>44 mm Hg
PO_2 (Room air)	Normal	>60 mm Hg	<60 mm Hg
pH	Respiratory alkalosis	Pseudo normal	Respiratory acidosis

*PEF, peak expiratory flow; PCO_2, partial pressure of carbon dioxide; PO_2, partial pressure of oxygen.

Tests (Table 33–1)

1. Laboratory tests are done to confirm diagnosis, assess severity, determine prognosis, and rule out other disease states.
2. One must establish bronchospasm, determine reversibility, and classify based on severity.
3. The following tests may be useful for diagnosis:
   a. Pulmonary function tests: used to confirm airway obstruction based on standard tables. *Reversibility* is defined as an increase in forced expiratory volume at 1 second (FEV_1) of 15 per cent or more following two puffs of a β-adrenergic agonist.
   b. Methacholine challenge test: a provocative test in which a patient inhales a bronchoconstricting agent (methacholine)
   c. Exercise stress test: useful in documenting exercise-induced bronchospasm (EIB)
4. The following tests may aid in the diagnosis:
   a. Complete blood count: May rule out other diagnoses and detect eosinophilia in atopic patients.
   b. IgE: May indicate allergic asthma
   c. Sputum examination: May show eosinophils or Curschmann's spirals (mucus casts of respiratory tree).
5. The following tests may aid in the acute evaluation:
   a. Wright peak flow measurement: useful in monitoring response to therapy or for early deterioration; measured value is compared to predicted normal or to patient's personal best value; convenient and cost-effective. Peak flow measurement is utilized for monitoring but *not* for diagnosis.
   b. Pulse oximetry: Monitors oxygen saturation when patient is in distress; convenient and cost-effective.
   c. Chest film: indicated to rule out diseases such as pneumonia, pneumothorax, or congestive heart failure
   d. Arterial blood gas measurement: indicated in severe cases; normal or elevated alveolar partial pressure of CO_2 (P_aCO_2) with acidosis indicates respiratory compromise/failure.
   e. Sinus films: Sinusitis may be a precipitating cause.
   f. Serum theophylline level: indicated if patient is taking theophylline

Key Test

Pulmonary function testing; increase in FEV_1 after a β-agonist

Diagnosis and Differential Diagnosis

1. Diagnosis
   a. Detailed medical history, including allergy history
   b. Careful exam focusing on respiratory system and chest exam
   c. Pulmonary function tests
   d. Special tests as indicated

2. Differential diagnosis
   a. Upper airway obstruction/foreign body
   b. Bronchitis/pneumonia/bronchiolitis
   c. Chronic obstructive lung disease
   d. Tumor/neoplasm
   e. Pulmonary embolism
   f. Congestive heart failure
   g. Vocal cord dysfunction
   h. Viral lower respiratory tract infection

Classification

1. Mild intermittent asthma
   a. Mild asthma symptoms once or twice weekly
   b. Nighttime asthma two or fewer times per month
   c. Pulmonary function tests are 80 per cent or more of predicted normal
   d. Peak expiratory flow (PEF) variability less than 20 per cent
2. Mild persistent asthma
   a. Symptoms more than two times per week but less than once per day
   b. Nighttime asthma more than two times per month
   c. Pulmonary function tests 80 per cent or more of predicted normal

   d. PEF variability 20 to 30 per cent
3. Moderate persistent asthma
   a. Daily asthma symptoms *with* two or more exacerbations per week
   b. Nighttime asthma more than once per week
   c. Pulmonary function tests more than 60 and less than 80 per cent of predicted normal
   d. PEF variability more than 30 per cent
4. Severe persistent asthma
   a. Continual symptoms with frequent exacerbations
   b. Frequent nighttime asthma
   c. Pulmonary function tests 60 per cent or less of predicted normal
   d. PEF variability more than 30 per cent

Treatment

The treatment strategy has changed from reactive therapy to proactive management (see Tables 33–2 through 33–4).

1. Mild intermittent asthma
   a. No daily medication for long-term control
   b. Short-acting bronchodilator (inhaled β_2-agonist) as needed for symptoms
2. Mild persistent asthma
   a. One of the following as a daily medication for long-term control:

TABLE 33–2. MEDICATION DOSAGES FOR QUICK RELIEF

Medication	Dosage Form	Adult Dose	Child Dose
Short-Acting Inhaled β_2-Agonists			
Metered-dose inhalers			
Albuterol, albuterol HFA (Proventil)	90 μg/puff, 200 puffs	2 puffs tid–qid	2 puffs tid–qid
Pirbuterol (Maxair)	200 μg/puff, 400 puffs		
Terbutaline (Brethine)	200 μg/puff, 300 puffs		
Nebulizer Solution			
Albuterol (Proventil)	5 mg/ml (0.5%)	1.25–5 mg (0.25–1 ml) in 2–3 ml of saline q4–8h	0.05 mg/kg (minimum 1.25 mg, maximum 2.5 mg) in 2–3 ml of saline q4–6h
Anticholinergics			
Metered-dose inhaler			
Ipratropium (Atrovent)	18 μg/puff, 200 puffs	2–3 puffs q6h	1–2 puffs q6h
Nebulizer Solution			
Ipratropium (Atrovent)	0.25 mg/ml (0.025%)	0.25–0.5 mg q6h	0.25 mg q6h
Systemic Corticosteroids			
Methylprednisolone	2-, 4-, 8-, 16-, 32-mg tablets	Short-course "burst": 40–60 mg/d as single or 2 divided doses for 3–10 d	Short-course "burst": 1–2 mg/kg/d, maximum 60 mg/d, for 3–10 d
Prednisone	1-, 2.5-, 5-, 10-, 20-, 25-mg tabs; 5 mg/ml, 5 mg/5 ml		

TABLE 33–3. MEDICATION DOSAGES FOR LONG-TERM CONTROL

MEDICATION	DOSAGE FORM*	ADULT DOSE	CHILD DOSE
Systemic Corticosteroids			
Methylprednisolone	2-, 4-, 8-, 16-, 32-mg tablets	7.5–60 mg daily in a single dose or qod as needed for control	0.25–2 mg/kg daily in single dose or qod as needed for control
Prednisone	1-, 2.5-, 5-, 10-, 20-, 25-mg tablets; 5 mg/ml, 5 mg/5 ml	Short-course "burst": 40–60 mg/d as single or 2 divided doses for 3–10 d	Short course "burst": 1–2 mg/kg/d, maximum 60 mg/d, for 3–10 d
Cromolyn and Nedocromil			
Cromolyn (Intal)	MDI, 1 mg/puff	2–4 puffs tid–qid	1–2 puffs
	Nebulizer solution, 20 mg/ampule	1 ampule tid–qid	1 ampule tid–qid
Nedocromil (Tilade)	MDI, 1.75 mg/puff	2–4 puffs bid–qid	1–2 puffs bid–qid
Long-Acting β_2-Agonists			
Salmeterol (Serevent)	MDI, 21 μg/puff, 60 or 120 puffs	2 puffs q12h	1–2 puffs q12h
	DPI, 50 mg/blister	1 blister q12h	1 blister q12h
Methylxanthines			
Theophylline	Liquids Sustained-release tablets and capsules	Starting dose 10 mg/kg/d up to 300 mg maximum; usual maximum 800 mg/d	Starting dose 10 mg/kg/d; usual maximum: $\geq$1 year of age: 16 mg/kg/d <1 year: 0.2 (age in weeks) + 5 = mg/kg/d
Leukotriene Modifiers			
Zafirlukast (Accolate)	20-mg tablet	40 mg daily (1 tablet bid)	40 mg daily (>age 12 yr) (1 tablet bid)
Zileuton (Zyflo)	300-mg tablet 600-mg tablet	2,400 mg daily 600 mg tablet qid	1200–2400 mg daily (>age 12 yr) 300- to 600-mg tablet qid
Montelukast (Singulair)	10-mg oral tablet 5-mg chewable tablet	10 mg daily	5 mg daily (>age 6 yr)

*DPI, dry powder inhaler; MDI, metered-dose inhaler.

TABLE 33–4. DAILY DOSAGES FOR INHALED CORTICOSTEROIDS

DRUG*	LOW DOSE	MEDIUM DOSE	HIGH DOSE
Adults			
Beclomethasone dipropionate DS (Vanceril, Beclovent), 84 μg/puff	168–504 μg (2–6 puffs)	504–840 μg (6–10 puffs)	>840 μg (>10 puffs)
Budesonide turbuhaler (Pulmicort), 200 μg/dose	200–400 μg (1–2 inhalations)	400–600 μg (2–3 inhalations)	>600 μg (>3 inhalations)
Fluticasone (Flovent)	88–264 μg	264–660 μg	>600 μg
MDI: 44, 110, 220 μg/puff	2–6 puffs of 44 μg or 2 puffs of 110 μg	2–6 puffs of 110 μg	>6 puffs of 110 μg or >3 puffs of 220 μg
DPI: 50, 100, 250 μg/dose	2–6 inhalations of 50 μg	3–6 inhalations of 100 μg	>6 inhalations of 100 μg or >2 inhalations of 250 μg
Children			
Beclomethasone dipropionate DS (Vanceril, Beclovent) 84 μg/puff	84–336 μg (1–4 puffs)	336–672 μg (4–8 puffs)	>6732 μg (>8 puffs)
Budesonide turbuhaler (Pulmicort) 200 μg/dose	100–200 μg	200–400 μg (1–2 inhalations)	>400 μg (>2 inhalations)
Fluticasone (Flovent)	88–176 μg	176–440 μg	>440 μg
MDI: 44, 110, 220 μg/puff	2–6 puffs of 44 μg	4–10 puffs of 44 μg or 2–4 puffs of 110 μg	>4 puffs of 110 μg or >2 puffs of 220 μg
DPI: 50, 100, 250 μg/dose	2–4 inhalations of 50 μg	3–6 inhalations of 100 μg	>4 inhalations of 100 μg or >2 inhalations of 250 μg

*DPI, dry powder inhaler; MDI, metered-dose inhaler.

(1) Anti-inflammatory medication (inhaled low-dose corticosteroid or cromolyn [Intal] or nedocromil [Tilade] in children)

(2) Sustained-release theophylline

(3) Consider zafirlukast (Accolate) or zileuton (Zyflo) (≥age 12 years) or montelukast (Singulair) (≥age 6 years)

b. Short-acting bronchodilator (inhaled β_2-agonist) as needed for symptoms

3. Moderate persistent asthma

   a. Daily medication for long-term control

(1) Anti-inflammatory inhaled corticosteroid (medium dose) *or*

(2) Inhaled corticosteroid (low-medium dose) and long-acting bronchodilator (long-acting inhaled β_2-agonist, sustained-release theophylline, or long-acting β_2-agonist tablets)

(3) If needed, add

   (a) Inhaled corticosteroid (medium-high dose) *AND*

   (b) Long-acting bronchodilator (as above)

b. Short-acting bronchodilator (inhaled β_2-agonist) as needed for symptoms

4. Severe persistent asthma

   a. Daily medications for long-term control

(1) Anti-inflammatory inhaled corticosteroid (high dose) *AND*

(2) Long-acting bronchodilator (long-acting β_2-agonist, sustained-release theophylline, or long-acting β_2-agonist tablets *AND*

(3) Corticosteroid tablets or syrup

b. Short-acting bronchodilator (inhaled β_2-agonist) as needed for symptoms

c. Consider consultation.

Specific Classes of Medications

The two classes of therapy are short-term relief medications and long-term control medications.

1. β-Adrenergic agonists

   a. Mainstay "rescue" medication used to treat bronchospasm

   b. Useful as prophylaxis for those with EIB

   c. Long-acting forms used as long-term control medication

   d. Indicated in all age groups

   e. Dosage forms: injectable (subcutaneous), oral liquid, oral tablets (short-acting and extended-release), inhalation (metered-dose inhaler [MDI] or nebulizer solution), inhaled powder, and long-acting MDI. May be given via endotracheal tube in emergency situations.

   f. Examples: albuterol (Proventil), terbutaline (Brethine), metaproterenol (Alupent), salmeterol (Serevent)

2. Methylxanthines

   a. Used as long-term control medication

   b. Less usage now with more effective medications and fewer drug interactions

   c. Useful in selected patients or those with nocturnal symptoms

   d. Inexpensive, but blood-level monitoring adds to cost

   e. Dosage forms: intravenous and oral (tablets and liquid)

   f. Examples: aminophylline, theophylline (Theo-Dur, Slo-Phyllin), dyphylline (Lufyllin)

3. Anticholinergics

   a. Not officially indicated for asthma, but selected patients with chronic obstructive lung disease and asthma may respond

   b. Used as a rescue medication

   c. Dosage forms: MDI and nebulizer

   d. Examples: ipratropium (Atrovent)

4. Leukotriene-modifying agents

   a. Indicated in mild, persistent asthma

   b. Used as a long-term control medication

   c. Useful in selected adult patients and age-specific pediatric groups

   d. Agent of choice in those with aspirin-sensitive asthma

   e. Dosage forms: oral tablets, chewable tablets

   f. Examples: zafirlukast (Accolate), zileuton (Zyflo), montelukast (Singulair)

5. Cromolyn

   a. Used as a long-term control medication

   b. Useful as anti-inflammatory agent, especially in children

   c. Effective as prophylaxis in EIB. (Albuterol and cromolyn taken together prior to exercise are 95 per cent effective in preventing EIB.)

   d. Dosage forms: MDI, inhaled powder, nebulizer solution

   e. Examples: cromolyn sodium (Intal), nedocromil (Tilade)

6. Glucocorticoids (systemic and inhaled)

   a. Main anti-inflammatory agent

   b. May be used as long-term control treatment or as a bolus/burst "rescue" medication.

When used as a burst medication, a tapering schedule is not necessary.

c. Dosage forms: intravenous, intramuscular, oral tablets and liquids, and MDIs

d. Examples: methylprednisolone, hydrocortisone, prednisone, prednisolone, steroid MDIs

Key Treatment

- β-Agonist
- Anti-inflammatory agent
- Leukotriene blocker

Diet

Avoid food allergens in those with specific food allergies

Activity

1. Encourage exercise and normal activity.
2. Control baseline asthma and premedicate those patients with EIB.

Immunizations

Administer pneumonia vaccine and yearly influenza immunizations.

Patient Education

1. Educate patients and their families. Develop guidelines for self-treatment versus physician consultation.
2. Emphasize the proper use of MDIs with a spacer device.

3. Most infectious exacerbations are due to viruses and do not require antibiotics.
4. Remove/avoid allergens (dust mites, pollens) and irritants (cigarette smoke, occupational chemicals).

Follow-Up

1. Asthmatic patients should be seen on scheduled intervals. Mild intermittent asthma patients can be seen every 3 to 6 months; those with more serious disease should be seen every 1 to 3 months.
2. Educate the patient to self-monitor peak flow measurements on a regular basis and report major deviations from baseline. Normal diurnal peak flow variation is 5 per cent. Peak flow measurements in asthmatics are best in the mid-afternoon and worst in the early morning.
3. Teach patient to adjust medications in response to changes.

Bibliography

Guidelines for the Diagnosis and Management of Asthma: Expert Panel Report II (NIH Publication no 97-04061). Bethesda, MD, National Institutes of Health, 1997.

Lemanske RF, Buesse WW: Asthma. JAMA 1997;278: 1855–1873.

McFadden ER Jr: Asthma. In Fauci AS, Braunwald E, Isselbacher KJ, et al (eds): Harrison's Principles of Internal Medicine, 14th ed, pp 1419–1426. New York, McGraw-Hill, 1998.

Nelson HS: Drug therapy: beta-adrenergic bronchodilators. N Engl J Med 1995;333:499–506.

O'Byrne PM, Israel E, Drazen JM: Antileukotrienes in the treatment of asthma. Ann Intern Med 1997;127:472–480.

Szefler SJ, Chambers CV: Diagnosis and management of asthma. Am Fam Physician 1995;Monogr 2.

34 Bronchitis

Richard A. Gleckman

Infectious bronchitis refers to two separate entities: acute infectious bronchitis and the exacerbation of chronic bronchitis.

Acute Infectious Bronchitis

Etiology

Acute infectious bronchitis, an inflammatory condition of the bronchi, is caused most commonly by a virus (rhinovirus, coronavirus, respiratory syncytial virus, adenovirus, influenza A and B, parainfluenza) and less frequently *Mycoplasma pneumoniae, Chlamydia pneumoniae, Bordetella pertussis, Bordetella parapertussis*, and *Legionella* species.

Symptoms

1. Acute infectious bronchitis is an isolated event clinically expressed as cough, with or without sputum production, chest discomfort, and fever.
2. Some patients will experience wheezing that resembles asthma, and others manifest shortness of breath.

Key Symptoms

- Cough
- Chest discomfort

Clinical Findings

1. Hoarseness suggests bronchitis caused by *C. pneumoniae*.
2. A paroxysmal, barking cough that is worse at night and interferes with completing a sentence suggests illness caused by *Bordetella* species.
3. Concomitant impressive constitutional symptoms (shaking chills, elevated temperatures, fatigue, sweats, and muscle aches) imply influenza.
4. Recurrent episodes raise a concern for human immunodeficiency virus (HIV) infection.

Laboratory Tests

1. Tests are usually not indicated. A chest radiograph should be obtained, however, for patients with profound constitutional symptoms, dyspnea, rales, rigors, pleurisy, or persistent fever/cough.
2. Diagnostic studies for *M. pneumoniae* (culture, elevated serum immunoglobulin M titer, acute or convalescent sera demonstrating fourfold rise in titer, antigen detection by polymerase chain reaction [PCR]); *C. pneumoniae* (microimmunofluorescent assay, tissue culture, PCR); and *B. pertussis* (cough plate culture; serology, including PCR) are not routinely recommended, are expensive, and are not readily available.

Key Test

Neither blood nor sputum analyses are indicated.

Differential Diagnosis

The differential diagnosis includes noninfectious disorders (environmental irritants, angiotensin-converting enzyme inhibitors) and infectious illness (pneumonia, sinusitis). In the HIV-infected patient the disease can resemble chest radiograph–negative tuberculosis or *Pneumocystis carinii* pneumonia.

Treatment

1. Agents are prescribed to suppress cough and reduce constitutional complaints. During an epidemic of influenza A, amantadine (Symmetrel) or rimantadine (Flumadine) should be prescribed within 48 hours of the onset of symptoms. They are more effective than aspirin or acetaminophen. These medications should not be prescribed to pregnant patients, however. Patients with wheezing are candidates for inhaled bronchodilator therapy with albuterol.
2. Theoretically a macrolide (erythromycin, clarithromycin, azithromycin) could be beneficial, because it could prevent the transmission of *Bordetella* species and because disease caused by *M. pneumoniae, C. pneumoniae*, and *Bordetella* species can be associated with protracted symptoms. However, there is no convincing evidence that a macrolide favorably influences the

course of bronchitis caused by *M. pneumoniae* or *C. pneumoniae.*

3. For most patients an antibiotic should not be prescribed. Antibiotics have no proven value, add to medical costs, foster the emergence of resistant organisms, and contribute to drug toxicity.

Key Treatment

- Symptomatic agents
- Antimicrobial not indicated

Follow-Up

1. If the patient fails to improve, confirm the diagnosis and exclude pulmonary disorders that are associated with persistent cough, such as pneumonia, lung abscess, tuberculosis, sarcoidosis, bronchiolitis obliterans with organizing pneumonia (BOOP), Wegener's granulomatosis, and cancer.

2. For the young adult with persistent cough and normal chest radiograph, rule out *Bordetella pertussis*–related bronchitis, because patients can infect children and adults and antimicrobial therapy (erythromycin or trimethoprim-sulfamethoxazole) is beneficial to accelerate the resolution of symptoms.

Acute Exacerbation of Chronic Bronchitis

Etiology

1. The organisms most commonly incriminated in acute exacerbation of chronic bronchitis (AECB) are viruses, *M. pneumoniae, Haemophilus influenzae, Haemophilus parainfluenzae, Streptococcus pneumoniae,* and *Moraxella (Branhamella) catarrhalis. Chlamydia pneumoniae* rarely causes AECB.

2. Not all exacerbations are caused by infectious organisms, however. AECB has been attributed to smoking, allergens, and occupational irritants.

Symptoms

1. The symptoms of AECB consist of an increase in fatigue, chest tightness, worsening cough, and dyspnea, accompanied by an increased volume and/or purulence of sputum. Some patients experience fever and/or hemoptysis.

2. The presence of rales can indicate chronic bronchitis, a superimposed pneumonia, or congestive heart failure (CHF).

Key Symptoms/Signs

- Worsening cough
- Increased dyspnea
- Sputum purulence

Laboratory Tests

1. There is no need to analyze the blood or sputum. Examination of sputum by Gram's stain smear or culture, or cytology is not usually useful because the findings during the acute exacerbation cannot consistently be distinguished from quiescent periods.

2. A chest radiograph is indicated when the patient appears ill, manifests new rales, or has findings that suggest CHF.

3. A blood gas determination would be appropriate for patients experiencing insomnia, agitation, or increasing dyspnea.

Key Test

There is no need to routinely assess the sputum or blood.

Differential Diagnosis

Additional disorders that need to be considered are pneumonia, CHF, tuberculosis, lung abscess, and lung cancer.

Treatment

1. After assessing the need for hospitalization, therapy consists of both an antimicrobial (for selective patients) and supportive care. Antimicrobials appear to have their greatest impact on the therapy of the patient experiencing a more "severe" exacerbation—not simply increased sputum or a change in the appearance of the sputum, but both of these features plus increased shortness of breath. Antimicrobials have accelerated the rate of clinical resolution and reduced the need for additional medication and/or return visits and hospitalization.

2. Clinicians have prescribed aminopenicillins, cephalosporins, carbacephem, fluoroquinolones, trimethoprim-sulfamethoxazole, and tetracyclines (Table 34–1). There is no documentation that one compound exerts superior efficacy. Features of the host and antimicrobial that would influence drug selection include the following: the patient's history of drug allergy, the

TABLE 34-1. ANTIMICROBIAL AGENTS

Macrolides
Erythromycin
Clarithromycin (Biaxin)
Azithromycin (Zithromax)
Dirithromycin (Dynabac)

Cephalosporins
Cefaclor (Ceclor)
Cefuroxime (Ceftin)
Cefixime (Suprax)
Cefprozil (Cefzil)
Cefpodoxime proxetil (Vantin)
Ceftibuten (Cedax)

Carbacephem
Loracarbef (Lorabid)

Aminopenicillins
Ampicillin
Amoxicillin
Amoxicillin-clavulanate (Augmentin)
Bacampicillin (Spectrobid)

Fluroquinolones
Ciprofloxacin (Cipro)
Ofloxacin (Floxin)
Lomefloxacin (Maxaquin)
Levofloxacin (Levaquin)
Sparfloxacin (Zagam)
Grepafloxacin (Raxar)
Trovafloxacin (Trovan)

Tetracylines
Doxycycline (Vibramycin)
Minocycline (Minocyn)
Tetracycline
Trimethoprim-sulfamethoxazole (Bactrim, Septra)

---

drug's track record, the drug's potential to initiate untoward events or undesirable drug-drug interactions, the drug's spectrum of activity, the ease of compliance, and the drug's cost.

3. Trimethroprim-sulfamethoxazole (Bactrim, Septra) and doxycycline appear to be appealing drugs. They inhibit the growth of the majority of bacteria incriminated in the exacerbation of chronic bronchitis, are an appropriate selection for the penicillin-allergic patient, are prescribed twice daily, are relatively safe compounds, have an established track record, and are inexpensive antimicrobials.

   a. With regard to trimethoprim-sulfamethoxazole, some patients develop hypersensitivity reactions (fever, rash) or gastrointestinal untoward events, and there is a risk of interaction when there is co-administration with warfarin, cyclosporine, phenytoin, methotrexate, and oral hypoglycemic agents. In addition, older patients are at greater risk of experiencing trimethoprim-sulfamethoxazole–induced blood dyscrasias and hyperkalemia.

   b. Doxycycline has a potential to cause gastrointestinal toxicity. This antibiotic has also produced esophageal ulcerations and strictures (particularly in elderly patients) and, rarely, hepatitis, rashes, and photosensitivity. The drug should not be prescribed to patients who receive antacids, ferrous sulfate, or cimetidine.

   c. Treatment with either of these compounds can be restricted to approximately 1 week.

4. Ancillary treatment consists of encouraging smoking cessation. The use of a bronchodilator, such as ipratropium or a β-adrenergic sympathomimetic agent, may confer some additional benefit. The value of drinking copious fluids or

taking an expectorant is undocumented. Patients usually clinically improve within 4 days and achieve complete resolution of the exacerbation within 2 weeks.

Follow-Up

When a patient fails to demonstrate any improvement within 5 days, the clinician should consider the following:

1. Incorrect diagnosis (perhaps pneumonia, neoplasm, or CHF)

2. An issue of compliance

3. Inappropriate antimicrobial selection (organism resistant to the medication prescribed)

4. Diminished antimicrobial bioavailability (the co-administration of iron, antacids, dideoxyinosine, and multivitamins with zinc decreases the absorption of tetracyclines and fluoroquinolones)

5. Excessive bronchospams and/or bronchial secretions

Prevention

1. Patients with chronic bronchitis are candidates for an annual influenza immunization as well as pneumococcal vaccine, although the value of pneumococcal vaccine for these patients is controversial.

2. Another potential preventive measure is to offer the patient antibiotic prophylaxis, with an agent such as tetracycline, ampicillin, amoxicillin, or trimethoprim-sulfamethoxazole prescribed once per day either four times a week or daily during the winter. The published scientific data are very "soft" in this regard, however. Antibiotic prophylaxis should be restricted to the patient who experiences four or more exacerbations per year.

Bibliography

Ball P, Harris JM, Lowson D, et al: Acute infective exacerbations of chronic bronchitis. Q J Med 1995;88: 61–68.

Ball P, Make B: Acute exacerbations of chronic bronchitis. Chest 1998;113:199S–204S.

Gleckman R: Acute bronchitis. In Rakel RE (ed): Conn's Current Therapy, pp 211–213. Philadelphia, WB Saunders Company, 1998.

MacKay DN: Treatment of acute bronchitis in adults without underlying lung disease. J Gen Intern Med 1996;11:557–562.

Roessingh PH, van Loon AM, Lammers JWJ, et al: Viral and atypical pathogens as causes of type 1 acute exacerbations of chronic bronchitis. Clin Microbiol Infect 1997;3:513–514.

35 Bronchiectasis

Bennet M. Wang

Etiology

Bronchiectasis (from the Greek *bronchus* for windpipe and *ektasis* for a stretching) is characterized by the abnormal and permanent dilatation and distortion of the pulmonary airways. Before the development of antibiotics and childhood immunizations, bronchiectasis was a common clinical disorder. Although less common now, bronchiectasis remains an important condition to recognize and manage appropriately. A variety of congenital and acquired processes can cause bronchiectasis.

1. Congenital
   a. Cystic fibrosis (see Bibliography)
   b. Immunodeficiency syndrome (e.g., hypogammaglobulinemia)
   c. Disorders of cilia structure and/or function
      (1) Primary ciliary dyskinesia (recurrent sinopulmonary infections, bronchiectasis, male infertility)
      (2) Kartagener's syndrome (situs inversus, sinusitis, bronchiectasis)
      (3) Young's syndrome (chronic sinopulmonary infections, bronchiectasis, obstructive azoospermia)
   d. α_1-Antitrypsin deficiency
   e. Developmental abnormalities
      (1) Swyer-James syndrome (unilateral hyperlucent lung)
      (2) Tracheobronchomegaly
2. Acquired
   a. Infection (severe bronchiolitis, necrotizing pneumonias)
      (1) Viral: measles, influenza
      (2) Bacterial: pertussis, mycoplasma
      (3) Mycobacterial: tuberculosis, mycobacteria other than *M. tuberculosis* (see Bibliography)
      (4) Fungal: allergic bronchopulmonary aspergillosis
   b. Endobronchial obstruction
      (1) Tumor
      (2) Foreign body

Symptoms

1. Chronic productive cough is the most common symptom.

2. The sputum is characteristically thick and tenacious, often mucoid, and becoming more purulent with exacerbations.
3. Hemoptysis, arising from dilated bronchial vessels, can sometimes produce large-volume and even life-threatening bleeding.
4. Nonspecific dyspnea, wheezing, and pleuritic chest pain can also be present.

Key Symptoms

- Recurrent productive cough
- Mucoid and purulent sputum
- Hemoptysis

Clinical Findings

1. Persistent moist crackles, often in the lower lung fields, can be present.
2. Focal inspiratory and/or expiratory wheezes can suggest foreign body aspiration and endobronchial narrowing or obstruction.
3. Clubbing of the fingers and hypoxemia can be seen with longstanding bronchiectasis.

Key Signs

- Moist crackles in lower lung fields
- Focal inspiratory/expiratory wheezes

Tests

1. Chest radiographs classically can show dilated and thickened airways that appear like parallel lines ("tramtracks") or as ring shadows and cystic spaces on cross section. Irregular peripheral opacities may represent mucous plugs and areas of atelectasis.
2. Chest computerized tomography (CT) scanning with thin sections ("high-resolution" CT) has high sensitivity and specificity for bronchiectasis and has replaced bronchography. Bronchial wall thickening and dilatation and obstructive

effects in the airways are the key findings on high-resolution CT scans.

3. Pulmonary function testing commonly reveals irreversible airflow obstruction.

4. Sputum analysis for Gram's stain, culture and sensitivity, fungal, and acid-fast bacilli studies can help direct antimicrobial therapy.

5. Advanced testing in selected individuals
    a. Sweat chloride and/or DNA mutation analysis for cystic fibrosis
    b. Immunoglobulin (Ig) quantitation (total and IgG subclasses)
    c. Total IgE level and serology tests for aspergillosis
    d. Sinus CT scan or plain films
    e. Cilia structure and function testing

Key Tests

- Standard chest radiograph
- High-resolution CT scan of chest
- Sputum stains and cultures

Differential Diagnosis

Recurrent sputum production and/or recurrent pulmonary infiltrates may be secondary to other causes, including the following:

1. Chronic bronchitis
2. Recurrent aspiration
3. Immunodeficiency states
4. Endobronchial obstruction without actual bronchiectasis
5. Bronchiolitis obliterans with organizing pneumonia (BOOP)
6. Incompletely treated pneumonias

Treatment

1. Antimicrobial drugs are the mainstay for both the prevention and treatment of bronchiectasis. The agent of choice is best directed by the sputum culture results:
    a. For mixed flora: amoxicillin, doxycycline, or trimethoprim-sulfamethoxazole
    b. For staphylococcal or pseudomonas species: as directed by sensitivity results
    c. For mycobacteria other than *M. tuberculosis*: multidrug regimens for many months (see Bibliography)

d. Antimicrobial agents are typically given during acute exacerbations; for frequent, chronic symptoms, antibiotics can be given on a regular basis (e.g., for the first 1 or 2 weeks each month).

2. Mobilization and clearing of secretions by chest physical therapy with postural drainage, humidification, use of mucolytics, and other measures can be helpful.

3. Bronchodilators can help those patients with bronchospasm and airflow obstruction.

4. Specific agents (e.g., immunoglobulin, recombinant human DNase) can be useful in certain cases.

5. Surgery is generally reserved for individuals with localized bronchiectasis who fail medical therapy or who have life-threatening hemoptysis (see Bibliography)

Key Treatment

- Antimicrobial agent(s)
- Bronchodilators
- Mobilization of secretions
- Surgery in selected patients

Follow-Up

Bronchiectasis can lead to the following complications: recurrent pneumonia, empyema, pneumothorax, lung abscess, and hemoptysis. Referral to a pulmonary specialist is appropriate in these instances. Overall, the prognosis for bronchiectasis in the current antibiotic era is favorable, with low mortality and controllable morbidity.

Bibliography

For more information on bronchiectasis, see
Luce JM: Bronchiectasis. In Murray JF, Nadel JA (eds): Textbook of Respiratory Medicine, 2nd ed, pp 1398–1417. Philadelphia, WB Saunders Company, 1994.
Nicotra MB: Bronchiectasis. Semin Respir Infect 1994;9: 31–40.
For more information on cystic fibrosis, see
Aitken ML, Fiel SB: Cystic fibrosis. Dis Mon 1993;39:1–52.
For more information on mycobacteria other than M. tuberculosis, *see*
American Thoracic Society: Diagnosis and treatment of disease caused by nontuberculous mycobacteria. Am J Respir Crit Care Med 1997;156:S1–S25.
For more information on surgery for bronchiectasis, see
Agasthian T, Deschamps C, Trastek VF, et al: Surgical management of bronchiectasis. Ann Thorac Surg 1996; 62:976–980.

36 Chronic Obstructive Pulmonary Disease

John M. Heath

Etiology

1. Chronic obstructive pulmonary disease (COPD) refers to a group of diseases that have in common symptomatic airflow obstruction.

2. Clinical manifestations are either chronic bronchitis or emphysema.

   a. Emphysema: loss of elasticity in distal portions of lung aveoli

   b. Chronic bronchitis: terminal bronchial pathology of smooth muscle hypertrophy and excess inflammatory secretions

3. Cigarette smoking is related to over 90 per cent of obstructive lung disease, although only 20 per cent of smokers will develop obstructive symptoms of chronic airflow obstruction. Unclear what predisposes a smoker to develop COPD.

4. COPD is fourth leading cause of death in United States.

5. COPD-related mortality trends expected to increase for those population groups whose smoking prevalence increased two to three decades ago (e.g., women and minorities) and among elderly smokers who are now surviving long enough to develop symptomatic airflow obstruction.

Symptoms

1. Principal features are cough, sputum production, dyspnea.

   a. Dyspnea may initially occur only with exertion and limits activities.

   b. Cough with sputum production *must* occur on a repeated basis over a prolonged time to make a distinction between COPD and acute infectious bronchitis.

2. Psychological aspects of COPD include those shared by many chronic diseases: depression, social isolation, withdrawal.

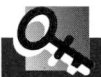

Key Symptoms

- Breathlessness
- Productive Cough

Clinical Findings

1. Airflow limitation resulting in prolonged expiration with decreased airflow and percussive hyperresonance

2. Bronchial hyperreactivity findings include bilateral wheezing or ronchi.

3. Classic descriptions of a "blue bloater" and "pink puffer" relate to late stages of COPD.

   a. Blue bloater: Progressive right-sided heart failure resulting from hypoxemia and pulmonary artery hypertension can cause peripheral edema and cyanosis.

   b. Pink puffer: Failing respiratory muscle strength in emphysematous patients results in their only being able to puff to maintain resting ventilation.

4. Wide variation in clinical course of illness due in part to exacerbations of underlying disease as well as to coexisting diseases, often smoking-related, that impact upon COPD.

Key Signs

- Prolonged expiration
- Decreased airflow

Laboratory Tests

1. Diagnosis is made clinically—no specific laboratory features are diagnostic.

2. Pulmonary function tests (PFTs) show characteristic patterns of airway flow.

   a. Responsiveness to inhaled β-agonists during PFTs important to determine role of this therapy.

   b. Rate of deterioration of obstructive findings can be improved by smoking cessation and may be smoking cessation tool for symptomatic smokers.

3. Radiologic findings in emphysema include bullous dilatation of terminal airways and relative hyperlucency of peripheral lung fields.

Key Test

- Pulmonary function tests

Differential Diagnosis

1. α_1-Antitrypsin deficiency with dyspnea, cough, and wheeze
   a. Suspect in a symptomatic nonsmoker
   b. PFTs reveal little reversibility of obstruction in response to inhaled β-agonists, along with a decreased carbon monoxide diffusing capacity.
   c. Diagnosis is confirmed by low serum levels of α_1-antitrypsin.
2. Cystic fibrosis: genetic abnormality presenting generally at younger ages with obstructive airway symptoms along with gastrointestinal disease

Treatment

Goal of therapy is to reduce airway obstruction by inducing bronchodilation, reducing airway inflammation, and reversing hypoxemia and its secondary effects.

Medication

1. Bronchodilatory therapy with inhaled β_2-adrenoreceptor agonists produces rapid response of smooth muscle airway tissue and relieves air hunger.
   a. Albuterol (Ventolin, Proventil), and other similar short-duration agents provide immediate relief when bronchospasm is causing symptomatic dyspnea.
   b. Longer acting preparations such as salmeterol (Serevent), can be used for maintenance and are dosed twice daily.
2. Inhaled anticholinergic agents such as ipratropium bromide (Atrovent), also induce bronchodilation as well as reduce airway inflammatory secretions.
   a. Maintenance therapy for chronic bronchitis secretion control
   b. First-line therapy for those COPD patients whose clinical response and PFTs do not demonstrate improvement with β-agonists
   c. Can be combined with β-agonists and dosed simultaneously.
3. Glucocorticoids are mainstay of therapy for acute exacerbations.
   a. Act by decreasing airway inflammatory reactions as well as enhancing bronchial reactivity to β-adrenergic stimulation.

   b. Variable responsiveness among COPD patients between acute episodes when used as maintenance therapy, when combined with above measures
4. Preferred medication delivery for all three of these agents is by inhalation route using metered-dose inhaler (MDI).
   a. High therapeutic index despite suboptimal technique in using devices by most COPD patients
   b. Spacer devices can improve actual drug delivery into the airway. Avoids chlorofluorocarbons in the pressurized MDI cannister.
5. Nebulization is an alternative route if patient unable to manage MDI
6. Oral theophylline was prior mainstay of therapy, although it has a narrow therapeutic range.
   a. Actions extend beyond respiratory smooth muscle actions to include immunomodulatory actions.
   b. Role for both refractory patients and those unable to use inhaler therapies
7. Antibiotics remain controversial in chronic bronchitis.
   a. Evidence of direct infectious role in triggering acute exacerbations often lacking.
   b. Fever may be related to airway inflammatory mediators.
   c. Less than 50 per cent of samples taken with protected-tip bronchoscopic culture techniques from the airway segments appearing inflamed identified an offending organism
   d. Antibiotics used for febrile bronchitis episodes with altered sputum characteristics
   e. Macrolide antibiotics most effective against common respiratory pathogens.
8. Oxygen is critical for patients with documented hypoxemia (partial pressure of O_2 <60 mm Hg).
   a. Dose expressed as flow rate of liters/minute.
   b. Duration of at least 18 hours/day for impact on overall mortality
   c. Supplied by concentrator, compressed gas, liquid oxygen reservoir
   d. Delivery device: nasal cannula, demand-flow device, or mask
   e. Although daytime use provides symptomatic relief, use during sleep is critical because nocturnal hypoxemia is associated with cardiac arrhythmias and pulmonary hypertension.
9. Surgical resection of bullous areas of emphysematous lung to allow greater expansion of functioning areas of the lung is receiving greater interest.

Diet

1. Increased respiratory effort to overcome obstructive forces requires enhanced calories.
2. Adequate hydration is critical to allow mucus expectoration.

Activity

1. Pulmonary rehabilitation can improved respiratory muscle tone and strength. Components include breathing resistance training, use of accessory respiratory muscles to aid in breathing, and improvement in aerobic capacity.
2. Few objective changes in actual pulmonary function are documented, although there is enhanced overall physical functioning and improved quality of life.

Patient Education

1. Smoking cessation is single most important element in longitudinal management of COPD.
2. Proper technique for inhaler use, monitoring respiratory efforts, and facilitating expectoration can be accomplished with input from respiratory therapy professionals.

Key Treatment

- Airway anti-inflammatory agents
- Bronchodilators
- Correct hypoxia

Follow-Up

1. Close communication with patient and caregiver during the start of acute exacerbations may help avoid unnecessary hospitalizations.
2. End-stage disease management requires advance directive discussions about the patient's wishes regarding the use of mechanical ventilation, cardiopulmonary resuscitation, and other invasive, life-prolonging interventions.

Bibliography

Celli BR: Standards for the optimal management of COPD: a summary. Chest 1998;113(Suppl 4):283S–287S.

Ikeda A, Nishimura K, Izumi T: Pharmacological treatment in acute exacerbations of chronic obstructive pulmonary disease. Drugs Aging 1998;12:129–137.

Lu CC: Bronchodilator therapy for chronic obstructive pulmonary disease. Respirology 1997;2:317–322.

Takasugi JE, Godwin JD: Radiology of chronic obstructive pulmonary disease. Radiol Clin North Am 1998; 36:29–55.

Wise RA: Changing smoking patterns and mortality from chronic obstructive pulmonary disease. Prevent Med 1997;26:418–421.

37 Pulmonary Function Testing

M. David Stockton

Indications

Just as a chest radiograph provides a "static" examination of lung function, spirometry provides a "dynamic" assessment. Pulmonary function testing provides a quantitative index of lung function based on air flow rates and lung volumes and is used in

1. Diagnostic testing: Assessment of type and severity of lung dysfunction
   a. Obstructive airway disease
   b. Restrictive airway disease
   c. Mixed disorders
2. Screening evaluations
   a. Medical surveillance of occupational exposures
   b. Early detection of smoking effects
   c. Respirator use clearance
   d. Preoperative pulmonary evaluations
3. Periodic serial testing
   a. Tracking the course of lung disease
   b. Assessing response to therapy
   c. Compliance with governmental occupational health regulations
4. Disability determinations

Contraindications

1. Absolute contraindications are rare, and often testing can proceed with care and close observation of the patient.
2. Relative contraindications to pulmonary function testing are few, but include
   a. Severe acute asthma
   b. Acute unexplained chest pain or recent myocardial infarction
   c. History of pneumothorax
   d. Extensive pulmonary bullae or blebes
   e. Accelerated hypertension
   f. History of vasovagal syncope

Equipment

1. There are two basic types of spirometers, differing only in whether the volume or flow of air is measured. They produce comparable information for categorization and assessment of lung function.
   a. Flow-sensing spirometer (pneumotachometer)
      (1) Measures air flow against time
      (2) Used in most primary care office settings
      (3) Can be electronically coupled with a computer to generate
         (a) Written reports
         (b) Graphs
         (c) Comparisons with data from standardization tables
         (d) Stored serial measurements
   b. Volume-displacement spirometer
      (1) Measures the displacement of air volume
      (2) Several mechanical designs available
2. Minimum standards for spirometers
   a. American Thoracic Society (ATS) recommendations in *Standards of Spirometry—1994 Update*: Specify accuracy criteria regarding airflow volume and time measurements.
   b. National Institute of Occupational Safety and Health (NIOSH) recommendations published in 1981 in the agency's *Manual of Spirometry in Occupational Medicine*
3. Equipment must be calibrated daily to validate accuracy. Computer-generated results and interpretations should periodically be cross checked manually.

Precautions

In addition to avoiding known contraindications, careful observation of the patient for signs of fatigue or lightheadedness is required when multiple measurements are necessary to obtain an acceptable study.

Technique

1. Technicians performing spirometry must be well trained and familiar with the specific equipment used and fundamentals of spirometry. Optimally, they are certified in accordance with Occupational Safety and Health Administration (OSHA) requirements for technicians.

2. Patient preparation includes
   a. Accurate measurement of height (in stocking feet) and weight
   b. Understanding of the importance of proper testing technique, including performance of maximum inspiration and expiration with sustained effort
   c. Smoking immediately prior to testing is discouraged.
3. Testing
   a. Testing occurs in the standing position.
   b. Nose clips are applied.
   c. A deep inspiration followed by a maximal forced expiration for a minimum of 6 seconds and until a 2-second plateau of maximum flow is achieved
   d. Acceptable readings require
      (1) A smooth start to the test
      (2) Absence of coughing, hesitation, and intratest breathing
   e. Between three and eight sequential measurements (tests) may be necessary to obtain a maximal respiratory effort. Submaximal effort results in a high false-positive rate for abnormal spirometry patterns.
4. Results: The three most important derived parameters are the forced vital capacity (FVC), the forced expiratory volume in 1 second (FEV_1), and the FEV_1/FVC ratio. By examining these parameters, the physician can make an initial assessment of respiratory flow status. Spirometric tracings indicate a pattern of air flow and volume suggestive, but not diagnostic, of a specific disease (Table 37–1).
   a. FVC
      (1) *Definition*: the maximal air volume rapidly and forcefully exhaled after a maximum inspiratory effort
      (2) *Spirometric tracing*: As plotted on a time-volume graph, the upper flat portion of the tracing represents the FVC (Fig. 37–1A).
      (3) *Significance*: When this value is reduced over the predicted value, it is suggestive of disorders that inhibit maximum expansion of the lungs (Fig. 37–1B). A decrease in the FVC indicates a restrictive disease pattern and involves a loss in the number of functional alveolar units. Restrictive diseases include interstitial lung disease, asbestosis, and other causes of pulmonary fibrosis.
   b. FEV_1
      (1) *Definition*: the volume of air that can be expired during the first second of forced expiration
      (2) *Spirometric tracing*: Draw a straight line up from the point where time equals 1 second. The point where this straight line intersects the tracing is the FEV_1 (Fig. 37–1C).
      (3) *Significance*: used to calculate FEV_1/FVC ratio
   c. FEV_1/FVC ratio
      (1) *Definition*: the FEV_1 expressed as a percentage of the FVC
      (2) *Spirometric value*: usually equal to 75 per cent or greater of the total expired volume
      (3) *Significance*: Smaller percentages than

TABLE 37–1. SPIROMETRY PATTERNS

	FVC	FEV_1	FEV_1/FVC
Normal	Normal	Normal	Normal
Obstructive	Normal	Low	Low
Restrictive	Low	Normal	Normal
Mixed	Low	Low	Low

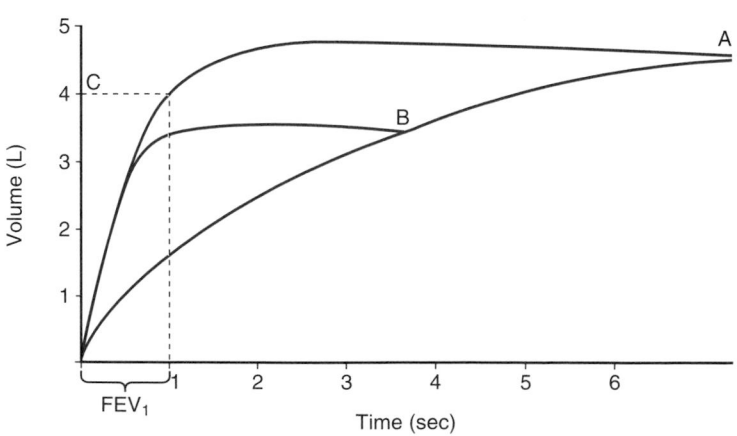

Figure 37–1 Spirometric tracings used in the assessment of respiratory flow status. *A*, Forced vital capacity (FVC): normal. *B*, FVC: restrictive pattern. *C*, Forced expiratory volume in 1 second (FEV_1; 80 per cent of FVC): "normal" pattern.

75 per cent of the total measured at 1 second of expiration suggest an "obstructive pattern." Pulmonary diseases with obstructive patterns are characterized by diminished air flow and include asthma, chronic bronchitis, emphysema, bronchiolitis, or reactive airway disease, such as from occupational exposures.

   d. Mean forced expiratory flow (FEF_{25-75})

     (1) *Definition*: mean forced expiratory flow during the middle of FVC.

     (2) *Spirometric tracing*: see Figure 37–2

     (3) *Significance*: Suggests flow measurements in the small airways (those <2 mm in diameter). The FEF_{25-75} is a highly variable test, however, and cannot be used as a single diagnostic variable but must be interpreted in context with the testing pattern as a whole.

   e. In certain disease states, such as acute severe asthma, the FEV_1 and FVC are both decreased along with the FEV_1/FVC ratio, suggesting a mixed obstructive/restrictive disorder. This term, however, should be reserved for only conditions that result in extensive lung failure, such as advanced silicosis.

5. Source and use of reference values: Predicted normal values for all tests mentioned above are based on the expected values taken from epidemiologic studies where spirometry is performed on a large number of subjects who are free of respiratory disease and who are nonsmokers.

   a. Lung function relative to predicted value is expressed as a percentage.

   b. By convention, 80 per cent of the standard value is used as the cutoff value for the la-

TABLE 37–2. NIOSH RECOMMENDED LOWER LIMITS OF NORMAL FOR SPIROMETRY

FVC	80% of predicted
FEV_1	80% of predicted
$FEV_1/FVC\%$	70

Data from National Institute of Occupational Safety and Health. In Horvath EP Jr (ed): Manual of Spirometry in Occupational Medicine, pp 29–30. Cincinnati, National Institute of Occupational Safety and Health, 1981.

beling of abnormal pulmonary function test results when compared to "normal" values (Table 37–2).

   c. Variables such as age, height, sex, and race are independent factors that affect these predicted normal values, and must be factored into any interpretation (i.e., norms for the black population are 15 per cent lower than those for whites). Many computerized spirometers offer a race adjustment in the set-up menu.

   d. Reference values vary according to the testing lab and how the equipment is programmed. Whatever source values are used must always be documented in the written report. Selected reference values should conform to the recommendations made by the ATS in 1991.

   e. For any individual tested, the most meaningful interpretation is the comparison of data from previous values collected over time.

6. Advanced pulmonary testing: Spirometry is a screening test that may suggest the need for more definitive diagnostic studies, such as flow-volume loops, diffusion capacity of carbon monoxide in the lung (DL_{CO}), biopsies, bronchoalveolar lavage, and other procedures.

   a. Flow-volume loop measurements are helpful in diagnosing upper airway obstruction. Available on most computerized machines, this test is a more physiologic measurement of lung function representative of the respiratory cycle, and can produce characteristic patterns suggestive of laryngeal and tracheal lesions. It is especially helpful for determining intrathoracic or extrathoracic airway dynamics and finding the site of airway obstruction.

   b. The single-breath diffusion capacity of carbon monoxide (DL_{CO}) estimates the gas transfer across the alveolar-capillary interface and is helpful in the diagnosis of emphysema or diffuse infiltrated lung disease.

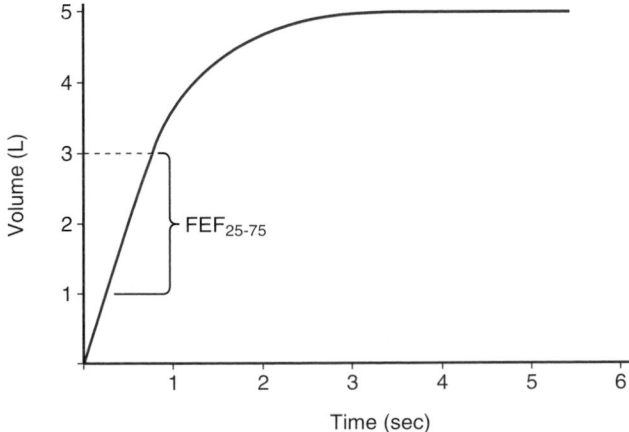

Figure 37–2 Mean forced expiratory flow in the middle of FVC (FEF_{25-75}).

The test is particularly helpful in further evaluation of the initial finding of restrictive patterns. In patients with acquired immunodeficiency syndrome, the DL_{CO} is a highly sensitive screening test for possible *Pneumocystis carinii* pneumonia, although it lacks specificity.

c. Postbronchodilator testing can assist in predicting reversible airway obstructive disease and is helpful in assessing response to therapeutic intervention with bronchodilators. An increase of 12 per cent or greater over baseline in FEV_1 and FVC, in addition to an absolute change of 200 ml, is required to consider a bronchodilator response positive.

Follow-Up

1. Medical surveillance in the occupational health setting includes both regulated (OSHA) and nonregulated periodic testing of worker exposure to substances such as asbestos, coke oven emissions, or cotton. Normally, FEV_1 and FVC decline at a rate of 20 to 30 ml/year. The ATS suggests that trend analysis revealing an annual per cent change of greater that 10 per cent in FEV_1 or FVC be considered a significant change. Pre– and post–work shift testing is often performed to evaluate pulmonary symptoms with possible occupational etiologies, and requires a 5 per cent change to warrant further action.

2. Respirator fitness testing: According to the new OSHA 1910.134 respiratory protection standards, effective April 1998, workers with a FEV_1 or FEV_1/FVC ratio of less than 70 per cent of predicted normals should be denied clearance for wearing respirators in the work setting because of impaired airway resistance and the resultant increased work of breathing. Fit testing should be performed on the preplacement examinations and at periodic medical surveillance examinations.

3. Disability determinations: Patients seeking disability as a result of pulmonary disease must meet the 1993 American Medical Association criteria published in *Guide to the Evaluation of Permanent Impairment*. A summary of the parameters found on spirometric examination required for disability are found in Table 37–1.

Bibliography

American Medical Association: Guide to the Evaluation of Permanent Impairment, 4th ed, pp 159–167. Chicago, American Medical Association, 1993.

American Thoracic Society: Lung function testing: selection of reference values and interpretive strategies. Am Rev Respir Dis 1991;144:1202–1218.

American Thoracic Society: Standardization of spirometery—1994 update. Am Rev Respir Dis 1995;152:1107–1136.

Mahler DA, Horowitz MB: Pulmonary function testing. In Bone RC (ed): Pulmonary and Critical Medicine, pp 1–20. St. Louis, Mosby–Year Book, 1998.

National Institute of Occupational Safety and Health. In Horvath EP Jr (ed): Manual of Spirometry in Occupational Medicine, pp 29–30. Cincinnati, National Institute of Occupational Safety and Health, 1981.

Indications

Arterial blood sampling provides the means for determining the pH, partial pressures of oxygen (p_aO_2) and carbon dioxide (pCO_2), bicarbonate, and oxygen saturation of hemoglobin. Arterial blood is required if the true effectiveness of the cardiovascular system is to be assessed. Venous blood is affected by a variety of factors, including the degree of tissue oxygen extraction, blood flow, and poor circulation. Arterial blood sampling may be necessary in the following conditions:

1. Assessing both the presence and severity of hypoxia of any etiology
2. Evaluating acid-base abnormalities
3. Assessing the need for home oxygen in patients with chronic obstructive pulmonary disease or cor pulmonale
4. Measuring carboxyhemoglobin in patients exposed to smoke inhalation
5. Calculating the content of arterial oxygen and delivery of oxygen to tissues
6. Obtaining a blood sample when an attempt at venipuncture is unsuccessful in either obese or edematous patients

Contraindications

There are no absolute contraindications to arterial puncture. Relative contraindications include the following:

1. Coagulopathy, including thrombolytic therapy
2. Severe peripheral vascular disease with poor collateral circulation
3. Trauma or infection at the site of arterial puncture

Preparation

1. If the patient is conscious, explain what the procedure is, and that it will be uncomfortable. Most well-informed patients cooperate well during the procedure.
2. Some institutions may require informed consent from patients for any invasive procedure; if so, explain the risks, benefits, and alternative options to the procedure.
3. The radial artery is the preferred site for arterial puncture because it is superficial and easily accessible. Other sites in order of preference are the femoral and brachial arteries.

a. The brachial artery is a large artery palpable at the cubital fossa. It divides into the larger ulnar artery and smaller radial artery. The radial and ulnar branches of brachial artery supply blood to the hand through the superficial palmar arch. The radial artery runs down the anterior radial aspect of the forearm and is easily palpated at the wrist in a longitudinal groove just medial to the distal radius.

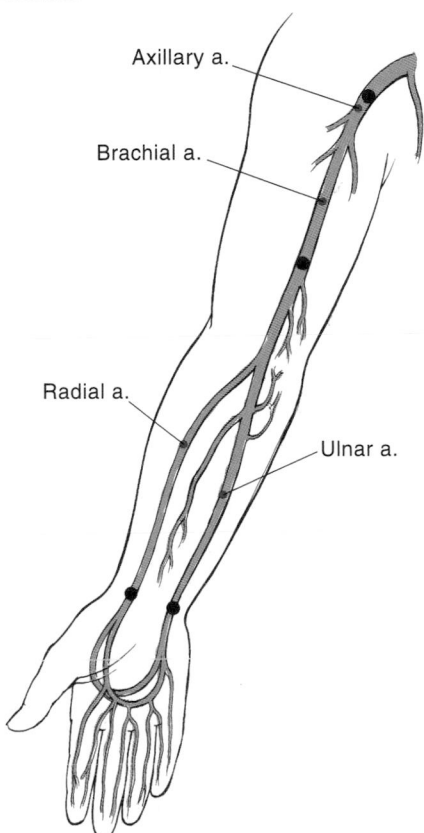

Axillary a.

Brachial a.

Radial a.

Ulnar a.

b. The femoral artery is the continuation of the external iliac artery as it runs beneath the inguinal ligament. The femoral artery passes at the midpoint between the anterior superior iliac crest and pubic symphysis. The femoral vein lies medial to the artery in the femoral sheath.

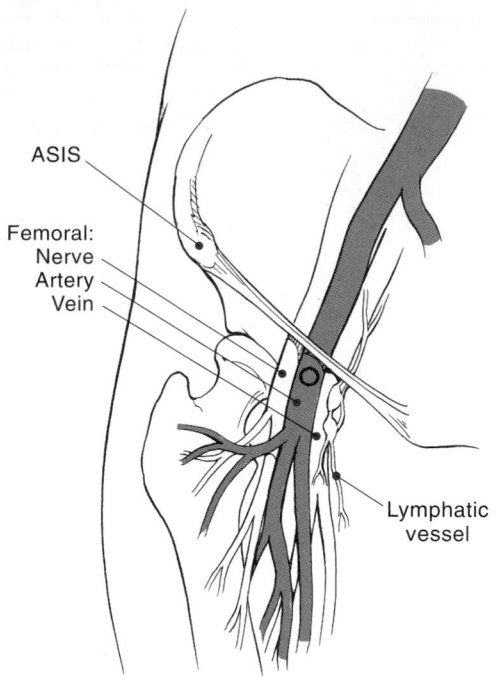

ASIS

Femoral:
Nerve
Artery
Vein

Lymphatic
vessel

Equipment

1. Sterile gloves
2. Rolled towel
3. A cup with ice for blood sample transport
4. Patient's ID label
5. Arterial blood gas request form for laboratory
6. Arterial blood gas kit, which contains a 2-ml heparinized syringe attached to a 25-gauge needle, alcohol pads, iodophor pads, 2×2 sterile gauze pads, and a Band-Aid.

Anesthesia

Experienced persons may not use a local anesthetic for an arterial puncture. If desired, 2% lidocaine so-lution may be injected at the site of puncture using a 1-ml syringe attached to a 25-gauge needle.

> **Important**
> Do not add epinephrine solution to lidocaine for prolonged anesthetic effect because it can cause digital ischemia as a result of its vasoconstrictive effect.

Precautions

1. Sterile gloves should be worn because it is prudent. The objective is to prevent transmission of bloodborne diseases and to minimize infection.
2. Perform Allen's test to assess the adequacy of collateral circulation.
   a. Place the patient's arm on the bedside table, supporting the wrist with a rolled towel. Have the patient clench the fist.
   b. Using the middle and index fingers of each hand, exert pressure on both radial and ulnar arteries.
   c. Without releasing the pressure, have the patient unclench fist. If the palm shows blanching, blood flow is inadequate.
   d. Release the pressure on the ulnar artery. Check to see whether the palm begins to turn pink in less than 6 seconds. If it takes longer than 15 seconds to turn pink, flow may be inadequate. Choose an alternate site for arterial puncture.

Technique

1. Rest the patient's arm on bedside table, supporting the wrist with rolled towel. Palpate the radial artery.
2. Prepare the site with an iodophor solution. Next wipe the area using alcohol and let the puncture site air dry.
3. Anesthetize with 2% lidocaine if you anticipate difficulty in completing the procedure.
4. Locate the artery with index and middle fingers of nondominant hand while holding the heparinized syringe in the other hand.
5. Puncture the skin at a 45-degree angle, with beveled edge of the needle facing up; advance the needle slowly.

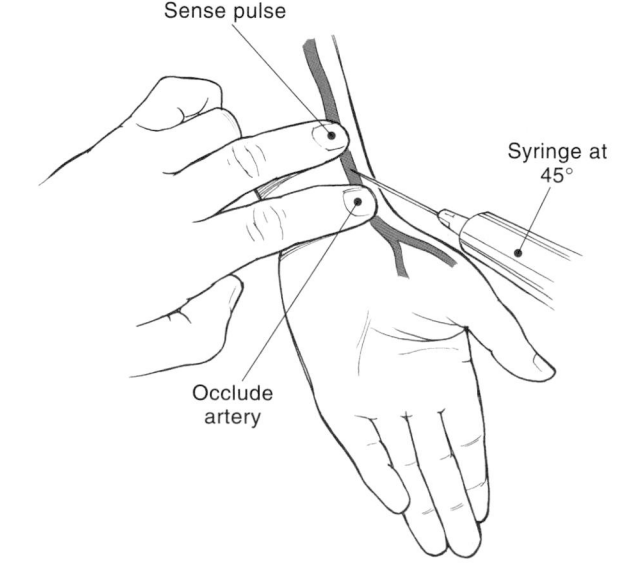

Sense pulse

Syringe at 45°

Occlude artery

When the needle punctures the artery, blood will flush in to syringe.

6. Collect about 2 to 3 ml of blood in the syringe.
7. Withdraw the syringe slowly.
8. Apply firm pressure over the puncture site using 2×2 gauze for 5 minutes. After pressure is released, cover the site with a Band-Aid if there is no bleeding.

Follow-Up

1. Expel all air bubbles from syringe to prevent falsely high pO_2. Blood may be spilled out of syringe while expelling air bubbles; if so, wipe blood off the syringe.
2. Handle blood gas samples carefully. Attach patient's ID label to syringe before placing it in an ice cup. Deliver sample as quickly as possible for an analysis.
3. Dispose of all sharp objects properly to prevent accidental needle sticks.
4. Never ask the patient to apply pressure over the puncture site. The patient may not apply enough pressure, or not for a long enough time, which can lead to bleeding and/or hematoma formation.
5. It is always important to check for the presence of pulse, bleeding, or hematoma at puncture site after 10 minutes.

Bibliography

Franklin C: The technique of radial artery cannulation. J Crit Illness 1995;10:424–432.

In Gomella LG (ed): Bedside procedures: Clinician's Pocket Reference, 8th ed, pp 219–292. East Norwalk, CT, Appleton & Lange, 1997.

Kaye WE, Dubin WG: Vascular cannulation. In Taylor RW, Civetta JM, Kirby RR (eds): Techniques & Procedures in Critical Care, pp 183–218. Philadelphia, JB Lippincott Company, 1990.

Marino PL: Vascular access. In: The ICU Book, pp 53–75. Baltimore, Williams & Wilkins, 1998.

Seneff M: Arterial line placement and care. In Rippe JM, Irwin RS, Fink MP, et al (eds): Procedures and techniques in Intensive Care Medicine, pp 36–47. Boston, Little, Brown, 1995.

Seneff M: Arterial line placement and care. In Rippe JM, Irwin RS, Fink MP, et al (eds): Intensive Care Medicine, 3rd ed, pp 36–47. Boston, Little, Brown, 1996.

Indications

1. Continuous noninvasive monitoring of arterial oxyhemoglobin saturation by trained personnel during mechanical ventilation, conscious sedation, general anesthesia, or as a screen for oxygenation status in emergency or ambulatory care departments, or within the home.

2. Noninvasive monitoring of arterial oxyhemoglobin saturation by trained personnel during ambulance transport or transport from the intensive care unit to operating room, recovery room, or radiology, and during procedures utilizing conscious sedation, including bronchoscopy and endoscopy.

3. Noninvasive monitoring of oxyhemoglobin saturation by trained personnel during exercise, including for the determination of oxygen supplementation needs in a patient who desaturates with activity.

Contraindications

1. Ongoing need for measurement of pH, partial pressure of carbon dioxide (pCO_2), total hemoglobin, or abnormal hemoglobin concentrations.

2. Known or significant risk for carboxyhemoglobinemia*

3. Known or significant risk for methemoglobinemia*

4. Intravenous administration of methylene blue, indigo carmine, and indocyanine green dyes

5. Reduced accuracy: severe peripheral vascular disease with ischemic digits, severe hypotension and/or use of high dose of vasopressor agents (low perfusion states), severe hypothermia, cardiopulmonary arrest, conditions of venous congestion

6. Inability to maintain probe on digit (e.g., uncooperative patient)

7. Magnetic resonance imaging: Probe-specific burns have been reported; evaluate manufacturer's instructions.

8. Oxygen saturation below 70 per cent where significant variation exists between oximeters.

9. Excessive skin pigmentation where results are unreliable (follow manufacturer's instructions)

10. Extremes of hyperbilirubinemia where results may be unreliable (follow manufacturer's instructions)

11. Nail polish/artificial fingernails (follow manufacturer's recommendations)

12. Incidents where the heart rate recorded by electrocardiographic monitoring disagrees with sensed pulse from oximetric equipment

13. Inappropriate probe/instrument compatibility; could lead to potential electrical shock or burns of involved area

Preparation

1. Ensure that appropriate personnel, knowledgeable of limitations of the application of oximetry, are available to operate equipment.

2. Explain the procedure to any conscious patient and ask that he or she cooperate in leaving the probe on the finger or other site to be utilized.

3. Digit or other site to be utilized should be clean and warm and have good perfusion.

4. Probe should be connected to oximeter and stabilized on digit. In the case of a combative or confused patient, consider risks for strangulation or harm from probe connectors, wiring.

5. Ensure that power source (battery) or electrical connections/supply are functional and safe.

6. Universal precautions should be followed at all times; for single-use probes, disposal of contaminated probes should be according to universal precautions. Multiuse probes should be cleaned according to manufacturer's instructions between use.

Equipment

1. Oximetry probe
2. Oximeter
3. Electrical supply unless device is battery operated

Anesthesia

Not required

Precautions

1. Be aware of the limitations of the procedure; for example, carboxyhemoglobinemia and other conditions listed above in "Contraindications" can lead to an overestimation of oxygenation status of the patient.

2. Be aware that the accuracy of oximeters may only be within 3 to 4 per cent (95 per cent con-

---

*May be considered for use in these cases after obtaining an arterial blood gas with *measured* oxygen saturation for comparison and/or after definitive treatment for the condition of carboxyhemoglobinemia.

fidence), such that a measurement of 94 per cent could be associated with a true saturation between 90 and 98 per cent, with significant variance in partial pressure of oxygen (p_aO_2). Currently available pulse oximeters are accurate when saturations are in the range of 80 to 100 per cent. If used during mechanical ventilation for monitoring, at least one simultaneous measurement of arterial blood gas oxygen saturation (measured oxygen saturation, not calculated), should be compared to pulse oximetry results for an estimation of accuracy.

3. Evaluate manufacturer's instructions regarding accuracy, standardization, and quality control of equipment.
4. Be aware that pulse oximetry is not reliable to monitor adequacy of *ventilation*.

Technique

1. Oximetry operating principles
   a. Many times each second, the oximeter passes red and infrared light into the sensor site and determines absorption; the absorption during the arterial pulsation is reflective of absorption by arterial blood, nonpulsatile blood, and tissue. Measurements of absorption taken in the nonpulsatile period are reflective of nonpulsatile blood and tissue. Through correcting the arterial pulsation absorption for the nonpulsatile period absorption, the oximeter determines red and infrared absorption of the arterial pulsation blood.
   b. Because of the variance between oxyhemoglobin and deoxyhemoglobin, the oxygen saturation is reported as the ratio of corrected absorption at each wavelength. This type of measurement is *not* reflective of dyshemoglobins.
   c. The manufacturer's instructions for each instrument should be examined for accuracy, whether or not dyshemoglobin is measured, and quality control procedures.

2. All instruments should be utilized and maintained according to the specific manufacturer's instructions.
3. Hypoxemia is generally considered to be present when the *measured oxygen saturation* is less than 90%. Given the limitations of the accuracy of oximetry (see "Precautions") consider performing an arterial blood gas, when clinically indicated, whenever the pulse oximeter measures less than 92 per cent.

 ## Bibliography

American Association of Respiratory Care: Pulse oximetry: American Association of Respiratory Care clinical practice guidelines. Respir Care 1991;36:1406–1409.

Bozeman WP, Myers RAM, Barish RA: Confirmation of pulse oximetry gap in carbon monoxide poisoning. Ann Emerg Med 1997;30:608–611.

Mendelson Y: Pulse oximetry: theory and applications for noninvasive monitoring. Clin Chem 1992;38:1601–1607.

Roberts JR, Hedges JR: Clinical Procedures in Emergency Medicine, 3rd ed, pp 85–90. Philadelphia, WB Saunders Company, 1998.

Venkatesh B, Hendry S-P: Continuous intra-arterial blood gas monitoring. Intensive Care Med 1996;22:818–828.

Wahr JA, Tremper KK: Noninvasive oxygen monitoring techniques. Crit Care Clin 1995;11:199–217.

38 Interstitial Lung Disease

Muhammad K. Zaman

Etiology

1. Diverse, with nearly 200 disease entities sharing common clinical, physiologic, imaging, and pathologic features. Idiopathic pulmonary fibrosis, sarcoidosis, collagen-vascular disease–associated interstitial lung disease, cryptogenic organizing pneumonia, and hypersensitivity pneumonitis constitute more than two thirds of all cases, whereas other entities, such as pulmonary alveolar proteinosis, are distinctly rare.

2. Classification (partial list)
   a. Unknown etiology
      (1) Sarcoidosis
      (2) Idiopathic pulmonary fibrosis
      (3) Cryptogenic organizing pneumonia
      (4) Eosinophilic granuloma
      (5) Wegener's granulomatosis
      (6) Pulmonary hemorrhage syndromes
      (7) Eosinophilic pneumonia
      (8) Pulmonary alveolar proteinosis
   b. Occupational and environmental exposure
      (1) Chemical fumes and gases
      (2) Organic dusts (pneumoconioses)
      (3) Inorganic dusts (hypersensitivity pneumonitis)
   c. Collagen-vascular disease
      (1) Rheumatoid arthritis
      (2) Scleroderma
      (3) Systemic lupus erythematosus
      (4) Polymyositis and dermatomyositis
      (5) Mixed connective tissue disease
      (6) Sjögren's syndrome
   d. Drug- or treatment-induced
      (1) Cytotoxic drugs
      (2) Noncytotoxic drugs
      (3) Radiation
      (4) Oxygen toxicity
   e. Infectious: clinically resemble true interstitial lung disease
      (1) *Pneumocystis* pneumonia
      (2) Viral and atypical pneumonias
      (3) Mycobacterial and fungal pneumonias
   f. Neoplastic: clinically resemble true interstitial lung disease
      (1) Lymphangitic carcinomatosis
      (2) Bronchoalveolar cell carcinoma
      (3) Pulmonary lymphoma

Symptoms

1. Progressively worsening dyspnea on exertion is the most common symptom.
2. Cough, usually nonproductive, may be prominent in diseases that are more bronchocentric.
3. Chest pain is uncommon but may be of pleuritic nature.
   a. Pleural involvement (e.g., collagen diseases)
   b. Pneumothorax (e.g., eosinophilic granuloma)
4. Hemoptysis is uncommon and suggests alveolar hemorrhage syndromes, underlying carcinoma, pulmonary embolism, bronchiectasis, mycetoma, and lymphangiomyomatosis.
5. Fever with acute presentation: Consider infection, acute idiopathic pulmonary fibrosis, acute eosinophilic pneumonia, hypersensitivity pneumonitis, and cryptogenic organizing pneumonia.

Key Symptoms

- Chronic progressive dyspnea
- Nonproductive cough

Clinical Findings

1. Look for history of the following:
   a. Occupational and environmental exposure
   b. Exposure to drugs or radiation
   d. Presence of multisystem disease
   e. Mineral oil–based nosedrops
   f. Gastroesophageal reflux
   g. Tobacco exposure
      (1) Inductive in eosinophilic granuloma and respiratory bronchiolitis
      (2) Protective in hypersensitivity pneumonitis and sarcoidosis
   h. Family history (e.g., familial pulmonary fibrosis)

2. Physical examination
   a. Bibasilar end-inspiratory dry "Velcro" crackles
      (1) Most characteristic finding; correlates with fibrosis; common in idiopathic pulmonary fibrosis
      (2) Often absent in sarcoidosis and other granulomatous diseases
   b. Clubbing
      (1) Indicates advanced fibrosis
      (2) Particularly common in idiopathic pulmonary fibrosis
      (3) May indicate complicating carcinoma
   c. Cutaneous and joint involvement: collagen disease, sarcoidosis
   d. Cyanosis: late sign of advanced disease

Key Signs

- Bibasilar inspiratory crackles
- Clubbing
- Associated cutaneous or joint involvement

Tests

1. Chest radiographs—and comparison with previous films
   a. Vast majority (90 per cent) have abnormal chest radiographs
      (1) Reticulonodular bilateral interstitial pattern is most common.
      (2) Air bronchograms and air alveolograms suggest active disease.
      (3) Honeycombing suggests extensive fibrosis.
   b. Adenopathy: sarcoidosis, lymphoma
   c. Nodules: granulomatous disease, silicosis, neoplasm
   d. "Radiographic negative of pulmonary edema": eosinophilic pneumonia
   e. Kerley B lines: pulmonary edema, lymphangitic carcinomatosis
   f. Pleural disease: collagen-vascular disease, asbestosis
   g. Pneumothorax: eosinophilic granuloma, advanced fibrosis
   h. Upper lobe predominance: sarcoidosis, silicosis, eosinophilic pneumonia
2. High-resolution computerized tomographic scan is an evolving technique and is not recommended for routine use. It is useful for the following purposes:

a. Detects early interstitial lung disease with normal chest radiograph.
b. Assesses the extent, distribution, and severity of disease.
c. Offers clues to differentiate various interstitial lung diseases by morphologic criteria.
d. Guides site of lung biopsy.
3. Gallium-67 scanning is not recommended for routine evaluations.
4. Serology
   a. Routine battery of serologic tests is not recommended.
   b. Serology for collagen-vascular disease, pulmonary-renal syndromes, and muscle function studies as clinically indicated.
   c. Studies of hepatic, hematologic, and renal function are useful in some diseases.
   d. Always consider human immunodeficiency virus serology.
5. Pulmonary function testing (spirometry, lung volumes, and diffusing capacity for carbon monoxide)
   a. Routinely performed as baseline and followed at intervals
   b. May be abnormal with normal chest radiograph.
   c. Classically reveals restrictive disease with decreased forced vital capacity, diffusing capacity for carbon monoxide, total lung capacity, and compliance with normal flow.
   d. Obstructive disease with decreased forced expiratory volume in 1 second and forced vital capacity in some diseases
   e. Valuable in determining the presence and severity of disease and monitoring the progression of disease and response to therapy.
6. Arterial blood gas analysis
   a. Most commonly reveals mild hypoxemia and respiratory alkalosis.
   b. Carbon dioxide retention is rare even in late stages.
   c. Exercise desaturation may occur in the absence of resting hypoxemia and may be the most sensitive marker of disease severity and progression.
7. Bronchoscopic studies: Should be the initial diagnostic procedure for most patients except those in whom the cause is known.
   a. Bronchoalveolar lavage (BAL)
      (1) Procedure of choice for assessment of infectious entities
      (2) Based on the number and percentage of neutrophils, lymphocytes, or eosino-

phils, the interstitial lung disease may be subcategorized and the differential diagnosis narrowed.

(3) Increased lymphocytes suggest response to corticosteroid therapy; increased eosinophils coupled with increased neutrophils suggest a lack of such response in idiopathic pulmonary fibrosis.

b. Transbronchial biopsy

(1) Small sample size limits diagnostic utility, except in granulomatous diseases

(2) Combined with BAL, can diagnose most infectious and neoplastic diseases.

8. Open lung biopsy or open thoracoscopic lung biopsy

a. Allows large tissue sample for adequate evaluation of airways, alveoli, and vessels.

b. Should be performed if expected result will alter patient therapy or outcome.

Key Tests

- Chest radiographs and comparison with previous films

- Pulmonary function tests

- Bronchoscopy with BAL and biopsy

- Open lung biopsy

Differential Diagnosis

Infectious and neoplastic diseases that resemble true interstitial lung diseases (see classification) must be excluded by appropriate tests.

Treatment

1. Depends on the ultimate diagnosis and the activity of disease—inflammatory versus end-stage fibrosis versus mixed histology.

2. Avoid known exposures in all cases.

3. Always stop smoking.

4. Corticosteroids: Initial drug of choice for most noninfectious, non-neoplastic interstitial lung diseases when treatment is indicated. The usual starting dose is 1 mg/kg/day of prednisone except in sarcoidosis (0.5 mg/kg/day). Response is good in granulomatous, vasculitic, and inflammatory processes.

5. Cytotoxic medications: when steroids fail or as initial therapy with steroids when BAL cytology suggests unresponsiveness to steroids (see above). Azathioprine (Imuran) and cyclophosphamide (Cytoxan) are commonly used, but controlled trials are lacking.

6. Lung transplantation for selected end-stage patients

Key Treatment

Drug of Choice	Alternative Therapy
• Corticosteroids	• Cytotoxic agents

Follow-Up

1. Frequency depends on diagnosis and treatment.

2. Subjective and serial radiographic scoring

3. Serial pulmonary function testing, arterial blood gas analysis, or exercise saturation

4. Cardiopulmonary exercise testing in selected cases

5. Deterioration is usually due to disease progression, but one should think of congestive heart failure, bronchoalveolar cell carcinoma, pulmonary embolus, and infectious pneumonia.

Bibliography

For more in-depth information on all clinical aspects of interstitial lung disease, see
Raghu G (ed): Interstitial lung diseases: Semin Respir Crit Care Med 1993;14:323–416 and 1994;15:1–96.
For more information on the immunopathogenetic approach to interstitial lung disease, see
Crystal RG, Bitterman PR, Rennard SI, et al: Interstitial lung diseases of unknown cause: disorders characterized by chronic inflammation of the lower respiratory tract. N Engl J Med 1984;310:154–166, 235–244.
For more information on the clinicopathologic correlation of interstitial lung disease, see
Fulmer JD, Katzenstein AA: The interstitial lung diseases. Pulmonary Crit Care Med 1993;2(M-1):1–15.
For more information on an overview of sarcoidosis, see
Izumi T: Sarcoidosis. Pulmonary Crit Care Med 1993; 2(M-5):1–9.
For more information on clinical overview, see
Schwarz MT: Approach to the understanding, diagnosis, management of interstitial lung disease. In Schwarz MI, King TE (eds): Interstitial Lung Disease, 3rd ed, pp 1–30. Hamilton, Ontario, BC Decker, 1998.

39 Pneumonia

Mary E. O'Brien

Etiology

Pneumonia is an acute infection of the lung parenchyma and may be described as segmental, lobar, or interstitial. It currently represents the sixth leading cause of death in the United States. Infants, the elderly, smokers, alcoholics, institutionalized individuals, cognitively impaired patients, and those with chronic obstructive pulmonary disease (COPD), heart disease, dysphagia, or immune dysfunction are especially at risk.

1. Common causes
   a. Bacterial: *Streptococcus pneumoniae, Staphylococcus aureus, Haemophilus influenzae, Mycoplasma, Legionella, Moraxella catarrhalis, Mycobacterium tuberculosis, Mycobacterium avium* complex, enteric gram-negatives (*Escherichia coli, Proteus, Klebsiella, Serratia*)
   b. Viral: influenza A, parainfluenza, adenovirus, respiratory syncytial virus, rhinovirus
   c. Fungal: *Histoplasma capsulatum, Cryptococcus neoformans*
   d. Parasitic: *Pneumocystis carinii, Toxoplasma gondii*
   e. Chlamydial: *Chlamydia psittaci* (psittacosis), *Chlamydia trachomatis*
2. Uncommon causes
   a. Bacterial: group A β-hemolytic streptococci, *Nocardia, Actinomyces, Franciscella tularensis* (tularemia)
   b. Viral: varicella, measles, rubella, Epstein-Barr virus, enterovirus, *Hantavirus*, cytomegalovirus, herpes simplex
   c. Fungal: *Coccidioides immitis, Blastomyces dermatitidis*, mucormycoses
   d. Rickettsial: *Coxiella burnetii* (Q fever)

Symptoms

Typical symptoms of pneumonia include fever, fatigue, chills, cough, dyspnea, and pleuritic chest pain. Sputum production varies with the causative agent. Associated symptoms may point toward specific etiologies:

1. Headache: *Mycoplasma*, psittacosis, tularemia
2. Diarrhea: legionnaires' disease
3. Myalgias: viruses, psittacosis, tularemia
4. Bullous myringitis: *Mycoplasma*
5. Blood-tinged sputum: *Pneumococcus, M. tuberculosis*

WARNING

Frail, elderly patients with pneumonia may present with confusion and lethargy alone.

 Key Symptoms

- Fever
- Cough
- Dyspnea

Clinical Findings

1. Typical findings
   a. Fever (or hypothermia in the frail elderly)
   b. Rales, rhonchi
   c. Egophony (E to A changes)
   d. Purulent sputum
   e. Pallor
   f. Tachypnea
   g. Tachycardia
2. Unusual findings
   a. Right upper quadrant tenderness
   b. Pharyngeal injection and exudates
   c. Cervical lymphadenopathy
   d. Conjunctivitis
   e. Pleural rub
   f. Hypotension
   g. Septic arthritis
   h. Meningitis

WARNING

Risk factors for a poor outcome include respiratory rate greater than 30 breaths/minute, hypotension, advanced age, altered mental status, partial pressure of O_2 less than 50 mm Hg, and extrapulmonary involvement.

- Fever

- Purulent sputum

- Leukocytosis

Laboratory Tests

1. The diagnosis of pneumonia requires a new or progressive infiltrate on chest radiograph plus two of the following:
   a. Fever
   b. Purulent sputum
   c. Leukocytosis
2. Bacterial pneumonias typically show a leukocytosis with a shift to the left.
3. Viral pneumonias often reveal a white blood cell (WBC) count of less than 5000/mm^3.
4. Additional tests
   a. Gram's stain of sputum
   b. Sputum cultures
   c. Blood cultures
   d. Arterial blood gases: hypoxemia, respiratory alkalosis

Key Tests

- Chest radiograph

- WBC count

- Sputum culture

Differential Diagnosis

The greatest diagnostic challenge in the setting of pneumonia is determining the causative organism. Occasionally, the clinical picture may be confused by underlying COPD, asthma, autoimmune disorders, or malignancy (postobstructive pneumonia). Several uncommon conditions may initially present as a community-acquired pneumonia:

1. Chemical pneumonitis: smoke inhalation, toluene in plastics
2. Hypersensitivity pneumonitis
   a. Bagassosis (sugar cane mold)
   b. Farmer's lung (moldy hay)
   c. Humidifier lung
   d. Bird fancier's lung
   e. Byssinosis (cotton)
   f. Silicosis (quartz, sandblasting, pottery workers)
3. Granulomatous disease: sarcoidosis
4. Infectious illnesses: psittacosis, tularemia, Q fever, cytomegalovirus, tuberculosis
5. Pulmonary embolism or infarction

Treatment

Medical

The treatment of pneumonia must often begin with empiric antibiotic coverage until culture and sensitivity results become available.

1. Outpatient, otherwise healthy
   a. Azithromycin (Zithromax), 500 mg PO day 1, then 250 PO qd × 4 days
   b. Clarithromycin (Biaxin), 500 mg PO q12h for 7 to 10 days
   c. Erythromycin, 500 mg PO qid for 7 to 10 days
   d. Doxycycline (Vibramycin), 100 mg PO bid for 7 to 10 days
2. Outpatient, over 60 or with associated illness
   a. Fluoroquinolone with enhanced activity against *S. pneumoniae*
      (1) Trovafloxacin (Trovan) 200 mg PO qd
      (2) Levofloxacin (Levaquin) 500 mg PO qd
      (3) Grepafloxacin (Raxar) 600 mg PO qd
   b. Second-generation cephalosporin plus a macrolide
3. Inpatient, stable
   a. Ceftriaxone (Rocephin), 1 to 2 gm IV q24h
   b. Fluoroquinolone with enhanced activity against *S. pneumoniae* (levofloxacin, trovafloxicin)
   c. Add a macrolide if *Legionella* suspected
4. Inpatient, seriously ill
   a. Ceftriaxone (Rocephin), 1 to 2 gm IV q12 to 24h plus aminoglycoside
   b. Fluoroquinolone plus aminoglycoside
   c. Antipseudomonal penicillin, piperacillin-tazobactam (Zosyn) 3.357 gm IV q6h or metronidazole (Flagyl)
   d. Add clindamycin (Cleocin), 600 mg IV q8h, for suspected aspiration
   e. Vancomycin (Vancocin), 500 to 1000 mg IV q12h for suspected *S. aureus*, in patients from nursing homes, or for suspected resistant *S. pneumoniae*.
5. Additional measures
   a. Increased oral or intravenous fluids.
   b. Chest physiotherapy, incentive spirometry
   c. Nasal oxygen
   d. Analgesics for pleuritic pain, headache

e. Acetaminophen for fever greater than 101°F

f. Expectorants

g. Cough suppressants if necessary for rest or chest pain

h. Nutritional measures: increase fruit and vegetables; avoid dairy products; consider multivitamin, vitamins C and E.

i. Balance rest with mild activity to prevent serious deconditioning.

Patient Education

In addition to the above measures, patients should be cautioned to wash their hands often and avoid unnecessary exposure to crowds, especially during winter months. Fatigue often lingers considerably longer than many people expect. Normal strength and endurance may not be recovered for 6 months or more in patients who have been ill with pneumonia.

Key Treatment

- A macrolide or fluoroquinolone with enhanced activity against *S. pneumoniae*

- Coverage for gram-negative organism in hospital settings

- Treat for 7 to 10 days.

Follow-Up

1. It has often been observed that patients with pneumonia show clinical signs of improvement (or deterioration) 24 to 36 hours before corresponding changes are discernible on chest radiograph. Resolution of fever and tachypnea generally correlate well with recovery, although elderly patients may be afebrile or even hypothermic in frank sepsis.

2. Failure to respond may be due to severe debilitation, malnutrition, immunosuppression, resistant organisms, or a noninfectious process. In the face of persistent or worsening symptoms, antibiotic coverage should be expanded to include gram-negative organisms, anaerobes, and methicillin-resistant *S. aureus*.

3. A follow-up chest radiograph is usually appropriate 6 to 12 weeks after diagnosis.

4. Patients with uncomplicated recovery

   a. Chest radiograph in 6 to 12 weeks

   b. Influenza and pneumonia vaccines

5. Patients with delayed or complicated recovery

   a. Augment antibiotic coverage

   b. Consider bronchoscopy

   c. Assess nutritional parameters and immune function

   d. Consider computerized tomography of chest

Bibliography

American Thoracic Society: Hospital-acquired pneumonia in adults: diagnosis, assessment of severity, initial antimicrobial therapy, and preventive strategies. A consensus statement, American Thoracic Society, November 1995. Am J Respir Crit Care Med 1996;153:1711–1725.

Bartlett JG, Breiman RF, Mandell LA, et al: Community-acquired pneumonia in adults: guidelines for management. Infectious Diseases Society of America. Clin Infect Dis 1998;26:811–838.

Farber MO: Managing community-acquired pneumonia: factors to consider in outpatient care. Postgrad Med 1999;105:106–113.

Kohler RB: Severe pneumonia: when and why to hospitalize. Postgrad Med 1999;105:117–129.

Levinson ME: Pneumonia, including necrotizing pulmonary infections. In Fauci AS, Braunwald E (eds): Harrison's Principles of Internal Medicine, 14th ed, pp 1437–1445. New York, McGraw-Hill, 1998.

Stein GE, Havlichek DH: New oral antimicrobials for resistant respiratory tract infections. Postgrad Med 1998;103:67–76.

40 Atelectasis

Atelectasis means imperfect expansion and denotes a state of airlessness of the lung. Atelectasis is best defined as collapse or loss of volume of a lung, lobe, or segment.

Classification

1. *Obstructive (resorption) atelectasis* (most common) occurs on occlusion of the main stem, lobar, or segmental bronchus by intraluminal obstruction or extrinsic bronchial compression. The involved portion diminishes in volume and becomes radiopaque as air distal to the obstruction is absorbed into the capillary blood, usually within 18 to 24 hours. Resorption rate is accelerated when a gas mixture containing a high concentration of oxygen is inspired. If concurrent transudation of capillary blood and fluid occurs, the volume loss is minimal or nil. The fluid-filled, airless lung appears intensely radiopaque (the "drowned lung"). Adequate collateral alveolar ventilation and collateral air drift distal to the site of total bronchial occulsion can prevent atelectasis.

2. *Relaxation atelectasis (passive)* is the result of unopposed elastic recoil of the lung that occurs in the presence of an intrathoracic space-occupying lesion, such as pneumothorax or pleural effusion. The collapsed lung is not airless.

3. *Contraction (cicatrization) atelectasis* occurs when pulmonary fibrosis leads to a diminution of lung volume and to radiopacification. In contrast to the uniform opacification of obstructive atelectasis, pockets of air trapped within fibrotic areas are often visible.

4. *Adhesive (nonobstructive) atelectasis*, or diffuse microatelectasis, is alveolar collapse caused by intra-alveolar changes; it occurs despite a patent bronchus. Although the mechanism is unclear, surfactant loss or dysfunction occurring after diffuse alveolar injury probably plays a dominant role. The resulting impairment of alveolar surface tension–lowering ability facilitates alveolar collapse. Continuous small-tidal-volume breathing, low end-expiratory volume, and removal of alveolar nitrogen are other factors responsible for microatelectasis seen in low lung

compliance states, postoperatively with diaphragmatic dysfunction, and during mechanical ventilation. Although peripheral, linear, plate-like densities caused by subsegmental atelectasis may be seen on the chest radiograph, volume loss without radiopacification is the hallmark. When diffuse radiopacification occurs, it is due to concomitant alveolar edema or the formation of hyaline membranes seen in diffuse alveolar injury states.

Etiology

Obstructive Atelectasis

1. Endobronchial obstruction
   a. Mucous plugs
      (1) Bronchial asthma
      (2) Allergic bronchopulmonary aspergillosis
      (3) Cystic fibrosis
      (4) Chronic bronchitis
      (5) Postoperative state
      (6) Postintubated state
   b. Endobronchial neoplasm
      (1) Bronchogenic carcinoma
         (a) Squamous cell
         (b) Small cell
      (2) Bronchial adenoma—carcinoid tumor
      (3) Endobronchial metastasis, primary
         (a) Kidney
         (b) Breast
         (c) Colon
      (4) Endobronchial lymphoma
   c. Foreign body
   d. Infection
      (1) Endobronchial tuberculosis
      (2) Broncholithiasis
         (a) Tuberculosis
         (b) Histoplasmosis
2. Extrinsic bronchial compression
   a. Neoplasm
      (1) Lung carcinoma
         (a) Large cell
         (b) Adenocarcinoma

202 • III Respiratory Diseases

(2) Mediastinal tumors

    (a) Thymoma

    (b) Teratoma

    (c) Germ cell tumors

b. Cardiovascular: compression of left lower lobe bronchus by aneurysm of ascending aorta, by enlarged left atrium in mitral stenosis

3. Trauma: tracheobronchial rupture secondary to blunt anterior chest wall injury

4. Congenital: bronchial atresia: left upper lobe bronchus

5. Tracheobronchial cartilage disorders, dynamic airway occlusion

    a. From relapsing polychondritis

    b. From tracheobronchomegaly

    c. From tracheomalacia

Relaxation Atelectasis

1. Large pleural effusion
2. Pneumothorax
3. Expanding bullae

Contraction Atelectasis

Pulmonary fibrosis caused by

1. Tuberculosis
2. Silicosis
3. Sarcoidosis

Adhesive Atelectasis

1. Diffuse alveolar injury caused by

    a. Toxic fume inhalation

    b. Gastric acid aspiration

    c. Endotoxin injury

2. Prolonged ventilatory support

Atelectasis from mucous plugging as in asthma and the postoperative state, airway occlusion from bronchogenic carcinoma, compression as a result of a large pleural effusion, and diffuse microatelectasis resulting from surfactant dysfunction constitute the more common causes of atelectasis. Extrinsic mass compression, endobronchial tuberculosis, and pulmonary fibrosis are less common causes, and congenital bronchial atresia, tracheobronchial rupture, and tracheobronchial cartilage disorders are rare causes.

Symptoms

1. Primarily those of the responsible underlying disease rather than atelectasis itself
2. Cough and exertional dyspnea from altered lung compliance and hypoxia
3. Dyspnea at rest when a whole lung collapses acutely

Key Symptoms

- Cough
- Exertional dyspnea
- Acute dyspnea at rest

Clinical Findings

Signs of atelectasis reflect the decreased ventilation in the involved area and the ipsilateral mediastinal shift as a result of the reduced lung volume. Hypoxia results from increased venous admixture because of perfusion of non-ventilated alveoli. Reduced lung compliance leads to hyperventilation and respiratory alkalosis. Extensive atelectasis, however, can cause hypoventilation and respiratory acidosis.

Key Signs

- Decreased chest wall movement
- Impaired chest percussion note
- Decreased vocal fremitus
- Decreased vocal resonance
- Decreased or absent breath sound
- Ipsilateral tracheal shift
- Tachypnea, tachycardia, hypoxia
- Hyperventilation and respiratory alkalosis
- Hypoventilation and respiratory acidosis

Tests

1. In most instances, diagnosis can be made by chest radiography. The lateral view is essential to recognize middle lobe and lingular atelectasis, whereas the apical lordotic view visualizes well the collapsed right middle lobe.

2. Not only can computerized tomographic (CT) scanning establish the diagnosis of atelectasis, but it can also show the endobronchial tree, lung parenchyma, and mediastinum and thereby help determine the cause.

3. Fiberoptic bronchoscopy under local anesthesia provides excellent visualization of the endobronchial tree, allowing for biopsy and aspiration of endobronchial and parabronchial lesions.

Diagnostic Chest Radiographic Signs

1. Major signs

    a. Displacement of the respective interlobar septum or fissure

b. Radiopacity of the atelectatic segment, lobe, or entire lung

2. Minor signs

 a. Displacement of the hilum in the direction of the atelectatic lobe

 b. Ipsilateral shift of mediastinal structures (e.g., trachea and heart)

 c. Elevation of the ipsilateral hemidiaphragm

 d. Compensatory hyperaeration of the adjacent lung parenchyma

 e. Crowding of ribs as a result of a decrease in size of the thoracic cage.

3. Demonstration of volume loss by adjoining interlobar septum or fissure displacement is essential to the diagnosis.

4. Displacement of the hilum is also a useful sign of volume loss. The hilum is displaced upward in upper lobe atelectasis and downward in lower lobe atelectasis.

Radiographic Appearance

1. *Right upper lobe atelectasis* is best visualized on a posteroanterior (PA) chest radiograph as an inverted triangular opacity in the right upper zone. The minor fissue is displaced superiorly and medially.

2. *Left upper lobe atelectasis* is also best visualized on a PA chest radiograph. The opacity seen is less intense and less well demarcated and appears as a hazy density over the left upper and midzone that obliterates the left mediastinal and cardiac border. When the lingular bronchus is patent, the left cardiac border remains well defined.

3. *Right middle lobe atelectasis* is best seen on the lateral chest radiograph as a band density, formed by the displaced minor and major fissures, extending from the hilum to the base of the sternum. The collapsed right middle lobe appears as a paracardiac spiculated opacity on an apical lordotic chest radiograph.

4. *Lower lobe atelectasis* is best identified on a PA chest radiograph as a retrocardiac triangular opacity that obliterates the margin of the diaphragm. In the case of the left lower lobe, the outer margin of the descending thoracic aorta is also obscured. On the lateral view, the collapsed lower lobe is seen as a faint opacity in the paravertebral region and obscures the involved hemidiaphragm.

5. *Right middle and lower lobe atelectasis* is seen on the PA film as an opacity in the right midzone and base silhouetting the cardiac border and hemidiaphragm. On lateral view, the opacified atelectatic lung and adjoining cardiac shadow form a band density that extends across the chest, covering the midzones and base of the lung.

6. *Total lung atelectasis* is characterized by opacification of the entire hemithorax and marked ipsilateral shift of mediastinal structures.

Special Radiographic Signs

1. *S sign of Golden*: refers to the convex appearance of the outer margin of the atelectatic right upper lobe when the proximal portion of the displaced minor fissure is pushed outward by a tumor.

2. *Double lesion sign of Felson*: refers to atelectasis of more than one lobe that cannot be explained by a single endobronchial occlusive lesion, as in right upper and right middle lobe atelectasis. This radiographic finding is suggestive of a non-neoplastic cause for the atelectasis.

3. *Open bronchus sign of Felson*: refers to atelectasis in the presence of a patent proximal airway and confirms a non-neoplastic cause.

4. *Comet tail sign*: seen in round atelectasis; a lesion that presents as a round or helical pleural-based density, densest at its periphery, with contiguous pleural thickening. The regional bronchovascular structures can be seen bundled together and curving into the mass, resembling a comet tail. This "comet tail" sign is best visualized on CT scanning, which often also demonstrates an air bronchogram in the central part of the mass and oligemic hyperinflated parenchyma adjacent to the mass. Pleural thickening and fibrosis as seen in asbestosis, causing contraction of adjacent lung parenchyma, and lung tissue initially compressed by pleural effusion and later becoming adherent to the parietal pleura, are possible mechanisms for the development of round atelectasis.

Key Tests

- Chest radiography—PA, lateral, and apical lordotic views
- CT scan of the chest
- Fiberoptic bronchoscopy

Differential Diagnosis

1. Encapsulated pleural effusion: Interlobular effusion in the right major fissure can resemble right middle lobe atelectasis on a lateral chest radiograph. A loculated pleural effusion can mimic right middle and lower lobe atelectasis on a PA chest radiograph.

2. Displaced or dilated right brachiocephalic vein:

Can appear on the PA film as atelectasis of the right upper lobe, especially when the minor fissure is not seen.

3. Left pulmonary ligament abnormalities: Thickening of or fluid accumulation in the left pulmonary ligament can be misdiagnosed as left lower lobe atelectasis on a PA radiograph.

4. Bronchogenic carcinoma in patients with round atelectasis: Bronchogenic carcinoma and round atelectasis resemble each other on the conventional chest radiograph. In most instances, additional chest radiographic views and CT scanning of the chest will establish the diagnosis.

Treatment

Lung expansion is best achieved by treating the underlying disease and correcting the mechanisms responsible for volume loss. Modalities include the following:

1. Chest physiotherapy—to facilitate high-volume breaths and the expectoration of airway secretions. It is both preventive and therapeutic, especially in critically ill patients and postoperative state, and includes the following:

   a. Deep-breathing exercises and incentive spirometer use

   b. Directed cough using the forced expiration technique

   c. Postural drainage, manual chest percussion and vibration

   d. Use of mechanical devices to provide high-frequency oscillation at the mouth and/or the chest wall

   e. Bronchodilator therapy

   f. Humidification of inspired air

   g. Use of mucolytic agents, such as iodinated glycerol, by mouth or nebulized acetylcysteine (Mucomyst) or recombinant human DNase (Dornase Alfa). The role of mucolytic agents is not clear. Acetylcysteine can cause bronchospasm. The use of Dornase Alfa to cleave extracellular DNA from degenerating polymorphonuclear cells and to convert the gelatinous sputum to a more liquid form has shown promise in patients with cystic fibrosis.

   h. Possible use of nebulized or intratracheally instilled artificial surfactant in diffuse microatelectasis

   i. Endotracheal intubation to facilitate vigorous airway suctioning with isotonic saline solution instilled into airways

2. Positive pressure breathing

   a. Continuous positive airway pressure by face mask

   b. Positive end-expiratory pressure in patients on mechanical ventilation

These techniques enable the recruitment of alveoli in states of diffuse microatelectasis and thereby increase functional residual capacity, help prevent atelectasis, and improve gas exchange. Positive pressure of 5 to 10 cm H_2O is usually adequate. The risks of positive-pressure breathing, such as barotrauma, hypotension, gastric distention, and aspiration, are the drawbacks.

3. Bronchoscopy

   a. Fiberoptic: Indication is re-expansion of lung in recurrent atelectasis, especially in postintubated states; also used for foreign-body removal.

   b. Rigid: method of choice for endobronchial foreign-body removal

4. Surgery: removal of the resectable neoplasm by thoracotomy

5. Endoscopic laser therapy

   a. Curative for benign endobronchial neoplasm

   b. Palliative for nonresectable malignant tumors

6. Radiotherapy: may restore airway patency in radiosensitive tumors. In most patients, the intent of radiation is palliation.

7. Chemotherapy: most effective in re-establishing airway patency in lymphoma and small cell carcinoma

Key Treatment

- Chest physiotherapy
- Positive-pressure breathing

Bibliography

Celli BR: Physiologic and mechanical aids to lung expansion. Clin Chest Med 1993;14:257–260.

Fraser RG, Paré JAP, Paré PD, et al: Parenchymal atelectasis. In Fraser RG, Paré JAP, Paré PD, et al (eds): Diagnosis of Diseases of the Chest, 3rd ed, vol 1, pp 472–537. Philadelphia, WB Saunders Company, 1988.

Gamsu G: Atelectasis and bronchial obstruction. In Moss A, Gamsu G, Genant HC (eds): Computed Tomography of the Body, 2nd ed, vol 1, pp 27–32. Philadelphia, WB Saunders Company, 1992.

Goldin JA, Wang KP, Keith FM: Intensive care and fiberoptic bronchoscopy, foreign body removal and laser therapy. In Murray JM, Nadel JA (eds): Textbook of Respiratory Medicine, 2nd ed, vol 1, pp 737–769. Philadelphia, WB Saunders Company, 1994.

Salathe M, O'Riordan TG, Wanner A: Treatment of mucociliary dysfunction. Chest 1996;110:1048–1057.

Webb WR: Atelectasis. In Rakel RE (ed): Conn's Current Therapy, pp 157–159. Philadelphia, WB Saunders Company, 1994.

41 Pulmonary Embolism

C. Gregory Elliott

Etiology

Thrombi that move from the deep veins to obstruct pulmonary arteries cause the symptoms, signs, and laboratory abnormalities of acute pulmonary embolism. The thrombi are the result of a complex interplay between (1) venous stasis, (2) tissue trauma, and (3) hypercoagulability (referred to as Virchow's triad). Often venous thrombi are secondary to a precipitating event such as recent surgery or trauma. Venous thrombosis and pulmonary embolism are idiopathic when a precipitating event is not present. Idiopathic pulmonary embolism may be the earliest sign of previously undetected cancer.

Symptoms

Shortness of breath is the most common symptom of acute pulmonary embolism. Patients may also complain of chest pain that is made worse by deep breathing. Less frequently, cough, syncope, or hemoptysis accompany acute pulmonary embolism.

Key Symptoms

- Dyspnea
- Chest pain accentuated by deep breathing

Clinical Findings

Typical findings

1. Tachypnea (respiratory rate >20 breaths/minute)
2. Tachycardia (heart rate >100 beats/minute)
3. Pleural friction rub
4. Accentuated pulmonic second sound
5. Fever

Key Signs

- Tachypnea
- Tachycardia
- Pleural friction rub

Laboratory Tests

The diagnosis of acute pulmonary embolism requires confirmation by objective testing. The tests may image the pulmonary circulation or identify a source of thromboemboli in the lower extremities.

1. A normal lung perfusion scan excludes pulmonary embolism. Lung perfusion and ventilation scan patterns that have a high probability of being associated with angiographic proof of pulmonary embolism can confirm the diagnosis.

WARNING

There is a high probability that lung scans cannot diagnose acute pulmonary embolism when pretest clinical suspicion is low or when prior pulmonary embolism has occurred.

---

2. Pulmonary arteriography is the definitive diagnostic test.
3. Fast computerized tomography of the chest with contrast enhancement of pulmonary vessels permits recognition of central pulmonary emboli but misses peripheral pulmonary emboli (i.e., those in subsegmental pulmonary arteries).
4. Compression ultrasonography of the legs permits treatment of venous thromboembolism if deep vein thrombi are identified. When this test is negative, it must be repeated over a 2-week interval to exclude proximal propagation of calf vein thrombi.

Key Tests

- Lung perfusion scan
- Pulmonary arteriography
- Spiral computerized tomography

Differential Diagnosis

The differential diagnosis of pulmonary embolism includes a variety of cardiopulmonary disorders that cause the symptoms commonly caused by pulmonary embolism.

1. Pneumonia

2. Pulmonary edema
3. Exacerbation of chronic obstructive pulmonary disease(s)
4. Cardiac arrhythmia

Treatment

The treatment of acute pulmonary embolism usually aims to prevent recurrent pulmonary embolism. Treatments that aim to immediately remove acute pulmonary emboli are reserved for more severely affected patients.

1. To prevent recurrent pulmonary embolism
   a. Unfractionated heparin titrated to produce a therapeutic prolongation of the activated partial thromboplastin time within the first 24 hours of treatment, overlapped with warfarin titrated to produce an international normalized ratio (INR) between 2.0 and 3.0.
   b. Low-molecular-weight heparins are effective for the treatment of venous thromboembolism.
   c. Vena cava filter placement when anticoagulants are contraindicated, when serious bleeding complicates anticoagulant therapy, or for selected high risk patients
2. To lyse massive pulmonary embolism in the patient with shock or cardiac arrest
   a. Tissue plasminogen activator: 100 mg intravenously over 2 hours; *or*
   b. Streptokinase: 250,000 IU intravenous bolus followed by 100,000 IU/hour infused for 24 hours; *or*
   c. Urokinase: 4400 IU/kg intravenous loading dose followed by 4400 IU/kg/hour infused for 12 hours

Patient Education

1. Patients should be made aware of the symptoms of recurrent venous thromboembolism, including dyspnea, pleuritic-type chest pain, or syncope.
2. Patients should understand that the principal risk of anticoagulants is bleeding, and that such bleeding may cause serious or fatal complications. Patients also should be taught the signs of internal bleeding, such as weakness or melena.
3. Patients must understand the importance of regular monitoring of the anticoagulant effects of warfarin. They also should understand that many factors, especially diet and the concomitant use of other medications, can alter their response to warfarin.
4. Patients capable of becoming pregnant should understand that warfarin can cause birth defects.

Key Treatment

- Heparin in a dose sufficient to produce a therapeutic anticoagulant effect
- Other choices (e.g., low-molecular-weight heparin, thrombolysis, or vena caval filter) depend upon the clinical situation (see text).

Follow-Up

Follow-up is essential for patients with acute pulmonary embolism. The physician must ensure that anticoagulation continues for at least 3 months. In addition, the physician should monitor patients for complications of acute pulmonary embolism or its treatment, such as bleeding, recurrence, or the appearance of an associated malignancy.

Bibliography

ACCP Consensus Committee on Pulmonary Embolism: Opinions regarding the diagnosis and management of venous thromboembolic disease. Chest 1996;109:233–237.

ACCP Consensus Committee on Pulmonary Embolism: Opinions regarding the diagnosis and treatment of venous thromboembolic disease. Chest 1998;113:499–504.

Elliott CG: Pulmonary embolism. Curr Pulmonol 1995; 16:51–85.

Goldhaber SZ: Pulmonary embolism. N Engl J Med 1998;339:93–104.

42 Acute Respiratory Distress Syndrome

Richard H. Snyder

Etiology

1. Predisposition to development of acute respiratory distress syndrome (ARDS): any disease process resulting in a systemic inflammatory response
2. Pathogenesis
   a. A diffuse inflammatory injury occurs to the lungs.
   b. Inflammatory injury results in fluid leaking into lung parenchyma.
3. Common processes leading to ARDS
   a. Sepsis
   b. Trauma
   c. Pancreatitis
   d. Drowning
   e. Multiple blood transfusions
   f. Pulmonary aspiration
   g. Multiple fractures
   h. Bypass surgery
   i. Burns
   j. Head injury

Symptom

Progressive acute shortness of breath

Key Symptom

Shortness of breath

Clinical Findings

1. Dyspnea
2. Tachycardia
3. Tachypnea
4. Signs of respiratory muscle fatigue
   a. Intercostal retractions
   b. Paradoxical chest and abdominal movement
5. Rales

Key Signs

- Dyspnea
- Tachypnea
- Intercostal retraction
- Rales

Differential Diagnosis

1. Cardiogenic pulmonary edema
2. Hydrostatic pulmonary edema
3. Pneumonia
4. Acute pulmonary embolism

Diagnostic Criteria for ARDS

- Acute onset
- Bilateral chest radiographic infiltrates
- Pulmonary artery occlusion pressure <18 mm Hg
- Impaired oxygenation regardless of positive end-expiratory pressure (PEEP) concentration
- Alveolar partial pressure of oxygen–to–fractional concentration of oxygen in inspired gas (p_aO_2/FiO_2) ratio <200 torr

Laboratory Tests

1. Arterial blood gases
   a. Severe refractory hypoxemia
   b. Normal to low partial pressure of carbon dioxide (pCO_2) initially
   c. Increased pCO_2 as dead space increases later in the disease process
2. Swan-Ganz catheter
   a. Normal to elevated cardiac output
   b. Wedge pressure less than 18 mm Hg
   c. Elevated pulmonary arterial pressures later on in the disease if pulmonary hypertension develops
3. Chest radiograph
   a. Initially may be normal.
   b. Within 24 hours of disease onset, bilateral pulmonary infiltrates develop.

Key Test

Arterial blood gases

Treatment

1. Must treat and control underlying illness.
2. Maintain optimal fluid balance. Use the minimum amount of fluid to maintain adequate cardiac vascular performance and renal function without fluid overloading patient.
3. Use vasopressors as necessary to support cardiovascular function.
4. Patient positioning: Prone positioning may have a role in optimizing ventilation-perfusion ratio.
5. Mechanical ventilation
   a. Mainstay of therapy
   b. Use PEEP to recruit atelectatic alveoli. PEEP in the range of 15 to 20 cm H_2O often needed.
   c. Use lower tidal volumes to prevent lung injury.
      (1) Use 6 to 8 ml/kg.
      (2) May need to use permissive hypercapnea.
   d. Inverse ratio and pressure-limited ventilation may be helpful.
   e. Goal is to reduce FiO_2 to levels less than 70 per cent while maintaining tissue oxygenation.

Key Treatment

Mechanical ventilation

Prognosis

1. Mortality 50 to 90 per cent
2. Survivors
   a. Lung mechanics return to normal.
   b. Not uncommon for pulmonary gas exchange abnormalities to persist.
   c. Survivors should live normal lives.

Bibliography

Connelly KG, Repine E: Markers for predicting the development of acute respiratory distress syndrome. Annu Rev Med 1997;118:129–145.

Fulkerson WJ, MacIntyre N, Stamler J, et al: Pathogenesis and treatment of adult respiratory distress syndrome. Arch Intern Med 1996;156:29–38.

Kollif MH, Schuster DP: The acute respiratory distress syndrome. N Engl J Med 1995;332:27–37.

Luce JM: Acute lung injury and the acute respiratory distress syndrome. Crit Care Med 1998;26:369–376.

Schuster DP: Identify patients with ARDS: time for a different approach. Intensive Care Med 1997;23:1197–1203.

Indications
1. Airway protection in patients at risk of airway compromise
2. Maintenance of patent airway
3. Facilitation of pulmonary toilet
4. Application of positive-pressure ventilation
5. Maintenance of adequate oxygenation
   a. Predictable fraction of oxygen in inspired air
   b. Positive end-expiratory pressure

Contraindications
1. Operator unskilled in airway management or endotracheal intubation
2. Extensive trauma to facial, oropharyngeal, laryngeal, or cervical spine regions (relative)

Preparation
1. Determine which method of intubation is appropriate for the patient.
2. Ensure airway management equipment is checked and functional (see "Equipment").
   a. Laryngoscope light source is working and the blade fits snugly.
   b. Endotracheal tube cuff does not leak.
3. Establish secure venous access, preferably with at least one 18-gauge IV cannula. Prepare all drugs that may potentially be necessary (see "Anesthesia").
4. Clear the airway of
   a. Foreign bodies
   b. Loose bodies (i.e., bridges, dentures)
   c. Excess secretions
5. Preoxygenate the patient with 100% oxygen by mask for 5 minutes. If time is of the essence, four vital capacity breaths are adequate for nitrogen washout in healthy lungs.
6. If there is inadequate ventilation, insert an oro- or nasopharyngeal airway, have an assistant apply cricoid pressure (Sellick's maneuver), and ventilate manually with a bag-valve mask until you are ready to intubate.
7. Attach a blood pressure and cardiac monitor if possible, as well as a pulse oximeter if available.
8. A fully stocked and prepared crash cart, as well as assistants trained in cardiopulmonary resuscitation or airway management, should preferably be available on standby.

Equipment
1. Bag-valve mask with oxygen source attachment, and assorted mask sizes
2. Two laryngoscope handles and blades (MacIntosh—curved, Miller—straight). A size 3 blade is used for the average adult.
3. Endotracheal tubes (size 7 to 8 mm for the average female, size 8 to 9 mm for the average male). A size 6-mm tube should be available in the event that the larger tube cannot be passed. Tubes should have low-pressure, high-volume cuffs.

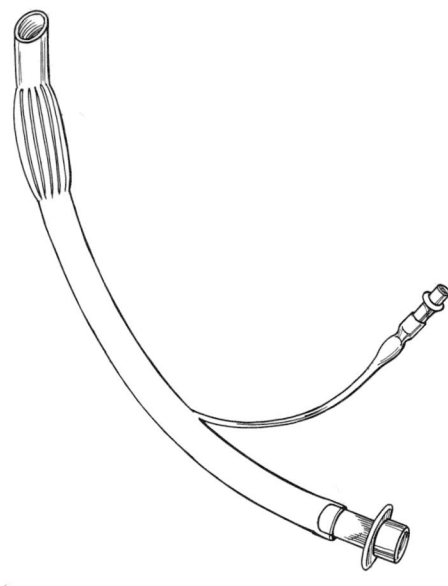

4. Assorted sizes of oropharyngeal (Guedel or Berman) and nasopharyngeal airways
5. Stylet (lubricated) in a "hockey-stick" formation
6. Magill forceps: for the removal of foreign objects or to aid in the insertion of the tip of the endotracheal tube into the larynx
7. Suction equipment: a rigid (Yankauer) and soft-tipped suction catheter
8. Water-soluble lidocaine jelly (2%) for lubrication of stylet. Lubricating the endotracheal tube is not recommended because the lubricant may irritate the larynx.
9. Adhesive or cloth tape to secure the endotracheal tube
10. A 10-ml syringe to inflate the endotracheal tube cuff

Anesthesia
1. In the unconscious patient, drugs are not usually required for endotracheal intubation. Ventilation and intubation, with the use of Sellick's maneuver, should be performed without delay.
2. A rapid-sequence (or "crash") intubation is used in the patient at risk for regurgitation or

aspiration during intubation. This implies rapid IV administration of a sedative-hypnotic and a fast-acting muscle relaxant, with or without a narcotic agent.

3. Medications most often used include the following:
   a. Sedative-hypnotics
      (1) Propofol, 2.5 mg/kg intravenously. This can cause a large drop in blood pressure and should not be used in hemodynamically unstable patients. The patient may experience discomfort with rapid administration of this agent.
      (2) Thiopental, 2 to 5 mg/kg intravenously. This is a very smooth and safe induction agent in most patients, but may cause a drop in blood pressure as a result of histamine release.
      (3) Etomidate, 0.2 to 0.3 mg/kg. This is the most cardiovascularly stable of the induction agents, but can cause local pain on injection.
   b. Neuromuscular blocking agents
      (1) Succinylcholine, 1 to 1.5 mg/kg intravenously. This is a depolarizing muscle relaxant and is a commonly used agent. Side effects include arrythmias and postoperative myalgias.
      (2) Rocuronium, 0.6 to 1.2 mg/kg intravenously. This is a new nondepolarizing muscle relaxant that is fast acting and of short duration.
   c. Additional agents include
      (1) Fentanyl, 3 to 5 μg/kg intravenously. This decreases the autonomic response to intubation.
      (2) Lidocaine, 1.5 mg/kg intravenously. This decreases airway reactivity and arrythmias during intubation, therefore offering a protective effect in patients with cardiovascular and central nervous system disease.
4. Intubation of the awake patient allows the patient to breathe spontaneously and leaves the airway reflexes intact. It may be performed using a combination of mild sedation, a topical anesthetic, and/or a narcotic analgesic. This technique is particularly recommended if a difficult intubation is suspected, the patient has a full stomach, or the patient's condition is so poor that even a small amount of induction agent may cause cardiovascular collapse. Agents commonly used are
   a. Lidocaine 4% topical spray. This is sprayed onto the tongue and posterior pharynx. Spraying the larynx is not recommended because this decreases airway reflexes and may result in aspiration.
   b. Midazolam, 1- to 2 mg boluses incrementally, or other short-acting benzodiazepine. This is a sedative as well as an amnesic agent.
   c. Fentanyl, 1 to 3 μg/kg, or morphine, 2- to 5-mg bolus intravenously. These often help facilitate the procedure.
   d. An anticholinergic agent, such as glycopyrrolate 0.1 to 0.4 mg/kg intravenously. This helps decrease airway secretions and prevent bradycardia.

Precautions

1. Drugs used to facilitate intubation may cause unwanted effects, such as arrythmias and hemodynamic instability. Use drugs with which you are familiar.
2. Laryngoscopy and intubation are potent stimulators of the autonomic nervous system. Patients with cardiovascular and central nervous system disease, in whom these effects may be detrimental, should have measures taken to minimize these effects.

WARNING
- Muscle relaxants should only be used by those skilled in airway management.
- Have an emergency backup plan for failed intubation.

Technique

1. Check all equipment, and ensure it is functioning correctly.
2. Position the patient in the "sniffing position." This is done by performing a jaw thrust or chin lift, extending the head at the atlanto-occipital joint and flexing the neck, thus aligning the oral, pharyngeal, and laryngeal axes. A folded towel under the occiput helps provide neck flexion. Ensure all foreign objects, such as dentures and bridges, have been removed from the oral

cavity. It is advisable to have an assistant trained in Sellick's maneuver, which may be applied once laryngeal reflexes have been lost.

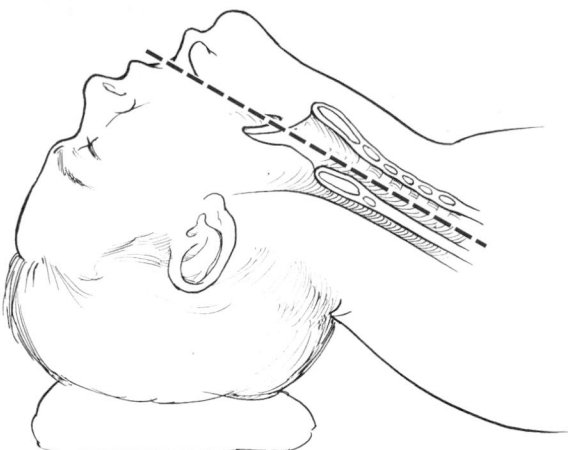

3. Sellick's maneuver consists of firm backward and downward pressure applied to the cricoid cartilage with the thumb and third finger. The index finger rests on the cricothyroid membrane.

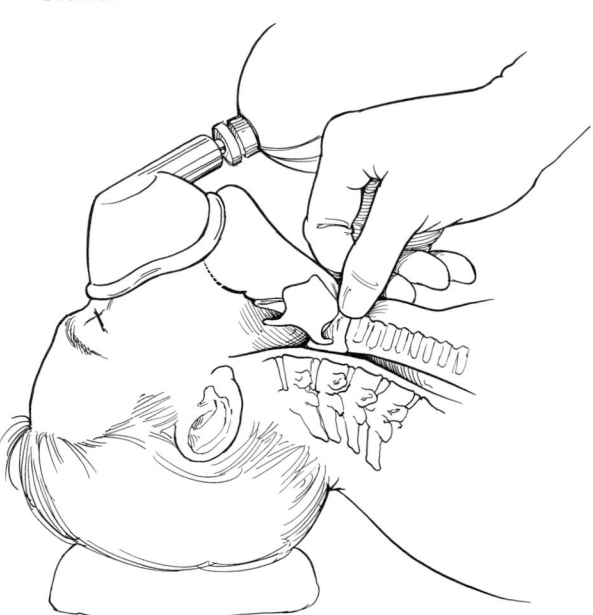

4. Place the laryngoscope in the left hand and insert it into the right side of the mouth. Sweep it across the midline, pushing the tongue to the left. A curved blade (Macintosh) is generally easier to use in less experienced hands, and should be inserted into the vallecula.

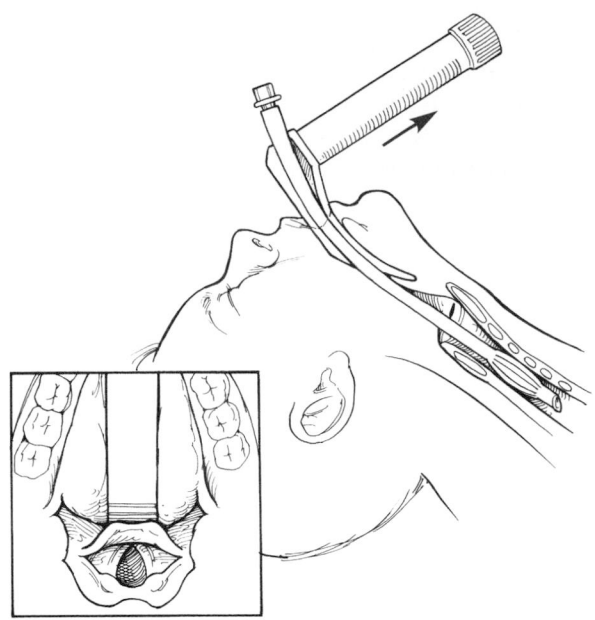

When using a straight blade (Miller), insert the tip to just below the epiglottis.

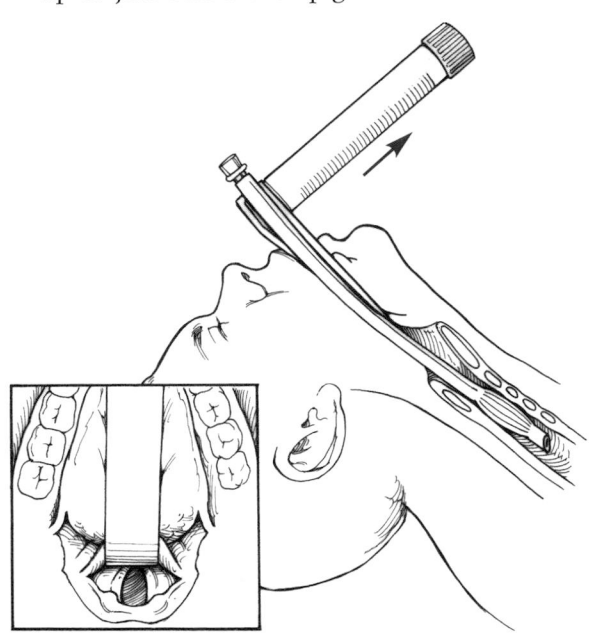

5. Lift the laryngoscope in a forward and upward manner, keeping the wrist stiff to avoid using the teeth as a fulcrum, until the vocal cords are visible. Avoid trapping the lips and tongue between the blade and teeth. If it is difficult to visualize the vocal cords, Sellick's maneuver will help bring an anterior larynx into view.

6. While maintaining view of the vocal cords, insert the endotracheal tube between them, until the tip of the cuff is 2 to 3 cm below the cords. Remove the laryngoscope and inflate the cuff with enough air to prevent an air leak during positive-pressure ventilation. If it is difficult to insert the endotracheal tube because of an anterior larynx, a stylet in the shape of a hockey

stick may be lubricated and inserted into the tube. Be sure the tip of the stylet does not protrude from the distal end. Remove the stylet once the cuff has been inflated. Generally the 21-cm mark in a female and the 23-cm mark in a male should be in line with the lower central incisors, thus helping to place the endotracheal tube in its correct position 3 to 4 cm above the carina.

7. Check for correct tube placement by observing for symmetry of chest wall expansion, auscultation of equal breath sounds in the anterior chest and absence of breath sounds in the epigastrium. A decrease of breath sounds in the left chest may indicate intubation of the right main-stem bronchus, and the tube should be pulled back 2 to 3 cm and rechecked. Maintenance of adequate hemoglobin saturation over a few minutes as documented on a pulse oximeter, as well as a typical capnograph tracing showing carbon dioxide return, are also useful in assessing correct tube placement.

8. Secure the tube to the skin over the maxilla using adhesive tape. In patients with beards or facial dressings, cloth tape often works better.

Follow-Up

1. A chest radiograph should be taken to confirm correct tube placement.

2. Ensure the tube is securely tied in place and has not shifted.

3. Monitor respiratory parameters frequently to ensure tube has not moved or become obstructed.

Bibliography

Eskuri SA: Complications of endotracheal intubation. In Faust RJ (ed): Anesthesiology Review, 2nd ed, pp 551–552. New York, Churchill Livingstone, 1994.

Marino PL: The ventilator-dependent patient. In The ICU Book, 2nd ed, pp 449–467. Baltimore, Williams & Wilkins, 1998.

Morgan GE Jr, Mikhail MS: Airway Management. In Morgan GE Jr, Mikhail MS (eds): Clinical Anesthesiology, 2nd ed, pp 50–72. East Norwalk, CT, Appleton & Lange, 1996.

Pfenninger JL, Fowler GC: Endotracheal Intubation: Procedures for Primary Care Physicians, pp 452–463. St. Louis, Mosby–Year Book, 1994.

Stone DJ, Gal TJ: Airway management. In Miller RD (ed): Anesthesia, 4th ed, vol 2, pp 1403–1435. New York, Churchill Livingstone, 1994.

43 Ventilator Support

John I. Kennedy, Jr.

Mechanical ventilation is a powerful tool that can provide support for respiratory function, allowing time for other therapy to yield its effect. The decision to use this tool must be made with careful reflection on the prognosis of the underlying disease and consideration of advance directives.

Indications and Goals

1. Respiratory failure: primary indication for ventilator support. Respiratory failure may take two forms that sometimes can coexist.
   a. Hypoxemic respiratory failure results when oxygenation is impaired by ventilation-perfusion imbalance, shunt, or diffusing impairment.
   b. Hypercapnic respiratory failure results from alveolar hypoventilation. A number of mechanisms may produce this result.
      (1) Decreased central nervous system drive may result in hypoventilation. A common example of this mechanism is sedative drug overdose.
      (2) Neuromuscular weakness (pump failure) can also result in hypoventilation. This may be due to primary neuromuscular diseases (e.g., myasthenia gravis, Guillain-Barré syndrome) or fatigue from increased workload (e.g., asthma, chronic obstructive pulmonary disease).
2. Relief of severe respiratory distress
3. Prevention or treatment of atelectasis
4. To permit the use of heavy sedation or neuromuscular blockade
5. To decrease intracranial pressure by therapeutic hyperventilation
6. To decrease oxygen consumption (e.g., in severe acute respiratory distress syndrome [ARDS], cardiogenic shock)
7. To stablize the chest wall (e.g., severe flail chest)

Modes

1. Standard modes
   a. Assist/control (A/C): In this mode, a predetermined volume is delivered when an inspiratory effort is sensed by the ventilator or whenever the respiratory rate falls below the backup rate. If large tidal volumes are used and/or tachypnea is present, respiratory alkalosis may develop, requiring the use of sedation or rebreathing dead space.
   b. Intermittent mandatory ventilation (IMV): Breaths of preset volume are delivered to the patient at the set rate. In contrast to A/C, the patient may also inspire spontaneously without assistance from the ventilator, with the rate and tidal volume being determined by the patient's effort. Some ventilators supply gas for the spontaneous breaths by way of a demand valve that can result in increased work of breathing.
   c. Pressure support ventilation: This mode may be used alone or, more commonly, in conjunction with IMV. In contrast to A/C and IMV, no volume is set. When an inspiratory effort is sensed, airway pressure is brought to the preset level and maintained until the patient's inspiratory flow rate falls. The delivered volume is therefore determined by the combination of the pressure setting, patient effort, and respiratory system compliance.
2. Additional (nonstandard) modes
   a. Pressure control ventilation (PCV): PCV differs from A/C and IMV by virtue of being pressure-limited rather than volume-limited. When an inspiratory effort is sensed (or rate falls below the preset value), flow is supplied until the preset pressure is reached. PCV limits peak airway pressure and may produce salutary effects on gas exchange in some patients (e.g., those with ARDS). The advantages of this mode may reside in the characteristics of the flow waveform (i.e., decelerating rather than square wave flow pattern). Thus, volume-cycled ventilation with a decelerating flow waveform may produce similar effects. PCV has also been used in conjunction with inverse ratio ventilation (PC-IRV), primarily in the support of severe ARDS. Mean airway pressure is increased in PC-IRV, and significant levels of intrinsic positive end-expiratory pressure (auto-PEEP) are typically produced. Thus the risk for barotrauma appears to be increased.
   b. High-frequency ventilation (HFV): Deliver-

ing low tidal volumes at very high rates (60 to 3000/minute), HFV may be useful in selected cases of refractory hypoxemia or with bronchopleural fistulas. Results have been more promising in pediatric patients than in adults.

c. Noninvasive ventilation using occlusive masks (i.e., nasal or full-face masks) can be effective in respiratory failure from neuromuscular disease or kyphoscoliosis and in some patients with chronic obstructive pulmonary disease. Improvements in these masks and their use make noninvasive support an attractive option, especially for patients who may improve rapidly with treatment. However, some patients tolerate the masks poorly, and aspiration may be a risk.

d. Alternative modes of ventilator operation include airway pressure release ventilation, proportional assist ventilation, and mandatory minute ventilation. The advantages and roles of these modes remain to be defined. Ventilation with the patient in prone position may improve oxygenation in some patients with ARDS. Partial liquid ventilation with perfluorocarbon compounds appears to be useful in some infants, but its utility in adults remains undefined.

Ventilator Settings

1. Fraction of inspired oxygen (FiO_2): In almost all situations, the initial FiO_2 should be 1.00. Subsequent downward adjustments in FiO_2 may then be made, guided by arterial blood gas analysis or pulse oximetry. The usual goal is to maintain alveolar partial pressure of oxygen (p_aO_2) equal to or greater than 60 mm Hg and oxygen saturation equal to or greater than 90 per cent with FiO_2 equal to or less than 0.50.

2. Tidal volume and rate: These parameters determine the minimum minute ventilation received. Most experts now recommend moderate tidal volumes of 5 to 8 ml/kg to minimize overdistention of alveoli and reduce the risk of barotrauma. The rate usually should be set in a physiologic range (8 to 16 breaths/minute). In patients with tachypnea, the work of breathing may be reduced by setting the rate at 2 to 4 breaths/minute below the spontaneous rate.

3. Flow rates; inspiratory/expiratory (I:E) ratio: Some ventilators allow flow rate to be set as an independent parameter. On other machines, the I:E ratio can be set, and the flow rate depends on the ventilatory rate, tidal volume, and I:E ratio. An inspiratory flow rate of 60 L/minute is adequate in most patients. Higher flow rates (80 to 100 L/minute) are often helpful in patients with severe airflow obstruction, allowing more time for expiration. When the I:E ratio must be set, typical settings are 1:3 or 1:2 (inspiratory per cent = 25 to 33).

4. Sensitivity of the ventilator should be adjusted to allow the patient to trigger the ventilator with the lowest pressure that avoids autotriggering of the machine. This can usually be accomplished at about -2 cm H_2O.

5. PEEP may improve p_aO_2 in some situations, particularly when terminal respiratory units are prone to collapse (e.g., ARDS), allowing FiO_2 to be reduced to nontoxic levels. Alternatively, PEEP may be adjusted in an effort to maximize systemic oxygen transport. The definition of optimal PEEP remains controversial. PEEP should be applied in increments of 2 to 5 cm H_2O and the response assessed promptly after each increase. When severe airflow obstruction exists or when IRV is used, auto-PEEP may develop. Auto-PEEP may go unrecognized and can contribute to hemodynamic compromise and respiratory distress.

Complications

1. Artificial airway complications: Endotracheal tubes may become kinked or occluded by secretions. These devices may also produce injury to the upper airway. Securing the tube so that movement is limited and using the lowest cuff pressure that achieves adequate seal help to minimize injury.

2. Ventilator malfunction: Modern ventilators are remarkably efficient and trouble-free, but problems do occur. Whenever a patient develops distress on the ventilator, it is prudent to assume that there is a malfunction and remove the patient from the machine and manually ventilate. The ease with which the patient is ventilated and the initial response to manual ventilation can provide important information in a matter of seconds.

3. Barotrauma: Disruption of alveoli from overdistention can lead to pneumomediastinum, subcutaneous emphysema, pneumoperitoneum, and pneumothorax. Of these, only pneumothorax is typically associated with important hemodynamic effects. Pneumoperitoneum may raise concern about a possible ruptured intra-abdominal viscus but is otherwise benign. Careful attention should be paid to limiting pressure and volume delivered in an effort to minimize the risk of barotrauma.

4. Cardiovascular effects: Intrathoracic pressure becomes elevated with positive-pressure venti-

lation, impeding venous return to the heart. This can result in significant decreases in cardiac output, which may be manifested as hypotension. Renal hypoperfusion and hepatic congestion may also result.

5. Infection: Nosocomial pneumonia is an important and serious complication of ventilator support. Elevating the patient's head and avoiding elevation of gastric pH may reduce the risk of ventilator-associated pneumonia. Prompt weaning and extubation are the most important preventive maneuvers.

Weaning

1. Timing: Selecting the appropriate time involves the assessment of multiple factors, including the following:

   a. Underlying disease: The initial problem should be improved or stabilized.

   b. Level of consciousness: The patient should be awake, alert, and cooperative. Sedative medications should be withheld before planned weaning.

   c. Gas exchange: p_aO_2 should be greater than or equal to 60 mm Hg, with FiO_2 less than or equal to 0.40.

   d. Ventilatory mechanics: Multiple parameters have been used to predict successful weaning, such as vital capacity and negative inspiratory force. Respiratory rate divided by tidal volume (L) less than 100 may be the best single parameter.

2. Techniques: A variety of approaches have been used for discontinuing ventilator support. Traditional weaning involves allowing the patient to breath spontaneously by way of a T-tube gas supply for a period of time (up to 2 hours) while observing for distress or desaturation. Alternatively, progressive reduction in IMV and/or pressure support may be used. The relative advantages of different approaches are unproven. Consistently utilizing a standardized protocol for weaning probably shortens the time on mechanical ventilation. The physician should be prepared to reinstitute support if needed.

Bibliography

For a more detailed general overview of ventilator support, see
Tobin MJ: Mechanical ventilation. N Engl J Med 1994; 330:1056–1061.

For detailed, specific recommendations and guidelines on ventilator support, see
Slutsky AS: Mechanical ventilation. Chest 1993;104: 1833–1859.

For more information about newer modes of ventilation, see
MacIntyre NR: New modes of mechanical ventilation. Clin Chest Med 1996;17:411–421.

For more information about techniques of noninvasive ventilation, see
Hillberg RE, Johnson DC: Noninvasive ventilation. N Engl J Med 1997;337:1746–1752.

For more information about discontinuation of ventilator support, see
Lessard MR, Brochard LJ: Weaning from ventilatory support. Clin Chest Med 1996;17:475–489.

Indications

1. Prolonged need for ventilatory support by way of an endotracheal tube
2. Need for ventilatory support in a patient who cannot be safely intubated nasally or orally or who poorly tolerates an orotracheal or a nasotracheal tube
3. Obstruction of the airway in which oral or nasal intubation of the trachea cannot be performed. Examples include tumor; bilateral vocal cord paralysis; laryngeal fracture; subglottic, glottic, or supraglottic stenosis; and laryngeal edema or hematoma.
4. Prolonged need for tracheobronchial toilet

Contraindications

1. Cricothyrotomy when laryngeal fracture is suspected
2. Cricothyrotomy in cases of subglottic airway obstruction
3. Acute inflammation of the trachea and coagulopathy are relative contraindications to elective tracheostomy.

Preparation

1. Ensure all necessary equipment is available to perform the procedure.
2. Have suction, electrocautery, and adequate lighting available.
3. A shoulder roll, 3 to 7 inches in diameter, is placed beneath the patient's shoulders, hyperextending the neck. This greatly facilitates tracheostomy and cricothyrotomy, as well as tracheostomy tube changing.
4. The skin is washed, dried, and painted with antiseptic solution.

Equipment

1. Tracheostomy tube
   a. A tube with a cuff that can be inflated after insertion prevents the flow of blood from the fresh tracheotomy/cricothyrotomy wound into the airway as well as allowing for positive-pressure ventilation.
   b. If no tracheostomy tube is available, a standard endotracheal tube is an emergency substitute.
2. An emergency tracheostomy tray should include an appropriate assortment of retractors, clamps, scalpel handle and blades, suction cannulas and catheters, tracheal hooks, tracheal dilators, sponges, towels, suture material, needles, syringes, and local anesthetic.

Anesthesia

The skin and subcutaneous tissues are infiltrated with lidocaine 1% with epinephrine for local anesthesia and vasoconstriction to decrease bleeding. Tracheostomy and cricothyrotomy can be performed with or without general anesthesia; however, in an emergent situation where the trachea cannot be intubated from above the larynx, the patient must not be significantly sedated.

Precautions

1. Creating a surgical airway in a prepared environment with experienced personnel is preferred.
2. Palpate the neck carefully for landmarks and pathology that may impede the surgical procedure (i.e., a high-riding innominate artery crossing the desired tracheostomy site, a thyroid isthmus mass, or deviation of the trachea caused by tumor or previous surgery).

Technique

Cricothyrotomy

1. Make a 4-cm vertical incision through the skin into the subcutaneous fat in the midline of the neck from the thyroid notch to the bottom of the cricoid cartilage.

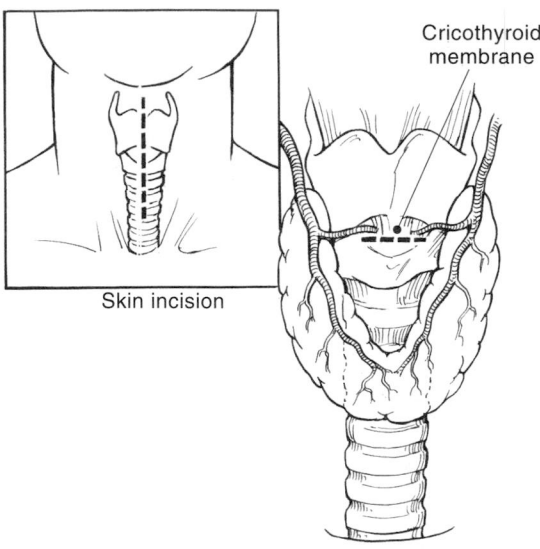

Cricothyroid membrane

Skin incision

2. Separate the investing cervical fascial and strap muscles in the midline, vertically exposing the cricoid cartilage and thyroid lamina.

3. Incise cricothyroid membrane with a horizontal incision, insert a curved Kelly clamp into the airway, and open it to create an adequate lumen to accept the tube. Insert tube into the lumen of the airway.

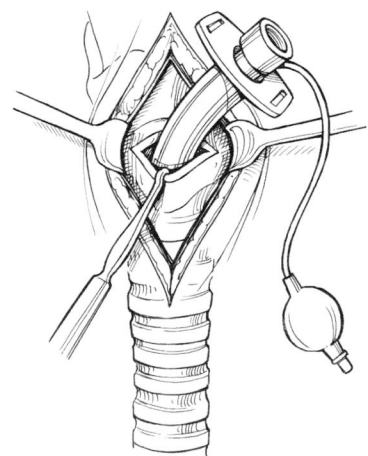

Tracheostomy

1. Create a transverse incision 4 cm in length, midway between the cricoid cartilage and the sternal notch and carry it through the skin and subcutaneous fat to the deep cervical fascia.

2. Dissect through the investing fascia, then between the sternohyoid muscles and sternothyroid muscles in the midline to expose the thyroid isthmus.

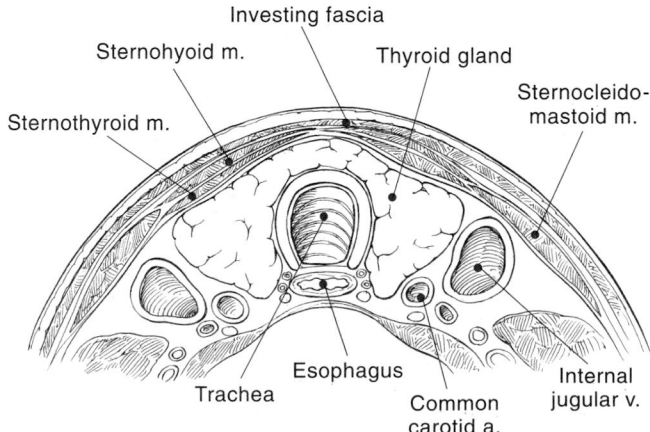

Investing fascia

Sternohyoid m.

Thyroid gland

Sternocleido-mastoid m.

Sternothyroid m.

Esophagus

Internal jugular v.

Trachea

Common carotid a.

3. The thyroid isthmus usually overlies the optimal tracheostomy site. It can be retracted superiorly after ligating or cauterizing the inferior thyroid plexus of veins. Alternatively, clamp and divide the thyroid isthmus and apply a suture ligature.

4. The tracheal hook hooks the cricoid cartilage or the first tracheal ring to retract the trachea superiorly and anteriorly.

5. Identify the second or third tracheal ring and make 5- to 7-mm horizontal cuts above and below it. Clamp the segment of tracheal ring and remove a 5- to 7-mm portion of this anterior ring.

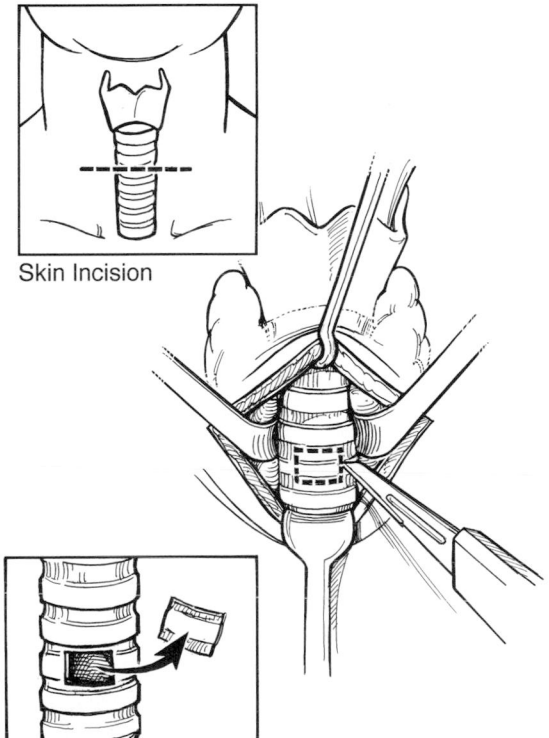

Skin Incision

6. Using a clamp or tracheostomy dilator, gently dilate the tracheal hole. If the tracheostomy is still too small, the horizontal incisions of the trachea can be extended.

7. If an endotracheal tube is present, partially withdraw it so it does not interfere with passage of the tracheostomy tube into the tracheostomy site. This allows the team to readvance the tube and ventilate the patient if insertion of the tube is unsuccessful.

8. Insert the tracheostomy tube with obturator in place into the airway, and inflate the cuff. Remove the obturator, insert the inner cannula of the tracheostomy tube, connect the ventilating tubing, and inflate the cuff.

9. Ausculate the chest bilaterally for air movement.

10. Place tracheostomy ties around the patient's neck and secure them tight enough so that only two fingers can be inserted between the tracheostomy ties and the patient's neck.

PEARLS

- The retraction can alter the location of the trachea. Palpate the trachea! If the location of the trachea remains uncertain, aspirate for air with a needle and syringe.

- Patients often have pain despite an initial infiltration with local anesthesia. Use additional local anesthetic intraoperatively.

- Adequate hemostasis should be attained at each step in tracheostomy.

- The superoanterior stabilization of the trachea by the tracheal hook helps to prevent collapse of the trachea and "false passage" of the endotracheal tube into the soft tissues of the mediastinum during tube insertion.

- Decannulation in the perioperative period can be life-threatening. Do not use Velcro straps in the first week. Use permanent 3-0 or larger sutures to secure the face plate of the tracheostomy tube to the skin of the anterior neck in addition to applying tracheostomy ties. Remove the sutures at 1 week.

- Although not described here, percutaneous dilation tracheostomy is a reasonable and effective alternative to this description of a classic tracheostomy. It is not a reasonable alternative tracheostomy for patients who cannot be intubated from the mouth or nose.

Follow-Up

1. Obtain postoperative chest radiographs in all difficult or emergency procedures.

2. Postoperative hemorrhage is usually controlled with oxidizing packing agents or standard packing gauze.

3. Massive bleeding from the tracheostomy site requires surgical intervention.

4. Standard nursing care of tracheostomy tubes includes cleaning of the inner cannula, cleaning of the tracheostomy site, irrigation and suctioning of the trachea, changing of the tracheostomy sponge dressing, and changing of the tracheostomy ties.

5. If the patient requires more than a 1-week duration of endotracheal tube support, an emergent cricothyrotomy should be converted to a standard tracheostomy.

6. Permanent decannulation should not be performed until the patient's upper airway has been assessed to be normal.

Bibliography

Brofeldt BT, Panacek EA, Richards JR: An easy cricothyrotomy approach: the rapid four-step technique. Acad Emerg Med 1996;3:1060–1063.

Loré JM Jr: Tracheostomy. In Loré JM Jr (ed): An Atlas of Head and Neck Surgery, 3rd ed, pp 811–818. Philadelphia, WB Saunders Company, 1988.

Myers EN, Stool SE, Johnson JT (eds): Tracheostomy. New York, Churchill Livingstone, 1985.

Powell DM, Price PD, Forrest LA: Review of percutaneous tracheostomy. Laryngoscope 1998;108:170–177.

Seid AB, Gluckman JL: Tracheostomy. In Paparella MM, Shumrick DA, Gluckman JL, et al (eds): Otolaryngology, 3rd ed, pp 2429–2437. Philadelphia, WB Saunders Company, 1991.

44 Pneumothorax

Joshua O. Benditt

Etiology

1. Pneumothorax (air within the pleural space) is classified etiologically as either spontaneous (occurring without immediate antecedent trauma) or traumatic. Spontaneous pneumothorax is further divided into either primary (occurring in a previously healthy person) or secondary (occurring in a person with an underlying and predisposing condition).

2. Spontaneous pneumothorax
   a. Primary
   b. Secondary
      (1) Pulmonary diseases
         (a) Airway diseases
            (i) Chronic obstructive pulmonary disease
            (ii) Bronchiectasis
            (iii) Asthma
            (iv) Cystic fibrosis
         (b) Interstitial diseases
            (i) Interstitial pulmonary fibrosis
            (ii) Sarcoidosis
            (iii) Collagen vascular diseases
            (iv) Pneumoconioses
         (c) Infections
            (i) Pneumonia (bacterial, fungal, and parasitic)
            (ii) Lung abscess
            (iii) Tuberculosis
         (d) Neoplastic
            (i) Lung cancer
            (ii) Metastatic cancer
      (2) Extrapulmonary causes
         (a) Catamenial pneumothorax (related to menses)
         (b) Esophageal rupture
         (c) Drug abuse (e.g., inhaled use of marijuana and cocaine)
         (d) Neonatal pneumothorax

3. Traumatic
   a. Iatrogenic (e.g., central line placement)
   b. Noniatrogenic (e.g., stab wound to chest)

Symptoms

1. Predominant symptoms are chest pain that is localized to the side of the pneumothorax (usually pleuritic in nature) and dyspnea.

2. The severity of symptoms is related to the size of the pneumothorax, being more severe in larger pneumothoraces.

3. Rarely, the patient may be asymptomatic.

Key Symptoms

- Chest pain
- Dyspnea

Clinical Findings

1. The physical findings are related to the size of the pneumothorax. The larger the pneumothorax, the more likely physical indications are to be found.

2. Physical findings
   a. Respiratory system
      (1) Decreased or absent breath sounds
      (2) Normal or hyperresonant chest percussion note
      (3) Unilateral enlargement of the chest
      (4) Absent tactile fremitus
      (5) Tracheal deviation (away from the side of the pneumothorax) in tension pneumothorax
   b. Cardiac system
      (1) Tachycardia
      (2) Hypotension (in tension pneumothorax)

Key Signs

- Hyperresonant chest percussion note
- Decreased or absent breath sounds
- Tachycardia

Tests

1. Chest radiography is the most important test in

evaluating pneumothorax. The radiographic appearance is a sharp line representing the lung edge that usually runs parallel to the chest wall and is separated from it by a radiolucent area without lung markings, which represents air in the pleural space.

   a. Small pneumothoraces may be difficult to diagnose.

   b. In a complete pneumothorax, the radiographic appearance is a grapefruit-sized opacity at the hilum.

2. An arterial blood gas analysis should be obtained in more severe pneumothoraces (greater than 20 per cent of the volume of the hemithorax) or in patients with underlying lung disease. In these situations, significant hypoxemia may be present secondary to intrapulmonary shunting.

3. Electrocardiographic abnormalities

   a. Left-sided pneumothoraces can present with findings that mimic an acute anterior non–Q-wave myocardial infarction.

     (1) Right axis deviation

     (2) Decreased R-wave amplitude in the precordial leads

     (3) Decreased QRS complex amplitude

     (4) Precordial T-wave inversion

   b. These changes should normalize if the electrocardiogram is taken in the upright position.

Key Test

Chest radiography

Differential Diagnosis

1. Lung-related disorders

   a. Pleuritis

   b. Pneumonia

   c. Pulmonary embolus

   d. Exacerbation of chronic obstructive pulmonary disease or asthma

   e. Pulmonary infarct

2. Chest wall–related

   a. Rib fracture

   b. Herpes zoster that affects a thoracic dermatome

   c. Bursitis of the shoulder

3. Cardiovascular system–related

   a. Pericarditis or pericardial effusion

   b. Myocardial infarction

   c. Dissecting aortic aneurysm

   d. Myocarditis

4. Intra-abdominal processes

   a. Cholecystitis

   b. Pancreatitis

   c. Perforated peptic ulcer

   d. Subphrenic abscess

Treatment

1. All patients should initially receive high-flow oxygen to increase the rate of resorption of air from the pleural space.

2. Observation alone

   a. Mild symptoms or asymptomatic

   b. No significant underlying lung pathology

   c. Pneumothorax less than 15 per cent of the volume of the hemithorax

3. Needle aspiration of pneumothorax

   a. Moderate symptoms

   b. Pneumothorax greater than 15 per cent of the volume of the hemithorax

4. Tube thoracostomy

   a. Significant respiratory distress

   b. Significant underlying lung pathology

   c. Bilateral pneumothoraces

   d. Traumatic pneumothorax (especially with hemothorax)

5. Tension pneumothorax (pleural air under positive pressure with potential for hemodynamic compromise) requires the following:

   a. Emergent placement of a large-bore (14-gauge) catheter in the second intercostal space on the affected side for decompression of the thorax

   b. Tube thoracostomy after the thorax is decompressed with the 14-gauge catheter

Key Treatment

Emergent decompression of the tension pneumothorax with a large-bore catheter

Follow-Up

1. The patient treated with observation or needle aspiration

   a. Follow-up chest radiography in 6 hours. If the pneumothorax has not enlarged, the patient can go home.

   b. Follow-up chest radiography in 24 hours

2. The patient treated with tube thoracostomy
   a. Admit to hospital
   b. Follow-up chest radiography immediately after a chest tube is placed
   c. Follow-up chest radiography in 24 hours
3. Recurrent pneumothoraces may require definitive surgical therapy (e.g., bullectomy, pleurodesis).

Bibliography

Jantz MA, Pierson DJ: Pneumothorax and barotrauma. Clin Chest Med 1994;15:75–92.

Light R: Pneumothorax. In Murray JF, Nadel JA (eds): Textbook of Respiratory Medicine, 2nd ed, vol 2, pp 2193–2208. Philadelphia, WB Saunders Company, 1994.

Massard G, Thomas P, Wihlm JM: Minimally invasive management of first and recurrent pneumothorax. Ann Thorac Surg 1998;66:592–599.

McEwen JI: Pleural disease. In Rosen P, Barkin RM (eds): Emergency Medicine—Concepts and Clinical Practice, 3rd ed, vol 2, pp 1121–1139. St Louis, Mosby-Yearbook, 1992.

Wait MA, Estera A: Changing clinical spectrum of spontaneous pneumothorax. Am J Surg 1992;164:528–531.

Indications

1. Pneumothorax—either secondary to trauma or spontaneous—causing respiratory distress
2. Hemothorax
3. Large pleural effusion causing respiratory distress
4. Empyema

Contraindications

1. Small pneumothorax that is not causing respiratory distress and is followed with serial chest radiographs
2. Pleura adherent to the chest wall
3. Coagulopathy (relative contraindication)

Preparation

1. Explain the procedure to the patient and obtain informed consent.
2. Place the patient in the lateral decubitus position with the involved side up.
3. Prepare and drape the area of the fifth or sixth intercostal space in the midaxillary line. The midaxillary line is used because it is the least muscular part of the thorax.

Equipment

1. Skin preparation (e.g., povidone-iodine [Betadine])
2. Sterile gloves, mask, goggles, and fenestrated drape
3. 22-gauge, 1½-inch needle with 10-ml syringe
4. Lidocaine 1%, 20 ml
5. No. 10 scalpel blade and handle
6. Curved clamp
7. Chest tube: type and size depend on the purpose and preference
   a. Pneumothorax: No. 22 to No. 24 French straight
   b. Hemothorax or pleural effusion: No. 32 to No. 36 French straight or right-angle
8. Multichamber water-seal suction

9. Needle holder
10. Skin suture
11. Suture scissors
12. Petroleum gauze
13. Sterile sponges
14. Elastic adhesive bandage

Anesthesia

1. Use a 22-gauge, 1½-inch needle to infiltrate the subcutaneous tissue in a wheal with lidocaine 1%. This should be done along the top edge of the involved rib to avoid the neurovascular bundle that lies inferiorly.
2. Slowly advance the needle, infiltrating along the costal periosteum and down to the parietal pleura with 5 to 10 ml of lidocaine.
3. The pleural space is reached when air or fluid can be aspirated.

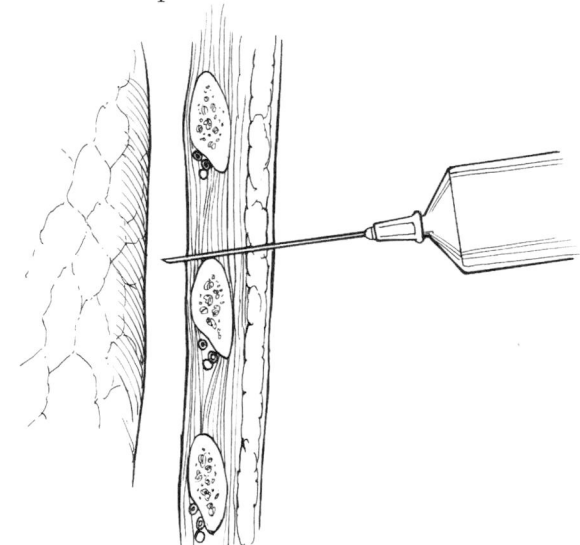

Precautions

1. Do not go lower than the fifth intercostal space to avoid perforation of the diaphragm or splenic or hepatic injury.
2. Avoid using trocars for this procedure because their use can increase the risk of injury to the pulmonary parenchyma.

Technique

1. Make a small incision through skin, fat, and muscle just superior to the lower rib of the interspace.

2. Use a curved clamp to enlarge the incision and perforate into the pleural space. Avoid lung injury by gripping the clamp so that the distance from hand to tip is just greater than the chest wall thickness. A gush of blood and/or air is to be expected on perforating the pleura.

3. Insert a finger to enlarge the tract and to confirm entry into the pleural space. Palpate the pleural surface to clean away adhesions and clots, and to confirm that the lung is not adherent to the chest wall.

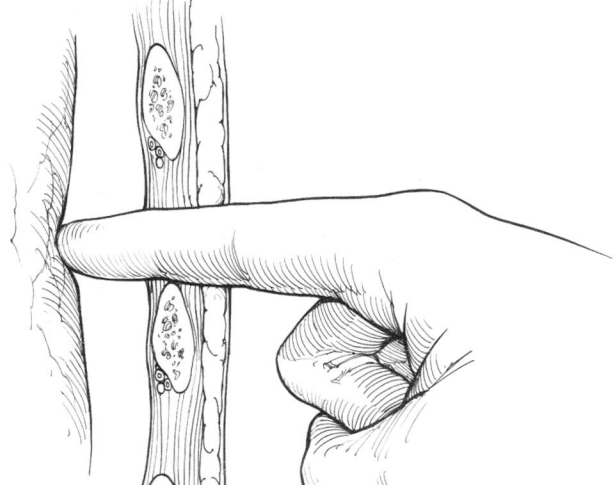

4. Grasp the chest tube with the clamp and guide it into the pleural space. Direct the tube posteriorly and toward the apex for a pneumothorax. For fluid drainage, the tube is directed posteriorly to reside in the most dependent position possible. Ensure that all drainage holes are inside the pleural space.

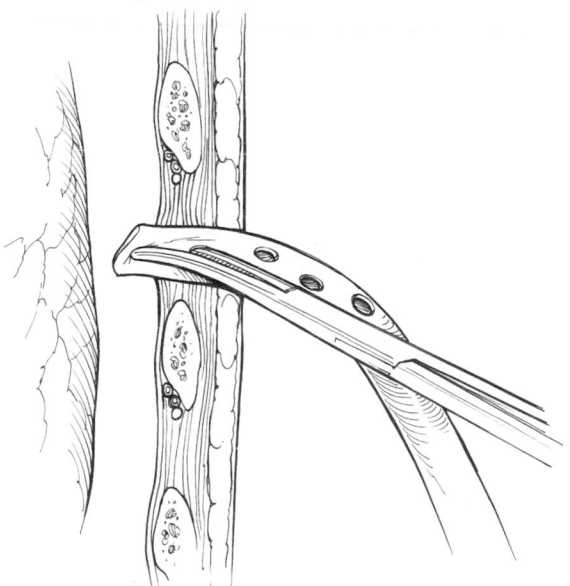

5. Attach the tube to a multichamber water-seal suction with 20 cm H_2O suction and tape the connections.

6. Have the patient cough to confirm that bubbles form at the water-seal level to ensure proper tube placement and patency of the system.

7. Place a suture through the skin and knot, leaving long ends to wrap and tie securely around the tube.

8. Place petroleum gauze around the tube exit site to make an airtight seal. Apply a split 2 × 2 sponge around the tube and apply benzoin to the surrounding skin. Place two strips of 1-inch tape over the sponge, allowing the tape to self-adhere for about 1 inch at the level of the tube. Secure the tube to these pieces of tape with additional tape. Ensure that the tube stays in place by adding tape strips perpendicular to the initial strips.

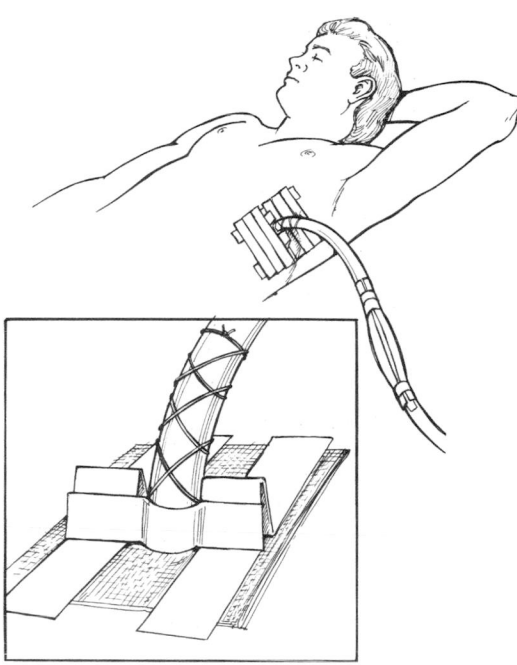

Follow-Up

Obtain a chest radiograph to confirm the position of the tube and to assess resolution of the pneumothorax or hemothorax.

 Bibliography

Arsenio JA, Barton JM, Worsetler LA, et al: Trauma: a systemic approach to management. Am Fam Physician 1988;38:96–104.

Miller AC, Harvey JE: Guidelines for the management of a spontaneous pneumothorax. Br Med J 1993;307: 114–116.

In Moore EE, Mattox KL, Feliciano DV (eds): Trauma, 2nd ed, pp 361–362. East Norwalk, CT, Appleton & Lange, 1991.

Spillane RM, Shepard JD, DeLuca SA: Radiographic aspects of pneumothorax. Am Fam Physician 1995;51: 459–464.

Tomlinson MA, Treasure T: Insertion of a chest drain: how to do it. Br J Hosp Med 1997;58:248–252.

45 Pleural Effusions

Linda L. Kuribayashi

Etiology

The accumulation of fluid in the pleural space can result from a number of mechanisms.

1. Increased hydrostatic pressure (e.g., congestive heart failure)
2. Decreased oncotic pressure (e.g., nephrotic syndrome with hypoalbuminemia)
3. Increased capillary permeability (e.g., pneumonia)
4. Decreased lymphatic drainage (e.g., carcinoma, tuberculosis)
5. Entry of fluid from a source outside the pleura (e.g., blood from trauma, chyle from rupture of the thoracic duct, crystalloid from a misplaced central line)

Symptoms

1. May be asymptomatic
2. Dyspnea
3. Pleuritic chest pain
4. Cough (often nonproductive)
5. Symptoms secondary to associated illnesses

Key Symptoms

- Often asymptomatic
- Dyspnea
- Pleuritic chest pain
- Cough

Clinical Findings

1. Physical examination reveals dullness to percussion, decreased fremitus, and decreased breath sounds at the location of the effusion.
2. Radiographic examination reveals a homogeneous density.
   a. Chest radiographs: Free-flowing pleural fluid responds to gravity and causes blunting of the costophrenic angle. A meniscus sign is frequently present.
   b. Lateral decubitus radiographs: Small amounts of free-flowing pleural fluid can be seen layered along the dependent portion of the chest wall. Loculated pleural effusions do not change position.
   c. Computerized tomography: Small pleural effusions can be visualized and aspirated under computerized tomographic guidance.
   d. Ultrasonography: Loculated effusions can be located and aspirated using ultrasound guidance.

Key Signs

- Dullness to percussion
- Decreased breath sounds

Tests

1. Pleural fluid analysis
   a. General appearance (e.g., pus would indicate empyema, a milky appearance may indicate a chylothorax, clear yellow fluid is consistent with transudates and some exudates)
   b. Protein: Leakage of protein into the pleural space occurs with inflammation. A pleural fluid protein-serum protein ratio greater than 0.5 is characteristic of an exudate (see Table 45–1).
   c. Lactate dehydrogenase (LDH): A pleural fluid LDH–serum LDH ratio greater than 0.6 is consistent with an exudate. An absolute pleural fluid LDH greater than 200 IU is another criterion for an exudate.
   d. Cell count and differential
      (1) Leukocytosis: Elevated white blood cell count ($>1000/\mu l$) indicates inflammation and can be associated with infection, connective tissue disease, and pulmonary

TABLE 45–1. CRITERIA FOR DIAGNOSING AN EXUDATE

One of the following:
1. Pleural fluid protein/serum protein > 0.5
2. Pleural fluid LDH/serum LDH > 0.6
3. Pleural fluid LDH > 200 IU

infarction. The presence of pus indicates empyema.

    (2) Red blood cell count: Grossly hemorrhagic effusions are associated with trauma, carcinoma, pulmonary infarction, and tuberculosis.

  e. Culture and smear: bacterial, acid-fast bacillus, and fungal

  f. pH: Low pH (<7.30) is associated with empyema, carcinoma, connective tissue disease, tuberculosis, and esophageal rupture.

  g. Glucose: Low glucose level (pleural fluid glucose–serum glucose ratio <0.5) is seen more frequently in rheumatoid pleuritis and empyema.

  h. Amylase: Elevated amylase level (pleural fluid amylase–serum amylase ratio >2) is associated with pancreatitis and esophageal rupture.

  i. Cytology: Can be diagnostic for carcinoma, systemic lupus erythematosus (LE cells)

  j. Lipids: Elevated lipid levels are seen with chylothorax.

2. Pleural biopsy (closed or open) can be diagnostic for carcinoma and granulomatous infections.

3. Bronchoscopy can help diagnose carcinoma and infectious causes in pleural effusions in which the diagnosis is still unclear after thoracentesis.

4. Thoracoscopy can help localize pleural disease and improve biopsy yield.

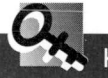

Key Test

Thoracentesis is the definitive test.

Differential Diagnosis

1. Transudates
  a. Congestive heart failure
  b. Cirrhosis with ascites
  c. Nephrotic syndrome
  d. Hypoalbuminemia
  e. Peritoneal dialysis
  f. Superior vena cava obstruction
  g. Subclavian catheter misplacement
  h. Early mediastinal carcinoma (rare)
  i. Pulmonary embolism (rare)
  j. Constrictive pericarditis
  k. Atelectasis

2. Exudates
  a. Parapneumonic effusion
    (1) Bacterial (including tuberculosis)
    (2) Viral
    (3) Fungal
    (4) Parasitic
  b. Empyema
    (1) Bacterial (including tuberculosis)
    (2) Fungal
  c. Pulmonary embolism and infarction
  d. Carcinoma
  e. Uremia
  f. Post–myocardial infarction
  g. Trauma (hemothorax)
  h. Connective tissue disease
    (1) Rheumatoid arthritis
    (2) Systemic lupus erythematosus
  i. Gastrointestinal
    (1) Pancreatitis
    (2) Esophageal rupture
    (3) Liver abscess
  j. Drug reactions (e.g., nitrofurantoin, dantrolene [Dantrium])
  k. Meigs' syndrome
  l. Chylothorax
  m. Sarcoidosis

Treatment

1. The primary treatment is therapy for the underlying disease process.

2. Unstable patients with severe dyspnea may require therapeutic thoracentesis in addition to treating the underlying cause. Removal of more than 1.5 liters of pleural fluid during a single thoracentesis is associated with the risk of re-expansion pulmonary edema.

3. Occasionally drainage by way of chest tubes or other surgical drainage procedures is required (e.g., empyema).

4. Recurrent, symptomatic pleural effusions in which the underlying disease process cannot be adequately treated (e.g., cancer) may benefit from pleurodesis.

Key Treatment

Treatment of the underlying disease process

Follow-Up

1. Appropriate follow-up is determined by the underlying cause.

2. Serial chest radiographs are often helpful in evaluating treatment response.

Bibliography

Berkman N, Kramer MR: Diagnostic tests in pleural effusion—an update. Postgrad Med J 1993;69:12–18.

Light RW: Pleural effusions. In Murray JF, Nadel JA (eds): Textbook of Respiratory Medicine, 2nd ed, vol 2, pp 2164–2192. Philadelphia, WB Saunders Company, 1994.

Mattison LE, Coppage L, Alderman DF, et al: Pleural effusions in the medical ICU: prevalence, causes, and clinical implications. Chest 1997;111:1018–1023.

Muller NL: Imaging the pleura. Radiology 1993;186:297–309.

Vices M, Porcel JM, Vicente de Vera M, et al: A study of Light's criteria and possible modifications for distinguishing exudative from transudative pleural effusions. Chest 1996;106:1503–1507.

Thoracentesis is literally the "puncture of the thorax." It is a relatively safe procedure with low morbidity, and also has considerable diagnostic and therapeutic importance.

Indications
1. Diagnosis of a new pleural effusion or one of unknown etiology (diagnostic)
2. Drainage of a pleural effusion in a symptomatic patient (therapeutic)
3. Drainage of a small pneumothorax (therapeutic)

Contraindications
1. Patient refusal or inability to cooperate with the procedure
2. Overlying soft tissue infection at the point of skin puncture
3. Coagulopathy (relative contraindication)

Preparation
1. Confirm the diagnosis of a pleural effusion or small pneumothorax with radiographs (posteroanterior and lateral chest radiographs are required, with decubitus films if necessary). Approximately 300 ml of fluid is necessary to visualize a pleural effusion on a chest radiograph.
2. Ultrasound may be helpful in localizing the pleural effusion if it is small and difficult to detect clinically or with radiographs.
3. Obtain the patient's informed consent prior to the procedure.

Equipment
A commercial tray such as the Pleura-Seal Thoracentesis Kit may be used, or the following items can be assembled for the procedure:
1. 10-ml Luer-Lok syringe
2. 25-gauge 1-inch needle: for intradermal and subcutaneous anesthesia
3. 22-gauge 1½-inch needle: for intercostal and pleural anesthesia
4. Antiseptic solution (povidone-iodine solution [Betadine])
5. Sterile 4 × 4-inch gauze pads
6. Sterile gloves
7. Sterile fenestrated drape
8. Nonfenestrated sterile drape
9. 10 ml of 1% lidocaine
10. Two curved clamps
11. Three specimen collection tubes
12. 14-gauge 2-inch needle with optional intracath: for fluid removal
13. 18-gauge 2-inch needle: for air removal
14. One three-way stopcock
15. 60-ml Luer-Lok syringe
16. Tubing set with an aspiration/discharge device and collecting bag, *or*
17. Tubing set with an 18-gauge needle and a vacuum bottle
18. Adhesive bandage

Anesthesia
Anesthesia is provided using a local injection of 10 ml of 1% lidocaine with infiltration of the skin, intercostal muscle, and parietal pleura.

Precautions
1. Provide supplemental oxygen before, during, and after the procedure.
2. The approach of the needle into the pleural space should be over the top of the rib just below the level of the effusion. This will ensure that you avoid traumatizing the intercostal neurovascular bundle that lies inferior to each rib.
3. Be cautious not to penetrate the visceral pleura and induce a pneumothorax.
4. Thoracentesis performed below the eighth intercostal space carries the risk of peritoneal perforation.
5. Removal of more than 1500 ml of pleural fluid may infrequently result in the development of re-expansion pulmonary edema.

Technique
1. Place the patient in an upright seated position, leaning forward over a Mayo stand. Locate the pleural effusion by finding dullness to percussion of the chest, loss of tactile fremitus, and decreased breath sounds. Mark the upper and lower margins of the effusion. The entry into the pleural cavity will be over *either* the uppermost rib below the level of the effusion, or the eighth rib, whichever is lowest, and approxi-

mately midway between the posterior axillary line and the paraspinous muscles.

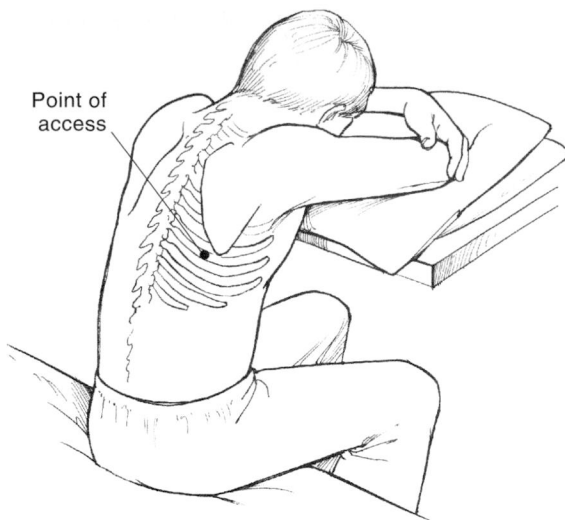

Point of access

The location of entry may be marked with a skin marker, or by indentation of the skin with the needle cap.

2. Prepare the site of entry using an antiseptic solution, don sterile gloves, and place the fenestrated drape on the back of the patient. The nonfenestrated drape can be placed on the bed or on a Mayo stand in close proximity. Draw 1% lidocaine into a 10-ml syringe and administer both intradermally and subcutaneously using the 25-gauge needle. By changing to a 22-gauge needle on the same syringe, deeper anesthesia can then be administered. As the needle is advanced, it should be "walked" over the rib.

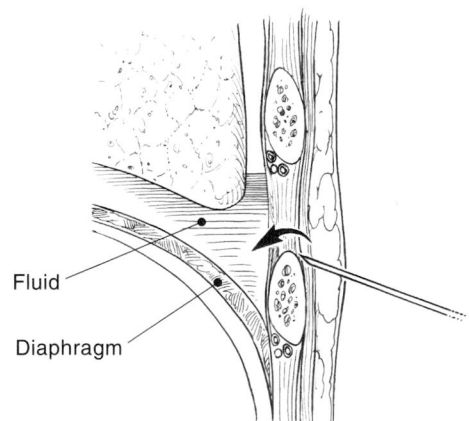

Fluid

Diaphragm

Continue to aspirate as you advance the needle, and, when fluid is returned, mark the depth of the needle at the skin by placing a curved clamp on the needle.

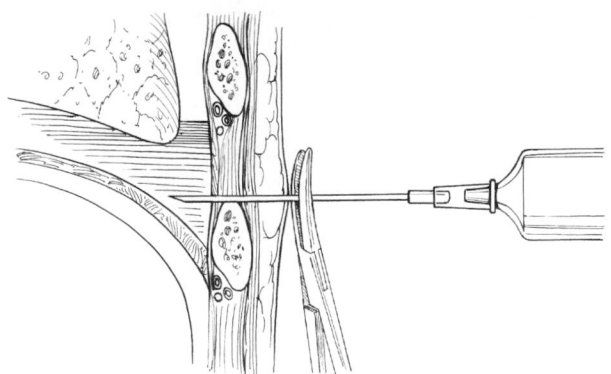

If no fluid is obtained, you may attempt the same procedure at the next higher intercostal space. If air is returned, attempt the procedure at the next lower intercostal space.

3. Two common techniques can now be used to drain fluid from the pleural space. First, using a 14-gauge needle, place the second curved clamp on the needle at the same depth as the clamp that was placed on the 22-gauge needle used to inject the lidocaine. Insert the 14-gauge needle at the entry site, being careful to aspirate as you advance the needle until pleural fluid is returned. At this point, remove the syringe and thread a catheter through the needle into the pleural space.

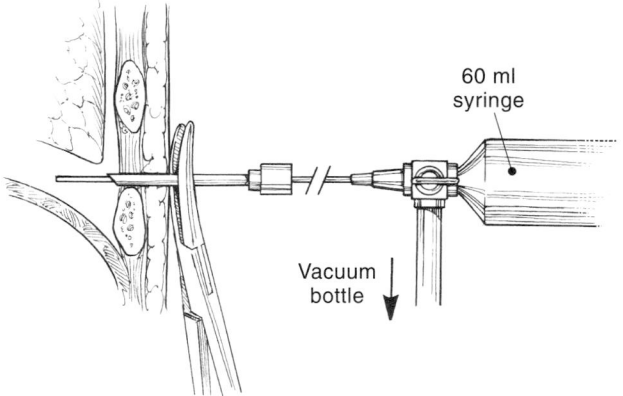

60 ml syringe

Vacuum bottle

Alternatively, an introducer needle with an overlying catheter can be introduced at the entry site and advanced until fluid is returned. The catheter can then be advanced over the introducer into the pleural space. Remove the introducer while the catheter remains in the pleural space.

4. Attach a 60-ml syringe to either system and obtain pleural fluid for analysis. If a larger effusion is present, a tubing system can be attached via an 18-gauge needle to a vacuum bottle. Not more than 1500 ml of pleural fluid should be removed in any single procedure.

5. Upon completion of the thoracentesis, remove the needle or catheter while the patient is ex-

haling, and place an adhesive dressing over the site of entry.

> **Note**
>
> For the removal of air in a patient with a small pneumothorax, the patient should be in the supine position with the head of the bed elevated approximately 30 to 45 degrees. The approach should then be directed at the second intercostal space, just lateral to the mid-clavicular line, because this minimizes the potential for traumatizing the internal mammary vessels.

Follow-Up

1. Obtain a stat chest radiograph after any attempted thoracentesis in order to assess for an iatrogenic pneumothorax, which occurs in 5 to 20 per cent of procedures.

2. Encourage slow, deep respirations.

3. Supplemental oxygen should be continued because of possible hypoxemia, which occurs secondary to a ventilation-perfusion mismatch in the newly expanded lung.

4. Watch for signs of blood loss resulting from hemothorax.

5. Send pleural fluid for appropriate studies and analysis:

   a. To differentiate a transudative process from an exudative process, obtain both pleural fluid and serum for lactate dehydrogenase and protein levels.

   b. If an exudate is present, consider the following additional studies: glucose, amylase, pH, cell count and differential, Gram's stain, aerobic and anaerobic cultures, tuberculosis and fungal cultures, acid-fast stain, and cell cytology assessment.

   c. To demonstrate if a hemothorax is present on a grossly bloody pleural fluid sample, the hematocrit of the pleural fluid should be greater than 50 per cent of that of the peripheral blood. Placement of a thoracostomy tube is indicated if the volume of the hemothorax is greater than 300 ml.

6. Instruct the patient to look for signs and symptoms of pneumothorax, bleeding, recurrence of effusion, and infection.

Bibliography

Anderson WM, Light RW: Invasive diagnostic procedures. In George RB, Light RW, Matthay MA, et al (eds): Chest Medicine: Essentials of Pulmonary and Critical Care Medicine, 3rd ed, pp 92–96. Baltimore, Williams & Wilkins, 1995.

Mathisen DJ, Head JM: General thoracic emergencies. In Wilkins EW (ed): Emergency Medicine, 3rd ed, pp 611–612, 1021–1022. Baltimore, Williams & Wilkins, 1989.

Quigley RL: Thoracentesis and chest tube drainage. Crit Care Clin 1995;11:111–126.

Ruhl TS: Thoracentesis. In Pfenninger JL, Fowler GC (eds): Procedures for Primary Care Physicians, pp 477–484. St. Louis, Mosby–Year Book, 1994.

Vander Salm TJ: Thoracentesis. In Vander Salm TJ (ed): Atlas of Bedside Procedures, 2nd ed, pp 239–250. Boston, Little, Brown, 1988.

46 Rib Fractures

R. Michael Morse

Etiology

1. Most rib fractures are a result of excessive stress on the rib cage either from external traumatic forces or from internal stress such as spasmodic coughing.
2. Ribs may fracture spontaneously without a clear stressful event if osteoporosis or metastatic lesions compromise their strength.

Symptoms

1. Rib fractures present as localized pain at the fracture site. The pain is aggravated by breathing, coughing, and physical activity, particularly involving use of the arms, and is relieved by rest.
2. Other symptoms may result from direct complications or from associated injuries. Increasing dyspnea, postural syncope or near-syncope, or more generalized chest or abdominal pain should always lead to further evaluation.

Key Symptoms

- Local pain with inspiration or cough
- Local pain with change in position

Clinical Findings

1. Most patients with simple rib fractures have normal vital signs and moderate local tenderness at the site(s) of fracture.
2. Those with displaced fractures may also have a palpable deformity and local crepitus.
3. Rib fractures may be complicated by pneumothorax, hemothorax, or cardiovascular injury. These patients typically have findings of tachycardia, tachypnea, hypotension, shock, decreased or absent breath sounds, or dullness to percussion on the side of the injury.
4. Chest trauma can also cause injury to the heart, resulting potentially in a new heart murmur.
5. The lung underlying chest trauma may suffer from contusion.
6. Severe injuries may result in a flail chest. In this condition, a segment of the chest wall is completely surrounded by fractures, resulting in paradoxical respiration where an area of the chest retracts instead of expands with inspiration. The combination of flail chest, underlying lung contusion, and the consequent inability to clear pulmonary secretions can markedly increase the work of breathing. This places the patient at risk for ventilatory failure.
7. Fractures of the first or second rib require clinical assessment for injury of the adjacent neurovascular structures. Fracture of the first rib accompanied by one or more additional rib fractures places the individual at high mortality risk.
8. Fractures of the 9th through 12th ribs should alert the physician to evaluate for underlying injury to adjacent abdominal organs.

Key Signs

- Local pain with palpation
- Local deformity or crepitus with palpation
- Local pain with chest compression

Tests

1. With severe injuries and underlying organ damage, arterial blood gases or pulse oximetry may reflect reduced oxygenation.
2. Internal bleeding will eventually result in reduction of hemoglobin and hematocrit.
3. Imaging studies
   a. Fractures believed to be single, low risk, and uncomplicated based on history and physical examination do not require radiologic confirmation unless a definitive diagnosis is necessary.
   b. Radiography has a 50 per cent sensitivity. Thus at least half of rib fractures will not be seen on x-ray films.
   c. In small studies, ultrasound has been shown to be significantly more sensitive than radiography but is rarely indicated. Small pleural effusions and hematomas are also detected more often with ultrasound.
   d. More severe pathology is adequately diag-

nosed on routine chest radiograph. Of particular importance is widening of the mediastinum secondary to bleeding from injuries to the heart and aorta.

   e. Vascular compromise or injury associated with fractures of the first or second rib requires angiography.

Key Tests

- Radiographs
- Other tests as indicated for associated injuries

PEARLS

- Radiograph not necessary with clinically diagnosed, single low-risk fractures

- Fractures or dislocation of cartilage will have all signs and symptoms of fracture without radiographic evidence

---

Differential Diagnosis

1. Rib fractures are categorized as single or multiple, displaced or nondisplaced, and complicated (by associated injuries) or uncomplicated.

2. Rib fractures may also lead to evaluation for predisposing conditions such as osteoporosis or metastatic cancer.

3. Children with chest trauma are of particular concern. Because of the incomplete ossification of the ribs, they have a more flexible chest wall structure. Therefore, in the absence of rib fracture, children are more likely than adults to suffer severe underlying organ damage. All children with significant chest trauma, regardless of the absence of rib fracture, require careful evaluation. Those *with* rib fractures should be of particular concern because this represents a significantly greater traumatic force than necessary for a similar fracture in an adult.

4. Patients may also have dislocations of ribs from attached cartilage anteriorly or from the vertebrae posteriorly. Cartilaginous dislocations are detected only by ultrasound.

Treatment

1. Once the patient has been evaluated and treated for emergent associated injuries and complications, the major goal for further therapy is pain relief.

   a. Provides patient comfort.

   b. Improves decreased ventilatory function secondary to painful respiration. This is particularly important in the elderly, those with chronic lung disease, and those with significant underlying lung injury, all of whom are at increased risk for hypoxia and pneumonia.

   c. Acetaminophen, nonsteroidal anti-inflammatories, aspirin, or oral narcotic preparations usually provide adequate pain relief for outpatients.

   d. Initial excellent local anesthesia can be obtained with intercostal nerve blocks (see Procedure following this chapter). This can be repeated several times during the initial first days of recovery. Care must be taken to avoid pneumothorax or intravascular injection of the intercostal arteries or veins.

2. Although restrictive devices such as rib belts or chest taping will relieve pain, they are generally not recommended because of assumed risk of complications such as pneumonia from restricting ventilatory function. This risk has not been demonstrated in a well-controlled, randomized clinical trial. Nevertheless, in low-risk, otherwise healthy patients with uncomplicated fractures, local taping often provides a splinting effect and pain relief with minimal respiratory compromise (Fig. 46–1).

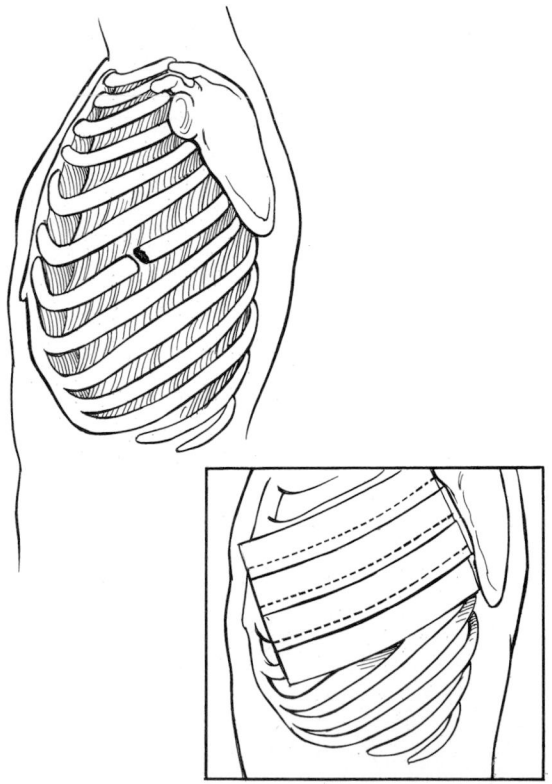

Figure 46–1 Local taping of uncomplicated rib fracture.

a. The area is prepped with tincture of benzoin and the nipple area is protected with gauze.

b. Approximately 30-cm-long strips of 2-inch cloth tape are applied in an overlapping fashion parallel to the ribs.

c. The area beginning one to two ribs below the fracture site to one to two ribs above the fracture site is firmly taped.

d. Increased pain relief, but also increased restriction of respiratory movement, can be obtained by placing the tape more horizontally.

Key Treatment

- Analgesia

- Intercostal nerve block

- Taping

WARNING

- **Always evaluate for associated injuries**

- **High-risk patients include**
  –Children
  –Steering wheel injury
  –Multiple or displaced fractures
  –Fractures of ribs 1, 2, 3, 9, 10, 11, or 12
  –Hemodynamically unstable

- **Chest taping or rib belts may increase risk of pneumonia**

Bibliography

Connolly JF: Injuries to the thoracic cage. In Connolly FJ (ed): DePalma's The Management of Fractures and Dislocations, pp 500–522. Philadelphia, WB Saunders Company, 1981.

Mayberry JC, Trunkey DD: The fractured rib in chest wall trauma. Chest Surg Clin North Am 1997;7:239–261.

Vukick DJ, Markovchick V: Thoracic trauma. In Rosen P, Barkin R (eds): Emergency Medicine: Concepts and Clinical Practice, 4th ed, pp 514–526. St. Louis, Mosby–Year Book, 1998.

Wilson RF, Walt AJ: Management of Trauma: Pitfalls and Practice, 2nd ed, pp 320–323. Baltimore, Williams & Wilkins, 1996.

Wisner DH: Trauma to the chest. In Sabiston DC, Spencer FC (eds): Surgery of the Chest, 6th ed, pp 459–462. Philadelphia, WB Saunders Company, 1996.

Indications

1. Surgical procedures of the chest wall or upper abdominal wall
2. Postoperative pain relief after thoracotomy or upper abdominal surgery (such as cholecystectomy). Improves cough and respiratory function.
3. Pain relief after rib fracture or dislocation of the costochondral junction
4. Pain relief for acute herpes zoster: Less consistent benefit for postherpetic neuralgia; may transiently increase pain.

Contraindications

1. Hypersensitivity to local anesthetic. Reactions are usually to epinephrine or preservatives. Hypersensitivity to the amide-type local (e.g., lidocaine, bupivacaine) anesthetics is rare.
2. Respiratory compromise such that the small risk of pneumothorax is unacceptable
3. Injections through areas of infection may spread infection to deeper structures. Often the nerve may be blocked successfully at a site proximal to the infection.

Equipment

1. Local anesthetic solution (with or without epinephrine), 5 ml for each segment to be blocked
2. Antiseptic solution
3. Syringe, 5 or 10 ml, with 22-gauge 1½-inch needle: A short-bevel needle improves the tactile feedback during needle placement and reduces the risk of pneumothorax.

Precautions

1. Do not exceed toxic dose of local anesthetic (4.5 mg/kg for lidocaine, 7 mg/kg for lidocaine with epinephrine, and 3 mg/kg for bupivacaine). Toxic reactions are more common after intercostal nerve blocks than when an equivalent dose of local anesthetic is injected at other sites. The proximity of intercostal blood vessels results in particularly rapid absorption of local anesthetic into the bloodstream.
2. The intercostal nerves lie in close proximity to intercostal vessels and the pleura, so careful aspiration for the presence of blood or air is essential.

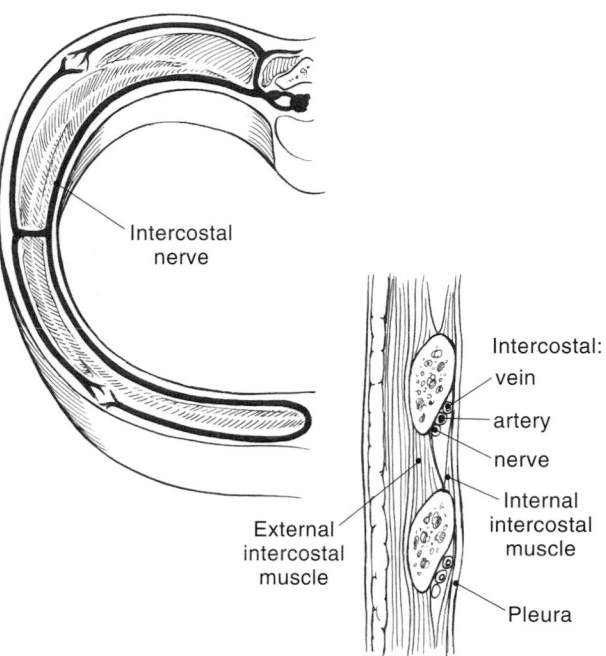

3. Local anesthetic may spread proximally, resulting in a sympathetic blockade when intercostal nerves are blocked near their origin. If multiple levels are blocked, hypotension may result.
4. The intercostal muscles are accessory muscles of respiration, so patients with severe chronic obstructive pulmonary disease may not tolerate blocks at multiple levels.

WARNING

- **Measures should be taken to detect pneumothorax in all patients following intercostal blocks.**

- **An inadvertent subarachnoid injection and resulting extensive spinal anesthesia can result if the needle is introduced near the vertebrae or directed toward the midline.**

Technique

1. Place the patient in the lateral position with the arm raised to displace the scapula laterally.

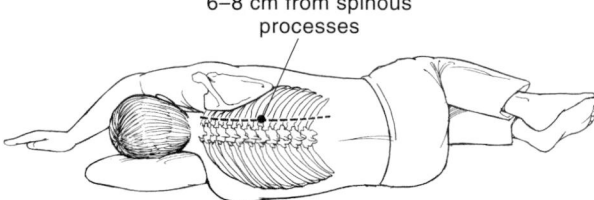

6–8 cm from spinous processes

The seated position with arms raised may be preferable for bilateral intercostal blocks. The posterior portions of ribs T5 and below are exposed and can be palpated. Usually the scapula and muscles make the first four ribs inaccessible. Injection should never be made unless the rib can be palpated. This allows exposure and palpation of the ribs as far cephalad as T5. This allows injection at the angle of the rib proximal to the lateral perforating branch at the mid-axillary line.

2. Prepare the skin with antiseptic solution and palpate the position of the rib. Raise a skin wheal overlying the lower (caudal) border of the rib approximately 6 to 8 cm lateral to the spinous process of the thoracic vertebrae.

3. Use the nondominant hand to displace the skin wheal slightly cephalad.

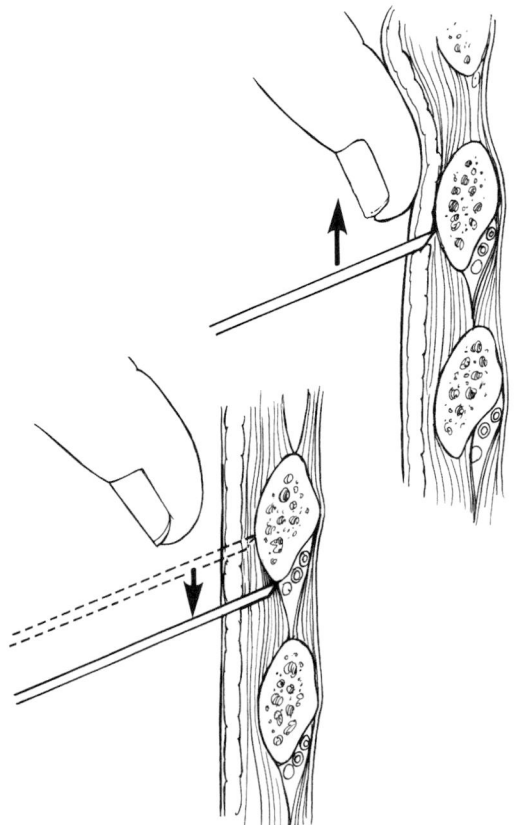

Introduce the needle through the skin wheal perpendicular to the skin until it impinges on the lower border of the rib.

4. Withdraw the needle slightly. Allow the skin to return toward its normal position and walk the needle off the lower edge of the caudal margin of the rib. Then advance the needle 2 to 3 mm beyond the caudal margin of the rib and carefully aspirate for blood or air prior to injection. A cough may indicate pleural puncture and is reason to withdraw the needle. Inject 3 to 5 ml of local anesthetic.

5. A sufficient number of levels must be blocked to produce the desired area of anesthesia. Anesthesia over the sternum will require bilateral blocks. In addition, one additional level above and below must be blocked to account for overlap in the dermal distribution of intercostal nerves. When multiple levels are blocked, the total dose of local anesthetic can easily exceed toxic doses. Using more dilute solutions of anesthetic and reducing the volume injected at each level can help keep the total dose injected within safe limits.

6. It is crucial to allow 5 to 10 minutes for the anesthetic to diffuse and the block to become complete before a surgical incision is made. This time can be spent preparing the skin, draping, and organizing the instruments.

Follow-Up

Patients should be observed for signs and symptoms of

1. Pneumothorax (typical incidence 1 per cent)
2. Local anesthetic toxicity: metallic taste, tinnitus, slurred speech, seizure, cardiac arrest (in order of appearance and severity)

Bibliography

Bonica JJ, Butler SH: Local anesthesia and regional blocks. In Wall PD, Melzack R (eds): Textbook of Pain, pp 1014–1016. New York, Churchill Livingstone, 1994.

Ferrera PC, Chandler R: Anesthesia in the emergency setting: part II. Head and neck, eye and rib injuries. Am Fam Physician 1994;50:797–800.

Henthorn TK, Krejcie TC: Postoperative pain management. In Tollison CD, Satterthwaite JR, Tollison JW (eds): Handbook of Pain Management, 2nd ed. Baltimore, Williams & Wilkins, 1994, pp 616–617.

Rung GW, Marshall WK: Nerve blocks in the critical care environment. Crit Care Clin 1990;6:343–367.

Yokoyama M, Mizobuchi S, Nakatsuka H, et al: Comparison of plasma lidocaine concentrations after injection of a fixed small volume in the stellate ganglion, the lumbar epidural space, or a single intercostal nerve. Anesth Analg 1998;87:112–115.

47 Cancers of the Larynx and Lung

Sandra K. Willsie

Cancer of the Larynx

Etiology

1. Tobacco smoking and consumption of alcohol (synergistic risks)
2. Toxic or industrial exposures (prolonged)
   a. Metal or wood dusts
   b. Asbestos
   c. Hair dyes; paint, diesel, or gasoline fumes
3. Squamous cell carcinoma of the larynx accounts for about 95 per cent of all cases. Less than 5 per cent of cases are sarcomas, lymphomas, cylindromas, melanomas, or metastatic adenocarcinomas.

Symptoms

1. The most frequent presenting symptom is hoarseness or muffled voice.
2. Cough—typically nonproductive, with or without dyspnea
3. Dysphagia or odynophagia, with or without neck swelling or pain
4. Otalgia (referred pain to the ear) may occur late in the course

Key Symptoms

• Hoarseness	• Otalgia
• Odynophagia	• Cough

Clinical Findings

1. Cervical adenopathy, particularly the jugular chain
2. Fixation of the cricoid, hyoid, or thyroid cartilages
3. Stridor signifying laryngeal obstruction
4. Indirect laryngoscopy (lighted mirror) examination may reveal laryngeal irregularity, mass, edema (99 per cent of lesions are in the glottic or supraglottic location).

Key Signs

• Cervical adenopathy	• Hemoptysis
• Stridor or respiratory distress	• Fixation of hyoid, cricoid, or thyroid cartilages

Tests

1. Direct laryngoscopy with biopsy is the examination of choice.
2. Because 15 per cent of patients may have a second primary, direct laryngoscopy should be combined with bronchoscopy and esophagoscopy.

Key Test

Inspection with biopsy is the only definitive test.

Differential Diagnosis

1. Hoarseness from other causes, including laryngeal edema, lymphatic obstruction from abscess or neoplasia, and chronic laryngitis from overuse, tobacco abuse, or syphilis
2. Upper airway obstruction from infection, cord paralysis, or thyroid enlargement

Treatment

1. Treatment of laryngeal carcinoma varies, depending on the stage of disease. Staging is by tumor, node, metastasis (TNM) classification.
2. Treatment of limited disease (squamous cell carcinoma)
   a. Carcinoma in situ: vocal cord stripping or laser ablation
   b. Localized: surgical removal or radiation (90 per cent 5-year cure rate for T1 lesions)
   c. Subglottic or transglottic lesions: total laryngectomy with lymph node dissection. Consider adjunctive preoperative or postoperative radiation therapy.
3. For locally advanced lesions, experimental chemotherapy protocols should be considered ver-

sus radiation therapy with surgical extirpation following.

4. Speech rehabilitation. Many patients need subsequent speech therapy.

Key Treatment

Laryngeal Carcinoma: Treatment of Limited Disease (Squamous Cell Carcinoma)

- Carcinoma in situ: vocal cord stripping or laser ablation

- Localized: surgical removal or radiation

- Subglottic or transglottic lesions: total laryngectomy with lymph node dissection

Follow-Up

Patients should be advised to abstain from alcohol and tobacco use. Regular follow-up to look for recurrence and new lesions is necessary.

Cancer of the Lung

Etiology

1. Tobacco smoking (85 per cent of cases); secondhand smoke (implicated in 15 to 20 per cent)

2. Ionizing radiation: radon daughters

3. Occupational exposures: may be additive or synergistic with tobacco—asbestos, chromium, nickel, hydrocarbons, chloromethyl ether

4. Less well-established risks: air pollution, vitamin A and E deficiencies, cigar or pipe use

Symptoms

1. Symptoms associated with bronchogenic carcinoma are often related to the cell type, location of the tumor, or rapidity of metastases—local and systemic.

2. Symptoms confined to the lung: cough, hemoptysis, hoarseness, wheezing, dyspnea, sputum production with or without fever related to postobstructive pneumonitis, chest pain

Key Symptoms

• Cough	• Dyspnea
• Hemoptysis	• Weight loss
• Chest pain	• Fever
• Hoarseness	

Clinical Findings

1. Disease confined to the chest includes stridor, hoarseness, changes on examination related to atelectasis, consolidation, diaphragm paralysis or effusion, superior vena caval obstruction (cyanosis, engorgement of neck veins and lack of pulsations, enlarged neck circumference), and pericardial disease or tamponade.

2. Findings related to regional or distant metastases include adenopathy (particularly supraclavicular or scalene nodes), Horner's syndrome (supracervical ganglia involvement with miosis, ptosis, anhidrosis), and organ-specific findings.

3. Evidence of paraneoplastic syndromes or ectopic hormone production

Key Signs

• Stridor	• Adenopathy
• Hemoptysis	• Horner's syndrome
• Clubbing	• Hoarseness
• Superior vena cava syndrome	

Tests

1. Chest radiograph presentation classically varies according to cell type. (*Note:* This does not hold true in all cases.)
    a. Central lesions: squamous cell carcinoma or small cell carcinoma (SCC)
    b. Peripheral lesions: adenocarcinoma, large cell carcinoma, bronchoalveolar cell carcinoma
    c. Cavitation: squamous cell, large cell
    d. Early mediastinal, hilar involvement: SCC

2. Sputum cytology: Negative results do not rule out carcinoma; more likely to be positive with central, endobronchial tumors.

3. Bronchoscopy: considered when sputum cytology is nondiagnostic (biopsies, needle aspiration, or lavage can be performed) and in cases of occult carcinoma (sputum cytology is positive with normal chest radiograph) preoperatively to rule out silent synchronous lesions

4. Percutaneous needle aspiration: helpful, particularly in patients with large or peripheral lesions and with negative cytology who are inoperative or not bronchoscopy candidates because of the extent of disease

5. Pleural fluid should be sampled when present and sent for cytology, pH, cell counts, lactate dehydrogenase, and protein.

6. Rarely mediastinal exploration or open biopsy is needed for diagnosis.

Key Test

The only definitive test is biopsy!

Differential Diagnosis

1. Includes other diseases with similar symptomatology or chest radiograph appearance: granulomatous disease, including mycobacterial and fungal diseases and sarcoidosis; hamartomas; carcinoid tumors

2. Metastatic disease to the lung from other sites: breast, gastrointestinal tract, genitourinary tract, germ cell carcinomas, sarcomas, head and neck cancers, melanoma

Treatment

1. Treatment of bronchogenic carcinoma varies according to cell type, stage of disease (TNM classification), premorbid condition, and underlying lung function.

   a. Cell types: SCC and non–small cell carcinoma (NSCC). NSCC includes squamous cell, adenocarcinoma (including bronchoalveolar cell), large cell, and adenosquamous.

   b. SCC, regardless of stage, is almost always treated with chemotherapy. In the event of SCC with a solitary pulmonary nodule, excision may be performed first followed by chemotherapy.

   c. NSCC treatment is highly dependent on stage of disease.

      (1) Surgical resection is the treatment of choice for a solitary nodule or localized disease in the patient who has adequate pulmonary reserve with stage I to IIIa disease. In patients who are not surgical candidates, radiation therapy may be considered (15 to 20 per cent curative stage I disease).

      (2) Stage IIIb or IV may be considered for palliative radiation therapy or experimental chemotherapy protocols. (Chemotherapy is of uncertain benefit in NSCC. It is generally limited to young patients with good performance status; however, referral to a medical oncologist should be considered in all cases.) Neoadjunctive therapy with chemother-apy with or without radiation therapy before attempted resection in stage IIIb or IV may be considered.

2. Malignant pleural effusions associated with bronchogenic carcinoma should be initially treated with therapeutic thoracentesis (if symptomatic). If there is symptomatic improvement but effusion recurs (particularly if rapid reaccumulation), pleurodesis should be considered. Pleurodesis is most likely to be effective if the pH of the fluid is greater than 7.3.

Key Treatment

Bronchogenic Carcinoma

- SCC is almost always treated with chemotherapy. SCC with a solitary pulmonary nodule should be excised and then treated with chemotherapy.

- NSCC treatment depends on the stage of disease. Surgical resection is the treatment of choice for a solitary nodule or localized disease in a patient who has adequate pulmonary reserve with stage I to IIIa disease. In patients who are not surgical candidates, radiation therapy may be considered. Stage IIIb or IV may be considered for palliative radiation therapy or experimental chemotherapy protocols.

- Malignant pleural effusions associated with bronchogenic carcinoma should be initially treated with therapeutic thoracentesis (if symptomatic). If there is symptomatic improvement but effusion recurs, pleurodesis should be considered.

Follow-Up

Close follow-up with periodic clinical examination and chest radiography should be performed to evaluate for recurrence or progression of disease.

Bibliography

Abolhoda A, Liu D, Brooks A, et al: Prolonged air leak following radical upper lobectomy. Chest 1998;113:1507–1510.

Dockery DW, Trichopoulos D: Risk of lung cancer from environmental exposure to tobacco smoke. Cancer Causes Control 1997;8:333–345.

McKenna JP, Fornataro-Clerici LM, McMenamin PG, Leonard RJ: Laryngeal carcinoma: diagnosis, treatment and speech rehabilitation. Am Fam Physician 1991;44:123–129.

Mountain CF: Revisions of the International System for Staging Lung Cancer. Chest 1997;111:1710–1717.

Silbey GS: Radiotherapy for patients with medically inoperable Stage I nonsmall cell lung carcinoma—a review. Cancer 1998;82:433–438.

48 Metastatic Cancer of Unknown Origin

Jai H. Joshi

Overview

1. Cancers of unknown origin are biopsy-proven metastatic neoplasms with histology that is inconsistent with a primary at the biopsy site. They account for about 5 per cent of cancers.

2. Patients with this diagnosis have generally fared poorly in the past (median survival less than 6 months). Recently, however, prolonged survival has been documented in certain subgroups treated with specific therapies. Identification of these treatable subgroups using recently available diagnostic techniques such as immunoperoxidase staining, electron microscopy, and cytogenetics is crucial. It is equally important to refrain from using costly, unrewarding, and futile diagnostic and/or therapeutic interventions in subgroups for which no therapy is available.

3. Patients with cancers of unknown origin usually present with symptoms and signs referable to the multiple sites of metastatic disease—the liver, lungs, lymph nodes, and bone. Most patients also have constitutional symptoms, such as anorexia, weight loss, and fatigue.

4. The need for obtaining adequate tissue whenever this diagnosis is considered is paramount. Open biopsy is preferable to fine-needle aspiration, and re-biopsy is mandatory whenever there is any question about the adequacy of biopsy material.

5. Findings on routine light microscopic examination of biopsy material provide a practical classification of these cancers into four groups: adenocarcinoma, squamous carcinoma, poorly differentiated carcinomas, and undifferentiated neoplasms. Most (60 per cent) are adenocarcinomas, a third (30 per cent) are carcinomas that are poorly differentiated, 5 per cent are squamous carcinomas, and 5 per cent are undifferentiated neoplasms.

    a. For undifferentiated neoplasms and poorly differentiated carcinomas, additional pathologic study is required. Rendering a specific diagnosis is important because lymphomas and germ cell tumors are highly curable when identified and specifically treated.

    b. Patients with well-differentiated adenocarcinoma and squamous carcinoma do not require additional pathologic study, except as a means of identifying treatable adenocarcinomas of the ovary, breast, and prostate. For these and squamous carcinomas of the head and neck, major palliation can be achieved, even in metastatic disease. For most other patients with adenocarcinoma, there is no effective therapy.

Undifferentiated Neoplasms

1. Light microscopy histology displays no lineage characteristics in this group, so that differentiation into even general neoplastic categories such as carcinoma, lymphoma, melanoma, and sarcoma is impossible. Based on the extent of differentiation, these "anaplastic" neoplasms (i.e., that lack differentiation) may be further divided into undifferentiated and poorly differentiated neoplasms.

2. Additional pathologic study (Table 48–1) with immunoperoxidase staining, electron microscopy, and cytogenetics is mandatory because it results in specific diagnosis of treatable cancers in most patients.

    a. Two thirds have a diagnosis of non-Hodgkin's lymphoma established when leukocyte common antigen can be demonstrated in tissue by immunoperoxidase staining using monoclonal antibodies. The presence of this antigen distinguishes lymphoma from essentially all other undifferentiated tumors.

    b. Cytogenetic analyses demonstrating chromosomal translocations or immunoglobulin gene rearrangements are additionally helpful.

    c. With the implementation of chemotherapy regimens such as CHOP (cyclophosphamide, doxorubicin, vincristine, and prednisone), many patients with lymphoma diagnosed in this manner enjoy prolonged disease-free survival.

Poorly Differentiated Carcinomas

Histopathology

This heterogeneous group is distinctive in that it possesses well-defined clinical characteristics and is treatment-responsive. Epithelial features on light mi-

TABLE 48-1. ADDITIONAL PATHOLOGIC STUDIES

Tumor	Finding
Immunoperoxidase Staining	
Lymphoma	LCA(CD45) +; B-, T-cell markers/antigens +; (EMA ±; all other stains −)
Carcinoma	Epithelial stains (i.e., keratin and EMA) +; (LCA, S-100, vimentin −)
Sarcoma	Mesenchymal stain (i.e., vimentin) +; (epithelial stains −)
	Rhabdomyosarcoma: desmin +; myosin +
	Angiosarcoma: factor VIII antigen +
	Leiomyosarcoma: myosin +
Melanoma	S-100, HMB-45 antigen +; (epithelial stains −; mesenchymal vimentin +; NSE often +)
Neuroendocrine tumors	NSE, chromogranin +; (epithelial stains +)
Germ cell tumor	hCG, AFP +; (epithelial stains +)
Prostate cancer	PSA +; (epithelial stains +)
Breast cancer	ER, PR +; (epithelial stains +)
Thyroid cancer	Thyroglobulin +
	Medullary carcinoma of the thyroid: calcitonin +
Electron Microscopy	
Adenocarcinoma	Intercellular and intracellular lumina and surface microvilli
Squamous carcinoma	Desmosomes and prekeratin filament bundles in cytoplasm
Carcinoma	Desmosomes
Lymphoma	
Melanoma	Premelanosomes
Neuroendocrine tumors	Secretory granules
Sarcoma	Actin-myosin filaments (rhabdomyosarcoma)
Cytogenetics	
Germ cell tumors	Isochromosome 12p; 12q(−)
Lymphoma	Chromosomal translocations t(14:18); t(8:14)
Ewing's sarcoma	t(11:22)
Molecular Biology	
Lymphoma	Immunoglobulin (B-cell lymphomas), T-cell receptor gene
	(T-cell lymphomas) rearrangements
Neuroblastoma	*myc* oncogene
Breast carcinoma	HER-2/*neu*

Abbreviations: +, positive result; −, negative result; AFP, α-fetoprotein; EMA, epithelial membrane antigen; ER, estrogen receptor; hCG, human chorionic gonadotropin; HMB-45, human melanoma black 45; LCA, leukocyte common antigen; NSE, neuron-specific enolase; PR, progesterone receptor; PSA, prostate-specific antigen.

croscopy define the histologic criterion for inclusion in this group.

1. In poorly differentiated, or *anaplastic, carcinoma*, the presence of epithelial features is the only lineage determinant.

2. In poorly differentiated *adenocarcinoma*, minimal adenomatous differentiation is additionally present. This implies rudimentary gland formation or strong positivity with the histochemical stain for mucin in what otherwise is poorly differentiated carcinoma. Clearly definable glandular formation, however, must be absent because cases involving lesions with well-formed glandular structures, ducts with lumina, and mucin evident from hematoxylin-eosin staining are classified as adenocarcinomas.

3. In poorly differentiated *small cell carcinoma* (*questionable neuroendocrine*), there is a cellular monotony of small cells with high nuclear/cytoplasmic ratios and displaced nuclear chromatin.

Clinical Features

1. The clinical features that define this group include a younger age of patients, a short (less than 30-day) onset period, rapid progression, and tumor located predominantly in mediastinal, retroperitoneal, or peripheral (neck, axillary, or inguinal) lymph node groups. These findings are present in 50 per cent of patients.

2. In others, the tumor may be located predominantly in the lung (with multiple lung masses on chest radiography and nonrevealing fiberoptic bronchoscopy results), or patients may have multiple sites of disease involvement without predominance at any one site.

Treatment

1. *All* patients in this group should be treated with a chemotherapy regimen that combines cisplatin and etoposide, with or without adding bleomycin to the combination. More than 60 per cent respond, at least 25 per cent have complete responses, and most of the complete responders remain disease-free for periods in excess of 5 years, almost tantamount to "cure."

2. Specific subgroups identified with additional pathologic study are even more likely to respond.

   a. Patients with undiagnosed *germ cell tumors* constitute one such subgroup. This diagnosis generally remains elusive until cytogenetic studies identify the highly specific isochromosome abnormality that involves the short arm of chromosome 12 (i12p). Nonetheless, germ cell tumors should be suspected in young men who present with metastatic poorly differentiated carcinoma of unknown origin, regardless of the level of serum chorionic gonadotropin β-subunit and α-fetoprotein and even in the absence of the the abnormal karyotype. With empirical treatment with cisplatin-based chemotherapy, excellent treatment responses and survival have been observed (50 per cent complete responses with 30 per cent having prolonged disease-free survival).

b. Another subgroup with excellent prognosis is *neuroendocrine carcinoma*. This diagnosis is best established by electron microscopy (demonstrating neurosecretory granules). Positive immunoperoxidase staining for neuron-specific enolase and chromogranin is additionally helpful. Although tumors with varying clinical manifestations (from the indolent carcinoid to anaplastic small cell carcinoma) are included in the category, when neuroendocrine carcinoma masquerades as poorly differentiated carcinoma, it behaves aggressively and demonstrates a responsiveness to cisplatin-based chemotherapy.

3. Other diagnoses in cisplatin responders include malignant thymoma, melanoma, and lymphoma.

a. *Malignant thymoma* should be considered in patients with predominant mediastinal disease.

b. *Melanoma* has been diagnosed retrospectively in cisplatin responders based on immunoperoxidase staining and electron microscopy findings. Accordingly, when melanoma is suggested in patients with poorly differentiated carcinoma, they should not be excluded from cisplatin-based chemotherapy trials because they may have uniquely sensitive tumors.

c. *Lymphomas* can resemble anaplastic carcinoma when examined by light microscopy. Lymphomas even stain positively with epithelial markers on immunoperoxidase staining. Because the distinction between carcinoma and lymphoma can consequently affect treatment and survival, immunoperoxidase staining for leukocyte common antigen should be routinely used in all patients with poorly differentiated carcinoma.

Adenocarcinoma

1. Metastatic adenocarcinoma of unknown origin is the largest (60 per cent) group. Compared with patients having poorly differentiated carcinomas, these patients have different clinical characteristics, no extant effective therapy, and a dismal prognosis. At presentation, they have widespread metastatic disease (to the liver, lungs, and bone) and a poor performance status and are generally much older; accordingly, they should receive supportive care alone.

2. The histologic qualification for inclusion in this group is the demonstration of clearly definable glandular formation on light microscopy. This group does not include patients with poorly or moderately differentiated adenocarcinoma. This distinction is crucial. The hopeless prognosis of this group applies only to those with clearly definable glandular formation, not to those with rudimentary glandular formation or mucin positivity alone.

Diagnosis of Treatable Forms

At autopsy, the most common primary sites of origin are the pancreas and lung. Because neither is treatable, attempts to find the primary are not worthwhile, and previously published large series have amply documented the futility of aggressive diagnostic testing in the pursuit of that goal. Therefore, only attempts at identifying treatable adenocarcinomas of the breast, ovary, prostate, and thyroid are appropriate. Unlike their frequency in the general population, these treatable adenocarcinomas are rare in this group. Nonetheless, given the potential therapeutic implications of such a discovery, women should be evaluated for a possible breast or ovarian primary and men for an occult prostate primary. A thyroid primary should be excluded in either sex.

1. Additional pathologic study with immunoperoxidase staining should be pursued. Adenocarcinoma of the breast is suggested with the presence of gross cystic fluid protein or estrogen and progesterone receptors. Prostate-specific antigen (PSA) and prostate acid phosphatase staining of tissue identify prostatic adenocarcinoma. Thyroglobulin positivity identifies the thyroid as the site of origin.

2. Radiologic evaluations should include mammography for breast cancer and either an abdominopelvic computerized tomographic (CT) scan or a pelvic ultrasound for ovarian cancer. The evaluation for a prostatic primary should include an abdominal CT scan, a bone scan, and serum PSA determinations.

3. Treatable adenocarcinomas of the breast, ovary,

and prostate can also be diagnosed with the recognition of specific clinical syndromes.

a. Women with enlarged axillary nodes and adenocarcinoma on biopsy represent one such syndrome. These women should be treated as are patients with stage II breast cancer, regardless of the presence of a lesion on examination or mammography and irrespective of estrogen and progesterone receptor status in the biopsied axillary node. They should undergo modified radical mastectomy or receive breast irradiation to reduce the risk of local recurrence. In addition, they should receive adjuvant systemic hormonal (tamoxifen) chemotherapy to reduce their risk of metastatic disease.

b. Women with malignant ascites represent the second treatable syndrome. After surgical debulking, these patients should receive cisplatin-based chemotherapy as would those with metastatic ovarian adenocarcinoma, regardless of the presence of a pelvic mass and even if normal ovaries were found at laparotomy.

c. The third syndrome involves men with osteoblastic bone metastasis. Regardless of serum PSA levels and tissue immunoperoxidase staining, these patients should be treated with hormonal therapy as are men with metastatic (stage D) prostate cancer.

Squamous Carcinoma

Squamous carcinomas of unknown origin present with neck, axillary, or inguinal adenopathy. Each presentation has specific recommendations in regard to the extent of diagnostic evaluations and therapies that may be required.

1. In patients with squamous carcinoma who present with *cervical adenopathy*, the head and neck are the most likely primary sites (especially if the patient is a heavy smoker or alcohol consumer), followed by the lungs.

a. Diagnostic evaluation should include a complete otolaryngologic examination and chest radiography, followed by panendoscopy (laryngoscopy, nasopharyngoscopy, and esophagoscopy) and a CT scan of the head and neck to identify submucosal lesions not visualized by endoscopy. If no primary is found, blind biopsies of the nasopharynx, piriform sinuses, base of the tongue, and tonsils should be obtained. If CT scanning of the chest uncovers a lung primary, bronchoscopy should be performed. It is not necessary to search below the diaphragm for a primary.

b. When no primary is found, treatment should generally involve radiation therapy to the involved cervical chain combined with prophylactic irradiation of the nasopharynx, oropharynx, and larynx (the likely occult primary sites). In addition, the contralateral uninvolved neck should also be irradiated. Radiation should be administered in the same dose and fields as in patients with known primary head and neck cancers. Five-year survival rates of 30 to 50 per cent have been documented with this approach. The preference for irradiation over surgery is based on a higher relapse rate with surgery alone.

2. Patients who present with *supraclavicular adenopathy* generally fare poorly because most have squamous carcinoma of the lung. The diagnostic evaluation for this group should include CT scanning of the chest and bronchoscopy. Again, it is not necessay to search below the diaphragm for a primary.

3. Squamous carcinoma presenting with *inguinal adenopathy* is usually the result of metastases from an occult primary in the perineal or anorectal area. Attempts to identify them are appropriate. When no primary is found, inguinal lymph node dissection with or without irradiation is the treatment of choice. Long-term survival has been documented with this treatment approach.

4. When an occult primary squamous carcinoma is found at other sites (e.g., brain, liver, or bone), the lung is the most likely site of origin, and this is usually obvious on chest radiography. When chest radiography is unrevealing, further studies should not be undertaken because no effective therapy exists for metastatic squamous carcinoma of the lung.

ACKNOWLEDGMENT: For his succinct and prompt reviews of this article and his many excellent suggestions, I recognize the contributions of my son, Amit Joshi.

 Bibliography

Hainsworth JD, Greco FA: Carcinoma of unknown primary site. In Stein JH (ed): Internal Medicine, 3rd ed, pp 1180–1184. Boston, Little, Brown, 1990.

Hainsworth JD, Greco FA: Treatment of patients with cancer of an unknown primary site [review]. N Engl J Med 1993;329:257–263.

Hainsworth JD, Greco FA, Johnson DH, et al: Cisplatin-based combination chemotherapy in the treatment of poorly differentiated carcinoma and poorly differentiated adenocarcinoma of unknown primary site: results of a 12-year experience. J Clin Oncol 1992;10:912.

National comprehensive cancer network: NCCN practice guidelines for occult primary tumors. Oncology 1998; 12:226–309.

Raber MN, Abbruzzese JL, Frost P, et al: Unknown primary tumors. Curr Opin Oncol 1992;4:3.

49 Oncologic Emergencies

Alison Grann

Although many consequences are associated with cancer, there are five oncologic emergencies that the primary care physician and house officer should look for when evaluating the patient with cancer.

Hypercalcemia

Etiology

Different tumors produce hypercalcemia by way of different mechanisms.

1. Parathyroid hormone–related peptide: most common mediator of cancer-related hypercalcemia.
   a. Gene mapped to short arm of chromosomes 11 and 12.
   b. Commonly found in squamous cell cancers of the lung, head, and neck and in breast cancer
   c. Increased renal absorption of calcium, increased bone absorption of calcium secondary to osteoclast activation, hypophosphatemia, phosphaturia
2. Bone metastasis
   a. Many tumors; common in breast cancer
   b. Increased bone destruction leads to increased calcium levels.
3. Increased production of 1,25-dihydroxycholecalciferol
   a. Seen in lymphomas, myelomas, and occasionally solid tumors
   b. Increased gut absorption of calcium leads to hypercalcemia.
4. Cytokines: formerly known collectively as osteoclast activating factor; now known to be multiple and to include interleukin-1, tumor necrosis factor, and others
   a. Seen in myeloma and other tumors
   b. Increased bone resorption caused by cytokines and impaired renal function secondary to increased calcium levels

Symptoms

Dependent on how quickly hypercalcemia develops

1. General: weakness, lethargy, pruritus

2. Gastrointestinal: anorexia, nausea, vomiting, constipation, acute pancreatitis
3. Renal: polydipsia and polyuria, dehydration, nephrocalcinosis
4. Cardiovascular: bradycardia, prolonged P-R interval, shortened Q-T intervals, wide T wave, arrhythmias
5. Neuromuscular: muscle weakness, hyporeflexia, confusion, psychosis, seizure, obtundation, coma

Clinical Findings

1. Renal failure
2. Hyporeflexia
3. Hypotonia
4. Stupor
5. Coma
6. Ventricular arrhythmias

Tests

1. Serum calcium: Must check albumin because 50 per cent of serum calcium is bound to protein and only free ionized calcium is active.
2. Serum phosphate: low in patients with parathyroid hormone–related peptide
3. Alkaline phosphate: elevated with bone metastasis
4. Electrolytes, blood urea nitrogen, creatinine
5. Electrocardiography: prolonged P-R interval, shortening of Q-T interval, broadening of T waves, heart block, asystole, atrial and ventricular arrhythmias.

Treatment

1. Treat underlying disease
2. Vigorous hydration with normal saline
3. Intermittent use of furosemide (Lasix) once the patient is well hydrated, to balance fluid intake with urine output
4. Monitor for volume overload or worsening dehydration.
5. Monitor cardiovascular status.
6. Biphosphonates: many types, each administered differently; most commonly used drugs
   a. Pamidronate (Aredia): newest compound; 60 to 90 mg IV over 2 to 4 hours

b. Binds to hydroxyapatite in bone and prevents bone from being broken down.
   c. No significant toxicity
   d. Second-line therapy after intravenous hydration unless the patient is extremely symptomatic and calcitonin is indicated
 7. Calcitonin: 6 to 8 IU/kg IM q6h
   a. Increases urinary excretion of calcium and decreases bone resorption.
   b. Second-line therapy after intravenous hydration if the patient is extremely symptomatic and calcium must be lowered quickly
   c. Limited use secondary to tachyphylaxis; can cause hypophosphatemia
 8. Glucocorticoids: 200 to 300 mg of hydrocortisone or its equivalent
   a. Decreases intestinal calcium absorption and inhibits bone resorption.
   b. Response may be delayed up to 1 week
   c. Many adverse effects
   d. Not optimal therapy
   e. Patients with nonhematologic cancer do not respond.
 9. Plicamycin (mithramycin): 25 μg/kg of body weight infused over 8 to 12 hours
   a. Inhibits ribonucleic acid synthesis of osteoclasts.
   b. Hepatic and renal toxicity; thrombocytopenia; hemorrhagic diathesis
   c. Not first-, second-, or third-line therapy
 10. Gallium nitrate (Ganite): 100 to 200 mg/m² body surface area over 24 hours
   a. Decreases bone resorption
   b. Chief toxicity is hypophosphatemia.
 11. Phosphate causes many complications and should rarely if ever be used.
 12. Dialysis: if therapies above do not work

Superior Vena Cava Syndrome

Etiology
Caused by partial or complete obstruction of blood flow through the superior vena cava to the right atrium
 1. Mechanism of obstruction
   a. Compression
   b. Thrombosis
   c. Fibrosis
   d. Invasion
 2. Most (80 to 95 per cent) of superior vena cava syndrome is caused by a mediastinal cancer, leading to compression of the superior vena cava.

Symptoms
Typically develop over 3 to 4 weeks
 1. Swelling of face, trunk, and upper extremities
 2. Dyspnea
 3. Cough
 4. Hoarseness
 5. Dysphagia
 6. Nausea
 7. Headache
 8. Visual changes
 9. Chest pain

Clinical Findings
 1. Neck vein distention
 2. Facial edema plethora
 3. Tachypnea
 4. Cyanosis

Tests
 1. Chest radiography
 2. Computerized tomographic scan with contrast
 3. Unless impeding airway obstruction or intracerebral hemorrhage, obtain tissue.

Treatment
 1. Position patient upright, and maintain adequate oxygenation.
 2. Obtain tissue diagnosis.
 3. Diuretics
 4. Steroids
 5. Radiation therapy or chemotherapy

Spinal Cord Compression

Etiology
 1. Occurs when metastasis to vertebral body or pedicle enlarges and compresses underlying dura or vertebral body collapses and compresses dura.
 2. Most common in thoracic spine; if not in thoracic then lumbosacral > cervical

Symptoms
Depend on level of spinal cord involved
 1. Back pain in 95 per cent of patients
 2. Motor and sensory symptoms
 3. Autonomic dysfunction with bowel or bladder incontinence

Clinical Findings
Dependent on level of cord involved; localized back pain

Tests

1. Detailed neurologic examination
2. Plain radiography
3. Magnetic resonance imaging scan of spine
4. Myelography if magnetic resonance imaging is not available.

Treatment

Key to effective management is to initiate treatment before neurologic deficits develop.

1. High-dose steroids: dexamethasone (Decadron), 10 mg, intravenously followed by 4 to 24 mg qid
2. Radiation therapy
3. Surgical decompression: for patients without known cancer, those who have received maximal radiation, and those whose condition deteriorates during radiation, spinal instability, or compression by bone.
4. Rarely chemotherapy
5. Sometimes surgery followed by radiation

Tumor Lysis Syndrome

Etiology

1. Occurs in patients who have a tumor that is extremely sensitive to chemotherapy as a result of rapid release of intracellular contents into bloodstream.
2. Classically seen in patients with Burkitt's lymphoma, non-Hodgkin's lymphoma, acute lymphoblastic leukemia, and acute myelogenous leukemia
3. Characterized by syndrome of hyperuricemia, hyperkalemia, hyperphosphatemia, and hypocalcemia

Symptoms and Clinical Findings

Secondary to electrolyte abnormalities and renal failure

1. Tetany
2. Ventricular arrhythmias
3. Renal failure
4. Nephrocalcinosis
5. Lethargy
6. Nausea
7. Vomiting
8. Muscle cramps

Tests

1. Serum electrolytes (Na^+, K^+, Ca^{2+}, HCO_3^-)
2. Uric acid
3. Calcium
4. Albumin
5. Creatinine
6. Blood urea nitrogen
7. Phosphate

Treatment

1. Prevention is essential
2. Vigorous intravenous hydration before and during chemotherapy
3. Alkalinize urine with $NaHCO_3$ for first few days of therapy.
4. Oliguric patients with bulky tumors may require dialysis during induction of chemotherapy.
5. Allopurinol before chemotherapy
   a. Decreases incidence of uric acid nephropathy.
   b. Causes xanthine nephropathy.
6. Monitor electrolytes every 3 to 4 hours, adjust frequency based on findings.

Fever and Neutropenia

Etiology

Acute leukemia, intensive chemotherapy, or radiation therapy may cause neutropenia in an already immunocompromised host.

1. Worry when absolute neutrophil count is less than 500.
2. Typically, no organism is identified, but the organisms most commonly isolated are *Pseudomonas* species, *Staphylococcus* species, *Enterobacter* species, *Candida* species, *Clostridium difficile*, and *Aspergillus*.

Symptoms

1. Fever (may be only symptom)
2. Cough
3. Dysuria
4. Urinary frequency or urgency
5. Tenderness over indwelling catheter
6. Perianal pain
7. Nausea
8. Vomiting
9. Diarrhea
10. Abdominal pain

Clinical Findings

1. May find only fever
2. Pay special attention to lung examination, indwelling catheter site, perirectal area, skin, and perianal examination.

Tests

1. Blood culture
2. Urinalysis and culture
3. Chest radiography
4. Sputum culture

Treatment

1. Without immediate antibiotics, at least 50 per cent of febrile neutropenic patients die as a result of infection.
2. Empiric antibiotics with an aminoglycoside in combination with an extended-spectrum penicillin or third-generation cephalosporin
3. If there is clinical suspicion of line infection, begin vancomycin (Vancocin) immediately. If the patient remains febrile after 48 hours on only gram-negative coverage, then add vancomycin.
4. If there is suspected anaerobic infection or persistent fever after 3 to 5 days, add metronidazole (Flagyl).
5. After 7 days of persistent fever, add amphotericin B (Fungizone).
6. Consider granulocyte colony-stimulating factor.
7. Once the absolute neutrophil count is higher than 500, the patient is afebrile for 48 hours, and all cultures are negative, discontinue antibiotics.

B Bibliography

American Society of Clinical Oncology: Recommendations for the use of hematopoietic colony-stimulating factors: evidence based, clinical practice guidelines. J Clin Oncol 1994;12:2471–2508.

Arrambide K, Toto RD: Tumor lysis syndrome. Semin Nephrol 1993;13:273–280.

Freifeld AG, Pizzo PA, Walsh TJ: Infections in the cancer patient. In DeVita VT Jr, Hellman S, Rosenberg SA (eds): Cancer: Principles and Practice of Oncology, 5th ed, pp 2659–2704. Philadelphia, Lippincott-Raven, 1997.

Sepkowitz KA, Brown AE, Armstrong D: Empirical therapy for febrile neutropenic patients: persistence of susceptibility of gram-negative bacilli to aminoglycoside antibiotics. Clin Infect Dis 1994;19:810–811.

Talcott JA, Siegel RD, Finberg R, et al: Risk assessment in cancer patients with fever and neutropenia: a prospective, two-center validation of a prediction rule. J Clin Oncol 1992;10:316–322.

Yahalom J, Fuller BG, Heiss J, et al: Oncologic emergencies. In DeVita VT Jr, Hellman S, Rosenberg SA (eds): Cancer: Principles and Practice of Oncology, 5th ed, pp 2469–2522. Philadelphia, Lippincott-Raven, 1997.

50 Tuberculosis

Seiji Yamada

Etiology

Mycobacterium tuberculosis (MTB) is a bacillus transmitted by respiratory droplets from the cough of people with active pulmonary or upper airway tuberculosis (TB).

1. Epidemiology
   a. Associated with crowded workplace and housing conditions
   b. World epidemiology: estimated one third of the people in the world infected; estimated 8 million cases of active TB and 3 million deaths in the world yearly
   c. U.S. epidemiology: A resurgence of TB in the late 1980s was attributed to increased cases in foreign-born persons, the human immunodeficiency virus/acquired immunodeficiency syndrome (HIV/AIDS) epidemic, and multidrug-resistant (MDR) TB. The number of cases has been declining for the period 1992–1997. The case rate in foreign-born persons is four to five times that of the general population.
2. Natural history: After infection is contracted, can progress to primary disease or remain asymptomatic for years until debility or an impaired immune system leads to reactivation.

Symptoms of Pulmonary TB

1. Respiratory: chronic productive cough, hemoptysis, pleuritic chest pain, dyspnea
2. Systemic: anorexia, weight loss, night sweats, fevers and chills, fever of unknown origin
3. Extrapulmonary: back pain, lower extremity weakness (spine, Pott's disease), headache, meningeal signs, altered mental status (meningitis), flank pain, hematuria, dysuria (genitourinary infection), abdominal pain, distention (peritonitis)

Key Symptoms

- Chronic productive cough
- Hemoptysis
- Fever and chills
- Poor appetite and weight loss
- Night sweats
- Chest pain

Clinical Findings

1. Respiratory disease
   a. Parenchymal involvement: rales, rhonchi
   b. Extensive cavitary disease: amphoric breath sounds
   c. Pleural disease: signs of pleural effusion
2. Systemic: weight loss and fever
3. Extrapulmonary: fever (miliary TB), lower extremity weakness (spine), meningeal signs (meningitis), flank tenderness (kidney), enlarged lymph nodes (especially in the cervical nodes [scrofula]), abdominal tenderness (peritonitis)

Key Signs

- Rales, rhonchi
- Fever
- Lymphadenopathy
- Amphoric breath sounds
- Weight loss

Laboratory Tests

1. Chest radiograph: infiltrate in apical, posterior aspects of upper lobe, superior aspects of lower lobe; cavitation; miliary pattern in disseminated TB. Immunosuppressed patients may have atypical findings.
2. Sputum or bronchoscopically obtained samples (or gastric aspirate) for acid-fast bacilli (AFB). Collect three specimens on 3 days, following infection control precautions.
3. Sputum mycobacterial culture: Traditional methods take 6 to 12 weeks; BACTEC methods in liquid media give results within 10 to 14 days.
4. Rapid testing on sputum: polymerase chain reaction, DNA probe
5. Perform drug susceptibility testing on all initial isolates. Repeat for patients failing to respond and those with positive cultures after 2 months of therapy.
6. A positive purified protein derivative (PPD) skin test is useful, but test may be negative if the patient is immunosuppressed. Consider anergy testing if immunosuppression is suspected (see Ch. 51, PPD Testing).

7. Consider genitourinary TB in sterile pyuria.

Key Tests

- Chest radiograph
- PPD
- Sputum for AFB stain, culture, rapid testing (if available)

Differential Diagnosis

1. A variety of acute and chronic lung diseases must be differentiated from TB. Making a diagnosis of TB depends upon maintaining a high index of suspicion.

2. Nontuberculous mycobacterial infection is often seen in patients with chronic obstructive pulmonary disease. In advanced AIDS in North America and Europe, *Mycobacterium avium-intracellulare* is more common than MTB.

Treatment

Report cases of active TB to local or state health authorities so that case-finding and PPD testing of contacts can be performed.

WARNING

Consider respiratory isolation for hospital patients in whom the diagnosis is suspected, until sputum smears are demonstrated to be negative for AFB.

Medication for Active TB

1. Short-course (6-month) regimen, with initial quadruple drug therapy: isoniazid (INH), rifampin (RIF), pyrazinamide (PZA), and either ethambutol (EMB) or streptomycin (SM) (see Table 50–1). Adjust regimen according to susceptibility. If the isolate is susceptible to INH/RIF, give 2 months of four drugs, then 4 months of INH/RIF. Add pyridoxine (10 to 25 mg daily) for patients at risk for vitamin deficiency.

WARNING

- **Avoid PZA and SM (VIIIth nerve toxicity) in pregnancy.**
- **Avoid EMB in children too young to be monitored for changes in visual acuity.**

---

2. Consider directly observed treatment for all. Predicting adherence to therapy is difficult. Options for 6-month intermittent directly observed treatment

   a. Four drugs daily for 8 weeks, then INH/RIF two to three times per week for 16 weeks

   b. Four drugs daily for 2 weeks, then two times per week for 6 weeks, then INH/RIF for 16 weeks

   c. Four drugs three times per week for 6 months

3. Baseline tests in adults: liver enzymes, bilirubin, blood urea nitrogen/creatinine, complete blood count with platelets, uric acid (elevated by PZA), vision testing (EMB optic neuritis), auditory testing (SM)

4. If drug resistance is suspected, start with alternative regimen.

5. If isolate is resistant to INH only, discontinue INH, continue RIF/PZA/(EMB or SM) for 6 months or use RIF/EMB for 12 months.

6. For MDR TB, add at least three new drugs to which isolate is susceptible, obtain consultation.

WARNING

Never add a single drug to an ineffective regimen.

TABLE 50–1. FIRST-LINE TB MEDICATIONS

DRUG	DAILY DOSAGE		TWICE- AND THRICE-WEEKLY DOSAGE	
	Children*	Adults (max.)	Children	Adults (max./dose)
Isoniazid	10–20 mg/kg	5 mg/kg (300 mg)	20–40 mg/kg	15 mg/kg (900 mg)
Rifampin	10–20 mg/kg	10 mg/kg (600 mg)	10–20 mg/kg	10 mg/kg (600 mg)
Pyrazinamide	15–30 mg/kg (2 gm)		50–70 mg/kg (4 gm for twice weekly, 3 gm for thrice weekly)	
Ethambutol	15–25 mg/kg		50 mg/kg for twice weekly, 25–30 mg/kg for thrice weekly	
Streptomycin	20–40 mg/kg	15 mg/kg (1 gm)	25–30 mg/kg (1.5 gm)	

*≤12 yrs. old.

7. Bone and joint TB, miliary TB, and TB meningitis in children should be treated for 12 months.

8. Initiate treatment in infants as soon as the diagnosis is suspected.

Medication for TB Prophylaxis (Positive PPD)

1. High-priority candidates who should receive prophylactic therapy regardless of age
   a. Persons with suspected or confirmed HIV infection
   b. Persons recently exposed to active TB
   c. Those with chest radiograph indicative of previous TB and history of inadequate treatment
   d. People with high-risk medical conditions
   e. Persons who inject drugs
   f. Recent PPD converters

2. Lower priority candidates who should receive prophylactic therapy if they are under 35 years of age
   a. People from countries with endemic TB
   b. Medically indigent people
   c. Long-term care residents
   d. Children under 4 years of age

3. Daily INH regimen (plus pyridoxine for those at risk for vitamin deficiency)
   a. Six months in adults
   b. Nine months in children and HIV-infected persons
   c. Twelve months if history of silicosis or chest radiograph with old TB (or INH/RIF for 4 months)

4. Consider prophylaxis with RIF if history of exposure to INH-resistant TB.

5. For high-risk candidates in institutions, consider twice-weekly directly observed preventive therapy with INH

6. If adherence difficult to ensure, consider daily RIF (600 mg) plus PZA (20 mg/kg) for 2 months.

Activity

1. Hospitalized patients should be placed in respiratory isolation if the diagnosis is suspected.

2. Patients may need to be hospitalized in order to initiate treatment and render the patient non-infectious (usually after 2 to 3 weeks).

WARNING

Failure to adhere to prescribed regimens leads to treatment failure and the development of drug resistance. Directly observed therapy is the only proven method of ensuring adherence.

Patient Education

1. For patients from different social and cultural backgrounds, eliciting patient knowledge, attitudes, and practices about TB may be of utility.

2. Enlist the aid of outreach workers sharing the patient's culture and language.

3. Educate the patient about the medications, their side effects, and rationale for adherence to therapy.

 Key Treatment

- Hospitalize and isolate patients with active pulmonary TB until the patient is noninfectious.

- Initial therapy should be with a four-drug regimen.

Follow-Up

1. Strict adherence to treatment regimens must be ensured.

2. Clinical evaluation at least monthly to monitor for side effects of medications. INH, RIF, and PZA are hepatotoxic. Patients must be educated about the symptoms of hepatitis. Liver functions should be monitored. Monitor vision with EMB. Monitor hearing with SM.

3. Patients with HIV may respond slowly or inadequately.

4. Facilitate access to TB services, comprehensive health services, and social services.

 ## Bibliography

Bayer R, Stayton C, Desvarieux M, et al: Directly observed therapy and treatment completion for tuberculosis in the United States: is universal supervised therapy necessary? Am J Public Health 1998;88:1052–1058.

Centers for Disease Control and Prevention: Core Curriculum on Tuberculosis: What the Clinician Should Know, 3rd ed. Atlanta, Centers for Disease Control and Prevention, 1994.

Farmer P: Social scientists and the new tuberculosis. Social Sci Med 1997;44:347–358.

Gordin F, Chaisson R, Matts J, et al: A randomized trial of 2 months of rifampicin (RIF) and pyrazinamide (PZA) versus 12 months of isoniazid (INH) for the prevention of tuberculosis (TB) in HIV-positive (+), PPD+ patients [Abstract]. 5th Conference on Retroviruses and Opportunistic Infections. Chicago IL, 1998. *http://www.retroconference.org/abstracts/abstracts/latebrekers/lb5.htm.*

Halsey N, Coberly J, Desormeaux J, et al: Randomised trial of isonizid versus rifampicin and pyrazinamide for prevention of tuberculosis in HIV-1 infection. Lancet 1998;351:766–792.

Zuber PL, McKenna MT, Binkin NJ, et al: Long-term risk of tuberculosis among foreign-born in the United States. JAMA 1997;278:304–307.

51 Tuberculin Skin Testing

Nancy E. Neff

The tuberculin skin test (TST) is an important tool in both diagnosis and prevention of tuberculosis (TB). High sensitivity makes it more useful than chest radiograph in identifying *Mycobacterium tuberculosis* infection. Chemoprophylaxis with isoniazid of tuberculin reactors is an effective method of preventing active disease. A positive TST by itself does *not* indicate active disease.

Key Concept

Tuberculin positive	↗ negative chest radiograph = tuberculosis *infection*
	↘ positive chest radiograph = tuberculosis *disease*

1. TST positivity to purified protein derivative (PPD)

   a. Indication of presence of *M. tuberculosis* bacilli (dormant but potentially viable)

   b. Adequate cell-mediated immunity manifesting in a delayed hypersensitivity reaction

   c. Risk of reactivation of disease is greatest in the first few years after conversion, particularly in young children, adolescents, the elderly, and immunologically impaired hosts.

2. Tuberculin skin tests

   a. Multiple prong (tine) test: no longer recommended

   b. Mantoux test using intradermal injection of PPD recommended by Centers for Disease Control and Prevention (CDC).

   c. Mantoux technique (Fig. 51–1)

   (1) Tuberculin syringe fitted with short-bevel, ½-inch, 26- to 27-gauge needle

   (2) Withdraw 0.1 ml of PPD (5 tuberculin units [TUs]).

   (3) With bevel up, insert needle into forearm dermis and inject material, producing a bleb or "wheal" about 6 to 10 mm with *peau d'orange*.

   (4) If no bleb, injection was probably subcutaneous. Repeat in another location at least 5 cm distant (or in other forearm); otherwise risk of false-negative reading.

   d. Dose: intermediate strength: 5 TUs

   e. Interpretation: A designated-trained health care worker should read the TST at 48 to 72 hours (up to 1 week) after administration. It is *not recommended* that the client/parent or other health care worker interpret the results.

   (1) With forearm slightly flexed, check for induration visually and by palpation.

   (2) If induration felt, take a ballpoint pen to measure size (lightly draw a line on the skin into the indurated area, stopping when resistance is felt). Measure the transverse diameter of the reaction, recording it in millimeters.

   (3) Induration, not erythema, is significant. Erythema has *no* diagnostic significance. Vesiculation is always considered a positive reaction.

   (4) False negatives occur in 5 to 10 per cent of cases.

Symptoms

The majority of persons screened by TST will be asymptomatic.

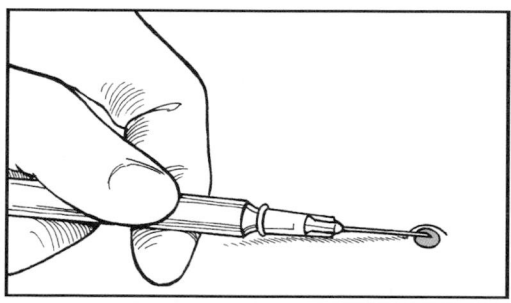

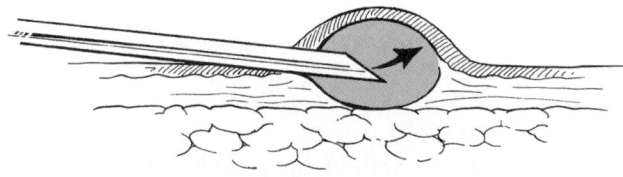

Figure 51–1 Mantoux technique for tuberculin skin testing.

High-Risk Individuals Who Should Receive TST

- Close contacts of known or suspected infectious TB cases (includes health care workers)

- Chest radiograph or clinical findings suggestive of TB

- Human immunodeficiency virus (HIV) infection or other immunosuppressive conditions (chronic steroids)

- Medical conditions (diabetes mellitus, Hodgkin's or lymphoproliferative disease, chronic renal disease, silicosis, or malabsorption)

- Immigrants from Latin America, Africa, Middle East, or Asia

- Residents of long-term care facilities (prisons, nursing homes)

- Injection drug users and alcoholics

- Medically underserved low-income populations

Screening Recommendations for Children

Annual
High risk
Every 2 to 3 Years
Exposed to individuals in following categories: HIV infected, homeless, institutionalized, users of illicit drugs, migrant farm workers, immigrants from endemic areas
At Ages 1, 4 to 6, and 11 to 16 Years
Low risk who live in high-risk areas

Key Points

- For children, the greatest risk of TB infection or disease is from close contact with an active case. For early detection and prevention of disease, contact investigation is more important than routine TST.

- *Routine* screening of low-risk populations is *not* cost effective.

Clinical Findings

1. Criteria for a positive TST are given in Table 51–1.
2. If TST positive, evaluate for presence of active disease (see Ch. 50, Tuberculosis).

Two-Step TST

1. Initial negative PPD in a high-risk individual whose sensitivity to tuberculin has waned over time. Administration of a single TST will boost immunologic memory, causing a second TST to react as positive and the individual to falsely be considered a recent converter.
2. Commonly used in screening health care workers and elderly nursing home residents
3. Determination if future positive reactions are due to booster phenomenon or to new conversion
4. *Procedure*: Repeat PPD 1 to 4 weeks after initial injection; record these results as the individual's baseline.

Differential Diagnosis

Causes of False-Positive and False-Negative TSTs

False Positives	*False Negatives*
- Prior bacille Calmette-Guérin (BCG) vaccination	- Early TB infection
	- Overwhelming TB
- Atypical mycobacterial infection	- Improper techniques
	- Anergic states
- Improper techniques	- Newborns and infants less than 3 months of age
- Hypersensitivity to PPD constituents	- Severe illnesses
- Cellulitis	- PPD within 2 months of measles-mumps-rubella vaccination or actual measles/mumps infection
- Arthus reaction	

Laboratory Tests
See Ch. 50.

Treatment
See Ch. 50.

Anergy Testing in Immunosuppressed Patients

1. CDC does not recommend *routine* anergy skin testing in conjunction with TST in screening programs for *M. tuberculosis* infection among HIV-infected persons.
2. If anergy skin testing is elected in order to assess an individual's risk for TB
   a. Use the two Food and Drug Administration–approved antigen controls by Mantoux method (mumps and *Candida*)
   b. Interpret reactions, with diameters of 5 mm or greater induration being considered positive.

TABLE 51–1. CRITERIA FOR A POSITIVE TUBERCULIN SKIN TEST

Induration ≥ 5 mm	Induration ≥ 10 mm	Induration ≥ 15 mm
HIV infection	Homeless, indigent population	Low risk
Close contacts of infectious TB cases	Immigrants from endemic areas	
Fibrosis or infiltrate on chest radiograph	Diabetes, renal failure, gastrectomy, other chronic disease	
Immunosuppression	Residents of long-term care facilities	
	Injection drug users, alcoholics	
	Health care workers	
	Infants, children <4 yr	

BCG Vaccination

1. BCG is live attenuated strain of *Mycobacterium bovis* used to prevent TB in endemic areas; efficacy is from 0 to 80 per cent—overall about 50 per cent. Increased efficacy demonstrated with intradermal injection.

2. Produces a positive TST initially (induration is generally ≤10 mm); the response diminishes with time (>3 years).

Key Point

Prior BCG vaccination is *never* a contraindication to TST.

3. Induration of 10 mm or greater signifies a positive TST and consideration of chemoprophylaxis is worthwhile (if indicated by other parameters and after active disease excluded). The larger the reaction, the greater the probability of TB infection.

4. Some individuals with a history of recent (<3 years) or repeated intradermal BCG vaccination may have persistent positive TST (>10 mm induration). Consideration of chemoprophylaxis should be made on the likelihood of exposure to active TB cases.

5. Although not indicated in United States (because of low incidence of new TB), BCG may be considered in populations at high risk for multi-drug-resistant TB (homeless, health care workers, and workers in institutions).

6. A major research effort to develop a more effective vaccine against TB is ongoing.

WARNING

BCG vaccination is contraindicated in immunosuppressed persons, including those with HIV infection.

Follow-Up

1. Frequency of repeat TST has not been determined for adults and should be based on clinical assessment of an individual's risk.

2. If an individual with an initial negative TST has close contact with an active case of TB, consider chemoprophylaxis and repeat TST in 3 months.

Special Note

TST should not be repeated in individuals with previously significantly positive skin test.

Bibliography

Centers for Disease Control and Prevention: Anergy skin testing and preventive therapy for HIV-infected persons: revised recommendations. MMWR Morb Mortal Wkly Rep 1997;46(RR-15):1–10.

Driver CR, Valway SE, Cantwell MF, et al: Tuberculin skin test screening in schoolchildren in the United States. Pediatrics 1996;98:97–102 (with comment by Starke JR: Tuberculosis skin testing: new schools of thought. Pediatrics 1996;98:123–125).

Hoft DF, Tennant JM: Persistence and boosting of Bacille Calmette-Guérin-induced delayed hypersensitivity. Ann Intern Med 1999;131:32–36.

McCollostor PJ, Neff NE: Outpatient management of tuberculosis. Am Fam Physician 1996;53:1579–1586.

Starkey RD: Tuberculin testing placement and interpretation. AAOHN J 1995;43:371–375.

U.S. Preventive Services Task Force: Screening for tuberculous infection—including Bacille Calmette-Guérin immunization. In: Guide to Clinical Preventive Services, 2nd ed, pp 277–286. Baltimore, Williams & Wilkins, 1996.

Indications

When spontaneous sputum is unavailable and one of the following is suspected

1. Infectious
   a. Mycobacterial disease
   b. *Pneumocystis* pneumonia
   c. Bacterial infection
   d. Fungal infection
2. Neoplastic
   a. Bronchogenic carcinoma
   b. Metastasis to lungs

Contraindications

1. No absolute contraindication
2. Altered mental status and extreme dyspnea are relative contraindications.
3. Defer sputum induction in patients with untreated pneumothorax.

Preparation

1. Patient instruction: The patient must understand the technique, particularly the need for deep coughing to produce sputum. Written instructions are particularly helpful.

Patient Instructions for Sputum Induction

You are requested to provide a sputum sample that contains secretions that collect in your lungs. This sample must not contain saliva or material from your mouth or throat. It is important that the sputum is produced by several very deep coughs.

This sputum will be analyzed to find out the cause of your respiratory symptoms. It is important to follow these steps so that the sputum you produce is useful.

Clean your mouth thoroughly. Vigorously brush your teeth, gums, and tongue and the back of your mouth. Then rinse your mouth repeatedly; next, make a grunting sound to clear your throat of any material.

Deeply inhale the aerosol spray. After you clean your mouth, you will be asked to breathe in a mist of salt water through a mask for 15 minutes. Breathe slowly and deeply, and inhale as much mist as possible. Try to avoid coughing during this period.

Cough forcefully. After you have inhaled mist for 15 minutes, you will be asked to cough repeatedly as hard as you can. After several deep coughs, spit out the sputum into the cup provided. Try not to swallow before you spit! Also, please try to avoid retching or vomiting during these cough efforts.

The key thing to remember is to cough as hard and as deeply as you can. Shallow coughs produce saliva and secretions from the mouth and throat that cannot be used to make a diagnosis.

---

2. Sputum induction suite: A single-patient room, a designated sputum induction room, or a sputum induction cubicle is recommended to avoid transmission of airborne pathogens. Personnel involved in sputum induction should use respiratory precautions.

Equipment

1. Standard jet nebulizer
2. Compressed gas source (oxygen or air)
3. Corrugated wide-bore plastic tube
4. Face mask or face tent
5. Hypertonic saline solution (3% or 5%): 2 to 4 oz
6. Sputum collection cups

Precautions

1. Maintain oxygenation if the patient is hypoxemic.
2. Use respiratory precautions for contagious infections (e.g., mycobacteria).

WARNING

Use respiratory precautions to prevent transmission of airborne pathogens such as *Mycobacterium tuberculosis*.

Technique

1. Tell the patient what is involved in obtaining a good sputum sample. Explain the difference between spitting and grunting (which often yield throat contents) and deep coughing.
2. The patient should be allowed to read and understand the written instructions provided (see "Patient Instructions for Sputum Induction").
3. Additional verbal reinforcement by a health care worker is usually necessary during the induction. It must be made clear that, unless the patient cooperates fully and coughs forcefully, this procedure is unlikely to be successful and, in some cases, fiberoptic bronchoscopy will be necessary to make the diagnosis.

Cleaning of Oropharynx

1. The patient should brush the teeth, gum surfaces, roof of the mouth, and surface of the tongue as far back as possible.
2. This should be followed by repeated rinsing of the mouth with water and expectoration of material from the throat.

Inhalation of Hypertonic Saline

1. Prolonged inhalation of an aerosol of hypertonic saline is usually necessary to induce sputum. Patient should be sitting upright and asked to inhale an aerosol generated by a standard jet nebulizer. A saline solution (2 to 3 oz of 3% to 5%) is used in the nebulizer and aerosolized by connecting the nebulizer to a gas source. Compressed air can be used, but, if the patient is hypoxic, oxygen can be used as the gas source to maintain an oxygen saturation level of greater than 90 per cent.
2. The nebulizer bottle is connected to a wide-bore tube, which in turn is connected to a face mask. The flow rate is set at 8 to 10 L/min. This high-output nebulization of saline is continued for 10 to 15 minutes while the patient breathes slowly and deeply through the mouth and nose. Coughing should be discouraged at this point.

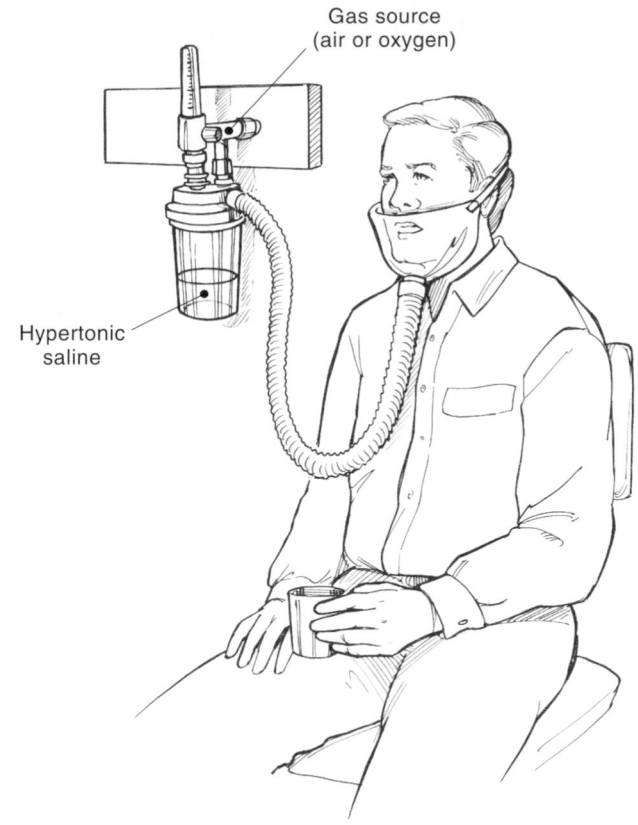

Gas source (air or oxygen)

Hypertonic saline

Sputum Collection and Processing

Obtaining the Specimen

1. After the patient has inhaled the aerosolized saline for at least 10 minutes, the mask is removed and the patient is instructed to expel saliva from the mouth and throat, which is discarded. A voluntary cough should then be initiated by the patient under the active supervision and encouragement of a health care worker. This person may be a physician, pulmonary function technologist, respiratory therapist, or any other person trained in the technique of sputum induction.
2. Several successive cough efforts in a stepladder manner (rapid, sequential coughs with brief pauses) are usually followed by forceful expectoration of the sputum, which is then collected in a specimen cup.
3. The patient should be encouraged to maintain forceful sequential cough efforts and not to swallow the sputum as it is raised in the throat. Several separate cough efforts should be attempted by the patient, and all sputum thus produced should be collected in one or more sputum cups.

4. If no sputum is obtained, inhalation of nebulized saline is resumed for 10 to 15 more minutes, after which coughing efforts should again be attempted. This process can be repeated once again, but if sputum cannot be obtained after two or three attempts, the induction should be terminated.

Processing the Specimen

The specimen should be stained and cultured as indicated, using standard techniques.

Follow-Up

At the end of the induction procedure, the patient is given a container and instructed to collect any subsequent sputum resulting from a deep cough. This sputum may be analyzed for appropriate pathogens or cells if initial samples are nondiagnostic.

Bibliography

For more information on the technique of sputum processing, see

Zaman MK, Wooten OF, Subrahmanya B, et al: Rapid noninvasive diagnosis of *Pneumocystis carinii* from induced liquefied sputum. Ann Intern Med 1988;109:7–10.

For more information on the use of sputum for the diagnosis of tuberculosis, see

Finch D, Beaty CD: The utility of a single sputum specimen in the diagnosis of tuberculosis: comparison between HIV-infected and non-HIV-infected patients. Chest 1997;111:1174–1179.

For more information on the use of sputum for bacterial infection, see

Lipinski EM, Flakas ED, Taylor BC: An evaluation of some methods of collecting sputum from patients with bronchitis and emphysema. Am Rev Respir Dis 1964; 89:760–764.

For more information on prevention of nosocomial tuberculosis during sputum induction, see

Centers for Disease Control and Prevention: Guidelines for the Prevention of *Mycobacterium tuberculosis* in health care facilities. MMWR Morb Mortal Wkly Rep 1995;43(RR-13):33–36.

52 Coccidioidomycosis

Diana S. Dark

Etiology and Epidemiology

1. Coccidioidomycosis is caused by a tissue dimorphic fungus, *Coccidioides immitis*. It grows in the soil as a mold. Infection is caused by inhalation of airborne, infective arthroconidia that grows in tissues as an endosporulating spherule. When the spherule ruptures, it releases endospores that migrate through lymphatics to form additional spherules in tissue at local and distant extrapulmonary sites.

2. *Coccidioides immitis* is endemic in specific geographic areas that have short, intense rainy seasons followed by hot and dry conditions.

3. Coccidioidomycosis is found only in the Western Hemisphere. Areas of highest endemicity are the southern San Joaquin River valley in California and southern Arizona, hence the popular term for the primary pulmonary manifestation of coccidioidomycosis, valley fever. Increasingly, cases are being recognized outside the endemic areas. They occur in travelers who have visited an endemic area, or as reactivations of infections acquired earlier in former residents of endemic areas, or as infections acquired from fomites from endemic areas (fruit, cotton, and landfills are documented sources of infection).

4. Disease can occur at any age; however, most cases occur in late childhood through early middle age and show a slight male preponderance.

5. In the United States alone, about 100,000 persons are infected annually.

Symptoms

Primary Infection

1. Most (60 per cent) of those infected have asymptomatic infections or illness indistinguishable from ordinary upper respiratory tract infections.

2. Forty per cent develop symptoms of a primary infection 1 to 3 weeks after exposure. These infections resemble a lower respiratory tract infection and/or systemic illness with some or all of the following symptoms: cough, sputum production, chest pain, malaise, headache, fever, chills, night sweats, anorexia, weakness, and arthralgias.

a. These infections are usually mild and passed off by the patient as an influenza-like illness.

b. In about one fourth of the symptomatic cases, the manifestations are more severe and include pleuritic chest pain. Most resolve uneventfully.

3. About 5 per cent of those infected have pulmonary residua, most commonly a pulmonary nodule or cavity.

4. A small number of patients develop acute progressive pneumonia, which often is fatal, or progress to chronic pulmonary disease.

5. About 0.5 per cent of patients develop disseminated (extrapulmonary) disease, which may involve almost any organ. This development is more common in an immunocompromised host.

Chronic Pulmonary Coccidioidomycosis

1. Acute pneumonia may progress to chronic pulmonary disease, usually of a cavitary nature. Patients with diabetes or with compromised immunity are more likely to develop this condition. The disease may wax and wane over many years.

2. Bronchiectasis may result from acute severe disease or chronic disease.

Disseminated Disease

1. Disseminated coccidioidomycosis occurs in patients who are at high risk:

a. Patients immunosuppressed as a result of steroid or cytotoxic therapy for cancer

b. Patients who have had organ transplantation

c. Patients with human immunodeficiency virus infection

d. Patients with other risk factors, including dark-skinned races, extremes of age, male sex, and diabetes mellitus

2. Muscles, tendons, bones, and joints may be involved in disseminated disease.

3. Meningitis may develop and usually occurs within 6 months after the primary infection. It may also appear acutely with the primary infection. Space-occupying central nervous system lesions are rare.

4. The skin is a common target for dissemination. Skin lesions can also result from direct inoculation with contaminated materials.

Key Symptoms

- Fever
- Nonproductive cough
- Pleuritic chest pain
- Arthralgias
- Atypical skin rash (20 per cent of patients)

Clinical Findings

Acute Coccidioidomycosis

1. Chest radiograph shows single or multiple areas of patchy pneumonitis. Hilar adenopathy is found in 20 per cent of cases. Necrosis of parenchymal lesions is common and eventually may form a characteristic thin-walled cavity.

2. Skin manifestations of primary illness are predominantly erythema nodosum and erythema multiforme.

3. Arthritis is seen in association with primary coccidioidomycosis. The ankle is the most commonly and most severely involved joint. The arthritis is usually symmetric and self-limited; it is known as "desert rheumatism" and represents an immune complex reaction, not disease dissemination.

Chronic Pulmonary Coccidioidomycosis

1. Cavitary lesions are usually seen on chest radiographs.
2. Pulmonary fibrosis can occur.
3. Cavities can become superinfected with bacteria or *Aspergillus* or, occasionally, rupture, causing empyema or pneumothorax.

Disseminated Coccidioidomycosis

1. Dissemination may involve the skin, soft tissues, bones and joints, the genitourinary system, and the central nervous system.
2. Signs depend on the organ system involved.
3. Cutaneous coccidioidomycosis can present variably as papules, pustules, plaques, nodules, ulcers, abscesses, or large proliferative lesions.

Key Signs

- Single or multiple areas of patchy pneumonitis on chest radiograph
- Hilar adenopathy (20 per cent of cases)
- Paratracheal and superior mediastinal adenopathy may signal dissemination.

Laboratory Tests

Acute Coccidioidomycosis

1. Knowledge of a patient's history of exposure through travel or residence in the endemic area is helpful.

2. Diagnosis can be confirmed by culture of the fungus on appropriate laboratory media. DNA probe identification of a suspected isolate may be helpful.

3. If a satisfactory sputum sample cannot be obtained, bronchoscopy or lung biopsy may be indicated.

4. Cultures of *C. immitis* represent a severe biologic hazard, and suspect isolates should be handled only by experienced laboratories that are prepared to deal with them.

5. The complement fixation test with *C. immitis* reacting with immunoglobulin G (IgG) antibody is the benchmark diagnostic test and becomes positive 2 to 6 weeks after infection.

6. There is growing experience with serum immunoglobulin M precipitins, which can be demonstrated by tube precipitin, latex agglutination, or immunodiffusion method. These antibodies occur 1 to 3 weeks after onset of the symptoms of primary infection in 75 per cent of cases and disappear within 4 months. More laboratories are becoming experienced with this method.

7. Coccidioidin skin testing has been widely used. However, a positive skin test does not necessarily connote acute disease, only prior infection.

Chronic Pulmonary Coccidioidomycosis

Serum titers are often high in patients with extensive chronic pulmonary disease but typically are low or absent in the presence of a solitary lung nodule or a single, thin-walled cavity.

Disseminated Coccidioidomycosis

1. The height of the IgG titer tends to parallel the extent of hematogenous dissemination.

2. A titer exceeding 1:16 is usually indicative of disseminated disease. However, there can be variation among laboratories. Regardless of the

laboratory, failure of the titer to fall during therapy of disseminated disease has an ominous prognosis.

3. Detection of complement-fixing antibody in cerebrospinal fluid is usually indicative of coccidioidal meningitis and remains the single most useful diagnostic test for that condition.

4. Biopsy material that shows a granulomatous histopathologic response to infection and contains characteristic spherules with evidence of endosporulation may also confirm the diagnosis.

5. It is more difficult to obtain positive cultures from urine, blood, gastric aspirates, pleural effusions, and peritoneal fluid.

Key Tests

- Culture of sputum or biopsy material

- Demonstration of positive complement fixation test in serum or cerebrospinal fluid

Differential Diagnosis

Coccidioidomycosis should be differentiated from other granulomatous diseases, such as tuberculosis and histoplasmosis.

Treatment

1. Acute pulmonary coccidioidomycosis: low risk for dissemination. Patients at low risk for dissemination need no therapy other than observation.

2. Acute pulmonary coccidioidomycosis: high risk for dissemination or disseminated disease

   a. Patients with pulmonary disease at high risk for dissemination

      (1) Fluconazole (Diflucan), 400 to 800 mg/day, or itraconazole (Sporanox), 200 mg twice a day with food

      (2) Alternative therapy: amphotericin B (Fungizone), 0.6 to 1.0 mg/kg/day intravenously for 7 days, then 0.8 mg/kg

every other day; total dose 2.5 gm or more

      (3) Duration of therapy is unclear—usually 9 to 12 months

   b. Relapse rate after therapy for disseminated disease is 15 to 25 per cent.

3. Meningitis in adults

   a. Amphotericin B intravenously as for pulmonary infections above plus 0.1 to 0.3 mg/day intrathecally by way of a reservoir device

   b. Alternative therapy: fluconazole, 400 to 600 mg/day orally indefinitely. Amphotericin B intrathecally is often added.

Key Treatment

Pulmonary and Extrapulmonary Disease

- **Drug of Choice:** fluconazole, 400 to 800 mg/day

- **Alternative Drugs:** itraconazole, amphotericin B

Meningitis in Adults

- **Drug of Choice:** amphotericin B intravenously and intrathecally

- **Alternative Drugs:** fluconazole orally plus amphotericin B intrathecally

Follow-Up

Because the relapse rate is fairly high, patients must be followed closely long term. Immunocompromised patients may need extended duration of therapy.

Bibliography

Coccidioidomycosis—United States, 1991–1992. MMWR Morb Mortal Wkly Rep 1993;42:21–24.

Einstein HE, Johnson RH: Coccidioidomycosis: new aspects of epidemiology and therapy. Clin Infect Dis 1993;16:349–356.

Galgiani JN: Coccidioidomycosis. Curr Clin Top Infect Dis 1997;17:188–204.

Stevens DA: Coccidioidomycosis. N Engl J Med 1995; 332:1077–1082.

53 Histoplasmosis

Dave G. Muthali

Etiology

The etiologic agent of histoplasmosis is *Histoplasma capsulatum*, a dimorphic fungus (i.e., exists in filamentous form and yeast form) endemic in the Ohio and Mississippi River valleys. The infection occurs by inhalation of small microconidia (2 to 5 μm) or yeast (3 to 4 μm) into the lungs by human beings.

Symptoms and Clinical Findings

1. Acute pulmonary histoplasmosis: Presents like acute flu-like illness after heavy-dose inhalation, and is self-limited. Symptoms are fever, chills, myalgias, nonproductive cough, anorexia, headache, chest pain.

2. Chronic pulmonary histoplasmosis: This type is characterized by slowly progressing disease with atypical infiltrates and cavities in the lungs. Common underlying disease is chronic obstructive pulmonary disease. Symptoms are cough, chest pain, dyspnea, weakness, fatigue, fever sweats, and weight loss. Cavities may be multiple, rarely may lead to bronchopleural fistula.

3. Disseminated histoplasmosis: Major predisposing factors in acquired immunodeficiency syndrome; however, other immune system–compromising disease also seen to predispose. Infection spreads outside the lungs: central nervous system (CNS) (chronic meningitis, brain lesions); oropharynx; gastrointestinal tract (ulcer, polyps); skin (maculopapular, necrotic); adrenal (Addison's disease is uncommon [<10% of cases]).

4. Other manifestations
   a. Mediastinal fibrosis
   b. Mediastinal granuloma
   c. Pericarditis
   d. Rheumatologic manifestation: erythema nodosum
   e. Arthritis/arthralgia
   f. Choroiditis: visual loss

Key Symptoms and Signs

- "Flu"-like illness
- Chronic symptoms with underlying lung disease
- CNS, gastrointestinal skin involvement

Laboratory Tests (see Table 53–1)

1. Histoplasma antigen assay
   a. Detection of *Histoplasma* antigen in blood, urine, bronchoalveolar lavage fluid, cerebrospinal fluid.
   b. Provides rapid diagnosis; results available in 1 to 2 days (see Table 53–1).

2. Fungal stain
   a. Bone marrow using Wright's stain has the highest yield; peripheral blood smear stain has low yield.
   b. The yield is better in disseminated histoplasmosis.

TABLE 53–1. SUMMARY OF DIAGNOSTIC TEST RESULTS IN HISTOPLASMOSIS

Test	Positive (%) Self-limited	Cavitary	Disseminated
Antibody			
Immunodiffusion	75	100	63
Complement fixation	89	93	63
Either immunodiffusion or complement fixation	99	100	71
Antigen detection	40–75*	21	92
Culture	15	85	85

*Seventy-five per cent with diffuse pulmonary infiltrates (J. Wheat, unpublished data, 1995).
From Williams B, Fojtasek M, Connolly-Stringfield P, et al: Diagnosis of histoplasmosis by antigen detection during an outbreak in Indianapolis, Ind. Arch Pathol Lab Med 1994;118:1205–1208. Copyright 1994 American Medical Association, with permission.

3. Fungal cultures
   a. This provides a low yield and delayed results. Agian, the highest yield is in disseminated histoplasmosis with bone marrow specimen.
   b. Multiple sputum cultures are recommended because of the lower yield in cavitary histoplasmosis.
4. Serology: Complement fixation test is most sensitive. A titre of 1:32 has the greatest significance, but titres of 1:8 to 1:16 should be interpreted with caution (see Table 53–1).
5. Histoplasmin skin test: not useful

Note

Antigen level declines during the first year after treatment and increases during relapse.

Note

False-positive results may arise with patients with other dimorphic fungi. Antibodies and antigen level decline after recovery and may increase with relapse. These level changes could be used to monitor the response to therapy.

 Key Test

- Complement fixation test is most sensitive.
- Cultures provide highest yield with disseminated disease.
- Multiple sputum cultures are recommended for cavitary disease.

Differential Diagnosis

1. Acute pulmonary histoplasmosis may mimic other bacterial and viral infections. The prodrome mimics influenza or any other febrile illness. Exposure to large doses of fungus spores is pertinent historic data that need to be elicited.
2. Chronic pulmonary histoplasmosis presents like tuberculosis and other dimorphic fungal infections. Chest radiographic appearance may mimic tuberculosis and cancer. Other constitutional symptoms are similar to tuberculosis. Weight loss and night sweats are present in all of the above illnesses.
3. High index of suspicion is necessary to diagnose histoplasmosis. Occupational history (e.g., chicken coop cleaners, tree cutters, chimney cleaners, and people involved in the demolition of old buildings) should be explored, even if

such an exposure is in the distant past. Life in the endemic belt and length of such stay are also important factors in the history.

Management

Antifungal Therapy (see Table 53–2)

1. Amphotericin B: 0.7 mg/kg/day for 1 week, thereafter, every other day if symptoms improve for 2 to 4 months. The treatment of choice for the initial period of 3 to 7 days. Later may be changed to itraconazole (Sporanox), or ketoconazole (Nizoral), for patients with moderate to severe infection (i.e., disseminated histoplasmosis, meningitis) (see Table 53–2).
2. Itraconazole or ketoconazole 200 to 400 mg PO daily may be given to patients with mild to moderate infection; however, itraconazole is proven to be superior to ketoconazole. Itraconazole is effective in 85 to 100 per cent of disseminated histoplasmosis cases and also is effective in chronic pulmonary histoplasmosis.

Note

- Itraconazole and ketoconazole should be taken with food or acid beverages.
- Histamine$_2$ blockers and omeprazole should be avoided.
- Liver enzyme inducers such as rifampin, rifabutin, phenytoin, and phenobarbital should be avoided because itraconazole and ketoconazole are eliminated solely by the liver.

Patient Education

1. This disease, unlike tuberculosis, does not spread from person to person by droplet infection; therefore, respiratory isolation is not warranted.
2. The therapy regimen of ketoconazole and itraconazole lasts for 12 months for disseminated

TABLE 53–2. INDICATIONS FOR ANTIFUNGAL THERAPY

INDICATED	NOT INDICATED
Acute pulmonary histoplasmosis with respiratory failure or prolonged symptoms	Acute self-limited pulmonary disease, rheumatologic pericarditis
Mediastinal granuloma with symptomatic obstruction	Fibrosing mediastinitis
Disseminated histoplasmosis	Sarcoid-like disease
Chronic pulmonary histoplasmosis	Presumed ocular disease

From Gorbach SL, Bartlett JG, Blacklow NR (eds): Infectious Diseases, 2nd ed. Philadelphia, WB Saunders Company, 1998, with permission.

histoplasmosis and longer for chronic pulmonary histoplasmosis; the duration of the course is 3 months for acute pulmonary histoplasmosis. Physician needs to work closely with the patient in order to ensure completion of therapy.

Prevention

People in occupations that involve soil sample collection, building demolition, chicken coop cleaning, and tree cutting should wear masks and respirators as recommended by the Centers for Disease Control and Prevention.

Follow-Up

The drug therapy is long term (between 3 months and 1 year) in most instances; therefore, close follow-up on the compliance and adverse reactions needs to be done as long as the patient is under therapy. For patients on amphotericin B, baseline renal function, and, for patients who are on itraconazole, baseline liver function, potassium, and triglycerides need to be established and these values monitored during therapy.

Bibliography

Bennett JE: Antifungal agents. In Hardman JG, Gilman AG, Limbird LE (eds): Goodman & Gilman's The Pharmacological Basis of Therapeutics, 9th ed, pp 1175–1190. New York, McGraw-Hill, 1996.

Sutliff WD: Histoplasmosis cooperative study: chronic pulmonary histoplasmosis treated with and without amphotericin B. Am Rev Respir Dis 1964;89:641.

U.S. Department of Health, Education and Welfare: Histoplasmosis Control: Decontamination of Bird Roosts, Chicken Houses and Other Point Sources. Washington, DC, U.S. Department of Health, Education and Welfare, 1990.

Wheat JH: Histoplasma. In Gorback SL, Bartlett JG, Blacklow NR (eds): Infectious Diseases, 2nd ed, pp 2335–2343. Philadelphia, WB Saunders Company, 1998.

Williams B, Fojtasek M, Connolly-Stringfield P, et al: Diagnosis of histoplasmosis by antigen detection during an outbreak in Indianapolis, Ind. Arch Pathol Lab Med 1994;118:1205–1208.

54 Blastomycosis

Dennis J. Baumgardner

Etiology

1. Causative agent: *Blastomyces dermatitidis*, a dimorphic fungus that infects humans and animals
2. Endemic areas: North America (southeastern United States, Ohio and Mississippi River basins to Colorado, and Canada around Great Lakes), Africa, India
3. Risk factors: residence or visitation in a highly endemic area, especially along waterways; excavation
4. Acquisition: Except for rare inoculation disease, spores are inhaled from environment; transition to yeast form occurs in the lungs; no person-to-person or zoonotic spread (sexual and vertical transmission has been reported)

Symptoms

1. Age: All ages are affected; peak in fourth and fifth decades.
2. Sex: Moderate male predominance may reflect differential exposure.
3. Pulmonary forms
   a. Acute pneumonia
      (1) Asymptomatic disease (like histoplasmosis) is common.
      (2) Mild or self-limited
      (3) Moderate to severe
   b. Chronic pneumonia
   c. Overwhelming disseminated pulmonary infection, often including adult respiratory distress syndrome

Clinical Findings

1. Physical pulmonary findings are nonspecific.
2. May have erythema nodosum
3. By extension or spread may involve respiratory tree, pericardium or myocardium, mediastinum
4. Disseminated disease
   a. Often not temporally related to lung disease
   b. Skin: most commonly involved
      (1) Verrucous form: sharp, raised, serpiginous border above subcutaneous abscess. Center often crusted with black dots. Tends to be on exposed peripheral areas.
      (2) Ulcerative form: often heaped borders, exudate
   c. Bone and joint: nonspecific presentation; vertebrae, ribs, skull, long bones, pelvis most commonly affected.
   d. Genitourinary: prostatitis and epididymoorchitis most common; female genital tract less common
   e. Central nervous system: epidural, cranial abscess; meningitis. Lumbar puncture not sensitive for diagnosis.
   f. Involvement of virtually every organ system and tissue has been reported. Subcutaneous abscesses and other cold abscesses may be involved.
5. Increasingly recognized as a severe disease in patients who are immunocompromised or who have acquired immunodeficiency syndrome; often disseminated.

Key Symptoms

Pulmonary Disease

- Cough (87 per cent)
- Fatigue (82 per cent)
- Fever (71 per cent)
- Weight loss (65 per cent)
- Chest pain (63 per cent)
- Night sweats (62 per cent)
- Myalgias (41 per cent)
- Hemoptysis (17 per cent)

From the author's series of 78 pulmonary blastomycosis patients from highly endemic northern Wisconsin, reported, in part, in Baumgardner et al. (1992).

Key Signs

Chest Radiograph

- No diagnostic patterns
- Air space findings most common; also mass, interstitial, miliary; often multiple lobes
- Chronic disease more apt to present as lung mass
- May have nodules, satellite lesions, cavitation, effusions, adenopathy
- Radiographic and clinical pictures often do not correlate.

Laboratory Tests

1. Potassium hydroxide 10% and/or Calcofluor White wet preparations are useful for sputum and exudates; fungal stains are useful for most specimens.
2. Culture is definitive but takes days to weeks.
3. Older serology (complement fixation, immunodiffusion) often is unreliable, but newer antigen tests (enzyme immunoassay, radioimmunoassay) continue to be improved and may become routinely useful.

Key Tests

Prompt, reasonably sensitive diagnosis afforded by microscopic examination of sputum, exudate, or other clinical material for yeast forms (generally 8 to 15 μm) with single, broad-based (4- to 5-μm) buds.

Differential Diagnosis

1. Prompt diagnosis depends on a high index of suspicion (and travel history, if nonendemic area).
2. Pulmonary disease: other fungal and pathogenic actinomycetes, especially histoplasmosis (overlapping endemic areas); tuberculosis; lung cancer; community-acquired pneumonia; sarcoidosis; silicosis; other
3. Skin disease: skin cancer, keratoacanthoma, other infections and conditions
4. Other sites: various infectious, neoplastic, and granulomatous disease

Treatment

Medication

1. Itraconazole (Sporanox), 200 mg/day orally after a full meal; may increase to 300 or 400 mg/day if needed. Efficacy is better than that of ketoconazole, with less toxicity but higher cost. Obtain baseline liver function tests and follow clinically for signs of hepatic dysfunction. Avoid terfenadine (Seldane), astemizole (Hismanal), and cisapride (Propulsid). Use for 6 months.
2. Ketoconazole (Nizoral), 400 mg/day orally with breakfast. Increase to 600 or 800 mg/day in 2 to 4 weeks if no response. Avoid any medication that reduces gastric acid. Nausea, vomiting, and headaches may occur (also hormonal abnormalities at higher doses); hepatocellular damage may occur (obtain baseline liver function tests and monitor while on therapy). Avoid terfenadine (Seldane) and astemizole (Hismanal). Take for minimum of 6 months.

3. Fluconazole (Diflucan) not considered equivalent to itraconazole, and higher doses (400 to 800 mg/day) must be used; other new azoles not fully tested.
4. Amphotericin B (Fungizone), total dose of 2000 mg. Use 1-mg test dose and then rapidly increase to 35 to 50 mg/day. Avoid dehydration. Premedicate with acetaminophen with or without antihistamines and/or meperidine. Monitor blood pressure during infusion, anemia, kidney and liver dysfunction, electrolytes and magnesium imbalance, and gastrointestinal, thrombophlebitic, and other adverse effects.
5. Pediatrics, pregnancy: usually supportive care and amphotericin B. Consult current literature.

Diet

As tolerated. Support respiratory muscles.

Activity

As tolerated.

Patient Education

1. Advise the patient who has a history of blastomycosis to always inform the physician when ill because reactivation may occur.
2. Patients who reside or visit in a highly endemic area should know the signs and symptoms to report to the physician.
3. The use of a respirator mask when excavating in a highly endemic area is recommended but of unproven benefit.

Key Treatment

- Asymptomatic or mild acute, nonpleural pulmonary disease, stable or improving: no treatment, careful observation
- Mild to moderate acute pulmonary; chronic progressive pulmonary; extrapulmonary (non–central nervous system) disease: itraconazole
- Life-threatening or central nervous system infection; noncompliance, immunocompromise, or failure of oral therapy: amphotericin B

Follow-Up

1. Fatalities still occur, but they should be minimized by prompt diagnosis in normal hosts.
2. The prognosis, after recovery, is generally good.
3. Observe for noncompliance with oral medication.
4. Be aware that reactivation may occur regardless of the severity of the initial infection or completion of a full course of therapy.

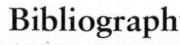

Bibliography

Al-Doory Y, DiSalvo AF (eds): Blastomycosis. New York, Plenum Medical Book Company, 1992.

Baumgardner DJ, Buggy BP, Mattson BJ, et al: Epidemiology of blastomycosis in a region of high endemicity in North Central Wisconsin. Clin Infect Dis 1992;15: 629–635.

Blastomycosis. Semin Respir Infect 1997;12:187–267. (entire September issue)

Chapman SW: *Blastomyces dermatitidis*. In Mandell GL, Bennett JE, Dolin R (eds): Principles and Practice of Infectious Diseases, 4th ed, pp 2353–2365. New York, Churchill Livingstone, 1995.

Pappas PG: Blastomycosis. In Rakel RE (ed): Conn's Current Therapy, pp 201–202. Philadelphia, WB Saunders Company, 1997.

55 Sarcoidosis

George Allen Tindol, Jr.

Etiology

1. Sarcoidosis, a multisystemic disease of unknown etiology, most commonly affects the lungs, lymph nodes, eyes, and skin. Genetic susceptibility in the host, plus one or more unknown environmental triggers, combine to activate the cell-mediated component of the immune system.

2. Lesions are characterized histologically as noncaseating granulomas.

3. The disease typically affects young adults in the third and fourth decades of life, and occurs more frequently in certain geographic and/or ethnic groups: for example, the lifetime risk for African Americans is 2.4 per cent, compared with 0.85 per cent for white Americans. Mortality rates are similar among races.

Symptoms and Clinical Findings

1. Although the lungs are involved in at least 90 per cent of patients, only approximately half of patients with pulmonary disease are symptomatic. Pulmonary symptoms include dyspnea, dry cough, and pleuritic chest pain. Clubbing of digits is rare. Progressive pulmonary failure is the most common cause of death in sarcoidosis.

2. Skin lesions occur in approximately 25 per cent of patients, and include lupus pernio (indurated violaceous lesions principally on the cheeks, nose, lips, and ears), skin plaques, maculopapular eruptions, subcutaneous nodules, erythema nodosum, alopecia, and erythema multiforme.

   a. Granuloma formation in an old scar or tattoo is characteristic.

   b. Erythema nodosum is a marker of good prognosis, and patients with erythema nodosum, bilateral hilar lymphadenopathy, and polyarthralgias (Löfgren's syndrome) have the best prognosis.

3. Ocular lesions occur in approximately 25 per cent of patients. Anterior uveitis, the most common manifestation, classically presents as rapid onset of blurred vision, photophobia, and excessive lacrimation, usually clearing spontaneously within a year. It is important to note that sarcoidosis is a preventable cause of blindness; treatment with topical or systemic corticosteroids is usually effective.

4. Nontender, freely moveable lymphadenopathy, especially cervical lymphadenopathy, is common. Splenomegaly occurs in less than one fourth of patients.

5. Of neurologic manifestations, which occur in approximately 5 to 15 per cent of patients with sarcoidosis, cranial neuropathies are most common. A peripheral VIIth nerve palsy (Bell's palsy) is the most common single lesion, and may be bilateral in one third of cases. The optic nerve is the second most commonly involved cranial nerve, leading to blurred vision, visual field deficits, pupillary abnormalities, and papilledema. Sarcoidosis may also cause aseptic meningitis, seizures, and peripheral neuropathy.

6. Head and neck manifestations (approximately 10 per cent of patients) include painless parotid swelling and involvement of the upper respiratory tract, particularly the nasal mucosa.

7. Polyuria and polydipsia may stem from sarcoid involvement of the pituitary and hypothalamus, or from hypercalcemia, hypercalciuria, and nephrogenic diabetes insipidus. Sarcoidosis may also cause hyperprolactinemia and the galactorrhea-amenorrhea syndrome.

8. Complete heart block leading to syncope is the most common presentation of cardiac involvement of sarcoidosis. Ventricular tachycardia and premature ventricular contractions are next most common. Electrocardiography may reveal ventricular arrhythmias in up to 22 per cent of patients with sarcoidosis. Sudden death is the most common cause of death in patients with cardiac involvement, followed by progressive heart failure.

9. Hypercalcemia is present in 10 per cent of patients with sarcoidosis, whereas hypercalciuria is three times more frequent. The abnormalities of calcium metabolism are the result of increased synthesis of 1,25-dihydroxyvitamin D_3 (calcitriol) by the epithelioid sarcoid granulomas, and enhanced absorption of calcium from the gastrointestinal tract. Hypercalcemia

and hypercalciuria in patients with sarcoidosis can lead to impaired renal function, nephrolithiasis, nephrocalcinosis, and chronic renal failure.

10. Acute sarcoid arthritis is a commonly described syndrome characterized by symmetric polyarthritis, with spontaneous resolution within months in most patients. Chronic sarcoid arthritis is a rare, usually nondestructive, polyarthritis that usually occurs in association with chronic cutaneous sarcoidosis.

11. Although symptomatic muscle involvement in sarcoidosis is rare, asymptomatic granulomas in skeletal muscle biopsies are frequent.

 Key Symptoms

- Asymptomatic; diagnosed on routine chest radiograph
- Dyspnea
- Cough (nonproductive)
- Retrosternal chest pain
- Arthralgia/myalgia

 Key Signs

- Lymphadenopathy
- Skin lesions
- Uveitis

Tests

1. Findings on chest radiograph are classified as follows: stage 0 (normal); stage I (bilateral hilar lymphadenopathy without pulmonary infiltrates); stage II (bilateral hilar lymphadenopathy plus pulmonary infiltrates); stage III (pulmonary infiltrates without hilar lymphadenopathy); stage IV (extensive fibrosis). Chest computerized tomography (CT) scan may reveal mediastinal adenopathy, parenchymal fibrosis, and infiltrates not visualized on chest radiograph, but is nonspecific and not required in routine diagnosis or follow-up. High-resolution CT may be useful for assessing activity of disease in patients who are in stage II or stage III and in selecting areas for diagnostic biopsy.

2. Pulmonary function studies reveal reductions in lung volumes (vital capacity and total lung capacity) and reduced carbon monoxide diffusion capacity (DL_{CO}). Gas exchange is preserved and hypoxemia is rare until late in the course. There is frequently poor correlation with the extent of the disease on chest radiograph, with the chest radiograph appearing much worse than the pulmonary function tests (PFTs).

3. Involved tissue, either from surgical removal of an accessible lymph node or transbronchial biopsy, is necessary for diagnosis. The absence of an infectious process, such as tuberculosis or fungal, bacterial, or protozoal infections, must be demonstrated by appropriate stains and cultures.

4. The serum level of angiotensin-converting enzyme (ACE) is elevated in approximately 60 per cent of patients but is nonspecific and has no prognostic value. Although serial values may grossly reflect activity of disease in some patients, they are not an accurate reflection in many others. ACE inhibitors may interfere with the test result.

5. Bronchoalveolar lavage aspirate typically reveals a lymphocytic alveolar infiltrate; it has been a valuable research tool but has little clinical or prognostic value.

6. Typical cerebrospinal fluid findings in sarcoidosis include an elevated protein concentration, lymphocytosis, and low glucose.

7. Cutaneous anergy, as demonstrated by a negative tuberculin skin test and control, is a common finding.

8. Hypercalciuria may be present with or without hypercalcemia.

9. Nephrocalcinosis may be evident on renal ultrasound.

10. Gallium scan correlates with active inflammatory processes and may indicate systemic involvement outside the lungs, but does not predict prognosis or responsiveness to therapy.

11. Rhythm, conduction, and repolarization abnormalities appear on electrocardiograms in approximately half of patients with sarcoid cardiac involvement. If pulmonary disease has progressed to extensive lung fibrosis and pulmonary hypertension, electrocardiogram may show signs of cor pulmonale.

12. In the Kveim-Siltzbach test, an antigenic extract prepared from the spleens of patients with known sarcoidosis is injected intradermally. A positive test is defined by the presence of typical sarcoid granulomata on biopsy 4 to

6 weeks later. In the era of concern for transmitting blood-borne infections, the feasibility of this test has been questioned, and it is now primarily of historic interest.

Key Tests

- Chest radiography
- Pulmonary function testing
- Tissue biopsy, with acid-fast bacillus and fungal cultures (negative)
- Electrocardiogram if cardiac involvement suspected

Differential Diagnosis

1. Chief among the differential diagnoses of sarcoidosis are berylliosis and fungal infections such as histoplasmosis.
2. Sarcoidosis has been described concurrently with tuberculosis, systemic lupus erythematosus, rheumatoid arthritis, Sjögren's syndrome, spondyloarthritis, and human immunodeficiency virus.
3. Mycobacterial infection has been linked with sarcoidosis but never conclusively proven as the etiologic agent.

Treatment

Approximately 75 per cent of patients will undergo a spontaneous remission or have mild, stable disease not requiring treatment. Indications for systemic treatment of sarcoidosis include severe ocular, neurologic, or cardiac manifestations; disfiguring skin lesions; malignant hypercalcemia; symptomatic or progressive (based on serial PFTs) stage II pulmonary disease; and stage III pulmonary disease.

Medication

1. Corticosteroids, although not curative, are the drugs of choice to suppress disease; initially 30 to 40 mg of prednisone daily, slowly tapered as tolerated over 6 to 12 months, usually relieves symptoms, suppresses inflammation, slows formation of new granuloma, and resolves existing granuloma. Normalization of hypercalcemia and improvement in pulmonary function tests has been demonstrated. Alternate-day therapy is usually effective and may decrease the adverse effects of treatment; however, daily treatment may improve compliance.

2. Alternative drugs include methotrexate for patients who are refractory to corticosteroids or who have severe skin lesions, arthritis, or refractory ocular manifestations. Folic acid should be administered concurrently with methotrexate. Routine hematologic, liver, and renal function tests should be performed. Both female and male patients should employ adequate birth control methods because all cytotoxic agents used to treat sarcoid are teratogenic.
3. Chloroquine (Aralen), hydroxychloroquine (Plaquenil), and ketoconazole (Nizoral) have been effective in treating the hypercalcemia associated with sarcoidosis, and cyclosporine (Sandimmune) may be useful in treating refractory neurosarcoidosis.
4. Inhaled corticosteroids may be effective in mild sarcoidosis characterized chiefly by cough and bronchial inflammation and hyperreactivity.

Key Treatment

Drugs of Choice: corticosteroids

Alternative drugs	*Indication*
• Methotrexate	• Pulmonary symptoms refractory to corticosteroids
• Hydroxychloroquine	
	• Severe skin involvement
	• Hypercalcemia
	• Chronic skin lesions

Follow-Up

1. Asymptomatic patients with bilateral hilar lymphadenopathy (stage I) but without extrapulmonary involvement have an approximately 80 per cent chance of spontaneous remission within 2 years, and therefore should be left untreated. A chest radiograph should be repeated initially every 3 months and then every 6 months until the outcome of the disease is established.
2. When patients are being treated for pulmonary involvement, their course should be monitored by spirometry, diffusion capacity, chest radiograph, and (possibly) serum ACE level.
3. Following initial electrocardiogram, Holter monitoring, exercise testing, and, when indicated, thallium scanning, patients with sarcoid cardiac involvement should receive yearly cardiologic evaluation.

Bibliography

 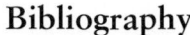

Baughman RP, Lower EE: Steroid-sparing alternative treatments for sarcoidosis. Clin Chest Med 1997;18: 853–864.

Costabel U, Teschler H: Biochemical changes in sarcoidosis. Clin Chest Med 1997;18:827–841.

Kimani AP, Aguayo SM: Sarcoidosis: an overview for the primary care physician. Compr Ther 1998;24:20–25.

Lynch JP, Kazerooni EA, Gay SE: Pulmonary sarcoidosis. Clin Chest Med 1997;18:755–785.

Newman LS, Rose CS, Maier LA: Sarcoidosis. N Engl J Med 1997;336:1224–1234.

Pollack CV, Jorden RC: Recognition and management of sarcoidosis in the emergency department. J Emerg Med 1993;11:297–308.

Sharma OP: Cardiac and neurologic dysfunction in sarcoidosis. Clin Chest Med 1997;18:813–825.

Sharma OP: Pulmonary sarcoidosis and corticosteroids. Am Rev Respir Dis 1993;147:1598–1600.

56 Sleep Apnea

Lee K. Brown

Etiology

1. The respiratory disturbances associated with sleep vary by *degree*.
   a. Apnea: the cessation of airflow at the nose and mouth for 10 seconds or longer
   b. Hypopnea: a reduction in airflow at the nose and mouth
2. In addition, apneas or hypopneas may vary by *mechanism*.
   a. Obstructive: The resistance of the upper airway increases.
   b. Central: Respiratory effort is reduced or ceases.
   c. Mixed: a period of central apnea followed by several obstructed breaths. These have the same clinical implications as purely obstructive events.
3. Following generally accepted usage, the asymptomatic disorder is defined as *sleep apnea* (central or obstructive); *sleep apnea syndrome* (central or obstructive) is diagnosed when symptoms occur. In addition, the upper airway resistance syndrome has recently been described and is regarded as a variant of obstructive sleep apnea syndrome. In this disorder, upper airway caliber is diminished during sleep, and respiratory effort increases to maintain normal airflow. The increased effort results in recurrent arousal from sleep (termed *respiratory effort–related arousal*) and produces daytime sleepiness in a manner similar to obstructive sleep apnea syndrome.
4. Central sleep apnea syndrome is a relatively uncommon entity most frequently associated with congestive heart failure or central nervous system disease. The following discussion concentrates on obstructive sleep apnea syndrome. With rare exceptions, the obstruction occurs at the oropharyngeal and/or hypopharyngeal level. Several mechanisms may contribute.
   a. Reduced upper airway caliber, caused by the following:
      (1) Obesity (collections of adipose tissue have been demonstrated adjacent to the airway)
      (2) Adenotonsillar hypertrophy (usually in children)
      (3) Mandibular deficiency (e.g., micrognathia or retrognathia)
      (4) Macroglossia (frequently associated with hypothyroidism)
      (5) Upper airway tumors (rare)
   b. Excessive pressure across the collapsible segment, most frequently attributed to nasal obstruction
   c. Activity of the muscles of the upper airway insufficient to maintain patency. Electromyographic studies have demonstrated reduced electrical activity of these muscles during apneas, consistent with a defect in respiratory control. The exact nature of this respiratory control instability is not known.

Symptoms

Symptoms may be either nocturnal (during sleep) or diurnal (during wakefulness).

1. Nocturnal
   a. Snoring, usually described as intermittent or *resuscitative*. Noise is produced between apneas, when large breaths are drawn through an airway that is still somewhat narrowed (almost universal).
   b. Abnormal motor activity, reflecting episodes of asphyxiation. The patients flail out and throw the bedcovers off and may sit up or get out of bed (common).
   c. Nocturia (or even enuresis), a manifestation of diuresis and natriuresis possibly caused by increased elaboration of atrial natriuretic factor (common).
   d. Symptoms of gastroesophageal reflux, presumably from the negative intrapleural pressures developed during obstructed breaths (relatively common).
   e. Self-reported nocturnal awakenings are uncommon, despite the fact that each respiratory event is generally terminated by an arousal. Occasionally, insomnia may be a presenting complaint.
2. Diurnal
   a. Excessive daytime sleepiness. Causation may be the nocturnal sleep disruption or hypoxemia (common).
   b. Cognitive impairment, including poor mem-

ory, and personality changes; correlates best with nocturnal hypoxemia (common).

c. Morning headache or nausea, probably of cerebrovascular origin, resulting from nocturnal hypercapnia (common).

Key Symptoms

- Snoring
- Excessive daytime sleepiness

Clinical Findings

Although a variety of physical findings may be associated with obstructive sleep apnea syndrome, none of them are specific to the disorder. They include the following:

1. Obesity
2. Macroglossia, usually associated with hypothyroidism
3. Enlarged, low-lying, edematous, or erythematous uvula
4. Narrow oropharynx, or oropharyngeal edema or erythema
5. Adenotonsillar enlargement (more common in children)
6. Retrognathia or micrognathia
7. Upper airway tumors
8. Systemic hypertension
9. Signs of pulmonary hypertension or cor pulmonale
10. Plethora

Tests

1. Polysomnography is the test of choice and is diagnostic if more than five obstructive apneas or hypopneas occur per hour of sleep (respiratory disturbance index >5) during at least 6 hours of nocturnal sleep. Daytime nap studies are discouraged because rapid-eye-movement (REM) sleep (which is associated with the most severe and at times the only respiratory events) seldom occurs during these studies. Unattended polysomnography in the home may be performed using portable equipment. Some systems are well validated, but all suffer from the unattended nature of the recording and some offer only a limited subset of the signals collected during a laboratory study. The following signals are recorded during the standard laboratory polysomnogram:

   a. Electrophysiologic indices of sleep stage (electroencephalogram, electro-oculogram, electromyogram)

   b. Electromechanical indices contrasting respiratory effort with actual ventilation (chest and/or abdominal movement; airflow at the nose and mouth)

   c. Consequences of apneic events, including electrocardiogram and pulse oximetry

2. Multiple sleep latency test (MSLT), a test of daytime somnolence performed by recording sleep staging parameters during four or five nap opportunities during the daytime. A nocturnal polysomnogram must always precede an MSLT. Reduced mean sleep latency (average time to fall asleep for all nap opportunities) indicates pathologic sleepiness and is used to assess the efficacy of treatment. The MSLT may be diagnostic of another disorder that causes hypersomnolence, the narcolepsy syndrome.

3. Several standard laboratory tests are useful in the overall management of these patients.

   a. Arterial blood gas analysis may reveal daytime hypercapnia, indicating coexisting pickwickian (obesity-hypoventilation) syndrome.

   b. Chest radiography and electrocardiography may reveal signs of pulmonary hypertension or cor pulmonale.

   c. Serum thyroid-stimulating hormone assay may detect unsuspected hypothyroidism.

4. Other specialized tests of use in selected patients include the following:

   a. Fiberoptic examination of the upper airway to rule out obstructing tumors

   b. Cephalometric radiography, useful in defining the anatomy of the upper airway when surgical treatment is contemplated

Key Test

Polysomnography

Treatment

Treatment is generally recommended for any patient with a respiratory disturbance index (number of apneas plus hypopneas per hour of sleep) greater than 20 because this has been associated with increased mortality. Symptomatic patients with fewer respiratory events may also be treated.

1. Nasal continuous positive airway pressure (nasal CPAP), which holds the upper airway open by a pneumatic splint effect. A tight-fitting nasal mask is attached to a flow generator, incorporating a positive end-expiratory pressure valve or other means to maintain positive airway pressure. Nasal "pillows," which fit into the

nares, may be more comfortable than the mask in some patients. Nasal CPAP is the most satisfactory treatment available. Problems with this therapy include the following:

   a. Patient compliance. Patients only use the device about 4 to 5 hours per night on average; some patients may not use the device at all or use it only on some nights.

   b. Nasal irritation or rhinitis. This problem can be minimized by

      (1) Humidification

      (2) Intranasal steroids (e.g., beclomethasone)

      (3) Intranasal disodium cromoglycate

   c. Barotrauma, of theoretical concern whenever positive-pressure therapy is used, has been exceedingly rare.

2. Oral appliances, including a mandibular advancement orthotic (Snore Guard and others) and tongue-retaining devices, have been of benefit in selected patients.

3. A variety of surgical procedures have been advocated.

   a. Uvulopalatopharyngoplasty (either conventional or laser-assisted) improves oropharyngeal patency and almost always eliminates snoring. However, obstructive sleep apnea syndrome is cured (defined as respiratory disturbance index <20) in only about one half of patients, probably because of persistent hypopharyngeal obstruction. No preoperative clinical indicators of response are known.

   b. Tonsillectomy and adenoidectomy may be of benefit when significant hypertrophy is present.

   c. Maxillofacial reconstruction, an aggressive therapy, is usually reserved for patients who fail nasal CPAP and uvulopalatopharyngoplasty. These procedures are designed to achieve the following:

      (1) Increase the size of the bony skeleton enclosing the tongue, using techniques such as inferior sagittal osteotomy of the mandible or maxillomandibular osteotomy

      (2) Put traction on the base of the tongue, usually by hyoid myotomy and suspension

4. Protriptyline (Vivactil) and fluoxetine (Prozac) are nonsedating antidepressant agents that suppress REM sleep, when the most severe apneas characteristically occur, and may increase the tone of upper airway muscles. They are occasionally of benefit in selected patients.

5. Weight reduction may be of significant benefit in the obese patient.

6. Sleep position training. Some patients exhibit apneas predominantly in the supine position and can be induced to avoid this position by sewing a tennis ball into the back of the pajama top or through the use of electronic sensors that alarm when the patient is supine.

 Key Treatment

Nasal CPAP

 Bibliography

ASDA Polysomnography Task Force: The indications for polysomnography and related procedures. Sleep 1997; 20:423–487.

Brown LK: Sleep apnea syndromes: overview and diagnostic approach. Mt Sinai J Med 1994;61:99–112.

Kaplan J, Staats BA: Obstructive sleep apnea syndrome. Mayo Clin Proc 1990;65:1087–1094.

Kryger MH: Management of obstructive sleep apnea. Clin Chest Med 1992;13:481–492.

Rapoport DM: Treatment of sleep apnea syndromes. Mt Sinai J Med 1994;61:123–130.

57 Common Cardiovascular Symptoms

SYMPTOM CHEST PAIN

Vaskar Mukerji

Chest pain is a common symptom encountered by physicians. The causes of chest pain range from serious, potentially life-threatening diseases to relatively minor disorders that pose no threat to life but produce recurrent aggravating symptoms. Every patient complaining of chest pain should be carefully investigated. In particular, it is important not to miss the presence of serious heart disease, because the consequences of such a mistake could be disastrous. Nevertheless, the vast majority of patients coming to a physician's office with chest pain are not having an acute myocardial infarction. A working knowledge of the various conditions that may cause chest pain is crucial for the appropriate management of these patients.

Differential Diagnosis

Cardiovascular

1. Coronary artery disease
   a. Acute myocardial infarction
   b. Unstable angina pectoris
   c. Stable angina pectoris
   d. Prinzmetal's angina
2. Valvular heart disease
   a. Mitral valve prolapse
   b. Aortic stenosis
3. Hypertrophic cardiomyopathy
4. Pericarditis
5. Aortic dissection

Noncardiac

1. Pulmonary: tracheobronchitis, pneumonia, pleurisy, pulmonary embolism, lung cancer
2. Esophageal: reflux, spasm
3. Rheumatologic: fibromyalgia, costochondritis, Tietze's syndrome, arthritis (rheumatoid or osteoarthritis), injury to chest wall, spinal disease
4. Neurologic: cervical or thoracic radiculopathy, herpes zoster
5. Psychiatric conditions: panic disorder, generalized anxiety, agoraphobia and other phobias,

depression, somatization, conversion, malingering, and Munchausen's syndrome
6. Breast conditions
7. Referred pain from abdominal viscera

Refer to Ch. 61, Coronary Artery Disease; Ch. 62, Myocardial Infarction; Ch. 66, Cardiomyopathy; Ch. 69, Aortic Dissection; and Ch. 71, Pericarditis.

History: Key Questions to Ask

1. What precipitates and what relieves the chest pain?
2. What is the character of the pain (location, radiation, quality, intensity, duration, frequency)?
3. Are there any associated symptoms?

Coronary artery disease primarily affects elderly and middle-aged individuals, with a predilection for males. Typically the chest pain of angina pectoris occurs with exertion, anxiety, or exposure to cold and is relieved with rest or sublingual nitroglycerin. Frequently, it is accompanied by dyspnea, diaphoresis, or fatigue. Patients commonly describe the pain as a dull substernal or precordial pressure sensation radiating down the left arm or to the neck. Others describe a burning, squeezing, or tight sensation. Some patients refer to their symptom as discomfort rather than pain. Usually, an anginal episode lasts less than 15 minutes. If the pain is severe, is not relieved by sublingual nitroglycerin, and lasts more than 15 minutes, myocardial infarction should be suspected. In general, when coronary artery disease is being considered, the patient should also be questioned to determine the presence of cardiac risk factors such as smoking history, hypertension, hyperlipidemia, and diabetes.

Chest pain from other causes may be recognized by its "atypical" presentation, which may vary considerably from the preceding description. In pericarditis, the pain may be relieved with a change in position. Chest pain occurring after meals or on reclining may be indicative of gastroesophageal reflux. The presence of cough or other upper respiratory symptoms is suggestive of pulmonary disease. In rheumatologic conditions the pain may be exacerbated by upper body movements.

Clinical Findings

1. Fourth heart sound
2. Systolic click
3. Murmur—systolic or diastolic
4. Friction rub
5. Findings suggestive of noncardiac disease

Many patients with chest pain have a normal physical examination. These include patients with coronary artery disease, esophageal disorders, or psychiatric disorders. The characteristic systolic murmur can be heard in hypertrophic cardiomyopathy and in aortic stenosis. A diastolic murmur in a patient with severe chest pain may signal involvement of the aortic valve in a patient with aortic dissection. A friction rub may be heard with pericarditis. A systolic click with or without a systolic murmur may accompany mitral valve prolapse. A fourth heart sound is commonly heard in patients with coronary artery disease but may also be heard in some healthy individuals and with conditions that cause ventricular hypertrophy. The presence of abnormal breath sounds or rales or rhonchi on auscultation of the lungs suggests pulmonary disease. Musculoskeletal tenderness and pain with movement of the shoulders or spine suggest rheumatologic chest pain.

Tests

1. Chest radiograph
2. Electrocardiogram
3. Echocardiogram
4. Stress test: graded exercise test with or without thallium (or sestamibi) scintigraphy, dipyridamole thallium test, dobutamine stress test, exercise echocardiography
5. Cardiac catheterization
6. Blood tests for myocardial injury: creatine kinase (CK) and CK-MB or troponin T or I.
7. Tests to identify some noncardiac causes of chest pain: esophageal manometry and pH monitoring, upper endoscopy, psychometric testing, specific blood tests (complete blood count, sedimentation rate, rheumatoid factor).

The chest film is useful in the diagnosis of pulmonary conditions as well as musculoskeletal disorders affecting the vertebral spine and rib cage. On the electrocardiogram, ST segment depression suggests myocardial ischemia, whereas acute ST segment elevation may be diagnostic of myocardial infarction. Transient ST segment elevation during episodes of chest pain occurs with Prinzmetal's angina. Exercise testing is indicated for stable patients with occasional chest pain. The use of thallium (or sestamibi) scintigraphy or echocardiography with exercise testing improves the reliability of the study. For patients who cannot exercise, the dipyridamole thallium test is a useful alternative. Myocardial injury can be detected by the presence of CK-MB or troponin (T or I) in the blood. Pericarditis, mitral valve prolapse, and hypertrophic cardiomyopathy can be identified with echocardiography. Coronary angiography provides the most accurate definition of the coronary anatomy and is also very useful in the diagnosis of valvular disorders and hypertrophic cardiomyopathy.

Management

The management of chest pain should be directed toward the primary disorder causing the symptom.

1. Medications used for coronary artery disease: nitrates, β-blockers, calcium channel blockers, aspirin or other oral platelet inhibitors (dipyridamole, ticlopidine, clopidogril). For patients having an acute myocardial infarction, thrombolytic agents should be considered: tissue plasminogen activator (t-PA), reteplase, streptokinase or anisoylated plasminogen-streptokinase activator (APSAC, anistreplase). The GPIIb/IIIa receptor blockers (abciximab, eptifibatide, tirofiban) can be administered intravenously to inhibit platelet aggregation in certain acute situations.
2. Coronary artery interventions: percutaneous transluminal coronary angioplasty, coronary stenting, rotational atherectomy (rotablation), directional coronary atherectomy, or laser
3. Coronary artery bypass surgery or surgery for other specific conditions (valve disease, recurrent pericardial effusion, etc.)
4. Noncardiac causes of chest pain: Refer to specific chapters.

Follow-Up

1. All patients with coronary artery disease should be followed clinically, as well as with some of the tests listed, for an indefinite period, to detect recurrence or progression of disease. Periodic adjustment of their medical regimen is necessary.
2. Most patients with chest pain and angiographically normal coronary arteries continue to complain of chest pain and physical disability, even with extended follow-up. Every effort should be made to identify and treat the cause of their chest pain.

Bibliography

Mukerji B, Alpert MA, Mukerji V: Musculoskeletal causes of chest pain. Hosp Med 1994;30:26–39.

Mukerji V, Beitman BD, Alpert MA: Chest pain and angiographically normal coronary arteries. Tex Heart Inst J 1993;20:170–179.

O'Rourke RA: Diagnostic approach to the patient with chest pain compatible with definite or suspected angina pectoris. In Sobel BE (ed): Medical Management of Heart Disease, pp 4–22. New York, Marcel Dekker, 1996.

Proudfit WL: Chest pain: angina pectoris and related states. Heart Dis Stroke 1992;1:5–10.

Richter JE: Gastroesophageal reflux disease as a cause of chest pain. Med Clin North Am 1991;75:1065–1080.

SYMPTOM SYNCOPE

Ward M. Brown

Syncope is commonly defined as the transient loss of consciousness, often with the loss of postural tone, followed by spontaneous recovery without the need for resuscitative interventions. Syncope may be experienced by 30 to 50 per cent of all people at some point in their lives and accounts for approximately 3 per cent of all emergency department visits as well as at least 1 per cent of all hospital admissions. Syncope is generally of cardiovascular origin.

Differential Diagnosis

1. Neurocardiogenic vasodepressor dysfunction (NVD)—also called vasovagal reaction, vasodepressor syncope, and neurally mediated syncope—includes postmicturition syncope, carotid sinus syncope, cough syncope, heat syncope, and postprandial syncope.
2. Orthostatic hypotension
3. Tachyarrhythmias
   a. Ventricular arrhythmias
      (1) Ventricular tachycardia (VT)
      (2) Ventricular fibrillation (VF)
   b. Supraventricular arrhythmias
      (1) Atrial fibrillation with a rapid ventricular response
      (2) Atrioventricular (AV) nodal re-entrant tachycardia (AVNRT)
      (3) Pre-excitation processes (with atrial fibrillation/flutter)
4. Bradyarrhythmias/conductive disorders
   a. AV block
      (1) Complete heart block
      (2) Mobitz II

   b. Sinus bradycardia—profound (heart rates <40 beats/min)
5. Other cardiac/vascular processes
   a. Aortic stenosis
   b. Hypertrophic cardiomyopathy (hypertrophic obstructive cardiomyopathy, idiopathic hypertrophic subaortic stenosis)
   c. Pulmonary embolus
   d. Pulmonary hypertension

NVD accounts for the majority of syncopal episodes experienced in the general population. If one includes light-headedness, wooziness, and near-syncope, NVD is the cause of some of the most common complaints that bring patients to medical attention. NVD is most often seen in patients with normal left ventricular (LV) function and no structural heart disease; these latter characteristics make NVD primarily a problem of younger people. The ventricular arrhythmias are seen most often in patients with abnormal LV function (ejection fractions <40 per cent) and/or patients with structural heart disease and metabolic abnormalities. Ventricular arrhythmias can have devastating consequences and require a thorough investigation. The high prevalence of LV dysfunction and/or structural heart disease and ischemic heart disease among older patients accounts for the high prevalence of ventricular arrhythmias in this age group.

The other processes mentioned warrant consideration if the physical examination is abnormal (i.e., findings of aortic stenosis), the electrocardiogram (ECG) is abnormal (i.e., pre-excitation or conductive abnormality), or NVD and ventricular arrhythmias are ruled out.

Refer to Ch. 41, Pulmonary Embolism; Ch. 61, Coronary Artery Disease; Ch. 66, Cardiomyopathy; Ch. 72, Sinus Rhythms and Ectopic Beats; Ch. 73, Supraventricular Tachyarrhythmias; Ch. 74, Ventricular Tachyarrhythmias; and Ch. 75, Atrioventricular Block and Sick Sinus Syndrome.

History: Key Questions to Ask

1. What were you doing when the event occurred?
2. Did you actually lose consciousness (black out)?
3. Did you fall and hurt yourself?
4. How long were you out?
5. Did you lose control of your bladder or bowel?
6. Was there any seizure-like activity noted?
7. Was there any chest pain, palpitation, change in vision, or nausea before or immediately after the event?
8. Has this ever happened before?

Knowing the events surrounding the syncopal episode can help to direct the subsequent evaluation and possible treatment. For example, if the syncope occurred during micturition in a male, even though this may be a variant of NVD, addressing a potential prostate problem may be curative. Other questions that help to determine the possible severity of the syncopal problem and thus the urgency of evaluation are: Was the person able to anticipate the event and thereby prevent injury? Or was there little or no warning of the event with resultant injury? Syncope that has occurred many times before and happens with warning probably requires less urgent assessment than that which has happened without warning and has resulted in injury.

Clinical Findings

1. General appearance
2. Presence or absence of orthostatic changes
3. Evidence of aortic stenosis or hypertrophic cardiomyopathy
4. Evidence of LV dysfunction

The general appearance of the patient will help in narrowing the differential diagnosis of syncope. For example, a well-nourished young person is much more likely to have NVD than an elderly individual with a sternotomy scar. The other findings, such as those listed above, render evidence of specific diagnoses. Evidence of LV dysfunction suggests a propensity to malignant ventricular arrhythmias (VT/VF), although it is not diagnostic for them.

Tests (see Fig. 57–1)

1. ECG: Helps to identify or rule out conductive abnormalities/pre-excitation.

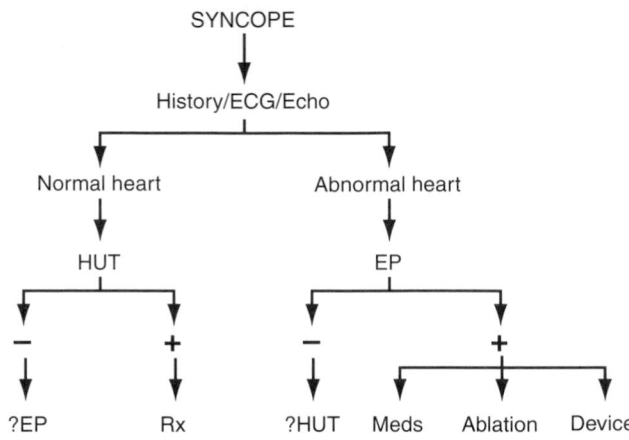

Figure 57–1 Algorithm for the diagnostic testing of a patient with syncope. Ablation, radiofrequency ablation therapy; Device, automatic implantable cardiodefibrillator (see text) or permanent pacemaker; ECG, electrocardiography; Echo, echocardiography; EP, electrophysiology testing; HUT, head-up tilt table testing; Rx, medication and/or hydration.

2. Echocardiogram: a good method of assessing LV function and valvular state
3. Signal-averaged ECG: In the absence of conductive abnormality on the ECG, the signal-averaged ECG (SAECG) can help predict the tendency toward VT. The SAECG is most predictive in patients with ejection fractions less than 40 per cent.
4. Head-up tilt table test: very useful test in patients with ejection fractions greater than 40 per cent in whom NVD is suspected
5. Electrophysiologic testing: test of choice in patients suspected of having a tachyarrhythmia as the cause of syncope, especially for AVNRT and VT/VF
6. Holter monitoring and electroencephalograms are generally of very low yield and are not indicated in the initial evaluation of syncope.

Management

Of NVD

1. Maintain hydration/advise caution when changing position
2. β-Blockers (divided-dose cardioselective β-blockers appear to work best)
3. Disopyramide (Norpace)
4. Theophylline preparations
5. Anticholinergic agents (e.g., transdermal scopolamine)
6. Fludrocortisone acetate (Florinef Acetate)
7. Serotonin reuptake inhibitor (e.g., fluoxetine [Prozac]) for patients refractory to β-blockers and/or theophylline

Of VT/VF

1. Treat/remove underlying ischemic heart disease if possible.
2. Treat metabolic abnormalities.
3. Consider automatic implantable cardiodefibrillator (AICD).

PEARLS

- Syncope primarily is associated with a cardiovascular problem, *not a neurologic disease.*

- NVD is most common in patients without structural heart disease.

- VT/VF is most common in patients with structural heart disease.

Bibliography

Benditt D: Clinical approach to diagnosis of syncope: an overview. Cardiol Clin 1997;May:165–176.

Day SC: Evaluation and outcome of emergency room patients with transient loss of consciousness. Am J Med 1982;73:15–23.

Eagle KA: Evaluation of prognostic classifications for patients with syncope. Am J Med 1985;79:455–460.

Kapoor WN: Diagnostic evaluation of syncope. Am J Med 1991;90:91–106.

Kosinski D: A reliable method of diagnosing neurocardiogenic syncope. Contemp Intern Med 1998;10:10–16.

Kosinski DJ: Neurocardiogenic syncope: a review of pathophysiology, diagnosis, and treatment. Cardiovasc Rev Rep 1993;June:22–29.

Sra JS: Unexplained syncope evaluated by electrophysiologic study and head-up tilt test. Ann Intern Med 1991;114:1013–1019.

1. In patients with asymptomatic coronary atherosclerosis, the first symptom of acute cardiac ischemia is sudden death in about 25 per cent. Thirty to 40 per cent of patients with a sudden-death event do not have heart disease.

2. People over 65 years of age make up the majority of patients experiencing out-of-hospital cardiac arrests.

3. The mechanism of cardiac arrest in patients with heart disease is usually ventricular fibrillation and/or ventricular tachycardia. Patients without heart disease are more likely to have pulseless electrical activity (PEA) or asystole. Patients with neurologic problems, sepsis, and hemorrhage usually have a drop in blood pressure and develop progressive slowing of the heart rhythm. These patients then go into either PEA or asystole. If a patient goes into PEA or ventricular fibrillation and no resuscitation is begun, they will usually deteriorate into asystole in 10 to 20 minutes.

4. Time is critical when a patient has a cardiac arrest. Four critical factors affect the outcome: time, defibrillation, cardiopulmonary resuscitation (CPR), and administration of epinephrine.

   a. Studies show that 93 per cent of long-term survivors of outside-of-the hospital cardiac arrest were witnessed in cardiac arrest and had ventricular fibrillation. Thus, it is apparent that time to defibrillation is the most important determinant of survival; time to CPR and time to administration of epinephrine also are important.

   b. Defibrillation is not effective and not indicated for PEA and asystole; therefore, time to CPR and time to advanced cardiac life support (epinephrine) are the critical elements.

   c. The shorter each of these key intervals is, the greater is the chance of survival.

5. The chain of survival (early access, early CPR, early defibrillation, early care) should be initiated immediately for all patients in cardiac arrest.

   a. Early access allows the necessary equipment to reach the victim. Outside the hospital, this means notifying the emergency medical services for the region, usually calling 911.

Note

- Not all areas have the 911 emergency telephone system; in these locations, a 7- or 10-digit emergency number must be called.

- There are two types of 911 systems, regular and enhanced. The enhanced 911 system identifies the calling party's address, speeding an emergency response and minimizing errors. (An enhanced 911 system does not get the address if the call is made on a cellular telephone.)

---

   b. The techniques of CPR are divided into four sets of skills labeled A, B, C, and D. A = airway, B = breathing, C = circulation, and D = defibrillation.

   c. The first step in resuscitation is to recognize that the patient is unconscious. Gently shake the victim and ask if he or she is okay. More than one code has been called because someone was soundly asleep. Once the patient is determined to be unresponsive, proceed in a rapid yet controlled manner.

Technique

A: Airway

1. Open the airway.
   a. Have the victim lying on his or her back on a flat, firm surface.
      (1) If the victim is in a chair or lying on the abdomen, you must position the victim on his or her back. Do so quickly while protecting the head and neck.
      (2) If the victim is on a soft bed, place a backboard under the victim or move him or her to the floor or other hard surface.

   b. With the unconscious victim lying on the back, the airway is easily obstructed by the tongue. To relieve the possible obstruction of the airway in victims who do not have a potential neck injury, tilt the head back by one of two easy methods:
      (1) *Head tilt/chin lift method*: Place one hand on the victim's forehead and the other hand on the patient's mandible and carefully tilt the head back so that the head is extended. Be certain that the hand that is on the mandible is not pressing against the base of the tongue

between the two sides of the mandible, because this could close the airway by moving the tongue toward the roof of the mouth. Tilt the head so that the long shaft of the mandible is vertical. This maneuver will usually pull the base of the tongue away from the posterior pharynx. This technique allows the rescuer to control the airway and to be in a proper position to ventilate the patient if needed without other assistance.

(2) *Jaw thrust with a head tilt*: Stand over the head of the victim (at the head of the bed). Place your fingers on each angle of the mandible. Tilt the head back so that the shaft of the mandible is vertical. Use your fingers to move the jaw forward, opening the airway. Because this technique uses both hands, ventilation of the patient often requires a second rescuer.

  (a) In victims with potential neck injury, do not tilt the head but hold it in-line and use the jaw thrust to open the airway.

  (b) In a trauma victim, it may require one rescuer to hold in-line traction on the head, a second rescuer to perform the jaw thrust, and a third rescuer to ventilate the patient.

2. Adjuncts for maintaining an open airway in the unconscious patient

  a. Oropharyngeal and nasopharyngeal airways

  (1) Both of these adjuncts should be of a size that they will reach the posterior pharynx and hold the tongue away from the posterior pharynx:

    (a) Oropharyngeal airways should be 100 mm in length for large adults, 90 mm in length for medium-sized adults, and 80 mm in length for small adults.

    (b) Nasopharyngeal airways should have an internal diameter of 8.0 to 9.0 mm for large adults, 7.0 to 8.0 mm for medium-sized adults, and 6.0 to 7.0 mm for small adults.

    (c) A rough guide to determine the size of an oropharyngeal airway is that it should extend from the lips to the ear lobe; a nasopharyngeal airway should be able to reach from the nostril to the ear lobe.

  (2) Insert an oropharyngeal airway into the mouth by placing it halfway in upside down and then twisting it 180 degrees while pushing it into the mouth so that the tip wraps around the base of the tongue and ends up in the posterior pharynx, holding the tongue away from the posterior pharynx with the end phalange just outside of the mouth touching the lips.

  (3) Place a nasopharyngeal airway through the nose into the posterior pharynx. Slide it across the nasal portion of the roof of the mouth into the posterior pharynx. Often this airway meets resistance when it is almost to the base of the tongue; a jaw thrust will allow the airway to be passed posterior to the base of the tongue into the proper position. The end phalange should be against the nostril.

  b. Endotracheal intubation with either oral or nasal tracheal intubation. Oral tracheal intubation is preferred during cardiac arrest because it is often quicker and easier to perform.

  c. Tracheostomy or cricothyrotomy

> **Note**
> Endotracheal intubation and surgical airways should be used only by rescuers trained in those techniques.

3. Once the airway is open in the unresponsive patient, you should then assess ventilation.

B: Breathing

1. Determine if the victim is breathing.

  a. Hold the head in the opened airway position described above and place your cheek close to the victims mouth and nose, looking toward the victim's chest.

  b. In this position, listen for breath sounds, try to feel air movement against your cheek, and watch for 3 to 5 seconds to see if there is rise and fall of the chest

2. If the victim is breathing, maintain an open airway while assessing the reasons for unconsciousness. There are many situations where a victim may be unconscious with an obstructed airway and may still be breathing; these include sedation or anesthesia, postictal status after a seizure, and a stroke, among others.

  a. If the patient is able to breathe on his or her own and the condition is very transient, merely holding the airway open may be adequate.

  b. If the victim does not quickly recover, roll him or her onto the side so that the tongue does not fall against the posterior pharynx. This also reduces the risk of aspiration of gastric contents into the pulmonary tree.

c. If the victim must be kept on the back, an airway adjunct may be used; however, watch to make sure the victim does not aspirate if vomiting should occur.

    (1) Generally, oropharyngeal or nasopharyngeal airways are used when it is believed that recovery will occur relatively soon and the risk of aspiration is thought to be low.

    (2) If there is risk of aspiration or the person may be unresponsive and unable to control the airway for a prolonged period, endotracheal intubation is the best method for maintaining the airway and preventing aspiration.

3. If you do not hear, feel, or see evidence of breathing, begin artificial ventilation.

a. Close the victim's nose and seal your mouth to the victim's mouth. If you are using the head tilt/chin lift method of opening the airway, close off the nose using the thumb and index finger of the hand on the forehead to gently squeeze the nose shut. Then place your mouth over the victim's mouth in order to ventilate him or her.

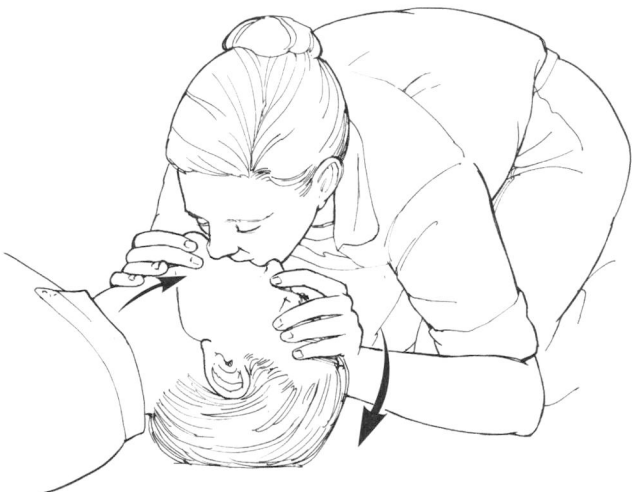

b. An alternative to mouth-to-mouth is mouth-to-nose. Hold the mouth shut with the thumb and index finger of the hand controlling the mandible and seal your mouth around the victim's nose. If the patient has a tracheostomy, hold the mouth and nose closed and put your mouth to the stoma to ventilate the patient.

c. An alternative method of ventilating the victim is to use a jaw thrust and have a second rescuer provide ventilation by squeezing the nose and sealing their mouth over the victim's mouth.

4. Then deliver two full breaths to the victim while

maintaining proper head position and closure of the nose. Make sure that the chest rises and falls with the ventilation and listen for exhalation of air from the victim.

5. If the chest does not rise and fall, reposition the head and airway to make sure that it is open. The most common reason for being unable to ventilate the patient is that the airway is not adequately opened. A foreign object or tumor may be obstructing the airway.

a. In the unconscious victim, if you cannot ventilate the patient after repositioning the airway, open the mouth by grasping the tongue and jaw with one hand and sweeping the fingers of the other hand into the mouth to see if there is an object that can be grasped.

b. If a laryngoscope is available, this may be used to quickly see if there is an object within reach of a pair of forceps or clamps that can be withdrawn. Many times the foreign object is down the trachea at the bifurcation.

c. If the obstructing object is not in the pharynx, perform abdominal thrusts:

    (1) Sit astride the victim at the level of the hips or beside the victim.

    (2) Place the heel of your hand halfway between the umbilicus and the xiphoid process perpendicular to the midline of the body with the second hand on top of the first.

    (3) Give up to five thrusts pushing down and toward the head at a 45-degree angle hoping to dislodge the object.

    (4) Check the mouth as before to see if the object can be grasped and attempt ventilation.

    (5) Repeat this process until you are able to ventilate the patient.

    (6) If the cause of the obstruction is laryngospasm or a laryngeal or pharyngeal tumor, a cricothyrotomy may be performed.

6. To prevent disease transmission, use barrier types of devices and adjuncts to ventilate the patient.

a. A piece of cloth may provide minimal protection; however, it quickly can become moist, allowing bacterial transmission through the cloth, and it probably would not stop viral transmission at all.

b. There are products available that can fit in the pocket or billfold and provide better protection. These are plastic types of materials with very small pores that allow gas transmission but not bacterial or viral transmission.

c. A pocket mask, similar to that found on a bag-valve mask device, can be sealed over the mouth and nose. It is best used in conjunction with a jaw thrust maneuver to open the airway. The device has a mouthpiece so that the rescuer can breathe into the mask using the mouthpiece. The newer versions have a non-rebreathing valve system so that exhaled air from the victim does not come back to the rescuer, providing some degree of isolation from the victim. Some of these devices have a port so that supplemental oxygen can be provided. Place the mask over the mouth and nose to provide a seal. Use the third, fourth, and fifth fingers to hold the jaw forward with the jaw thrust, and the thumb and index finger to hold the mask to the victim's face. Then give two full breaths through the mouthpiece. The use of a pocket mask is the only method where a single rescuer can use the jaw thrust and ventilate the victim unassisted.

d. A bag-valve mask is probably the most widely used method of initial ventilation for the victims in emergency situations. A single rescuer can use the head tilt/chin lift method with the bag-valve mask.

(1) Place the mask over the mouth and nose to seal the airway.

(2) Use the third, fourth, and fifth fingers to hold the mandible in order to maintain the proper head tilt.

(3) Place the thumb and index finger on either side of the ventilation port to hold a tight seal.

(4) Squeeze the bag to deliver air into the victim. Oxygen can be attached to the bag with a reservoir so that nearly 100% oxygen can be delivered.

(5) Disadvantages:

(a) Even with practice, the rescuer can usually ventilate only with about 750 ml or less of air or oxygen using this device; it is recommended that the volume of ventilation be at least 800 ml and up to 1200 ml of air or oxygen. This device at best delivers the minimum amount of ventilation needed.

(b) It is easy to squeeze the bag too forcefully, opening the esophagus and forcing air or oxygen into the victim's stomach and making aspi-

ration more likely. It takes a great deal of skill to hold the head in the proper position, have a tight seal around the mask, and perfectly squeeze the bag so that an adequate volume can be given to the patient without forcing air into the stomach. Practice with this technique is required for it to be an effective adjunct during cardiac arrest.

(6) For the novice rescuer, mouth-to-mouth or mouth-to-mask ventilation is a better technique to ensure adequate ventilation.

7. Endotracheal intubation: Because each of the adjuncts mentioned above has limitations, it is recommended that endotracheal intubation be performed very early during a cardiac arrest.

a. It should be performed as soon as practical if the victim has asystole or PEA.

b. If the victim has ventricular fibrillation, endotracheal intubation is recommended after the first three attempts at defibrillation if a defibrillator is immediately available.

c. A bag-valve system connected to an endotracheal tube is a very effective method of ventilating a patient with nearly 100% oxygen without the problems with other systems.

8. Once the victim has been ventilated, quickly assess the circulation.

C: Circulation

1. Assess the circulation by feeling for the carotid pulse for 5 to 10 seconds. Do not use the radial pulse because the victim may be in shock and the radial pulse may not be palpable even without a cardiac arrest.

2. If a pulse is present, check the victim's blood pressure.

3. If the victim has adequate circulation but is not breathing on his or her own, continue artificial ventilation with a ventilation every 5 seconds or 12 times/min. If the patient was not previously intubated, endotracheally intubate and place him or her on a ventilator. Continue to assess the problem with the patient and treat the patient appropriately.

4. If the victim does not have a pulse, start artificial circulation promptly by compressing the chest.

a. To find the appropriate position for closed-chest compression:

(1) Position yourself so that you are beside the lower half of the chest.

(2) Place your hand that is closest to the vic-

tim's abdomen on the lower rib cage and slide your hand along the lower rib until it reaches the notch that is formed by the junction of the rib cage and the sternum (your fingers should be between the lower rib and the xiphoid process).

(3) Place the heel of your hand on the lower sternum 1 to 2 fingerbreadths above the top of the notch that you have identified with your fingers between the lower rib and xiphoid process.

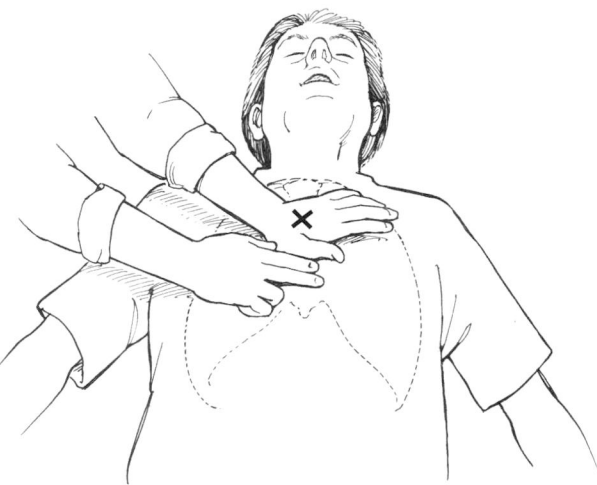

The heel of your hand should touch only the sternum, and the axis of the heel of your hand should be the same as the long axis of the sternum. Take care not to touch the ribs with the palm of your hand or your fingers.

(4) Place your other hand on top of the first hand. Your shoulders should be directly over the sternum.

b. Compress the sternum 1½ to 2 inches using the weight of your upper body rather than your arms.

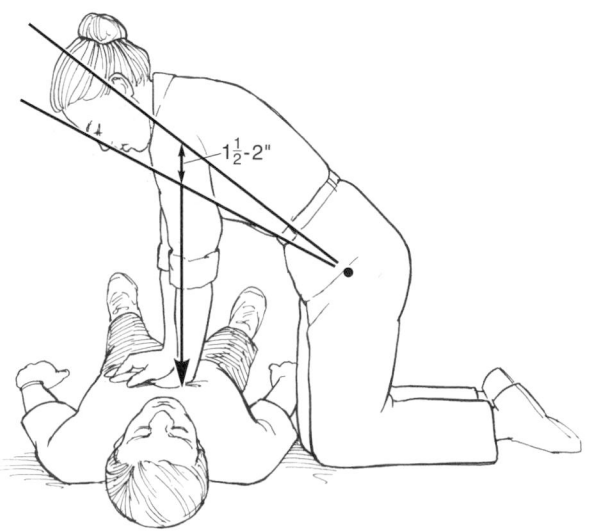

You should be doing most of the work by bending from your hips. If you use your arms to do the work, you will quickly tire.

c. Compression of the sternum should be a rhythmical compression and relaxation without removing the heels of the hands from the victim's sternum. The compression and relaxation phases should be roughly equal; you do not want to jab the sternum sharply but rather squeeze the chest, allowing time for the pressure to cause blood flow, not just a sharp pulse.

d. Cardiac compressions should be done at a rate of 80 to 100 times per minute; because you will be pausing for ventilation, this will allow the actual number of compressions delivered to be at least 60 in 1 minute.

5. These techniques can be performed with one, two, or more rescuers. The sequences are slightly different if there is one rescuer or two rescuers performing CPR. If the defibrillator is present, assess the rhythm to see if ventricular fibrillation or ventricular tachycardia is present with the cardiac arrest.

D: Defibrillation

1. If ventricular fibrillation/ventricular tachycardia is present, attempt rapid defibrillation with up to three initial shocks of 200 joules, 200 to 300 joules, and 360 joules if a shock is not successful in converting the rhythm.

2. After the first three shocks, proceed to the other steps of cardiac arrest management. The technique of defibrillation is discussed in the procedure following Chapter 63.

One-Rescuer CPR

When there is a single rescuer, cardiac compressions are done in sets of 15 followed by two breaths or ventilations. The rescuer performs 15 chest compressions and then returns to perform ventilation. The rescuer does not change position but leans toward the victim's head, quickly reopens the airway, and gives two full breaths as before. After the breaths, the rescuer again finds the notch between the ribs and the xiphoid process, places the hands on the victim's sternum as before, and begins another set of 15 compressions. After the rescuer performs four sets of 15 compressions and two ventilations (about 1 minute), he or she should reassess the carotid pulse. If there is no pulse, the process continues until a defibrillator and other advanced cardiac life support (ACLS) equipment arrives.

The entire sequence for a single rescuer is as follows:

1. Determine unconsciousness (gently shake the patient and ask if he or she is okay).

2. If unconscious, open the **Airway**.

3. Once the airway is open, assess **Breathing** (look, listen, and feel for respiration).

4. If no breathing, give two full breaths.

5. After delivering two full breaths, assess **Circulation** (check carotid pulse).

6. If no pulse, find the proper landmarks and begin chest compressions.

7. Perform 15 chest compressions.

8. Reopen airway and give two full breaths.

9. Continue giving 15 compressions followed by two full ventilations.

10. Check the pulse after 1 minute and every few minutes therafter.

11. Check rhythm as soon as defibrillator is available and defibrillate if indicated.

12. Continue until the rhythm is restored or you assess that the victim will not respond to ACLS protocols.

Two-Rescuer CPR

When there are two rescuers present, the recommended ratio of compressions to ventilation is 5:1. One rescuer should be positioned for ventilation and one for chest compression. The person performing chest compression should perform five chest compressions and pause for the second rescuer to give one full breath. They continue at the 5:1 ratio but otherwise perform in a manner similar to single-rescuer CPR. They need to make all of the same assessments as for single-rescuer CPR and should check pulses at 1 minute and every few minutes thereafter.

Drug Therapy

1. Epinephrine is the most important drug during cardiac arrest.

   a. Intravenous (IV) access is needed so that epinephrine and possible other drugs can be given.

   b. The IV fluid should not contain glucose; hence, the most widely used fluid during cardiac arrest is normal saline run at a keep-open rate.

   c. The IV dose of epinephrine is 1 mg of 1:10,000 dilution.

   d. If no IV access is available and the patient is intubated, epinephrine can be given down the endotracheal tube in a dose 2 to 2½ times the IV dose flushed with 10 ml of normal saline.

   e. Repeat the same dose of epinephrine every 3 to 5 minutes until a perfusing rhythm is restored.

   f. Higher doses of epinephrine have been proposed and are allowed by American Heart Association guidelines; however, seven large prospective randomized trials in adults have shown no benefit of high-dose epinephrine.

2. Other drugs

   a. Antiarrhythmic agents for ventricular fibrillation or ventricular tachycardia.

   b. Atropine, sodium bicarbonate, or calcium chloride may benefit selected patients. Proper administration of these agents is covered in the American Heart Association material on ACLS.

Ventricular Fibrillation

Ventricular fibrillation (also pulseless ventricular tachycardia) should be treated aggressively. The major portion of the treatment protocol is as follows:

1. Determine unresponsiveness.

2. If no defibrillator is immediately available, begin CPR.

3. As soon as a defibrillator is available, defibrillate at 200 joules, 200 to 300 joules, and 360 joules. (If the patient converts at any time, change to the appropriate algorithm.)

4. Begin CPR and intubate the patient; begin an IV of normal saline.

5. Administer epinephrine 1 mg 1:10,000 IV push (2 to 2.5 mg down an endotracheal tube).

6. Defibrillate at 360 joules (you can give stacks of three shocks of 360 joules).

7. Administer an antiarrhythmic agent (lidocaine, bretylium, amiodarone, magnesium sulfate, or procainamide).

8. Repeat the epinephrine and antiarrhythmic agent after 3 to 5 minutes.

9. Repeat defibrillation after each administration of epinephrine or antiarrhythmic agent.

Pulseless Electrical Activity

1. Most of the salvage from PEA is determined by reversing the cause of the PEA. Causes are multiple:

   a. Hypoxia (hypoventilation): Administration of oxygen with ventilation may be of benefit.

   b. Hypovolemia: Administration of volume is appropriate if this may be the etiology.

   c. Hyperkalemia from renal failure, diabetes, or iatrogenic causes: Administration of calcium chloride, insulin and glucose, and sodium bicarbonate may be of benefit.

   d. Cardiac tamponade: Treat with pericardiocentesis.

   e. Tension pneumothorax: Treat with needle pleural decompression.

   f. Drug overdose: Give specific therapy.

g. Pre-existing acidosis from renal failure or diabetes: Administer sodium bicarbonate.

h. Massive myocardial infarction or massive pulmonary emboli: potentially treatable with invasive techniques

i. Hypothermia can present with PEA and is potentially reversible.

2. The major portion of the treatment of PEA is as follows:

a. Recognize unresponsiveness.

b. Begin CPR and intubate the patient; begin an IV of normal saline.

c. Administer epinephrine 1 mg 1:10,000 IV push (2 to 2.5 mg down an endotracheal tube).

d. If the rate of the rhythm is less than 60 beats/min, administer atropine 1 mg.

e. Assess for a treatable cause of PEA and treat the cause if possible.

f. Repeat the epinephrine every 3 to 5 minutes.

Asystole

Asystole is often a late finding after ventricular fibrillation or PEA. Therefore, you need to be certain that the rhythm is not ventricular fibrillation; the recommendation is that you confirm asystole in two leads. If the rhythm in either lead appears to be ventricular fibrillation, treat the patient for ventricular fibrillation. The victim may have deteriorated from PEA; thus you should consider and treat, if present, any of the potentially treatable causes of PEA.

The major portion of the treatment of asystole is as follows:

1. Recognize unresponsiveness.

2. Begin CPR and intubate the patient; begin an IV of normal saline.

3. Consider using an external pacemaker (rarely effective).

4. Administer epinephrine 1 mg 1:10,000 IV push (2 to 2.5 mg down an endotracheal tube) and atropine 1 mg.

5. Assess for a treatable cause of asystole (same as PEA) and treat the cause if possible.

6. Repeat the epinephrine every 3 to 5 minutes.

Technique for the Heimlich Maneuver

1. Purpose: To remove a foreign body obstructing the airway: often a large piece of meat, but can be another object in a person with impaired swallowing.

2. Common causes include eating after drinking alcohol, while talking, or with a neurologic deficit.

3. If the person is conscious, assess whether he or she has an adequate cough.

a. If the cough is adequate, observe the patient closely.

b. If the patient does not have an adequate cough and cannot speak, consider doing the Heimlich maneuver.

4. If the patient is sitting or standing, position yourself behind the victim. Place your arms around the victim, make a fist and place the thumb of your fist halfway between the navel and the xiphoid process.

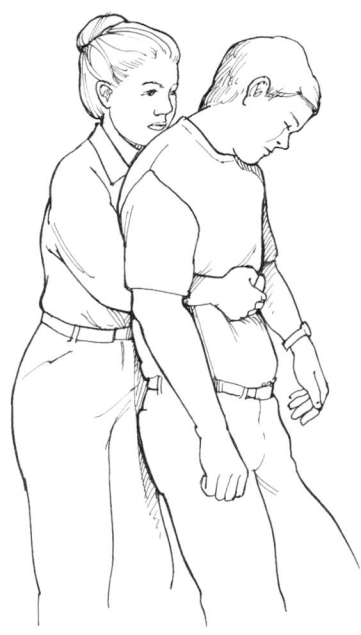

Place your second hand on top of the first and pull toward yourself and upward.

5. If this does not dislodge the obstruction, try again repeatedly and with more vigor until the obstruction is dislodged or the patient loses consciousness.

6. If the victim becomes unconscious, lay the victim on the ground and proceed as discussed above under the CPR section for airway and breathing.

 ## Bibliography

American Heart Association: BLS for Healthcare Providers. Dallas, TX, American Heart Association, 1997.

Brown CG, Martin DR, Pepe PE, et al: A comparison of standard-dose and high-dose epinephrine in cardiac arrest outside the hospital. N Engl J Med 1992;327: 1051–1055.

Cummins RO (ed): Textbook of Advanced Cardiac Life Support. Dallas, TX, American Heart Association, 1997.

Emergency Cardiac Care Committee and Subcommittee, American Heart Association: Guidelines for cardiopulmonary resuscitation and emergency cardiac care. JAMA 1992;268:2171–2302.

Woodhouse SP, Cox S, Boyd P, et al: High dose and standard dose adrenaline do not alter survival, compared with placebo, in cardiac arrest. Resuscitation 1995;30: 243–249.

SYMPTOM PALPITATIONS

James D. Alexander

Palpitations are the unpleasant sensation of an abnormal heartbeat or rhythm. They may be described as extra heartbeats, missed heartbeats, or a fluttering feeling in the chest. These symptoms may or may not be associated with a true electrical abnormality or cardiac arrhythmia. Palpitations are the second most common reason for referral to a cardiologist, exceeded only by chest pain.

Differential Diagnosis

Potential Arrhythmias

1. Sinus tachycardia
2. Atrial fibrillation/atrial flutter
3. Multifocal atrial tachycardia
4. Supraventricular tachycardia (SVT)
5. Ventricular tachycardia
6. Wolff-Parkinson-White (WPW) syndrome or other re-entrant tachycardia
7. Premature atrial or ventricular contractions
8. Sick sinus syndrome

Associated Conditions

1. Anxiety disorder
2. Panic attacks
3. Hyperthyroidism
4. Pheochromocytoma
5. Anemia
6. Mitral valve prolapse
7. Stress
8. Electrolyte imbalances
9. Increased adrenergic tone

History

1. The key to establishing a diagnosis is to characterize the palpitations, including their rate and rhythm. Many practitioners have the patient tap out the rhythm on a tabletop. The frequency and duration of the episodes should also be described. In this way, the physician can narrow down significantly the potential rhythms.
2. Additional symptoms that may be elicited
   a. Syncope/near-syncope
   b. Chest pain
   c. Shortness of breath
   d. Throat fullness
   e. Provoking factors: stress, caffeine, smoking, alcohol, exercise
   f. Symptoms suggestive of anxiety or depression
   g. Symptoms suggestive of hyperthyroidism
3. Further areas that should be reviewed
   a. Diet history
      (1) Caffeine intake
      (2) Foods that are associated with symptoms (e.g., monosodium glutamate, chocolate)
   b. Smoking history
   c. Medication history
      (1) Over-the-counter decongestants
      (2) Adrenergic and anticholinergic medications
      (3) Illicit drugs (e.g., cocaine)

Key Questions

- Can you tap out the rhythm or fluttering you feel in your chest?

- Do you feel any chest pain or shortness of breath during your palpitations?

- Do you feel dizzy or light-headed, or even pass out, when you have symptoms?

- Are there any particular triggers to your symptoms?

Clinical Findings

1. A thorough cardiac examination must be performed, with emphasis on
   a. Rate and regularity of the heart rhythm
   b. Murmurs
   c. Midsystolic click suggestive of mitral valve prolapse
2. The thyroid gland should be evaluated for signs of nodularity or a goiter.
3. A brief mental status assessment should also be performed for signs suggestive of depression or anxiety.

Diagnostic Tests

1. A 12-lead electrocardiogram (ECG) with rhythm strip is the initial test of choice and is

widely available in medical offices. The test is ideally performed while the patient is having symptoms. A normal rate and rhythm when palpitations are present is highly suggestive of a noncardiac cause (e.g., a psychosomatic etiology). Heart rates under 140 beats/min when symptoms are present are usually identified as sinus tachycardia and suggest a benign course.

2. Frequently, palpitations will not occur during the office evaluation. An extended evaluation in the patient's natural environment is possible through Holter monitors and event monitors. If symptoms occur daily, a 24- or 48-hour Holter monitor recording should be performed. If symptoms are less frequent (e.g., only several times a month), a continuous loop event monitor for 2 weeks will be more successful at capturing potential cardiac arrhythmias when a patient has symptoms. In either test, the patient should record when symptoms occur and the tracing will be reviewed for any recorded abnormality.

3. Additional tests to consider
   a. Complete blood count: to rule out anemia
   b. Thyroid-stimulating hormone level: to rule out hyperthyroidism
   c. Electrolytes: if on diuretic medication
   d. Chest radiograph: to evaluate cardiac size and shape
   e. Echocardiogram: if murmurs or click is found on physical examination
   f. Treadmill stress test: if symptoms triggered by exercise
   g. Electrophysiologic testing in consultation with a cardiologist: for unexplained or sustained arrhythmias

Management

1. Patient education and lifestyle modification are often the interventions performed on the first office visit.
2. Reassurance about the benign nature of palpitations is vital to alleviate many patients' apprehensions. Reassurance is most appropriate for patients with mild symptoms, no syncope, and a negative initial work-up.

Medication

1. β-Blockers, digoxin, or other antiarrhythmics are not indicated unless a sustained tachyarrhythmia, such as atrial fibrillation or SVT, is diagnosed on ECG or Holter monitor.
2. β-Blockers may be considered in idiopathic inappropriate sinus tachycardia, but all secondary causes must be ruled out and side effects may outweigh the benefits.

3. Calcium channel blockers are specifically contraindicated in WPW.
4. Avoid over-the-counter decongestants.
5. Appropriate antidepressant or anxiolytic may be initiated if depression or anxiety is considered the cause of the palpitations.

Diet

1. Decrease or abstain from caffeine.
2. Abstain from alcohol.
3. Abstain from any foods that trigger symptoms.

Activity

1. Avoid situations and stressors that trigger symptoms.
2. Exercise is contraindicated only where it triggers palpitations or syncope.

Education

1. Smoking cessation counseling should be provided if appropriate.
2. Where stress, anxiety, or depression appears to be the inciting cause, appropriate counseling may be initiated. Biofeedback therapy may also be useful.
3. A cardiology referral may be necessary for patients with
   a. Sustained tachyarrhythmias (SVT, ventricular tachycardia)
   b. Atrial fibrillation and a candidate for cardioversion
   c. Symptomatic WPW
   d. Persistent idiopathic sinus tachycardia with syncope or near-syncope
   e. Abnormality on echocardiogram

Follow-Up

Palpitations accompanied by syncope, near-syncopal episodes, or chest pain require an expedited work-up. For benign etiologies or in cases where no etiology is found, symptoms may wax and wane. Patients can be followed with periodic reassurance or re-evaluated if new symptoms develop.

PEARLS

- Tapping out the rhythm of the palpitations can narrow down the possible arrhythmias involved.
- Heart rates under 140 beats/min during symptoms usually suggest a benign etiology.
- Decreasing stimulants in the patient's diet is a simple intervention that can be done on the first visit.
- Occasional premature heartbeats are harmless and require no treatment other than reassurance.

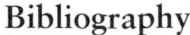

Bibliography

Bennett DH: Cardiac Arrythmias: Practical Notes on Interpretation and Treatment, 5th ed. London, Butterworth-Heinemann, 1997.

Fogoros RN: Antiarrhythmic Drugs: A Practical Guide. Boston, Blackwell Science, 1997.

Lee RJ, Shinbane JS: Inappropriate sinus tachycardia: diagnosis and treatment. Cardiol Clin 1997;15:599–605.

Mayou R: Chest pain, palpitations and panic. J Pyschosom Res 1998;44:53–70.

Zimetbaum PJ, Josephson ME: Evaluation of patients with palpitations. N Engl J Med 1998;338:1369–1373.

Zimetbaum PJ, Kim KY, Josephson ME, et al: Diagnostic yield and optimal duration of continuous-loop event monitoring for the diagnosis of palpitations: a cost effectiveness analysis. Ann Intern Med 1998;128:890–895.

SYMPTOM LEG EDEMA

Ralph Weber

Edema is an increase in the amount of interstitial fluid. Its basic determinants are *filtration* (arterial end) and *reabsorption* (venous end) at the capillary bed.

1. Four factors influence development of edema

   a. Hydrostatic pressure in capillaries and interstitial tissue

   b. Colloid osmotic pressure in plasma and interstitial tissue

   c. Permeability of capillary walls

   d. Alterations (obstruction) of lymphatic flow

2. The above processes are often modified by renal sodium retention.

3. Three types of leg swelling occur according to content (i.e., water, lymph, or fat) (Table 57–1).

   a. Systemic edema (main component[s] similar to normal interstitial fluid)

   b. Lymphedema (chief component is protein)

   c. Lipedema (principal component is fat)

4. The distribution of edema (unilateral vs. bilateral) is useful in diagnosis.

Differential Diagnosis

1. *Bilateral (systemic) edema* may be secondary to

   a. Cardiac dysfunction (e.g., congestive heart failure [CHF])

   b. Renal dysfunction (e.g., nephritic or nephrotic)

   c. Hepatic dysfunction (e.g., cirrhosis) or, more rarely, hepatic vein thrombosis (Budd-Chiari syndrome) and portal vein thrombosis

   d. Metabolic dysfunction (e.g., protein deficiency)

   e. Endocrine dysfunction (e.g., Cushing's disease, thyroid disease)

   f. Physiologic (e.g., pregnancy, salt overload)

   g. Idiopathic cyclic edema (after other edema causes excluded): usually only in women ages 20 to 40 years; tends to involve upper extremities as well as lower; tends to have self-limited course of a few months to several years.

   h. Lipedema: symmetric nonpitting fat deposition in buttocks and legs but sparing feet in women

   i. Microvascular capillary "leak" syndromes

TABLE 57–1. GENERAL FEATURES OF EDEMA

	SYSTEMIC EDEMA	LYMPHEDEMA	LIPEDEMA
Water and sodium retention	Increased	Normal	Normal
Distribution			
Bilateral	+	±	+
Foot and/or leg	Both	Both	Legs only
Toes involved before foot	−	+	−
Skin appearance			
Pitting, soft	+	*	−
General thickening	−	+	−
Toe fold thickening (Stemmer's sign)	−	+	−
Decreased with elevation of part	+	−	−

Symbols: +, present; −, absent; *, soft only if very recent onset.
Data from Spittel JA Jr, Schirger A: Edema, peripheral. In Taylor RB (ed): Difficult Diagnosis. Philadelphia, WB Saunders Company, 1985:130.

(e.g., exposure to temperature extremes, angioneurotic edema)

2. *Unilateral (regional) edema* may be secondary to

    a. Venous disease: intrinsic (e.g., acute deep venous thrombosis [DVT], chronic venous insufficiency [CVI]); extrinsic (e.g., tumor, pressure of overlying iliac artery); traumatic interruption (e.g., surgical ligation, plication, insertion of filter)

    b. Lymphedema: congenital (primary) or acquired (secondary). Most common causes are postphlebitic syndrome, tissue injury after surgery/radiation, or underlying tumor. Less frequent causes are parasitic inflammations (e.g., filariasis, lymphogranuloma venereum), syphilis, and granulomatous disease, especially tuberculosis.

    c. Miscellaneous: most often the result of bacterial inflammation (e.g., cellulitis, deep tissue abscess, osteomyelitis), especially with sickle cell disease or neuropathies, as in diabetics. Occasional causes include muscle (e.g., gastrocnemius) rupture, congenital and acquired vascular disorders, compartment syndromes.

Refer to Ch. 65, Chronic Heart Failure; Ch. 76, Varicose Veins; Ch. 77, Deep Venous Thrombosis; Ch. 98, Cirrhosis; Ch. 143, Acute Renal Failure; Ch. 144, Chronic Renal Failure; Ch. 145, Glomerulonephritis; Ch. 177, Hypothyroidism; and Ch. 181, Cushing's Syndrome/Disease.

History: Key Questions to Ask

1. Onset? Measured in hours to days: acute (e.g., cellulitis, DVT, compartment syndrome, gastrocnemius rupture) versus chronic (e.g., systemic process, medication, chronic venous insufficiency, lymphedema)

2. Clinical course and localization? This is usually characterized as intermittent (recurrent) versus constant.

3. Quality of pain? Painless (systemic causes or lymphedema) versus painful (cellulitis, ruptured gastrocnemius, ruptured Baker's cyst, compartment syndrome, DVT)

4. Associated systemic symptoms?

    a. Fever and chills suggest cellulitis, lymphangitis, or venous thrombosis.

    b. Symptoms associated with CHF (e.g., dyspnea, orthopnea, paroxysmal nocturnal dyspnea) suggest cardiac origin.

    c. Glomerulosclerosis and/or nephritis (e.g., history of recent streptococcal sore throat, recurrent cystitis, hypertension, changes in ocular fundi, urinalysis, blood urea nitrogen/creatinine, and serum albumin) offer a renal pathogenesis.

    d. Signs of acute or chronic liver disease (e.g., hepatitis, alcoholism, axillary hair loss, palmar erythema, icterus, spider telangiectasias, gynecomastia, hepatomegaly, splenomegaly, abdominal wall collateral veins, ascites, or abnormal liver function tests) are all suggestive of hepatic etiology of edema formation.

5. Medications? These include diazoxide, minoxidil, hydralazine, calcium channel blockers, α- and β-receptor blockers, reserpine, guanethidine, nonsteroidal anti-inflammatory drugs, carbenicillin, amantadine, lithium, phenothiazines, thioridazine, monamine oxidase inhibitors, corticosteroids, testosterone, estrogen, and progesterone. Alcohol and other substance abuse? Diet faddism?

6. Endocrine diseases? These include Cushing's syndrome, thyroid dysfunction (pretibial "myxedema"), and thickened pretibial and/or foot skin during treatment of Graves' disease.

7. Miscellaneous factors? Pregnancy, salt overload, sudden cessation of laxative or diuretic abuse, carbohydrate-loading–induced antinatriuresis (diet enthusiasts after weekend binge), prolonged dependent positioning, impaired ambulation resulting from severe joint or neurologic disease (paraplegia).

Clinical Findings

1. Distribution: bilateral—smaller number of diseases, usually systemic; unilateral—larger number of diseases, usually regional

2. Location of swelling: calf or thigh only without feet or ankles—local cause within involved muscle groups (ruptured muscle, trauma, aneurysm, hematoma, sarcoma), or sparing of feet (lipedema)

3. Appearance of overlying skin: red (with or without tender streaks suggestive of cellulitis, phlebitis, lymphangitis); reddish-blue (DVT); slightly cyanotic and bilateral (suggestive of CHF); venous "stars" (denoting local stasis with elevated venous pressure); ecchymosis (suggestive of trauma, ruptured muscle)

4. Pitting: suggestive of systemic cause; mobility of nonchronic (i.e., <3 months in duration) pitting edema a function of tissue viscosity related to fluid protein content. When edema "pits" with little resistance and recovery is seen in less than 30 to 40 seconds, hypoproteinemia generally is present. *However*, if edema is chronic (>3

months), interstitial tissue fibrosis and scarring may produce prolonged pitting even if hypoproteinemia is present.

Tests

1. Serum electrolytes and biochemistry profile (including liver function tests, serum albumin, total protein, blood urea nitrogen, and creatinine)
2. Urinalysis (routine and microscopic)
3. Chest radiograph
4. Echocardiogram to assess cardiac dysfunction (prn)
5. Thyroid function tests to rule out thyroid dysfunction (prn)
6. Duplex Doppler or venography to rule out DVT (prn)

Management

1. General
   a. Diuretics, dietary manipulation of salt and water, vasodilators, and digoxin are prescribed (see Chs. 60 and 130).
   b. Angiotensin-converting enzyme inhibitors sometimes are helpful in the treatment of idiopathic cyclic edema, in addition to reassurance.
   c. Elastic compression with stockings, physical therapy, and intermittent pneumatic compression may be useful.
2. Specific: Treatment depends on the cause of the edema.
   a. DVT: anticoagulation with heparin followed by warfarin.
   b. CVI: sclerotherapy used in selected patients.

Surgical management (ligation/stripping of incompetent perforator veins, venous reconstruction to bypass isolated obstruction or to interpose a functioning valve segment in a patent deep venous system) is applicable to less than 25 per cent of patients *only* after studies determine site and degree of valve dysfunction or obstruction. Surgical therapy usually is limited to patients with severe (grade III) CVI.

   c. Treatment of edema caused by lymphatics is usually medical to remove as much fluid as possible (compression with stockings, physical therapy, and intermittent pneumatic compression). If medical therapy fails, palliative surgery is considered. Two types are available: excisional (debulking) and microvascular reconstruction (lymphovenous anastomosis or lymph vessel transplant).
   d. For miscellaneous inflammatory causes, antibiotics are prescribed. Abscess and osteomyelitis may warrant surgery in selected patients.

Bibliography

Abraham WT, Schrier RW: Body fluid volume regulation in health and disease. Adv Intern Med 1994;39:23–47.

Ciocon JO, Fernandez BB, Ciocon DG: Leg edema. Geriatrics 1993;48:34–45.

Powell AA, Armstrong MA: Peripheral edema. Am Fam Physician 1997;55:1721–1726.

Ruschaupt III WF: The swollen limb. In Young JR, Graor RA, Olin JW, et al (eds): Peripheral Vascular Diseases, pp 639–650. St. Louis, Mosby, 1991.

Seller RH: Swelling of legs. In Seller RH: Differential Diagnosis of Common Complaints, 3rd ed, pp 335–341. Philadelphia, WB Saunders Company, 1996.

SYMPTOM CLAUDICATION

Fernando F. Stancampiano

The term *claudication* derives from the Latin word *claudicare*, "to limp." In addition to its negative impact on ambulation, this condition is frequently associated with occlusive disease in other vascular areas, such as the coronary or extracranial arteries. As revealed by the Framingham study, men with intermittent claudication (IC) have a higher annual mortality rate than their normal counterparts (39/1000 vs. 10/1000), mostly because of a high incidence of myocardial infarction and stroke. Although IC is usually the consequence of insufficient arterial blood supply to the lower extremities caused by arteriosclerosis obliterans (ASO), patients with lumbar canal stenosis often present with similar complaints; the latter condition is referred to as *pseudoclaudication.*

Differential Diagnosis

1. ASO
2. Lumbar canal stenosis and disk disease (pseudoclaudication)
3. Embolic disease
4. Buerger's disease
5. Vasculitis (Takayasu's disease, giant cell arteritis)
6. Drugs (ergot derivatives)
7. Phlegmasia (ileofemoral vein thrombosis with secondary arterial insufficiency)
8. Metabolic disease (homocystinuria)
9. Miscellanea (adventitial cyst, entrapment syndromes, fibromuscular dysplasia, reflex sympathetic dystrophy, persistent sciatic artery)

Although numerous medical and surgical conditions mimic the clinical presentation of IC, ASO of the lower extremities and aortoiliac territories is the most common etiology. Typically, patients with pseudoclaudication have pain while standing and need to change position in order to get relief, whereas, in those with IC, the simple interruption of exercise is sufficient to abort the symptoms within minutes. Obvious findings consistent with ASO do not rule out pseudoclaudication, because both frequently coexist. Patients with pseudoclaudication may experience relief upon leaning forward ("shopping cart sign"). Patients with vasculitis often have "ischemic-looking" ulcers in atypical locations.

History

1. Pain in the lower extremities (buttocks, calves)
2. Symptoms may be unilateral or bilateral.
3. Claudication occurs with exercise and is relieved within a few minutes by resting.
4. A decrease in the claudication threshold correlates with progression of the disease.
5. Evidence of ischemia at rest is a reflection of increased severity.

At the time the diagnosis of IC is made, a significant proportion of patients are known to have coronary and/or cerebrovascular disease. These patients commonly have a history of diabetes mellitus, tobacco abuse, and other risk factors for heart disease.

Clinical Findings

1. Diminished/absent pulses
2. Arterial bruits (femoral, Hunter's canal)
3. Diminished temperature in the affected limb(s)
4. Ischemic ulcers
5. Dependent rubor/edema
6. Pallor on elevation
7. Muscle weakness/atrophy

Most patients with IC have absent or markedly diminished palpable pulses; however, a normal examination does not rule out the disease. Blood flow studies usually reveal one or more localized abnormalities. The typical ischemic ulcer is painful, well circumscribed, and usually located in the distal portion of the toes, interdigital areas (kissing ulcers), or pressure sites (ASO and trauma). In severe cases, atrophy and ischemic neuropathy may develop. Dependent edema and rubor tend to occur late in the course of the disease and seem to be markers of a threatened limb.

Tests

1. Arteriogram (aortogram with "runoffs")
2. Ankle/brachial systolic blood pressure index (ABI)
3. Pulse volume recordings (PVRs)
4. Other tests: plethysmography, magnetic resonance imaging, digital subtraction angiography, duplex scanning
5. Risk stratification: myocardial perfusion studies, coronary angiogram, carotid duplex scanning

Most cases can be diagnosed accurately on the basis of a detailed history and physical examination, combined with noninvasive methods. The simple application of basic Doppler techniques (ABI) provides valuable information regarding the severity of the disease. IC is usually associated with an ABI of between 0.5 and 0.9. An ABI of less than 0.3 frequently correlates with ischemic rest pain and impending necrosis. In PVRs, partially inflated blood pressure cuffs sense volume changes in limb segments, which are subsequently transduced and displaced as waveforms. The same techniques can be used to document the outcome of a revascularization procedure. The angiographic evaluation of the lower extremities is not indicated in every patient but becomes more valuable when a surgical intervention is considered. Some institutions now plan angioplasty and even revascularization surgery on the basis of duplex imaging alone. Myocardial infarction significantly contributes to the postoperative mortality among patients who undergo aortofemoral or femoropopliteal reconstruction. Therefore, the status of the coronary circulation should be evaluated in all patients by means of a coronary angiogram or noninvasive nuclear techniques (Dipyridamole 201-Tl or SestaMIBI, 82-Rb positron emission tomography scanning, dobutamine echocardiography). Findings consistent with high ischemic risk warrant myocardial revascularization before surgery in the lower extremities.

Management

1. Conditioning exercises
2. Smoking cessation
3. Pharmacologic treatment
4. Revascularization procedures: angioplasty, stent placement, surgery

It is well documented that a training program of walking exercises improves resting blood flow, reduces the onset of claudication symptoms, and increases maximal walking time. Unfortunately, the use of vasodilating drugs has yielded disappointing results. Most vasodilators reduce systemic blood pressure and increase collateral vessel resistance. The current literature does not support their widespread use. Many of the drug trials have methodologic flaws, and only show modest improvement in walking distance. Pentoxifylline (Trental) has been extensively used. Initially introduced as a vasodilator, it was subsequently reclassified as a rheologic agent. Cilostazol appears to be a promising option. Patients with IC should be considered for treatment with antiplatelet agents such as aspirin or clopidogrel (Plavix), because these drugs reduce the risk of ischemic stroke, myocardial infarction, and vascular death. The most important operative indications for lower extremity ischemia include ischemic rest pain or tissue loss (ulceration and/or gangrene), disabling claudication, and lack of response to an adequate trial of medical therapy. Ongoing trials are aimed at defining the role of therapeutic angiogenesis (use of endothelial growth factors to promote the development of collateral circulation).

Patient Education

1. Lifestyle modification: smoking cessation, exercise
2. Foot care: daily inspection, skin care
3. Use of professionally customized shoes/orthotics

PEARLS

- Consider non-ASO causes of IC in patients with atypical features.

- Objectively assess the patient's functional capacity and status of the circulation in the lower extremities (PVRs).

- Provide positive feedback to reinforce lifestyle changes.

- Try to establish the proper timing for a surgical intervention.

Bibliography

Bergqvist D, Karacagil S: Femoral artery disease. Lancet 1994;343:773–778.
Brand F, Abbott R, Kannel W: Diabetes, intermittent claudication, and risk of cardiovascular events: the Framingham Study. Diabetes 1989;38:504–509.
Golledge J: Lower-limb arterial disease. Lancet 1997;350: 1459–1465.
Porter J: Chronic lower extremity ischemia. Curr Probl Surg 1991;28:3–179.
Yeager R: Nonatherosclerotic claudication. Semin Vasc Surg 1993;6:24–35.

SYMPTOM **SHOCK**

Benjamin H. Chadi

Shock is defined as the *state of hypoperfusion of vital organs associated with hypotension and a critical prognosis*. Ohm's law regarding flow in a circuit:

Flow = (Pressure gradient afferent-efferent)/

(Resistance in vascular bed)

is valid for a local vascular bed, individual organs, and the circulatory system as a whole. Areas of higher resistance, such as the kidneys and stenosed coronary arteries, require a higher perfusion pressure (blood pressure) for flow to occur. Above this minimal pressure, many organs such as the brain can autoregulate blood flow to maintain a relatively constant perfusion at varying blood pressures. Differential shunting occurs as a result of nonuniform regulation of blood flow in different vascular territories.

Reduced organ perfusion can occur because of an inadequate blood volume (hypovolemic), a loss of vascular resistance (distributive), inability to generate a pressure (cardiogenic), or block to flow in the circuit (obstructive).

Differential Diagnosis

Hypovolemic (Loss of Preload)

1. Acute hemorrhage or blood loss (gastrointestinal, trauma, surgery, anticoagulants)

2. Dehydration resulting from fever, vomiting, diarrhea, nasogastric suction, diabetic ketoacidosis, peritonitis

3. Intravascular depletion caused by third spacing, including postsurgical states and hypoalbuminemia

4. Adrenal insufficiency, pheochromocytoma

Distributive (Generalized Systemic Vasodilatation)

1. Sepsis: bacterial (gram-positive, gram-negative), fungal, rickettsial (Rocky Mountain spotted fever), and toxins (toxic shock)

2. Anaphylaxis: drug reaction—penicillins; stings of bees, wasps, scorpions; snakebites

3. Neurogenic: spinal shock—trauma, anesthesia; vagotonic—related to procedures, sight of blood

4. Drugs: α-blockers, β-agonists, and vasodilators, including nitroprusside, captopril, nifedipine, sildenafil, and nitroglycerin

5. Other vascular shunts, such as arteriovenous (AV) malformations and AV fistulas

Cardiogenic (Low Cardiac Output Resulting From Right or Left Ventricular Pump Failure)

1. Myocardial infarction with large areas of myocyte necrosis or right ventricular infarction in

the setting of reduced preload (due to nitrates or diuretics)

2. Acute myocardial ischemia in a large area, a sign of left main or severe three-vessel coronary artery disease

3. Cardiomyopathy with progressive pump failure

4. Ischemia associated with hypotension of another cause, including coronary steal due to arterial vasodilators

5. Acute coronary spasm (Prinzmetal's angina or related to drugs, cocaine)

6. Tachyarrhythmias (ventricular or supraventricular tachycardia [VT or SVT]) with inadequate time for chamber filling or loss of vasoconstrictor reflexes

7. Bradyarrhythmias, including heart block

8. Ventricular free wall rupture

9. Ventricular septal defect (postinfarction)

10. Papillary muscle necrosis with acute mitral regurgitation

11. Congenital heart disease with associated sepsis

12. Severe valvular heart disease (aortic or mitral stenosis) or idiopathic hypertrophic subaortic stenosis (IHSS) or supravalvular stenosis with inability to increase cardiac output (CO) in response to stress (e.g., infection, vasodilator)

Obstructive (Massive Increase in Afterload)

1. Aortic dissection with obliteration of true lumen

2. Pericardial tamponade

3. Pulmonary embolism

4. Tension pneumothorax

5. Valvular obstruction: prosthesis malfunction, prolapse of atrial myxoma, or valve obstruction by ball valve thrombus

---

Refer to Ch. 62, Myocardial Infarction; Ch. 63, Cardiac Arrest; Ch. 64, Acute Pulmonary Edema (Heart Failure); Ch. 65, Chronic Heart Failure; Ch. 66, Cardiomyopathy; Ch. 70, Endocarditis; Ch. 72, Sinus Rhythms and Ectopic Beats; Ch. 73, Supraventricular Tachyarrhythmias; Ch. 74, Ventricular Tachyarrhythmias; Ch. 75, Atrioventricular Block and Sick Sinus Syndrome; Ch. 210, Anaphylaxis; and Ch. 248, Bacteremia/Sepsis.

History

1. Hypotension: fatigue, dizziness, syncope

2. Poor perfusion: slow mentation, decreased urination, decreased appetite

3. Etiology: infection, fever, new drug, hypersensitivity, sting, heart attack, chest pain, shortness of breath, trauma, bleeding, melena, diarrhea, fluid losses

Clinical Findings

1. Hypotension: systolic blood pressure less than 90 mm Hg except when there is severe vasoconstriction and low output with cardiogenic shock, or a unilateral pulse deficit in aortic dissection

2. Pulse: Tachycardia occurs with fever, pain, hypoxia, hyperthyroidism, or stress (adrenaline). Tachycardia increases CO (= stroke volume × heart rate), increases myocardial oxygen demand (and ischemia in coronary stenosis), and shortens diastole (and ventricular filling time). Very rapid heart rates can significantly reduce stroke volume, cardiac output, and blood pressure. Bradycardia may symptomatically drop cardiac output, as in the sick sinus syndrome. In high-grade and complete heart blocks, atrioventricular dissociation further impairs ventricular filling. In hypervagotonia such as with vasovagal syncope, carotid sinus hypersensitivity, or the Bezold-Jarisch reflex noted in inferior myocardial infarction, a vasodepressor component (vasodilation) frequently accompanies the cardioinhibitory component (bradycardia), resulting in hypotension. Peripheral vasodilation alone (without bradycardia) causes orthostatic hypotension in the Shy-Drager syndrome.

3. Fever: in sepsis, anaphylaxis, and adrenal insufficiency

4. Organ hypoperfusion: cold, clammy skin (except for distributive shock, in which skin is warm), pallor or cyanosis, poor mentation, decreased bowel sounds, oliguria

5. Jugular veins: flat in hypovolemic and distributive shock (<6 cm H_2O); distended in cardiogenic and obstructive shock (>8 cm H_2O)

6. Pulmonary rales, edema, effusion: in cardiogenic or obstructive shock; in acute respiratory distress syndrome or pneumonia in any type of shock

7. Heart sounds

   a. Distant in tamponade

   b. Loud P_2 in pulmonary hypertension

   c. Delayed A_2 in aortic stenosis

   d. S_3 and diffuse impulse in cardiogenic

   e. S_4 and prominent impulse in obstructive

   f. Murmurs of mitral regurgitation, IHSS, aortic stenosis, aortic insufficiency, ventricular septal defect

g. Rub (two- or three-component) of pericarditis
h. Pericardial knock of constriction
i. Diastolic tumor plop of myxoma
j. Muffling of metallic prosthetic valve clicks
k. Bruit over vascular shunt or AV malformation

Tests

Shock must be diagnosed immediately and its cause determined accurately, so that lifesaving therapy can be initiated immediately to correct the reversible causes of this otherwise rapidly fatal state. Monitoring, diagnosis, and therapy often have to occur simultaneously, with frequent updates and rapid response and action necessary by health care personnel. The duration of hypotension measured in minutes and hours often determines the degree and reversibility of organ system damage and sequelae. Tests include the following.

1. Electrocardiography: Evaluate for VT, SVT, heart blocks, ST elevations of acute infarction, spasm, pericarditis, ST depressions of ischemia, Q waves of old infarctions, new right axis in pulmonary embolism, right-sided chest leads for right ventricular (RV) infarction.

2. Chest roentgenogram: Evaluate for cardiomegaly, progressive enlargement in tamponade, evidence of pulmonary congestion, dilated aortic arch in dissecting aneurysm, pulmonary vascular plethora in septal defects, effusions in heart failure, pulmonary embolism, and other states.

3. Complete blood count: Hematocrit drops after hydration in acute blood loss; hemoconcentration in dehydration; leukocytosis, left shift, and toxic granulations in sepsis; thrombocytopenia or coagulopathies in bleeding diatheses; and schistocytes in disseminated intravascular coagulation.

4. Arterial blood gases and electrolytes: Rule out and correct hypoxia, respiratory and metabolic acidosis, hyper- and hypokalemia, natremia, calcemia, magnesemia, and glycemia, whether primary or secondary to the shock. Consider naloxone (Narcan) and flumazenil (Mazicon).

5. Blood cultures for aerobic, anaerobic, acid-fast, and fungal organisms

6. Urinalysis and culture: pyuria, casts in urosepsis, acute tubular necrosis

7. Assays: creatine kinase and MB elevation in myocardial infarction; elevated lactate dehydrogenase levels in myocardial infarction and hemolysis (prosthetic valve dysfunction); documentation of serum amylase and lipase, renal and hepatic function including albumin, and phosphorus; serum cortisol and drug levels; plasma vasopressin level (reduced in septic shock)

8. Echocardiography with Doppler: Evaluate pericardial effusion and diastolic right atrial, RV collapse in tamponade with respiratory variation in the mitral and aortic flow Doppler tests; evaluate for a cardiomyopathy with generalized hypokinesis or for infarctions with focal wall motion abnormalities; calculate pulmonary artery pressures and CO, valve function, chamber sizes, and septal defects.

9. Transesophageal echocardiography can diagnose pulmonary artery thromboembolus, aortic dissection, septal defects, and congenital heart diseases.

10. Ventilation-perfusion scanning for pulmonary embolism and gallium or white blood cell scanning for abscess

11. Cardiac catheterization
   a. Arterial line to monitor blood pressure
   b. Central venous line to monitor right heart (central venous) pressure
   c. Swan-Ganz catheterization to evaluate pulmonary artery pressures and pulmonary capillary wedge pressure (PCWP, left heart preload), with measurements of CO by thermodilution or Fick (oxygen uptake) methods and calculation of systemic vascular resistance
   d. Oximetry with oxygen saturations from the central vein compared to the pulmonary artery oxygen saturations, with a significant step-up indicating a left-to-right shunt
   e. Coronary angiography to evaluate location and severity of coronary stenoses and occlusion of vessels in acute infarctions with evidence of reperfusion or ongoing necessity for acute revascularization
   f. Left ventriculography to evaluate function, regurgitation
   g. Aortography to evaluate for dissection, regurgitation
   h. Pulmonary angiography to evaluate for thromboembolism
   i. Fluoroscopic evaluation of prosthetic valve function

12. Continuous monitoring of vital signs, blood pressure, oxygen saturations, and electrocardiography (ECG) for arrhythmias.

Management

Medical Therapy

Treatment depends on cause. Control of the airway and oxygen may be necessary.

1. Hypovolemic
   a. Find source of blood loss and stop bleeding (vascular compression, endoscopy, surgery if necessary; consider platelets or fresh frozen plasma). Large-bore intravenous lines are used for fluid support (saline, packed red blood cells, albumin).
   b. Monitor blood pressure, hematocrit, central venous pressure, rales, PCWP (in cardiomyopathy), oxygen delivery (DO$_2$), and oxygen consumption (VO$_2$).
2. Distributive
   a. Intravenous saline and fluids are given to replete intravascular volume; then consider dopamine and vasopressors (norepinephrine, phenylephrine, metaraminol, methoxamine) via central line.
   b. Antibiotics for sepsis (consider antifungal drug if patient is already on several broad-spectrum antibiotics, especially for more than one to two weeks and especially if immunocompromised). Consider vasopressin infusion (0.01 to 0.04 U/min) in septic shock.
   c. Give antihistamines (H$_1$ and H$_2$) and steroids for anaphylaxis. Consider atropine for vagotonia.
   d. Search for and remove source of infection, including infected catheters and abscesses.
3. Cardiogenic
   a. Relieve ischemia (oxygen, aspirin, heparin). Consider nitrates, morphine, and low dose metoprolol (Lopressor).
   b. Perform thrombolysis of acute infarction (less successful in shock). Intra-aortic balloon counterpulsation with emergency angioplasty, coronary stenting, or bypass surgery is recommended in the setting of an acute myocardial infarction and ongoing chest pain or hemodynamic instability.
   c. Perform valve repair or replacement in acute papillary muscle rupture with mitral regurgitation, and surgical repair of ventricular free wall rupture or septal defects.
   d. For heart failure, titrate inotropes to cardiac output. Dobutamine, amrinone, and milrinone may cause vasodilation and hypotension. Avoid digoxin or isoproterenol in the acute infarct setting (increases myocardial oxygen demand). In end stage, consider stronger β-agonists (epinephrine).
   e. Optimize preload.
   f. Antiarrhythmic therapy and rapid cardioversion are used to treat unstable ventricular tachycardia and primary SVT (treat underlying cause; look for hypovolemia). Monitor for blood pressure response to IV saline boluses and infusions in tamponade and acute right ventricular infarction. Remove vasodilators (nitrates) contributing to hypotension. Avoid calcium blockers in hypotension or treat overdose with intravenous calcium.
   g. For long-term treatment, consider need for diuretics, nitrates, angiotensin-converting enzyme inhibitors, digoxin, and β-blockers.
4. Obstructive: Immediate removal of the cause of obstruction is imperative.
   a. Pulmonary embolectomy or prolonged thrombolytic infusion for pulmonary embolism
   b. Aortic root and arch repair for type I aortic dissection
   c. Pericardiocentesis at bedside using ECG with a grounded V lead attached under asepsis to the needle (and ideally echo or fluoroscopic guidance) for tamponade

Supportive Therapy

1. Diet: nothing by mouth; low-cholesterol/low-salt diet when tolerated
2. Activity: bed rest immediately; gradual ambulation after treatment
3. Patient education: Condition is critical unless rapidly reversed.

Follow-Up

1. Intensive care unit care with (invasive) hemodynamic monitoring until blood pressure, systemic vascular resistance, and CO have normalized off drips
2. Meticulous attention to line sterility with frequent replacement (every 3 to 4 days) to avoid superinfection
3. Observe for recovery of function of brain, kidneys, and intestine as shock resolves.

B Bibliography

Berger PB, et al: Impact of an aggressive invasive catheterization and revascularization strategy on mortality in patients with cardiogenic shock in the Global Utilization of Streptokinase and Tissue Plasminogen Activator for Occluded Coronary Arteries (GUSTO-I) trial: an observational study. Circulation 1997;96:122–127.

Califf RM, Bengston JR: Cardiogenic shock. N Engl J Med 1994;330:1724–1730.

Effron MB, Chernow B: Shock. In Rubenstein E, Federman D (eds): Scientific American Medicine, 1:III:1–12. New York, Scientific American, 1992.

Hinshaw LB: Sepsis/septic shock: participation of the microcirculation: an abbreviated review. Crit Care Med 1996;24:1072–1078.

Reid IA: Role of vasopressin deficiency in the vasodilation of septic shock. Circulation 1997;95:1108–1110.

Shoemaker WC, et al: Resuscitation from severe hemorrhage. Crit Care Med 1996;24:125–235.

Weil MH, von Planta M, Rackow EC: Acute circulatory failure (shock). In Braunwald E (ed): Heart Disease: A Textbook of Cardiovascular Medicine, 4th ed, pp 569–587. Philadelphia, WB Saunders Company, 1992.

Indications

To gain peripheral intravenous access for the infusion of fluids, blood, or medicine.

Contraindications

Peripheral intravenous infusion cannot be used when hypertonic solutions such as total parenteral nutrition are needed. This requires central venous access.

Preparation

1. All materials should be gathered and set up before beginning the procedure.
2. Gloves should always be worn when starting an intravenous infusion.

Equipment

1. Intravenous cannula: catheter over-the-needle type or a butterfly needle
   a. 14 to 21 gauge common for adults
   b. 21 to 27 gauge common for infants and small children
2. Intravenous fluid
3. Intravenous tubing
4. Tape: preterm in the sizes needed
5. Alcohol or povidone-iodine swab
6. Tourniquet (surgical Penrose tubing works well)
7. Latex gloves

Extra Equipment for Infants and Children

8. Arm board (tongue blades padded and taped together work well for infants.)
9. Clear intravenous site protector (*Tip*: The catheter package may be cut in half and placed over a successful intravenous site.)
10. Rubber band (cut) works as a tourniquet on infants.
11. Neonatal transilluminator (a high-intensity light that shines through the hands of infants) (optional)

Anesthesia (Optional)

1. 1% Lidocaine without epinephrine
2. EMLA (eutectic mixture of a local anesthetic) cream (2.5% lidocaine, 2.5% prilocaine)

Precautions

1. Intravenous cannulation should be avoided on an extremity with compromised circulation or lymph drainage, such as an arm on the side on which a mastectomy has been performed.
2. An intravenous catheter should not be placed through an active infection in the skin or distal to a thrombosed vein.
3. Avoid using vessels over a joint.
4. Minimize the time the tourniquet is applied.
5. Take care not to cannulate arteries for intravenous infusions.
6. Take care not to secure intravenous tubing or arm board too tightly.

Technique

1. Locate a site
   a. Usually the upper extremity is the site of choice. The forearm

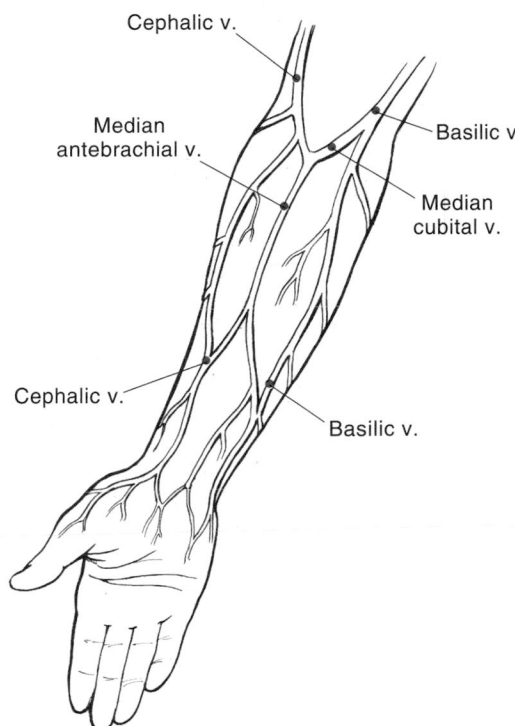

or the dorsum of the hand

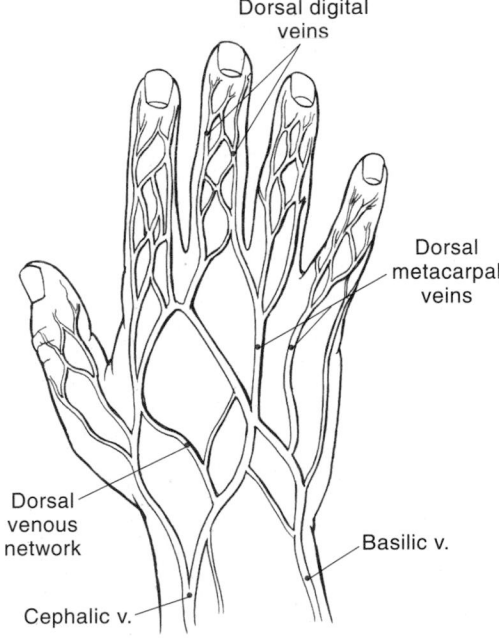

is commonly used. It is best to choose a distal site so that if the intravenous line infiltrates, it can be restarted more proximally.

   b. In infants it is sometimes necessary to use scalp veins because they are large and easily accessible.

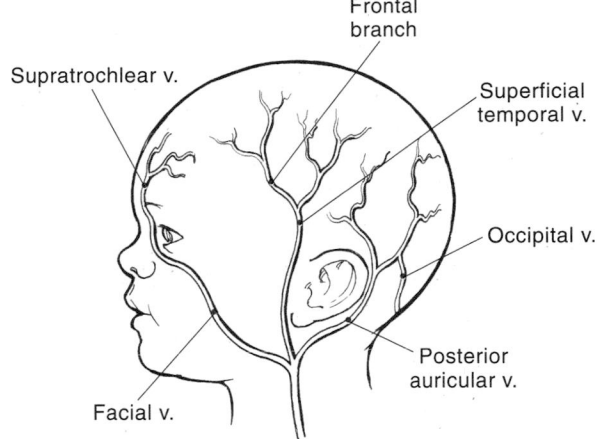

A patch of hair may need to be shaved to readily expose the veins.

> **WARNING**
>
> **Avoid using the lower extremity in adults because there is an increased risk of thrombophlebitis.**

2. Apply tourniquet: Firmly apply the tourniquet proximal to the chosen site of insertion. Be careful to not apply so tightly as to cut off arterial blood flow.
3. Clean site: Clean the insertion site with alcohol or povidone-iodine.
4. Anesthesia (optional): For large-bore intravenous catheters (14 to 18 gauge), you may wish to infuse a small amount of 1% lidocaine subdermally. Be careful not to infuse into a vein or infuse so much that it distorts the anatomy. Another anesthetic is EMLA cream, which may be applied under occlusive dressing at the site of choice for 1 hour prior to IV insertion. This is especially helpful for young children.

> **WARNING**
>
> **EMLA cream should not be used in any infant less than 1 month old nor in infants less than 12 months old who are receiving methemoglobin-inducing agents (see package insert).**

5. Insert:
   a. Stabilize the distal portion of the chosen vein with the thumb of your free hand while grasping the extremity.

b. Insert the chosen over-the-needle catheter into the skin directly over the vein or just parallel to it with the bevel up at approximately a 30-degree angle to the skin for adults (approximately 20 degrees for infants).

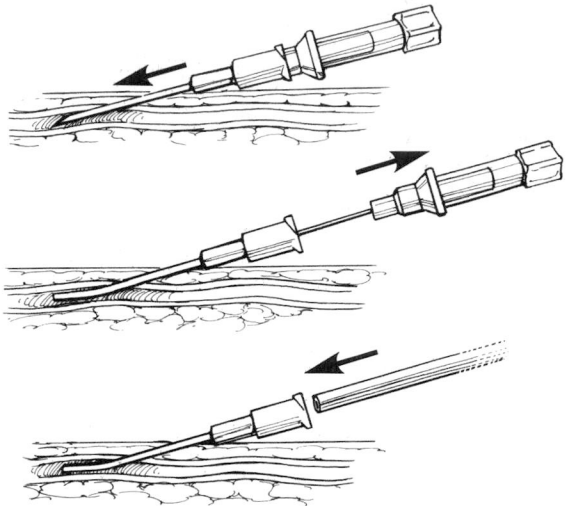

Then direct the tip of the needle into the vein until blood is seen in the flash chamber. Advance a few more millimeters to ensure that the catheter tip is completely in the lumen of the vein.

> **Note**
> Penetration of the skin and vein is often carried out in two steps. Penetration of both in one motion seldom works except in large, stable veins.

c. While stabilizing the needle, gently rotate and push the catheter over the needle into the vein.

d. Remove the tourniquet and then remove the needle from the catheter.

> **WARNING**
>
> **Never push the needle back into the catheter or pull the catheter back over the needle as this may shear off the catheter tip, causing a catheter embolism.**

6. Connect tubing: After ensuring there is no air in the tubing, connect the intravenous tubing to the catheter hub. Allow the intravenous fluid to gently flow into the vein while observing the site for any induration that may indicate improper catheter placement.

7. Secure the site:
   a. Secure the catheter and intravenous tubing to the patient with the pretorn tape. (*Note:* Never let go of a successful intravenous line until it is secured in place.)
   b. With infants and children, consider utilizing a clear plastic site protector and an arm board.

Follow-Up

1. Check the site at least daily if not more often for induration, swelling, or signs of infection and to ensure that the line is functioning properly.
2. The intravenous site should be changed every 72 hours to lessen the risk of infection and formation of a thrombus. This can be extended to 96 hours with close observation in those patients with difficult intravenous access.

Tips to Increase Your Success

1. Make yourself comfortable (sit if possible). This tip alone brings the most success.
2. Place the extremity in a dependent position below the level of the heart to increase vasodilation.
3. Warm the extremity with a heating pad or a warm, moist towel.
4. Firmly stroke the vein. This causes vasodilation and is more comforting to the patient than slapping the vein.
5. Raise the patient's legs above the level of the heart to make more blood available to fill the veins in the arm.
6. Use the help of an assistant and/or the aid of a restraining device such as a papoose board for the child too young to cooperate.

Bibliography

Astra USA: EMLA cream. In Physicians' Desk Reference, 52nd ed, pp 549–552. Montvale, NJ, Medical Economics Company, 1998.

Chaneides L, Hazinski MF (eds): Vascular access. In Textbook of Pediatric Advanced Life Support, pp 5-1–5-17. Chicago, American Heart Association, 1994.

Cummins RO (ed): Intravenous techniques. In Textbook of Advanced Cardiac Life Support, pp 6-1–6-13. Chicago, American Heart Association, 1997.

Grant HD, Murray RH, Bergeron JD, et al: Assisting in IV therapy (Appendix). In Brady Emergency Care, 7th ed, pp 743–745. Englewood Cliffs, NJ, Prentice-Hall, 1995.

Nettina SM: IV therapy. In The Lippincott Manual of Nursing Practice, 6th ed, pp 56–71. Philadelphia, Lippincott-Raven Publishers, 1996.

Simon RR, Brenner BE: Vascular procedures. In Retford DC (ed): Emergency Procedures and Techniques, 3rd ed, pp 380–445. Baltimore, Williams & Wilkins, 1994.

58 Hypertension

Carlos R. Herrera

Etiology

1. Hypertension occurs in 10 to 20 per cent of persons ages 25 to 45 years and 30 to 40 per cent of persons ages 55 to 74 years.

2. Risk factors include excessive dietary salt and calories consumed and stress. It is more prevalent in African Americans, in those who are overweight, and in those who have a family history of hypertension.

3. The major system affecting blood pressure is the renin-angiotensin pathway. Renin, from the juxtaglomerular apparatus, leads to the formation of angiotensin I, which is converted in the lungs to a powerful vasoconstrictor, angiotensin II.

4. The leading pathophysiologic hypotheses are

   a. Stress and high sodium intake lead to high sympathetic activity and high renin/angiotensin, which lead to sodium reabsorption and elevated blood pressure.

   b. Kaplan states abnormalities in the renin-angiotensin system, peripheral vascular resistance, and cell membrane function have been documented. Obesity and insulin resistance worsen hypertension.

Symptoms

1. Patients are typically asymptomatic. They may have headaches, dizziness, vertigo, visual problems, malaise, chest pain, dyspnea, claudication, sweating, tremors.

2. Occasionally neurologic symptoms are seen: numbness or weakness of extremities, diplopia, eyelid weakness, decreased visual acuity, slurred speech, altered mental status.

Clinical Findings

1. *Retinal:* thickened arterial walls, compression of a vein where an artery crosses it, blurred disk margins, focal areas of white exudate

2. *Cardiac:* lateral displacement of point of maximal impulse, third and fourth heart sounds

3. *Neurologic:* cranial nerve palsies, focal weakness or numbness, altered mental status

4. *Vascular:* decreased peripheral pulses; femoral, abdominal, or carotid bruits

5. *Secondary hypertension:* edema, striae, truncal obesity, hyperpigmentation, numbness of extremities, foot ulcers, muscle weakness, tachycardia

Laboratory Tests

1. *Blood pressure measurement:* The patient should be asked to return three to five times to verify measurements. For proper measurement, the patient should sit at rest for 5 minutes in a quiet room. The clothing should be removed from the arm and not bunched up along the deltoid. Use the proper-sized blood pressure cuff and bell of the stethoscope.

2. The basic work-up is electrolytes, blood urea nitrogen, creatinine, calcium, albumin, liver profile, cholesterol, urine analysis for leukocytes and protein, and electrocardiogram for left ventricular hypertrophy.

3. Patients with renal insufficiency, creatinine greater than 1.2 mg/dl, may warrant 24-hour urine collection for protein and creatinine, renal ultrasonography, renal nuclear scan, or captopril renin stimulation test (measure peripheral renin after oral captopril). In patients with progressively worsening renal function, renal arteriograms and renal vein renin determination may be necessary to document the need for renal artery angioplasty or surgery.

4. Other atypical presentations may be widely fluctuating blood pressure or electrolyte abnormalities, indications for a computerized tomography scan of the adrenal glands in search of pheochromocytoma or adrenal tumors, respectively. Several 24-hour urine collections for catecholamine and metanephrines occasionally are helpful in detecting a pheochromocytoma. A dexamethasone suppression test may be indicated in a person with hypokalemia and striae to rule out Cushing's syndrome.

5. Ambulatory blood pressure monitoring is indicated when the patient has episodic, fluctuating blood pressures, difficult-to-control blood pressure, hypotensive symptoms with medications, or autonomic dysfunction.

Differential Diagnosis

1. *Temporary condition:* pain, anxiety, alcohol use, improper blood pressure measurement
2. *Renal hypertension:* nephrosclerosis, interstitial nephritis (which can be caused by prolonged hypertension), medications, diabetes, collagen-vascular disease, infection, or ischemia (Ch. 143, Acute Renal Failure; Ch. 144, Chronic Renal Failure)
3. *Renovascular disease,* such as fibromuscular dysplasia and atherosclerotic plaque obstruction
4. *Endocrine hypertension* includes many conditions, but the most common are aldosteronism, Cushing's disease, pheochromocytoma, and oral contraceptive use (see Part X, Metabolic and Endocrine Diseases).

Treatment

Medication

1. Consider history of medication intolerance and cost of medications.
2. *First-line agent:* diuretic, angiotensin-converting enzyme (ACE) inhibitor, or calcium channel blocker. If hypertension not controlled on a first-line medication, then maximize dose; if still not controlled, then switch to another agent. If continued poor control, then add another first-line agent. In asymptomatic patients allow 2 to 4 weeks between dose changes or switches for complete efficacy.
   a. *Diuretics:* hydrochlorothiazide or chlorthalidone, 12.5 to 50 mg by mouth daily (higher doses of these diuretics may frequently cause hypokalemia and hyponatremia); or indapamide, 2.5 to 5 mg by mouth daily. (These are frequently combined with potassium-sparing diuretics such as spironolactone.) Diuretics are preferred in the elderly. *Adverse effects:* hypokalemia, dehydration, hyperlipidemia.
   b. *ACE inhibitors:* enalapril, 2.5 to 20 mg by mouth twice a day, lisinopril, 2.5 to 40 mg by mouth daily; fosinopril, 5 to 40 mg by mouth daily, quinapril, 10 to 80 mg by mouth daily; ramipril, 1.25 to 2.5 mg by mouth daily. *Adverse effects:* use with caution in patients with renal insufficiency and congestive heart failure, hyperkalemia, facial swelling, cough, reversible renal failure.
   c. *Calcium channel blockers;* nifedipine XL, 30 to 120 mg/day by mouth; diltiazem CD, 180 to 360 mg/day by mouth; verapamil SR, 120 to 480 mg/day by mouth; amlodipine, 2.5 to 10 mg/day by mouth; felodipine, 5 to 20 mg/day by mouth. *Adverse effects:* bradycardia, pedal edema, cardiac failure with verapamil, tachycardia, orthostatic hypotension, constipation.
3. *Second line:* β-blockers, clonidine, doxazosin, terazosin, and methyldopa
4. *Acute treatment:* Attempt to give long-acting agent as above if patient is asymptomatic and pressure is less than 210/120. Clonidine 0.1 mg by mouth every 2 hours until pressure is below 180/110; or captopril, 12.5 mg by mouth every hour. Intravenous therapy is needed only for unstable angina or acute stroke situations.

WARNING

Be careful! Do not lower blood pressure rapidly below 140/80!

Diet

Patients should eat less salt, cholesterol, and calories. The amount of meat on the plate should be about the size of a deck of cards and the rest of the plate vegetables and starch. Insist on multiple visits with nutritionist.

Activity

Daily exercise helps with weight loss, reduces stress, and improves cardiovascular performance. Walking, stretching while sitting, and water aerobics are good ways to start sedentary patients on an exercise program.

Patient Education

Hypertension can be prevented. Once present, it results in a lifelong battle with diet, exercise, and medications. Small, long-term dietary changes are preferable. Crash or fad diets are dangerous. Blood pressure should be monitored at home or by visits to the local pharmacy.

WARNING

Avoid wide fluctuation of blood pressure. This may cause an acute stroke or medication intolerance owing to dizziness, palpitations, and pain.

Key Treatment

First-line agent: diuretic, ACE inhibitor, or calcium channel blocker

Follow-Up

1. The goal of therapy is to reduce pressure below 140/90 without adverse effects.
2. If blood pressure is above 140/90 and below 160/100, institute behavioral therapy (low-salt diet, exercise, weight reduction) and check blood pressure every 2 months.
3. If blood pressure is above 160/100 and below 180/110, follow every 2 weeks, until controlled; more frequent follow-up if renal damage is progressing. If cardiac ischemia or neurologic phenomena occur, then hospitalize.

4. If blood pressure is above 180/110, follow weekly; if above 210/120, hospitalize or follow daily as an outpatient.

 Bibliography

Black HR: Treatment of mild hypertension. The more things change . . . . JAMA 1993;6:757–759.

Joint National Committee on Prevention, Detection, Evaluation, and Treatment of High Blood Pressure: The sixth report of the Joint National Committee on Prevention, Detection, Evaluation, and Treatment of High Blood Pressure. Arch Intern Med 1997;157: 2413–2446.

Kaplan NM: Clinical Hypertension, 7th ed. Baltimore, Williams & Wilkins, 1998.

Mulrow CD, Cornell JA, Herrera CR, et al: Hypertension in the elderly: implications and generalizability of randomized trials. JAMA 1994;272:1932–1938.

Rimmer JM, Gennari FJ: Atherosclerotic renovascular disease and progressive renal failure. Ann Intern Med 1993;118:712–719.

59 Hyperlipidemia

David Dovnarsky

Etiology

1. Primary hyperlipidemia: genetic disorders of lipoprotein metabolism
2. Secondary hyperlipidemia
   a. Excess dietary intake of fat, calories, or alcohol
   b. Concurrent illnesses
   c. Medications

Symptoms

1. No symptoms until significant atherosclerosis has developed late in course of disease; then may include
   a. Angina
   b. Claudication
   c. Amaurosis fugax, weakness, or numbness (symptoms of transient ischemic attack or stroke)
2. Extreme elevations of triglycerides (>1000 mg/dl) may cause abdominal pain resulting from pancreatitis.

Clinical Findings

Xanthomas may be present on extensor tendons and xanthelasmas present periorbitally in familial cases.

Laboratory Tests

1. Lipid profile (total cholesterol, high-density lipoprotein [HDL], estimated low-density lipoprotein [LDL], and triglycerides) or random cholesterol may be used for screening.
   a. Screening is recommended every 5 years in all adults.
   b. Screening is controversial in children.
2. If initial test abnormal, lipid profile recommended and at least two readings averaged to make treatment decision.

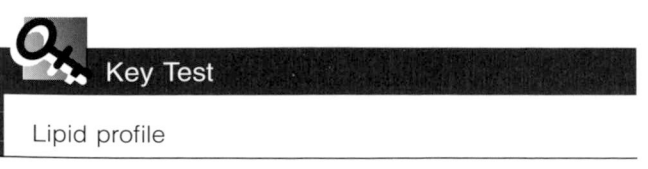

Key Test

Lipid profile

Differential Diagnosis

Secondary causes of hyperlipidemia should be considered and treated. These include

1. Obesity
2. Hypothyroidism
3. Diabetes mellitus
4. Nephrotic syndrome or uremia
5. Drugs
   a. Corticosteroids
   b. Diuretics
   c. β-Blockers
   d. Oral contraceptives
   e. Alcohol

Treatment

1. Goals for cholesterol levels are noted in Table 59–1. Goals for LDL cholesterol (Table 59–2) are set on the basis of the presence of other risk factors for coronary heart disease (CHD) and other atherosclerotic conditions (stroke, peripheral vascular disease) (Table 59–3) in combination with the LDL.
2. Classification of triglyceride levels is normal, less than 200 mg/dl; borderline, 200 to 400 mg/dl; high, greater than 400 mg/dl.
3. Treatment of hypertriglyceridemia is more controversial. Medication may be considered if diet and exercise fail and levels remain greater than 400 mg/dl. Medication is strongly recommended for levels over 1000 mg/dl to prevent pancreatitis.

TABLE 59–1. INITIAL CLASSIFICATION BASED ON TOTAL CHOLESTEROL AND HDL CHOLESTEROL LEVELS

CHOLESTEROL LEVEL	INITIAL CLASSIFICATION
Total Cholesterol	
<200 mg/dl (5.2 mmol/L)	Desirable blood cholesterol
200–239 mg/dl (5.2–6.2 mmol/L)	Borderline–high blood cholesterol
≥240 mg/dl (6.2 mmol/L)	High blood cholesterol
HDL Cholesterol	
<35 mg/dl (0.9 mmol/L)	Low HDL cholesterol

TABLE 59–2.   TREATMENT DECISIONS BASED ON LDL CHOLESTEROL LEVEL

Patient Category	Initiation Level	LDL Goal
Dietary Therapy		
Without CHD and with fewer than two risk factors (see Table 59–3)	≥160 mg/dl (4.1 mmol/L)	<160 mg/dl (4.1 mmol/L)
Without CHD and with two or more risk factors	≥130 mg/dl (3.4 mmol/L)	<130 mg/dl (3.4 mmol/L)
With CHD	>100 mg/dl (2.6 mmol/L)	≤100 mg/dl (2.6 mmol/L)
Drug Treatment		
Without CHD and with fewer than two risk factors	≥190 mg/dl (4.9 mmol/L)	<160 mg/dl (4.1 mmol/L)
Without CHD and with two or more risk factors	≥160 mg/dl (4.1 mmol/L)	<130 mg/dl (3.4 mmol/L)
With CHD	≥130 mg/dl (3.4 mmol/L)	≤100 mg/dl (2.6 mmol/L)

Diet

Diet is the mainstay of therapy and should be used initially in all cases.

1. A step 1 diet (total fat ≤30 per cent of total calories, <300 mg cholesterol, 8 to 10 per cent saturated fat) should be tried for 3 to 6 months.
2. If target is not reached, consider step II diet (consult dietitian) or medication.

Activity

Exercise program should be recommended routinely unless contraindicated; minimum recommendations of 20 to 30 minutes of aerobic exercise three times a week. Exercise has been shown to reduce triglycerides and increase HDL cholesterol.

Medication

1. Drug of choice: 3-hydroxy-3-methylglutaryl coenzyme A (HMG CoA) reductase inhibitors (Table 59–4) (decrease total, LDL cholesterol; atorvastatin also decreases triglycerides) are generally well tolerated. Follow liver function tests at 6 and 12 weeks, then every 6 months, and, if greater than three times normal, discontinue drug (1 to 2 per cent). Myopathy can occur but is very uncommon. Recent studies demonstrate reduced cardiovascular morbidity and mortality with use of these agents.
2. Alternative drugs
   a. Bile acid sequestrants: cholestyramine (Questran), one to three 4-gm doses twice daily (decreases LDL cholesterol). Gastrointestinal side effects may limit use; may increase triglycerides.
   b. Niacin: nicotinic acid 1 to 3 gm tid; start with 100 mg tid (decreases total, LDL cholesterol; decreases triglycerides; increases HDL cholesterol). Side effects include flushing and gastrointestinal distress. Dose should be increased gradually. Aspirin taken before dose may reduce side effects. Follow liver function tests.
   c. Fibric acid derivatives: gemfibrozil (Lopid) 600 mg bid (decreases triglycerides; increases HDL, decreases LDL cholesterol).
   d. Probucol (Lorelco) 500 mg bid (decreases total, LDL, HDL cholesterol). May prolong Q-T interval.
   e. Estrogen replacement therapy, e.g., conjugated estrogen (Premarin) 0.625 mg daily (decreases LDL, increases HDL, increases TG) should be considered in postmenopausal women.
   f. Combinations of medications may be used for resistant cases.

Patient Education

1. Explain link between hyperlipidemia and atherosclerosis.
2. Make patient aware of asymptomatic nature of condition until disease has progressed.

TABLE 59–3.   RISK STATUS BASED ON PRESENCE OF CHD RISK FACTORS OTHER THAN LOW-DENSITY LIPOPROTEIN CHOLESTEROL

Positive Risk Factors
Age, years
   Male ≥45
   Female ≥55 or premature menopause without estrogen replacement therapy
Family history of premature CHD (definite myocardial infarction or sudden death before 55 years of age in father or other male first-degree relative, or before 65 years of age in mother or other female first-degree relative)
Current cigarette smoking
Hypertension (blood pressure ≥140/90 mm Hg confirmed by measurements on several occasions or taking antihypertensive medication)
Low HDL cholesterol (<35 mg/dl [0.9 mmol/L] confirmed by measurements on several occasions)
Diabetes mellitus

Negative Risk Factors
High HDL cholesterol (≥60 mg/dl [1.6 mmol/L])

TABLE 59–4. HMG CoA REDUCTASE INHIBITORS

Generic Name	Trade Name	Initial Dose	Maximal Dose
Atorvastatin	Lipitor	10 mg qd	80 mg qd
Cerivastatin	Baycol	0.3 mg qd	0.3 mg qd
Fluvastatin	Lescol	20 mg qd	40 mg bid
Lovastatin	Mevacor	20 mg qd	80 mg qd or divided bid
Pravastatin	Pravachol	20 mg qd	40 mg qd
Simvastatin	Zocor	10 mg qd	40 mg qd

3. Stress compliance with diet, exercise, and medication (if used).

4. Discuss concomitant CHD risk factor reduction (smoking cessation, control of diabetes and hypertension).

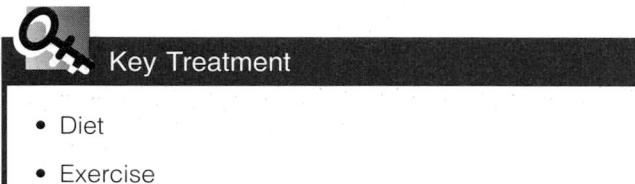

Key Treatment

- Diet

- Exercise

Follow-Up

1. If screening test is normal, rescreen in 5 years.

2. If treatment is initiated, follow cholesterol or lipid profile every 3 to 6 months based on results and particular regimen used.

3. Monitor compliance with diet and medication because this is often key to successful treatment.

Bibliography

Cholesterol Lowering in the Patient with Coronary Heart Disease: Physician Monograph (NIH Publication no. 97-3794). Bethesda, MD, National Institutes of Health, 1997.

Expert Panel on Detection, Evaluation and Treatment of High Blood Cholesterol in Adults: Summary of the second report of the National Cholesterol Education Program (NCEP) Expert Panel on Detection, Evaluation and Treatment of High Blood Cholesterol in Adults (Adult Treatment Panel II). JAMA 1993;269:3015–3023.

NIH Consensus Development Panel on Triglyceride, High-Density Lipoprotein, and Coronary Heart Disease: Triglyceride, high-density lipoprotein, and coronary heart disease. JAMA 1993;269:505–510.

Rakel RE, Schaefer EJ: Clinical Advances in Lipid Management in Family Practice. AAFP Video CME Program, 1997.

Report of the National Cholesterol Education Program Expert Panel on Detection, Evaluation and Treatment of High Blood Cholesterol in Adults. Arch Intern Med 1988;148:36–69.

60 Exercise Prescribing

Jane E. Corboy

Definition

1. Fitness: a general term describing a level of cardiovascular function that results in increased energy reserves for optimum performance and well-being
2. Endurance: the ability to work for long periods of time and resist fatigue
   a. Muscular endurance: specific muscle groups' endurance
   b. Cardiovascular endurance: total body endurance
3. VO_{2max} (maximum volume of oxygen consumption; maximum aerobic power): the capacity of the oxygen transport system
   a. Other terms include maximum oxygen uptake, cardiovascular endurance capacity, aerobic capacity.
   b. Mathematical definition of VO_2 maximum is

   Cardiac output $\times$ A $-$ VO_2

   (arteriovenous oxygen difference)

   or

   Heart rate [HR] $\times$ stroke volume $\times$ A $-$ VO_2

4. Conditioning: an increase in energy capacity through exercise that produces adaptation of the cardiovascular system and muscle

Benefits of Exercise (Indications)

1. Cardiovascular effects
   a. Myocardial
      (1) Increased stroke volume and cardiac output
      (2) Decreased myocardial oxygen demand at rest
      (3) Increased tolerance for given workload
   b. Peripheral vascular
      (1) Increased capillary flow
      (2) Decreased peripheral vascular resistance
      (3) Decreased resting blood pressure
   c. Oxygen-carrying capacity
      (1) Increased blood volume and hemoglobin
      (2) Enhanced muscle extraction of oxygen
2. Musculoskeletal effects
   a. Muscle-tendon unit
      (1) Increased blood flow to muscle
      (2) Increased muscle strength
      (3) Increased tolerance for a given workload
   b. Bones-joints
      (1) Increased bone mass with weight-bearing exercise
      (2) Increased blood flow to synovium
3. Metabolic/endocrine effects
   a. Glucose metabolism
      (1) Increased muscle utilization of glucose (non–insulin-dependent transport)
      (2) Decreased blood glucose levels
   b. Lipid metabolism
      (1) Increased utilization of triglycerides
      (2) Increased levels of high-density lipoprotein cholesterol
      (3) Lowered levels of total cholesterol
      (4) Improved overall lipid profile
4. Obstetric-gynecologic effects
   a. Labor and delivery
      (1) Improved tolerance of labor
      (2) Shortened first and second stages of labor
   b. Gynecologic effect: lessened dysmenorrhea
5. Psychological effects
   a. Improved sense of well-being
   b. Stress reduction

Risks of Exercise

1. Cardiovascular risks
   a. Patients with ischemic heart disease
      (1) Precipitation of angina or prolonged ischemia
      (2) Precipitation of arrhythmia
   b. Patients with structural heart disease
      (1) Hypertrophic cardiomyopathy: sudden death resulting from arrhythmia
      (2) Marfan's syndrome: aortic dissection
2. Musculoskeletal risks
   a. Acute effects
      (1) Muscle soreness
      (2) Traumatic injury: sprains, contusions, etc.
   b. Chronic effects: overuse injuries

3. Endocrine-metabolic: Patients with *uncontrolled* diabetes, thyroid disease, and the like may have worsened control because of increased autonomic activity with exercise.

4. Obstetric-gynecologic risks
   a. Obstetric
      (1) Decreased exercise tolerance with advanced pregnancy
      (2) Decreased uterine blood flow during exercise
      (3) Thermal stress on fetal development
      (4) Uterine contractions after exercise may increase risk of premature labor
      (5) Risks to fetus with high-intensity exercises
   b. Gynecologic: amenorrhea
      (1) Only occurs with combination of intense exercise and weight loss (to below 10% body fat)
      (2) May *increase* risk of osteoporosis/stress fractures

5. Psychological risks
   a. Obsessive-compulsive disorder
   b. Anorexia equivalent

Exercise Prescription Technique

Assessment

1. Assess current fitness level
   a. History
   b. Physical
   c. Exercise testing: patients with more than two coronary risk factors or symptoms suggestive of cardiovascular disease, if planning vigorous exercise

2. Assess motivation for exercise
   a. Medical
   b. Social
   c. Psychological

3. Assess barriers to exercise
   a. Medical
      (1) Health conditions
      (2) Medications
   b. Social/work-related
   c. Concerns

Prescription

1. Be specific when giving prescriptions. *A written prescription increases patient adherence to program.*

2. Mnemonic
   a. *Frequency*
   b. *Intensity*
   c. *Timing* (duration)
   d. *Type* of exercise
   e. *Energizing* (warm-up)
   f. *Relaxing* (cool-down)

3. Frequency: 3 to 5 days per week

4. Intensity
   a. Exercise at 50 to 85 per cent of maximum heart rate (MHR), which can be estimated as (220 − age) or measured via exercise testing
   b. Calculation of target HR range
      (1) Method 1

$$\left.\begin{array}{l}(MHR) \times 50\% \\ (MHR) \times 85\%\end{array}\right\} = \text{target HR range}$$

      (2) Method 2

$$\left.\begin{array}{l}(MHR - \text{resting HR}) \times 50\% + \text{resting HR} \\ (MHR - \text{resting HR}) \times 85\% + \text{resting HR}\end{array}\right\}$$

$$= \text{target HR range}$$

      Method 2 gives a narrower range and is better for patients with higher fitness levels

      For Methods 1 and 2: count pulse for 6 seconds and multiply by 10
      (3) Method 3: rating of perceived exertion (see Table 60–1); *best for patients who are familiar with the feeling of appropriate intensity of exercise*

5. Duration: 15 to 60 minutes
   a. The aerobic portion should be at least 15 minutes.
   b. The lower the intensity, the longer the duration needed.

6. Type of exercise depends on goals, but most adults need balance of the four goals listed below.

TABLE 60–1. RATING OF PERCEIVED EXERTION SCALE

3. Extremely light	
5. Very light	
7. Light	
9. Rather light	
11. Neither light nor hard	
13. Rather hard	"Conversational pace"
15. Hard	
17. Very hard	Target HR zone
19. Extremely hard	

Use of the scale: The exercise level associated with the "rather hard" to "very hard" rating of exertion generally correlates with the target heart rate zone. This range is also the pace at which most people can carry on a conversation with moderate breathlessness.

a. *Increased cardiovascular endurance*: aerobic exercise
   (1) Uses large muscle groups in continuous rhythmic manner
   (2) Examples: walking, jogging, bicycling (stationary or regular), swimming, aerobic dance, cross-country skiing, rowing, rope jumping
b. *Increased flexibility*: stretching
   (1) Sustained static stretches, no bouncing
   (2) Major target areas are hamstrings, quadriceps, calves, and low back
c. *Increased muscle strength*: resistance training
   (1) High tension, low repetition
   (2) May create anaerobic environment; avoid Valsalva maneuver
d. *Increased muscle endurance*: light weights or gravity
   (1) Low tension, high repetition
   (2) "Sport-specific"
   (3) "Cross-training" using different aerobic activities will increase endurance in different muscle groups.

7. Warm-up
   a. Five minutes of light exercise
   b. Five minutes of gentle stretching
8. Cool-down: similar to warm-up activities, but increased stretching to decrease soreness later

Modifications for Particular Illnesses or Health Conditions (Precautions)

1. Cardiovascular disease
   a. Angina—stable
      (1) Exercise at 5 to 10 beats under HR at which angina occurs ("ischemic threshold")
      (2) Use nitroglycerin
      (3) Supervised programs
   b. Hypertension: Avoid isometric exercise. Aerobic and low resistance exercise beneficial.
   c. Valvular disease: Mild to moderate OK after valve repair or replacement. Anticoagulants; no contact sports.
   d. Cardiac medications:
      (1) β-Blockers: Blunt HR response.
      (2) Diuretics may increase risk of dehydration, hypokalemia, and muscle cramps
   e. Peripheral vascular disease: Claudication limits exercise.
      (1) Exercise increases functional capacity.
      (2) Walk to onset of pain, rest, then resume
2. Pulmonary disease
   a. Chronic obstructive pulmonary disease: Exercise improves functional capacity; mainly walking.
   b. Exercise-induced asthma: worse with cold weather, dry air. May need to pretreat with cromolyn or β-adrenergic inhalers, leukotriene receptor antagonists.
3. Musculoskeletal disability
   a. Arthritis—severe: May prefer swimming, non-weight-bearing exercise, but either aerobic or resistance training improves function. Emphasize importance of stretching and range-of-motion exercises
   b. Spinal cord injury: Wheelchair sports, arm exercises have different cardiovascular response (lower muscular efficiency so higher oxygen consumption than with leg exercises)
4. Metabolic-endocrine
   a. Diabetes
      (1) Type 1: Adjust insulin dose/exercise/medications to avoid hypoglycemia.
      (2) Type 2: Chronic, be sure to emphasize foot care, no ballistic exercises with retinopathy.
   b. Obesity: Start with lower intensity to minimize musculoskeletal injuries.
5. Pregnancy
   a. Avoid exercise in patients with vaginal bleeding, history of premature deliveries, incompetent cervix.
   b. Avoid supine position after 20th week of pregnancy.
   c. Avoid core temperature over 102° F (39° C) throughout pregnancy.

Bibliography

For more general information on exercise prescription, see
ACSM position stand on the recommended quantity and quality of exercise for developing and maintaining cardiorespiratory and muscular fitness, and flexibility in adults. Med Sci Sports Exerc 1998;30:975–991.
For more information on exercise in pregnancy, see
Wang TW, Apgar BS: Exercise during pregnancy. Am Fam Physician 1998;57:1846–1852, 1857.
For more information on psychological effects of exercise, see
Scully D, Kremer J, Meade M, et al: Physical exercise and psychological well being: a critical review. Br J Sports Med 1998;32:111–120.
For more information on exercise in hypertension, see
Petrella RJ: How effective is exercise training for the treatment of hypertension? Clin J Sport Med 1998;8:224–231.

61 Coronary Artery Disease

William H. Winkler

Epidemiology and Etiology

1. Atherosclerotic coronary artery disease (CAD) is the leading cause of death in the United States, claiming nearly 500,000 victims each year. Although the *rate* of death from CAD declined 22 per cent in the decade from 1985 to 1995, the actual *number* of deaths decreased by only 2.8 per cent.

2. African American men have a 49.4 per cent higher death rate from CAD than do white men. There is an even greater disparity among women, with African American women having a 67.2 per cent higher death rate than white women.

3. Premenopausal women have an incidence of CAD 80 per cent lower than that of men of the same age. By 10 years after menopause, however, the gap narrows considerably. Women are more likely to present with chest pain as an initial manifestation of CAD, whereas men are more likely to present initially with myocardial infarction or sudden death.

4. CAD is highly lifestyle dependent. Known risk factors such as tobacco use, hyperlipidemia, elevated blood pressure, and diabetes mellitus can be modified by changes in diet, exercise, counseling, and medical management. Other risk factors, such as age, male sex, and family history, cannot, of course, be altered.

Symptoms

1. Angina pectoris (Latin for "a tightening of the chest") is the classic symptom of myocardial ischemia. It has been called "the heart crying out for help." Angina is the result of increased oxygen demand by the myocardium, decreased ability of the coronary circulation to supply oxygenated blood to the myocardium, or, most commonly, a combination of both.

2. Myocardial oxygen demand is dictated by heart rate, ventricular wall tension (as measured by ventricular systolic pressure and wall thickness), and the state of myocardial contractility. Myocardial oxygen supply depends upon the patency of the coronary arteries and the oxygen-carrying capacity of the blood. Imbalance between myocardial oxygen supply and demand results in angina.

3. Angina is often described as squeezing, burning, heavy, or tight, seldom as sharp or stabbing. A patient who depicts the sensation by holding a clenched fist against the epigastrium or sternum is giving an important clue to the diagnosis of angina.

4. Angina is frequently provoked by exertion, strong emotions, cold exposure, or a large meal. Exertional angina typically begins after a well-defined period of exercise and persists for a predictable period after cessation of the exercise. Most attacks of angina last 10 minutes or less. Anginal discomfort may radiate to the neck, jaw, shoulders, or arms.

5. Some patients with CAD (especially patients with diabetes) may not experience typical anginal symptoms. These patients, however, may experience exertional dyspnea out of proportion to their level of exertion. Appearance of new-onset exertional dyspnea in patients with the presence of risk factors should raise the clinician's index of suspicion for the presence of CAD.

Key Symptom

Chest pain with exercise

Clinical Findings

1. The diagnosis of CAD is largely based upon a careful and focused medical history. Clinical findings, if present, may help to confirm the clinician's suspicions, but their absence does not rule out the diagnosis of CAD.

2. Examination of a patient during an attack of angina may disclose signs of left ventricular dysfunction, the most common of which are a fourth heart sound and a precordial bulge palpated at the cardiac apex. Decreased blood flow to a papillary muscle resulting in temporary valvular dysfunction may provoke a transient murmur characteristic of the involved valve.

3. The clinician should search for physical findings often found in association with CAD, including elevated blood pressure, atherosclerotic changes in the retinal arteries, deposition of lipids

around the eyes and in the skin, bruits in the carotid or femoral arteries, decreased peripheral pulses, and the abdominal bruit and pulsatile mass suggestive of abdominal aortic aneurysm.

Laboratory Tests

1. Resting electrocardiography is of limited value in the diagnosis of CAD. Findings suggestive of old myocardial infarction establish the diagnosis of CAD, but approximately 50 per cent of CAD patients at rest will have a normal electrocardiogram.

2. Stress electrocardiography is more useful for establishing the diagnosis of CAD. It has a sensitivity of approximately 70 per cent and a specificity approaching 90 per cent. The preferred test is the treadmill electrocardiogram. Stress testing is more likely to produce false-positive results in women, patients on digitalis therapy, and patients with electrolyte disturbances, left ventricular hypertrophy, or intraventricular conduction disturbances.

3. Radioisotope imaging can be a helpful diagnostic tool in patients with strong risk factors for CAD, a suggestive history, and equivocal results from exercise testing.

   a. Exercise thallium testing in combination with 12-lead stress electrocardiography increases the sensitivity of diagnosis 15 per cent above stress electrocardiography alone.

   b. Pharmacologic stress testing with adenosine or dipyridamole combined with radioisotope imaging can be used to evaluate patients who are unable to exercise. The sensitivity and specificity of this combination of examinations is similar to that of exercise thallium testing, about 85 per cent and 90 per cent, respectively.

4. Coronary angiography is the gold standard for the diagnosis of CAD. In addition, angiography identifies anatomic and functional aspects of CAD that allow the clinician to choose between medical and surgical therapy. Angiography carries an acceptably low (approximately 0.1 per cent) mortality rate when performed by an experienced operator in an institution where at least six procedures a week are performed.

Key Tests

- Stress electrocardiography
- Radioisotope imaging
- Coronary angiography

Differential Diagnosis

Any structure innervated by thoracic dermatomes one through six can produce symptoms similar to angina pectoris. Again, a careful and focused history can narrow the list of possible diagnoses. Clinically, the most important possibilities include

1. Cardiovascular: myocardial infarction, vasospastic (Prinzmetal's) angina, congestive heart failure, aortic or mitral valve disease, and aortic aneurysm

2. Pulmonary: pulmonary embolus, pneumothorax, and pleurisy

3. Gastrointestinal: cholecystitis, esophageal reflux or spasm, gastritis, and peptic ulcer disease

4. Musculoskeletal: costochondritis, cervical or thoracic radiculopathy, chest wall trauma, and intercostal muscle strain or spasm

5. Psychologic: hyperventilation syndrome, panic attack

Treatment

1. The goal of treatment of CAD is restoration and preservation of myocardial perfusion and reduction of morbidity and mortality from myocardial ischemia and infarction. Stratification of patients into risk categories can aid in the selection of appropriate therapies.

2. Risk factor modification benefits patients of every risk category.

   a. *Complete and permanent cessation of tobacco use is the most important single modification a patient with CAD can accomplish.*

   b. Attainment of ideal body weight reduces systemic blood pressure.

   c. Aggressive lowering of serum lipids reduces the risk of new or secondary coronary events.

   d. Control of hypertension is thought to be the primary driving force behind the reduction in mortality rates from CAD.

   e. Although tight control of diabetes is a laudable goal for other reasons, no evidence to date has shown it to improve CAD morbidity or mortality.

3. Patients at *low risk* (disease of any single vessel except the left main) can be managed with medical therapy.

   a. Antiplatelet therapy with aspirin, 81 to 325 mg daily, or clopidogrel (Plavix), 75 mg daily in patients unable to tolerate aspirin, reduces the risk of myocardial infarction by inhibiting aggregation of platelets on atherosclerotic plaques in the coronary arteries.

b. Antianginal agents: All decrease myocardial oxygen demand (see "Symptoms").

   (1) β-Blockers reduce heart rate and myocardial contractility in the resting state as well as blunting exercise-induced tachycardia. β-Blockers should be used with caution, if at all, in patients with asthma, diabetes, or peripheral vascular disease. If β-blockers must be discontinued, tapering the dose will reduce the risk of myocardial infarction or worsened angina. Some authorities recommend β-blockers as first-line antianginal therapy. Side effects of β-blockers include decreased ventricular function, blunted response to hypoglycemia, bronchospasm, reduced peripheral perfusion, depression, and nightmares.

   (2) Calcium channel blockers increase peripheral arteriolar dilatation, thereby reducing blood pressure and afterload. Some calcium channel blockers also reduce heart rate. Recent research suggests increased cardiovascular mortality associated with short-acting calcium channel blockers; however, no such association appears to exist with sustained-release agents. Side effects of calcium channel blockers include atrioventricular delay or block, pedal edema, headache, and constipation.

   (3) Nitrates reduce ventricular preload and afterload as well as dilating epicardial coronary arteries. Short-acting nitrates are used for episodic therapy. Long-acting nitrates can be used prophylactically, but tolerance develops rapidly unless a daily 10- to 12-hour nitrate-free interval is included. Other antianginal agents should be used during the nitrate-free interval. Side effects of nitrates include headache, tachycardia (which can be ameliorated by the concomitant use of β-blockers or calcium channel blockers), and hypotension.

4. Patients at *moderate risk* are those with two-vessel disease and normal left ventricular function. This subgroup usually benefits from revascularization. The choice between percutaneous transluminal coronary angioplasty (PCTA) and coronary artery bypass grafting (CABG) is based upon operator experience and patient preference because no clear-cut outcome or cost advantage can be demonstrated for either approach.

5. Patients at *high risk* are those with left main artery disease or three-vessel disease and left ventricular dysfunction. This group clearly benefits from CABG revascularization. Some patients with left main artery disease may be candidates for minimally invasive bypass surgery.

Key Treatment

- Risk factor modification
- β-Blockers
- Nitrates
- Calcium channel blockers

Follow-Up

1. Most patients with CAD can benefit from cardiac rehabilitation. Benefits of cardiac rehabilitation include development of collateral coronary circulation, optimization of body weight, reduction in serum lipids and blood sugar, reduction of arterial blood pressure, and improvement in a general sense of well-being.

2. Secondary prevention efforts are aimed at control of the same risk factors mentioned in "Treatment" above.

Bibliography

Alexander RW, Schlant RC, Fuster V (eds): The Heart, 9th ed, pp 1127–1618. New York, McGraw-Hill, 1998.

DeGowin RL: Diagnostic Examination, 6th ed, pp 232–248. New York, McGraw-Hill, 1994.

Gutstein DE, Fuster F: Management of stable coronary artery disease. Am Fam Physician 1997;56:99–106.

Solomon AJ, Gersh BJ: Management of chronic stable angina: medical therapy, percutaneous transluminal coronary angioplasty, coronary artery bypass graft surgery: lessons from the randomized trials. Ann Intern Med 1998;128:216–223.

Staniforth AD: Evidence based treatment of chronic stable angina. Int J Cardiol 1998;63:21–25.

Indications

1. Assisting in the evaluation and diagnosis of chest pain
2. Screening for ischemic heart disease in asymptomatic patients at risk
3. Evaluating dysrhythmias that may be exacerbated with stress
4. Determining exercise capacity and generating exercise programs
5. Establishing prognosis of patients with ischemic heart disease*
6. Evaluating antianginal or antihypertensive therapy*
7. Evaluating patients after myocardial infarction*

Contraindications

1. Evolving myocardial infarction, unstable angina, or uncontrolled heart failure
2. Uncontrolled hypertension
3. Cardiomyopathy, myocarditis, pericarditis, or suspected aortic aneurysm
4. Recent embolic phenomena (cerebral, pulmonary, or systemic)
5. Severe aortic stenosis or idiopathic hypertrophic subaortic stenosis
6. Rapid dysrhythmias or conduction defects greater than first-degree heart block
7. Patient unwilling or unable to give informed consent

Preparation

1. Choose patients carefully. Thoroughly explain procedure, risks, and benefits.
2. Have informed consent document signed by patient.
3. Evaluate for signs of heart failure or pericarditis.
4. Determine predicted end point. This could be limited by symptoms or heart rate. Maximal ($220 -$ age) or submaximal (maximal $\times$ 85 per cent) heart rates can be used.

Equipment

1. Treadmill: Those with varying speeds and grade are preferred.
2. Monitor: Three-lead continuous monitoring preferred.
3. Electrocardiogram (ECG) machine: Twelve leads preferred.
4. Emergency resuscitation kit: Rapid access to advanced cardiac life support (including medications and defibrillation) is necessary.

Technique

1. Obtain pretest resting 12-lead ECG in both supine and standing positions, along with a baseline heart rate and blood pressure. Obtain hyperventilation ECG.
2. Demonstrate to the patient the method for starting the exercise test.
3. Have the patient begin exercising, increasing speed or grade of exercise (depending on protocol) at 3-minute intervals.
4. During the last minute of each 3-minute stage, record a 12-lead ECG, heart rate, and blood pressure. Likewise, ask the patient to rate his or her exertion on a scale of 0 to 10 (0 being no exertion and 10 being maximal exertion).
5. Stop the test for any of the following reasons:
   a. Patient is unwilling or unable to continue (exhaustion, severe dyspnea, chest pain).
   b. Significant ST segment deviation (2 mm or more horizontal, downsloping, or delayed upsloping ST segment depression or ST segment elevation)

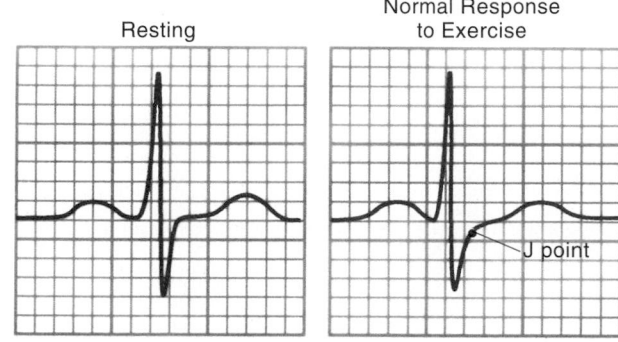

Resting · Normal Response to Exercise · J point

*These indications carry a higher risk, and consultation with a cardiologist should be considered.

Upsloping ST Depression

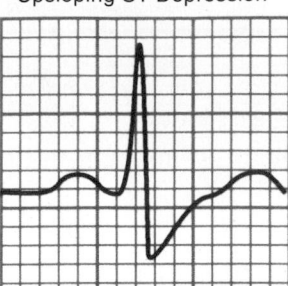

Horizontal ST Depression

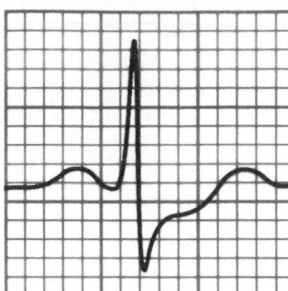

Downsloping ST Depression

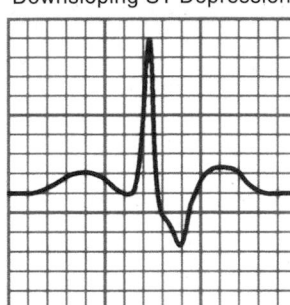

ST Elevation

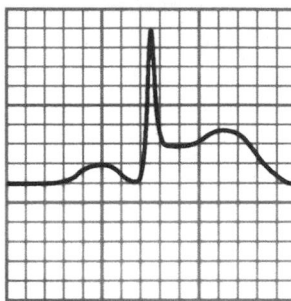

   c. Appearance of bundle-branch block or any exercise-induced heart block or dysrhythmia (including atrial fibrillation or flutter, ventricular tachycardia or fibrillation, second- or third-degree heart block)

   d. Ventricular premature contractions induced or exacerbated by exercise (>25 per cent of beats)

   e. Decreasing systolic blood pressure with increasing workload

   f. Development of acute chest pain

   g. Significant hypertension (>240/110 mm Hg)

6. Record ECG, heart rate, and blood pressure immediately upon termination of test while patient is standing or walking (slowing down).

7. Obtain ECG, heart rate, and blood pressure readings at 2, 5, and 10 minutes after termination of test.

8. Monitor patient until full recovery from any precipitated ischemia.

Follow-Up/Interpretation

1. Evaluate the entire test when reporting the results. Note the blood pressure and heart rate response, the amount of work performed in metabolic equivalents (METs), any dysrhythmias, any symptoms, and finally the presence or absence of ECG changes.

2. ECG criteria suggestive of a positive test include

   a. Horizontal or downsloping ST depression greater than 1 mm.

   b. J-point depression and upsloping ST depression that does not return to baseline within 80 msec

   c. Any J-point or ST elevation greater than 1 mm

3. Note that the normal ECG response to exercise is a depressed J point with the ST segment returning to baseline within 80 msec. The baseline is considered to be the PQ junction, and the J point is considered the junction of the QRS complex and the ST segment.

4. Other criteria suggestive of ischemia include hypotension, frequent exercise-induced ectopy, or exercise-induced angina.

Bibliography

Chaitman B: Exercise stress testing. In Braunwald E (ed): Heart Disease: A Textbook of Cardiovascular Medicine, 4th ed, pp 161–179. Philadelphia, WB Saunders Company, 1992.

Evans CH, Karunaratne HB: Exercise stress testing for the family physician: Part I. Performing the test. Am Fam Physician 1992;45:121–132.

Evans CH, Karunaratne HB: Exercise stress testing for the family physician: Part II. Interpretation of results. Am Fam Physician 1992;45:679–688.

Marriott HJL: Coronary insufficiency. In Practical Electrocardiography, 8th ed, pp 455–464. Baltimore, Williams & Wilkins, 1988.

62 Myocardial Infarction

Edgar Lichstein

Etiology

Myocardial infarction usually is the result of thrombus formation in an epicardial coronary artery, initiated by ulceration of a plaque, that releases thrombogenic factors and causes vasoconstriction. This may occur early in the morning, when catecholamine levels are high, or unexpectedly at any time. Triggers, such as physical or emotional stress, may cause the initial plaque rupture. Aortic dissection with dissection of a coronary artery, coronary spasm, and embolism from endocarditis are less common causes of myocardial infarction. Cocaine use may cause myocardial infarction by inducing coronary artery spasm.

Symptoms

1. Pain
   a. Persistent pressing or squeezing sensation in the substernal region, with radiation to the left shoulder, arm, neck, or jaw
   b. Radiation to the left arm and hand is usually noted on the inner aspect, and in the ulnar distribution.
   c. May only be noticed in the neck and the lower jaw, commonly with occlusions of the right coronary artery.
   d. Typically crescendo in onset, lasts more than 30 minutes, and is not relieved by rest or nitroglycerin
   e. Accompanying symptoms include diaphoresis, weakness, shortness of breath, nausea, and vomiting.
2. Approximately 25 per cent of patients have myocardial infarctions that are unrecognized clinically, and detected only by appearance of pathologic Q waves on the electrocardiogram. This is more common in patients with diabetes.
3. Myocardial infarction in the elderly may present differently. The patient may note sudden shortness of breath or worsening heart failure. Occasionally, the patient may present with acute confusion and disorientation, which is a sign of decreasing cardiac output.

Key Symptoms

- Pressing substernal chest pain
- Diaphoresis
- Weakness
- Dyspnea

Clinical Findings

1. General appearance
   a. Anxious, restless, diaphoretic, and pallid
   b. The patient may clutch the fist over the sternum (Levine's sign).
   c. Dyspnea, if the patient is in congestive heart failure *or* pink frothy sputum, if the patient has pulmonary edema
2. Vital signs
   a. Heart rate may vary from bradycardia, usually with inferior wall infarction, to tachycardia, which may be due to increased sympathetic tone caused by anxiety or possibly decreased cardiac output.
   b. Blood pressure is usually normal or low, especially if there is extensive heart damage. If the patient is anxious, and normal heart function has been maintained, blood pressure may be elevated.
   c. Irregular pulse, resulting from ventricular ectopic beats, or occasionally periods of atrial fibrillation
3. Cardiovascular examination
   a. The neck veins are usually flat at 30 degrees, unless the patient is in biventricular failure.
   b. Palpation of the precordium
      (1) Usually normal
      (2) The point of maximum impulse may be diffuse, with a sustained or lifting impulse, especially if there has been a large amount of myocardial damage.
   c. Auscultation
      (1) The first heart sound (S_1) may be soft.
      (2) The aortic component of the second heart sound (S_2) may be soft if the blood pressure is low. The pulmonic component of S_2 may be increased if there is pulmonary congestion.

(3) A fourth heart sound (S_4) is frequently heard.

(4) A third heart sound (S_3) may be heard if there is extensive myocardial damage and congestive heart failure.

(5) A blowing holosystolic murmur may be heard at the apex as a result of mitral regurgitation related to papillary muscle dysfunction. This murmur, with heart failure, may be the sign of papillary muscle rupture.

(6) A harsh systolic murmur at the upper left sternal border may indicate ventricular septal rupture.

(7) Pericardial friction rubs are rarely heard in the early stages of myocardial infarction but may be heard after 24 hours. The rub may have three components, but occasionally only a systolic or diastolic component is heard and is confused with a cardiac murmur.

Key Signs

- Diaphoresis
- Pallor
- Bradycardia, tachycardia, or irregular pulse
- Fourth heart sound (S_4)

Laboratory Tests

1. Electrocardiogram (ECG)

   a. The ECG usually shows ST segment elevation early after the onset of chest pain. As the infarction evolves, the ST segment returns toward normal, the T wave inverts, and pathologic Q waves develop in the areas of infarction.

   b. Myocardial infarctions are categorized as either Q wave or non–Q wave infarctions. The term *non–Q wave* replaces the older terms *subendocardial* and *nontransmural*.

   c. An ECG taken while the patient is actually having chest pain that shows absolutely no abnormalities is useful in ruling out myocardial ischemia.

2. Enzymes: Serial measurement of the MB isoenzyme of creatine kinase (CK-MB) is the current standard for measuring myocardial necrosis. The diagnosis of myocardial necrosis may usually be excluded by CK-MB samples that remain negative for 12 hours or more.

3. Lactate dehydrogenase (LDH): LDH usually peaks in 3 to 5 days and therefore is used diagnostically only when the patient presents several days after an episode of chest pain. The presence of necrosis is indicated by the ratio of LDH_1 (cardiac fraction) to LDH_2 being greater than 1.

4. Troponin T and troponin I: Troponins T and I are more specific and sensitive than CK-MB. They are released with myocardial necrosis at approximately the same time as CK-MB, and may be in the serum for up to 3 weeks. Troponin T is currently the best marker for definitive diagnosis in myocardial infarction. It appears in the serum within 6 to 9 hours of the onset of symptoms and remains abnormal for 4 to 10 days.

5. Echocardiography: The two-dimensional echocardiogram, which can establish the diagnosis by showing segmental wall motion abnormalities, is particularly useful if a baseline echocardiogram showing no abnormalities is present for comparison.

Key Tests

- Electrocardiogram
- LDH
- CK-MB (serial)
- Troponin T

Differential Diagnosis

1. Acute pericarditis: The pain is usually sharp, intensified with inspiration, and usually worse when the patient is supine. A pericardial friction rub may be heard. The ECG frequently shows ST segment elevation in all leads, with no reciprocal depression.

2. Aortic dissection: The pain is described as tearing and very severe and usually reaches peak intensity immediately. The pain may radiate straight through to the back. Physical examination may reveal aortic regurgitation or absence of a peripheral pulse.

3. Pulmonary embolism: The pain is sudden in onset and usually described as pleuritic. It is frequently accompanied by rapid heart beat and shortness of breath.

4. Pleurisy: The pain is sharp and increased with inspiration, and usually changes with position.

5. Gastrointestinal pain: usually in the epigastric and occasionally in the substernal region. It is frequently described as burning. It may be as-

sociated with belching and is not relieved by sublingual nitroglycerin.

6. Musculoskeletal pain: usually sharp but may be dull. The pain is located in various parts of the anterior chest, and its location and severity may vary. It is frequently intensified by motion and palpation and is not relieved by sublingual nitroglycerin.

Treatment

1. Oxygen should be administered as soon as possible.

2. Chewable aspirin, 160 to 325 mg, as soon as possible if no contraindications

3. Sublingual nitroglycerin if there is ST elevation, followed by intravenous nitroglycerin if evidence of myocardial ischemia persists

4. If pain persists, morphine, 2 to 5 mg, given intravenously

5. Coronary re-perfusion: This is usually done with thrombolytic therapy if there is no contraindication. Occasionally, emergent percutaneous transluminal coronary angioplasty, or even coronary bypass surgery, may be performed. One of three thrombolytic drugs is used: These are alteplase (tissue plasminogen activator), anistreplase (anisoylated plasminogen-streptokinase activator complex), and streptokinase. These are given as outlined in Table 62–1. Contraindications to thrombolytic therapy include

    a. Active bleeding

    b. Suspected aortic dissection

    c. Prolonged or traumatic cardiopulmonary resuscitation

    d. Recent head trauma or known intracranial neoplasm

    e. Diabetic retinopathy or other hemorrhagic ophthalmic conditions

    f. Pregnancy

    g. Previous allergic reaction to thrombolytic agents

    h. Significant systolic and diastolic hypertension

    i. Definite history of hemorrhagic cerebrovascular accident

6. Heparin: Heparin is used as an adjunct to thrombolytic therapy and is also useful to prevent left ventricular mural thrombus. Newer antithrombin agents, such as hirudin, are being evaluated.

7. β-Blockers: Decrease mortality after myocardial infarction. They are indicated for all patients unless such contraindications as significant obstructive pulmonary disease, significant heart failure, hypotension, high-degree atrioventricular (AV) block, and significant bradycardia are present. Metoprolol (Lopressor), 25 mg bid, is started as soon as possible and then increased to 50 mg bid if tolerated.

8. Angiotensin-converting enzyme (ACE) inhibitors: Reduce mortality after myocardial infarction by preventing ventricular remodeling and cardiac failure. This should be given to all patients who have some decrease in ejection fraction. This therapy should be initiated within the first 24 hours unless the patient is hypotensive.

9. Calcium channel blockers: The first-generation calcium channel blockers, diltiazem, verapamil, and nefedipine, are usually not used after acute myocardial infarction. They are specifically contraindicated if there is any evidence of pulmonary venous congestion or a decreased ejection fraction.

Diet

1. A light or liquid diet should be given for the first 24 hours.

2. Low-salt diet if the patient is hypertensive or if there is any evidence of heart failure

3. A low-fat, low-cholesterol diet is important to emphasize for the future.

Activity

The patient is usually kept in bed for 24 hours in a monitored unit, and then allowed to gradually ambulate in a monitored unit for at least another 48 hours. Patients are usually discharged at the end of 5 days if there are no complications.

TABLE 62–1. THROMBOLYTIC REGIMENS

"Front-Loaded" or "Accelerated" Infusion of Alteplase (Activase)
Aspirin, 325 mg, chewed and swallowed
Alteplase:
　15-mg IV bolus, *followed by*
　Infusion of 0.75 mg/kg (not to exceed 50 mg) over a 30-min period, *followed by*
　Infusion of 0.5 mg/kg (not to exceed 35 mg) over the next 1 hr
Heparin 5000 U IV, followed by infusion at 1000 U/hr

Streptokinase
Aspirin, 325 mg, chewed and swallowed
Streptokinase, 1.5 million U IV infusion over a 1-hour period
Heparin 5000 U IV, followed by IV infusion at 1000 U/hr, starting after SK infusion

Anistreplase (Eminase)
Aspirin, 325 mg, chewed and swallowed
Anistreplase, 30 U IV over 2–5 min

Key Treatment

- Oxygen
- Aspirin
- Thrombolytic agent
- β-Blocker
- ACE inhibitor
- Morphine

Predischarge Assessment

1. Ventricular function is usually assessed by echocardiogram.

2. Coronary angiogram is done in patients having recurrent chest pain or heart failure. Acute mitral regurgitation and ventricular septal defect are also indications for angiography.

3. Submaximal stress test on day 4 or 5, prior to discharge. Pharmacologic stress with either persantine or dobutamine and echocardiographic or thallium imaging may be done in patients who cannot exercise because of skeletal or pulmonary problems. A coronary angiogram is done if the patient has a positive submaximal exercise test.

4. A full-symptom limited stress test, usually with thallium, is done 6 to 8 weeks after myocardial infarction, prior to the patient returning to full normal activities.

Complications

1. Arrhythmia

   a. Ventricular premature beats are common. Prophylactic lidocaine is no longer recommended, and is only used with sustained or symptomatic ventricular arrhythmia or in patients with frequent asymptomatic, nonsustained ventricular tachycardia.

   b. Episodes of atrial fibrillation or paroxysmal atrial tachycardia are usually treated by controlling the heart rate with a β-blocker.

   c. Sinus bradycardia is frequently seen early after acute inferior wall myocardial infarction, and is usually due to increase in vagal tone. If the patient is symptomatic, atropine may be given. A temporary pacemaker is rarely needed.

   d. Second-degree or third-degree AV block at the AV node may be seen after inferior wall myocardial infarction. No therapy is required if the patient is asymptomatic. The block always reverts in a matter of hours to days. A temporary pacemaker is only indicated if the patient is symptomatic.

   e. Second-degree or complete AV block, associated with bundle-branch block and acute anterior myocardial infarction, is due to block below the AV node, is associated with a high mortality, and should always be treated with immediate insertion of a temporary and then a permanent pacemaker.

2. Congestive heart failure: Increased intravascular volume is treated with preload-reducing agents such as diuretics and nitrates. ACE inhibitors should be given to all patients with decreased ejection fractions. Digoxin has been found to be useful only in patients with persistent symptomatic heart failure.

3. Acute myocardial regurgitation resulting from papillary muscle rupture: This is a sudden and catastrophic event. The patient has a systolic murmur of mitral regurgitation and develops pulmonary edema. This is an indication for urgent angiography and urgent cardiac surgery.

4. Cardiogenic shock: Cardiogenic shock is associated with a high mortality. An intra-aortic balloon catheter is inserted as an interim measure until the patient can have coronary reperfusion, which is done with either urgent angioplasty or bypass surgery.

5. Ventricular septal rupture: Occurs in 2 per cent of patients, has a high mortality, and usually occurs 5 to 7 days after infarction. It presents with abrupt cardiac failure or shock and a holosystolic murmur along the left sternal border, frequently accompanied by a thrill.

6. Right ventricular infarction: Associated with inferior wall infarction and results in inadequate left ventricular preload and low cardiac output. It should be suspected in a patient with inferior wall infarction, hypotension, increased jugular venous pressure, and clear lung fields. If suspected, the patient should have volume replacement, and diuretics should be avoided.

7. Thromboembolism: Usually detected by echocardiogram in large anterior wall myocardial infarctions. These patients should be placed on heparin and then warfarin for three months.

8. Pericarditis: It is only seen in patients with transmural infarction, and occurs between the second and fifth day. The patient develops pleuritic pain, and usually has a pericardial friction rub.

Bibliography

GUSTO II Angioplasty Substudy Investigators: A clinical trial comparing primary coronary angioplasty with tissue plasminogen activator and recombinant hirudin with heparin for acute myocardial infarction. N Engl J Med 1997;336:1621–1928.

Hennekens CH, Albert CM, Godfried SL, et al: Adjunctive drug therapy of acute myocardial infarction: evidence from clinical trials. N Engl J Med 1996;335:1660–1667.

Pfeffer MA: ACE inhibitors in acute myocardial infarction—patient selection and timing. Circulation 1998;97:2192–2194.

Ryan TJ, Anderson JL, Antman EM, et al: ACC/AHA guidelines for the management of patients with acute myocardial infarction: executive summary: a report of the American College of Cardiology/American Heart Association Task Force on Practice Guidelines (Committee on Management of Acute Myocardial Infarction). Circulation 1996;94:2341–2350.

White HD, Van der Werf F: Thrombolysis for acute myocardial infarction. Circulation 1998;97:1632–1646.

63 Cardiac Arrest

Kenneth A. Ballew

Etiology

1. The incidence of sudden cardiac death in the United States is approximately 300,000 per year.
2. Coronary artery disease is the most common cause of sudden cardiac death. Cardiac arrest is the initial manifestation of coronary disease in 20 to 25 per cent of patients with coronary artery disease.
   a. Chronic ischemia with or without underlying myocardial scarring
   b. Acute myocardial infarction (MI): Only 20 per cent of out-of-hospital cardiac arrests are associated with acute MI.
   c. Congenital coronary artery anomalies
3. Left ventricular hypertrophy
4. Obstructive hypertrophic cardiomyopathy
5. Chronic congestive heart failure
6. Prolonged Q-T interval syndrome
   a. Congenital
   b. Drug-induced (antiarrhythmics, psychotropics)
7. Wolff-Parkinson-White syndrome
8. Toxic/metabolic/electrolyte disturbances
9. Proarrhythmic medications (encainide, flecainide)
10. Pulmonary embolism

Symptoms

Some patients may have prodromal symptoms such as chest pain, palpitations, dyspnea, fatigue, and lightheadedness up to several months prior to the onset of cardiac arrest.

Key Symptoms

- Chest pain
- Palpitations
- Dyspnea
- Fatigue
- Lightheadedness

Clinical Findings

1. Unresponsiveness
2. Pulselessness
3. Apnea or agonal respirations
4. Pallor or cyanosis

Key Signs

- Unresponsiveness
- No pulse
- Apnea or agonal respirations
- Pallor or cyanosis

Laboratory Tests

1. Electrocardiography: Findings include
   a. Ventricular fibrillation or ventricular tachycardia (VF/VT)
   b. Pulseless electrical activity (electromechanical dissociation)
   c. Asystole
2. Consider the following toxic, electrolyte, or metabolic disturbances as the cause of arrest:
   a. Hypoxia
   b. Hypokalemia or hyperkalemia
   c. Hypomagnesemia
   c. Acidosis
   d. Drug overdose
   e. Proarrhythmic medications

Key Test

Electrocardiography

Differential Diagnosis

1. Foreign body aspiration ("cafe coronary")
2. Vasovagal syncope
3. Seizure

Treatment

Basic Life Support

1. Assess responsiveness.
2. Activate emergency medical system.
3. Assess airway, breathing, and circulation. If airway obstruction is present, dislodge the object

using the Heimlich maneuver (see Ch. 57, Procedure: Cardiopulmonary Resuscitation).

4. If the patient is apneic and pulseless and does not have airway obstruction, initiate cardiopulmonary resuscitation (CPR).

5. Consider precordial thump if the arrest is witnessed, the patient is pulseless, and a defibrillator is not immediately available.

6. Begin advanced cardiac life support when the necessary equipment becomes available. Cardiac rhythm determines the treatment system that should be used.

Advanced Cardiac Life Support

1. VF and pulseless VT

   a. Immediate defibrillation prior to intubation or establishment of intravenous access is crucial to success. Defibrillation should begin using 200 joules and, if needed, be repeated in rapid succession at 300 and 360 joules.

   b. If the patient remains in VF/VT after three defibrillations, then intubate and place intravenous access.

   c. Epinephrine 1:10,000, 1.0 mg intravenous push; repeat defibrillation at 360 joules. Repeat epinephrine followed by defibrillation every 3 to 5 minutes for continued VF/VT. If the initial dose of epinephrine does not convert VF/VT, give:

   d. Lidocaine, 1.5 mg/kg intravenous push. After 30 to 60 seconds, defibrillate at 360 joules. Repeat lidocaine and defibrillation after 3 to 5 minutes if unsuccessful. Once spontaneous circulation is restored, start a continuous infusion of lidocaine at 2 to 4 mg/min. If the patient remains in VF/VT, give:

   e. Bretylium (Bretylol), 5 mg/kg intravenous push. After 1 to 2 minutes defibrillate at 360 joules. If the patient remains in VF/VT after 5 minutes, give bretylium, 10 mg/kg, and repeat defibrillation. Once spontaneous circulation is restored, bretylium can be given as a continuous infusion at 1 to 2 mg/min.

2. Pulseless electrical activity (electromechanical dissociation)

   a. Intubate and obtain intravenous access.

   b. Identify and treat underlying cause of arrest:

      (1) Hypovolemia

      (2) Hypoxia

      (3) Cardiac tamponade

      (4) Tension pneumothorax

      (5) Hypothermia

      (6) Pulmonary embolism

      (7) Drug overdose

      (8) Hyperkalemia

      (9) Acidosis

      (10) Massive myocardial infarction

   c. Epinephrine, 1.0 mg intravenous push

   d. For bradycardia give atropine, 1.0 mg intravenous push.

3. Asystole

   a. Intubate and obtain intravenous access.

   b. Confirm asystole in more than one lead.

   c. Consider possible causes:

      (1) Hypoxia

      (2) Hyperkalemia or hypokalemia

      (3) Acidosis

      (4) Drug overdose

      (5) Hypothermia

   d. Epinephrine, 1.0 mg intravenous push; repeat every 3 to 5 minutes.

   e. Atropine, 1.0 mg intravenous push; repeat after 5 minutes.

Key Treatment

- Basic life support
- Assess responsiveness
- Assess airway, breathing, circulation (A, B, C)

- Initiate CPR if patient is apneic and pulseless and does not have airway obstruction
- Consider precordial thump if arrest is witnessed and patient is pulseless

Follow-Up

1. Initial management of cardiac arrest survivors includes stabilization of cardiac rhythm and hemodynamics. Provide supportive treatment of organ damage caused by cardiac arrest.

2. Further management is designed to prevent recurrence and depends on the underlying cause of the arrest.

3. For cardiac arrest unassociated with acute MI or other reversible causes

   a. Evaluate coronary artery anatomy with cardiac catheterization.

   b. Assess cardiac function with echocardiography.

   c. Treat coronary artery disease:

      (1) Aspirin

      (2) β-Blocker and other antianginal therapy

      (3) Percutaneous transluminal coronary angioplasty

      (4) Coronary artery bypass graft surgery

d. Treat congestive heart failure with angiotensin-converting enzyme inhibitors.

e. Most survivors of cardiac arrest not due to myocardial infarction or reversible causes will require placement of an implantable cardioverter-defibrillator (ICD). The utility of electrophysiology study in this setting is unclear.

f. Some patients may benefit from amiodarone with or without an ICD.

4. For cardiac arrest due to reversible causes, generally, electrophysiologic testing and chronic antiarrhythmic therapy are not required. Treat underlying cause of arrest:

a. Acute myocardial infarction

b. Toxic/metabolic/electrolyte disturbances

c. Pulmonary embolism

Bibliography

For more information on the management of sudden cardiac death survivors, see

Domanski MJ, Zipes DP, Schron E: Treatment of sudden cardiac death: current understandings from randomized trials and future research directions. Circulation 1997;95:2694–2699.

Pinski SL, Trohman RG: Implantable cardioverter-defibrillators: implications for the nonelectrophysiologist. Ann Intern Med 1995;122:770–777.

For more information on in-hospital cardiac arrest, see

Ballew KA, Philbrick JT: Causes of variation in reported in-hospital cardiopulmonary resuscitation survival: a critical review. Resuscitation 1995;30:203–215.

For more information on CPR and advanced cardiac life support, see

Ballew KA: Cardiopulmonary resuscitation. BMJ 1997; 314:1462–1465.

Emergency Cardiac Care Committee and Subcommittees, American Heart Association: Essentials of ACLS. In Cummins R (ed): Textbook of Advanced Cardiac Life Support. Dallas, American Heart Association, 1997.

Indications
1. Termination of life-threatening ventricular arrhythmias
   a. Ventricular tachycardia
   b. Ventricular fibrillation
   c. Ventricular flutter
2. Termination of supraventricular tachyarrhythmias (with hemodynamic compromise)
3. Termination of refractory supraventricular tachycardia (such as atrial fibrillation)

Contraindication
The contraindication is termination of atrial fibrillation with severe digitalis toxicity. The toxicity should be alleviated before cardioversion-defibrillation.

Preparation

1. The defibrillator should be inspected regularly.
2. The defibrillator should be plugged into a standard electrical outlet that is appropriately grounded.
3. The electrocardiogram (ECG) should be monitored to determine the arrhythmia and to rule out artifact. Presence or absence of a palpable pulse and blood pressure should be confirmed.
4. For elective cardioversions, the electrolytes and hematologic laboratory values should be checked and should preferably be within normal limits.
5. Patients with an organized arrhythmia (such as ventricular tachycardia or ventricular flutter) or a more benign arrhythmia such as supraventricular tachycardia (atrial fibrillation) should receive defibrillation synchronized to the R wave of the QRS complex, which is known as cardioversion. These more organized arrhythmias require lower energies to convert as compared with the more disorganized arrhythmias such as ventricular fibrillation.
6. Defibrillation conducting gel should be available for use with paddles; skin patches suitable for defibrillation can be used as an alternative.

Equipment
1. Standard external defibrillator
2. Skin patches or defibrillator paddles
3. Conducting gel
4. ECG leads
5. Advanced cardiac life support equipment

Anesthesia
1. During hemodynamically significant arrhythmia (cardiac arrest), anesthesia is not necessary because the patient is unconscious.
2. During more stable arrhythmias, patients should be appropriately sedated, with close monitoring of their oxygen saturation, respiratory rate, heart rate, and blood pressure. Anesthesia should be administered according to the recommendations of an anesthesiologist.

Precautions
1. Conducting gel and/or skin patches should be placed in discrete areas over the chest (not in continuity with one another). This is to prevent sparking between the cathode and anode.
2. The operator should avoid contact with the patient as well as touching a metal surface during defibrillation. The operator may shout "All clear" before defibrillation.
3. The defibrillator must be inspected regularly to make sure that it will function appropriately. The hospital's biomedical engineering service should be able to provide this function as a standard of care.

WARNING

To perform defibrillation or cardioversion requires the delivery of high direct-current energy to the patient. It is essential that the operator or medical personnel not be in physical contact (other than through defibrillation paddles) with the patient or the electrical equipment during delivery of high-voltage energy. The person performing defibrillation should make sure the paddles are well separated.

Technique
1. The technique of external transthoracic cardioversion-defibrillation requires placement of either skin patches or defibrillation paddles in an anterior or posterior location. We routinely place the posterior skin patch between the two scapulae and the anterior patch over the left ventricular apex. This is to encompass

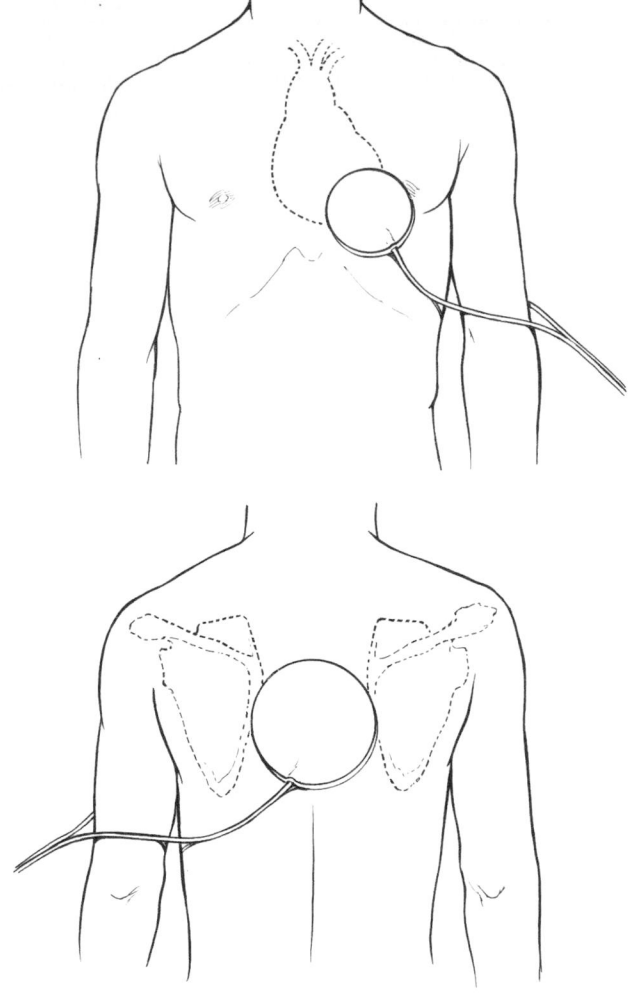

For cardioversion of atrial arrhythmias (including atrial fibrillation and atrial flutter), a more midline anterior and posterior patch placement is preferable. If one configuration fails multiple times, an alternative configuration can be utilized.

2. The defibrillator is turned on and the ECG is monitored.

3. The arrhythmia is verified, perhaps by a true 12-lead ECG as well as hemodynamic data (i.e., pulse and blood pressure).

4. Before defibrillation or cardioversion, the defibrillator ECG strip should be activated to record data, and the defibrillator should be charged to the appropriate energies.

5. Hemodynamically significant ventricular tachyarrhythmias require shocks of the order of 200, 300, and 360 joules as per advanced cardiac life support protocols. Termination of atrial fibrillation requires lower energy levels of the order of 100 joules initially. Atrial flutter may be terminated by as low as 25 joules. If unsuccessful, higher energies can be utilized.

6. The defibrillator capacitors are charged before delivery of direct-current energy. This can be performed either via the paddles or via the defibrillator box itself. Once fully charged, the operator makes sure that all personnel move away from the patient and that all metal is removed from the area around the patient's bed. Defibrillation is then performed by pressing the button to discharge the capacitor.

7. After defibrillation, the ECG is then checked to determine whether there is termination of the arrhythmia as well as return of the vital signs (i.e., heart rate and blood pressure) toward normal.

8. If unsuccessful, further delivery of direct energy can be performed according to advanced cardiac life support protocols.

9. If it is an elective and not an emergency case and there is hemodynamic stability, anesthesia should be used. This helps minimize the discomfort to the patient of the direct-current shocks.

10. If the arrhythmia is not terminated by maximal energies (for treatment of refractory ventricular tachyarrhythmias), emergency rescue techniques should be considered. These techniques include applying pressure over the patches or paddles (active compression defibrillation), sequential defibrillation using two different defibrillators, emergency intracardiac defibrillation, and transesophageal defibrillation. Each of these methods facilitate the de-

as much of the myocardium as possible in order to perform a successful defibrillation. Alternatively, skin paddles can be placed over the anterior chest as well as lateral precordium.

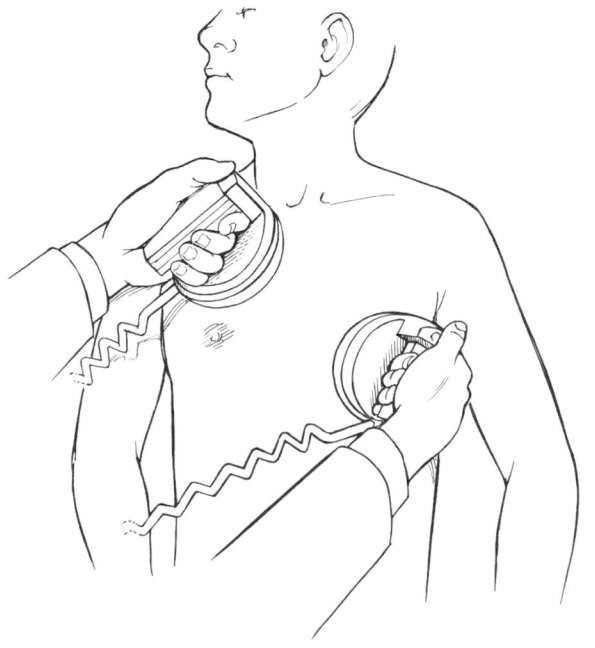

livery of high direct-current energy in proximity to the myocardium using a standard defibrillator.

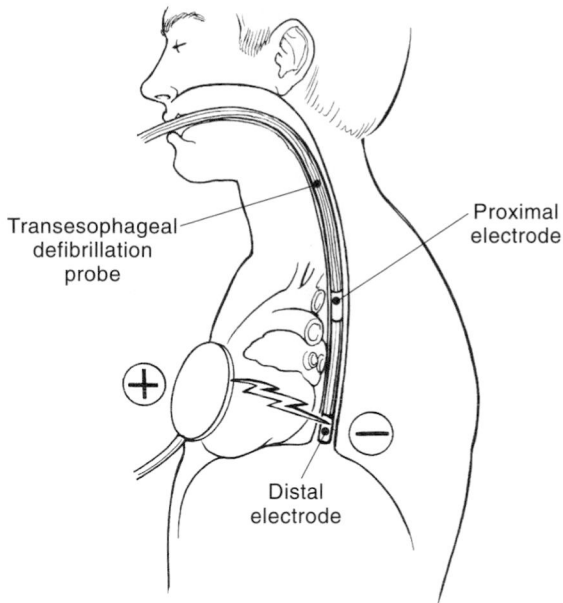

Transesophageal defibrillation probe

Proximal electrode

Distal electrode

Follow-Up

1. For all patients in the setting of significant ventricular tachyarrhythmias, critical care monitoring in an appropriate hospital facility is required. For termination of more benign arrhythmias, such as atrial fibrillation and atrial flutter, monitoring for at least a 3-hour period by trained advanced cardiac life support nursing personnel is also prudent.

2. An appropriate 12-lead ECG should be obtained, as well as follow-up by the patient's physician.

Bibliography

Cohen TJ, Ibrahim B, Denier D, et al: Active compression cardioversion for refractory atrial fibrillation. Am J Cardiol 1997;80:354–355.

Cohen TJ, Scheinman MM, Pullen BT, et al: Emergency intracardiac defibrillation for refractory ventricular fibrillation during routine electrophysiology study. J Am Coll Cardiol 1991;18:1280–1284.

Defibrillation. In Cummins R (ed): Advanced Cardiac Life Support, pp 4-1 to 4-22. Dallas, American Heart Association, 1994.

Eisenberg MS, Copass MD, Hallstrom AP, et al: Treatment of out-of-hospital cardiac arrests with rapid defibrillation by emergency medical technicians. N Engl J Med 1980;302:1379–1383.

Weaver WD, Copass MK, Bufi D, et al: Improved neurologic recovery and survival after early defibrillation. Circulation 1984;69:943–948.

64 Acute Pulmonary Edema (Heart Failure)

David E. Gutstein

Etiology
1. Definition: a sudden cardiac event with overwhelming effects on left ventricular function. This results in an acute decline in cardiac output, insufficient perfusion, and acute pulmonary congestion.
2. Precipitating factors
   a. May arise from acute myocardial infarction, ischemia, acute mitral regurgitation or ventricular septal defect, aortic dissection causing acute aortic insufficiency, cardiac rupture, arrhythmia, or pulmonary embolus.
   b. Ischemia and infarction decrease cardiac output and compliance, resulting in increased left ventricular filling pressures and pulmonary edema, without changing total blood volume.

Symptoms
1. May develop over the course of several minutes or less, reflecting a sudden decompensation of pump function.
2. The most profound symptom of acute heart failure is acute dyspnea, or sudden onset of respiratory distress.
3. May be accompanied by chest pain, palpitations, diaphoresis, cough productive of frothy sputum, and a feeling of impending doom.

Key Symptoms

- Sudden, extreme dyspnea
- Pink, frothy sputum
- Diaphoresis

Clinical Findings
1. Patients may appear grossly cyanotic, with diaphoretic, cold, and clammy skin.
2. Acute onset of hypertension and tachycardia
3. Jugular venous distention
4. New heart sounds, such as third heart sound (S_3) or a new murmur
5. Pulmonary rales and rhonchi. Presence of pulmonary wheezes is referred to as "cardiac asthma."

6. May rapidly progress to signs of respiratory failure and shock

Key Signs

- Tachycardia
- Cyanosis
- Jugular venous distention
- Third heart sound (S_3)
- Pulmonary rales

Diagnostic Tests
1. Hematocrit, blood urea nitrogen, and creatinine: to rule out concomitant anemia and renal failure
2. Arterial blood gas and oxygen saturation: to quantitate extent of respiratory failure, assess oxygenation
3. Electrocardiogram: to evaluate for arrhythmia, ischemia, or infarction
4. Chest radiograph: Signs of heart failure include vascular redistribution, interstitial pulmonary edema, and alveolar edema. Film may also reveal other sources of dyspnea (e.g., pneumonia, pneumothorax). Increased cardiothoracic ratio suggests acute exacerbation of chronic congestive heart failure (CHF).
5. Echocardiogram: may reveal mitral regurgitation or ventricular septal defect in the patient with a new systolic murmur; shows focal wall motion abnormalities, pericardial effusion, and overall left ventricular function.
6. Right-heart (Swan-Ganz) catheterization: to assess pulmonary artery pressures and cardiac output, rule out left-to-right shunt, quantitate response to therapy
7. Cardiac catheterization: to evaluate coronary arteries

Key Tests

- Arterial blood gas
- Chest film
- Electrocardiography

Differential Diagnosis

Conditions that may imitate aspects of acute heart failure include reactive airway diseases (e.g., asthma, chronic obstructive pulmonary disease), pneumonia, pneumothorax, re-expansion pulmonary edema, adult respiratory distress syndrome, high-altitude pulmonary edema, neurogenic pulmonary edema, pulmonary embolus, eclampsia, and heroin overdose.

Treatment

Medication

Treatment of "flash pulmonary edema" revolves around improving hemodynamics by reversing ischemia, reducing preload and afterload, and improving cardiac contractility.

1. Supplemental oxygen: may require mechanical ventilation for respiratory failure

2. Nitrates: intravenous nitroglycerin drip starting at 20 μg/min. Hold for hypotension.

3. Morphine: reduces preload. Start with 2 mg intravenously (IV); may repeat once or twice every few minutes. Hold for hypotension.

4. Diuretics: limited role in true ischemic flash pulmonary edema, but useful in acute-on-chronic exacerbations of heart failure. Furosemide (Lasix) may be used, starting at 20 mg IV. Hemodialysis or ultrafiltration may be needed to treat heart failure complicated by anuria.

5. Afterload reduction: in patients with systolic blood pressure greater than 100 mm Hg, start angiotensin-converting enzyme inhibitor (e.g., IV enalapril, initially at 1.25 mg). Alternatively, IV nitroprusside may be used, especially for hypertension that is difficult to control (start at 0.3 μg/kg/minute and titrate up as needed).

6. Digoxin (Lanoxin): useful for slowing rapid atrial fibrillation in the setting of heart failure or shock

7. β-Blockers and calcium channel blockers: contraindicated in decompensated CHF, but useful for rate control in rapid atrial fibrillation in patients with normal ventricular function

8. Inotropes: used in refractory heart failure with poor cardiac output but systolic blood pressure greater than 100 mm Hg.
   a. Dobutamine (Dobutrex): Increases contractility, decreases systemic vascular resistance. Start at 2 to 6 μg/kg/minute.
   b. Phosphodiesterase inhibitors (e.g., amrinone [Inocor], milrinone [Primacor]): Effects similar to those of dobutamine. For milrinone, load 50 μg/kg, then maintain on 0.375 to 0.75 μg/kg/minute.

9. Pressors: for acute heart failure with severe hypotension refractory to above measures
   a. Dopamine: "Alpha-range" (10 to 20 μg/kg/minute) stimulates systemic vasoconstriction. "Beta-range" (5 to 10 μg/kg/minute) has inotropic and chronotropic effects. "Renal dose" dopamine (2 to 3 μg/kg/minute) may improve diuresis in oliguric patients unresponsive to diuretics by dilating renal vascular beds.
   b. Norepinephrine: acts as a vasoconstrictor, positive inotrope, and chronotrope. Start at 1 to 4 μg/minute. Oten used in combination with dopamine when hypotension does not respond to dopamine alone.

10. Intra-aortic balloon pump and left ventricular assist device: indicated for cardiogenic shock refractory to inotropes. Useful for stabilizing patient before definitive procedure (e.g., revascularization or transplant).

11. Revascularization: Thrombolysis is indicated for stabilizing heart failure in the setting of acute myocardial infarction. Many practitioners prefer primary angioplasty for the treatment of acute myocardial infarction complicated by heart failure or cardiogenic shock, when available.

Diet

Should include salt restriction initially. Maintenance diet depends on cause of initial event and presence of underlying risk factors.

Activity

Bed rest should be observed during treatment of acute event. Patients are often more comfortable in the sitting position during the event.

Key Treatment
• Supplemental oxygen   • Morphine
• Nitrates

Follow-Up

1. Prevention of recurrent events: Must emphasize medical compliance, avoidance of smoking, and attention to other correctable cardiac risk factors. A full ischemic work-up, including cardiac catheterization, followed by revascularization with angioplasty or bypass surgery, may be necessary. The use of an implantable cardioverter-defibrillator or a pacemaker may be needed to

prevent recurrence of events precipitated by tachy- or bradyarrhythmias.

2. Monitoring: close observation after stabilization. If the nature of the underlying heart disease is unknown, careful work-up may reveal a correctable lesion.

3. Complications: Watch for signs of recurrent acute heart failure, development of chronic heart failure, dehydration secondary to diuresis, electrolyte abnormalities, and drug toxicity.

4. Prognosis: Acute heart failure continues to carry a high mortality, especially in the elderly.

Bibliography

Braunwald E, Colucci WS, Grossman W: Clinical aspects of heart failure: high output heart failure; pulmonary edema. In Braunwald E (ed): Heart Disease: A Textbook of Cardiovascular Medicine, 5th ed, pp 445–470. Philadelphia, WB Saunders Company, 1997.

Levin TN: Acute congestive heart failure: the need for aggressive therapy. Postgrad Med 1997;101:97–111.

McGhie AI, Goldstein RA: Pathogenesis and management of acute heart failure and cardiogenic shock: role of inotropic therapy. Chest 1992;102(Suppl 2):626S–632S.

65 Chronic Heart Failure

David E. Gutstein

Etiology

1. Definition: Chronic heart failure on the basis of severe systolic dysfunction is marked by the failure of the heart to pump blood sufficiently to meet the metabolic needs of the tissues. Injury to the heart may cause loss of functioning myocardium. Compensatory mechanisms, including cardiac hypertrophy and neurohumoral processes, exert adverse long-term effects. Alternatively, abnormalities in ventricular relaxation (i.e., diastolic dysfunction) or valvular function may lead to pulmonary or systemic congestion.

2. Epidemiology: Four to 5 million Americans have chronic heart failure. Incidence increases with age and is higher in men than in women. Almost 1 million heart failure hospitalizations are recorded yearly in the United States. The most common cause of heart failure in the United States is coronary artery disease.

3. Precipitating factors
   a. Injuries to the myocardium that may lead to chronic heart failure include myocardial infarction, toxins (e.g., alcohol, cytotoxic drugs), viral myocarditis, hypertensive or valvular heart disease, hypertrophy, congenital lesions, amyloidosis, hemochromatosis, pregnancy-related disorders, lipid storage disorders, dietary deficiencies (e.g., selenium and thiamine deficiencies), and idiopathic dilated cardiomyopathy.
   b. Factors that may suddenly exacerbate chronic heart failure include medical or dietary noncompliance, uncontrolled hypertension, myocardial infarction, ischemia, valvular disorders, infection, arrhythmia, renal failure, anemia, pulmonary embolus, and thyrotoxicosis.

Symptoms

1. Chronic heart failure develops over a protracted period of time, with symptoms reflecting long-standing whole-body fluid overload.
2. Dyspnea on exertion is the most common initial symptom.
3. Orthopnea is the most sensitive clinical indicator of high filling pressures.
4. Other symptoms include fatigue, paroxysmal nocturnal dyspnea, nocturia, confusion, ankle edema, nausea, and right upper quadrant abdominal pain.

Key Symptoms

- Dyspnea on exertion
- Orthopnea
- Fatigue
- Edema
- Paroxysmal nocturnal dyspnea

Clinical Findings

1. Tachycardia and hypotension are common chronically; pulse pressure decreases as cardiac index declines.
2. Jugular venous distention with hepatojugular reflux
3. Signs of cardiomegaly; third heart sound (S_3); regurgitant systolic murmurs; laterally displaced apical impulse
4. Pulmonary rales with dullness at the bases
5. Hepatomegaly and ascites
6. Edema, cyanosis, and cachexia

Key Signs

- Jugular venous distention
- Third heart sound (S_3)
- Pulmonary rales
- Edema

Diagnostic Tests

1. Blood tests: to rule out anemia, renal failure, hepatic and thyroid abnormalities
2. Electrocardiogram: abnormal in most advanced chronic heart failure patients, showing conduction abnormalities, infarct patterns, atrial arrhythmias, or ventricular ectopy
3. Chest film: Signs of chronic heart failure include cardiomegaly, vascular redistribution, pleural effusions, and occasionally frank pulmonary edema.
4. Pulmonary function testing: may reveal pulmonary source of dyspnea.

5. Exercise testing: evaluates for the presence of underlying ischemia; analysis of expired gas provides an accurate indication of overall cardiac function and carries prognostic value.

6. Echocardiography, radionuclide angiography: Both estimate ejection fraction and evaluate wall motion; echocardiography also evaluates chamber sizes and valves and estimates pulmonary pressures.

7. Electrophysiologic studies: used to evaluate serious ventricular arrhythmias

8. Cardiac catheterization (with hemodynamics, coronary angiography, and occasionally endomyocardial biopsy): used to evaluate suspected coronary artery disease, refractory advanced chronic heart failure, unstable patients, nonischemic dilated cardiomyopathy, and heart transplant candidates

 Key Tests

- Electrocardiogram
- Chest film
- Echocardiogram

Treatment

Medication

The following discussion refers to treatment of heart failure resulting predominantly from systolic dysfunction.

1. Diuretics: Improve symptoms and hemodynamics. Loop diuretics include furosemide (Lasix), which is commonly started at 20 mg/day orally. Furosemide may be combined with another class of diuretic in refractory cases (e.g., metolazone [Zaroxolyn], 2.5 to 5 mg orally 30 minutes before furosemide).

2. Digoxin (Lanoxin): Improves symptoms; no significant effect on mortality. Maintenance doses of digoxin range from 0.125 to 0.25 mg/day orally in most patients (reduce dose in renal failure).

3. Angiotensin-converting enzyme (ACE) inhibitors: Long-term treatment improves symptoms, hemodynamics, and survival. Example: enalapril (Vasotec), 2.5 to 20 mg orally twice daily. The role of angiotensin II receptor blockers in heart failure is currently under study.

4. Isosorbide dinitrate (Isordil) and hydralazine (Apresoline): Combination vasodilator treatment confers greater survival benefit than placebo but less than enalapril.

   a. Isosorbide: 10 to 40 mg orally three to four times daily.

   b. Hydralazine: 10 to 60 mg orally four times daily.

5. β-Blockers: Prolong survival and improve symptoms in chronic heart failure despite potentially worsening ventricular function initially. Therapy with carvedilol is started at a low dose (3.125 mg orally twice daily) and increased gradually under close supervision.

6. Anticoagulation: recommended in patients at high risk for thromboembolism, such as those with atrial fibrillation or a prior history of thromboembolism

7. Antiarrhythmic agents: Most not recommended in patients with abnormal left ventricular function, because of risk of proarrhythmia. Amiodarone has lowest proarrhythmic risk and appears safe for use in heart failure patients.

8. Calcium channel blockers: Certain calcium blockers (i.e., amlodipine and felodipine) do not appear to worsen survival in patients with systolic dysfunction. However, other calcium blockers have proven harmful in patients with heart failure.

9. Short-term intravenous therapy for refractory heart failure

   a. Nitroprusside (Nipride): combined with intravenous diuretics, hemodynamic monitoring for 24 to 48 hours; oral vasodilator is added as nitroprusside is tapered. Start at 10 μg/minute, increase by 5 to 10 μg/minute every 5 minutes to a maximum of 300 μg/minute. Adverse effects include hypotension and thiocyanate toxicity (especially in renal failure).

   b. "Dobutamine holiday": short-term (48 to 72 hours) infusion of dobutamine (Dobutrex) or phosphodiesterase inhibitor (e.g., amrinone [Inocor], milrinone [Primacor]) to improve cardiac function while oral medications are adjusted. Also used to maintain patients with end-stage heart failure awaiting cardiac transplantation.

10. Left ventricular assist device: increasingly used as a temporizing measure for patients awaiting cardiac transplantation who cannot be sustained with medical therapy alone.

11. Revascularization: Coronary artery bypass grafting provides survival benefit when compared with medical therapy in selected patients

with poor systolic function and underlying multivessel coronary artery disease.

12. Implantable cardioverter-defibrillator: effective in the treatment of recurrent life-threatening ventricular arrhythmias

13. Cardiac transplantation: This may be a consideration in advanced heart failure that is not amenable to other surgical or medical therapy. Improves 5-year survival to nearly 80 per cent. Selection criteria tend to be fairly strict.

14. Other surgical approaches include the "Batista operation," which reduces left ventricular volume by removal of a segment of left ventricle wall and is currently under investigation.

15. Diastolic dysfunction: Treatment of heart failure resulting from diastolic dysfunction, in patients with normal systolic function, differs substantially from the treatment for systolic dysfunction. Goals of treating isolated diastolic dysfunction include improving left ventricular relaxation and relieving pulmonary congestion. As a result, several of the interventions discussed above (e.g., diuretics, digoxin, inotropes) may be inappropriate for treatment of the patient with diastolic dysfunction.

Diet

Weight loss, salt restriction, and abstention from alcohol are the rule. Limit fluid intake to less than 2 L/day.

Activity

Bed rest is required only during treatment of decompensated chronic heart failure.

Patient Education

1. Moderate regular exercise, being careful not to provoke dyspnea. Avoid isometric exercise.

2. Avoid smoking.

3. Regular influenza and pneumococcal vaccines

4. Explaining rationale of medical therapy may help to improve patient compliance.

Key Treatment

- Diuretics
- Digoxin
- ACE inhibitors
- β-Blockers

Follow-Up

1. Prevention: ACE inhibitors have been shown to reduce the risk of developing heart failure in patients with asymptomatic left ventricular dysfunction and after myocardial infarction. Digoxin reduces the need for recurrent hospitalizations. β-Blockers slow progression of heart failure. Secondary prevention in coronary artery disease patients with antiplatelet agents and aggressive lipid management helps improve survival even in patients with abnormal ventricular function.

2. Monitoring: Close follow-up is required if the patient is to be maintained as an outpatient.

3. Complications: These include atrial and ventricular arrhythmias, thromboembolic events, pulmonary infections, acute decompensation, electrolyte abnormalities, dehydration from overzealous diuresis, and drug toxicity.

4. Prognosis: Mortality rate remains high. Predictors of poor outcome include an ejection fraction less than 20 per cent, ischemic etiology, ventricular arrhythmias, serum sodium less than 130 mEq/L, poor functional class, low cardiac index, and high filling pressures.

Bibliography

Baker DW, Konstam MA, Bottorf M, et al: Management of heart failure: pharmacologic treatment. JAMA 1994;272:1361–1366.

Cohn JN: The management of chronic heart failure. N Engl J Med 1996;335:490–498.

Gheorghiade M, Bonow RO: Chronic heart failure in the United States: a manifestation of coronary artery disease. Circulation 1998;97:282–289.

LeJemtel TH, Sonnenblick EH, Frishman WH: Diagnosis and management of heart failure. In Alexander RW, Schlant RC, Fuster V (eds): Hurst's The Heart, Arteries and Veins, 9th ed, pp 745–782. New York, McGraw-Hill, 1998.

Schlant RC, Sonnenblick EH, Katz AM: Pathophysiology of heart failure. In Alexander RW, Schlant RC, Fuster V (eds): Hurst's The Heart, Arteries and Veins, 9th ed, pp 687–726. New York, McGraw-Hill, 1998.

Indications

1. Hypotension: rapid administration of large volume of fluids/blood
2. Code blue: emergency central venous access for drugs/fluids
3. Insertion of Swan-Ganz catheter
4. Central venous pressure measurement
5. Total parenteral nutrition
6. Hemodialysis
7. Inotropic agents
8. Poor peripheral access

Contraindications

1. Thrombocytopenia
2. Coagulopathy or patient on anticoagulants
3. Uncooperative or combative patient

Preparation

1. Obtain informed consent from the patient after explaining the risks and possible complications. In the case of a minor or an incompetent patient, get the consent from a parent or guardian or person having power of attorney.
2. Position: For the internal jugular or subclavian insertion, the patient should be in Trendelenburg's position with the feet elevated at 15 degrees and the head turned contralaterally at about 45 degrees. For a femoral line, patient should be supine with the leg in external rotation.
3. Part preparation: Insertion site should be cleaned with povidone-iodine in circular manner.

Equipment

Currently available disposable central line kits are well equipped with the necessary items. The key items include

1. Sterile gloves, drapes
2. Sterile prep solution
3. Syringes (5, 10 ml)
4. Needles (21, 25 gauge)
5. Lidocaine, 1%
6. 18-gauge insertion needle (new kits have a 10-ml syringe with an introducing needle)
7. Flexible-tip guidewire; J wire
8. Central venous catheter (mostly triple lumen)
9. Dilator
10. Scalpel with No. 11 blade
11. 2-0 Silk suture, hemostat
12. Saline flushes
13. Antibiotic ointment
14. Sterile dressings

Anesthesia

Usually performed under local anesthesia (1% lidocaine without epinephrine)

Precautions/Complications

1. Arterial puncture
2. Bleeding, hematoma
3. Pneumothorax
4. Dysrhythmias
5. Air embolism
6. Malpositioning
7. Infection
8. Thrombosis
9. Cardiac tamponade from erosion through cardiac chambers
10. Fragmentation and embolism of a guidewire

Technique

Insertion of a catheter over a guidewire into a central vein by Seldinger technique

1. Identification of landmarks
   a. Internal jugular: Identify the triangle formed by medial end of clavicle and two heads (sternal and clavicular) of sternocleidomastoid muscle. Internal jugular vein lies lateral to the carotid artery.
   b. Subclavian line: Locate the junction between medial third and middle third of the clavicle.
   c. Femoral line: Femoral vein runs parallel and medial to the femoral artery, below the inguinal ligament at a midpoint between anterior superior iliac spine and the symphysis pubis.
2. Flush all the ports of the catheter to check for its patency.
3. Maintain aseptic conditions and follow Occupational Safety and Health Administration guidelines for blood and body fluid precautions.
4. Anesthetize the insertion site with 1% lido-

caine using 25-gauge needle. To anesthetize deeper structures, use 21-gauge needle. This needle can also be used to locate the vein.

5. Locate the vein

   a. Internal jugular: Palpate the carotid artery. Insert needle with a syringe at the apex of the triangle at an angle of 45 degrees to the skin and advance it slowly toward the ipsilateral nipple. Maintain gentle aspiration while advancing the needle.

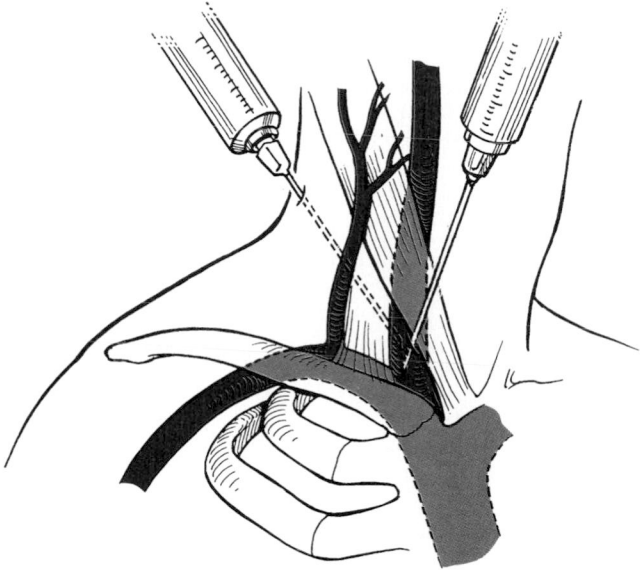

Alternatively, in a posterior approach the needle is inserted in the posterior border of sternocleidomastoid, about 5 cm above the clavicle and directed anteriorly and inferiorly to reach the vein.

   b. Subclavian line: Insert the needle 1 cm below the junction of the middle and medial thirds of the clavicle, directing it toward the suprasternal notch. Advance the needle just under the clavicle. Try to keep the needle horizontal to avoid a pneumothorax.

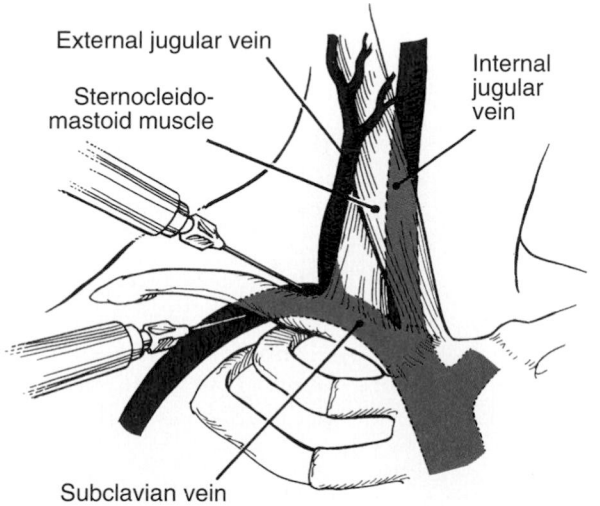

External jugular vein

Sternocleido-mastoid muscle

Internal jugular vein

Subclavian vein

The subclavian vein can also be approached by a supraclavicular technique.

   c. Femoral line: Insert the needle at an angle of 45 degrees to the skin, medial to the femoral artery and 2 to 3 cm below the inguinal ligament. Once the vein is entered, bring the needle parallel to the skin.

6. When a good flow of blood is obtained in the syringe (Fig. A), detach it from the insertion needle and pass the guidewire through the needle (Fig. B). The tip of the J wire is aimed toward the heart. It should pass without significant resistance. Then remove the needle while holding the wire carefully (Fig. C).

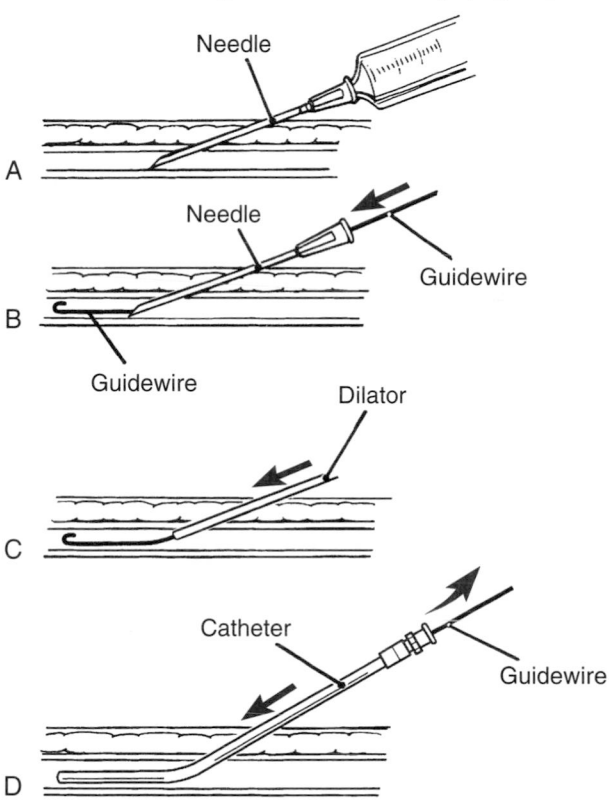

Needle

Needle

Guidewire

Guidewire

Dilator

Catheter

Guidewire

7. Enlarge the puncture site with a scalpel.

8. Pass the dilator over the guidewire for about 3 to 4 cm to dilate the subcutaneous tissue. Then remove the dilator.

9. Now, advance the central venous catheter over the guidewire into the vein for a length of 15 cm and remove the wire (Fig. D).

10. Aspirate blood from all the ports to confirm venous placement and flush with saline.

11. Suture the catheter to the skin.

12. Apply antibiotic ointment at the puncture site and dress the skin with sterile dressing.

13. Finally, a chest radiograph should be obtained to confirm the placement of the catheter into the superior vena cava and to rule out pneumothorax.

WARNINGS

- If carotid artery is punctured, withdraw the needle immediately and compress the site for at least 10 minutes.

- Never lose control of the guidewire.

- In case of unsuccessful attempt on one side, do not try on the opposite side without confirming the absence of pneumothorax by checking a chest radiograph.

Bibliography

Agee KR, Balk RA: Central venous catheterization in the critically ill patient. Crit Care Clin 1992;8:677–686.

Chen H, Foster CL: Central venous access. In Chen H, Sola JE, Lillemore KL (eds): Manual of Common Bedside Surgical Procedures, pp 30–48. Baltimore, Williams & Wilkins, 1996.

Donnelly JF, Passmore JM: Central venous catheter insertion. In Pfenninger JL, Fowler CG (eds): Procedures for Primary Care Physicians, pp 300–318. St. Louis, Mosby, 1994.

Johnson JC: Complications of vascular access devices. Emerg Med Clin North Am 1994;12:691–705.

McGee WT, Ackerman BL, Rouben LR, et al: Accurate placement of central venous catheters: a prospective randomized multicenter trial. Crit Care Med 1993;21: 1118–1123.

Indications

In general, Swan-Ganz catheter (or pulmonary artery flotation catheter) monitoring of patients should only be done when the stability of a patient's condition or intravascular volume status cannot be determined adequately by clinical means or when clinical evidence suggests their condition is deteriorating. Indications for hemodynamic monitoring have expanded to include a number of conditions:

1. Acute myocardial infarction complicated by severe heart failure, mechanical lesions (i.e., mitral regurgitation, ventricular septal rupture, tamponade), recurrent ischemia
2. Multiorgan failure resulting from a variety of conditions: trauma, sepsis, massive embolism, extensive burns, renal failure, respiratory failure
3. Heart failure
   a. to assess ventricular function at rest with stress or with therapeutic intervention
   b. to distinguish specific causes of heart failure
4. Before, during, and after surgery in high-risk cardiac patients
5. As an aid to diagnosing constrictive pericarditis and restrictive cardiomyopathy
6. As a research tool for objective clinical monitoring
7. To monitor therapeutic interventions
8. Unclear volume status

Contraindications

1. No absolute contraindications exist to hemodynamic monitoring with Swan-Ganz catheters; however, access problems and the potential to do harm require that this technique be performed only after careful review of the potential benefit to the patient. Heparin-bound catheters should not be used in patients with heparin sensitivity or a history of heparin-induced thrombocytopenia.
2. Relative contraindications include
   a. Coagulopathy
   b. Susceptibility to arrhythmia
   c. Recent permanent pacemaker implantation
   d. Pulmonic stenosis
   e. Left bundle-branch block: Catheter placement may be done if a temporary transvenous pacer is placed or a transcutaneous pacer is at the patient's bedside during the time of catheter flotation.

> **WARNING**
>
> **Potential complications include, but are not limited to, pneumothorax, infection, hemorrhage, arterial cannulation, air embolism, knotting of catheter tubing intravascularly, and arrhythmias.**

Preparation

Before inserting the Swan-Ganz catheter, it is important to choose the appropriate equipment needed and prepare the patient for insertion.

1. Access to the venous circulation can be gained by percutaneous cannulation of the subclavian, internal jugular, external jugular, antecubital, or femoral vein.
2. The site of cannulation chosen depends on the experience of the operator, the urgency of the situation, and the accessibility of the site. The preferred site of cannulation is the right internal jugular (RIJ) vein, which can be cannulated with relative ease with a minimal rate of complications and provides the most direct path to the right atrium.
3. The area should be prepped and draped using aseptic technique and the patient placed in Trendelenberg position (if tolerated) at the time of venous cannulation.

Equipment

1. Catheter
   a. Each port of the catheter should be tested for patency by flushing with normal saline, and the balloon should be inflated with 1 to 1.5 ml of air to test for integrity.
   b. A number of different Swan-Ganz balloon flotation catheters exist; however, the size 7 French triple-lumen 110-cm catheter with 1.5-ml balloon capacity is the most common. It is marked at 10-cm intervals, with small black rings and a thicker black ring at 50 cm.
   c. The tip contains a thermistor for measuring temperature, and this should be checked by attaching the catheter thermistor connector to the monitor and determining if it is correctly reading room temperature.

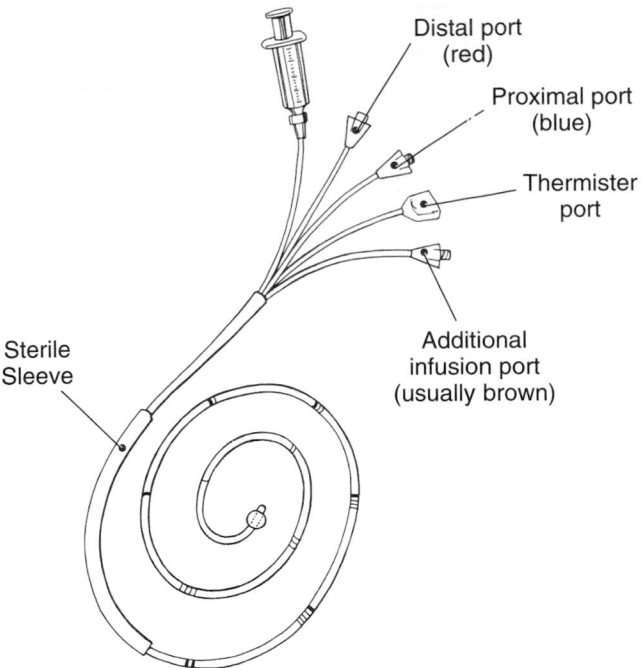

Distal port (red)

Proximal port (blue)

Thermister port

Sterile Sleeve

Additional infusion port (usually brown)

2. Dilator sheath
3. Three-way stopcock
4. Pressure tubing and normal saline
5. Transducers
6. 18-gauge Cook needle and No. 22 gauge finder needle
7. Sterile gown/gloves/drape
8. 1% lidocaine
9. J-tipped guidewire and No. 11 blade scalpel
10. Towel dips, suture material, syringes
11. Electrocardiograph, pressure and temperature monitoring equipment
12. Atropine
13. Defibrillator unit

> **WARNING**
>
> **It is important to have all the necessary equipment on hand and have tested all the ports of the Swan-Ganz catheter prior to use.**

Anesthesia

Local anesthesia (2 to 4 ml of 1% lidocaine) is given at the site of cannulation.

Precautions

1. Strict aseptic technique is mandatory, especially because the overall risk of catheter-related bacteremia is approximately 1 per cent.
2. Sterile gloves, gown, cap, and mask with eye-shield should be worn.
3. The area surrounding the site of cannulation should be covered with a large sterile drape to prevent contamination of the long pulmonary artery catheter.

> **WARNING**
>
> **When the catheter is passed from the right atrium (RA) through the right ventricle (RV) to the pulmonary artery (PA), the balloon should always be inflated and passage should be done quickly to limit the risk of arrhythmias.**

Technique

1. Position the patient in the supine position and zero the pressure transducer at midaxillary level.
2. If there is an existing central venous catheter, the Swan-Ganz catheter introducer sheath can be placed over a guidewire change of the existing catheter. If there is no central venous access, the Swan-Ganz catheter introducer sheath should be placed using a method similar to that used to place a central venous catheter. The only difference is that the dilator is placed in the Swan-Ganz catheter introducer sheath and then passed over the guidewire.
3. Secure the catheter introducer sheath by suturing it to nearby skin.
4. Attach a three-way stopcock to the distal port of the Swan-Ganz catheter.
5. Attach a 6-foot pressure tube to the stopcock and have an assistant attach the opposite end of the 6-foot pressure tubing to the pressure transducer, which then attaches to the monitor.
6. Flush the tubing and distal catheter port, making sure to remove all bubbles.
7. Use saline-filled syringes to flush the remaining ports and leave the remaining syringes attached.
8. Put the catheter protective sleeve over the catheter without expanding it.
9. Check the zero position of the transducer by holding the catheter tip at the midaxillary line to see if the monitor reads zero. If it does not, re-zero the transducer.
10. Check the pressure transducer function by gently tapping the tip of the catheter and observing appropriate artifact waves on the monitor.
11. Pass the catheter into the introducer sheath 20 cm, then inflate the balloon.

12. If unable to inflate the balloon, advance the catheter 2 cm and reattempt inflation. If this is unsuccessful, remove the catheter and recheck the balloon.

13. Advance the catheter with the balloon inflated, observing the pressure tracings as the balloon passes through the RA, RV, and PA. The PA is usually reached within 40 to 50 cm if the RIJ is cannulated (see tracing below).

14. With the balloon still inflated, advance slowly into the PA until a pulmonary capillary wedge pressure (PCWP) tracing is obtained (see tracing below).

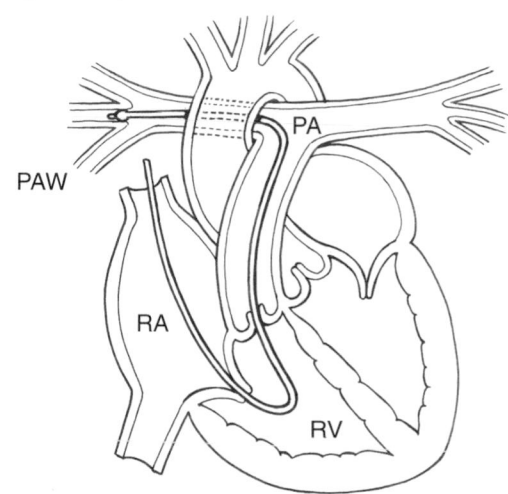

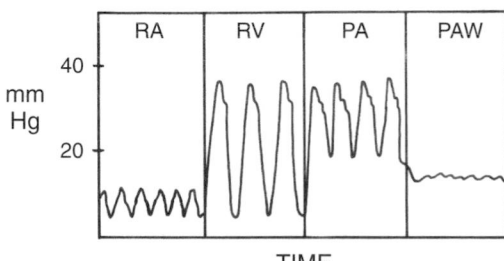

TIME

15. Deflate the balloon and look for the reappearance of a PA tracing. If a wedge tracing is still seen, withdraw the catheter a few centimeters until a PA tracing is seen.

16. Reinflate the balloon and a pulmonary artery wedge (PAW) tracing should occur. Repeat the above until the optimal catheter position is obtained.

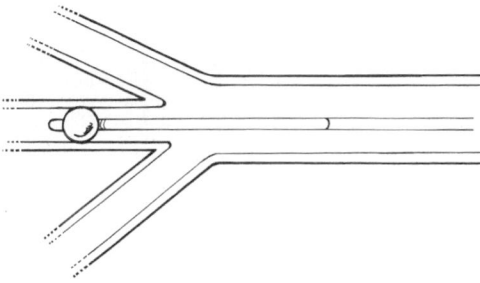

17. Expand catheter sleeve to cover entire external portion of the catheter.

18. Apply dressing.

Follow-Up

1. Obtain a chest radiograph to confirm positioning of the catheter in the lower lung zone (zone 3).

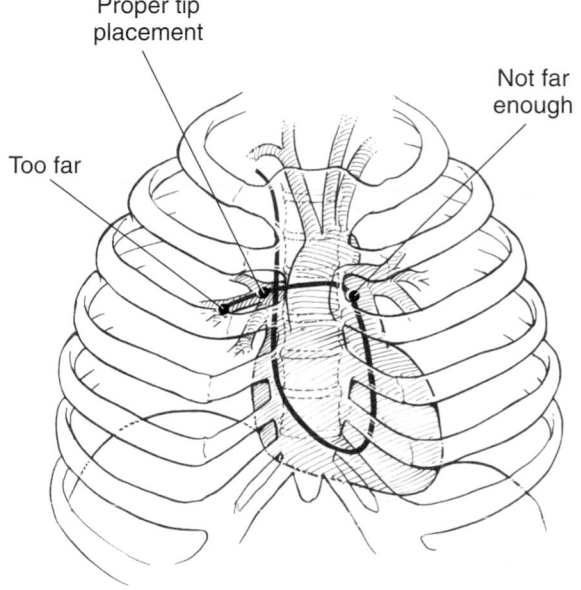

Proper tip placement

Not far enough

Too far

2. Measure all pressures when the intrathoracic pressures are closest to zero—during end expiration—regardless of whether the patient is spontaneously breathing or on mechanical ventilation.

3. Measuring cardiac output (CO) is rapid and easy using the thermodilution technique. Inject 5 to 10 ml of cold saline rapidly and smoothly and the monitor computer calculates the CO. The average of three measurements should be obtained.

TABLE 65–1. INTERPRETATION OF HEMODYNAMIC FINDINGS IN SWAN-GANZ MONITORING

	NORMAL	CARDIOGENIC SHOCK	SEPSIS: "WARM"	CHRONIC CHF	PULM. HTN, PE	LOW VOLUME	TAMPONADE	MR	SHUNT/ VSD	RV INFARCT
RA (=CVP) (mm Hg)	5	10–20	5	10–15	10–15	2	20	10	10–20	10–20
RV (mm Hg)	25/5	40–50/10–20	30/5	40/10–15	50/10	20/2	30/20	40–50/10	40/20–20	25/10–20
PA (mm Hg)	25/10; mean 15	40–50/25; mean 30	30/10; mean 17	40/20; mean 27	50/20; mean 30	20/5; mean 10	30/20; mean 23	40–50/30; mean 37	40/20; mean 27	25/10–15
PAW (mm Hg)	<10	25	10	20	10	5	20	30 Large V waves	20 Large V waves	10
AO (mm Hg)	120/80; MAP 93	80/50; MAP 60	80/50; MAP 60	100/60; MAP 73	120/80; MAP 93	80/50; MAP 60	90/70; MAP 77	120/80; MAP 93	120/80; MAP 93	100/60; MAP 73
CO (L)	5–8	3–4	8–10	4	5	8*	5	4–5	5	4–5
CI (L/m²)	2.5–4.2	<2.0	>4–5	>2	2.5	4*	2.5	2–2.5	2.5	2–2.5
PA sat. (Sat %)	67–75	60	75	60	67	65	67	60	75–80	65
SVR (Dynes-sec-cm⁵)	700–1600 (<2 Wood units)	Usually high	200–400	1200 Normal to high	1300 High	580*	900	Normal to high	Variable low	Normal to high
PVR (Dynes-sec-cm⁵)	80–130 (<2 Wood units)	Usually high	Usually low	140 (1.75 Wood units)	319 (4 Wood units)	50 (<1 Wood unit)	48 (<1 Wood unit)	Normal to high	Normal to low	Normal to high

Abbreviations: AO, aortic output; CHF, congestive heart failure; CI, cardiac index; CO, cardiac output; CVP, central venous pressure; Pulm. HTN, pulmonary hypertension; MAP, mean arterial pressure; MR, mitral regurgitation; PA, pulmonary artery pressure; PA sat., pulmonary artery saturation; PAW, pulmonary artery wedge pressure; PE, pulmonary embolism; PVR, pulmonary vascular resistance; RA, right atrial pressure; RV, right ventricular [pressure]; SVR, systemic vascular resistance; VSD, ventricular septal defect.

* = Highly variable.

4. Computer calculation of the systemic vascular resistance can then be obtained by entering the CO, the blood pressure, and RA pressure.

5. Table 65–1 summarizes hemodynamic findings in various conditions.

ACKNOWLEDGMENT: A special thanks to J. E. Atwood, M.D., for supplying the table and for his expert advice.

Bibliography

Amin DK, Shah PK, Swan HJC: The Swan Ganz catheter. J Crit Illness 1986;1:24–45 and 1:40–61.

Mermel LA, Maki DG: Infectious complications of Swan-Ganz pulmonary artery catheters. Am J Respir Crit Care Med 1994;149:1020–1036.

Sharkey SW: Beyond the wedge: clinical physiology and the Swan-Ganz catheter. Am J Med 1987;87:111–122.

Warren J: Pulmonary Artery Catheterization. In Jastremski MS, Dumas M, Peñalver L (eds): Emergency Procedures, pp 306–312. Philadelphia, WB Saunders Company, 1992.

66 Cardiomyopathy

Benjamin H. Chadi

Etiology

Cardiomyopathies, heart muscle diseases associated with cardiac dysfunction, may be of unknown cause (primary or idiopathic) or due to specific causes (secondary). They are now categorized into six overlapping groups:

1. Dilated cardiomyopathy (DCMP): dilatation and impaired (left or bi-) ventricular contraction with nonspecific histology, presenting usually with progressive heart failure. Arrhythmias, thromboembolism, and sudden death occur commonly and at any stage.

   a. Idiopathic

   b. Familial/genetic

      (1) X-linked: dystrophin gene in Duchenne and Becker muscular dystrophy (Xp21)

      (2) Autosomal dominant

      (3) Autosomal recessive

      (4) Sporadic

   c. Viral and immune

   d. Alcoholic/toxic

   e. Other cardiovascular disease in which the degree of dysfunction cannot be explained by the degree of (ischemic) damage or loading conditions (fluid status) (see item 6 below)

2. Hypertrophic cardiomyopathy (HCMP): hypertrophy of the left (LV) and/or right ventricle (RV), particularly of the septum (asymmetric), with normal or reduced ventricular volume; commonly associated with intracavitary systolic pressure gradients and, on histology, myocyte hypertrophy and disarray. Arrhythmias and premature sudden death are common.

   a. Predominantly familial, autosomal dominant, with mutations in genes for sarcomeric contractile proteins

      (1) β-Myosin heavy chain (chromosome 14)

      (2) Cardiac troponin T (chromosome 1)

      (3) α-Tropomyosin (chromosome 15)

      (4) Myosin-binding protein C (chromosome 11)

   b. Unknown, heritable, or sporadic, including de novo transmissible mutations

3. Restrictive cardiomyopathy (RCMP): restriction in filling and reduction in diastolic ventricular volume without systolic dysfunction

   a. Idiopathic myocardial fibrosis (interstitial)

   b. Associated with other diseases

      (1) Endomyocardial fibrosis without eosinophilia

      (2) Endomyocardial fibrosis with eosinophila (Löffler's disease)

         (a) Hypersensitivity states (e.g., tryptophan)

         (b) Parasitic infestations

         (c) Eosinophilic leukemia

      (3) Infiltrative disorders

         (a) Amyloidosis

         (b) Hemochromatosis

         (c) Sarcoidosis

4. Arrhythmogenic RV cardiomyopathy: a rare disorder; progressive fibrofatty myocardial replacement generally beginning focally in the RV with subsequent global RV and some LV involvement, sparing the septum. Arrhythmias and sudden death are a common presentation, especially in the young.

   a. Familial: common

      (1) Autosomal dominant, incomplete penetrance

      (2) Recessive

   b. Unknown

5. Unclassified cardiomyopathy: cases not readily classified as above

   a. Fibroelastosis

   b. Noncompacted myocardium

   c. Systolic dysfunction with minimal dilatation

   d. Mitochondrial involvement (Kearns-Sayre syndrome)

6. Specific cardiomyopathies: associated with other cardiac or systemic disorders

   a. Ischemic: DCMP out of proportion to the infarction/coronary disease

   b. Valvular: ventricular dysfunction out of proportion to the abnormal load of the lesions (regurgitation/stenosis)

   c. Hypertensive: left ventricular hypertrophy (LVH) with features of DCMP or RCMP and heart failure

d. Inflammatory: myocarditis
   (1) Idiopathic
   (2) Autoimmune: collagen-vascular diseases (systemic lupus erythematosus [SLE], polyarteritis nodosa [PAN], progressive systemic sclerosis, Churg-Strauss syndrome)
   (3) Infectious
       (a) Parasitic: Chagas' disease, caused by *Trypanosoma cruzi*; schistosomiasis, trichinosis, toxoplasmosis
       (b) Fungal, bacterial, rickettsial (leptospirosis), spirochetal
       (c) Viral: adenovirus, coxsackievirus, cytomegalovirus, echovirus, and human immunodeficiency virus
e. Metabolic
   (1) Hormonal: thyrotoxicosis, pheochromocytoma, adrenal insufficiency, myxedema, acromegaly, diabetes mellitus, and disturbances of potassium metabolism
   (2) Nutritional deficiencies: thiamine (beriberi), selenium (Keshan's disease), L-carnitine, kwashiorkor, and magnesium
   (3) Storage diseases: iron (hemochromatosis), glycogen, and other syndromes (Hurler's and Refsum's) and diseases (Niemann-Pick, Hand-Schüller-Christian, Fabry-Anderson, Morquio-Ullrich)
   (4) Amyloidoses: primary, secondary, familial, hereditary cardiac, senile, and familial Mediterranean fever
f. Other
   (1) General system disease: connective tissue disorders (SLE, PAN, rheumatoid arthritis, scleroderma, dermatomyositis), infiltrations, and granulomas (sarcoidosis, leukemia)
   (2) Muscular dystrophies: myotonic, Duchenne, and Becker-type
   (3) Neuromuscular: Friedreich's ataxia, Noonan's syndrome, lentiginoses
   (4) Toxicity and sensitivity reactions: alcohol, catecholamines, anthracyclines (doxorubicin, daunorubicin), radiation, and miscellaneous
g. Peripartum: May first manifest in pregnancy or after delivery.

Symptoms
1. Heart failure: dyspnea on exertion and later at rest; subsequently paroxysmal nocturnal dyspnea, orthopnea, pedal edema, and right upper quadrant abdominal tenderness in acute hepatic congestion
2. Arrhythmias: palpitation, tachycardia, syncope
3. Chest discomfort, cough, hemoptysis
4. Low output state with fatigue, decreased mentation, skin and gut hypoperfusion, and decreased urination
5. Embolisms: pulmonary, peripheral vasculature (stroke, renal and splenic infarcts)

Key Symptoms

- Dyspnea on exertion
- Fatigue
- Orthopnea

Clinical Findings
1. History: family, alcohol, toxins, viral syndrome, residence in tropics or South America (Chagas' disease)
2. Examination
   a. Tachycardia with narrow pulse pressure resulting from low output with pulsus alternans in end stage
   b. Jugular venous distention more than the normal 6- to 8-cm vertical height above the right atrial (RA) level (manubriosternal junction at the midaxillary line)
   c. Crackles, pedal edema, hepatomegaly, and ascites (quantify)
   d. Cardiomegaly with point of maximal impulse laterally displaced and enlarged diffusely (in DCMP) or more forceful (in HCMP)
   e. Parasternal lift and heave with mitral regurgitation or with pulmonary hypertension
   f. Loud P_2 and reversed split S_2 in pulmonary hypertension
   g. Diastolic gallops: S_3 early filling and S_4 atrial kick
   h. Holosystolic murmurs of mitral regurgitation (apical to axillary or left sternal) and tricuspid regurgitation (parasternal, louder with inspiration). A harsh midsystolic murmur may be evidence of obstruction in HCMP.

Key Signs

- Tachycardia
- Pedal edema
- Rales
- Cardiomegaly

Laboratory Tests

1. Electrocardiogram: normal or abnormal.
   a. Arrhythmias: atrial and ventricular ectopies, sinus tachycardia, atrial fibrillation
   b. Increased voltage and left axis deviation in LVH; right ventricular hypertrophy (RVH) and right axis deviation in pulmonary hypertension and right heart failure; low voltage in amyloid, sarcoid, hemochromatosis, and hypothyroidism (also with chronic obstructive pulmonary disease [COPD] and obesity); electrical alternans in pericardial tamponade
   c. Conduction abnormalities and bundle-branch blocks (BBBs), generally LBBB in DCMP, RBBB in Chagas' disease, and complete heart block in muscular dystrophies
   d. Left atrial (LA) abnormality caused by left atrial hypertrophy or dilatation, commonly with mitral valve or LV disorders; RA abnormality in right arterial enlargement or hypertrophy, as with severe tricuspid regurgitation or pulmonary hypertension and RV failure
   e. Q waves of infarction or mimic
   f. ST/T changes of infarction, ischemia, pericarditis, myocarditis, electrolyte imbalance
   g. Prolonged Q-T interval

2. Chest radiograph
   a. Cardiomegaly with an enlarged cardiac silhouette resulting from dilatation, hypertrophy, or effusion; enlargement of LA, RA, and RV chambers
   b. Increased pulmonary vascular redistribution, interstitial and alveolar edema, Kerley B lines, and perihilar infiltrates

3. Doppler and echocardiography
   a. Wall thickness: markedly increased septal thickness, often with evidence of dynamic outflow tract obstruction in HCMP. A ground-glass texture often accompanies the wall thickening in infiltrative disorders such as amyloidosis. Ventricular hypertrophy commonly accompanies hypertensive disorders and aortic stenosis. Apical thrombus and cavity obliteration occur in endomyocardial disease. RVH commonly accompanies pulmonary hypertension.
   b. Wall motion abnormalities: usually hypercontractile in HCMP; reduced ejection fraction with global or *local* wall motion abnormalities in DCMP.
   c. Chamber size: LA enlargement is the rule in all forms of cardiomyopathy. The LV cavity size is small in HCMP and RCMP but dilated in DCMP. The RV may dilate in right heart failure.
   d. Pericardial disease: the presence of an effusion and, if large, evidence for tamponade and chamber collapse
   e. Valvular evaluation: systolic anterior motion (SAM) of the anterior mitral leaflet in HCMP with systolic closure of the aortic valve evidence dynamic outflow obstruction. Color Doppler can localize the outflow gradient, and continuous-wave Doppler can quantitate its severity. Mitral regurgitation may be due to SAM in HCMP or to a dilated mitral annulus in DCMP. Pulmonary artery systolic pressure (P; millimeters of mercury) can be reliably calculated from the peak tricuspid regurgitation velocity (v; meters/second) by the modified Bernoulli equation

$$(P \text{ in } RV - P \text{ in } RA = 4v^{**}2)$$

   Diastolic dysfunction, restriction, and differentiation from pericardial diseases can be inferred from Doppler velocity tracings.
   f. The presence of congenital heart disease and shunts or abnormal flows (such as atrial septal defect, patent ductus arteriosus) can be evaluated.
   g. Specific evaluations include contrast injection and transesophageal echocardiography for better resolution of pathologic features, as in HCMP, or to evaluate LA thrombus, anomalous pulmonary venous return, patent foramen ovale. Provocative maneuvers such as use of nitroglycerin for amyl nitrite are used to provoke the outflow gradient in HCMP. Stress echo/Doppler to evaluate for ischemia or changes in a valvular or subvalvular gradient with exercise.

4. Radionuclide studies
   a. Multiple gated acquisition blood pool scan (radionuclide ventriculography): ejection fraction
   b. Stress thallium: rule out ischemic etiology, infarction

5. Cardiac catheterization
   a. Right heart to evaluate RA, pulmonary, and wedge pressures (LV preload); cardiac output by thermodilution or Fick; oximetry to evaluate for right-to-left shunt; and calculations of systemic and pulmonary vascular resistance
   b. Left heart catheterization to evaluate intracavitary pressures and evaluate gradients

(HCMP or valve stenosis) by simultaneous measurements and by pullback

   c. Coronary angiography to evaluate coronary disease, including intravascular ultrasound of suspicious lesions

   d. Ventriculography and aortography to evaluate ejection fraction and valvular regurgitation

   e. Provocation of gradient in HCMP by vasodilators, inotropes, or post–premature ventricular complexes

   f. Myocardial biopsy to rule out infiltrative disorders, myocarditis, transplant rejection, and drug toxicity

6. Blood tests

   a. Antistreptolysin-O titer (rheumatic heart disease), Chagas' titers

   b. Westergren erythrocyte sedimentation rate (myocarditis)

   c. Creatine kinase (CK) MB isoenzyme (acute myocardial infarction, myocarditis, neuromyopathies); CK MM isoenzyme (elevated in muscular dystrophies)

   d. Screen for toxins, including cocaine, alcohol.

   e. Thyroid function tests. Screen for pheochromocytoma.

Key Tests

- Electrocardiogram
- Chest radiograph
- Echocardiogram

Differential Diagnosis

1. Cardiac disorders mimicking heart muscle disease

   a. Valvular regurgitation, stenosis

   b. Pericardial constriction, tamponade, pericarditis

   c. Congenital heart diseases: atrial septal defect, anomalous pulmonary venous return, cor triatriatum, ventricular septal defect, tetralogy of Fallot

   d. Cor pulmonale resulting from pulmonary hypertension associated with any etiology, including idiopathic, collagen-vascular disease, recurrent pulmonary embolism, COPD, methotrexate

2. Noncardiac disorders: acute pulmonary embolism, acute respiratory distress syndrome, COPD, pneumonias, renal failure with hypervolemia, hypoalbuminemia

Treatment

Medication

1. Diuretics to decrease preload in DCMP with evidence of congestion. Loop diuretics such as furosemide or bumetanide can be used alone or in combination with thiazides or metolazone. Closely monitor and supplement potassium. Restrict free water intake in hyponatremia. Potassium-sparing diuretics (e.g., aldactone, ameloride) improve survival.

2. Vasodilators can increase cardiac output and survival in DCMP. The angiotensin-converting enzyme inhibitors such as captopril and enalapril can be titrated to blood pressure and help conserve potassium. Angiotensin receptor blockage may also improve survival, but should be avoided in pregnancy. Isordil and hydralazine have documented efficacy. Vasodilators can worsen the dynamic obstruction in HCMP.

3. Digitalis increases inotropic state, improves ejection fraction, and improves symptoms in DCMP, without causing hypotension. It can control the ventricular response to atrial fibrillation. It should be avoided in infiltrative cardiomyopathy of amyloid and in HCMP. Because of a narrow therapeutic index and risk for potentially life-threatening arrhythmias and toxicity, it should be monitored. Digibind Fab anti-digitalis antibodies can be used acutely in the management of intoxication.

4. Pure β-blockers such as metoprolol and the mixed β-blocker carvidelol may exacerbate heart failure in DCMP but, if tolerated (begin at low doses and gradually increase as blood pressure allows), increase survival. β-Blockers improve diastolic filling parameters in HCMP.

5. Calcium channel blockers: The vasodilators amlodipine and nifedipine may treat ischemia in DCMP without exacerbating congestive heart failure. Verapamil and diltiazem with negative inotropic and chronotropic effects improve ventricular filling in HCMP.

6. Pacemaker insertion may be necessary preventively in cardiomyopathies that progress to heart block (Kearns-Sayre syndrome and some muscular dystrophies). Dual-chamber pacing has shown promise in reducing the outflow tract gradient in HCMP.

7. Surgical considerations include coronary revascularization, mitral valve replacement, myomectomy for HCMP with obstruction, thrombectomy with endocardial stripping for eosinophilic endomyocardial disease, and transplant in end-stage DCMP.

8. Anticoagulation therapy in atrial fibrillation, in

DCMP, and in RCMP reduces risk for thromboembolism.

9. Anti-inflammatory agents may be given in eosinophilic endocardial disease, but their efficacy has not been documented in myocarditis, in which 50 per cent of patients may improve spontaneously.

10. The role of the implantable defibrillator is being defined. Automatic implantable defibrillators improve survival in patients with ventricular tachycardia or high risk of sudden death.

Diet

1. Lower sodium (2 gm/day, or 500 mg in severe cases), optimize nutrition, avoid alcohol and cardiotoxins.

2. Nutrition, thiamine, selenium, potassium, magnesium, and L-carnitine for specific deficiencies

Activity

1. Avoid heavy lifting, vigorous exertion, and hot weather.

2. Maintain a mild daily aerobic exercise regimen to improve muscle conditioning, peripheral blood flow, exercise tolerance.

Education

1. Symptoms and signs of heart failure (edema, dyspnea, loss of appetite, rapid weight gain, or stable weight with anorexia)

2. Measure body weight daily and record.

3. Salt content of foods (fresh or frozen vs. processed, pickled, canned)

4. Importance of fluid balance: Water intake is generally controlled by thirst related to dietary salt intake. An adequate urinary output and brisk response to diuretic are critical to maintain homeostasis. A lack of urine output may relate to renal disease, urinary obstruction, or worsening heart failure, with gut edema and poor diuretic absorption along with poor renal

perfusion and resultant potential for serious hyperkalemia and digitalis toxicity. Anuria needs emergent evaluation.

5. Role of diarrhea in causing potassium loss or as a manifestation of hyperkalemia

6. Signs of hypokalemia including leg cramps, arrhythmias

7. Need to monitor prothrombin time on warfarin and electrolytes regularly and digoxin level periodically.

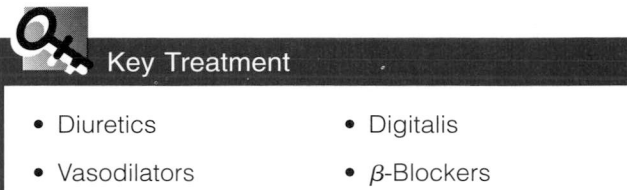

Key Treatment

- Diuretics
- Digitalis
- Vasodilators
- β-Blockers

Follow-Up

Depends on the specific etiology, preventive therapy, and severity of heart failure.

Bibliography

Kushwaha SS, Fallon JT, Fuster V: Restrictive cardiomyopathy. N Engl J Med 1997;336:267–276.

Leiden JM: The genetics of dilated cardiomyopathy: emerging clues to the puzzle. N Engl J Med 1997;37:1080–1081.

Richardson P, McKenna W, Bristow M, et al: Report of the 1995 World Health Organization/International Society and Federation of Cardiology Task Force on the Definition and Classification of Cardiomyopathies. Circulation 1996;93:841–842.

Rudkey SM, Ratliff NG, Young JB: Cardiomyopathy and myocardial failure. In Topol EJ (ed): Textbook of Cardiovascular Medicine, pp 2215–2246. Philadelphia, Lippincott-Raven, 1998.

Spirito P, Seidman CE, McKenna WJ, et al: The management of hypertrophic cardiomyopathy. N Engl J Med 1997;336:775–785.

Wynne J, Braunwald E: The cardiomyopathies and myocardites: toxic, chemical, and physical damage to the heart. In Braunwald E (ed): Heart Disease: A Textbook of Cardiovascular Medicine, pp 1404–1463. Philadelphia, WB Saunders Company, 1997.

67 Mitral Valve Diseases

Sherif F. Nagueh

Mitral Regurgitation

Etiology

1. Mitral valve prolapse (most common cause)
2. Ischemic heart disease with papillary muscle dysfunction
3. Infective endocarditis
4. Rheumatic fever
5. Congenital
6. Drugs (ergot alkaloids, anorectic drugs)
7. Marfan's syndrome
8. Systemic lupus erythematosus
9. Hypertrophic cardiomyopathy
10. Trauma (ruptured chordae tendinae)

Symptoms

1. Pulmonary congestion symptoms: exertional dyspnea, orthopnea, paroxysmal nocturnal dyspnea
2. Systemic congestion symptoms: edema, epigastric discomfort related to hepatic congestion
3. Low output symptoms: fatigue, weakness
4. Symptoms caused by dysrhythmias: palpitations, presyncope, syncope
5. Symptoms of the disease causing mitral regurgitation (MR): exertional chest pain, arthritis and arthralgias, fever, chest trauma, rheumatic fever during adolescence, ingestion of diet pills or ergot alkaloids for migraine

Key Symptoms

- Exertional dyspnea
- Orthopnea
- Paroxysmal nocturnal dyspnea

Clinical Findings

1. Apical displacement of the left ventricular (LV) apex
2. Bibasilar rales
3. Enlarged, tender liver
4. Edema of the lower extremities
5. Increased jugular venous pressure

6. Apical systolic murmurs: usually holosystolic that radiate to the axilla but may at times radiate to the base with diseases of the posterior mitral leaflet; mitral valve prolapse murmurs are usually of a more brief duration
7. Additional sounds and murmurs: apical S_3, opening snap, aortic murmurs in patients with rheumatic heart disease

Key Signs

- Enlarged left ventricle with a downward displacement of the apex
- Apical holosystolic murmur that radiates to the axilla

Tests

1. Chest radiograph: No specific findings for MR. Patients may have left atrial and/or LV enlargement, pulmonary congestion with prominent hilar vessels and pleural effusion (usually right-sided).
2. Electrocardiogram (ECG): No specific findings for MR; however, it may have signs of left atrial enlargement and/or LV hypertrophy. Most frequent arrhythmia is atrial fibrillation.
3. Echocardiography: Most valuable test in evaluating patients with known or suspected MR. It provides valuable data, including left atrial size, LV size and function, severity of MR, and pulmonary artery pressures. Furthermore, it can assess the hemodynamic significance of other valvular lesions.
4. Cardiac catheterization: Needed prior to surgery for MR to assess for coronary artery disease. It is also helpful in occasional cases with discrepancy between the clinical and the echocardiographic assessment of MR severity. Patients with severe MR usually have an enlarged left ventricle as well as increase in LV filling pressures.

Differential Diagnosis

1. Aortic stenosis: ejection systolic murmur usually loudest at upper right sternal border, aortic component of S_2 frequently diminished. In older

patients aortic stenosis murmur may be loudest inside the apex.

2. Tricuspid regurgitation: holosystolic murmur loudest at lower left sternal border and increases with inspiration; "v" waves may also be detected in the jugular veins and systolic expansion of the liver.
3. Ventricular septal defect: holosystolic murmur loudest at lower left sternal border; no significant respiratory variation; may be associated with a thrill in the same location.
4. Infundibular pulmonary stenosis isolated or as part of tetralogy of Fallot: ejection systolic murmur maximum at left sternal border, usually with signs of right ventricular hypertrophy as parasternal lift and prominent "a" wave in jugular venous pulse

Treatment

Asymptomatic patients with normal ventricular function do not need medical or surgical therapy, but should be followed closely for the development of symptoms and/or LV enlargement or dysfunction (indications for surgery).

Surgery
1. Indications
   a. Symptomatic patients with normal ejection fraction (EF)
   b. Symptomatic patients with early evidence of systolic dysfunction (EF 50 to 60 per cent; end-systolic dimension ≥45 mm)
   c. Asymptomatic patients with early evidence of systolic dysfunction (EF 50 to 60 per cent; end-systolic dimension ≥45 mm)
   d. Atrial fibrillation (paroxysmal or permanent) with normal LV EF
   e. Asymptomatic patients with normal ventricular function and pulmonary artery systolic pressure greater than 50 mm Hg at rest, or greater than 60 mm Hg with exercise
   f. Symptomatic or asymptomatic patients with LV EF of 30 to 50 per cent (or end-systolic dimension of 50 to 55 mm)
2. Types of surgery
   a. Mitral valve repair: preserves LV function and allows patient in sinus rhythm to avoid anticoagulants.
   b. Mitral valve replacement, with or without chordal preservation; chordal preservation is preferable because it may decrease the likelihood of postoperative LV dysfunction.

Medical Therapy
1. In patients with atrial fibrillation, anticoagulants are needed to prevent systemic thromboembolic events, aiming for an international normalized ratio of 2 to 3.
2. In patients with atrial fibrillation, rate slowing with digoxin and/or β-blockers/calcium channel blockers is needed to allow for an adequate diastolic filling period.
3. Conversion to sinus rhythm with electric or pharmacologic means may also be attempted, although the likelihood of success with atrial fibrillation of greater than 1 year is low.
4. Symptomatic patients with inoperable severe MR: digoxin, diuretics, and vasodilators may provide symptomatic relief. This is particularly helpful in patients with annular dilatation and LV systolic dysfunction.

Diet
In patients with pulmonary congestion, salt and water restriction are mandatory.

Activity
Asymptomatic patients should have no limitations on their physical activity; however, when symptoms develop, their activity should be limited to a level that is not associated with dyspnea.

Patient Education
1. Patients should be educated about the need for endocarditis prophylaxis, and the importance of early reporting of pulmonary congestion symptoms.
2. Those in atrial fibrillation should be instructed about the risks of bleeding or thromboembolic events with an unsatisfactory Coumadin dose.

Mitral Valve Prolapse

This is the most common cause of mitral regurgitation in the United States. It may be associated with significant degrees of MR. Its causes include

1. Myxomatous degeneration of the mitral valve
2. Marfan's syndrome
3. Collagen diseases

Symptoms
Patients are frequently asymptomatic, with abnormal findings only detected on auscultation or echocardiographic examination. Symptoms include

1. Chest pain
2. Anxiety
3. Fatigue
4. Other symptoms similar to those present with significant MR (see above)

Clinical Findings

1. Mid-systolic click
2. Mid- to late systolic apical murmur

The onset of the click and the duration of the murmur are dependent on the ventricular volume. With a larger ventricular size, the mitral leaflets prolapse later into the left atrium, leading to a delayed onset of the click and a shorter duration of the murmur (e.g., with a supine position or squatting). Standing and Valsalva maneuver result in clinical findings opposite to those described above through a reduction in LV volume.

3. Other signs related to left and right ventricular enlargement with severe degrees of MR (see above)

Key Signs

Apical systolic click and murmur of varying onset and duration dependent on patient's position

Tests

1. The chest radiograph and ECG have no specific findings for this disease. In advanced cases of MR, findings similar to those described above (under MR) may be present.
2. The definitive diagnosis is established by echocardiography. In addition to seeing the prolapse, one can determine the thickness of the mitral valve leaflets, the presence or absence of flail scallops of the leaflets, and the significance of MR (if present). The presence of leaflet redundancy and chordal disease are other important features that should be ascertained.

Treatment

1. Asymptomatic patients
   a. Reassurance of benign prognosis in patients with minimal thickness of valve leaflets and mild degrees of MR
   b. *Endocarditis prophylaxis* is not needed in patients with isolated systolic clicks and normal valves on echocardiography; however, it is indicated in
      (1) Patients with the characteristic click-murmur auscultatory findings
      (2) Patients with apical systolic click and leaflet thickening (>5 mm), elongated chordae, left atrial enlargement, and/or LV dilatation
      (3) Patients with apical systolic click and echocardiographic features of mitral valve prolapse and MR

   c. Follow up at intervals for possible progression of disease. More frequent follow-up (once a year) is needed in those with structurally abnormal valves and/or significant degrees of MR. Other patients can have their clinical evaluation at 2- to 3-year intervals or sooner should symptoms develop.
2. Symptomatic patients
   a. Patients with chest pain or anxiety symptoms may benefit from β-blockers and cutting their intake of caffeinated and alcoholic beverages.
   b. Aspirin is indicated in
      (1) Patients in sinus rhythm without clots who have had transient ischemic attacks
      (2) Patients who had stroke with contraindications to anticoagulants
      (3) Patients in atrial fibrillation and low risk for thromboembolic events (i.e., no history of embolic events, no hypertension, no history of heart failure, and age <65 years)
   c. Coumadin is indicated in
      (1) Patients with atrial fibrillation and high risk of thromboembolic events
      (2) Patients who suffered stroke
      (3) May also be considered for patients with transient ischemic attacks despite aspirin.
   d. When severe MR is present, the approach is similar to that described under management of MR of other etiologies.

Mitral Stenosis

Etiology

1. Rheumatic fever: long latent period from rheumatic fever to symptoms of mitral stenosis; most frequent lesion in women with rheumatic heart disease
2. Left atrial myxoma: higher incidence in women; may also be associated with MR.
3. Parachute mitral valve: congenital malformation associated with a single papillary muscle

Symptoms

Normal valve area is 4 to 6 cm². Patients with valve area of 1.5 cm² or more may have symptoms only with exertion, pregnancy, fever, or atrial fibrillation. Valve areas of 1 cm² or less are associated with symptoms at rest. Survival of untreated patients in class III or IV with pulmonary hypertension is less than 3 years.

1. Pulmonary congestion symptoms: exertional dyspnea, orthopnea, paroxysmal nocturnal dyspnea, or frank pulmonary edema

2. Systemic congestion symptoms: edema, epigastric discomfort related to hepatic congestion

3. Low output symptoms caused by severe stenosis and/or severe pulmonary hypertension with increased pulmonary vascular resistance: fatigue, weakness

4. Symptoms caused by arrhythmias; most common is atrial fibrillation: palpitations, presyncope, syncope

5. Systemic thromboembolism: transient ischemic attacks, stroke, peripheral arterial embolism

6. Pulmonary embolism: sudden onset of dyspnea, chest pain, hemoptysis

7. Chest pain: May be due to concomitant coronary disease, right ventricular hypertrophy and ischemia, or pulmonary embolism.

Key Symptoms

- Pulmonary congestion symptoms
- Systemic thromboembolic disease
- Symptoms of atrial arrhythmias

Clinical Findings

1. Lateral displacement of the apex (outside the midclavicular line)

2. Right ventricular hypertrophy and enlargement: parasternal lift, prominent "a" wave in jugular venous pulse

3. Pulmonary hypertension: loud P_2 sometimes even palpable, narrow split S_2, diastolic murmur of pulmonic regurgitation (the "Graham-Steel" murmur)

4. Accentuated S_1 with preserved mobility of valve leaflets; with severe calcification and restricted mobility S_1 is diminished.

5. Opening snap: again only with mobile leaflets; present in very early diastole just after P_2 and before any other diastolic heart sounds.

6. Mitral diastolic murmur: rumbling murmur best heard in left lateral position with the bell of the stethoscope. If sinus rhythm is still present, it will have presystolic accentuation, which is absent with atrial fibrillation. This murmur is very much localized to the apex, and careful auscultation is mandatory to elicit this sign. The duration and not the intensity signify the severity of mitral stenosis (i.e., longer and not nec-

essarily louder murmurs occur with severe mitral stenosis).

7. Systemic congestion signs: enlarged tender liver, ascites, edema of lower limbs

8. With pulmonary hypertension and right ventricular dilatation, signs of tricuspid regurgitation may be present: left sternal border holosystolic murmur that increases with inspiration, prominent "v" wave in jugular venous pulse, and systolic expansion of the liver

Key Signs

- Loud S_1
- Opening snap
- Mitral diastolic rumble
- Signs of pulmonary hypertension

Tests

1. Chest x-ray: left atrial enlargement; pulmonary venous congestion, including findings of alveolar and interstitial pulmonary edema and signs of right ventricular enlargement

2. ECG: P mitrale (wide P wave in limb leads), P pulmonale (tall P wave in limb leads), and signs of right ventricular hypertrophy in V_1 and V_2. Patients may also have coarse atrial fibrillation waves.

3. Echocardiography: *two-dimensional echocardiography with Doppler* is the cornerstone for establishing the diagnosis, assessing the severity of the lesion and the response to mechanical interventions. Valuable data can be readily available, including the gradient across the stenotic valve, valve area, pulmonary artery pressures, and right ventricular size and function. Concomitant valvular lesions can also be readily detected. Furthermore when the severity of the stenosis is in question, an exercise bike study can determine the changes in the transvalvular gradient and pulmonary artery pressures with exercise and thus the possible contribution of mitral stenosis to symptoms of exertional dyspnea.

4. Cardiac catheterization: Should not be performed for routine hemodynamic information. In the vast majority of cases satisfactory data are readily obtained with Doppler echocardiography. In the older population with possible coronary artery disease, coronary angiography is needed prior to planned mechanical interventions (if indicated).

Differential Diagnosis

1. Left atrial myxoma: Echocardiography confirms the diagnosis.
2. Cor triatriatum: Echocardiography confirms the diagnosis.
3. Austin-Flint murmur: an apical diastolic murmur with severe aortic regurgitation; patients usually have the peripheral signs of severe aortic regurgitation as well as the early diastolic decrescendo murmur of aortic regurgitation. If patients are given amyl nitrite, which lowers the systemic vascular resistance and causes reflex tachycardia, the Austin-Flint murmur decreases in intensity, whereas the mitral stenosis murmur becomes louder.
4. Tricuspid diastolic murmurs: May be due to tricuspid stenosis or severe regurgitation. In either case, signs of the corresponding lesion can help establish the diagnosis.
5. Pulmonary hypertension of other etiologies: interstitial lung disease, obstructive airway disease, and pulmonary vascular disease

Treatment

1. Asymptomatic patients
   a. Patients with valve area greater than 1.5 cm^2 may be followed at regular intervals for the development of symptoms and/or progression of mitral stenosis. Patients will need repeat echocardiography with changes in their symptoms or signs.
   b. Patients with valve area of 1.5 cm^2 or less should be evaluated for possible percutaneous valvotomy if they have pliable leaflets and pulmonary hypertension (pulmonary artery systolic pressure >50 mm Hg at rest or >60 mm Hg with exercise).
   c. Endocarditis prophylaxis
   d. Rheumatic fever prophylaxis in children and adolescents
2. Symptomatic patients
   a. *Medical therapy*: The only definitive treatment for mitral stenosis is percutaneous or surgical relief of the obstruction. Medical therapy may be of value in selected cases who refuse interventions or are deemed inoperable. If pulmonary congestion symptoms are present, patients usually benefit from diuretic therapy. Also, in the presence of faster heart rates, rate slowing with calcium blockers or β-blockers, which prolong the diastolic filling period, is indicated. Digoxin is helpful in cases of atrial fibrillation and/or right or left ventricular systolic dysfunction.
   b. *Atrial fibrillation*: Management includes rate control with digoxin, β-blockers, and/or calcium channel blockers. If hemodynamic instability is present, emergent synchronized cardioversion is needed. To maintain sinus rhythm, one may resort to antiarrhythmic drugs (usually low efficacy in sinus rhythm maintenance in the presence of significant mitral stenosis). Before and 3 to 4 weeks after cardioversion, patients should be on anticoagulants.
   c. *Prevention of embolic events*: Long-term anticoagulation is indicated in the presence of atrial fibrillation. This has been shown to reduce the incidence of systemic and pulmonary thromboembolic events. Patients with prior embolic events should also receive anticoagulants.
   d. *Percutaneous valvotomy*
      (1) A large balloon (or two balloons) is introduced into the left atrium (through transseptal puncture), advanced across the mitral valve, and then inflated. This results in splitting the commissural fusion and therefore increasing the mitral valve area. The outcome is satisfactory with low risk and high success in centers with a large experience.
      (2) Contraindicated with left atrial clots or severe MR. Patients with pliable, mildly thickened leaflets with little calcification and limited subvalvular fusion derive the most benefit from this procedure.
      (3) Complications include development or increased severity of MR, development of an atrial septal defect (related to the puncture of the interatrial septum), embolic events, and ventricular perforation (rare).
   e. *Surgery*: Commissurotomy (closed or open) or valve replacement. Mitral valve replacement is a viable alternative for patients who are poor candidates for percutaneous valvotomy (patients with markedly thickened, immobile leaflets with multiple areas of calcification and significant subvalvular pathology) and is the only treatment recommended for patients with concomitant severe MR. Valve replacement usually carries a low risk in younger patients without significant functional limitation.

Diet

In patients with pulmonary congestion, salt and water restriction are usually needed.

Activity

1. Asymptomatic patients with valve areas of 1.5 cm^2 or less should limit their physical activity because physical activity is associated with increased transvalvular flow rate and shortening of the diastolic filling period (because of the increase in heart rate). Consequently, left atrial pressure increases, with worsening of the pulmonary congestion symptoms.

2. Symptomatic patients should limit their activity to a level that is not associated with dyspnea.

Patient Education

1. Importance of endocarditis prophylaxis

2. Importance of rheumatic fever prophylaxis in children and young adolescents

3. Compliance with and close surveillance of anticoagulant regimen (including patients with mechanical valves)

4. Technique of determining the pulse rate and prompt reporting of irregular irregularity, which may denote the onset of atrial fibrillation

Bibliography

Bonow RO, Carabello B, de Leon AC Jr, et al: Guidelines for the management of patients with valvular heart disease: executive summary: a report of the American College of Cardiology/American Heart Association Task Force on Practice Guidelines (Committee on Management of Patients with Valvular Heart Disease). Circulation 1998;98:1949–1984.

Bruce CJ, Nishimura RA: Clinical assessment and management of mitral stenosis. Cardiol Clin 1998;16:375–403.

Dajani AJ, Taubert KA, Wilson W, et al: Prevention of bacterial endocarditis: recommendations by the American Heart Association. Circulation 1997;96:358–366.

Enriquez-Sarano M, Schaff HV, Orszulak TA, et al: Valve repair improves the outcome of surgery for mitral regurgitation: a multivariate analysis. Circulation 1995;91:1022–1028.

Palacios IF: Percutaneous mitral balloon valvotomy for patients with mitral stenosis. Curr Opin Cardiol 1994;9:164–175.

68 Aortic Valve Disease

Anil Shah

Aortic Stenosis

Etiology

1. Congenital aortic stenosis (major cause in patients under age 30)
2. Congenital bicuspid valve (progressive sclerosis occurs with age)
3. Rheumatic aortic stenosis (usually accompanied by disease of the mitral valve)
4. Calcific aortic stenosis (most common cause in patients older than age 60)

Symptoms

Paucity of symptoms occur until valve area of less than 1 cm^2.

1. Angina: Left ventricular hypertrophy causes increase in oxygen demand and reduction of oxygen delivery.
2. Syncope: commonly associated with exercise
3. Congestive heart failure (CHF): initially diastolic failure; may progress to systolic dysfunction.

> **WARNING**
>
> **Once symptoms begin, life expectancy is significantly decreased.**

Key Symptoms

- Angina
- Syncope
- CHF

Clinical Findings

1. Harsh crescendo-decrescendo murmur heard best at base with radiation to carotids
2. Absent aortic component of second heart sound with severe stenosis
3. Carotid impulses are diminished and delayed: pulsus parvus et tardus.
4. Sustained forceful apical impulse

Key Signs

- Systolic murmur
- Pulsus parvus et tardus

Laboratory Tests

1. Electrocardiogram (ECG): left ventricular hypertrophy (most common finding), left atrial enlargement, intraventricular conduction delay, left axis deviation
2. Chest radiograph: left ventricular predominance (without gross cardiomegaly), calcification of aortic cusps and/or annulus, poststenotic dilatation of the ascending aorta, and pulmonary vascular congestion (in the presence of heart failure)
3. Echocardiography: concentric left ventricular hypertrophy and thickening with or without calcification of the aortic cusps with decreased separation. Doppler gradient across the aortic valve (greater than 50 mm in severe cases). Valve area calculation of less than 0.8 cm^2 consistent with critical stenosis.
4. Radionuclide scanning: Gated blood pool scanning gives an accurate assessment of left ventricular function. Time to peak filling is often delayed.
5. Cardiac catheterization: direct measurement of valvular gradient; angiography to exclude concomitant coronary artery disease

Key Tests

- ECG
- Chest radiograph
- Echocardiogram
- Cardiac catheterization

Differential Diagnosis

1. Aortic sclerosis (not associated with absent A$_2$ or diminished carotid pulses)
2. Mitral regurgitation (holosystolic murmur at apex)
3. Pulmonic stenosis (ejection murmur loudest at left sternal border)

4. Hypertrophic obstructive cardiomyopathy (ejection murmur at left sternal border, prominent pulses with bifid quality)

Treatment
1. Medical (drugs)
   a. Diuretics if CHF present
   b. Antibiotic prophylaxis for dental and surgical procedures

---

WARNING

Avoid vasodilators; may result in profound and irreversible hypotension.

---

2. Valvuloplasty: Small improvements in valve area result in significant symptom improvement. High restenosis rate within a year of procedure. Bridge procedure in patients needing noncardiac surgery with critical stenosis; palliative procedure in symptomatic patients who are poor surgical candidates.
3. Surgery: definitive therapy in symptomatic patients. Reduced systolic function not a contraindication to surgery. Bioprosthetic or metal valves; latter requires lifetime anticoagulation.

Diet
Sodium restriction if CHF present

Activity
Moderate limitation (no competitive exercise in significant cases)

Patient Education
1. Strict compliance with diet and medication
2. Adherence to prothrombin time (PT) evaluation (warfarin [Coumadin] needed with mechanical valve)

Key Treatment	
• Diuretics	• Valvuloplasty
• Salt restriction	• Surgery

Follow-Up
1. Serial echocardiography
2. PT checks with mechanical valve (aim for an international normalized ratio [INR] of 3 to 4)

Aortic Regurgitation

Etiology
1. Rheumatic fever
2. Endocarditis
3. Congenital valvular deformities (e.g., bicuspid valve)
4. Collagen-vascular disorders (e.g., ankylosing spondylitis, systemic lupus erythematosus)
5. Myxomatous degeneration (e.g., Marfan's syndrome)
6. Aortic dissection
7. Trauma

Symptoms
1. Dyspnea
2. Paroxysmal nocturnal dyspnea and orthopnea
3. Edema (if biventricular failure present)
4. Chest pain and rarely syncope

Key Symptoms
• Dyspnea
• Edema

Clinical Findings
Acutely may result in pulmonary edema; chronic state may be tolerated for decades.
1. High-pitched decrescendo diastolic murmur at aortic area; radiates along left sternal border
2. Rapid and forceful carotid upstrokes with dramatic collapse (Corrigan's pulse)
3. Wide pulse pressure
4. Head bobbing with each systole (de Musset's sign)
5. Prominent pulsations of skin capillaries (Quincke's pulse)
6. Hill's sign (significantly higher popliteal artery pressure than brachial pressure)
7. Duroziez murmur (to-and-fro murmur heard over the femoral artery)
8. Displaced and hyperdynamic point of maximum impulse
9. Third or fourth heart sound (S_3 or S_4)

Key Signs
• Diastolic murmur
• Wide pulse pressure

Laboratory Tests
1. ECG: left ventricular hypertrophy and ST segment–T wave changes

2. Chest radiograph: cardiomegaly (in chronic cases), pulmonary vascular congestion, aortic root dilatation, and "double-lumen" sign when aortic dissection present

---

PEARL

Computerized tomography or magnetic resonance imaging can be invaluable in diagnosing dissection.

---

3. Echocardiography: left ventricular chamber dilatation (chronic cases); systolic function abnormality (may be hyperdynamic in acute cases, poor in decompensated chronic cases); diastolic fluttering of anterior leaflet of the mitral valve; Doppler estimation of degree of regurgitation (range: mild to severe)
4. Radionuclide studies: ejection fraction, stroke volume index (degree of regurgitation). Serial studies and exercise studies may help decide timing of elective valve replacement.
5. Cardiac catheterization: elevated left ventricular diastolic pressure; root flush for quantification of degree of regurgitation (1+ to 4+); coronary angiography

Key Tests

- ECG
- Radionuclide scan
- Chest radiograph
- Cardiac catheterization
- Echocardiogram

Differential Diagnosis
1. Pulmonic regurgitation (left ventricular prominence not seen)
2. Patent ductus arteriosus (continuous murmur heard in diastole and systole)

Treatment
1. Medical (drugs)
   a. Afterload-reducing agents (e.g., ACE inhibitors, nifedipine)
   b. Digitalis
   c. Diuretics
   d. Endocarditis prophylaxis
2. Surgical: Valve replacement is only surgical option. Indications are symptomatic patients with chronic regurgitation, severe acute regurgitation, progressive reduction in systolic function, end-systolic dimensions of left ventricle greater than 55 mm via echocardiogram, ejection fraction below 55 per cent, and failure to increase ejection fraction with exercise.

Diet
Salt restriction

Activity
Moderate restriction

Patient Education
1. Explain risks of Coumadin (needed with mechanical valve).
2. Stress prothrombin (PT) checks.

Key Treatment

- Afterload reduction
- Digoxin
- Diuretics
- Surgery

Follow-Up
1. Serial echocardiography
2. PT checks (aiming for INR of 3 to 4)

Bibliography

Braunwald E: Valvular heart disease. In Braunwald E (ed): Heart Disease: A Textbook of Cardiovascular Medicine, 5th ed, pp 1035–1053. Philadelphia, WB Saunders Company, 1997.

Carabello BA, Crawford FA: Valvular heart disease. N Engl J Med 1997;337:32–41.

Dajani AS, Taubert KA, Wilson W, et al: Prevention of bacterial endocarditis: recommendations by the American Heart Association. JAMA 1997;277:1794–1801.

Frank S, Johnson A, Ross J: Natural history of valvular aortic stenosis. Br Heart J 1973;35:41.

Morton MJ, Rahimtoola SH: How to follow patients with prosthetic heart valves. J Cardiovasc Med 1980; 5:475.

Scognamiglio R, Rahimtoola SH, Fasoli G, et al: Nifedipine in asymptomatic patients with severe aortic regurgitation and normal left ventricular function. N Engl J Med 1994;331:689–694.

69 Aortic Dissection

Thomas P. Power

Aortic dissection occurs when blood accumulates within the media of the aorta, causing separation of the intima from the adventitia. The usual initiating event is tearing of the intima and migration of the blood into the media. Rarely, rupture of the vasa vasorum within the media may lead to dissection without intimal tearing. In either case, blood tracks within and dissects the media, creating a false lumen. Aortic dissection may occur at any age (mean age is 59 years), and the ratio of males to females is 3:1. Aortic dissections are classified as follows:

1. Based on the anatomic location
   a. Proximal (type A): those dissections that involve, but are not necessarily limited to, the ascending aorta
   b. Distal (type B): those dissections whose involvement is limited to the distal aorta
2. Based on the age of the dissection
   a. Acute dissections are those that have occurred within the preceding 2 weeks.
   b. Chronic dissections are more than 2 weeks old.

Etiology

Although the exact cause of aortic dissection is not known, it is usually associated with an abnormality of the media. The following conditions predispose to aortic dissection:

1. Hypertension
2. Congenital disorders (Marfan's syndrome, Ehlers-Danlos syndrome, Turner's syndrome, aortic coarctation)
3. Trauma (including iatrogenic trauma)
4. Inflammatory conditions (relapsing polychondritis, giant cell arthritis)
5. Pregnancy (third trimester)

Symptoms

1. Chest pain is the cardinal symptom of aortic dissection. It occurs in 89 per cent of proximal dissections and 97 per cent of distal dissections. The pain is severe, described as tearing or ripping, and is usually of sudden onset. It may migrate to the neck, jaw, arms, or back, and migration of the pain is usually associated with progression of the dissection.

2. Syncope occurs considerably less frequently than chest pain. It may be due to severe pain or hypotension, as would occur with aortic rupture or pericardial tamponade. Occasionally syncope occurs before any pain is perceived and is therefore the presenting symptom.

3. Dyspnea as a presenting symptom is unusual; however, if specifically sought on history it is usually present. It may be related to cardiac tamponade, cardiac failure, or the presence of a large pleural effusion.

4. Alteration of mental status is not uncommon but is often subtle and overshadowed by chest pain. It may be due to impaired cerebral perfusion (hypotension or cerebral vessel involvement) or to the effects of previously administered narcotics.

Key Symptoms

- Chest pain: sudden, severe, tearing or ripping
- Syncope

Clinical Findings

1. Blood pressure changes. If all patients with aortic dissection are considered, hypertension is more common than hypotension at the time of presentation. However, patients with proximal dissection more commonly present with hypotension than with hypertension, and in these cases pericardial tamponade and aortic rupture must be considered. Occasionally, because of branch vessel involvement in the dissection, the cuff blood pressure may not reflect the true intra-arterial blood pressure (pseudohypotension).

2. Pulse deficits occur in about 50 per cent of patients with proximal aortic dissection and are considerably less common in distal dissection. Their presence is highly suggestive of this diagnosis. Pulse deficits are the result of either an intimal flap, which overlies and occludes the origin of a branch vessel, or propagation of the dissection into the lumen of the branch vessel.

3. Aortic valvular regurgitation, with its associated physical signs, occurs in approximately

two thirds of patients with proximal aortic dissection. The presence of new aortic regurgitation in a patient with chest pain should lead one to strongly suspect aortic dissection. It should be remembered, however, that the clinical picture of acute aortic regurgitation, such as occurs with dissection, is often much less dramatic than that of chronic regurgitation. The first heart sound is often diminished due to premature closure of the mitral valve (related to the rapid rise in left ventricular diastolic pressure). The diastolic murmur may be heard best at the right sternal border, in contradistinction to pure valvular regurgitation, in which it is heard best to the left of the sternum. Aortic regurgitation is the usual cause of cardiac failure in both acute and chronic aortic dissection.

4. Neurologic deficits are found in 36 per cent of proximal and 6 per cent of distal dissections. Global changes result from hypotension, whereas focal signs are due to aortic branch vessel involvement (cerebral vessels, spinal arteries) or peripheral ischemic neuropathy.

5. Pericardial rub is a rare finding in aortic dissection but, when present, is an ominous sign because it is often followed by pericardial tamponade.

6. Tracheal tug caused by traction on the left main bronchus during systolic expansion of the dissected aorta is also a rare but interesting sign.

Key Signs

- Hypertension
- Pulse deficit
- Aortic insufficiency

Laboratory Tests

Whenever aortic dissection is suspected, no time should be wasted in confirming the diagnosis because the mortality increases with time to treatment. Chest radiograph (showing widening of the mediastinum, left pleural effusion) and electrocardiogram (showing sinus tachycardia, low voltage) will often show abnormalities consistent with aortic dissection, but they are never diagnostic. Therefore the most easily available, most accurate, and safest test should be chosen. This choice will differ from patient to patient and from institution to institution.

1. Echocardiography: Transthoracic and transesophageal (TEE) echocardiography are now available in most hospitals. Neither requires the use of intravenous contrast agents and both can be performed at bedside. TEE is particularly helpful in visualization of the true and false lumens, the intimal flap, and the presence of associated aortic regurgitation. It can often identify the site and extent of dissection and determine the degree of involvement of the proximal coronary arteries.

2. Computerized tomographic (CT) scanning has been used since 1979 in diagnosis of aortic dissection and is now widely available. Sensitivity and specificity are high, and alternative diagnoses are often evident in those who do not have aortic dissection. However, CT scanning necessitates transportation of the patient and the use of intravenous contrast agents. It is not particularly useful in identification of associated aortic regurgitation or coronary artery involvement.

3. Aortography was considered the gold standard for diagnosis of aortic dissection, and it is still commonly used. It is particularly useful in the determination of the extent of dissection and the degree of branch vessel involvement (including the coronary arteries). Aortic regurgitation can also be identified. However, aortography is invasive, and large volumes of contrast agent are sometimes required. It necessitates transportation of the patient and assembly of a team to perform the procedure.

4. Magnetic resonance imaging (MRI) has the highest sensitivity and specificity for diagnosis of aortic dissection. However, monitoring of patients during imaging is difficult, and imaging times may be prohibitively long for unstable patients. MRI may be most useful in the diagnosis of chronic aortic dissection in stable patients or in long-term follow-up of treated patients. However, this technology is not available in many hospitals.

Key Tests

- TEE
- CT scan

Differential Diagnosis

1. Myocardial infarction (MI) is important in the differential diagnosis of aortic dissection for two reasons:

    a. Administration of thrombolytic therapy to a patient with aortic dissection may have disastrous consequences.

    b. One to 2 per cent of proximal aortic dissections extend into the proximal coronary arteries and cause MI. Therefore, an electrocardiogram consistent with acute MI does not exclude the diagnosis of aortic dissection.

2. Aortic valvular regurgitation without dissection
3. Nondissected aortic aneurysm
4. Pericarditis
5. Musculoskeletal chest pain
6. Mediastinal tumors

Treatment

Initial Treatment

Mortality from untreated aortic dissection is high and increases incrementally with time. Prompt diagnosis and treatment are therefore of utmost importance. Treatment should begin as soon as the diagnosis is suspected. The aim of initial pharmacologic therapy is to prevent extension of the dissection by reducing shear force on the aorta during systole.

1. β-Blockers (e.g., propranolol, 1 mg intravenously q5 min) should be administered until the pulse rate is 60 to 70 beats/minute.
2. This should be followed by nitroprusside (25 μg/min intravenously) until the systolic blood pressure is reduced to 100 to 120 mm Hg.
3. Analgesia (morphine sulfate, 3 to 5 mg intravenously q10 min prn) will also help to reduce systolic shear forces.

Definitive Therapy

Definitive therapy depends on the site and age of the aortic dissection. All patients with acute proximal dissection should be referred for immediate surgical correction. Chronic proximal dissection, if complicated (e.g., extension, aneurysm formation, aortic regurgitation) should also be treated surgically. Distal dissections, both acute and chronic, should be treated medically if uncomplicated and referred to surgery if complications arise. Patients with Marfan's syndrome should be treated surgically regardless of the site or age of their dissection. Medical treatment consists of rigorous blood pressure control. It must continue indefinitely for all patients, including those who have undergone surgical correction, as there is a continued risk of re-dissection.

Key Treatment

- β-Blockers
- Surgery

Follow-Up

All patients who survive to be discharged from the hospital require careful lifelong follow-up. Physical examination, chest film, and noninvasive imaging should be performed at 3-month intervals for the first year and twice yearly thereafter. The choice of imaging modality is dependent on availability of technology and expertise.

Bibliography

Cigarroa JE, Isselbacher EM, DeSanctis RW, Eagle KA: Diagnostic imaging in the evaluation of suspected aortic dissection. N Engl J Med 1993;328:35–43.

Crawford ES: The diagnosis and management of aortic dissection. JAMA 1990;264:2537–2541.

Nienaber CA, von Kodolitsch Y, Nicolas V, et al: The diagnosis of thoracic aortic dissection by noninvasive imaging procedures. N Engl J Med 1993;328:1–9.

Slater EE, DeSanctis RW: The clinical recognition of dissecting aortic aneurysm. Am J Med 1976;60:625–633.

Treasure T: Imaging the dissected aorta. Br Heart J 1993; 70:497–498.

70 Endocarditis

Michael S. Bronze

Infective endocarditis (IE) denotes infection of the endocardial surface of the heart, including the valves, septal defects, and the mural endothelium. The designations of acute and subacute endocarditis are often used, but a classification based on the microbiologic etiology is preferable because it has implications for course, complications, and appropriate therapy.

Etiology/Epidemiology

1. Microbiology
   a. Causes of IE are diverse (see Table 70–1).
   b. Less common causes of IE include the following:
      (1) HACEK bacterial group (species of *Haemophilus, Actinobacillus, Cardiobacterium, Eikenella,* and *Kingella*)
      (2) Anaerobes: *Chlamydia, Rickettsia, Brucella, Legionella*
      (3) Viruses (echovirus, coxsackievirus, adenovirus)
   c. Culture-negative IE occurs in 3 to 5 per cent of patients and may be related to
      (1) Prior exposure to antibiotics
      (2) Fastidious organisms or nonbacterial cause (viral or fungal)
      (3) Indolent tricuspid valve disease
2. Frequency of cardiac valve involvement in IE
   a. Per cent isolated: mitral valve >aortic >tricuspid >pulmonic
   b. 3 to 5 per cent have simultaneous left and right heart valves involved
   c. 30 to 35 per cent have concomitant mitral and aortic valve involvement
3. Estimated risk for IE resulting from underlying cardiac lesion
   a. Increased risk
      (1) Prosthetic heart valve
      (2) Congenital heart disease
         (a) Patent ductus
         (b) Ventricular septal defect
         (c) Bicuspid aortic valve
         (d) Coarctation of aorta
      (3) Rheumatic valvular disease
      (4) Mitral valve prolapse with regurgitation
      (5) Prior endocarditis
      (6) Marfan's syndrome
      (7) Isolated valve dysfunction
      (8) Acquired valvular stenosis
      (9) Acquired valvular insufficiency
   b. Low to negligible risk
      (1) Coronary artery disease
      (2) Syphilitic aortitis
      (3) Permanent cardiac pacemaker
      (4) Atrial septal defect
      (5) Mitral valve prolapse without regurgitation

Symptoms

1. The symptoms of IE are the manifestations of the following factors:
   a. The infectious process on the valve leading to valve disruption
   b. Bland or septic emboli
   c. Bacteremia and metastatic infections
   d. Circulating immune complexes
2. They are protean and include fever, chills, sweats, weight loss, malaise, fatigue, and dyspnea.

TABLE 70–1. COMMON CAUSES OF INFECTIVE ENDOCARDITIS

NATIVE VALVE	PROSTHETIC VALVE	IV DRUG ABUSE
Streptococci	Staphylococci	Staphylococci
Staphylococci	Streptococci	Streptococci
Gram-negative rods	Gram-negative rods	Gram-negative rods
	Fungi	Fungi

Clinical Findings

1. Similar to the symptomatology, clinical signs of IE demonstrate varying levels of sensitivity and specificity. Major physical findings include fever (90 to 95 per cent), heart murmur (>80 per cent), embolic phenomena, and signs of congestive heart failure.

2. Less common findings may include splenomegaly, retinal lesions (Roth's spots), signs of metastatic infection (pneumonia, meningitis), and cutaneous signs including splinter hemorrhages, Osler's nodes, Janeway lesions, and petechiae.

Key Signs

- Fever

- Heart murmur

Pathologic Findings

1. Cardiovascular findings may include intracardiac suppuration (valve ring abscess, valvular perforation and rupture, myocardial abscess), valvular stenosis caused by large vegetations, systemic embolization, and mycotic aneurysms.

2. Kidney involvement is common and may consist of renal abscess, renal embolization with infarction, or glomerulonephritis.

3. The central nervous system involvement includes cerebral infarction resulting from embolization, cerebral vasculitis, cerebritis or abscess, meningitis, or intracranial/subarachnoid hemorrhage caused by ruptured mycotic aneurysms.

Laboratory Tests

1. Routine laboratory findings may include
   a. Normocytic anemia (>70 per cent)
   b. Elevated ESR (>90 per cent)
   c. Leukocytosis, monocytosis (>25 per cent)
   d. Proteinuria, pyuria, hematuria (<65 per cent)
   e. Positive blood cultures (>93 per cent)

2. Echocardiography may be useful both as a diagnostic tool and for prognosis. For the diagnosis of IE, the current debate is whether to use transthoracic (TTE) or transesophageal (TEE) echocardiography.

a. Studies suggest that
   (1) TTE has a lower sensitivity but a highly acceptable specificity. A negative TTE does not exclude the diagnosis of IE.
   (2) TEE has improved sensitivity but may have a higher false-positive rate. Uses of TEE may include prosthetic valve endocarditis, confirming the diagnosis of IE in a patient with a negative TTE, and detecting intracardiac suppurative complications such as perivalvular ring abscesses.

b. The role of echocardiography in assessing prognosis has been the focus of several studies, especially those involving patients with right-sided IE. Echocardiographic evidence of large vegetations may indicate an increased risk of embolization, valve disruption with congestive heart failure, and a more prolonged febrile course. However, the presence of visible vegetations by echocardiography does not imply the need for surgery in all cases, treatment failure if the vegetations persist, or the specific organism involved (i.e., fungal).

3. Ancillary imaging tests with anecdotal support, but undefined clinical utility, include gallium-67, gallium–single-photon emission computerized tomography, or indium radionuclide scans.

Key Tests

- Echocardiogram

- Sedimentation rate

Treatment

Antibiotic Therapy

1. Antibiotic therapy for IE should include the following:
   a. Use of parenteral antibiotics that ensure sustained drug levels
   b. Long-term administration, usually for 4 to 6 weeks, to reduce the risk of relapse
   c. Use of synergistic combinations to achieve a bactericidal effect
   d. Selection of antibiotics dictated by the isolated organism and the determined minimum inhibitory concentration (MIC) and minimum bactericidal concentration for the antibiotics used

2. Streptococcal infective endocarditis: Treament of IE caused by streptococci should take into consideration whether the organism is penicillin-

sensitive (MIC <0.2 μg/ml) or pencillin-resistant (MIC >0.5 μg/ml). Streptococci considered to be penicillin-sensitive include most viridans streptococci, *S. bovis*, and group A streptococci, and exclude the group D enterococci.

a. "Penicillin-sensitive"

10 to 20 million units of penicillin G IV daily for 4 weeks (may also include 2 weeks of gentamicin, 1 mg/kg q8h)

or

10 to 20 million units penicillin G IV daily plus gentamicin 1 mg/kg (not to exceed 80 mg IV q8h) for 2 weeks*

or, if penicillin-allergic

Vancomycin, 15 mg/kg IV q12h for 4 weeks

*Two-week course is designed for patients with streptococci with MIC to penicillin ≤0.1 μg/ml in the absence of impaired renal function, complicated course, prosthetic valve IE, or a tolerant strain.

b. "Pencillin-resistant" (includes enterococci)

20 million units penicillin G IV daily plus gentamicin, 1 mg/kg q8h for 6 weeks

or

Ampicillin, 2 gm IV q6h, plus gentamicin for 6 weeks

or

Vancomycin, 15 mg/kg IV q12h, plus gentamicin for 6 weeks

3. Staphylococcal infective endocarditis

a. Recommended regimens should take into consideration that most strains are resistant to penicillin G and may be resistant to methicillin or oxacillin. Antibiotic regimens may include those presented in the following box.

TABLE 70–2. RECOMMENDED ENDOCARDITIS PROPHYLAXIS BY UNDERLYING CARDIAC CONDITION AND PROPOSED PROCEDURES

Underlying Cardiac Conditions
Recommended

High risk	Prosthetic heart valve
	Previous endocarditis
	Complex cyanotic congenital heart disease
Moderate risk	Acquired or congenital valvular heart disease
	Hypertrophic cardiomyopathy
	Mitral valve prolapse with murmur
	Most forms of congenital heart disease
Not recommended	Isolated secundum ASD
	Repaired ASD, VSD, or patent ductus arteriosus
	Previous CABG, cardiac pacemaker
	Mitral valve prolapse without murmur
	Functional heart murmur

Proposed Procedures

Recommended	Dental extractions, implants, root canal
	Periodontal surgery, scaling, dental cleaning
	Tonsillectomy ± adenoidectomy
	Rigid bronchoscopy, respiratory tract surgery
	Esophageal sclerotherapy, dilation
	ERCP, biliary or intestinal tract surgery
	Prostatic surgery, cystoscopy
	Removal of infected intrauterine device
Not recommended	Flexible bronchoscopy even with biopsy
	Gastrointestinal endoscopy even with biopsy
	Transesophageal echocardiography*
	Vaginal hysterectomy or delivery*
	Cesarean section
	Insertion of intrauterine device[†]
	Urinary or urethral catheterization[†]
	Sterilization or therapeutic abortion[†]
	Cardiac catheterization, PTCA, pacemaker

Abbreviations: ASD, atrial septal defect; CABG, coronary artery bypass grafting; ERCP, endoscopic retrograde cholangiopancreatography; PTCA, percutaneous transluminal coronary angioplasty; VSD, ventricular septal defect.
*Optional for high-risk patients.
[†]Implies uninfected tissues or urine.
Modified from Dajani AS, Taubert KA, Wilson W, et al: Prevention of bacterial endocarditis: recommendations by the American Heart Association. Circulation 1997;96:358–366. Copyright 1997 American Medical Association, with permission.

Nafcillin, 1.5 to 2.0 gm IV q4h for 4 to 6 weeks, plus gentamicin, 1 mg/kg IV q8h for 5 to 7 days

or

Vancomycin, 15 mg/kg IV q12h, plus rifampin, 300 mg PO q12h for 4 to 6 weeks, plus gentamicin for 5 to 7 days

or

Cephalothin, 2 gm IV q6h for 4 to 6 weeks, plus gentamicin for 5 to 7 days

---

b. Recently a 2-week regimen consisting of nafcillin and tobramycin has been shown to be effective in uncomplicated right-sided endocarditis caused by methicillin-sensitive *S. aureus* in intravenous (IV) drug abuse–associated IE.

4. Enteric gram-negative bacillus–associated infective endocarditis: Treatment of IE caused by gram-negative aerobic bacilli (e.g., *Escherichia coli, Klebsiella* species, *Proteus* species, *Pseudomonas* species, *Serratia* species) should be dictated by antimicrobial sensitivities. Regimens typically include a cephalosporin or expanded-spectrum penicillin combined with an aminoglycoside continued for 6 weeks. Left-sided endocarditis caused by *Pseudomonas* or *Serratia* species may require a combined medical-surgical approach for cure.

5. Prosthetic valve endocarditis: Prosthetic valve endocarditis (PVE) is often divided into "early" (within 60 days of surgery) or "late" (after 60 days).
   a. Early PVE is most commonly caused by *Staphylococcus epidermidis*, *S. aureus*, *Streptococcus* species, and gram-negative bacilli.
   b. Late PVE is most often associated with viridans streptococci, but can also be due to *Staphylococcus* species, enterococci, and gram-negative bacilli.
   c. Antimicrobial therapy should be based on antimicrobial sensitivities of the isolated organism, but initial therapy should include vancomycin and gentamicin plus rifampin pending results of cultures.

6. Endocarditis in IV drug users: The most commonly isolated organisms include *S. aureus*, streptococci including the enterococci, gram-negative bacilli, and fungi. Empiric coverage pending results of cultures should include nafcillin (or vancomycin) plus gentamicin. Some would advocate adding pencillin or ampicillin for added coverage of enterococci.

TABLE 70–3. ANTIBIOTIC REGIMENS FOR PROPHYLAXIS

ANTIBIOTIC	ADULT	CHILD
Dental, Oral, Respiratory, or Esophageal Procedures*		
No ampicillin allergy		
Amoxicillin	2.0 gm PO	50 mg/kg PO, *or*
Ampicillin	2.0 gm IM/IV	50 mg/kg IM/IV
Ampicillin allergic (choose one):		
Clindamycin	600 mg PO/IV	20 mg/kg PO/IV
Cephalexin/cephazolin	2.0 gm PO/IV	50 mg/kg PO/IV
Azithromycin	500 mg PO	
Genitourinary/Gastrointestinal Procedures*		
No ampicillin allergy		
High risk[†]		
Ampicillin *plus*	2.0 gm IM/IV	50 mg/kg IM/IV
Gentamicin[‡]	1.5 mg/kg IM/IV	1.5 mg/kg IM/IV
Moderate risk		
Amoxicillin	2.0 gm PO	50 mg/kg PO, *or*
Ampicillin	2.0 gm IM/IV	50 mg/kg IM/IV
Ampicillin allergic		
High risk		
Vancomycin *plus*	1.0 gm IV	20 mg/kg IV
Gentamicin[‡]	1.5 mg/kg IM/IV	1.5 mg/kg IM/IV
Moderate risk		
Vancomycin	1.0 gm IV	20 mg/kg IV

*Oral dose given 1 hour prior and IM/IV dose 30 minutes prior to procedure.
[†]Dose of ampicillin (or amoxicillin) and gentamicin should be repeated in 6 hours.
[‡]Gentamicin dose not to exceed 120 mg.
    Modified from Dajani AS, Taubert KA, Wilson W, et al: Prevention of bacterial endocarditis: recommendations by the American Heart Association. Circulation 1997;96:358–366. Copyright 1997 American Medical Association, with permission.

Indications for Surgical Intervention in Infective Endocarditis

Generally accepted indications for surgical therapy in IE include

1. Progressive congestive heart failure
2. Recurrent major embolization
3. Uncontrolled infection or resistant infection (e.g., fungal)
4. Extravalvular intracardiac suppuration (e.g., ring abscess)
5. Selected patients with prosthetic valve endocarditis

Endocarditis Prophylaxis

1. Patients with known cardiac conditions predisposed to the development of IE or patients with previous episodes of IE who undergo certain invasive procedures should be given antibiotic prophylaxis to prevent endocarditis.
2. The decision to recommend prophylaxis is based on the risk of bacteremia from the procedure and the type of underlying cardiac condition (Table 70–2). These conditions and procedures and the recommended antibiotic regimens have been clearly delineated by the American Heart Association (Table 70–3).

Bibliography

Birmingham GD, Rahko PS, Ballantyne F: Improved detection of infective endocarditis with transesophageal echocardiography. Am Heart J 1992;123:774–781.

Dajani AS, Taubert KA, Wilson W, et al: Prevention of bacterial endocarditis: recommendations by the American Heart Association. Circulation 1997;96:358–366.

Durack DT, Lukes AS, Bright DK, and the Duke Endocarditis Service: New criteria for diagnosis of infective endocarditis: utilization of specific echocardiographic findings. Am J Med 1994;96:200–209.

McKinsey DS, Ratts TE, Bisno AL: Underlying cardiac lesions in adults with infective endocarditis: the changing spectrum. Am J Med 1987;82:681–688.

Scheld WM, Sande MA: Endocarditis and intravascular infections. In Mandell GL, Bennett JE, Dolin R (eds): Principles and Practice of Infectious Diseases, 4th ed, pp 740–783. New York, Churchill Livingstone, 1995.

71 Pericarditis

Vishwanatha S. Nadig

Pericarditis, the inflammatory response of the pericardium, results from diverse etiology. It could take the form of acute pericarditis, pericardial effusion, or constrictive pericarditis. Acute pericarditis has an incidence of 2 to 6 per cent. It affects men more than women and adults more than children.

Etiology

1. Acute pericarditis: Important causes of acute pericarditis include infections, myocardial infarction, cardiac surgery, malignancy, uremia, autoimmune disorders, and radiation (Table 71–1).
2. Constrictive pericarditis: usually a complication of acute pericarditis. Common causes of constrictive pericarditis are idiopathic (42 per cent), cardiac surgery (29 per cent), radiotherapy (13 per cent), tuberculosis, uremia, and rheumatoid arthritis.

Symptoms

1. Acute pericarditis: Classically presents with a sharp, intermittent, retrosternal chest pain relieved by sitting up and leaning forward. Pain typically radiates to superior border of scapula but may radiate to neck or arms, simulating myocardial ischemia. Pericardial effusion resulting from acute pericarditis may cause symptoms by compression of adjoining structures (hoarseness, dysphagia, and dyspnea) or by decreasing cardiac output (oliguria and dizziness).
2. Constrictive pericarditis: Thick fibrocalcific scar in constrictive pericarditis limits cardiac output, resulting in symptoms of right-sided heart failure with ascites and peripheral edema. Ninety per cent of patients also experience dyspnea, orthopnea, and cough as a result of left ventricular failure.

Key Symptoms

Acute Pericarditis	Constrictive Pericarditis
• Sharp retrosternal chest pain with pleuritic quality	• Exertional dyspnea, orthopnea
• Radiation to superior scapular border	• Cough
	• Ascites and peripheral edema

Clinical Findings

1. Acute pericarditis
   a. Pericardial friction rub is the characteristic sign of acute pericarditis. This is a high-pitched, superficial scratching sound with systolic, diastolic, and presystolic components. Rub is best heard adjacent to lower left sternal border. Patients who develop atrial fibrillation may lose the presystolic component.
   b. Nonspecific signs include low-grade fever, tachycardia, and tachypnea.
   c. Large pericardial effusion results in absent apical impulse, faint heart sounds, crackles over lung bases, and *Ewart's sign* (dullness on percussion over inferior angle of scapula).
2. Constrictive pericarditis
   a. Signs of right-sided failure: increased jugular venous distention, hepatomegaly, peripheral edema, and ascites
   b. With inspiration the neck veins become more prominent (Kussmaul's sign).
   c. Early diastolic pericardial knock best heard

TABLE 71–1. ETIOLOGY OF PERICARDITIS

1. Idiopathic
2. Infectious agents
   a. Viral: coxsackie, varicella, influenza, human immunodeficiency virus, hepatitis B viruses
   b. Bacterial: *Staphylococcus, Streptococcus, Mycobacterium, Pneumococcus, Gonococcus*
   c. Fungal: *Histoplasma, Candida, Blastomyces*
   d. Parasitic: *Echinococcus, Cysticercus,* ameba
3. Autoimmune disorders: systemic lupus erythematosus, rheumatic fever, rheumatoid arthritis, and polyarteritis nodosa
4. Neoplasms: lung cancer, breast cancer, lymphoma-leukemia
5. Radiation
6. Uremic pericarditis
7. Hypersensitivity: post–myocardial infarction, postsurgical
8. Drugs: procainamide, hydralazine, methysergide, penicillins, and the like
9. Miscellaneous: myxedema, chylopericardium, sarcoidosis, amyloidosis, regional enteritis

along left sternal border is characteristic of constrictive pericarditis.

Key Signs

Acute Pericarditis	Constrictive Pericarditis
• Pericardial friction rub	• Jugular venous distention
• Tachycardia	• Positive Kussmaul's sign
	• Pericardial knock, right ventricular failure

Laboratory Tests

1. Electrocardiography (ECG): Four stages of ECG changes are classically described in acute pericarditis.

   a. Stage I: ST segment elevation in all leads except aVR and V1, which show reciprocal ST segment depression.

   b. Stage II and Stage III: PR segment depression is seen approximately 2 weeks after the onset of disease. This is followed by T wave inversion.

   c. Stage IV: Normalization of ST and PR segment and T wave changes observed usually 4 weeks after the onset of disease.

2. Routine laboratory tests: Leukocytosis and an elevated erythrocyte sedimentation rate are seen in acute pericarditis. Routine laboratory tests will be normal in constrictive pericarditis.

3. Radiography

   a. Chest radiograph: entirely normal in acute pericarditis; may show enlarged cardiac shadow if there is a moderate-sized pericardial effusion. Chest radiographic findings in patients who have constrictive pericarditis include pulmonary edema (85 per cent), pleural effusion (85 per cent), left atrial enlargement (85 per cent), cardiomegaly (65 per cent), and calcification (43 per cent).

   b. Computerized tomography and magnetic resonance imaging may aid in diagnosis of constrictive pericarditis.

4. Cardiac catheterization: very useful in differentiating constrictive pericarditis and cardiac tamponade from restrictive cardiomyopathy

   a. In cardiac tamponade, pulmonary wedge and left ventricular pressures are elevated. On jugular venous examination, X descent is preserved in the absence of Y descent.

   b. In constrictive pericarditis, a dip-and-plateau configuration (square root sign) is classically seen on the ventricular tracings. The diastolic pressures in all four cardiac chambers will be equal.

5. Echocardiography is the gold standard for diagnosing pericardial effusion. Echocardiography can detect as little as 20 ml of fluid in the pericardial space. Moderate effusions (>300 ml) demonstrate an echo-free space both posterior and anterior to the left ventricular wall. Collapse of the right ventricular and right atrial cavities during diastole is the characteristic echocardiographic finding in cardiac tamponade. In constrictive pericarditis, M-mode echocardiography demonstrates multiple dense echoes (indicative of calcification) and two parallel lines (representing two pericardial layers) separated by clear space.

6. Pericardiocentesis with pericardial biopsy as a diagnostic tool is rarely indicated. Fluid should be examined for tuberculosis, neoplasia, and autoimmune disorders.

Key Tests

Acute Pericarditis	Constrictive Pericarditis
• ECG: diffuse ST segment depression, PR segment depression, T wave inversion	• ECG: low voltage in all the leads, P mitrale
• Echocardiogram: pericardial effusion	• Chest radiograph: ring calcification, cardiomegaly
	• Cardiac catheterization: square root sign, equalization of diastolic pressures in all four chambers

Differential Diagnosis

1. Acute pericarditis: Accurate clinical examination together with appropriate diagnostic tests will help to distinguish acute pericarditis from other acute chest pain syndromes (dissecting aneurysm, acute coronary syndromes, pneumothorax, pulmonary infarction, and esophageal rupture).

2. Constrictive pericarditis: Clinically it is very difficult to distinguish constrictive pericarditis from restrictive cardiomyopathy. Echocardiography and cardiac catheterization will aid in differentiating these two conditions.

Treatment

1. Acute pericarditis: Patients presenting with acute pericarditis should be monitored as inpatients to exclude acute coronary syndromes or other fatal chest pain syndromes. Nonsteroidal anti-inflammatory drugs (NSAIDs) including indomethacin, ibuprofen, and aspirin, will achieve adequate analgesia. If pain persists beyond 48 hours, a different analgesic should be prescribed. Steroids should be used with caution because sudden steroid withdrawal may result in recurrent disabling chest pain. Treatment of underlying cause of pericarditis should be pursued.

2. Constrictive pericarditis: Total pericardiectomy remains the only effective therapy for constrictive pericarditis. Even though cardiac hemodynamics may not return to normal, 90 per cent of patients will experience significant symptomatic improvement within 6 months. Because of significant perioperative mortality (up to 14 per cent), elderly patients should be managed conservatively. Inadequate response to surgery is usually due to incomplete removal, extension to epicardium, or involvement of myocardium.

Diet

There are no dietary restrictions for acute pericarditis or constrictive pericarditis.

Activity

Patients with acute pericarditis need adequate bed rest until their pain abates. Constrictive pericarditis patients who experience significant dyspnea should not exert themselves until after the surgery.

Patient Education

Patients should be forewarned against potential complications of acute pericarditis, such as recurrences, cardiac tamponade, and constrictive pericarditis.

Key Treatment

Acute Pericarditis	Constrictive Pericarditis
NSAIDs: aspirin, indomethacin	Surgery: pericardiectomy

Follow-Up

1. Acute pericarditis: Acute pericarditis is a self-limiting disease with complete remission within 4 to 6 weeks. Recurrent pericarditis is the most common complication (28 per cent) followed by cardiac tamponade and chronic pericarditis. Initial clinical follow-up should be as frequent as every 2 weeks. Prompt echocardiography is warranted if there is any early sign of tamponade.

2. Constrictive pericarditis: Majority of patients (90 per cent) achieve symptomatic relief within 2 to 6 months. Postsurgical follow-up is needed to identify remaining 10 per cent who fail to improve because of above-mentioned causes. Frequent monitoring is also required for elderly patients who are managed conservatively.

Bibliography

For more information on acute pericarditis, pericardial effusion, and cardiac tamponade, see

Lorrell BH: Pericardial disease. In Braunwald E (ed): Heart Disease, 5th ed, pp 1479–1534. Philadelphia, WB Saunders Company, 1997.

Shabetai R: Disease of the pericardium. In Schlant RC, Alexander RW (eds): The Heart, pp 1647–1674. New York, McGraw Hill, 1994.

For more information on constrictive pericarditis, see

Fowler NO: Constrictive pericarditis: new aspects. Am J Cardiology 1982;50:1014–1017.

Restrictive cardiomyopathy or constrictive pericarditis? [editorial]. Lancet 1987;2:372.

Shabetai R: Diseases of pericardium. Cardiol Clin 1990; 8:621–622.

72 Sinus Rhythms and Ectopic Beats

Milind R. Dhond

A cardiac arrhythmia is a rhythm other than normal sinus rhythm. Cardiac arrhythmias can be caused by the spectrum of cardiac disease: ischemic, hypertensive, valvular, inflammatory, congenital, or primary myocardial disease. In addition, noncardiac diseases (pulmonary or metabolic abnormalities), drugs (e.g., digoxin, diuretics, sympathomimetics, psychotropic agents), and the postoperative state are frequently arrhythmogenic.

The key to the diagnosis of cardiac arrhythmias is a systematic approach to interpretation of the electrocardiogram (ECG), as outlined in Table 72–1.

Sinus Rhythms

Normal Sinus Rhythm
This is the normal rhythm of the heart at a rate of 60 to 100 beats/minute (bpm).

ECG Features
1. P wave upright in leads II, III, and aVF, inverted in aVR (axis 15 to 75 degrees)
2. PR interval is 0.12 to 0.20 second. A QRS complex follows each P wave (1:1 conduction).
3. Constant PP and PR intervals

Sinus Bradycardia
1. Defined as sinus rhythm at a rate less than 60 bpm.
2. Caused by a decrease in the normal rate of discharge of the sinoatrial (SA) node.
3. Can be a physiologic alteration in trained athletes as a result of increased vagal tone.
4. Pathologic causes include sinus node disease, inferior myocardial infarction, hypothyroidism, elevated intracranial pressure, or drugs (β-adrenergic blockers or certain calcium channel blockers).

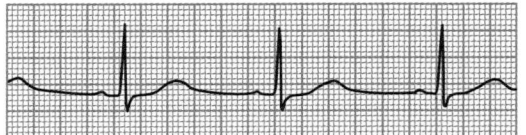

Sinus Bradycardia

ECG Features
1. P wave rate is less than 60 bpm, with constant PP and PR intervals.

2. P wave vector is normal.
3. Each P wave is followed by a QRS complex (1:1 conduction).

Treatment
1. Only indicated for hemodynamic compromise or symptoms
2. Atropine sulfate intravenously (IV) in 0.5- to 1.0-mg boluses
3. Isoproterenol IV at 1 to 4 μg/minute
4. Calcium chloride 10% IV in 100- to 500-mg boluses in cases of calcium channel blocker toxicity
5. Glucagon IV in 2- to 4-mg boluses in cases of β-blocker toxicity

Sinus Tachycardia
1. Defined as sinus rhythm at a rate greater than 100 bpm.
2. Caused by an increase in the normal rate of discharge of the SA node.
3. Can be a physiologic response in conditions that increase sympathetic nervous system tone, such as exercise, pain, or anxiety.
4. Pathologic causes include hypovolemia, cardiac failure, pulmonary embolism, fever, thyrotoxicosis, or drugs (e.g., sympathomimetic agents, dihydropyridine calcium channel blockers, cocaine).

TABLE 72–1. APPROACH TO ECG INTERPRETATION

P Wave Analysis
- Are P waves present? At what rate? Is the PR interval normal?
- Do the P waves have a normal morphology and axis? (e.g., are they upright in the inferior leads?)
- Is atrial fibrillation or atrial flutter present?

QRS Analysis
- What is the QRS rate? Is each QRS complex associated with a P wave (1:1 conduction)?
- Is the P wave before, after, or part of the QRS complex?
- Is the QRS complex narrow or wide?

Interval Analysis
- Are the PP, PR, RR, and QT intervals normal? (*Note*: Familiarity with normal values is essential.)

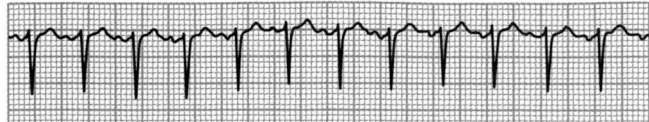

Sinus Tachycardia

ECG Features

1. P wave rate is 100 to 160 bpm, with constant PP and PR intervals.
2. P wave vector is normal.
3. Each P wave is followed by a QRS complex (1:1 conduction).

Treatment

1. Treatment, if indicated, is directed at the underlying cause.
2. Rarely β-blockers may be used to reduce the heart rate.

Sinus Arrhythmia

1. Related to a reflex decrease in vagal tone caused by inspiration and a reflex increase in vagal tone during expiration, resulting in an increase in heart rate during inspiration and a decrease during expiration.
2. A normal phenomenon in young individuals; occasionally occurs in the elderly.
3. Accentuated by digoxin.

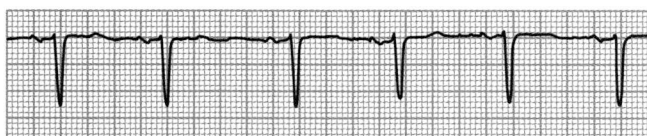

Sinus Arrhythmia (Variable R–R interval)

ECG Features

1. Each P wave is followed by a QRS complex (1:1 conduction).
2. Normal P wave vector
3. Cyclical increase and decrease in the PP interval with respiration
4. PP interval does not vary by more than 0.16 second.

Treatment

No specific treatment required.

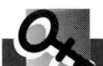

Ectopic Beats

An ectopic beat is defined as an impulse arising outside the sinus node. If the ectopic beat is earlier than the next anticipated sinus beat, it is a premature ectopic beat; if it occurs later than the next sinus beat, it is an escape ectopic beat. It can be an atrial, junctional, or ventricular ectopic beat, depending on its site of origin.

Atrial Ectopic Beats

1. This ectopic form results from a premature atrial impulse that originates within the atria but outside the SA node.
2. Most atrial ectopic beats (AEBs) conduct normally through the atrioventricular node (AV) and into the ventricles.
3. If the impulse is early, it may encounter the AV node when it is partially or totally refractory. Partial refractoriness of the AV node leads to prolongation of the PR interval, while complete refractoriness leads to a nonconducted (or blocked) AEB.
4. Partial or complete refractoriness affecting one of the bundle branches can lead to "phasic aberrant ventricular conduction," or a P wave followed by a QRS complex with a bundle-branch block (BBB) pattern (usually a right BBB).
5. Premature AEBs may be caused by increased sympathetic drive, smoking, alcohol, fatigue, or drugs (e.g., β-agonists, theophylline).

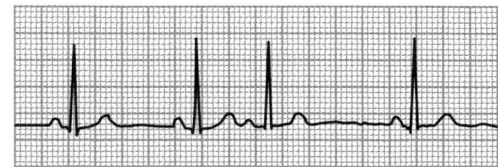

Atrial Ectopic Beat (3rd beat is AEB)

ECG Features

1. P wave is premature and morphologically abnormal.

2. PR interval may be prolonged by a partially refractory AV node.

3. P wave may not have QRS complex after it (completely refractory node). (*Note*: P wave may be superimposed on the preceding T wave.)

4. QRS morphology is normal or may have a BBB pattern.

Treatment

1. Usually benign, requiring no specific treatment.

2. If very frequent, β-blockers can be used to decrease atrial automaticity.

Junctional Ectopic Beats

1. This beat originates from an ectopic focus arising in the AV junction or bundle of His. It is not possible to distinguish between the two types on the surface ECG. Premature junctional beats are, by definition, earlier than the next anticipated sinus beat.

2. The junctional ectopic impulse may depolarize both the atria (by retrograde conduction) and the ventricle (by antegrade conduction), leading to a premature QRS complex with normal morphology. If aberrant conduction is present, the QRS complex will be wide.

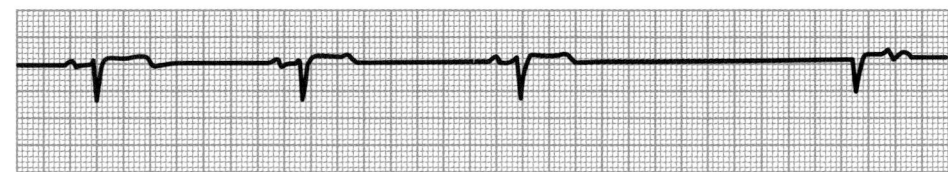

Junctional Ectopic (Escape) Beat
(Fourth beat is junctional escape with P wave appearing after QRS complex)

ECG Features

1. P wave precedes, follows, or is concealed in the QRS complex (if the P wave precedes the QRS complex, it is inverted in the inferior leads).

2. QRS complex is premature but has normal morphology.

3. QRS complex is followed by an incomplete compensatory pause.

Treatment

Uncommon and typically benign; usually no specific treatment indicated.

Ventricular Ectopic Beats

1. Ventricular ectopic beats (VEB) arise in the Purkinje cells of the left or right ventricle and may be due to enhanced automaticity, a re-entry mechanism, or after-depolarizations.

   a. Those arising in the right ventricle have a left BBB morphology; those arising in the left ventricle have a right BBB morphology.

   b. VEB arising from the same focus (unifocal) have the same QRS morphology and coupling interval with the preceding normal QRS complex.

   c. Those arising from different ventricular foci (multifocal) have differing QRS morphologies and coupling intervals.

2. The ectopic beat can occur early or late in the cardiac cycle.

   a. When it occurs early and is superimposed on the T wave of the preceding complex, it is referred to as an "R-on-T" beat. Because the vulnerable period (interval during which a stimulus can produce repetitive ventricular firing) of the ventricle occurs during the T wave, R-on-T beats are capable of initiating ventricular tachycardia and fibrillation, especially in the presence of underlying cardiac disease.

   b. Late VEB may occur even after the next P wave, and can sometimes be mistaken for premature atrial beats.

3. *Bigeminy* is the term given to VEB that follow each sinus beat; *trigeminy* describes VEB that follow every two sinus beats.

4. VEB can be benign or may be caused by structural heart disease, drugs, or metabolic abnormalities. Frequent multifocal or R-on-T VEB are commonly related to underlying cardiac disease and may be associated with increased cardiac events and mortality.

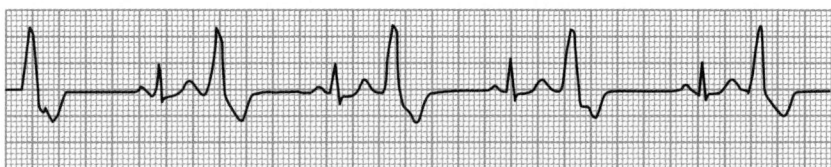

Ventricular Ectopic Beats (Unifocal)
(Bigeminal rhythm with alternating VEBs)

ECG Features

1. Wide QRS complex (≥0.12 second) usually followed by compensatory pause
2. ST-T wave of VEB abnormal (abnormal depolarization → abnormal repolarization).

Treatment

1. Indicated for symptoms or when high-grade, postmyocardial infarction (e.g., three or more consecutive VEB)
2. Lidocaine IV in 50- to 100-mg bolus, then infusion at 1 to 2 mg/minute
3. β-Blockers may be effective in symptomatic individuals.

Escape Beats

1. Usually arise when there is a pause or slowing of the dominant rhythm. The site of origin is the next highest subsidiary pacemaker tissue.
2. Usually junctional in origin, but ventricular escape beats can occur.

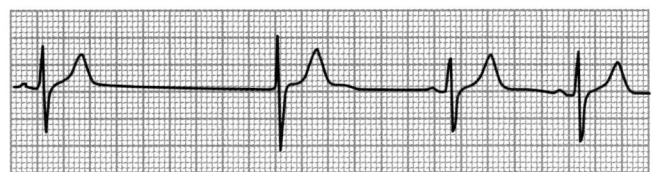

Sinus Arrest With Junctional Escape Beat (second beat)

ECG Features

1. QRS similar to sinus rhythm (junctional escape beat).
2. QRS similar to VEB (ventricular escape beat).
3. Coupling interval greater than cycle length of dominant rhythm.

Treatment

No treatment except for the underlying cause of the bradycardia

Bibliography

Amsterdam EA: Premature beats. In Rakel RE (ed): Conn's Current Therapy, pp 265–268. Philadelphia, WB Saunders Company, 1997.

Bennet DH: Cardiac Arrhythmias, 3rd ed. London, Wright, 1989.

Charles RG, Marshall AJ: Arrhythmias. In Cardiology, pp 1–45. Oxford, England, Heinemann, 1989.

Heger JW, Fernando Roth R, Niemann JT, et al: Arrhythmias. In Cardiology, 3rd ed, pp 30–76. Baltimore, Williams & Wilkins, 1994.

Zipes DP: Specific arrhythmias: diagnosis and treatment. In Braunwald E (ed): Heart Disease, 5th ed, pp 640–704. Philadelphia, WB Saunders Company, 1997.

73 Supraventricular Tachyarrhythmias

Milind R. Dhond

A supraventricular tachycardia (SVT) is defined as a tachycardia that arises above the bundle of His. The two main mechanisms for SVT are re-entry or enhanced automaticity. The re-entrant type of SVT is usually initiated by an ectopic beat and tends to have a sudden onset and termination (i.e., it is paroxysmal). Conversely, the less common, enhanced automaticity type of SVT is more sustained and characterized by a gradual increase in heart rate. SVT can be broadly divided into those involving the atria (atrial tachycardia, flutter, and fibrillation) and those involving the atrioventricular (AV) junction (junctional, AV node re-entry, and AV re-entry).

Atrial Tachycardia

1. Atrial tachycardia has an atrial rate of 150 to 200 beats/minute (bpm).
2. Can result from enhanced automaticity or re-entry. A sudden onset preceded by an atrial ectopic beat suggests a re-entry mechanism.
3. The P wave is abnormal and, when it is irregular and has three or more different morphologies, the arrhythmia is termed *multifocal atrial tachycardia* (MAT). MAT is typically associated with a rapid, irregular ventricular response.
4. Because of the rapid atrial rate in atrial tachycardia not all atrial beats are conducted to the ventricles, and varying degrees of AV block may occur (see AV block below).
5. Atrial tachycardia is frequently associated with chronic lung disease, metabolic abnormalities, or drugs (e.g., digitalis, sympathomimetic agents).

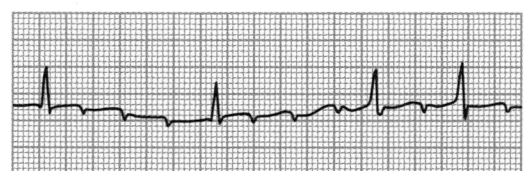

Atrial Tachycardia With Variable AV Conduction

Electrocardiographic (ECG) Features

1. P wave rate 150 to 200 bpm.
2. QRS rate equal to, or less than, atrial rate if AV block present.
3. Three or more P wave morphologies suggest MAT.

Treatment

1. Stop digoxin or other cardiac-stimulating drug if toxicity suspected.
2. AV nodal blocking agents such as calcium-channel blockers (CCB) or β-blockers
3. Treat underlying condition.
4. Rarely, rapid atrial pacing (RAP) or direct current (DC) cardioversion may be required.

Atrial Flutter

1. A regular atrial rate of 250 to 350 bpm, usually with a significant AV conduction deficit (e.g., 2:1, 3:1, 4:1).
2. Usually associated with structural heart disease; common postoperatively following thoracotomy.
3. Atrial depolarizations (flutter waves) have a "sawtooth" pattern and are best seen in ECG lead V1 or the inferior leads.
4. Diagnostically, carotid sinus massage (CSM) or IV adenosine may be used to increase the degree of AV block and help to distinguish flutter waves.

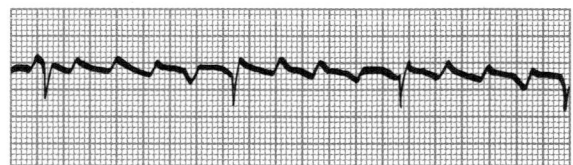

Atrial Flutter With 4:1 AV Conduction

ECG Features

1. Atrial rate 250 to 350 bpm ("sawtooth" pattern)
2. AV conduction deficit (typically 2:1) usually present.
3. The ventricular rate is not regular if the AV conduction deficit varies.
4. Diagnostic maneuvers include CSM and IV adenosine, 6 mg (up to 18 mg).

Treatment

1. AV nodal blockers to reduce ventricular rate (CCB, β-blockers; digoxin less effective)
2. DC cardioversion or RAP for hemodynamic compromise

Atrial Fibrillation

1. The most common sustained arrhythmia
2. Results from disorganized atrial electrical activity (rate 350 to 600 bpm) without effective atrial contraction. Because of the refractory period of the AV node, not all atrial impulses are conducted to the ventricles and the ventricular rate usually does not exceed 200 bpm.
3. Ventricular rates of greater than 250 bpm suggest the presence of a concealed bypass tract through which the impulses are being conducted to the ventricles.
4. Usually caused by structural heart disease. Noncardiac causes include thyrotoxicosis, pulmonary embolism, alcohol abuse, or the postoperative state.
5. Because of the significant risk of systemic embolization, almost all cases (except lone atrial fibrillation, i.e., no structural heart disease, in patients <65 years old) require anticoagulation.
6. Tends to occur in younger patients with less cardiovascular disease and fewer co-morbid conditions. The risk of stroke is probably less, but co-morbid conditions should be considered in assessing the indications for anticoagulation.

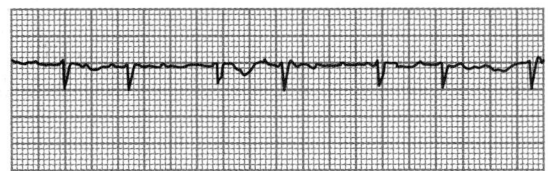

Atrial Fibrillation

ECG Features

1. No P waves, irregularly irregular QRS complexes.
2. Undulations of baseline; occasionally flat baseline between each QRS-T wave group may be seen.
3. QRS rate usually less than 200 bpm.

Treatment

Management can be selected from several options, depending on the individual factors in each case.

1. Conversion to normal sinus rhythm (NSR)
   a. Treatment with 3 to 6 weeks of anticoagulation prior to, and following, chemical or electrical cardioversion; *or* transesophageal echocardiography demonstrating absence of atrial thrombi, followed by electrical cardioversion and short-term (3 to 6 weeks) anticoagulation
   b. Treatment with amiodarone, sotalol, or propafenone should be considered prior to electrical cardioversion to facilitate conversion to NSR.

   c. Chronic prophylaxis with one of these agents will be required in most patients with structural heart disease to maintain NSR.
   d. Treat underlying cause (e.g., thyrotoxicosis) before cardioversion.
2. Long-term anticoagulation and ventricular rate control in chronic atrial fibrillation with CCB or β-blocker (digoxin in patients with poor left ventricular function)
3. Emergency electrical cardioversion in patients with hemodynamic compromise
4. Paroxysmal atrial fibrillation without structural heart disease and co-morbid conditions can be treated with aspirin, 325 mg/day. In the older patient with structural heart disease and co-morbid conditions (e.g., hypertension, left ventricular dysfunction, diabetes mellitus), consideration should be given to initiating Coumadin therapy.

Junctional Tachycardia

1. Results from enhanced automaticity of the AV junction; tends to have a gradual onset (non-paroxysmal).
2. Associated with digoxin toxicity
3. If the junctional tachycardia activates both the atria and ventricles, there is an inverted P wave associated with each QRS complex. If no retrograde atrial activation occurs, the atrial activity is independent of the QRS activity and AV dissociation is present.

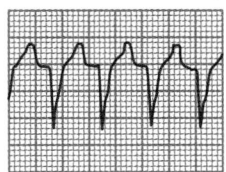

Junctional Tachycardia
(P waves not seen)

ECG Features

1. QRS complex normal/slightly prolonged.
2. QRS rate 100 to 160 bpm.
3. P wave inverted, precedes or follows QRS complex (retrograde atrial activation).
4. AV dissociation (no retrograde atrial activation)

Treatment

1. Stop digoxin if toxicity suspected; correct electrolyte abnormalities.
2. If hemodynamically stable, no treatment usually needed.

AV Nodal Re-Entrant Tachycardias (AVNRT)

1. Caused by a re-entry circuit occurring entirely within the AV node at a rate of 150 to 250 bpm

2. Sudden onset and termination
3. Often preceded by a premature atrial ectopic beat with a prolonged PR interval.
4. Usually occurs in patients with no structural heart disease.
5. Accounts for the great majority of SVT originating in junctional or AV nodal tissue.

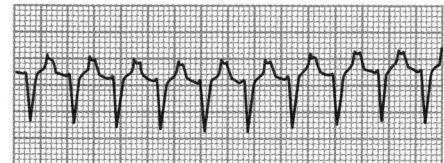

AV Nodal Reentry Tachycardia
(P wave superimposed on T wave)

ECG Features

1. QRS rate 150 to 250 bpm, narrow QRS complex
2. QRS complex prolonged ($\geq$0.12 second) if pre-existing bundle-branch block or aberrant conduction.
3. Inverted P waves seen in or after QRS complex (P waves can sometimes appear as "pseudo R-prime" in V1).

Treatment

1. Acutely: CSM, IV adenosine, CCB, β-blocker, or digoxin
2. DC cardioversion or RAP
3. Prevention with oral CCB, β-blocker, digoxin; rarely requires amiodarone, sotalol, or propafenone.
4. Definitive therapy with selective radiofrequency ablation of AV nodal tissue

AV Re-Entrant Tachycardia (AVRT)

1. Usually cause by re-entry over a retrogradely conducting (extranodal) accessory pathway and has rates of 200 bpm or higher. A common type is the Wolf-Parkinson-White (WPW) syndrome, with antegrade and retrograde conduction over an accessory pathway.
2. If antegrade conduction occurs through the bypass tract during sinus rhythm, a "delta" wave is seen on the ECG. If only retrograde conduction is possible through the bypass tract, the QRS complex will appear normal during NSR and is termed an AVRT with a concealed bypass tract.

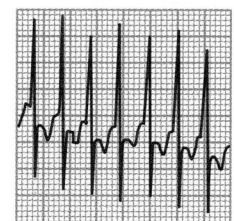

AV Reentrant Tachycardia
(no P waves seen)

ECG Features

1. QRS complex normal or with "delta" wave, rate greater than 200 bpm.
2. Inverted P waves may be seen in or after the QRS complex (concealed bypass tract).
3. Beat-to-beat variation in amplitude of QRS complex (usually in bypass tract)

Treatment

1. CSM, IV adenosine, CCB, or β-blocker (caution in WPW because these agents may slow conduction in AV node and enhance conduction in bypass tract)
2. DC cardioversion or RAP
3. Definitive treatment is radiofrequency ablation.

Bibliography

Amsterdam EA: Premature beats. In Rakel RE (ed): Conn's Current Therapy, pp 265–268. Philadelphia, WB Saunders Company, 1997.

Bennet DH: Cardiac Arrhythmias, 3rd ed. London, Wright, 1989.

Charles RG, Marshall AJ: Arrhythmias. In Cardiology, pp 1–45. Oxford, England, Heinemann, 1989.

Heger JW, Fernando Roth R, Niemann JT, et al: Arrhythmias. In Cardiology, 3rd ed, pp 30–76. Baltimore, Williams & Wilkins, 1994.

Laupacis A, Albers G, Dalen J, et al: Antithrombotic therapy in atrial fibrillation. Chest 1998;114:579S–589S.

Zipes DP: Specific arrhythmias: diagnosis and treatment. In Braunwald E (ed): Heart Disease, 5th ed, pp 640–704. Philadelphia, WB Saunders Company, 1997.

74 Ventricular Tachyarrhythmias

Ezra A. Amsterdam

1. Ventricular tachycardias (VT) are defined as three or more ventricular ectopic beats occurring at a rate of 100 to 250 beats/minute (bpm).
2. Can be monomorphic or polymorphic (e.g., torsades de pointes)
3. The mechanism is usually re-entry but it can also be increased automaticity or after-depolarizations.
4. Usually occurs in patients with structural heart disease (see Ch. 72, Sinus Rhythms and Ectopic Beats) as well as the post–cardiac surgery state, drug toxicity, or electrolyte abnormalities. The latter two can cause a prolonged QT interval, which promotes VT.
5. A relatively benign form of VT is accelerated idioventricular rhythm (AIVR), which is non-paroxysmal and due to enhanced automaticity. This usually occurs as an escape rhythm (rate 60 to 100 bpm) during sinus rate slowing and requires no treatment. AIVR is common in the first 48 hours after acute myocardial infarction, is usually benign, and is typically self-limited.

Monomorphic VT

1. The most common type of VT
2. Characterized by wide but uniformly shaped QRS complexes in a regular rhythm
3. The atria may be retrogradely activated and an inverted P wave may be seen (usually concealed) in the QRS complex
4. Retrograde atrial conduction may not occur, in which case the sinus node fires independently of the VT and at a slower rate (atrioventricular [AV] dissociation). Evidence of this can be seen by the presence of *independent P waves* and capture or fusion beats.
   a. A *capture beat* is due to a normally conducted atrial impulse activating the ventricle before the next anticipated ventricular impulse from the VT. It appears as a narrow QRS complex in the VT.
   b. A *fusion beat* is due to simultaneous activation of separate regions of the ventricle by both the normal atrial impulse and the ventricular focus, leading to a QRS complex that is a blend of the two.
5. The above features aid in differentiating VT from supraventricular tachycardia with aberrant conduction.
6. VT commonly causes hemodynamic compromise and is potentially lethal if not terminated.

Electrocardiographic (ECG) Features

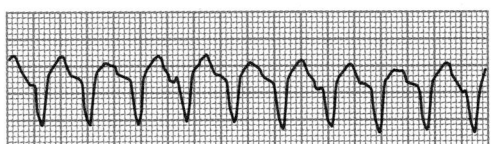

Monomorphic Ventricular Tachycardia

1. QRS complex longer than 0.12 second, with uniform morphology.
2. Independent P waves (AV dissociation)
3. Fusion or capture beats

Treatment

1. IV lidocaine, 50- to 100-mg bolus, followed by a continuous infusion (1 to 2 mg/minute)
2. IV procainamide or IV amiodarone as second-line agents
3. Direct current (DC) cardioversion for hemodynamic compromise
4. Consider overdrive ventricular pacing.
5. Long-term therapy consists of oral antiarrhythmics, implantable cardioverter-defibrillator, or radiofrequency ablation.

Polymorphic VT (Torsades de Pointes)

1. Usually occurs at faster rates (200 to 250 bpm), with QRS complexes of differing morphologies that "twist" around the baseline.
2. Defined as a polymorphic VT associated with a prolonged QT interval prior to the VT.
3. Caution is required in treating this arrhythmia because it can be exacerbated by antiarrhythmic drugs.
4. In addition to structural heart disease, this type of VT is promoted by conditions that prolong the QT interval, such as bradycardia (e.g., sinus node dysfunction or AV block), as well as congenital QT prolongation, type I antiarrhythmic agents, hypokalemia, or tricyclic antidepressants.

ECG Features

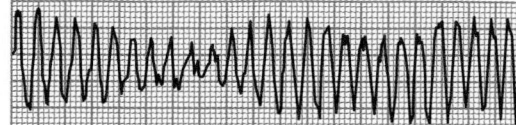

Torsades de Pointes

1. Prolonged QT interval prior to VT
2. QRS complexes of differing amplitude "twisting" about the baseline.

Treatment

1. IV magnesium sulfate, 1 to 2 gm over several minutes

2. Treat underlying electrolyte abnormalities (hypokalemia, hypomagnesemia).
3. Discontinue antiarrhythmic drugs.
4. Ventricular pacing.
5. Atropine, isoproterenol.

Ventricular Fibrillation

1. A terminal arrhythmia reflecting complete absence of any organized electrical activity of the ventricles
2. Associated with absence of effective cardiac contractile function
3. Frequently follows degeneration of VT.

ECG Features

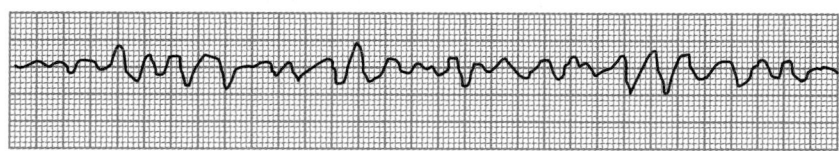

Ventricular Fibrillation

Coarse, undulating baseline with no recognizable wave forms

Treatment

Emergency cardiopulmonary resuscitation and electrical cardioversion

Bibliography

Amsterdam EA: Premature beats. In Rakel RE (ed): Conn's Current Therapy, pp 265–268. Philadelphia, WB Saunders Company, 1997.

Bennet DH: Cardiac Arrhythmias, 3rd ed. London, Wright, 1989.
Charles RG, Marshall AJ: Arrhythmias. In Cardiology, pp 1–45. Oxford, England, Heinemann, 1989.
Heger JW, Fernando Roth R, Niemann JT, et al: Arrhythmias. In Cardiology, 3rd ed, pp 30–76. Baltimore, Williams & Wilkins, 1994.
Zipes DP: Specific arrhythmias: diagnosis and treatment. In Braunwald E (ed): Heart Disease, 5th ed, pp 640–704. Philadelphia, WB Saunders Company, 1997.

75 Atrioventricular Block and Sick Sinus Syndrome

Ezra A. Amsterdam

Atrioventricular Block

1. Atrioventricular block (AV) is due to failure of normal conduction between the atria and ventricles, with block occurring in the AV node, bundle of His, bundle branches, or a combination of these sites.
2. It may be caused by structural heart disease or drug toxicity.

First-Degree AV Block

1. Benign but may progress to higher degrees of block depending on the etiology
2. The site of block is usually in the AV node but can occasionally occur in the bundle of His.

Electrocardiographic (ECG) Features

1. PR interval prolonged (>0.20 second).
2. Each P wave is followed by QRS complex.

Treatment

No treatment indicated.

Second-Degree AV Block

This consists of two types: Mobitz I (Wenckebach), with block occurring at the AV node, and Mobitz II, with block occurring in the His-Purkinje system.

1. Mobitz I block
   a. Characterized by progressive prolongation of the PR interval leading to a P wave not conducted to the ventricle (dropped beat).
   b. If two sinus beats with gradual PR prolongation are followed by a dropped beat, 3:2 block is present. This leads to the occurrence of "group beating."
   c. Can be caused by physiologically increased vagal tone; digoxin, β-blocker, or calcium channel blocker toxicity; or inferior myocardial infarction (MI) causing AV node ischemia and/or vagotonia (Bezold-Jarisch reflex).
2. Mobitz II block
   a. Characterized by intermittent failure of conduction of sinus impulses to the ventricles with no prior prolongation of the PR interval.
   b. Can be caused by structural heart disease, extensive anterior MI, and degenerative conduction system disease (Lev's disease).

c. Because it involves the Purkinje system and bundle branches, it is associated with a wide QRS complex and with progression to third-degree AV block, Stokes-Adams attacks, and sudden death.

ECG Features

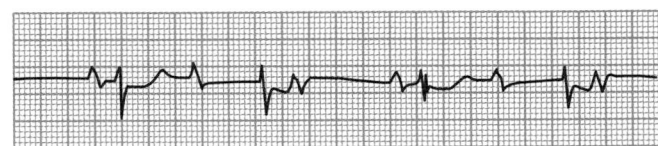

Second–Degree Mobitz I Heart Block (Wenckebach) (Progressive PR interval prolongation with non-conducted third P wave)

1. Mobitz I
   a. PR interval gradually lengthens before dropped beat; QRS complex narrow or wide.
   b. "Group beating"

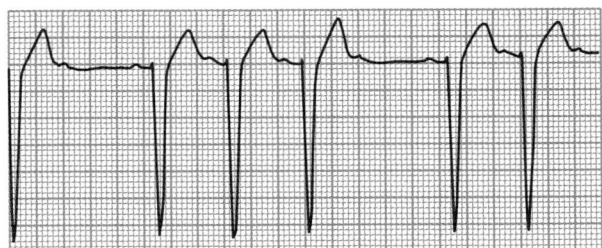

Second–Degree Mobitz II Heart Block (Non-conducted first and fifth P waves, no PR prolongation)

2. Mobitz II
   a. Intermittent loss of conduction of P wave, no PR interval prolongation
   b. QRS complex wide.

Treatment

1. Mobitz I
   a. Usually no treatment needed.
   b. If hemodynamically unstable, consider IV atropine sulfate, 0.5 mg prn.
   c. Discontinue AV nodal blocking drugs.
2. Mobitz II: Requires temporary or permanent cardiac pacing.

Third-Degree AV Block

1. Occurs when there is total interruption of conduction from atria to ventricles.

2. If the level of the block is at the AV node, a stable junctional escape pacemaker usually initiates ventricular contraction at a rate of 40 to 60 beats/minute (bpm).

3. If the level of the block is at the bundle branch–Purkinje system, the subsidiary pacemaker is idioventricular, with a rate of 20 to 40 bpm, and is less stable.

ECG Features

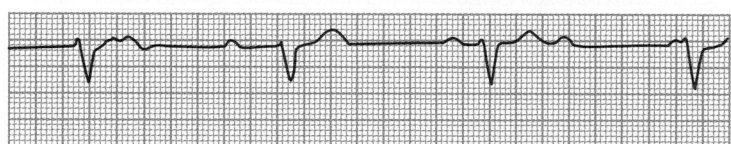

Third–Degree Heart Block
(P wave rate slower than QRS rate with P waves dissociated from QRS complexes)

1. Narrow QRS complex at 40 to 60 bpm indicates block at AV node level.
2. Broad QRS complex (≥0.12 second) at 20 to 40 bpm indicates block below His bundle.
3. P waves unrelated to QRS complex and at faster rate than QRS complex

Treatment

1. Block at AV node level: May require temporary or permanent pacemaker.
2. Block below His bundle: Usually requires permanent pacemaker.

Sick Sinus Syndrome

1. Usually due to idiopathic fibrosis of the sinoatrial node (SAN)
2. Rhythm disturbances include inappropriate sinus bradycardia, *sinus arrest* (absence of P wave is due to failure of impulse generation by the SAN), *sinoatrial exit block* (SAN is functional but impulse cannot emerge to depolarize atrium), and atrial ectopic beats (AEB).
3. If there are associated paroxysms of atrial fibrillation or flutter leading to episodes of tachy-

cardia alternating with bradycardia, the arrhythmia complex is termed the *brady-tachy syndrome*.

ECG Features

Intermittent sinus bradycardia, sinus pause, sinus arrest, sinoatrial exit block, atrial fibrillation, atrial flutter, AEB

Treatment

Cardiac pacing is required.

 Bibliography

Amsterdam EA: Premature beats. In Rakel RE (ed): Conn's Current Therapy, pp 265–268. Philadelphia, WB Saunders Company, 1997.

Bennet DH: Cardiac Arrhythmias, 3rd ed. London, Wright, 1989.

Charles RG, Marshall AJ: Arrhythmias. In Cardiology, pp 1–45. Oxford, England, Heinemann, 1989.

Heger JW, Fernando Roth R, Niemann JT, et al: Arrhythmias. In Cardiology, 3rd ed, pp 30–76. Baltimore, Williams & Wilkins, 1994.

Zipes DP: Specific arrhythmias: diagnosis and treatment. In Braunwald E (ed): Heart Disease, 5th ed, pp 640–704. Philadelphia, WB Saunders Company, 1997.

76 Varicose Veins

William M. Simpson, Jr.

Etiology

1. An inherited defect almost certainly plays a major role in the development of varicosities.
2. Periods of high venous pressure related to prolonged standing or heavy lifting are contributing factors.
3. Highest incidence in women who are or have been pregnant.
4. Secondary varicosities develop as a result of obstruction (from neoplasm—fibroids, fetus, ovarian tumors, etc.) or valve damage secondary to thrombophlebitis.
5. Arteriovenous fistulas (congenital or acquired) are also associated with venous varicosities.

Symptoms

1. Dull, aching heaviness or feeling of fatigue on standing
2. Not necessarily correlated with number or size of varicosities.
3. Leg cramps at night, often relieved by elevation of the legs
4. Itching from an associated dermatitis may occur.

Key Symptoms

- Leg ache, heaviness, or fatigue
- Nocturnal leg cramps

Clinical Findings

1. Dilated, tortuous, elongated veins
2. Located beneath the skin of the thigh and leg
3. Generally readily visible in the individual on standing
4. In very obese patients, palpation may be required to locate symptomatic veins.
5. Edema, worsening as the day progresses, usually resolving overnight
6. Chronic venous stasis may progress to persistent edema, skin hyperpigmentation, and ulceration (usually proximal to the medial malleolus).

7. Some authorities consider significant pigmentation and ulceration to be rare except in the postphlebitic state.

Key Signs

- Dilated tortuous veins
- Edema

Tests

1. Tap test: Percuss at the top of a vein, feel how far down its length the tap is transmitted. Normally tap is interrupted by competent veins.
2. Trendelenburg test: With patient supine, raise leg, place two fingers on saphenofemoral junction (5 cm below and medial to the femoral pulse). Patient stands with fingers in place. If veins fill from below, deep or communicating valve leaks exist. Release fingers—if veins are rapidly filled, saphenofemoral valve incompetence.

Key Test

Trendelenburg test

Differential Diagnosis

1. Pain or discomfort secondary to arthritis, radiculopathy, or arterial insufficiency should be distinguished from that associated with varicose veins.
2. Primary varicose veins must be distinguished from those related to obstruction in the pelvis or retroperitoneum.
3. Congenital venous malformations and arteriovenous fistulas may be distinguished by their chronicity and bruit with thrill, respectively.

Treatment

1. Patient education: Avoid prolonged standing, use support stockings (preferably support pantyhose to avoid compression of most proximal venous structures), lose weight, regular walking.

2. Injection therapy: also referred to as compression sclerotherapy; becoming more widely used for medium and small varicose veins. Ultrasound-guided treatment of larger varices of the saphenofemoral and saphenopopliteal junctions has been successful, particularly in Europe. Injection of the sclerosing solution into the varicosed vein is followed by a period of compression of the segment, resulting in obliteration of the vein.

3. Surgical measures

   a. The mainstay of treatment of varicose veins has been high ligation, stripping, and excision. It remains the most commonly performed procedure for varicose veins in the United States.

   b. Venous segments not demonstrated to be incompetent and varicosed should not be ligated or removed (they may be needed as artery grafts later in life).

   c. Ambulatory phlebectomy is an alternative to high ligation and stripping. Performed through small incisions (1 to 5 mm) parallel to the long axis of the leg; veins are delivered through the incisions by specially designed hooks. The vein is then divided between mosquito clamps. Very good cosmetic results are reported from this procedure, performed in the office under local anesthesia.

Key Treatment

- Support stockings
- Sclerotherapy
- Surgical stripping

Follow-Up

1. Despite extensive and careful sclerotherapy or surgery, additional varicosities may develop and previously treated varicosities may recur.

2. Secondary tissue changes may not completely regress.

3. Exercise and optimization of weight continue to be important even after definitive therapy.

Bibliography

Boccalon H, Janbon C, Saumet J, et al: Characteristics of chronic venous insufficiency in 895 patients followed in general practice. Int Angiol 1997;16:226–234.

Butie A: Clinical examination of varicose veins. Dermatol Surg 1995;21:52–56.

Goldman M, Bergan J: Ambulatory Treatment of Venous Disease: An Illustrative Guide. St. Louis, CV Mosby Company, 1996.

Johnson M: Treatment and prevention of varicose veins. J Vasc Nurs 1997;15:97–103.

Olivencia J: Changing trends in varicose vein treatment. Iowa Med 1996;86:203–204.

Indications

1. Desire for improvement in appearance of the leg
2. Symptom relief; may also lead to improvement in restless legs syndrome.
3. Prevention of complications
4. The technique of sclerotherapy is most appropriate for treatment of small varicose veins (<6 mm in diameter) and telangiectasias.

Contraindications

1. Recent thrombophlebitis (deep or superficial)
2. Arterial insufficiency
3. Known allergy to sclerosant
4. Inability to ambulate because of age or illness
5. Anticoagulation
6. Active infection
7. Pregnancy
8. Severe systemic disease (relative, depending on severity)
9. Obesity (relative)

Preparation

1. Perform a complete history and physical examination, including use of medications that affect bleeding or clotting and personal and family history of vascular disorders.
2. Identify presence of saphenofemoral, saphenopopliteal, or perforator incompetence by maneuvers such as Brodie-Trendelenburg and Perthes' tests (see Bibliography or standard physical examination texts).
3. Order noninvasive venous studies (photoplethysmography, duplex or venous Doppler) to evaluate competence and patency of the deep venous system and perforators if the patient has signs of venous hypertension, including edema, ulceration, large-size (4-mm diameter) veins, extensive spider telangiectasias, veins in the groin or popliteal fossa, rapidly progressing veins, or a history of deep venous thrombosis. These studies are not necessary prior to treatment of limited, scattered telangiectasias less than 1 mm.
4. Identified reflux at the saphenofemoral and saphenopopliteal junctions or perforators should be repaired surgically or by an experienced sclerotherapist prior to treatment of superficial varicosities. If the primary problem is not corrected, secondary varicosities will recur rapidly.
5. Document location and size of varicosities to be treated. Examples of office forms are given in sources listed in the Bibliography.

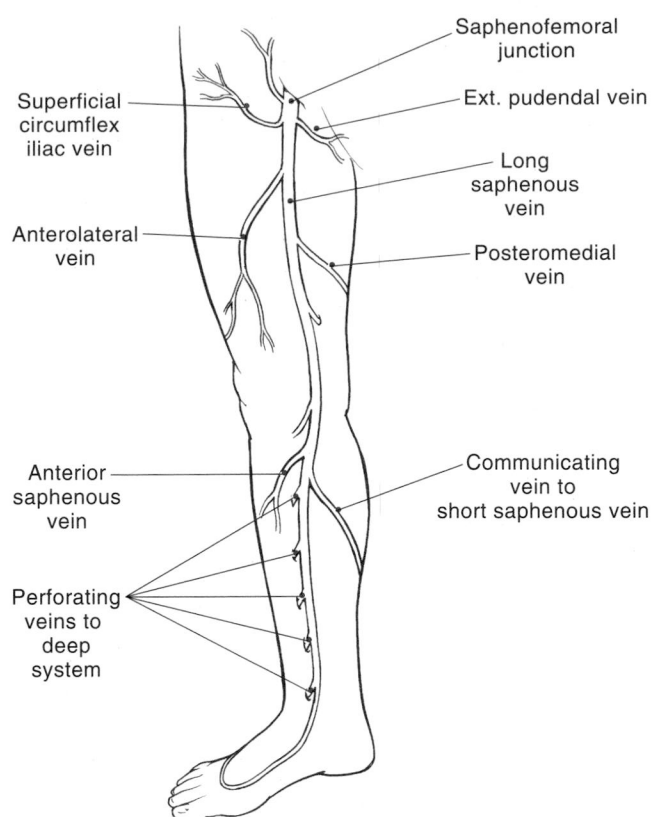

MAJOR SUPERFICIAL VEINS OF LOWER EXTREMITY–ANTERIOR

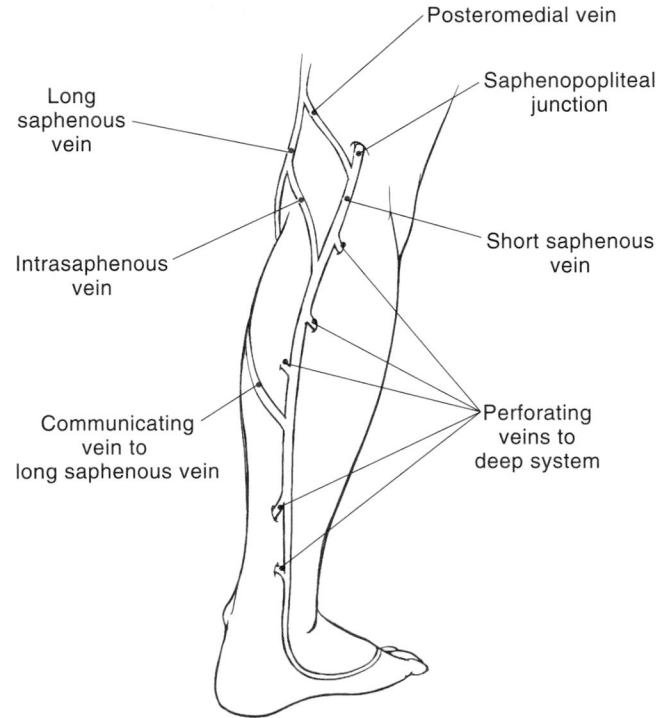

MAJOR SUPERFICIAL VEINS OF LOWER EXTREMITY–POSTERIOR

6. Educate the patient regarding realistic expectations and requirements for postprocedure care. Veins will gradually fade over weeks after treatment. Some veins will require multiple treatments. New varicosities may develop.

7. Measure for support hose if needed postprocedure.

Equipment

Several sclerosants are in use in the United States and Europe. Discussion of their individual properties is beyond the scope of this chapter. Use of hypertonic saline for telangiectasias is well accepted and is described here. The operator should be familiar with the risks and benefits of various solutions.

1. Sclerosant: 30-ml vial of hypertonic saline 23.4%

2. 2% *plain* lidocaine

3. 1-ml tuberculin syringes

4. 30-gauge, 0.5-inch needles; some operators prefer a needle bent to 30 degrees.

5. Gauze pads with paper tape
6. Clear antiseptic solution
7. High-intensity light
8. Graduated compression stocking, class I or II (not over-the-counter hose), to cover treatment areas with veins greater than 1 mm in diameter

Anesthesia

Lidocaine mixed with sclerosant. Hypertonic saline causes short-term burning and/or cramping.

Precautions

1. Hyperpigmentation occurs in up to 10 per cent of patients and fades over 1 year. It is more frequent in patients with a history of hyperpigmented scars.

2. Telangiectatic matting develops in 1 to 3 per cent of patients but can be treated with further injections.

3. Extravasation of sclerosant can cause ulceration and scarring

Technique

1. Inject 2 ml of 2% plain lidocaine into vial of saline.

2. Prepare 1-ml tuberculin syringes with injection solution prior to beginning procedure.

3. Have patient lie flat on examining table.

4. Begin at highest point of reflux and work down the leg.

5. Apply antiseptic solution. Enter vein with needle bevel down. Magnification and bright light assist in accurate placement.

   a. If intraluminal position is in doubt, do not inject.

   b. Inject slowly, monitoring tip of needle continuously.

   c. Stop injecting at once if bleb forms at needle tip, signifying extravasation.

   d. Do not inject more than 0.5 ml per injection site.

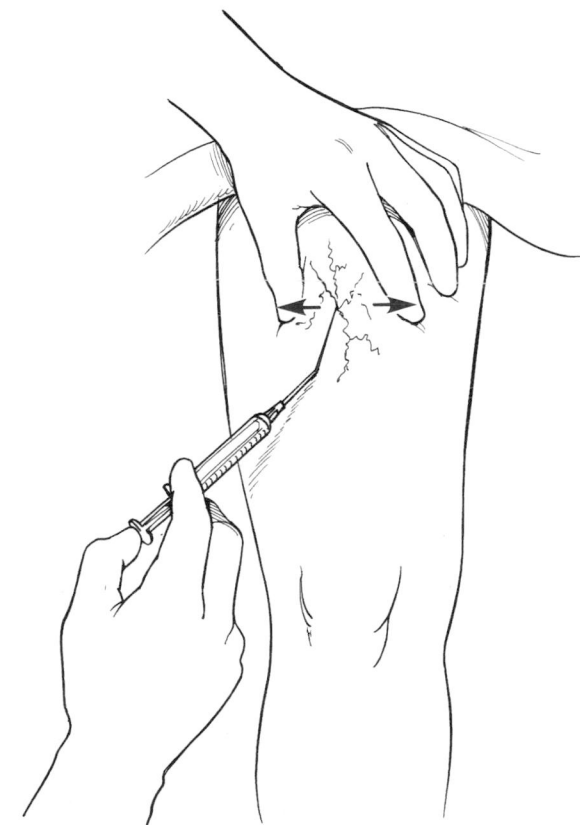

6. Correct injection leads to temporary blanching of vein followed by appearance of erythema around vein and refilling.

7. Withdraw needle. Tape stacked gauze pads over site to apply pressure while injecting other sites.

Follow-Up

1. No compression is needed for telangiectasias less than 1 mm in diameter.

2. Compression of larger vessel to maximize sclerosant contact with vessel wall and to decrease formation of intraluminal clot will lead to superior outcomes.

3. Patient should apply graded compression stockings before standing and keep them on continuously for 3 days. Bathing is not recommended during this period.

4. Patient should wear compression hose during sleep for at least 2 weeks, including while showering.

5. Usual daily activities are permitted, but patient should elevate legs as much as possible and do no exercise in first 2 weeks.

6. Chronic use of compression hose, especially during prolonged standing, may delay formation of new varicosities.

7. Evaluate patient and consider repeat sclerosis for remaining varicosities in 2 weeks. Some veins may require two to four treatments.

Bibliography

American Academy of Dermatology: Guidelines of care for sclerotherapy treatment of varicose and telangiectatic leg veins. J Am Acad Dermatol 1996;34:523–528.

Baccaglini U, Spreafico G, Castoro C, et al: Sclerotherapy of varicose veins of the lower limbs: consensus of the North American Society of Phlebology. Dermatol Surg 1996;22:883–889.

Green D: Sclerotherapy for the permanent eradication of varicose veins: theoretical and practical considerations. J Am Acad Dermatol 1998;38:461–475.

Pfeifer JR: Sclerotherapy. In Pfenninger JL, Fowler GC (eds): Procedures for Primary Care Physicians, pp 63–75. St. Louis, Mosby–Year Book, 1994.

Weiss RA: Evaluation of the venous system by Doppler ultrasound and photoplethysmography or light reflection rheography before sclerotherapy. Semin Dermatol 1993;12:78–87.

Weiss RA, Goldman MP: Advances in sclerotherapy. Dermatol Clin 1995;13:431–445.

77 Deep Venous Thrombosis

David J. Tanaka

Etiology

1. Virchow, in 1856, cited three factors that lead to thrombosis.
   a. Stasis: Common causes of stasis are
      (1) Bed rest secondary to illness or surgery
      (2) Prolonged sitting on a plane or automobile
      (3) Paralysis or paresis
   b. Vessel wall injury or abnormality
      (1) The most common cause is hip or knee surgery. Hip or knee replacement without deep venous thrombosis (DVT) prophylaxis is associated with approximately 50 per cent incidence of postoperative DVTs.
      (2) Chemical (chemotherapeutic, radiocontrast, or blood pressor) agents or infectious agents
   c. Hypercoagulability
      (1) Activated protein C resistance (factor V Leiden): This is the most common inherited hypercoagulable state in Caucasians; rare in Asian and African populations.
      (2) Antithrombin III, protein C, and protein S deficiencies
      (3) Dysfibrinogenemia
      (4) Antiphospholipid antibodies (lupus anticoagulant), sometimes indicated by an increased activated partial thromboplastin time (aPTT)
      (5) Trauma and surgery
2. Other risk factors
   a. Advancing age
   b. Pregnancy and pharmacologic doses of estrogen
   c. Malignancy—especially adenocarcinoma of lung, breast, and viscera
   d. Polycythemia

Symptoms

Symptoms of DVT are often nonspecific. Many DVTs are asymptomatic.

1. Pain in a limb along the distribution of the deep venous system, made worse by standing or walking and better with rest and elevation
2. Swelling of the lower extremity sometimes associated with varicosities, edema, and/or cyanosis

Key Symptoms

- Pain along the distribution of the deep venous system
- Swelling

Clinical Findings

Physical examination for DVT is insensitive and nonspecific. Proximal DVTs are associated with an approximately 50 per cent incidence of pulmonary embolism, which is often asymptomatic.

1. Swelling of the affected lower extremity above or below the knee: This can be verified by measuring and comparing extremity circumferences; greater than 3 cm in symptomatic leg measured 10 cm below the tibial tuberosity
2. Unilateral edema (greater in the symptomatic leg)
3. Homan's sign (calf pain on dorsiflexion of the foot with the knee slightly flexed)
   a. This is present in only 10 to 20 per cent of cases of DVT.
   b. This is also seen with any cause of calf inflammation.
4. Fever has been found in patients with proximal DVT, possibly secondary to unappreciated polmonary embolism.

Key Signs

- Entire leg swelling
- Calf swelling more than 3 cm when compared with the asymptomatic leg (measured 10 cm below the tibial tuberosity)
- Pitting edema (greater in the symptomatic leg)
- Collateral superficial veins (nonvaricose)

Laboratory Tests

1. There are no blood tests for DVT.
2. Noninvasive tests
   a. Ultrasonography is the initial test of choice in a symptomatic patient without a prior history of DVT. Impedance plethysmography (IPG) is not as specific as ultrasound, but may be more useful in the evaluation of patients for possible recurrent DVT.
   b. The tests utilizing ultrasonography are real-time ultrasonography, duplex scanning, and color-flow Doppler ultrasonography. The criterion used to diagnose DVTs by these methods is the failure of the venous lumen, as identified by real-time ultrasound, to fully collapse under gentle pressure from the transducer probe.
      (1) Duplex scanning and color-flow Doppler add Doppler information to assist in identifying the venous system.
      (2) Ultrasonography by real-time, duplex, or color-flow Doppler has sensitivities and specificities of 90+ per cent.
      (3) They are all more operator dependant than IPG.
      (4) Ultrasonography may not be as useful as IPG in the evaluation of recurrent DVT because the affected veins remain incompressible in many cases.
3. Ascending contrast venography: This is the gold standard for the diagnosis of DVT. Venography does have many disadvantages:
   a. Approximately 10 per cent of studies will be inadequate or unable to be performed.
   b. The test causes a DVT in approximately 2 to 3 per cent of studies.
   c. There is the risk of a hypersensitivity reaction.
   d. the test is uncomfortable for the patient.
   e. The test may cause renal insufficiency or congestive heart failure in susceptible patients.
   f. The test is the most costly of the diagnostic tests for DVT.
4. Diagnostic strategy: Stratify probabilities by risk factors, symptoms, and signs (see Table 77–1), then use ultrasonography and/or venography to diagnose or rule out DVT (see Fig. 77–1).

Key Tests

- Noninvasive tests: Ultrasound—real-time ultrasonography, duplex scanning, color-flow Doppler ultrasonography

- Ascending contrast venography: gold standard for diagnosis of DVT

Differential Diagnosis

1. Cellulitis
2. Superficial thrombophlebitis and lymphangitis
3. Ruptured popliteal synovial membrane or cyst (Baker's): The main difference between this and a DVT is that a ruptured cyst usually occurs in the setting of an arthritic knee.
4. Muscle strain or rupture (plantaris or gastrocnemius muscles): The mechanism of injury is the main differentiating clue between these disorders and DVTs.
5. Postphlebitic syndrome: This is usually a chronic disorder but can present with symptoms similar to an acute DVT.

TABLE 77–1. SIMPLIFIED CLINICAL MODEL*

CLINICAL PARAMETER	SCORE
Active cancer (treatment ongoing or within previous 6 months or palliative)	1
Paralysis, paresis, or recent plaster immobilization of the lower extremities	1
Recently bedridden for >3 days or major surgery within 4 weeks	1
Localized tenderness along the distribution of the deep venous system	1
Entire leg swelling	1
Calf swelling by >3 cm when compared with the asymptomatic leg (measured 10 cm below the tibial tuberosity)†	1
Pitting edema (greater in the symptomatic leg)	1
Collateral superficial veins (nonvaricose)	1
Alternative diagnosis as likely or greater than that of deep vein thrombosis	−2

*Scoring method: high probability if score is 3 or greater; moderate if score is 1 or 2; and low if score is 0 or less.
†In patients with symptoms in both legs, the more symptomatic leg was used.
From Anand SS, Wells PS, Hunt D, et al: Does this patient have deep venous thrombosis? JAMA 1998;279:1094–1099. Copyright 1998 American Medical Association, with permission.

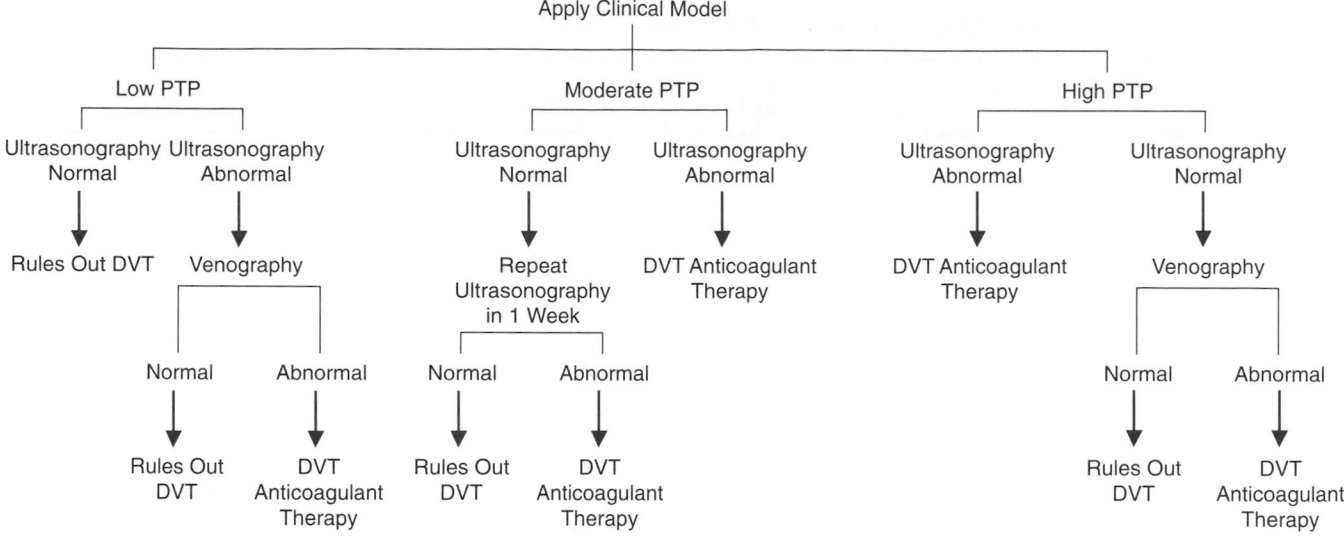

Figure 77–1 Suggested diagnostic approach in patients with suspected DVT. PTP, pretest probability. (From Anand SS, Wells PS, Hunt D, et al: Does this patient have deep venous thrombosis? JAMA 1998;279:1094–1099. Copyright 1998 American Medical Association, with permission.)

Treatment

1. Unfractionated heparin (traditional therapy)
2. Low-molecular-weight heparin
   a. Many advantages over unfractionated heparin (see Bibliography for more information)
      (1) More predictable anticoagulant response because of less binding to plasma proteins and to proteins released from activated platelets and endothelial cells
      (2) Better bioavailability at low doses because of less binding to endothelium
      (3) Dose-independent clearance mechanism because of less binding to macrophages
      (4) Longer half-life because of less binding to macrophages and endothelium
      (5) Lower incidence of heparin-induced thrombocytopenia because of less binding to platelets and PF4 (tetrameric protein released during platelet activation)
      (6) Possible lower incidence of osteoporosis because of less binding to osteoclasts and reduced activation
   b. Some patients with DVT may be treated as outpatients.
   c. Not yet approved by Food and Drug Administration for treatment of DVT
3. Initiate unfractionated heparin therapy with a 5000- to 10,000-U intravenous bolus and start maintenance infusion at 1300 U/hour. Check aPTT at 6 hours to keep aPTT between 1.5 and 2.5 times control (see Tables 77–2 and 77–3).

WARNING

Failure to achieve an adequate anticoagulant response (aPTT > 1.5 times control) is associated with a 20 to 25 per cent recurrence of venous thromboembolism.

TABLE 77–2. GUIDELINES FOR ANTICOAGULATION

DISEASE	GUIDELINE
Suspected	Obtain baseline aPTT, PT, CBC
	Check for contraindication to heparin therapy
	Give heparin, 5000 U IV and order imaging study
Confirmed	Re-bolus with heparin 5000–10,000 U IV and start maintenance infusion at 1300 U/hr (heparin, 20,000 U in 500 ml D$_5$W, infused at 33 ml/hr)
	Check aPTT at 6 hr to keep aPTT between 1.5 and 2.5 times control (blood heparin level, 0.2 to 0.4 U/ml)
	Check platelet count daily
	Start warfarin therapy on day 1 at 5 to 10 mg and then administer warfarin daily at estimated daily maintenance dose
	Stop heparin therapy after 4 to 7 days of joint therapy when INR is 2.0 to 3.0 without heparin therapy
	Anticoagulate with warfarin for 3 months at an INR of 2.0 to 3.0 (longer treatment should be given to patients with ongoing risk factors or recurrent thrombosis)

Abbreviations: aPTT, activated partial thromboplastin time; CBC, complete blood count; D$_5$W, 5 per cent dextrose in water; INR, international normalized ratio; PT, prothrombin time.

Adapted from Hyers TM, Hull RD, Weg JG: Antithrombotic therapy for venous thromboembolic disease. Chest 1995; 108(Suppl):335S–351S.

TABLE 77–3. HEPARIN: MONITORING AND ADJUSTING DOSAGE*

APTT (sec)[†]	RATE CHANGE (ml/hr)	DOSE CHANGE (U/24 hr)	ADDITIONAL ACTION	NEXT APTT
≤45	+6	+5760	Re-bolus with 5000 U	4–6 hr
46–54	+3	+2880	None	4–6 hr
55–85[‡]	0	0	None	Next morning[§]
86–110	−3	−2880	Stop infusion after 1 hr	4–6 hr after restart
>110	−6	−5760	Stop infusion after 1 hr	4–6 hr after restart

*Initial dosing: loading: 5000 to 10,000 U; maintenance infusion: 1300 U/hr (aPTT in 4 to 6 hr). A starting bolus of 5000 to 10,000 U is given IV followed by IV infusion of 1300 U/hr (heparin: 20,000 U in 500 ml D_5W at approximately 33 ml/hr). The concentration of heparin is 40 U/ml. When aPTT is checked at 6 hr or longer, steady-state kinetics can be assumed. Dosage adjustments are made according to the protocol.

[†]Normal aPTT range with Dade-Actin FS reagent of 27 to 35 seconds.

[‡]The therapeutic range of 55 to 85 is roughly equivalent to a plasma heparin concentration range of 0.2 to 0.4 U/ml by protamine titration or to 0.35 to 0.7 U/ml by inhibition of factor Xa. The therapeutic range will vary with different aPTT reagents and coagulation timers. Thus the therapeutic range should be determined in every laboratory.

[§]During the first 24 hr, repeat aPTT in 4 to 6 hr. Thereafter, monitor aPTT daily unless it is outside the therapeutic range.

Adapted from Hyers TM, Hull RD, Weg JG: Antithrombotic therapy for venous thromboembolic disease. Chest 1995;108(Suppl): 335S–351S, with permission.

a. The main risk of heparin therapy is bleeding and thrombocytopenia. Thrombocytopenia associated with thrombosis, often arterial is seen less commonly.

b. Osteoporosis is a risk for more prolonged heparin therapy.

4. Coumarin compounds: Warfarin or dicumarol, oral anticoagulants, may be started once the heparin is therapeutic (usually day 1). The anticoagulant effect of coumarin compounds is measured by the prothrombin time and the international normalized ratio (INR). The therapeutic range for the INR is 2.0 to 3.0.

   a. Start warfarin therapy on day 1 at 5 to 10 mg and then administer at estimated daily maintenance dose (see Table 77–2).

   b. Anticoagulate with warfarin for 3 months at an INR of 2.0 to 3.0 (longer treatment should be given to patients with ongoing risk factor or recurrent thrombosis).

WARNING

Acetaminophen at usual/therapeutic doses has been found to increase warfarin effect. Patients initiating or using high doses of acetaminophen should have their prothrombin time/INR monitored closely.

Alternative Treatments

1. Inferior vena caval interruption

   a. The major indication is the presence of a proximal DVT in a patient in whom anticoagulation is contraindicated.

b. Less common indications are

   (1) Recurrent thromboembolism despite adequate anticoagulation

   (2) The presence of a large, free-floating caval thrombus

   (3) Chronic recurrent embolism with pulmonary hypertension

2. Thrombolytic agents: Thrombolytic agents have the theoretical advantage of lysing the thrombus and hopefully preserving the venous valves. There is conflicting evidence that thrombolytics may decrease the incidence of postphlebitic syndrome. Because of the increased risk of bleeding and inadequate evidence of benefit, thrombolytics cannot be routinely recommended at this time.

Special Cases

1. Isolated calf venous thrombosis should be treated with anticoagulation for 3 months. If anticoagulation is not given, serial noninvasive studies of the lower extremity should be performed for 10 to 14 days to assess for proximal extension of the thrombus.

2. Patients with recurrent thromboembolism or continuing risk factor (hypercoagulable state) should be treated indefinitely.

Diet

The diet should contain a consistent amount of vitamin K (70 to 140 μg) during warfarin therapy.

1. Avoid substantial changes in diet.

2. Avoid foods high in vitamin K:

   a. Liver

b. Tea (green)

c. Green leafy vegetables: broccoli, brussels sprouts, cauliflower, chick peas, kale, spinach, turnip greens

d. Lettuce, cabbage, asparagus, and green beans are OK.

Activity

1. During hospitalization, the affected extremity should be elevated as much as possible and the patient may ambulate as tolerated. After discharge, the patient should gradually resume normal activities but avoid prolonged sitting or standing.

2. Avoid any contact sport that exposes the patient to risk of serious injury during warfarin therapy.

Patient Education

1. Patient compliance is critical for effective and safe anticoagulation.

2. Patients should alert their doctor if they have any unusual bleeding (excessive bleeding from gums, nose, vagina, etc.; hematuria, melena, or excessive bruising).

3. Medication

   a. Patients should check their warfarin tablets and take exactly as prescribed.

   b. Warfarin should be taken at the same time every day.

   c. All new medicines or changes in medicines should be reported to their doctor immediately.

4. Patients need to inform their doctor if they are planning on becoming or have become pregnant.

5. Any travel should be discussed with the doctor in advance.

Key Treatment

- Low-molecular-weight heparin or unfractionated heparin

- Warfarin

Follow-Up

1. Patients need to have regular prothrombin/INR testing to monitor warfarin therapy.

2. Noninvasive venous testing is not routinely done after an acute DVT. If postphlebitic syndrome is suspected, noninvasive venous studies can document the degree and location of venous insufficiency.

Bibliography

For more information on the treatment DVT, see
Hyers TM, Agnelli G, Huyll RD, et al: Antithrombotic therapy for venous thromboembolic disease. Chest 1998;114(Suppl):561S–578S.

For more information on heparin and low-molecular-weight heparin therapy, see
Hirsh J, Warkentin TE, Raschke R, et al: Heparin and low-molecular weight heparin: mechanism of action, pharmacokinetics, dosing considerations, monitoring, efficacy, and safety. Chest 1998;114(Suppl):489S–510S.

For more information on warfarin therapy, see
Hirsh J, Dalen JE, Anderson DR, et al: Oral anticoagulants: mechanism of action, clinical effectiveness, and optimal therapeutic range. Chest 1998;114(Suppl):445S–469S.

For more information on the diagnosis of DVT, see
Anand SS, Wells PS, Hunt D, et al: Does this patient have deep venous thrombosis? JAMA 1998;279:1094–1099.

For more information on low-molecular-weight heparin in the treatment of DVT, see
Litin SC, Heit JA, Mees KA: Use of low-molecular-weight heparin in the treatment of venous thromboembolic disease: answers to frequently asked questions. Mayo Clin Proc 1998;73:545–551.

78 Peripheral Arterial Disease

Chris Goerdt

Etiology and Epidemiology

1. Atherosclerosis causes the majority of peripheral arterial disease (PAD).

2. PAD most commonly involves the lower extremities and presents after the fifth decade of life.

3. Approximately 1 to 2 per cent of the adult population and 10 per cent of those over age 70 have symptomatic disease.

4. Risk factors: smoking (most important), diabetes, hyperlipidemia, and hypertension

5. Ten per cent of patients with lower extremity PAD also have high-grade carotid artery stenoses and 50 per cent have high-grade coronary artery stenoses.

6. Progressive deterioration occurs in 15 to 20 per cent of patients, but less than 5 per cent require an amputation. Smoking and diabetes markedly increase the risk of deterioration and the need for surgery.

7. The presence of lower extremity PAD determined by an ankle/brachial systolic blood pressure ratio less than 0.9 more than triples the risk of mortality for both symptomatic and asymptomatic patients. Cardiovascular diseases cause 80 per cent of the deaths.

8. Other less common causes include
   a. Arteritis (connective tissue diseases, giant cell arteritis, Takayasu's disease)
   b. Thromboangiitis obliterans (Buerger's disease)
   c. Raynaud's disease
   d. Artery entrapment

9. Symptoms of abrupt onset, digit or upper extremity involvement, or in a person less than 40 years of age suggest an uncommon etiology.

Symptoms

1. Intermittent claudication is the hallmark symptom.
   a. Produces cramping, pain, weakness, or numbness in affected muscles (calf discomfort is most common but may also occur in buttock, thigh, or foot)
   b. Predictably produced by walking a specific speed and distance; relieved by resting within about 5 minutes

2. Rest pain occurs in advanced disease.
   a. Involves the foot, usually distal to the metatarsals (nocturnal metatarsalgia)
   b. Aggravated by leg elevation or cool temperature

3. Approximately 50 per cent of patients with clinically evident lower extremity PAD are asymptomatic.

4. Nocturnal leg cramps and "cold feet" usually do not indicate PAD.

Key Symptoms

- Intermittent claudication
- Rest pain

Clinical Findings

1. Diminished or absent pulses. Dorsalis pedis pulse is congenitally absent in approximately 8 per cent of normal individuals. The posterior tibial pulse should be palpable.

2. Arterial bruits

3. Arterial insufficiency: dry, scaly, atrophic skin; extremity hair loss, brittle nails, and dependent rubor

4. Ischemic ulcers that are painful, dry, and pale, and often have a black necrotic crust. Ulcers usually occur on the heels or toes.

5. Gangrene

6. Lower extremity pallor within 1 minute after leg elevation to 60 degrees and return of color delayed more than 15 seconds after lowering

7. Rest pain, ischemic ulcers, or gangrene, especially with a resting ankle systolic pressure of 50 mm Hg or less, indicate limb-threatening ischemia.

Key Signs

- Diminished pulse
- Arterial bruit
- Ischemic ulcer
- Pallor with elevation

Laboratory Tests

1. Ankle/brachial index (ABI)
   a. Noninvasively assesses lower extremity arterial insufficiency by determining ratio of ankle to brachial systolic blood pressures measured by a Doppler device; can be performed at the bedside.
   b. Abnormal ratio less than 0.9, moderate disease less than 0.8, severe disease less than 0.6, and less than 0.4 associated with ulcers and gangrene
   c. A 20 per cent decrease in ABI postexercise indicates disease and is useful if resting ABI is normal and yet patient has symptoms suggesting PAD.
   d. Ankle pressures in diabetics may be falsely elevated secondary to medial calcinosis of arteries.
2. Special procedures
   a. Plethysmography
      (1) Measures pulse-volume waveforms and toe pressures
      (2) Useful in patients with diabetes who may have falsely elevated ankle pressures or disease confined to distal arterial beds
   b. Transcutaneous oxygen tension measurements
      (1) Assess tissue perfusion and viability
      (2) Also useful in patients with diabetes (see above)
   c. Angiography is the "gold standard" for the diagnosis of anatomic disease; used when considering an interventional procedure.

Key Test

Ankle/brachial index

Differential Diagnosis

1. Arthritis
2. Lumbar spinal stenosis (pseudoclaudication)
   a. Symptoms produced by walking or prolonged standing
   b. Relieved by flexing spine (sitting)
3. Herniated lumbar disk
4. Peripheral neuropathy
5. Muscle cramps
6. Restless legs syndrome
7. Shin splints
8. Venous claudication
   a. Edema and venous stasis are present
   b. Typically produces rest pain as well
9. Other arterial diseases: arteritis, thromboangitis obliterans, Raynaud's disease, artery entrapment.

Treatment

1. Management of PAD without limb-threatening ischemia
   a. Smoking cessation
   b. Control of diabetes, hyperlipidemia, and hypertension
   c. Regular walking for 30 minutes a day has improved walking distance more than any drug treatment and is as beneficial as angioplasty.
   d. Special attention to foot care (see below)
   e. Optimize treatment of concurrent medical conditions (e.g., congestive heart failure, chronic obstructive pulmonary disease).
   f. Weight loss
2. Prompt surgical referral for consideration of arterial bypass, angioplasty, thrombolysis (for acute ischemia), or amputation for critical leg ischemia (rest pain, ischemic ulcers, or gangrene). A concomitant resting ankle systolic pressure of 50 mm Hg or less or a toe systolic pressure of 30 mm Hg or less worsens the prognosis.

Medication

1. Aspirin prevents myocardial infarctions, strokes, and deaths in patients with PAD.
2. Clopidogrel (Plavix), 75 mg orally once daily, is an antiplatelet drug that is marginally more effective than aspirin in preventing vascular events in patients with cardiovascular disease. It is much more expensive than aspirin but less expensive and safer than ticlopidine (Ticlid).
3. Pentoxifylline (Trental), 400 mg tid, has shown only modest clinical efficacy.

Diet

As determined by risk factor status

Activity

Regular walking, cycling, or stair climbing

Patient Education

1. Inspect and wash feet daily.
2. Check water temperature before washing feet (avoid very hot water).
3. Dry between toes to prevent maceration.
4. Apply moisturizing lotion to feet.
5. Keep nails trimmed.

6. Wear comfortable shoes.
7. Regularly inspect shoes for foreign bodies.
8. Do not smoke.
9. Do not walk barefoot.
10. Do not treat corns or calluses yourself.
11. Do not use heating pads on feet.

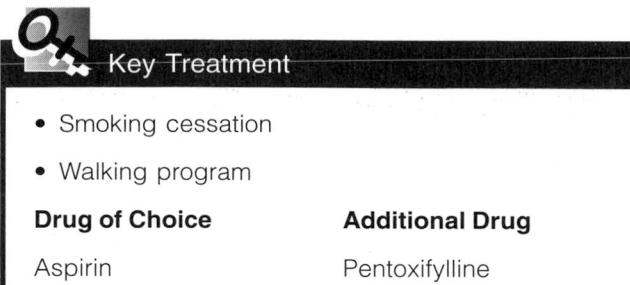

Key Treatment

- Smoking cessation
- Walking program

Drug of Choice	Additional Drug
Aspirin	Pentoxifylline

Follow-Up
As needed for control of risk factors

Bibliography

Golledge J: Lower-limb arterial disease. Lancet 1997;350: 1459–1465.

Newman AB, Sutton-Tyrrell K, Vogt MT, Kuller LH: Morbidity and mortality in hypertensive adults with a low ankle/arm blood pressure index. JAMA 1993;270: 487–489.

Porter JM: Chronic lower extremity ischemia. Part 1. Curr Probl Surg 1991;28:11–92.

Spittell JA: Diagnosis and management of occlusive peripheral arterial disease. Curr Probl Cardiol 1990;15: 7–35.

Wilt TJ: Current strategies in the diagnosis and management of lower extremity peripheral vascular disease. J Gen Intern Med 1992;7:87–102.

79 Raynaud's Phenomenon

Jeffrey F. Minteer

Epidemiology and Etiology

1. Affects 3 to 5 per cent of male and 4 to 9 per cent of female population.
2. It is estimated that fewer than 50 per cent ever seek medical attention.

Primary Raynaud's Phenomenon (PRP)

1. Affects younger age group (15 to 20 years old); only 24 per cent present after age 20.
2. Predominance of women (60 to 90 per cent)
3. Origin of vasospasm unknown but probably multifactorial; associated with increased sympathetic tone and/or increased sensitivity or density of α_2 receptors under central sympathetic influence; if severe, may have characteristics of endothelial damage.
4. Distinction from a connective tissue disorder is of questionable value because the interval between onset of symptoms and the diagnosis of a collagen disease is 3 to 16 years (11.5 years on average).

Secondary Raynaud's Phenomenon (SRP)

1. Affects older age group (over 35); less sex difference
2. Associated with endothelial damage, intimal proliferation, fixed vascular obstruction, or inflammation resulting in release of vasospastic substances such as thromboxane and endothelin-1
3. Sixty per cent of Raynaud's phenomenon cases occurring beyond age 60 are atherosclerotic in origin.
4. Also associated: hard red cells, activated platelets, increased plasma viscosity, decreased fibrinolysis
5. Seen in 90 per cent of patients with systemic sclerosis (SS) (80 per cent present with Raynaud's), 85 per cent of those with mixed connective tissue disease, 10 to 44 per cent with systemic lupus erythematosus (SLE), 20 per cent with Sjögren's syndrome, 5 per cent with rheumatoid arthritis (RA)
6. Can be caused by drugs such as bleomycin and vincristine (see "Differential Diagnosis"); usually resolves after drug is discontinued.

Symptoms

Primary Raynaud's Phenomenon

Seventy per cent of all cases

1. Classic triphasic color changes: pallor → cyanosis → rubor; usually two are required, pallor and cyanosis being the most common (best to use the Maricq's standard color chart to get accurate history).
2. Bilateral, episodic attacks of well-demarcated pallor followed by cyanosis and rubor brought on by cold exposure or emotional stress; affects fingers (one or more but may spare the thumb) more often than toes; lasts 15 to 30 minutes after rewarming.
3. May also affect toes, earlobes, lips, or tip of nose.
4. May also give rise to complaints of tingling and burning sensations during reperfusion.

Secondary Raynaud's Phenomenon

1. Similar color changes (cyanosis more prominent)
2. May be unilateral.
3. Symptoms of precipitating disease such as sicca symptoms, dysphagia, photosensitivity, skin lesions, joint pain, telangiectasias; history of more than 5 years in high-risk occupations such as use of vibratory tools
4. Symptoms tend to be more severe with rapid progression.

Key Symptoms

- Episodic triphasic color changes
- Precipitated by cold, emotional stress

Clinical Findings

Primary Raynaud's Phenomenon

1. Pallor: vasospasm in response to cold or emotional stress
2. Cyanosis: stagnated blood flow in dilated capillaries
3. Rubor: accumulation of vasodilating agents in ischemic tissue
4. Normal examination when patient is not having symptoms; normal pulses

Secondary Raynaud's Phenomenon

1. May see digital pitting scars or gangrene.
2. May see signs of primary disease such as peri-ungual telangiectasias, sclerodactyly, arthritis, signs of carpal tunnel syndrome, decreased peripheral pulses, or signs of thoracic outlet syndrome.

Key Signs

- Color changes in response to cold
- Digital pitting scars

Laboratory Tests

1. Basic tests to exclude precipitating cause (all normal in primary Raynaud's phenomenon)
   a. Antinuclear antibodies (ANA), sedimentation rate, complete blood count
   b. Wide-field capillary microscopy of the nail folds (apply immersion oil to nail base and observe with 10× magnification and inverted microscope eyepiece): capillary loss and enlarged, tortuous capillary loops
   c. Abnormal ANA and microscopy identify 95 per cent of those who will develop SS but SS not inevitable; 28 per cent with abnormal capillaries develop SS in 6 years.
2. Expanded work-up—if there are suggestive symptoms/signs or abnormal screening tests (i.e., sedimentation rate greater than 20, ANA greater than 1:100, or abnormal nail fold capillaries)
   a. Anti–double-stranded DNA, anti-centromere antibody (ACA), anti–topoisomerase I (anti-Sc1-70)
   b. For signs of increased viscosity (cyanosis predominates clinical picture) add serum protein electrophoresis, cold agglutinins, cryoglobulins.
   c. Add vascular studies if obstruction indicated.
   d. Add nerve conduction studies if nerve entrapment suggested.
   e. Pulmonary diffusion or esophageal motility studies if subclinical SS suspected
3. No method of testing reliably reproduces the characteristic syndrome.

Key Tests

- Antinuclear antibodies, erythrocyte sedimentation rate
- Nail fold microscopy

Proposed Criteria for Diagnosis of PRP

1. Attacks episodic with acral pallor or cyanosis
2. Strong and symmetric pulses
3. No evidence of peripheral pitting, gangrene, or ulcerations
4. Normal nail fold capillaries
5. ANA under 100
6. Westergren erythrocyte sedimentation rate under 20 mm/hour

Differential Diagnosis: Secondary Causes

1. Systemic rheumatic disorders: 20 per cent of all causes of Raynaud's phenomenon
   a. SS: suggested by signs/symptoms, abnormal nail fold capillaries, and high ANA (speckled) with positive anti-Sc1-70 or ACA. Most common connective tissue disease causing Raynaud's phenomenon: 80 per cent present with Raynaud's as the first symptom, 90 per cent have Raynaud's
   b. SLE (+ anti–double-stranded DNA), RA (? association): dermatomyositis, mixed connective tissue disease, Sjögren's (29 per cent), and possible association with SS-like syndrome associated with silicone breast implants
2. Occupational
   a. Vibration white finger: 90 per cent of loggers; carpal tunnel syndrome; does not develop while using tool but with cold exposure.
   b. Polyvinyl chloride
3. Drugs or chemicals
   a. β-Blockers (? evidence acutely), ergotamine, narcotics, birth control pills, sympathomimetics, imipramine, bromocriptine, α-interferon
   b. Heavy metals, caffeine
   c. Chemotherapy: bleomycin, vincristine, vinblastine—20 to 40 per cent
4. Occlusive arterial disease: thromboangiitis obliterans, peripheral vascular disease, thoracic outlet syndrome, steal syndrome following dialysis shunting
5. Hyperviscosity diseases: polycythemia, cryoglobulinemias, paraproteinemias, thrombocytosis
6. Other causes: reflex sympathetic dystrophy, infections, malignant disease, cerebrovascular accident, polio, syringomyelia, pulmonary hypertension, hypothyroidism—48 per cent; Lyme disease
7. Nonspecific syndromes

a. Blue toe syndrome: cyanotic lesions with dependent mottling from emboli, thrombosis, or vasculitis

b. Erythromelalgia: red, warm, and painful feet made worse by warm temperatures and improved on aspirin; occurs in idiopathic myeloproliferative disorder, autoimmune disease, pregnancy, and use of vasodilator drugs.

8. Associated conditions: possibly indicate systemic vasospasm

   a. Sixty-one per cent of PRP patients have migraine syndromes.

   b. Forty-seven per cent of PRP patients have atypical chest pain, especially those with aura-associated migraines (67 per cent).

   c. Forty-one per cent of females with fibromyalgia have PRP.

Treatment

Medication

Forty to 66 per cent of patients benefit but rarely obtain complete relief. Drug therapy for patients unresponsive to patient education measures or signs of severe disease (e.g., ulcers/gangrene)

1. Vasodilating drugs

   a. Calcium channel blockers: nifedipine (Procardia), 30 to 60 mg/day or prior to precipitating events (e.g., 10 mg orally before cold exposure); others may be useful. Two thirds of patients so treated have decrease in symptoms. Work better for primary disease in sustained-release form.

   b. ACE inhibitors, peripheral vasodilators (controversial)

   c. Serotonin receptor antagonist: ketanserin (not available in the United States) affects vasoconstriction and platelet aggregation.

2. Drugs that alter prostaglandin metabolism

   a. Prostacyclin analogue: iloprost (not available in the United States) improved signs and symptoms in 47 per cent of patients who failed nifedipine; drug-induced hypercoagulable state a concern.

   b. Intravenous infusion of prostaglandin E_1 (alprostadil) is useful in severe acute attacks.

3. Rheologic agents

   a. Aspirin, 80 mg/day, if there is high risk of digital vessel occlusion

   b. Pentoxifylline (Trental), 400 mg three times daily; no long-term studies

Surgery

1. Cervical sympathectomy does not affect long-term course of disease and is a last resort in SRP unresponsive to medications.

2. Digital sympathectomy has shown some success in healing digital ulcers.

Diet

Fish oil supplements: substrate for cyclooxygenase, antiaggregative effects on platelets, no clinical support as yet

Patient Education

1. Dress appropriately in the cold.

2. Stop smoking, reduce caffeinated beverages.

3. Avoid over-the-counter sympathomimetics.

4. Biofeedback for stress-induced symptoms (one third are stress related, with 92 per cent response rate).

Key Treatment

- Patient education
- Nifedipine

Follow-Up

1. Prognosis in PRP: 38 per cent stable, 36 per cent improved, 16 per cent worse, 10 per cent disappear over a 6- to 10-year follow-up.

2. Ten to 30 per cent of those with PRP are diagnosed with a connective tissue disease within 6 to 8 years.

3. The risk of progression of PRP to SRP is high when

   a. Onset occurs after 20 years of age.

   b. Patient has intense, painful attacks and/or digital ulcers.

   c. Attacks are asymmetric.

   d. The ANA is positive and/or nail fold capillaries are abnormal.

 ## Bibliography

Adee AC: Managing Raynaud's phenomenon: a practical approach. Am Fam Physician 1993;47:823–829.

Klippel JH: Raynaud's phenomenon. Arch Intern Med 1991;151:2389–2393.

Merritt WH: Comprehensive management of Raynaud's syndrome. Clin Plast Surg 1997;24:133–159.

Ohtsuka T, Ishikawa H: Statistical definition of nail fold capillary pattern in patients with systemic sclerosis. Dermatology 1994;188:286–289.

Waller PA, Leroy EC: Raynaud's phenomenon and connective tissue disease. J South Carolina Med Assoc 1993;89:536–542.

Wigley FM: Raynaud's phenomenon. Curr Opin Rheumatol 1993;5:773–784.

80 Gastrointestinal Symptoms

| SYMPTOM | **ABDOMINAL PAIN** | *William Y. Huang* |

Abdominal pain is a common condition seen by physicians. In most cases, evaluation of the patient with abdominal pain should consist of a thorough history, a careful physical examination and appropriately selected diagnostic tests.

The patient may present in different ways. The pain can be severe and acute, requiring an urgent evaluation in the hospital. The pain may be chronic, still requiring a methodical evaluation, but less urgently in the outpatient setting. In some patients, the pain resolves before a diagnosis is made. In other patients, the pain persists and is difficult to diagnose because of a normal evaluation.

Differential Diagnosis

1. Cardiac: myocardial ischemia/infarction, pericarditis
2. Respiratory: pneumonia, pulmonary embolus, pneumothorax, pleuritis
3. Gastrointestinal
   a. Inflammatory (e.g., cholecystitis, pancreatitis, appendicitis, diverticulitis)
   b. Vascular (e.g., mesenteric ischemia, ruptured abdominal aortic aneurysm)
   c. Mechanical (e.g., small bowel obstruction caused by adhesions)
   d. Neoplastic (e.g., carcinoma of the colon or pancreas)
   e. Abdominal wall (e.g., musculoskeletal strain, rectus sheath hematoma)
4. Genitourinary: urinary tract infection, ureteral stone passage, prostatitis
5. Gynecologic: ovarian cyst, ruptured ectopic pregnancy, pelvic inflammatory disease, tubo-ovarian abscess, threatened abortion
6. Metabolic: diabetic ketoacidosis, porphyria, sickle cell crisis

History: Key Questions to Ask

1. General questions: location of pain, radiation of pain, severity and quality of pain, precipitating or aggravating factors, alleviating factors, duration and frequency of pain, associated symptoms and progression of symptoms
2. Medical history
   a. Medical (especially cardiovascular disease, gastrointestinal disorders)
   b. Surgical (especially abdominal surgery or pelvic surgery)
   c. Medications and allergies
3. Social history: tobacco/alcohol/substance abuse and sexual history
4. Review of systems
   a. Constitutional: fever, weight change
   b. Cardiac: chest pain, shortness of breath, radiation of pain, diaphoresis
   c. Respiratory: fever, cough, sputum production, wheezing, shortness of breath
   d. Gastrointestinal: decreased appetite, nausea and/or vomiting (bloody, bilious, feculent), change in bowel habits, constipation, diarrhea, jaundice, hematochezia
   e. Urinary: dysuria, hematuria, hesitancy, urgency, frequency of urination
   f. Gynecologic: menstrual history, contraceptive use, vaginal discharge or bleeding
   g. Psychiatric (especially if chronic pain): anxiety or depression, emotional trauma

Clinical Findings

1. General
   a. Appearance of the patient (ill-appearing, presence of distress, most comfortable position)
   b. Vital signs (presence of fever, tachycardia, or hypotension)
2. Chest: character of breath sounds in all lung fields; presence of rales, rhonchi, or rubs
3. Cardiovascular: character of heart sounds and pulses; presence of murmurs or rubs
4. Abdomen
   a. Inspection: presence of distention, scars, hernias, protuberant abdomen

b. Auscultation: character of bowel sounds, presence of bruits

c. Percussion: loss of normal hepatic dullness, presence of shifting dullness. Use light percussion to check for rebound rather than palpation.

d. Palpation: Start palpating with light pressure *away* from the area of tenderness. Palpate entire abdomen saving the area of tenderness for last. Presence of masses (pulsatile or non-pulsatile), tenderness (diffuse or localized), rigidity, guarding, Murphy's sign.

5. Genitourinary

a. Inguinal area: presence of hernia or lymphadenopathy

b. In males

(1) Scrotum: Presence of testicular masses or tenderness

(2) Prostate: especially note consistency and presence of tenderness

c. In females

(1) Vagina: presence of bleeding or discharge

(2) Cervix: appearance, presence of motion tenderness or discharge

(3) Uterus: abnormal size, masses or tenderness

(4) Adnexa: size of ovaries if palpable; presence of other masses or tenderness

6. Rectal: presence of tenderness or masses, stool for occult blood

7. Back: presence of costovertebral angle or flank tenderness

8. Skin: presence of lesions such as herpes zoster or fistulas

Diagnostic Tests

1. Laboratory tests (order selected tests rather than a routine battery of tests)

a. Complete blood count with differential

(1) Anemia may suggest a bleeding lesion in the gastrointestinal tract.

(2) An elevated white blood cell count with a shift to the left may confirm suspicion of an infectious or inflammatory process (e.g., appendicitis).

b. A urinalysis may indicate a urinary tract infection or suggest passing of a stone.

c. A serum or urine pregnancy test diagnoses pregnancy.

d. Liver function tests are helpful in suspected cases of hepatic or biliary disease.

e. Amylase or lipase may confirm inflammation of the pancreas.

2. Radiologic tests

a. A chest radiograph may reveal a lower lobe pneumonia or signs of a perforated abdominal viscus.

b. A flat and upright abdominal x-ray series may show signs of a small bowel obstruction.

c. A barium enema may be used in stable patients to detect the cause of a large bowel obstruction. It may reduce some cases of intussusception and sigmoid volvulus.

d. An intravenous pyelogram may show a ureteral stone.

e. An ultrasound of the abdomen/pelvis is helpful in cases of suspected cholelithiasis/cholecystitis and in females with pelvic pain. It may clarify cases of suspected appendicitis but is not recommended as a routine test for this condition.

f. A radionuclide scan (e.g., hepato-iminodiacetic acid scan) can confirm cases of acute cholecystitis.

g. A computerized tomographic scan of the abdomen/pelvis can diagnose patients with a perforated viscus, intra-abdominal neoplasm, appendicitis, diverticulitis, mesenteric ischemia, pancreatitis, aneurysm, or intestinal obstruction.

3. Other tests

a. Upper endoscopy may reveal esophagitis or peptic ulcer disease or neoplasm.

b. Flexible sigmoidoscopy or colonoscopy may show the cause of a colonic obstruction (e.g., carcinoma) or changes of inflammatory bowel disease.

c. Laparoscopy may clarify in female patients with lower quadrant pain whether they have appendicitis or a gynecologic condition (ovarian cyst, tubal pregnancy, salpingitis).

Management

Depends on the condition of the patient and the cause of the pain.

Medication

1. Recent studies show that pain medication is helpful in patients with acute abdominal pain and does not hinder the diagnostic process.

2. Histamine$_2$ blockers or proton pump inhibitors help patients with reflux esophagitis or peptic ulcer disease.

3. Appropriate antibiotics are needed in patients

with infectious causes such as pelvic inflammatory disease.

Diet

Patients with acute abdominal pain should take nothing by mouth and be given intravenous fluids until their condition improves. Patients with nonacute abdominal pain may eat a regular diet but are advised to avoid foods that aggravate their condition (e.g., fatty foods in patients with gallstones). A high-fiber diet may help those with irritable bowel syndrome.

Activity

Patients with acute abdominal pain should be kept at bed rest until their condition improves and their diagnosis is clear. Patients with nonacute abdominal pain may continue their normal activities, but may wish to rest during episodes of severe pain.

Patient Education

Patients should be instructed on the nature of their disease, the treatment plan, and exacerbating and ameliorating factors.

Follow-Up

Patients with acute pain may require follow-up every few minutes to every few hours until their condition is stable and the diagnosis is clear. Patients with nonurgent pain should be followed regularly until the diagnosis is clear and they are improving.

PEARLS

- Determine the urgency of the situation. Patients with hemodynamic instability require resuscitation. Patients with severe pain require immediate evaluation.

- Use diagnostic tests selectively to pursue diagnoses suggested by the history and physical.

- The nature of the pain may change. A patient with acute appendicitis may initially present with vague, periumbilical pain, but later on develop pain that is localized in the right lower quadrant.

- A therapeutic patient-physician relationship is important in patients with chronic, functional abdominal pain. Focus of the patient visits should be on helping the patient understand and control his or her symptoms.

Bibliography

American College of Emergency Physicians: Clinical policy for the initial approach to patients presenting with a chief complaint of nontraumatic acute abdominal pain. Ann Emerg Med 1994;23:906–922.

Drossman DA: Chronic functional abdominal pain. Am J Gastroenterol 1996;91:2270–2281.

Glasgow RE, Mulvihill SJ: Abdominal pain, including the acute abdomen. In Feldman M, Sleisenger MH, Scharschmidt BF (eds): Gastrointestinal and Liver Disease: Pathophysiology/Diagnosis/Management, 6th ed, vol 1, pp 80–89. Philadelphia, WB Saunders Company, 1998.

Martin RF, Rossi RL: The acute abdomen—an overview and algorithms. Surg Clin North Am 1997;77:1227–1243.

Silen W: Cope's Early Diagnosis of the Acute Abdomen, 19th ed. New York, Oxford University Press, 1996.

SYMPTOM NAUSEA AND VOMITING

John B. Pope

1. *Nausea* is an ill-defined and unpleasant, although not painful, sensation generally perceived in the pharynx and upper abdomen. It is usually accompanied by hypersalivation and the desire to vomit, or the feeling that vomiting is imminent. It may be brief or quite prolonged and sometimes occurs in waves. *Retching* refers to forceful rhythmic contractions of the respiratory and abdominal musculature that sometimes precedes vomiting. *Vomiting* is the forceful expulsion of gastric contents through the mouth.

2. Although generally regarded clinically as undesirable side effects, nausea and vomiting may have evolved as a survival function for eliminating potentially toxic substances from the gastrointestinal tract. This function may be triggered by various toxins recognized by sensors in the upper gut and central nervous system. The initiation and coordination of these events involves complex neurochemical interactions involving specific areas of the brain, including the vomiting center of the lateral reticular formation and the chemoreceptor trigger zone (CTZ) in the area postrema in the floor of the fourth ventricle.

3. Although generally self-limited, nausea and vomiting may be severe or protracted, leading

to serious complications such as dehydration, hypokalemia, metabolic alkalosis, aspiration pneumonitis, malnutrition, dental caries, ruptured esophagus (Boerhaave's syndrome), or mucosal tears with hemorrhage (Mallory-Weiss syndrome).

Differential Diagnosis

Nausea and vomiting are manifestations of a large number of disorders not limited to the digestive system or abdomen.

1. Acute infectious diseases: Virtually any infection (bacterial, viral, parasitic) can stimulate nausea and vomiting. These symptoms are common in children with systemic infections not directly involving the gastrointestinal (GI) tract.
2. Acute abdominal emergencies: appendicitis, cholecystitis, pancreatitis, peritonitis, intestinal obstruction, visceral inflammation, perforation, ischemia
3. Drugs and toxins: Many different classes of drugs and various toxins may stimulate the CTZ or directly irritate the stomach mucosa, triggering nausea (nonsteroidal anti-inflammatory drugs, digitalis, morphine, erythromycin, azathioprine, enterotoxins).
4. Intracranial disease: Increased central nervous system pressure may cause vomiting, sometimes projectile.
5. Pregnancy: usually confined to the first trimester but may be prolonged or severe
6. Psychogenic: anorexia nervosa, bulimia, emotional upset
7. Gastric retention: gastroparesis, dysmotility, pyloric obstruction
8. Metabolic and endocrine disorders: diabetic ketoacidosis, adrenal insufficiency, thyrotoxicosis, uremia, hypercalcemia, acute renal failure
9. Chronic indigestion: peptic ulcer disease, aerophagia
10. Labyrinthine disorders: acute labyrinthitis, Ménière's disease
11. GI bleeding: blood in the stomach may stimulate vomiting
12. Cardiac disease: congestive heart failure, myocardial infarction
13. Pain: more often associated with nausea than with frank vomiting

History

1. Timing and character of vomitus: helpful in delineating cause
   a. Early morning vomiting: pregnancy, alcoholic gastritis, uremia
   b. Feculent vomitus: gastrocolic fistula, distal intestinal obstruction
   c. Projectile vomiting: increased intracranial pressure, pyloric stenosis
   d. Bilious vomitus: Increased bile may indicate obstruction below ampulla of Vater.
   e. Blood vomitus: GI bleeding
2. Associated symptoms
   a. Vertigo and tinnitus: Ménière's disease, labyrinthitis
   b. Relief of abdominal pain with vomiting: peptic ulcer disease
   c. Early satiety: gastroparesis
   d. Weight loss: malignancy
3. Food ingestion
   a. Potential toxin ingestion
   b. Vomiting during or soon after eating: psychogenic cause
   c. Delayed vomiting after eating: obstruction or dysmotility
   d. Vomiting old food: impaired gastric emptying
   e. Vomiting undigested food: esophageal or Zenker's diverticulum
4. Recent use of medications
5. Other close contacts similarly affected
6. Unusual stressors, emotional upset, depression

Clinical Findings

1. Abdominal tenderness, rebound, guarding, distention, abnormal bowel sounds (hyperactive, diminished, or absent)
2. Intravascular volume depletion: bradycardia, hypotension, skin pallor
3. Anorexia, weight loss, wasting
4. Altered autonomic activity: diarrhea, increased perspiration, hypersalivation
5. Hematemesis, coffee-ground emesis, feculent emesis
6. Dental caries
7. Projectile vomiting

Tests

1. Plain radiographs: may suggest intestinal obstruction
2. Upper GI series: can assess motility and mucosa of proximal GI tract
3. Esophagogastroduodenoscopy: obstruction, mucosal aberrations
4. Gastric emptying scans: gastric paresis

5. Computerized tomography of the brain: intracranial disorders
6. Pregnancy test
7. Electrolytes: useful for assessing volume and electrolyte status

Management

1. Correction of the underlying cause
2. Antiemetics for symptom alleviation—effectiveness variable
3. Prevention and treatment of complication development

Medication

Because of complexity of the neurophysiologic process in vomiting, it may not be possible to find a single agent that is effective for all emetic stimuli.

1. Antihistamines (dimenhydrinate, promethazine): useful in inner ear dysfunction
2. Anticholinergics (scopolamine): useful for motion sickness
3. Phenothiazines (prochlorperazine [Compazine], chlorpromazine [Thorazine]): useful for mild symptom relief but fraught with side effects (sedation, hypotension, Parkinson-like symptoms)
4. Butyrophenones (haloperidol [Haldol], droperidol [Inapsine]): useful in cytotoxic drug-induced vomiting
5. Dopamine antagonists (metaclopromide [Reglan]): useful in gastric and small bowel stasis and prophylaxis for chemotherapy-induced nausea and vomiting
6. 5-Hydroxytryptamine type 3 antagonists (ondansetron [Zofran], granisetron [Kytril], dolasetron): excellent in cytotoxic drug–induced and radiation-induced vomiting
7. Cannabinoids (tetrahydrocannabinol)
8. Corticosteroids: useful in conjunction with other agents
9. Benzodiazepines (particularly lorazepam [Ativan]): useful as adjunct therapy for anticipatory nausea or vomiting.

Diet

1. Avoid all foods for several hours; irritable stomachs respond to food with nausea and vomiting.
2. Nausea may be reduced by sucking on hard candy or popsicles, particularly in children.
3. Begin frequent, small quantities of clear liquids and slowly advance diet as tolerated.

Activity

Avoid excessive activity and overheating.

Patient Education

1. Hematemesis or other evidence of GI bleeding needs prompt medical attention.
2. Frequent or prolonged vomiting (particularly in children) may result in dehydration.
3. Persistent vomiting during pregnancy should be investigated.
4. Numerous drugs have nausea as a common side effect.

Follow-Up

1. Most cases of nausea and vomiting are mild and self-limited and require no specific follow-up once the underlying etiology is identified and corrected.
2. Follow-up, when required, should be tailored to the individual case on the basis of cause, severity, and risk of complication development.

PEARLS

- A careful history is the most important factor in determining etiology.

- Assess volume status with history of frequent or prolonged vomiting.

- Check stool for occult blood with history of hematemesis (unwitnessed).

- Obtain pregnancy test with history of vomiting and amenorrhea.

Bibliography

For more information on nausea and vomiting, see
Cooke CE: Oral ondansetron for preventing nausea and vomiting. Am J Hosp Pharm 1994;51:763–771.
Friedman LS, Isselbacher KJ: Anorexia, nausea, vomiting, and indigestion. In Wilson JD, Braunwald E, et al (eds): Harrison's Principles of Internal Medicine, 12th ed, pp 251–253. New York, McGraw-Hill, 1991.
Kousen M: Treatment of nausea and vomiting in pregnancy. Am Fam Physician 1993;48:1279–1284.
For more information on antiemetics, see
Axelrod RS: Antiemetic therapy. Compr Ther 1997;23: 539–544.
For more information on the physiology of nausea and vomiting, see
Andrews PLR: Physiology of nausea and vomiting. Br J Anaesth 1992;69(Suppl 1):2S–19S.

1. Swallowing is a clinically complex process involving as many as 40 steps in three stages. The voluntary oral phase (1 second) propels a liquid or solid bolus into the pharynx, initiating a peristaltic wave. The involuntary pharyngeal phase (1 second) moves the bolus from the pharynx across the upper esophageal sphincter (UES), and the involuntary esophageal phase (8 to 10 seconds) moves the bolus through the esophagus and across the lower esophageal sphincter (LES) to the stomach.

2. Dysphagia is the subjective sensation of difficulty swallowing. Up to 7 per cent of people experience dysphagia at some time. Up to 10 per cent over age 50 are affected by it. Most do not consult a physician. About 30 to 60 per cent of nursing home patients and up to 25 to 30 per cent of patients on general medical wards have dysphagia. Neuromuscular conditions account for about 80 per cent of cases, cerebrovascular accidents (CVA) being the most common. Dysphagia contributes to significant morbidity and mortality because of aspiration pneumonia or hospitalizations. It also lowers quality of life via isolation and meal-related anxiety.

Differential Diagnosis

Dysphagia implies obstruction or physiologic dysfunction and is classified as oropharyngeal or esophageal. Here, categorization is meant to provide a framework for causes of dysphagia, hence defining a differential diagnosis.

Oropharyngeal Dysphagia

1. Neuromuscular
   a. Central: CVA, head injury, Parkinson's disease, multiple sclerosis, Huntington's chorea, Alzheimer's disease, brain stem tumors, amyotrophic lateral sclerosis, bulbar palsy, pseudobulbar palsy, familial dysautonomia
   b. Peripheral: neuropathies (diabetes mellitus, lead poisoning), myasthenia gravis
   c. Skeletal muscle: polymyositis, dermatomyositis, muscular dystrophy (myotonic dystrophy, oculopharyngeal dystrophy), steroid myopathy, metabolic myopathy (hypo- or hyperthyroidism), alcoholic myopathy, systemic lupus erythematosus
2. Infectious/inflammatory: diphtheria, chronic meningitis, syphilis, Lyme disease, poliomyelitis, rabies, tetanus, botulism, pharyngitis, retropharyngeal abscess, stomatitis

3. Salivary: Sjögren's syndrome (poor salivation), drugs that reduce salivary flow (anticholinergics, antihistamines, phenothiazines)
4. Obstructive/mechanical
   a. Intrinsic: local neoplasm, proximal esophageal webs and rings, Zenker's diverticulum, surgical resection or trauma of oropharynx or larynx, radiation injury (neuromuscular or salivary gland damage), rheumatoid cricoarytenoid arthritis, UES dysfunction (cricopharyngeal achalasia or fibrosis), enlarged thyroid
   b. Extrinsic: anterior mediastinal masses, cervical spondylosis, vertebral osteophytes

Esophageal Dysphagia

1. Neuromuscular (motility): achalasia (peristaltic dysfunction of the LES), diffuse esophageal spasm, scleroderma, collagen disorders, hypertensive LES, Chagas' disease, amyloidosis; alcohol-, diabetes-, drug-, and gastroesophageal reflux disease (GERD)–related motility disorders
2. Obstructive (mechanical)
   a. Intrinsic: peptic strictures, rings (Schatzki's), webs, carcinomas, diverticula
   b. Extrinsic: mediastinal compression, osteoarthritis, foreign bodies

History

Dysphagia is not always obvious. Patients may give clues to the specific diagnosis, but they may be ignorant of their problem, gradually accommodate to it, or not think it worthy of reporting. Therefore, it is important just to ask if there is any trouble swallowing. For example, the elderly may present with pneumonia and be unaware of dysphagia because of hypesthesia of the larynx or trachea. Thorough questioning of the patient and caregivers can reveal causes and guide work-up and management.

1. Oropharyngeal problems include difficulty with mastication or initiating the swallow.
   a. Is there mouth dryness (decreased salivation)?
   b. Does a cough accompany the swallow (indicating an unprotected larynx)? Frequent throat clearing or choking may be related to attempts at clearing the larynx.
   c. Are there speech disorders or a "gargle" voice during or after meals, nasal regurgitation, or nasal speech (resulting from palate weakness)?
   d. Where does the food get stuck? Patients may

be capable of localizing oropharyngeal symptoms above the sternal notch and esophageal discomfort to the substernal area. Other signs or symptoms should support this. For instance, a Zenker's diverticulum may present as discomfort at the pharynx, but questions of breathing difficulty, insomnia, regurgitation, and halitosis should follow.

2. Esophageal problems are associated with "food sticking" in the throat after a swallow.

   a. Does the difficulty occur with solids, liquids, or both?

   b. Are symptoms intermittent or have they increased in frequency?

   c. Is there heartburn, snoring, weight loss, a respiratory symptom, or chest pain? Noncardiac chest pain suggests a motility abnormality, reflux, malignancy, or inflammation.

   d. Mechanical obstruction is indicated by symptoms, at onset, that occur with intake of only solid foods, although this may progress to trouble with soft foods and later liquids. Solids causing only intermittent problems suggest a ring, versus rapid progression toward thinner textures, which may signal cancer (particularly over age 50 and/or with weight loss). Progression past solids, with heartburn present, suggests peptic stricture.

   e. Solids *and* liquids causing dysphagia at its onset indicate a motility disorder. Here, intermittent symptoms associated with chest pain imply diffuse esophageal spasm, whereas gradually worsening symptoms associated with heartburn point to scleroderma. Gradually worsening symptoms associated with respiratory symptoms suggests achalasia.

3. Is there pain with swallowing (*odynophagia*), which implies an inflammatory process? Dysphagia is usually painless.

4. Is there a longer lasting, constant "lump in the throat" often relieved during a swallow? This defines *globus*, a distinct sensation not to be confused with dysphagia, although the two can occur together. *Globus hystericus* is probably a misnomer because these patients tend to be depressed or obsessive rather than hysterical. Organic disease, especially GERD, should be ruled out before a psychological diagnosis is given.

5. Are there other neurologic symptoms, such as gait disturbance, speech disorder, facial droop, or hoarseness? Has eating become a slower process?

6. Are there other medical problems, such as diabetes, or habits such as smoking or alcohol?

7. What medications are taken, including nonsteroidal anti-inflammatory drugs and antacids? Was sufficient fluid taken with pills? "Pill esophagitis" is caused by local mucosal injury.

Clinical Findings

1. General observations: patient's posture, weight, voice quality, and speech

2. Oral: dentition, structures such as palate, lesions and dryness in mucous membranes

3. Neck: palpate and inspect for masses, lymph nodes, thyromegaly

4. Neurologic: cranial nerves, especially sensory function of V, IX, and X and motor function of V, VII, X, XI, and XII. Observing mastication and swallow may reveal problems.

Further examination should be based on history or suspicion of concomitant disease (e.g., atrophy, the tremor of Parkinson's disease, the ptosis of myasthenia gravis, or the skin and hair changes of thyroid disease). Usually, the only physical signs of esophageal dysphagia relate to systemic scleroderma or manifestations of the CREST syndrome (calcinosis, Raynaud's phenomenon, esophageal dysmotility, sclerodactyly, and telangiectasia). Generally, physical examination is of limited value in the diagnosis of dysphagia.

Tests

1. A modified barium swallow or videofluoroscopy is usually the most valuable first step. Swallowing function, aspiration, and reflux may be seen, as well as intrinsic and extrinsic obstructions. Speech pathologists should evaluate the patient prior to the exam to determine aspects of swallowing that need assessment and the barium texture to be administered. It is wise to explore how the exam is performed at the local institution as there can be variability in administration. Static barium swallow is mainly limited to obstruction and mucosal lesion.

2. Laryngoscopic or endoscopic evaluation may be necessary. Advantages include direct view of the swallowing process, mucosa, erosions, neoplasm, and foreign bodies.

3. Manometry, utilized if other abnormalities are not found, assesses peristaltic pressure wave amplitude patterns of swallowing that can distinguish disease-specific patterns.

4. Blood work is seldom indicated unless history and physical examination suggest a systemic etiology, such as collagen-vascular, hypothyroid, or muscular disease.

Management

Specific therapies, including myotomy and drugs, have been developed to treat underlying entities such as Zenker's diverticulum, Parkinson's disease, and myasthenia gravis, to name a few, so the specific diagnosis can be critical. Nonspecific treatment by speech pathologists to establish safe oral routes by altering deglutition reflex, sensory enhancement, dietary modification, and postural maneuvers have made significant improvements in the management of degenerative neurologic diseases. Primary care physicians have the opportunity to coordinate the multidisciplinary team that is often necessary to diagnose and treat dysphagia and to minimize the discouragement experienced by their patients.

PEARLS

- The presence or absence of a gag reflex indicates little about swallowing function.

- Speech pathologists help in the diagnosis and treatment of dysphagia.

- Dysphagia is seldom purely psychogenic.

Bibliography

Castell DO: Approach to the patient with dysphagia. In Yamada T (ed): Textbook of Gastroenterology, 2nd ed, pp 638–647. Philadelphia, JB Lippincott Company, 1995.

Koch W: Swallowing disorders: diagnosis and therapy. Med Clin North Am 1993;77:571–582.

Logemann J: Screening, diagnosis and management of neurogenic dysphagia. Semin Neurol 1996;16:319–327.

Paterson WG: Dysphagia in the elderly. Can Fam Physician 1996;42:925–932.

Trate DM, Parkman HP, Fisher RS: Dysphagia: evaluation, diagnosis and treatment. Prim Care 1996;23:417–432.

SYMPTOM HEARTBURN AND INDIGESTION

Holli K. Neiman

1. Heartburn or indigestion is a pain or discomfort centered in the upper abdomen. It is a burning feeling behind the breastbone that may move into the throat. It is extremely common, accounting for 2 to 5 per cent of all family practice consultations. Approximately 25 per cent of the U.S. population is affected, 4 to 7 per cent of them with daily symptoms.

2. Less than 50 per cent of affected patients consult a physician. Many people consider these common symptoms a fact of life.

3. Heartburn is caused when stomach acid moves up from the stomach into the esophagus. There may be a sour taste in the mouth. Factors involved include decreased lower esophageal sphincter tone, decreased mucosal resistance, delayed gastric emptying, and increased acid clearance time.

4. *It may be difficult to distinguish heartburn from angina; some patients have exercise-induced heartburn.*

5. *The frequency of heartburn does not correlate well with the complications of reflux.*

Differential Diagnosis

1. Gastrointestinal
   a. Gastroesophageal reflux disease
   b. Gastroduodenal ulcer
   c. Gastric cancer
   d. Hiatal hernia
   e. Esophageal motility disorder
   f. Irritable esophagus
   g. Functional dyspepsia
   h. Irritable bowel syndrome
   i. Gallbladder disease
   j. Esophageal spasm
   k. Mallory-Weiss tear
   l. Pancreatitis
2. Vascular
   a. Angina
   b. Coronary artery disease
   c. Microvascular angina
3. Other
   a. Pregnancy
   b. Uremia
   c. Pulmonary tuberculosis
   d. Hypercalcemia
   e. Diabetes mellitus
   f. Migraine

g. Viral esophagitis

h. Moniliasis of the esophagus

History: Key Questions to Ask

1. When? What exacerbating factors?

   a. Time of day (night vs. daytime symptoms)

   b. Relation to food, especially caffeine, fried or greasy, spicy, citrus, carbonated beverages, peppermint, chocolate, coffee, garlic, tomato, onion

   c. Relation to position (lying down or bending over)

   d. *Nocturnal symptoms more predictive of reflux complications.*

2. How long?

   a. When did symptoms start?

   b. How long do symptoms last?

3. Lifestyle issues

   a. Smoking

   b. Alcohol use

   c. Excess weight

4. Medication use? Many medications decrease lower esophageal sphincter tone.

   a. Heart and blood pressure medications: calcium channel blockers, nitrates, α-adrenergic antagonists

   b. Nonsteroidal anti-inflammatory drugs and salicylates

   c. Asthma medications: theophylline, β_2-agonists

   d. Anticholinergics

   e. Antidepressants

   f. Progesterone

   g. Antibiotics

   h. Digitalis

   i. Potassium or iron supplements

   j. Corticosteroids

5. Alleviating factors: What makes it better?

   a. Relief with eating: Consider ulcer.

   b. Relief with position change

   c. Relief with medication

6. Associated diseases: diabetes mellitus

7. Associated symptoms

   a. Nausea and vomiting

   b. Water brash

   c. Dysphagia

   d. Early satiety

   e. Bloating

   f. Cough

   g. Shortness of breath

Clinical Findings

1. Clinical findings are frequently minimal, but may include

   a. Epigastric tenderness

   b. Halitosis

   c. Dental disease (erosion of enamel)

   d. Cough

2. Warning or alarm signs indicate a need for prompt evaluation of the symptoms. These signs include

   a. Weight loss

   b. Signs of blood loss or anemia

   c. Recurrent vomiting

   d. Dysphagia

   e. Abdominal mass

   f. Lymphadenopathy

3. Other associated findings may include

   a. Hoarseness

   b. Shortness of breath

   c. Choking

   d. Wheezing

   e. Recurrent pneumonitis

   f. Subglottic stenosis

Diagnostic Tests

The use of diagnostic testing in the patient with heartburn or indigestion is somewhat controversial, and the decision to test, as well as which tests to perform, should be individualized depending on presentation, associated signs and symptoms, and response to interventions.

1. Endoscopy

   a. Can rule out gastroduodenal ulceration, reflux esophagitis, gastric cancer.

   b. Is superior to radiography in establishing diagnosis, targeting therapy, and reassuring patients.

   c. Cannot confirm dysmotility disorder or reflux as the cause of symptoms.

   d. Indications:

      (1) Patient older than 45 to 50 years of age with new-onset symptoms

      (2) Symptoms failed to respond to empiric therapy.

      (3) Symptoms are persistent or refractory.

      (4) *Promptly if warning or alarm symptoms are present or develop*

2. Barium studies

   a. Insensitive for mild inflammation but highly specific for severe inflammation

   b. Barium swallow helpful with associated dysphagia

3. Provocative tests
   a. Edrophonium (Tensilon): used to evoke symptoms during manometry
   b. Acid perfusion (Bernstein) test: detection of reflux in addition to dysmotility
   c. Esphageal balloon distention: increases the sensitivity of provocative testing.
4. Motility studies
   a. Can be done as ambulatory test.
   b. Helpful if associated symptoms of early satiety, bloating, nausea, and vomiting are present.
5. Twenty-four–hour pH monitoring
   a. Greater sensitivity and specificity than provocative tests
   b. Indicated when manometry and provocative tests are not differentiating the cause of the symptoms or when therapeutic medical trial has failed
6. *Helicobacter pylori*
   a. Role in nonulcer dyspepsia not proven.
   b. Controversy over best method to use for evaluation of infection
      (1) Biopsy: Requires endoscopy; can do urease test and get results in a shorter time.
      (2) Serology: helpful in determining infection (at some time), but not in following response to therapy, because titers do not fall for 4 to 6 months. Acute and convalescent sera must be analyzed together.
      (3) Breath test: better indicator of current infection and can be used to check for eradication after therapy (wait at least 1 month).

Management

The American Gastrointestinal Association offers four options for treatment in their position statement (Gastroenterology 1998;114:579):

1. Empiric medical therapy with antisecretory or prokinetic drug
2. Diagnostic evaluation, preferably with endoscopy
3. Testing for *H. pylori* infection and, if positive, endoscopy to look for ulcers or cancer
4. Testing for *H. pylori* and treating all positive cases with antibacterial therapy

Medication

Many patients use antacids and histamine$_2$ (H$_2$) blockers for symptomatic relief. If a patient is using an over-the-counter medication more than two times per week, a physician should be consulted.

1. Antacids—with or without alginate
2. H$_2$ blockers: Need to dose adequately to inhibit daytime and nighttime acid secretion.
   a. Cimetidine (Tagamet)
   b. Ranitidine (Zantac)
   c. Famotidine (Pepcid)
   d. Nizatidine (Axid)
3. Prokinetic agents: Increase lower esophageal sphincter pressure and accelerate gastric emptying.
   a. Bethanechol (Urecholine): cholinergic agonist
   b. Metaclopramide (Reglan): dopaminergic and cholinergic agonist
   c. Cisapride (Propulsid): Enhances acetylcholine release from postganglionic nerve endings; serotonin type IV agonist.
   d. Erythromycin: uncertain role
4. Sucralfate (Carafate)
   a. Acts as a buffer and adherent.
   b. Results are variable
   c. May augment response to H$_2$ blocker.
5. Proton pump inhibitors: Irreversibly and noncompetitively inactivate parietal cell H$^+$/K$^+$-ATPase, inhibiting basal and stimulated acid production.
   a. Omeprazole (Prilosec)
   b. Lansoprazole (Prevacid)
   c. *For long-term therapy, more cost effective than H$_2$ agents, related to better healing and decreased complications*
6. Combination therapy: Results not consistently proven. Can use H$_2$ blocker with prokinetic or sucralfate.

Diet

1. Several small meals per day, rather than three large meals
2. Avoid alcohol.
3. Avoid foods that irritate stomach.

Activity

Lifestyle modification

1. Smoking cessation
2. Decrease alcohol intake.
3. Raise head of bed 6 in or sleep on foam wedge.
4. No food for 3 to 4 hours before going to bed or lying down
5. Weight loss if overweight
6. Avoid lying on right side.

Patient Education

1. The patient needs to be aware of the etiology of the symptoms, their own exacerbating factors, and how to avoid those factors.

2. Stress the importance of lifestyle modifications in controlling symptoms.

3. The patient should be aware of warning/alarm symptoms and should consult the physician promptly if these should occur.

4. If the patient has other medical problems, a review of any medications that may exacerbate the symptoms is needed.

Follow-Up

1. Follow-up depends on the patient's response to treatment. Some patients respond to short-term medical therapy and require no further treatment, as-needed treatment, or only bedtime use of H_2 blockers or antacids.

2. Follow-up 4 to 8 weeks after therapy is initiated is appropriate to determine response.

3. If endoscopy has been performed, there is no need to repeat it, unless new alarm symptoms develop that require investigation or symptoms worsen.

Bibliography

American Gastroenterological Association Medical Position Statement: evaluation of dyspepsia (approved AGA governing board 11/8/97). Gastroenterology 1998;114:579–581.

Camilleri M: Nonulcer dyspepsia: a look into the future. Mayo Clin Proc 1996;71:614–622.

Fass R, Hixson LJ, Ciccolo ML, et al: Contemporary medical therapy for gastroesophageal reflux disease. Am Fam Physician 1997;55:205–212.

Johnson DA: Gastroesophageal reflux disease: long-term management strategies. Consultant 1997;7:1833–1844.

Larsen RR: Gastroesophageal reflux disease, gaining control over heartburn. Postgrad Med 1997;101:181–187.

SYMPTOM ACUTE UPPER GASTROINTESTINAL BLEEDING

Zobair M. Younossi

Acute upper gastrointestinal (GI) bleeding is estimated to result in 250,000 to 300,000 hospitalizations each year. The mortality rate from upper GI bleeding has remained stable at about 10 per cent. This stable rate has been interpreted as an improvement (considering the aging population), which in turn may be a reflection of recent advances in endoscopic, medical, or surgical therapies.

The prognosis of upper GI bleeding depends largely on the source of bleeding and the clinical status of the patient. Variceal bleeding, peptic ulceration, and stigmata of recent hemorrhage (active arterial "spurting," visible vessel, and fresh blood clot) all are associated with higher morbidity and risk for rebleeding. Patient characteristics that are important prognostic factors include older patients (more than 60 years of age), hemodynamic instability, and presence of multisystem failure.

Differential Diagnosis

The sources of upper GI bleeding are summarized in order of occurrence in Table 80–1.

> Refer to Ch. 84, Peptic Ulcer Disease.

History

The history may suggest the time of onset of bleeding, its severity, and possible causes.

1. A history of syncope and hematochezia in the presence of coffee-ground emesis would indicate severe bleeding.

2. A medication history, especially drugs such as nonsteroidal anti-inflammatory drugs, would provide clues to drug-induced gastropathy or gastric ulcers as the possible source of bleeding. The use of anticoagulants is important as well.

3. A history of recurrent ulcers (especially duodenal) should raise the suspicion of a gastrinoma as the possible factor.

4. Duodenal ulcers are almost always associated with *Helicobacter pylori* infection.

TABLE 80–1. SOURCES OF GASTROINTESTINAL BLEEDING, IN ORDER OF OCCURRENCE

	FREQUENCY (%)
1. Peptic ulcer (duodenal and gastric)	33–51
2. Esophageal and gastric varices	23–33
3. Mallory-Weiss tear	3–10
4. Gastric or duodenal erosion	1–19
5. Angiomata	0–7
6. Neoplasm	1–5
7. Dieulafoy's lesion	1.3
8. Aortoenteric fistula	<1
9. Hematobilia	<1
10. Ménétrier's disease	<1

Modified from Jensen DM (ed): Severe nonvariceal upper GI hemorrhage. Gastrointest Endosc Clin North Am 1991;1:211, with permission.

5. Heavy ethanol consumption can be associated with portal hypertension resulting in esophageal or gastric variceal bleeding.

6. A Mallory-Weiss tear may result from retching and vomiting.

7. A history of aortic stenosis or chronic renal failure should raise suspicion for angiomata.

8. Abdominal aortic surgery remains important as a source of gastrointestinal bleeding via an aortoenteric fistula.

Clinical Findings

1. Vital signs may provide important information about the severity of blood loss. Tachycardia, hypotension, or hypovolemic shock all indicate severe, acute blood loss. The presence of orthostatic changes suggests a 20 per cent or greater blood volume loss. In those who lose over 40 per cent of their blood volume, hypovolemic shock may result.

2. Skin examination may provide evidence of the amount of blood loss (pallor of the skin) and suggest a possible etiology. Spider angiomata, palmar erythema, icterus, splenomegaly, or ascites may suggest chronic liver disease and possible variceal bleeding. Telangiectasia of the lip and perioral area suggests Osler-Weber-Rendu syndrome.

3. Nasogastric lavage provides important information in clinical assessment. The severity of bleeding can be estimated by examining nasogastric aspirate and stool color. Aspiration of bright red blood by nasogastric tube indicates active bleeding and is associated with higher mortality.

4. Clinical indices such as the Baylor Bleeding Score (see Saeed et al, 1995) help to identify patients at high risk.

Tests

1. All patients with significant GI bleeding should have blood sent for type and crossmatch, hemoglobin/hematocrit, prothrombin time, partial thromboplastin time, platelet count, electrolytes, urea nitrogen, creatinine, and liver enzymes. Although the initial hematocrit is important in determining the baseline oxygen-carrying capacity, it poorly reflects the degree and severity of blood volume loss because it takes 24 to 48 hours to equilibrate the intravascular volume.

2. An electrocardiogram in the elderly and in those with coronary artery disease may indicate ischemia related to severe anemia. Barium studies in the setting of acute upper GI bleeding are of little value. Endoscopy (both diagnostic and therapeutic) has contributed significantly in the management of patients with upper GI bleeding.

Management

1. Patients must undergo a rapid clinical evaluation with concomitant resuscitative measures. Those with significant bleeding should have two large-bore intravenous lines and should be admitted to the intensive care unit for close monitoring and administration of an appropriate amount of fluids to correct the volume loss. Central venous access may be used for resuscitation and monitoring. Blood transfusion may be required depending on the volume of blood loss, age of the patient, presence of concomitant cardiorespiratory disease, and presence of continued bleeding. A reduction in oxygen-carrying capacity in those with hemoglobin below 10 gm/dl, especially the elderly, may be crucial. If coagulopathy is present, fresh frozen plasma and vitamin K should be given. Patients receiving massive blood replacement may require platelet transfusion and, rarely, calcium supplementation.

2. In those with active bleeding, airway protection is needed to avoid aspiration of blood and gastric contents. This can usually be accomplished with continuous suction and elevation of the head of patient's bed. Endotracheal intubation to reduce the risk of aspiration must be considered in those with active massive hematemesis and in those with mental status changes or shock.

3. In the recent past the role of emergency endoscopy as a diagnostic and therapeutic tool has been well recognized. Endoscopy, when available, should be considered in all patients with upper GI bleeding. It may be reasonable to omit endoscopy in patients with terminal illness and minor bleeding *or* in whom the decision to withdraw care has been made. In those presenting with upper GI bleeding, a source can be found in 95 per cent of patients. The timing of endoscopy is important, and, in this respect, patients may be divided into three groups:

   a. Those with evidence of active hemorrhage. This group should have emergent endoscopy performed as soon as they are hemodynamically stabilized.

   b. Those with acute, self-limited bleeding without active bleeding. This group can have endoscopy within 24 hours unless they are suspected of having portal hypertension or aortoenteric fistula or have re-bled after initial stabilization.

c. Those with chronic blood loss. Patients with chronic blood loss can have elective endoscopy.

Unless urgent endoscopy is indicated, there is now a growing consensus among endoscopists to avoid middle-of-the-night endoscopies because of the possibility of suboptimal support. The value of endoscopy is not only to determine the source of blood loss but also to provide therapeutic and prognostic assistance in managing these patients. The Baylor Bleeding Score (see Saeed et al, 1995) can help to predict those patients at high risk for rebleeding. In patients with active bleeding with a negative endoscopy or those with uncontrollable bleeding, angiography may provide diagnostic and therapeutic assistance.

4. Surgical consultation in patients with significant upper GI bleeding may be necessary to coordinate the management appropriately. Further treatment depends on the source of the bleeding, the most common being peptic ulcer (see Ch. 84, Peptic Ulcer Disease) and esophageal varices. Current approaches to the latter entity are addressed here.

Variceal Bleeding

1. Variceal hemorrhage is one of the most expensive nonmalignant digestive diseases in the United States. Bleeding varices occur when the portal-hepatic vein pressure gradient exceeds 12 mm Hg. The risk of death ranges between 20 and 80 per cent per bleeding episode.

2. Endoscopic therapy, with esophageal band ligation or sclerotherapy, has been shown to successfully control active bleeding in over 90 per cent of patients. It also reduces the acute mortality and rebleeding rate from varices. Although there are a variety of sclerosant agents, 1 to 2 per cent sodium tetradecyl sulfate is used in most centers for sclerotherapy. Multiple intravariceal and sometimes paravariceal injections may be required to achieve hemostasis. The complication rate of sclerotherapy is between 10 and 30 per cent and the mortality rate is 0.5 to 2.0 per cent. These complications include esophageal perforation, ulceration, stricture, and stenosis in addition to pleural effusion and mediastinitis.

3. The advent of new multiple band ligators allows for efficient and effective banding of esophageal varices. As compared to sclerotherapy, esophageal band ligation has lower rebleeding rates, slightly improved mortality, faster variceal obliteration, and lower complication rates. In most centers, band liga-

tion has become the endoscopic method of choice.

4. Infusion of vasopressin with a combination of nitroglycerin can result in a reduction of portal flow and a decrease in portal-systemic pressure gradient which results in a reduction in variceal bleeding. The initial dose of vasopressin ranges between 0.1 and to 0.4 units/minute, which can be gradually increased to 0.8 units/minute. Concomitant use of nitroglycerin is required as either an infusion or a patch. Vasopressin administration should only be given in the intensive care unit setting, where blood pressure and electrocardiographic monitoring is available.

5. Use of intravenous octreotide (Sandostatin) (a somatostatin analogue) has been shown to reduce the risk of rebleeding without significant side effects. Somatostatin is shown to decrease intestinal blood flow by 25 per cent (variceal pressure by 35 per cent) with no change in pulse rate, arterial pressure, or cardiac index. The dose of octreotide is an initial bolus of 50 μg followed by an infusion of 50 μg/hour for 5 days. In most centers, octreotide is the preferred agent for variceal hemorrhage.

6. Transjugular intrahepatic portal-systemic shunt (TIPS) has become an important alternative for patients with recurrent variceal bleeding and those who failed endoscopic therapy. This is a radiologically placed shunt that allows for direct reduction of the portal-systemic gradient and results in control of bleeding in 98 per cent of patients. The main complication of TIPS is portosystemic encephalopathy, which is usually controlled with medications such as lactulose. Shunt stenosis is a problem that results mainly from neointima formation within the shunt; occurring 6 to 12 months following placement of TIPS.

7. Surgical placement of shunts reduces portal flow and pressure, and represents a valuable treatment option in patients with repeated variceal bleeding. Emergent surgical shunts can be associated with high mortality. The types of surgical shunts depend on the amount of portal flow that is diverted. Total shunts are those shunts that divert all portal flow, such as portocaval shunts. More selective shunts, such as the distal splenorenal shunt or other partial shunts, may have the advantage of allowing some portal perfusion of hepatic parenchyma while decompressing the portal hypertension. In patients with advanced liver disease and repeated variceal bleeding, liver transplantation should be considered.

8. Balloon tamponade, using either a Sengstaken-Blakemore or Minnesota tube (with gastric and esophageal balloons) or a Linton tube (with gastric balloon only) may be a useful temporizing measure in patients with esophagogastric variceal bleeding. Familiarity with the use of these devices is important to avoid complications such as esophageal perforation, necrosis, and asphyxiation. Recent advances in endoscopic, medical, and surgical treatment of variceal bleeding has resulted in reduced reliance on balloon tamponade.

Bibliography

Grace ND: Diagnosis and treatment of gastrointestinal bleeding secondary to portal hypertension. Am J Gastroenterol 1997;92:1081–1091.

Jutabha R, Jensen DM: Management of upper gastrointestinal bleeding in the patient with chronic liver disease. Med Clin North Am 1996;80:1035–1068.

LaBrecque DR (ed): Portal hypertension. Clin Liver Dis 1997;1:45–128.

Rollhauser C, Fleischer DE: Nonvariceal upper gastrointestinal bleeding: an update. Endoscopy 1997;29:91–105.

Saeed ZA, Ramirez FC, Hepps KS, et al: Prospective validation of the Baylor Bleeding Score for predicting the likelihood of rebleeding after endoscopic hemostasis of peptic ulcers. Gastrointest Endosc 1995;41:561–556.

Indications

1. Diagnostic evaluation and possible treatment for upper gastrointestinal bleeding
2. Obstruction of small bowel or gastric outlet obstruction
3. Lavage for poisoning or overdose and administration of oral antidote
4. Enteral feeding

Contraindications

1. Maxillofacial trauma or basilar skull fracture: tube may enter the cranium.
2. Bilateral nasal obstruction: oral route may be used.
3. Recent surgery to the nose, pharynx, esophagus, or stomach
4. Use caution in patients with a bleeding diathesis.

Equipment

1. Use the proper tube for the situation: Salem sump tube (16 to 18 Fr) for drainage of air and liquids; large-bore tube (Ewald) by oral route for overdose; specialized small-bore tubes for enteral nutrition
2. Lubricant, topical anesthetic, and topical vasoconstrictor
3. Emesis basin, 30- to 60-ml syringe with catheter tip
4. Gloves, goggles, gown, and protective sheet

5. Suction tube, tonsilar tip, and suction device
6. Tape and benzoin

Anesthesia

1. Xylocaine jelly, solution, and spray
2. Topical vasoconstrictor such as phenylephrine or cocaine

Precautions

1. Aspiration of gastric contents may cause aspiration pneumonia. Risk of this complication is high with enteral feeding (20 to 50 per cent) and may be decreased by placement of a feeding tube into the duodenum.
2. Injury to nasal mucosa may cause epistaxis.
3. Inadvertent tracheal intubation may occur and is identified by coughing, choking, and difficulty in talking. These signs are less apparent with small-bore feeding tubes.
4. Lung injury and pneumothorax may occur if enteral feeding tubes with weighted tip and/or metal stylet are passed into the trachea.
5. Vigorous attempts at passage can cause perforation of the esophagus (rare).

WARNING

In a patient with altered mental status, tracheal intubation may occur without typical signs.

Technique

1. Place the patient in the sitting position or left lateral decubitus with neck flexed (if no C-spine injury) to make esophageal passage more direct and avoid tracheal intubation.
2. Measure the distance from the patient's ear to umbilicus to estimate the required length of tube to be inserted.

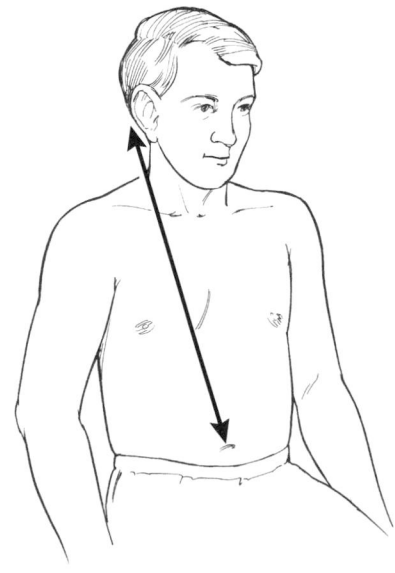

3. Select the most patent nostril and apply topical anesthetic and vasoconstrictor to nasal mucosa. Apply Xylocaine jelly to the tube.

4. Have suction ready to remove emesis or secretions, especially in obtunded patients.

5. Gently insert the tube directed toward the occiput; have the patient swallow when the tube is felt on the back of the throat (15 to 20 cm); sipping water through a straw may help.

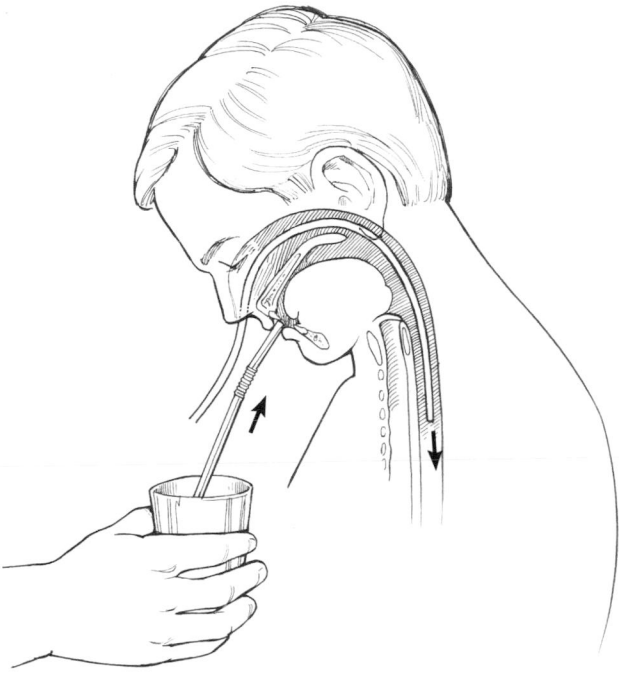

6. If passage into the mouth or coiling occurs, chill the tube with ice to increase its rigidity and help eliminate this problem. The tube can also be stiffened by passing lubricated gastroscope biopsy forceps through the lumen to within 2 cm of the tip, then closing the jaws tightly when stiffness is desired in the oropharynx.

7. If excessive gagging occurs, spray the patient's throat with Xylocaine.

8. Insert the tube to the level of the stomach as previously measured (usually 40 to 50 cm).

9. Instill air with a 30- to 60-ml syringe and listen over the stomach for passage of air.

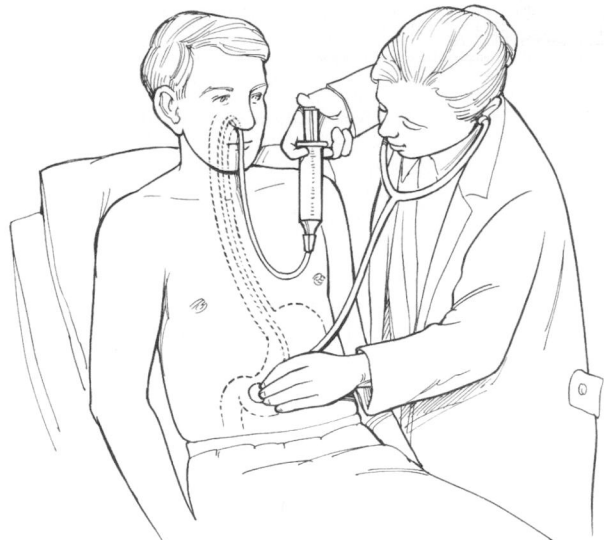

Aspiration of gastric contents and pH of aspirate (usually <5) can be used to help confirm placement.

10. Secure tube with tape and benzoin to the nose, avoiding pressure to the nostril.

11. Radiographic confirmation of placement is mandatory if any substance is to be administered through the tube or if the tube is to be left in place for any length of time.

12. Enteral feeding tubes with weighted tip may pass into the duodenum by placing the patient on the right side for 8 to 24 hours. Active passage into the pylorus using a tube with wire stylet can be performed. Duodenal location is indicated by aspiration of bile and/or aspirate with a pH over 7. Fluoroscopic, sonographic, or endoscopic methods may be needed to achieve placement in the duodenum. Position is confirmed with radiographs.

Follow-Up

1. Check periodically to confirm proper tube functioning by observing continued accumulation of gastric fluids in the collection bottle.

2. If the tube becomes blocked, instill 20 to 30 ml of air into the sump channel to free the tube from gastric mucosa. If blockage persists, inject air or a small amount of normal saline into the main lumen. If blockage recurs, reposition the tube.

3. Periodically check for pressure necrosis of the nose and reposition the tube if necessary.

4. Remove the tube as soon as feasible to avoid complications of prolonged use. Potential problems include gastric erosion with hemorrhage, perforation of stomach or intestine, sinusitis, otitis, pharyngitis, and laryngeal obstruction from subglottic stenosis.

Bibliography

Campbell B: A novel method of nasogastric tube insertion. Anaesthesia 1997;52:1234.

Hernandez-Socorro CR, Marin J, Ruiz-Santana S, et al: Bedside sonographic-guided versus blind nasoenteric feeding tube placement in critically ill patients. Crit Care Med 1996;24:1690–1694.

Sagar PM, Kruegener G, MacFie J: Nasogastric intubation and elective abdominal surgery. Br J Surg 1993; 79:1127–1131.

Wrenn K: The lowly nasogastric tube: still appropriate after all these years (at times). Am J Emerg Med 1993; 11:84–89.

Zaloga GP: Bedside method for placing small bowel feeding tubes in critically ill patients. Chest 1991;100: 1643–1646.

SYMPTOM ACUTE DIARRHEA

Marilee C. S. Cole

Most episodes of acute diarrhea are mild and self-limited. Of the fewer than 10 per cent of cases that come to the physician's attention, most simply require symptomatic oral rehydration.

Differential Diagnosis

1. Infectious diarrhea
   a. Viral diarrhea
   b. Bacterial diarrhea
      (1) *Campylobacter jejuni*: often in college students, day care centers; from poultry
      (2) *Salmonella*: from contaminated beef, poultry, milk, raw eggs
      (3) *Shigella*: in day care centers, Native American reservations, areas of food and water contamination, homosexual males
      (4) Enterohemorrhagic *Escherichia coli*: in nursing homes, in the severely debilitated; from undercooked beef
      (5) Staphylococcal food poisoning: from unrefrigerated meat and cream-based foods
      (6) *Clostridium difficile*: with exposure to antibiotics
      (7) *Vibrio parahaemolyticus*: from exposure to raw or partially cooked seafood
      (8) Consider *Yersinia entercolitica, Vibrio cholerae, Clostridium perfringens, Bacillus cereus*, enterotoxigenic *E. coli, Aeromonas hydrophila, Plesiomonas shigelloides, Cyclospora, Mycobacterium avium-intracellulare* (MAI), sexually transmitted diseases under special circumstances.
   c. Protozoa
      (1) *Giardia lamblia*: in day care centers, travelers, campers, homosexual males, and the immunocompromised
      (2) *Entamoeba histolytica*: predominantly in homosexual males and travelers to the tropics
      (3) *Cryptosporidium*: in young children, in the immunocompromised (such as those with acquired immunodeficiency syndrome), and from contaminated water
2. Drugs
   a. Laxatives: phenolphthalein, magnesium citrate, senna, bisacodyl, lactulose, castor oil, milk of magnesia, polyethylene glycol purge
   b. Antibiotics: erythromycin, clindamycin, cephalosporins, penicillins
   c. Antiarrhythmics: quinidine, digitalis
   d. Diuretics: furosemide, thiazide
   e. Other drugs: over-the-counter headache remedies, nonsteroidal anti-inflammatory drugs, gold, magnesium-containing antacids, thyroid medications, theophylline, stimulants, enemas, misoprostol, colchicine, anticholinesterase inhibitors, methyldopa, chemotherapy
3. Dietary items: lactose, caffeine, sorbitol, mannitol, fructose, sucrose, diet colas
4. Diverticulitis, inflammatory bowel disease
5. Toxins: heavy metals, insecticides, mushrooms
6. Intestinal ischemia

> Refer to Ch. 266, Giardiasis; and Ch. 267, Amebiasis.

History

1. Description of diarrhea: onset, duration, frequency, character of stools (soft, watery, bloody, mucous), associated nausea, vomiting, abdominal pain, tenesmus
2. Systemic symptoms: fever, chills, rigors, dry mouth, dizziness, decreased urine output, weight loss
3. Dietary history 48 hours before symptoms: ingestion of rice, milk, meat, uncooked or poorly cooked fish/seafood, untreated water, unrefrigerated cream-based food, caffeine
4. Sexual history: homosexuality, multiple sex partners, sex with intravenous drug users, oral/anal sex, sexually transmitted diseases

5. Social history: exposure to day care center, nursing home, mental institution, poultry processing, military, travel abroad, camping, industrial toxins, farms/insecticides, Native American reservations

6. Medications: especially antibiotics

7. Medical history: sickle cell anemia, gastrectomy, thyroid disorder, malignancy, radiation, immunosuppression, malaria

Clinical Findings

1. Vital signs: temperature, blood pressure, pulse, orthostasis

2. Skin: turgor, mucous membranes, rash, erythema nodosum

3. Abdomen: distention, tenderness, bowel sounds, splenomegaly, liver, appendicitis, rectal discharge, fissures

4. General: arthritis, lymphadenopathy

Tests

1. Stool examination for white cells or blood: on moderately symptomatic patients with fever, abdominal pain, tenesmus, dehydration, passage of 6 or more unformed stools in 24 hours or illness more than 48 hours' duration

2. Stool cultures: on those patients with white cells, blood, or mucus in stool, fever, abdominal pain (use rectal swab if no stool sample is available)

3. Stool for ova and parasites: for severe or persistent diarrhea (tetracycline, sulfonamides, castor oil, magnesium hydroxide, barium, hypertonic saline, soap, tap water, bismuth, kaolin, and antiprotozoals interfere with the examination)

4. Blood tests: electrolytes; blood cultures for high fever, rigors

5. Additional tests (as indicated by type of patient and type of exposure)

   a. Day care centers: stool enzyme-linked immunosorbent assay (ELISA) for *G. lamblia*, modified acid-fast, *C. difficile* toxin, *E. coli* serotype 0157:H7

   b. Travelers: Enterotoxigenic *E. coli* toxin, *V. cholerae* (alert the laboratory); duodenal aspirate/stool ELISA for *G. lamblia*, modified acid-fast (*Cryptosporidium*)

   c. Antibiotics: *C. difficile* toxin

   d. Immunosuppressed patients: modified acid-fast, human immunodeficiency virus (HIV), MAI, cytomegalovirus, herpes simplex virus

   e. Food poisoning: culture food, vomitus, feces

   f. Seacoast: thiosulfate citrate bile salts (*Vibrio parahaemolyticus*)

   g. Weight loss: stool ELISA for *G. lamblia*, ameba titers

   h. Unexplained fever: *Yersinia enterocolitica* (alert lab)

   i. Nursing home or hospital: enterohemorrhagic *E. coli* serotype 0157, *C. difficile* toxin

6. Sigmoidoscopy: reculture and perform biopsy in undiagnosed diarrhea.

Management

1. Fluid replacement

   a. Minimally dehydrated: "drink lots of fluids" (except with vomiting, ileus)

   b. Moderately dehydrated: oral replacement therapy with glucose and electrolytes (e.g., Pedialyte, Gatorade) to 1000 ml/hour

   c. Severely dehydrated: intravenous hydration with Ringer's lactate with potassium supplement in emergency department

2. Adsorbant: Kaopectate improves stool form.

3. Antidiarrheal agents: After removing lactose and caffeine from the diet in an afebrile patient with nonbloody diarrhea without fecal leukocytes, the following agents are useful:

   a. Antimotility agent: loperamide (Imodium), 4 mg orally to begin and 2 mg orally after each unformed stool to five doses per day

   b. Antisecretory agent: bismuth subsalicylate (Pepto Bismol), 2 tablets q30 min for eight doses; AVOID in HIV-positive patients.

4. Antimicrobials

   a. *Campylobacter jejuni*: ciprofloxacin (Cipro), 500 mg, or erythromycin stearate, 500 mg orally bid ×5 days, or azithromycin, 500 mg ×3 days; start before fourth day of illness for severe illness

   b. *Clostridium difficile*: metronidazole (Flagyl), 500 mg orally tid for 10 days (avoid in pregnancy); vancomycin, 125 to 250 mg orally qid for 5 to 10 days for severe or persistent disease if the offending antibiotics cannot be stopped.

   c. Enterohemorrhagic *E. coli*: Antibiotics withheld.

   d. Enterotoxigenic *E. coli* (traveler's diarrhea): ciprofloxacin 500 mg, norfloxacin 400 mg, or ofloxacin 300 mg orally bid for 3 to 5 days

   e. *Entamoeba histolytica*: metronidazole, 750 mg orally tid for 10 days, followed by iodoquinol, 650 mg orally tid for 20 days to eliminate the cyst phase (do not use if patient is allergic to iodine)

   f. *Giardia lamblia*: metronidazole, 250 mg orally qid for 7 days (avoid in pregnancy), or quinacrine HCl (Atabrine), 100 mg orally tid for 7 days, or albendazole, 400 mg orally for 5 days

   g. *Salmonella enteritidis*: Treat only if immunocompromised, bacteremic, or younger than 1 year with ciprofloxacin, 500 mg orally bid for 7 days, or trimethoprim-sulfamethoxazole (TMP/SMX), 160 mg TPM/800 mg SMX orally bid for 5 days (adult dosage).

   h. *Shigella*: if acquired in the United States, TMP/SMX, 160 mg TMP/800 mg SMX orally bid for 3 to 5 days; if acquired outside the United States, ciprofloxacin 500 mg or norfloxacin (Noroxin) 400 mg orally bid for 3 to 5 days

Prevention

1. Vaccines: typhoid, cholera, shigella, rotavirus
2. Travelers: "Boil it, cook it, peel it, or forget it."
3. Prophylaxis for travelers to underdeveloped countries consists of bismuth subsalicylate (Pepto Bismol), 2 tablets (total 524 mg) orally qid for up to 3 weeks.
4. In day care centers: handwashing after each diaper change

PEARLS

- Be sure to ask the patient to describe the frequency, liquidity, and character of the stools, because patients often misdiagnose any change in bowel habits as diarrhea.

- Look for *G. lamblia* in lactose-intolerant patients.

- Patients on oral hypoglycemic agents should avoid TMP/SMX because it may lead to hypoglycemia.

B Bibliography

Cheney C: Acute infectious diarrhea. Med Clin North Am 1993;77:1169–1196.

DuPont H: Guidelines on infectious diarrhea in adults. Am J Gastroenterol 1997;92:1962–1973.

Kelly C: *Clostridium difficile* colitis. N Engl J Med 1994; 330:257–262.

Kozicki M: Boil it, cook it, peel it, or forget it: does this rule prevent travelers' diarrhoea? Int J Epidemiol 1985; 14:169–171.

Mac Kenzie W: A massive outbreak in Milwaukee of *Cryptosporidium* infection transmitted through the public water supply. N Engl J Med 1994;331:161–167.

Patterson J: The pre-travel medical evaluation: the traveler with chronic illness and the geriatric traveler. Yale J Biol Med 1992;65:317–327.

SYMPTOM CHRONIC DIARRHEA

Marilee C. S. Cole

Chronic diarrhea lasts longer than 3 to 4 weeks and may be continuous or episodic. With the advent of acquired immunodeficiency syndrome (AIDS), chronic diarrhea is an increasingly common and often difficult complaint to manage.

Differential Diagnosis

1. Irritable bowel syndrome
2. Diet and medications (see preceding symptom, Acute Diarrhea)
3. Infection: *Giardia lamblia, Entamoeba histolytica, Campylobacter*, salmonella, *Clostridium difficile, Cryptosporidium, Mycobacterium avium-intracellulare, Isospora*, Cytomegalovirus, *Microsporidium*
4. Malabsorption: pancreatic insufficiency, bacterial overgrowth, gluten-sensitive enteropathy (celiac disease), ileal resection
5. Carcinoma of the bowel or pancreas
6. Inflammatory bowel disease: ulcerative proctitis, ulcerative colitis, Crohn's disease; ischemic colitis; radiation colitis; diverticulitis
7. Metabolic: hyperthyroidism, diabetes mellitus, hypoadrenalism
8. Peptide-induced gastrinoma, vasoactive intestinal polypeptide (VIP) tumor, carcinoid, villous adenoma, thyroid medullary carcinoma
9. Laxative abuse
10. Fecal impaction—especially in nursing home patients on tricyclic and anticholinergic medications
11. Psychiatric: depression, anxiety/panic, somatization

Refer to Ch. 86, Colorectal Cancer; Ch. 89, Crohn's Disease, Ch. 90, Ulcerative Colitis; Ch. 91, Irritable Bowel Syndrome; Ch. 94, Fecal Impaction; Ch. 101, Pancreatic Carcinoma; Ch. 266, Giardiasis; and Ch. 267, Amebiasis.

History

This is key to differentiating irritable bowel syndrome, the most common cause of chronic diarrhea, from the less common forms of chronic diarrhea. Irritable bowel syndrome is characterized by frequent, incomplete evacuations and daytime diarrhea (often alternating with constipation), typically beginning in adolescence and exacerbated by stress.

1. Abdominal symptoms: age at onset; chronicity, frequency and character of stools (color, mucus, blood); presence of abdominal pain, bloating, flatulence, incontinence; inciting and ameliorating factors (time of day, foods, medicines, stress, fasting)
2. General: fever, weight loss, flushing, joint aches
3. Travel history, work history
4. Medical history: diverticulosis, diabetes mellitus, radiation therapy, ileal resection, anorectal surgery
5. Medications: Consider laxative abuse, opioid withdrawal (for complete list see preceding symptom, Acute Diarrhea).
6. Sexual history: homosexuality, human immunodeficiency virus (HIV) status
7. Endocrinologic: salt craving, heat intolerance, polyuria, polydipsia, polyphagia
8. Psychiatric: increased stress, eating disorders, history of physical or sexual abuse

Clinical Findings

1. General: racial group, flushing, lymphadenopathy
2. Vital signs: fever, tachycardia
3. Eye, ear, nose, and throat: iritis, aphthous ulcers, parotid enlargement, loss of tooth enamel
4. Neck: thyroid swelling
5. Abdomen: tenderness, presence of right lower quadrant mass, perirectal fistula
6. Skin: erythema nodosum, dermatitis herpetiformis, dorsum of hand roughened, larva currens
7. Extremity: arthritis, bone fractures
8. Neurologic: peripheral or autonomic neuropathy, tetany

Tests

Before launching into an extensive evaluation, eliminate infectious causes of diarrhea. In one study, 38 per cent of patients thought to have inflammatory bowel disease had infectious diarrhea instead.

1. Exclude acute causes (see preceding symptom, Acute Diarrhea)
2. Exclude lactose intolerance by lactose restriction or lactose tolerance test
3. Flexible sigmoidoscopy, preferably without enema prep, for culture and biopsy (or colonoscopy)
4. Plain film of abdomen: for pancreatic calcifications, obstruction
5. Air contrast barium enema (except with severe ulcerative colitis or Crohn's disease of the colon to avoid toxic megacolon)
6. Upper gastrointestinal series with small bowel follow-through to evaluate for Crohn's, celiac, and Whipple's disease
7. Blood tests: potassium, calcium, cholesterol, albumin, fasting blood sugar, 2-hour postprandial blood sugar, thyroxine, 8 AM cortisol, amylase, iron, prothrombin time, immunoglobulins, sedimentation rate, eosinophil count, vitamin B_{12}, HIV
8. Malabsorption work-up (for weight loss with good appetite)
   a. A 72-hour fecal fat (abnormal if greater than 6 gm/day on 80- to 100-gm fat diet)
   b. D-Xylose absorption (abnormal if less than 4.5 gm/5-hour urine collection after ingesting 25 gm D-xylose orally)
   c. Schilling or breath test for bacterial overgrowth
   d. Small bowel biopsy, aspirate, culture
   e. Bentiromide test for pancreatic function
   f. Gluten sensitivity screen—especially for gliadin antibody
9. Stool volume, electrolytes, osmolality (especially after fasting)
10. Therapeutic trials
    a. Restricted diets (e.g., gluten)
    b. Antibiotics (e.g., tetracycline, metronidazole)
11. Heavy metals: arsenic, mercury, lead, cadmium
12. Urine 5-hydroxyindoleacetic acid, plasma gastrin, calcitonin, VIP, glucagon, somatostatin
13. Stool alkalinization for identification of laxative phenolphthalein use/abuse

Management

1. As for acute diarrheas: hydrate, eliminate causative medicines and foods, treat underlying infections, use antimotility agents when necessary (see preceding symptom, Acute Diarrhea)
2. Irritable bowel syndrome: adequate fluids and dietary fiber, stress reduction, sympathetic physician, psyllium, antispasmodics such as dicyclomine (Bentyl), 10 mg orally tid
3. Lastose-intolerant patients: add lactase supplement when ingesting lactose or remove lactose

from diet; maintain dietary calcium intake with yogurt, lactose hydrolyzed milk (Lactaid), or calcium carbonate tablets (Tums)

4. Malabsorption
   a. Pancreatic insufficiency: pancreatic enzyme (Pancrease), 1 to 2 capsules with each meal and 1 with snack
   b. Bacterial overgrowth: antibiotics—for example, trimethoprim-sulfamethoxazole (TMP/SMX [Bactrim DS]), 160 mg TMP/800 mg SMZ orally bid
   c. Celiac disease: avoid wheat, barley, rye flours

5. Inflammatory bowel disease
   a. Ulcerative proctitis: mesalamine (Rowasa), 2- to 4-gm enema, or hydrocortisone, 100 mg retention enema (Cortenema) at bedtime for 21 days
   b. Ulcerative colitis: sulfasalazine (Azulfidine), or mesalamine, 1 gm orally qid; if refractory, use prednisone, 60 mg orally daily until remission. Consider immunomodulators (for mild to moderate: 6-mercaptopurine [Purinethol], or azathioprine [Imuran]; for severe: short-course cyclosporine [Sandimmune]).
   c. Crohn's disease: as per ulcerative colitis, sulfasalazine or mesalamine, then prednisone (budesonide* 9 mg, with fewer systemic effects, has been used as an alternative to prednisone 60 mg), plus antibacterial (metronidazole), vitamin supplement with folic acid, antimotility agent, occasionally elemental diet (Ensure), smoking cessation

6. Diabetes mellitus: clonidine, octreotide (Sandostatin)
7. Chronic secretory diarrhea: octreotide
8. Intractable diarrhea: cholestyramine

---

*Not yet available in the U.S. (used in Canada).

PEARLS

- Think Crohn's disease in the elderly with nonspecific symptoms and an indolent course. Time to diagnosis in one study was three times longer in the elderly than in younger patients with Crohn's disease (6.4 versus 2.4 years).

- Prepare a homemade hydrocortisone enema (cheaper than the expensive commercial preparations) by blending 100 mg hydrocortisone hemisuccinate in 60 ml of safflower oil.

- In patients with Crohn's disease the incidence of smoking is greater than that of the general population, whereas in ulcerative colitis it is less.

- A majority of AIDS patients have had at least one diarrheal episode. Symptomatic treatment of stool culture–negative AIDS-related diarrhea is both efficacious and cost-effective.

Bibliography

Greenberger N: Diagnostic approach to the patient with chronic diarrheal disorder. Dis Mon 1990;36:131–179.
Grimm I: Inflammatory bowel disease in the elderly. Gastroenterol Clin North Am 1990;19:361–389.
Jernigan J: Parasitic infections of the small intestine. Gut 1994;35:289–293.
Johanson J: Efficient management of diarrhea in the acquired immunodeficiency syndrome (AIDS). Ann Intern Med 1990;112:942–948.
Moses P: Inflammatory bowel disease. Postgrad Med 1998;103:77–102.
Nolte F: Practical considerations in the laboratory diagnosis of bacterial enteric infections. Am J Clin Pathol 1994;101:S14–S17.

SYMPTOM CONSTIPATION

Andrew M. D. Wolf

1. Epidemiology: Constipation is the most common digestive complaint in the United States, affecting over 4.5 million people or 2 per cent of the population. It is two to three times more common in women, and there is a marked increase in constipation after age 65, but this is a consequence of co-morbidity, environmental influences, and over-reporting, not of the aging process itself. Between 2 and 3 million people use laxatives regularly in the United States, with potentially damaging consequences and an annual expenditure approaching $400 million for over-the-counter (OTC) laxatives alone.

2. Definition: The generally accepted standard is fewer than three stools per week. Passage of hard small stools, straining, and sense of incomplete evacuation are often included in the definition.

3. Etiology (see Table 80–2).

History
1. Clarify "constipation": stool frequency, consis-

TABLE 80-2. CAUSES OF CONSTIPATION

Health habits	Neurologic
Low fiber/fluid intake	Parkinson's disease
Inactivity	Dementia
Medications	Multiple sclerosis
Anticholinergics (tricyclics, neurolep- tics, anti-Parkinson)	Spinal cord lesions
Antihypertensives (verapamil, diuret- ics, clonidine)	Autonomic neuropathy (esp. diabetes mellitus, pseudo-obstruction)
Narcotics	Hirschsprung's disease
Antacids (with aluminum or calcium)	Psychiatric
Iron	Depression
Bile resins	Endocrine/metabolic
Sympathomimetics	Hypothyroidism
Chronic stimulant laxative use	Pregnancy/premenstrual
Irritable bowel syndrome	Hypercalcemia
Structural lesions	Hypokalemia
Tumor	Uremia
Stricture	
Hemorrhoids	
Fissure	
Rectocele	
Descending perineum syndrome	

tency, straining; many patients are preoccupied with their bowels but are not constipated.

2. Onset: Recent onset raises possibility of significant pathology, especially tumor.

3. Associated symptoms: Abdominal pain can suggest irritable bowel syndrome or tumor; hematochezia, reduced caliber, and tenesmus can suggest structural lesion (tumor, hemorrhoids, fissure, stricture); constitutional symptoms can suggest malignancy or endocrine or metabolic causes; depressive symptoms may suggest a psychiatric etiology.

4. Sexual history: As many as 50 per cent of women with functional gastrointestinal (GI) complaints have been victims of sexual abuse.

5. Medication history (see Table 80-2): Be sure to ask about OTC laxative use, because this may well contribute to chronic constipation ("cathartic" or atonic colon).

6. Brief diet/exercise screen: adequate fiber, fluids, activity

Key Questions to Ask
1. What does the patient mean by "constipation?"
2. When did symptoms begin?
3. Any associated GI symptoms?
4. Any constitutional symptoms?
5. What medications?

Clinical Findings
1. Abdominal examination: Check for tenderness, masses.
2. Rectal examination: Examine for anal tone (rule out neurologic lesion), trauma (especially in children and adolescents), hemorrhoids, fissure, stricture/stenosis, rectocele, tumor, impaction, and occult blood.

3. General examination: Look for signs of hypothyroidism and neurologic disease.

Tests
1. Blood tests: Recent onset of severe constipation warrants checking serum potassium, calcium, and thyroid-stimulating hormone. Chronic laxative users should have a complete set of electrolytes, blood urea nitrogen, and creatinine in view of the potential metabolic sequelae.

2. Endoscopy: Most middle-aged or older patients with recent onset of significant constipation should undergo flexible sigmoidoscopy at a minimum to rule out colorectal carcinoma. This may also detect other structural lesions (see above) and melanosis coli, suggestive of chronic stimulant laxative abuse. Severe constipation, concomitant abdominal pain, occult blood in the stool, and constitutional symptoms generally dictate the need for full colonoscopy or addition of barium enema to the sigmoidoscopy.

3. Radiography: Plain abdominal films are not routinely indicated but can occasionally be useful to confirm the diagnosis by demonstrating feces throughout the colon. Barium enema may also be necessary, as discussed above.

4. Colonic transit time/motility studies: rarely indicated. Reserve for instances of severe constipation unresponsive to treatment, when the results will alter management approach.

Management

1. First treat fecal impaction if present.
2. Nonpharmacologic treatment should be mainstay of therapy.
   a. Ensure adequate fluid intake (1500 ml minimum).
   b. Ensure adequate dietary fiber intake: bran cereal, beans, vegetables, fruit (14 gm crude fiber, 30 gm dietary fiber per day).
   c. Ensure adequate physical activity.
   d. Bowel retraining: Patient should attempt to defecate at the same time daily within 10 to 15 minutes of a meal (to utilize the gastrocolic reflex); may require daily suppository or enema at first.
3. Pharmacologic treatment (Table 80–3)
   a. Bulk-forming laxatives: should be used preferentially for long-term management of ambulatory patients but may be ineffective in bed-bound patients.
   b. Osmotic agents: preferred second-line agents because they are less toxic than other alternatives
   c. Stool softeners: useful when straining should be avoided (e.g., hemorrhoids, myocardial infarction), but have no effect on stool frequency and are greatly overprescribed.
   d. For refractory constipation: A regimen including bisacodyl suppositories or enemas once or twice a week, together with a daily osmotic laxative, is generally safe and effective; chronic stimulant laxatives are a last resort because of potential long-term toxicity. An oral colon washout solution (e.g., 250 to 500 ml of polyethylene glycol) is effective and safe for periodic use if obstruction has been excluded. Consider referral at this point for specialized testing (e.g., defacography, anorectal manometry).
   e. Cisapride, a GI prokinetic drug, may be useful for slow-transit constipation but has not yet been approved for this indication.

PEARLS

- Check the list of medications for constipating drugs.

- New onset of significant constipation requires lower GI evaluation.

- Mainstays of treatment are adequate fluids, fiber, and exercise.

- Bulk-forming laxatives should be first-line, followed by osmotic agents.

- Stool softeners have little or no laxative effect; they simply soften stool.

TABLE 80–3. COMMON LAXATIVES

CATEGORY NAME (EXAMPLES)	ADULT DOSE	POTENTIAL ADVERSE EFFECTS/COMMENTS
Bulk-forming		
Psyllium (Metamucil)	1 tsp qd–tid	Bloating, gas, obstipation if taken without fluids
Methylcellulose (Citrucel)	1 tbsp qd–tid	Bloating, gas, but less than with psyllium
Stool softeners		Mucosal irritation; no evidence for true laxative effect
Docusate sodium (Colace)	50–500 mg qd	
Docusate calcium (Surfak)	240 mg qd	
Osmotic		
Lactulose	15–60 ml/day	Bloating, cramps, flatulence
Sorbitol (70%)	30–60 ml/day	Same as lactulose, much less expensive
Glycerin	1 suppository	Occasional rectal irritation
Saline		
Magnesium hydroxide (Milk of Magnesia)	30–60 ml	Cramping, diarrhea, dehydration, ↑ Mg in elderly and renal disease
Sodium phosphate (Fleet Enema, Phospho-Soda)	PO: 20–30 ml Enema: 1–2/wk	Dehydration, ↑ phosphate in renal disease
Stimulants		Electrolyte imbalance, ? "cathartic" (atonic) colon (the risk of cathartic colon is uncertain)
Bisacodyl (Dulcolax)	1–3 tabs, 1 suppository (max. 3/wk)	
Senna (Senokot)	2 tabs at hs	
Cascara	1 tab at hs	
Lubricants		
Mineral oil	15–45 ml PO or by enema	Fat-soluble vitamin malabsorption, lipoid pneumonia if aspirated

Bibliography

Camilleri M, Thompson WG, Fleshman JW, Pemberton JH: Clinical management of intractable constipation. Ann Intern Med 1994;121:520–528.

Lennard-Jones JE: Constipation. In Feldman M, Scharschmidt BF, Sleisenger MH (eds): Sleisenger & Fordtran's Gastrointestinal and Liver Disease: Pathophysiology/Diagnosis/Management, 6th ed, vol 1, pp 174–197. Philadelphia, WB Saunders Company, 1998.

Marshall JB: Chronic constipation in adults: how far should evaluation and treatment go? Postgrad Med 1990;88:49–63.

Romero Y, Evans JM, Fleming KC, Phillips SF: Constipation and fecal incontinence in the elderly population. Mayo Clin Proc 1996;71:81–92.

Wald A: Constipation and fecal incontinence in the elderly. Gastroenterol Clin North Am 1990;19:405–418.

Indications

1. Constant anal pain of sudden onset
2. Ulceration or rupture of the thrombosed hemorrhoid
3. Failure of medical treatment and persistence of symptoms

> **IMPORTANT**
>
> **The pain associated with a thrombosed hemorrhoid often resolves after 48 hours. The clot is gradually absorbed over 7 to 10 days. When this does not occur or the patient desires immediate relief, excision is an option.**

Contraindications

1. Absolute: if thrombosed hemorrhoid is internal (above dentate line)
2. Relative
   a. Bleeding or clotting disorder
   b. Associated infection

Preparation

1. Patient is placed either in the lateral Sims position or jackknife position.
2. Assistant to adequately expose the entire thrombosed hemorrhoid
3. The anal area is cleansed with povidone-iodine.

Equipment

1. No. 15 or No. 11 blade
2. Adson's forceps with teeth
3. Straight hemostat
4. Curved iris scissors
5. 10-ml syringe
6. 27-gauge 1¼-in needle
7. Electrocautery and/or Monsel's solution

Anesthesia

1. 0.5% bupivacaine in 1:200,000 epinephrine with 1:10 sodium bicarbonate, USP 8.4 per cent
   a. The sodium bicarbonate is mixed with the bupivacaine just before surgery to avoid precipitation.
   b. By alkalinizing the solution, one can prevent the burning pain of the anesthetic.
   c. Slow infiltration of the anesthetic will also decrease the pain of injection.
2. The area surrounding the base of the thrombosed hemorrhoid is infiltrated just beneath the skin, raising a slight wheal circumferentially.
3. Adequate time is allowed (2 to 4 minutes) for the anesthetic to take effect.

Precautions

1. If the patient is hypertensive, the blood pressure should be checked following anesthesia.
2. Failure to anesthetize completely around the hemorrhoid may result in pain with the excision.
3. Failure to completely remove the clot may result in prolonged postoperative bleeding and continuing pain.

Technique

1. After exposure of the hemorrhoid, the incision is planned. The type of excision depends on the size of the hemorrhoid and the amount of skin that can be safely removed.
   a. For hemorrhoids 2 cm or larger, a radial elliptical (fusiform) incision over the top of the hemorrhoid can be made using the curved iris scissors and Adson's forceps or blade.

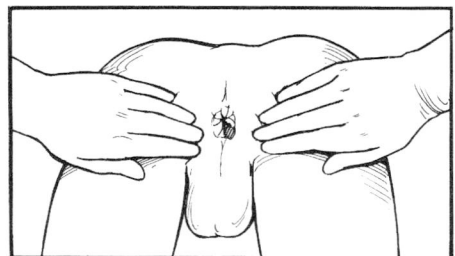

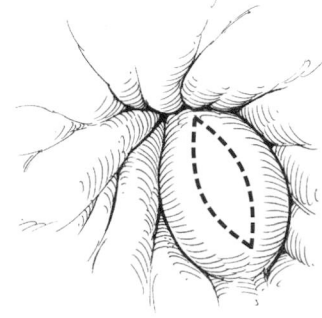

b. For hemorrhoids less than 2 cm, the entire hemorrhoid can be excised using the curved iris scissors and Adson's forceps, again utilizing a radial elliptical (fusiform) excision.

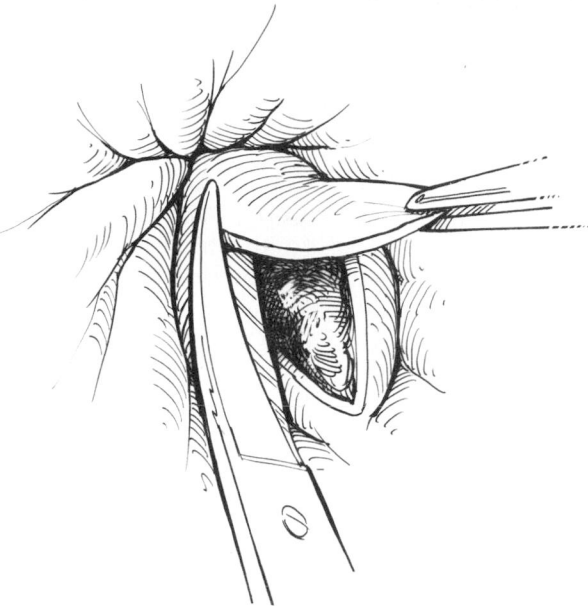

c. Express the clot by applying pressure laterally. Determine whether the entire clot has been removed by palpating over the area. If any clot remains, a straight hemostat may be used to open up any remaining clotted veins.

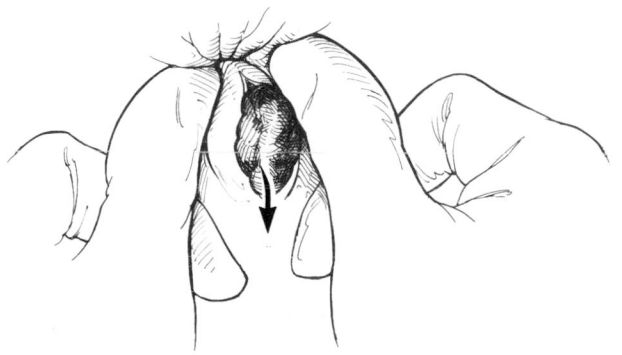

2. Hemostasis can be achieved with pressure, Monsel's solution, and/or electrocautery.

3. Packing is not required.
4. A dressing of 4 × 4s and a large pad can be applied. This should be left on for at least 4 hours.

Follow-Up

1. The patient is instructed to begin warm sitz baths twice a day, no sooner than 4 hours after the surgery, and continue these for 7 to 10 days.
2. Stool softeners
3. Analgesia in the form of acetaminophen plus propoxyphene hydrochloride can be given for the first few days following surgery. After that, acetaminophen should be all that is required.

IMPORTANT

If a stronger narcotic, such as hydrocodone or oxycodone, is required, the patient should be warned about its potential for causing constipation.

---

4. The patient is to report any bleeding that soaks through the dressing in the first 24 hours. Subsequently, the bleeding should gradually stop over 5 to 7 days. If it begins heavier than before, the physician must be notified.
5. Anoscopy and flexible sigmoidoscopy are recommended in 2 weeks.

 Bibliography

Corman ML: Colon and Rectal Surgery, 3rd ed, pp 77–78. Philadelphia, JB Lippincott Company, 1993.

Grosy CR: A surgical treatment of thrombosed external hemorrhoids. Dis Col Rect 1990;249–250.

Janicke DM, Pundt MR: Anorectal disorders [review]. Emerg Med Clin North Am 1996;14:757–788.

Salvati EP, Eisenstat TE: Hemorroidal disease. In Zuidema G (ed): Shackelford's Surgery of the Alimentary Tract, 4th ed, vol IV, pp 330–343. Philadelphia, WB Saunders Company, 1996.

SYMPTOM RECTAL BLEEDING   *Arthur H. Herold*

The complaint of rectal bleeding must be taken seriously. The severity of bleeding does not relate to the significance of the underlying pathology, and the same types of lesions can produce extremes in bleeding rates. The physician must first determine whether the rectal bleeding has produced hemodynamic compromise. Such patients require resuscitation and stabilization first before searching for the cause. However, episodes of rectal bleeding are usually self-limiting, and the evaluation can be carried out in a timely, methodical manner. Determining the site (upper gastrointestinal [GI], small bowel, colorectal) takes precedence over identifying the source. The frequency of causes of rectal bleeding is influenced by the patient's age, whether a particular study is conducted on inpatients or outpatients, and whether the bleeding is occult, small, or massive.

Differential Diagnosis

1. Colorectal diseases (80 to 85 per cent)
   a. Diverticulosis
   b. Angiodysplasia
   c. Neoplasms
      (1) Colon cancer
      (2) Colonic polyps
   d. Inflammatory bowel disease
      (1) Ulcerative colitis
      (2) Crohn's colitis
   e. Anorectal disorders
      (1) Hemorrhoids
          (a) External
          (b) Internal
      (2) Anal fissure (fissure in ano)
      (3) Anal fistula (fistula in ano)
      (4) Rectal prolapse
      (5) Neoplasms
          (a) Rectal carcinoma
          (b) Rectal polyps
      (6) Proctitis
          (a) Ulcerative
          (b) Infectious
      (7) Cryptitis
      (8) Draining perirectal abscess, pilonidal cyst
      (9) Dermatologic conditions
   f. Colitis
      (1) Ischemic
      (2) Infectious
      (3) Radiation
2. Upper GI tract (10 per cent)
   a. Duodenal ulcer
   b. Erosive gastritis
   c. Mallory-Weiss tear
   d. Esophagitis
   e. Gastric ulcer
   f. Esophageal varices
   g. Neoplasm
   h. Biliary or pancreatic duct bleeding
3. Small intestine diseases (5 per cent)
   a. Neoplasms
   b. Crohn's disease
   c. Aortoenteric fistula
   d. Angiodysplasia
   e. Meckel's diverticulum
   f. Intussusception
4. Systemic conditions (rare)
   a. Anticoagulation therapy
   b. Thrombocytopenia
   c. Histiocytosis
   d. Amyloidosis
   e. Vasculitis
   f. Elastic tissue diseases
5. Trauma (uncommon)
   a. External abdominal
   b. Rectal

> Refer to Ch. 83, Gastritis; Ch. 84, Peptic Ulcer Disease; Ch. 86, Colorectal Cancer; Ch. 88, Intussusception; Ch. 90, Ulcerative Colitis; Ch. 92, Diverticulitis; and Ch. 93, Hemorrhoids.

History

1. Character of blood: color, consistency, amount, frequency, duration
   a. Hematochezia
      (1) Bright red: usually a distal colorectal or anorectal source. Can be a proximal GI hemorrhage if brisk and associated with increased colonic motility.
          (a) On toilet paper, dripping into toilet, typically limited amounts, especially with defecation: probably a perianal source
          (b) Coating a normal stool: Consider a lesion in the anal canal.
          (c) Streaking or mixed with a formed stool: Suggests rectosigmoid or descending colon lesion.
      (2) Maroon stools: Source may be proximal colon, small intestine, or distal colon if associated with constipation.
   b. Melena (sticky, jet-black, tarry, foul-smelling stools)
      (1) Do not confuse with
          (a) Clotted blood, which will turn water red
          (b) Iron or bismuth ingestion
          (c) Dark but normal stools
      (2) Source
          (a) Significant upper GI bleeding (oral cavity, esophagus, stomach, or duodenum)
          (b) May be lower GI hemorrhage if colonic motility is slow.
   c. Occult blood loss: The patient may present with symptoms of anemia (orthostasis, syncope, dyspnea on exertion, angina, fatigue, or pallor) but usually is asymptomatic.

2. Pain with bleeding
   a. Absent: consider diverticulosis, angiodysplasia, internal hemorrhoids, esophageal varices
   b. Abdominal
      (1) Epigastric (may radiate into chest): upper GI source, such as peptic or gastric ulcer, esophagitis, Mallory-Weiss tear. Typical symptoms include hematemesis or vomiting, history of aspirin, nonsteroidal anti-inflammatory drugs (NSAIDs), alcohol, or tobacco use; peptic ulcer disease.
      (2) Periumbilical: small bowel. Think ischemic bowel if there is a history of vascular or coronary artery disease.
      (3) Hypogastric: colonic lesions
      (4) Suprapubic: rectosigmoid lesion
      (5) Generalized (but may be upper, mid, or lower abdominal): ruptured abdominal aortic aneurysm (AAA) with aortoenteric fistula. (Patient is catastrophically ill, has tearing back pain during dissection.) A fistula is most likely to follow prior AAA repair and be painless.
      (6) Left lower quadrant: descending colon or sigmoid lesions
      (7) Crampy with gas and bloating: inflammatory bowel disease
      (8) Colicky: intussusception
   c. Sacral: rectal lesions
      (1) Sharp, knife-like after bowel movement: anal fissure
      (2) Constant throbbing: perirectal abscess, acute thrombosed external hemorrhoids
3. Change in bowel habits with bleeding
   a. Constipation
      (1) Chronic: hemorrhoids
      (2) Recent progressive: distal colonic annular constricting carcinoma
      (3) Voluminous hard stool with pain: anal fissure
   b. Diarrhea
      (1) Frequent bloody bowel movements, small amounts ± mucus, weight loss: inflammatory bowel disease
      (2) With pus: infectious colitis or proctitis
   c. Tenesmus: anorectal lesions such as proctitis or neoplasm
   d. Discharge, mucopurulent ± blood ± stool ± foul odor: proctitis, draining perirectal abscess/cryptitis, fistula in ano, pilonidal cyst
   e. Change in shape of stool, decreased caliber, or flat spot: anal or rectal carcinoma

   f. Sensation of rectal fullness, incomplete evacuation, or recognition of rectal mass present: rectal carcinoma or hemorrhoids
4. History of systemic disease, anticoagulation therapy, aspirin, or NSAID use or symptoms of metastasis such as weight loss, anorexia, abdominal bloating or swelling, malnutrition; history of AAA repair
5. History of trauma, abuse (child, sexual, spouse), insertion of foreign objects into the rectum, or anal intercourse

The clinician must be suspicious that an underlying lesion has been unmasked when rectal bleeding occurs in an anticoagulated patient, especially if the patient is not overly anticoagulated.

Clinical Findings
1. Degree of blood loss: Evaluate general appearance and vital signs.
   a. Chronic (pallor, tachycardia, postural hypotension): carcinoma
   b. Acute
      (1) Massive (altered mental status, hypotension, shock, gross evidence of blood loss rectally ± abdominal distention): bleeding ulcer, varices, angiodysplasia, diverticulosis, ruptured AAA
      (2) Minimal (stable vital signs): anorectal conditions, carcinoma
2. Abdominal examination
   a. Distended: ruptured aneurysm
   b. Pulsating mass: aneurysm
   c. Tender epigastrium: ulcers
   d. Hepatomegaly: metastatic colon cancer
   e. Ascites: metastatic colon cancer
   f. Sausage-shaped mass right side: intussusception
   g. Diffuse mild tenderness without guarding: colitis
   h. Left lower quadrant tenderness: sigmoid colon lesion
   i. Mass along course of colon: colon cancer
   j. Hyperactive bowel sounds: colitis, obstruction
3. Rectal examination
   a. Anal inspection: Spread the buttocks vigorously with patient in left lateral position.
      (1) External hemorrhoids, prolapsing internal hemorrhoids, and carcinoma should be apparent.
      (2) Draining sinus tract: superior—pilonidal cyst; perianal—fistula in ano
      (3) Tear in anal skin parallel to anal canal,

superior or inferior ± sentinel tag: anal fissure

b. Digital examination

(1) Perianal mass deep in buttocks with surrounding erythema and inflammation: perirectal abscess

(2) Pain with insertion of digit into anal canal: anal fissure

(3) Stenosis of anal canal: constricting anal carcinoma

(4) Solid mass in rectum: rectal carcinoma

4. Confirmation of bleeding

a. Inspect toilet or bed pan for color and amount. If stool just eliminated, Hemoccult-test sample if presence of blood is doubtful.

b. Rule out bleeding from the vagina or urethra in women.

c. Inspect underclothes and buttocks. The presence of blood in a continent patient suggests bleeding external to the anal sphincter.

d. Inspect sample during rectal examination for presence of melena, maroon-colored blood, or bright red blood.

e. Hemoccult-test stool sample from rectum regardless of appearance

Tests

1. Laboratory

a. Complete blood count

(1) Anemia: may be present when GI blood loss has been subacute or chronic and significant.

(2) Normal blood count: present when bleeding has been acute and massive because plasma volume has not equilibrated, or chronic lesions with insignificant blood loss

b. Serum iron, total iron-binding capacity, ferritin: helpful to confirm iron deficiency when patient has anemia and GI blood loss is suspected but not confirmed

c. Chemistry studies: useful if a systemic process is suspected, such as inflammatory bowel disease or metastatic carcinoma

d. Fecal occult blood test: If the patient is stable and GI blood loss is questionable, give the patient three cards to collect samples at home. Hand out instructions to minimize false-positive or false-negative test results.

2. Anoscopy

a. Should be performed during the initial physical examination

b. Rules out lesions of the anus and anal canal, such as hemorrhoids or fissures

3. Proctosigmoidoscopy: The clinician must be trained before attempting this procedure.

a. Examines the rectum, sigmoid, and sometimes part of the descending colon

b. Useful to rule out left-sided colorectal lesions such as polyps, proctitis, colitis, and carcinoma, when brisk bleeding is not present

4. Colonoscopy: ideally inspects the entire colon

a. Limited value if lower GI bleeding is acute and massive or patient is unprepped

b. Used to diagnose slow bleeding lesions to include polyps, diverticula, angiodysplasia, carcinoma, or colitis

c. May be useful in patients with active lower GI bleeding who are hemodynamically stable after resuscitation. A colon prep is required.

5. Arteriography

a. Best initial test if bleeding is rapid (must be at least 0.5 to 1.0 ml/min)

b. Allows rapid localization and possible treatment of a briskly bleeding lesion, such as diverticula, angiodysplasia, carcinoma, and lesions proximal to the colon.

c. Has high complication rate.

6. Technetium-99m–labeled red blood cell scintigraphy

a. Order for intermittent bleeding if the patient is stable and recurrent bleeding is anticipated within 30 hours; delayed images can be obtained.

b. Slowly bleeding lesions (as low as 0.1 ml/min) can be seen to include diverticula or angiodysplasia.

c. More useful than technetium-99m sulfur colloid scan because this radionuclide is rapidly cleared, making it a poor technique for diagnosing intermittent bleeding

7. Barium enema: Do not order when vigorous bleeding is present.

a. Diagnostic for space-occupying lesions larger than 1 cm, such as polyps and carcinoma

b. Can detect moderately advanced inflammatory bowel disease.

c. Cannot detect actual sites of bleeding, such as angiodysplasia or bleeding from diverticulosis.

d. Order this test only after performing sigmoidoscopy or if colonoscopy does not visualize the cecum.

8. Nasal gastric tube insertion
   a. Should be done first if the patient has rectal bleeding, is hemodynamically compromised, and is suspected of having an upper GI bleed.
   b. Positive findings are active bleeding, gross blood, blood clots or "coffee grounds." Otherwise do not Hemoccult-test other materials because a traumatic insertion can produce a positive result.
9. Esophagogastroduodenoscopy: Order this test if
   a. Lower GI work-up is unrevealing
   b. Nasogastric tube insertion is positive
   c. Nasogastric tube insertion is negative but clinically an upper GI bleed is suspected
10. Enteroclysis: radiography of the small intestine using controlled infusion of contrast via a nasogastric tube inserted into the duodenum
    a. Order for evaluation of chronic GI bleeding when work-up of the upper GI tract and colon has not revealed the source.
    b. Low-yield test but can diagnose Meckel's diverticulum, Crohn's ileitis, and small bowel cancers.
11. Miscellaneous tests
    a. Meckel's radionuclide scan: most useful in the evaluation of lower GI bleeding in children and adolescents; positive in only 60 per cent of cases
    b. Plain films of the abdomen: usually not helpful but can show an ileus from ischemic colitis or severe inflammatory bowel disease, calcification of an abdominal aneurysm, or free air from a perforated viscus.
    c. Enteroscopy: Allows for endoscopic evaluation of the small bowel, coagulation of angiodysplasias, and biopsy of neoplasms in the jejunum.
    d. Intraoperative endoscopy: useful for patients with active bleeding in whom preoperative studies have failed to document a bleeding source

For patients older than age 50 with nonurgent rectal bleeding, order colonoscopy, because diverticulosis and angiodysplasia are high in the differential diagnosis. Middle-aged adults may have the colon assessed with fiberoptic flexible sigmoidoscopy and air-contrast barium enema in lieu of colonoscopy. Young adults may be evaluated with just sigmoidoscopy if a source is found, such as anorectal lesions, or if there is a reasonable explanation for the bleeding.

Management

1. General
   a. Resuscitate hemodynamically compromised patients.
   b. Looking for the source of bleeding may occur concomitantly with attempts to stabilize the patient.
   c. Even if bleeding has stopped, anticipate rebleeding.
2. Upper GI bleeding
   a. Must treat urgently because upper GI bleeding that produces rectal bleeding will be massive.
   b. See other sections of the book for treatment of specific diseases of the upper GI tract.
3. Lower GI bleeding
   a. Urgent therapy: continuous bleeding or recurrent bleeding that has required more than 3 units of blood
   b. Elective therapy
      (1) In about 80 per cent of acute lower GI bleeding cases, bleeding will stop spontaneously.
      (2) Most patients with anorectal conditions
   c. Colonoscopic therapies
      (1) Employs various probes, forceps, or lasers
      (2) Used initially for angiodysplasia, diverticula, polyps, or small carcinoma
   d. Angiographic techniques
      (1) Intra-arterial vasopressin or embolization
      (2) Used for bleeding from angiodysplasia or diverticula that is massive or unresponsive to colonoscopic therapies
   e. Surgical treatment: usually a segmental or subtotal colectomy
      (1) For patients with large-volume blood loss (≥ 6 units of blood), actively or recurrently, who have failed colonoscopic or angiographic treatment
      (2) Patients with multiple lesions (angiodysplasia or diverticula) not amenable to colonoscopic or angiographic treatment
      (3) Patients with cancers
      (4) Obscure and uncontrolled colonic bleeding
   f. Specific conditions: see appropriate section under "Gastrointestinal Diseases."

PEARLS

- The volume of bleeding is not related to the significance of the underlying lesion.

- The color and consistency of the blood depend on GI motility. Do not rely solely on the blood's appearance as an indicator of the level from which it is coming.

- Be skeptical of attributing rectal bleeding to just a benign anorectal source in adults 50 or more years of age, even if active bleeding is seen from such lesions in this area.

- Middle-aged adults are also susceptible to colon cancer. Do not rule it out solely because of age less than 50.

Bibliography

Cello JP, Slivka A, Wolfe M: Lower gastrointestinal bleeding. In Taylor MB (ed): Gastrointestinal Emergencies, pp 493–513. Baltimore, Williams & Wilkins, 1997.

Edmundowicz SA, Zuckerman GR: Gastrointestinal bleeding. In Dunagan WC, Ridner ML (eds): Manual of Medical Therapeutics, 26th ed, pp 280–289. Boston, Little, Brown, 1989.

Friedman LS (ed): Lower gastrointestinal bleeding. Gastroenterol Clin North Am 1994;23:1.

Marshall JB: Acute gastrointestinal bleeding. Postgrad Med 1990;87:63–70.

Peterson WL: Obscure gastrointestinal bleeding. Med Clin North Am 1988;72:1169–1176.

81 Stomatitis

Etiology

1. Stomatitis represents a spectrum of inflammatory changes of the oropharynx, typically ulcerative or vesicular.
2. Causes are multiple and may be *primary*, such as local infections or trauma in the oral cavity, or *secondary*, such as oral manifestations of systemic diseases. Often, no cause can be identified.

   a. The etiologic agent is unknown in the most common ulcerative oral lesion aphthous stomatitis ("aphtha" means "ulcer"). Proposed factors have included streptococcal and herpetic infections, minor dental trauma, stress, menstruation, and nutritional deficiencies, to name a few, but none have withstood rigorous analysis.

   b. Viral-induced oral infections are common. Herpes simplex virus type 1 causes several distinct oral diseases, among them acute herpetic gingivostomatitis and herpes simplex labialis ("cold sores"). Coxsackie A viruses cause at least two clinical entities: (1) herpangina and (2) hand-foot-and-mouth disease. Many of the childhood viral exanthems (rubella, rubeola, varicella) present with oral lesions.

   c. Other infectious causes include syphilis, tuberculosis, deep fungal infections, *Mycoplasma pneumoniae*, cytomegalovirus, and anaerobic bacteria.

   d. Stomatitis may reflect systemic disease, particularly inflammatory bowel disease, collagen vascular disease, Behçet's syndrome, Kawasaki's disease, erythema multiforme, and immunosuppressive conditions such as human immunodeficiency virus (HIV) infections.

   e. Other etiologies include trauma (from biting or ill-fitting dentures), irritants (aspirin, nicotine), chemotherapy, and carcinoma. Xerostomia (dry mouth) can be related to medications, radiation therapy, or Sjögren's syndrome.

Symptoms

1. Aphthous ulcers or "canker sores" are painful and can recur four or more times a year.
2. Stomatitis caused by viral infections has classic prodromal phases of fever, chills, myalgias, arthralgias.
3. Any stomatitis can be disabling and cause anorexia.

Key Symptoms

- Oral pain

- May have systemic symptoms: fever, chills, malaise, anorexia, arthralgias

Clinical Findings

1. Aphthous stomatitis (or "canker sores") is characterized by its painful and recurring nature. Aphthous ulcers are rarely found on oral mucosa that is bound to periosteum, such as the attached gingiva and hard palate; this provides an important distinction from herpetic ulcers. There are three variants.

   a. The *minor* form (80 per cent) is usually a solitary oval ulcer measuring less than 1 cm in diameter and lasting 7 to 10 days. Most patients are young.

   b. *Major* ulcers (10 per cent) are multifocal and ragged and may be up to 2 cm in diameter; these frequently last up to 6 weeks, may scar, and are often immediately followed by a recurrent ulcer. This is the more common form in acquired immunodeficiency syndrome (AIDS).

   c. *Herpetiform* ulcers (10 per cent) are so named because the papulovesicular lesions are grouped, simulating herpex simplex infections.

2. In *acute primary herpetic gingivostomatitis*, the patient is usually young and toxic-appearing with the classic viral prodrome, followed in 24 to 48 hours by mucosal vesicles, which quickly rupture and coalesce into large, painful ulcers associated with gingivitis, a white coating on the tongue, and regional lymphadenopathy. The acute phase rarely lasts more than a week. Recurrent episodes, commonly known as *herpes labialis*, or "cold sores," are characterized by

81 Stomatitis • 421

single or multiple 2- to 4-mm vesicles around the vermilion border of the lip, frequently following prodromal "itchiness" or "tingling," and rupturing in 36 to 48 hours to form crusts. Frequency of recurrences varies and may be influenced by sunlight, cold, and stress.

Key Signs

- Oral vesicles or ulcers
- Fever
- Lymphadenopathy
- Toxic appearance (in herpetic infections)

Laboratory Tests

1. Diagnosis of aphthous stomatitis is clinical.
2. Herpes infection can be confirmed by titers in acute and convalescent sera and by cytology showing giant cells with viral inclusion bodies.
3. Suspected syphilitic lesions can be sampled by smear for darkfield microscopy.
4. Biopsy may be required where tuberculous, fungal, or carcinomatous etiologies are considered.

Differential Diagnosis

Aphthous ulcers must be differentiated from acute herpetic gingivitis, traumatic ulcers, allergy, and ulcerations caused by systemic disease.

1. Ulcerations caused by herpes simplex virus infections usually follow constitutional symptoms and rupture of vesicles.
2. Ask about other gastrointestinal symptoms (inflammatory bowel disease), ocular or genital symptoms (Behçet's syndrome), or HIV risk factors.
3. Traumatic and aphthous ulcers are clinically and histologically identical and are distinguished by anatomic relation to irritating structures.
4. Allergic lesions tend to be diffuse and do not ulcerate.
5. Xerostomia may also be painful; mucosa appears reddened and dry.

Treatment

1. Palliative therapy for aphthous stomatitis may include gentle rinsing with saline solution and topical viscous lidocaine (3 ml of 2% solution held in the mouth for 1 to 2 minutes before meals). Diphenhydramine solution, sometimes mixed with Kaopectate, is also analgesic.
2. Five per cent amlexanox oral paste (Aphthasol) applied qid accelerates healing and resolution of pain of aphthous ulcers.

3. Antibacterial washes (tetracycline mouthwash or chlorhexidine gluconate oral rinse [Peridex]) may diminish secondary bacterial infection.
4. Topical steroids provide relief for aphthous but not viral stomatitis. Dry the lesion first, then apply triamcinolone cream 0.1% every 4 to 6 hours mixed with, or followed by, Orabase to affix the steroid. Use systemic or locally injected steroids only in severe cases.
5. Topical acyclovir (5%) may help herpes labialis. Consider oral acyclovir during the prodrome.
6. Thalidomide may be helpful in major aphthous ulcers associated with AIDS.
7. Treat other infections (e.g., syphilis, tuberculosis) as appropriate.

Diet

1. Avoid hot, acidic, irritating foods or toothpastes. Encourage fluid intake.
2. Role of iron, vitamin B_{12}, and folate supplementation is not clear; consider checking levels.

Patient Education

1. Probably a role in aphthous stomatitis for stress reduction.
2. Patients with herpesvirus infection need to understand they are infectious.

Key Treatment

- Amlexanox oral paste
- Steroid cream applied locally

Follow-Up

Perform biopsy on any ulcer that fails to heal spontaneously in 10 to 14 days.

Bibliography

Eversole LR: Inflammatory diseases of the mucous membranes. Part 1: Viral and fungal infections; Part 2: Immunopathologic ulcerative and desquamative diseases. CDA (California Dental Association) J 1994;22:52–66.

Khandwala A: Five percent amlexanox oral paste, a new treatment for recurrent minor aphthous ulcers. Oral Surg Oral Med Oral Pathol Oral Radiol Endod 1997; 83:222–230.

MacPhail LA: Oral ulceration in HIV infection: investigation and pathogenesis. Oral Dis 1997;3(Suppl 1): 190–193.

Rogers RS III: Common lesions of the oral mucosa: a guide to diseases of the lips, cheeks, tongue, gingivae. Postgrad Med 1992;91:141–148, 151–153.

Woo SB: Recurrent aphthous ulcers: a review of diagnosis and treatment. J Am Dent Assoc 1996;127:1202–1213.

82 Gastroesophageal Reflux Disease

Stephen A. Brunton

Etiology

1. Predominantly a motility disorder with an incompetent lower esophageal sphincter (LES) allowing retrograde flow of stomach contents into esophagus; may also have delayed gastric emptying and impaired esophageal clearance.
2. Hiatal hernia is present in approximately 80 per cent of people with reflux esophagitis, although approximately half of all people with hiatal hernia have no reflux.

Symptoms

1. The predominant symptom is heartburn (pyrosis), which may be associated with regurgitation, water brash, and odynophagia. Other symptoms that may reflect dysmotility include early satiety, abdominal fullness, bloating, and belching.
2. Atypical symptoms include chest pain or symptoms referable to the respiratory tract, such as cough, laryngitis, or wheezing.

Key Symptoms

Typical	Atypical
• Heartburn	• Chest pain
• Regurgitation	• Cough
• Water brash	• Laryngitis

Clinical Findings

The physical examination is nonspecific and usually is negative.

Laboratory Tests

1. Radiographs: Upper gastrointestinal (GI) series may be helpful to detect sequelae of gastroesophageal reflux disease (GERD), such as ulcerations and stricture; however, it has limited usefulness in diagnosing GERD without complications.
2. Upper GI endoscopy: useful for evaluation of GERD sequelae such as esophagitis, ulceration, and stricture; essential for identification of Barrett's esophagus (columnar metaplasia of esophageal squamous epithelium) or as a screen for adenocarcinoma
3. Bernstein test—provocative test for GERD: Dilute HCl alternating with normal saline dripped above LES and correlated with symptoms; highly sensitive but has low specificity
4. A 24-hour esophageal pH monitor: definitive diagnostic test correlating symptoms with periods of time that pH is less than 4 above LES

Key Tests

- Upper GI film series
- Upper GI endoscopy
- Acid Bernstein test
- 24-hour esophageal pH monitor

Differential Diagnosis

1. Peptic ulcer disease: Pain may be epigastric and is often relieved by food.
2. Coronary ischemia: It is essential to rule out central chest pain of cardiac origin. GERD and coronary ischemia may coexist, and the pain of GERD may aggravate ischemia.

Treatment

1. Phase 1
   a. Dietary modifications
      (1) Weight loss in obese
      (2) Decrease in food with high fat content
      (3) Avoidance of citrus fruits, tomato-based products, coffee (caffeinated and decaffeinated), onions, chocolate, and peppermint.
   b. Smoking cessation
   c. Elevation of the head of the bed
   d. Avoiding late or large evening meals
   e. Modifying or stopping medications that decrease LES pressure, including theophylline, anticholinergics, nitrates, calcium channel blockers, progesterone-containing birth control pills
   f. Antacids

2. Phase 2
   a. Histamine$_2$ (H$_2$) antagonists
      (1) Cimetidine (Tagamet), 400 mg bid
      (2) Famotidine (Pepcid), 20 mg bid
      (3) Nizatidine (Axid), 150 mg bid
      (4) Ranitidine (Zantac), 150 mg bid
   b. Prokinetic agents
      (1) Cisapride (Propulsid), 10 to 20 mg qid or 20 mg bid
      (2) Metoclopramide (Reglan), 10 to 20 mg qid
3. Phase 3—proton pump inhibitor: omeprazole (Prilosec), 20 mg qd, or lansoprazole (Prevacid), 15 mg qd; other proton pump inhibitors being evaluated: rabeprazole, perprazole, pantoprazole
4. Phase 4—surgery: Laparoscopic techniques result in reduced morbidity and shorter hospital stays. Nissen fundoplication most frequently utilized.

Patient Education

Patients should follow guidelines as listed in phase 1 treatment.

Key Treatment

- Phase 1: Lifestyle modification and antacids
- Phase 2: H$_2$ antagonist or prokinetic agent or combination
- Phase 3: Proton pump inhibitor
- Phase 4: Surgery

Follow-Up

GERD is a lifelong, irreversible condition. The patient should be re-evaluated regularly to assess therapeutic progress. GERD sequelae, such as esophagitis, stricture, or Barrett's esophagus, require intensive lifelong follow-up.

Bibliography

Champion GL, Richter JE: Atypical presentation of gastroesophageal reflux disease: chest pain, pulmonary, and ear, nose, throat manifestations. Gastroenterologist 1993;1:18–33.

Devault KR, Castell DO: Guidelines for the diagnosis and treatment of GERD. Arch Intern Med 1995;155:2165–2173.

Fass R, Nixson LJ, Ciccolo ML, et al: Contemporary medical therapy for gastroesophageal reflux disease. Am Fam Physician 1997;55:204–212.

Hixson LJ, Kelly CL, Jones WN, et al: Current trends in the pharmacotherapy for gastroesophageal reflux disease. Arch Intern Med 1992;152:717–723.

Richter JE: Gastroesophageal reflux disease. In Winawer SJ (ed): Management of Gastrointestinal Diseases, pp 2–44. New York, Gower, 1992.

83 Gastritis

John B. Pope

Etiology

Inflammatory changes of the gastric mucosa are classified by histology, pathogenesis, or clinical associations, and may result from various causes.

1. *Helicobacter pylori*–associated gastritis: the major etiologic agent in chronic gastritis
   a. May result in acute inflammation with evolution into chronic superficial gastritis and ultimately chronic atrophic gastritis with intestinal metaplasia, or ulceration.
   b. Over 80 per cent of chronic gastritis is associated with this organism.
   c. Pathogenesis unclear but may involve altered mucosal integrity secondary to secretion of potentially toxic enzymes or chemicals.
   d. May promote development of peptic ulcer disease or gastric cancer.
2. Non–*H. pylori* infectious gastritis
   a. Bacterial: Any gastric bacterial infection may lead to gastritis.
      (1) Syphilis—secondary and tertiary: May cause superficial gastritis to transmural infiltration.
      (2) *Mycobacterium* species: Uncommon but may cause ulceration, transmural inflammation, or even fibrosis of gastric antrum.
      (3) *Clostridium* and *Escherichia*: May cause emphysematous gastritis (wall gas).
      (4) *Streptococcus*, *Staphylococcus*, *E. coli*, and *Proteus*: May cause a severe purulent gastritis known as phlegmonous gastritis.
   b. Viral (e.g., cytomegalovirus, herpesvirus): Occurs more frequently in immunocompromised hosts.
   c. Fungal (e.g., *Candida*, histoplasmosis, mucormycosis): usually seen in immunocompromised host, although rarely
   d. Parasitic: also more common in immunocompromised host
      (1) *Strongyloides stercoralis*: common worldwide; rarely affects stomach
      (2) Anisakiasis: an unusual cause of clinical acute gastritis
3. Noninfectious granulomatous gastritis
   a. Crohn's disease: Clinically significant gastric disease is relatively uncommon.
   b. Sarcoidosis: Although gastrointestinal involvement is rare, the stomach is most frequently affected.
   c. Eosinophilic: extensive infiltration causing wall thickening and fibrosis
4. Mucosal irritants: Generally cause chronic superficial gastritis, but the gastritis may be acute with severe erosion and hemorrhage.
   a. Alcohol: Depletes epithelium of extracellular mucus and intracellular mucus glycoproteins, producing gastric mucosal injury.
   b. Nonsteroidal anti-inflammatory drugs (NSAIDs): positively linked to chronic gastritis and gastric ulcer
5. Autoimmune disease: Causes chronic atrophic gastritis.
   a. Exclusive distribution in the gastric corpus and fundus; *H. pylori* rarely seen.
   b. Found in 20 per cent of patients with pernicious anemia
   c. Genetic link with autosomal dominant mode of inheritance
   d. Characterized by parietal cell and intrinsic factor autoantibodies, hypergastrinemia, and eventual hypochlorhydria
6. Stress-induced gastritis: damage from gastric secretions as a result of increased mucosal susceptibility from conditions of extreme physical stress
   a. True incidence disputed; may be 80 to 100 per cent of critically ill patients evaluated endoscopically.
   b. Characterized by multiple shallow erosions of proximal stomach
7. Alkaline reflux gastritis: reflux of alkaline secretions into the gastric remnant
   a. Incidence may range from 5 to 35 per cent of patients with operations obliterating sphincteric function of pylorus—most commonly Billroth II.
   b. May rarely occur in patients without gastrobiliary surgery who have reduced pyloric pressure and abnormal sphincteric response to gastrointestinal stimulation.

c. Pathogenic mechanism uncertain but may involve motility disorders and cytotoxic effects of bile and pancreatic enzymes on susceptible mucosa.

8. Miscellaneous gastritis
   a. Gastric ischemia: sometimes seen with vasculitis and atheromatous embolization, but generally not recognized
   b. Ménétrier's disease: entity of unknown cause characterized by marked mucosal hypertrophy with pseudopolypoid, thickened rugal folds; protein-losing gastropathy with hypoalbuminemia; and foveolar (gastric pit region) hyperplasia
   c. Gastric antral vascular ectasia: uncommon entity characterized by dilated antral vasculature with fibrin thrombi and fibromuscular hyperplasia
   d. Hypersecretory: Zollinger-Ellison syndrome with hypergastrinemia
   e. Physical causes
      (1) Corrosive: Cardia and pylorus commonly affected with scarring and obstruction.
      (2) Irradiation: 1600 rads can produce marked deep gastritis.

Symptoms

1. Acute gastritis: Symptoms usually mild if present and may include epigastric pain, nausea/vomiting, flatulence, excess salivation, headache, malaise.
2. Chronic gastritis
   a. Frequently asymptomatic
   b. Symptoms usually nonspecific, and likelihood of symptoms may increase with depth of inflammatory involvement.
      (1) Chronic abdominal pain, usually epigastric in location
      (2) Vague dyspepsia or mild ulcer-like symptoms
      (3) Nausea, anorexia
      (4) Malodorous breath

Key Symptom

Epigastric pain (chronic gastritis is frequently asymptomatic)

Clinical Findings

Significant clinical findings are frequently absent but may include

1. Hematemesis, bloody nasogastric aspirate, or other evidence of gastrointestinal bleeding
2. Abdominal tenderness
3. Bloating, emesis, and other findings of delayed gastric emptying
4. Intravascular volume depletion and shock may be seen in stress gastritis

Key Sign

Epigastric tenderness (clinical findings are frequently absent in chronic gastritis)

Laboratory Tests

1. Endoscopy with biopsy: gold standard diagnostic test providing macroscopic and histologic confirmation of inflammation, modalities for detection of etiologic agents, and evidence of complication development
2. Upper gastrointestinal radiographic study: typical radiographic features useful in diagnosis and delineation of specific etiologies
3. Nasogastric aspirate: useful in detection of bleeding, bile reflux, and infections
4. Vitamin B_{12}, gastrin, and pepsinogen levels may be affected in severe atrophic gastritis.
5. *Campylobacter*-like organism test: useful in confirming presence of *H. pylori*.
6. Serum or whole blood antibodies to *H. pylori*: least invasive and least expensive. Undetectable antibody levels beyond the first year of therapy may confirm cure of *H. pylori* in initially seropositive subject.
7. Urea breath tests (^{13}C and ^{14}C): sensitive for detection of *H. pylori* and useful in determining eradication; however, time consuming and expensive
8. *H. pylori* stool antigen test: highly sensitive, specific
9. [^{13}C]urea blood test: sensitive, specific, simple; not yet commercially available
10. *H. pylori* vaccine: currently in Phase II trials

Key Test

Endoscopy coupled with history is the best diagnostic test

Differential Diagnosis

1. Peptic ulcer disease
2. Nonulcer dyspepsia

3. Gastroparesis
4. Gastric carcinoma and lymphoma
5. Gastroesophageal reflux disease
6. Pancreatitis

Treatment

1. General treatment for acute gastritis includes
   a. Removal of mucosal irritants
   b. Treatment of underlying etiologic agents
   c. Acidification prevention
2. Severe hemorrhage in acute stress gastritis is managed with a variety of surgical and nonsurgical therapies; prevention is most important.
3. Treatment of chronic gastritis is variable depending on the etiology.
   a. General treatment would include avoidance of potential etiologic agents.
      (1) Eradication of underlying infectious agents (e.g., *H. pylori* triple therapy)
      (2) Treatment of underlying chronic diseases (e.g., Crohn's disease, sarcoidosis)
      (3) Avoidance of potentially etiologic drugs and foods (e.g., NSAIDs, spices)
   b. Specific symptoms may be treated with antacids, acid antisecretory drugs, mucosal protective drugs, or gastric motility stimulants; response is variable.
   c. Surgical therapy may be necessary in alkaline reflux gastritis.

Medication

1. Combination of tetracycline, 500 mg four times a day, or amoxicillin, 500 mg four times a day, *plus* metronidazole, 250 mg four times a day, *plus* bismuth subsalicylate, 524 mg four times a day for 14 days, has efficacy approaching 90 per cent against *H. pylori* infection (see Table 83–1 for regimens approved by the Food and Drug Administration [FDA]).
2. Antacids, histamine$_2$-blockers, omeprazole (Prilosec), and sucralfate (Carafate) are useful with hypersecretion.

Diet

Avoidance of spicy foods

Patient Education

1. Avoidance of alcohol, tobacco, and excessive NSAID use

TABLE 83–1. FDA-APPROVED *HELICOBACTER PYLORI* TREATMENT OPTIONS AND RETAIL COST

1. Omeprazole (Prilosec) 40 mg qd + clarithromycin (Biaxin) 500 mg tid ×2 wk, then omeprazole 20 mg qd ×2 wk	$245.00
2. Ranitidine bismuth citrate (RBC) 400 mg bid + clarithromycin 500 mg tid ×2 wk, then RBC 400 mg bid ×2 wk	$192.00
3. Bismuth subsalicylate (Pepto Bismol) 525 mg qid + metronidazole (Flagyl) 250 mg qid + tetracycline 500 mg qid* ×2 wk + histamine$_2$ receptor antagonist therapy as directed ×4 wk	$95.00
4. Lansoprazole (Prevacid) 30 mg bid + amoxicillin 1 gm bid + clarithromycin 500 mg bid ×14 d	$170.00
5. Lansoprazole 30 mg tid + amoxicillin 1 gm tid ×14 d†	$163.00
6. Omeprazole 20 mg bid + clarithromycin 500 mg bid + amoxicillin 1 gm bid ×10 d	$164.00

*Although not FDA-approved, amoxicillin has been substituted for tetracycline for patients in whom tetracycline is not recommended.
†This dual-therapy regimen has restrictive labeling. It is indicated for patients who are either allergic or intolerant to clarithromycin or for infections with known or suspected resistance to clarithromycin.

2. Chronic gastritis is a risk factor for the development of peptic ulcer disease.
3. Atrophic gastritis is associated with an increased risk of gastric cancer.

Follow-Up

The benefit of surveillance endoscopy for chronic gastritis has not been established.

Bibliography

For more information on Helicobacter pylori *infection, see*
Dunn BE, Cohen H, Blaser MJ: *Helicobacter pylori*. Clin Microbiol Rev 1997;10:720–741.
Feldman MD, Cryer B, Lee E, et al: Role of seroconversion in confirming cure of *Helicobacter pylori* infection. JAMA 1998;280:363–365.
Unge P: What other regimens are under investigation to treat *Helicobacter pylori* infection? Gastroenterology 1997;113:S131–S148.
For more information on stress gastritis and acute hemorrhagic gastritis, see
Chamberlain CE: Acute hemorrhagic gastritis. Gastroenterol Clin North Am 1993;22:843–873.
Durham RM, Shapiro MJ: Stress gastritis revisited. Surg Clin North Am 1991;71:791–810.
For more information on specific types of gastritis, see
Lichtenstein JE: Inflammatory conditions of the stomach and duodenum. Radiol Clin North Am 1993;31:1315–1333.

84 Peptic Ulcer Disease

George T. Fantry

Etiology

1. *Helicobacter pylori* infection.
   a. The major cause of chronic active gastritis and the primary etiologic factor in peptic ulcer disease (PUD)
   b. Associated with 90 per cent of duodenal ulcers and 75 per cent of gastric ulcers
   c. Cure of *H. pylori* improves the healing rate and markedly decreases the recurrence rate of peptic ulcers, altering the natural history of the disease.
2. Nonsteroidal anti-inflammatory drugs (NSAIDs)
   a. May cause gastric or duodenal ulcers; addition of steroids potentiates risk.
   b. Account for the majority of *H. pylori*–negative ulcers
3. Stress: severe physiologic stress such as burns, central nervous system trauma, surgery, severe medical illness
4. Hypersecretory states (uncommon): gastrinoma (Zollinger-Ellison [ZE] syndrome or multiple endocrine neoplasia type I), antral G cell hyperplasia, systemic mastocytosis, basophilic leukemias
5. Rare causes: viral (herpes, cytomegalovirus), radiation or chemotherapy, vascular insufficiency (crack cocaine), duodenal obstruction
6. Diseases associated with PUD: cirrhosis, chronic pulmonary disease, renal failure, renal transplantation

Pathogenesis

1. The pathogenesis of PUD is related to an imbalance between the normal protective factors and injurious factors.
   a. Offensive factors: *H. pylori* (most important factor), acid, pepsin, smoking, ethanol, bile acids, NSAIDs, aspirin, steroids, stress
   b. Defensive factors: mucus, bicarbonate, mucosal blood flow, prostaglandins, alkaline tide, hydrophobic layer, restitution, epithelial renewal

Symptoms

Symptoms may vary from classic symptoms to vague symptoms to symptoms related to complications of PUD.

1. Epigastric pain
   a. Gnawing or burning
   b. Occurs 1 to 3 hours after meals.
   c. Relieved by food or antacids
   d. May occur at night.
   e. May radiate to back (consider penetration).
2. Nausea
3. Vomiting (may be related to partial or complete gastric outlet obstruction)
4. Dyspepsia (belching, bloating, distention, fatty food intolerance)
5. Heartburn
6. Chest discomfort
7. Anorexia, weight loss
8. Hematemesis or melena (resulting from gastrointestinal bleeding)

Key Symptoms

- Epigastric burning pain
- Dyspepsia

Clinical Findings

In uncomplicated PUD, clinical findings are few and nonspecific.

1. Epigastric tenderness
2. Guaiac-positive stool (resulting from occult blood loss)
3. Melena (resulting from acute or subacute gastrointestinal bleeding)
4. Succussion splash (resulting from partial or complete gastric outlet obstruction)

Key Sign

Epigastric tenderness

Laboratory Tests

1. Routine laboratory tests in most patients with uncomplicated PUD are usually not helpful.
2. Diagnostic studies

a. Upper gastrointestinal endoscopy with antral biopsy: superior sensitivity and specificity, allows for detection of *H. pylori*.

b. Upper gastrointestinal series

3. Detection of *H. pylori* infection (essential in all patients with peptic ulcers)

a. Endoscopic tests (invasive): rapid urease test (best endoscopic diagnostic test), histopathology, culture (not sensitive or routinely available)

b. Nonendoscopic tests (noninvasive): urea breath test, serum *H. pylori* antibodies

4. Special studies

a. Serum gastrin: useful in recurrent, refractory, or complicated PUD and in patients with a family history of PUD to screen for ZE syndrome

b. Secretin stimulation test: used to distinguish ZE syndrome from other conditions with a high serum gastrin, such as achlorhydria, antisecretory therapy

c. Measurement of acid secretion: not useful in routine evaluation of PUD

Key Test

Endoscopy, diagnostic test for *H. pylori*

Differential Diagnosis

1. Gastroesophageal reflux disease
2. Nonulcer dyspepsia, gastroduodenitis
3. Drug-induced dyspepsia (theophylline, digitalis, caffeine)
4. Biliary tract disease
5. Pancreatitis
6. Musculoskeletal (back-gut syndrome)
7. Gastric cancer, duodenal cancer, pancreatic cancer
8. Crohn's disease
9. Other infectious and infiltrative lesions of the stomach and duodenum: giardiasis, sarcoidosis, tuberculosis, syphilis, Ménétrier's disease, lymphoma, *Mycobacterium avium* complex

---

WARNING

Elderly patients are more likely to be asymptomatic and have an increased risk of complications such as gastrointestinal bleeding, particularly if taking NSAIDs.

Treatment

ALL patients with peptic ulcers and *H. pylori* infection should be treated with a regimen to cure *H. pylori* (10 to 14 days), followed by ulcer therapy for an additional 2 to 6 weeks depending on which therapeutic agent is chosen. Considerations when choosing a regimen include effectiveness, compliance, side effects, drug interactions, and cost. NSAID-induced ulcers should be treated with cessation of NSAIDs and an appropriate course of standard ulcer therapy. Gastric ulcers may require a longer course of therapy than duodenal ulcers.

Helicobacter pylori *Treatment*

1. Triple therapy: treatment of choice; duration of therapy 10 to 14 days, cure rate of 85 to 90 per cent

a. Proton pump inhibitor (PPI)–based triple therapy

(1) Omeprazole (Prilosec), 20 mg bid, or lansoprazole (Prevacid), 30 mg bid

(2) Clarithromycin (Biaxin), 500 mg bid

(3) Metronidazole (Flagyl), 500 mg bid or amoxicillin 1 gm bid

b. Bismuth-based triple therapy

(1) Bismuth subsalicylate (Pepto Bismol), 2 tablets qid

(2) Metronidazole, 250 to 500 mg tid

(3) Tetracycline, 500 mg qid

2. Dual therapy: not recommended as first-line therapy; duration of therapy 2 weeks, variable cure rate approximately 75 to 80 per cent

a. PPI-based dual therapy

(1) Omeprazole, 20 mg bid, or lansoprazole, 30 mg bid

(2) Clarithromycin, 500 mg tid, or amoxicillin, 1 gm bid

b. Bismuth-based

(1) Ranitidine bismuth citrate (Tritec), 400 mg bid

(2) Clarithromycin, 500 mg tid

Antisecretory Ulcer Therapy (Acid-Dependent)

1. Histamine$_2$ (H$_2$) receptor antagonists (H$_2$RA)

a. Inhibit acid secretion by blocking H$_2$ receptors on parietal cells.

b. Equal efficacy in equivalent doses: healing rate of 70 to 80 per cent at 4 weeks, 90 to 95 per cent at 8 weeks

c. Therapeutic regimen

(1) Cimetidine (Tagamet), 400 mg bid or 800 mg hs ×6 to 8 weeks

(2) Famotidine (Pepcid), 20 mg bid or 40 mg hs ×6 to 8 weeks

(3) Nizatidine (Axid), 150 mg bid or 300 mg hs ×6 to 8 weeks

(4) Ranitidine (Zantac), 150 mg bid or 300 mg hs ×6 to 8 weeks

2. Proton pump inhibitors (PPIs)

a. Inhibit the parietal cell H^+/K^+-ATPase pump, the final common pathway in acid secretion.

b. Achieve a healing rate of 80 to 100 per cent at 4 weeks, significantly greater than H₂RA.

c. Therapeutic regimen

(1) Omeprazole, 20 mg qd ×4 weeks

(2) Lansoprazole, 15 mg qd ×4 weeks

3. Prostaglandins

a. Inhibit acid secretion by decreasing generation of cyclic AMP in the parietal cell in response to histamine stimulation.

b. Primary role is as a prophylactic agent to prevent NSAID-induced ulcers (see below). Not recommended as routine therapy for PUD; use may be limited by side effects.

c. Prophylactic regimen: misoprostol (Cytotec), 100 to 200 μg bid to qid

Cytoprotective Ulcer Therapy (Enhances Mucosal Defense, Acid-Independent)

1. Sucralfate

a. Healing rates comparable to those with H₂RA

b. Therapeutic regimen: sucralfate (Carafate), 1 gm qid or 2 gm bid ×6 to 8 weeks

2. Antacids (multiple aluminum-, magnesium-, and calcium-based antacids are available)

a. Moderate- to high-dose antacids result in healing rates comparable to those with H₂RA.

b. Tablet and liquid forms are equally effective; four-times-a-day dosing is adequate.

c. Therapeutic regimen: antacid 1 hour pc and hs ×6 to 8 weeks

Diet

No special diet required.

Patient Education

1. Smoking cessation

2. Avoid NSAID and aspirin use.

3. Avoid heavy alcohol use.

4. Stress reduction counseling may be helpful in individual cases but not routinely needed.

Key Treatment

Treatment of Choice	Adjunctive Therapy
• Anti–*H. pylori* therapy	• PPIs
	• H₂RA
	• Sucralfate, antacids

Follow-Up

1. Endoscopy is required to document healing of gastric ulcers to rule out gastric cancer.

2. Documentation of *H. pylori* cure with a noninvasive test, such as the urea breath test, is appropriate in patients with complicated ulcers

Prevention

1. *H. pylori*–associated ulcers

a. Cure of *H. pylori* results in a decrease in ulcer recurrence rate from 60 to 90 per cent to less than 10 per cent per year.

b. Maintenance therapy with half-standard doses of H₂RA at bedtime should be considered in patients with recurrent, refractory, or complicated ulcers, particularly if cure of *H. pylori* has not been documented.

2. NSAID-induced ulcers

a. Prophylactic therapy should be considered in patients requiring chronic, daily NSAID therapy who are older than 60, have a history of peptic ulcer disease or a complication such as gastrointestinal bleeding, or have significant co-morbid medical illnesses.

b. Prophylactic regimen: Misoprostol (see above), high-dose H₂RA twice daily, and once-daily PPI therapy have been shown to prevent gastric and duodenal ulcers.

Bibliography

For more information on etiology, pathogenesis, diagnosis, and treatment of peptic ulcer disease, see

Peterson WL, Graham DY: *Helicobacter pylori.* In Sleisenger MH, Fordtran JS (eds): Gastrointestinal Disease, 6th ed, vol 1, pp 604–619. Philadelphia, WB Saunders Company, 1997.

Soll AH: Peptic ulcer and its complications. In Sleisenger MH, Fordtran JS (eds): Gastrointestinal Disease, 6th ed, vol 1, pp 620–678. Philadelphia, WB Saunders Company, 1997.

For more information on the epidemiology, pathogenesis, diagnosis, treatment, and prevention of H. pylori *infection, see*

Proceedings of the American Digestive Health Foundation International Update Conference on *Helicobacter pylori*. Gastroenterology 1997;113:S1–S170.

For more information on treatment of H. pylori *and peptic ulcer disease, see*

Salcedo JA, Al-Kawas F. Treatment of *Helicobacter pylori* infection. Arch Intern Med 1998;158:842–851.

Soll AH: Medical treatment of peptic ulcer disease: practice guidelines. JAMA 1996;275:622–629.

In general, an upper gastrointestinal (GI) endoscopy is indicated if a change in patient management is probable or management would be altered based on the results of the endoscopy; if an empiric trial of therapy has been unsuccessful; or as an initial evaluation as an alternative to radiologic studies.

Indications

1. Upper abdominal distress persisting after an appropriate trial of therapy
2. Upper abdominal distress suggesting serious organic disease
3. Dysphagia or odynaphagia
4. Esophageal reflux symptoms persisting or recurring after appropriate therapy
5. Persistent nausea or vomiting of unknown cause or unexplained weight loss
6. When GI pathology might modify management of another disease process
7. Abnormal or nonspecific radiographic findings
    a. Suspected tumor, polyp, or bezoar
    b. Gastric or esophageal ulcer
    c. Stricture or obstruction
8. GI bleeding
    a. Stable acute upper GI bleed, for determination of site
    b. Chronic iron deficiency anemia when colonoscopy is negative
    c. Positive fecal occult blood when colonoscopy is negative
9. Surveillance endoscopy for
    a. Barrett's esophagus
    b. Gastric polyp or familiar polyposis
10. Biopsy or culture of duodenal tissue or fluid
11. Foreign body removal

Contraindications

1. Known or suspected perforation of esophagus or stomach
2. When unable to obtain adequate patient cooperation
3. History of bleeding disorder
4. Previous bleeding in the esophageal varices
5. Unstable cardiorespiratory status
6. Severe obstruction or stricture

Potential Complications

1. Cardiorespiratory compromise (usually from medication)
2. Bleeding
3. Infection
4. Mucosal injury or perforation of GI tract
5. Vocal chord injury
6. Aspiration

Preparation

1. Obtain informed consent: Include the nature of the procedure, reasons for the procedure, risks and complications, what the benefits would be as well as alternatives to the procedure.
2. The patient should take nothing by mouth for 6 to 8 hours (longer if impaired gastric emptying is suspected). Patient should arrive 1 hour prior to the procedure.
3. Patient's cardiorespiratory status, including pulse, blood pressure, and oxygen saturation, should be assessed prior to the procedure and monitored throughout. It is helpful to have continuous pulse oximetry available, but most important is to have a qualified assistant closely monitoring the patient's status.
4. Intravenous (IV) access may be obtained but is not critical if no IV medications will be used.

Medications

Although IV access is helpful, some patients will tolerate the procedure with topical anesthetic only. When using IV medications, a combination of narcotic and benzodiazepine is used most frequently. Simethicone, 40 to 80 mg, can be given orally before the procedure or through the biopsy port of the scope during the procedure, or added to the wash water to reduce gastric bubbles.

1. Topical anesthetics
    a. Viscous lidocaine 2%, gargle and swallow
    b. Benzocaine 20% spray (Hurricaine)
    c. Benzocaine 14% plus tetracaine, 2% (Cetacaine)
2. Narcotics
    a. Meperidine (Demerol), 10 to 75 mg IV
    b. Fentanyl (Sublimaze), 0.05 to 0.1 mg IV
    c. Butorphanol (Stadol), intranasal or 1.0 to 2.0 mg sprayed via syringe (1.0 mg per spray)
3. Benzodiazepines
    a. Diazepam (Valium), 2 to 10 mg IV
    b. Midazolam (Versed), 1 to 5 mg IV
    c. Triazolam (Halcion), 0.25 to 0.5 mg administered PO one-half hour prior to procedure
4. Antagonists
    a. Naloxone (Narcan), 0.4 mg
    b. Flumazeril (Romazicon), 0.2 mg

Equipment

1. Fiberoptic endoscope or videogastroscope (diameter of 8 to 10 mm and length of 104 cm)
2. Light source
3. Camera source
4. Biopsy forceps
5. Pulse oximeter
6. Suction equipment and tubing
7. Oxygen with nasal cannula
8. *Campylobacter*-like organism (CLO) test and specimen containers
9. Oral introducer
10. Crash cart supplies

Technique

1. Patient should take nothing by mouth for 6 to 8 hours, IV access (if required) should be obtained, and any questions reviewed with the patient. Vital signs should be obtained and pulse oximeter applied.
2. With the patient in the sitting position, the oral cavity and teeth should be examined and any dentures removed.
3. Posterior pharynx is sprayed with benzocaine and/or 15 ml viscous lidocaine is administered and the patient is asked to gargle and then swallow. Patient is placed in the left lateral recumbent position and IV medications are given.
4. An oral introducer is placed over the scope and the lubricated tip of the endoscope is introduced with a gentle curve over the posterior aspect of the tongue.
5. The scope is advanced to approximately 16 to 18 cm or to area of first resistance, which will be at the cricopharyngeal muscle. This can be identified as the slit-like opening just posterior to the arytenoid cartilage and the vocal cords. This is also a good opportunity to look for masses or abnormalities around the hypopharynx or vocal cords (see figure of vocal cords in Rhinolaryngoscopy procedure).
6. The patient is asked to swallow repeatedly until the scope passes naturally into the esophagus. Alternative methods include directing the scope with two fingers in the oral cavity, or direct visualization as the scope passes the entire route.

7. Slight insufflation is helpful as the scope is passed through the esophagus, visualizing for any mucosal abnormalities. It is important to view the esophagus on the way in because the scope irritation can obscure the original mucosa. At approximately 40 cm from the incisors, the squamocolumnar junction or Z line will be visualized. Patient is asked to sniff at this point to help identify diaphragmatic level and/or hiatal hernia (if the diaphragm is greater than 2 cm from the Z line, a hiatal hernia is likely). This is also an area to inspect closely for signs of esophagitis or neoplastic change.
8. The scope is passed through the junction into the stomach, where air should be insufflated and stomach juices suctioned.

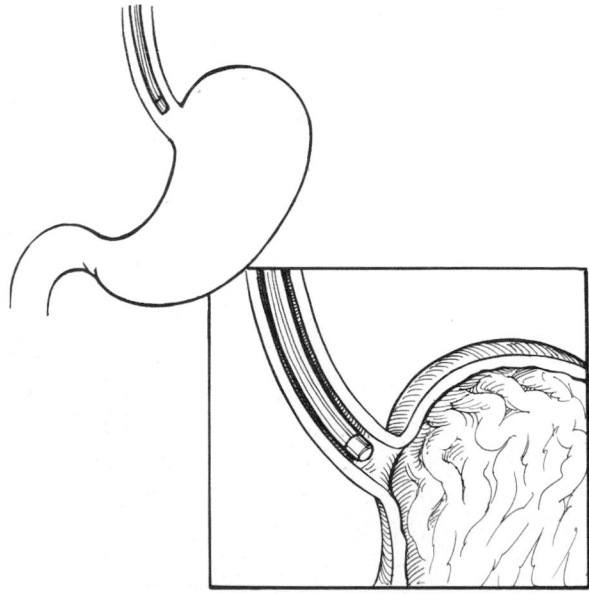

With a brief look for gross abnormalities within the body of the stomach, the scope should be advanced along the lesser curve to the region of the angularis incisura. As the scope progresses, the pyloric sphincter should become quickly visible.

9. The endoscope should be guided through the pyloric sphincter and into the duodenal bulb. It may be necessary to watch several of the peristaltic contractions to appropriately time advancing through the pylorus.

10. Once in the duodenum, the scope should be advanced down and to the right, sometimes with a series of advancements and withdrawals, to completely visualize the duodenum, paying special attention to the bulb or first portion.

11. The scope is then straightened and withdrawn through the pylorus and, once it is back in the antrum, should be retroflexed, allowing for good visualization of the lesser curvature (a location where ulcers frequently occur) as well as the cardia and fundus regions. Retroflexion is critical to completely visualize the gastric mucosa.

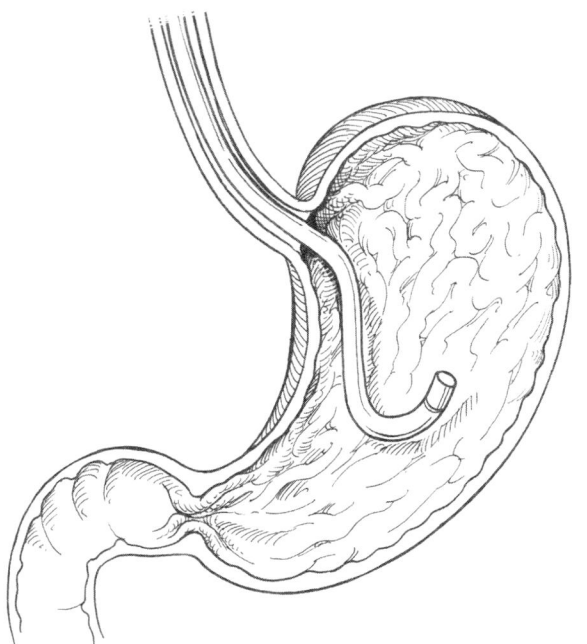

12. Samples for cultures, cytology, or *Helicobacter pylori* testing can be obtained at this time. A CLO test for *H. pylori* can be done with biopsy material from healthy-appearing mucosa in the antrum for the best yield (saline or water lavage may be needed to more accurately visualize a lesion).

13. The scope is then withdrawn through the esophagogastric junction, again visualizing this area and continuing to withdraw as the hypopharynx is visualized.

14. The patient should be observed for 30 minuters prior to leaving the hospital or office, and should be instructed not to drive for the remainder of the day.

Follow-Up

1. Any specific medication changes or follow-up instructions are best given in writing as well as verbally to the patient and family.

2. The patient should be seen in 2 to 4 weeks to review any pathology reports and to assess how symptoms are changing.

Bibliography

Norris TE: Esophagogastroduodenoscopy. Prim Care 1997;24:327–340.

Phenninger JL, Fowler GC (eds): Procedures for Primary Care Physicians. St. Louis, CV Mosby Company, 1994.

Pierzchajlo RPJ, Ackermann RJ, Vogel RL: Esophagogastroduodenoscopy performed by a family physician: a case series of 793 procedures. J Fam Pract 1998;46: 41–46.

Pope JB, Mayeaux EJ Jr, Harper MB: Effectiveness and safety of esophagogastroduodenoscopy in family practice: experience at a university medical center. Fam Med 1995;27:506–511.

Silverstein FE, Tytgat GNJ: Gastrointestinal Endoscopy, 3rd ed. London, Mosby-Wolfe, 1997.

85 Appendicitis

Bonnie P. Malvea

Acute appendicitis (inflammation of the vermiform appendix) commonly occurs in the age group 10 to 19 years, although it can occur at any age. Approximately 250,000 cases of appendicitis occur in the United States annually. Males have a slightly higher rate than females (1.4:1) for all age groups.

Etiology

1. Luminal obstruction is usually the initial event in the pathogenesis of appendicitis. It may be caused by any one of the following:
   a. A fecalith
   b. Lymphoid hyperplasia of the appendix
   c. Primary or metastatic tumors of the appendix (adenocarcinoma or carcinoid)
   d. Worms (oxyuriasis [pinworm] or roundworm)
   e. Foreign bodies or inspissated barium from previous studies
   f. In some cases no obvious cause is found.
2. Luminal obstruction causes retention of mucosal secretion and leads to inflammation of the appendix as follows:
   a. Accumulation of mucosal secretion
   b. Increasing intraluminal pressure
   c. Impaired lymphatic drainage and compromised vascular supply
   d. Mucosal ulceration and bacterial infection
   e. Inflammation of the appendix: May proceed to abscess formation, gangrene, and rupture. Inflammation may in some cases resolve spontaneously with or without treatment.

Symptoms

The following symptoms occur in most patients:
1. Vague abdominal discomfort
2. Abdominal pain (periumbilical, epigastric, or right lower quadrant)
3. Anorexia
4. Nausea and vomiting
5. Constipation or mild diarrhea

Following a period of abdominal discomfort, patients experience acute abdominal pain located in the epigastrium or periumbilical area. They become anorectic and have nausea and vomiting. In the elderly

patient, abdominal pain may be minimal or even absent. In very young children, fussiness or refusal to feed, with vomiting and diarrhea, may be signs suggestive of acute appendicitis. Repeated examination and careful evaluation of their condition are necessary because rupture of the appendix takes place early, with increased morbidity and mortality.

Key Symptoms

- Right lower quadrant abdominal pain
- Anorexia
- Nausea and vomiting

Clinical Findings

1. Fever: Initially, temperature may be normal. Usually a moderate increase from 100°F to 101°F may be seen in most cases. Fever above 101°F may indicate a complication (abscess or gangrene). Temperature may be normal in the elderly.
2. Abdominal pain: The most significant feature of acute appendicitis. Location of the pain may depend on the anatomic position of the appendix. Usually pain is felt in the periumbilical or epigastric area and within a few hours may localize to the right lower quadrant of the abdomen.
3. Rebound tenderness: Palpation of the right lower quadrant of the abdomen may elicit tenderness and cause "muscle guarding." Keeping the examining hand depressed until the patient gets used to the pressure and suddenly releasing the pressure causes a sudden increase in tenderness and a "grimace" by the patient.
4. Rovsing's sign: Deep palpation of the *left* lower abdominal quadrant causes pain to be felt in the *right* lower quadrant.
5. Obturator sign: With patient lying supine, flexing the right hip and leg and rotating them internally causes pain in the right lower quadrant of the abdomen as a result of irritation of the internal obturator muscle.
6. Psoas sign: With the patient lying in the left lateral position, extending the right thigh at the hip increases pain in the right lower abdominal

quadrant as a result of irritation of the psoas muscle.

Key Signs

- Right lower abdominal rebound tenderness
- Fever
- Positive Rovsing's sign

Laboratory Tests

The following laboratory tests should be done in all patients suspected of having acute appendicitis.

1. Complete blood count (CBC): May be normal in the early stages, but usually a modest increase in the white blood cell (WBC) count (10,000 to 15,000) is seen, with a left shift. WBC count may be normal in the elderly and immunocompromised patients.
2. Serum creatinine, blood urea nitrogen (BUN), amylase
3. Urinalysis: May be normal or may show a few WBC or red blood cells if the appendix abuts the ureter or bladder.
4. A urine pregnancy test should be done in all reproductive-age females.

Key Laboratory Tests

- CBC with differential
- Amylase, BUN, and creatinine
- Urinalysis and urine pregnancy test

Imaging

1. Plain abdominal radiograph: signs suggestive of appendicitis
   a. Identification of fecalith or presence of gas in the appendix
   b. Distention of ileum, cecum, or ascending colon or the presence of air-fluid levels
   c. Loss of cecal shadow
   d. Free intraperitoneal air or fluid
2. Barium enema
   a. Signs suggestive of appendicitis
      (1) Incomplete or nonvisualization of appendix
      (2) Irregularity of the appendiceal lumen
      (3) Extrinsic mass effect on the cecum or terminal ileum

b. Because of frequency of technical failures resulting in nondiagnostic study, barium enema may be of limited use in evaluating appendicitis
3. Ultrasonography (US)
   a. Primary criteria for diagnosis of appendicitis by US
      (1) Identification of fecalith in the appendiceal lumen
      (2) Noncompressible appendix 7 mm or greater in anteroposterior diameter
   b. Other signs suggestive of appendicitis by US
      (1) Loss of echogenic submucosal ring
      (2) Gas bubbles in the lumen
      (3) Presence of loculated fluid collection
   c. Ultrasonography has a high sensitivity and specificity, but needs specialized equipment and trained personnel. When available, it is the study of choice for evaluating patients suspected of having appendicitis as well as female patients with inflammatory problems of the right fallopian tube or with ovarian pathology.
4. Computerized tomography (CT)
   a. Diagnosis of appendicitis by CT is made when
      (1) Abnormal appendix is identified by CT
      (2) An appendicolith is identified in association with a right lower quadrant abscess
   b. CT is reported to have a high sensitivity and specificity. Recent studies indicate the use of focused appendiceal CT has reduced costs of patient care by its high accuracy in evaluating patients with appendicitis and reducing the number of unnecessary appendectomies.

Key Imaging Tests

- US
- Focused appendiceal CT

Differential Diagnosis

1. A detailed discussion of the differential diagnosis is beyond the scope of this chapter. A good history, a careful physical examination (including a rectal and a pelvic examination), essential laboratory tests, and imaging studies will help in establishing a correct diagnosis in most cases.
2. The following should be considered in differential diagnosis: mesenteric adenitis, acute cho-

lecystitis, Meckel's diverticulitis, acute pancreatitis, inflammatory bowel disease, perforated duodenal ulcer, ileitis, incarcerated inguinal hernia, acute salpingitis, tubo-ovarian abscess, ovarian torsion, rupture ovarian cyst, torsion of ovarian cyst, ruptured tubal pregnancy, ureteral calculus, acute pyelonephritis, perinephric abscess, endometriosis, aortic dissection

Treatment

Treatment for acute appendicitis is appendectomy by abdominal laparotomy or by laproscopic surgery. Patients with suspected acute appendicitis must be hospitalized. Early surgical consultation should be sought. Delay in diagnosis in very young children and the elderly may lead to perforation and increased morbidity and mortality.

1. Intravenous fluid (lactated Ringer's solution and 5% dextrose in water) should be given to correct dehydration and electrolyte deficits.
2. Antibiotics are given to cover aerobic and anaerobic bacteria.
   a. Prophylaxis before surgery for all adult patients: 2 gm cefoxitin or cefotetan given before surgery results in significant reduction in wound infections.
   b. In cases of perforation or gangrenous appendicitis, clindamycin with gentamycin or metronidazole is given to cover *Bacteroides fragilis* infection.
3. Indications for laproscopic surgery
   a. Patients with atypical history of physical findings
   b. Women with a possibility of gynecologic disease

Key Treatment

- Surgery (appendectomy)
  - Laparotomy
  - Laproscopic

4. Prognosis
   a. Outcome for acute appendicitis with early recognition and prompt surgical treatment is excellent.
   b. Mortality in unruptured appendicitis is reported to be 0.1 to 0.2 per cent in general population. Mortality rate for ruptured appendicitis is 3 to 5 per cent.
   c. Mortality in elderly patient, where diagnosis is delayed and rupture takes place early, is 15 per cent.
   d. In pediatric age group below age 2, mortality may be high because of early rupture and delayed diagnosis.
   e. Acute appendicitis may resolve spontaneously without treatment and may recur (recurrent appendicitis).

Bibliography

Adiss DJ, Shaffer N, Fowler BS, Tauxe RV: The epidemiology of appendicitis in the U.S. Am J Epidemiol 1990;132:910–925.

Faye CL: Ultrasonography of the acute abdomen. Radiol Clin North Am 1992;30:389–404.

Graffeo CS, Counselman FL: Appendicitis. Emerg Med Clin North Am 1996;14:653–671.

Rao PM, et al: Effect of computed tomography of the appendix on treatment of patients and use of hospital resources. N Engl J Med 1998;338:141–146.

Sabiston DC Jr: The Biological Basis of Modern Surgical Practice, 15th ed. Philadelphia, WB Saunders Company, 1997.

Tintinalli JE: Emergency Medicine: A Comprehensive Study, 3rd ed. New York, McGraw Hill, 1992.

86 Colorectal Cancer

Heather Rossi

Epidemiology

1. Geography: Colorectal cancer is common in the United States, Australia, New Zealand, Scandinavia, and Western Europe. The disease is relatively uncommon in Asia, Africa, and South America.
2. Statistics
   a. In 1995, there were an estimated 138,200 cases of colorectal cancer with 55,300 deaths.
   b. The incidence increases with age and is uncommon in those less than 40 years old.
   c. The incidence rises rapidly after age 50.
   d. In the United States, there has been an increase of 0.3 per cent in incidence; however, there has been a decrease in whites of 1.6 per cent and an increase in nonwhites of 26.6 per cent.
   e. Mortality has decreased 15.5 per cent overall, with a 17.6 per cent decrease in white patients and a 12.4 per cent increase in African Americans.
   f. Improved survival is seen across the board, probably because of improved surgical techniques, adjuvant chemotherapy, radiotherapy, and early detection.

Etiology

The exact cause of colorectal cancer is unknown. However, genetic and environmental factors have been implicated.

1. Genetic predisposition: It is estimated that approximately 10 per cent of colorectal cancers occur in patients with a genetic predisposition.
   a. Hereditary nonpolyposis colorectal cancer (Lynch's syndrome)
      (1) Comprises approximately 5 to 6 per cent of all cases of colorectal cancer. A mutation in chromosome 2 has been identified; the result is an inability to repair errors in DNA replication. Patients with this genetic alteration have an 80 per cent probability of developing colorectal cancer during their lifetimes.
      (2) This syndrome should be suspected if a family has
         (a) Three relatives with confirmed colorectal cancer and one individual is a first-degree relative of the other two
         (b) Two generations afflicted with colorectal cancer
         (c) At least one case of cancer diagnosed before age 50
         (d) No evidence of familial polyposis.
      (3) Two variations have been described.
         (a) Lynch's syndrome I: autosomal dominant, young age at onset, cancer usually occurring in the proximal colon, and a high rate of synchronous or metachronous cancer.
         (b) Lynch's syndrome II: the above features also with a family history of endometrial, gastric, and urothelial cancer.
      (4) Screening at-risk, nonaffected family members can be accomplished with either *genetic* or *clinical* (endoscopic) methods.
         (a) Genetic screening is performed by identifying the exact mutation in an affected relative, then testing at-risk members by direct gene sequencing of a peripheral blood sample.
         (b) Clinical screening is performed with colonoscopy beginning between age 20 and 25 or 10 years before the age of the youngest affected relative and is repeated at 1- to 3-year intervals. The age at which to discontinue colonoscopy has not been determined.
   b. Familial adenomatous polyposis (FAP) is characterized by the presence of more than 100 adenomatous polyps in the colon.
      (1) FAP includes
         (a) Gardner's syndrome: colonic polyps, epidermal inclusion cysts, osteomas, desmoid tumors, papillary thyroid cancer
         (b) Turcot's syndrome: colonic polyps and brain tumors
      (2) Autosomal dominant pattern of inheritance except Turcot's syndrome, which

may be autosomal recessive or dominant with incomplete penetrance.

(3) Genetic defect present on chromosome 5 causes a loss of tumor suppressor function normally present.

(4) One hundred per cent of patients with defective gene will develop cancer of the colon if left untreated.

(5) Screening at-risk family members can be done with commercially available genetic testing or with proctosigmoidoscopy beginning at puberty and repeated annually until age 40.

c. Acquired somatic defects account for the majority of colorectal cancers. Neoplasia develops after multiple mutations have occurred that allow normal colonic epithelium to progress to adenoma and ultimately to carcinoma. Volgelstein proposed a genetic model for colorectal tumorigenesis. Mutational activation of an oncogene (permits uncontrolled regulation and continued stimulation) is followed by inactivation of multiple suppressor genes (act to inhibit cell proliferation and tumorigenicity) (Fig. 86–1). The mutations allow for uncontrolled growth in varying degrees.

2. Environmental factors: Epidemiologic data implicate important environmental components.

a. Risk factors: diets high in red meat and saturated fat, obesity, cigarette smoking, alcohol consumption

b. Protective factors: high fiber diet, physical activity, aspirin or nonsteroidal anti-inflammatory agents

3. Premalignant conditions

a. Ulcerative colitis: Patients with total colonic involvement and disease of long duration are at high risk. The incidence for such patients is approximately 1 per cent per year after 10 years. Surveillance with annual or every-other-year colonoscopy with biopsies for dysplasia are generally advised beginning after 7 to 10 years of disease.

b. Crohn's disease: The incidence of neoplasia is approximately 7 per cent over 20 years. Patients with colonic strictures have a higher incidence at the stricture site.

Screening

Accepted guidelines for the patient who lacks an inherited genetic cancer predisposition or inflammatory bowel disease are as follows, beginning at age 50:

1. Yearly fecal occult blood test *and* flexible sigmoidoscopy every 5 years, or

2. Colonoscopy every 10 years, or

3. Double-contrast barium enema every 5 to 10 years

4. A digital examination is mandatory with each of the above.

Symptoms

1. Subacute presentation

a. Right colon tumors tend to cause occult bleeding and anemia.

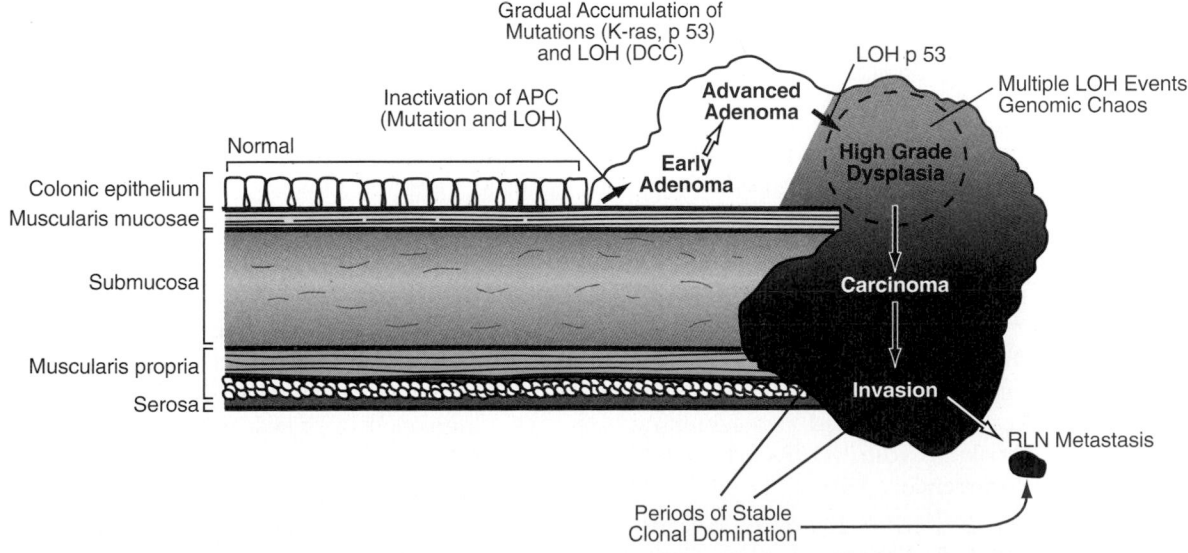

Figure 86–1 A model of genetic events in colorectal carcinogenesis. (From Boland CR, Sato J, Appelman HD, et al: Microallelotyping defines the sequence and tempo of allelic losses at tumour suppressor gene loci during colorectal cancer progression. Nature Med 1995;1:903, with permission.)

b. Tumors of the narrower left-sided colon tend to cause abdominal pain with a change in bowel habits and the passage of bright red blood per rectum.

c. Less commonly, weight loss and fever occur.

2. Acute presentation

a. Complete or partial obstruction

b. Perforation

Key Symptom

Lower abdominal pain

Clinical Findings

1. Dark or tarry stools
2. Iron deficiency anemia with resultant fatigue, palpitations, or dizziness
3. Abdominal mass
4. Metastatic disease may present with ascites, pruritus and jaundice, hemoptysis

Key Signs

- Tarry stools
- Anemia
- Abdominal mass

Laboratory Tests

The definitive diagnosis is made by endoscopy (flexible sigmoidoscopy or colonoscopy) or double-contrast barium enema. Other tests are useful to evaluate the extent of the disease.

1. Chest radiograph to rule out pulmonary metastasis
2. Computerized tomography to inspect for metastatic liver disease
3. Serum carcinoembryonic antigen (CEA): Nonspecific, not intended to be used as a screening tool; used primarily to follow for early detection of tumor recurrence.
4. Rectal ultrasound is used to determine if transanal excision of selected tumors is appropriate (small size, minimal penetration, no sign of nodal metastases).

Key Tests

- Fecal occult blood test
- Double-contrast barium enema
- Sigmoidoscopy
- Colonoscopy

Treatment

The objective in treatment of colorectal cancer is to surgically remove or ablate the diseased segment of bowel, mesentery with associated lymphatics, and any organs involved by direct extension.

1. Surgical treatment: Bowel must be properly prepared with bowel purging and antibiotics.

a. The approach is to remove the cancerous bowel, mesentery, and lymphatics while preserving arterial supply to the remaining colon.

b. Patients with obstructing lesions require initial fluid resuscitation. Emergent surgery in unprepared bowel usually mandates a stoma.

c. Perforated lesions usually require resection of involved area with colostomy.

d. Patients with hereditary nonpolyposis colorectal cancer should undergo subtotal colectomy and ileorectal anastomosis because of the risk of metachronous cancer (40 per cent at 10 years) if treated only with segmental colectomy.

e. Patients with FAP are treated with subtotal colectomy and ileorectal anastomosis or total proctocolectomy and ileoanal anastomosis if the rectum has innumerable polyps.

2. Staging and prognosis are related to depth of wall penetration, lymph node involvement, and distant metastases. Staging is described by either modified Dukes' or tumor-node-metastasis (TNM) classification (Table 86–1).

3. Adjuvant therapy is indicated in the following instances:

a. For patients with Dukes' C colon adenocarcinoma, 5-fluorouracil and levamisole (Ergamisol) or leucovorin (Wellcovorin) have improved both disease free and overall survival.

b. For patients with Dukes' B or C rectal carcinoma, postoperative combined-modality therapy with radiation and chemotherapy improves both disease-free and overall survival.

TABLE 86-1. COMPARISON OF TNM AND DUKES' STAGING SYSTEMS FOR COLORECTAL CANCER

STAGE	TNM DESIGNATION*			DUKES' DESIGNATION
0	Tis	N0	M0	—
I	T1	N0	M0	A
	T2	N0	M0	
II	T3	N0	M0	B
	T4	N0	M0	
III	Any T	N1	M0	C
	Any T	N2, N3	M0	
IV	Any T	Any N	M1	D

Abbreviations: Tis, tumor in situ; T1, tumor invades submucosa; T2, tumor invades muscularis propria; T3, tumor invades through muscularis propria; T4, tumor invades serosa ± adjacent organs; N0, negative lymph nodes; N1, one to three positive nodes; N2, more than three positive nodes; N3, positive nodes on vascular trunk; M0, no distant metastases; M1, distant metastases.

From Winawer SJ: Tumors of the colon and rectum. In Rakel RE (ed): Conn's Current Therapy 1999, p 532. Philadelphia, WB Saunders Company, 1999, with permission.

c. The use of preoperative radiation for rectal cancers is controversial but may be beneficial in rendering large, bulky tumors resectable. Such therapy *may* lower recurrence rates and, when combined with chemotherapy, *may* improve survival. Clinical studies are in progress.

Key Treatment

Surgical removal

Follow-Up

The majority of recurrences occur within 5 years of surgery, with 80 per cent occurring by 2 years.

1. Follow-up recommendations
   a. History, physical examination, stool evaluation for occult blood, and CEA every 3 months for 2 years, then every 6 months for 2 years, then annually.

   (1) CEA is helpful if initially elevated and returns to normal.
   (2) An increase of CEA greater than 5 mg/ml requires investigation.

   b. Colonoscopy is performed 1 year after surgery, then every 3 years thereafter. Barium enema should be performed if colonoscopy was unsuccessful in evaluating the entire colon.

2. Treatment of recurrent disease.
   a. Local recurrence: Attempt cure by resection.
   b. Distant metastases
      (1) Tend to involve liver, lung, bone, and brain.
      (2) Liver metastases develop in 35 to 50 per cent of patients with colorectal cancer.
      (3) Ten to 20 per cent of patients with liver metastases may benefit from resection, with 5-year survival of 25 per cent.
      (4) Relative contraindications to resection
         (a) Positive porta-hepatis nodes
         (b) Extrahepatic metastases
         (c) More than four hepatic metastases
      (5) For unresectable systemic disease, chemotherapy is used with limited success.

Bibliography

Boland CR: Colorectal neoplasia, part I: the scientific basis for current management. Gastroenterol Clin North Am 1996;25:717–858.

Boland CR: Colorectal neoplasia, part II: diagnosis and treatment. Gastroenterol Clin North Am 1996;26:1–139.

Cohen A: Surgical consideration in patients with cancer of the colon and rectum. Semin Oncol 1991;18:381–386.

Makela T, Laitinen SO, Kaitraluoma M: Five-year follow-up after radical surgery for colorectal cancer: results of a prospective randomized trial. Arch Surg 1995;130:1062–1067.

Metzger U, Gross TH, Honegger HP: Adjuvant treatment for colorectal cancer: "state of the art" messages from recent trials. Eur J Surg Oncol 1995;21:342–356.

The techniques used in flexible sigmoidoscopy and colonoscopy are similar. The following information, except as noted, is pertinent to both. Many of the subtle techniques would require too lengthy a discussion. This procedure guide is intended as a complement to supervised, hands-on training. Additional reading is encouraged.

Indications

1. Rectal bleeding
2. Unexplained lower abdominal symptoms
3. Equivocal or abnormal barium enema
4. Unexplained chronic diarrhea
5. Cancer surveillance: Sigmoidoscopy is recommended for routine screening every 5 years for patients over age 50. Colonoscopy should be performed if stool is guaiac positive or if there is a family history.

Contraindications

1. Absolute contraindications
   a. Patient refusal
   b. Patient moribund
   c. Known or suspected perforation
   d. Unstable cardiac condition
   e. Unavailability of resuscitation
2. Relative contraindications
   a. Respiratory insufficiency
   b. Diagnosis already established
   c. Fulminant colitis

Patient Preparation

1. Informed consent is necessary for these procedures. Videotapes and patient handouts are available and are very useful in answering the patient's questions.
2. Preprocedure instructions: sigmoidoscopy
   a. Most physicians now prepare patients for flexible sigmoidoscopy by having the patient take only clear liquids the day before the procedure. Magnesium citrate, 10 oz, is given at approximately 5:00 PM (after work), followed by three Dulcolax tablets 2 hours later. The patient then takes nothing by mouth after midnight for AM procedure.
   b. While Fleet's enemas can be used to prepare patients for flexible sigmoidoscopy, studies have shown that such preparation is inferior to oral preparation. Fleet's enemas can also on occasion cause proctitis. For the patient who comes to the office unprepped, two

Fleet's enemas 20 minutes apart will usually enable the physican to visualize the rectum and part of the sigmoid.
   c. In order to avoid discoloration of the colon mucosa, it is best for the patient to avoid iron and red gelatin preparations the day before the procedure.
3. Preprocedure instructions: colonoscopy
   a. In addition to the flexible sigmoidoscopy preparation (2.a. above), the patient will need to drink at least 4 liters of colon prep solution (GoLYTELY or Colyte). The prep solution can be drunk the evening of the day prior to the procedure, but a cleaner colon is achieved by having the patient drink the solution early in the morning on the day of the procedure. Enough solution must be ingested to ensure no particles in the "stool."
   b. Other preparations, including Fleet Phospha-Soda, have been used, but none is superior to the preceding prep.
4. Antibiotics
   a. Artificial heart valves, valvular deformity with stenosis or insufficiency, and previous subacute bacterial endocarditis demand antibiotic coverage appropriate to the patient's allergies. Amoxicillin and gentamicin are often used. If there is penicillin sensitivity, vancomycin is usually substituted for amoxicillin.
   b. The diagnosis of mitral valve prolapse without valvular damage does not demand antibiotics.

Equipment

Flexible sigmoidoscopes are available in 35- and 60-cm sizes. After the practitioner becomes facile, he or she will want the 60-cm scope in order to visualize up to the sigmoid–descending colon junction (rarely further in the normal colon). When purchasing a scope, keep in mind

1. Small-diameter and stiff scopes may make it easier to pass the instrument, but operator expertise and use of minimal air is what decreases patient discomfort.
2. A biopsy channel is important if biopsies of mucosa and polyps are planned. The biopsy channel increases cost and difficulty of cleansing.
3. The ease in which air, water, and suction are used is an important consideration.
4. Video scopes are more expensive but give excellent pictures and allow easy documentation.

5. The scopes must be cleaned thoroughly, first with soap and water using brushing technique described by the manufacturer, and then soaked with a chemical solution recommended by the manufacturer. (Proper venting of the room used to clean the scopes is important for the health of the personnel as recommended by the Occupational Safety and Health Administration.)

6. For colonoscopies you must also have oxygen, vital sign and O_2 saturation monitors, IV equipment, and resuscitation equipment.

Anesthesia

1. Flexible sigmoidoscopy

   a. Usually medication is not needed for flexible sigmoidoscopy.

   b. Remember, the length of the scope introduced is determined by patient comfort and preparation, not by the length of the instrument.

2. Colonoscopy

   a. Some degree of conscious sedation is usually needed for most patients undergoing colonoscopy.

   b. Patient reaction to medication is extremely variable.

   c. The patient must be monitored by an individual other than the endoscopist in addition to monitoring by pulse oximeter and vital sign monitoring.

   d. Medications often used

      (1) Midazolam (Versed), 3 to 5 mg IV, titrated in 0.5-mg increments

      (2) Meperidine (Demerol), 50 to 100 mg IV, titrated in 12.5- to 25-mg increments; or morphine, 5 to 10 mg IV, titrated in 1- to 2-mg increments; or other medication such as fentanyl have been used by those with experience with those medications.

      (3) Reversal agents (naloxone [Narcan] and flumazenil [Mazicon]) should be available.

   e. The physician should be familiar with the medication used, side effects, monitoring, and resuscitation.

Technique

1. Check equipment to be sure light, water, air, and suction are in working order.

2. Reassure the patient and begin sedation if needed.

3. Perform digital rectal examination with the patient lying on the left side with the right knee flexed.

4. Lubricate the distal 2 to 3 cm of the scope and insert the scope 5 to 10 cm, visualizing the lumen and advancing the scope, always keeping the lumen in the center of the view and not forcing the instrument.

   a. Loss of visualization of the lumen and blanching of the mucosa suggest impending perforation, and the scope should be partially withdrawn in order to visualize the lumen before proceeding. Use the air sparingly to keep the lumen inflated. Water is effective to cleanse the lens.

   b. Observe for mucosal irregularities and polyps, biopsying any suspicious mucosa or lesion. The finding of an adenomatous polyp (tubular ademona), especially if greater than 5 mm, demands that the patient undergo entire colonoscopy. Hyperplastic polyps, in contrast, do not demand colonoscopy. Random biopsies may be appropriate if you suspect colitis even if the mucosa visualized has a normal appearance.

5. A thorough examination includes the following.

   a. Rectum: Retroverting the scope is the best method to visualize the distal rectum.

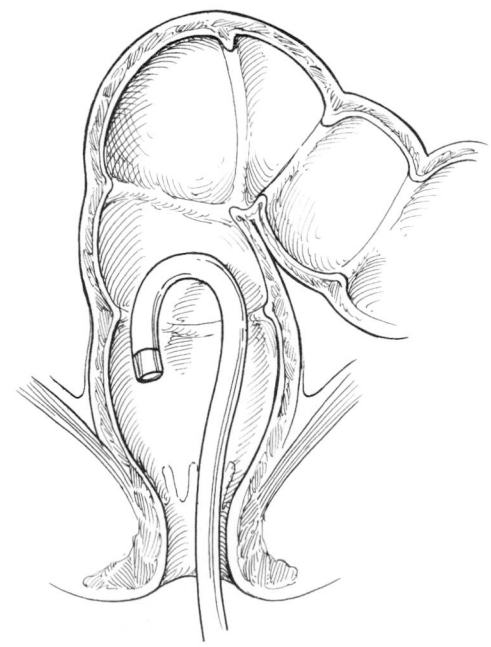

This is accomplished by rotating the large wheel counterclockwise when 10 to 15 cm of the scope has been introduced. Gently advance the scope while torquing the scope clockwise. This should bring the scope into position to view the internal sphincter. Continue the torquing motion and slight withdrawal in order to obtain an excellent view of the rectum. This maneuver is usually done at the end of the examination.

b. Sigmoid: The sigmoid frequently has multiple curves and is the most likely place for loop formation and for diverticula. A "blind" curve should not be "pushed through" but can usually be negotiated by torquing the instrument while simultaneously withdrawing it several centimeters. Large diverticula could be mistaken for the lumen of the bowel, with resultant perforation if pressure is applied.

c. Descending colon (reached with colonoscopy): The descending colon is reached at about 55 cm and is often difficult to negotiate because of a sharp angle at the junction of the descending and sigmoid colon. Because of the patient's left lateral decubitus position, there is usually fluid remaining in the descending colon. The descending colon ends at the splenic flexure, where there is another sharp turn.

d. Transverse colon: The transverse colon usually has a triangular lumen and is usually easier to intubate with the patient on the back. The hepatic flexure is often confused with the cecum. Loop formations can also occur in the transverse colon.

e. Ascending colon: The ascending colon often has bile-stained liquid. The wall is thinner than the rest of the colon. The cecum has a bird's foot appearance, and the ileocecal valve should be identified. If enteritis is suspected, intubation of the terminal ileum should be performed.

6. Alpha loops, often formed when a moderate amount of redundant bowel is present, commonly occur in the sigmoid colon.

a. A loop usually becomes evident when there is paradoxical movement of the scope. Paradoxical movement is occurring if the scope seems to be withdrawing as it is being advanced. Loops make passage of the scope more difficult and increase discomfort for the patient.

b. Reduction of an alpha loop is usually achieved by torquing the scope in a clockwise direction while withdrawing.

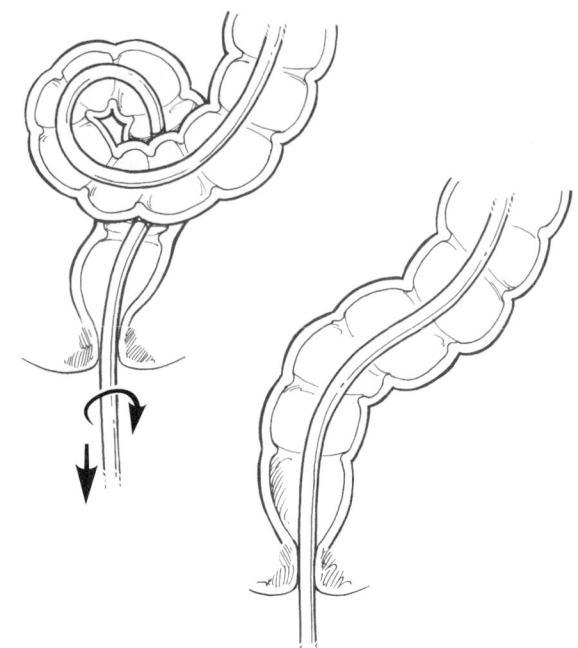

This often takes several attempts. A reverse alpha loop requires counterclockwise torquing of the scope.

c. After reduction to avoid recurrence of the loop the intestine should be telescoped on the scope. This is achieved by gently catching the side of the bowel wall with the tip of the scope and withdrawing as the scope is torqued.

7. Counter-pressure: Abdominal counter-pressure by an assistant or by the physician is a useful technique in colonoscopy to help advance the scope. While the patient is lying on the back or even on the left side, pressure may be applied in the left lower quadrant or where a loop of scope is encountered.

8. Patient positioning: There is no rule that the patient must remain in the left lateral decubitus position when the scope is advanced. Although this is the most useful position for examination of the left colon, moving the patient onto the back or even the right side will often straighten out a sharp corner of bowel and allow easier advancement.

9. Complications

a. Complications are infrequent if the examination is gentle and not rushed. Complications are more apt to occur with physician inexperience, poor colon preparation, and patient intolerance of pain, "forcing" the physician to use too much medication.

b. Perforations can usually be avoided by terminating the procedure rather than forcing the scope.

c. Bleeding may be encountered when biopsy or polypectomy is performed.

d. Explosion can occur when cautery is used in the poorly prepped colon. Cautery can also cause immediate or late perforations.

Follow-Up

1. Sedated patients should be observed by competent personnel until stable, awake, and coordinated. Sedated patients must not drive home.

2. Written findings and recommendations should be given to the patient with specific instructions regarding a phone number to call if fever, increasing pain, bleeding, or other complications occur. It is best to include findings and date of follow-up.

Bibliography

Cappell MS: An illustrated guide to flexible sigmoidoscopy. Hosp Med 1995;Feb:28–42.

Hawes RH, Lehman GA, O'Conner KW, et al: Effect of instrument diameter on the depth of penetration of fiberoptic sigmoidoscopes. Gastrointest Endosc 1988; 34:28.

Schertz RD, Baskin WN, Frakes JT: Flexible fiberoptic sigmoidoscopy training for primary care physicians: result of a five year experience. Gastrointest Endosc 1989;35:316.

Sharma VK, Chockalingham S, Clark V, et al: Randomized, controlled comparison of two forms of preparation for screening flexible sigmoidoscopy. Am J Gastroenterol 1997;92:809.

Wong RC, Van Dam J: The technique of flexible sigmoidoscopy. J Crit Illness 1994;9:797.

87 Small and Large Bowel Obstruction

Robert M. Gerbo

Etiology

Small Bowel

1. Adhesions are the most common cause.
2. Neoplasm, with the primary origin more likely to be from an intra-abdominal site such as the colon, stomach, pancreas, or ovary
3. Hernia, especially an abdominal wall hernia (i.e., inguinal, femoral, umbilical, ventral, or incisional)
4. Other causes include inflammatory bowel disease, volvulus, intussusception, gallstones, foreign body, bezoar, intestinal worms, traumatic injury, radiation injury, meconium, endometriosis, and congenital intrinsic lesions.
5. There frequently may be more than one cause.

Large bowel

1. Cancer is the most common cause.
2. Volvulus
3. Diverticulitis usually only causes partial obstruction.
4. Other causes include inflammatory bowel disease, benign tumors, fecal or barium impaction, and congenital disorders such as Hirschsprung's disease.

Symptoms

1. Cramping abdominal pain may be localized or diffuse. Severe, constant pain suggests strangulation.
2. Nausea and vomiting are common and in a distal obstruction may even be feculent. However, vomiting may not occur at all in a large bowel obstruction.
3. Obstipation occurs with complete obstruction, although feces distal to the obstruction may still pass.
4. Bloating and distention occur late.

Key Symptoms

- Cramping abdominal pain
- Vomiting
- Obstipation

Clinical Findings

1. Tenderness is common. Severe tenderness and rigidity suggest strangulation or perforation.
2. Abdominal distention may be mild or severe.
3. Bowel sounds may be high-pitched and "tinkling" or absent.
4. Gross or occult fecal blood may be present.
5. Fever is suggestive of strangulation or perforation.
6. Signs of dehydration may also be present.

Key Signs

- Tenderness
- "Tinkling" or absent bowel sounds
- Distention

Laboratory Tests

1. Laboratory tests are of no diagnostic value. Leukocytosis may not be present. Chemistries may indicate dehydration.
2. Plain abdominal radiographs (supine and upright) typically demonstrate dilated loops of bowel and air-fluid levels in a stepladder fashion.
   a. Gas is usually absent distal to the obstruction.
   b. In large bowel obstruction, the small bowel will also be dilated if the ileocecal valve is incompetent.
   c. Free air beneath the diaphragm is an ominous sign indicating bowel perforation.

> **WARNING**
>
> **Free air beneath the diaphragm on radiograph indicates bowel perforation, and emergent surgical consultation should be obtained.**

3. In equivocal cases, contrast studies (barium or water-soluble medium) confirm the diagnosis. Water-soluble contrast is safer if perforation oc-

curs. Computerized tomography may also be helpful.

4. With a suspected large bowel obstruction and a "nonsurgical" abdomen, endoscopy can confirm diagnosis and aid in determining etiology.

Key Tests

- Radiography (supine and upright)
- Contrast studies

Differential Diagnosis

1. Small versus large bowel obstruction
   a. Symptoms of large bowel obstruction are slower to develop.
   b. Abdominal films show dilated colon in large bowel obstruction.
2. Paralytic (adynamic) ileus occurs with recent abdominal surgery, peritonitis, abdominal or spinal trauma, and other associated illnesses.
   a. The pain is constant and mild, and there is abdominal distention.
   b. Radiographs show gas in both the small and large bowel.
   c. Contrast studies are useful in equivocal cases.
3. Pseudo-obstruction is a chronic, recurring syndrome of signs and symptoms of bowel obstruction caused by abnormal gastrointestinal (GI) motility and not a mechanical obstructing lesion.
   a. Secondary causes are numerous and include collagen vascular disease, amyloidosis, various neurologic and endocrine disorders, drugs, and multiple miscellaneous entities.
   b. Primary causes are characterized as familial or sporadic.
   c. Contrast studies exclude a mechanical obstructing lesion.
4. Mesenteric vascular occlusion is usually due to emboli or atherosclerosis of the mesenteric vasculature.
   a. A history of cardiac disease and/or a thromboembolic event is common with severe abdominal pain.
   b. Arteriography confirms the diagnosis.
   c. The bowel may appear dusky in color on colonoscopy.

Treatment

1. Begin with nasogastric (NG) tube decompression and intravenous fluids. There has been de-

bate regarding the use of long intestinal tubes, which are more difficult to place.

2. Obtain surgical consultation, because nearly all complete obstructions require operative intervention.
3. Endoscopy can be an option in some nonacute settings (i.e., no peritoneal signs).
   a. In malignant large bowel obstruction, endoscopic dilatation and decompression, as well as laser fulguration, are options.
   b. Detorsion of a volvulus endoscopically is frequently successful, but the recurrence rate is high and surgical treatment is definitive.
   c. Endoscopic removal of some foreign bodies and gallstones
   d. More studies are needed regarding the use of endoscopically placed colonic stents.

Medication

1. Broad-spectrum antibiotic coverage against gram-positive, gram-negative, and anaerobic organisms should be considered in the perioperative period.
2. Use of cathartics or other GI stimulants proximal to a bowel obstruction may result in perforation and should therefore be avoided. Enemas are safer but still require caution.

WARNING

Use of cathartics or other GI stimulants proximal to an obstruction may result in perforation.

Diet

Nothing by mouth (NPO) status should be maintained.

Activity

Bed rest is advised while the patient is acutely ill.

Patient Education

1. Being NPO and having an NG tube are uncomfortable, but hopefully these measures will prevent perforation, which could result in life-threatening infection.
2. Perforation of the bowel is a risk of both surgical and endoscopic procedures.
3. If primary reanastomosis is not possible at the time of bowel resection, an ostomy will be performed with the possibility of reanastomosis at a later date.

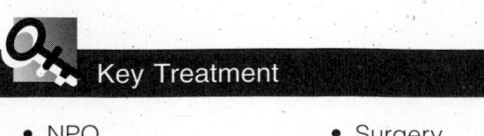

Key Treatment

- NPO
- NG suction
- Surgery

Follow-Up

1. Monitor for signs and symptoms of recurrence at follow-up visits.

2. After resection for colon cancer, examination of stool for occult blood, colonoscopy, and carcinoembryonic antigen levels should be used to monitor for recurrence.

Bibliography

Bass KN, Jones B, Bulkley GB: Current management of small-bowel obstruction. Adv Surg 1997;31:1–34.

Dorudi S, Berry AR, Kettlewell MGW: Acute colonic pseudo-obstruction. Br J Surg 1992;79:99–103.

Holder WD Jr: Intestinal Obstruction. Gastroenterol Clin North Am 1988;17:317–340.

McGregor JR, O'Dwyer PJ: The surgical management of obstruction and perforation of the left colon. Surg Gynecol Obstet 1993;177:203–208.

88 Intussusception

Eileen M. Reickert

Etiology

Intussusception is defined as the telescoping of a proximal bowel segment into the adjacent distal segment. This process leads to bowel obstruction, ischemia, infarction, and perforation.

1. Intussusception can occur in both children and adults, although only 5 per cent of cases occur in adults.
2. The most common cause in the pediatric group is idiopathic, with no specific identifiable lead point.
3. Adult intussusception is usually associated with a primary pathologic cause. Most cases of adult intussusception have a demonstrable lead point.
4. In children, most cases are of ileocolic intussusception, although involvement of any part of the small and large bowel has been described in both children and adults.

Common Causes

Pediatric	Adult
• Idiopathic	• Tumors (65 per cent of cases)
• Hyperplasia of lymphoid tissue	• Meckel's diverticulum
• Meckel's diverticulum	• Postoperative complications (intestinal tube removal, adhesions)

Symptoms

Intussusception can occur at any age; however, 60 to 80 percent of cases occur in children less than 2 years of age, with a peak incidence at 6 months of age.

1. Pediatric patients
   a. Intermittent 10- to 30-minute bouts of colic and crying fits followed by periods of exhaustion and fatigue
   b. During restless periods the child pulls the legs to the abdomen in crampy pain.
   c. Vomiting is common, particularly in young infants.
   d. Diarrhea may be present and does not exclude the diagnosis. Currant jelly stools may be passed.
   e. Complete obstruction is a later occurrence.
2. Adult patients
   a. The presentation is often atypical.
   b. Symptomatology may be acute or chronic and can include abdominal pain, weight loss, vomiting, and/or rectal bleeding.
   c. The diagnosis is often delayed until laparotomy.

Key Symptoms

- Vomiting
- Intermittent colic and lethargy
- Blood in stools

WARNING

The complete constellation of classic symptoms is often absent. Early diagnosis is essential because delays in treatment increase morbidity and mortality. A high clinical index of suspicion is mandatory.

Clinical Findings

1. Abdominal examination in children often reveals a sausage-shaped, nontender mass in the right upper quadrant or epigastrium.
2. Focal or diffuse peritonitis may be present.
3. Rectal prolapse of the intussuscepted intestine may occur.
4. Stool is usually Hemoccult-positive.

Key Signs

- Abdominal mass
- Hemoccult-positive stools

Laboratory Tests

Early diagnosis is the key to successful therapy.

1. If the diagnosis is strongly suspected, the patient should undergo immediate evaluation and treatment. The definitive diagnostic and therapeutic test is a contrast (barium or air) enema.
2. For the patient with an unclear diagnosis, other radiographic evaluation may be employed.
   a. Plain films, if obtained, may reveal a soft-tissue mass at the site of intussusception, abnormal gas pattern, or obstruction.
   b. Ultrasonography is a useful screening test for patients with atypical symptoms or contraindications to contrast studies (peritonitis, sepsis, or longstanding obstruction).
      (1) Ultrasonographic findings suggestive of intussusception include the doughnut and pseudokidney signs.
      (2) A nondiagnostic ultrasound test does not rule out intussusception.
   c. Computerized tomography has also been used in patients with atypical symptoms. A target lesion can be identified. This modality offers no improvement over ultrasound.

Key Tests

- Abdominal ultrasound: doughnut or pseudokidney sign
- Air or barium contrast enema—gold standard

Differential Diagnosis
1. Gastroenteritis
2. Volvulus
3. Malrotation
4. Adhesions
5. Tumor

Treatment
1. Prior to attempted reduction, the patient should be fluid-resuscitated and nasogastric NG tube decompression performed.
2. Antibiotics should be administered to prevent sepsis. Ampicillin, gentamicin, and clindamycin provide adequate coverage.
3. Mild sedation may be given.
4. Surgical involvement is mandatory prior to attempted reduction. A surgeon should be available during the procedure in case of complications.
5. The primary diagnostic and therapeutic test for children is a contrast enema (barium or air).
   a. The study identifies the process, and a pressure-controlled reduction of the intussusception can be attempted if the patient is stable and does not need an immediate operation.
   b. If contrast enema fails, or peritonitis and/or perforation is identified, then the patient should undergo laparotomy for definitive management.
6. Adult patients should not undergo pressure-controlled reduction but instead primary laparotomy because of the high incidence of associated pathologic lesions.
7. After reduction, the patient is usually admitted for 24 hours of observation and given antibiotics.
8. After nonoperative reduction, meals may be started the following morning. After operative reduction, meals are started as bowel function returns.
9. There are no specific activity restrictions for patients with intussusception once treated.

Patient Education
1. Intussusception is a relatively common cause of obstruction in the infant and child, although it is quite rare in the adult.
2. Contrast enema reductions are successful 70 to 95 per cent of the time.
3. Failure rate for contrast reductions increases with longer symptomatology.
4. Mortality is rare (<1 per cent) and is usually secondary to delayed diagnosis, hypovolemia, and sepsis.
5. In pediatric patients the risk of early recurrence is approximately 6 per cent.
6. For adult patients, the course and prognosis of their disease relates to the etiologic factors. These factors are usually clear postlaparotomy.

Key Treatment

All
- Intravenous fluid resuscitation
- NG tube decompression
- Antibiotics
- Surgical consult

Pediatric
- Contrast enema (barium or air) with pressure-controlled reduction
- If reduction fails, laparotomy with reduction or resection

Adult
- Primary laparotomy after resuscitation

Follow-Up

In pediatric patients, no specific follow-up is required after resolution of symptoms. Adult follow-up plan is determined after causative factors are determined.

Bibliography

Ein SH, Stephens CA: Intussusception: 354 cases in 10 years. J Pediat Surg 1971;6:16–27.

Losek JD, Fiete RL: Intussusception and the diagnostic value of testing for occult blood. Am J Emerg Med 1991;9:1–3.

Reijnen HAM, Joosten HJ, deBoer HH: Diagnosis and treatment of adult intussusception. Am J Surg 1989; 158:25–28.

Swischuk LE, Hayden CK, Boulden T: Intussusception: indications for ultrasonography and an explanation of the doughnut and pseudokidney signs. Pediatr Radiol 1985;15:388–391.

Young DG: Intussusception. In O'Neill JA (ed): Pediatric Surgery, 5th ed, vol 2, pp 1185–1198. St. Louis, CV Mosby Company, 1998.

89 Crohn's Disease

Stephen P. James

Etiology

1. Cause is unknown, but is probably multifactorial.

   a. Environmental: More common in industrial countries, with rapid increase in prevalence in 20th century (currently 20 to 40/100,000); relative risk higher in smokers.

   b. Bacterial products: Products of intestinal flora thought to contribute to intestinal inflammation; no unique infectious agent has been identified.

   c. Genetic: There is a familial tendency and high concordance in twins; it is more common in Jews and non-Jewish Caucasians.

   d. Immunologic factors: No unique immunologic abnormality has been identified, but disease appears to be immunologically mediated.

2. Pathogenesis: Inflammatory lesions may be present anywhere in alimentary tract. There are characteristic patterns of disease.

   a. Ileocolonic Crohn's disease (40 per cent of patients): tendency to form strictures in ileum, fistula formation, abdominal abscess, perirectal disease

   b. Colonic Crohn's disease (granulomatous colitis, Crohn's colitis, 30 per cent of patients): Inflammation may occur anywhere in colon with skip areas that distinguish it from ulcerative colitis.

   c. Small bowel Crohn's disease (regional ileitis, 30 per cent of patients): tendency to form strictures, obstruction

   d. Upper gastrointestinal (GI) Crohn's disease (less than 5 per cent of patients): Inflammatory lesions of esophagus, stomach, and duodenum may resemble acid-peptic disease.

Symptoms

Symptoms are highly variable depending on site and severity of lesions.

1. Diarrhea (absence does not preclude diagnosis)
2. Abdominal pain
3. Fatigue
4. Weight loss
5. Rectal pain, hematochezia, purulent discharge from fistula
6. Fever
7. Growth failure (children)
8. Nausea, vomiting, dyspepsia
9. Arthralgias (joint swelling uncommon)
10. Skin ulcers (pyoderma gangrenosum), skin nodules (erythema nodosum)
11. Painful aphthous mouth ulcers
12. Visual changes (iritis)
13. Jaundice

Key Symptoms

- Diarrhea
- Abdominal pain
- Fatigue
- Weight loss

Clinical Findings

Clinical findings are highly variable depending on location and severity of lesions. Some patients have no physical findings.

1. Abdominal tenderness
2. Abdominal mass
3. Abdominal distention (with partial obstruction)
4. Hyperactive bowel sounds (with partial obstruction)
5. Fever
6. Perineal fistulas with purulent drainage
7. Rectal abscess
8. Mouth ulcers
9. Extraintestinal manifestations (all relatively uncommon)

   a. Eye: episcleritis, iritis, uveitis

   b. Skin: erythema nodosum, pyoderma gangrenosum

   c. Joints: swelling, tenderness

   d. Hepatic: hepatomegaly, splenomegaly, jaundice

Key Signs

- Highly variable
- Some patients may have no physical findings
- Abdominal tenderness
- Abdominal mass
- Fistulas
- Perirectal abscess

Laboratory Tests

Routine laboratory tests are helpful as a clue to underlying inflammatory disease and to assess complications of severe diarrhea, bleeding, or malabsorption.

1. Complete blood count: anemia, leukocytosis, thrombocytosis
2. Electrolytes, blood urea nitrogen, creatinine: metabolic acidosis, prerenal azotemia
3. Sedimentation rate: useful for monitoring response to therapy
4. Liver function tests: Abnormal values suggest pericholangitis or sclerosing cholangitis.
5. Nutritional status: albumin, prealbumin, vitamin B_{12}
6. Stool
   a. Leukocytes, occult blood often present.
   b. Exclude bacterial pathogens, parasites, *Clostridium difficile* toxin.
7. Blood cultures: for suspected sepsis.
8. Special studies are required to make the diagnosis and for potential complications.
   a. Colonoscopy
      (1) Diagnose colonic and terminal ileal Crohn's disease; biopsies mandatory.
      (2) Define extent and severity of colonic disease
      (3) Screen for colon cancer in longstanding colonic Crohn's

---

WARNING

In severely ill patients with abdominal abscess, small bowel obstruction, toxic megacolon, or suspected perforation, bowel preparations or invasive procedures may precipitate marked deterioration or complication and should be either avoided or used with extreme caution.

---

   b. Upper GI and small bowel series
      (1) For diagnosis of upper GI Crohn's disease, strictures, fistulas

      (2) Small bowel enteroclysis may provide better definition
   c. Abdominal, pelvic computerized tomography with oral contrast
      (1) Define abdominal mass, abscess, ureteral obstruction
      (2) Identify abdominal fistulas
   d. Abdominal ultrasound
      (1) Hydronephrosis resulting from oxalate stones
      (2) Gallstones associated with bile salt deficiency
   e. Upper GI endoscopy: for diagnosis, biopsy of suspected upper GI Crohn's disease

Key Tests

- Stool examination
- Colonoscopy with biopsy
- Upper GI and small bowel series

Differential Diagnosis

1. Irritable bowel syndrome
2. Other forms of colitis: ulcerative colitis, infectious colitis, pseudomembranous colitis, ischemic colitis, radiation colitis, lymphocytic colitis
3. Other causes of hematochezia: hemorrhoids, colorectal cancer, diverticular disease, ischemic colitis
4. Other causes of diarrhea
5. Other causes of small bowel narrowing, obstruction, inflammation: infectious ileitis (*Mycobacterium*, *Yersinia*, *Actinomyces*), lymphoma, carcinoma, nonsteroidal anti-inflammatory drugs, adhesions, intussusception, celiac disease
6. Other causes of right lower quadrant pain: appendicitis, pelvic inflammatory disease, ovarian mass, nephrolithiasis
7. Other causes of gastric or duodenal inflammation: peptic ulcer disease, Zollinger-Ellison syndrome, adenocarcinoma

Treatment

The disease and its complications are highly variable, and treatment must be tailored to the particular location and severity of disease. There is no universal prescription for therapy. Some symptoms may be due to obstruction, abscess, or fistulas that will not respond to anti-inflammatory therapy and require surgical intervention.

Medication

1. Metronidazole (Flagyl), 250 mg qid: for colonic, fistulous disease; other antibiotics have been used in uncontrolled trials (ciprofloxacin).
2. 5-Acetylsalicylic acid drugs: sulfasalazine (Azulfidine), olsalazine (Dipentum), mesalamine (Asacol, Pentasa). Used for mild disease of colon or terminal ileum or as adjunct to prednisone. Mesalamine is useful for small bowel disease.
3. Corticosteroids
   a. Forty to 60 mg/day of prednisone orally for acute exacerbations tapered over approximately 2 months
   b. Low continuous dose may be required for maintenance.
   c. Intravenous steroids for severe exacerbations
   d. Avoid with septic complications, abscess, fistulas.
4. Immunosuppressive/immunomodulatory drugs
   a. Azathioprine (Imuran), 2 to 2.5 mg/kg/day, or 6-mercaptopurine (Purinethol), 1 to 1.5 mg/kg/day: indicated as steroid-sparing agents; primary therapy for fistulous disease; long delay before onset of action (2 to 6 months)
   b. Methotrexate: for severe, unresponsive disease
   c. Cyclosporine: for severe, unresponsive disease
5. Adjunctive therapy
   a. Antidiarrheals: diphenoxylate-atropine, loperamide; 1 to 2 tablets two to four times daily
   b. Vitamin B_{12}: monthly by injection for extensive ileal disease or prior ileal resection
   c. Cholestyramine: 4 gm one to two times daily for bile salt–induced diarrhea
   d. Infliximab (Remicade): for severe disease or refractory fistulas

Surgery

Indicated for major complications: obstruction, pyogenic abscess, fistulas unresponsive to medical therapy, perforation, toxic megacolon, cancer, refractory disease, severe hemorrhage. Surgery is not curative; therefore, it should be conservative.

Diet

1. Low-residue diet when obstructive symptoms present
2. Oral elemental diet or total parenteral nutrition for severe unresponsive disease or growth retardation
3. Lactose-free diet if lactase deficient

Patient Education

1. Careful education as to realistic expectations required for this chronic relapsing disease and side effects of therapy
2. Special problems: pregnancy, childhood Crohn's disease, genetic counseling
3. Patient educational materials are available through Crohn's and Colitis Foundation of America, 386 Park Avenue South, 17th Floor, New York, NY 10016 (Web site: *www.ccfa.org*).

Key Treatment

No universal prescription for therapy

Follow-Up

Prognosis is for lifelong relapsing and remitting disease that may require frequent follow-up.

1. After initial evaluation and definition of disease extent, adjustment of therapy can often be made by careful symptom assessment and examination. Reevaluation of procedures may be necessary if a major complication is suspected or if there is a lack of expected response to therapy.
2. Steroids and immunosuppressive drugs should be tapered to lowest possible dose.
3. Surgical therapy should be offered for intractable symptoms resulting from fixed stricture, fistulas, severe unresponsive disease. Majority of patients require surgery at some time during course.
4. Colon cancer surveillance by colonoscopy should be considered with longstanding colonic disease (more than 10 years). Screening Hemoccult cards and flexible sigmoidoscopy are not useful.
5. Emotional support is required, but psychiatric evaluation is indicated only for major psychiatric diagnosis.

Bibliography

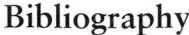

For general references on Crohn's disease, see
Hanauer SB: Inflammatory bowel disease. N Engl J Med 1996;334:841–848.
Hanauer SB, Meyers S: Management of Crohn's disease in adults. Am J Gastroenterol 1997;92:559–566.

For more information on nutritional therapy, see
O'Sullivan MA, O'Morain CA: Nutritional therapy in Crohn's disease. Inflamm Bowel Dis 1998;4:45–53.

For more information on surgery for Crohn's disease, see
Glotzer DJ: Surgical therapy for Crohn's disease. Gastroenterol Clin North Am 1995;24:577–596.

For more information on treatment of children with Crohn's disease, see
Grand RJ, Ramakrishna J, Calenda KA: Therapeutic strategies for pediatric Crohn disease. Clin Invest Med 1996;19:373–380.

For more information on medical treatment of Crohn's disease, see
Feagan BG, Rochon J, Fedorak RN, et al: Methotrexate for the treatment of Crohn's disease: The North American Crohn's Study Group investigators. N Engl J Med 1995;332:292–297.
Pearson DC, May GR, Fick GH, et al: Azathioprine and 6-mercaptopurine in Crohn disease: a meta-analysis. Ann Intern Med 1995;123:132–142.
Sutherland LR, Martin F, Bailey RJ, et al: A randomized, placebo-controlled, double-blind trial of mesalamine in the maintenance of remission of Crohn's disease: the Canadian Mesalamine for Remission of Crohn's Disease Study Group. Gastroenterology 1997;112:1069–1077.
Targan SR, Hanauer SB, van Deventer SJ, et al: A short-term study of chimeric monoclonal antibody cA2 to tumor necrosis factor alpha for Crohn's disease: Crohn's Disease cA2 Study Group. N Engl J Med 1997;337:1029–1035.

90 Ulcerative Colitis

Bruce D. Greenwald

Etiology

Cause is unknown, but it is probably multifactorial.

1. Environmental: more common in Scandinavian countries, Great Britain, North America
2. Genetic: familial tendency, increased concordance in twins, more common in Jews and non-Jewish Caucasians
3. Immunologic: No unique abnormality identified at this time. Anti-colon antibodies are present, but their significance is uncertain.

Symptoms

1. Diarrhea: usually small volume (200 ml/day or less), can be bloody
2. Hematochezia
3. Abdominal pain or cramping
4. Fever: seen in more severe cases
5. Weight loss
6. Fatigue
7. Proctitis symptoms
   a. Tenesmus (straining without passing stool)
   b. Rectal urgency
   c. Constipation
8. Extracolonic symptoms (45 per cent of cases)
   a. Joints: arthralgias and arthritis
   b. Skin
      (1) Erythema nodosum: tender red nodules, most commonly on the anterior lower legs
      (2) Pyoderma gangrenosum: painful ulcers, usually on extremities
   c. Eyes: pain or burning, blurred vision, photophobia, scleral injection

Key Symptoms

- Diarrhea
- Rectal bleeding
- Abdominal cramping

Clinical Findings

Some patients may have no physical findings.

1. Abdominal tenderness
2. Hematochezia or heme-positive stools
3. Severe disease
   a. Fever
   b. Tachycardia
   c. Malnutrition and dehydration
   d. Abdominal distention
4. Extracolonic manifestations
   a. Eyes: uveitis, iritis, episcleritis
   b. Skin: erythema nodosum, pyoderma gangrenosum
   c. Joints: arthritis, often migratory, affecting large joints; usually nondestructive.
   d. Hepatic: jaundice, hepatomegaly, splenomegaly

Key Signs

- Rectal bleeding
- Abdominal tenderness

Laboratory Tests

Blood tests may be normal in mild or moderate colitis.

1. Complete blood count (CBC): anemia, leukocytosis, thrombocytosis
2. Electrolytes: prerenal azotemia
3. Sedimentation rate: elevated in severe disease
4. Liver function tests: elevated alkaline phosphatase or bilirubin suggests associated pericholangitis, sclerosing cholangitis
5. Albumin, prealbumin, transferrin: May be low.
6. Stool studies
   a. Leukocytes: frequently present
   b. Occult blood: frequently present
   c. Culture, ova, and parasites, *Clostridium difficile* toxin: done to exclude other causes of colitis.

> **Note**
> Culture of *Yersinia*, *Campylobacter*, and *Escherichia coli* O157:H7 must be specifically requested in many labs when sending stool cultures.

7. Abdominal radiograph: Look for colonic distention in severe disease.

8. Special studies are required to make the diagnosis and assess for complications.

   a. Colonoscopy
      (1) Define extent and severity of disease. Obtain stool for culture and biopsies to exclude other causes of colitis.
      (2) Screen for colon cancer in patients with longstanding disease.

   b. Barium enema: less sensitive in mild disease

WARNING

In severely ill patients, especially with colonic distention, bowel preparations or invasive procedures may precipitate marked deterioration or complication and should be either avoided or used with extreme caution.

---

   c. Upper gastrointestinal and small bowel series: to exclude a diagnosis of Crohn's disease

Key Tests

- Stool examination
- Colonoscopy with biopsy

Differential Diagnosis

Ulcerative colitis is a diagnosis of exclusion. Other causes of colitis must be excluded before this diagnosis is made.

1. Irritable bowel syndrome
2. Infectious colitis
   a. Bacteria: *Shigella, Salmonella, Yersinia, Campylobacter, E. coli* O157:H7
   b. Parasites: *Entamoeba histolytica, Giardia lamblia*
3. Ischemic colitis
4. Drug-induced—especially antibiotics
5. Diverticulitis
6. Colon cancer
7. Crohn's disease
8. Radiation colitis
9. Human immunodeficiency virus–associated diarrhea

Treatment

Medication

1. Mild to moderate attack
   a. Proctitis: mesalamine suppositories (Rowasa) 500 mg, hydrocortisone suppositories (Anusol-HC) 25 mg, or hydrocortisone foam (Cortifoam) bid to tid
   b. Left-sided colitis: mesalamine enemas (Rowasa) 4 gm or hydrocortisone enemas (Cortenema) 100 mg qhs to bid
   c. Left-sided and pancolitis
      (1) 5-Aminosalicylic acid (5-ASA) preparations: Studies have shown that response to therapy is dose-related, but the benefits of higher doses may be offset by increased side effects, especially with sulfasalazine.
         (a) Sulfasalazine, 1 to 1.5 gm qid (should also give folic acid, 1 mg daily)
         (b) Mesalamine (Asacol), 800 to 1600 mg tid
         (c) Mesalamine (Pentasa), 1 gm qid
      (2) Prednisone, 40 to 60 mg once daily, or equivalent: Use for more severe disease.

2. Severe attack: Patients with fever, dehydration, or severe diarrhea should be hospitalized.
   a. Methylprednisolone, 20 to 30 mg intravenously (IV) tid *or*
   b. Adrenocorticotropic hormone, 80 units daily either intramuscularly or as continuous IV infusion. (*Note*: Efficacy greatest with first attack or in those who have never received corticosteroids.)
   c. Intravenous antibiotics to cover bowel flora

3. Maintenance therapy: Goal is to prevent relapse of disease. Most patients should be placed on maintenance therapy after an acute attack.
   a. Steroids are ineffective as maintenance therapy.
   b. Proctitis: mesalamine suppositories, 500 mg at bedtime or bid; may be tapered weekly to every other night, then every third night, until the lowest dose maintaining remission is found.
   c. Left-sided colitis: Mesalamine or steroid enemas may be tapered as described above for suppositories; oral aminosalicylates as described below for pancolitis.
   d. Pancolitis: Studies have shown that maintenance of remission is dose-related, but the benefits of higher doses may be offset by increased side effects, especially with sulfasal-

azine. The dose needed to attain remission should be used to maintain remission.

    (1) Sulfasalazine, 1 to 1.5 gm qid (should also give folic acid, 1 mg daily)
    (2) Mesalamine (Asacol), 400 to 1200 mg bid to tid
    (3) Olsalazine (Dipentum), 500 to 1000 mg bid

4. Immunosuppressive therapy
    a. Indicated for refractory colitis: patients unable to reduce their dose of steroids below prednisone 5 to 10 mg daily (or equivalent) or those suffering from sequelae from chronic steroid use.
    b. Drugs: equal efficacy and cost
        (1) Azathioprine: initial dose 100 to 150 mg once daily, increase up to 2.5 mg/kg, *or*
        (2) 6-Mercaptopurine: initial dose 50 mg once daily, increase up to 1.5 mg/kg
    c. Two to 6 months of treatment may be needed until an effect is seen.
    d. Complications of therapy include pancreatitis (usually seen within the first month), leukopenia, allergic reactions, hepatitis.
    e. CBC with differential should be monitored monthly. Liver function tests should be monitored quarterly.

WARNING

Immunosuppressive agents should only be prescribed by practitioners experienced in their use.

---

5. Antimotility agents (loperamide [Imodium], diphenoxylate [Lomotil]) should be used with caution.

Diet

1. Diet is ineffective as primary therapy. Elemental diets are ineffective as treatment of ulcerative colitis.
2. Total parenteral nutrition and bowel rest may be needed during severe attacks of acute colitis because of incapacitating diarrhea, abdominal pain, nausea, and vomiting.
3. Nutritional supplementation may be needed for malnutrition. Oral supplements can be used.
4. Foods that induce diarrhea, such as large amounts of raw fruits and vegetables, caffeine, and spicy foods, should be avoided during acute attacks.

Surgery

1. Surgery is curative in ulcerative colitis.

2. Indications
    a. Colon perforation or obstruction
    b. Toxic megacolon
    c. Severe disease refractory to intensive inpatient medical therapy for 3 to 7 days
    d. Intractable or refractory disease
    e. Colon cancer or high-grade dysplasia

Patient Education

1. Ulcerative colitis is a chronic disease with variable course. Surgery is curative.
2. Pregnancy planning should begin prior to conception.
3. Patients are at increased risk for colorectal cancer, especially those having disease beyond the rectum for greater than 10 years.
4. Patient educational materials available through Crohn's and Colitis Foundation of America (386 Park Avenue South, 17th Floor, New York, NY 10016-8804; phone 1-800-932-2423; e-mail *info@ccfa.org*; Internet *www.ccfa.org/*).

Pregnancy

Corticosteroids and sulfasalazine are safe and have been widely used during pregnancy. 5-ASA drugs have been less well studied but are likely safe. Limited data exist on use of immunosuppressive drugs during pregnancy. Surgery should be performed for unequivocal conditions but carries a risk of postoperative spontaneous abortion.

Follow-Up

1. After initial evaluation and definition of disease extent, adjustment of therapy can often be made by careful symptom assessment and physical examination. Re-evaluation with endoscopy or barium enema may be necessary if a major complication is suspected or a lack of expected response to therapy is noted.
2. Steroids should be tapered by 5 to 10 mg/week until 20 mg, then 5 mg/week, and halted within 3 months of initiation.
3. Colon cancer surveillance by colonoscopy is necessary in patients with disease for greater than 10 years extending beyond the rectum.
4. Emotional support required, but psychiatric consultation indicated only for major psychiatric diagnosis.

B | Bibliography

Korelitz BI: Inflammatory bowel disease and pregnancy. Gastroenterol Clin North Am 1998;27:213–224.
Kornbluth A, Sachar DB: Ulcerative colitis practice guidelines in adults. Am J Gastroenterol 1997;92:204–211.
Robinson M: Optimizing therapy for inflammatory bowel disease. Am J Gastroenterol 1997;92:12S–17S.

$\mathbf{91}$ Irritable Bowel Syndrome

Fred M. Sutton, Jr.

Etiology

1. Definition: Irritable bowel syndrome (IBS) is a functional gastrointestinal disorder attributed to the intestines and associated with symptoms of pain and altered defecation and/or symptoms of bloatedness and distention.

2. Epidemiology: Studies from Western countries indicate that 15 to 20 per cent of patients suffer from IBS and most do not seek medical attention for their symptoms. In Western countries, 75 per cent of patients with IBS seen by a physician are female. In countries such as India and Sri Lanka, male patients predominate.

3. Pathophysiology: Certain motility and sensory abnormalities are found in patients with IBS as a group, and these distinguish them from healthy individuals.

    a. Various stimuli, including stress, meals, and peptides, alter colonic or small intestinal motor response.

    b. It is presumed that pain symptoms in patients with IBS are due to hyperactivity.

    c. These patients also have reduced sensory thresholds for stimuli such as rectal and ileal distention.

    d. Evidence that balloon distention at certain points in the small and large intestine reproduces pain confirms the gut as the site of the symptom.

Symptoms

Criteria for IBS include continuous or recurrent symptoms for at least 3 months.

1. Abdominal pain or discomfort relieved by defecation or associated with a change in the frequency or consistency of stool, *and/or*

2. An irregular pattern of defecation at least 25 per cent of the time—three or more of the following:

    a. Altered stool frequency

    b. Altered stool form: hard or loose, watery stool

    c. Altered stool passage: straining or urgency, feeling of incomplete evacuation

    d. Passage of mucus

    e. Bloating or feeling of abdominal distention

Key Symptoms

- Alternating diarrhea and constipation
- Abdominal pain relieved by defecation
- Abdominal bloating
- Passage of mucus

Clinical Findings

1. The physical examination in most patients with IBS is generally normal.

2. Physical examination may reveal tenderness in the area of the colon in patients with the spastic colon variety of IBS. In patients with small bowel involvement, pressure over the umbilicus or epigastrium may precipitate symptoms.

3. Most patients with IBS are between the ages of 20 and 50.

4. Patients with IBS commonly have a past history of multiple illnesses, such as allergies, headache, kidney disease, joint symptoms, and, in women, dyspareunia.

Key Sign

Normal physical examination findings

Laboratory Test

1. Laboratory studies are generally normal in IBS. The diagnosis should be suspected based on the patient's symptoms and by excluding organic diseases. There are no definitive tests for a diagnosis of IBS.

2. A minimal evaluation would consist of a complete blood count and erythrocyte sedimentation rate (ESR).

3. If diarrhea is a predominant symptom, stool samples for leukocytes, culture for enteric pathogens, and examination for ova and parasites should be pursued.

4. A urinalysis should be obtained because urinary tract symptoms can mimic functional gastrointestinal disease.

5. Sigmoidoscopy offers little diagnostic information unless there is suspicion of inflammatory bowel disease. In patients with IBS, air insufflation during sigmoidoscopy often reproduces their symptoms.

6. Roentgenographic studies of the small bowel or colon are generally not indicated with typical IBS symptoms. If the patient has had symptoms for more than 3 months or is over age 45, a barium enema or colonoscopy should be performed.

Key Tests

- Normal complete blood count
- Normal ESR
- Stool negative for leukocytes, blood
- Pain reproduced by sigmoidoscopy

Differential Diagnosis

1. Malignancies such as colon cancer; inflammatory diseases such as Crohn's disease or ulcerative colitis; infectious diseases such as infectious colitis, diverticulitis, and parasitosis; and ischemic diseases of the gastrointestinal tract

2. Diarrhea as the predominant symptom may be due to lactase deficiency, laxative abuse, malabsorption, and hyperthyroidism.

3. Constipation as the predominant symptom may be due to hypercalcemia, hypothyroidism, and medication side effects.

4. Epigastric and periumbilical pain may be due to peptic, biliary, gastric, or pancreatic disease.

Treatment

The key to successful management of IBS is a positive diagnosis, which depends on identifying certain symptom patterns.

1. Constipation predominant
   a. Review dietary history
   b. Therapeutic trial
      (1) Increase fiber: Start with 1 tablespoon psyllium per day or twice a day. Alternatives include polycarbophil or methylcellulose.
      (2) Osmotic laxative
      (3) Stool softener
      (4) Prokinetic agents: trial of cisapride (Propulsid), 20 mg twice daily
2. Diarrhea predominant

a. Review dietary history. Eliminate sorbitol products; consider lactose intolerance.
b. Consider lactose histamine$_2$ breath test.
c. Therapeutic trial
   (1) Loperamide (Imodium), 2 to 4 mg every 6 to 8 hours
   (2) Diphenoxylate (Lomotil), 2.5 to 5 mg every 4 to 6 hours
d. Fiber
3. Pain/gas/bloating predominate
   a. Review diet history.
   b. Plain abdominal radiography
   c. Therapeutic trial
      (1) Anticholinergics: dicyclomine (Bentyl), 10 to 20 mg 30 to 45 minutes before meals four times a day; hyoscyamine
      (2) Antidepressants: amitriptyline HCl (Elavil), or doxepin (Sinequan), starting with 25 to 50 mg hs and gradually increased to 75 to 150 mg hs as tolerated. Fluoxetine (Prozac), 20 mg as single daytime dose, is less sedating.
      (3) Prokinetic agents: cisapride, 10 to 20 mg daily
      (4) Psychiatric intervention employing biofeedback, psychotherapy, or hypnosis is an alternative for patients with IBS refractory to standard therapeutic measures.

Diet

1. If certain products such as lactose, caffeine, fatty foods, alcohol, sorbitol, or beans are associated with symptoms, they can be eliminated to see if symptoms abate.

2. Fiber results in improvement of constipation and abdominal pain.

Activity

Low physical activity has been reported as an association with constipation.

Patient Education

1. A positive physician-patient interaction is associated with a reduced number of return visits for IBS-related symptoms.

2. Certain acute situations seem to precipitate attacks of IBS. These include acute illnesses, severe financial demand, loss of a job, a serious family crisis, or death of a close friend or relative.

3. Many patients with IBS come from families in which other members have the syndrome, suggesting that symptoms may be a learned behavior.

4. It is usually helpful to explain that IBS is a real disorder in which the intestine is overly sensitive to various stimuli such as food, hormonal changes (menses), and stress.

5. Make the patient aware that, although chronic, the symptoms do not indicate serious illness, require surgery, or shorten life expectancy.

6. Setting realistic goals is extremely important.

7. The patient needs to concentrate on functioning as normally as possible and not on eliminating all symptoms.

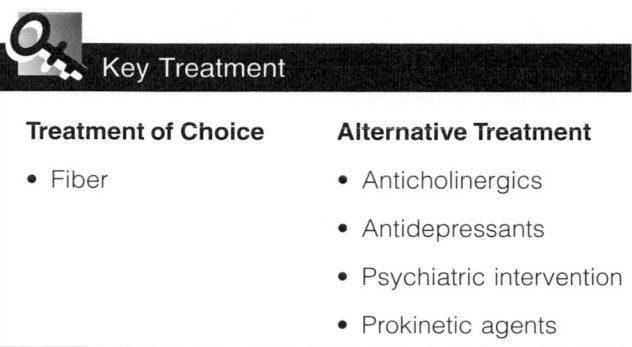

Key Treatment

Treatment of Choice	Alternative Treatment
• Fiber	• Anticholinergics
	• Antidepressants
	• Psychiatric intervention
	• Prokinetic agents

Follow-Up

1. Prevention
   a. High-fiber diet and prophylactic use of medications
   b. Regular exercise

c. Avoid products that aggravate symptoms.

2. Monitoring
   a. Periodic evaluation for a change in symptoms, particularly diarrhea
   b. Regular physician visits early in treatment to reassure the patient

3. Prognosis
   a. A diagnosis of IBS persists over time, and most patients continue to have symptoms several years following the initial diagnosis.
   b. Up to 30 per cent of patients with IBS resort to alternative medicine.
   c. IBS does not predispose one to more serious diseases or shorten one's life expectancy.

Bibliography

AGA Medical Position Statement: Irritable bowel syndrome. Gastroenterology 1997;112:2118–2119.

Brannan DP, Drossman DA: Toward a new understanding of irritable bowel syndrome. Contemp Intern Med 1991;9:73–91.

Camilleri M, Prather CM: The irritable bowel syndrome: mechanisms and a practical approach to management. Ann Intern Med 1992;116:1001–1008.

Drossman DA, Thompson WG: The irritable bowel syndrome: review and a graduated multicomponent treatment approach. Ann Intern Med 1992;116:1009–1016.

Owens DM, Nelson DK, Talley NJ: The irritable bowel syndrome: long-term prognosis and the physician-patient interaction. Ann Intern Med 1995;122:107–112.

92 Diverticulitis

Michael Jon Brooks

Etiology

1. Pre-existing diverticulosis
   a. Diverticulosis is a herniation of mucosa through the muscular wall of the colon, typically located where nutrient arteries penetrate the muscularis propria (Fig. 92–1).
   b. Diverticulosis develops secondary to increased intraluminal pressures that likely results from insufficient intake of dietary fiber.
2. Microperforation and inflammation of a diverticulum

Symptoms

1. Abdominal pain
   a. Constant in nature
   b. Typically left lower quadrant (LLQ) in location but may be diffuse.
2. Fever
3. Altered bowel habits
   a. Constipation most often
   b. Diarrhea in some cases
4. Nausea/vomiting
   a. Mechanical causes
      (1) Localized edema/inflammation-induced obstruction
      (2) Abscess causing obstruction
      (3) Spasm
   b. Systemic causes
      (1) Sepsis
      (2) Electrolyte abnormalities
5. Malaise
6. Urinary complaints
   a. Dysuria/frequency; secondary to adjacent bladder inflammation
   b. Pneumaturia; secondary to colovesical fistula

Key Symptoms

- Constant abdominal pain, LLQ or diffuse
- Fever
- Altered bowel habits
- Nausea and vomiting
- Malaise

Clinical Findings

1. Mild/moderate abdominal tenderness (common); more often localized to LLQ
2. Severe abdominal tenderness: "acute abdomen" (uncommon)
   a. Caused by diffuse peritonitis
   b. Abdominal guarding and rebound often present.
   c. May represent frank perforation.
   d. Surgical emergency
3. Temperature over 38° C (100.4° F)
4. Abnormal bowel sounds
   a. Usually hypoactive
   b. May be high-pitched/tinkling with impending or early intestinal obstruction.
   c. May be absent (ileus) with complete obstruction or frank perforation.
5. Guaiac-positive stools
   a. Commonly seen
   b. Frank bleeding is rare.
6. Leukocytosis (>12,000 μl) with "left shift"
7. Abdominal mass: may be palpated in the presence of significant abscess or inflammation.

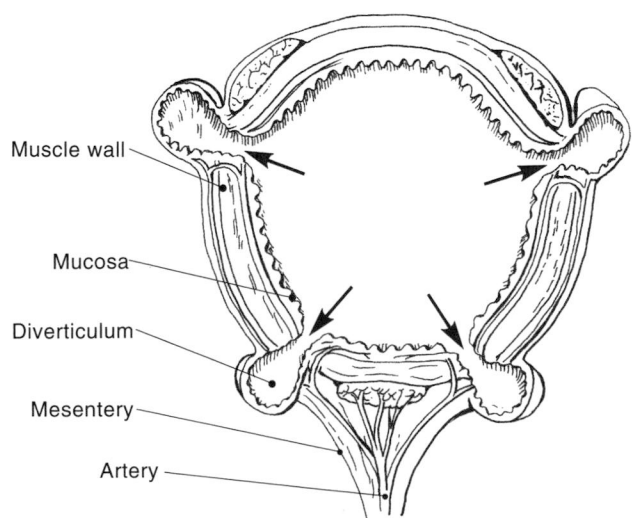

Figure 92–1 Schematic cross section of the colonic wall showing sites of formation of diverticula at points of the vasa recta.

Muscle wall
Mucosa
Diverticulum
Mesentery
Artery

Key Signs

- Abdominal tenderness (LLQ usually; ±rebound)
- Temperature >38° C (100.4° F)
- Hypoactive bowel sounds
- Guaiac-positive stools
- Abdominal mass (palpable abscess/inflammation
- Leukocytosis

Laboratory Tests

1. Complete blood count with differential: Generally reveals leukocytosis with left shift.
2. Plain films of abdomen
   a. Signs of obstruction
      (1) Distended bowel loops with abrupt end
      (2) Air-fluid interfaces
   b. Signs of perforated viscus (rare); free air under diaphragm
   c. Ileus (common)
   d. Extracolonic gas pattern suggestive of pericolic abscess.
3. Computerized tomography (CT) scan of abdomen and pelvis
   a. Diagnostic test of choice in most institutions
   b. Very sensitive for delineation of diverticular pericolic abscess versus nondiverticular causes of abdominal symptomatology
4. Barium enema (BE) with water-soluble contrast material
   a. Safe and effective to diagnose diverticulitis
   b. Yields less information concerning extracolonic pathology.
5. Abdominal ultrasonography
   a. Noninvasive, safe; may be technically difficult to perform.
   b. Usually provides less information than CT or BE.
6. Endoscopy: Role is limited in acute diverticulitis.

7. Urinalysis: Presence of pyuria or hematuria may signify colovesical fistula.
8. Erythrocyte sedimentation rate: almost always elevated

Key Tests

- CT scan of abdomen + pelvis or BE (single contrast) with water-soluble contrast material
- Complete blood count with differential
- Abdominal radiographs

Differential Diagnosis

1. Intestinal ischemia
   a. Usually in patient with diffuse arteriosclerotic vascular disease
   b. Most consistent finding is pain out of proportion to examination.
2. Cancer of colon: Frequently diagnosed with endoscopic biopsy after resolution of acute abdominal process.
3. Intestinal obstruction
4. Appendicitis
5. Pyelonephritis
6. Inflammatory bowel disease
7. Tubo-ovarian abscess: seen in younger, sexually active women
8. Sigmoid volvulus
9. Pancreatitis: Elevated amylase and lipase should be noted.

Treatment

1. Hospitalization: required in a majority of patients
2. Surgical evaluation: Should be obtained early in hospital course.
3. Outpatient therapy is effective in selected patients
   a. Mild abdominal pain/tenderness
   b. Tolerates liquid diet, no evidence of obstruction
   c. Low-grade fever/mild leukocytosis (<12,000/μl)
   d. Failure to improve after 24 to 36 hours indicates need for inpatient treatment.
4. Nasogastric intubation for decompression if distention develops

Medication

1. Amoxicillin–clavulanate potassium (Augmentin), 875/125-mg tablet q12h for 2 weeks, or ciprofloxacin (Cipro), 500 mg bid, plus metronidazole (Flagyl), 500 mg tid

2. Broad-spectrum parenteral antibiotics in more severe cases

   a. Ampicillin + aminoglycoside + metronidazole

   b. Ampicillin-sulbactam (Unasyn)

   c. Ticarcillin-clavulanate (Timentin)

   d. Imipenem-cilastatin (Primaxin)

3. Intravenous (IV) hydration

4. Analgesics

Diet

1. Liquid diet during treatment of mild/outpatient cases

2. Nothing by mouth (NPO)/bowel rest in hospitalized patients with acute disease

3. Initial low residue diet with stool softener after resolution of acute inflammation

4. Gradual increase of dietary fiber to achieve 25 to 35 gm/day

Patient Education

1. Maintenance of adequate dietary fiber intake after recovery is essential (25 to 35 gm/day).

   a. High-fiber cereals

   b. Fresh fruits/vegetables

   c. Legumes

2. Adequate fluid intake in association with dietary fiber is important to prevent constipation and bloating.

3. Low dietary fat intake is also prudent.

Key Treatment

- Hospitalization in majority of patients

- NPO/bowel rest

- IV hydration

- Parenteral broad-spectrum antibiotics

- Surgical evaluation (or intervention if indicated)

- Outpatient therapy with liquids and oral antibiotics in mild cases

Follow-Up

1. Colonoscopy approximately 1 month after recovery to evaluate extent of disease and/or associated conditions.

   a. Rule out malignancy.

   b. Rule out stricture.

2. Alternatively, BE or CT with rectal contrast may be used in follow-up evaluation.

3. Recurrent attacks are common (up to 30 per cent).

   a. Patient awareness of presenting signs and symptoms is essential.

   b. Surgical resection of diseased segment may become necessary to prevent recurrence.

Bibliography

Ferzoco LB, Raptopoulos V, Silen W: Acute diverticulitis. N Engl J Med 1998;338:1521–1526.

Freeman SR, McNally PR: Diverticulitis. Med Clin North Am 1993;77:1149–1167.

Jones DJ: ABC of colorectal disease and diverticular disease. Br Med J 1992;304:1435–1437.

Rothenberger DA, Wiltz O: Surgery for complicated diverticulitis. Surg Clin North Am 1993;73:975–990.

Schoetz JD: Uncomplicated diverticulitis: indications for surgery and surgical management. Surg Clin North Am 1993;73:965–974.

93 Hemorrhoids

Mark H. Belfer

Hemorrhoids are anal "cushions" consisting of redundant rectal mucosa, venous and arterial plexuses, smooth muscle, and connective tissue in the submucosa of the anal canal. These are not just "varicose veins," although venous drainage from hemorrhoids is into the portal venous system. Three quarters of all patients have hemorrhoids at some time during their life, most after age 50. They occur in almost one third of pregnant patients but otherwise are uncommon under age 25. Hemorrhoids are a source of considerable pain and suffering, but usually symptoms will respond to conservative medical therapy.

Etiology

1. Shearing force caused by defecation of a large stool
2. Constipation and straining at defecation; diarrhea may also cause hemorrhoids.
3. A familial tendency has been noted for predisposition to hemorrhoidal development.
4. Some believe portal venous hypertension from congestive heart failure, pelvic neoplastic disease, or pregnancy may increase the likelihood of hemorrhoid formation.

Symptoms

1. Rectal bleeding (occasionally associated with pain) is usually bright red and intermittent; hemorrhoids are probably the number one cause of lower gastrointestinal bleeding.

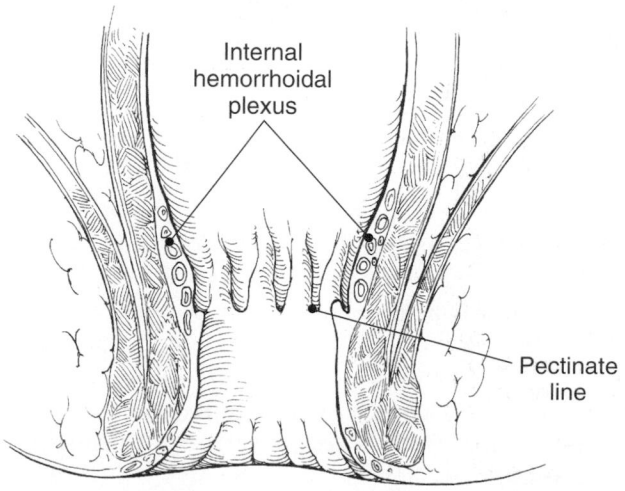

Figure 93–1 Hemorrhoidal veins above the pectinate line.

2. Internal hemorrhoids are painless unless they extend distal to the pectinate (dentate) line or strangulation occurs in a prolapsed internal hemorrhoid.
3. Sensation of "fullness" in anal canal
4. External hemorrhoids may be painful, especially if thrombosed.
5. Palpable mass protruding from anus
6. Pruritis or burning sensation in the perianal area
7. Fecal soilage and mucus accumulation
8. Pain during and after defecation

Key Symptoms

- Rectal bleeding, usually painless
- Fecal soilage
- Anal pruritis
- Palpable lump in perianal area that may or may not be painful

Clinical Findings

1. Internal hemorrhoids ("piles" or anal cushions) are located at and just proximal to the pectinate line (a circumferential row of glands approximately 1 in proximal to the anal verge). The rectal mucosa is insensitive to pain and is composed of glandular epithelium (Fig. 93–1). External hemorrhoids are located at the anal verge, distal to the pectinate line. The tissue is sensitive to pain and is composed of squamous epithelium (perianal skin). External hemorrhoids are usually painless and soft and may be blue in color if thrombosed.
2. Thrombosis occasionally occurs in external hemorrhoids, causing significant pain. Patients usually complain of a painful lump in the perianal area. If thrombosis occurs in internal hemorrhoids, pain also may be severe.
3. External and internal hemorrhoids are usually located at the right anterior, right posterior, and left lateral quadrants of the anal canal.
4. Internal hemorrhoidal classification (Fig. 93–2)

a. Grade I: A swollen, bulky anal cushion protrudes into the lumen of the anal canal but does not prolapse below the pectinate line.

b. Grade II: A medium-sized anal cushion drops below the pectinate line with straining (e.g., with defecation) but disappears spontaneously after straining.

c. Grade III: Prolapse of a larger sized anal cushion is noted upon straining and must be manually replaced to disappear.

d. Grade IV: Irreducible prolapse of a larger sized anal cushion outside the anus.

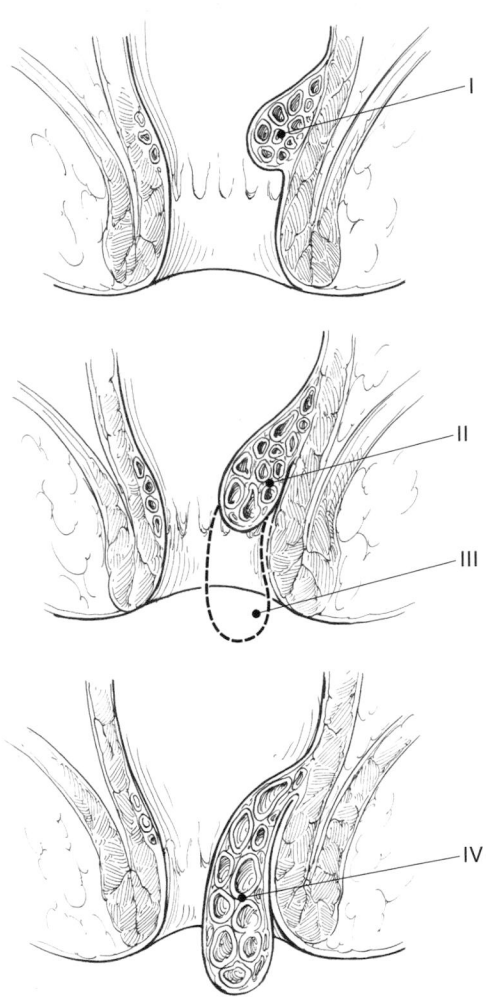

Figure 93–2 Primary hemorrhoidal groups.

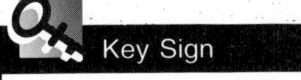

Hemorrhoids are noted within the anal canal or prolapsed outside of the anus

Tests

1. Anoscopy and a digital rectal examination should always be performed.

2. Flexible sigmoidoscopy should ideally be done to evaluate for other pathology in the distal colon, especially if symptom onset is new or if the patient is over age 50. Consider colonoscopy if bleeding is significant.

3. Coagulation testing (e.g., partial thromboplastin time and prothrombin time) should be obtained if surgical therapy is contemplated or if bleeding is significant.

Key Tests

- Anoscopy
- Digital rectal examination
- Sigmoidoscopic examination

Differential Diagnosis

1. Inflammatory bowel disease with proctitis
2. Rectal neoplasia (i.e., polyps or anal carcinoma)
3. Anal fissures
4. Anal fistula
5. Perianal abscess
6. Anal skin tags
7. Prolapse of rectal mucosa, especially in elderly

Treatment

1. For *external hemorrhoids* or *grade I hemorrhoids*: analgesic ointment; stool softeners (e.g., Colace or Surfak); bulk-forming agents; acetaminophen or ibuprofen for analgesia

2. Several options may be utilized for treatment of *grades II and III internal hemorrhoids*.

   a. Rubber band ligation (banding) is very effective 70 to 90 per cent of time for grades II and II because it decreases the bulk of the hemorrhoidal plexus more effectively.

   b. Injection sclerotherapy (submucosally above the dentate line; not intraluminal) is effective for grades II and III.

   c. Infrared photocoagulation is effective in grades I and II, occasionally in grade III.

   d. Bipolar diathermy (above the pectinate line) has been shown to be effective.

   e. Laser therapy with CO_2 laser for grades I, II, and III hemorrhoids is effective therapy, but expensive and not considered superior to other methods.

   f. Cryotherapy is no longer recommended because of untoward side effects (e.g., anal discharge).

3. *Grade IV hemorrhoids*: For the 10 per cent of

patients with grade IV disease, surgical three-quadrant hemorrhoidectomy may be necessary. Surgery should be reserved for grade IV hemorrhoids or for those patients with grade III disease who have failed more conservative treatment. This requires general or spinal anesthesia.

4. For *thrombosed external hemorrhoids*, either surgical evacuation of the clot within the hemorrhoid or complete excision of the hemorrhoid may be undertaken in the office.

Medication

1. Psyllium supplementation (bulk-forming agents, e.g., Metamucil) and stool softeners.

2. Laxatives may be required for severe constipation.

3. Topical preparations for local inflammation and itching (hydrocortisone-containing preparations [e.g., Proctofoam-HC] used two to three times daily). Avoid suppositories because they are not considered effective. Avoid using cortisone-containing preparations for more than 2 weeks to avoid anal tissue atrophy.

4. Anesthetic creams and ointments used externally for pain may be useful (e.g., lidocaine 2.5% to 5% ointment applied three times daily).

5. Systemic analgesics may be necessary for painful, thrombosed hemorrhoids, although one must take care not to *cause* constipation through use of narcotic analgesics.

6. Consider subacute bacterial endocarditis prophylaxis on an individualized basis.

Diet

A high-fiber diet with increased fluid consumption is advisable.

Activity

Bed rest may be necessary, especially after nonconservative (e.g., surgical) treatment measures.

Patient Education

1. Avoid direct pressure. If sitting is necessary (e.g., at work), consider a donut-shaped pillow or ring. Avoid prolonged sitting on the toilet or straining at stool to prevent recurrences of hemorrhoids.

2. Warm sitz baths three to four times daily.

3. There is no convincing evidence for the efficacy of Preparation H at this time.

Key Treatment

- Stool softeners

- Topical analgesic and anti-inflammatory creams or ointments

- Moist heat

- High-fiber diet

- Rubber band ligation, infrared photocoagulation, sclerotherapy, laser therapy, and surgical management reserved for patients where conservative treatment failed.

Bibliography

Barnett JL, Raper SE: Hemorrhoids. In Yamada T (ed): Textbook of Gastroenterology, 2nd ed, vol 2, pp 2029–2032. Philadelphia, JB Lippincott Company, 1995.

Janicke DM, Pundt MR: Anorectal disorders. Emerg Med Clin North Am 1996;14:757–788.

MacRae HM, McLeod RS: Comparison of hemorrhoidal treatments: a meta-analysis. Can J Surg 1997;40:14–17.

Pfenninger JL, Surrell J: Nonsurgical treatment options for internal hemorrhoids. Am Fam Physician 1995;52:821–834.

Salvati EP, Eisenstat TE: Hemorrhoidal disease. In Zuidema GD (ed): Shackelford's Surgery of the Alimentary Tract, 4th ed, vol 4, pp 330–343. Philadelphia, WB Saunders Company, 1996.

Sclerotherapy

Indications

Sclerotherapy has come and gone in the medical armamentarium. Because of variable outcomes and the availability of more definitive therapy, management of internal hemorrhoids by sclerotherapy should be limited to grade I and grade II (occasionally grade III) hemorrhoidal masses.

Contraindications

1. Allergy to the sclerosant solutions
2. Coagulopathy or any medical condition that would contraindicate intervention

Technique: Sclerotherapy

1. The patient assumes either a jackknife or a left lateral Sims' position. The discomfort of sclerotherapy is primarily secondary to the introduction of the anoscope required for visualization and tissue manipulation. Most intraoperative discomfort can be alleviated by the topical application of lidocaine (Xylocaine) jelly to the anal tissues and the anoscope.

2. The anoscope (I prefer a Fansler or Fansler-Ives anoscope) is inserted, and the hemorrhoid to be treated is selected.

3. Sclerosis is achieved by the submucosal injection of a sclerosing solution of quinine and urea hydrochloride or 5 per cent phenol in peanut oil using a 30-gauge needle proximally at three sites. Injection of approximately 0.2 to 1.5 ml is usually sufficient for each hemorrhoid. Total sclerosant volume injected when using solutions containing quinine should not exceed 3.0 ml.

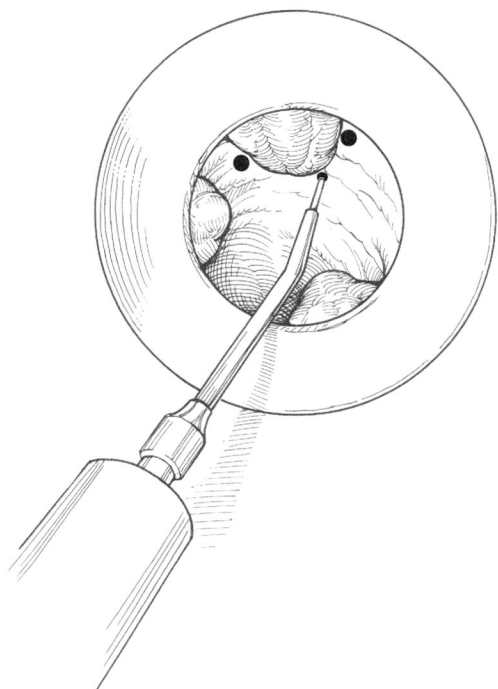

4. It is crucial that sclerosing injections be placed submucosally adjacent to the hemorrhoid to be treated and that they not be injected intravascularly.

 Key Points

- Primarily indicated for grade I and grade II hemorrhoids

- Occasionally indicated for grade III hemorrhoids

- Inject with 30-gauge needle.

- Inject sclerosant submucosally, not intravascularly.

- Inject only one hemorrhoid at each visit.

- Space successive treatments 3 to 4 weeks apart.

Complications

1. Long-term success with sclerotherapy is variable because recanalization may occur after a brief interval.
2. The procedure may be uncomfortable, and allergic reactions to sclerosing materials are not uncommon.
3. Sloughing, burning, and thrombosis are among the most common complications reported.

Postoperative Instructions

1. The patient is advised to use stool softeners (fiber and/or surface tension–decreasing agents) temporarily and is instructed in dietary and toilet habit modification.
2. Significant bleeding, fever, and unusual pain are to be immediately reported to the physician.

Infrared Coagulation

This technique, accomplished above the dentate line, requires no anesthesia. It uses an instrument that generates infrared energy with a halogen light source. The radiant energy produced is conducted to the surgical site by means of a quartz rod. The heat produced "spot welds" the mucosa to the muscularis in the tissues adjacent to the internal hemorrhoidal plexus, causing obliteration of the hemorrhoidal vein complex. Following the use of the infrared coagulator, the overlying redundant mucosal tissue shrinks because it is no longer being distracted and distended by the underlying bulging hemorrhoidal vein system. The infrared coagulation technique does not produce slough of tissue, bleeding, or stenosis.

Indications

Infrared coagulation therapy is appropriate for grades I, II, and III hemorrhoids.

Contraindications

Coagulopathy or any medical condition that would contraindicate surgical intervention

Technique: Infrared Coagulation

1. The patient assumes the left lateral Sims' or jackknife position.
2. The anal canal is lubricated with Xylocaine jelly, as is the Fansler of Fansler-Ives anoscope, which is inserted to permit visualization of the hemorrhoid to be treated.
3. The infrared coagulator is set for 1.0 to 1.5 seconds.
4. The tip of the coagulator is lightly pressed against the tissues just proximal to the hemorrhoid.

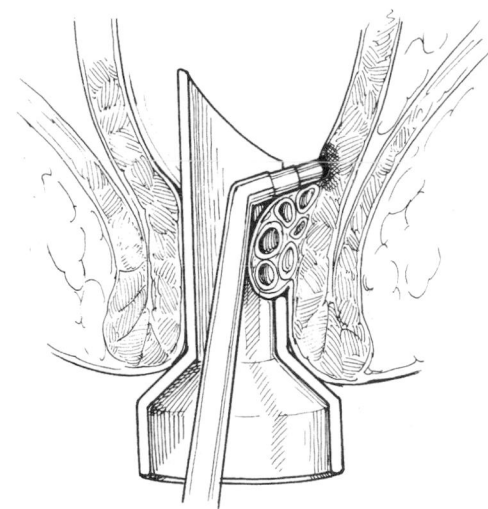

5. The coagulator is energized.
6. Repeat the process five to seven times in the area above the hemorrhoid, leaving a 2-mm untreated tissue bridge between treatment sites. Only one hemorrhoid is treated at each session.

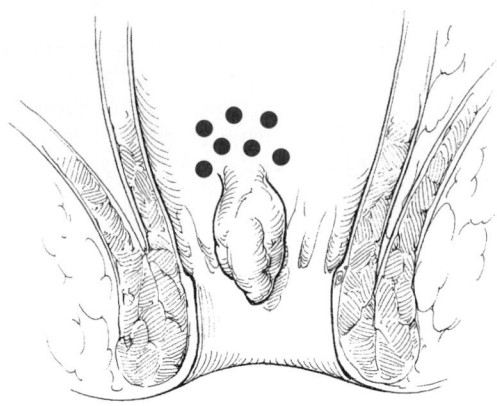

• Place all IRC "welds" above dentate line.

• Place all IRC "welds" just above the hemorrhoid in diamond or triangle pattern.

• Leave 2 to 3 mm untreated tissue between "welds."

• Treat only one hemorrhoid at each visit.

• Space successive treatments every 10 to 14 days.

7. Successive treatments may be undertaken, one hemorrhoid at a time, every 10 to 14 days.

Key Points

• Indicated for grades I, II, and III hemorrhoids

• The most common inspiratory reserve capacity (IRC) setting is 1.5 seconds.

Complications

Rare postoperative pain and bleeding have been reported.

Postoperative Instructions

1. The patient is advised to use stool softeners (fiber and/or surface tension–decreasing agents) temporarily and is instructed in dietary and toilet habit modification.

2. Significant bleeding, fever, and unusual pain are to be immediately reported to the physician.

Banding Ligation

1. Rubber ring banding ligation is a procedure that ablates the internal hemorrhoidal mass through the application of a constricting rubber ring, which is intended to produce ischemia and painless sloughing of the hemorrhoid in 7 to 10 days. Banding should be performed on only one hemorrhoidal mass at a time. If more than one hemorrhoid is to be banded, at least 14 to 21 days should intervene between the banding procedures. Because banding is intended to be done on lesions that lie above the pectinate line, anesthesia is not required for this procedure. However, if tissues below the pectinate line are included in the rubber band ligature, severe pain will be instantly produced.

2. Banding, if properly performed, is at worst uncomfortable. Most complaints are referable to the introduction of the anoscope required for visualization and tissue manipulation. Most intraoperative discomfort is alleviated by the topical application of Xylocaine jelly to the anal tissues and the anoscope.

Indications

Banding is appropriate for grades II and III and some grade IV internal hemorrhoids.

Contraindications

Coagulopathy and certain medical conditions would contraindicate surgical intervention.

Technique: Banding Ligation

1. The patient assumes either a jackknife or left lateral Sims' position.

2. The Fansler or Fansler-Ives anoscope is inserted, and the hemorrhoid to be treated is selected. The hemorrhoidal banding instrument is "loaded" with two rubber rings.

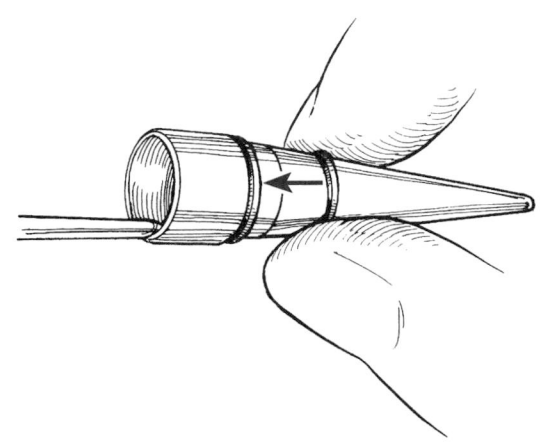

3. An alligator forceps is inserted through the banding instrument, and the hemorrhoid is grasped and placed under tension.

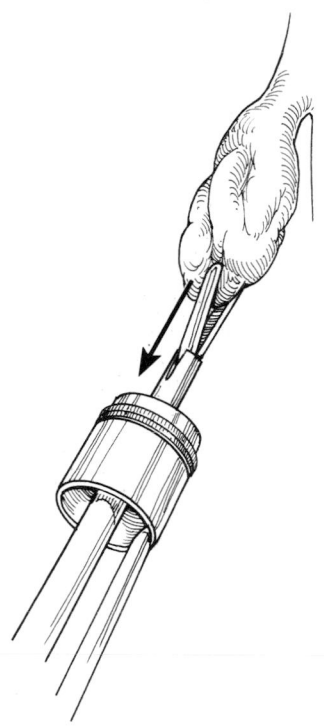

4. The banding instrument is advanced to the base of the hemorrhoid and the two rubber ring ligatures are simultaneously placed. Care must be taken to grasp and band the hemorrhoid above the dentate line or pain will be produced.

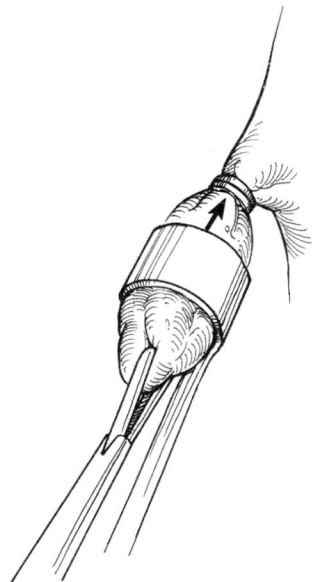

5. Only one hemorrhoid is banded at each visit. Patients who have more than one hemorrhoid will require multiple banding visits that should be spaced about 3 to 4 weeks apart.

Key Points

- Most useful for grade II and grade III hemorrhoids.

- May be occasionally used for grade IV hemorrhoids.

- Place all bands above the dentate line.

- Place two bands on each hemorrhoid.

- Treat only one hemorrhoid at each visit.

- Space successive treatments at 3- to 4-week intervals.

Complications

1. Common complications of the banding technique most frequently reported include ulceration, slipping or breaking of the rubber ring ligature, and pain.

2. Rarely, brisk bleeding that may require surgical intervention to establish hemostasis occurs at the time of slough.

3. Patients who have not undergone anticoagulation or have known coagulopathies may be at higher risk if they experience any postoperative bleeding.

Postoperative Instructions

1. The patient is advised to use stool softeners (fiber and/or surface tension–decreasing agents) temporarily and is instructed in dietary and toilet habit modification.

2. Significant bleeding, fever, and unusual pain are to be immediately reported to the physician.

 Bibliography

American Society for Colon and Rectal Surgeons, Standards Task Force: Practice parameters for anorectal surgery. Dis Colon Rectum 1991;34:285.

Corman M: Colon and Rectal Surgery, 3rd ed. Philadelphia, JB Lippincott Company, 1993.

Dodi G, Pirone E: Sclerotherapy and elastic ligation of hemorrhoids. Ann Ital Chir 1995;66:769.

MacRae HM, McLeod RS: Comparison of hemorrhoid treatments: a meta-analysis. Can J Surg 1997;40:14–17.

Polglase AL: Hemorrhoids: a clinical update. Med J Aust 1997;167:85.

94 Fecal Impaction

Aubrey L. Knight

Etiology

1. Definition: a large, firm, immovable mass of stool in the colon resulting from incomplete evacuation of feces. The impaction is usually found in the rectum but can occur in the more proximal segments of the colon.

2. Epidemiology: The elderly are at particular risk as a result of several physiologic changes that occur with aging.

   a. The total colonic transit time in elderly individuals with constipation has been shown to be prolonged.

   b. There is a decline in internal sphincter tone and external sphincter and pelvic muscle strength with aging.

   c. Subsets of elderly persons with a history of constipation or fecal impaction may have increased or decreased rectal tone. Those with increased rectal tone tend to have difficult, painful passage of hard fecal pellets. Similar rectal physiology is evident in irritable bowel syndrome. Those with decreased rectal tone require a higher volume of rectal distention to achieve sphincter relaxation and may be asymptomatic.

3. Risk factors

   a. Institutionalized elderly: This occurrence is sometimes referred to as the "terminal reservoir syndrome" and is primarily the result of immobility and a failure to respond appropriately to the urge to defecate. The gastrocolic reflex requires physical activity for its initiation.

   b. Depression

   c. Hypothyroidism

   d. Localized or generalized neurologic disorders

   e. Individuals with painful rectal conditions such as anal fissures and hemorrhoids

   f. Diet lacking in fiber or in fluids

   g. Hypokalemia and hypercalcemia

   h. Medications, such as stimulant laxatives, opiates, iron, aluminum-containing antacids, psychoactive substances, and drugs with anticholinergic potential

   i. Infants with congenital bowel obstruction caused by stenosis, atresia, or Hirschsprung's disease

Symptoms

1. The major symptoms of fecal impaction are abdominal pain and distention; the pain is frequently postprandial.

2. Paradoxically, a predominant symptom may be fecal incontinence. This is frequently misinterpreted and mistreated as diarrhea, which can worsen the problem.

3. Other symptoms include nausea, vomiting, anorexia, headache, confusion, urinary frequency and incontinence, and tenesmus.

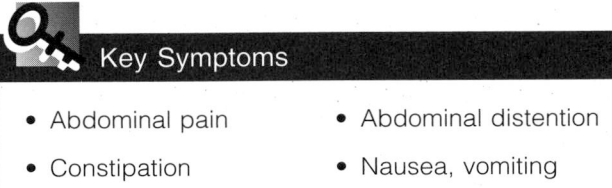

Key Symptoms

- Abdominal pain
- Abdominal distention
- Constipation
- Nausea, vomiting
- Fecal incontinence
- Confusion

Clinical Findings

1. On physical examination, one might expect to see a low-grade fever, tachycardia and tachypnea, and elevated blood pressure.

2. There may be signs of dehydration and weight loss.

3. A mass of stool may be palpable in the left lower quadrant or rectal vault.

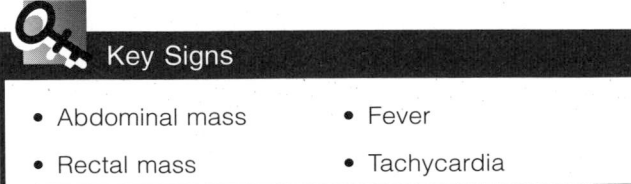

Key Signs

- Abdominal mass
- Fever
- Rectal mass
- Tachycardia

Laboratory Tests

1. The diagnosis can usually be made by careful history and physical examination. There are no specific laboratory tests, but the white blood

cell count may be elevated; there may be hypokalemia and laboratory values consistent with dehydration.

2. The stool may be positive for occult blood.

3. Plain abdominal films will identify the stool or signs of obstruction when the physical examination is unrevealing. Barium enema or sigmoidoscopy may identify rectosigmoid masses that are contributory.

Key Test

Plain abdominal radiographs

Differential Diagnosis

1. Irritable bowel syndrome
2. Carcinoma of the colon
3. Inflammatory colonic conditions

Treatment

1. Treatment of established fecal impaction involves first clearing the bowels with gentle manual fragmentation and removal of the fecal mass.

2. Enemas and suppositories may be of additional value in clearing the bowels.

3. Proximal masses may be fragmented with a water jet directed through a flexible sigmoidoscope.

4. Rarely, laparotomy is necessary.

Medications

1. There is no drug of choice for the acute treatment of fecal impaction.

2. When gentle digital evacuation is not completely successful, bisacodyl suppositories or enemas with mineral oil, tap water, or sodium phosphate may be of value. Soap suds enemas should be avoided in this situation because they may produce mucosal damage.

3. Poorly absorbed isosmotic solutions (GoLYTELY, Colyte) taken orally may be of further value.

Diet

1. Persons with fecal impaction should be maintained on a high-fiber diet.

2. A minimum intake of 1500 ml/day of fluid is recommended. This should be increased in summer.

Activity

Increased regular activity is an important aid in the initial therapy of fecal impaction and in the prevention of reimpaction.

Patient Education

1. Avoid irritant laxatives and hot water or soap enemas.

2. Establish a regular toilet time.

3. Recognize the importance of exercise, diet, and fluids.

4. Monitor bowel habits because reimpaction is likely.

Key Treatment

Treatment of Choice	Alternative Treatment
• Manual disimpaction	• Isosmotic fluids orally (GoLYTELY, Colyte)
• Bisacodyl suppository	
• Enemas	

Follow-Up

1. Prevention

   a. High-fiber diet, ± fiber supplements

   b. Adequate fluid intake

   c. Regular exercise

   d. Establish a regular toilet time and evoke the gastrocolic reflex, if necessary.

   e. Stool-softening agents (e.g., Colace), if needed.

   f. Periodic suppositories or enemas

2. Monitoring

   a. Periodic rectal examination

   b. Bowel movements less often than every second to third day signify the possibility of reimpaction.

3. Complications of fecal impactions include urinary tract infections, bowel obstruction, perforation, rectal bleeding, stercoral ulcers, volvulus, and weight loss. Rectovaginal fistulas have been described in elderly women and dystocia in pregnant women.

4. Prognosis

   a. Mortality is highest in the very old.

   b. Patients with a history of impaction have a higher likelihood of reimpaction. Following a bowel regimen becomes very important.

Bibliography

Hariri D, Gurwiz JH, Minaker KL: Constipation in the elderly. J Am Geriatr Soc 1993;41:1130–1140.

Norton RA: Gastrointestinal disorders in the aged. In Reichel W (ed): Care of the Elderly: Clinical Aspects of Aging, 4th ed, p 202. Baltimore, Williams & Wilkins, 1995.

Wald A: Constipation and fecal incontinence in the elderly. Gastroenterol Clin North Am 1990;19:405–418.

Williams ME: Complete Guide to Aging and Health, pp 356–357. New York, Harmony, 1995.

Wilson JAP, Rogers EL: Gastroenterologic disorders. In Cassel CK, Cohen EB, Meier DE, et al (eds): Geriatric Medicine, 3rd ed, pp 647–648. New York, Springer-Verlag, 1996.

95 Common Hepatobiliary Symptoms

Neonatal jaundice is very common, with a prevalence of about 60 to 80 per cent. In most healthy term neonates, it is benign and self-limited. Clinicians must differentiate physiologic from pathologic jaundice and prevent kernicterus. Higher bilirubin levels in breast-fed infants are usually due to infrequent or ineffective breast-feeding in the first week and breast milk jaundice beyond the second week. In either case, discontinuation of breast-feeding is rarely necessary.

Differential Diagnosis

Differentiate conjugated (direct) from unconjugated (indirect) hyperbilirubinemia (defined as >15 per cent direct bilirubin).

1. Early onset (first week of life)—unconjugated
   a. Physiologic jaundice: onset after 24 hours, peak at 3 to 5 days; aggravating factors include prematurity, maternal diabetes, Asian or Native American background, bruising/cephalhematoma, male sex.
   b. Starvation jaundice: infrequent/ineffective feedings
   c. Pathologic jaundice: onset often before 24 hours
      (1) Hemolysis: ABO or Rh incompatibility; hereditary spherocytosis
      (2) Sepsis
      (3) Hereditary defects in bilirubin conjugation: Crigler-Najjar syndrome, Gilbert's syndrome
      (4) Drugs that displace bilirubin from albumin
2. Early onset (first week of life)—conjugated
   a. Neonatal hepatitis: hepatitis A, B, or C; STORCH (syphilis, toxoplasmosis, rubella, cytomegalovirus, herpesvirus)
   b. Postasphyxia
   c. Congenital heart disease; congestive heart failure
   d. Drug-induced cholestasis

3. Late onset (beyond first week of life)—unconjugated
   a. Breast milk jaundice
   b. Pathologic jaundice
      (1) ABO incompatibility
      (2) Hypothyroidism
      (3) Glucose-6-phosphate dehydrogenase (G6PD) deficiency
      (4) Intestinal obstruction
4. Late onset—conjugated
   a. Biliary atresia
   b. Liver disease
   c. Extrahepatic obstruction
   d. α_1-Antitrypsin deficiency
   e. Inborn errors of metabolism: galactosemia, Gaucher's disease, glycogen storage disease
   f. Cystic fibrosis

Unconjugated hyperbilirubinemia in the neonate can be due to increased bilirubin production, decreased bilirubin delivery or uptake by the hepatocyte, decreased hepatic storage, decreased conjugation, or increased enterohepatic recirculation. Only *free* unconjugated bilirubin (i.e., not bound to albumin because of saturation of or displacement from binding sites) can cross the blood-brain barrier and cause kernicterus. Conjugated hyperbilirubinemia can be caused by extrahepatic obstruction or intrahepatic disturbances.

History: Key Questions to Ask
1. Infant history
   a. History of asphyxia or birth trauma?
   b. Prematurity or small for gestational age?
   c. Time of first feed; feeding frequency and efficacy
   d. If breast-fed, use of supplements—formula, water? Use of pacifiers?
   e. Passage of meconium and stooling frequency
   f. Color of stools; frequency and color of voids
   g. Was there bruising or cephalohematoma?

h. Blood type and Rh

i. Has baby received any medications?

2. Maternal history

a. Was there significant prenatal illness or infection?

b. Duration of labor and delivery

c. Was oxytocin used for augmentation or induction?

d. History of maternal diabetes?

e. Ethnic background (bilirubin usually higher in Asian babies; Asian or Mediterranean babies may have G6PD)

f. Family history of neonatal jaundice?

g. Medications used during labor?

In many otherwise healthy neonates, early-onset hyperbilirubinemia is due to reabsorption of unconjugated bilirubin via the enterohepatic circulation as a result of inadequate caloric intake. In breast-fed babies, maternal-infant separation, formula or water supplementation, and pacifier use can interfere with the milk supply. Ineffective latching-on and/or suckling may cause suboptimal intake. Both the frequency (at least 8 to 12 feedings/24 hours) and the efficacy of feedings must be evaluated.

In late-onset jaundice, pathologic causes must be ruled out. In a thriving breast-fed baby with no pathologic signs or symptoms, the likely diagnosis is breast milk jaundice, which is benign and gradually decreases over several weeks.

Clinical Findings

1. Extent of visible jaundice

2. Degree of alertness

3. Appropriateness for gestational age

4. Feeding and sucking ability

5. Signs of dehydration

6. Pallor; petechiae

7. Bruising or cephalhematoma

8. Hepatosplenomegaly

Diagnostic Tests

1. Total and direct bilirubin (may not be necessary with mild physiologic jaundice)

2. Blood type and Rh; direct Coombs' test

3. Complete blood count with differential, reticulocyte count

4. Other diagnostic studies as indicated by clinical condition

Treatment

1. Early onset

a. Prevention in many cases involves appropriate breast-feeding management: early and frequent feedings, avoidance of mother-infant separation, avoidance of unnecessary supplements and pacifiers, maternal education, careful evaluation of positioning and latching-on.

b. Management depends on the age of onset, the rapidity of the rise in serum bilirubin, and the presence of risk factors such as prematurity, hemolysis, or hypoxia. The current American Academy of Pediatrics (AAP) recommended threshold bilirubin levels are shown in Table 95–1 (thresholds are lower in premature or sick babies).

c. The AAP discourages interruption of breast-feeding in the healthy jaundiced neonate. Interruption risks decreased maternal milk supply, untimely weaning, and possible sensitization of atopy-prone babies to foreign (cow or soy) proteins. If formula supplements must be used, give in a way least likely to interfere with breast-feeding (cup, syringe, or supplemental feeding tube are preferable to bottles).

d. Whenever possible, continue breast-feeding during phototherapy (a fiberoptic phototherapy unit allows continued breast-feeding without interruption of phototherapy).

2. Late onset

a. If pathologic causes are ruled out and breast

TABLE 95–1. MANAGEMENT OF HYPERBILIRUBINEMIA IN THE HEALTHY TERM NEWBORN

AGE (hr)	TSB LEVEL mg/dl (μmol/L)*			
	Consider Phototherapy[†]	Photo-therapy	Exchange Transfusion if Intensive Phototherapy Fails[‡]	Exchange Transfusion and Intensive Phototherapy
≤24[§]	—	—	—	—
25–48	≥12 (170)	≥15 (260)	≥20 (340)	≥25 (430)
49–72	≥15 (260)	≥18 (310)	≥25 (430)	≥30 (510)
>72	≥17 (290)	≥20 (340)	≥25 (430)	≥30 (510)

*TSB, total serum bilirubin.

[†]Phototherapy at these TSB levels is a clinical option, meaning that the intervention is available and may be used *on the basis of individual clinical judgment.*

[‡]Intensive phototherapy should produce a decline of TSB of 1 to 2 mg/dl within 4 to 6 hours, and the TSB level should continue to fall and remain below the threshold level for exchange transfusion. If this does not occur, it is considered a failure of phototherapy.

[§]Term infants who are clinically jaundiced at 24 hours old or less are not considered healthy and require further evaluation.

Modified from American Academy of Pediatrics, Subcommittee on Hyperbilirubinemia: Practice parameter: management of hyperbilirubinemia in the healthy term newborn. Pediatrics 1994; 94:558–565. Copyright 1994 American Academy of Pediatrics, with permission.

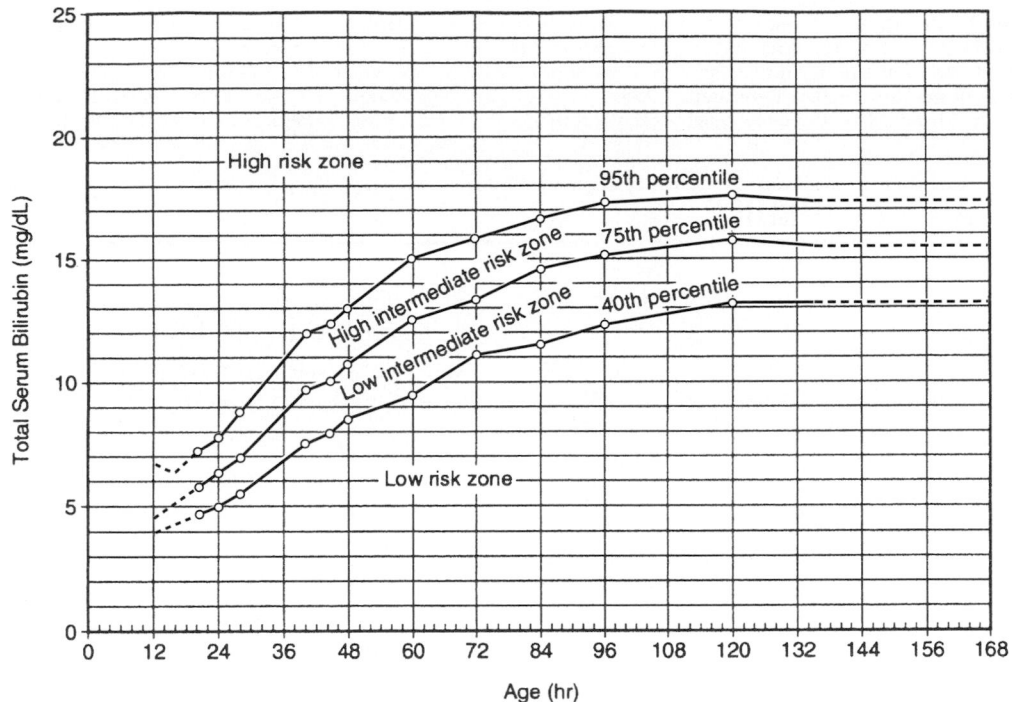

Figure 95–1 Risk designation of term and near-term well newborns based on their hour-specific serum bilirubin values. The high-risk zone is designated by the 95th percentile track. The intermediate-risk zone is subdivided to upper- and lower-risk zones by the 75th percentile track. The low-risk zone has been electively and statistically defined by the 40th percentile track. (Dotted extensions are based on <300 total serum bilirubin values/epoch.) (From Bhutani VK, Johnson L, Sivieri EM: Predictive ability of a predischarge hour-specific serum bilirubin for subsequent significant hyperbilirubinemia in healthy term and near-term newborns. Pediatrics 1999; 103:6–14, with permission.)

milk jaundice is diagnosed, continue breast-feeding, with or without supplementation and phototherapy. Pumping and scalding mother's milk is an alternative to formula supplementation.

b. Discontinuation of breast-feeding is rarely necessary and carries the same risks as earlier discontinuation (see above).

Patient Education

1. Reassure parents about the benign nature of the condition.

2. Reassure mothers that there is nothing wrong with their milk or with their baby.

Follow-Up

Frequency of repeat bilirubin levels and clinical evaluations varies with the severity of the jaundice, presence of concomitant illness, and the response to treatment.

In a recent study, hour-specific total serum bilirubin level before discharge was predictive of significant hyperbilirubinemia based on a nomogram for near term healthy neonates in the first week of life who were direct Coombs' negative (Fig. 95–1). Use of such a screening nomogram may identify high-risk newborns for appropriate follow-up, while avoiding

unnecessary repeat bilirubin measurements in the low-risk group.

PEARLS

- Early-onset jaundice in a breast-fed baby is *not* breast milk jaundice—it is *lack-of-breast-milk* jaundice.

- Water supplements are *not indicated*—they may actually aggravate jaundice.

- Discontinuation of breast-feeding is rarely necessary regardless of the cause of the jaundice.

Bibliography

American Academy of Pediatrics, Subcommittee on Hyperbilirubinemia: Practice parameter: management of hyperbilirubinemia in the healthy term newborn. Pediatrics 1994;94:558–565.
Bhutani VK, Johnson L, Sivieri EM: Predictive ability of a predischarge hour-specific serum bilirubin for subsequent significant hyperbilirubinemia in healthy term and near-term newborns. Pediatrics 1999;103:6–14.
Gartner LM: Neonatal jaundice. Pediatr Rev 1994;15: 422–432.

Guthrie RA, Auerbach KG: Jaundice and the breastfeeding baby. In Riordan J, Auerbach KG (eds): Breastfeeding and Human Lactation, 2nd ed, pp 375–391. Sudbury, MA, Jones and Bartlett Publishers, 1999.

Martinez JC, Maisels MJ, Otheguy L, et al: Hyperbilirubinemia in the breastfed newborn: a controlled trial of four interventions. Pediatrics 1993;91:470–473.

Newman TB, Maisels MJ: Evaluation and treatment of jaundice in the term newborn: a kinder, gentler approach. Pediatrics 1992;89:809–818.

SYMPTOM ADULT JAUNDICE

Angela J. Shepherd

Jaundice (icterus) is a yellow discoloration of the skin, mucous membranes, and plasma caused by staining by bile, the red pigment product of heme metabolism. It is clinically noted in adults when the serum bilirubin exceeds 2.5 to 3.0 mg/dl. It is often the first and sometimes the sole manifestation of liver disease, and frequently is best detected in the sclera.

Anatomically, elevated bilirubin is prehepatic, hepatic, or posthepatic. Prehepatic jaundice is due to excess production of bilirubin (e.g., hemolysis). In hepatic jaundice, elevated serum bilirubin is caused by dysfunction of liver cells (e.g., faulty uptake, metabolism or excretion of bilirubin). Posthepatic jaundice results from interference with the removal of bilirubin from the hepatobiliary system (e.g., obstruction of the common bile duct).

Differential Diagnosis
1. Prehepatic
   a. Hemolytic anemias or reactions
   b. Resolving large hematomas
2. Hepatic
   a. Gilbert's syndrome (asymptomatic)
   b. Hepatitis (viral, autoimmune, and alcoholic)
   c. Hepatic cirrhosis
   d. Drug-induced cholestasis
   e. Wilson's disease
3. Posthepatic
   a. Gallstones
   b. Carcinoma of the biliary duct
   c. Sclerosing cholangitis
   d. Pancreatitis
   e. Pancreatic neoplasm
   f. Ascending cholangitis

History
A good history is essential in the quest for determining the etiology of jaundice.
1. Alcohol exposure
   a. Alcohol use points toward alcoholic hepatitis and/or cirrhosis.
   b. Bartenders and liquor salesmen may have occupational exposure to alcohol and may develop alcoholic hepatitis/cirrhosis.
2. Bodybuilders who have taken androgens may be at risk for androgen-induced cholestasis.
3. Patients with gallstones may report a history of postprandial colic.
4. Patients with tumors may report longstanding, dull abdominal pain.
5. Hepatitis exposure
   a. Day care workers who are exposed to feces need to be considered at risk for hepatitis A.
   b. Medical workers with exposure to needles may be at risk for hepatitis B and C.
   c. Asians, those from developing countries (or those who have visited such), intravenous drug abusers, prostitutes, male homosexuals, and nonmonogamous heterosexuals who do not practice safe sex may be at risk for hepatitis B exposure.
   d. Hepatitis patients may report malaise, "flu-like" symptoms, and anorexia.
6. Surgical history is important because those patients may be at risk for having a retained stone in the biliary tree, postsurgical bile duct stricture, or pancreatitis from operative pancreatic trauma.
7. A history of prior blood transfusions is important in assessing risk for hepatitis C because, in most institutions, hepatitis C was not specifically tested for by blood banks until the 1990s. Screening of donors for elevated alanine transaminase (ALT) began in 1986, so those who received blood prior to those times may be at increased risk.
8. Numerous drugs can potentially cause jaundice. Classes of drugs that should be asked about include: anesthetics, neurospychotropics, anticonvulsants, analgesics (acetaminophen, nonsteroidal anti-inflammatory agents), oral hypoglycemics, oral contraceptives, anabolic steroids, antibiotics, antituberculosis agents, cardiovascular agents, and antineoplastic agents.

Key Questions
1. How much alcohol do you drink per day?
2. What is your occupation?
3. Have you felt sick?
4. Are you at risk for hepatitis B?
5. Have you had abdominal surgery in the past?

6. Did you have a blood transfusion prior to 1986?

7. What drugs do you take now and have you taken in the recent past?

Clinical Findings

1. General
   a. Depression
   b. Cachexia
   c. Fever
2. Skin
   a. Yellow discoloration of skin, sclera, and mucous membranes
   b. Bruises
   c. Excoriations from scratching
   d. Spider angiomas
   e. Red hands
3. Abdomen
   a. Ascites
   b. Splenomegaly
   c. Right upper quadrant or epigastric mass
   d. Palpable gallbladder
   e. Positive Murphy's sign
   f. Hepatomegaly
4. Excrement
   a. Chalky white stool
   b. Tea-colored urine
5. Miscellaneous
   a. Joint inflammation
   b. Testicular atrophy
   c. Gynecomastia

Diagnostic Tests

1. First line
   a. Liver function tests: bilirubin, aspartate transaminase (AST), alanine aminotransferase (ALT), gammaglutamyl transpeptidase, alkaline phosphatase, lactate dehydrogenase, urinalysis, complete blood count
   b. ALT may be useful in differentiating alcoholic from viral hepatitis because ALT is much lower than AST in alcoholic hepatitis.
2. Second line (as indicated by results of the above)
   a. Hepatitis studies: hepatitis A virus (HAV), hepatitis B surface antigen (HBsAg), hepatitis C virus (HCV)
   b. Cytomegalovirus and Epstein-Barr virus tests
   c. Abdominal ultrasound
   d. Prothrombin time
   e. Antinuclear antibodies

3. Third line
   a. Computerized tomography (CT) scan of abdomen
   b. Liver biopsy
   c. Endoscopic retrograde cholangiopancreatography (ERCP)

Management (See Also Sections for Specific Hepatobiliary Diseases)

1. Diet: no alcohol, sufficient carbohydrate and calories
2. Activity: bed rest only during the acute initial phase if hepatitis suspected; avoidance of strenuous exercise
3. Medications
   a. Cholestyramine, 1 packet or scoop one to four times daily, to bind bilirubin and decrease pruritis
   b. Antihistamines (diphenhydramine [Benadryl] 25 mg q6h, or hydroxyxine [Atarax] 10 to 25 mg q6h) may be helpful in symptomatic treatment of pruritis.
4. Surgery: General surgical consultation may be indicated for posthepatic (obstructive) causes of jaundice.
5. Patient education: discussion regarding transmission of hepatitis if indicated (hand washing after bowel movements and after contact with infected patients, abstinence from sexual activity and instruction in safe sex practices)
6. Close follow-up is indicated until resolution and/or definitive diagnosis is made.

PEARLS

- Although jaundice infrequently represents a medical emergency, the notable exception is jaundice accompanied by fever, leukocytosis, rigors, and hypotension—signs suggesting ascending cholangitis and septicemia.

- The major causes of jaundice according to age and gender are
  - In young adults: viral hepatitis
  - In males over 50: malignant obstruction of the biliary tree
  - In females over 30: choledocholithiasis
  - In middle adulthood (both sexes): drug-induced liver disease and cirrhosis
  - Middle aged and older men: alcoholic liver disease, pancreatic cancer, hepatoma, primary hemochromatosis
  - Women: primary biliary cirrhosis, chronic active hepatitis, choledocholithiasis, carcinoma of the gallbladder

---

Bibliography

Knauer CM: Liver, biliary tract & pancreas. In Tierney LM Jr, McPhee FJ, Papadakis MA (eds): Current Medical Diagnosis and Treatments, pp 503–513. Norwalk, CT, Appleton & Lange, 1993.

Lumeng L, O'Connor KW: Differential diagnosis of jaundice. In Osstrow JD (ed): Bile Pigments and Jaundice, pp 475–523. New York, Marcel Dekker, 1986.

Palmer KR: Jaundice. In Bouchier IAD, Ellis H, Fleming PR (eds): French's Index of Differential Diagnosis, 13th ed, pp 314–330. Oxford, England, Butterworth-Heinemann, 1996.

Schiff L: Jaundice: a clinical approach. In Schiff L, Schiff ER (eds): Diseases of the Liver, 7th ed, pp 334–340. Philadelphia, JB Lippincott Company, 1993.

Zimmerman HJ, Ishak KG: General aspects of drug-induced liver disease. Gastroenterol Clin North Am 1995;24:739–745.

SYMPTOM ASCITES

Todd A. May

Ascites is the pathologic accumulation of fluid in the peritoneal cavity, usually caused by chronic parenchymal liver disease, malignancy, heart failure, infection, or nephrotic syndrome. Evaluation of ascitic fluid yields diagnostic and prognostic information that guides therapy.

Differential Diagnosis

1. Gaseous distention of the bowel, including ileus and bowel obstruction
2. Obesity
3. Massive tumor (e.g., lymphoma, ovarian, hepatic, and uterine tumors)

Etiology

1. Portal hypertension from cirrhosis, hepatitis, hepatic vein obstruction (Budd-Chiari syndrome), portal vein thrombosis: 80 to 85 per cent
2. Malignancy, especially with peritoneal carcinomatosis: 10 per cent
3. Heart failure: 3 per cent
4. Tuberculosis, nephrogenous (dialysis-related), pancreatic, biliary, nephrotic syndrome, serositis, myxedema: 1 per cent or less

History: Key Questions to Ask

1. Increase in abdominal girth? With or without pain/discomfort?
2. Recent weight gain or loss?
3. Fever and abdominal discomfort?
4. History of alcoholism and/or intravenous drug use?
5. History of jaundice, hepatitis, liver disease, gastrointestinal bleeding, or encephalopathy?
6. History of heart failure or myocardial infarction?
7. Risk factors for viral hepatitis?
8. History of renal, thyroid, pancreatic, biliary, or connective tissue disease?

The increase in abdominal girth found in the cirrhotic typically is painless until tense ascites develops.

Ascites associated with malignancy and infection may cause abdominal pain.

Clinical Findings

1. Abdominal examination
   a. Abdominal distention
   b. Bulging flanks, flank dullness, shifting dullness (~1500 ml), fluid wave
2. Signs of chronic liver disease (absence does not exclude cirrhosis)
   a. Jaundice
   b. Palmar erythema, spider angiomas, caput medusae
   c. Gynecomastia, testicular atrophy
   d. Parotid enlargement
3. Other extra-abdominal signs
   a. Peripheral edema: liver or heart disease
   b. Jugular venous distention, gallop rhythm, pulsatile liver: heart failure
   c. Kussmaul's sign, pulsus paradoxus: constrictive pericarditis
   d. Periumbilical nodule or Virchow's node: malignancy
   e. Edema of hands, face: nephrotic syndrome

The strongest indicators of the presence of ascites are shifting dullness, demonstration of a fluid wave, and peripheral edema. However, the physical examination is not always reliable in making the diagnosis of ascites; radiologic confirmation may be required. Extra-abdominal findings often provide evidence for the underlying cause of ascites.

Diagnostic Tests

1. Paracentesis and ascitic fluid analysis
   a. Screening tests
      (1) Cell count with differential to rule out infection: Polymorphonuclear leukocytes >250 cells/mm^3 presumes bacterial peritonitis; predominance of lymphocytes or monocytes suggests other conditions, including tuberculosis.

(2) Fluid culture: highest yield when blood culture bottles are inoculated with 10 ml of ascitic fluid at the bedside

(3) Albumin concentration for serum-ascites albumin gradient (SAAG)

(a) High SAAG (≥1.1 gm/dl): Ascites is portal hypertension–related (e.g., cirrhosis, vascular obstruction, congestive heart failure, fulminant hepatic failure).

(b) Low SAAG (<1.1 gm/dl): Ascites is not portal hypertension–related (e.g., peritoneal carcinomatosis, tuberculosis, pancreatic or biliary ascites, nephrotic syndrome).

b. Selected tests (not routine)

(1) Total protein, glucose, and lactate dehydrogenase have limited value.

(2) Cytology has low sensitivity unless peritoneal carcinomatosis is present.

(3) Acid-fast bacilli smear and culture when indicated by risk factors or clinical findings

(4) Amylase when pancreatic ascites suspected (tea-colored ascites)

2. Serum tests: complete blood count with platelets, liver panel, renal panel, albumin, coagulation studies

3. Urinary sodium: Measure initially at diagnosis and serially to assess effects of therapy.

4. Selective imaging (not routine)

a. Abdominal ultrasound: sensitive to 100 ml; can detect hepatocellular carcinoma, liver metastases, Budd-Chiari syndrome, and uterine/ovarian masses. May be used to guide paracentesis.

b. Abdominal computerized tomography: highly sensitive for detecting liver metastases and pancreatic disease

c. Chest radiograph: May reveal evidence of tuberculosis or heart failure.

d. Echocardiogram: Obtain when cardiac cause is suspected.

Ascitic fluid analysis provides the most vaulable diagnostic information. The SAAG is 97 per cent accurate in determining if portal hypertension is present. Paracentesis should be performed in all cases, without the use of blood products, unless there is frank bleeding or disseminated intravascular coagulation.

Management

Cirrhosis/Portal Hypertension

1. Diet

a. Sodium restriction to 2000 mg/day (88 mmol/day) or less

b. Abstain from alcohol.

c. Fluid restriction only when hyponatremia is severe (e.g., serum sodium < 120 mmol/L)

2. Medication/procedures

a. Oral diuretics are effective for 90 per cent of patients. Start with spironolactone 100 mg and furosemide 40 mg once daily. Increase to maximum 400 mg/day spironolactone and 160 mg/day furosemide as needed. (Caution: Overvigorous diuresis may lead to orthostatic hypotension, prerenal azotemia, and the hepatorenal syndrome.)

b. A single 4- to 6-L therapeutic paracentesis can be performed for patients with tense ascites.

3. Activity

a. Bed rest has not been demonstrated to be beneficial.

b. Elevation of lower extremities while at rest may help mobilize peripheral edema.

4. Patient education

a. Education in preparing or obtaining a diet limited to 88 mmol/day of sodium; referral to a nutritionist is highly recommended.

b. Abstain from alcohol.

c. Avoid nonsteroidal anti-inflammatory drugs.

5. Monitoring therapy

a. Monitor weight daily with goal of loss of 1 kg/day with peripheral edema and 0.5 kg/day without.

b. Serial monitoring of urinary sodium excretion to ensure a negative sodium balance is helpful in determining the optimal diuretic dose and assessing dietary compliance.

c. Periodic serum electrolytes, blood urea nitrogen, and creatinine

Refractory Ascites

1. Only 10 per cent of patients with cirrhosis and ascites are truly refractory to standard therapy.

2. Serial therapeutic paracenteses (up to 5 L) can be performed every 2 weeks as needed.

3. Liver transplantation can be considered.

4. Peritoneovenous shunt (e.g., LeVeen or Denver) or transjugular intrahepatic portosystemic stent-shunt (TIPS) might be considered (high failure and complication rates).

Malignancy

Median survival varies by tumor of origin, ranging from several days to several months. Some malignancies respond to systemic therapies (e.g., ovarian, lymphoma), so accurately establishing the origin may be important. Palliative measures to maximize comfort are essential.

1. Symptomatic paracentesis: serial large-volume (4- to 6-L) pericenteses as needed for relief of symptoms

2. Oral diuretics: May be tried but generally ineffective.

3. Chemotherapy—systemic and intraperitoneal: Can provide palliative benefits and sometimes improves survival.

4. Peritoneovenous shunt: Recommended for non-gastrointestinal malignancies when treatment options fail and prognosis is more than 3 months. Associated complications and morbidity limit its use.

5. Novel treatments: Immunotherapy, radioimmunotherapy, intraperitoneal radiocolloids, and matrix metalloproteinase inhibitors have shown some promise.

Other Causes

Other causes of ascites require therapies directed at the underlying pathophysiology.

1. Heart failure: sodium restriction, diuretics, afterload reducers (e.g., angiotension-converting enzyme inhibitors), inotropes

2. Tuberculosis: appropriate antibiotics

3. Pancreatic, biliary: stents, surgical repair

4. Serositis: anti-inflammatory agents

5. Myxedema: levothyroxine replacement

Bibliography

McHutchinson JG: Differential diagnosis of ascites. Semin Liver Dis 1997;17:191–202.

Parsons SL, Watson SA, Steele RJC: Malignant ascites. Br J Surg 1996;83:6–14.

Runyon BA: Care of patients with ascites. N Engl J Med 1994;330:337–342.

Runyon BA: Management of adult patients with ascites caused by cirrhosis: American Association for the Study of Liver Diseases Practice Guidelines. Hepatology 1998;27:264–272.

Williams JW, Simel DL: Does this patient have ascites? How to divine fluid in the abdomen. JAMA 1992;267:2645–2648.

1. *Ascites* is the abnormal accumulation of fluid within the abdominal cavity and *paracentesis* is an invasive procedure to remove this fluid for both therapeutic and diagnostic purposes. Epidemiologic studies have shown that formation of ascites is most commonly related to parenchymal liver disease (about 80 per cent), whereas another 5 per cent may involve a mixed pattern of liver disease and an abdominal malignancy. Less frequent causes of ascitic fluid collections are heart failure, tuberculosis, pancreatitis, myxedema, and nephrotic syndrome.

2. Patients with ascites may complain of weight gain, increasing abdominal girth, and shortness of breath, especially in the recumbent position.

3. Evidence of flank dullness on physical examination should lead to evaluation of shifting dullness in the abdomen. It has been estimated that 1500 ml of ascitic fluid need to be present in order to detect shifting dullness. The presence of a fluid wave is a less sensitive indicator of ascites. Studies have reported that abdominal ultrasonography has been able to detect at least 100 ml of fluid in the abdomen.

Indications

1. Ascitic fluid analysis is valuable in helping to pinpoint the etiology of ascites.

2. Paracentesis is especially important to perform because up to 25 per cent of patients admitted with ascites have evidence of peritonitis.

Contraindications

An underlying coagulopathy is rarely a contraindication to performing paracentesis. Some patients with coagulopathies are given fresh frozen plasma and/or platelets before or during the procedure to lessen the likelihood of bleeding. There are no data to support giving blood products to prevent hematoma formation and, in fact, transfusing such products places the patient at increased risk for developing post-transfusion hepatitis.

Preparation

1. Once a site has been chosen, a sterile field should be established.

2. Although use of sterile gloves is essential, a mask, gown, and hat are not required.

3. The area should be disinfected with an iodine-based solution, and local anesthetic should be infiltrated into the skin and deeper tissues.

Equipment

1. 60-ml syringe
2. 1.5-in 22- or 18-gauge needles
3. 1 liter evacuated collection bottle and sterile plastic tubing (if a therapeutic paracentesis is being done)
4. Three sterile drapes
5. Iodine solution

Anesthesia

Use a 1% lidocaine solution without epinephrine.

Technique

1. The site of needle insertion depends on the amount of ascites. It is often recommended that the needle be introduced approximately 2 fingerbreadths cephalad and 2 fingerbreadths medial to the anterosuperior iliac spine—whichever quadrant is most dull to percussion. Because the lower quadrants can be highly vascular, an alternative side is in the midline, caudad to the umbilicus. Because patients may have a neurogenic bladder or bladder outlet obstruction, it is recommended that the bladder be emptied before use of a midline approach to avoid bladder puncture.

2. Needles should never be introduced into a highly vascular area, into an area midline cephalad to the umbilicus, or through or within several centimeters of scar tissue. Such placements put the patient at risk of vessel puncture and subsequent hematoma formation or a perforated viscus adherent to a surgical scar.

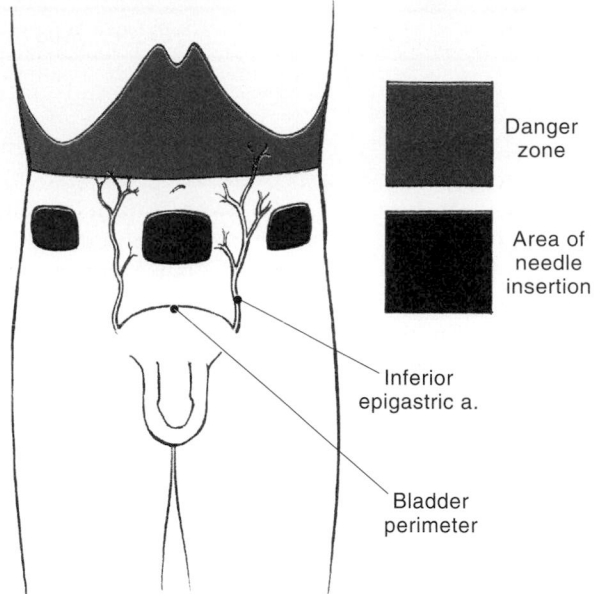

Danger zone

Area of needle insertion

Inferior epigastric a.

Bladder perimeter

3. When the area has been prepped, the needle should be introduced in a "Z" track to prevent leakage of ascitic fluid when the needle is removed. This is done by retracting the skin caudally before inserting the needle and then releasing the skin when the peritoneum is entered. The needle should be advanced in small increments (about 5 mm) and aspirated intermittently to ensure that the tip does not enter a blood vessel.

Fluid Analysis

1. *Cell count*: A pre-diuresis elevation of the ascitic fluid white blood cell (WBC) count greater than 250 cells/mm^3 is seen in episodes of spontaneous bacterial peritonitis with a left shift. Lymphocytic predominance occurs in cases of tuberculosis peritonitis and peritoneal carcinomatosis. In cases of a bloody fluid, 1 polymorphonuclear leukocyte is subtracted for every 250 red blood cells present. If the corrected WBC count is greater than 250 cells/mm^3, the fluid is presumed to be infected.

2. *Albumin*: Ascitic fluid albumin should be measured the same day as the serum albumin. When the ascitic fluid value is subtracted from the serum value, the physician obtains the serum-ascites albumin gradient (SAAG). The SAAG is determined by oncotic-hydrostatic balance. Portal hypertension produces a high hydrostatic pressure gradient between the portal bed and the ascitic fluid.

   a. A SAAG value greater than 1.1 gm/dl is consistent with portal hypertension and is associated with cirrhosis, liver metastatis, hepatic failure, alcoholic hepatitis, the Budd-Chiari syndrome, cardiac ascites, portal vein thrombosis, myxedema, fatty liver of pregnancy, or veno-occlusive disease.

   b. SAAG values less than 1.1 gm/dl are frequently associated with peritoneal carcinomatosis, biliary ascites, pancreatic ascites, tuberculous ascites, the nephrotic syndrome, bowel obstruction with infarct, postoperative lymphatic leakage, or serositis seen in connective tissue disease.

3. *Culture*: Studies have shown that bedside inoculation of ascitic fluid is superior to laboratory inoculation. Although the majority of cases of spontaneous bacterial peritonitis (SBP) are due to a monomicrobial infection, it is imperative to obtain both aerobic and anaerobic cultures.

Adjunctive Testing

1. *Protein*: This test has largely been replaced by the SAAG determination. It is noteworthy that patients with extremely low protein ascites have been found to be predisposed to develop SBP.

2. *Amylase*: Patients with pancreatitis or gut perforation exhibit elevated amylase levels, usually three to five times serum concentrations.

3. *Tuberculosis Testing*: Tuberculous peritonitis is often associated with negative standard cultures of ascitic fluid and a mononuclear predominance of total WBCs from the ascites. However, studies have shown that laparoscopy with histologic analysis of biopsy samples is more sensitive than culture of the ascitic fluid and smear testing for acid-fast bacilli.

4. *Cytology*: Ascitic fluid cytologic analysis is proved most sensitive in cases of peritoneal carcinomatosis. This analysis is less sensitive in conditions where tumor cells do not line the peritoneal cavity (e.g., hepatoma or lymphoma).

5. *Triglycerides*: Suspicion of chylous ascites usually arises when the ascitic fluid is milky white or cloudy. This is further supported by triglyceride levels of more than 200 mg/dl, sometimes as high as 1000 mg/dl.

6. *Bilirubin*: If the ascitic fluid bilirubin is greater than or equal to 6 mg/dl and elevated more than that found in the serum, this can indicate a biliary or upper gastrointestinal tract perforation. A dark-brown ascitic fluid is often seen in such cases.

 Bibliography

Buckley SE, Herrera JL: Management of ascites. Compr Ther 1995;21:195–199.

Habeeb KS, Herrera JL: Management of ascites. Postgrad Med 1997;101:191–200.
Runyon BA: Care of patients with ascites. N Engl J Med 1994;330:337–341.
Runyon BA: Paracentesis of ascitic fluid: a safe procedure. Arch Intern Med 1986;146:2259–2261.

Runyon BA, Montano AA, Akriviadis EA, et al: Comparison of the utility of the serum-ascites albumin gradient to the exudate/transudate concept in the differential diagnosis of ascites. Hepatology 1992;16:15A.

SYMPTOM ABNORMAL LIVER FUNCTION TESTS

Jason Chao

Abnormal biochemical liver function tests are commonly discovered in asymptomatic individuals. Although liver disease is often present, it is also common for patients to have results outside the "normal" range because of statistical chance. Liver disease may also be far advanced without any elevation in liver function tests. Most liver or biliary tract disease manifests in one of two pathologic and biochemical patterns: parenchymal necrosis or cholestasis.

Differential Diagnosis

1. Patients with minor elevations in liver function tests (less than threefold) and no risk factors by history or physical examination are at low risk of significant liver pathology and may have follow-up liver testing in 1 to 3 months. Patients with chronic (more that 6 months) or major elevations in liver function tests should undergo further testing without delay.

2. Parenchymal liver disease typically causes elevated serum levels of alanine transaminase (ALT, or SGPT) and aspartate transaminase (AST, or SGOT). Lactate dehydrogenase is a less sensitive and less specific marker of liver cell damage. Gammaglutamyl transpeptidase is a more specific indicator of liver pathology but is also often elevated when cholestasis is present.

   a. Alcohol-induced hepatitis: Alcoholism is a lethal but treatable disease that may be first detected by abnormal liver tests.

   b. Chronic viral hepatitis B or C: Acute viral hepatitis A is self-limited. Patients with hepatitis B or C need to be followed for chronic hepatitis.

   c. Toxin-induced and drug-induced hepatitis

   d. Obesity: Some morbidly obese patients may develop liver disease with hepatosteatonecrosis.

   e. Hemochromatosis: This treatable autosomal recessive disease may occur as a spontaneous mutation without a family history. There is an excess accumulation of iron in the liver and other organs. Transaminases are usually only moderately elevated.

   f. Autoimmune hepatitis. This disease primarily affects women between the ages of 20 and 40 years. Transaminases are quite elevated. *Less common.*

   g. Wilson's disease. This should be considered in patients less than 40. There is an excess accumulation of copper that leads to liver failure and neurologic symptoms if untreated. *Less common.*

   h. α_1-Antitrypsin deficiency: Many patients with this autosomal recessive disease do not have chronic obstructive pulmonary disease at the time of diagnosis.

3. *Cholestatic or biliary tract disease is suggested by alkaline phosphatase (ALP) levels greater than three times normal or elevated bilirubin. ALT and AST are usually less than three times normal.*

   a. Biliary tract obstruction: Extrahepatic structural or mechanical obstruction of the bile ducts is most commonly due to choledocholithiasis, biliary stricture, pancreatic or periampullary carcinoma, pancreatitis, or biliary atresia.

   b. Drug-induced cholestasis

   c. Congestive heart failure: Older patients may present with right-sided heart failure and jaundice.

   d. Intrahepatic cholestasis of pregnancy

   e. Hemolytic anemias and ineffective erythropoiesis, such as thalassemias

   f. Gilbert's and Crigler-Najjar syndromes cause isolated hyperbilirubinemia.

   g. Hepatobiliary neoplasms: Primary benign and malignant tumors of the liver, gallbladder, and extrahepatic bile ducts, and metastatic tumors to the liver, may cause cholestasis.

   h. Primary biliary cirrhosis: Typical patients are middle-aged females with very high serum ALP levels.

   i. Primary sclerosing cholangitis: This chronic, progressive disease is more common in middle-aged males with elevated serum ALP levels. Most patients also have inflammatory bowel disease. It may be difficult to differentiate from a cholangiocarcinoma.

Refer to Ch. 96, Hepatitis; Ch. 99, Gallstones and Cholecystitis; Ch. 100, Pancreatitis; Ch. 101, Pancreatic Carcinoma; and Ch. 344, Alcoholism.

History

1. Look for symptoms of liver disease, including fatigue, pruritus, jaundice, and bruising.
2. Detailed alcohol intake history: Under-reporting is common among alcoholics, so a sensitive yet thorough history of alcohol consumption is necessary. Verification of the history by family or friends may be necessary.
3. Occupational or home chemical exposure to hepatotoxins: Household toxins include carbon tetrachloride, chloroform, heavy metals, and phosphorus.
4. Risk factors for viral hepatitis: blood transfusions, needle-stick injury, injection drug use, contact with patient with known hepatitis, unsafe sexual practices
5. Family history of liver disease
6. Past and current medications
   a. Drug-induced hepatitis: acetaminophen, amiodarone, anesthetic agents, isoniazid, ketoconazole, nitrofurantoin, penicillins, sulfonamides, tetracyclines, methyldopa, procainamide, quinidine, propylthiouracil, niacin, vitamin A, disulfiram, dantrolene, methotrexate, carbamazepine, phenytoin, valproic acid
   b. Drug-induced cholestasis: androgens, estrogens, carbamazepine, clavulanic acid, diazepam, disulfiram, erythromycin estolate, haloperidol, oral hypoglycemics, penicillamine, phenothiazines, propoxyphene.

Clinical Findings

1. Liver size and tenderness
2. Ascites
3. Encephalopathy

Tests

1. Further testing should be chosen selectively based upon the history and pattern of abnormal test results.
2. Serologic tests for hepatitis A, B, and C, Epstein-Barr virus, and cytomegalovirus for viral hepatitis
3. Elevation of serum iron, transferrin saturation, and ferritin may detect hemochromatosis.
4. Low serum ceruloplasmin and elevated 24-hour urinary excretion of copper may detect Wilson's disease.

5. Low serum α_1-antitrypsin level may detect α_1-antitrypsin deficiency. These patients often have an abnormal serum protein electrophoresis.
6. Elevated immunoglobulin G and autoimmune markers such as antinuclear antibodies and anti–smooth muscle antibodies help identify autoimmune hepatitis. Other markers of collagen-vascular disease may be absent.
7. Anti-mitochondrial antibodies are usually present in patients with primary biliary cirrhosis.
8. For parenchymal liver disease, hepatic imaging with ultrasound or computerized tomography may be helpful.
9. Liver biopsy should be reserved for those with persistent elevations greater than three times normal.
10. Conjugated and unconjugated bilirubin determination in cholestatic liver disease helps differentiate causes of jaundice.
11. Prothrombin time may be prolonged in both hepatocellular and cholestatic liver disease.
12. Ultrasonographic imaging of the liver and biliary tract is recommended for initial radiologic evaluation of cholestatic liver disease.
13. Endoscopic retrograde cholangiopancreatography (ERCP) or percutaneous transhepatic cholangiography (PTC) may be necessary if extrahepatic obstruction is suspected.

Management

1. Alcohol and other hepatotoxic drugs should be avoided.
2. The underlying cause for elevated biochemical liver function tests will determine further treatment.

PEARLS

- Most hepatocellular dysfunction causes the AST/ALT ratio to remain less than 1, except for alcoholic liver disease, which typically raises the ratio to greater than 2.

- Although alcoholic liver disease is very common, other treatable causes of liver disease may coexist.

- Elevated ALP may originate from bone, placenta, or bowel, rather than liver.

- If the prothrombin time is prolonged, administration of a single dose of parenteral vitamin K may dramatically improve the prothrombin time in obstructive disease.

Bibliography

For more information on the causes of abnormal liver tests, see

Herrera JL: Abnormal liver enzyme levels: the spectrum of causes. Postgrad Med 1993;93:113–116.

For more information on the evaluation of abnormal liver tests, see

Moseley RH: Evaluation of abnormal liver function tests. Med Clin North Am 1996;80:887–906.

For more information on the usefulness of liver biopsy, see

VanNess MM, Diehl AM: Is liver biopsy useful in the evaluation of patients with chronically elevated liver enzymes? Ann Intern Med 1989;111:473–478.

For more information on obesity and abnormal liver tests, see

Palmer M, Schaffner F: Effect of weight reduction on hepatic abnormalities in overweight patients. Gastroenterology 1990;99:1408–1413.

96 Viral Hepatitis

Christi A. Matteoni

Management of viral hepatitis has seen some major changes, and therefore knowledge of the various types is important. At least seven major viruses have been identified and cause the majority of disease: hepatitis A (HAV), hepatitis B (HBV), hepatitis C (HCV), hepatitis D or the delta agent (HDV), hepatitis E (HEV), hepatitis G (HGV), and transfusion-transmitted virus (TTV) (Table 96–1). Infection from these agents may clinically range from asymptomatic to a rapid fulminant course.

Hepatitis A

Epidemiology
1. Hepatitis A is seen worldwide, and its prevalence is related to sanitation, quality of the water supply, and age of the subject. Ninety per cent of persons exposed will become infected. In areas of high endemicity, most persons are infected at a young age. In areas of low endemicity, such as the United States, the highest infection rates are seen in day care centers and residential institutions.
2. The most common risk factor is personal contact with another individual that is HAV infected.

Clinical Manifestations and Diagnosis
1. The common prodromal symptoms include fatigue, anorexia, nausea and vomiting, and abdominal pain. Less common symptoms include arthralgias, myalgias, diarrhea, fever, and headaches.
2. Jaundice and dark urine occur in most patients within 1 to 2 weeks of the prodrome.
3. Mild hepatomegaly and tenderness occur in 85 per cent, splenomegaly in 15 per cent, and posterior cervical adenopathy in 15 per cent.
4. HAV has fewer extrahepatic manifestations than HBV (Table 96–2).
5. Transaminase levels are commonly greater than 500 IU/L, with peak hyperbilirubinemia occurring later and bilirubin levels generally less than 10 mg/dl.
6. Older patients tend to have more severe disease. Pregnancy does not increase the risk for severity, but patients with chronic liver disease, such as HBV or HCV, are more at risk for fulminant hepatitis.
7. Detecting HAV immunoglobulin M (IgM) in the serum makes the diagnosis, but only 25 per cent of patients have detectable IgM beyond 6 months.

Treatment and Prevention
1. Treatment is predominantly supportive. Patients with prolonged prothrombin times and changes in mental status need to be hospitalized and considered for liver transplantation.

TABLE 96–1. CLINICAL FEATURES OF VIRAL HEPATITIS

	HAV	HBV	HCV	HDV	HEV	HGV	TTV
Transmission	Oral	Percutaneous, sexual	Percutaneous, sexual	Percutaneous	Oral	Percutaneous	Transfusion
Incubation (days)	15–49	60–180	14–160	21–45	15–60	14–35	Unknown
Fulminant	<1%	<1%	Unknown	2–7.5%	<1%, higher in pregnant women	Unknown	Unknown
Chronic infection	No	<5% adults	80–90%	Superinfection 80%, co-infection <5%	No	Yes	Yes
Diagnostic tests							
Acute	Anti-HAV IgM	HBsAg, anti-HBc IgM	HCV RNA	Anti-HDV IgM	Anti-HEV IgG	HGV RNA	Not available
Chronic	No	HBsAg, anti-HBc IgG	Anti-HCV	Anti-HDV IgG	No	HGV RNA	Not available

TABLE 96–2. EXTRAHEPATIC MANIFESTATIONS

HAV	HBV	HCV
Evanescent rash	Acute	Membranoproliferative glomerulonephritis
Arthralgias	Serum sickness–like syndrome	Essential mixed cryoglobulinemia
Leukocytoclastic vasculitis	Polyarteritis nodosa	Porphyria cutanea tarda
Glomerulonephritis	Neuropathy (mononeuritis)	Leukocytoclastic vasculitis
Arthritis	Renal disease	Mooren corneal ulcers
	Cutaneous vasculitis	Lichen planus
	Arthritis	Idiopathic pulmonary fibrosis
	Raynaud's phenomenon	Rheumatoid arthritis
	Chronic	
	Membranoproliferative glomerulonephritis	
	Type II mixed essential cryoglobulinemia	
	Guillain-Barré syndrome	
	Polyneuropathy	

2. Travelers to endemic areas should be advised to avoid drinking water or beverages with ice or eating uncooked shellfish or unpeeled fruits and vegetables.

3. Vaccination
   a. Passive immunoprophylaxis with immune globulin is recommended for travelers to endemic areas for a duration less than 2 weeks and household contacts.
   b. Vaccination with either Havrix or Vaqta, both formalin-inactivated viral particles, can generate greater than 95 per cent protective antibodies within 4 weeks of immunization. The schedule and dose for adults over 18 years is Havrix, 1440 ELISA units/1.0 ml at 0 and 6 to 12 months, or Vaqta, 50 units/ 0.5 ml at 0 and 6 to 12 months.
   c. Hepatitis A vaccination has an excellent safety profile, but its safety in pregnant women needs to be determined.
   d. Candidates for vaccination include travelers to endemic areas, children in communities with high rates of infection, homosexual men, injection drug users, and persons with chronic liver disease.

Hepatitis B

Epidemiology
1. HBV is a common disease with a global prevalence of 5 per cent. High prevalence is seen in Southeast Asia, the Philippines, the Middle East, Africa, and parts of South America. Prevalence is lowest in the United States, Canada, Australia, northern Europe, and the southern part of South America.
2. Transmission is parenteral, with viral particles detectable in body fluids including saliva and semen. Sexual transmission is the most common mode in countries of low prevalence but vertical transmission is the most common cause worldwide. Intravenous drug use is an important mode for transmission. Transfusion-associated infection is 1:50,000 per unit transfused.

Clinical Manifestations and Diagnosis
1. Acute
   a. Markers of acute infection (hepatitis B surface antigen [HBsAg], hepatitis B early antigen [HBeAg], and HBV DNA) can be detected at 6 weeks after exposure and may be present before symptoms. At the onset of symptoms, antibody to hepatitis B core antigen (anti-HBc IgM) becomes positive. The last marker to become positive is anti-HBs, which indicates resolving infection and development of immunity.
   b. Biochemically, the transaminase levels are generally greater than 500 IU/L, with alanine transaminase (ALT) generally greater than aspartate transaminase (AST), and bilirubin ranges from 5 to 10 mg/dl.
   c. Fulminant hepatic failure is the most serious complication of acute HBV, occurring in 1 per cent of patients.
   d. Extrahepatic manifestations are seen commonly, with 25 per cent of patients experiencing arthralgias and rashes (Table 96–2).
2. Chronic
   a. HBsAg, HBeAg, and HBV DNA may remain positive at least 6 months, with anti-HBc IgM almost undetectable after 6 months. Anti-HBc immunoglobulin G (IgG) persists indefinitely. There may be spontaneous

loss of HBeAg and HBV DNA but rarely HBsAg.

b. Chronic disease is also associated with extrahepatic manifestations (Table 96–1).

c. The risk of chronic infection ranges from 1 to 12 per cent in adults and up to 90 per cent in those who had a neonatally acquired infection.

d. Prognosis of chronic HBV is determined by whether or not there is active viral replication and the degree of histologic damage. Fortunately, many "healthy carriers" (HBsAg$^+$ with normal liver enzymes, no active viral replication and minimal abnormality on the liver biopsy) have normal transaminase levels and minimal if any histologic change. Of the 1 to 12 per cent who are chronic carriers, 50 per cent will have active viral replication (HbeAg and/or HBV DNA positivity), and 15 to 20 per cent of these patients may develop cirrhosis within 5 years.

Treatment and Prevention

1. Supportive care is the treatment option for acute infection. Interferon-α (IFN-α) is approved by the Food and Drug Administration (FDA) for chronic infection, but the response rate (clearance of HBeAg and HBV DNA) is only 35 per cent. Clearance of all markers and development of anti-HBs occurs in approximately 6 per cent. Treatment for 4 months with 5 million units subcutaneously daily or 10 million units three times a week is indicated. Pretreatment variables associated with a sustained loss of virus include high transaminase levels, low HBV DNA level, short duration of infection, and active hepatitis histologically.

2. Passive immunoprophylaxis with hepatitis B immune globulin is recommended after sexual or needle-stick exposure and in all infants born to HBsAg-positive mothers, along with vaccination. Genetically engineered Recombivax HB and Engerix-B have replaced the plasma-derived vaccine, Hepatavax B, in the United States. Approximately 95 to 99 per cent of immunocompetent individuals develop anti-HBs after three intramuscular doses. For adults over 20 years, the dose of Recombivax HB is 10 μg/1.0 ml and that of Engerix-B 20 μg/1.0 ml. Both should be given at 0, 1 to 2, and 4 to 6 months. These are among the safest of vaccines and there are no contraindications in pregnancy. Candidates include all infants and all children under 11 not previously vaccinated and those individuals at increased risk.

Hepatitis C

Epidemiology

1. Marked geographic differences in prevalence exist, but it is estimated that the worldwide prevalence is 1 per cent and the general U.S. population prevalence is 1.8 per cent. Blood donor screening has resulted in a decline in the number of transfusion-related cases. The risk is 0.6 per cent per patient or 0.03 per cent per unit transfused.

2. Intravenous drug use is the most common cause identified. The prevalence of HCV in hemodialysis patients is up to 45 per cent, and seroconversion rates for health care workers with a needle stick are 0 to 4 per cent. Sexual transmission is infrequent but does occur in less than 5 per cent of cases.

Clinical Manifestations and Diagnosis

1. Rarely is acute infection identified. For those with chronic HCV, the most common complaint is fatigue. Other symptoms include abdominal discomfort, nausea, anorexia, and depression. Table 96–2 lists the extrahepatic manifestations.

2. Second-generation assays have improved sensitivity and specificity. Viral detection and quantitation can be accomplished with polymerase chain reaction (PCR) amplification or branched-chain DNA (bDNA) assays.

3. Infection with HCV persists in most patients who were infected. Disease progression is silent, and at least 2 decades are required before patients develop clinically significant disease.

4. HCV is the most common indication for liver transplantation. Recurrence after transplantation is nearly universal, but only 10 per cent of patients develop severe recurrence.

Treatment and Prevention

1. Treatment is recommended for those patients with no contraindications and who are at greatest risk for progressive liver disease. These patients may have persistently elevated serum ALT, HCV RNA positivity, and/or histologic evidence of inflammation, necrosis, and fibrosis. Patients with decompensated cirrhosis should not be treated; liver transplantation evaluation should be considered.

2. IFN-α alone or in combination with ribavirin (Virazole) has been approved for patients with HCV.

a. The standard dose is 3 million units subcutaneously three times a week. The dose of ribavirin is weight dependent but ranges from 1000 to 1200 mg/day. Treatment is given for 6 to 12 months.

   b. Normalization of ALT and sustained loss of HCV RNA define efficacy. The rates of sustained virologic response are approximately 40 per cent. Pretreatment variables that indicate a favorable response to therapy include HCV genotype 2 or 3, low HCV RNA levels, and the absence of cirrhosis on liver biopsy.

   c. The majority of patients have flu-like symptoms early in the course of therapy. Giving the medication at nighttime or premedicating with acetaminophen may be helpful. Severe side effects such as suicidal ideation, acute cardiac or renal failure, or autoimmune thyroid disease are seen in less than 2 per cent of patients. The major side effect of ribavirin is hemolytic anemia, which may mandate a dosage reduction. Hemoglobin should be checked at two and four weeks after therapy is started and then again as clinically indicated. Ribavirin is considered a teratogen and all patients should practice an effective contraceptive method.

3. Continued education of risk groups and screening of blood products, as well as organs and body fluids, remain our best tools at present. Investigative efforts to develop a vaccine for HCV continue.

Hepatitis D

1. The delta agent (HDV) requires HBV in order to spread from cell to cell. Areas of high prevalence are Italy, Eastern Europe, Columbia, Venezuela, and western Asia.

2. The transmission of HDV is similar to that of HBV. HDV can be a superinfection on established HBV infection, or a patient could have an acute co-infection with both HBV and HDV. Patients with co-infection generally have a complete recovery but are more likely to experience a fulminant course than those with HBV alone. Greater than 80 per cent of patients with superinfection will develop chronic progressive liver disease.

3. Anti-HDV IgM is positive in early acute infection and may persist for long periods of time in those with chronic disease. One test that may distinguish acute co-infection from superinfection is the presence of anti-HBc IgM.

4. Acute infection requires supportive care, with transplantation consideration for those with fulminant disease. Chronic HDV may benefit from IFN-α therapy. There are no factors that

will predict which patients may respond to therapy. Prevention of percutaneous routes of transmission (i.e., intravenous drug use) with education and behavior modification is the goal.

Hepatitis E

1. HEV is associated with epidemics wherein people were exposed to fecally contaminated water. The attack rate is only 1 to 10 per cent, and the overall fatality is less than 4 per cent. However, pregnant women in the third trimester are at a definite risk for HEV, with the fatality rate nearly 20 per cent.

2. The first phase (prodromal and preicteric) is characterized by fever and malaise in 95 to 100 per cent of patients. The icteric phase is characterized by jaundice, anorexia, nausea and vomiting, abdominal pain, and peak serum transaminase levels.

3. Most clinical laboratories do not perform testing for HEV. Diagnosis is generally made after exclusion of other illnesses.

4. Most patients do well with no chronic sequelae. Treatment is supportive, with liver transplantation evaluation for those with fulminant disease. Travelers to endemic areas are advised to avoid drinking water and beverages with ice and eating uncooked shellfish and unpeeled fruits and vegetables.

Hepatitis G (HGV or GBV-C) and Transfusion-Transmitted Virus (TTV)

1. Hepatitis G was identified in patients with clinically significant non-A, non-B hepatitis that was not HCV. The virus is now characterized as another RNA virus that is similar to but distinct from HCV. TTV is a newly discovered virus that is transmitted through transfusion. Although viremia is common, liver disease has not been proven.

2. HGV is common in blood donors regardless of whether or not there is ALT elevation.

3. Clinical manifestations, natural history, and pathogenesis for HGV have not been characterized. PCR is the means by which diagnosis can be made.

Bibliography

Koff RS: Hepatitis A. Lancet 1998;351:1643–1649.
Lee WM: Hepatitis B virus infection. N Engl J Med 1997; 337:1733–1745.

Lemon SM, Thomas DL: Vaccines to prevent viral hepatitis. N Engl J Med 1997;336:196–204.

McHutchison JG, Gordon SC, Schiff ER, et al: Interferon alfa-2b alone or in combination with ribavirin as initial treatment for chronic hepatitis C. N Engl J Med 1998; 339:1485–1492.

NIH Consensus Statement: Management of hepatitis C. 1997;15:1–41.

Sjogren MH: Serologic diagnosis of viral hepatitis. Med Clin North Am 1996;80:929–956.

Terrault NA, Wright TL: Viral hepatitis A through G. In Feldman M, Scharschmidt BF, Sleisenger MH (eds): Gastrointestinal and Liver Disease: Pathophysiology/Diagnosis/Management, 6th ed, pp. 1123–1170. Philadelphia, WB Saunders Company, 1998.

97 Hyperbilirubinemia

Michael David Bernstein

Etiology

Unconjugated (Indirect) Hyperbilirubinemia

1. Overproduction of bilirubin
   a. Hemolysis, intravascular: disseminated intravascular coagulation (DIC)
   b. Hemolysis, extravascular
      (1) Hemoglobinopathies
      (2) Enzyme deficiencies, such as glucose-6-phosphate deficiency
      (3) Autoimmune hemolytic anemias
   c. Ineffective erythropoiesis
   d. Hematoma
   e. Blood transfusions
2. Hereditary unconjugated hyperbilirubinemia
   a. Gilbert's syndrome (autosomal dominant)
   b. Crigler-Najjar syndrome type I (autosomal recessive)
   c. Crigler-Najjar syndrome type II (autosomal dominant)
3. Drugs
   a. Chloramphenicol: neonatal hyperbilirubinemia
   b. Vitamin K: neonatal hyperbilirubinemia
   c. 5β-Pregnane-$3\alpha,20\alpha$-diol: cause of breast milk jaundice

Conjugated (Direct) Hyperbilirubinemia

1. Inherited disorders
   a. Dubin-Johnson syndrome (autosomal recessive)
   b. Rotor syndrome (autosomal recessive)
2. Hepatocellular diseases and intrahepatic causes
   a. Viral hepatitis and autoimmune hepatitis
   b. Alcoholic hepatitis
   c. Drug-induced hepatitis: isoniazid (INH), nonsteroidal anti-inflammatory drugs (NSAIDs), trimethoprim-sulfamethoxazole (Bactrim), zidovudine
   d. Cirrhosis
   e. Drug-induced cholestasis: perchlorperazine, haloperidol (Haldol), estrogens
   f. Sepsis
   g. Postoperative jaundice
   h. Infiltrative liver disease: tumor, abscesses (pyogenic, amebic), tuberculosis (TB), parasites (*Toxoplasma*), *Pneumocystis carinii* pneumonia, *Echinococcus*
   i. Primary biliary cirrhosis
   j. Primary sclerosing cholangitis (PSC)
3. Extrahepatic causes
   a. Gallstone disease
   b. Pancreatitis-related stricture
   c. Pancreatic head tumor
   d. Cholangiocarcinoma
   e. PSC

Production and Elimination

Bilirubin is a waste product of heme metabolism, largely produced in the spleen, where senescent red blood cells are destroyed. The bilirubin is bound to albumin and transported to the liver, where it is taken up and conjugated with glucuronic acid by the enzyme uridine diphosphoglucuronyl transferase (UDPGT). It is then excreted into the bile. Hyperbilirubinemia can result from overproduction, failure of conjugation, or failure to excrete into bile at the level of the canaliculus or the common bile duct.

1. Indirect hyperbilirubinemia is usually the result of overproduction of bilirubin.
2. Hemolysis: Either intravascular as in DIC or extravascular as in hemolytic anemia. Transfusions of blood and resorbing hematomas also can increase bilirubin levels. The total bilirubin level rarely rises above 4 mg/dl in these states.
3. Gilbert's disease is a probable autosomal dominant disease characterized by indirect hyperbilirubinemia caused by a deficiency of UDPGT. Inadequate conjugation of bilirubin leads to decreased elimination in bile and accumulation of indirect bilirubin. Levels range from 1 to 6 mg/dl. The disease is usually asymptomatic, but overt jaundice can occur at times of stress, such as starvation, intercurrent disease, or alcohol consumption. The diagnosis is made by excluding hemolysis or intrinsic liver disease. Phenobarbital will rapidly decrease serum indirect bilirubin level, but treatment is unnecessary because the disease has an excellent prognosis.

4. Crigler-Najjar syndrome type I is inherited as an autosomal recessive disease. It is manifested by the onset of severe indirect hyperbilirubinemia 3 to 4 days after birth. Levels of indirect bilirubin are in the range of 20 to 50 mg/dl. Bilirubin encephalopathy or kernicterus usually leads to death within the first year. The disease is caused by complete or near-complete deficiency of UDPGT with failure to excrete unconjugated nonpolar bilirubin into the bile. A lack of response to phenobarbital is characteristic. Definitive treatment is liver transplantation. Phototherapy, which converts bilirubin into more polar excretable photoisomers, done over a 12-hour period may serve as temporary therapy (see Fig. 95–1).

5. Crigler-Najjar syndrome type II is a probable autosomal dominant inherited disease characterized by deficiency of UDPGT but associated with less severe indirect hyperbilirubinemia than in type I. Bilirubin levels range between 7 and 20 mg/dl. Type II is responsive to phenobarbital treatment (60 to 180 mg/day) with a rapid decline in plasma bilirubin level. The diagnosis rests on exclusions of intrinsic liver disease or hemolysis and a dramatic response to administration of phenobarbital. Unlike type I disease, type II disease has an excellent prognosis. It rarely requires treatment except in the newborn with seriously rising bilirubin levels (see Fig. 95–1).

6. Physiologic jaundice results from deficient UDPGT activity in the first week of life combined with increased destruction of red blood cells, leading to indirect hyperbilirubinemia in the newborn. This is usually benign and resolves by the first week of life.

7. Breast milk jaundice is a benign disease that results either from a β-glucuronidase that metabolizes bilirubin diglucuronide or a fatty acid in breast milk that inhibits UDPGT.

8. Post-transfusion and hematoma resorption: Indirect hyperbilirubinemia results from overproduction of unconjugated bilirubin that overwhelms the conjugating system. Intrinsic liver disease must be excluded.

9. Familial conjugated hyperbilirubinemia
   a. Dubin-Johnson syndrome, an autosomal recessive disease, is associated in Iranian Jews with factor VII deficiency. Dubin-Johnson syndrome results from defective secretion of conjugated bilirubin. Characteristically, the liver appears black due to accumulation of a black pigment contained in lysosomes. The plasma bilirubin level approaches 2.5 mg/dl but can rise as high as 20 mg/dl. Typically, total urine coproporphyrin levels are normal or slightly increased, and there is a reversal in the ratio of urinary coproporphyrin I to coproporphyrin III, with greater coproporphyrin I levels. Additional findings include a nonvisualizing oral cholecystogram (OCG) and a second peak in sulfobromophthalein plasma levels 45 to 90 minutes after intravenous injection. Phenobarbital may lower bilirubin levels in some patients. Patients are generally asymptomatic, and prognosis is excellent.
   b. Rotor syndrome is an autosomal recessive disease that is similar to Dubin-Johnson syndrome in course and treatment. In contrast, however, black pigment does not accumulate, OCG is visualized, and the sulfobromophthalein curve, while abnormal, does not show a second plasma peak. Urinary coproporphyrin levels are increased, and the ratio is less dramatically reversed than in Dubin-Johnson syndrome.

10. Hepatocellular disease (Table 97–1)
    a. Hepatitis A, B, C, D, E, or G and autoimmune hepatitis: liver cell destruction with rise in aspartate transaminase (AST)/alanine transaminase (ALT) (SGOT/SGPT) to 10 to 50 times the upper limit of normal and possible jaundice with bilirubin ranging from 0 to 20 mg/dl, mostly direct
    b. Drugs such as acetaminophen, INH, NSAIDs: same as above
    c. Alcohol: with AST 6 to 10 times the upper limit of normal and ALT 2 to 3 times the upper limit of normal, with increased bilirubin related to liver cell destruction
    d. Ischemic hepatitis: very high transaminase levels, 100 times the upper limit of normal, with increased bilirubin

11. Cholestatic disease
    a. Drugs such as phenothiazines, sulfonylureas, allopurinol, and estrogens: alkaline phosphatase 5 to 10 times the upper limit of normal
    b. Viral, such as cytomegalovirus, Epstein-Barr virus, hepatitis C, and cholestatic hepatitis A: alkaline phosphatase 5 to 10 times the upper limit of normal
    c. Infiltrative disease, such as TB, lymphoma, *Mycobacterium avium-intracellulare*, hepatoma, metastatic carcinoma, or sarcoid, diagnosed by liver biopsy: alkaline phosphatase 5 to 10 times the upper limit of normal
    d. Gram-negative sepsis

TABLE 97–1. GENERAL LABORATORY FINDINGS IN DIRECT HYPERBILIRUBINEMIA (APPROXIMATES THAT MAY BE SEEN)

DISEASE	BILIRUBIN (mg/dl)	ALKALINE PHOSPHATASE (U/L)	AST (IU/L)	ALT (IU/L)	ALBUMIN (gm/dl)
Alcoholic liver disease	0–20	5–10 × nl	5–6 × nl	2 × nl	nl or ↓
Acute viral hepatitis and autoimmune hepatitis	0–20	2–3 × nl	10–50 × nl	10–50 × nl	nl
Drug-induced cholestasis	0–20	5–10 × nl	5–10 × nl	5–10 × nl	nl
Common bile duct obstruction	0–20	5–10 × nl	nl to 2–3 × nl	nl to 2–3 × nl	nl
Malignant bile duct obstruction	0–20	5–20 × nl	nl to 1.5–2 × nl	nl to 1.5–2 × nl	nl
Primary biliary cirrhosis	0–20	1.5–20 × nl	nl	nl	nl or ↓
PSC	0–20	1.5–20 × nl	nl	nl	nl or ↓
Ischemic hepatitis	0–20	3–5 × nl	20–50 × nl	20–50 × nl	nl

Abbreviations: ALT, alanine transaminase; AST, aspartate transaminase; nl, normal; PSC, primary sclerosing cholangitis.

e. Primary biliary cirrhosis, diagnosed by antimitochondrial antibodies and liver biopsy

12. Extrahepatic cholestasis

a. Gallstone disease: Ultrasound and computerized tomographic (CT) findings show dilated common bile duct with possible stones. Generally, alkaline phosphatase is 5 to 10 times the upper limit of normal, with smaller elevations of AST and ALT and a bilirubin less than 20 mg/dl. Endoscopic retrograde cholangiopancreatography (ERCP) is the "gold standard" for visualization of stones in the common bile duct. Magnetic resonance cholangiopancreatography (MRCP), which is both sensitive and specific for common bile duct stones, may become the initial test of choice for choledocholithiasis in the future.

b. Benign strictures of intra- and extrahepatic ducts: Examples include PSC and pancreatitis-related strictures. Alkaline phosphatase is disproportionately elevated in relation to AST and ALT. ERCP is diagnostic.

c. Neoplasm: cholangiocarcinoma, Klatskin tumors, pancreatic carcinoma; usually high alkaline phosphatase out of proportion to AST and ALT. Diagnosis is made with aid of CT scan, ultrasound, and ERCP.

 ## Bibliography

Jansen PL, Oude Elfeink RP: Hereditary conjugated hyperbilirubinemia in Wistar rats: a model for the study of ATP-dependent hepatocanalicular organic ion transport. Adv Vet Sci Comp Med 1993;37:175–195.

Lidofsky S, Scharschmidt BF: Jaundice. In Feldman M, Scharschmidt BF, Sleisenger MH (eds): Sleisinger and Fordtran's Gastrointestinal and Liver Disease: Pathophysiology/Diagnosis/Management, 6th ed, pp 220–232. Philadelphia, WB Saunders Company, 1998.

Polin RA: Management of neonatal hyperbilirubinemia: rational use of phototherapy. Biol Neonate 1990; 58(Suppl 1):32–43.

Schiff ER, Schiff L: Diseases of the Liver. Philadelphia, JB Lippincott Company, 1993.

Zakim D, Boxer TD: Hepatology: A Textbook of Liver Disease. Philadelphia, WB Saunders Company, 1990.

98 Cirrhosis

Goutham Rao

Etiology

Cirrhosis refers to the process characterized by fibrosis through which the normal architecture of the liver is gradually replaced by structurally abnormal nodules. It is the response by the liver to a wide variety of inflammatory, toxic, and metabolic insults.

1. Common causes
   a. Alcohol: by far the most common cause of cirrhosis in the United States
   b. Infectious hepatitis B and C: Hepatitis B is a common cause of cirrhosis in many other parts of the world
2. Less common causes
   a. Other drugs and toxins such as isoniazid and methotrexate
   b. Autoimmune diseases such as primary biliary cirrhosis, which affects mostly middle-aged women
   c. Metabolic disorders such as hemochromatosis, Wilson's disease, and α_1-antitrypsin deficiency
   d. Other uncommon causes such as Budd-Chiari syndrome and chronic right heart failure

Symptoms

Unfortunately, no set of symptoms is specific for cirrhosis. Some patients are asymptomatic, and their disease is detected incidentally with the aid of physical findings and specific laboratory tests. Many patients present with nonspecific symptoms, including fatigue, malaise, and abdominal pain. Others manifest symptoms of chronic liver disease, including pruritus and jaundice.

Key Symptoms

General	Symptoms Common to Other Liver Diseases
• Fatigue	• Pruritus
• Malaise	• Jaundice
• Abdominal pain	

Clinical Findings

There is no single clinical finding or constellation of findings that are diagnostic of cirrhosis. As in the case of symptoms, patients with cirrhosis often present with findings consistent with chronic liver disease. Some findings are specific to particular etiologies. Kayser-Fleischer corneal rings, for example, are found only in patients with Wilson's disease. Signs of chronic liver disease that may be present in patients with cirrhosis include spider nevi, palmar erythema, gynecomastia, and testicular atrophy. If portal hypertension is present, splenomegaly, ascites, esophageal varices, and prominence of the veins of the abdominal wall (caput medusa) may be evident. The cirrhotic liver itself is usually enlarged except in the very advanced stages of disease, when it is shrunken in size. It is firm or even very hard in consistency.

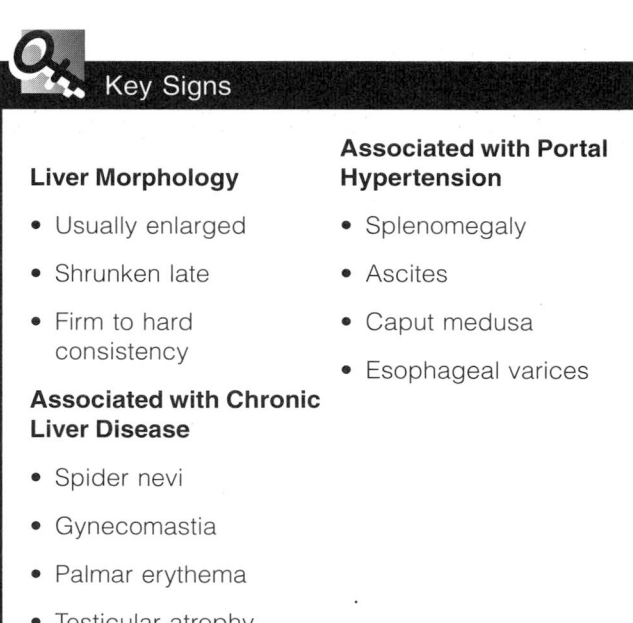

Key Signs

Liver Morphology	Associated with Portal Hypertension
• Usually enlarged	• Splenomegaly
• Shrunken late	• Ascites
• Firm to hard consistency	• Caput medusa
Associated with Chronic Liver Disease	• Esophageal varices
• Spider nevi	
• Gynecomastia	
• Palmar erythema	
• Testicular atrophy	

Laboratory Tests

1. Liver cirrhosis is ultimately a histologic diagnosis. Liver biopsy with pathology examination, therefore, remains the gold standard diagnostic test. It also helps pinpoint the cause of cirrhosis. In hemochromatosis, for example, excess iron is found in bile duct cells and hepatocytes. Liver biopsy should be undertaken with care in patients with coagulation abnormalities.

2. Imaging studies may reveal findings compatible with liver cirrhosis. Ultrasound with color Doppler imaging, for example, can be used to detect changes in blood flow associated with portal hypertension, ascites undetectable by physical examination, and increased echogenicity. Computerized tomography (CT) and magnetic resonance imaging (MRI) also play a role in diagnosis. MRI is useful in distinguishing focal hepatic lesions, such as metastases, from cirrhosis.

3. A decreased serum albumin level and prolonged prothrombin time are serum abnormalities characteristic of cirrhosis. The serum bilirubin is elevated in jaundiced patients. Levels of the liver enzymes aspartate transaminase (AST), alanine transaminase (ALT), and alkaline phosphatase are usually elevated in cirrhotic patients, depending upon the etiology of cirrhosis and the stage of disease.

4. Other laboratory tests are employed to determine the cause of cirrhosis when it is not apparent. In Wilson's disease, for example, the serum ceruloplasmin level is reduced. In hemochromatosis, the serum ferritin is elevated.

Key Tests

- Liver biopsy
- Ultrasound with color Doppler
- CT
- MRI
- Serum albumin
- Prothrombin time
- Serum bilirubin
- AST
- ALT
- Alkaline phosphatase

Differential Diagnosis

Some clinical features associated with cirrhosis are also found in other conditions. The differential diagnosis, therefore, depends upon the presentation.

1. Ascites: also found in right heart failure, pancreatic disease, malignancy, lymphatic obstruction and hepatic vein thrombosis

2. Bleeding esophageal varices: Other causes of upper gastrointestinal bleeding (e.g., bleeding ulcers) should be considered.

3. Hepatic encephalopathy: The encephalopathy associated with liver failure in cirrhotic patients can be confused with other causes of mental impairment, including dementia, drugs, and renal failure.

Treatment

Treatment of cirrhosis should target the underlying cause (e.g., abstinence from alcohol for alcoholic cirrhosis, phlebotomy for hemochromatosis) to preserve hepatic function and prevent complications. Complications include bleeding varices, ascites, spontaneous bacterial peritonitis, hepatorenal syndrome (renal failure associated with cirrhosis), hepatic encephalopathy, hepatocellular carcinoma, and malnutrition. Several treatments are available for complications if they arise. Surgical treatments include placement of a transjugular intrahepatic portosystemic shunt (TIPS) for treatment of esophageal varices. Liver transplantation remains an ultimate treatment for selected patients.

Medication

1. Ascites: spironolactone (Aldactone), initial dose of 50 to 100 mg PO bid and up to 400 mg/day to promote diuresis; furosemide (Lasix), 40 to 160 mg PO qd in patients unresponsive to spironolactone alone

2. Esophageal varices: propranolol (Inderal), or nadolol (Corgard), in doses that do not cause bradycardia, can be used as prophylaxis against bleeding.

3. Spontaneous bacterial peritonitis: cefotaxime (Claforan), IV 2 gm q6h as initial therapy

4. Hepatic encephalopathy
   a. Lactulose, 30 mL three or four times daily
   b. Neomycin, 500 to 1000 mg PO q6h
   c. Metronidazole (Flagyl) (alternative to neomycin), 250 mg three or four times daily

Diet

Protein-calorie malnutrition is common among patients with advanced liver disease. Nutritional supplementation by enteral formulas may be necessary. Encephalopathic patients, however, benefit from a low-protein (2 gm/day or less) diet. Patients with ascites should restrict their salt intake to 2 gm/day or less. Alcohol should be completely avoided in all patients.

Activity

No standard activity restrictions are recommended for any patients with cirrhosis. Bed rest is recommended for patients with severe ascites.

Patient Education

1. Patient education should be designed with the specific etiology of cirrhosis in mind. Patients

with alcoholic cirrhosis, for example, should not only be told to abstain from alcohol but also directed to appropriate treatment programs for alcoholism. Patients with infectious hepatitis should be encouraged to practice "safer sex" and to avoid sharing needles for intravenous drugs. Information about hepatotoxic medications (e.g., large doses of acetaminophen) should be provided.

2. In general, patients need to understand that liver cirrhosis is a serious condition with devastating consequences that requires careful monitoring. Close follow-up with their physician should be very much encouraged, especially with the onset of new symptoms. Patients should weigh themselves daily and record weights in a diary to be reviewed by their physician.

Key Treatments

- Avoidance or removal of cause of cirrhosis

- Spironolactone for ascites

- Propranolol or nadolol for esophageal varices

- Lactulose and/or neomycin for hepatic encephalopathy

- Enteral formula supplementation if indicated for malnutrition

Follow-Up

Patients who are stable and have no complications should be followed up at least once per year for clinical examination and monitoring of liver function tests. Unstable patients and those with complications, such as severe ascites, encephalopathy, varices, and hepatorenal syndrome, require more frequent clinical and laboratory monitoring—as often as once per week depending on the patient's condition.

Bibliography

Fitz G: Systemic complications of liver disease. In Feldman M, Scharschmidt BR, Sleisenger MH, (eds): Gastrointestinal and Liver Disease. Pathophysiology/Diagnosis/Management, 6th ed, pp 1334–1354. Philadelphia, WB Saunders Company, 1998.

Keeffe EB: Cirrhosis of the liver. In Dale DC, Federman DD (eds): Scientific American Medicine CD-ROM. New York, Scientific American, 1998.

McGuire BM, Bloomer JR: Complications of cirrhosis: why they occur and what to do about them. Postgrad Med 1998;103:209–224.

Schuppan D, Strobel D, Hahn EG: Hepatic fibrosis—therapeutic strategies. Digestion 1998;59:385–390.

Williams EJ, Iredale JP: Liver cirrhosis. Postgrad Med J 1998;74:193–202.

99 Gallstones and Cholecystitis

Michael H. Kleinman

Etiology

Gallbladder pathology encompasses a handful of diseases that may originate with gallstones or in the absence of gallstones. Over 400,000 cholecystectomies are performed in the United States each year for various indications.

1. Cholelithiasis
   a. Seventy per cent cholesterol-based
      (1) Caused by stasis plus nucleating agents
      (2) Predisposing factors: obesity, estrogen, pregnancy, genetics (Pima Indians)
   b. Thirty per cent pigment-based
      (1) Bilirubinate polymer (hemoglobin breakdown) and calcium salts
      (2) Predisposing factors: cirrhosis, hemolysis (sickle cell disease, thalassemia, spherocytosis, prosthetic valves)
2. Noncalculous gallbladder dysfunction (i.e., biliary dyskinesia)
   a. May comprise 10 per cent of gallbladder disease.
   b. Poorly understood; may have several etiologies, including adhesions, anatomic variations.
3. Acalculous cholecystitis
   a. Five per cent of gallbladder disease
   b. Usually in elderly or diabetic patients
   c. Strongly associated with underlying vascular disease
   d. Often precipitated by unrelated surgery or critical illness
4. Carcinoma of the gallbladder
   a. Only 1 per cent of patients with gallstones
   b. Should *not* be used as an excuse for surgery.
   c. Calcified gallbladders are thought to have a higher risk of carcinoma and *should* be removed.

Symptoms

Symptoms of gallbladder disease are variable. Most patients who develop symptoms experience more frequent and severe attacks over time, leading to the need for cholecystectomy.

1. Postprandial bloating
2. Vague, poorly localized abdominal discomfort
3. Biliary colic: postprandial epigastric or right upper quadrant (RUQ) pain, waxing and waning in severity
   a. Radiates to the right back or tip of right scapula.
   b. Pronounced nausea, often with vomiting

WARNING

Epigastric pain radiating straight through to the back may represent biliary colic, but can also be caused by common duct obstruction or pancreatitis.

---

4. Acute cholecystitis
   a. May present with symptoms of biliary colic.
   b. Persistent pain
   c. Fever
   d. Leukocytosis
   e. Caused by obstruction of the cystic duct, usually with superimposed bacterial infection (*Escherichia coli*, *Klebsiella*, *Enterococcus*, and *Clostridium*)
5. Chronic cholecystitis
   a. May be minimally symptomatic.
   b. Nausea, vomiting, postprandial bloating, colicky pain, pain radiating to the back or tip of right scapula
6. Biliary dyskinesia: symptoms are similar to those of biliary colic or chronic cholecystitis.

Key Symptoms

- RUQ/epigastric pain
- RUQ/epigastric tenderness
- Fever

Clinical Findings

Classic Findings of Biliary Colic/Cholecystitis

1. Epigastric/RUQ tenderness
2. Specific tenderness over the gallbladder fundus just medial to the anterior axillary line
3. Exquisite tenderness of gallbladder fundus on palpation (Murphy's sign)
4. Progressive disease results in increased tenderness with guarding and rebound in the RUQ.

Atypical Findings

1. Spontaneous reduction in tenderness may represent
   a. Interposition of omentum between the inflamed gallbladder and the parietes
   b. Infarction of the gallbladder
2. Jaundice
   a. Most often occurs with common duct obstruction.
   b. Can occasionally occur with acute cholecystitis.
   c. If associated with fever, chills, hypotension, or change in mental status, one should suspect ascending cholangitis.

Key Signs

- Epigastric/RUQ tenderness
- Specific tenderness over the gallbladder fundus just medial to the anterior axillary line
- Exquisite tenderness of gallbladder fundus on palpation (Murphy's sign)

Laboratory Tests

1. The following should permit creation of a differential diagnosis of gallbladder disease (see Table 99–1).
   a. Complete blood count
   b. Liver function tests
   c. Amylase
2. Marked elevation of transaminases (>1000 IU) usually indicates hepatic injury rather than biliary tract disease
3. Mild elevations of bilirubin *may* reflect acute cholecystitis, but common duct stones or Gilbert's syndrome must be considered.

Diagnostic Tests

1. Plain abdominal films may detect gallstones but generally are not useful.
2. Ultrasound of gallbladder and biliary tree
   a. Is 95 per cent accurate in detection of gallstones.
   b. Is only 65 per cent accurate in detection of common duct stones.

TABLE 99–1.   LABORATORY TEST FINDINGS IN GALLBLADDER DISEASE

	WBC	TRANSAMINASES	ALKALINE PHOSPHATASE	TOTAL BILIRUBIN	DIRECT BILIRUBIN	AMYLASE
Biliary dyskinesia	N	N	N	N	N	N
Biliary colic		N	N	N	N	N
Acute cholecystitis	↑	↑	↑	N, sl ↑	N	N
Common duct obstruction	N, ↑	↑	↑↑	↑↑	↑↑	N
Ascending cholangitis	↑↑	↑	↑↑	↑ or ↑↑	↑ or ↑↑	N
Acute hepatitis	N, sl ↑	↑↑↑	↑↑	↑↑	↑	N
Gallstone pancreatitis	N, ↑, ↑↑	↑	↑	↑	N	↑↑↑
Gilbert's syndrome	N	N	N	sl ↑	N, sl ↑	

Abbreviations: N, normal; sl, slight; WBC, white blood cell count.

c. Thickening of the gallbladder is a variable finding not necessarily associated with acute disease.

3. Oral cholecystogram: imaging of the gallbladder via accumulation of iopanoic acid (dye) in the bile and hence the gallbladder; has significant false-positive and false-negative rates.

4. Nuclear biliary scanning (hepato-iminodiacetic acid [HIDA] or similar scan): the test of choice to establish the diagnosis of acute cholecystitis

   a. Radioactive isotopes (imidoacetic acid derivatives) are accumulated by the liver and excreted via the biliary tree.

   b. With normal bile circulation the gallbladder is seen promptly.

   c. If the cystic duct is obstructed, the gallbladder fails to visualize.

   d. If the gallbladder fails to visualize over 4 hours, the test is 98 per cent sensitive for acute cholecystitis.

   e. If the radiolabeled tracer fails to empty into the duodenum, common duct obstruction should be assumed until proven otherwise.

5. Fractional excretion HIDA scan is the best test of gallbladder function and biliary dyskinesia. The test begins as a routine HIDA scan. After the gallbladder is visualized, the patient is given a dose of cholecystokinin analogue (Kinevac). This stimulates gallbladder contraction, and an ejection fraction (per cent) is calculated.

   a. If the patient's ejection fraction is less than 35 per cent *and* injection of Kinevac is associated with biliary colic, cholecystectomy will alleviate symptoms in about 80 per cent of patients.

   b. A diminished gallbladder ejection fraction *without* elicitation of symptoms on injection of cholecystokinin is not sufficiently correlated with gallbladder disease to justify cholecystectomy.

6. Endoscopic retrograde cholangiopancreatography (ERCP)

   a. Not generally useful in detection of cholelithiasis

   b. Does allow evaluation of the common bile duct where associated biliary tract disease is suspected.

7. Intravenous cholangiography is no longer used because of risks posed by intravenous contrast.

8. Percutaneous transhepatic cholangiography (PTC) is not of specific value for gallstones or intrinsic gallbladder disease, but is used to delineate and decompress the extrahepatic biliary tree in cases of obstruction.

9. Magnetic resonance cholangiopancreatography (MRCP) uses magnetic resonance imaging to view the biliary tree. Not yet as accurate as ERCP, but may make possible *noninvasive* evaluation of the biliary tree as techniques are refined.

 Key Tests

- Ultrasound defines gallbladder anatomy
- HIDA scan—Best test for gallbladder function
  —Best test for acute cholecystitis

Differential Diagnosis

A variety of other visceral pathology can mimic gallbladder disease. Because the gallbladder is a foregut organ, it shares innervation with several other foregut organs.

1. Diseases for which similar presentation is common

   a. Esophageal spasm

   b. Esophagitis

   c. Gastritis

   d. Gastric or duodenal ulcer disease

   e. Pancreatitis

   f. Hepatitis

   g. Acute hepatic congestion resulting from right heart failure or Budd-Chiari syndrome

   h. Hepatic tumors, including hepatic adenoma

2. Diseases for which similar presentation is possible, not rare

   a. Angina

   b. Aortic dissection

   c. Aortic aneurysm

   d. Appendicitis (RUQ appendix either anterior or retrocecal)

   e. Pleurisy

   f. Right lower lobe pneumonia

   g. Pyelonephritis

Treatment

1. The otherwise healthy patient with asymptomatic gallstones should not undergo cholecystectomy.

2. Certain patients who are at higher risk for complications or tend to present with advanced disease should be considered for cholecystectomy.

   a. Young children with gallstones

   b. Diabetics

   c. Sickle cell disease patients

3. Patients who are undergoing other major abdominal surgery should be considered for cholecystectomy. There is substantial risk of new-onset gallbladder disease in previously asymptomatic patients in the postoperative period.

4. Patients with minimal symptoms may be considered for treatment with ursodiol (Actigall) and low-fat diet. Ursodiol is only effective in dissolution of cholesterol stones and requires a lengthy course of treatment. Risks and benefits of ursodiol should be discussed thoroughly with the patient, just as one would discuss the risks and benefits of surgery.

5. Purgative regimens may have a role in evacuating gallstones, but results have not been demonstrated widely enough for these to be accepted as standard therapy.

6. Cholecystectomy is the treatment of choice for symptomatic gallstones.
   a. Cholecystectomy is now performed laparoscopically in 90 per cent of cases.
      (1) Complication rates, while higher initially, are now about the same as for open cholecystectomy.
      (2) Most serious complications are bile leak, common duct injury, and visceral injury.
      (3) Blood vessel injury with embolism or hemorrhage also occurs.
      (4) Mortality rate for cholecystectomy is about 0.5 per cent, mostly in older patients with other medical problems and/or advanced gallbladder disease.
   b. Advantages of laparoscopic cholecystectomy
      (1) Earlier hospital discharge
      (2) Decreased postoperative pain
      (3) Reduced visible scars
      (4) Early return to normal activities

WARNING

Laparoscopic cholecystectomy is *not* minor surgery, nor is it painless. Patients should be informed of risks and expected postoperative course, just as with open surgery.

---

   c. In pregnancy, laparoscopic surgery may increase risk to the patient because of diminished operative space and to the fetus because of hypercarbia-induced acidosis.

7. Acute cholecystitis/biliary sepsis requires proper resuscitation prior to surgery.

   a. Nothing by mouth
   b. Vigorous hydration
   c. Broad-spectrum antibiotic coverage
      (1) Minimal to moderate symptoms: first- or second-generation cephalosporin
      (2) Significant toxicity, higher risk: ampicillin–clavulanic acid or other advanced penicillin derivative
   d. Surgical consultation
   e. Medication for pain: Demerol preferred over morphine because morphine causes spasm of the sphincter of Oddi

8. Cholecystostomy, done surgically or percutaneously, is reserved for patients with acute cholecystitis believed to be at very high risk for surgery. These procedures risk missing gangrenous changes and perforation with continued sepsis.

9. Gallbladder lithotripsy has been used to fragment stones and facilitate their dissolution. It is not widely available.

10. Methylterbutyl ether (MTBE) has been very effective in dissolving gallstones but requires direct instillation (by PTC or ERCP) and has potential for serious side effects if the chemical escapes the biliary tree.

Follow-Up

1. Patients who defer cholecystectomy should be followed at intervals and given warnings regarding the significance of increasing symptoms.

2. Patients who undergo uncomplicated cholecystectomy require no particular follow-up beyond the postsurgical period, traditionally 1 month.

3. Signs of early complications of cholecystectomy include jaundice, fever, persistent vomiting, abdominal distention, guarding, and rebound. Prompt re-evaluation by a surgeon is essential.

Bibliography

MacFadyen BV, Vecchio R, Ricardo AE, et al: Bile duct injury after laparoscopic cholecystectomy. Surg Endos 1998;12:315–321.

Nahrwold DL: Acute cholecystitis. In Sabiston DC (ed): Textbook of Surgery, 15th ed, pp 1126–1131. Philadelphia, WB Saunders Company, 1997.

Nahrwold DL: Chronic cholecystitis and cholelithiasis. In Sabiston DC (ed): Textbook of Surgery, 15th ed, pp 1132–1139. Philadelphia, WB Saunders Company, 1997.

Nahrwold DL: Cholangitis. In Sabiston DC (ed): Textbook of Surgery, 15th ed, pp 1140–1145. Philadelphia, WB Saunders Company, 1997.

Schwesinger WH, Diehl AK: Changing indications for laparoscopic cholecystectomy: stones without symptoms and symptoms without stones. Surg Clin North Am 1996;76:493–504.

100 Pancreatitis

C. S. Pitchumoni

Acute Pancreatitis

Etiology

1. Nearly 90 per cent of clinically acute pancreatitis is secondary to alcoholism or gallstone disease. Alcoholic pancreatitis is histologically chronic.

2. Rare causes include abdominal trauma, infections (mumps and other viral diseases), hyperlipidemias, hypercalcemia, drugs (thiazide, furosemide, valproic acid, dideoxyinosine sulfonamides, pentamidine, and azathioprine), postendoscopic pancreatography, and ductal abnormalities (pancreas divisum).

Symptoms

The primary symptom is *abdominal pain* in the epigastrium and left upper quadrant, radiating to the back, associated with nausea and vomiting, aggravated by eating food and partially relieved by sitting up and leaning forward, lasting for hours to days.

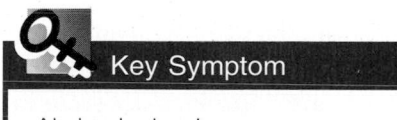

Key Symptom

Abdominal pain

Clinical Findings

1. Physical examination findings include a low-grade fever, tachycardia, tachypnea, and basal consolidation of the lung and minimal pleural effusion on the left side.

2. Bowel sounds are often feeble or totally absent in view of paralytic ileus.

3. Low blood pressure, rapid thready pulse, diaphoresis, and tachypnea indicate shock.

4. Rare findings include jaundice (common bile duct compression), distention of the abdomen, and a bluish discoloration of flanks (Grey-Turner sign) or of the periumbilical region (Cullen's sign).

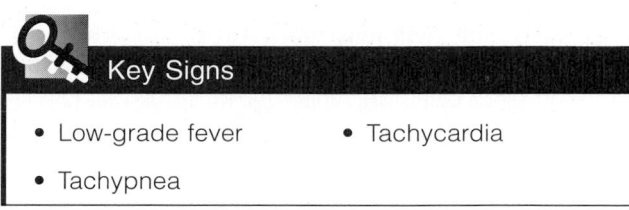

Key Signs

- Low-grade fever
- Tachycardia
- Tachypnea

Laboratory Tests

1. Serum amylase elevation
   a. Greater than four times normal is suggestive of acute pancreatitis.
   b. May be high in other conditions, such as acute cholecystitis, mesenteric thrombosis, intestinal obstruction, and perforated peptic ulcer.
   c. Does not correlate with prognosis.
   d. In hyperlipidemic pancreatitis, may not be appreciable.

2. Urine amylase levels are neither sensitive nor specific.

3. Serum lipase elevation is delayed but is more specific than amylase.

4. Routine blood counts and biochemical tests: Hemoglobin, hematocrit, leukocyte count, blood glucose, serum calcium, blood urea nitrogen, creatinine, liver function tests, and blood gas studies assist in the prognostic evaluation.

Radiologic Studies

1. Plain film of the abdomen in the upright position helps to exclude perforated peptic ulcer or intestinal obstruction. A dilated loop of jejunum (sentinel loop) or transverse colon (colon cutoff sign) is nonspecific.

2. Abdominal sonogram identifies gallbladder stones and the size of the common bile duct.

3. Computerized tomographic (CT) scan of the abdomen: The size of the pancreas, extent of necrosis, and the number and size of fluid collections help in the diagnosis and in assessing the prognosis.

Key Tests

- Plain film of abdomen
- CT scan of abdomen
- Abdominal sonogram

Prognosis

An uncomplicated acute pancreatitis subsides with conservative measures in 48 to 72 hours. Mortality is nearly 5 per cent.

Treatment

1. Total elimination of oral feedings (NPO) until pain subsides
2. Nasogastric tube aspiration of the stomach in all patients except in mild pancreatitis
3. Intravenous fluids to maintain fluid and electrolyte balance. (Intravenous calcium may be needed if there is hypocalcemia.)
4. Parenteral analgesics to relieve pain. Meperidine (Demerol), 75 to 100 mg intramuscularly q4h, is recommended.
5. Parenteral broad-spectrum antibiotics in severe biliary pancreatitis.
6. Surgical treatment when diagnosis is not clear, abscess is suspected, or no relief with conservative treatment. In gallstone-induced pancreatitis, cholecystectomy is to be performed during the same admission but only after the pancreatitis subsides.
7. Endoscopic papillotomy with stone extraction when common bile duct is dilated and a stone is impacted in the distal duct, and when ascending cholangitis is suspected.
8. Other complications of acute pancreatitis, such as pancreatic necrosis (sterile necrosis versus infected necrosis), pseudocyst, and pancreatic abscess, need prompt diagnosis and appropriate treatment.

Key Treatment

- NPO until pain subsides
- Nasogastric tube aspiration of stomach
- Intravenous fluids
- Parenteral analgesics

Chronic Pancreatitis

Etiology

Secondary to alcoholism (80 gm of alcohol per day for more than 15 years); rarely, idiopathic, hereditary, or tropical (in Afro-Asian countries attributed to nutritional deficiency).

Symptoms and Clinical Findings

1. Abdominal pain is recurrent, epigastric, radiating to the back, lasting for hours to days, and often precipitated by drinking alcohol.
2. Steatorrhea when 90 per cent of the pancreas is destroyed
3. Diabetes mellitus: a late manifestation, brittle in nature. Hypoglycemic episodes may be fatal.
4. Other complications include obstructive jaundice, pseudocyst, pancreatic ascites, pleural effusion, gastrointestinal bleeding (peptic ulcer, varices), and malnutrition (malabsorption, poor eating habits, and alcoholism).

Key Symptom

Recurrent abdominal pain

Key Sign

Epigastric tenderness

Tests

Laboratory Tests

1. Blood tests are not useful. Amylase or lipase elevations occur only in acute exacerbations.
2. Duodenal aspiration after intravenous secretin administration to estimate the volume and bicarbonate of pancreatic secretion (secretin test) is not practical.

Radiologic Tests

1. Flat-plate abdominal radiograph may reveal calculi; pathognomonic but notable only in a minority of patients.
2. Endoscopic retrograde cholangiopancreatography (ERCP): Dilated main pancreatic duct with strictures and intraductal filling defects and prominent side branches indicates chronic pancreatitis.
3. CT scan of abdomen may show calculi, ductal abnormalities, and pseudocyst.
4. Magnetic resonance cholangiopancreatography (MRCP) shows pancreatic and ductal morphology.

Other Tests

Miscellaneous tests: Chymex test and stool chymotrypsin levels helpful only in the diagnosis of exocrine insufficiency.

Key Tests

- Flat-plate abdominal radiograph
- ERCP
- CT scan
- Secretin stimulation test

Treatment

Symptomatic for pain, steatorrhea, and diabetes. Complications such as pseudocyst and pancreatic ascites may need surgery.

1. Pain
   a. Abstinence from alcohol
   b. Non-narcotic analgesics such as acetaminophen or aspirin
   c. Narcotic analgesics (fear of addiction)
   d. A low-fat diet/antioxidant supplementation
   e. Therapy with large doses of pancreatic extracts
   f. Endoscopic papillotomy, stent placement in selected cases, helpful in some patients
   g. Surgical treatment when the preceding measures fail
2. Steatorrhea: Oral enzyme supplements with meals, low-fat diet, and medium-chain triglyceride supplementation.

3. Diabetes: Calorie restriction is not needed, but insulin is to be administered only in small doses at frequent intervals.

Key Treatment

- Abstinence from alcohol
- Analgesics
- Pancreatic enzyme for steatorrhea
- Small doses of insulin for diabetes
- Surgery in selected cases

Bibliography

For more information on acute and chronic pancreatitis, see

Banks PA: Acute and chronic pancreatitis. In Feldman M, Scharschmidt BF, Sleisenger MH (eds): Sleisenger and Fordtran's Gastrointestinal and Liver Disease: Pathophysiology/Diagnosis/Management, 6th ed, vol I, pp 809–862. Philadelphia, WB Saunders Company, 1998.

For more information on complications of acute pancreatitis, see

Agarwal N, Pitchumoni CS: Acute pancreatitis: a multisystem disease. Gastroenterologist 1993;1:115–128.

For more information on management of acute pancreatitis, see

Banks PA: Practice guidelines in acute pancreatitis. Am J Gastroenterol 1997;92:337–386.

For more information on management of pain in chronic pancreatitis, see

Barnett JL, Owyang C: Medical management of chronic pancreatitis. In Howard J, Idezuki Y, Ihse I, et al (eds): Surgical Diseases of the Pancreas, 3rd ed, pp 335–341. Baltimore, Williams & Wilkins, 1998.

101 Pancreatic Carcinoma

Martin H. Poleski

Etiology

1. Ductal adenocarcinomas are responsible for 90 per cent of pancreatic cancers. The remaining cancers are of endocrine, connective tissue, acinar cell, epidermoid, and mixed cell origin. This chapter will consider the ductal cell cancers.

2. The incidence of pancreatic duct adenocarcinoma in the United States is approximately 10 per 100,000, with a male-to-female ratio of 1.3:1. Overall 2-year survival is 10 per cent; 5-year survival is 3 per cent. In surgical series 5 to 22 per cent of patients have resectable tumors; of these people, 15 per cent may survive 5 years.

3. Risk factors
   a. Cigarette smoking: relative risk of 1.5
   b. Diet high in fat and/or meat, low in vegetables and fruits
   c. Chronic pancreatitis of any origin, such as alcohol, familial: standardized incidence ratio of 26.3
   d. Diabetes mellitus
   e. Exposure chronically to 2-naphthylamine, benzidine, and gasoline derivatives
   f. Age greater than 60 years

Symptoms

1. Pain is usually the earliest symptom of the disease. The pain can be vague and may be diagnosed initially as nonulcer dyspepsia. More characteristic is discomfort in the back or abdomen that is worsened by lying or relieved by sitting or crouching.

2. Weight loss and/or depression may be present with or without the pain.

3. The onset of jaundice is also characteristic, since a majority of tumors occur in the head of the pancreas.

4. New onset of glucose intolerance may begin a year before diagnosis, and up to 80 per cent of patients are glucose-intolerant to some degree.

5. Other less common and nonspecific symptoms include anorexia, nausea, vomiting, and weakness.

6. Superficial thrombophlebitis (Trousseau's sign) occurs in less than 5 per cent of patients but occurs with other malignancies.

7. Obstruction of the pancreatic duct may lead to the onset of acute pancreatitis.

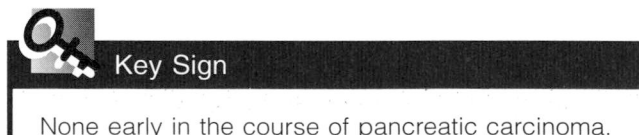

Key Symptoms

- Abdominal pain
- Weight loss
- Pruritus
- Jaundice
- New-onset diabetes

8. Variceal hemorrhage is very rare and occurs with invasion or compression of the splenic or portal veins.

Clinical Findings

1. Most patients who present early in the course of the disease have no physical findings.

2. If the common bile duct is obstructed as a result of a mass in the head of the pancreas, jaundice and scleral icterus may be found. In this situation, the gallbladder may be palpated 30 per cent of the time (Courvoisier's sign). Those with prolonged or marked jaundice may have excoriations and lichenification of the skin as a result of persistent scratching.

3. Hepatomegaly may be found in association with jaundice or in advanced disease may signify the presence of metastases.

4. Ascites or peripheral edema may be a sign of portal hypertension or peritoneal metastases.

Key Sign

None early in the course of pancreatic carcinoma.

Laboratory Tests

1. Routine blood tests in patients with early cancer may be normal. Laboratory studies that are frequently abnormal include elevated glucose, lipase, and amylase levels, all of which can also be elevated with benign diseases such as acute or chronic pancreatitis. Alkaline phosphatase and transaminases are often abnormal but are

nonspecific because they are often abnormal in a variety of hepatobiliary disorders.

2. No sensitive or specific serologic marker is available to aid in screening or diagnosis of pancreatic cancer. Mucinous glycoproteins such as CA 19-9 may be elevated (>37 units/ml) in 75 per cent of pancreatic cancers but are often elevated in other gastrointestinal malignancies, acute and chronic pancreatitis, and about 6 per cent of normal individuals. CA 19-9 levels greater than 70 units/ml in people suspected of having pancreatic cancer have a positive predictive value of 59 per cent and a negative predictive value of 92 per cent. CA 50 is another muciglycoprotein with sensitivity and specificity very similar to that of CA 19-9.

3. Ultrasonography (US) is the best initial diagnostic imaging test in patients suspected of pancreatic cancer. It is noninvasive, results in no radiation exposure, and can detect lesions as small as 2 cm, as well as pancreatic and bile duct dilations and hepatic metastases. It is also cheaper than the alternative, computerized tomography (CT). CT is better at staging pancreatic cancer and providing better definition of the tumor and its invasion of surrounding structures. CT depends less on the patient's body habitus or the operator's experience. If diagnosis is still in doubt after US and CT, endoscopic retrograde cholangiography (ERCP) and pancreatography may be performed. Magnetic resonance imaging has no significant advantage over CT. Angiography is no longer used as a diagnostic test for pancreatic cancer, although some surgeons use it to assess resectability and vascular anatomy preoperatively.

Key Tests

- US should be initial imaging study in suspected pancreatic cancer—75 per cent sensitivity, 85 per cent specificity.

- US- or CT-guided percutaneous needle biopsy can be done to confirm diagnosis in those who are not surgical candidates.

- Preoperative pancreatic biopsy to confirm cancer is controversial.

Differential Diagnosis

1. Chronic pancreatitis
2. Cholecystitis
3. Irritable bowel syndrome
4. Other causes of jaundice, hepatitis
5. Retroperitoneal lymphoma or sarcoma
6. Carcinoma of the duodenum
7. Common bile duct stones and strictures
8. Peptic ulcer disease
9. Depression
10. Ampullary carcinoma
11. Metastatic disease to the pancreas and/or retroperitoneum

Treatment

1. Surgery is the only form of curative therapy available for pancreatic cancer. Unfortunately, only 10 to 15 per cent of tumors are surgically resectable. Recent studies suggest that, of those patients who have successful resection, about 30 per cent are alive at 2 years and approximately 17 per cent at 5 years. Staging of pancreatic cancer to determine resectability requires the use of high-resolution CT scanners using a thin-section collimation (5 to 7 mm), an orally administered contrast agent to opacify the upper gastrointestinal tract, and acquisition of the scan at the dynamic phase of contrast enhancement with injection of a bolus of 150 to 180 ml of 60 per cent iodinated contrast material. This technique maximizes detection of the pancreatic tumor, as well as identification of hepatic metastases and vascular involvement. CT is almost 100 per cent accurate in predicting unresectability and 70 per cent accurate in predicting resectability. Because of the latter figure, some surgeons begin pancreatectomy with laparoscopy to detect occult metastases to the liver, peritoneum, and so on. Pancreatoduodenectomy (Whipple's operation) is still the most popular surgical technique. Total pancreatectomy is much less frequently used; occasionally, a distal pancreatectomy may be possible.

2. Some centers advocate the addition of pre- or postoperative radiotherapy with or without chemotherapy, usually 5-fluorouracil. Intraoperative radiotherapy also has been used. Chemoradiotherapy may delay or prevent local recurrence, but it is unclear whether it improves survival. Gemcitabine (Gemzar) is approved for the treatment of advanced pancreatic cancer.

3. Lesions of most patients are unresectable. Palliation of jaundice may be accomplished with a cholecystojejunostomy or choledochojejunostomy; duodenal obstruction can be bypassed with a gastrojejunostomy. Mean survival after palliative surgery is 5 to 6 months. Those patients whose projected survival is less than 3 months because of advanced disease, or who have other factors that increase their surgical

risk, can have jaundice relieved with stents. These can be placed endoscopically (ERCP). This technique is more comfortable for the patient than percutaneously placed stents. Stents may become blocked or infected and are replaced every 2 to 3 months on average.

4. *Pain management* is an important aspect of pancreatic cancer palliation. Pain often can be managed initially with acetaminophen or nonsteroidal anti-inflammatory drugs (NSAIDs). More severe pain requires the adequate use of narcotics such as morphine or codeine. Pain medications should be used on a regular basis and in combination, such as NSAIDs and codeine. In some patients, intraoperative or percutaneous neurolytic celiac plexus block can be effective in controlling pain.

5. Malabsorption may be a problem with mild to moderate steatorrhea. Pancreatic enzyme therapy with meals in an adequate dose to abolish diarrhea is usually successful.

Key Treatment

Surgery is the only curative therapy.

Bibliography

For general reference, see
Rosewicz S, Wiedenmann B: Pancreatic carcinoma. Lancet 1997;349:485–489.

For more information on the classification, see
Cubilla AL, Fitzgerald PJ: Classification of pancreatic cancer (nonendocrine). Mayo Clin Proc 1979;54:449–452.

For more information on risk factors, see
Lowenfels AB, Maisonneuve P, Cavallini G: Pancreatitis and the risk of pancreatic cancer. N Engl J Med 1993; 328:1433–1437.

For more on the methods of staging and imaging techniques, see
Rivera JA, Fernandez-del Castillo C, Warshaw AL: The preoperative staging of pancreatic adenocarcinoma. Adv Surg 1996;30:97–122.

For more on surgery and adjuvant therapy, see
Carmichael J, Fink U, Russell RC: Phase II study of gemcitabine in patients with advanced pancreatic cancer. Br J Cancer 1996;73:101–105.
Spitz FR, Abbruzzese JL, Lee JE: Preoperative and postoperative chemoradiation strategies in patients treated with pancreaticoduodenectomy for adenocarcinoma of the pancreas. J Clin Oncol 1997;15:928–937.

102   Common Reproductive Symptoms

SYMPTOM   NIPPLE DISCHARGE   *Elana Nudel Kripke*

Nipple discharge is a common office complaint. It is incumbent upon the primary care physician to determine whether it requires medical or surgical intervention. Initially one must distinguish between *spontaneous* discharge and *nonspontaneous* discharge (i.e., requiring manipulation to produce). Only spontaneous discharge is clinically significant. Evaluation is based on the type of discharge: milky (galactorrhea), purulent, nonbloody, or bloody.

Galactorrhea

Differential Diagnosis
1. Normal
2. Drugs: Common culprits are oral contraceptives, tricyclic antidepressants, tranquilizers, and cannabis.
3. Hyperthyroidism or hypothyroidism
4. Pituitary adenoma: Patient will have elevated prolactin levels. Prolactin level will be normal in the first three diagnoses listed. Nonpathologic galactorrhea can occur during puberty as well as during pregnancy. It can continue after pregnancy for months or years. Pituitary adenomas can cause infertility.

Refer to Ch. 124, Contraception; Ch. 177, Hypothyroidism; Ch. 178, Hyperthyroidism; and Ch. 184, Hyperprolactinemia.

History
1. Is the patient pubertal?
2. Careful reproductive history: pregnancy, infertility, lactation, menses
3. History of visual disturbances, headaches, and/or neurologic symptoms may suggest adenoma.
4. Medications?
5. Palpitations, weight change, changes in skin or hair may suggest thyroid disease.

Clinical Findings
1. Bilateral milky discharge
2. Visual field cut (with a pituitary adenoma)
3. Stigmata of thyroid disease

Tests
1. Prolactin level
2. Pregnancy test
3. Computerized tomography scan with contrast or magnetic resonance imaging of head with attention to sella turcica *if* patient has a significantly elevated prolactin level

Management
1. Observation alone (if normal prolactin level)
2. Bromocriptine for persistent galactorrhea not secondary to an adenoma
3. Referral to an endocrinologist

Purulent Discharge

A purulent discharge is almost always noted during lactation or pregnancy and secondary to bacterial infection, usually staphylococcal. Physical examination may reveal elevated temperature, erythema, and fluctuance, as well as purulent discharge. A sample should be sent for culture, and treatment with appropriate antibiotics should be instituted. If an abscess is suspected, treatment by incision and drainage is appropriate; biopsy of the abscess wall should be obtained to rule out malignancy.

Nonbloody Discharge

This includes green, brown, and yellow heme-negative discharge. It is the most common discharge and is usually benign. Patients first notice it on their bras or nightgowns or secondary to manipulation of the breast. It often occurs in association with menses.

Differential Diagnosis
1. Duct ectasia: The discharge from benign ectasia is usually from multiple ducts.
2. Carcinoma (rarely)

History

1. Breast manipulation?
2. Relation to menses?

Clinical Findings

1. Breasts are examined to determine which duct or ducts are secreting.
2. Breasts are palpated for underlying breast mass.

Tests

1. Mammogram: Should be done in women past 30 years of age or with strong family history of breast cancer.
2. Cytologic examination of fluid
3. Galactogram

Management

1. Advise patient to decrease breast manipulation.
2. If findings on palpation, mammogram, or cytologic examination are positive, prompt referral to a surgeon is appropriate.
3. Surgical transection of the mammary ducts is an option if work-up is negative and the discharge interferes with the patient's life.

Bloody Discharge

Sanguineous, serosanguineous, or clear hemepositive discharge is indicative of cancer until proved otherwise.

Differential Diagnosis

1. Intraductal papilloma
2. Duct ectasia
3. Carcinoma

Refer to Ch. 104, Breast Cancer

Clinical Findings and Tests

1. Prompt surgical referral
2. Mammogram
3. Cytologic examination of fluid

Management

1. Excisional biopsy of any mass
2. Excision of offending duct for pathologic evaluation if no mass is found

Follow-Up

If work-up is negative

1. Monthly breast examination for 1 year
2. Biannual mammograms for 1 year

PEARLS

- Bloody discharge is cancer until proved otherwise.

- Nipple discharge in *men* is cancer until proved otherwise.

- Discharge that is from multiple ducts or bilateral is rarely cancer.

- Breast cancer rarely presents as isolated nipple discharge.

- *Bilateral* discharge is usually normal or secondary to endocrine disorders or drugs.

- *Unilateral* discharge should raise suspicion of neoplasm or infection—consider surgical consultation.

Bibliography

King E, Goodson W: Discharges and secretions of the nipple. In Bland K, Copeland E (eds): The Breast, pp 61–67. Philadelphia, WB Saunders Company, 1991.

Leis HR Jr: Management of nipple discharge. World J Surg 1989;13:736–742.

State D: Nipple discharge in women. Postgrad Med 1991; 89:65–68.

Taber SW: The clinical challenge of nipple discharge. J Ky Med Assoc 1996;94:387–392.

SYMPTOMS DYSMENORRHEA

Stephen Paul

Pain with menstruation is reported to be the most frequent reason for which young females seek medical help. Dysmenorrhea is found to be the leading cause of absenteeism for adolescent females, in addition to contributing to a significant loss of working hours. The reported prevalence is from 30 to 80 per cent, with between 10 and 18 per cent of young females experiencing pain severe enough to restrict daily activities, including missing work or school.

Dysmenorrhea is divided into primary and secondary dysmenorrhea according to history, clinical findings, etiology, and treatment.

Differential Diagnosis

1. Primary dysmenorrhea
2. Secondary dysmenorrhea
   a. Endometriosis

b. Complications of pregnancy
   (1) Ectopic
   (2) Spontaneous abortion
   (3) Incomplete abortion
c. Pelvic inflammatory disease (PID)
d. Intrauterine device (IUD)
e. Ovarian cysts
f. Tumors
   (1) Adenomyosis
   (2) Fibroids: myomata uteri, leiomyoma
   (3) Malignant
g. Adhesions
   (1) Postoperative, dilatation and curettage
   (2) Endometriosis
   (3) Infections
h. Obstruction of the cervix
   (1) Congenital
   (2) Polyps
   (3) Submucous fibroids
   (4) Infection
   (5) Postprocedural: electrocautery, cryotherapy, conization, radiation
i. Congenital malformations
   (1) Müllerian duct
   (2) Bicornate uterus
   (3) Septate uterus
   (4) Rudimentary uterine horn
   (5) Cervical stenosis
j. Pelvic congestion

Primary dysmenorrhea is noted for having a typical history (see below) in the absence of clinical findings or pelvic pathology. The pathophysiology of primary dysmenorrhea is related to an increase in prostaglandin $F_{2\alpha}$ ($PGF_{2\alpha}$) concentration in the endometrial lining shed during menstruation, resulting in increased myometrial resting tone and pressures, frequency of contractions, uterine hypoxia, and smooth muscle contractions. Prostaglandin concentrations with resulting endometrial effects are greater in women with dysmenorrhea than in asymptomatic women.

Secondary dysmenorrhea is associated with pelvic pathology. Increase in prostaglandin concentration is also reported in association with IUD use and in some cases of endometriosis and uterine fibroids.

Refer to Ch. 107, Endometrial Cancer; Ch. 109, Ovarian Cancer; Ch. 112, Pelvic Inflammatory Disease; Ch. 119, Endometriosis; Ch. 122, Ectopic Pregnancy; and Ch. 124, Procedure; IUD Insertion and Removal.

History

1. Complete menstrual history
2. Family history of dysmenorrhea
3. Sexual history, including method of contraception
4. Description of pain, including
   a. Temporal relationship of pain to age at menarche
   b. Temporal relationship (onset, duration, intensity) of pain to menses
   c. Quality, whether pain is referred elsewhere
5. Associated symptoms such as nausea, vomiting, diarrhea, headache, dizziness, or fatigue
6. Limitation of daily activities
7. Previous treatment attempts and results
8. Risk factors increasing duration, severity, and occurrence of dysmenorrhea include early age at menarche and long menstrual periods. Smoking and alcohol increase the length and duration of dysmenorrhea.

Primary dysmenorrhea becomes symptomatic after ovulation, often after the first few menstrual cycles after menarche. Eighty per cent of symptomatic females develop dysmenorrheic symptoms within the first 3 years after menarche. Incidence of primary dysmenorrhea is greatest in the teens and early twenties and declines with increasing age. The pain of primary dysmenorrhea typically begins 1 to 2 hours before menstrual flow and lasts several hours to 1 to 2 days, often decreasing with menstrual flow. The pain is usually a diffuse, dull ache centered in the midline lower abdomen, just above the pubis, often radiating to the lower back and/or anterior thighs. Symptoms of nausea, vomiting, diarrhea, headache, dizziness, or fatigue are often associated with primary dysmenorrhea.

Secondary dysmenorrhea is typically noted either with the first menstrual cycles after menarche (congenital problems) or much later, usually after age 25. The pain of secondary dysmenorrhea often begins a few days before menstrual flow and lasts longer. Pain from secondary dysmenorrhea is atypical, sometimes chronic, and varies in description and temporal relationships depending on the etiology. With endometriosis the pain is often deep and aching and may radiate to the rectum or the perineum, many times increasing with each successive cycle, and is often associated with dyspareunia, menorrhagia, or infertility. The pain with PID is often greatest premenstrually and decreases with menses. Pain secondary to IUD use appears after placement of the IUD. Cervical obstruction is noted for scant menstrual flow with pain throughout menses. Fibroids usually affect women in their forties and are associated with menorrhagia. Menorrhagia is also associated with endometriosis, tumors, PID, and polyps.

Clinical Findings

1. Primary dysmenorrhea
   a. Physical findings are normal.
   b. Pelvic examination may not be necessary in non–sexually active adolescents with a typical history.
2. Secondary dysmenorrhea: Pelvic examination is recommended for
   a. Non–sexually active females with an atypical history
   b. All sexually active females
   c. Rule out
      (1) Endometriosis (best performed in late luteal phase), painful nodules in posterior cul de sac, restricted uterine motion
      (2) Infection (bilateral adnexal and cervical motion tenderness with discharge)
      (3) Placement and location of IUD
      (4) Pelvic mass, uterine enlargement
      (5) Adhesions (restricted uterine motion)
      (6) Cervical obstruction and abnormalities (inability to pass a small probe)
      (7) Pelvic congestion (engorged pelvic vasculature, uterine enlargement and tenderness)
      (8) Congenital malformations

Tests (If Clinically Indicated)

These tests are recommended to identify specific pelvic pathology if clinically indicated by history and physical examination. A therapeutic trial of medication is often recommended first, with the following tests employed after failure of trial of treatment, unless clinically indicated.

1. Pregnancy test
2. Papanicolaou smear
3. Cultures with sensitivities (include gonorrhea and chlamydia)
4. Pelvic ultrasound
5. Exploratory laparoscopy
6. Hysterosalpingogram
7. Hysteroscopy

Pap smear is used to rule out cancer. Cultures are utilized to identify infection in PID. Pelvic ultrasound is used to look for pregnancy, fibroids, and other tumors, ovarian cysts, and congenital malformations. Invasive tests are recommended only after noninvasive tests and trial of treatments are exhausted. Exploratory laparoscopy is the diagnostic test for endometriosis and other pelvic pathology. Hysterosalpingogram and hysteroscopy are used to identify abnormalities in the uterus such as polyps, adhesions, tumors, and congenital malformations.

Management

1. Primary dysmenorrhea
   a. Medication (see below)
   b. Transcutaneous electrical nerve stimulation (TENS) unit
   c. Investigational methods not approved or not conclusively proven by randomized, blinded clinical trials
      (1) Calcium channel blockers
      (2) Osteopathic manipulative treatment
      (3) Clonidine
      (4) Acupuncture
      (5) Transdermal nitroglycerin
      (6) Fish oil (ω-3 polyunsaturated fatty acids)
2. Secondary dysmenorrhea
   a. Trial of medication (see below)
   b. Treat cause—correct and/or treat underlying pathology
   c. Surgery is reserved for intractable, severely debilitating pain as last resort; caution patient as to risks versus benefits of surgical procedure.
      (1) Presacral neurectomy
      (2) Laster ablation of uterosacral nerves/ligaments

Medication

1. The nonsteroidal anti-inflammatory medications (NSAIDs) (prostaglandin inhibitors)
   a. Benefits
      (1) Summary of clinical trials reports successful alleviation of symptoms in 56 to 100 per cent.
      (2) Suppress $PGF_{2\alpha}$ synthesis, which decreases $PGF_{2\alpha}$ concentration in endometrium, resulting in decrease in uterine contractility and pressures, an increase in platelet aggregation, and a decrease in menstrual blood lost
      (3) May be helpful in pain associated with IUDs, endometriosis, and fibroids.
   b. Instructions
      (1) Take with first symptoms or with onset of menstrual flow.
      (2) Allow 3- to 6-month trial.
      (3) If poor response, change to NSAID of different family.
   c. Medication and dosages

(1) Naproxen (Naprosyn), 500 then 250 mg q6–8h (longer duration of action)

(2) Naproxen sodium (longer duration *and* rapid onset)

    (a) Anaprox, 550 then 275 mg q6–12h

    (b) Aleve, 440 then 220 mg q6–12h

(3) Ibuprofen (Motrin), 400 mg q6–8h

(4) Fenamates (also block action of $PGF_{2\alpha}$ at target organs)

    (a) Mefenamic acid (Ponstel), 500 then 250 mg q6–8h

    (b) Meclofenamate sodium (Meclomen), 100 then 50 to 100 mg q6–8h

(5) Other NSAIDs

d. Contraindications: currently pregnant or a history of hypersensitivity reaction to NSAIDs, bronchospasm, peptic ulcer disease, gastrointestinal bleeding

e. Side effects: nausea, gastrointestinal discomfort and/or bleeding, dizziness, visual disturbances, hemolytic anemia, rash, tinnitus

2. Oral contraceptives (low-dose combination)

a. Benefits

(1) Reported to be 80 to 90 per cent effective

(2) Ideal if patient desires contraception

(3) Inhibit ovulation

(4) Decrease concentration of $PGF_{2\alpha}$ in menstrual fluid, decreasing uterine contractions and amount of menstrual flow

b. Medication and dosage—oral contraceptive of choice

c. Contraindications and side effects as per oral contraceptive guidelines

Activity

1. No conclusive evidence with regard to exercise.

2. Aerobic exercise has been recommended, and it does not appear to worsen symptoms.

Patient Education

1. See above (medications) for instructions on treatment options. Patients should be reassured of diagnosis and response to treatment. Understanding and empathy for psychological impact of disability from symptoms should be noted, along with encouraging the patient to resume normal activities.

2. Pamphlet: *Dysmenorrhea* (publication no. APO46, 1985). Available from the American College of Obstetricians and Gynecologists, 600 Maryland Avenue SW, Suite 300 East, Washington, DC 20024-2588. May leave requests by e-mail through their Web site: *www.acog.org.*

3. Griffith HW: Dysmenorrhea (Menstrual Cramps). In Instruction for Patients, 6th ed, p 143. Philadelphia, WB Saunders Company, 1998.

4. Web sites: *www.AAFP.org/patientinfo/pelvicpa. html*; *www.acog.org*; *www.thriveonline.com*; *www.womens-health.com*; *www.intelihealth. com.*

PEARLS

- *Primary dysmenorrhea* is noted for onset 6 to 18 months after menarche in the teens and early twenties. The pain starts 1 to 2 hours before menses, lasts 1 to 2 days, and is typically a dull ache in lower abdominal midline radiating to low back/anterior thighs and associated with nausea, vomiting, diarrhea, headache, dizziness, or fatigue.

- *Secondary dysmenorrhea* occurs with first menses or later, often in women older than age 25. The pain begins earlier and lasts longer than the pain in primary dysmenorrhea.

- Dysmenorrhea associated with menorrhagia, dyspareunia, infertility, vaginal discharge, or IUD use warrants further work-up.

- Warning women to start NSAID treatment only with onset of menstrual flow will help prevent potential teratogenic effects of NSAIDs used during pregnancy.

- Counseling women using oral contraceptives of the benefit of decreased symptoms of dysmenorrhea may increase compliance.

Follow-Up

1. Assess effectiveness and/or side effects of treatment; change family of medications if necessary.

2. Investigate possible complications

a. Decrease in daily activities secondary to symptoms may lead to depression or anxiety.

b. Sexually transmitted diseases

c. Infertility secondary to pathology in secondary dysmenorrhea

Bibliography

For more information on risk factors for dysmenorrhea, see

Harlow SD, Park M: Longitudinal study of risk factors for occurrence, duration and severity of menstrual cramps in a cohort of college women. Br J Obstet Gynaecol 1996;103:1134–1142.

For more information on dysmenorrhea, see
Menstrual problems and common gynecological concerns: dysmenorrhea. In Hatcher RA, Trussell J, Stewart F, et al: Contraceptive Technology, 17th ed, pp 96–99. New York, Irvington Publishers, 1998.

For more information on the treatment of dysmenorrhea, see
Kaplan B, Rabinerson D, Lurie S, et al: Clinical evaluation of a new model of a transcutaneous electrical nerve stimulation device for the management of primary dysmenorrhea. Gynecol Obstet Invest 1997;44: 225–259.

For more information on treatment of dysmenorrhea with nonsteroidal anti-inflammatories, see
Dawood MY: Nonsteroidal antiinflammatory drugs and reproduction. Am J Obstet Gynecol 1993;169:1255–1265.

SYMPTOM AMENORRHEA

Carol A. Baase

Amenorrhea is the absence of menstruation in a woman of reproductive age. *Primary amenorrhea* occurs when there is no menses by the age of 16. In *secondary amenorrhea*, there is an absence of periods for 6 months in a woman in whom normal menstruation had been established.

Differential Diagnosis

1. Pregnancy: the most common explanation for amenorrhea

2. Menopause: symptoms include hot flashes, night sweats, and vaginal dryness. The follicle-stimulating hormone (FSH) and luteinizing hormone (LH) levels are elevated.

3. Hypothalamic amenorrhea, including

   a. Functional amenorrhea caused by a failure of the LH surge that is required for ovulation. The FSH level and estrogen stimulation are normal. A progesterone challenge test induces withdrawal bleeding. This pattern can be caused by emotional stress, concurrent illness, sudden weight loss, or increase in exercise and will usually resolve on its own.

   b. Amenorrhea associated with anorexia causes a more severe disruption of the hypothalamic-pituitary axis. There is loss of LH release, and estrogen secretion is low. A progesterone challenge test does not induce a withdrawal bleed. Normal menstrual function is resumed with weight gain.

   c. Athlete's amenorrhea is characterized by hypothalamic suppression and a hypoestrogenic state. The progesterone challenge test fails to induce a withdrawal bleed. Energy expenditure (stress) and level of body fat both have critical roles contributing to the amenorrhea.

4. Hyperprolactinemia accounts for up to 20 per cent of the cases of secondary amenorrhea. Prolactin inhibits the release of gonadotropin-releasing hormone from the hypothalamus, resulting in the cessation of FSH and LH release.

Only about one third of women with high prolactin levels will have galactorrhea. Causes of hyperprolactinemia include

   a. Prolactin-secreting adenomas

   b. Idiopathic hyperprolactinemia: clinically indistinguishable from adenoma except there is no tumor

   c. Hypothyroidism

   d. Drug-induced hyperprolactinemia: phenothiazines, thioxanthenes, and other dopamine antagonists

5. Other pituitary lesions are less common, but amenorrhea may be the first clue of their existence. Headache and visual defects are late signs of an expanding mass. Pituitary ischemia and infarction (Sheehan's syndrome) develop in the setting of an obstetric hemorrhage.

6. Polycystic ovarian disease (Stein-Leventhal syndrome) is characterized by amenorrhea, hirsutism, infertility, and obesity. The ovaries are enlarged, with increased stroma and a thickened capsule. Anovulation is caused by increased secretion of androgen, which is converted to estrogen in adipose tissue. This hyperestrogenic state stimulates the pituitary to secrete an elevated LH:FSH ratio, leading to further anovulation. A progesterone challenge test induces a withdrawal bleed.

7. Asherman's syndrome is generally the result of overly vigorous curettage, which results in intrauterine scarring with destruction of the endometrium.

8. Structural abnormalities typically cause primary amenorrhea and include an imperforate hymen, absence of the cervix or uterus, and absence of the vagina.

9. Chromosomal abnormalities can produce problems with gonadal development. Examples include Turner's syndrome (45,XO) and mosaicism.

10. Endocrine disorders: These include uncontrolled diabetes mellitus, severe hypo- and hyperthyroidism, and Cushing's syndrome.

Refer to Ch. 121, Menopause; Ch. 128, Pregnancy; Ch. 177, Hypothyroidism; Ch. 184, Hyperprolactinemia; and other endocrine disorders in Part X.

History

A detailed history should include

1. Menstrual history, including age of menarche, character of normal cycles, pattern and timing of periods. This is helpful in determining anovulatory periods because they tend to be irregular in interval, duration, and amount of flow.

2. Any prior pregnancies or abortions

3. History of sexual activity, contraception use, and any pregnancy symptoms

4. Changes in exercise and eating habits

5. Medications and drug use

6. Emotional stressors

7. Physical symptoms, including headache, breast discharge, changes in body hair pattern, and symptoms of thyroid and adrenal disease

8. Family history of a problem similar to the patient's

Clinical Findings

1. Assessment of weight and height, in search of possible anorexia, polycystic ovary disease, or genetic disorder

2. Breast development and other secondary sexual characteristics, assessing for hormonal presence

3. Body hair distribution and virilization

4. Breast examination, seeking evidence of galactorrhea or darkening of the areola (occurring in pregnancy)

5. Assessment of visual fields for possible pituitary tumor

6. Pelvic examination, looking specifically for any clitoromegaly, intact patent vagina, appearance of cervix, presence and size of uterus, and size of ovaries

Tests

1. Pregnancy test: All patients should have pregnancy ruled out before proceeding further.

2. Prolactin assay should be done early in all cases of secondary amenorrhea. If elevated, computerized tomography (CT) or magnetic resonance imaging (MRI) is warranted.

3. Progestin challenge test: Administer medroxyprogesterone acetate (Provera), 10 mg orally once daily for 5 days. After stopping the medication, the patient will either bleed or not bleed within 2 to 7 days.

   a. Bleeding confirms that there is adequate endogenous estrogen and that the amenorrhea is caused by anovulation. If the prolactin is normal and there is no galactorrhea, further evaluation is not needed.

   b. If there was no withdrawal bleeding, further testing is needed.

4. Estrogen/progestin cycle: Administer 2.5 mg conjugated estrogen daily for 21 days. Add medroxyprogesterone acetate, 10 mg daily, for the last 5 days. Absence of withdrawal bleeding confirms that there is an end-organ problem (e.g., Asherman's syndrome, cervical obstruction).

   If there is withdrawal bleeding, proceed with

5. FSH: If this is elevated, the diagnosis is ovarian failure (menopause).

   If the FSH is normal or low, proceed with

6. CT scan or MRI to rule out a pituitary tumor. If normal and the prolactin is low, the diagnosis is hypothalamic amenorrhea with a hypoestrogenic state.

7. Chromosomal evaluation is reserved for those patients with ovarian failure who are under 30 years of age or for those with evidence of a genetic disorder.

Management

Anovulatory Amenorrhea

1. Medication

   a. Monthly administration of a progestational agent (10 mg medroxyprogesterone acetate daily for 10 days) every 1 to 2 months to prevent hyperplasia of the endometrium *or*

   b. Oral contraceptive pill for younger patients

2. Patient education

   a. Treatment for induction of ovulation is available, and fertility can be achieved.

   b. Use of the progestational agent alone does not provide contraceptive protection should ovulation occur.

Hyperprolactinemic Amenorrhea

1. Medication: Bromocriptine (Parlodel), 2.5 mg daily, to reduce the prolactin level and often control or reduce the adenoma

2. Patient education: Fertility can be achieved with the use of bromocriptine.

Hypoestrogenic Amenorrhea

1. Medication

   a. Oral contraceptives for younger patients *or*

   b. Conjugated estrogen, 0.625 mg daily, days 1 through 25; add medroxyprogesterone acetate, 10 mg, days 16 through 25.

2. Patient education
   a. Advise about the risk of developing osteoporosis and encourage adequate calcium intake.
   b. Encourage those with amenorrhea secondary to inadequate fat stores to gain weight.

Follow-Up

1. All patients should be followed annually to review any problems or concerns.
2. Patients with hyperprolactinemia should have annual prolactin level testing and radiologic evaluation of the pituitary.

PEARLS

- Always rule out pregnancy before proceeding with an amenorrhea evaluation.

- Use the stepwise approach to evaluate all amenorrhea and a cause will be determined in the majority of patients.

- Tailor management decisions according to the cause of amenorrhea.

Bibliography

For more information on amenorrhea, see
Kiningham R, Apgar B, Schwenk T: Evaluation of amenorrhea. Am Fam Physician 1996;53:1185–1194.
Scherzer W, McClamrock H: Amenorrhea. In Berek J (ed): Novak's Gynecology, 12th ed, pp 809–832. Baltimore, Williams & Wilkins, 1996.
Speroff L, Glass R, Kase N: Clinical Gynecological Endocrinology and Infertility, 5th ed, pp 401–456. Baltimore, Williams & Wilkins, 1994.
For more information on amenorrhea in athletes, see
Kolnick AA: "Female athlete triad" risk for women. JAMA 1993;270:921–923.
Marshall L: Clinical evaluation of amenorrhea in active and athletic women. Clin Sports Med 1994;13:371–387.

SYMPTOM | **ABNORMAL VAGINAL BLEEDING**   *Diane K. Beebe*

Abnormal vaginal bleeding may result from gynecologic lesions, structural abnormalities, infections, hormonal disturbances, or underlying systemic disease. Causes may differ depending on age group.

Differential Diagnosis

1. Prepubertal age group
   a. Vulvovaginitis
   b. Vaginal trauma may result from three causes:
      (1) Accidents from a fall on a sharp object
      (2) Foreign bodies
      (3) Sexual abuse
   c. Urologic abnormalities, such as urethral prolapse
   d. Ovarian tumors: Two thirds are benign.
      (1) Follicular cysts
      (2) Juvenile granulosa cell tumors
      (3) Carcinomas, such as embryonal cell, are rare.
   e. Vaginal
      (1) Tumors, most commonly benign
      (2) Polyps and hymenal tags
   f. Hormonal stimulation
      (1) Menstruation secondary to precocious puberty
      (2) Exogenous estrogen exposure, most commonly oral contraceptive ingestion
2. Reproductive age group
   a. Pregnancy
      (1) Early: spontaneous abortion, ectopic pregnancy, gestational trophoblastic disease (hydatidiform mole), lesions of the cervix or vagina
      (2) Late: placenta previa (usually bright red, painless bleeding) and abruptio placentae (usually dark red, painful bleeding)
      (3) Trauma (motor vehicle accidents, domestic abuse, falls)
   b. Hormonal abnormalities
      (1) Dysfunctional uterine bleeding
      (2) Endocrine diseases
         (a) Ovarian dysfunction or tumor
         (b) Hyper- or hypothyroidism
         (c) Diabetes mellitus
         (d) Pituitary dysfunction
         (e) Adrenal dysfunction or tumor
   c. Infections: endometrial or cervical

d. Uterine pathology
   (1) Leiomyoma: most common benign neoplasm of the uterus. Submucosal leiomyomas are more likely to bleed than intramural ones because of disruption of endometrial vasculature.
   (2) Endometrial polyps
   (3) Neoplasms
   (4) Use of an intrauterine contraceptive device
e. Cervical polyps, lacerations, and carcinoma
f. Vaginal trauma, neoplasia, and atrophy
g. Vulvar atrophy and neoplasia
h. Underlying systemic disease
   (1) Coagulopathies: thrombocytopenia, von Willebrand's disease, or vitamin K deficiency
   (2) Hepatic disease
   (3) Renal disease
i. Medications: steroids, anticoagulants, oral contraceptives, anti-inflammatory agents, major tranquilizers and neuroleptics, chemotherapeutic agents, digitalis, phenytoin
j. Nutritional factors such as obesity, iron deficiency anemia, vitamin C deficiency

3. Postmenopausal age group
   a. Hormonal disturbances
   b. Cervical lesions, including carcinoma
   c. Endometrial lesions, most benign

Refer to Ch. 106, Cervical Cancer; Ch. 107, Endometrial Cancer; Ch. 108, Dysfunctional Uterine Bleeding; Ch. 110, Vaginitis; Ch. 121, Menopause; Ch. 122, Ectopic Pregnancy, Ch. 124, Contraception; Ch. 128, Pregnancy; Ch. 131, First Trimester Bleeding; Ch. 132, Third Trimester Bleeding; Ch. 133, Postpartum Hemorrhage; and Part X, Metabolic and Endocrine Diseases

---

History
1. Pattern of bleeding (onset, duration)
2. Medical illness such as thyroid, renal, liver, or blood disorders, history of bleeding or easy bruising
3. Gynecologic history, such as previous or recent gynecologic disorders or infections, last menstrual period, menstrual history, associated moliminal symptoms, contraceptive use, and sexual history
4. In young children, sexual abuse questioning and access to exogenous estrogens
5. Drug use

Important Patterns of Abnormal Uterine Bleeding

- Menorrhagia: excessively heavy or prolonged menstrual bleeding
- Metrorrhagia: irregular intermenstrual bleeding
- Polymenorrhagia: menses at less than 21-day regular intervals
- Menometrorrhagia: regular but excessive uterine bleeding

Clinical Findings
1. Vital signs, especially blood pressure, pulse, and weight
2. Thyroid examination
3. Hirsutism or stria may suggest adrenal disease.
4. Petechia or ecchymosis for evidence of bleeding disorders
5. Cervical abnormalities such as polyps or lesions
6. Uterine size to suggest fibroids or pregnancy

Tests
1. Blood analysis
   a. Complete blood count and platelet count
   b. Human chorionic gonadotropin
   c. Thyroid functions
   d. Prolactin, follicle-stimulating hormone, luteinizing hormone
   e. Renal/hepatic studies
2. Tissue sampling
   a. Cervical: Pap smear, biopsy
   b. Endometrial: biopsy, dilatation and curettage, hysteroscopy-directed
3. Imaging
   a. Pelvic sonogram
   b. Transvaginal ultrasonography
   c. Saline infusion sonohysterography
   d. Computerized tomography
   e. Magnetic resonance imaging
   f. Hysterosalpingography

Management
1. Perineal hygiene, particularly in prepubertal age group
2. Antibiotics for bacterial organisms present
3. Hormonal therapy
   a. Combination oral contraceptives: for acute bleeding, 4 pills daily for 4 days, then 3 pills daily for 3 days, followed by routine oral contraceptives for several months
   b. Oral progestins (medroxyprogesterone ace-

tate), 10 mg daily for the first 10 days of each month on a cyclic basis. For active bleeding, 10 mg three times a day.

   c. Intravenous estrogen, 25 mg q4–6h for four to six doses, usually resolves bleeding within 24 hours.

   d. Gonadotropin-releasing hormone agonists (leuprolide, naferelin) for pituitary-gonadal suppression in chronic anovulatory bleeding, followed by cyclic low-dose estrogen and progestin

4. Danazol for endometriosis, 200 to 400 mg twice daily for 3 to 6 months

5. Nonsteroidal anti-inflammatory drugs for pain as well as reduction of blood loss

6. Transfusion for hemorrhage or a hemodynamically unstable patient

7. Surgery

   a. Dilatation and curettage

   b. Endometrial ablation for refractory anovulatory bleeding

   c. Hysterectomy for uterine fibroids, endometrial hyperplasia, refractory anemia, or bleeding

---

PEARLS

- In the prepubertal age group, bleeding is most commonly associated with vulvovaginitis.

- In the nonpregnant reproductive age group, dysfunctional uterine bleeding, a diagnosis of exclusion, is most common.

- Postmenopausally, hormonal disturbances, followed by cervical and uterine abnormalities, are most common.

Bibliography

Brenner PF: Differential diagnosis of abnormal uterine bleeding. Am J Obstet Gynecol 1996;175:766–769.

Fishman A, Paldi E: Vaginal bleeding in premenarchal girls: a review. Obstet Gynecol Surv 1991;46:457–460.

Kenney A: Abnormal vaginal bleeding in young women. Int J STD AIDS 1997;8:82–87.

Long CA, Cowan BD: Abnormal uterine bleeding. In Jacobs AJ, Gast MJ (eds): Practical Gynecology, pp 158–164. Reading, MA, Appleton & Lange, 1994.

Weiss RM: The management of abnormal uterine bleeding. Hosp Pract 1992;Oct:55–78.

SYMPTOM VAGINAL DISCHARGE

Jennifer R. Kessmann

Vaginal discharge, whether physiologic or pathologic, is one of the most common presenting complaints in gynecology practices. Vaginitis, although frequently caused by infection, often has a noninfectious etiology. Establishing an accurate diagnosis can often be difficult but is imperative for treatment success. Using a combination of clues from the history and findings from the exam will help the practitioner to accurately diagnose and treat vaginal discharge.

Many different factors play a role in maintaining the delicate ecosystem found within the vagina. Adequate estrogen levels and a pH less than 4.5 create an environment for the growth of lactobacilli. Lactobacilli produce hydrogen peroxide and lactic acid, which inhibit the growth of other pathogenic bacteria. Discovering factors that have disrupted this acidic environment can be very beneficial in preventing problems in the future.

Differential Diagnosis

Infectious

1. Bacterial vaginosis (*Gardnerella vaginalis*, *Haemophilus*, *Corynebacterium*): etiologic agent in 50 per cent of cases of vaginitis

2. *Candida*: etiologic agent in 20 to 25 per cent of cases; 80 per cent caused by *C. albicans*, 15 to 20 per cent caused by *C. glabrata* or *C. tropicalis*

3. Trichomoniasis: cause in 15 to 20 per cent of cases

4. *Mycoplasma* or *Ureaplasma*

5. Herpes simplex or human papillomavirus

6. Nonspecific vaginitis: caused by group A streptococcus, *Staphylococcus*, *Escherichia coli*, enterococci; more common in the prepubescent female

7. *Neisseria gonorrhoeae*, chlamydia cervicitis

8. Pinworm vaginitis

9. Retained foreign body with secondary infection

10. Idiopathic ulceration with human immunodeficiency virus (HIV) infection

Noninfectious

1. Allergy/hypersensitivity/contact dermatitis

   a. Deodorant hygiene products: tampons, pads, toilet paper, and soaps

b. Contraceptives: latex condoms and spermicides

c. Medications/treatment creams: povidone-iodine douches, topical antimycotic creams

2. Desquamative inflammatory vaginitis
3. Atrophic vaginitis
4. Erosive lichen planus
5. Collagen vascular disease, Behçet's syndrome, pemphigus syndromes
6. Idiopathic vaginitis
7. Physiologic discharge

History

1. Duration of symptoms
2. Color, odor, consistency of discharge
3. Any new sexual contacts
4. Last menstrual period
5. Pruritus
6. Self-treatment attempts
7. Chronic diseases

Symptoms and Clinical Findings

The symptoms and clinical findings in the most common types of infectious vaginitis are shown in Table 102–1.

Tests (See Also Table 102–1)

1. Wet prep: In bacterial vaginosis, more than 10 to 20 per cent of the squamous cells are clue cells. Yeast, spores, and pseudohyphae are found in candidiasis, and motile protozoans are found in trichomoniasis (60 to 80 per cent sensitive in symptomatic patients). Trichomonads may be nonmotile and more ovoid with hypertonic saline. False positives occur with Pap smear readings in trichomoniasis.

2. PH: The normal pH of the vagina is 4.0. In candidiasis, the pH consistently remains less than 4.5. If the pH is greater than 4.5, consider trichomoniasis or bacterial vaginosis. In the postmenopausal female, when the pH is neutral, consider atrophic vaginitis.

3. Application of 10% KOH: A positive "whiff" test (fishy, amine odor when KOH applied) can be found in bacterial vaginosis. This test can also be positive in trichomoniasis.

4. Appropriate cultures
   a. *Candida albicans*: Nickerson's media at room temperature for 24 hours. (remember that *Candida* can be normal flora.)
   b. *Trichomonas vaginalis*: tricholt or Diamond's media
   c. *Neisseria gonorrhoeae*: chocolate agar
   d. Culture of no value in bacterial vaginosis.
   e. Consider aerobic cultures in prepubescent female with discharge.

5. Immunofluorescence studies can detect chlamydia in the office.

6. Consider colposcopy of vagina when no cause can be found.

Management

1. Identify etiology and begin treatment or remove offending agent.
2. Treat sexual partner in trichomoniasis, chlamydia, and *N. gonorrhoeae*.
3. Evaluate for possible systemic cause of the vaginitis.
4. In cases of recurrent *Candida* (considered more than four episodes per year), consider screening for diabetes and HIV. Yield is usually low.

Medications/Treatment (See Also Table 102–2)

1. Bacterial vaginosis: Consider metronidazole, either oral or intravaginal; clindamycin 2% vaginal cream; or oral clindamycin.

2. Trichomoniasis: Metronidazole (Flagyl) 2-gm single dose or 500 mg PO bid for 7 days for patient and partner. Both regimens are 90 to 95 per cent effective, and treating asymptomatic patients is beneficial.

TABLE 102–1. CHARACTERISTICS OF INFECTIOUS VAGINITIS

	BACTERIAL VAGINOSIS	TRICHOMONIASIS	CANDIDIASIS
Symptoms	Malodorous, purulent discharge	Malodorous, purulent discharge; dyspareunia	Pruritis, dyspareunia, soreness
Color of discharge	Gray/thin	Greenish or yellow/green, frothy/thin	Thick, white, clumpy
Examination	Discharge adherent in nondependent portions of vagina	Erythema of labia; "strawberry" cervix in 10%	Erythema and edema of labia
Wet prep	>20% of squamous cells are clue cells; absence of lactobacilli; positive "whiff" test with KOH	Motile trichomonads (60% of cases); may be nonmotile if hypertonic saline used	Budding yeast forms and pseudohyphae with KOH in 60–70%
pH	>4.5	5–7	>4.5

TABLE 102-2. TREATMENT OPTIONS IN THE NONPREGNANT FEMALE

Etiology	Treatment Options
Bacterial vaginosis	Metronidazole (Flagyl), 500 mg PO bid for 7 d (78% effective)
	Metro Gel 0.75%, 5 gm intravaginally bid for 5 d (75% effective)
	Clindamycin (Cleocin) 2% cream, 5 gm bid for 7 d (82% effective)
	or (alternate regimens)
	Metronidazole, 2 gm PO as single dose (less effective)
	Clindamycin, 300 mg bid for 7 d
Candidiasis	Topical azole drugs for 3 or 7 d (80–90% effective)
	Fluconazole (Diflucan), 150 mg PO as single dose
	Oral ketoconazole (Nizoral) or itraconazole (Sporanox) for 14 d with resistant cases
	Topical gentian violet 1% applied in office q wk for 2–3 wk
Trichomoniasis	Metronidazole, 2 gm PO single dose
	Metronidazole, 500 mg bid for 7 d (both regimens 90–95% effective)

3. Candidal vaginitis: Topical azole drugs (e.g., clotrimazole vaginal cream 1% [Myclex-7, Gyne-Lotrimin] or miconazole vaginal cream 2% [Monistat 7]) are effective in 80 to 90 per cent of cases. Oral fluconazole (Diflucan) as a single dose is also effective. Severe or recurrent candidiasis may require 10 to 14 days of a topical or oral azole.

4. Atrophic vaginitis: Oral or topical estrogens are very effective, but onset of action can be delayed.

Activity

1. Avoid sexual activity until patient and partner are cured.

2. Change damp clothing promptly after swimming or exercising.

Patient Education

1. Avoid tight-fitting clothing; wear cotton garments.

2. Avoid chemical irritants. Use showers rather than tub baths.

3. Discourage douching and using perfumes in the vaginal area.

4. Reinforce importance of completing entire course of medication.

5. Change tampons and sanitary napkins frequently.

Follow-Up

1. Consider reculturing in cases of chlamydia and *N. gonorrhoeae* to ensure cure.

2. If sexually transmitted disease found, counsel on prevention of other such diseases and consider further testing.

PEARLS

- Vaginal discharge/vaginitis may be caused by mixed agents.

- The most common causes include bacterial vaginosis (50 per cent), candidiasis (20 to 25 per cent), and trichomoniasis (15 to 20 per cent).

- The mere presence of *Candida* and/or *Gardnerella* does not always make either the etiologic agent because these can be normal flora in the reproductive age group.

- Bacterial vaginosis and trichomoniasis have been associated with premature delivery in pregnant females.

WARNINGS

- **Advise no alcohol for 48 hours after metronidazole.**

- **Creams (imidazole and clindamycin) weaken latex condoms.**

- **Oral fluconazole together with oral hypoglycemics may cause hypoglycemia.**

Bibliography

Centers for Disease Control and Prevention: 1998 Guidelines for the treatment of sexually transmitted diseases. MMWR Morb Mortal Wkly Rep 1998;47(RR-1):1–111.

Droegemueller W: Vaginitis. In Mishell DR, Stenchever MA, Droegemueller W, et al (eds): Comprehensive Gynecology, pp 624–635. St. Louis, CV Mosby Company, 1998.

Eschenbach DA: Diagnosis and treatment of vaginitis. In Stenchever MA (ed): Office Gynecology, 3rd ed, pp 317–340. St. Louis, CV Mosby Company, 1996.

Farrington PF: Pediatric vulvo-vaginitis. Clin Obstet Gynecol 1997;40:135–140.

Sobel JD: Vaginitis. N Engl J Med 1997;337:1896–1903.

Chronic pelvic pain (CPP) is a frequently encountered clinical symptom that is difficult to assess and treat. A careful, detailed history along with a problem-directed examination is necessary to appropriately diagnose and manage these patients. A multidisciplinary approach is often appropriate because this symptom may challenge even the best clinicians.

Differential Diagnosis

1. Endometriosis
2. Pelvic adhesions
3. Pelvic inflammatory disease (PID)
4. Musculoskeletal disorders
5. Urinary tract disease: infection, nephrolithiasis
6. Gastrointestinal tract disorders: irritable bowel syndrome (IBS), diverticular disease, inflammatory bowel disease
7. Dysmenorrhea
8. Other gynecologic disorders: ovarian cysts, mittelschmerz
9. Psychological: somatization disorder

History: Key Questions to Ask

1. Onset, location, character, radiation of pain?
2. Aggravating factors: standing, driving, climbing stairs, sexual intercourse?
3. Associated bowel or bladder symptoms?
4. Correlation with menstrual cycle phases?
5. Prior diagnostic tests and surgical procedures?
6. Prior sexual abuse?
7. Prior gynecologic history: vaginal deliveries, abortion, PID?

Careful attention to the chronologic course of pain is important. Endometriosis often begins as early dysmenorrhea, then progresses to constant pain that is worse with sexual intercourse. Adhesions often cause a positional pain aggravated by climbing stairs or driving. Spasm of the levator muscle often causes a "falling out" sensation.

It is also important to assess the patient's psychological response to pain. Her relationship with family and friends, degree of physical activity, and work productivity should be determined. A formal depression scale or psychological profile may be helpful in assessing the patient's quality of life and coping mechanisms.

Clinical Findings

The examination may be problem-directed if a more detailed examination has been done recently.

1. Observe gait, posture, and movement to examination table.
2. Note surgical scars.
3. Identify superficial abdominal muscle spasm or tenderness.
4. Exclude organomegaly, abdominal tenderness, or masses.
5. Determine lower extremity reflexes.
6. Piriformis muscle spasm is suggested when pain occurs with external rotation of a straightened leg.
7. Note ability to voluntarily relax vaginal introitus muscles, exclude disease.
8. Inspect cervix for signs of infection, malignancy, or intrauterine device use.
9. Determine size, mobility, and tenderness of uterus and ovaries with bimanual examination.
10. Palpation of nodules in the cul-de-sac or uterosacral ligaments suggests endometriosis.
11. Palpate coccyx, note whether levator muscles are relaxed.
12. Palpate anterior vaginal wall and urethra, determine if adnexal mass is present.
13. Perform rectovaginal examination to exclude nodularity of uterosacral ligaments, rectovaginal lesions.

Diagnostic Tests

1. Urinalysis: interstitial cystitis, urethritis, nephrolithiasis
2. Complete blood count: leukocytosis, anemia
3. Stool for occult blood and white blood cells
4. Plain film of abdomen: nephrolithiasis, free air
5. Cervical culture, test for gonorrhea and chlamydia
6. Ultrasound
   a. Pelvic ultrasound: May help to confirm suspicions found on clinical examination; incidental findings common.
   b. Abdominal ultrasound: gallstones, intra-abdominal mass, ascites
7. Colonoscopy: selected patients, dependent on clinical history and patient's risk for occult disease
8. Cystourethroscopy: if urologic origin suspected
9. Diagnostic laparoscopy: Rule out infection, neoplasm; confirm adhesions or endometriosis; map if future surgery planned.

Management

Patients with CPP have often reached a point of despair and hopelessness that influences the doctor-patient relationship. Physicians should maintain a nonjudgmental attitude and consider the emotional burden placed on the patient with this difficult symptom. Most CPP is multifactorial, so the physician should avoid identifying a specific cause because unsuccessful treatment erodes the patient's ability to manage the psychological aspect of chronic pain. Instead, the physician should focus on therapies directed at areas identified by careful history and examination and selected diagnostic tests.

Medication

1. Nonsteroidal anti-inflammatory drugs on scheduled basis
2. Muscle relaxants
3. Oral contraceptives: primary dysmenorrhea, endometriosis
4. Stool softeners: anticholinergics if increased bowel motility, IBS
5. Antidepressants: amitriptyline, nortriptyline, trazodone. Consider coexisting sleep disorder.
6. Anxiolytics
7. Suppressive antibiotics for chronic urethritis
8. Local anesthetics, nerve block: superficial abdominal muscle spasm
9. Danazol, gonadotropin-releasing hormone, oral contraceptives, progestogens for endometriosis

Diet

1. High fiber, increased fluids for IBS
2. Limit caffeine
3. Identify aggravating foods (chronic cystitis)

Other

Transcutaneous electrical nerve stimulation (TENS) units

Activity

Encourage progressive activity program: walking, bicycling.

Patient Education

1. Basic anatomy instruction
2. Pelvic relaxation and distraction techniques
3. Void after intercourse if appropriate
4. Teach pain scale, medication and activity log use.
5. Management of stress, coping skills, goal setting
6. Sleep hygiene

Follow-Up

Patients with CPP should be seen at a regular interval (1 to 2 months) during the first 6 months of therapy, then at 6-month intervals if stable. Encourage more frequent visits if necessary because of symptom exacerbation.

PEARLS

- Endometriosis often begins as early dysmenorrhea and progresses to constant pain that is worse with sexual intercourse. Nodules are often palpated in the cul-de-sac.

- Adhesions often cause a positional pain made worse by climbing stairs or driving.

- Spasm of the levator muscles often causes a falling out sensation.

- Piriformis spasm is suggested when pain occurs with external rotation of a straightened leg.

- Psychological counseling should be considered a cornerstone of treatment, with referral for specific therapy (sexual abuse, marital counseling) as indicated.

- Recent studies indicate a multidisciplinary nonsurgical approach may offer the best long-term prognosis.

Bibliography

Lipscomb GH, Ling FW: Chronic pelvic pain and dysmenorrhea. In Ransom SB, McNeeley SG Jr (eds): Gynecology for the Primary Care Provider, pp 99–111. Philadelphia, WB Saunders Company, 1997.

Longstreth GF: Irritable bowel syndrome and chronic pelvic pain. Obstet Gynecol Surv 1994;49:505–507.

McDonald JS: Management of chronic pelvic pain. Obstet Gynecol Clin North Am 1993;20:817–838.

Milburn A, Reiter RC, Rhomberg AT: Multidisciplinary approach to chronic pelvic pain. Obstet Gynecol Clin North Am 1993;20:643–661.

Steege JF: Office assessment of chronic pelvic pain. Clin Obstet Gynecol 1997;40:554–563.

Vulvar pruritus is defined as intense itching of the female external genitalia. It is estimated that approximately 10 per cent of private-practice gynecologic patients have this as their chief complaint. More commonly, it is a symptom indicating underlying local or systemic disease. Idiopathic vulvar pruritus is not uncommon; it is however, primarily a diagnosis of exclusion. From the outset of the patient's presentation, the physician should attempt to differentiate vulvar pruritus from pain (vulvodynia) and also the role of the itch-scratch cycle (i.e., itching leading to excoriations and skin changes, which in turn cause more itching) in the cause of the patient's complaints.

Differential Diagnosis

In order of likelihood, from anecdotal evidence

1. Vulvovaginitis
   a. Fungal: Candidiasis
   b. Bacterial: *Gardnerella vaginalis*, gonorrhea, syphilis, chlamydia, others
   c. Protozoal: trichomoniasis
   d. Viral: human papillomavirus causing condyloma accuminata and herpes simplex
2. Essential pruritus/localized neurodermatitis
3. Contact dermatitis: irritant, allergic and atopic
4. Atrophic vaginitis: secondary to estrogen deprivation
5. Urinary tract infection
6. Vulvar vestibulitis
7. Non-neoplastic epithelial disorder
   a. Lichen sclerosus et atrophicus
   b. Squamous cell hyperplasia
   c. Other dermatoses: psoriasis, lichen simplex chronicus
8. Vulvar neoplasia
   a. Vulvar intraepithelial neoplasia
   b. Carcinoma (in situ and invasive malignancy)
9. Seborrheic dermatitis
10. Fecal soilage secondary to anal incontinence
11. Parasitic infestations: crab lice, pinworms, scabies or other insect bites
12. Neurogenic/psychiatric
13. Fox-Fordyce disease resulting from apocrine sweat gland occlusion
14. Associated systemic conditions
    a. Diabetes
    b. Drug hypersensitivity
    c. Gout
    d. Pellagra
    e. Pregnancy
    f. Sjögren's syndrome
    g. Lymphoma
    h. Leukemia
    i. Hepatic or renal disease
    j. Carcinomatosis or polycythemia

History: Key Questions to Ask

1. When did the symptoms begin, and is there any variation of the symptoms with sanitary or tampon use, menses, sexual activity, or vaginal cleansing routines?
2. Where else is the patient itching or has a rash?
3. What treatment has been or is presently being tried?
4. Are there psychogenic/marital stresses?

Clinical Findings

1. Visible skin changes (vulvar area especially)
2. Note color; look for warts, tumors, ulcers, and scaling.
3. Do entire cutaneous examination, and check pubic hair if indicated.
4. Check for vaginal or anal discharge.
5. Colposcopic and histologic changes

Tests

1. Examination of skin and vulvar/anal region
2. Wet mount of vaginal secretions: Check for trichomoniasis and clue cells (indicative of bacterial vaginosis).
3. KOH of vaginal secretions: Rule out fungal infection.
4. Colposcopy before and after acetic acid application if indicated
5. Biopsy of all suspicious-looking lesions
6. Urinalysis with microscopy to check for bacteriuria and glycosuria; send culture if indicated.
7. Scotch tape test: Rule out pinworm, if indicated.
8. Complete blood count if indicated to check for blood dyscrasias
9. Chemistry panel: Check the glucose (do 1-hour glucose tolerance test if indicated) and for values indicating uremia and hepatobiliary problems.
10. Patch testing if indicated for contact dermatitis: for allergy testing

Management

1. Outpatient medical management and appropriate local excision is the usual. In general, patient should suspend all previous treatments and implement the indicated patient education instructions.
2. Inpatient care is reserved for intractable cases requiring ethanol injection or Mering procedure (vulvar undercutting causing denervation).
3. Some investigators have recommended laser to vaporize the vulvar epidermis or Grenz-ray therapy.

Medication

1. Symptomatic
   a. Hydroxyzine (Atarax, Vistaril), 25 to 50 mg tid to qid and hs
   b. Doxepin (Sinequan, Adapin), 25 to 50 mg bid to tid
   c. Amitriptyline (Elavil), 25 mg qhs
   d. Topical lidocaine (Xylocaine)
   e. Ice packs at night as needed
   f. Crotamiton cream (Warn patients that they will have initial burning.)
2. For chronic or idiopathic vulvar pruritus
   a. Topical steroids: 1% to 2.5% hydrocortisone cream apply twice daily. Initially, it may be necessary to start therapy with a more potent steroid, for example, triamcinolone ointment (Kenalog) (0.025%), clobetasol propionate (Temovate), 0.05% for approximately 3 months, or fluocinolone ointment (Synalar) (0.025%), but therapy should be switched to hydrocortisone once improvement is noted so as to avoid anogenital atrophy.
   b. Subcutaneous injection of triamcinolone acetonide (Kenalog)—for intractable cases—depends on comfort and expertise of practitioner.
3. Systemic steroids may be used in very acute self-limiting cases.

Diet

Avoidance of certain foods is advocated: those that contain caffeine; also, tomatoes and peanuts.

Activity

As tolerated

Patient Education

1. Avoid possible irritants: douches, perfumed soaps and body powders or lotions, fabric softeners and detergents, rubber condoms and diaphragms.
2. Observe regular but not overzealous perineal hygiene. Can wash anogenital area with hypoallergenic cleansing lotion and afterward apply hypoallergenic emollient cream.
3. Avoid tight-fitting clothes or nylon pantyhose; instead, wear loose-fitting cotton underwear.
4. Notify sexual partner to obtain treatment if experiencing similar symptoms.
5. Sitz baths (tepid water at 98° F) with a few drops of water-dispersible oil or tar emulsion as necessary.

Follow-Up

1. Need to monitor progress of therapy closely because some of the treatments can accentuate symptoms.
2. Also need to be aware of the 1 to 5 per cent malignant potential of vulvar dystrophies and that the most common presenting symptom of vulvar carcinoma is pruritus.
3. Gynecology and/or dermatology consult may be needed for specific cases.
4. The majority of patients can be managed with success on an outpatient basis with conservative medical management. With recurrent symptoms after different therapies, the possibility of a psychogenic basis should be more thoroughly investigated.

PEARL

The primary symptoms of vulvar and vaginal neoplasms is itching.

Bibliography

ACOG Technical Bulletin Number 139: Vulvar dystrophies. Int J Gynecol Obstet 1991;35:269–273.

Bornstein J, Pascal B, Abramovici H: The common problem of vulvar pruritus. Obstet Gynecol Surv 1993;48:111–118.

Kelly RA, Foster DC, Woodruff JD: Subcutaneous injection of triamcinolone acetonide in the treatment of chronic vulvar pruritus. Am J Obstet Gynecol 1993;169:568–570.

Nyirjesy P: Vulvar diseases. In Lepport PC, Howard FM (eds): Primary Care for Women, pp 218–222. Philadelphia, Lippincott-Raven Publishers, 1997.

Pincus SH: Vulvar dermatoses and pruritus vulvae. Dermatol Clin 1992;10:297–308.

Acute scrotal pain and/or mass is one of the most anxiety-provoking problems that present to the physician's office. With the similar symptoms and multitude of diagnoses, it is imperative to systematically and accurately diagnosis scrotal pain and/or mass. An accurate diagnosis can prevent a lapse of time before treatment that would potentially lead to infertility.

Differential Diagnosis

1. Testicular torsion: 1 in 4000 males younger than 25 years
2. Epididymitis, acute or chronic: treatment is age dependent
3. Torsion of the testicular appendix: blue dot sign
4. Orchitis, viral: associated parotitis
5. Testicular tumor: most common cancer in men from 15 to 45 years of age
6. Hydrocele (85 per cent of all asymptomatic patients), epididymal cyst
7. Varicocele (15 per cent of all males), spermatocele, granuloma
8. Trauma: testicular laceration, hematoma, and hematohydrocele
9. Renal colic, nephrolithiasis: flank to groin pain
10. Inguinal hernia, incarcerated hernia
11. Acute appendicitis, dissection of aortic aneurysm, Henoch-Schönlein purpura
12. Referred pain from the hip, back, and pelvic floor

History: Key Questions to Ask

Routine genital and urologic history plus

1. Is there pain? When did the pain start? Was it sudden or gradual? Any trauma?
2. Can you point to the area of most intense pain? Adenopathy?
3. Is there a mass that you feel? Or a change in the size of the testicle/scrotum?
4. Are you sexually active? Are you using safe sex practices? Homosexuality?
5. Do you have any dysuria, urethral discharge, frequency, urgency, or hematuria?
6. Do you have any nausea, vomiting, abdominal pain, fever?
7. Any past history of cryptorchidism, nephrolithiasis, cancer, or viral illness?

Testicular torsion and appendix testis torsion occur abruptly and are painful because of ischemia of the corresponding organ. Epididymitis, hernia incarcer-

ation, and orchitis have a more gradual onset of pain. Testicular tumor is usually painless, as are hydrocele, varicocele, and cysts.

Clinical Findings

THINK TORSION in any painful testicle.

1. Testicular torsion
   a. Pain, swelling, with or without fever, occasional nausea and vomiting
   b. Nontransillumination of the testicle
   c. Cremastric reflex (ipsilateral elevation of the testicle with stroking of the medial aspect of the thigh) absent.
   d. Positive Prehn's sign: increased pain with testicle elevation to the pubic bone
2. Epididymitis
   a. Swelling, fever, pain, associated with discharge
   b. Negative Prehn's sign: pain relieved with elevation of the testicle above pubic bone
   c. Nontransillumination of the testicle
3. Torsion of the appendix testis
   a. Pain without fever, nausea and vomiting
   b. Blue dot sign: Scrotal skin tightened over testicle causes "blue dot."
   c. Transillumination of testicle highlights the blue dot
4. Incarcerated hernia
   a. Painful nonreducible mass, nontransillumination, nausea and vomiting
   b. No bowel sounds heard in scrotum; abdominal pain likely.
5. Inguinal hernia
   a. Nonpainful reducible mass with bowel sounds, nontransillumination
   b. Infant inguinal hernias are corrected urgently; high risk of incarceration.
6. Varicocele (bag of worms)
   a. Swelling, no pain, nontransillumination; patient may be infertile.
   b. Provocative maneuvers will accentuate mass (Valsalva maneuver)
7. Orchitis (preceded by viral illness)
   a. Pain, swelling, fever, nontransillumination, nausea and vomiting
   b. Negative Prehn's sign: pain relieved with elevation of the testicle above the pubis
8. Hydrocele
   a. Painless swelling that transilluminates

b. May spontaneously resolve; clear fluid is usually aspirated

c. May have associated inguinal hernia; needs to be corrected early.

9. Epididymal cyst
   a. Nonpainful swelling/mass at the epididymis
   b. May be aspirated (usually clear fluid); no treatment needed.

10. Spermatocele: nonpainful swelling/mass that transilluminates

11. Testicular tumor
    a. One to 2 per cent of all malignant tumors in men
    b. Nonpainful palpable mass on or in the testicle, nontransillumination; swelling may be involved (feels like hard lump on a hard-boiled egg)

12. Nephrolithiasis/renal colic
    a. Flank pain that radiates into the groin and testicle on the involved side
    b. Scrotal tenderness, hematuria

Diagnostic Tests

1. Complete blood count: elevated with epididymitis, orchitis
2. Culture for chlamydia and gonorrhea: always try first to isolate organism
3. Urinalysis and urine culture and sensitivity second
4. Abdominal radiographs to include flat plate and upright
5. Scrotal ultrasound, testicular ultrasound, color Doppler evaluation
   a. Ultrasound is 100 per cent sensitive for tumor.
   b. Color Doppler not 100 per cent sensitive in torsion, operator dependent, probably the best method for evaluation of torsion.
6. Nuclear scintigraphy of the testicle: good test for torsion, but, if clinically likely, do not delay treatment to obtain test.

Management

1. Torsion of the testicle: Diagnostic testing should not delay surgical exploration in a suspected torsion.
   a. Urologic emergency: Requires immediate referral to a surgeon.
   b. Manual detorsion can be attempted in the outpatient setting. If attempting closed manual detorsion, the physician is looking at the patient in the anatomic position (from the foot of the bed). The testicle should be ro-

tated in the same fashion as opening a book: the patient's left testicle is turned in a clockwise direction and the right testicle is turned in a counterclockwise direction.

   c. Surgical detorsion and bilateral orchioplexy is indicated within the first 4 to 6 hours to prevent infarction and infertility.

2. Torsion of the appendix testis
   a. Analgesia, scrotal elevation, and bed rest
   b. Surgical exploration if diagnosis uncertain

3. Epididymitis
   a. First, urethral cultures for *Neisseria gonorrhoeae* and *Chlamydia trachomatis*
   b. Second, urine cultures and sensitivity
   c. Patient less than 35 years, sexually active: Treat for *N. gonorrhoeae* and *C. trachomatis*
      (1) Ceftriaxone (Rocephin), 250 mg IM in a single dose *PLUS*
      (2) Doxycycline (Vibramycin), 100 mg orally twice a day for 10 days
      (3) If allergic, Ofloxacin (Floxin), 300 mg twice daily for 10 days
   d. Azithromycin (Zithromax), 2 gm PO single dose, 1 gm PO for urethritis
   e. Patient over 35 years, monogamous: treat for *Escherichia coli*, enterococcus, *Pseudomonas*, proteus
      (1) Ciprofloxin (Cipro), 500 mg orally bid for 10 days
      (2) Trimethoprim-sulfamethoxazole (Bactrim), 160/800 mg orally bid for 10 days
      (3) If systemically ill, add an aminoglycoside IV.

4. Nephrolithiasis: pain control, hydration, straining of urine to test for type of stone

5. Varicocele
   a. If infertile, consider varicocelectomy; otherwise no treatment.
   b. Acute onset: Consider retroperitoneal neoplasm causing renal vein thrombosis.

6. Epididymal cyst, spermatocele, and hydrocele
   a. Ultrasound: to rule out neoplasm
   b. No treatment needed; aspirate if painful.

7. Testicular tumor: seminoma most common
   a. Urgent ultrasound and surgical consultation
   b. All males should be taught self-evaluation of their testicles at an early age.

Follow-Up

1. Epididymitis: Recheck if no improvement; may want to rule out syphilis.

2. Orchitis: occasional testicular atrophy, infertility, and minimal elevated risk of tumor

3. Hernias: Re-examine at annual examination.

Bibliography

Centers for Disease Control and Prevention: 1998 Guidelines for the treatment of sexually transmitted diseases. MMWR Morb Mortal Wkly Rep 1998;47(RR-1):1–118.

Horstman WG: Scrotal imaging. Urol Clin North Am 1997;24:653–671.

Junnila J: Testicular masses. Am Fam Physician 1998;57:685–692.

Rabinowitz R, Hulbert WC: Acute scrotal swelling. Urol Clin North Am 1995;22:101–105.

Schneider RE: Male genital problems. In Tintinalli JE (ed): Emergency Medicine, 4th ed, pp 532–539. New York, McGraw-Hill, 1996.

103 Fibrocystic Breast Disease

Susan B. Arjmand

Etiology

Fibrocystic breast disease (FBD) is a general term for a variety of benign breast findings that include cysts, lumpy breasts, mastodynia, and nipple discharge. It is the most common cause of breast abnormalities in women under the age of 50. FBD is an exaggerated response of the cyclic breast changes that normally occur in the menstrual cycle. During ovulation and just before menstruation, hormone levels change and can cause fluid retention, sometimes resulting in cysts. Usually tender, they decrease or disappear within 1 to 2 days of menses onset.

Symptoms

1. May be asymptomatic.
2. More commonly results in pain, especially preceding menses.
   a. May last from a few days to 2 to 3 weeks of each cycle.
   b. May radiate to shoulder and arm or may be localized.
   c. More common in upper and outer quadrants of breasts
3. Breast engorgement
4. Occasionally see nipple discharge.

Key Symptoms

Cyclic breast pain

Clinical Findings

1. Generalized lumpiness. May contain smooth, tense, or fluctuant masses (cysts).
2. Usually symmetric
3. Diffuse thickening that blends into adjacent tissue; not well-demarcated
4. Tenderness on examination

> **WARNING**
>
> FBD may be difficult to distinguish from benign or malignant tumors. Generally, tumors have a more discrete shape. Cysts and benign tumors have smooth surfaces; carcinomas may have a more irregular, ill-defined surface.

Key Signs

- Breast thickening or lumpiness
- Tenderness

Laboratory Tests

1. Clinical examination
2. Thyroid-stimulating hormone, prolactin (if galactorrhea)
3. If mass or cyst, imaging studies or aspiration biopsy/cytology. The decision depends on patient's age, risk factors, nature of the lump, availability and reliability of procedures.

Differential Diagnosis

1. Pain: intercostal neuralgia, stretching of Cooper's ligaments, costochondritis, cholelithiasis, intermittent mild ischemia, gastroesophageal reflux, Pancoast's tumor
2. Lumps: malignancy
3. Skin changes: malignancy, eczema
4. Discharge: malignancy, galactorrhea, medications, exercise

Treatment

1. Rule out the possibility of malignancy using appropriate diagnostic measures, if indicated.
2. Reassure patient that, although 100 per cent resolution of FBD is unlikely, significant symptomatic improvement is possible.
3. Symptomatic pain relief with analgesics
4. Well-fitted support bra (day and night if necessary)
5. Dietary restriction of salt and methylxanthines
6. Vitamin E and A supplements; some anecdotal supportive evidence but physiologic basis unclear
7. Mild diuretic premenstrually
8. Oral contraceptives
9. For more severe cases, danazol, 200 to 400 mg daily for 3 to 6 months

Key Treatment

- Rule out breast cancer.

- Reassurance

- Symptomatic relief with medication and dietary modification

Follow-Up

1. If conservative treatment fails, consider medications that alter hormonal function (i.e., oral contraceptives or danazol). Know that, if oral contraceptives are used, a patient may not see results for at least a year. If danazol is selected, be mindful of significant side effects (nausea, mood change, virilization) and cost. Also, there is a significant chance of recurrence when treatment is discontinued.

2. If a suspicious area is recalcitrant to treatment or if a discrete mass is evident, a biopsy should be considered. Breast cancer risk is increased for FBD with atypia. Mammograms are used for screening; ultrasound can differentiate cysts from solid lesions. Aspiration cytology is useful to diagnose cysts and solid lesions.

3. If nipple discharge is present, consider whether it is unilateral or bilateral. Spontaneous or provoked? What is the color and consistency? If unilateral, spontaneous, and serosanguinous, consider malignancy and proceed with histologic evaluation.

4. Regular breast self-examination and frequent follow-up is critical because FBD can make the physical examination and mammogram difficult to interpret.

5. The course is benign but chronic and recurring. Patient education and reassurance is important.

 ## Bibliography

Astuto A, Chou P, Otero D, et al: Gynecology. In Rucker LM (ed): Essentials of Adult Ambulatory Care, p 500. Baltimore, Williams & Wilkins, 1997.

Freeman J: Fibrocystic breast disease. In Dambro M, Griffith J (eds): Griffith's Five Minute Clinical Consult, pp 394–395. Baltimore, Williams & Wilkins, 1998.

London W, Connolly J, Schmitt S, et al: A prospective study of benign breast disease and the risk of breast CA. JAMA 1992;267:941–944.

Marchant D: The breast. In Scott J, DiSaia P, Hammond C, et al (eds): Danforth's Obstetrics and Gynecology, 7th ed, pp 696–698. Philadelphia, JB Lippincott Company, 1994.

Margolese R: The palpable breast lump: information and recommendations to assist decision-making when a breast lump is detected. Can Med Assoc J 1998;159(3-Suppl).

104 Breast Cancer

Martha S. Grayson

Epidemiology

1. Breast cancer is the most common nonskin malignancy in the United States, with 178,700 projected new cases in 1998. It is estimated that one in eight women will develop breast cancer in their lifetimes.
2. Approximately 435,000 deaths in women will be attributable to breast cancer in 1998. Only lung cancer has a higher cancer mortality in women.
3. Although black women have a lower overall incidence of breast cancer, mortality rates are higher. This is attributed to black women having a more advanced stage of disease at diagnosis as well as a lower relative survival rate for each stage.

Etiology

1. The etiology of breast cancer is a complex interplay between hormonal factors, genetics, and lifestyle. Fewer than half of all breast cancer cases can be attributed to known risk factors.
2. The most important risk factor for breast cancer is age, with increasing incidence with increased age.
3. A family history should be taken to identify any first-degree relatives with breast cancer and the age at which they were diagnosed. A first-degree relative with premenopausal breast cancer increases a woman's risk three- to fourfold.
4. Length of menstruation, including dates of menarche and menopause, as well as age of first pregnancy are important factors in the assessment of risk. First pregnancies prior to age 20 reduce the risk of breast cancer to 50 per cent that of a nulliparous woman, menopause 10 years earlier than the national mean reduces risk by 35 per cent, and late menarche (16 years vs. 12) reduces risk by 40 to 50 per cent.
5. There is controversy about lifestyle factors, such as diet and exercise, and their correlation with breast cancer risk. Serum estradiol levels have been significantly decreased when postmenopausal women changed their diet from average to low-fat. However, it has not been shown that this correlates with a decreased risk of breast cancer.
6. There is some evidence that physical activity can reduce breast cancer risk. The recommended types, amount, and frequencies have yet to be determined.
7. There is an increased relative risk of breast cancer (1.3 to 1.6) with alcohol intake. This risk increases with increasing amounts of alcohol consumption.
8. Genetic syndromes account for about 5 per cent of all breast cancers, which usually occur at younger ages. Women who inherit a mutation in *BRCA1* or *BRCA2* have a 56 to 85 per cent lifetime risk of breast cancer. The prevalence of these mutations is higher in individuals of Ashkenazi Jewish descent compared to the general population.
9. Women with a history of atypical hyperplasia on previous breast biopsy have a fourfold greater risk of developing breast cancer compared to women without such a previous biopsy.
10. There is a relationship between exposure to radiation and breast cancer, especially during childhood or adolescence. Women treated for Hodgkin's disease prior to age 16 had a 35 per cent chance of developing breast cancer by age 40. The vast majority of these cancers develop within the field of radiation.
11. There are data to suggest that there is an increased risk of breast cancer with hormone replacement therapy, but the studies are controversial. The risk is not significantly different for women with a family history of breast cancer compared to those without a family history.
12. There have been ongoing trials on the use of tamoxifen in preventing breast cancer. A preliminary report from the Breast Cancer Prevention Trial was released in April 1998 that stated that there was a 45 per cent reduction in the incidence of breast cancer among women randomized to receive prophylactic tamoxifen.

Symptoms

1. Breast cancer is increasingly being detected in the asymptomatic phase by screening mammography.

2. Cancer may present as a single painless lump. A woman should be questioned about how long the lump has been present and any changes in size or tenderness. Premenopausal women should be asked about the association of symptoms with the menstrual cycle.

3. Patients may present with a variety of symptoms that are also present in benign breast disease, such as increased nodularity, breast tissue thickening, pain, soreness, increased sensitivity, and changes in the appearance of the skin, nipples, or areola.

4. Nipple discharges should be evaluated and are more suspicious if they are spontaneous, unilateral, confined to one duct, and clear, serous, or bloody.

Key Symptoms

- Asymptomatic
- Painless lump
- Nipple discharge
- Increased nodularity or thickening
- Changes in skin

Clinical Findings

1. A firm solitary breast mass is suspicious. The size and location of the mass and whether there is fixation to the skin should be noted. The overlying skin should be inspected for inflammation, peau d'orange, or ulceration.

2. Lymph nodes in the axilla and supraclavicular region should be examined for size, consistency, and mobility.

3. Each nipple should be gently squeezed for evidence of discharge. Sequential compression should be done to locate the duct or area involved.

Key Signs

- Solitary breast mass
- Unilateral nipple discharge
- Enlarged, palpable lymph nodes

Laboratory Tests

Screening

1. The goal of screening is to detect breast cancer in its earliest and most treatable stage. Screening consists of a combination of breast self-examination (BSE), clinical breast examination (CBE), and mammography.

2. Monthly BSE is frequently advised, but the evidence from randomized trials has not shown a decrease in mortality. BSE should be considered as a supplement to CBE and mammography.

3. CBE should be performed as part of the routine physical examination for all women. Ten to 25 per cent of all palpable breast masses may not be detected by mammography.

4. There has been considerable debate about the age at which to start and stop screening mammograms. Pooled data from randomized controlled trials shows the most convincing evidence for the benefit of annual screening mammography for women ages 50 to 69, with a 25 to 30 per cent reduction in mortality. A recent meta-analysis from eight randomized trials of mammogram screening shows an 18 per cent reduction in breast cancer mortality in women who entered the trials at age 40 to 49. Based on these findings, the American Cancer Society now recommends annual mammography for women starting at age 40. In addition, they state no age limit at which screening should be terminated. The decision to screen older women should be based on co-morbidity.

Diagnosis

Laboratory tests to evaluate a woman with a palpable breast mass consist of the following:

1. Diagnostic mammography: utilized to evaluate the surrounding breast tissue and opposite breast for nonpalpable cancers. In general, this is not performed on women less than 35 years of age.

2. Ultrasound: utilized to distinguish cystic from solid masses. A mass not visualized on ultrasound should be assumed to be solid.

3. Fine-needle aspiration: if nonbloody fluid is aspirated and the mass is completely resolved, no further evaluation is necessary. The false-negative rate for fine-needle aspiration of a solid mass can be as high as 20 per cent.

4. Stereotactic biopsy: mostly used with abnormalities found on mammogram, such as clustered microcalcifications or a new finding on mammogram that is considered to be low risk.

5. Open surgical biopsy (lumpectomy): the complete pathologic assessment of breast tissue.

6. Newer diagnostic tests are being studied, such as magnetic resonance imaging and positron emission tomography, but are not yet recommended for screening or diagnosis at this time.

Key Tests

- Mammography
- Ultrasound
- Fine-needle aspiration
- Stereotactic biopsy
- Surgical biopsy

Differential Diagnosis

1. Fibroadenomas and fibrocystic changes are the two most common forms of breast disease presenting with a palpable lump. Fibroadenomas are usually firm and freely movable, with sharp borders. Fibrocystic changes are usually bilateral, vary with the menstrual cycle, and more common in the upper outer quadrants.

2. Nipple discharges that are bilateral or multiductal and either milky, green, or black may be indicative of galactorrhea and may require an endocrine evaluation.

Treatment

1. Breast cancer is treated by a combination of surgery, radiation, chemotherapy, and/or hormonal therapy. Selection of treatment is based on patient age, tumor stage (size and axillary lymph node involvement), menopausal status, overall health, and patient preference.

2. Pathologic characteristics of the primary tumor, including estrogen and progesterone receptor status, histologic classification, tumor necrosis, and measures of proliferative capacity (thymidine labeling index, S-phase analysis utilizing flow cytometry), also influence prognosis and treatment selection.

3. Options for surgery include mastectomy, mastectomy with reconstruction, and breast-conserving surgery with radiation. Reconstruction can be accomplished with a saline-filled artificial implant or a rectus muscle flap.

4. Long-term studies have shown equivalent survival with either modified radical mastectomy or breast-conserving surgery plus radiation.

5. Axillary node dissection is utilized for staging but can be a source of lymphedema and residual arm discomfort. Several investigators are comparing the results of lymphatic mapping with sentinel node biopsy to complete axillary node dissection. Preliminary results show high concordance, which would eliminate the need for axillary dissection in many patients.

6. The need for adjuvant therapy, either chemotherapy or hormonal, is usually based on tumor stage, estrogen receptor status (positive or negative), and whether the patient is pre- or post-menopausal. In general, patients with tumors less than 1 cm and negative nodes are not candidates for systemic therapy. Combination chemotherapy and/or tamoxifen has been shown to decrease recurrences and increase survival for all groups of women with primary breast cancer. Tamoxifen has a greater benefit for women who are estrogen receptor–positive.

7. The recommended length of treatment with tamoxifen is 5 years. Tamoxifen is associated with a two- to sevenfold increased risk of endometrial cancer. Patients should be monitored with yearly pelvic examinations and be promptly evaluated for any irregular uterine bleeding.

8. Several national organizations provide information for patients with breast cancer, such as the National Alliance of Breast Cancer Organizations (NABCO) (212-719-0154; www.nabco.org), the Y-ME National Breast Cancer Organization (800-221-2141, English; 800-986-9505, Spanish; www.y-me.org), and Share (212-382-2111). Several of these organizations provide support groups, hot lines, or listings of resources geared to the breast cancer patient.

Key Treatment

- Surgery
- Radiotherapy
- Chemotherapy
- Hormonal therapy

Follow-Up

1. Recommended follow-up after treatment consists of a careful history and physical every 3 to 6 months for 3 years, then 6 to 12 months for the next 3 years, followed by annual checkups.

2. Monthly BSE and annual mammograms are recommended.

3. Periodic follow-up of asymptomatic patients with periodic chest radiographs, chemistries and serologic tests, and bone and liver scans have not been found to improve survival or overall quality of life.

Bibliography

American Society of Clinical Oncology: Recommended breast cancer surveillance guidelines. J Clin Oncol 1997;15:2149–2156.

Cady B, Steele GD, Morrow M, et al: Evaluation of common breast problems: guidance for primary care providers. CA Cancer J Clin 1998;48:49–63.

Fisher B, Anderson S, Redmond CK, et al: Reanalysis and results after 12 years of follow-up in a randomized clinical trial comparing total mastectomy with lumpectomy with or without irradiation in the treatment of breast cancer. N Engl J Med 1995;333:1456–1461.

Leitch AM, Dodd GD, Costanza M, et al: American Cancer Society guidelines for the early detection of breast cancer: update 1997. CA Cancer J Clin 1997;47:150–153.

Thune I, Brenn T, Lund E, et al: Physical activity and the risk of breast cancer. N Engl J Med 1997;336:1269–1275.

Indications

1. Palpable breast mass
2. Cystic or solid lesion of breast

Contraindications

1. Known bleeding disorder
2. Anticoagulant therapy

Preparation

1. History and physical examination
2. Informed consent

Equipment

1. Povidone-iodine (Betadine) or 70% alcohol solution
2. 10- or 20-ml syringe—standard or three-finger control
3. 1.5-inch 22-gauge needle
4. Glass slides (preferably poly-L-lysine–coated)
5. Cell filtration solution (i.e., Cytolyt for Cytospin or solution used in Thin Prep for Pap smear), if cell filtration equipment is available. This technique allows minimal in-office handling of specimen.
6. Slide fixative or 95% ethanol, depending on preference of cytopathologist
7. Diff Quick stain: optional if planning to view air-dried slides immediately
8. 1-inch 30-gauge needle (optional for anesthetic)
9. Lidocaine (Xylocaine) without epinephrine, 0.5 to 1 ml (optional for anesthesia)
10. 3-ml syringe (optional for local anesthetic)

Precautions

1. Hematoma is the most common complication.
2. Pneumothorax: rare
3. Acute mastitis: rare
4. Tumor growth in the needle track: theoretical risk but not observed with needle sizes used in this procedure. If cancer is present, the track will likely be excised or will be included in radiation therapy field of treatment.

Technique

1. Antiseptic preparation to skin over biopsy site with alcohol or povidone-iodine
2. Optional: lidocaine injection into dermis and subcutaneous tissue, being careful to avoid biopsy tissue. Anesthetic should be in 3-ml syringe with 30-gauge needle.
3. Use a three-finger control syringe or place a standard 10- or 20-ml syringe in pistol grip, if available.
4. Optional—withdraw plunger of syringe to 3- to 5-ml mark. This step avoids need to remove syringe after obtaining specimen for transport or slide preparation.
5. Place index and middle fingers of nonaspirating hand over mass, compressing structures over mass.
6. Spread fingers and press more firmly.

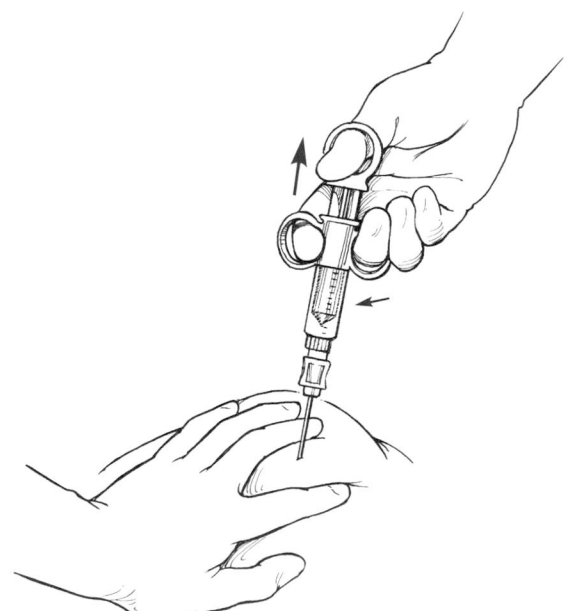

7. Introduce needle through skin and into mass. Move needle from side to side, and palpate mass. Mass should move with needle if proper placement is achieved.

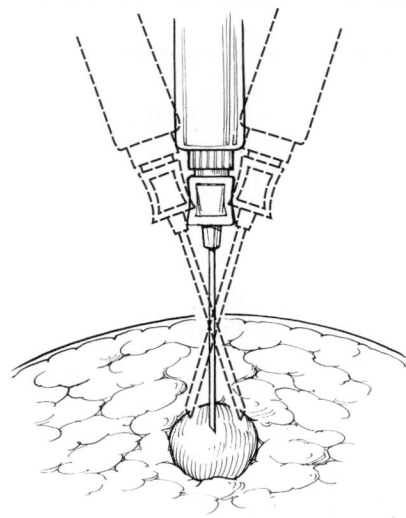

8. Apply negative pressure by withdrawing syringe plunger (see figure on p. 534).

9. Pass needle through mass 6 to 10 times, maintaining negative pressure. If fluid is obtained, remove all fluid and then re-examine for mass. If mass is present, repeat the procedure to obtain a biopsy specimen for evaluation.

> **Note**
> Tactile sensation (gritty [malignant] vs. soft, rubbery or fibrous [benign]) should be recorded to add sensitivity to the classic triad of clinical examination, fine-needle aspiration biopsy, and mammogram.

10. Upon completion of multiple passes, cellular material may be noted in the hub of the needle, although this is not necessary to have an adequate specimen.

11. Release negative pressure from syringe prior to removal from mass, then remove needle from lesion.

12. Apply pressure to areas for 1 to 2 minutes to minimize occurrence of hematoma.

13. If step 4 was omitted, remove syringe from needle and withdraw plunger to fill syringe with air.

14. If using cell filtration solution (i.e., Cytolyt or Thin Prep solution), contents of needle may be expressed into solution, and this can be sent for laboratory evaluation. Occasionally, solution may be drawn into syringe to ensure maximal yield of specimen when specimen is scant. If using Thin Prep technique, clearly label specimen as breast mass aspirate.

15. Slides can be prepared as with standard hematologic smear and fixed in 95% ethanol or fixative spray. Alternatively, "book-opening technique," with one air-dried and one fixed slide, may be used. (See Wilkinson and Bland [1990] for description of book-opening technique.)

Follow-Up

1. Positive results should be followed by open biopsy and definitive care.

2. Negative results should be evaluated. Acellular results may require rebiopsy or close clinical follow-up. Clinical suspicion of malignancy based on history and examination should be used to decide on further treatment or evaluation.

> **WARNING**
>
> Mammogram *may* be altered for up to 3 weeks after the procedure. Recent evidence shows this is not likely if proper precautions are taken for hematoma (pressure to site for 2 minutes).

> **WARNING**
>
> All laboratory preparation and handling should be discussed with individual reference laboratory and/or pathologist to maximize information obtained from procedure.

Bibliography

Editorial Opinion: the uniform approach to breast fine-needle aspiration biopsy. Am J Surg 1997;174:371.

Hindle WH, Chen EC: Accuracy of mammographic appearance after breast fine-needle aspiration. Am J Obstet Gynecol 1997;176:1286.

Hindle WH: The use of fine-needle aspiration in the evaluation of persistent palpable dominant breast masses. Am J Obstet Gynecol 1993;168:1814.

Kline TS: Fine-needle aspiration biopsy of the breast. Am Fam Physician 1995;57:2021.

Perez-Reyes N, Mulford OK, Rutkowski MA, et al: Breast fine-needle aspiration—a comparison of thin layer and conventional preparation. Am J Clin Pathol 1994;102:349.

Sirkin W, Auger M, Donat E, et al: Cytospins—an alternative method for fine-needle aspiration cytology of the breast—a study of 148 cases. Diagn Cytopathol 1995;13:266.

Wilkinson EJ, Bland JI: Techniques and results of aspiration cytology for diagnosis of benign and malignant diseases of the breast. Surg Clin North Am 1990;70:801.

Indications

The Papanicolaou (Pap) smear is used primarily to screen for cervical cancer. Opinions on the frequency of Pap smears are outlined below.

1. The U.S. Preventive Services Task Force has established the following screening guidelines:

   a. Pap smear should begin at age 18 or at the age of first sexual intercourse, whichever comes first.

   b. Between the ages of 18 and 65, Pap smears should be repeated every 1 to 3 years on the basis of risk factors for cervical cancer.

   c. After the age of 65, screening tests may be discontinued if previous smears have been consistently normal.

2. The American Cancer Society and the American College of Obstetricians and Gynecologists recommend annual Pap smears beginning at age 18 or at the age of first sexual intercourse, whichever occurs first. After three or more consecutive, satisfactory annual tests with normal findings, it can be performed less frequently if recommended by the physician. I favor annual Pap smears in women with one or more risk factors for cervical cancer.

Precautions

The Pap smear should not be obtained if the patient is menstruating or has douched within 24 hours.

Equipment for Conventional Technique

1. Vaginal speculum
2. One or two glass slides
3. Wooden cervical spatula
4. Cytobrush or cotton swab moistened with normal saline solution
5. Fixative (95% ethyl alcohol or commercial spray)
6. Gloves

Equipment for Thin Prep Technique

1. PreservCyt Solution vial
2. Cervical collection device

Conventional Technique

1. With an assistant in attendance and patient in lithotomy postion, insert an unlubricated speculum (water only) to expose the cervix, and gently wipe away any excessive discharge.

2. Insert the cytobrush or cotton swab into the cervical canal, rotate 360 to 720 degrees, and roll onto the glass slide.

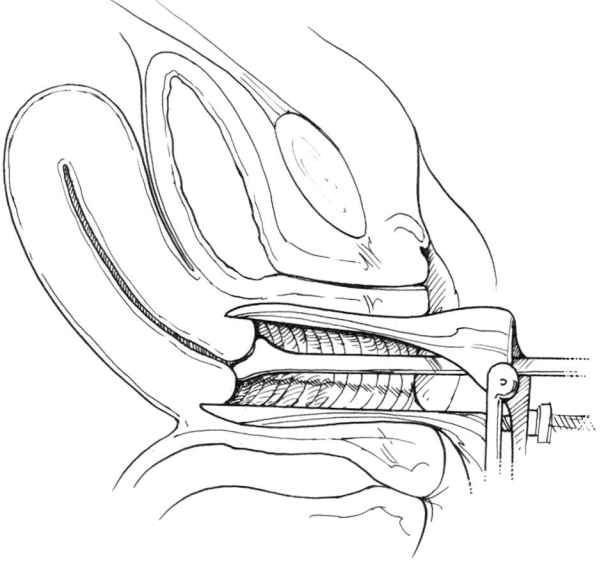

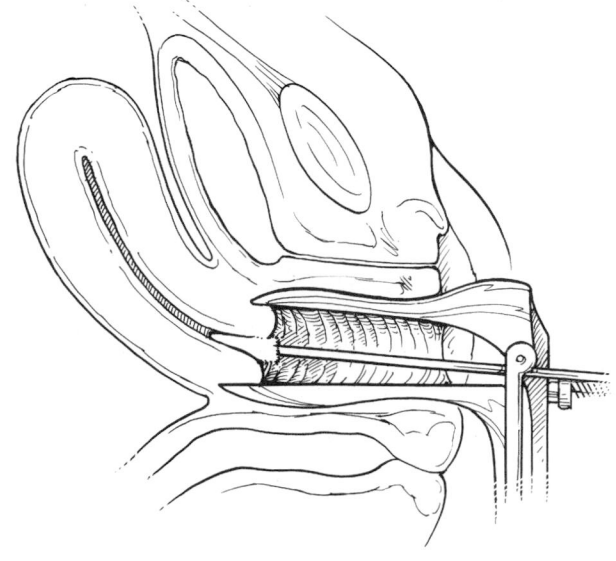

3. Rotate a wooden cervical spatula 360 degrees around the external os to obtain scraping from the squamocolumnar junction, and then roll onto the same or second slide, depending on the requirements of the cytopathologist.

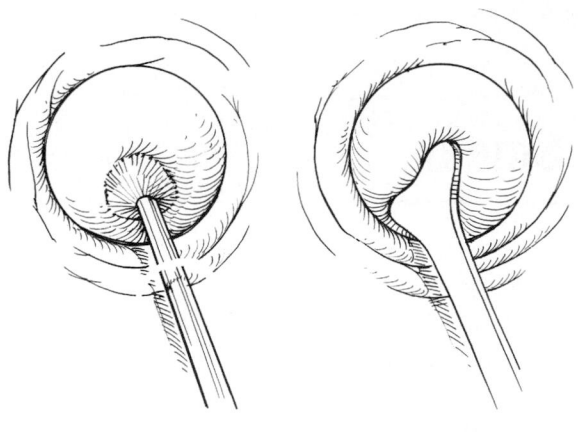

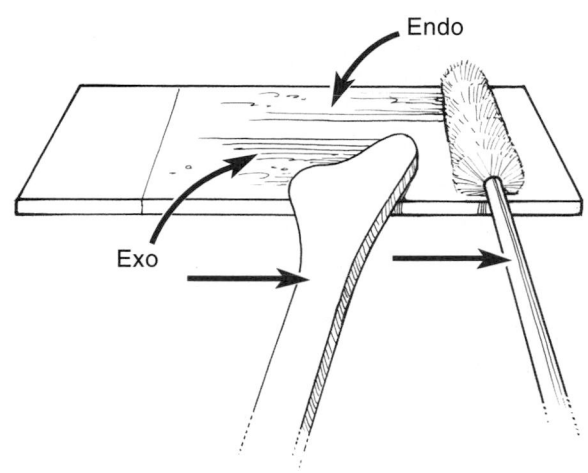

Endo

Exo

4. The slides must be fixed within 10 seconds or there will be drying artifacts.

5. Include with slides all pertinent clinical information, such as patient age, last menstrual period, type of contraceptive, and any previous diagnosis or treatment (e.g., biopsy, laser, radiation therapy).

Thin Prep Technique

The Thin Prep system is a new technique that is intended as a replacement for the conventional method. The patient's gynecologic sample is collected by a broom-type or endocervical brush-spatula combination collection device and immersed and rinsed in a vial filled with PreservCyt solution. The vial is then sent to a lab equipped with a Thin Prep Processor. This method improves specimen quality significantly and increases the cytologic diagnosis of cervical lesions.

Follow-Up

1. Forewarn the patient that she may experience some spotty vaginal bleeding.
2. Follow-up is indicated to inform the patient of the cytologic analysis. An appropriate appointment for the patient must be made if the results are abnormal.

Bibliography

Committee on Gynecologic Practice: Routine Cancer Screening (ACOG Committee Opinion), p 128. Washington, DC, American College of Obstetricians and Gynecologists, 1993.

Fink DJ: Change in American Cancer Society checkup guidelines for detection of cervical cancer. CA Cancer J Clin 1988;38:127–128.

Gall SA: Pap smears: do them right and every year—forever. Postgrad Med 1989;85:235–239.

Kurman RJ: Cervical cytology: Evaluation and Management of Abnormalities (ACOG Technical Bulletin), p 183. Washington, DC, American College of Obstetricians and Gynecologists, 1993.

Lee KR, Ashfaq R, Birdsong GG, et al: Comparison of conventional Pap smears and a fluid-based, thin-layer system for cervical cancer screening. Obstet Gynecol 1997;90:278–283.

U.S. Preventive Services Task Force: Screening for cervical cancer. Am Fam Physician 1990;41:853–857.

Etiology

A report of abnormalities on Pap smear may reflect either cervical pathology or technical inadequacies in obtaining or preserving the specimen. Pathologic abnormalities on routine Pap smear range from inflammation without atypia through atypia of increasing severity to carcinoma. Although many of these changes are associated with human papilloma virus (HPV), other causes are possible.

1. Infectious causes
    a. HPV (especially types 16, 18, 31, 33, 35)
    b. Bacterial vaginosis or trichomoniasis
    c. *Neisseria gonorrhoeae*
    d. *Chlamydia trachomatis*
    e. *Candida* and other fungal infections
    f. Herpes
2. Noninfectious causes
    a. Reparative changes
    b. Atrophic changes

Symptoms

Generally, abnormal Pap smears are not associated with symptoms. On occasion, however, women may report symptoms associated with lower genital tract disease.

1. Bleeding per vagina
2. Vaginal discharge
3. Dyspareunia
4. Lower abdominal pain

Risk Factors

1. Early onset of sexual activity
2. Multiple male sexual partners
3. Male partners with multiple partners
4. Smoking
5. Immunosuppression

Clinical Findings

Abnormal clinical findings noted during performance of Pap smear screening examination are usually limited. Special note should be made of findings associated with abnormal Pap smear results.

1. Genital warts
2. Vaginal discharge
3. Abnormal vulvar, vaginal, or cervical lesions
4. Cervical motion tenderness or adnexal tenderness on bimanual examination
5. Lower abdominal tenderness

Laboratory Tests

1. The key laboratory finding is the Pap smear report itself, reported most commonly using the Bethesda system, although some laboratories may use either the World Health Organization or Papanicolaou reporting systems (see Table 105–1). Typically 5 to 10 per cent of Pap smears will have squamous cell abnormalities, of which approximately 95 per cent will be atypical squamous cells of undetermined significance (ASCUS) or low-grade squamous intraepithelial lesions (LGSIL).
2. Other laboratory tests may have utility under some circumstances.
    a. Complete blood count: leukocytosis
    b. Gonorrhea/chlamydia testing by
       (1) Culture

TABLE 105–1. COMPARISON OF PAP SMEAR RESULTS REPORTING SYSTEMS

BETHESDA SYSTEM	WHO SYSTEM	PAPANICOLAOU SYSTEM
Normal	Normal	Class I
Benign epithelial changes (infection, reparative or atrophic)	Atypia	Class II
Atypical squamous cells of undetermined significance (ASCUS)	Atypia	Class II
Low-grade squamous intraepithelial lesions (LGSIL)	Mild dysplasia (HPV changes or CIN I)	Class III
High-grade squamous intraepithelial lesions (HGSIL)	Moderate dysplasia (CIN II) Severe dysplasia (CIN III) Carcinoma in situ	Class III/IV
Squamous cell carcinoma (SCC)	Invasive SCC	Class V

(2) Antigen detection/nucleic acid hybridization

c. Wet prep

d. Erythrocyte sedimentation rate

e. C-reactive protein

Differential Diagnosis

Although the report of an abnormal screening Pap smear requires follow-up for pathologic diagnosis, providers should be aware that the test is associated with both false-negative and false-positive results. Reports of false-negative rates range from 1 to 80 per cent (5 per cent in most carefully controlled studies). Reports of false-positive rates range from 0 to 8 per cent.

WARNING

Pap smear screening is associated with both false-positive and false-negative results and should be interpreted in light of patients' clinical history, associated risk factors, and findings on physical examination.

Treatment

1. Treatment for abnormal Pap smear involves confirmation of the diagnosis and identification of the underlying cause (Table 105–2). For those Pap smears showing benign epithelial changes, treatment should be directed to the underlying cause when that cause is identifiable.

   a. For infectious causes

      (1) Gonorrhea: ceftriaxone (Rocephin), 250 mg IM once; oral quinolones may also be used.

      (2) Chlamydia: doxycycline, 100 mg PO ×7 days; azithromycin may also be used.

      (3) Trichomonas: metronidazole (Flagyl), 2 gm PO once

      (4) Bacterial vaginosis: metronidazole gel; topical clindamycin may also be used.

   b. For noninfectious causes—atrophic changes: estrogen cream per vagina qhs for 2 or more weeks

2. Treatment of squamous epithelial changes requires an understanding of the significance of the abnormality noted, the natural history of dysplastic cervical changes, and assessment of the patient's willingness to follow up. Less severe lesions, which tend to progress slowly if at all, may be managed more conservatively in patients preferring a more conservative approach with whom close follow-up can be arranged.

Patient Education

Follow-up of abnormal Pap smears is strongly dependent on the cooperation of the patient; therefore, patient education is of critical importance. Patients must be fully informed to participate in treatment planning and to ensure appropriate follow-up as needed.

1. Risk factors for cervical pathology, including preventive measures for sexually transmitted disease

2. Significance of abnormality noted on Pap smear, including the possibility of progression

3. Risks and benefits of treatment options

4. Follow-up plans, including when and for what

Key Treatment

Indications for Colposcopy

- Dysplasia or cancer on Pap smear
- Suspicious visible lesion
- Repeated or unexplained atypia
- HPV
- Abnormal bleeding per vagina
- Diethylstilbestrol exposure in utero

TABLE 105–2.   TREATMENT AND FOLLOW-UP OF ABNORMAL PAP SMEAR RESULTS

DIAGNOSIS	TREATMENT	FOLLOW-UP
Benign cellular changes	Treat as noted in text	Repeat Pap smear in 3 to 6 mo. Repeated abnormalities should be referred for colposcopy.
ASCUS	Repeat Pap smear or referral for colposcopy	Pap smears q6mo for 2 yr, then annually if all results are normal. Repeated abnormalities should be referred for colposcopy.
LGSIL	Referral for colposcopy or repeat Pap smear in 3–6 mo	Pap smears q6mo for 2 yr, then annually if all results are normal. Repeated abnormalities should be referred for colposcopy.
HGSIL	Referral for colposcopy	Follow-up depends on colposcopic findings.

Contraindications for Colposcopy

- Patient refuses
- Cervicitis: contraindication for endocervical curettage (ECC)
- Heavy menses
- Pregnancy: relative contraindication to ECC and/or cervical biopsy

Follow-Up

As noted, patient education to ensure appropriate follow-up is important, especially for those patients who have chosen a conservative treatment plan. Because many abnormalities will resolve with treatment (infection or atrophy) or will regress spontaneously, follow-up with repeat Pap smear screening may be appropriate for patients who prefer conservative treatment and with whom cooperation with follow-up planning is anticipated.

Bibliography

Brotzman GL, Julian TM: The minimally abnormal Papanicolaou smear. Am Fam Physician 1996;53:1154–1162.

Cannistra SA: Cancer of the uterine cervix. N Engl J Med 1996;334:1030–1038.

Johnson BA: The colposcopic examination. Am Fam Physician 1996;53:2473–2482.

Nuovo J, Melnikow J, Palieschesky M: Management of patients with atypical and low grade pap smear abnormalities. Am Fam Physician 1995;52:2243–2250.

Shepherd JC, Fried RA: Preventing cervical cancer: the role of the Bethesda system. Am Fam Physician 1995;51:434–440.

Verdon ME: Issues in the management of human papillomavirus genital disease. Am Fam Physician 1997;55:1813–1822.

Indications

1. Abnormal Pap smear
   a. Chronic inflammation
   b. Atypical squamous cells of undetermined significance (ASCUS) persistent after treatment for inflammatory or reactive causes
   c. Atypical glandular cells of undetermined significance (AGCUS)
   d. Human papillomavirus effect: koilocytosis
   e. Low-grade squamous intraepithelial lesion (LGSIL)
   f. High-grade squamous intraepithelial lesion (HGSIL)
   g. Carcinoma in situ
   h. Repeated unexplained atypia
2. Visible or palpable cervical lesion
3. Vaginal or vulvar lesion
4. Anal condyloma
5. History of in utero diethylstilbestrol exposure
6. Follow-up of previously treated or high-risk patients

Contraindications: Most are relative and only postpone the procedure.

1. Active, inflammatory cervicitis
2. Uncooperative patient
3. Postmenopausal patient who is not on hormone replacement therapy
4. Heavy menses
5. Coagulopathy, or treatment with anticoagulants

Preparation

1. Informed consent
2. Explanation of procedure and all questions answered
3. Pregnancy test if needed

Equipment

1. Colposcope with blue/green filter

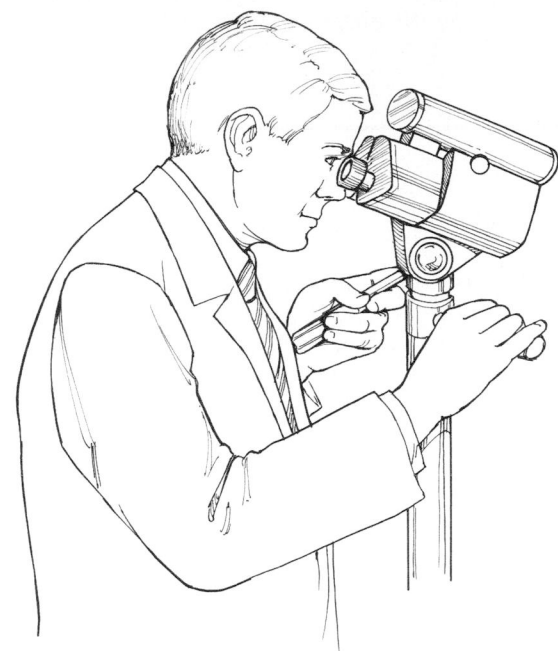

2. Vaginal speculum of appropriate size
3. Materials for Pap smear, if more than 6 weeks since last Pap done
4. Large swabs/OB-GYN applicators
5. 5% acetic acid solution (white vinegar)
6. Full-strength Lugol's iodine
7. Paste of Monsel's solution (ferric subsulfate)
8. Endocervical speculum
9. Endocervical curette (Kogan)
10. Biopsy forceps (Kevorkian, Tischler, baby Tischler)
11. Cotton- or rayon-tipped swabs
12. Ring forceps
13. 4 × 4-inch gauze
14. Single-tooth tenaculum: rarely used
15. Medicine or urine cups for solutions
16. Long needle holders and 3-0 chromic gut suture: rarely used
17. Biopsy containers

Anesthesia

None needed under normal circumstances.

1. Optional: Apply 20% benzocaine syrup or spray.
2. Can premedicate with nonsteroidal anti-inflammatory (NSAID) 30 minutes prior.
3. Can premedicate anxious patients with lorazepam.

Precautions

1. Pregnant patients: no endocervical curettage, caution with biopsies

2. Postmenopausal patients: May need estrogen priming to prevent atrophic friability.

3. Subacute bacterial endocarditis prophylaxis in appropriate patients

Technique

1. Perform bimanual examination for position and mobility of the cervix, depth of vagina, palpable abnormalities, size of uterus; visual examination of external genitalia for signs of condylomata. (Use acetic acid as necessary.)

2. Insert warmed speculum. Use largest size that is tolerated by patient. Vaginal sidewalls may be retracted by placing cut end of glove finger or finger cot over speculum before inserting.

3. Visualize cervix. Gently blot any cervical mucus away. Note areas of leukoplakia before applying acetic acid. Repeat Pap smear if indicated.

4. Apply 5% acetic acid to the entire portio of the cervix. Wait 1 to 2 minutes for the acetic reaction to occur. Note any areas of acetowhitening, mosaicism, punctation, abnormal vessels, or any other abnormality. (Vessel pattern is accentuated by viewing under blue or green filter.)

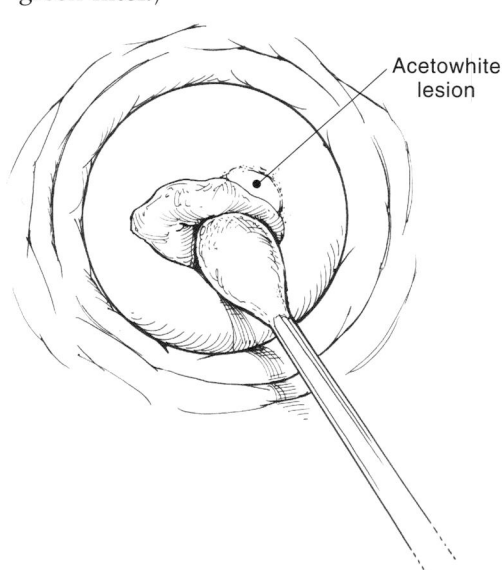

Acetowhite lesion

Reapply acetic acid if more than 5 minutes elapses. Grade lesions.

5. Assess adequacy of colposcopic examination.
   a. Entire squamocolumnar junction seen
   b. Entirety of lesions seen. Inspect endocervical canal if necessary.

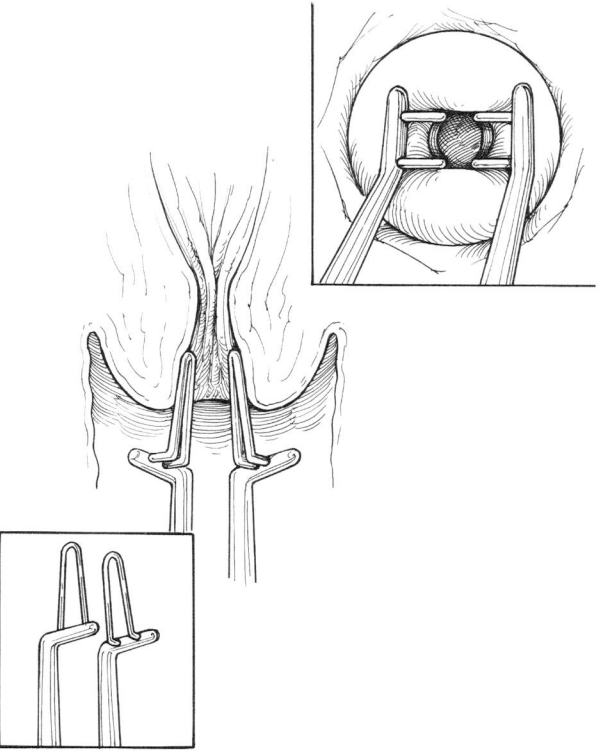

   c. Grade of lesions visualized corresponds to Pap smear report.

6. Confirm lesions with Lugol's iodine.

7. Perform endocervical curettage (nonpregnant patients only).

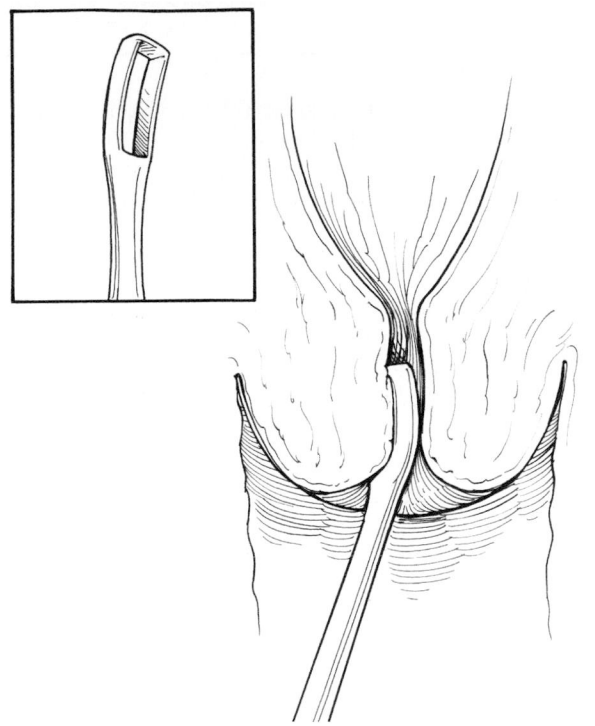

Biopsy posterior sites before anterior to prevent contamination of specimens with blood.

9. Apply Monsel's paste for hemostasis.
10. Examine vaginal sidewalls, using acetic acid as necessary.
11. Complete appropriate paperwork, including chart note with diagram of lesions and biopsy lab slips.

Follow-Up

Patient instructions include

1. Pelvic rest for 1 to 2 weeks
2. Expect black or dark bloody discharge and some cramping.
3. Take NSAIDs for pain.
4. Call for fever, purulent discharge, odor, pain, or bright red bleeding.
5. Make follow-up appointment to discuss biopsy results and treatment options.

Bibliography

American Academy of Family Physicians: Basic and Advanced Colposcopy for the Family Physician. Kansas City, MO, American Academy of Family Physicians, 1995.

Campion MJ, Ferris DG, di Paola FM, et al: Modern Colposcopy: A Practical Approach. Augusta, GA, Educational Systems, 1991.

Johnson BA: The colposcopic examination. Am Fam Physician 1996;53:2473–2482.

Newkirk GR: The colposcopic examination. In Pfenninger JL, Fowler GC (eds): Procedures for Primary Care Physicians, pp 616–639. St. Louis, Mosby-Year Book, 1994.

8. Take biopsies and send to lab in appropriate containers.

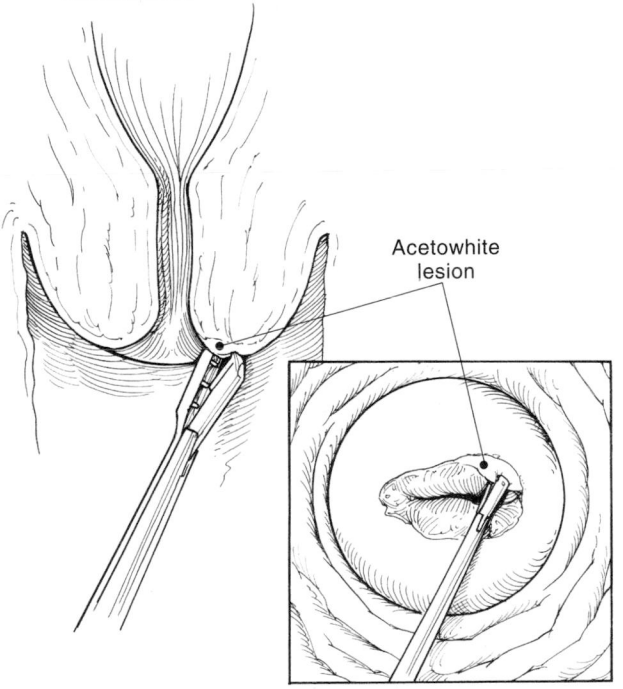

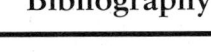

Acetowhite lesion

Cervical Biopsy

Indications
A biopsy should be taken from any visible abnormal lesion on the cervix.

Contraindications
1. Acute pelvic inflammatory disease or acute cervicitis
2. Coagulopathy (biopsy should be performed in a hospital setting)

Preparation
Obtain consent after patient is fully informed of procedure and its indications. May premedicate with nonsteroidal anti-inflammatory drug.

Equipment
1. Cervical biopsy punch (variety of styles and sizes; Eppendorfer, Tischler, Burke) (see previous procedure: Colposcopy)
2. 5% acetic acid
3. Monsel's paste or silver nitrate sticks
4. Labeled specimen container (10% neutral buffered formalin)
5. Skin hook, forceps
6. Cotton-tipped applicators, large and small

Anesthesia
1. No local anesthesia is typically used, although a paracervical block may be performed.
2. A nonsteroidal anti-inflammatory medication may be given prior to the procedure.

Precautions
Clinician should have adequate training, expertise, and understanding of cervical disease.

Technique
1. Insert the speculum. Apply acetic acid to the cervix to enhance visualization of the lesion.
2. Push biopsy forceps against the lesion site. Open forceps, push against tissue, close, and snip. Immediately place biopsy in specimen container (see preceding procedure: Colposcopy).
3. Obtain hemostasis via pressure, application of Monsel's paste, or cautery with silver nitrate.

Follow-Up
1. Patients are instructed to place nothing in the vagina (e.g., no douching, tampons, sex) for 2 weeks.
2. Patients should be seen for persistent bleeding or malodorous discharge.

LEEP (Loop Electrosurgical Excisional Procedure)

Indications
1. LEEP is a treatment option for cervical intraepithelial neoplasia (CIN) that entirely excises the lesion and transformation zone (TZ). Thin wire loop electrodes cut/coagulate tissue via high-frequency current.
2. LEEP can be used as a type of cervical conization procedure.
3. LEEP may be used to treat or remove superficial benign lesions (e.g., verrucae, nevi, keratoses).
4. Advantages/practical benefits of LEEP include
   a. Office procedure, low cost of equipment, quick excision time, relatively easy to learn
   b. Excellent patient acceptance, local anesthesia, minimal bleeding and pain, high cure rate
   c. Diagnosis of unsuspected microinvasive/invasive disease; all affected tissue and TZ removed (not destroyed), and submitted for histopathologic analysis.
   d. Simultaneous diagnosis/treatment of cervical lesion in single office visit for potentially noncompliant patients

Contraindications
1. Pregnancy
2. Acute cervicitis
3. Suspected invasive or microinvasive cancer
4. Abnormal Pap test without a biopsy confirmation or a colposcopically clear-cut CIN lesion
5. Coagulopathy

Preparation
1. Various options should be discussed with the patient and informed consent obtained.
2. Good colposcopic skills are required to identify the TZ, presence of disease, and complications.
3. Experience at a "hands-on" course prior to performing LEEP is highly recommended.

Equipment
1. Electrosurgical generator (with coagulate, cut, and blend modes) and a hand or foot switch
2. Loop (tungsten or stainless steel) and ball electrodes (variety of sizes and shapes)
3. Patient grounding pad

4. *Nonconductive* instruments (e.g., speculum, vaginal wall retractor, forceps, hooks)
5. Smoke evacuator, tubing, and filter system
6. Colposcope
7. 5% acetic acid, Lugol's iodine solution, Monsel's paste
8. 2% lidocaine (Xylocaine) with epinephrine (1:100,000); 27-gauge needles with extender or dental syringe
9. 10% neutral buffered formalin in container, pathology cassette for tissue specimen
10. Large gynecologic or rectal swabs, mask, gloves
11. Consent form, postprocedure information sheet
12. If needed: endocervical curette (for endocervical curettage [ECC]), long needle holder, and 2-0 Vicryl (for suturing)

Anesthesia

Infiltrate the cervix superficially with a total of 3 to 5 ml lidocaine at four to eight positions (3, 6, 9, and 12 o'clock and spaces between) at a distance of 3 mm beyond the TZ. A paracervical block is not needed.

Precautions

1. Morbidity/complications include
   a. Burns: inadvertent contact with active electrode, inadequate patient grounding, uninsulated instruments
   b. Bleeding: intraoperative or postoperative
   c. Injury: cautery, laceration, cervical stenosis (more common in postmenopausal patients)
   d. Infection: rare; occurs in 1 to 3 weeks, typically responds to antibiotics.
2. The smoke evacuator must be used and attached to the speculum.
   a. This helps to provide an unobstructed view.
   b. Viral particles in the plume are potentially contagious.
3. A depth of 5 mm or less at the 3 and 9 o'clock positions avoids cervical branches of the uterine arteries, which may bleed significantly. A depth of 7 to 8 mm is desirable at the center of the biopsy.

Technique: LEEP

1. Obtain informed consent; place patient in lithotomy position; apply ground pad; insert insulated, vented speculum. Use vaginal sidewall retractor as needed.
2. Perform colposcopy and apply acetic acid to cervix to delineate lesion; apply Lugol's solution to delineate TZ.
3. Anesthetize the cervix with lidocaine as described above.
4. Select the proper-sized loop based on the size of the TZ (a 20-mm wide by 8-mm deep loop is often adequate for a simple excision). Insert the loop onto the electrode handle.

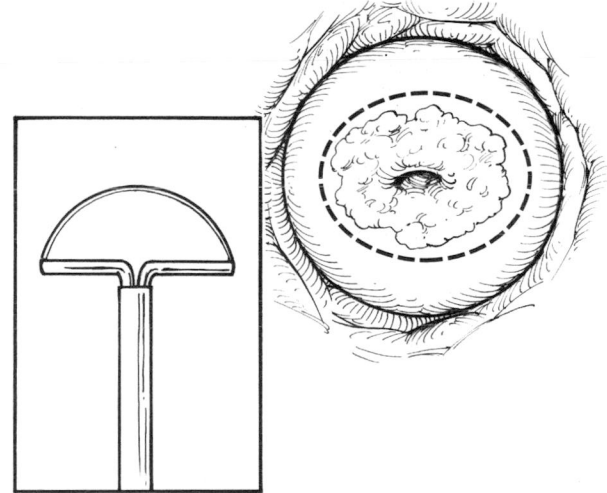

5. Make a test pass without power to ensure that loop chosen is the correct size and the vaginal walls are clear. Move either from side to side, top to bottom, or bottom to top, but avoid a backhanded pass.
6. Moisten the cervix with acetic acid before the excision.
7. Turn on the generator to the blended mode. Turn on the smoke evacuator.
8. Begin 3 to 5 mm lateral to the TZ and apply pressure to the loop to push it perpendicularly

into the tissue to a depth of 5 to 8 mm (or until the loop crossbar is reached).

9. Draw the loop across and underneath the tissue to 3 to 5 mm beyond the TZ on the opposite side. Bring the loop straight up and out of the tissue. (If the loop stalls during a pass, stop, turn off the unit, and remove and clean the loop. Reposition it and begin where you left off to complete the pass.)

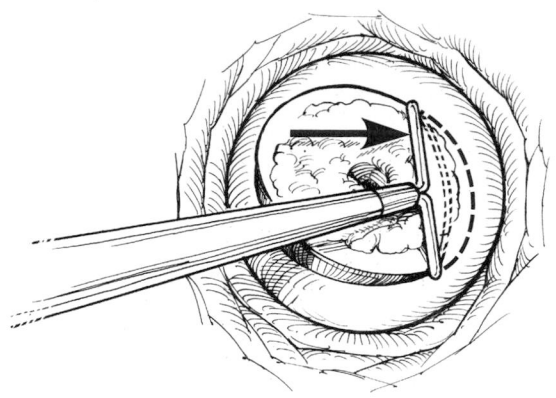

10. If a single pass does not encompass the entire TZ, it can be excised in several transverse strips.

11. Remove the tissue from the cervix, and mark it for orientation in a pathology cassette. Place in formalin.

12. Perform an ECC as indicated.

13. Insert the ball electrode into the handle. Set the electrosurgical generator to coagulation and lightly fulgurate the entire crater base. Treat all bleeding points. Spare the external os as much as possible.

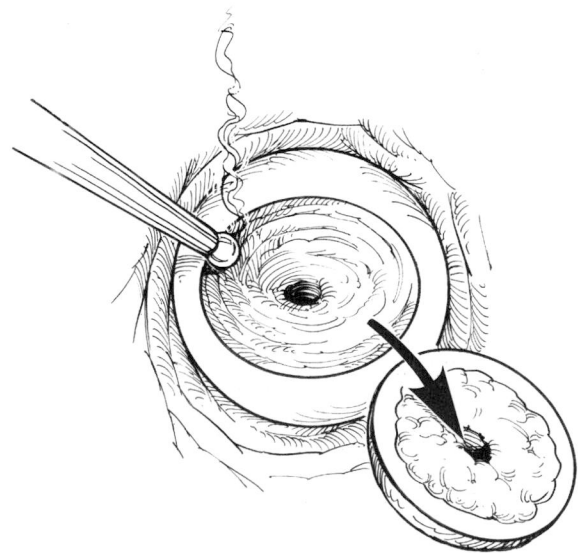

14. Apply a thick layer of Monsel's paste to the tissues. Remove the speculum after the bleeding has stopped. (Incidence of perioperative bleeding is approximately 1 per cent.)

15. A cone biopsy can be performed with a two-step LEEP approach. (See Bibliography for more detail.)

Follow-Up

1. An information sheet should make patients aware that
   a. Abdominal cramps may occur for a day or two.
   b. Brownish discharge will last for several weeks.
   c. No heavy lifting is recommended for 4 weeks.
   d. Nothing should be placed in the vagina for 4 weeks (no sex, tampons, etc.).
   e. The physician should be contacted in case of heavy bleeding or malodorous discharge.

2. Bleeding for more than a week should be evaluated. Heavy postoperative bleeding may occur several days to 3 weeks after the procedure. Treat with fulguration or Monsel's paste. Hospitalization is rare.

3. Follow-up should include colposcopy, Pap smear, and ECC at 4 to 6 months, then routine Pap smear every 3 to 4 months for the first year.

B Bibliography

Apgar BS, Wright TC, Pfenninger JL: Loop electrosurgical excision procedure for CIN. Am Fam Physician 1992;46:505–520.

Ferenczy A, Choukroun D, Arseneau J: Loop electrosurgical excision procedure for squamous intraepithelial lesions of the cervix: advantages and potential pitfalls. Obstet Gynecol 1996;87:332–337.

Mathevet P, Dargent D, Roy M, et al: A randomized prospective study comparing three techniques of conization: cold knife, laser and LEEP. Gynecol Oncol 1994; 54:175–179.

Mayeaux EJ, Harper MB: Loop electrosurgical excisional procedure. J Fam Pract 1993;36:214–219.

Prendiville W: Large loop excision of the transformation zone. Clin Obstet Gynecol 1995;38:622–639.

106 Cervical Cancer

Jim Nuovo

Etiology

Risk Factors

1. First sexual contact at a young age
2. Multiple sexual partners
3. A promiscuous male partner
4. History of genital warts
5. Smoking
6. Folate deficiency
7. Immunosuppression
8. Low socioeconomic status
9. A prolonged time since the last Pap smear (>5 years)

Human Papillomavirus Types and Extent of Cervical Disease

It had been suspected for a number of years that the agent responsible for the development of cervical cancer is contagious and sexually transmittable. The link between the human papillomavirus (HPV) and cervical cancer and its precursors (dysplasia) is strong. With the development of techniques in molecular biology allowing for the identification and classification of HPV, it has been possible to compare specific HPV types to the extent of cervical disease. The findings from this research include the following observations:

1. Infection with HPV is extremely common, and in fact HPV represents the most common viral sexually transmitted disease. HPV infects 10 per cent of the general population and up to 30 per cent of individuals presenting to sexually transmitted disease clinics.
2. HPV is a highly contagious disease.
3. Many patients with HPV will have "subclinical" disease, and there may be a long latency period between the time of infection and the expression of overt disease.
4. There has been an association between certain HPV types and the development of cervical cancer. HPV types 16, 18, 31, 33, 35, and 39 are particularly associated with an increased risk. However, patients infected with an oncogenic strain will not necessarily develop cervical cancer or dysplasia. Because of this problem, it remains unclear whether HPV testing is worthwhile.

Symptoms

1. Cervical cancer and dysplasia usually occur without symptoms. For this reason it is important to recommend that patients at risk for cervical cancer participate in periodic cytology screening.
2. Among women being screened for cervical disease with a Pap smear, approximately 90 to 95 per cent will be diagnosed as normal.
3. Because of extensive screening, most women who have cervical precancers are identified by the Pap smear at a stage where the lesion is easily eradicated. The 5-year survival rate is considerably better for women with local cervical cancer versus those with advanced disease (90 vs. 40 per cent). Therefore, the goal of screening is to detect precursors to cervical cancer and to provide an opportunity for the provider to prevent progression to invasive cancer.
4. The effectiveness of cervical cancer screening increases when Pap smear testing is performed more frequently. Aggressive (dysplastic) lesions are less likely to escape detection when the interval between smears is short.
5. Pap smear screening schedule recommendations have come from many groups. The recent recommendations from the U.S. Preventive Services Task Force encompasses many of the principles seen in other reports, that is, "testing should begin at the age when the woman first engages in sexual intercourse. Pap tests are appropriately performed at an interval of one to three years, to be recommended by the physician based on the presence of risk factors."
6. Another issue related to screening is that of false-negative examinations. The reported frequency has ranged from 20 to 45 per cent.
7. Two factors contributing to this problem include Pap smear technique and reliability of interpretation. Proper technique in the performance of a Pap smear is critical. The proper methodology is reviewed elsewhere in the text (see Procedure: Pap Smear).
8. The combined use of a cytobrush and Ayre spatula has been shown to improve the quality

of the submitted smear. A cytopathologist has over 50,000 epithelial cells to review on a given Pap smear slide. Only a small percentage of the cells may be abnormal on any given slide.

9. The criteria used to define an abnormal cell include

    a. Abnormal amount for nuclear chromatin

    b. Collection of chromatin clumps in the nucleus

    c. Increased nuclear size and nuclear/cytoplasmic ratio

    d. Increased mitotic activity and increased number of nuclei

10. These criteria are subject to problems with intra- and interobserver variability. In a study of the reproducibility of cytodiagnosis of Pap smears, it was shown that agreement between two cytopathologists was achieved 75 per cent of the time and, on re-review by the same pathologist, 80 per cent of the time. New automated technologies have become available that are designed to enhance the ability of the cytopathologist to detect cytologic abnormalities. Rigorous testing of these devices is underway.

11. In 1988, federal Pap smear legislation was enacted to improve the quality of Pap smear reporting and reduce the confusion in Pap smear terminology. Uniform standards were established in reporting cytology results. This new classification system was designated the Bethesda System. The new system has not been adopted by all pathologists, and therefore it is important to be able to compare the differences between the systems (see Ch. 105, Abnormal Pap Smear). Even with the Bethesda System, there remains confusion by family physicians as to how to manage an abnormal result. Melnikow et al. (1993) found that family physicians were more likely to misinterpret the results of a cytology report using the Bethesda System of nomenclature and were likely to overutilize colposcopy.

Key Symptoms

- Usually asymptomatic
- Postcoital bleeding
- Abnormal vaginal bleeding/discharge

Clinical Findings

1. In order to get a good cervical smear, direct visualization of the cervix during a Pap smear is an important part of the pelvic examination. However, cervical cancer and its precursors will not generally be detectable by direct inspection.

2. Colposcopy has been used to identify the specific abnormal areas, to determine the extent of a lesion, and to direct the biopsy to the areas of concern.

3. Some authors advocate acetic acid washes of the cervix as an adjunct to the Pap smear. Those patients who demonstrate areas of whitening would be advised to undergo colposcopy.

4. Cervicography, acetic acid washing followed by a standardized photograph of the cervix, has also been proposed. The "cervigram" is reviewed by an expert and recommendations follow as to whether the patient needs colposcopy. Because of their inherently high false-positive rates, it remains controversial as to whether either test offers an advantage over periodic Pap smears with colposcopy for those with dysplastic or atypical findings.

Key Sign

- Ulcerative/friable cervix

Laboratory Tests

The "laboratory test" in the evaluation of a patient for cervical cancer is the Pap smear report. Clarity in the reporting of Pap smear results has been an ongoing problem.

1. Systems used to report cytologic findings

    a. Class system (classes I through V)

    b. World Health Organization system (Normal; Atypical; Dysplasia—Mild, —Moderate and —Severe; Invasive Squamous Cell Carcinoma; and Adenocarcinoma)

    c. Cervical intraepithelial neoplasia (CIN) system (Normal; CIN I, II, or III; Invasive Squamous Cell Carcinoma)

    d. Bethesda System (Within Normal Limits; Epithelial Cell Abnormalities; Atypical Squamous Cells of Undetermined Significance, Squamous Intraepithelial Lesions [SIL]; Low-Grade, High-Grade SIL; Squamous Cell Carcinoma; and gland cell abnormalities).

2. Equivalent reports among the four systems

    a. Normal (Class I, Within Normal Limits)

    b. Atypia (Class II, Atypical, Atypical Squamous Cells of Undetermined Significance)

    c. Dysplasia (Class III, CIN I, Dysplasia—Mild, Low-Grade SIL)

d. Dysplasia (Class IV, CIN II or III, Dysplasia–Moderate to –Severe, High-Grade SIL)

e. Carcinoma (Class V, Carcinoma, Squamous Cell Carcinoma)

> **WARNING**
>
> There is confusion among physicians as to how to interpret Pap smear reports. All women with dysplasia (or the equivalent term) should undergo colposcopy. Women with atypia may be evaluated for infection and, if present, treated and have another Pap smear in 3 to 4 months. Persistent atypia warrants colposcopy.

Key Tests

- Pap smear
- Colposcopy

Differential Diagnosis

1. Dysplasia on a Pap smear must be investigated to rule out invasive carcinoma.

2. Atypia on a Pap smear may be produced by dysplasia, infection or repair of the cervix. Infectious processes that may produce atypia (other than HPV) include:

   a. Bacterial vaginosis
   b. *Candida*
   c. *Trichomonas*
   d. *Chlamydia trachomatis*
   e. *Neisseria gonorrhoeae*

3. In the post-menopausal patient hormone related atrophic changes may produce atypia as well.

Treatment

Dysplasia

1. All patients with a Pap smear demonstrating high-grade dysplasia are recommended to undergo an immediate colposcopic examination of the cervix.

2. The management of the patient after colposcopy is dependent on the specific findings. If dysplasia is found, the patient may undergo cryotherapy, laser ablation, low-voltage loop electroexcision, or cone biopsy. The appropriate treatment and follow-up will depend on the following parameters: lesion grade, size, and whether it involves the endocervical canal.

Atypia

1. In patients who have atypia or low-grade dysplasia on their Pap smear, there remains a great deal of controversy as to whether an immediate colposcopy is warranted.

2. One may choose to re-examine a patient with atypia to assess whether there is an ongoing infection. If an infection is discovered, the patient may be treated accordingly and the Pap smear repeated in 3 to 4 months.

3. In patients with low-grade dysplasia, the rate of spontaneous regression may be as high as 50 per cent. Therefore, repeat Pap smear is recommended in 4 to 6 months.

4. Patients with persistent abnormalities should undergo a colposcopic evaluation.

5. There are no data to suggest that cautious follow-up with repeat Pap smears will result in a delayed diagnosis with increased morbidity.

Cancer

1. Cervical cancer has a clinical staging system that routinely incorporates the following information:

   a. History and physical examination
   b. Biopsy
   c. Chest radiograph
   d. Intravenous pyelogram (IVP)
   e. Stool for occult blood

2. Often additional tests are done to further investigate abnormal results of these screening tests. They include

   a. Cystoscopy
   b. Urine cytology
   c. Sigmoidoscopy
   d. Barium enema
   e. Bone scan

3. Potentially useful tests include

   a. Computerized tomography scan (pelvis and abdomen)
   b. Laparoscopy
   c. Serum tumor markers: carcinoembryonic antigen (CEA)

4. Treatment for cervical cancer is dependent on the stage. The standard operation for microinvasive cancer is simple excision (cone biopsy). Patients with early-stage cancers should undergo radical hysterectomy with bilateral pelvic lymphadenectomy. Patients with later stage cancers often receive combined therapy with radiation (external beam and intracavity) followed by hysterectomy.

   a. Microinvasive cancers: The criteria for diagnosis of microinvasion are that the cancer penetrates less than 3 mm beneath the basement membrane and there is no lymph/vascular space involvement.

b. Early-stage cancers include

   (1) Stage I: The cancer is confined strictly to the cervix. Patients diagnosed with disease confined to the cervix have a 5-year survival of 91%.

   (2) Stage IIa: The cancer extends beyond the cervix, but it has not extended to the pelvic wall. The cancer involves the vagina, but not as far as the lower third. There is no parametrial involvement.

c. Later stage cancers include

   (1) Stage IIb: As stage IIa but with obvious parametrial involvement

   (2) Stage III: The cancer has extended to the pelvic wall. On rectal examination, there is no cancer-free space between the tumor and the pelvic wall.

   (3) Stage IV: The cancer has extended beyond the true pelvis or has clinically involved the mucosa of the bladder or rectum.

Key Treatment

- For microinvasive disease: cone biopsy

- For early-stage cancers: radical hysterectomy with bilateral pelvic lymphadenectomy

- For later stage cancers: radiation therapy (external beam and intracavity) followed by hysterectomy

Follow-Up

The appropriate follow-up for a patient with an abnormal Pap smear is dependent on the abnormality seen.

1. Dysplasia: Patients who have high-grade or persistent low-grade dysplasia should undergo a colposcopic examination. If dysplasia is detected on this examination, the patient should undergo the appropriate treatment. Follow-up for these patients will be more frequent (on av-

erage every 4 to 6 months for 1 to 2 years). Repeat colposcopy is done for recurrent abnormalities. If there is a marked discrepancy between the Pap smear and the colposcopy report (e.g., high-grade dysplasia on a Pap smear and a normal or nondiagnostic colposcopy report), a repeat colposcopy should be considered.

2. Atypia: Patients with atypia may be investigated for infection. If an infection is discovered, the patient should be treated and seen again for a Pap smear in 3 to 4 months. Persistent atypia warrants colposcopy.

3. Microinvasive disease: Patients with microinvasive disease should be followed with repeat Pap smear and colposcopy.

4. Cancer: Most recurrences occur within 2 years of treatment. Follow-up should include

  a. Repeat bimanual rectovaginal/abdominal examinations

  b. Palpation of inguinal lymph nodes

  c. Examination of abdomen and lower extremities

  d. Pap smear

  e. Yearly chest radiograph

  f. IVP every 6 months for 2 years

  g. Possibly CEA markers

Bibliography

For more information on cervical cancer screening, see
U.S. Preventive Services Task Force: Screening for cervical cancer. Am Fam Physician 1990;41:853–857.

For more information on the Pap smear test, see
Koss LG: The Papanicolaou test for cervical cancer detection: a triumph and a tragedy. JAMA 1989;261: 737–743.

For more information on the confusion in interpreting Pap smear reports, see
Melnikow J, Sierk A, Flocke S, et al: Does the system of Papanicolaou test nomenclature affect the rate of referral for colposcopy? A survey of family physicians. Arch Fam Med 1993;2:253–258.

For more information on the human papillomavirus, see
Reid R: Biology and colposcopic features of human papillomavirus-associated cervical disease. Obstet Gynecol Clin North Am 1993;20:123–151.

For more information on the management of patients with an abnormal Pap smear, see
Nuovo GJ: Cytopathology of the Lower Female Genital Tract: An Integrated Approach. Baltimore, Williams & Wilkins, 1994.

107 Endometrial Cancer

Daniel E. Brewer

Etiology

1. Endometrial cancer is the most common gynecologic cancer and the fourth most common cancer in women in the United States. It is the ninth most common cause of cancer death in American women.

2. Age is the most important risk factor. Median age of diagnosis is 61 years, with less than 5 per cent of cases occurring before age 40 and 20 per cent occurring before menopause. Incidence is 3.4:100,000 at less than age 50, 76:100,000 at greater than age 50.

3. Most risks other than age are related to unopposed estrogen stimulation of the endometrium (see Table 107–1).

4. Diabetes mellitus is less clear as a risk factor. This may be an association with obesity.

Symptoms

1. Postmenopausal bleeding is the cardinal symptom of endometrial cancer.

   a. Ninety per cent of endometrial carcinomas cause irregular perimenopausal or postmenopausal bleeding.

   b. Twenty per cent of patients with postmenopausal bleeding will have a pelvic carcinoma.

   c. "Postmenopausal bleeding" is defined as any vaginal bleeding 1 year or more after the last menstrual period.

2. In the case of a patient receiving estrogen replacement therapy, any nonmenstrual or intermenstrual bleeding should be considered suspicious.

3. If a woman is given a continuous estrogen/progesterone regimen, irregular bleeding can be tolerated for the first 6 months but should be investigated if it lasts longer than that.

4. Advanced cases with metastases may exhibit abdominal pain, pelvic pressure, hematuria, urinary frequency, constipation, rectal bleeding, or symptoms of abdominal obstruction.

Key Symptom

Postmenopausal bleeding

Clinical Findings

1. Pelvic examination and general physical examination will be normal in the majority of cases.

2. The presence of uterine fibroids should not prevent further evaluation.

3. Advanced disease may be associated with a pelvic or abdominal mass.

4. Because of the low overall incidence of disease and the high survival rates, screening in asymptomatic patients is not recommended.

Key Signs

None

Laboratory Tests

The standard evaluation is the Pap smear, endocervical curettage (to differentiate from cervical carcinoma), and tissue evaluation of the endometrium (endometrial biopsy or dilatation and curettage [D&C]). Transvaginal ultrasonography is an emerging technology used to avoid invasive evaluation.

1. D&C is the traditional test for initial diagnosis.

   a. Invasive procedure that requires general anesthesia or conscious sedation

   b. Now generally reserved for inadequate endometrial biopsy or when signs and symptoms are confusing

TABLE 107–1. RISK FACTORS FOR ENDOMETRIAL CANCER

RISK FACTOR	RELATIVE RISK
Polycystic ovary disease	5
Anovulatory infertility	4
Obesity	
20–50 lb above ideal body weight	3
>50 lb above ideal body weight	9
Family history of breast, colon, endometrial cancer	2
Late menopause (>52 years of age)	2
Early menarche	2
Unopposed postmenopausal estrogens	5–10
Postmenopausal estrogen/progesterone	0.5
Tamoxifen therapy	6

2. Endometrial biopsy
   a. Sensitivity is greater than 90 per cent compared to D&C.
   b. Small, flexible curettes cause less pain and make this an office procedure.
   c. May miss carcinoma that is confined to a polyp or localized in a small area of endometrium.
3. Transvaginal ultrasonography
   a. Sensitivity for endometrial cancer is greater than 90 per cent but specificity is around 50 per cent.
   b. This gives a negative predictive value (chance that patient with negative test does not, in fact, have cancer) of 99 per cent.
4. Hysteroscopy with biopsy: usually reserved for complicated cases or when the diagnosis is still in doubt after less invasive testing
5. Pap smear
   a. Not an effective tool to evaluate possibility of endometrial cancer, but should be done because of the chance of cervical cancer as the cause of bleeding.
   b. Presence of "endometrial cells" or "glandular abnormality" on Pap should lead to work-up for endometrial cancer.

Key Tests

- Endometrial biopsy
- Endocervical curettage
- Pap smear

Differential Diagnosis

1. Endometrial hyperplasia
   a. Simple (cystic) hyperplasia and complex (adenomatous) hyperplasia without atypia are generally not precursors to invasive cancer.
   b. Hyperplasia with atypia is potentially a premalignant lesion.
2. Atrophic endometrium
3. Endometrial or endocervical polyps
4. Submucous fibroids
5. Cervicitis or cervical cancer

Treatment

1. Total abdominal hysterectomy with bilateral salpingo-oophrectomy is the cornerstone of all potential curative therapies.
2. Staging of the tumor is done at the time of surgery (Table 107–2).

TABLE 107–2. SIMPLIFIED DEFINITIONS FOR FIGO STAGES AND PROGNOSIS WITH CORRECT TREATMENT

Classification	Description	5-Year Survival (%)
Stage 0	Hyperplasia with atypia or carcinoma in situ	100
Stage I	Carcinoma confined to the uterine corpus	
	IA, grade 1	98
	IC, grade 2	63
Stage II	Carcinoma extends into the cervix	55
Stage III	Carcinoma extends outside the uterus but not outside the true pelvis	28
Stage IV	Carcinoma extends beyond the true pelvis	9

3. Radiation therapy is recommended for all tumors greater than stage I and some stage I tumors based on pathologic grade.
3. Extensive metastases may also be treated with chemotherapy and/or progesterone-based hormonal manipulation.
4. Intravaginal radium treatment reduces the risk of vaginal cuff recurrence.

Patient Education

1. Emphasize importance of follow-up monitoring for patients who have risk for local recurrence.
2. Future use of estrogen products requires careful explanation of potential risk and benefits.

Key Treatment

Abdominal hysterectomy and salpingo-oophorectomy ± radiation treatment

Follow-Up

1. Although there are established protocols for follow-up of patients after treatment for endometrial carcinoma, there is no evidence that such follow-up reduces morbidity or mortality.
2. Follow-up efforts should be directed at early detection of local vaginal cuff recurrences, not metastatic disease. Pap smear of the vaginal cuff should be done every 6 months for the first 3 years and yearly thereafter (most recurrences occur in the first 3 years).
3. There is an association between endometrial cancer and cancer of the breast and bowel, so patients should receive the appropriate screening for those cancers.

4. Estrogen treatment after therapy for endometrial cancer remains controversial but is not absolutely contraindicated. Careful consideration of each individual case is required.

Bibliography

Berchuch A, Anspach C, Evans A, et al: Postsurgical surveillance of patients with FIGO stage I/II endometrial adenocarcinoma. Gynecol Oncol 1995;59:20–24.

Harras A (ed): Cancer: Rates and Risks, 4th ed (NIH publication No. 96-691). Bethesda, MD: National Institutes of Health, 1996.

Langer RD, Pierce JJ, O'Hanlan KA, et al for the PEPI investigators: Transvaginal ultrasonography compared with endometrial biopsy for the detection of endometrial disease. N Engl J Med 1997;337:1792–1798.

Shelly M: Endometrial biopsy. Am Fam Physician 1997; 55:1731–1736.

Speroff L, Glass RH, Kase NG: Dysfunctional uterine bleeding. In: Clinical Gynecologic Endocrinology and Infertility, 5th ed, pp 531–546. Baltimore, Williams & Wilkins, 1994.

108 Dysfunctional Uterine Bleeding

Lili Church

Etiology

1. Dysfunctional uterine bleeding (DUB) is defined as the bleeding manifestations of anovulatory cycles. There are many additional causes of abnormal vaginal bleeding, and DUB is a diagnosis of exclusion.

2. In a normal menstrual cycle, the endometrial lining is built up during the initial proliferatory phase primarily as a result of the effects of estrogen. Ovulation then occurs midcycle, followed by the secretory phase, during which the endometrial lining further develops and stabilizes as a result of the combined effect of both estrogen and progesterone. If ovulation does not occur, unopposed estrogen continues to stimulate the endometrial lining, causing it to thicken abnormally. In the relative absence of progesterone, however, this thickened lining is relatively unstable and results in intermittent partial sloughing of the endometrial lining.

3. Causes of DUB resulting from a thickened endometrium include:
   a. Perimenopause
   b. Puberty
   c. Polycystic ovarian disease (PCOD), or Stein-Leventhal syndrome
   d. Obesity
   e. Unopposed estrogen replacement therapy

4. Another pattern of anovulatory cycles causing DUB occurs when estrogen is low relative to progesterone. This results in a thin and unstable endometrial lining that similarly is prone to irregular bleeding. Causes of DUB resulting from a thinned endometrium include
   a. Progestins
      (1) Norethindrone "mini-pill" (Micronor, Nor-Q.D.)
      (2) Medroxyprogesterone acetate injection (Depo-Provera)
      (3) Levonorgestrel implants (Norplant)
   b. Some low-estrogen combination oral contraceptive pills (OCPs)

Symptoms

1. Dysfunctional bleeding pattern is typically amenorrhea with infrequent periods of heavy flow. In general, women whose DUB is caused by a thickened endometrium will have heavier bleeding and are at risk for acute hemorrhage. Although women with a thin endometrium similarly have irregular and unpredictable bleeding, the actual blood loss is usually small and inconvenient rather than dangerous, and requires no treatment.

2. Another risk of untreated anovulation is endometrial cancer. Endometrium that is chronically stimulated with a relative excess of estrogen is prone to developing proliferative hyperplasia. This may further progress into adenomatous hyperplasia and eventually endometrial cancer.

Key Symptoms

- Irregular heavy periods
- Intermittent spotting

Clinical Findings

Clinical presentation may be acute or chronic.

1. Acutely, DUB may present with
   a. Orthostatic changes in blood pressure and heart rate
   b. Pallor
   c. Vagina: large amount of blood in vault rapidly replaced with ongoing bleeding from cervical os
   d. Uterus: normal or enlarged (retained clots)

2. Chronically
   a. Stable blood pressure and heart rate
   b. Body habitus: may reflect underlying obesity or stigmata of PCOD
   c. Skin: pale or normal
   d. Vagina: small amount or absence of blood
   e. Uterus: normal

Key signs

- Pale skin
- Vaginal bleeding

Laboratory Tests

Tests obtained are individualized to each case, but may include

1. Pregnancy test
2. Hematocrit
3. Pap smear
4. Cervical cultures
5. Prothrombin time, partial thromboplastin time, platelets
6. Luteinizing hormone, follicle-stimulating hormone, thyroid-stimulating hormone, prolactin, testosterone
7. Endometrial biopsy is indicated in patients over age 40, and any patient with a prolonged history of irregular vaginal bleeding, such as a young patient with PCOD.
8. Hysteroscopy is helpful when other work-up fails to diagnose the abnormal bleeding. It is used to detect and excise endometrial polyps and submucosal fibroids, and to obtain directed biopsies.
9. Transvaginal ultrasound detects fibroids and endometrial polyps and assesses for a thickened endometrial stripe larger than 5 mm that may indicate hyperplasia or carcinoma.
10. Hysterosonography (hydrosonography), a newer modality with increased sensitivity, combines sonography with the infusion of fluid into the intrauterine cavity.

Note

The choice to utilize endometrial biopsy, transvaginal sonography, or a combination of these, must be made on an individual basis. The choice is dependent on patient history, symptoms, level of suspicion for malignancy, cost, test availability, and patient preference.

 Key Tests

- Hematocrit
- Pregnancy test
- Endometrial biopsy

Differential Diagnosis

There are many other causes of abnormal uterine bleeding in addition to anovulatory cycling. These must be assessed for and excluded before a patient is diagnosed to have DUB. This is accomplished by taking a careful history with particular attention to the timing and characteristics of the bleeding pattern, performing a physical examination, and utilizing individualized laboratory tests.

1. Hormonal
   a. Anovulation, that is, DUB: puberty, perimenopause, precursor to premature ovarian failure, anorexia, extreme stress, obesity, hypothyroidism, hyperprolactinemia, PCOD
   b. Breakthrough bleeding on exogenous hormones (e.g., combination or progestogen-only OCPs, Depo-Provera, Norplant, or hormone replacement therapy)
2. Anatomic and physiologic
   a. Cancer: vulvar, vaginal, cervical, endometrial, ovarian
   b. Polyps: cervical, endometrial
   c. Uterine fibroids: usually submucosal
   d. Pregnancy: miscarriage, ectopic, mole
   e. Ovulation
   f. Postpartum: retained placental tissue, atony, subinvolution
   g. Trauma: intercourse, foreign body, intrauterine device (IUD)
3. Infectious
   a. Cervicitis (e.g., chlamydia)
   b. Endometritis (e.g., postpartum)
   c. Pelvic inflammatory disease (e.g., gonococcal)
4. Hematologic: bleeding and coagulation disorders (e.g., von Willebrand's disease, idiopathic thrombocytopenic purpura, hemophilia, liver or renal failure)

Treatment

Treatment is determined by the severity and chronicity of bleeding.

Acute Treatment

1. Required if the patient is hemorrhaging, vital signs unstable, with anemia present or predictable.
2. Treatment options include
   a. Combination OCP qid for 7 days
   b. Combination OCP qid for 2 days, then tid for 2 days, then qd until 21-day pack is completed. (Then expect heavy bleeding several days after stopping pills. Warn the patient of this!)
   c. Intravenous conjugated estrogen (Premarin), 25 mg q2–4h
   d. Antiemetic medication if estrogens are given
   e. Dilatation and curettage (only when above fails). Avoid if possible in adolescents.

Subacute Treatment

Acute bleeding episode has already been controlled. If the endometrium is still estimated to be thickened overall, continued but controlled shedding is indicated with such treatment as combination OCP for 3 months. Many patients then resume normal ovulatory menstrual cycling on their own without further need for hormonal regulation. However, a significant number redevelop anovulation with resultant DUB and require chronic treatment.

Chronic Treatment

Chronic treatment usually is required when the patient has an underlying predisposing cause (e.g., perimenopause, PCOD, obesity) that results in ongoing abnormal bleeding. Treatment is aimed both at preventing complications of chronic blood loss and preventing endometrial cancer. This is accomplished by hormonally thinning (or surgically eliminating) the endometrial lining. Choice of treatment additionally depends on whether contraception is desired. Options include

1. Combination estrogen and progesterone
   a. OCPs
   b. Hormone replacement therapy
2. Progestins
   a. Medroxyprogesterone acetate tablets (Provera qmo 10 mg days 1 to 10)
   b. Medroxyprogesterone acetate tablets (Provera), 10 mg days 1 to 14 q3mo
   c. Norethindrone (Micronor), 2 mg, same timing as Provera
   d. Norethindrone "minipill" (Micronor, Nor-Q.D.), 0.35 mg qd
   e. Medroxyprogesterone acetate injection (Depo-Provera), 150 mg IM q3mo
   f. Levonorgestrel implants (Norplant)
   g. Progestin IUD (Progestasert)
   h. Progestins potentially used for DUB are micronized oral progesterone, progesterone patch, vaginal progesterone cream
3. Antiprostaglandins: As prostaglandin synthetase inhibitors, nonsteroidal anti-inflammatory drugs can be used to decrease endometrial bleeding. (*Note*: Drugs that treat the menorrhagia component of DUB do not prevent anovulation, and thus do not prevent metrorrhagia, endometrial hyperplasia, or endometrial cancer.)
   a. Mefenamic acid (Ponstel), 500 mg tid
   b. Ibuprofen (Motrin), 400 to 600 mg qid
   c. Naproxen (Naprosyn), 250, 375, or 500 mg bid

   d. Naproxen sodium (Anaprox), 550 mg, then 275 mg bid to qid
4. Clomiphene citrate (Clomid): used for women wanting to conceive
5. Androgenic steroids (Danazol, 100 to 200 mg bid): very selective criteria for use. In DUB, used to treat severe menorrhagia in patients who fail other hormonal treatments. Significant side effects.
6. Gonadotropin-releasing hormone agonists: very selective criteria for use. In DUB, used to treat severe menorrhagia in patients who fail other hormonal treatments and wish to retain fertility, in those with hematologic disorders, and in patients to thin the endometrial lining prior to endometrial ablation. With chronic use, creates a "medical menopause" with accompanying long-term complications that are only partially addressed by using estrogen and/or progesterone "add-back" therapy.
   a. Leuprolide acetate injectable (Lupron), 3.75 mg IM qmo
   b. Nafarelin acetate intranasal (Synarel), 1 spray (200 μg) bid in alternating nostrils
   c. Goserelin acetate subcutaneous implant (Zoladex), 3.6 mg IM q28d
7. Desmopressin: treatment for menorrhagia in patients with coagulation disorders such as von Willebrand's disease
   a. Desmopressin acetate (DDAVP) parenteral, 0.3 mg/kg in 50 ml normal saline IV over 15 to 30 minutes every 12 to 24 hours
   b. DDAVP nasal spray, 1.5 mg/ml: 150 μg for patients weighing less than 50 kg and 300 μg for patients weighing more than 50 kg; effective for up to 24 to 48 hours
8. Endometrial ablation
9. Myomectomy
10. Hysterectomy (last resort)

Key Treatment

- Combination OCPs
- Estrogen
- Progestins

Follow-Up

Close follow-up for DUB is important for both its acute and chronic presentations. DUB can be a recurrent problem for which patient education is particularly crucial. Treatment goals include

1. Stop acute bleeding, avert future episodes, prevent long-term complications, and replenish iron stores.
2. Identify and treat underlying cause of DUB.
3. Treat anemia, if present, with dietary and/or supplementary oral iron if indicated. Monitor for initial normalization of hematocrit and whether further chronic maintenance iron is required.
4. Monitor for treatment effectiveness, compliance, and side effects.
5. Change therapy as treatment goals change, such as a change in need for concurrent contraception.
6. Work with patients to develop mutual treatment goals.
7. Educate patients about warning symptoms and when to seek medical advice.
8. Consult gynecologist for DUB that remains unexplained or unresponsive to hormonal therapy.

Bibliography

Apgar BS: Dysmenorrhea and dysfunctional uterine bleeding. Prim Care 1997;24:161–178.

Ash SJ, Farrell SA, Flowerdew G: Endometrial biopsy in DUB. J Reprod Med 1996;41:892–896.

Chen BH, Giudice LC: Dysfunctional uterine bleeding. West J Med 1998;169:280–284.

Lavin C: Dysfunctional uterine bleeding in adolescents. Curr Opin Pediatr 1996;8:328–332.

Speroff L, Glass RH, Kase NG: Clinical Gynecologic Endocrinology & Infertility, 5th ed, pp 531–546. Baltimore, Williams & Wilkins, 1994.

Stabinsky SA, Einstein M, Breen JL: Modern treatments of menorrhagia attributable to dysfunctional uterine bleeding. Obstet Gynecol Surv 1999;54:61–62.

Towbin NA, Gviazda IM, March CM: Office hysteroscopy versus transvaginal ultrasonography in the evaluation of patients with excessive uterine bleeding. Am J Obstet Gynecol 1996;174:1678–1682.

Indications

Usually performed to rule out endometrial cancer or hyperplasia

1. Suspected anovulatory cycles and unopposed estrogen effect
2. Dysfunctional uterine bleeding in women over 35
3. Postmenopausal bleeding
4. Abnormal bleeding in women on estrogen and progesterone or tamoxifen
5. Periodically when unopposed estrogen has been prescribed for a woman with a uterus
6. Pap smear with normal endometrial cells in a postmenopausal woman or during the latter half of the cycle in a premenopausal woman
7. After treatment for endometrial hyperplasia
8. As part of work-up for infertility or recurrent miscarriages; sample on day 25 to 26 to test for a luteal-phase defect.

Contraindications

1. Acute pelvic infection (unless endometrial sampling is being used to confirm a diagnosis of endometritis)
2. Pregnancy
3. Bleeding disorders
4. Circumstances when dilatation and curettage (D&C) or hysteroscopy is preferable
   a. Abnormal uterine anatomy
   b. Inability to accomplish office endometrial aspiration
   c. Tissue insufficient for diagnosis on endometrial aspiration, with continued abnormal bleeding
   d. Endometrial hyperplasia that did not respond to treatment
   e. Pap smear with atypical or suspicious endometrial cells

Preparation

1. Timing: late luteal phase if cycling
2. Premedication may be helpful: nonsteroidal anti-inflammatory drug 1 hour beforehand.
3. Obtain informed consent.

Equipment

1. Endometrial sampling devices: When successful, all have equivalent yield of endometrial neoplasms.
   a. Flexible 3-mm plastic cannula (Pipelle from Unimar, Wilton, CT; or Z-Sampler from Zinnanti, Chatsworth, CA)
   b. Rigid 3-mm cannula with syringe for suction (e.g., Explora, Tis-U-Trap from Milex)
   c. Rigid cannula with mechanical suction (e.g., Vabra aspirator from Berkeley Medevices attached to electric suction pump)
   d. Less discomfort and risk from flexible aspiration devices
   e. Use 3-mm rigid cannula if unable to pass flexible one. Have both types available.
2. Other equipment for the procedure
   a. Vaginal speculum and light
   b. Pap smear sampling devices
   c. Endocervical curette
   d. Ring forceps
   e. Large swabs or small gauze with prep solution
   f. Tenaculum
   g. Benzocaine gel 20% (optional)
   h. Uterine sound (usually unnecessary)
   i. Scissors
   j. Specimen containers with fixative (10% buffered formalin)

Anesthesia

1. Usually none
2. Benzocaine gel may be applied to one lip of the cervix before tenaculum.
3. Paracervical anesthesia used rarely for exceptional cases (e.g., stenotic os)

Precautions

1. Consider a pregnancy test before endometrial sampling in premenopausal women.
2. Those at risk for bacterial endocarditis should have prophylactic antibiotics.
3. Ask about iodine allergy before using iodine to cleanse cervix.

Technique

1. Bimanual examination: Ascertain axis of endometrial cavity, uterine size and contour, adnexae.

2. Examine vulva, vagina, cervix. Obtain Pap smear with endocervical sampling to rule out extrauterine causes of abnormal bleeding.

3. Cleanse the cervix with povidone-iodine (Betadine), Zephiran, or other antibacterial solution, using large swabs or ring forceps and gauze.

4. Warn the patient of impending discomfort, usually "cramping."

5. Attempt to pass the flexible cannula through the internal cervical os. If this is unsuccessful, stabilize the cervix by grasping the anterior or posterior lip with a tenaculum and exert gentle countertraction.

6. With steady, controlled pressure, insert the flexible or rigid cannula through the internal cervical os to the depth of the endometrial cavity (typically 7 cm).

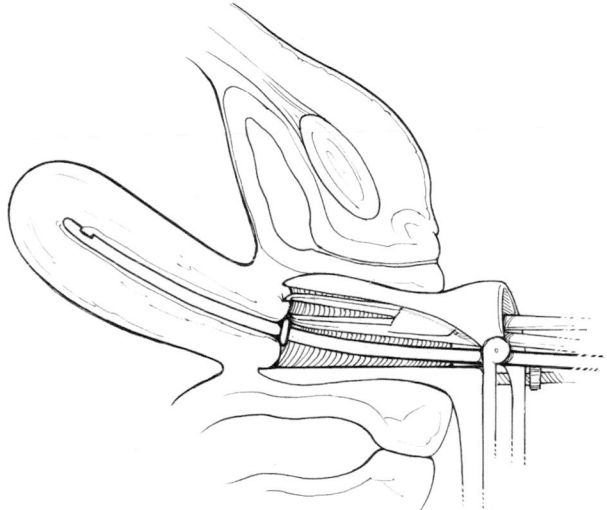

7. Flexible cannula (Pipelle or Z-Sampler)

   a. Apply suction by withdrawing the plunger most of the way. Do not allow the hole in the tip to emerge from the uterine cavity during aspiration or all suction will be lost.

   b. Rotate the cannula at least 360 degrees while moving it from side to side and gradually withdrawing it almost to the internal os. The area sampled will be a spiral. Make more than one pass in this fashion until the cannula is full or no more tissue enters the cannula.

   c. If it is full, continue the aspiration with a new Pipelle or Z-Sampler until no more tissue is obtained.

8. Rigid cannula (e.g., Explora)

   a. Apply suction on the attached syringe; lock plunger in position.

   b. Use an in-and-out motion while rotating the cannula, never withdrawing it completely from the endometrial cavity until sampling is complete. (Sample longitudinal strips of endometrium.)

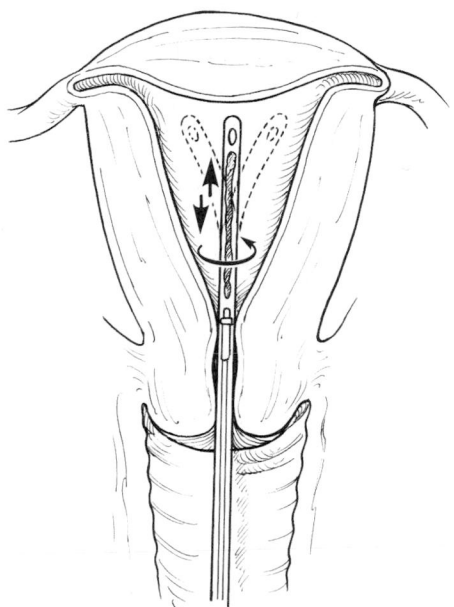

9. Using scissors, cut off the distal tip of the flexible cannula (rigid cannulae do not need to be cut). Expell the tissue sample into a container of fixative and send it for histologic examination.

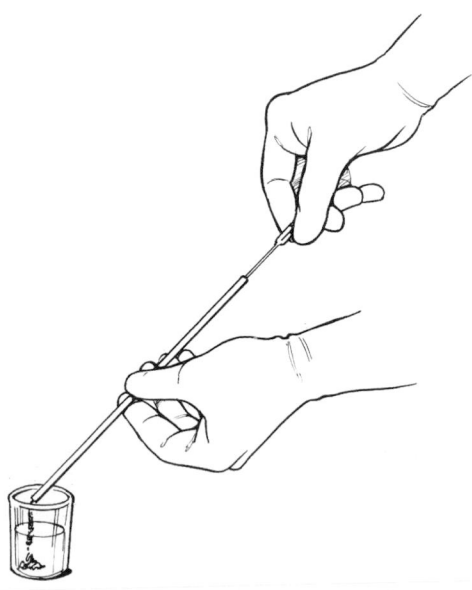

10. If a tenaculum was used, remove it and apply pressure to the site until hemostasis is achieved.

11. Remove the speculum.

12. Instruct the woman not to insert anything into her vagina for about 3 days, and to contact you for hemorrhage, pain, or signs of infection.

Follow-Up

Depends on the histologic diagnosis

1. "Insufficient tissue" may indicate atrophic endometrium: reassuring if technique was good and suspicion of endometrial cancer low. Otherwise, consider proceeding to hysteroscopy. Transvaginal ultrasound confirming a thin (<5-mm double thickness) endometrium *before* endometrial sampling is also reassuring and may obviate the need for biopsy.

2. Proliferative endometrium indicates unopposed estrogen effect. Cyclic or continuous progesterone may be indicated in premenopausal woman with anovulatory cycles.

3. Endometrial hyperplasia: May be a precursor to endometrial cancer.

   a. Adenomatous or cystic, without atypia: usually treated with cyclic or continuous progesterone. Repeat sampling after 2 to 3 months. If hyperplasia has not resolved, hysteroscopy is indicated.

   b. Atypical hyperplasia: cancer precursor; may be an indication for D&C and/or hysteroscopy, with or without progesterone treatment.

4. Endometrial carcinoma requires definitive treatment.

5. Polyp: usually benign; often missed with blind sampling (office biopsy or D&C). If found in a postmenopausal woman, consider hysteroscopy because of increased incidence of associated endometrial neoplasia.

Bibliography

Apgar BS, Newkirk GR: Endometrial biopsy. Prim Care 1997;24:303–326.

Chambers JT, Chambers SK: Endometrial sampling: When? Where? Why? With what? Clin Obstet Gynecol 1992;35:28–39.

Feldman S, Berkowitz RS, Tosteson ANA: Cost-effectiveness of strategies to evaluate postmenopausal bleeding. Obstet Gynecol 1993;81:968–975.

Rees MC: The uterus and the menopause. Baillieres Clin Obstet Gynaecol 1996;10:419–432.

Youssif SNM, McMillan DL: Outpatient endometrial biopsy: the Pipelle. Br J Hosp Med 1995;54:198–201.

Indications

1. Abnormal premenopausal and postmenopausal bleeding evaluation
2. Control dysfunctional uterine bleeding
3. Diagnostic evaluation for malignancies of uterus and endocervix
4. Failed or inconclusive endometrial biopsy
5. Pregnancy-related, such as abnormal postpartum bleeding; hydatidiform mole; incomplete, inevitable, or missed abortion; and termination

Contraindications

1. Pelvic infections without prior adequate antibiotic therapy
2. Pyometra that is best treated by simple transcervical drainage
3. Viable pregnancy
4. Medical status unstable for surgical procedure

Preparations

1. No eating or drinking by patient within 6 to 8 hours prior to surgery. An exception would be life-threatening hemorrhage.
2. An enema is strongly encouraged to remove any stool from rectal vault. The bladder is also emptied prior to call for surgery.
3. A complete blood count and urinalysis are recommended for all patients. Electrocardiography, coagulation studies, and chest radiographs are recommended depending on age, health status, or anesthesiologist.
4. Verify pregnancy status by last menstrual period, urine pregnancy test, and/or ultrasound.
5. Shaving of the perineum is not indicated.
6. Insertion of laminaria into the cervical canal 8 hours prior to the procedure may make the procedure less traumatic to the cervix.

Equipment

1. Speculum to visualize cervix, preferably a weighted posterior speculum
2. Single-tooth tenaculum(s) or clamp(s) to grasp and manipulate the cervix
3. Uterine sound with centimeter gradations to verify depth and position of uterus
4. Set of dilators, such as Hank-Bradley, Pratt, or Hegar
5. Curettes, of variable size and malleability, or vacuum suction curette
6. Narrow ring forceps for grasping polyps
7. Vaginal retractor

Anesthesia

1. General endotracheal intubation in surgery suite
2. Local paracervical block, with intravenous sedation, as office procedure

Precautions

1. Perforation of anteflexed or retroflexed uterus is more prevalent when position of uterus is unknown. Perforation can result in possible bowel trauma and uterine bleeding, especially with lateral perforation through uterine vessels.
2. A stenotic cervical canal can lend itself to difficult sounding and formation of a false channel and perforation.
3. A single-tooth tenaculum can result in a laceration of the cervix.
4. The pregnant uterus is subject to easy perforation secondary to the thinner musculature. Increased care and delicate use of the instruments must be maintained to reduce risk of perforation with any of the pregnancy-related indications.

Technique

1. The patient is placed in lithotomy position on the surgical table and anesthetized appropriately.
2. A bimanual examination is performed on the completely relaxed patient to identify uterine position, size, and mobility. Attention also should be given to the vagina, cul-de-sac, ovaries, ligaments, and any palpable lymph nodes for any abnormality.
3. Perineum, vagina, and vulva are cleaned with povidone-iodine or equivalent antiseptic solution.
4. The rectal area is covered with a sterile towel to decrease chance of contamination, and the remainder of the area, including the legs and abdomen, are draped in sterile fashion.
5. A red rubber catheter is inserted into the urethra to completely empty the bladder to reduce the risk of bladder trauma.

6. The weighted speculum is inserted posteriorly, and a retractor is inserted anteriorly. The cervix is then visualized fully and grasped anteriorly with a clamp or tenaculum. The anterior retractor can then be removed for better visualization.

7. The malleable uterine sound is passed through the undilated cervical canal, and depth and direction are noted.

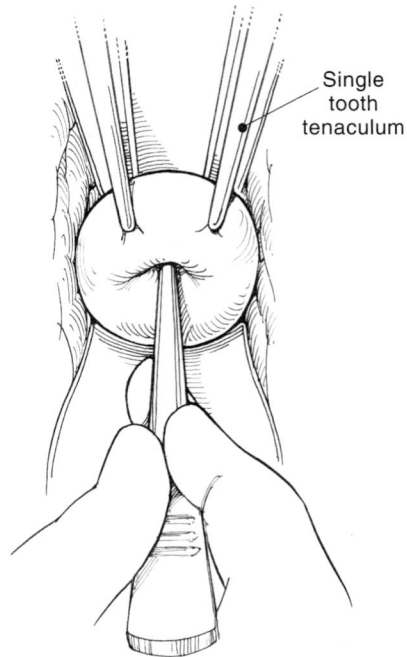

Single tooth tenaculum

The shape of the sound is altered prior to insertion according to the findings of the bimanual examination of the uterus. The sound is inserted to the uterine fundus, and the distance from the fundus to the external cervical os is measured to assess uterine depth. If the sound cannot pass through a stenotic cervix, a small dilator can be used.

8. The dilators are inserted sequentially into the canal to a diameter of 8 or 9 mm for ordinary curettes to adequately access the endometrium.

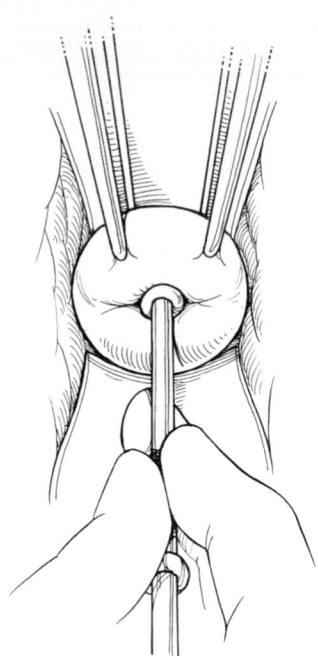

Each dilator can be lubricated with sterile water or a water-based lubricant. Dilation of the cervix past 10 mm in a woman of childbearing age may increase the risk of cervical incompetence during a subsequent pregnancy.

9. A narrow ring or polyp forceps is inserted into the uterine cavity, opened, rotated 90 degrees, and then closed before withdrawal to capture any intrauterine polyp growths.

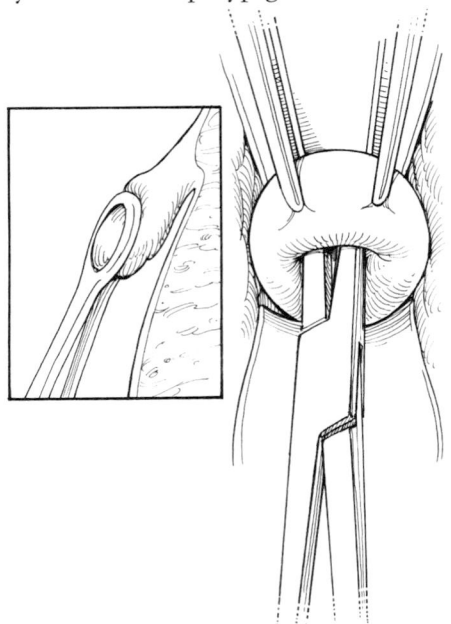

This is repeated until all quadrants have been evaluated, including the fundal area.

10. A medium-sized sharp curette or vacuum curette is introduced into the uterine cavity and is systematically curetted over all surfaces. Pressure is exerted only during the withdrawal phase to decrease risk of perforation. Periodic

withdrawal of the sharp curette from the uterus is recommended to collect any fragments currently removed from the endometrium.

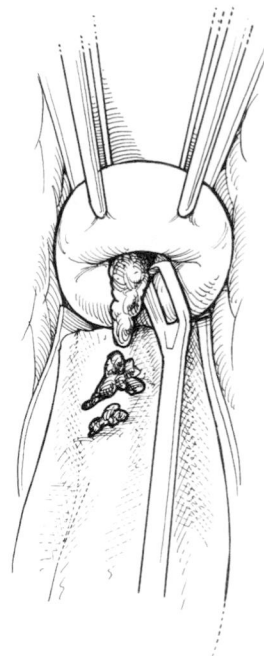

The physician should be aware of the feel of the curette against the endometrium, noting any variation in texture in a particular area of the uterine cavity. Repeat step 10 once.

11. The tissue specimens are placed in the appropriate preservative and sent to pathology for evaluation. Any unusual findings during the procedure should be communicated to the pathologist who will be evaluating the slides. Other information should include any previous findings, any current treatment, and a tentative diagnosis.

12. The tenaculum(s) is removed and the cervix monitored for a short period for any abnormal significant bleeding from the cervical os or the tenaculum trauma. If excessive uterine bleeding occurs, oxytocics such as Pitocin or Methergine may be used. If cervical bleeding occurs, application of gentle pressure to the cervix with the ring forceps should provide control. Electrocautery and suture closure are also options. Once bleeding is controlled, the posterior speculum is removed. The sterile drapes can then be removed and the patient placed in a supine position for transfer to the postanesthesia care unit (PACU).

13. The patient remains in the PACU until transfer to the outpatient department. Vital signs are monitored and the patient is observed for excessive bleeding or pain until the patient is sufficiently awake and tolerating liquids. The patient is then discharged home.

Follow-Up

1. Cramping can be expected for several days. The patient also should understand that slight bleeding, usually less than normal menses, will occur but will decrease with time.

2. Instructions include
   a. Nothing per vagina for 1 week to reduce chance of infection.
   b. Report any elevated temperature greater than 100.5°F.
   c. Report any increase in pain or vaginal bleeding and any malodorous vaginal discharge.

3. Follow-up in 7 to 10 days for pathology reports and further management plans for treatment.

Bibliography

Butler WJ: Normal and abnormal uterine bleeding. In Rock JA, Thompson JD (eds): Te Linde's Operative Gynecology, 8th ed, pp 453–476. Philadelphia, JB Lippincott Company, 1996.

Coulter A, Klassen A, MacKenzie IZ, et al: Diagnostic dilatation and curettage: is it used appropriately? BMJ 1993;306:236–239.

Deutchman ME, Hartman KJ: Postpartum pyometra: a case report. J Fam Pract 1993;36:449–452.

Hemminki E: Treatment of miscarriage: current practice and rationale. Obstet Gynecol 1998;91:247–253.

Hurt WG: Outpatient gynecologic procedures. Surg Clin North Am 1991;71:1099–1110.

Jurkovic D, Ross JA, Nicolaides KH: Expectant management of missed miscarriage. Br J Obstet Gynaecol 1998;105:670–671.

109 Ovarian Cancer

Lori A. Whittaker

Etiology

1. The cause of ovarian cancer is unknown, but several risk factors for the disease have been identified.

   a. A history of infertility of anovulatory cycles

   b. Use of infertility drugs

   c. Nulliparity or low parity

   d. Toxin exposure, such as perineal talc or asbestos exposure

   e. Genetic factors, such as a family history of breast or ovarian cancer. A woman with one first-degree relative with ovarian cancer has a 5 per cent lifetime risk and a woman with two first-degree relatives a 7 per cent lifetime risk of developing ovarian cancer, compared with a 1.4 per cent risk in the general population. There are at least three different inheritance patterns associated with ovarian cancer.

      (1) Hereditary site-specific ovarian cancer

      (2) Hereditary breast-ovarian cancer syndrome: associated with mutations in the genes *BRCA1* and, to a lesser extent, *BRCA2*. A woman with an inherited defect in *BRCA1* has a 40 per cent lifetime risk of developing ovarian cancer.

      (3) Lynch II syndrome: familial predisposition to breast, endometrial, colon, prostate, and ovarian cancers

2. Factors that *decrease* the risk for ovarian cancer include

   a. Oral contraceptive use

   b. Multiparity

   c. Tubal ligation

   d. Breast-feeding

   e. Hysterectomy

3. Classification based on cell type

   a. Epithelial cell tumors: more than 90 per cent of all ovarian cancers. Incidence increases with age.

   b. Germ cell tumors: most common in children or young adults

   c. Sex cord–stromal tumors; rare. Usually occur in postmenopausal women.

Symptoms

Symptoms of ovarian cancer are notoriously vague and nonspecific. Most women with early disease are asymptomatic. Symptoms usually herald more advanced disease, with large or disseminated tumor or ascites. Symptoms include

1. Abdominal bloating

2. Early satiety or anorexia

3. Dyspepsia

4. Pelvic pressure or pain

5. Frequent urination

6. Constipation

Key Symptoms

- Abdominal bloating
- Dyspepsia
- Early satiety or anorexia
- Pelvic pain or pressure

Clinical Findings

1. Pelvic mass detected on pelvic or rectovaginal examination

2. Abdominal distention or fullness from partial bowel obstruction, omental involvement, or ascites

3. Supraclavicular, axillary, inguinal, or umbilical lymph adenopathy

4. Pleural effusion

5. Cachexia

Key Signs

- Pelvic mass
- Abdominal distention
- Ascites
- Adenopathy

Laboratory Tests

1. Screening tests

   a. Pelvic exam

   b. Pelvic transvaginal ultrasonography

   c. Color-flow Doppler of ovarian vessels

d. Serum tumor markers (i.e., CA-125)

e. Genetic testing for the *BRCA1* gene

To date there is no evidence to indicate that routine screening for ovarian cancer in asymptomatic women results in earlier detection or decreased mortality, and it is not generally recommended. Despite lack of conclusive evidence, a consensus panel convened by the National Institutes of Health (NIH) in 1994 recommended that women at high risk for the disease, such as those with two or more first-degree relatives with ovarian cancer, be specifically targeted by a screening strategy that includes annual pelvic examination, CA-125 levels, and transvaginal pelvic ultrasound. The NIH panel also suggested that prophylactic oophorectomy by age 35 or the end of childbearing be considered in such women. As genetic testing for genes such as *BRCA1* becomes more widely available, such recommendations may be targeted more specifically to women with high-risk genetic mutations.

2. Preoperative staging tests in patients with suspected ovarian cancer

   a. Chest radiography

   b. Complete blood count and serum chemistry profile

   c. Intravenous pyelogram

   d. Cystoscopy

   e. Proctoscopy

   f. Barium enema

3. Surgery: A definitive tissue diagnosis is made by histology on a surgical specimen. The specimen is usually obtained at laparotomy, but in selected cases laparoscopy may be appropriate.

Key Tests

- Pelvic exam
- CA-125
- Transvaginal pelvic ultrasound
- Color flow Doppler of ovarian vessels

Differential Diagnosis

1. Benign pelvic masses

   a. Functional follicular or corpus luteum cyst

   b. Luteoma of pregnancy

   c. Benign germ cell neoplasm (e.g., dermoid cyst)

   d. Benign mesothelial ovarian tumor (e.g., serous cystoma or cystadenoma)

   e. Ovarian fibroma

   f. Endometriosis

   g. Tubo-ovarian abscess or cyst

2. Other pelvic or abdominal neoplasm

3. Ectopic pregnancy

Treatment

1. Surgery: All patients with suspected ovarian cancer should under laparotomy to accurately diagnose and stage the lesion, debulk the tumor, and relieve any bowel obstruction.

2. Postoperative therapy: Treatment following surgery is dependent upon the stage of disease at initial diagnosis. The FIGO classification system for ovarian cancer staging is found in the references.

   a. Early-stage disease (stage I [tumor confined to one or both ovaries], grade I [well-differentiated] and selected cases of grade II [moderately differentiated] disease): No further treatment is required. Five-year survival is greater than 90 per cent.

   b. Advanced disease (stage I, grade 2 or 3; stages II, III, and IV)

      (1) First-line therapy: six courses of cisplatin-based chemotherapy (e.g., cisplatin plus cyclophosphamide or cisplatin and paclitaxel) or three-drug combination of cisplatin, doxorubicin, and cyclophosphamide (CAP)

      (2) Second-line therapy and alternative agents

         (a) Radiotherapy

         (b) Intraperitoneal chemotherapy

         (c) Biologic response modifiers

         (d) Autologous bone marrow transplantation

         (e) Hormonal therapy

3. Palliative therapy

   a. Second debulking surgery

   b. Radiation therapy

   c. Nutritional support

   d. Drainage of ascites or pleural effusions

Key Treatment

- Surgery

Drugs of Choice

- Cisplatin and cyclophosphamide
- Cisplatin and paclitaxel
- Cisplatin, doxorubicin, and cyclophosphamide

Follow-Up
1. Second-look laparotomy to assess residual disease
2. Serial CA-125 levels

 ## Bibliography

Cannistra SA: Cancer of the ovary. N Engl J Med 1993; 329:1550–1559.

Gershenson DM, Tortolero-Luna G, Malpica A, et al: Ovarian intraepithelial neoplasia and ovarian cancer. Obstet Gynecol Clin North Am 1996;23:475–543.

Mann WJ: Diagnosis and management of epithelial cancer of the ovary. Am Fam Physician 1994;49:613–618.

National Institutes of Health: Ovarian cancer: screening, treatment and follow-up NIH Consensus Statement. 1994;12:1–30.

110 Vaginitis

Barbara D. Reed

Etiology

Vaginal symptoms are common in women, and are usually caused by infections of the vaginal vault. Common causes, in order of prevalence, are

1. Bacterial vaginosis
2. *Candida* vulvovaginitis
3. *Trichomonas* vaginitis

Symptoms

Typically, women present with complaints of vaginal discharge, itching, or odor. However, vaginitis can also be asymptomatic. Classic symptoms include

1. Bacterial vaginosis
   a. Moderate white discharge
   b. Possible fishy odor (often accentuated after vaginal exposure to semen)
2. *Candida* vulvovaginitis
   a. Itching and/or discomfort
   b. Discharge (may be absent)
   c. Swelling of the vulva may be present
3. *Trichomonas* vaginitis
   a. Moderate to copious thin discharge, occasionally foamy
   b. Possible fishy odor
   c. Discolored discharge suggests this diagnosis

Most women with vaginal symptoms do not present as a "classic" case, and *an accurate diagnosis cannot be based on symptoms and signs alone.*

Key Symptoms

- Vaginal discharge
- Vaginal and/or vulvar itching, irritation, or swelling
- Genital odor

Clinical Findings

1. Bacterial vaginosis
   a. White or yellow homogeneous discharge
   b. Fishy odor may be evident during examination.
   c. Erythema and swelling unlikely.
2. *Candida* vulvovaginitis
   a. White, thick, curd-like discharge (classic but usually absent)
   b. White creamy discharge, or no discharge at all, may be present.
   c. Erythema, swelling, and/or excoriations of vulva or vagina
3. *Trichomonas* vaginitis
   a. White, yellow, gray, or green thin discharge —occasionally foamy
   b. Fishy odor may be present.
   c. "Strawberry" cervix classic but rare.

Key Signs

- Bacterial vaginosis: white or yellow homogeneous discharge; fishy odor
- *Candida* vulvovaginitis: white, occasionally thick, discharge; erythema or swelling; no odor
- *Trichomonas* vaginitis: thin, foamy, discolored discharge; fishy odor

Laboratory Tests

In-office laboratory testing is critical for the accurate diagnosis of vaginal symptoms.

1. pH: Apply one drop of the vaginal specimen to pH paper and assess for a normal (≤ 4.5) or abnormal (>4.5) pH.
2. Normal saline preparation
   a. Vaginal discharge placed in 0.5 ml or more of normal saline (NS) in tube, applied to slide and examined immediately.
   b. Examine under low power and assess presence of organisms with flagellar motion (*Trichomonas vaginalis*).
   c. Examine under high power, assessing
      (1) Clue cells (epithelial cells studded with bacteria that obscure the edges of the cells)
      (2) Background flora: Long rods suggest normal *Lactobacillus* milieu, but predominate short or curved rods or cocci are abnormal and suggest a diagnosis of bacterial vaginosis. Very long rods (re-

sembling long filaments) suggest a diagnosis of lactobacilliosis.

3. KOH preparation
   a. Vaginal discharge placed directly on a slide.
   b. Add 1 to 2 drops of KOH to the specimen, and sniff to detect volatilized amines (fishy odor)—this is the "whiff test."
   c. Examine microscopically more than 3 minutes after preparation—first at low power to scan for hyphae or budding yeast forms, then confirm at high power.
   d. Identification of single (nonbudding) spherical forms is inaccurate for diagnosing yeast.
4. Culturing of vaginal discharge: If the diagnosis remains unclear, culturing of the vaginal discharge for yeast (Sabaurand's or Nickerson's media) and/or *Trichomonas* (modified Diamond's media) is imperative to avoid misdiagnosis and treatment.

Key Tests

- pH determination
- NS microscopic preparation
- KOH evaluation with whiff test
- Culturing of discharge if diagnosis uncertain

Diagnostic Criteria

1. Bacterial vaginosis: Amsel criteria—three out of four of the following: pH greater than 4.5, homogeneous discharge, positive "whiff" test for amines, and clue cells
2. *Candida* vulvovaginitis: pseudohyphae or budding yeast forms observed microscopically, or positive culture
3. *Trichomonas* vaginitis: Motile *T. vaginalis* observed on fresh NS preparation, or positive culture

Differential Diagnosis

Other causes of vulvovaginal symptoms include the following:

1. Cervicitis or pelvic inflammatory disease: Women with mucopurulent discharge from the cervical os or cervical motion tenderness should be tested further for *Chlamydia trachomatis* and *Neisseria gonorrhoeae*.
2. Allergic or irritant reactions: Assess for association to exposures, such as intravaginal treatments, genital hygiene products, soaps, sprays, or semen.

3. Atrophic vaginitis (caused by estrogen deficiency): May present with itching or irritation, discharge, and numerous white blood cells and parabasal cells on normal saline preparation.
4. Desquamative inflammatory vaginitis: associated with itching, dyspareunia, thin discharge, and necrotic epithelial cells on NS prep. May lead to adhesions and synechiae.
5. Lactobacilliosis: vaginal discharge and itching; characterized by very-long-chain lactobacilli on normal saline preparation.
6. Lesions on vulva associated with itching: including lichen panus, lichen sclerosis et atrophicus, or lichen simplex chronicus; diagnosed by biopsy
7. Vulvodynia or vestibulitis: more than 3 months of constant or intermittent vulvar/introital burning or irritation. Typically have pain with intercourse and/or tampon use, with no evidence of other vaginal/vulvar diagnosis. Typically women are tender to Q-tip probing of the vulva/introitus.
8. Unknown etiology

PEARL

The KOH preparation is positive for yeast cells in approximately one half of women with *Candida* vulvovaginitis—when in doubt, send a fungal culture.

Treatment

1. The treatment of vaginitis is specific to the etiology of the entity, and hence accuracy of diagnosis is imperative. Failure of response should be followed with re-evaluation prior to continued treatment.
2. Treatment of bacterial vaginosis and *Trichomonas* vaginitis is recommended in pregnancy to decrease the risks of adverse pregnancy outcomes, such as premature labor and low birth weight. Medication regimens marked with an asterisk below may be used in pregnancy.

Medications

1. Bacterial vaginosis
   a. Metronidazole (Flagyl or generic), 500 mg PO bid for 7 days or 250 mg tid for 7 days*
   b. Clindamycin 2% vaginal cream (Cleocin 2% vaginal), 5 gm intravaginally qd for 7 days
   c. Metronidazole 0.75% vaginal gel (MetroGel), 5 gm intravaginally bid for 5 days
   d. For resistant cases
      (1) Clindamycin (Cleocin) 300 mg PO bid

for 7 days (alternative treatment in pregnancy)

(2) Povidone-iodine (Betadine) gel or suppositories intravaginally bid for 14 to 28 days

2. *Candida* vulvovaginitis

a. Topical regimens

(1) Miconazole, 200-mg suppository (Monistat 3) intravaginally qd for 3 days; or 2% vaginal cream (Monistat 7), one applicatorful intravaginally qd for 7 days*; or 100-mg vaginal suppository intravaginally qd for 7 nights*

(2) Clotrimazole, 1% vaginal cream (Mycelex-7) or 100-mg vaginal tablet (Gyne-Lotrimin) intravaginally qd for 7 days*; or one 500-mg vaginal tablet (Mycelex-G) once

(3) Butoconazole 2% cream (Femstat 3 or Mycelex 3), one application intravaginally qd for 3 days

(4) Terconazole, 80-mg suppository of 0.8% vaginal cream (Terazol 3) intravaginally qd for 3 days; or 0.4% vaginal cream (Terazol 7) intravaginally qd for 7 nights

(5) Tioconazole 6.5% ointment (Vagistat-1 or Monistat-1), intravaginally once

b. Oral regimens

(1) Fluconazole (Diflucan), 150 mg PO once

(2) Itraconazole (Sporonox), 200 mg PO qd for 3 days

c. For recurrent or resistant cases

(1) Any of the above vaginal products extended from 7 days to 14 to 21 days

(2) Boric acid suppositories, 600 mg intravaginally twice daily for 14 days (as tolerated)

(3) Gentian violet vaginal staining once or twice per week

d. For prevention of recurrences

(1) Clotrimazole, 500-mg suppository intravaginally q mo

(2) Miconazole, 100-mg vaginal tablet twice weekly

(3) Ketoconazole, 400 mg PO qd for 5 days at beginning of menses

(4) Fluconazole, 150 mg PO monthly, or weekly if needed (data lacking)

3. *Trichomonas* vaginitis

a. Metronidazole, 500 mg PO bid for 7 days or 2 gm PO one time.* Treat both patient and partner(s).

b. For persistent or recurrent cases: metronidazole, 500 mg PO bid for 14 to 21 days, or 2 gm PO qd for 3 days. Add to either regimen one of the following: metronidazole, 0.75% gel 5 mg intravaginally bid for 5 days; or clotrimazole, 100-mg vaginal tablet intravaginally qd for 7 nights.

c. During lactation, use metronidazole, 2 gm PO once only, with discontinuation of breast-feeding for 24 hours only.

PEARL

Treating partners: Because *Trichomonas vaginalis* is sexually transmitted, the partner(s) of the women infected should also be treated. Controversy exists regarding the value of treating partners of women with bacterial vaginosis—consider this only in recurrent cases. No evidence supports treating partners of women with *Candida* vulvovaginitis.

Diet

Ingestion of culture-positive yogurt has been reported to decrease *Candida* vulvovaginitis recurrences. Although avoidance of sugars, alcohol, or yeast-containing products has been suggested, data are insufficient to support this, and any dietary manipulation should be observed for response and discontinued if ineffective.

Activity

Patients with *Trichomonas* vaginitis should abstain from intercourse until they and their partner(s) are treated.

Patient Education

1. The diagnosis of the cause of vaginitis is inaccurate if based on history, symptoms, and signs alone. Office examination and laboratory tests substantially increase the diagnostic accuracy.

2. If patients choose to self-treat for *Candida* vulvovaginitis using over-the-counter regimens, they should plan to come for medical evaluation if symptoms recur or only partially resolve.

Key Treatment

- Bacterial vaginosis: metronidazole or clindamycin —in oral or vaginal preparations

- *Candida* vulvovaginitis: intravaginal or oral antifungal medications

- *Trichomonas* vaginitis: metronidazole oral regimen

Follow-Up

1. Women with *Trichomonas* infection—a sexually transmitted infection—should be re-examined for cure 2 weeks following treatment.

2. Women with bacterial vaginosis or *Trichomonas* vaginitis who anticipate pregnancy may be treated even if asymptomatic, and should be re-evaluated for cure.

3. Women with *Candida* vulvovaginitis that recurs should be re-evaluated for other genital infections and repeat definitive diagnosis.

Bibliography

Centers for Disease Control and Prevention: 1988 Guidelines for treatment of sexually transmitted diseases. MMWR Morb Mortal Wkly Rep 1998;47:70–78.

Ferris DG, Hendrich J, Payne PM, et al: Office laboratory diagnosis of vaginitis: clinician-performed tests compared with a rapid nucleic acid hybridization test. J Fam Pract 1995;41:575–581.

Reed BD, Eyler A: Vaginal infections: diagnosis and management. Am Fam Physician 1993;47:1805–1818.

Sobel J: Vaginitis. N Engl J Med 1997;337:1896–1903.

Sobel JD, Faro S, Force RW, et al: Vulvovaginal candidiasis: epidemiologic, diagnostic, and therapeutic considerations. Am J Obstet Gynecol 1998;178:203–211.

111 Cervicitis

Carey Vinson

Etiology

1. *Chlamydia trachomatis* causes 30 to 60 per cent of cases.
2. *Neisseria gonorrhoeae*
3. A primary infection of herpes simplex virus may cause cervicitis along with genital herpes.
4. In up to half of cases, an etiology cannot be determined.
5. True prevalence is usually underestimated. Cervicitis has been found in 24 to 40 per cent of female patients in sexually transmitted disease (STD) clinics and 34 per cent of patients seen routinely at a university student health clinic.

Symptoms

1. Often, cervicitis is asymptomatic or symptoms are vague, but untreated infection can lead to pelvic inflammatory disease and infertility.
2. An increase in vaginal discharge
3. Vaginal bleeding or spotting, especially postcoital
4. Vague lower abdominal pain
5. Mild dyspareunia
6. Can be confused with vulvovaginitis

Key Symptoms

- Often asymptomatic
- Increased amount of vaginal discharge
- Postcoital bleeding

Risk Factors

1. Previous treatment for STD
2. New sexual partner
3. Male partner with urethritis

WARNING

- **Cervicitis should be considered a sexually transmitted disease.**
- **High risk of spread of infection to sexual partners**

- **Proximal extension of infection can cause endometritis, salpingitis, infertility, chorioamnionitis, and premature rupture of membranes in pregnancy.**

Clinical Findings

1. Cervical ectopy, the appearance of endocervical epithelium on the visible exocervix, is not cervicitis and is *not* pathologic.
2. Yellow or green mucopurulent cervical discharge
3. Cervical os friable, easily produces bleeding.
4. Edema of the columnar epithelium

Key Signs

- Cervical os discharge
- Friable cervix

Laboratory Tests

1. Gram's stain of cervical discharge
   a. Positive if more than 10 to 30 white blood cells (WBCs) per high-power field
   b. Gram-negative intracellular diplococci: gonorrheal cervicitis, but only 60 per cent sensitive
2. Thayer-Martin media culture: gonorrheal cervicitis
3. Enzyme-linked immunosorbent assay (ELISA): chlamydia cervicitis
4. Direct fluorescent antibody test for chlamydial antigens: chlamydia cervicitis
5. Nucleic acid hybridization test (DNA probe): chlamydia cervicitis

Key Tests

- Gram's stain of cervical discharge: greater than 10 to 30 WBCs per high-power field
- Gram's stain of cervical discharge: gram-negative intracellular diplococci—gonorrhea
- Gonorrhea culture
- Immunoassay test for chlamydia

Differential Diagnosis

1. Nonspecific bacterial vaginosis
2. *Trichomonas* vaginitis

Treatment

1. Sexual partner needs treatment.
2. Many patients have simultaneous chlamydial and gonorrheal infections.
3. Empiric treatment considered for suspected chlamydia and/or gonorrhea infections if area of high prevalence or patient might be difficult to locate for treatment.
4. Chlamydia
   a. Azithromycin (Zithromax), 1 gm orally one time
   b. Doxycycline (Vibramycin, Vibra-Tabs, Doryx), 100 mg orally twice daily for 7 days
   c. Erythromycin base (E-Mycin, Eryc, Ery-Tab), 500 mg orally four times daily for 7 days
   d. Erythromycin ethylsuccinate (EES, EryPed), 800 mg orally four times daily for 7 days
   e. Ofloxacin (Floxin), 300 mg orally twice daily for 7 days
   f. Pregnancy
      (1) Erythromycin base, 500 mg orally four times daily for 7 days
      (2) Amoxicillin (Amoxil, Wymox), 500 mg orally three times daily for 10 days
      (3) Erythromycin base, 250 mg orally four times daily for 14 days
      (4) Erythromycin ethylsuccinate, 800 mg orally four times daily for 7 days
      (5) Erythromycin ethylsuccinate, 400 mg orally four times daily for 14 days
      (6) Azithromycim, 1 gm orally one time only
5. Gonorrhea: Co-infection with chlamydia is common, favoring dual therapy.
   a. Chlamydia treatment regimens
      (1) Azithromycin (Zithromax), 1 gm orally one time
      (2) Doxycycline (Vibramycin), 100 mg orally two times daily for 7 days
   plus
   b. Gonorrhea treatment regimens
      (1) Ceftriaxone (Rocephin), 125 mg intramuscularly once
      (2) Cefixime (Suprax), 400 mg orally once
      (3) Ciprofloxacin (Cipro), 500 mg orally once
      (4) Ofloxacin (Floxin), 400 mg orally once

   c. Pregnancy
      (1) Ceftriaxone, 125 mg intramuscularly; or cefixime, 400 mg orally once
      (2) Spectinomycin (Trobicin), 2 gm intramuscularly once for women who cannot tolerate a cephalosporin
   plus
      (3) Erythromycin base (E-mycin, Eryc, Ery-tab), 500 mg orally four times daily for 7 days
      (4) Amoxicillin (Amoxil, Wymox), 500 mg orally three times daily for 7 days

Key Treatment

- Chlamydia cervicitis: azithromycin, 1 gm orally once; sexual partner needs treatment.
- Gonorrheal cervicitis: cefixime, 400 mg orally once plus azithromycin 1 gm orally once; sexual partner needs treatment.

Follow-Up

1. For chlamydia, no need to test for cure if treated with doxycycline or azithromycin. Test for cure at 3 weeks after completion of treatment with erythromycin. Retest if symptomatic after treatment.
2. For gonorrhea, no need to test for cure if treated with recommended regimens. Retest if symptomatic after treatment.
3. Test for other STDs.
   a. VDRL test for syphilis
   b. ELISA anti-HIV antibody test for human immunodeficiency virus
   c. Saline wet smear test of vaginal secretions for *Trichomonas* vaginitis

Bibliography

For more information on cervicitis, see
American College of Obstetricians and Gynecologists: Antibiotics and gynecologic infections (ACOG Educational Bulletin No 237, June 1997 [replaces no. 153, March 1991]). Int J Gynaecol Obstet 1997;58:333–340.
Centers for Disease Control and Prevention: 1998 Guidelines for treatment of sexually transmitted diseases. MMWR Morb Mortal Wkly Rep 1998;47(RR-1):1–118.
For more information on chlamydial cervicitis, see
Majeroni BA: Chlamydial cervicitis: complications and new treatment options. Am Fam Physician 1994;49:1825–1829.
Reddy SP, Yeturu SR, Slupik R: *Chlamydia trachomatis* in adolescents: a review. J Pediatr Adolesc Gynecol 1997;10:59–72.
For more information on gonorrheal cervicitis, see
Krowchuk DP: Sexually transmitted diseases in adolescents: what's new? South Med J 1998;91:124–131.

112 Pelvic Inflammatory Disease

Margaret Walsh

Pelvic inflammatory disease (PID) is a generalized term that refers to infection and inflammation of the female upper genital tract. PID presents as a broad spectrum of disorders that may include endometritis, salpingitis, tubo-ovarian abscess, and pelvic peritonitis.

Etiology
1. *Chlamydia trachomatis*
2. *Neisseria gonorrhoeae*
3. Aerobes
   a. *Escherichia coli*
   b. Group B streptococcus
   c. *Gardnerella vaginalis*
   d. *Haemophilus influenzae*
   e. *Mycobacterium tuberculosis*
4. Anaerobic
   a. *Peptococcus* species
   b. *Peptostreptococcus* species
   c. *Bacteroides* species
5. Mycoplasma
   a. *Mycoplasma hominis*
   b. *Ureaplasma urealyticum*

Symptoms
1. Asymptomatic
2. Lower abdominal pain
3. Vaginal discharge
4. Dyspareunia
5. Vomiting

Key Symptoms

- Lower abdominal pain
- Vaginal discharge

Clinical Findings
1. Lower abdominal tenderness
2. Vaginal discharge
3. Purulent endocervical discharge
4. Cervical motion tenderness
5. Adnexal tenderness

6. Fever of 38°C or higher
7. Adnexal mass
8. Leukocytosis of 10,500/mm^3 or greater
9. Sedimentation rate greater than 15 mm/hour
10. Laboratory evidence of gonococcal or chlamydial cervicitis
11. Elevated C-reactive protein

Key Signs

- Lower abdominal tenderness
- Adnexal tenderness
- Cervical motion tenderness
- Vaginal discharge

Laboratory Tests
1. Laparoscopy
2. Pregnancy test
3. Complete blood count (CBC)
4. Gonococcal/chlamydial cultures (endocervical, urethral, and rectal)
5. Transvaginal sonogram
6. Endometrial biopsy
7. Culdocentesis

Key Tests

- Laparoscopy—the only definitive test
- Pregnancy test
- CBC

Differential Diagnosis
1. Ectopic pregnancy
2. Appendicitis
3. Ovarian torsion
4. Endometriosis
5. Irritable bowel syndrome
6. Psychosomatic cause—abuse
7. Dyspareunia

8. Dysmenorrhea
9. Mittelschmerz
10. Adhesions
11. Anatomic abnormality
12. Malignancy

Treatment

Considerations
1. Cost
2. Patient acceptance
3. Antimicrobial susceptibility

Hospitalization Criteria
1. Appendicitis
2. Pregnant patient
3. Adolescent
4. Failed/unresponsive outpatient oral treatment
5. Questionable compliance
6. Severe illness
7. Tubo-ovarian abscess
8. Immunodeficient patient

Medication
1. Outpatient treatment
   a. Regimen 1
      (1) Ceftriaxone (Rocephin), 250 mg IM as one dose, or cefoxitin (Mefoxin), 2 gm IM, plus probenicid (Benemid), 1 gm PO
      (2) A cephalosporin plus doxycycline (Vibramycin), 100 mg PO bid ×14 days
   b. Regimen 2: ofloxin (Floxin), 400 mg orally bid ×14 days plus metronidazole (Flagyl), 500 mg orally bid ×14 days
2. Inpatient treatment
   a. Regimen 1
      (1) Cefoxitin (Mefoxin), 2 gm every 6 hours IV, or cefotetan (Cefotan), 2 gm IV every 12 hours, plus doxycycline (Vibramycin), 100 mg every 12 hours PO/IV
      (2) Re-evaluate for clinical improvement at 24 to 48 hours; if improvement in signs/symptoms is noted, may change to doxycycline 100 mg PO bid ×14 days.
   b. Regimen 2
      (1) Clindamycin (Cleocin), 900 mg IV every 8 hours plus gentamicin (Garamycin) loading dose IV/IM (2 mg/kg of body weight), followed by a maintenance dose (1.5 mg/kg) every 8 hours
      (2) Re-evaluate for clinical improvement in symptoms at 24 to 48 hours. If improvement noted, may switch to doxycycline 100 mg PO bid or clindamycin 450 mg qid ×14 days.

Prevention/Patient Education
1. Examination and treatment of all sexual contacts within 60 days preceding onset of symptoms in the patient
2. Sexual abstinence
3. Barrier methods of contraception
4. Anticipatory guidance regarding normal adolescent development to help educate about less risky behavior
5. Sexually transmitted diseases
6. Routinely screen patients for gonorrheal and chlamydial infection.
7. Presumptive antibiotic treatment

Key Treatment

- Outpatient—ceftriaxone plus probenicid
- Inpatient—cefoxitin plus doxycycline

Follow-Up
1. Look for improvement in clinical symptoms in patient within 72 hours after initiation of treatment.
2. If no improvement, consider additional diagnostic tests, surgical intervention.

Bibliography

Centers for Disease Control and Prevention: 1998 Guidelines for treatment of sexually transmitted diseases. MMWR Morb Mortal Wkly Rep 1998;47(No. RR-1).

McCormack WM: Pelvic inflammatory disease. N Engl J Med 1994;330:1115–1119.

Newkirk GR: Pelvic inflammatory disease: a contemporary approach. Am Fam Physician 1996;53:1127–1135.

Washington E, Berg A: Preventing and managing pelvic inflammatory disease: key questions, practices and evidence. J Fam Pract 1996;43:283–293.

113 Gonorrhea

Judith D. Kinzy

Etiology

Neisseria gonorrhoeae, a gram-negative diplococcus

Symptoms

1. Women are usually asymptomatic. Only 10 to 20 per cent will complain of vaginal discharge. Other symptoms include dyspareunia, lower abdominal discomfort, intermenstrual spotting, and menorrhagia.
2. Men may complain of urinary frequency and dysuria. Approximately 95 to 99 per cent have purulent urethral discharge, which may be eliminated or reduced with micturition.

Key Symptoms

- Vaginal or urethral discharge
- Urinary frequency
- Women usually asymptomatic
- Dysuria

Clinical Findings

1. Purulent urethral or cervical discharge
2. Red and swollen cervix or urethra
3. Tender and inguinal adenopathy

Key Signs

- Red and swollen cervix or urethra
- Tender inguinal adenopathy
- Purulent urethral or cervical discharge

Laboratory Tests

1. A stained smear of urethral exudate in men or endocervical smear in women may be diagnostic, particularly in patients with purulent drainage.
2. Cultures on selective media such as Thayer-Martin, Martin-Lewis, or NYC are essential in most women.

3. Nucleic acid hybridization (NAH) tests on cervical and urethral samples and polymerase chain reaction (PCR) on urine may be helpful.

Key Tests

- Gram's stain of purulent drainage
- NAH on cervical or urethral samples
- PCR on urine
- Culture on selective media

Differential Diagnosis

1. Nongonococcal urethritis
2. Traumatic urethritis
3. Herpes simplex
4. Foreign body
5. *Chlamydia trachomatis* infection
6. Prostatitis
7. *Gardnerella* vaginitis
8. *Candida albicans* infection

Treatment

1. Patients who have *N. gonorrhoeae* are often co-infected with *C. trachomatis*; therefore, it is recommended to treat for both.
2. Pharyngeal gonococcal infection may be more difficult to treat than uncomplicated gonococcal infections of the cervix, urethra, and rectum. Treatment recommendations are the same except cefixime 400 mg orally in a single dose is not recommended.

Medication

1. Drugs of choice for gonorrhea are cefixime (Suprax), 400 mg orally once, ceftriaxone (Rocephin), 125 mg IM once, ciprofloxacin (Cipro), 500 mg orally once, or ofloxacin (Floxin), 400 mg orally once, plus azithromycin (Zithromax), 1 gm orally once, or doxycycline (Vibramycin), 100 mg orally bid for 7 days, in order to treat concurrently for *Chlamydia*.
2. Treat sexual partner.

3. Ciprofloxacin and ofloxacin are contraindicated in pregnant and lactating women and in persons less than 18 years old.

Patient Education

Avoid sexual intercourse for 2 days after IM injection and for 5 days after oral medication.

Key Treatment

Drugs of Choice

- Cefixime, 400 mg orally once

- Ceftriaxone, 125 mg intramuscularly once

- Ciprofloxacin, 500 mg orally once

- Ofloxacin, 400 mg orally once

Plus (to Treat for Chlamydia)

- Azithromycin, 1 gm orally once

- Doxycycline, 100 mg orally bid for 7 days

Follow-Up

1. Patients do not need follow-up for uncomplicated gonorrhea if treated as above.

2. Repeat culture and sensitivity if the patient is thought to be noncompliant, if only one antibiotic was given, or if patient complains of persistent symptoms.

3. Sexual partners need to be seen for evaluation and treatment.

4. Avoid sexual intercourse until therapy is complete and symptoms have resolved.

Bibliography

Centers for Disease Control and Prevention: 1998 Guidelines for treatment of sexually transmitted diseases. MMWR Morb Mortal Wkly Rep 1998;47(RR-1):1–116.

Fiumara NJ: Pictorial Guide to Sexually Transmitted Diseases. New York, Cahners Publishing, 1989.

Lappa S, Moscicki AB: The pediatrician and the sexually active adolescent: a primer for sexually transmitted diseases. Pediatr Clin North Am 1997;44:1405–1445.

114 Chlamydia

Judith D. Kinzy

Etiology
Chlamydia trachomatis

Symptoms
1. Men complain of dysuria and/or discharge.
2. Women present with dysuria or frequency but often are asymptomatic.

Key Symptom

Dysuria

Clinical Findings
1. Urethritis and epididymitis are the most frequent manifestations of *C. trachomatis* infection in men.
2. Cervicitis, urethritis, endometritis, or salpingitis is seen most commonly in women.
3. Unexplained pyuria or culture-negative cystitis in sexually active women suggests chlamydia infection.

Key Signs

- Urethritis
- Culture-negative cystitis
- Epididymitis
- Cervicitis

Laboratory Tests
1. Culture in mammalian cell lines is the "gold standard."
   a. Use wire swabs with Dacron or cotton because the wood swabs are treated with chemicals that may interfere with the culture.
   b. Remove all secretions from cervix.
   c. Swab at least 1 to 2 cm into the endocervix in women and at least 2 to 3 cm into the urethra in men and then rotate for 10 to 30 seconds.

d. Initial diagnosis may be made by Gram's stain, leukocyte esterase test (LET) strip on first-void urine, by presence of mucopurulent or purulent discharge, or by demonstration of greater than 10 white blood cells per high-power field on first-void urine.
2. Nonculture diagnostic tests include direct fluorescent antibody (DFA) test, enzyme immunoassay (EIA), and DNA probe.
3. If initial screening is negative, then culture or nonculture diagnostic test should be done prior to initiation of treatment.
4. Nucleic acid amplification test on first void urine may be more sensitive than traditional culture techniques.

Key Tests

- Gram's stain and LET on urine for screening
- DFA test, EIA, and DNA probe
- Culture is the gold standard.

Differential Diagnosis
1. *Neisseria gonorrhoeae*
2. *Ureaplasma urealyticum*
3. Herpes simplex virus

Treatment
1. The drug of choice is azithromycin (Zithromax), 1 gm orally in a single dose, or doxycycline (Vibramycin), 100 mg orally bid for 7 days.
2. Alternative drugs
   a. Erythromycin base, 500 mg PO qid for 7 days
   b. Erythromycin ethylsuccinate, 800 mg orally qid for 7 days
   c. Ofloxacin (Floxin), 300 mg orally bid for 7 days
3. Doxycycline and ofloxacin are contraindicated in pregnancy.
4. Treat sexual partner.

Key Treatment

Drugs of Choice

- Azithromycin, 1 gm orally in a single dose

- Doxycycline, 100 mg PO bid ×7 days

Alternative Drugs

- Erythromycin base, 500 mg orally qid ×7 days

- Erythromycin ethylsuccinate, 800 mg orally qid for 7 days

- Ofloxacin, 300 mg orally bid for 7 days

Follow-Up

1. Patients need further testing only if symptoms persist or reinfection is suspected.

2. Treat most recent sex partner.

3. No intercourse for 7 days after treatment.

 ## Bibliography

Centers for Disease Control and Prevention: 1998 Guidelines for treatment of sexually transmitted diseases. MMWR Morb Mortal Wkly Rep 1998;47(RR-1):1–116.

Heath CR, Heath JM: *Chlamydia trachomatis* infection update. Am Fam Physician 1996;53:1085.

Lappa S, Moscicki AB: The pediatrician and the sexually active adolescent: a primer for sexually transmitted diseases. Pediatr Clin North Am 1997;44:1405–1445.

115 Lymphogranuloma Venereum

Judith D. Kinzy

Etiology

Invasive serovars L1, L2, or L3 of *Chlamydia trachomatis*

Symptoms

1. The primary lesion is a painless papule, vesicle, or erosion that heals after 2 to 3 days.
2. Heterosexual men complain of unilateral inguinal pain and swelling.
3. Women and homosexual men may complain of bloody diarrhea, abdominal pain, and perianal inflammation.

Key Symptoms

- Unilateral inguinal pain and swelling
- Bloody, mucopurulent diarrhea
- Abdominal pain
- Perianal inflammation

Clinical Findings

1. Heterosexual men present with tender inguinal and/or femoral lymphadenopathy that is usually unilateral. Initially the lymph nodes are hard, tender, and nonmovable. They become enlarged, elongated, and extremely painful. The overlying skin becomes dusky brown and adheres to the nodes. The skin breaks down to form multiple serosanguineous and purulent draining sinuses.
2. Women and homosexually active men may present with proctocolitis and/or hyperplasia of intestinal and perirectal lymph nodes that can result in fistulas and strictures.

Key Signs

- Unilateral tender lymphadenopathy
- Overlying dusky brown, adherent skin
- Proctocolitis

- Mucopurulent anal discharge
- Rectal strictures
- Rectovaginal strictures

Laboratory Tests

Diagnosis is made serologically or by exclusion of other causes of genital ulcers or inguinal lymphadenopathy.

Key Tests

- Lymphogranuloma venereum complement fixation test
- Microimmunofluorescent test
- Culture
- Direct fluorescent antibody

Treatment

Patients may require aspiration of lymphadenopathy through intact skin or incision and drainage to prevent inguinal or femoral ulceration.

Medication

1. The drug of choice is doxycycline, 100 mg orally twice a day for 21 days.
2. Alternative treatment is with erythromycin base, 500 mg orally four times daily for 21 days.
3. Doxycycline is contraindicated in pregnant women.

Key Treatment

Drug of Choice

- Doxycycline, 100 mg PO bid ×21 days

Alternative

- Erythromycin base, 500 mg PO qid ×21 days

Follow-Up

1. Patients should be followed clinically until signs and symptoms have resolved.
2. Sexual partners should be evaluated if contact has occurred within 30 days preceding the onset of symptoms.

Bibliography

Centers for Disease Control and Prevention: 1998 Guidelines for treatment of sexually transmitted diseases. MMWR Morb Mortal Wkly Rep 1998;47(RR-1):1–116.

Fiumara NJ: Pictorial Guide to Sexually Transmitted Diseases. New York, Cahners Publishing, 1989.

116 Granuloma Inguinale (Donovanosis)

Judith D. Kinzy

Etiology

Calymmatobacterium granulomatis

Symptoms

Painless, progressive, beefy-red ulcerative lesions of the genital, inguinal, or perianal areas

Key Symptom

Painless ulcers

Clinical Findings

1. The disease is rare in the United States but endemic in certain tropical and developing areas.
2. Patients present with highly vascular lesions without regional lymphadenopathy. The ulcers bleed easily on contact. They are described as having a "beefy, red appearance."

Key Signs

- Beefy, red ulceration
- No regional lymphadenopathy

Laboratory Tests

1. Diagnosis is made by the presence of dark-staining Donovan bodies on tissue crush preparation or biopsy. The organism cannot be cultured.
2. *Calymmatobacterium granulomatis* is found in large histiocytes and plasma cells. The organism stains bright red with bipolar staining and resembles a closed safety pin.
3. Smear and culture for gonorrhea.
4. Do blood test for syphilis.

Key Tests

- Tissue crush preparation or biopsy
- Rule out syphilis and gonorrhea

Treatment

1. Drugs of choice
   a. Trimethoprim-sulfamethoxazole, one double-strength tablet orally twice a day for a minimum of 3 weeks
   b. Doxycycline, 100 mg orally twice a day for a minimum of 3 weeks
2. Alternative drugs
   a. Ciprofloxacin, 750 mg orally twice a day for a minimum of 3 weeks
   b. Erythromycin base, 500 mg orally four times a day for a minimum of 3 weeks
3. Pregnant women should be treated with the erythromycin regimen.

Key Treatment

Drugs of Choice

- Trimethoprim-sulfamethoxazole DS, 1 PO bid ×3 weeks
- Doxycycline, 100 mg PO bid ×3 weeks

Alternatives

- Ciprofloxacin, 750 mg PO bid ×3 weeks
- Erythromycin base, 500 mg PO qid ×3 weeks

Follow-Up

1. Follow patients clinically until signs and symptoms have resolved.
2. Treat partners if sexual contact has occurred within 60 days of the patient's symptoms and if partner has signs and symptoms of the disease.

Bibliography

Centers for Disease Control and Prevention: 1998 Guidelines for treatment of sexually transmitted diseases. MMWR Morb Mortal Wkly Rep 1998;47(RR-1):1–116.

Fiumara NJ: Pictorial Guide to Sexually Transmitted Diseases. New York, Cahners Publishing, 1989.

117 Chancroid

Judith D. Kinzy

Etiology

Haemophilus ducreyi, a gram-negative streptobacillus

Symptoms

1. Men may complain of a painful ulcer or inguinal adenopathy.
2. Women may complain of symptoms unrelated to the ulcer, such as dysuria, dyspareunia, or hematochezia.

Clinical Findings

1. Deep necrotizing ulcerations are found on the shaft of the penis.
2. Tender unilateral lymphadenopathy is common.

Key Signs

- Deep necrotizing ulcers
- Tender inguinal lymphadenopathy

Laboratory Tests

1. Obtain smear and/or biopsy from undermined edges of lesion.
   a. Gram's stain reveals "schools of fish" or "railroad tracks."
   b. Culture on gonococcal agar or Mueller-Hinton agar. Sensitivity of culture is less than 80 per cent.
2. Probable diagnosis may be made if a patient has one or more painful genital ulcers and no evidence of *Treponema pallidum* or herpes simplex virus infection.

Key Tests

- Gram's stain of smear
- Culture

Differential Diagnosis

1. Syphilis
2. Herpes simplex
3. Lymphogranuloma venereum
4. Granuloma inguinale

Treatment

1. Drugs of choice
   a. Ceftriaxone (Rocephin), 250 mg IM once
   b. Erythromycin base, 500 mg PO qid ×7 days
   c. Azithromycin (Zithromax), 1 gm orally once
   d. Ciprofloxacin (Cipro), 500 mg orally bid for 3 days
2. Ciprofloxacin is contraindicated in pregnant and lactating women and for persons less than age 18.
3. Aspiration of fluctuant lymph nodes may be necessary to prevent rupture.
4. Avoid sexual activity for one week after treatment.

Key Treatment

Drugs of Choice

- Azithromycin, 1 gm PO once
- Ceftriaxone, 250 mg IM one time
- Erythromycin, 500 mg PO qid ×7 days
- Ciprofloxacin, 500 mg PO bid ×3 days

Follow-Up

1. Patients should be seen weekly until cure is achieved (re-examine 3 to 7 days after initiation of therapy).
2. Test for coexisting sexually transmitted diseases, including human immunodeficiency virus (HIV). Repeat HIV testing in 3 to 6 months.
3. Treat partners.
4. Uncircumcised men and HIV-infected patients may not respond as well to treatment as those who are circumcised or HIV-negative.

Bibliography

Centers for Disease Control and Prevention: 1998 Guidelines for treatment of sexually transmitted diseases. MMWR Morb Mortal Wkly Rep 1998;47(RR-1): 1–116.

Hoffman IF, Schmitz JL: Genital ulcer disease: management in the HIV era. Postgrad Med 1995;98(3):67–70, 73–76, 79–82.

118 Syphilis

Judith D. Kinzy

Etiology

Treponema pallidum

Symptoms

1. Primary syphilis presents as a chancre, a painless ulcer at the point of inoculation.
2. Secondary syphilis presents with rash, fever, malaise and lymphadenopathy 4 to 10 weeks after the chancre.

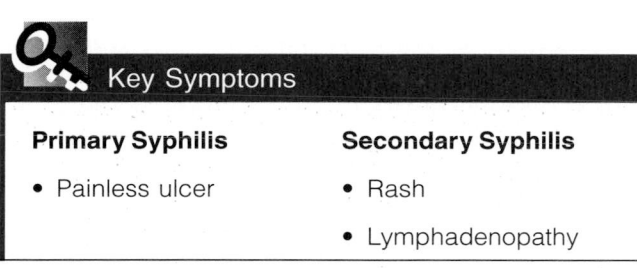

Key Symptoms

Primary Syphilis	Secondary Syphilis
• Painless ulcer	• Rash
	• Lymphadenopathy

Clinical Findings

1. Chancre is a painless solitary lesion with raised, well-defined borders and a clean, indurated base found in primary syphilis. Patients may have unilateral or bilateral regional nontender lymphadenopathy.
2. A macular, papular, annular, or follicular rash is the typical manifestation of secondary syphilis. Alopecia, condylomata lata, and shallow, painless ulcerations seen on the mucous membranes (called "mucous patches") are other clinical findings.

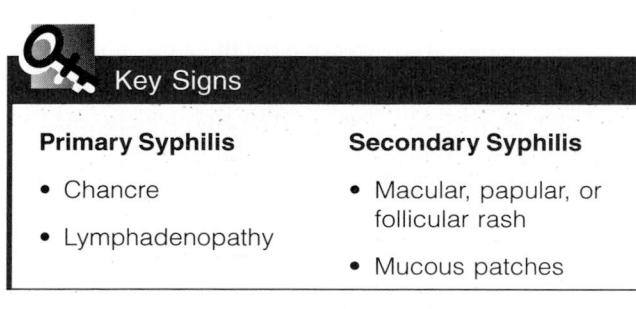

Key Signs

Primary Syphilis	Secondary Syphilis
• Chancre	• Macular, papular, or follicular rash
• Lymphadenopathy	• Mucous patches

Laboratory Tests

1. Rapid plasma reagin (RPR) and Venereal Disease Research Laboratory (VDRL) tests are recommended for screening. One can follow the response to therapy with these tests as titers diminish with treatment.
2. Fluorescent treponemal antibody absorption (FTA-Abs) and microhemagglutination assay for antibody to *T. pallidum* (MHA-TP) are more sensitive. These tests are not used for screening but are needed to verify a positive RPR or VDRL.

Key Tests

Screening	Verification (One Needed)
• RPR	• FTA-Abs
• VDRL	• MHA-TP

Differential Diagnosis

1. Primary syphilis
   a. Herpes simplex
   b. *Haemophilus ducreyi*
   c. Streptococci
   d. Staphylococci
   e. *Candida*
2. Secondary syphilis
   a. Pityriasis rosea
   b. Lichen planus
   c. Psoriasis
   d. Drug eruption
   e. Impetigo
   f. Chickenpox

Treatment

Medication

The drug of choice is penicillin G benzathine, 2.4 million units intramuscularly once. Alternatives for nonpregnant patients include doxycycline, 100 mg orally bid for 14 days, or tetracycline, 500 mg orally qid for 14 days. Treat sexual contacts.

Patient Education

Avoid sexual contact for 1 week after treatment.

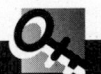
Key Treatment

Drug of Choice	Alternative Drugs
• Penicillin G benzathine, 2.4 million U IM	• Doxycycline, 100 mg PO bid × 14 days
	• Tetracycline, 500 mg PO bid × 14 days

Follow-Up

1. Follow VDRL or RPR titers. Successful treatment leads to a fourfold decrease in serum RPR at 6 months for primary syphilis and eightfold decline within 12 months with secondary syphilis.

2. Check for human immunodeficiency virus (HIV) because syphilis is linked with HIV.

Bibliography

Centers for Disease Control and Prevention: 1998 Sexually transmitted diseases treatment guidelines. MMWR Morb Mortal Wkly Rep 1998;47(RR-1):1–116.

Fiumara NJ: Pictorial Guide to Sexually Transmitted Diseases. New York, Cahners Publishing, 1989.

Hoffman IF, Schmitz JL: Genital ulcer disease: management in the HIV era. Postgrad Med 1995;98:67–70, 73–76, 79–82.

Hook EW, Marra CM: Acquired syphilis in adults. N Engl J Med 1992;326:1060–1069.

Lappa S, Moscicki AB: The pediatrician and the sexually active adolescent: a primer for sexually transmitted diseases. Pediatr Clin North Am 1997;44:1405–1045.

1. The Bartholin's (greater vestibular) glands are situated inferolaterally to the bulbocavernosus muscles. They lie beneath the urogenital diaphragm and are surrounded by dense fibromuscular tissue. In the absence of neoplasia or infection, these glands are approximately 1 cm in diameter and are usually nonpalpable.

2. The Bartholin's glands are tubuloalveolar glands that secrete a clear, viscous fluid responsible for lubricating the vaginal vestibule. Maximal secretion occurs during the late excitement and early plateau phases of sexual stimulation. Each gland secretes fluid into the vaginal introitus just lateral to the hymenal ring or its remnant at the 5 and 7 o'clock positions of the vestibule through a duct that is 1 to 2 cm in length. The duct and glandular acini are lined with transitional and mucous-secreting cuboidal epithelium, respectively. The duct opens into the vestibule, which is lined with nonkeratinized squamous epithelium.

3. When the orifice for the Bartholin's gland duct becomes occluded, a cyst or abscess may develop. The cyst or abscess occurs within the duct and generally *does not* involve the Bartholin's gland.

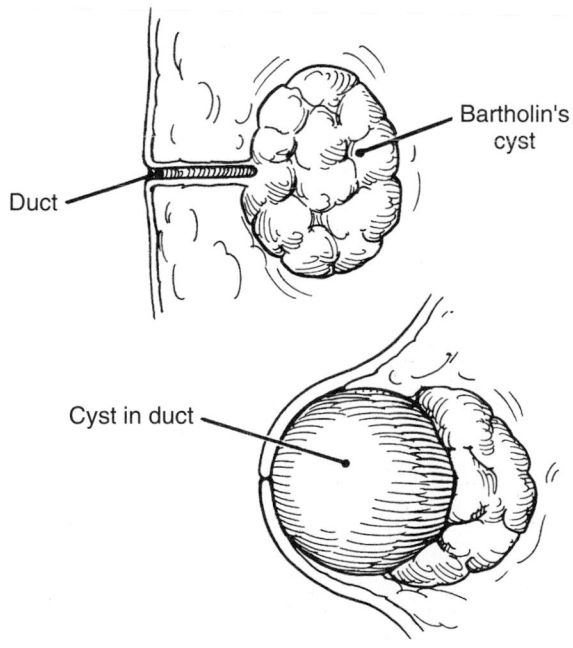

Differential Diagnosis

1. Bartholin's gland tumor

   a. The average patient age for a primary tumor of the Bartholin's gland is 50.

   b. Types of tumor include adenocarcinoma (40 per cent), squamous cell carcinoma (40 per cent), adenoid cystic carcinoma (15 per cent), adenosquamous carcinoma (<5 per cent), transitional cell carcinoma (<5 per cent), and other (<5 per cent). Squamous cell tumors may arise from metaplasia or from infiltration from vestibular squamous cell components. Metastatic neoplasms have also been identified. Solid benign tumors are rare.

   c. Malignant Bartholin's gland tumors constitute 1 per cent of all vulvar malignancies and have a low incidence (0.023 and 0.114 per 100,000 woman-years in pre- and postmenopausal women, respectively).

   d. If a tumor is suspected, biopsy or fine-needle aspiration should be considered. Tumor is suggested by a fixed, hard mass or persistent localized ulceration.

   e. Bartholin's gland cancers spread via lymphatics to the inguinal and pelvic lymph nodes. Treatment often necessitates radical vulvectomy. Automatic Bartholin's gland excision in postmenopausal females with glandular-ductal enlargement is no longer routine because of a high complication rate (bleeding, scarring, and dyspareunia, among others) and low incidence of cancer. Malignancy should, however, be ruled out if the enlargement does not drain or resolve with therapy or if there is a high index of suspicion.

2. Cyst formation in other glandular (sebaceous or inclusion cysts, mucinous cysts) or embryonic (wolffian duct cysts, Gartner's duct cyst, and cysts of the canal of Nuck) structures

3. Vulvar endometriosis. This is most frequently encountered in the region of the Bartholin's gland.

4. Vulvar tumors: lipoma, fibroma, fibromyoma, hidradenoma, angioma, sarcoma, granular cell myoblastoma, von Recklinghausen's tumor

5. Other: vulvar hematoma, ischiorectal abscess, accessory breast tissue, vaginal leiomyoma, and inguinal hernia

Etiology

1. The vestibular orifice of the Bartholin's gland duct may become occluded secondary to mucus plugging, inflammation, infection, or scarring. Scarring may result from chronic inflammation/infection or vulvar trauma (birth trauma, impact injury, posterior colporrhaphy). Bartholin's duct cysts progressively enlarge as the gland

continues to produce secretions with an occluded outlet.

2. For many years *Neisseria gonorrhoeae* was thought to be the leading microbial etiology for Bartholin's duct abscesses. Newer data have disproven this. Both commensal (streptococcus, staphylococcus, *Escherichia coli*, *Gardnerella vaginalis*, *Proteus mirabilis*, and anaerobic bacteria) and sexually transmitted (*N. gonorrhoeae*, *Chlamydia trachomatis*) organisms have been cultured from Bartholin's duct abscesses. Genital mycoplasmas do not appear to play a significant role.

3. Abscesses may be secondary to infection with a single organism or multiple organisms. Infection is most commonly polymicrobial and requires broad-spectrum antibiotics. Amoxicillin–clavulanic acid, clindamycin, azithromycin, and doxycycline, among others, can be used.

Symptoms

1. Cysts are typically fluctuant, nontender, and the patient may not even be aware of them. Small asymptomatic cysts in premenopausal women may not require therapy.

2. Abscesses are tender, fluctuant, and can distend the labia and vestibule. An abscess is often surrounded by indurated, erythematous tissue and causes the patient persistent discomfort. They may be accompanied by fever, chills, and purulent drainage if there is spontaneous rupture. These lesions are most frequently encountered in the 20- to 29-year age group. Women of high parity (≥4) or high gravidity (≥5) have the lowest risk.

3. Complications of a Bartholin duct abscess include gangrene, necrotizing fasciitis, toxic shock, and septic shock.

Management

Indications

A variety of methods have been developed for the management of Bartholin's duct cysts and abscesses. Simple incision and drainage is discouraged because of a 75 per cent recurrence rate. Of the methods with demonstrated efficacy, marsupialization and Word catheter placement are the most frequently used. They are equally effective. Placement of a Word catheter is easier to perform in the office setting and is presented here.

Preparation

Sterile procedure should be used. Prepare the cyst or abscess site with povidone-iodine or alcohol in iodine-allergic patients.

Equipment

1. A No. 11 scalpel blade
2. Cotton-tipped swab
3. Hemostat
4. Aerobic and anaerobic culture tubes
5. Culture materials for chlamydia and gonorrhea
6. A Word Bartholin Gland Catheter

Anesthesia

Infiltrate the overlying vestibular tissue with 1% or 2% lidocaine without epinephrine. Do not inject the anesthetic directly into the cyst/abscess cavity.

Technique

1. Make a stab incision in the cyst/abscess just lateral to the hymenal ring. It should be placed approximately where the duct outlet is situated. The incision should be just large enough to introduce the Word catheter tip.

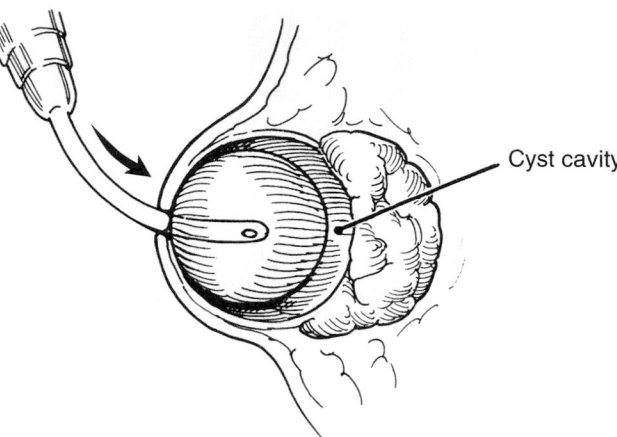

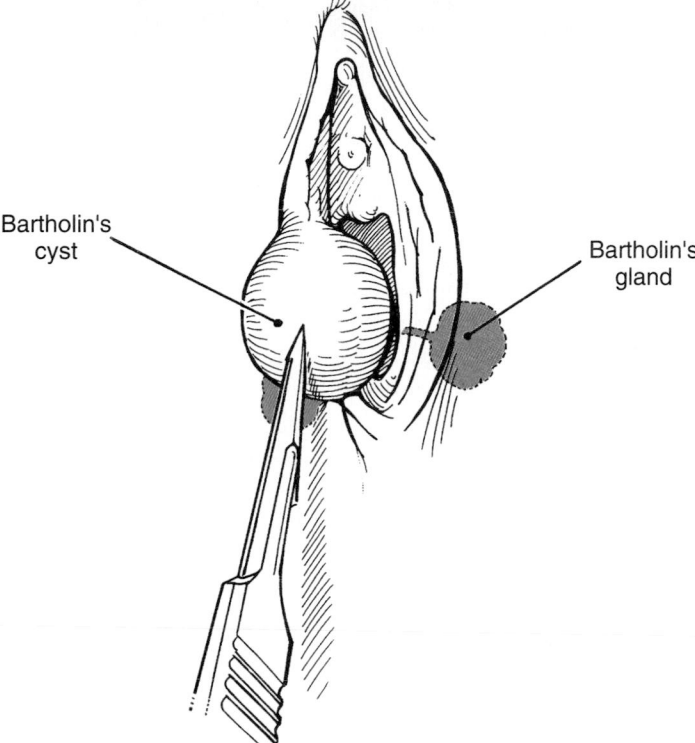

2. Submit the drainage fluid for routine culture and evaluate for chlamydial and gonorrheal infection. In the appropriate clinical setting, cultures of the cervix may also be indicated.

3. Decompress the cyst/abscess as much as possible.

4. Introduce a hemostat or cotton-tipped swab into the cavity and disaggregate loculations.

5. Once the top of the Word catheter is securely placed in the cavity, inflate the tip with 2 to 5 ml of water. If the volume injected causes pain, withdraw 1 or 2 ml and adjust tip size to ensure the patient's comfort.

6. The catheter port may be placed in the vagina to minimize the patient's awareness of its presence.

7. Leave the catheter in place for 4 to 6 weeks to allow epithelialization of the fistulous tract. Over time the cyst/abscess cavity will contract and resume its function as a duct.

Follow-Up

1. During the first 10 to 14 days after the procedure, the patient should take Sitz baths and begin a broad-spectrum antibiotic.

2. Opiate and/or nonsteroidal anti-inflammatory analgesics can be provided as needed for pain relief.

3. Abstinence from intercourse is advised until the catheter is removed or until vestibular/vaginal discomfort resolves.

Bibliography

Hill DA, Lense JJ: Office management of Bartholin gland cysts and abscesses. Am Fam Physician 1998; 57: 1611–1616.

Lee Y-H, Rankin JS, Alpert S, et al: Microbiological investigation of Bartholin's gland abscesses and cysts. Am J Obstet Gynecol 1977;129:150–153.

Visco AG, Del Priore G: Postmenopausal Bartholin gland enlargement: a hospital-based cancer risk assessment. Obstet Gynecol 1996;87:286–290.

Wilkinson EJ, Mullins DL: The vulva and vagina. In Silverberg SG, DeLellis RA, Frable WJ (eds): Principles and Practice of Surgical Pathology and Cytopathology, vol 3, pp 2411–2457. New York, Churchill Livingstone, 1998.

Word B: Office treatment of cyst and abscess of Bartholin's gland duct. South Med J 1968;61:514–518.

119 Endometriosis

Patricia A. Sereno

Etiology

1. Simply defined as the presence of functioning endometrial tissue outside of the uterus, which often leads to dysmenorrhea, dyspareunia, and infertility

2. Reported to have a prevalence of 15 per cent among fertile women and up to 50 per cent among infertile women

3. Affects women of reproductive age, with a mean age at the time of diagnosis of 25 to 29 years

4. Higher prevalence rates in Japanese women, and increased risk among women with first-degree relatives also diagnosed with the disease. No specific pattern of inheritance has been established.

5. The most widely accepted theory of pathogenesis is retrograde menstruation. It is known that, in the majority of women, menstrual tissue moves up through the fallopian tubes. In women with endometriosis, current theories suggest that changes in the immune and inflammatory regulatory systems allow for cell implantation along the peritoneum.

Symptoms

1. As a result of peritoneal inflammation, patients complain of chronic pelvic pain.

2. Two thirds of women will complain of dysmenorrhea, and most will complain of dyspareunia.

3. Infertility either is secondary to anatomic distortion or is a result of an as-yet undefined change in the uterine milieu. Proposed mechanisms for endometriosis-associated infertility include ovulatory dysfunction, altered follicle development, sperm phagocytosis, impaired fertilization, defective implantation, luteal-phase defects, and immunologic alterations.

4. Menstrual irregularities, including premenstrual spotting, menstrual hematuria, or rectal bleeding, can be found in patients with endometriosis.

5. It is important to remember that symptom severity and laparoscopic findings are poorly correlated, and some women, even with severe disease, may be asymptomatic.

Key Symptoms

- Dysmenorrhea
- Dyspareunia
- Infertility

Clinical Findings

1. Physical examination may be normal even with severe endometriosis.

2. Tender and inflamed areas are more easily found if examination is performed premenstrually.

3. With bimanual examination, patients may complain of cervical motion tenderness or tenderness with palpation of the vaginal cul-de-sac. Adnexal masses consistent with endometriomas of either ovary may also be palpable.

4. Rectovaginal examination may also reveal a nodularity consistent with seeding along the uterosacral ligaments.

Key Signs

- Tender adnexal masses
- Cervical motion tenderness
- Nodularity of the uterosacral ligaments

Laboratory Tests

1. The gold standard for diagnosis is laparoscopy. Treatment with ovarian suppressive therapy may result in the appearance of a "clean" peritoneum, but implants will reappear once therapy is discontinued. At the time of laparoscopy, because of the heterogeneous appearance of the disease, the surgeon should biopsy any suspicious areas.

2. Staging systems have attempted to correlate laparoscopy findings and patient symptoms, but have thus far not been proven reliable.

3. Ultrasound can be used to identify endometriomas, but cannot be used to differentiate between endometriomas and cysts from other

sources. Diagnostic accuracy can be improved with Doppler sonography.

4. Magnetic resonance imaging is being investigated for its use as a noninvasive technique for identifying and determining the location of endometriomas.

Key Test

- Laparoscopy

Differential Diagnosis

1. Adhesions from previous infection (i.e., pelvic inflammatory disease) or previous pelvic surgery
2. Ovarian cysts or tumors

Treatment

1. Treatment strategies in endometriosis seek to preserve fertility and maximize pain relief.
2. At the time of laparoscopy or laparotomy, visible implants may be ablated using either laser or thermal cautery. Adhesions may also be lysed. Endometriomas can be removed or drained.
3. To improve fertility, microsurgery on a distorted fallopian tube may also be attempted. Infertile patients are usually treated with ovarian stimulation and in vitro fertilization, although pregnancy rates among women with endometriosis are lower than those of women with other causes of infertility.
4. Hysterectomy with bilateral salpingo-oophorectomy eliminates pain in 90 per cent of affected women, but obviously is only an option for women not desiring future fertility. Discussions with these patients should include the increased risk of osteoporosis and cardiovascular disease. Options regarding future hormone replacement therapy should also be presented.

Medication

1. Analgesics
   a. Nonsteroidal anti-inflammatory agents may provide some relief when used either alone or in combination with other agents.
   b. Narcotic agents can be used to provide short-term pain relief, but prolonged use should be avoided because of their addictive potential.
2. Hormonal therapy
   a. Danazol (Danocrine), a derivative of 17_α-ethynyltestosterone

(1) Causes amenorrhea by suppressing luteinizing hormone (LH) and follicle-stimulating hormone (FSH).
(2) Dose: 200 to 400 mg PO bid
(3) Treatment for 6 months results in relief from pelvic pain in up to 90 per cent of women
(4) Treatment reduces the extent of implants in 60 per cent of women but does not have any effect on endometriomas larger than 3 cm in diameter. Pelvic adhesions are also not affected by treatment with this drug.
(5) Danazol has no effect on fertility.
(6) Up to 80 per cent of women will experience side effects with this drug.
   (a) Weight gain (20 to 30 lb), edema, acne, hot flashes, and uterine spotting.
   (b) Danazol has also been shown to have a reversible effect on lipoproteins. Low-density lipoprotein is increased by 14 to 41 per cent, and high-density lipoprotein is decreased up to 50 per cent during treatment.
   (c) Elevation of hepatic transaminases has been reported, and should be checked periodically throughout treatment.
b. Gonadotropin-releasing hormone (GnRH) agonists
   (1) Act by eliminating the GnRH pulse, resulting in the paradoxical down-regulation of the pituitary axis, and then a decrease in LH and FSH. Gonadal suppression causes a hypoestrogenic state, and the resulting amenorrhea is associated with pain relief in 70 to 90 per cent of women.
   (2) Doses for medications currently available in the United States include
      (a) Nafarelin (Synarel), 200 to 400 μg nasal spray bid
      (b) Lupreolide (Lupron), 3.75 mg IM every 28 days or 11.25 mg IM every 3 months
      (c) Goserelin (Zoladex), 3.6 mg IM every 28 days
   (3) Side effects are associated with the hypoestrogenic state and include hot flashes, vaginal dryness, headache, decreased libido, and mood swings.
   (4) Treatment also results in a 2 to 6 per cent reduction in bone mass, which lim-

its the use of these agents to 6 months of therapy. Early data do, however, suggest that the effects on bone mass are reversible.

(5) "Add-back therapy": To limit the side effects associated with GnRH agonists, small amounts of estrogen and progestins, or progestin alone, can be added to GnRH therapy without recurrence of pelvic pain.

c. Medroxyprogesterone acetate

(1) Acts by inhibiting FSH and LH, and thereby inhibiting ovulation.

(2) Results in an atrophic endometrium and relief of pain by causing menorrhea.

(3) Depot medroxyprogesterone acetate (Depo-Provera), 400 mg IM every 2 weeks for four doses, then every 4 weeks for 5 months

(4) Medroxyprogesterone acetate (Provera), 10 mg PO tid

(5) Side effects include bloating and irregular bleeding.

(6) Up to 90 per cent of women will have relief with progestin therapy with no long-term effect on fertility.

d. Estrogen-progestin combinations (oral contraceptive pills)

(1) Administration of continuous combination oral contraceptive pills for 6 to 9 months results in amenorrhea, although may require up to three tablets per day.

(2) Tablets should contain 30 to 35 μg ethinyl estradiol.

(3) Pain relief reported in 60 to 94 per cent of patients.

(4) Side effects include nausea, bloating, and breakthrough bleeding.

(5) This treatment is contraindicated in women with thromboembolic disease or significant hepatic disease.

e. Mifepristone (RU 486)

(1) RU 486 is an antiprogesterone and antiglucocorticoid that inhibits ovulation and alters endometrial proliferation.

(2) Early research suggests doses of 50 to 200 mg PO qd; however, further studies are needed before its widespread use.

(3) Side effects include hot flashes, fatigue, nausea, and transient transaminase elevation.

Patient Education

1. Physicians need to counsel their patients regarding the chronic nature of the disease and the significant incidence of infertility.

2. For information, patients may contact the Endometriosis Association of America at 1-800-992-3636, or by searching various web sites on the World Wide Web.

Key Treatments

- Nonsteroidal anti-inflammatory drugs
- GnRH agonists
- Progesterone
- Combination oral contraceptive pills

Bibliography

Brosens I: Endometriosis: current issues in diagnosis and medical management. J Reprod Med 1998;43:281–286.

Gargiulo AR, Hornstein MD: The role of GnRH agonists plus add back therapy in the treatment of endometriosis. Semin Reprod Endocrinol 1997;15:273–284.

Hemmings R: Combined treatment of endometriosis GnRH agonists and laparoscopic surgery. J Reprod Med 1998;43:316–320.

Olive DL (ed): Endometriosis. Obstet Gynecol Clin North Am 1997;22:219–465.

Ryan I, Taylor R: Endometriosis and infertility: new concepts. Obstet Gynecol Surv 1997;52:365–371.

120 Endometritis

Michael P. Rowane

Etiology

1. "Endometritis," inflammation of the endometrium, the decidual mucous membrane of the gravid uterus, is the most common postpartum infection, occurring in 1 to 3 per cent of vaginal deliveries and in 10 to 50 per cent of cesarean deliveries.
2. The cellular debris and the large raw area of placental insertion are excellent media. The cervicovaginal flora, with anaerobes and gram-negative organisms, are the most common causes.
3. Microorganisms
   a. Aerobic bacteria
      (1) Gram-positives
         (a) Group A, B, and D streptococci (30 per cent of group B are completely/partially involved)
         (b) Enterococci
         (c) *Staphylococcus aureus*
      (2) Gram-negatives
         (a) *Escherichia coli* (most common gram-negative)
         (b) *Gardnerella vaginitis*
         (c) *Neisseria gonorrhoeae* (2 to 8 per cent)
   b. Anaerobic bacteria (involved in 50 to 95 per cent of uterine puerperal infections)
      (1) *Bacteroides bivius* and other *Bacteroides* species
      (2) Peptostreptococci
      (3) Peptococci
      (4) *Proteus mirabilis*
   c. Other organisms
      (1) *Ureaplasma urealyticum*
      (2) *Mycoplasma hominis*
      (3) *Chlamydia trachomatis* (associated specifically with a late-onset postpartum endometritis)

Symptoms

1. *Fever*
   a. Occurs most commonly on the first or second postpartum day.
      (1) Oral temperature of greater than 38.5° C in the first 24 hours after delivery, *or*
      (2) Greater than 38.0° C for more than 6 consecutive days after first postpartum day.
   b. Fever can be a clue to involved organisms.
      (1) Less than 48 hours postpartum: Suspect gram-positive streptococci.
      (2) More than 48 hours postpartum: Suspect a mixed anaerobic and gram-negative infection.
2. *Chills* (Fever and chills occur more commonly in the late afternoon or evening.)
3. *Malaise*
4. *Abdominal pain*
5. Foul-smelling lochia
6. Symptoms of ileus (i.e., distention, constipation)

Key Symptoms

- Fever
- Malaise
- Abdominal pain
- Foul-smelling lochia

Clinical Findings

1. Temperature above 100.4° F: Fever, after excluding other causes, will remain as the most important criterion for the diagnosis of endometritis.
2. Tachycardia
3. Abdominal
   a. Tenderness in the lower abdomen without lateralization
   b. Infection of abdominal wound after cesarean section
   c. Fundal height same as uterus of normal puerpera
   d. Ileus with diminished/absent bowel sounds and distention
4. Pelvic
   a. Uterus soft and tender to palpation
   b. Inspect uterus for retained material or pyom-

etra, a collection of pus within the endometrial cavity.

   c. Adnexal mass (abscess vs. infected hematoma)

   d. May or may not have a foul-smelling lochia/discharge.

   e. Evaluate for infection of episiotomy.

5. Severe disease: high fever, abdominal tenderness, ileus, hypotension, and generalized sepsis

Key Signs

- Temperature above 100.4° F
- Soft, tender uterus

Laboratory Tests

1. Cervical/endometrial cultures

   a. Unfortunately, genital cultures are frequently contaminated and rarely indicate the infecting organism.

   b. May consider a culture of any wound infection, abscess, or hematoma.

2. Complete blood count (CBC) with differential: Leukocytosis may be seen, but difficult to interpret because of expected physiologic leukocytosis of the early puerperium.

3. Blood cultures and sensitivities ×2: Most helpful with suspected septicemia; positive in only 5 to 10 per cent of patients and rarely demonstrate a single causative agent

4. Electrolytes, blood urea nitrogen, and creatinine

5. Urinalysis, with urine culture and sensitivities

6. Chest radiograph: rarely of benefit unless signs and symptoms point to a possible pulmonary cause of the fever

7. Ultrasound (if considering pyometra)

Key Tests

- CBC with differential
- Blood cultures and sensitivities ×2
- Urinalysis, with urine culture and sensitivities

Differential Diagnosis

1. Genital source

   a. Infected mass, such as abscess and incisional hematoma

   b. Pelvic cellulitis

   c. Septic pelvic thrombophlebitis

2. Nongenital source

   a. Urinary tract infection

   b. Pneumonia (especially smokers and after general anesthesia)

   c. Intravenous phlebitis

   d. Appendicitis

   e. Viral syndrome

   f. Drug fever

   g. Breast engorgement

Risk Factors

1. Cesarean delivery

2. Prolonged rupture of membranes more than 12 to 24 hours (the major risk factor after cesarean section if more than 6 hours)

3. Intrapartum and postpartum anemia

4. Multiple vaginal examinations in labor (single predictor of prophylactic antibiotic failure following cesarean section)

5. Intrauterine pressure catheters (>8 hours)

6. Fetal scalp electrode monitoring

7. Pre-existing vaginitis/cervicitis

8. Operative vaginal deliveries

9. Prolonged labor (>8 hours)

10. Coitus near term

11. Indigent patients

12. Chorioamnionitis

13. Toxemia

14. Poor nutrition

15. Obesity

Treatment

1. General principles

   a. A short course of prophylactic antibiotics will significantly lower the risk of endometritis after a nonelective cesarean delivery.

   b. The prognosis of postpartum endometritis is excellent with prompt therapy.

   c. Delays in diagnosis may lead to complications (e.g., pelvic abscess or septic pelvic thrombophlebitis bacterial heparinase progressing to clots in pelvic vessels, with potential septic emboli).

   d. The choice of antibiotics for treatment depends on the suspected organisms and the severity of the disease.

   e. Initial therapy requires high-dose intravenous antibiotics.

   f. For patients with known risk factors or at high risk for infection at delivery, initial therapy is with two- or three-drug regimens, preferably including clindamycin. Equal efficacy seen with a single-agent intravenous infusion of broad-spectrum agent.

g. There are numerous acceptable antimicrobial regimens with broad-spectrum antimicrobial therapy as the mainstay.

h. Intravenous therapy until afebrile (<38° C [99.5° F]) and pain-free for 48 hours and asymptomatic.

i. Clindamycin is added if clinical/laboratory results suggest that *Bacteroides* species are involved.

j. Expect a prompt response to treatment. In the event of any persistent fever, consider alternate etiologies: pelvic abscess, wound infection, septic pelvic thrombophlebitis, inadequate antibiotic coverage, and retained placenta.

PEARLS

- In septic abortion, *Clostridium perfringens* may cause fulminate intravascular hemolysis.

- In postpartum patients with uncertain fever and/or pulmonary emboli, consider septic pelvic vein thrombophlebitis requiring heparin and antibiotics.

- Endometritis requires the same coverage as amnionitis and septic abortion.

- Abdominal wound infections are primarily responsible for persistent fever and therefore antibiotic failure.

- With high fever and hypotension soon after delivery, think of a group B streptococcal infection.

---

2. Surgical

a. Dilatation and curettage (D&C) of uterus if indicated (e.g., to remove retained products of conception)

b. Drainage of pyometra (ultrasound may assist/guide)

Medication

1. *Early postpartum*, first 48 hours: Two options to consider:

a. Doxycycline along with one of the following agents

(1) Cefoxitin (Mefoxin), 2 gm intravenously q6h

(2) Ticarcillin-clavulanate (Timentin), 3.1 gm intravenously q4–6h

(3) Imipenem-cilastatin (Primaxin), 0.5 to 1 gm q6h

(4) Ampicillin-sulbactam (Unasyn), 3 gm intravenously q6h

b. Clindamycin along with one of the following agents

(1) Gentamicin, 120 mg (2 mg/kg) intravenous piggyback (IVPB) then 80 mg (1.5 mg/kg) IVPB q8h (monitor peak and trough levels). (*Note*: Recent data support 1 mg/kg per dose as adequate.)

(2) Third-generation cephalosporin

c. After discharge, continue doxycycline or clindamycin.

2. *Late postpartum*, 48 hours to 6 weeks

a. Usually after vaginal delivery

b. Doxycycline, 100 mg q12h intravenously or orally for 14 days

3. *Postcesarean endometritis*: Clindamycin and gentamicin or ceftriaxone, 1 to 2 gm intravenously or intramuscularly q12–24h

4. *Alternative regimen*: Add one of the following agents to gentamicin:

a. Clindamycin, 900 mg intravenously q8h

b. Cefoxitin (Mefoxin), 2 gm intravenously q6h

c. Cefotetan (Cefotan), 2 gm intravenously q12h

d. Piperacillin-mezlocillin, 4 gm intravenously q6h

e. Ampicillin-sulbactam (Unasyn), 3 gm intravenously q6h

f. Ticarcillin-clavulanate (Timentin), 3.1 gm intravenously q4–6h

5. *Single-agent therapy* also has been successful with broad-spectrum agents such as ampicillin-sulbactam, imipenem-cilastatin, ticarcillin-clavulanate, cefoxitin, cefotetan, or ceftizoxime.

6. Discontinue nursing if using tetracyclines, because they are not recommended in nursing mothers.

Diet

1. Must encourage fluids.

2. Intravenous fluids if lacking adequate oral intake

3. Diet as tolerated

Activity

1. Mild to moderate endometritis: bed rest with limited activities (e.g., bathroom privileges)

2. Severe endometritis: bed rest

3. Increase activity as tolerated

Patient Education

1. Labor and delivery education/prevention
   a. The possibility of endometritis
   b. Avoid high-risk behavior.
   c. Need for last-trimester cultures
2. Stress that, with antibiotic therapy and supportive management, most patients are afebrile in a few days with complete resolution.

Key Treatment

Drugs of Choice (Multiple Options)

- Gentamicin
- Doxycycline
- Clindamycin
- Ampicillin-sulbactam
- Piperacillin-mezlocillin
- D&C of uterus if indicated

- Ticarcillin-clavulanate
- Imipenem-cilastatin
- Ceftizoxime
- Cefoxitin
- Cefotetan

Follow-Up

1. Hospitalize
2. The response to this therapy should be carefully monitored for 24 to 48 hours. Deterioration or failure to respond both clinically and on laboratory tests results requires a complete reevaluation.

3. Office follow-up within the first week of discharge
4. Inform patient of need to call with any complications.

Bibliography

For more information on endometritis and other obstetric emergencies, see
Benrubi GI: Obstetrical and Gynecological Emergencies, pp 156–159. Philadelphia, JB Lippincott Company, 1994.

For more information on endometritis in what most people consider the "Bible" of obstetrics, see
In Cunningham GF, MacDonald PC, Gant NF et al (eds): Infection and disorders of the puerperium. In Williams' Obstetrics, pp 547–558. Stamford, CT, Appleton & Lange, 1997.

For more information from a cooperative effort, see
American Academy of Pediatrics Committee on Fetus and Newborn and the American College of Obstetricians and Gynecologists Committee on Obstetric Practice: Guidelines for Perinatal Care, 4th ed, pp 144–146. Elk Grove Village, IL, American Academy of Pediatrics, 1997.

For more information on antimicrobial therapy in endometritis and other disorders, see
Gillbert DN, Moellering RC, Sande MA: Sanford Guide to Antimicrbial Therapy 1999, 29th ed. Vienna, VA, Antimicrbial Therapy, Inc, 1999.

For more information on a family-centered maternity care utilizing an evidence-based approach, see
Baxley E: Postpartum biomedical concerns. In Ratcliffe SD, Byrd JE, Sakornbut EL (eds): Handbook of Pregnancy and Perinatal Care in Family Practice Science and Practice, pp 431–434. Philadelphia, Hanley & Belfus, Inc, 1996.

121 Menopause

Shirley L. Dickinson

Definition/Epidemiology

1. Menopause is the cessation of menstruation as a result of the failure of ovarian follicular development in the presence of sufficient gonadotropin levels.
2. The perimenopause is characterized by a gradual decline in ovarian function and estrogen production.
   a. Declining estrogen levels result in the onset of increased rate of bone loss, previously believed to start only after complete cessation of menstruation.
   b. Patients may be asymptomatic during this period or complain of symptoms typical of the menopause.
3. The average age of menopause is 51.4 years, with the age range being 40 to 60 years. Smoking and high-altitude living accelerate the menopause.

Symptoms of Estrogen Deficiency

1. Prevalence
   a. Seventy-five to 80 per cent will experience some discomfort.
   b. Ten to 15 per cent have symptoms that interfere with daily functioning.
   c. Twenty-five per cent of women complain of symptoms lasting more than 5 years.
2. Menstrual cycle changes, including hypermenorrhea, oligomenorrhea, and finally amenorrhea
3. Genitourinary atrophy
4. Extragenital symptoms
   a. Hot flashes/vasomotor symptoms
   b. Psychological manifestations may occur before and 3 to 5 years after the menopause.
      (1) Insomnia, fatigue
      (2) Irritability, anxiety, depression
      (3) Memory loss, difficulty concentrating
   c. Skin thickness and collagen content are decreased, resulting in wrinkles.
   d. Osteoporosis and coronary heart disease (CHD) may be silent until 10 to 15 years after the onset of the menopause. At this point significant irreversible disease may be present.

Key Symptoms

- Vasomotor flushes
- Vaginal dryness
- Urinary stress incontinence
- Cystitis-like symptoms
- Insomnia
- Irritability
- Anxiety
- Memory loss

Clinical Findings

1. Urogenital atrophy can begin prior to and 3 to 5 years after the development of amenorrhea.
   a. Mucosa of the genitourinary tract is extremely sensitive to estrogen.
   b. *Vaginal atrophy:* resulting in dyspareunia, atrophic vaginitis, an increased susceptibility to bacterial vaginitis, or vaginal bleeding
   c. *Vulvar atrophy:* resulting in pruritus vulvae, loss of pubic hair, and labial atrophy
   d. *Atrophy of urethra and bladder trigone:* resulting in symptoms of cystitis or urgency incontinence
   e. *Atrophy of the pelvic floor muscles:* resulting in uterine prolapse, cystocele, and rectocele
2. Osteoporosis
   a. Affects one third of postmenopausal women in the United States.
   b. Results in a loss of bone strength, resulting in an increased susceptibility to fracture primarily of the hip, vertebrae, distal forearm, humerus, and pelvis.
   c. Accounts for significant morbidity and mortality.
      (1) Survivors of hip fractures are frequently severely affected and may become permanently disabled.
      (2) Mortality rate of hip fracture is 10 to 20 per cent within the first 6 months. Mortality is related either directly to the hip fracture or to surgical, embolic, or cardiopulmonary complications.
   d. Prevention in high-risk women includes early estrogen replacement, adequate calcium intake, and weight-bearing exercise.

3. Cardiovascular disease
   a. After the menopause there is a progressive increase in the incidence of CHD
   b. Estrogen results in a 50 per cent reduction in the incidence of CHD and related mortality.
      (1) Estrogen benefits the lipoprotein profile by increasing the high-density lipoprotein (HDL) cholesterol and decreasing low-density lipoprotein (LDL) and total cholesterol.
      (2) Acts directly at the coronary arteries, resulting in vasodilatation, and inhibits the development of atheromatous plaques.
      (3) Reduces platelet aggregation.
      (4) Antioxidant effects on LDL and total cholesterol.
      (5) Improves glucose metabolism, lowering circulating insulin levels
      (6) Reduces fibrinogen and plasminogen activator inhibitor levels, enhancing fibrinolysis.
   c. Estrogen is not currently recommended for the secondary prevention of CHD based on a recent randomized placebo controlled study (Heart and Estrogen/progestin Replacement Study—HERS). This study demonstrated an early increased risk of CHD events in postmenopausal women started on HRT with pre-existing CHD.
      (1) Women already receiving HRT should continue with treatment, as the number of CHD events did decrease after 4 and 5 years of therapy.
      (2) Postmenopausal women 60 to 70 years of age would benefit from a risk factor assessment regarding cardiac disease. If significant risk factors for CHD are present consider a cardiac evaluation for the presence of CHD prior to the initiation of HRT for the first time.
      (3) Only CCE/MPA in a continuous dose regimen was studied. Results might be different with unopposed estrogens (in hysterectomized women), alternative estrogen/progestin preparations, or a cyclic regimen. Further studies are needed to more definitively outline the role of estrogen in the secondary prevention of CHD.
4. Potential benefits of estrogen
   a. Alzheimer's disease–by delaying the onset and/or slowing the progression
   b. Prevention of colon cancer
   c. Prevention of stroke
   d. Improvement in postural balance

Key Signs

- Genitourinary atrophy
- Osteoporosis
- CHD

Laboratory Tests

In general, no tests are necessary to diagnose the menopause. Symptoms and clinical evidence should suffice. When necessary to confirm, the following tests can be done.

1. Follicle-stimulating hormone (FSH) and estradiol
   a. During the perimenopausal period, women have lower estradiol levels and rising FSH levels as the follicular phase begins to shorten.
   b. FSH levels in the postmenopausal range (>40 mIU/ml) can be seen despite continued menstrual bleeding.
   c. Decreasing estradiol levels result in early bone loss.
2. Luteinizing hormone (LH)
   a. During the perimenopausal period, LH levels remain in the high-normal range.
   b. Reaches a peak 1 to 3 years after the menopause, followed by a gradual decline.
3. Endometrial biopsy
   a. Baseline biopsy not necessary unless history of abnormal bleeding.
   b. Biopsy is indicated if breakthrough bleeding or heavy withdrawal bleeding occurs.
4. Transvaginal ultrasonography
   a. Endometrial stripe of less than 5 mm not associated with endometrial hyperplasia or cancer.
   b. Endometrial stripe of 5 mm or more has poor predictive value. Increased risk of hyperplasia or cancer requires pathologic tissue sample to confirm. Thickness of stripe not predictive of severity of diagnosis.

Key Tests

- FSH elevated
- LH normal to elevated

Treatment

1. Natural estrogens should be used for replacement therapy because synthetic estrogens have a profound hepatic stimulatory effect.
2. Oral estrogens undergo a first pass effect through the liver that is responsible for the beneficial effects on the lipoprotein profile. Transdermal estrogens bypass this first-pass effect and are the preferred route in patients with underlying hepatic disease.
3. Estrogen can be given either unopposed or in combination with a progestin. Unopposed estrogen should be reserved for hysterectomized women because of an increased incidence of endometrial hyperplasia and cancer.
4. Progestins
   a. Medroxyprogesterone acetate (MPA): synthetic estrogen with mild androgenic effects; most common progestin prescribed
      (1) Diminishes the estrogen-associated increase in HDL slightly.
      (2) No change in the estrogen-associated LDL and fibrinogen decrease.
   b. Micronized progesterone: natural progestin from soy and yam products. Produces excellent blood levels without the usual progestin side effects.
      (1) Increases HDL levels in combination with estrogen better than MPA.
      (2) Dose conversion: 5 mg MPA = 100 mg micronized progesterone.

Medication

See Table 121–1 for recommended dosages.

1. *Unopposed estrogen* is given on a continuous basis to hysterectomized women.
2. *Combination therapy* can be given either cyclically or continuously.
   a. *Cyclic therapy:* Results in the resumption of regular menses.
      (1) Traditional method: estrogen days 1 to 25, progesterone days 12 or 14 to 25. Results in resumption of symptoms for the 5 days off estrogen.
      (2) Current method: estrogen continuously, progesterone days 1 to 14
   b. *Continuous therapy:* Estrogen and progesterone given daily. Often results in irregular spotting for several months before the onset of amenorrhea. If the spotting is troublesome, the progesterone dose can be temporarily increased to achieve amenorrhea sooner.
3. *Progestin-only therapy* may be necessary in patients unable to take estrogens because of contraindications. Progestins can relieve vasomotor symptoms and are beneficial in maintenance of bone mass. Clonidine, 0.05 to 0.2 mg twice a day, is also beneficial.
4. Selective estrogen receptor modulators (raloxifene)
   a. Tissue-specific estrogens with estrogen and antiestrogen effects.
   b. Designed to preserve the beneficial effects of estrogens and to avoid the undesired effects on the reproductive organs.
   c. Acts positively on the bone to increase bone mineral density, although not as well as estrogens. Effect in preventing fractures is unknown.
   d. Cardiovascular effects include lowering total and LDL cholesterol and inhibition of LDL oxidation. HDL cholesterol and triglycerides are not affected. Effect on prevention of cardiovascular events requires further study.
   e. No stimulatory effect on the endometrium, thus can be administered without a progestin.
   f. Antagonistic effect on the breast, with preliminary results demonstrating a decrease in the risk of breast cancer.
   g. Not effective treatment for hot flashes. Hot flashes occur slightly more often in raloxifene-treated patients.

TABLE 121–1. ESTROGEN AND PROGESTERONE DOSAGES IN THE MENOPAUSE

CYCLIC		CONTINUOUS	PROGESTERONE ONLY
Estrogens	Progesterones		
Conjugated equine estrogen (CEE), 0.625 mg, estrone sulfate, 0.625 mg, estradiol, 1.0 mg, or transdermal estradiol, 0.05 mg days 1–25 or continuously	Medroxyprogesterone acetate (MPA), 5–10 mg, or micronized progesterone, 100–200 mg, for 14 days each month	CEE, 0.625 mg, estradiol, 1.0 mg, or transdermal estradiol, 0.05 mg *and* MPA, 2.5–5.0 mg, or micronized progesterone, 50–100 mg, daily	MPA, 20 mg daily, or depot MPA, 100 mg monthly

h. Excellent choice for patients needing prophylaxis against osteoporosis who are unable to tolerate estrogens because of side effects or specific contraindications.

i. Recommended for the prevention of osteoporosis, not the treatment of established disease.

Diet

1. *Calcium:* In order to maintain zero calcium balance, women on estrogen require 1000 mg/day of calcium. The average American diet contains 500 mg/day. Untreated women require 1500 mg/day. Calcium alone or in combination with exercise will *not* prevent osteoporosis.

2. Dietary calcium is better than supplemental calcium.
   a. Eight ounces of milk or yogurt = 300 mg calcium.
   b. Calcium citrate or calcium carbonate most bioavailable supplements.
   c. Test for bioavailability of supplemental calcium tablets: tablets should dissolve in vinegar within 30 minutes to be bioavailable.

3. Phytoestrogens: naturally occurring chemicals derived from plants with a structure similar to estrogens
   a. Found in soy products, cashews, peanuts, almonds, oats, corn, wheat, apples, and other high-fiber, whole-grain products in the form of isoflavones and lignans.
   b. Block the effects of excess estrogen stimulation on the breasts and uterus and may have a protective action.
   c. Asian women with a traditional high-soy, low-fat diet complain of minimal menopausal symptoms and have a lower rate of endometrial cancer.
   d. There is a lower incidence of breast and prostate tumors found in Asian populations whose soy-based diet contains high amounts of phytoestrogens.
   e. May have cardiovascular benefits as well.

Activity

Aerobic weight-bearing exercise should be done three to five times a week to benefit bone mineral density, improve balance, and reduce the number of falls.

Patient Education

1. Performance of breast self-examination every month.
2. Importance of regular mammograms
3. Importance of reporting any abnormal vaginal bleeding

4. Prior to the initiation of therapy, the patient should be well informed regarding the potential benefits and risks of therapy in order to make an informed choice regarding initiation of treatment.

Risks of Estrogen Replacement Therapy (ERT)

1. Endometrial cancer
   a. A four- to eightfold increase in the risk of developing endometrial cancer in users of unopposed therapy. Cancers that do develop are well differentiated and treatable.
   b. Increased risk persists for 5 to 10 years after discontinuing therapy.
   c. Addition of a progestin results in a significant reduction but does not eliminate the risk for endometrial cancer.

2. Breast cancer
   a. No conclusive evidence has demonstrated an *overall* increased risk; however, the risk may be increased with duration of use.
   b. Possible 30 per cent increased risk with estrogen use of more than 5 years based on some observational studies.
   c. Increased dosages of estrogen and parenteral or pellet forms may have an increased risk.
   d. Cancers in women who have used ERT are less advanced clinically than those in never-users; probably related to more frequent mammograms and clinical breast examinations.

3. Thromboembolic disease
   a. Three recent observational studies suggested a two- to threefold increased risk of deep venous thrombosis and pulmonary embolism, with the risk being confined to current short-term users.
   b. The incidence of idiopathic venous thromboembolism in the menopausal/postmenopausal age group is approximately 1 per 10,000 women per year. Thus the incidence may be increased to 3 per 10,000 women per year, a minimal increase.
   c. Biologic evidence argues against an increased thrombotic tendency with estrogen based on its effect on reducing plasminogen activator inhibitor and fibrinogen levels.

4. Hypertension
   a. Previously believed to be a problem; however, multiple studies have shown no significant difference in mean systolic or diastolic blood pressure (BP) with ERT.
   b. Idiosyncratic response with elevated BP may occur in 5 to 7 per cent of patients receiving conjugated equine estrogens. Changing to an

alternative preparation corrects the hypertension.

5. Headaches/migraines
   a. Estrogen may potentiate pre-existing headache or migraine syndromes.
   b. Changing preparations often results in improvement of symptoms.

Contraindications to Estrogens

1. Absolute
   a. Pregnancy
   b. Undiagnosed uterine bleeding
   c. Active thromboembolic disease
   d. Acute severe liver disease
2. Relative
   a. Personal history of estrogen-dependent tumor
   b. History of recurrent thromboembolic disease
   c. Chronic liver disease

Key Treatment

- Natural estrogens
- Natural progesterone or low-androgenic synthetic progestin
- Calcium, 1000 to 1500 mg/day
- Regular weight-bearing exercise

Follow-Up

1. Encourage patients to perform monthly breast self-examination.
2. Regular mammograms per recommended guidelines based on age and family history
3. Regular clinical breast examinations every 6 to 12 months
4. Endometrial biopsy if any abnormal bleeding on ERT

 ## Bibliography

Beresford S, Weiss NS, Voigt LF, et al: Risk of endometrial cancer in relation to use of oestrogen combined with cyclic progestagen therapy in postmenopausal women. Lancet 1997;349:458–461.

Daly E, Vessey MP, Hawkins MM, et al: Risk of venous thromboembolism in users of hormone replacement therapy. Lancet 1996;348:977–980.

Hulley S, Grady D, Bush T, et al: Randomized trial of estrogen plus progestin for secondary prevention of coronary heart disease in postmenopausal women. JAMA 1998;280:605–613.

Ingram D, Sanders K, Kolybaba M, et al: Case-control study of phytoestrogens and breast cancer. Lancet 1997;350:990–994.

Koh KK, Mincemoyer R, Bui MN, et al: Effects of hormone replacement therapy on fibrinolysis in postmenopausal women. N Engl J Med 1997;336:683–690.

Sidney S, Petitti DB, Quesenberry CP: Myocardial infarction and the use of estrogen and estrogen progestagen in postmenopausal women. Ann Intern Med 1997;127:501–508.

122 Ectopic Pregnancy

Robert J. Carr

Etiology

1. Definition: the implantation of a fertilized egg outside the uterine cavity
2. Incidence
   a. Two per cent of pregnancies in the United States
   b. Accounts for 9 to 13 per cent of all pregnancy-related deaths.
   c. Sixfold increase in the last 20 years largely as a result of increased prevalence of sexually transmitted diseases, frequency of sterilization procedures, delayed childbearing, and more successful clinical detection
3. Risk factors
   a. *High risk*: fallopian tube surgery, sterilization, previous ectopic pregnancy, diethylstilbestrol exposure in utero, intrauterine device use, and documented tubal pathology
   b. *Moderate risk*: infertility, previous genital infections, multiple sexual partners
   c. *Slight risk*: previous pelvic/abdominal surgery, cigarette smoking, vaginal douching, less than 18 years at first intercourse
   d. More than 50 per cent of patients with ectopics have no identified risk factors.
4. Location of ectopic implantation
   a. Fallopian tube (97 per cent)
   b. Abdomen, cervix, ovary (3 per cent)

Symptoms

Nonspecific and often misdiagnosed on initial presentation

1. Abdominal pain and amenorrhea are most common.
2. Vaginal bleeding (40 to 50 per cent)
3. Pregnancy-associated symptoms (nausea, vomiting, breast tenderness, fatigue)

Key Symptoms

- Abdominal pain with amenorrhea
- Vaginal bleeding (40 to 50 per cent)
- Pregnancy-associated symptoms

Clinical Findings

Also nonspecific and easily confused with other entities

1. Abdominal tenderness in about 75 per cent (with or without rebound)
2. Cervical motion tenderness in about 67 per cent
3. Palpable adnexal mass in only about 50 per cent
4. Hemodynamic compromise (orthostasis, hypotension, shock) in 20 per cent

Key Signs

- Abdominal tenderness
- Cervical motion tenderness
- Adnexal mass
- Hemodynamic compromise

Laboratory Tests

1. Hormonal tests
   a. *Quantitative β-human chorionic gonadotropin (β-hCG)*: produced by trophoblastic cells
      (1) Rises exponentially for first 38 days after ovulation.
      (2) Doubling time in normal early pregnancy ranges from 1.5 to 3.5 days
      (3) Doubling time is prolonged in both ectopics and abnormal intrauterine pregnancies (IUPs) as a result of impaired β-hCG production.
      (4) Less than 66 per cent increase in 48 hours represents ectopics or IUPs that are likely to abort.
   b. *Serum progesterone*: produced by corpus luteum
      (1) Significantly decreased in ectopic gestation compared to IUP
      (2) Not gestational age dependent
      (3) Less than 5 ng/ml is not compatible with normal pregnancy.
      (4) Greater than 25 ng/ml excludes an ectopic pregnancy with 98 per cent sensitivity.

2. Ultrasound
   a. Presumptive diagnosis through exclusion of an IUP in patients with a positive β-hCG
   b. Positive diagnosis by identification of an extrauterine fetus
   c. Transabdominal ultrasound
      (1) Can detect gestational sac of normal IUP when β-hCG level is 6000 to 6500 mIU/ml (discriminatory zone).
      (2) Most useful for presumptive diagnosis
   d. Transvaginal ultrasound
      (1) Can detect gestational sac of normal IUP when β-hCG level is 1500 to 2000 mIU/ml (discriminatory zone).
      (2) Allows earlier presumptive diagnosis (within 1 week of missed menses), as well as increased potential for direct visualization of extrauterine gestations.
3. Uterine curettage
   a. Useful when β-hCG is below discriminatory zone
   b. Differentiates ectopic pregnancy from abnormal intrauterine gestation (incomplete abortion).
   c. Indicated only when nonviable pregnancy has been documented by
      (1) Serum progesterone of 5 ng/ml or less, *or*
      (2) Absence of a rise in β-hCG after 2 days
   d. Diagnosis of a completed abortion is made after curettage by
      (1) Presence of chorionic villi in the curettage sample, *or*
      (2) Decrease in the β-hCG by 15 per cent or more 8 to 12 hours postprocedure
      If neither of these is present, a presumptive diagnosis of ectopic pregnancy can be made.
4. Culdocentesis
   a. Aspiration of nonclotted blood from the peritoneal cul-de-sac
   b. Less sensitive and specific than hormonal and ultrasonographic methods
   c. Use has largely been supplanted by the other methods listed above.

Key Tests

- Hormonal
  - Quantitative β-hCG
  - Serum progesterone
- Transvaginal ultrasound
- Uterine curettage if β-hCG is below discriminatory zone

Differential Diagnosis

Nonspecific symptoms are often confused with other pregnancy-related, gastrointestinal, or gynecologic causes of abdominal pain.

1. Pregnancy-related
   a. Threatened or incomplete abortion
   b. Normal pregnancy
2. Gastrointestinal
   a. Acute gastroenteritis
   b. Appendicitis/acute abdomen
   c. Inflammatory and infectious bowel diseases
3. Gynecologic
   a. Ovarian cyst
   b. Uterine fibroids
   c. Pelvic inflammatory disease

Treatment

Goal for most patients is to remove the ectopic pregnancy while preserving reproductive function.

Surgery

1. Treatment of choice in cases of rupture, hypotension, anemia, large ectopics (diameter >4 cm), or pain longer than 24 hours
   a. *Laparoscopic salpingostomy*: lowest cost, blood loss, and anesthesia requirements; shorter postoperative recovery
   b. *Laparotomy*: for hemodynamically unstable patients or when laparoscopic approach is technically too difficult
   c. *Salpingectomy*: in cases of uncontrollable hemorrhage, significant anatomic distortion, or recurrent ectopic pregnancy in the same tube, or if future pregnancies are not desired
2. Complications
   a. Persistence of viable trophoblastic tissue in tube (5 to 20 per cent)
   b. Secondary implantation of displaced trophoblast (rare)

Medication

1. Alternative to surgery for patients with smaller ectopics (<3 to 4 cm), stable or rising β-hCG levels, and no evidence of rupture
2. Treatment of choice when surgery is contraindicated
3. *Methotrexate*: folic acid antagonist
   a. Two regimens in common use:
      (1) *Variable dose*: 1 mg/kg IM given on al-

ternate days with leucovorin calcium (0.1 mg/kg) until the β-hCG demonstrates a fall of more than 15 per cent in 48 hours

(2) *Single dose*: 50 mg/m² IM with repeated dose if β-hCG on day 7 is greater than or equal to that on day 4; higher risk of persistent trophoblastic tissue

b. Side effects: transient pelvic pain at time of tubal abortion (3 to 7 days). Bone-marrow suppression, hepatotoxicity, stomatitis, pulmonary fibrosis, alopecia, and photosensitivity are unusual in short courses. Persistent trophoblastic tissue occurs in 4 to 8 per cent.

c. Contraindications: active hepatic, renal, or peptic ulcer disease; fetal cardiac activity; neutropenia; thrombocytopenia

Key Treatment

Surgery

- Laparoscopic salpingostomy

- Laparotomy/salpingectomy

Medical

- Methotrexate

Follow-Up

1. Surgical management
   a. Weekly postoperative β-hCGs until nonpregnant levels are achieved
   b. No intercourse, pelvic or transvaginal examinations until resolved

2. Medical management
   a. Weekly β-hCGs until nonpregnant levels are achieved
   b. No intercourse, pelvic or transvaginal examinations until resolved
   c. Avoid gas-producing foods (e.g., beans, cabbage).
   d. Avoid nonsteroidal anti-inflammatory drugs, penicillin, alcohol, and vitamins containing folic acid.
   e. Avoid sun exposure.

Bibliography

American College of Obstetricians and Gynecologists: Ectopic Pregnancy (Technical Bulletin no. 150). Washington, DC, American College of Obstetricians and Gynecologists, 1990.

Emerson DS, McCord ML: Clinician's approach to ectopic pregnancy. Clin Obstet Gynecol 1996;39:199–222.

Fylstra DL: Tubal pregnancy: a review of current diagnosis and treatment. Obstet Gynecol Surv 1998;53:320–328.

Pisarska MD, Carson SA, Buster JE: Ectopic pregnancy. Lancet 1998;351:1115–1120.

Simpson JL: Fetal wastage. In Gabbe SG (ed): Obstetrics: Normal and Problem Pregnancies, pp 732–735. New York, Churchill Livingstone, 1996.

123 Premenstrual Syndrome

Janet C. Lindemann

Etiology

1. "Premenstrual syndrome" (PMS) is the cyclic recurrence of a group of symptoms that peak premenstrually and disappear postmenstrually.
2. Although no cause has been clearly substantiated, PMS seems to be related to the interaction between hormonal events and neurotransmitter function, specifically serotonin.

Symptoms

1. Multiple and diverse symptoms including but not limited to
   a. Somatic (mastalgia, bloating, headache, pelvic pain, fatigue)
   b. Mood (irritability, depression, mood swings)
   c. Cognitive (poor concentration, confusion)
   d. Behavioral (social withdrawal, impulsiveness, appetite changes)
2. "Premenstrual dysphoric disorder" (PMDD), as defined in the *Diagnostic and Statistical Manual of Mental Disorders, Fourth Edition* (DSM-IV), requires the presence premenstrually of at least five symptoms (one of which must be mood-related), marked interference with social or occupational functioning, and must not be an exacerbation of an existing disorder.
3. The cyclic premenstrual timing of the symptoms is key. The patient's pattern is repetitive and demonstrates a peak of symptom severity immediately prior to menses and a symptom-free interval following menses.

Key Symptom

Cyclic recurrence of multiple symptoms premenstrually

Clinical Findings

There are no characteristic physical signs for PMS, but a complete physical examination should be performed to rule out other illnesses.

Laboratory Tests

1. The symptom diary is the essential test for PMS and should be kept prospectively for a minimum of 3 months (Fig. 123–1).

Month:	Jan.	Feb.	March		
1					
2					
3					
4					
5					
6		h			
7					
8					
9					
10					
11					
12					
13			H d		
14			H D		
15			H D		
16		D	H D		
17		H d	M d		
18	d	H D	M		
19	H d	H D	M		
20	D	M	M		
21	M D	M	M		
22	M D	M			
23	M h	M			
24	M				
25	M				
26	M				
27	M				
28					
29					
30					
31					

Key: M = menstruation

symbol	symptom
H	headache
D	depressive symptoms

Use capital letters for severe symptoms and small letters for mild symptoms.

Figure 123–1 Symptom diary. (From Lindemann JC: Premenstrual syndrome: a practical approach. Wis Med J 1984;83:30–32, with permission.)

2. No other laboratory tests are useful except to rule out other causes.

Key Test

A symptom diary is the key test for PMS.

Differential Diagnosis
1. Primary affective disorder
   a. Anxiety or depressive neuroses may have related physical symptoms and premenstrual exacerbation.
   b. Absence of symptoms will not be present postmenstrually.
2. Dysmenorrhea:
   a. Physical symptoms of pelvic cramping may begin premenstrually but peak during menses.
   b. Pelvic pain is rarely a symptom of PMS.
3. Menstrual migraine
   a. Vascular headache symptom complex with exacerbation premenstrually.
   b. Probably a separate disorder and responsive to migraine therapy.

Treatment

Medication
1. Selective serotonin reuptake inhibitor antidepressants, including fluoxetine (Prozac), 20 mg daily, sertraline (Zoloft), 50 to 150 mg daily, or paroxetine (Paxil), 20 mg daily, have been shown to significantly reduce PMS symptoms when used throughout the cycle.
2. The anxiolytic alprazolam (Xanax), 0.25 mg tid to qid, may be used effectively during the luteal phase only.
3. Gonadotropin-releasing hormone agonists, such as leuprolide (Lupron), eliminate ovulation and hormone production with limited effect on PMS symptoms.
4. Spironolactone (Aldactone), 25 mg qid, is effective for bloating symptoms.
5. Progesterone (oral or suppository), vitamins, and herbal and mineral preparations are of little benefit.

Diet
1. Patients should be encouraged to eat small, frequent meals that are high in complex carbohydrates to avoid sharp fluctuations in blood glucose concentrations.
2. Limit salt and caffeine.

Activity
Regular moderate exercise has been shown to be effective in alleviating symptoms.

Patient Education
1. Because patients may have preconceived notions about PMS from the lay media, it is essential to provide information based on medical studies.
2. The education that results from maintaining the symptom diary often reduces anxiety and other symptoms.

Key Treatment

SSRI antidepressant

Follow-Up
1. Initially, the patient needs to be seen every 3 months to make the diagnosis and monitor treatment.
2. Establish realistic expectations for symptom improvement.

Bibliography

For more information on diagnosis, see
Barnhart KT, et al: A clinician's guide to the premenstrual syndrome. Med Clin North Am 1995;79:1457–1472.
Campbell EM, et al: Premenstrual symptoms in general practice patients: prevalence and treatment. J Reprod Med 1997;42:637–646.

For more information on treatment, see
Freeman EW: Premenstrual syndrome: current perspectives on treatment and etiology. Curr Opin Obstet Gynecol 1997;9:147–153.
Freeman EW, et al: A double-blind trial of oral progesterone, alprazolam, and placebo in treatment of severe premenstrual syndrome. JAMA 1995;274:51–57.
Steiner M, et al: Fluoxetine in the treatment of premenstrual dysphoria. N Engl J Med 1995;332:1529–1534.

124 Contraception

Robert J. Woolley

Selecting a Contraceptive Method

1. The first consideration is permanent versus reversible contraception. If permanent contraception is desired, sterilization of either partner is the method of choice, if cost is not prohibitive.

2. If reversibility is desired, level of contraceptive efficacy is the next consideration. The couple must decide what degree of risk of failure their life situation can tolerate. Reversible contraception can be broadly grouped into high, medium, and low effectiveness.

    a. *High effectiveness*: Norplant, depot medroxyprogesterone acetate (DMPA), intrauterine device (IUD), progestin-only oral contraceptives (OCs), and combined oral contraceptives (COCs)

    b. *Medium effectiveness*: condoms, female condoms, cervical cap, diaphragm, and spermicides. (Appropriately selected combinations of these should be able to achieve effectiveness equivalent to the first category.)

    c. *Low effectiveness*: periodic abstinence, coitus interruptus. These can be recommended only in the very unusual circumstances in which all other methods are unacceptable to the couple; these will not be discussed further in this chapter.

3. Engage the patient in an honest evaluation of her ability to be consistently compliant with daily pill use or coitus-dependent actions (barrier methods). If this cannot be ensured, a long-acting method is to be strongly preferred.

4. Prepare for the patient a list of options in order of your customized recommendations for her, based on the preceding considerations. Discuss relative advantages, disadvantages, and costs, leaving the final decision to the patient. If condoms are not to be the primary contraceptive method, their use should be advised in addition to the primary method for any couple at risk of sexually transmitted disease (STD) transmission.

Male Sterilization

1. *Advantages*: Permanent, highly effective, no user action needed after azoospermia verified.

2. *Disadvantages*: Reversal expensive and inconsistently successful.

3. *Short-term complications*: less than 2 per cent incidence of infection, hematoma, sperm granuloma, and congestive epididymitis

4. *Long-term complications*: Possible consequences in essentially every organ system, especially cardiovascular disease, have been postulated, but none confirmed. Recent studies appear to show an increased lifetime risk of prostate cancer, but no plausible explanatory biological mechanism is available. At present, consensus is that this possibility need not deter patients from vasectomy.

5. *Failures*: Most are due to recanalization, usually within 6 weeks. This can be detected by semen analysis 6 to 10 weeks after procedure.

Female Sterilization

1. *Advantages*: Permanent, highly effective, no user action needed after procedure.

2. *Disadvantages*: Compared with male sterilization, cost, invasiveness, complications, and failure rate are all higher. Reversal is expensive and inconsistently successful. May leave visible scars.

3. *Short-term complications*: Occasional bleeding, infection

4. *Long-term complications*: When failure occurs, relative risk of ectopic pregnancy is increased. Hormonal and menstrual pattern changes have been reported, but a causal relationship has not been established.

Intrauterine Device

Note: This section describes the Copper-T 380A (Paragard) IUD. A progesterone-releasing IUD (Progestasert) is also available but is generally reserved for patients experiencing menorrhagia and will not be discussed herein.

1. *Mechanism*: Exact mechanism is uncertain, but primarily prevents fertilization, probably by immobilization of sperm by copper, as well as nonspecific foreign body reaction.

2. *Effectiveness*: 0.8 per cent typical first-year failure rate; 78 per cent 1-year continuation rate

3. *Advantages*: High effectiveness. No user action is required after insertion (although patient should check position monthly). Longest dura-

tion (10 years) and lowest annualized cost of any reversible contraception

4. *Disadvantages*: appropriate only for parous women in stable, monogamous relationships

5. *Risks*: Insertion occasionally causes uterine infection or perforation. STDs more likely to result in pelvic inflammatory disease (PID) with IUD in place. In case of failure, risk of ectopic pregnancy is increased, and risk of spontaneous abortion is 25 to 50 per cent.

6. *Side effects*: Increased menstrual bleeding and cramping, usually well tolerated; cause for removal in 10 to 15 per cent of patients. Intermenstrual bleeding is common in first few months.

7. *Contraindications*: nulliparity, risk for acquiring STD, uterine malformations or cancer, undiagnosed unusual vaginal bleeding.

8. *Insertion and removal*: See Procedure following this chapter.

Levonorgestrel Implants (Norplant)

1. *Mechanism*: Six subdermal 34-mm flexible Silastic capsules release levonorgestrel over 5 years. Levonorgestrel causes genital tract changes typical of the luteal phase: increased thickness of cervical mucus, decreased uterine tube motility, disorganized endometrium. Ovulation is only inconsistently suppressed.

2. *Effectiveness*: 0.9 per cent first-year failure with both typical and perfect use. One-year continuation rate is 85 per cent (highest of any reversible method). Body weight greater than 70 kg decreases effectiveness, estimated at a cumulative pregnancy risk of 7 per cent over 5 years. This is still better use-effectiveness than OCs or any barrier method and should not be considered a contraindication to use of Norplant.

3. *Advantages*: High effectiveness, long duration, high continuation rate, no user action needed after insertion.

4. *Disadvantages*: Frequent menstrual changes, high initial cost (although, if amortized over 3 or more years, comparable to OCs), requires minor surgical procedure to insert and remove.

5. *Risks*: No tumorigenic effect known or suspected. No known adverse effect on fetus in case of failure. No known adverse effect in infant if used during breast-feeding. Relative risk of ectopic pregnancy, in case of failure, may be increased. No permanent effect on fertility; serum levels are undetectable within 48 hours of removal. Minimal or no adverse effect on blood

pressure, carbohydrate metabolism, liver function tests, coagulation, or blood lipids.

6. *Side effects*

   a. Sixty per cent of women have significant changes in menstrual patterns. Bleeding may occur daily for first 6 to 9 months of use. Patient must be explicitly warned about this, because it is the leading cause of patient dissatisfaction. After this interval, irregular menses remain the rule, although the total amount of bleeding per year is about the same as without hormones. Many women regain a fairly regular pattern in third or fourth year, but this cannot be ensured.

   b. Headaches, mechanism unknown: If not relieved by standard analgesics, a common cause for Norplant removal.

   c. Weight gain or loss: Neither is clearly a direct effect of the hormone.

   d. Mastalgia, galactorrhea: More common when insertion occurs during lactation. Usually transitory; no treatment needed.

   e. Acne: Worst in first year. Treat in standard manner. (Antibiotics are not contraindicated.)

   f. Other: ovarian cysts, hirsutism, scalp hair loss, cervicitis, vaginitis, dizziness, abdominal pain, musculoskeletal pain, insertion-site pain or pigmentation. All are usually self-limited or, if severe or prolonged, treated by removal of the Norplant.

   g. *Prediction of side effects*: A 1- to 6-month trial of norgestrel progestin-only pills (Ovrette) may predict tolerance of Norplant side effects, but this theory has not been formally tested.

7. *Contraindications*: active thrombotic disease (although probably not worsened by Norplant), undiagnosed abnormal vaginal bleeding, active liver disease, current breast or genital tract cancer

8. *Drug interactions*: phenytoin and carbamazepine significantly reduce effectiveness of Norplant; their use should be considered a contraindication.

9. *Insertion and removal*: See Procedure following this chapter.

Depot Medroxyprogesterone Acetate (Depo-Provera)

1. *Mechanism*: Primary means of action is inhibition of ovulation by suppression of pituitary secretion of luteinizing hormone and follicle-stimulating hormone. DMPA also causes genital tract changes typical of the secretory phase

(e.g., thickened cervical mucus, decreased uterine tube motility).

2. *Effectiveness*: 0.3 per cent first-year failure rate with both typical and perfect use; 70 per cent first-year continuation rate

3. *Advantages*: High effectiveness. No user action is needed between injections. Use is undetectable to partner (a feature unique to this method). Can be given immediately postpartum; does not interfere with lactation. Probably protective against ovarian and endometrial cancer. Increases hemoglobin concentration. Inhibits sickling in sickle cell anemia.

4. *Disadvantages*: Return of fertility after last injection is variable: 50 per cent at 6 months, 75 per cent at 12 months, 85 per cent at 18 months, 95 per cent at 24 months. (Remainder have other causes of infertility.)

5. *Risks*: No known teratogenicity. No known carcinogenicity. Relative risk of ectopic pregnancy is increased in case of failure. Possible slight decrease in bone density with long-term use, although, if true, presumably reversible upon cessation of use. No adverse effects on glucose, lipids, or blood pressure.

6. *Side effects*: Menstrual irregularity is nearly universal; continued use usually leads to amenorrhea. About 1 in 200 women will require treatment for very heavy or prolonged bleeding; one COC pill (50 or 35 μg estrogen) daily for 14 days is usually adequate. Injection soon after childbirth usually causes prolonged (weeks), but not severe, postpartum bleeding. Weight gain of about 1 to 3 kg is common, but 20 to 40 per cent of patients lose weight. Premenstrual syndrome–like symptoms are common with first injection but resolve spontaneously and are less severe with subsequent shots.

7. *Contraindications*: none

8. *Drug interactions*: no known interaction with antibiotics or anticonvulsants

9. *Administration*: 150 mg injected deep intramuscularly (deltoid or gluteus). Peak serum levels occur within 24 hours. Plateau levels are maintained about 3 months, with gradual declines thereafter. First injection is ideally given in first 7 days of menstrual cycle, but it can be given at any time that the absence of pregnancy can be ensured. Subsequent doses are given every 3 months. A patient presenting up to 2 weeks beyond the scheduled date can be given her shot without fear of pregnancy.

Combined Oral Contraceptives

1. *Mechanism*: Primarily suppress ovulation by inhibition of gonadotropins. Secondarily, the progestin component produces genital tract changes of the luteal phase.

2. *Effectiveness*: 0.1 per cent first-year failure rate with perfect use; 3 per cent with typical use. One-year continuation rate is 72 per cent.

3. *Advantages*: Highly effective with proper use. Causes decreased rates of benign breast disease, endometriosis, dysmenorrhea, anemia, premenstrual syndrome, and ovarian and endometrial cancers. Can be used to treat benign menstrual irregularities, endometriosis, acne, and polycystic ovarian disease. Mild protective effect against PID

4. *Disadvantages*: Effectiveness is dependent on consistent daily use, which is difficult for many users, especially adolescents.

5. *Risks*

   a. Small adverse effect on lipid profile, but probably not atherogenic.

   b. Rare thrombotic effects (deep vein thrombosis, stroke, myocardial infarction). This is essentially limited to smokers and those with pre-existing (although often unknown) hypercoagulable state. In smokers over age 35, risk of death from this cause exceeds risk of death from accidental pregnancy, contraindicating COCs.

   c. Between 1 and 5 per cent of women develop hypertension, reversible with cessation of use. Previously controlled hypertension may worsen, but a trial of COCs may be attempted.

   d. *Reproductive system*: Relative risk of ectopic pregnancy is increased in case of failure. Possibly a slight (3 per cent) increase in lifetime risk of cervical cancer. Breast cancer risk probably not increased by COCs. Conflicting evidence on whether tricyclic preparations increase risk of functional ovarian cysts.

   e. *Hepatobiliary system*: Increased incidence of gallstones. Relative risks of hepatic adenoma and hepatocellular carcinoma are increased, but absolute risk is negligible.

   f. *Teratogenicity*: Several effects postulated, none confirmed.

   g. *Use during lactation*: No adverse effect on infant but may decrease quantity and quality of milk produced; progestin-only methods are preferred.

6. *Side effects*

   a. *Systemic*: Symptoms similar to early pregnancy (nausea, fluid retention, breast tenderness) may occur during first two to three cycles. Some women report libido changes, mood changes, and frank depression. Increased appetite may lead to weight gain, although weight loss is just as common.

b. *Reproductive tract*: Breakthrough bleeding common in first three cycles. Menstrual bleeding is often scant. Amenorrhea may occur occasionally; if for two or more consecutive cycles, test for pregnancy, and then consider change of COC formulation.

c. *Neurologic*: New onset of migrane with pill use requires discontinuation. Pre-existing common migranes are not necessarily a contraindication.

d. *Dermatologic*: Oily skin and exacerbation of acne are reported frequently, but most women show improvement in acne. Melasma and significant hair loss occur rarely.

7. *Contraindications*

a. *Absolute*: current or past thrombotic disease, cerebrovascular accident, coronary artery disease, breast cancer, genital tract cancer, or liver cancer; current pregnancy or impaired liver function

b. *Relative*: smoker over age 35, diabetes, undiagnosed abnormal vaginal bleeding, lactation

8. *Drug interactions*

a. *Antibiotics*: Rifampin and griseofulvin reduce contraceptive efficacy; barrier method should be added during their use. Contrary to common belief, other commonly used antibiotics do not exert any clinically significant effect on COC efficacy, and additional precautions are not needed.

b. *Anticonvulsants*: Phenytoin, carbamazepine, and barbiturates decrease COC efficacy. Alternative methods (such as DMPA) are preferred, although a 50-μg pill may be considered.

c. Other drugs whose effect may be altered by COCs and must be monitored: warfarin, thyroid hormone, corticosteroids (effect decreased); cyclosporine, tricyclic antidepressants, theophylline (effect increased)

9. *Prescribing information*

a. *Pill selection*: Clinical differences between formulations of low-dose pills (≤35 μg estrogen) are minimal. Selection can logically be made on the basis of cost (several generic formulations are available) and/or lowest total monthly hormone dose. Also, 28-day packs are to be preferred.

b. *Patient education*: Needs to emphasize consistency of use. Also include written information on when to start pills (Sunday start

seems to be easiest and most common method), side effects, missed pills, warning signs of dangerous complications.

c. *Follow-up*: If possible, give three or four sample packages, and then see patient again to check blood pressure, evaluate side effects, inquire about consistency of use. Encourage phone calls for problems or questions and have well-trained nurse to handle such calls.

Progestin-Only Pills

1. *Mechanism*: Primary mechanism is induction of genital tract changes of the luteal phase. Ovulation inconsistently suppressed.

2. *Effectiveness*: 0.5 per cent first-year failure rate with perfect use; 3 per cent with typical use. One-year continuation rate 72 per cent.

3. *Advantages*: Highly effective with consistent use. Progestin-only pills (POPs) eliminate estrogenic and thrombotic side effects and risks of COCs. Can be used immediately postpartum with no adverse effect on infant or lactation.

4. *Disadvantages*: Effectiveness dependent on consistent daily use, which is difficult for many users, especially adolescents. This is even more important with POPs than with COCs, a method more tolerant of occasional omissions.

5. *Risks*: Relative risk of ectopic pregnancy is increased in case of failure. No known carcinogenicity or teratogenicity. No thrombotic risks. Increased rate of functional ovarian cysts

6. *Side effects*: Menstrual irregularity indicates consistent or intermittent anovulation (and higher efficacy); many women continue having regular ovulatory cycles. Any of the other side effects listed for COCs may occur with POPs, but with much lower incidences.

7. *Contraindications*: undiagnosed irregular vaginal bleeding, current genital tract cancer, active liver disease

8. *Drug interactions*: None of clinical significance.

9. *Prescribing information*

a. *Pill selection*: Only two formulations are available in the United States (norethindrone 0.35 mg, norgestrel 0.075 mg); there is no compelling reason to prefer one over the other.

b. *Patient education*: Must emphasize consistency of use. Also stress that, unlike with COC, there are no monthly pill-free intervals and no placebo pills that can be ignored; pill ingestion is daily, without exception.

c. *Follow-up*: same as for COCs

Barrier Methods

1. *Male condoms*: 3 per cent first-year failure rate with perfect use; 12 per cent with typical use. Provide best protection against STDs. Recommend latex, prelubricated condoms and use of additional intravaginal spermicide (any form). During patient education, include information on consistency of use, method and timing of use, and lubrication use.

2. *Female condoms* (Reality): 5 per cent first-year failure rate with perfect use; 21 per cent with typical use. Instruct patient in consistency of use, proper insertion, and use of additional spermicide.

3. *Diaphragm*: 6 per cent first-year failure rate with perfect use; 18 per cent with typical use. Increases risk of urinary tract infections. Instruct patient in concurrent use of spermicide, timing of use, proper care of diaphragm. See Procedure following this chapter for fitting instructions.

4. *Cervical cap*: First-year failure rate 26 per cent (parous) or 9 per cent (nulliparous) with perfect use; 36 or 18 per cent, respectively, with typical use. No apparent effect on cervical dysplasia, as earlier feared. Can be left in up to 48 hours. Care is similar to that of a diaphragm. See source in Bibliography for fitting instructions.

5. *Spermicides*: 6 per cent first-year failure rate with perfect use; 21 per cent with typical use. Can be purchased without prescription in multiple forms: creams, gels, foams, suppositories, and film. All use either nonoxynol 9 (1% to 28%) or octoxynol 9 (1% to 3%), surfactants with similar properties. Instructions for proper use are different for each product. Can be combined with any other method to increase efficacy. May cause local irritation and increase risk of vaginal candidiasis.

Postcoital Contraception

1. *Oral contraceptives*: Give 2 tablets of Ovral, or 4 tablets of Lo-Ovral, Nordette, or Levlen, or 20 tablets of Ovrette as one dose; repeat 12 hours later. Initiate as soon as practicable after unprotected intercourse. Efficacy is proven with initiation as late as 72 hours after coitus, but there is no reason to withhold the prescription if the patient presents later, because it is not known how late treatment may be effective. With combined pills, nausea risk is 30 to 50 per cent; vomiting occurs in 15 to 25 per cent. Opinions are mixed as to whether a dose should be repeated if emesis occurs. Effectiveness is same but risk of nausea/vomiting much lower with the progestin-only pill (Ovrette). Either treatment reduces risk of pregnancy by about 74 per cent, to approximately 2 per cent. Older, high-dose estrogen regimens (including diethylstilbestrol) are no longer recommended.

2. *Danazol*: 600 mg as a single dose, repeated 12 hours later. Must be initiated within 72 hours of intercourse. Pregnancy risk after treatment is approximately 2.0 per cent. Side effects are similar to above but less frequent.

3. *IUD insertion*: Can be performed up to 5 days after intercourse and is the most effective available method (pregnancy rate 0.1 per cent). However, it is rare to find a woman in need of emergency postcoital contraception who is both a willing and suitable candidate for an IUD.

Bibliography

Choice of contraceptives. Med Lett 1995;37:9–12.

Contraceptives. In Drug Evaluations Subscription. Chicago, American Medical Association, Fall 1993.

Filshie M, Guillebaud J (eds): Contraception: Science and Practice. London, Butterworths, 1989.

Hatcher RA, Trussell J, Stewart F, et al: Contraceptive Technology, 17th ed. New York, Ardent Media, 1998.

Shoupe D, Haseltine FP (eds): Contraception. New York, Springer-Verlag, 1993.

Indications

1. For the prevention of pregnancy in women who are candidates for this barrier method
2. Intended for use in conjunction with appropriate spermicide
3. For patients who prefer not to use hormonal contraceptive methods and who may need some protection from sexually transmitted diseases (STDs)

Advantages

1. Simple to use and noninvasive
2. Can be used intermittently at a woman's discretion, allowing for more personal control
3. Does not require involvement of male partner
4. Reduced risk for some STDs if using spermicide
5. Not hormonal

Contraindications

1. Sensitivity or allergy to latex, natural rubber, or spermicide
2. Inability to fit because of vaginal stenosis, uterine prolapse, severe cystocele, rectocele, perineal relaxation, extreme anteversion or retroversion of the uterus
3. Inability to insert or remove diaphragm
4. History of toxic shock syndrome
5. Less than 6 weeks postpartum (or before uterus involutes)
6. History of recurrent urinary tract infections (UTIs), especially with use of diaphragm

Preparation

1. Patient selection and counseling: Assess if patient is a candidate for this method. Assess her ability and motivation for using diaphragm. Assess her risk of STDs. Discuss advantages and disadvantages including failure rate.
2. Perform complete medical and gynecologic history, including allergies.
3. Perform complete pelvic examination; note any pelvic abnormalities.
4. Demonstrate use of diaphragm to the patient with a model or illustration.

Equipment

1. Lubricating jelly
2. Examination gloves (sterile not required)
3. Written educational handouts with instructions and illustrations for patients
4. Clean set of diaphragm rings or full diaphragms for fitting: Most patients will fit sizes from 65 to 80 mm. Diaphragms are available in sizes 50 to 100 mm. Sizes increase in increments of 5 mm. Common diaphragm types:
   a. *Arcing spring*: sizes 55 to 95 mm (most commonly used in the United States). Molded natural rubber with one-piece spring and dome with firm ring. Easiest to insert. May be used in women with mild cystocele, rectocele, or retroversion of uterus. Bends in arc when the edges are pressed together.
   b. *Coil spring*: sizes 55 to 100 mm. Molded natural rubber with one-piece tension-adjusted coil spring and dome with soft flexible rim. Used for women with cervix in mid or anterior position and good pelvic support structures. May be used with an introducer. Remains in a straight line when the edges are pressed together.
   c. *Flat spring*: sizes 55 to 95 mm. Molded natural rubber one-piece spring and dome with soft rim and flat plane. Used for women with narrow pelvic shelf or nulliparous women. May be used with an introducer. Remains in a straight line when the edges are pressed together.
5. Cleaning solution for fitting rings and diaphragms and disinfectant for soaking them after each use. The manufacturer can provide more detailed instructions for this.

Precautions

1. Allergy or sensitivity to latex, natural rubber, or spermicide
2. Not all women can be fitted for a diaphragm; patient may need to return at a later date to attempt refitting.

Technique

1. Position patient in lithotomy position.
2. Measure the correct diaphragm size: Take your gloved hand, with the second and middle finger together and straight, and insert them into the patient's vagina. Touch your middle finger to the posterior fornix and then raise your hand

so that your index finger touches the pubic arch. Use your thumb to mark the point on your index finger when the pubic bone meets it.

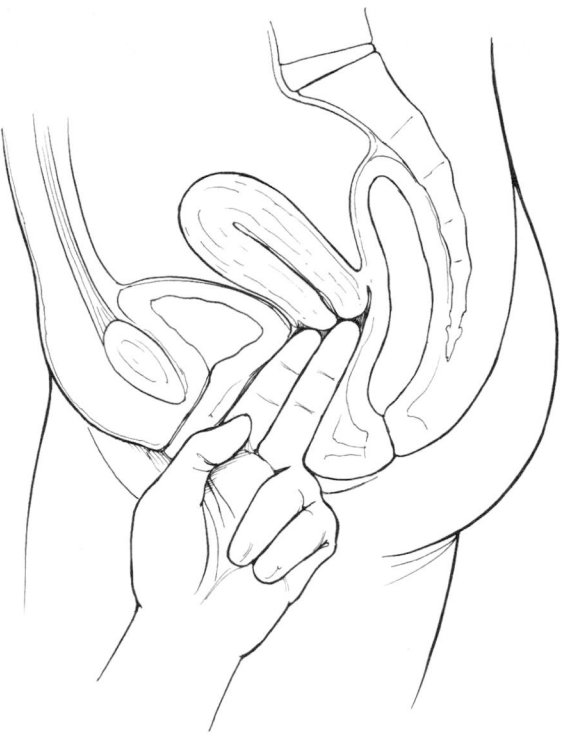

Hold your fingers in this same position while you remove them from the vagina.

3. Select the proper fitting ring/diaphragm: measure the distance between the end of your thumb on your index finger and the end of your middle finger. This should correspond to the approximate diameter of the size that fits best.

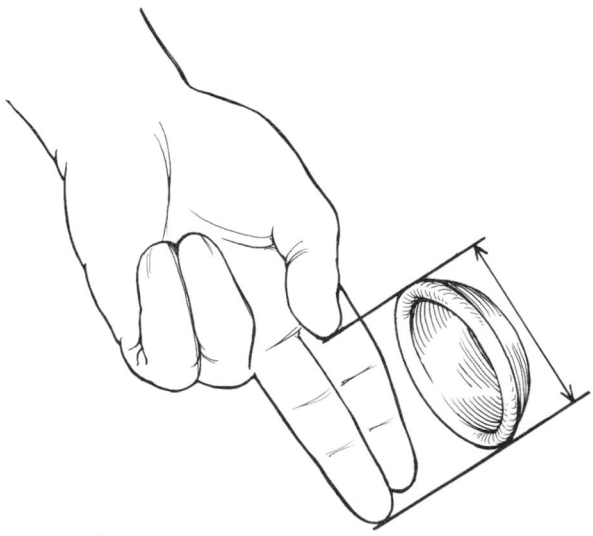

4. Insert the diaphragm: Apply lubricant liberally to the properly sized fitting ring/diaphragm rim. Pinch the edges of the ring or diaphragm rim together in half. Using your other gloved hand to hold the vulva open, insert the ring/dia-

phragm with the ring or rim facing up. Gently push the ring/diaphragm into the vagina toward the posterior fornix. Once in place, let the ring/diaphragm open and remove your fingers from the vagina.

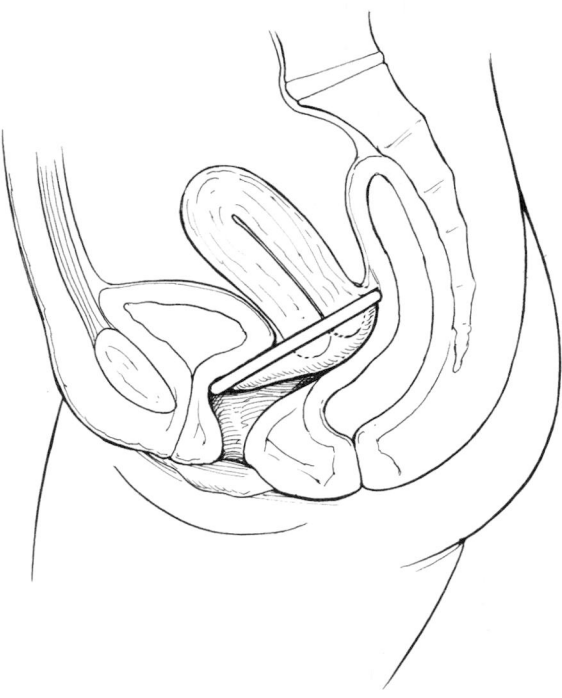

Check to be sure the ring is surrounding the cervix or the dome of the diaphragm is completely covering the cervix. Be sure the proximal ring/rim fits behind the pubic arch easily; you should be able to get just one finger width between the diaphragm and the pubic arch. If you are unable to put one finger between or the patient feels the diaphragm pressing anteriorly, try using one size smaller; if you can get more than one finger between them try one size larger.

5. Remove the fitting ring/diaphragm: Hook your index finger under the anterior edge and pull it out of the vagina.

6. Instruct the patient in the use of the diaphragm: Reinsert the diaphragm and have the patient get up and move around. She should not be able to feel the diaphragm in place. The practitioner should leave the room to allow her privacy. Have her feel the proper position of the ring around her cervix or the dome of the diaphragm covering it. Have her practice inserting the diaphragm properly and removing it. Check to be sure that she can insert it correctly.

7. Clean and disinfect the fitting rings/diaphragms. The manufacturer can supply further instructions on this.

8. Write a prescription for the spring type and proper size.

Follow-Up

1. Counseling is very important.
   a. Reinforce the instructions on use and care of the diaphragm, including the importance of correct insertion each time she has intercourse. Proper use includes putting spermicide in the dome of the diaphragm each time it is used.
   b. The diaphragm must be left in place at least 6 hours after intercourse and removed as soon after that as possible. It should not be left in longer than 24 hours to decrease chance of toxic shock syndrome, foul discharge, or vaginal ulceration.
   c. The patient should use additional vaginal spermicide if having intercourse more than once while the diaphragm is in place.
   d. Have the patient check for any deterioration or holes and refill her prescription if those occur.
2. Condoms are recommended in addition to the diaphragm if the patient is at risk for STDs.
3. The patient may have an increased risk of UTIs; prophylactic antibiotics with use may be necessary.
4. The patient should come for refitting if her weight changes more than 10 pounds or if she has a pregnancy, an abortion, or pelvic surgery.
5. Have the patient bring her diaphragm for routine visits to recheck the fit and be sure she is using it properly. Give her written handouts.
6. The practitioner or a trained health care advisor should be available by phone for any questions or problems that may arise.

Bibliography

Apgar B: Diaphragm fitting. In Pfenninger JL, Fowler GC (eds): Procedures for Primary Care Physicians, pp 750–756. St. Louis, Mosby, 1994.

Heaton CJ, Smith MA: The diaphragm. Am Fam Physician 1989;39:231–236.

Speroff L, Glass RH, Kase NG (eds): Clinical Gynecologic Endocrinology and Infertility, 6th ed, pp 997–1010. Baltimore, Williams & Wilkins, 1999.

Stewart F: Vaginal barriers. In Hatcher RA, Trussell J, Stewart F, et al (eds): Contraceptive Technology, 17th ed, pp 371–404. New York, Ardent Media, 1998.

Stifel EN, Anderson J: Contraception. In Rosenfeld JA (ed): Women's Health in Primary Care, pp 289–314. Baltimore, Williams & Wilkins, 1997.

Indications

Desire for contraception with a high level of effectiveness, easy compliance, and lack of hormonal influence

Contraindications

1. Pregnancy
2. Pelvic inflammatory disease
3. Uterine or cervical malignancy
4. Postpartum endometritis or infected abortion within the past 3 months
5. Undiagnosed vaginal bleeding
6. Polygamous sexual activity
7. History of a previous intrauterine device (IUD) that has not been removed

Preparation

1. Before insertion, the patient should give appropriate informed consent. A brochure is usually provided with the IUD that delineates the risks involved. Always review these risks and spend time answering any questions.
2. The optimal time to place an IUD is during the menses. Although this is the optimal time, it can safely be placed any day as long as the patient is not pregnant. Always check a pregnancy test and document its negativity prior to beginning the insertion.
3. Determine the patient's hemoglobin. A side effect of IUDs is increased menstrual flow. Should your patient experience this in the future, you will have a hemoglobin value established to aid in future management.
4. For added patient comfort, it helps to administer an analgesic or nonsteroidal anti-inflammatory drug (NSAID) prior to the procedure.

Equipment

1. Examination table with stirrups
2. Light source
3. Metal speculum
4. Antiseptic solution
5. Long cotton swabs
6. Uterine sound
7. IUD
8. Ring forceps
9. Scissors
10. Tenaculum

IUDs currently available in the United States are the copper-containing Tcu-380 A and the hormone-containing progesterone T. The copper IUD can stay in utero for 10 years, whereas the progesterone IUD is approved for 1 year of contraception. The Levonorgestrel (LNG 20) IUD is currently undergoing studies for use in the United States. It currently is used widely in 10 countries. It is more effective than other IUDs, its length of use is 5 years, and it is associated with less vaginal bleeding.

Anesthesia

NSAIDs are usually adequate analgesics. If stenosis is a problem or the patient is extremely uncomfortable during the procedure, a paracervical block using 1% lidocaine can be administered.

Precautions

1. If there is any suspicion that the patient may be pregnant, withhold the insertion until the next menses.
2. If an IUD has been placed in the past and not removed, do not place a new one until the old IUD is either removed or documentation exists (pelvic ultrasound or kidney-ureter-bladder film) that the old IUD is no longer in the patient (either intra- or extrauterine).
3. If the patient complains of abnormal genital bleeding, do not place an IUD until the etiology of the complaint is discovered.

Technique

1. After obtaining consent, a negative pregnancy test, and hemoglobin value, place the patient in the examination room and have her disrobe and drape from the waist down.
2. Position the patient in lithotomy position and set the table at a comfortable height. Perform a bimanual examination to determine uterine size and position.
3. Place the speculum into the vaginal vault, using the light source for adequate visualization. Once the speculum is in place, ensure the cervix is in the center of the field and the cervical os in view.

4. Cleanse the endocervix with an antiseptic solution

5. Place the tenaculum on the anterior lip of the cervix.

6. Dilate the cervical os with the uterine sound. Apply gentle pressure and forward the sound into the uterine cavity until it stops. The sound should not be forced into the uterus because this may cause a perforation. The uterine cavity should measure somewhere between 6 and 9 cm for the copper IUD and up to 10 cm for the progesterone IUD (Progestasert).

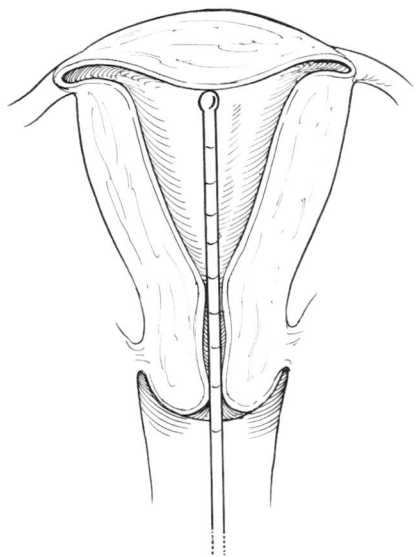

7. Prepare the IUD for insertion. This should be done in sterile conditions. Bend the arms of the copper-containing IUD downward and place them into the insertion tube. Do not bend the arms of the IUD earlier than 5 minutes prior to its insertion. If the insertion is prolonged, the arms will stay bent and not expand appropriately in the uterine cavity.

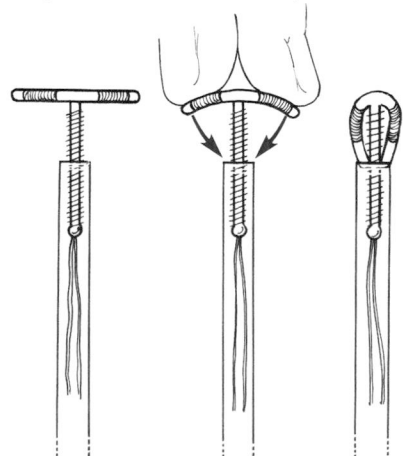

Adjust the movable flange on the outside of the insertion tube to match the distance the intrauterine cavity measured out to be with the

sound. Place the solid rod into the opposite side of the insertion tube and advance it until it touches the bottom of the IUD.

8. Introduce the loaded insertion tube through the cervical canal until the IUD comes in contact with the fundus of the uterus.

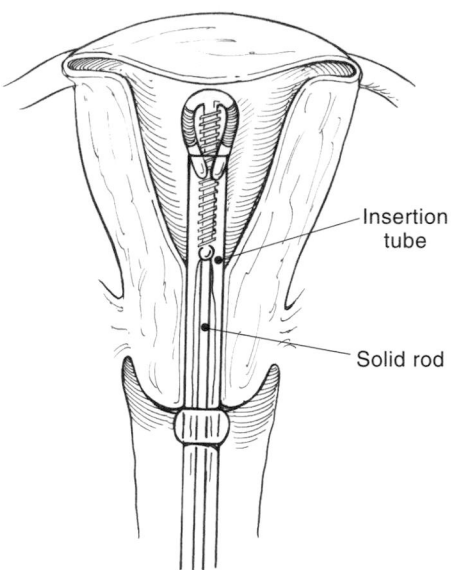

Insertion tube

Solid rod

The movable flange should now be at the cervix. Do not force the insertion.

9. To release the arms of the IUD, withdraw the insertion tube from the uterus while holding the solid rod stationary. This maneuver will release the arms.

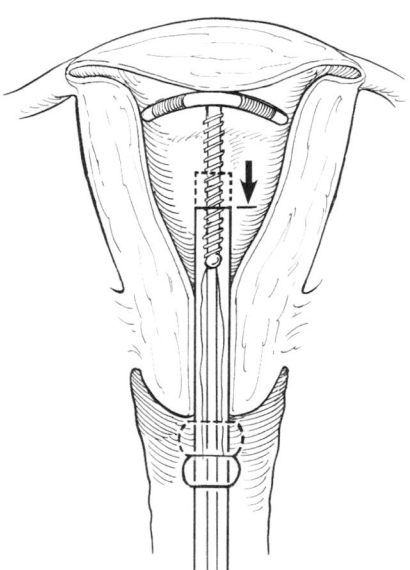

10. After the arms are released, move the insertion tube upward to push the IUD into the highest position within the uterus. This will ensure its position in the fundus.

11. Withdraw the solid rod while holding the insertion tube stationary. Now, withdraw the insertion tube.

12. Cut the threads 2.5 cm beyond the cervical os.

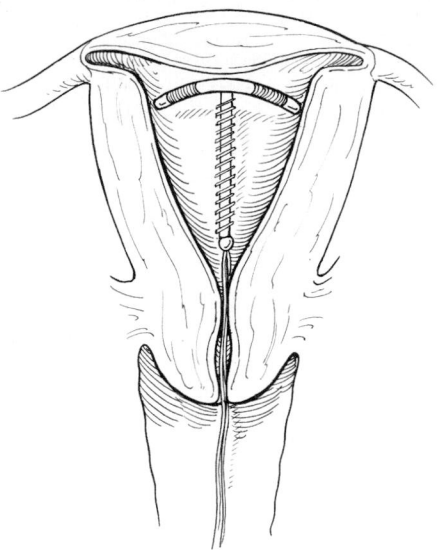

Follow-Up

1. Strings should be palpated monthly.
2. A return check-up should be scheduled after the next menses, or in 6 weeks.
3. The patient should report any missed periods.

IUD Removal

1. Place the patient in the lithotomy position.
2. Insert the speculum into the vagina and ensure the cervix is in view.
3. Locate the IUD strings protruding through the cervical os.
4. Take a ring forceps and pick up the strings.
5. Apply traction on the strings and pull the IUD out of the uterus.
6. Always show the removed IUD to the patient. This will remove any doubt from her mind whether the IUD was truly removed or not.
7. Examine the cervix for any lacerations or excessive bleeding.
8. Prescribe another form of contraception if the patient desires to continue avoiding pregnancy.

Bibliography

American College of Obstetricians and Gynecologists: The Intrauterine Device (ACOG Technical Bulletin No. 164). Washington, DC, American College of Obstetricians and Gynecologists, 1992.

Grimes DA (ed): Modern IUDs, Part 1. The Contraception Report, 1998;9(4).

Health Learning Systems: Intrauterine contraception. Little Falls, NJ, ParaGuard Speaker's Bureau, 1996.

Mishell DR Jr: Family planning. In Mishell DR Jr, Stenchever MA, Droegemueller W, et al (eds): Comprehensive Gynecology, 3rd ed, pp 330–339. St. Louis, Mosby, 1997.

World Health Organization: Mechanism of Action, Safety, and Efficacy of Intrauterine Devices (WHO Technical Report Series 753), pp 1–91. Geneva, World Health Organization, 1987.

Norplant Insertion

Procedure time of 10 to 15 minutes

Indications
1. A means of contraception for someone requiring reversibility but long-term effectiveness
2. Poorly compliant patient
3. Patient with contraindication to estrogen and therefore combined oral contraceptive

Contraindications
1. Pregnancy
2. Acute liver disease
3. Undiagnosed vaginal bleeding
4. Breast malignancy
5. Thromboembolic disorders

Preparation
1. Patient needs to sign informed consent form and needs full counseling on the risks of the procedure, the benefits, contraceptive efficacy, failure rate of 0.2 per cent, and alternative methods of contraception.

2. Patient also needs to be informed prior to insertion of the potential side effects of Norplant.

Equipment
1. A 6-ml syringe
2. A 22-gauge, 1.5-inch needle, for infiltrating anesthetic agent
3. An 18-gauge, 1-inch needle, for drawing up anesthetic agent
4. A 10-gauge, 2.75-inch trocar
5. Six Silastic Norplant implants
6. Scalpel with No. 11 blade

Anesthesia
Six milliliters of 1% lidocaine

Precautions
1. Ensure that the patient is not pregnant.
2. There may be diminished contraceptive effectiveness in patients who are taking antiseizure medications such as phenytoin or carbamazepine.

Technique: Norplant Insertion

1. Stencil a fan-like pattern on the medial surface of the arm 8 to 10 mm above the elbow crease.
2. Cleanse the area with antiseptic solution and drape with sterile drapes.
3. Using aseptic technique, draw 6 ml of 1% lidocaine into the syringe using an 18-gauge needle. Infiltrate six channels of 1 ml of anesthesia subdermally, each about 4.0 to 5.0 cm long, approximating the fan-shaped configuration, using the 22-gauge needle.
4. At the base of the fan, use the scalpel to make a 3.0-mm incision.
5. Insert the trocar with obturator in place through the incision (bevel up) into the subdermal plane, at a shallow angle of 30 degrees, and advance it up to the proximal notch.

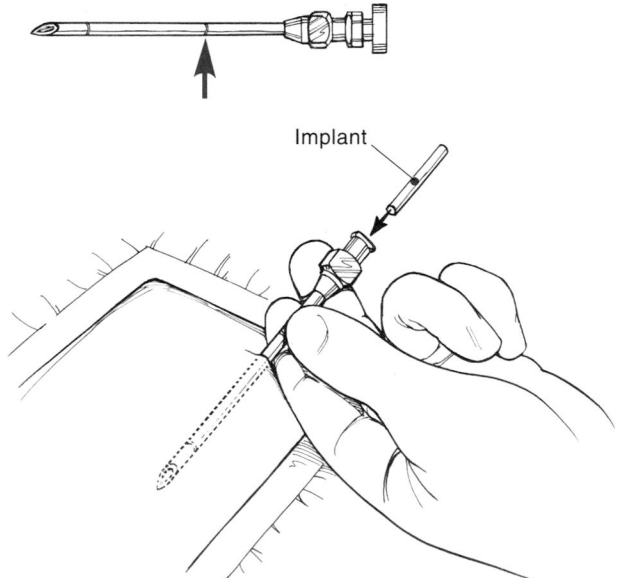

Implant

6. Remove the obturator and place the implant in the trocar. Replace the obturator and withdraw the trocar until the distal notch is visible. This leaves the implant in place.

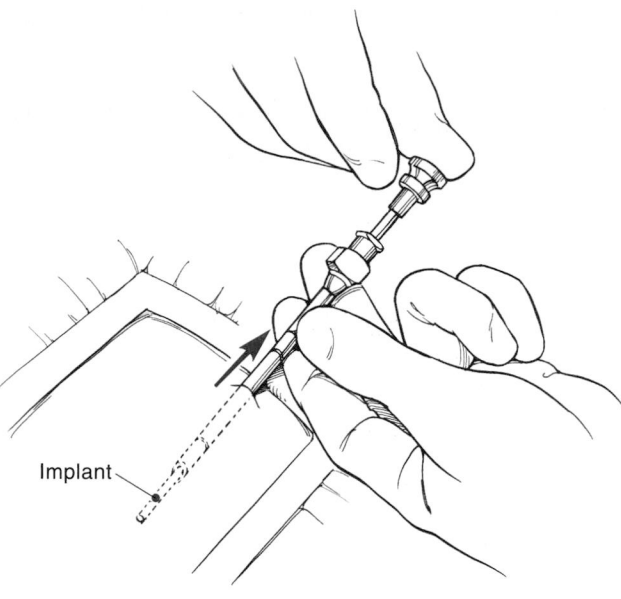

Implant

7. Repeat the procedure for the second through the sixth implants, following the fan-shape pattern traced on the skin.

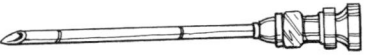

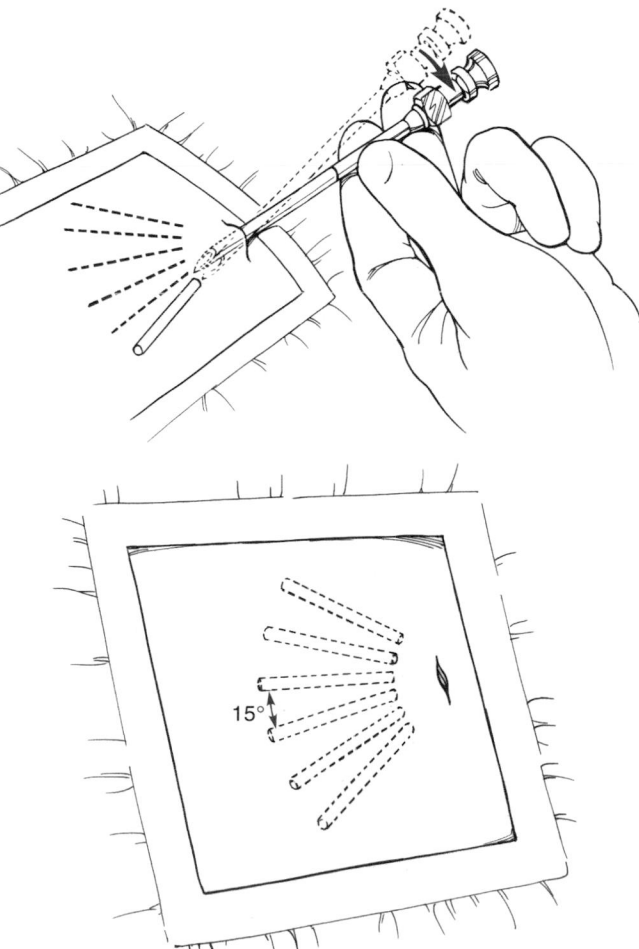

15°

8. Tell patients that some bruising and mild discomfort are normal, but they should report purulent drainage and excessive pain.

9. Finally, record a procedure note in the patient's chart detailing the location of the insert.

Norplant Removal

Whereas Norplant insertion is a simple procedure, removal is relatively more difficult and more time consuming. Many removal methods are described in the literature: the standard method developed by the Population Council and recommended by the distributor, the Emory method, the "U" technique, the pop-out method, the needle elevation method, and the hook traction method. As with anything in medicine, the existence of many methods means that no method is without drawbacks. Not all of the methods have been evaluated formally in clinical trials. The author prefers to use the Emory method. Procedure time is up to 30 minutes.

Equipment
1. Sterile surgical drapes
2. One pair of sterile gloves, free of talc
3. Antiseptic to clean the Norplant implant removal site
4. Local anesthetic
5. A 12-ml syringe and 22-gauge, 1½-inch needle
6. One No. 11 scalpel
7. Two mosquito Halstead forceps (one straight and one curved, 5 inches long)
8. One Adson tissue forceps, with 1 × 2 teeth
9. Butterfly bandages or other skin closures
10. Sterile gauze and compresses

Precautions
1. Inform patient that removal will take longer than the insertion procedure did.
2. Obtain signed informed consent.

Technique: Norplant Removal, Emory Method

1. *Draw up 6 ml of 1% lidocaine.*

2. Inject about 1 ml at the incision site and 0.75 ml underneath the lower (proximal) half of each implant.

3. *Make a superficial, horizontal incision about 1 cm long at the original incision site or close to the lower ends of the implants.*

4. If any of the implants have slid below the incision site, avoid damage to the implants, paying particular attention to making the incision superficial at that site.

5. The incision should not include the subcutaneous tissue.

6. *Introduce the curved mosquito forceps (5 inches long) into the incision and vigorously but gently dissect the subcutaneous tissues deep to the proximal ends of each implant for about 20 seconds.* (The Population Council Method suggests pushing the implant gently toward the incision until the tip is visible and to clear the fibrous sheath over the tip of the implant using the gauze or the scalpel.)

7. The dissection should be vigorous enough to break the tissue encapsulation under the implants. Avoid injuring the implants or traumatizing major vessels underneath.

8. While pushing the distal end of the implant toward the incision with the index finger, grasp the implant from underneath with the curved mosquito forceps.

9. Flip the curved mosquito forceps to bring the implant toward the incision.

10. At this juncture, the white surface of the implant is often noted.

11. With the help of the straight mosquito forceps, hold the implant, without holding any surrounding tissues.

12. Remove the curved mosquito forceps and pull the implant as the forceps is pulled out; clear it either with a piece of gauze or the Adson forceps.

13. Remove each of the implants in the same manner.

14. Clean the incision site with an antiseptic; apply Steri-Strips to close the incision and wrap it with a bandage.

15. Record a procedure note in patient chart.

Bibliography

Dunson TR, Amatya RN, Krueger SL: Complications and risk factors associated with the removal of Norplant implants. Obstet Gynecol 1995;85:543–548.

Hatasaka H: Implantable levonorgestrel contraception: 4 years of experience with Norplant. Clin Obstet Gynecol 1995;38:859–871.

Mastroianni L, Robinson JC: Contraception in the 1990s. Patient Care 1994;28:107–119.

Praptohardjo U, Wibowo S: The "U" technique: a new method for Norplant implants removal. Contraception 1993;48:526–536.

Sharma S, Hatcher R: The Emory Method: a modified approach to Norplant implant removal. Contraception 1994;49:551–556.

Shihata A, Salzetti RG, Schrepper FW, et al: Innovative technique for Norplant implant removal. Contraception 1995;51:83–85.

Indications

1. Vasectomy is a method of permanent sterilization for the male. It is a safe and frequently performed procedure in an outpatient setting, with local anesthesia, at less expense and risk than female tubal sterilization.

2. The prevasectomy conference with the patient, and ideally his spouse, is of paramount importance. At this conference the nature of the operation must be explained, with all of the attendant implications of permanent sterilization. It must be stressed to the patient that this should be considered an irreversible and permanent procedure. While vavovasostomy is technically feasible, its success rate (10 to 40 per cent) makes it a poor option. The risks, benefits, and alternatives must be discussed and documented with each patient.

Complications (Table 124–1)

1. The reported failure rate ranges from 0.1 to 5 per cent depending on the type of occlusive technique used. Intraluminal cautery with application of a medium hemoclip, after removal of a 1- to 2-cm segment of vas, has the lowest reported recanalization rate. The technique described here of crushing the vas ends with a hemostat and ligature with polyglactin (Vicryl) after excision of a 1- to 2-cm segment of vas deferens with fascial interposition, has less than a 1 per cent failure rate.

2. Informed consent must be documented in the patient's chart. Some states require separate consent forms for any sterilization procedure in addition to standard operative consent forms.

Contraindications

1. Individuals on chronic anticoagulation medications

2. Those who express any ambivalence concerning becoming sterile

3. Anatomic factors that preclude performing a vasectomy under local anesthesia. These patients may require referral for the procedure to be done with general anesthesia.

   a. Inability to palpate bilateral vasa through scrotal wall

   b. Individuals who have had prior scrotal content surgery or injury with resulting scarring that may require general anesthesia to allow adequate exploration of the scrotal sac to identify the vas

Preparation

After informed consent has been obtained, and the patient has been examined to determine that he is a suitable candidate for vasectomy under local anesthesia, he is given instructions on how to prepare for the procedure.

1. Avoid aspirin for at least 5 days prior to the procedure.

2. On the day of the procedure, the patient should shave his scrotum of any hair.

3. He should bring an athletic supporter to his appointment to wear postoperatively.

Equipment (Table 124–2)

For vasal occlusion, the equipment used depends on the technique that is chosen.

1. Ligature occlusion with polyglactin (Vicryl) or polyglycolic acid (Chromic) after crushing the vasal ends with a mosquito clamp

2. Thermal fine wire cautery intraluminal occlusion with or without hemoclip application

3. Hemoclip application alone

4. Any of the above combined with separation of the vasa into different tissue planes by fascial interposition. This involves covering either cut

TABLE 124–1. COMPLICATIONS OF VASECTOMY

COMPLICATION	RATE
Failure with recanalization	0.1–5%
Hematoma	2%
Infection/cellulitis	1–3%
Epididymitis	2%
Sperma granuloma	1–2%
Sperm antibodies	40–60%
Chronic orchalgia	0.01%

TABLE 124–2. EQUIPMENT FOR VASECTOMY

REQUIRED	OPTIONAL*
Sterile drapes and sponges	3-0 polyglactin (Vicryl) suture
Xylocaine 1% and bupivacaine 0.5%	Medium hemoclips and applicator
10-ml, 3-ring syringe and 25-gauge, ⅝-inch needle	Fine wire thermal cautery
No. 15 scalpel	Electrocautery unit
Allis clamps (2)	
Curved mosquito clamps (2)	
Toothed forceps	
Needle driver	
Suture scissors	
4-0 polyglactin (Vicryl) skin closure	

*Depending on vasal closure technique.

end of the vas with fascia and suturing the fascia closed.

5. Scrotal skin closure may be either with absorbable suture such as polyglactin (Vicryl) or plain gut, or by crimping the cut ends together with an Allis clamp for 1 to 2 minutes after the procedure is completed.

Anesthesia

1. Local anesthesia is either with lidocaine without vasoconstrictors, or a combination of half-and-half 1% lidocaine and 0.25% bupivacaine.

2. Preoperative medication for sedation can be given if so desired, such as short-acting benzodiazepine, either intravenously or orally. "Verbal anesthesia" has been successful in calming the anxious patient and can eliminate the need for sedation.

Technique

1. The patient is laid supine on the operating table. His groin, including the penis, is prepped with an antiseptic solution, such as povidone-iodine.

2. Use sterile drapes to isolate the scrotum and keep the penis out of the operating field.

3. Standing on the right side of the patient, examine the scrotum and its contents to identify the vasa bilaterally.

4. Use the three-finger technique to isolate the vas, starting first with the patient's left side.

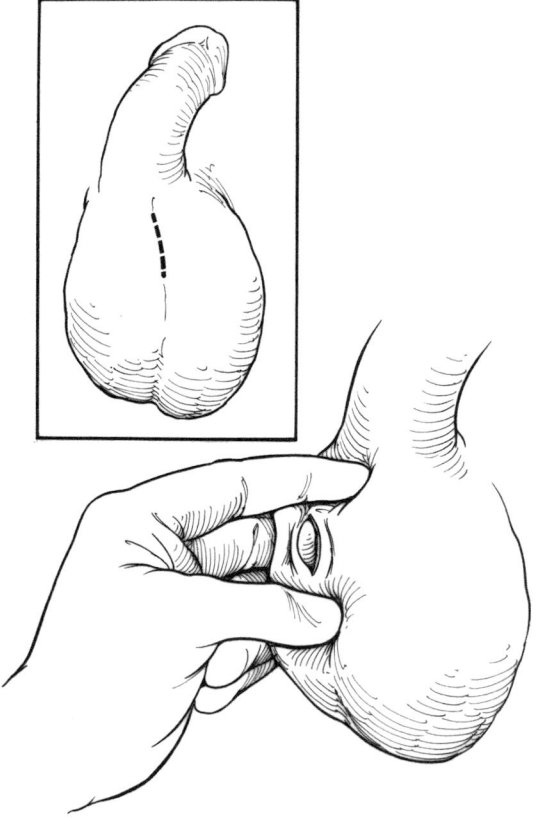

This involves draping the tube-like vas over the middle finger of your left hand while stretching the scrotal sac tautly with the thumb and index finger. Because the scrotal skin is loose, the vas can be moved over such that the midline of the scrotum overlies the vas so that only one incision is needed.

5. Apply local anesthesia to the skin overlying the vas with a 25-gauge needle. While still holding the vas, drive the needle through the skin and pierce the fascia sheath surrounding the vas. Inject anesthetic into this space. Successful vasal nerve block can be assessed by noting the patient's sensation of discomfort in the ipsilateral groin.

6. While still grasping the vas, use a No. 15 scalpel to make a 1-cm incision down through the midline of the scrotum. Identify the vas by rubbing over it with the closed end of an Allis clamp. Grasp the vas by opening the Allis clamp over it while pushing down on the finger over which the vas is draped. Grasp the surrounding sheath and vas securely and deliver through the skin incision.

7. Use the scalpel to incise the vasal sheath longitudinally and expose the vas.

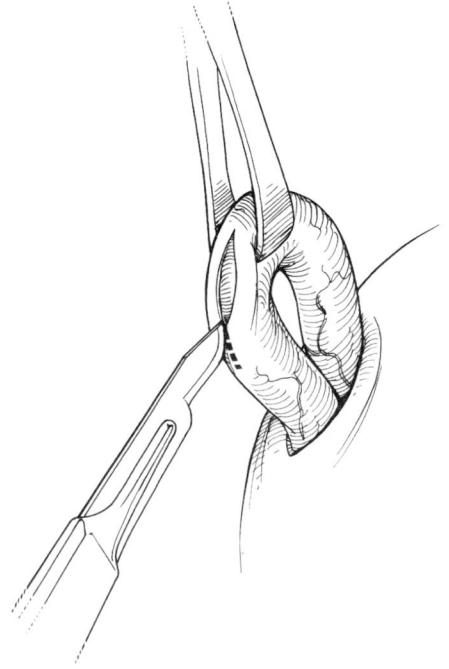

A second Allis clamp grasps the vas to bring it out of its sheath.

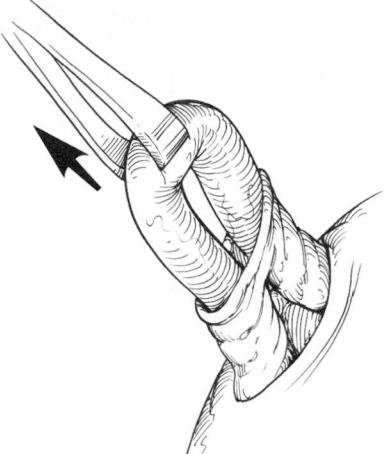

8. The next step depends on the type of occlusive technique. My technique is to use curved mosquito clamps to divide the connecting tissue attached to the vas, clamping the vas distally and proximally, and excising the intervening segment of 1 to 2 cm.

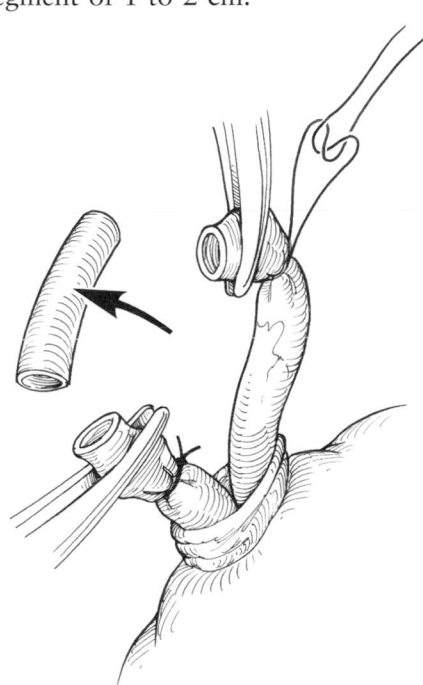

The cut ends are then tied with a ligature of 3-0 polyglactin (Vicryl). An optional step is to cover the cut end of the proximal vas with fascia, suturing the fascia closed over the vas with 3-0 polyglactin (Vicryl), thereby placing the two vas ends in different tissue planes.

9. Isolate the right vas with the three-finger technique, and adjust the scrotal skin so that the midline incision lies over the grasped vas. Repeat the procedure on the right vas.

10. Close the scrotal skin with 4-0 undyed poly-glactin (Vicryl) with a subcuticular stitch that closes the fascia of the scrotum.

Precautions

1. Postoperative instructions given to the patient include
   a. No heavy lifting (greater than 25 lbs) for 5 days
   b. No sexual intercourse for 5 days
   c. Place an ice pack on the scrotum for 20 minutes of each hour for the first 8 to 12 hours
   d. Pain medications can be prescribed, such as acetaminophen with codeine.
2. A semen sample must be brought to the laboratory for microscopic sperm analysis 15 to 20 ejaculations after the vasectomy. Two azoospermic specimens 4 weeks apart are considered proof of sterility. Until the patient is sterile, the couple must be counseled to use an alternative form of birth control to prevent pregnancy.

Postoperative Complications

1. Hematoma: If minor, can be handled with scrotal support and bed rest; if major, may require incision and drainage, with placement of Penrose drains in the scrotum.
2. Infection: skin cellulitis can be treated with antibiotics (dicloxacillin or cephalexin); epididymitis, a tender, erythematous, warm lump usually at the site of the cut end of the testicular vas, responds well to anti-inflammatory medication and antibiotics (doxycycline or sulfamethoxazole-trimethoprim).
3. Sperm granuloma: This occurs at the cut end of the testicular vas, often as a tender lump. It can be treated with anti-inflammatory medication. It is differentiated from epididymitis by its time of presentation, usually weeks to months after the vasectomy as opposed to days to a few weeks for epididymitis.

Bibliography

Alderman PM: Complications in a series of 1224 vasectomies. J Fam Pract 1991;33:579–584.

Davis JE: Male sterilization. Curr Opin Obstet Gynecol 1992;4:522–526.

Goldstein M: Surgery of male infertility and other scrotal disorders. In Walsh PC, Retik AB, Vaughan ED Jr, et al (eds): Campbell's Urology, vol 2, 7th ed, pp 1331–1377. Philadelphia, WB Saunders Company, 1998.

Greenberg MJ: Vasectomy technique. Am Fam Physician 1989;39:131–138.

Schmidt SS: Vasectomy by section, luminal fulguration and fascial interposition: results from 6248 cases. Br J Urol 1996;76:373–374.

No-scalpel vasectomy is a refined, less invasive approach to isolation and delivery of the vas deferens.

Background

In 1995, approximately 494,000 vasectomies were performed by 15,800 physicians in the United States. Nearly one-third (29 per cent) of vasectomies in 1995 were no-scalpel vasectomies. Family physicians performed 15 per cent of all vasectomies that year, the second leading specialty performing vasectomies. Twenty-eight per cent of vasectomies performed by family physician practices were no-scalpel vasectomies.

Benefits

The benefits of no-scalpel vasectomy, compared with traditional approaches, are as follows:

1. Up to 10 times fewer complications (bleeding, hematoma, infection)
2. Less intimidating to clients
3. Less intraoperative and postoperative pain
4. Reduced operative time
5. Faster recovery

Contraindications

1. For health or personal reason(s), client is unready or inappropriate for vasectomy.
2. Inability to identify and isolate both vasa

Preparation

1. Carefully select patients during a thorough prior consultation with the prospective couple.
2. A relaxed scrotum is key to a smooth procedure. Provide a warm room (76° to 80°).
3. Retract the penis upward onto the man's abdomen with a rubber band and clip.

4. Shave or clip the scrotal hair overlying the small operative area.
5. Wash the scrotum with a warm antiseptic solution.
6. Cover the prepared area with a sterile fenestrated drape.

Equipment

1. Extracutaneous ringed forceps ("ringed clamp"): used to fix the vas deferens
2. Surgical hemostat ("dissecting forceps"): used to puncture the scrotal skin, to spread underlying tissues, to dissect the sheath, and to deliver the vas deferens

Anesthesia: Vasal Nerve Block

1. Prepare a 10-ml syringe with 2% lidocaine without epinephrine attached to a 1.5-inch, 27-gauge needle.
2. Using the three-finger technique, isolate the right vas from the spermatic cord vessels to a superficial position under the median raphe, fixing the vas over the middle finger of the left hand and under the index finger and thumb.
3. Inject lidocaine to raise a 1-cm superficial skin wheal.
4. Fully advance the needle within the perivasal sheath. Gently aspirate to verify that the needle is not in a blood vessel, and then slowly inject 2 to 3 ml of lidocaine around the vas. Avoid multiple injections.
5. Similarly fix and anesthetize the left vas through the initial skin puncture.
6. Pinch the original skin wheal to reduce local edema.

Technique

1. Three-finger technique to isolate and fix the vas deferens
   a. Stand comfortably near the patient's scrotum on his right side, facing his head, and take one step backward toward his feet.
   b. The left thumb is placed to *indicate* the juncture of the middle and upper thirds of the median raphe, in an area free of blood vessels.
   c. The left middle finger *isolates* the vas from the spermatic cord and sweeps the vas from under the scrotum toward the raphe beneath the thumb.
   d. The left index finger further *stabilizes* the vas when placed slightly above the thumb.

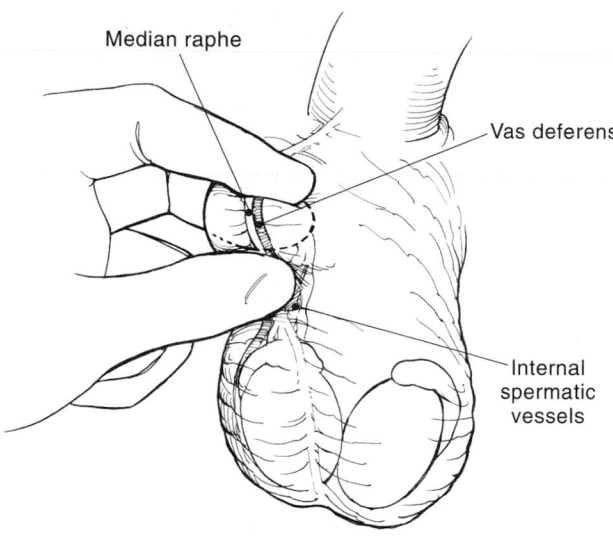

Median raphe

Vas deferens

Internal spermatic vessels

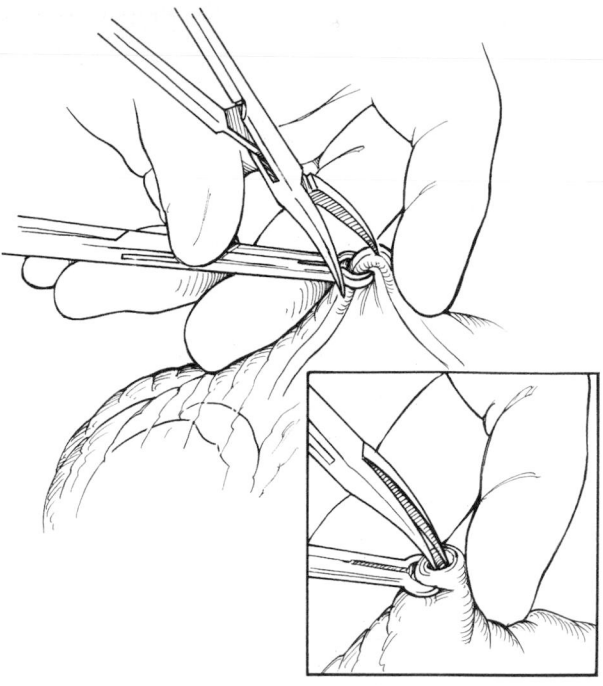

e. Upward pressure from the middle finger, combined with downward pressure from the index finger and thumb, creates a bend in the vas for better isolation and fixation.

f. To isolate the patient's left vas while standing on his right side, take one step toward the patient's head and turn the body to face his feet. Reach across the patient's abdomen with the left hand, and repeat the three-finger technique.

2. Surgical approach

a. Fix the right vas under the skin wheal with the left hand using the three-finger method.

b. Apply the ringed clamp perpendicularly with downward pressure, stretching the scrotal skin tightly over the vas and locking the entire vas within the clamp.

c. Place the ringed clamp in the left hand, lowering the handles to elevate the trapped vas, with the left index finger tightening the scrotal skin over the vas.

d. At the apex of the bend, pierce the scrotal skin, vas sheath, and vas wall down to the lumen at a 45-degree angle with the left blade of the dissecting forceps.

e. Using the same angle, introduce the closed tip of the dissecting forceps through the puncture to the same depth, and gently open and close the blades a few times, stretching and spreading all layers to fully expose the bare vas wall.

f. Skewer the vas wall at a 45-degree angle with the right blade of the dissecting forceps, and rotate the instrument 180 degrees, delivering the vas while the fixation clamp is simultaneously released.

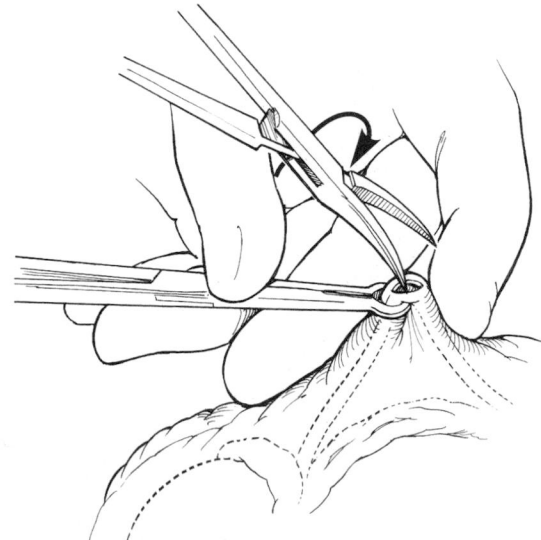

g. Grasp a partial thickness of the elevated vas at the crest of the loop with the ringed clamp.

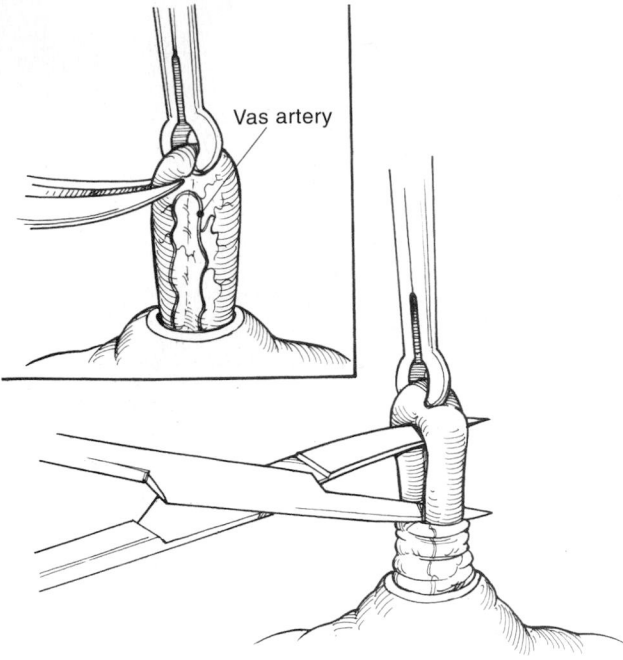

Vas artery

h. With one tip of the dissecting forceps facing upward, puncture the vas sheath just below the vas and above the vas artery. Reintroduce the closed tip of the forceps. Spread the tips to gently strip the sheath, including the vas artery, downward to yield a clean 1-cm segment of vas.

i. Occlude and divide the right vas using a conventional method.

j. Return the fully retracted ends of the right vas to the scrotum.

k. After isolating the left vas directly under the puncture using the three-finger technique, apply the ringed clamp around the puncture or directly grasp the vas and its sheath through the puncture site.

l. The remainder of the procedure is identical to that described for the right side.

m. Pinch the puncture site, and inspect for bleeding.

n. A Band-Aid may be used to cover the small wound; a supporter is worn for comfort.

o. Observe the patient for 30 minutes following the procedure for possible bleeding or hematoma.

Hands-on training is crucial to precisely learn and ultimately master this technique.

Follow-Up

1. Patient rests for 24 to 48 hours, using a cold pack.

2. With prior permission, call the day after the procedure to check patient's progress.

3. Have patient visit 1 week following the procedure to discuss normal recovery and to emphasize instructions regarding semen analysis and postprocedure contraception.

4. Obtain two absolutely azoospermic specimens 4 to 6 weeks apart.

Bibliography

AVSC International: No-Scalpel Vasectomy: An Illustrated Guide for Surgeons. Second edition. New York, AVSC International, 1997.

Haws JM, Morgan GT, Pollack AE, et al: Clinical aspects of vasectomies performed in the United States in 1995. Urology 1998;52:685–691.

Huber D: No-scalpel vasectomy: the transfer of a refined surgical technique from China to other countries. Adv Contracept 1989;5:517–218.

Li PS, Li SQ, Schlegel PN, et al: External spermatic sheath injection for vasal nerve block. Urology 1992;39:173–196.

Nirapathpongporn A, Huber D, Drieger JN: No-scalpel vasectomy at the king's birthday vasectomy festival. Lancet 1990;335:894–895.

125 Infertility

Keith A. Frey

Etiology

1. There are multiple cases of infertility, and interference with the conception process may occur at various sites in the male or female reproductive system. Consider more than one cause, because as many as 40 per cent of couples have more than one cause.
2. Common etiologies of infertility are listed in Table 125–1.

Symptoms

1. Symptoms are as varied as the etiologies.
2. It is crucial that the physician perform a detailed reproductive and sexual history and general review of systems (Table 125–2).

Clinical Findings

1. A thorough physical examination of each partner, with specific attention to the reproductive tract, is essential.
2. Observe for findings of structural abnormalities, endocrinopathy, and infection (Table 125–3).
3. Arrange a meeting with the couple early in the diagnostic work-up. This provides an important opportunity to review reproductive biology and the rationale for subsequent laboratory tests.

Laboratory Tests

1. Each couple must be evaluated by a series of routine laboratory tests and appropriately timed studies to evaluate each major reproductive factor that may cause infertility.
2. Routine laboratory tests for the male and female partners are listed in Table 125–3.
3. Basal body temperature recording provides valuable information regarding both the presence and timing of ovulation and the timing of key diagnostic studies (Table 125–4).
4. The comprehensive diagnostic survey can and should be completed for most couples in 3 to 6 months.

Differential Diagnosis

1. The results of the comprehensive diagnostic survey (history, physical examination, laboratory tests, and diagnostic studies) generally identify the factor(s) contributing to the couple's infertility.
2. The more common disorders, by reproductive category, include
   a. Male factors
      (1) Varicocele
      (2) Oligospermia/azoospermia
      (3) Disorders of sperm function or motility (asthenospermia)
      (4) Abnormalities of sperm morphology (teratospermia)
   b. Ovulatory dysfunction
      (1) Hypothalamic anovulation (e.g., psychogenic trauma, anorexia nervosa, pharmacologic agents)
      (2) Pituitary anovulation (e.g., pituitary tumors, ischemia, defects)
      (3) Ovulatory anovulation (e.g., ovarian dysgenesis, premature ovarian failure, ovarian tumors
      (4) Integrative anovulation (e.g., polycystic ovarian syndrome, nonpsychogenic weight disturbances)
   c. Tubal damage
      (1) Tubal damage or obstruction (following acute salpingitis)
      (2) Adnexal adhesions
   d. Endometriosis (leading to chronic inflammation and disruption of conception)
   e. Cervical mucus abnormalities (e.g., cervical infections, previous surgery or cautery, hormonal disruptions)

TABLE 125–1. CAUSES OF INFERTILITY IN COUPLES

ETIOLOGIC FACTORS	INFERTILE COUPLES
Male problems	35%
Tubal and pelvic pathology	35%
Ovulatory dysfunction	15%
Unexplained infertility	10%
Unusual problems	5%

Data from Petrie K, Frey KA: Preconception care/infertility. Monograph No. 234, Home Study Self-Assessment program. American Academy of Family Physicians, Kansas City, Nov. 1998.

TABLE 125-2. THE INFERTILITY WORK-UP IN OUTLINE: HISTORY (MALE, FEMALE, OR BOTH)

Marriage
Duration of infertility
Fertility in previous relationships
Frequency of intercourse
Sexual potency and techniques
Use of coital lubricants

Adult Illnesses
Acute viral or febrile illness in past 3 months
Mumps orchitis
Renal disease
Radiation therapy
Sexually transmitted disease
Radiation therapy
Stress and fatigue
Tuberculosis

Occupation and Habits
Exposure to radiation, chemicals, excessive heat (saunas, hot tubs, etc.)

Childhood Illness
Cryptorchidism
Timing of puberty

Surgery
Herniorrhaphy
Retroperitoneal surgery
Vasectomy

Drug Use
Alcohol, tobacco, and drugs
Alkylating agents
Hormones
Nitrofurantoin (Macrodantin)

Review of Symptoms
Focus on endocrine conditions (diabetes, thyroid disorders)

Gynecology
Coital frequency and techniques
Contraceptives used
Diethylstilbestrol use by mother
Douches and lubricants used
Exposure to radiation and chemicals
Fertility in previous relationships
Menarche
Menses (regularity and flow)
Mittelschmerz

From Frey KA: Infertility. In Mengel MB, Schwiebert LP (eds): Ambulatory Medicine: The Primary Care of Families, p 559. East Norwalk, CT, Appleton & Lange, 1993, with permission.

Treatment

1. Generally, treatment should not be initiated until the diagnostic evaluation is completed. Therapy should proceed at a rate that the couple finds comfortable.

2. Therapy for the specific disorders identified by the comprehensive diagnostic evaluation often can be initiated by the primary care physician. For detailed descriptions of specific treatment approaches, the reader is referred to the Bibliography.

3. The work-up, diagnosis, and treatment of infertility can precipitate intense emotional reactions. The physician should discuss such emotions as anger, guilt, self-doubt, depression, and grief with the couple. In addition, help the couple understand their motives for parenting. Assist the couple in the development of mutual support and an adaptive "couple-coping" style. Discuss sexual issues, and encourage the couple to nurture their intimacy. Help the couple broaden their support system, including self-help groups (e.g., RESOLVE [the National Infertility Organization]).

Follow-Up

1. The exact prognosis of infertility can be difficult to define because of the multiple potential causes.

2. Conception rates following specific therapy are favorable for most disorders.

TABLE 125-3. THE INFERTILITY WORK-UP (MALE AND FEMALE)

MALE		FEMALE	
Physical Examination	Routine Laboratory Tests	Physical Examination	Routine Laboratory Tests
Hair pattern	Complete blood count	Breast formation	Complete blood count
Genitalia	Semen analysis	Distribution of body fat	Pap smear
Meatus size and location	Abstinence of 2 days	Galactorrhea	Urinalysis and urine culture if indicated
Prostate and seminal vesicles	Masturbation into sterile vessel	Hair pattern (virilization)	At home test: basal body temperature
Scrotum	To lab (warm) within 2 hours	Height and weight	Measure temperature for 5–10 min orally before arising
Testicular size (≥4 cm in long axis)	Results:	Neurology	Measure temperatures throughout evaluation and treatment
Varicocele (standing and Valsalva maneuver)	Volume: 2–5 ml	Anosmia	Bring chart on each visit
Neurology	Liquefaction: complete within 30 min	Visual fields	Rubella immunity
Visual fields	Sperm count: 60–150 million/ml	Pelvis	
	Sperm motility: >60%	External genitalia	
	Morphology: >60% normal forms	Retrovaginal area (endometriosis)	
	2–3 tests as necessary	Uterus and adnexa	
	Urinalysis and urine culture if indicated	Vagina and cervix	

Modified from Frey KA: Infertility. In Mengel MB, Schwiebert LP (eds): Ambulatory Medicine: The Primary Care of Families, p 560. East Norwalk, CT, Appleton & Lange, 1993, with permission.

TABLE 125–4. THE INFERTILITY WORK-UP: FURTHER DIAGNOSTIC TESTS

Postcoital (Sims-Huhner) Test
Determines number and condition of sperm and their ability to penetrate cervical mucus
Performed around time of ovulation

Hysterosalpingogram (HSG)
Preferred test of tubal patency
Performed 2–6 days after cessation of menstrual flow
May enhance fertility temporarily

Laparoscopy
Performed if HSG unproductive or history of pelvic inflammatory disease
Permits examination of pelvic contents

Endometrial Biopsy
Determines if luteal-phase defect exists
Performed 2–3 days before expected menses
Informed consent required
Requires histologic dating

Serum Progesterone
May be an alternative to endometrial biopsy
Sample drawn 5–7 days after supposed ovulation
Serum level >6.5 ng/ml is compatible with ovulation

Modified from Frey KA: Infertility. In Mengel MB, Schwiebert LP (eds): Ambulatory Medicine: The Primary Care of Families, p 561. East Norwalk, CT, Appleton & Lange, 1993, with permission.

3. "Unexplained" infertility is the persistent inability to conceive after a comprehensive diagnostic assessment fails to identify a specific diagnosis. If an etiology is not apparent or treatment is unsuccessful, referral is warranted. The primary care physician also should discuss adoption options with the couple, and the costs involved in further infertility evaluation and treatment.

B Bibliography

Frey KA: Infertility. In Mengel MB, Schwiebert LP (eds): Ambulatory Medicine: The Primary Care of Families, pp 558–562. East Norwalk, CT, Appleton & Lange, 1993.

Jones WJ, Toner, JP: The infertile couple. N Engl J Med 1993;329:1710–1715.

Neumann PJ, Gharib SD, Weinstein MC: The cost of a successful delivery with in vitro fertilization. N Engl J Med 1994;331:239–243.

Petrie K, Frey KA: Preconception care/infertility. Monograph No. 234, Home Study Self-Assessment program. American Academy of Family Physicians, Kansas City, Nov. 1998.

RESOLVE National Infertility Organization: *www.resolve.org*

Speroff L, Glass RH, Kase NG: Clinical Gynecologic Endocrinology and Infertility, 6th ed. Baltimore, Williams & Wilkins, 1999.

126 Sexual Dysfunction in Men

Edward D. Kim

Etiology

1. Organic
   a. Vasculogenic: hypertension, smoking, atherosclerosis
   b. Endocrine: diabetes mellitus, hypogonadism, thyroid disorders
   c. Neurologic: multiple sclerosis, spinal cord injury, neuropathies, stroke
   d. Medication induced: antihypertensives, antihormonals, substance abuse, antidepressants, antipsychotics, anticholinergics
   e. Postoperative: prostate surgery, types of colon cancer surgery, spine surgery
   f. Anatomic deformity: Peyronie's disease, severe hypospadias
   g. Unspecified
2. Psychogenic
   a. Performance anxiety, fear of failure
   b. Marital discord
   c. Depression
   d. Psychiatric disturbance
3. Mixed organic and psychogenic

Symptoms

1. Erectile dysfunction is defined as the consistent inability to achieve or maintain an erection suitable for intercourse. Erectile dysfunction is one component of the male sexual response.
2. Phases of the male sexual response and common related disorders
   a. Arousal: poor libido
   b. Erection: erectile dysfunction
   c. Orgasm: anorgasmia
   d. Ejaculation: premature or delayed ejaculation
   e. Latency period: increased latency period

Key Symptoms

- Inability to achieve rigid erection
- Inability to maintain rigid erection
- Poor sexual desire

Clinical Findings

1. History
   a. Sexual history
      (1) Duration and onset
      (2) Degree of impairment: ability to have intercourse, quality of erections (per cent), problem of obtaining or maintaining erection
      (3) Sexual desire
      (4) Nocturnal erections and with masturbation
      (5) Nonsexual relationship with partner
      (6) Consider use of standardized erectile function questionnaire, such as the International Index of Erectile Function (IIEF)
   b. Medical and surgical history
   c. Family/social/medical history
      (1) Tobacco and alcohol use
      (2) Illicit drug use
      (3) Nitrate use, careful review of medications
   d. Review of systems
      (1) Cardiac risk factors, angina
      (2) Stress factors
2. Physical examination
   a. Secondary male characteristics: hair growth, muscle mass, fat distribution
   b. Penis: Peyronie's penile plaque, hypospadias
   c. Testes: size, nodules, masses
   d. Vascular: abdominal, inguinal, pedal pulses
   e. Neurologic: general status, brief motor/sensory examination
   f. Psychologic: depression, mood
   g. Other: digital rectal examination

Diagnostic Testing

1. Laboratory testing

Key Initial Lab Testing

- Serum testosterone
- Urinalysis

a. Serum testosterone

b. Urinalysis

c. Optional testing, as clinically indicated

    (1) Serum prolactin and free testosterone: if total testosterone is low

    (2) Serum electrolytes, blood urea nitrogen, creatinine, glucose/complete blood cell count, lipid profile, thyroid function tests, prostate-specific antigen: depending on patient age and medical condition

> **Note**
>
> Advanced testing of erectile dysfunction is generally not necessary during the initial evaluation and treatment of the impotent male. Testing may be obtained if the patient
>
> - Fails initial therapies
>
> - Desires further testing to understand why he is having a problem
>
> - Has a history highly suggestive of pelvic or perineal trauma as the etiology

2. Advanced testing

  a. Penile duplex ultrasonography

  b. Nocturnal penile tumescence monitoring

  c. Intracavernosal injection testing

  d. Pelvic arteriography

3. Other

Consider cardiac stress tests for men with significant cardiovascular disease. Sexual activity can precipitate cardiac ischemia.

Differential Diagnosis

1. Erectile dysfunction is often multifactorial in etiology.

2. Special attention should be directed toward identifying endocrine and psychological causes, because successful treatment of these underlying etiologies may restore normal spontaneous erectile function.

3. See "Etiology" for underlying causes.

Treatment

1. Specific medical

  a. Sildenafil citrate (Viagra)

    (1) First choice for the vast majority of men

    (2) A selective-type 5-phosphodiesterase inhibitor that improves erections

    (3) Avoid in men on nitrates and with significant cardiovascular disease.

    (4) Decreased dose is appropriate for men with severe hepatic or renal impairment, as well as for elderly men.

> **WARNING**
>
> **Sildenafil citrate should not be used in men using nitrates or with significant cardiovascular disease.**

  b. Intracavernous injection therapy

    (1) Prostaglandin E_1 (PGE-1) alone: Caverject, Edex

    (2) Combination therapy: papaverine, phentolamine, PGE

    (3) Erection onset in 5 to 10 minutes; detumescence in about 45 to 60 minutes

  c. Vacuum constriction devices

    (1) Effective but cumbersome

    (2) Works with constriction ring by causing venous engorgement

  d. MUSE intraurethral suppository

    (1) Active ingredient: alprostadil (synthetic PGE_1)

    (2) Limited by lack of rigid erections

  e. Hormonal replacement

    (1) Best if used for hypogonadal men

    (2) Much more effective for poor libido than poor erections

  f. Investigational oral therapies: apomorphine (Uprima), phentolamine (Vasomax)

  g. Yohimbine: not effective for organic erectile dysfunction

2. General medical

  a. Treat underlying conditions: diabetes, hypothyroidism, hypertension, depression

  b. Avoidance of detrimental factors: smoking, excessive alcohol use

3. Surgical

  a. Penile prosthesis (implant)

    (1) High patient and partner satisfaction

    (2) Malleable and inflatable types

    (3) Patients should try nonsurgical options first.

  b. Penile arterial revascularization: for traumatic injuries

  c. Venous ligation: nonstandard therapy

4. Psychiatric

  a. Counseling: sex therapy

  b. Psychotherapy

  c. Pharmacologic therapy

Key Treatment

- Sildenafil citrate (Viagra)
- Intracavernous injection, MUSE, vacuum device
- Penile prosthesis
- Treatment of underlying medical condition

Follow-Up

1. Compliance with vacuum devices, MUSE, and intracavernous injections may be as poor as 30 to 50 per cent at 1 year.
2. Initial follow-up with treatments should be conducted within several months of initiation. Thereafter, annual or semiannual visits should be advised.
3. If sildenafil citrate is unsuccessful as the first treatment choice, then vacuum devices, intracavernous injection therapy, and MUSE should be offered as the next forms of therapy.

4. If a penile prosthesis is placed, the patient should understand that use of noninvasive forms of therapy will not be effective.

Bibliography

Goldstein I, Lue TF, Padma-Nathan H, et al: Oral sildenafil in the treatment of erectile dysfunction. N Engl J Med 1998;338:1397–1404.

Linet OI, Ogrinc FG: The Alprostadil Study Group: Efficacy and safety of intracavernosal alprostadil in men with erectile dysfunction. N Engl J Med 1996;334:873–877.

Montague DK, Barada JH, Belker AM, et al: Clinical Guidelines Panel on Erectile Dysfunction: summary report on the treatment of organic erectile dysfunction. J Urol 1996;156:2007–2011.

Padma-Nathan H, Hellstrom WJG, Kaiser FE, et al: Treatment of men with erectile dysfunction with transurethral alprostadil. N Engl J Med 1997;336:1–7.

Rosen RC, Riley A, Wagner G, et al: The International Index of Erectile Function (IIEF): A multidimensional scale for assessment of erectile dysfunction. Urology 1997;49:822–830.

127 Sexual Function and Dysfunction in Women

A. E. Eyler

General Concepts

Differential Diagnosis

Sexual dysfunctions are classified by the phase of the sexual response cycle in which they manifest, and can be caused by a variety of medical, psychological, and relational etiologies, the most common of which are listed in Table 127–1.

History

1. Sexuality is a fundamental aspect of human self-concept in both health and illness. Issues regarding sexual functioning commonly present in primary care practice. However, many patients experience difficulty in raising concerns about their sexual health because of embarrassment or fear of censure or ridicule.

2. Questions regarding sexual relationships and functioning, offered in a calm and supportive manner, communicate the importance and acceptability of sexual health concerns, and often enable further discussion to occur. It is useful to include questions pertinent to the sexual history in the review of systems, especially the gynecologic and urologic portions, although some clinicians prefer to begin by asking relationship questions as part of the social history.

3. One example of a basic, "screening" sexual history is included in Table 127–2.

Diagnostic Interviewing: The Sexual Response Cycle

1. Clinical evaluation of sexual difficulties requires understanding of normal sexual physiology and functioning. Regardless of the nature of the sexual episode (solo or with a mate or casual partner) or method of stimulation employed, both women and men experience a characteristic series of physiologic stages as they approach orgasmic release.

2. The human sexual response cycle (SRC) was first described by Masters and Johnson in 1966. Understanding the SRC makes possible the description, diagnosis, and treatment of sexual dysfunctions.

   a. Masters and Johnson conceptualized the human sexual response cycle as consisting of four phases: *excitement*, *plateau*, *orgasm*, and *resolution*. The physiologic changes associated with the SRC (for women) are described in Table 127–3 and represented graphically in Figure 127–1.

   b. Helen Singer-Kaplan subsequently investigated sexual responsiveness from a more subjective, psychologically oriented perspective. She described the SRC as consisting of three phases: *desire*, *excitement*, and *orgasm*.

TABLE 127–1. SEXUAL DYSFUNCTIONS*

ETIOLOGIES	CLASSIFICATION
Drugs	Sexual desire disorders
Neurogenic	Sexual arousal disorders
Vascular	Orgasm disorders
Endocrine	Sexual pain disorders
Disability/illness/degenerative diseases	Sexual dysfunction, not
Psychologic/social	otherwise specified

*Data from Kaplan (1979) and the American Psychiatric Association (1994).

From Eyler AE: Sexuality issues and common sexual dysfunctions: evaluation and management in the primary care setting. In Knesper DJ, Riba MB, Schwenk TL (eds): Primary Care Psychiatry, p 375. Philadelphia, WB Saunders Company, 1997, with permission.

TABLE 127–2. THE (SCREENING) SEXUAL HISTORY

This is a very basic screening sexual history that can be routinely included in clinical encounters. Key questions include:

1. Sexual activity (type and frequency).
2. Sexual partners, if any, and their relationship to the patient.
3. Sexual orientation.
4. Satisfaction with sexual functioning as well as the existence and nature of any problem with sexual functioning.
5. Understanding of the health issues relevant to his or her sexual behavior and whether the patient has taken precautions (if applicable) to prevent injury, the transmission of infection, or undesired conception.
6. Conversely, understanding of the implications for his or her sexual functioning of his or her physical condition or therapeutic regimen.
7. Any anxieties, misconceptions, or questions that the patient may be willing to share about sexual issues or sexual functioning.
8. Any relevant past events, especially emotional, physical, or sexual abuse.

Data from Cheadle MJ: The screening sexual history. Clin Geriatr Med 1991;7:9–13. In Knesper D et al (eds): Primary Care Psychiatry. Philadelphia, WB Saunders Company, 1997, with permission.

TABLE 127-3. THE HUMAN SEXUAL RESPONSE CYCLE

Excitement
- Onset of vaginal lubrication
- Swelling of the glans clitoris; increase in shaft diameter
- Nipple erection; increase in breast size

- Engorgement of vaginal walls
- Swelling of labia minora
- Muscle tension; sex flush

Plateau
- Further engorgement of the outer vagina and labia
- Increase in muscle tension; sex flush (possible)
- Marked increase in heart rate, respiration, BP

- Retraction of the clitoris, under the clitoral hood
- Further nipple engorgement

Orgasm
- Strong muscular contractions in the outer vagina
- Strong, diffuse muscular contractions
- BP increase (as much as 1/3 above normal)
- Vocalization (possible)

- Contractions of uterus, anal sphincter
- Peak intensity of sex flush
- Doubling of HR, RR (possible)

Resolution
- Quick dispersion of vaginal engorgement
- Gradual decrease of breast and nipple size
- Muscular and psychological relaxation
- Return to usual color, size, position of vagina, labia, clitoris

- Return to normal of HR, RR, BP
- Disappearance of sex flush
- Sweating reaction (possible)

Abbreviations: BP, blood pressure; HR, heart rate; RR, respiratory rate.
Data from Masters WH, Johnson VE: Human Sexual Response. Boston, Little, Brown & Co, 1966. In Knesper D et al (eds): Primary Care Psychiatry. Philadelphia, WB Saunders Company, 1997, with permission.

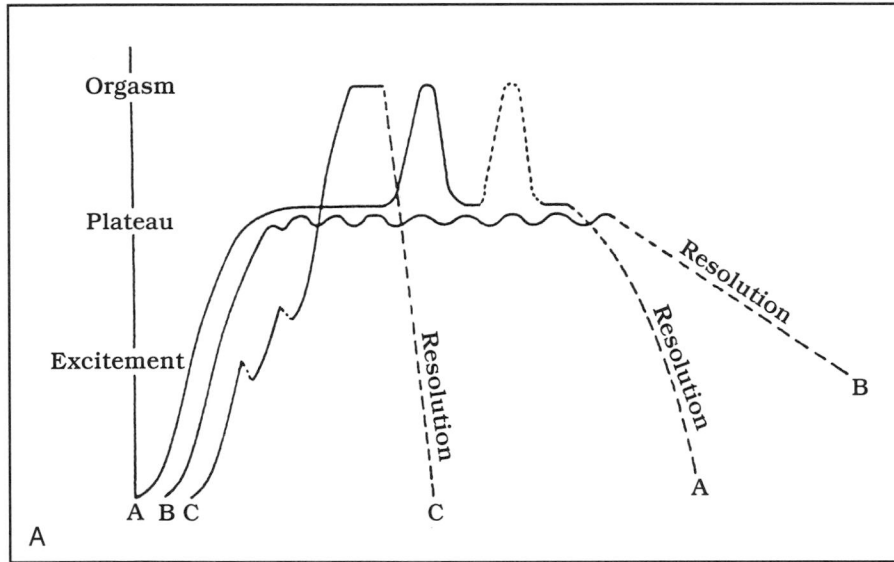

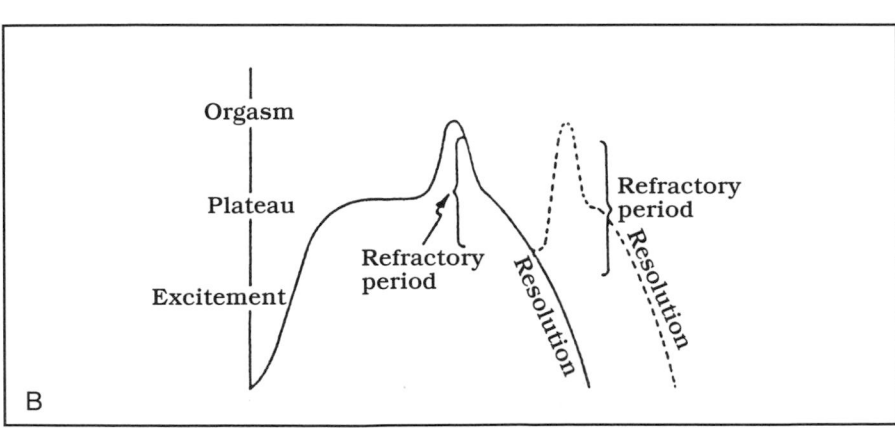

Figure 127–1 The female (*A*) and male (*B*) sexual response cycles. The phases of the response cycle are arbitrarily defined and differ considerably across individuals. Before the beginning of the response cycle is the phase of desire; this phase is not illustrated. The three illustrated phases are excitement, plateau, and orgasm. The length of the plateau phase is variable. For men with premature ejaculation, the plateau phase is usually quite brief; for women, a brief plateau phase may precede a very intense orgasm (illustrated by cycle C). Women may have multiple orgasms without dropping below the plateau phase. Most women are not multiorgasmic. Directly after ejaculation, most men enter a refractory period, when ejaculation is impossible. The male refractory period may last from minutes to hours. Women have no refractory period. The resolution phase for women is characterized by considerable variability. (Adapted from Kolodny RC, Masters WH, Johnson VE: Textbook of Sexual Medicine, 4th ed, pp 7–18. Boston, Little, Brown & Co, 1979, with permission.)

Desire is defined as "libido . . . the specific psychoneurological sensations that lead people to seek out sexual experiences, feel 'sexy' or sexually interested, or restless" (Kaplan, 1979).

c. For medical purposes, either schema is acceptable, as long as it can accommodate the clinical data. For example, dysfunctions that affect sexual desire or the plateau phase should be described in those terms. Many clinicians prefer to combine these two descriptions of the SRC for general use.

3. When discussing a specific sexual dysfunction, it is often useful to briefly educate the patient about the SRC, and to refer to it during the clinical discussion.

Physical Examination

1. Diagnosis of many sexual dysfunctions can be made through the interview alone. Nonetheless, in the absence of diagnostic certainty, a complete physical examination should be performed.

2. Areas of particular relevance to sexual functioning include the thyroid gland; cardiovascular and pulmonary systems; neurologic examination, including the sensory organs and mental status; genital, rectal, and urologic examinations; and dermal integrity.

Specific Sexual Disorders

Desire-Phase Disorders

Desire-phase disorders, in which the patient experiences a lower level of sexual desire than she would like or a loss of previous libido, often require referral to a sex therapist. Primary care physicians should evaluate and treat any related illness, such as depression or chronic fatigue.

Vaginismus (An Excitement Phase Disorder)

Vaginismus is an involuntary, usually painful, spastic contraction of the pelvic musculature surrounding the outer third of the vagina.

1. Complete: precluding intercourse, tampon insertion, or other vaginal penetration
2. Partial: resulting in dyspareunia or difficulty with other forms of vaginal penetration, including speculum examination
3. Situational: for example, occurring when intercourse is anticipated

Etiology

1. Idiopathic
2. Onset follows an episode (or episodes) of pelvic trauma, such as painful intercourse, sexual as-

sault, rough gynecologic examination, complicated episiotomy, vaginal infections or pelvic inflammatory disease, pelvic congestion, or pelvic surgery.
3. Childhood or adolescent sexual abuse may lead to vaginismus during adulthood.

Diagnosis

1. The diagnosis of vaginismus is generally made by history. Patients report the inability to engage in vaginal intercourse, or to use tampons or vaginal contraceptives, or the experience of pain and difficulty with intercourse, digital vaginal stimulation, or pelvic examination.

2. The physical examination may occasionally be revealing. Patients who demonstrate visible contraction of the pelvic floor musculature with anticipated speculum examination should be asked about dyspareunia, previous pelvic trauma, and other sexual concerns. Physical examination can also detect pertinent anatomic abnormalities, such as vaginal septae.

Treatment

1. It must be stressed that true vaginismus is not under the conscious control of the sufferer, and that *therapy must be directed at restoring this control under conditions that respect the autonomy of the patient and maintain safety from further trauma.*

a. At no time should the patient be encouraged to participate in activities that she perceives as uncomfortable, stressful, painful, or upsetting, regardless of the expectations of her partner.

b. If the patient expresses fear or anxiety (either verbally or physically), the pelvic examination may be deferred until a subsequent visit, at which time she can be accompanied by a supportive friend.

c. In severe cases, sedation may be necessary even for routine gynecologic examination.

2. Any physical abnormalities detected on pelvic examination, such as infections, should first be treated.

3. Next, the patient may begin self-treatment with size-graded vaginal dilators, gradually teaching her vagina to remain relaxed and to receive nonpainful, self-controlled penetration. Warmth and lubrication are helpful. The initial "dilator" employed should be of very small diameter in order to avoid triggering vaginal spasm (usually smaller than a tampon). (A graded set of dilators can be purchased from Syracuse Medical Devices, Inc., 214 Hurlburt Road, Syracuse, NY 13224.)

4. Referral to a sex therapist is often helpful, and treatment of post-traumatic stress disorder (PTSD) and other sequelae of past trauma may be crucial.

5. Follow-up over time is necessary.

Orgasmic Dysfunction

1. Orgasmic dysfunction refers to the inability to reach orgasm when desired.
   a. Primary inhibited orgasm: The patient has never (yet) experienced orgasm.
   b. Secondary inhibited orgasm: The dysfunction manifests after previous satisfactory orgasmic functioning.

2. Not included in this disorder is the inability to reach orgasm with vaginal intercourse, because fewer than 50 per cent of women are orgasmic without additional clitoral stimulation.

Etiology

1. Primary inhibited orgasm
   a. Lack of knowledge regarding female sexual anatomy and functioning
   b. Lack of prior self-stimulation
   c. Guilt feelings about sexuality, sexual fantasies, and sexual behavior (which occur frequently among women who have been raised with negative messages regarding sexuality or strict religious or cultural prohibitions, even if their behavior never violates these principles)
   d. Physical or sexual abuse

2. Secondary inhibited orgasm
   a. Other medical and psychological illnesses
   b. Lack of personal or partner knowledge regarding sexual functioning or technique
   c. Relationship problems
   d. Stressful life circumstances or preoccupations
   e. Substance abuse
   f. Dyspareunia
   g. Abuse.

Evaluation

1. The clinical history in cases of secondary inhibited orgasm should focus on the patient's perception of this dysfunction.
   a. Time and circumstances of onset
   b. Possible causes
   c. Effect on relationship(s)
   d. Treatment goals
   e. Physiologic functioning during sexual stimulation, including adequacy of lubrication and ability to sustain states of high arousal

f. Contributing factors: fatigue, depression, postpartum physical and social changes, preoccupation with other life issues, substance abuse, other medical illnesses
   g. Relationship issues: lack of tenderness or interest in nonintercourse stimulation/foreplay by the partner, early ejaculation, contraceptive responsibility, lack of privacy, other conflicts

2. In both primary and secondary inhibited orgasm, it is important to ask about past or current experiences of violence and victimization, including emotional (psychological), physical, and sexual abuse.

3. In most cases of orgasmic dysfunction, no specific physical examination or laboratory testing is necessary. Neurologic, gynecologic, or other examination may be suggested by the clinical history.

Treatment

Treatment of orgasmic dysfunction usually involves increasing knowledge and sexual options for the patient and partner.

1. Women experiencing primary inhibited orgasm often benefit from receiving information about female sexual anatomy and function. *For Yourself: The Fulfillment of Female Sexuality* (Barbach, 1976) is an excellent book to recommend for women who have not yet experienced orgasm. *How to Have an Orgasm . . . As Often as You Want* (Swift, 1993) is a bit more modern in perspective.

2. Masturbation is frequently helpful because it provides information about sexual responsiveness and preferred stimulations that can then be transferred to sexual situations with the partner. It should be kept in mind that many people who have been discouraged from masturbation for religious reasons will not be opposed to participating in this behavior in order to improve their orgasmic functioning or couple/marriage relationship.

3. Partner education is usually important, especially with regard to the importance of clitoral stimulation and adequate preintercourse lovemaking. Changing the focus of the relationship from intercourse to mutual pleasuring, spontaneity, and satisfaction can be crucial.

4. Referral for more in-depth therapy is indicated if the evaluation reveals significant relationship dysfunction, past abuse as an etiologic factor, or other severe medical or psychosocial complications.

Dyspareunia (Sexual Pain Disorder)

Dyspareunia refers to pain experienced immediately before, during, or after intercourse or other penetration.

Etiology

1. Anatomic or physiologic factors: vaginal septae, partial vaginismus, and inadequate lubrication
2. Relationship difficulties
3. Poor sexual technique
4. Rough or abusive partner
5. Emotional factors, such as religious conflicts and the sequelae of childhood abuse

Diagnosis

1. Diagnosis of dyspareunia is made by history and physical examination.
2. Useful questions include the onset, duration, and circumstances in which this problem has occurred; the location of the pain (superficial, deep, unilateral, bilateral, etc.); and whether it is specific to a particular partner or practice.
3. In addition to evidence of infection, vaginismus, or anatomic abnormality, physical examination may reveal evidence of trauma, such as introital fissuring and bruising of the medial thighs, because many women experiencing dyspareunia are in relationships with husbands or boyfriends in which tolerance of sexual roughness and insensitivity is expected.

Treatment

Treatment of dyspareunia depends on determination of its etiology, and usually requires clinical follow-up.

1. Treatment of physiologic causes, such as atrophic or infectious vaginitis, is often straightforward.
   a. The clinical management of vaginismus is discussed earlier in this chapter.
   b. In some cases, providing information regarding the importance of clitoral stimulation and adequate sex play before intercourse, as well as the option of using supplemental water-based lubrication, may be sufficient, especially if the pain is located in the distal vagina or introitus.
   c. "Deep" dyspareunia is often due to overvigorous penetration or excess cervical pressure, and may respond to simple educational interventions. (For example, many people do not realize that both penises and vaginas vary in length, and that, in cases in which the former is substantially longer, the vagina will not "stretch" to accommodate full penile engulfment; attempts to do so, however, will cause deep dyspareunia. Changing position to allow the woman to control the amount of cervical pressure may also be of crucial importance.)
2. In cases in which partner roughness or poor sexual technique is a factor, it is important to stress that no one should be required to tolerate sexual pain (and that this can lead to medical complications, such as vaginismus) and to clarify the patient's goals for the relationship. Referral for sex therapy for the couple may prove helpful; in other cases, the patient may be able to bring about change in the sexual relationship with sufficient information and assertiveness. If dyspareunia is the result of deliberate carelessness or abuse by the partner, ending the relationship may be the only viable option.

Sex Therapy Referrals

1. Referral to a sex therapist should be initiated whenever the care of the particular sexual dysfunction is beyond the knowledge and expertise of the treating physician, when significant couples issues are present, or at the request of the patient.
2. Other disorders that are identified during the diagnostic or therapeutic process (e.g., depression, PTSD from prior trauma) may also require the services of a mental health professional.
3. A list of certified sex therapists can be obtained from the American Association of Sex Educators, Counselors, and Therapists (AASECT) at the following address: AASECT, P.O. Box 238, Mount Vernon, IA, 52314-0238 (Phone: 1-319-895-8407; fax 1-319-895-6203).

Bibliography

American Psychiatric Association: Diagnostic and Statistical Manual of Mental Disorders, 4th ed. Washington, DC, American Psychiatric Press, 1994.

Barbach, LG: For Yourself: The Fulfillment of Female Sexuality. New York, Anchor/Doubleday, 1976.

Cheadle, MJ: The screening sexual history. Clin Geriatr Med 1991;7:9–13.

Eyler AE: Sexuality issues and common sexual dysfunctions: evaluation and management in the primary care setting. In Knesper DJ, Riba MB, Schwenk TL (eds): Primary Care Psychiatry, pp 367–386. Philadelphia, WB Saunders Company, 1997.

Janus SS, Janus CL: The Janus Report on Sexual Behavior. New York, John Wiley & Sons, 1993.

Kaplan HS: Disorders of Sexual Desire and Other New Concepts and Techniques in Sex Therapy. New York, Simon & Schuster, 1979.

Kolodny RC, Masters WH, Johnson VE: Textbook of Sexual Medicine. Boston, Little, Brown & Co, 1979.

Swift R: How to Have an Orgasm . . . As Often as You Want. New York, Carol and Graf Publishers, 1993.

128 Pregnancy

Diane D. Homan

Pregnancy should be a planned experience and, when possible, preconception counseling and good gynecologic health care should be provided. Family planning is the establishment of the preferred number and spacing of children. Effective family planning contributes to safe and healthy childbearing and helps reduce the incidence of maternal morbidity, low-birth-weight infants, and infant mortality. Numerous and complex variables influence pregnancy outcomes and infant mortality rates, including demographic, medical, physical, environmental, education, behavioral, and attitudinal factors. Early and regular prenatal care allows for early diagnosis of medical and/or social problems. Prenatal visits also provide the opportunity to educate on health promotion and parenting.

Symptoms

1. Some women notice only amenorrhea in early pregnancy; others have the following symptoms
   a. Breast tenderness
   b. Fatigue
   c. Nausea and/or vomiting
   d. Urinary frequency
   e. Constipation
   f. Emotional changes
2. Throughout the pregnancy, the common discomforts may include heartburn, shortness of breath, varicose veins, leg cramps, leukorrhea, hemorrhoids, backache, skin changes, and abdominal aches and pains.

Key Symptoms

- Breast enlargement and/or tenderness
- Fatigue
- Nausea and/or vomiting

History

Prenatal care should be documented in a good-quality prenatal record, which provides an accurate record of information. The American College of Obstetricians and Gynecologists (ACOG) has developed a comprehensive antepartum record presently available in version 4 (see Appendix, p 640).

1. Menstrual history and previous obstetric history: accurate dates of last normal menstrual period and previous menstrual period; recent contraceptive use; history of preterm labor as an important risk factor in subsequent pregnancies.
2. Past medical and surgical history: drug allergies, anesthetic complications, collagen-vascular disease, diabetes mellitus, hypertension, heart disease, infectious exposures, neurologic disease, psychiatric disease, pulmonary disease, renal disease, thyroid disease
3. Family history with genetic screening and teratology counseling: preferably obtained prior to conception
4. Social history: religious and cultural considerations; employment; social support system, including risk for domestic violence; habits, including smoking, alcohol, and illicit drug use

---

PEARLS

- Identify and initiate special care for obstetric, medical, and psychosocial risks.

- Avoid fetal exposure to teratogenic agents, including tobacco, alcohol, drugs, x-rays.

- Establish an accurate due date, when possible.

Clinical Findings

1. Dental evaluation: caries
2. Thyroid examination
3. Breast examination: abnormal masses
4. Cardiovascular examination: murmurs
5. Respiratory examination
6. Spine examination: scoliosis
7. Abdominal examination: fundal height, fetal movement
8. Pelvic examination: Chadwick's sign (cyanosis of the cervix); Hegar's sign (softening of the lower uterine segment); cervical examination for dilation, effacement, and uterine size; and evaluation of pelvic type and adequacy
9. Extremities: varicose veins, edema

Key Signs

- Amenorrhea
- Cervical changes
- Uterine enlargement

Laboratory Tests

1. Confirmation of pregnancy and establishment of gestational age

    a. Urine human chorionic gonadotropin (hCG) tests: available for home use; positive 10 days after impregnation

    b. Serum hCG tests: available both for qualitative and quantitative analysis when viability in question

    c. Ultrasound: for pregnancy confirmation and dating, when indicated

Key Tests

- hCG: urine or serum
- Ultrasound

2. Required testing

    a. Blood type, D (Rh) type, and antibody screen: for Rh-negative mothers, repeat D (Rh) antibody screen at 28 weeks and administer D immune globulin (RhIG)

    b. Complete blood count at initial visit and hemoglobin and hematocrit at 24 to 28 weeks and 32 to 36 weeks

    c. Serologic tests for rubella and syphilis (Venereal Disease Research Laboratory [VDRL] or rapid plasma reagin [RPR]), hepatitis B surface antigen

    d. Urinalysis and urine culture

    e. Papanicolaou smear

    f. Gonococcus and chlamydia cultures

    g. Maternal serum α-fetoprotein (MSAFP) or multiple markers screening: between 15 and 18 weeks' gestation; should be offered to all pregnant women

    h. Diabetes screening: 1-hour 50-gm glucola at 24 to 28 weeks' gestation; glucose tolerance test (GTT) if screen abnormal; may be done with initial labs if patient is high risk.

Diabetes Screening

- 1-hour 50-gm glucola: abnormal if above 130 mg/dl

- GTT: abnormal test if two or more values are abnormal

    –Fasting blood sugar, 105 mg/dl or less

    –1 hour, 190 mg/dl or less

    –2 hours, 165 mg/dl or less

    –3 hours, 145 mg/dl or less

---

i. Group B streptococcal vaginal-rectal culture: at 35 to 37 weeks; plan intrapartum antibiotic prophylaxis if colonization exists

---

Group B Streptococcal Colonization

- If the culture of the lower vagina and rectum returns positive

- If any urine culture is positive for group B streptococcus

- If the patient has had an infant with group B streptococcal sepsis

- If the patient presents in preterm labor or with preterm rupture of the membranes, treat prophylactically pending results of group B streptococcal vaginal-rectal culture.

---

3. Optional testing

    a. Infectious diseases: hepatitis C antibody, herpes simplex type II, human immunodeficiency virus (HIV) antibody, tuberculosis

    b. Genetic and chromosomal screening: cystic fibrosis, Down's syndrome, hemoglobinopathies, hemophilia, maternal metabolic disorder (including insulin-dependent diabetes or phenylketonuria), muscular dystrophy, sickle cell anemia, Tay-Sachs disease, mental retardation, autism

    c. Hemoglobin electrophoresis

    d. Illicit drug screen

    e. Ultrasound: to assess growth and development of the fetus

    e. Amniocentesis: advanced maternal age, genetic/chromosomal screening, fetal maturity

Key Laboratory Tests

Initial Labs

- Blood type, D (Rh) type, antibody screen
- Complete blood count
- Pap smear
- Rubella
- VDRL/RPR
- Urinalysis/culture
- Hepatitis B surface antigen
- Gonococcus/chlamydia cultures
- HIV counseling/testing
- Hemoglobin electrophoresis, when indicated
- Ultrasound, when indicated

15- to 18-Week Labs

- MSAFP/multiple markers
- Amniocentesis, when indicated and elected

24- to 48-Week Labs

- Hemoglobin/hematocrit
- Diabetes screen
- D (Rh) antibody screen, if Rh negative

32- to 36-Week Labs

- Hemoglobin/hematocrit
- Group B streptococcus culture (35 to 37 weeks)
- Ultrasound, when indicated
- VDRL/RPR, gonococcus, chlamydia, if indicated

Management

Medications

Medications should be taken during pregnancy only as specifically approved or prescribed by the physician. Whenever possible, nonpharmacologic remedies for common ailments are advised. Prenatal vitamins containing folic acid and iron are often recommended.

Diet

A balanced diet is recommended throughout pregnancy and should include four to five servings of dairy products, three or more servings of protein, four or more servings of fruits and vegetables, and three to six servings of grain daily.

1. Caloric needs increase by about 300 cal/day, depending on prepregnancy weight status.
2. Protein requirements are about 10 gm/day above nonpregnant needs.
3. Requirements for all vitamins, with special attention to folic acid, vitamin A, and vitamin C, are increased.
4. Iron and calcium are also required in pregnancy.
5. Water is important.
6. Caffeine and salt should be taken in moderation.
7. Fats and sweets should be kept to a minimum to prevent excess weight gain.

WARNING

Weight loss is not recommended during pregnancy.

Activity

All pregnant women should be physically active throughout pregnancy, unless a medical contraindication is identified, to maintain muscle tone, flexibility, and strength.

1. Most established exercise routines can be continued. As the uterus enlarges, activities that may lead to falls should be avoided.
2. Regular aerobic exercise is an important component of healthy pregnancy. Walking, stationary biking, and swimming provide safe exercise.
3. Avoid overheating, dehydration, discomfort, and fatigue.
4. Rest is as important as exercise.
5. Breathing exercises are taught to promote relaxation, provide contraction practice, and teach abdominal breathing.
6. Kegel exercises are designed to strengthen the pelvic floor muscles and allow for relaxation of these muscles for delivery.

Key Activities

- Regular aerobic exercise
- Breathing exercises
- Kegel exercises

Patient Education

A woman's interest in education during pregnancy changes as she progresses through per pregnancy.

Childbirth classes are encouraged for all first-time parents. Sibling classes should be considered when appropriate.

1. During the first trimester, most women are interested in learning more about themselves and the physical and emotional changes that result from the pregnancy.
   a. Expectations of care during the pregnancy
   b. Vaginal birth after cesarean section counseling, when appropriate
   c. Education of maternal health improvement: nutrition counseling; physical and sexual activity; lifestyle changes, including tobacco, alcohol, and drug cessation; environmental and work hazards, including toxoplasmosis precautions; travel; and management of the discomforts of pregnancy
2. As the pregnancy progresses, the woman's awareness of the fetus as a person increases. The educational focus becomes fetal growth and development, planning for the baby, and parenting.
   a. Childbirth classes
   b. Feeding preference: breast versus bottle
   c. Newborn safety, including car seat
   d. Circumcision
3. By the third trimester, women become introspective, with interest in the labor and delivery process as well as the needs of others in the family.
   a. Labor signs and course of labor
   b. Anesthesia plans
   c. Postpartum contraception, including tubal sterilization counseling, when appropriate

Follow-Up

Content of Prenatal Care

Visits during the prenatal period provide a unique opportunity to identify pregnancy complications early and to provide education and health maintenance education. For uncomplicated pregnancy, office visits are scheduled monthly until 28 weeks, then every 2 to 3 weeks until 36 weeks, then weekly until delivery. Office visit frequency can be increased appropriately should any complications develop. Each visit should include three components: (1) early and continuing risk assessment; (2) health promotion; and (3) medical, nutritional, and psychosocial interventions and follow-up.

1. Weight: weight gain of 10 pounds by 20 weeks, then 1 pound weekly until term
2. Blood pressure
3. Urine glucose/protein
4. Presence of edema
5. Fundal height: Uterine enlargement correlates closely with fetal growth throughout pregnancy. Fundal height reaches the umbilicus at 20 weeks' gestation and grows 1 cm weekly until term.
6. Fetal movement: Quickening occurs at 18 to 20 weeks; during last trimester, fetal movement should be perceived at least 10 times in 2 hours.
7. Fetal position and heart rate: detectable by Doppler at 10 to 12 weeks or by fetoscope at 16 to 20 weeks
8. Contractions: Braxton Hicks versus preterm labor
9. Cervical changes: dilation and effacement

Postpartum

Postpartum visit is normally scheduled 4 to 6 weeks after delivery to assess healing and restoration of the reproductive organs as well as to assess general adaptation and maternal and family responses to childrearing.

PEARL

The postpartum visit is an opportunity for

- Risk detection and health monitoring
- Health education, including family planning and contraception
- Assessment of psychosocial supports

Bibliography

American College of Obstetricians and Gynecologists: Exercise During Pregnancy and the Postpartum Period (Technical Bulletin no 189). Washington, DC, American College of Obstetricians and Gynecologists, 1994.

American College of Obstetricians and Gynecologists: Nutrition During Pregnancy (Technical Bulletin no 179). Washington, DC, American College of Obstetricians and Gynecologists, 1993.

Johnson TRB, Walker MA, Niebyl JR: Preconception and prenatal care. In Gabbe SG, Niebyl JR, Simpson JL, et al (eds): Obstetrics: Normal & Problem Pregnancies, 3rd ed, pp 161–184. New York, Churchill Livingstone, 1996.

Prenatal care. In Cunningham FG, MacDonald PC, Gant NF, et al (eds): Williams' Obstetrics, 20th ed, pp 227–250. Stamford, CT, Appleton & Lange, 1997.

Samuels M, Samuels N: Prenatal care and medical concerns. In The New Well Pregnancy Book. New York, Simon & Schuster, 1996.

ACOG Antepartum Record

Patient Addressograph

DATE _____

NAME _____

    LAST   FIRST   MIDDLE

ID # _____ HOSPITAL OF DELIVERY _____

NEWBORN'S PHYSICIAN _____ REFERRED BY_____

FINAL EDD_____ PRIMARY PROVIDER/GROUP _____

BIRTH DATE	AGE	RACE	MARITAL STATUS	ADDRESS:		
MONTH DAY YEAR			S M W D SEP			
OCCUPATION		EDUCATION		ZIP:	PHONE: (H)	(O)
☐ HOMEMAKER		(LAST GRADE COMPLETED)		INSURANCE CARRIER/MEDICAID #		
☐ OUTSIDE WORK						
☐ STUDENT	Type of Work					
HUSBAND/FATHER OF BABY:			PHONE:	EMERGENCY CONTACT:		PHONE:

TOTAL PREG	FULL TERM	PREMATURE	AB, INDUCED	AB, SPONTANEOUS	ECTOPICS	MULTIPLE BIRTHS	LIVING

MENSTRUAL HISTORY

LMP ☐ DEFINITE ☐ APPROXIMATE (MONTH KNOWN)   MENSES MONTHLY ☐ YES ☐ NO   FREQUENCY: Q _____ DAYS   MENARCHE _____ (AGE ONSET)

☐ UNKNOWN ☐ NORMAL AMOUNT/DURATION   PRIOR MENSES _____ DATE   ON BCP AT CONCEPT. ☐ YES ☐ NO   hCG + _____ / _____ / _____

☐ FINAL _____

PAST PREGNANCIES (LAST SIX)

DATE MONTH / YEAR	GA WEEKS	LENGTH OF LABOR	BIRTH WEIGHT	SEX M/F	TYPE DELIVERY	ANES.	PLACE OF DELIVERY	PRETERM LABOR YES / NO	COMMENTS / COMPLICATIONS

PAST MEDICAL HISTORY

	O Neg + Pos.	DETAIL POSITIVE REMARKS INCLUDE DATE & TREATMENT		O Neg + Pos.	DETAIL POSITIVE REMARKS INCLUDE DATE & TREATMENT
1. DIABETES			16. D (Rh) SENSITIZED		
2. HYPERTENSION			17. PULMONARY (TB, ASTHMA)		
3. HEART DISEASE			18. ALLERGIES (DRUGS)		
4. AUTOIMMUNE DISORDER			19. BREAST		
5. KIDNEY DISEASE / UTI			20. GYN SURGERY		
6. NEUROLOGIC/EPILEPSY					
7. PSYCHIATRIC			21. OPERATIONS / HOSPITALIZATIONS (YEAR & REASON)		
8. HEPATITIS / LIVER DISEASE					
9. VARICOSITIES / PHLEBITIS					
10. THYROID DYSFUNCTION			22. ANESTHETIC COMPLICATIONS		
11. TRAUMA/DOMESTIC VIOLENCE			23. HISTORY OF ABNORMAL PAP		
12. HISTORY OF BLOOD TRANSFUS.			24. UTERINE ANOMALY/DES		
	AMT/DAY PREPREG	AMT/DAY PREG	#YEARS USE	25. INFERTILITY	
13. TOBACCO				26. RELEVANT FAMILY HISTORY	
14. ALCOHOL					
15. STREET DRUGS				27. OTHER	

COMMENTS: _____

The American College of Obstetricians and Gynecologists, 409 12th Street, SW, PO Box 96920, Washington, DC 20090-6920

ACOG ANTEPARTUM RECORD (FORM A)

<table>
<tr><td colspan="2">SYMPTOMS SINCE LMP</td></tr>
<tr><td></td><td></td></tr>
<tr><td></td><td></td></tr>
<tr><td></td><td></td></tr>
<tr><td></td><td></td></tr>
<tr><td></td><td></td></tr>
</table>

GENETIC SCREENING/TERATOLOGY COUNSELING
INCLUDES PATIENT, BABY'S FATHER, OR ANYONE IN EITHER FAMILY WITH:

	YES	NO		YES	NO
1. PATIENT'S AGE ≥ 35 YEARS			12. MENTAL RETARDATION/AUTISM		
2. THALASSEMIA (ITALIAN, GREEK, MEDITERRANEAN, OR ASIAN BACKGROUND): MCV < 80			IF YES, WAS PERSON TESTED FOR FRAGILE X?		
3. NEURAL TUBE DEFECT (MENINGOMYELOCELE, SPINA BIFIDA, OR ANENCEPHALY)			13. OTHER INHERITED GENETIC OR CHROMOSOMAL DISORDER		
4. CONGENITAL HEART DEFECT			14. MATERNAL METABOLIC DISORDER (EG. INSULIN-DEPENDENT DIABETES, PKU)		
5. DOWN SYNDROME			15. PATIENT OR BABY'S FATHER HAD A CHILD WITH BIRTH DEFECTS NOT LISTED ABOVE		
6. TAY–SACHS (EG, JEWISH, CAJUN, FRENCH CANADIAN)			16. RECURRENT PREGNANCY LOSS, OR A STILLBIRTH		
7. SICKLE CELL DISEASE OR TRAIT (AFRICAN)			17. MEDICATIONS/STREET DRUGS/ALCOHOL SINCE LAST MENSTRUAL PERIOD		
8. HEMOPHILIA			IF YES, AGENT(S):		
9. MUSCULAR DYSTROPHY					
10. CYSTIC FIBROSIS			18. ANY OTHER		
11. HUNTINGTON CHOREA					

COMMENTS/COUNSELING: _____
_____
_____

INFECTION HISTORY	YES	NO		YES	NO
1. HIGH RISK HEPATITIS B/IMMUNIZED?			4. RASH OR VIRAL ILLNESS SINCE LAST MENSTRUAL PERIOD		
2. LIVE WITH SOMEONE WITH TB OR EXPOSED TO TB			5. HISTORY OF STD, GC, CHLAMYDIA, HPV, SYPHILIS		
3. PATIENT OR PARTNER HAS HISTORY OF GENITAL HERPES			6. OTHER (SEE COMMENTS)		

COMMENTS: _____
_____
_____ INTERVIEWER'S SIGNATURE _____

INITIAL PHYSICAL EXAMINATION

DATE _____ / _____ / _____   PREPREGNANCY WEIGHT _____   HEIGHT _____   BP_____

1. HEENT	☐ NORMAL	☐ ABNORMAL	12. VULVA	☐ NORMAL	☐ CONDYLOMA	☐ LESIONS
2. FUNDI	☐ NORMAL	☐ ABNORMAL	13. VAGINA	☐ NORMAL	☐ INFLAMMATION	☐ DISCHARGE
3. TEETH	☐ NORMAL	☐ ABNORMAL	14. CERVIX	☐ NORMAL	☐ INFLAMMATION	☐ LESIONS
4. THYROID	☐ NORMAL	☐ ABNORMAL	15. UTERUS SIZE	_____ WEEKS		☐ FIBROIDS
5. BREASTS	☐ NORMAL	☐ ABNORMAL	16. ADNEXA	☐ NORMAL	☐ MASS	
6. LUNGS	☐ NORMAL	☐ ABNORMAL	17. RECTUM	☐ NORMAL	☐ ABNORMAL	
7. HEART	☐ NORMAL	☐ ABNORMAL	18. DIAGONAL CONJUGATE	☐ REACHED	☐ NO	_____ CM
8. ABDOMEN	☐ NORMAL	☐ ABNORMAL	19. SPINES	☐ AVERAGE	☐ PROMINENT	☐ BLUNT
9. EXTREMITIES	☐ NORMAL	☐ ABNORMAL	20. SACRUM	☐ CONCAVE	☐ STRAIGHT	☐ ANTERIOR
10. SKIN	☐ NORMAL	☐ ABNORMAL	21. SUBPUBIC ARCH	☐ NORMAL	☐ WIDE	☐ NARROW
11. LYMPH NODES	☐ NORMAL	☐ ABNORMAL	22. GYNECOID PELVIC TYPE	☐ YES	☐ NO	

COMMENTS (Number and explain abnormals): _____
_____
_____ EXAM BY _____

ACOG ANTEPARTUM RECORD (FORM B)

NAME _____

LAST   FIRST   MIDDLE

DRUG ALLERGY:

RELIGIOUS/CULTURAL CONSIDERATIONS _____   ANESTHESIA CONSULT PLANNED   ☐ YES   ☐ NO

PROBLEMS/PLANS	MEDICATION LIST:	Start date	Stop date
1.	1.		
2.	2.		
3.	3.		
4.	4.		
5.	5.		
6.	6.		

EDD CONFIRMATION

INITIAL EDD:

LMP   ____ / ____ / ____   = EDD ____ / ____ / ____

INITIAL EXAM   ____ / ____ / ____ = ____ WKS = EDD ____ / ____ / ____

ULTRASOUND   ____ / ____ / ____ = ____ WKS = EDD ____ / ____ / ____

INITIAL EDD   ____ / ____ / ____   INITIALED BY _____

18–20-WEEK EDD UPDATE:

QUICKENING   ____ / ____ / ____   +22 WKS = ____ / ____ / ____

FUNDAL HT. AT UMBIL.   ____ / ____ / ____   +20 WKS = ____ / ____ / ____

FHT W/FETOSCOPE   ____ / ____ / ____   +20 WKS = ____ / ____ / ____

ULTRASOUND   ____ / ____ / ____   = ___ WKS = ____ / ____ / ____

FINAL EDD   ____ / ____ / ____   INITIALED BY _____

VISIT DATE (YEAR)	WEEKS GEST. (BEST EST.)	FUNDAL HEIGHT (CM)	PRESENTATION	FHR	FETAL MOVEMENT	PRETERM LABOR SIGNS/SYMPTOMS: +=PRESENT 0=ABSENT	CERVIX EXAM (DIL./EFF./STA.)	BLOOD PRESSURE	EDEMA	WEIGHT	URINE (GLUCOSE/ALBUMIN)	NEXT APPOINTMENT	PROVIDER (INITIALS)	COMMENTS:

PROBLEMS: _____

COMMENTS: _____

ACOG ANTEPARTUM RECORD (FORM C)

LABORATORY AND EDUCATION

INITIAL LABS	DATE	RESULT	REVIEWED
BLOOD TYPE	/ /	A B AB O	
D (Rh) TYPE	/ /		
ANTIBODY SCREEN	/ /		
HCT/HGB	/ /	_____ % _____ g/dL	
PAP TEST	/ /	NORMAL / ABNORMAL / _____	
RUBELLA	/ /		
VDRL	/ /		
URINE CULTURE/SCREEN	/ /		
HBsAg	/ /		
HIV COUNSELING/TESTING	/ /	☐ POS. ☐ NEG. ☐ DECLINED	

OPTIONAL LABS	DATE	RESULT
HGB ELECTROPHORESIS	/ /	AA AS SS AC SC AF ↑A$_2$
PPD	/ /	
CHLAMYDIA	/ /	
GC	/ /	
TAY–SACHS	/ /	
OTHER		

8–18-WEEK LABS (WHEN INDICATED/ELECTED)	DATE	RESULT
ULTRASOUND	/ /	
MSAFP/MULTIPLE MARKERS	/ /	
AMNIO/CVS	/ /	
KARYOTYPE	/ /	46, XX OR 46, XY / OTHER_____
AMNIOTIC FLUID (AFP)	/ /	NORMAL_____ ABNORMAL_____

24–28-WEEK LABS (WHEN INDICATED)	DATE	RESULT
HCT/HGB	/ /	_____ % _____ g/dL
DIABETES SCREEN	/ /	1 HOUR_____
GTT (IF SCREEN ABNORMAL)	/ /	_____FBS _____1 HOUR _____2 HOUR _____3 HOUR
D (Rh) ANTIBODY SCREEN	/ /	
D IMMUNE GLOBULIN (RhIG) GIVEN (28 WKS)	/ /	SIGNATURE _____

32–36-WEEK LABS (WHEN INDICATED)	DATE	RESULT
HCT/HGB (RECOMMENDED)	/ /	_____ % _____ g/dL
ULTRASOUND	/ /	
VDRL	/ /	
GC	/ /	
CHLAMYDIA	/ /	
GROUP B STREP (35–37 WKS)	/ /	

COMMENTS/ADDITIONAL LABS

PLANS/EDUCATION (COUNSELED ☐)

☐ ANESTHESIA PLANS _____
☐ TOXOPLASMOSIS PRECAUTIONS (CATS/RAW MEAT) _____
☐ CHILDBIRTH CLASSES _____
☐ PHYSICAL/SEXUAL ACTIVITY _____
☐ LABOR SIGNS _____
☐ NUTRITION COUNSELING _____
☐ BREAST OR BOTTLE FEEDING _____
☐ NEWBORN CAR SEAT _____
☐ POSTPARTUM BIRTH CONTROL _____
☐ ENVIRONMENTAL/WORK HAZARDS _____

☐ TUBAL STERILIZATION _____
☐ VBAC COUNSELING _____
☐ CIRCUMCISION _____
☐ TRAVEL _____
☐ LIFESTYLE, TOBACCO, ALCOHOL _____

REQUESTS _____
_____

TUBAL STERILIZATION   DATE   INITIALS
CONSENT SIGNED   _____ / _____ / _____   _____

AA128   12345/10987

PROVIDER SIGNATURE (AS REQUIRED) _____

ACOG ANTEPARTUM RECORD (FORM D)

NAME _____
              LAST   FIRST   MIDDLE

ID # _____

Supplemental Visits

VISIT DATE (YEAR)	WEEKS GEST. (BEST EST.)	FUNDAL HEIGHT (CM)	PRESENTATION	FHR	FETAL MOVEMENT	PRETERM LABOR SIGNS/SYMPTOMS: +=PRESENT O=ABSENT	CERVIX EXAM (DIL./EFF./STA.)	BLOOD PRESSURE	EDEMA	WEIGHT	URINE (GLUCOSE/ALBUMIN)	NEXT APPOINTMENT	PROVIDER (INITIALS)	COMMENTS:
														_____
														_____
														_____
														_____
														_____
														_____
														_____
														_____
														_____
														_____
														_____
														_____
														_____
														_____
														_____
														_____
														_____

Progress Notes

_____

_____

_____

_____

_____

_____

_____

_____

_____

_____

PROVIDER SIGNATURE (AS REQUIRED) _____

The American College of Obstetricians and Gynecologists, 409 12th Street, SW, PO Box 96920, Washington, DC 20090-6920

ACOG ANTEPARTUM RECORD (FORM E, *continued*)

Indications

1. Episiotomies do not decrease perineal trauma, prevent pelvic relaxation, improve postpartum perineal healing, or prevent fetal distress. Having an episiotomy increases the rate of perineal lacerations and trauma up to 50 times and predisposes women to third- or fourth-degree lacerations. Rectal injuries are 8.9 times more likely in women with episiotomies. Women without episiotomies have less postpartum pain and are more likely to resume sexual intercourse within 1 month. There has been no proven beneficial effect of episiotomies for the infant. Episiotomy rates have declined only 13 per cent in the last decade in the United States.

2. Episiotomies may help with the delivery of a large infant who has a shoulder dystocia.

Contraindications

Bleeding disorders and severe scarring on the perineum are contraindications.

Preparation

1. Sterile procedure should be maintained. The woman can be redraped after delivery.

2. The operator may wish to place a packing gauze in the vagina.

3. Inspect the cervix and vagina for lacerations after delivery, and stop bleeding, if possible.

4. The operator may need fresh sterile gloves after the delivery.

Equipment

1. Standard laceration repair equipment should be present, including pickups, long scissors, two needle holders, and 4×4 sponges.

2. In addition, the following specific equipment should be available: packing gauze, two Allis clamps, one Gelpi clamp, one ring forceps, a straight catheter, and lubrication.

3. Two to three packages of 3-0 or 2-0 synthetic absorbable suture material (Dexon or Vicryl). Compared with catgut, their use is associated with a 40 per cent decrease in short-term pain and need for analgesia.

4. For repair of fourth-degree lacerations, one package of absorbable 4-0 synthetic suture material is needed.

Anesthesia

1. Usually the anesthesia used for delivery is sufficient for repair of an episiotomy or lacerations.

2. Additional local anesthesia can be used. Lidocaine 1% or 2% without epinephrine infiltrated in the laceration may help immensely.

Technique

Episiotomy

1. Cut a midline episiotomy, if required, after the perineum is thinned by the pressure of the fetal head. The surgeon places index and middle fingers into the posterior vagina between the fetal head and the vagina, one finger on each side of the midline, and cuts between the fingers downward and posteriorly on the midline. One cut with scissors at this point will incise both the posterior wall of the vagina and the perineum from the posterior vaginal opening posteriorly toward but not into the rectal capsule.

2. Delivery usually occurs soon. If not, light pressure on the episiotomy incision with a 4×4 bandage will decrease the amount of bleeding.

Repair

1. Determine the depth and degree of episiotomy and lacerations. Lacerations are considered first-degree if only superficial skin or vaginal wall is torn and second-degree if the laceration extends into subcutaneous tissues down to fascia. A laceration is considered third-degree if it extends through the external anal sphincter and fourth-degree if it tears through into the rectal mucosa.

2. Repair of the second-degree episiotomy requires reconstruction in layers. Start with repair of the posterior vaginal wall. Place the first stitch approximately 1 cm proximal to the deepest extension of the episiotomy on the vaginal wall. Place the stitch 1 cm to each side of the midline defined by the episiotomy, and tie.

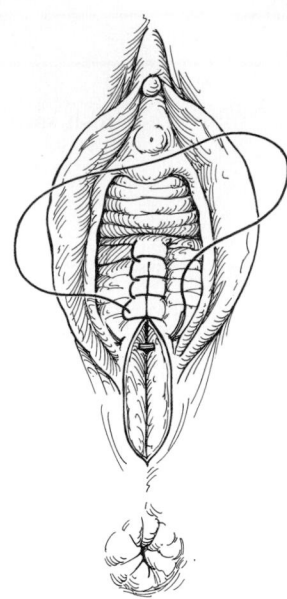

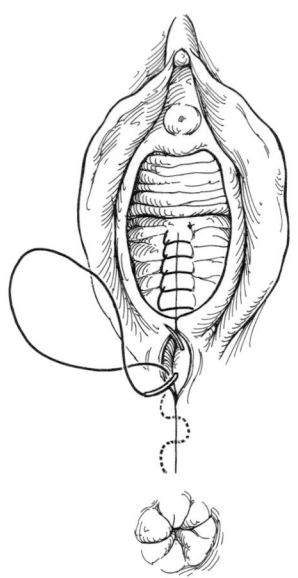

neum. Sew posteriorly down the perineum with a continuous nonlocking suture, bringing the edges together; the perineum should lie closed at the end of this layer. The final layer is sewn anteriorly toward the vagina as a subcuticular continuous layer. The last stitch is brought into the vagina and tied.

3. Using a continuous "locking" stitch, place sutures approximately 1 cm apart, each approximately 1 cm from the edge of the incision, working toward the introitus. Make the sutures shallow, approximately 0.5 cm below the posterior vaginal wall. Match the edges of the hymenal ring. Stop at the introitus, putting this suture down. Some experts choose to make a knot at this point.

4. Unless the episiotomy is very superficial or if there is a third- or fourth-degree laceration, the next step is to place three to four deep interrupted sutures using a new suture, bringing the edges of the perineum together. These stitches should be approximately 1 cm apart; the most posterior stitch should be 1 cm above the exterior anal sphincter.

First- and Second-Degree Lacerations

1. First- and second-degree periurethral lacerations are common and usually are easily repaired. If bleeding has stopped and the edges are less than 1 cm apart, no suturing is necessary. If the lacerations are larger or hemorrhaging, one or two figure-of-eight sutures should bring the edges together and are sufficient. If the lacerations are very close to the urethra or the urethra is swollen, a red rubber intermittent catheter can be placed in the urethra while stitching is done to prevent inadvertent closure of the urethra.

2. First- and second-degree lacerations of the posterior vaginal wall should be repaired before the episiotomy is repaired. Start the repair the same way as the repair of the episiotomy. Place the first stitch 1 cm deep or proximal to the furthest extension of the tear. Tie the first stitch, and then proceed with a locking continuous repair. The suture can be tied off before episiotomy repair or continued right into the episiotomy.

Third- and Fourth-Degree Lacerations

1. Use a Gelpi clamp to hold the laceration apart, and place one Allis clamp on each edge of the torn rectal sphincter.

2. Start the repair by suturing the anterior rectal wall, if needed, with a row of interrupted sutures of 4-0 synthetic absorbable suture. Carry the stitch submucosal to the mucosa of the an-

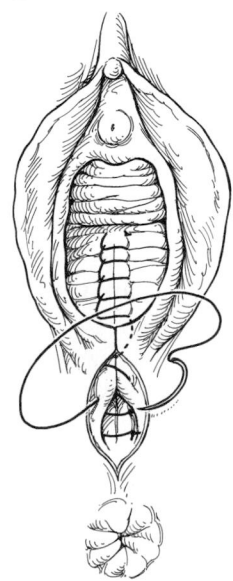

5. Then, taking up the first suture, bring the needle from the vagina under the hymen to the peri-

terior wall of the rectum to approximate the mucosa without the suture entering the rectal lumen.

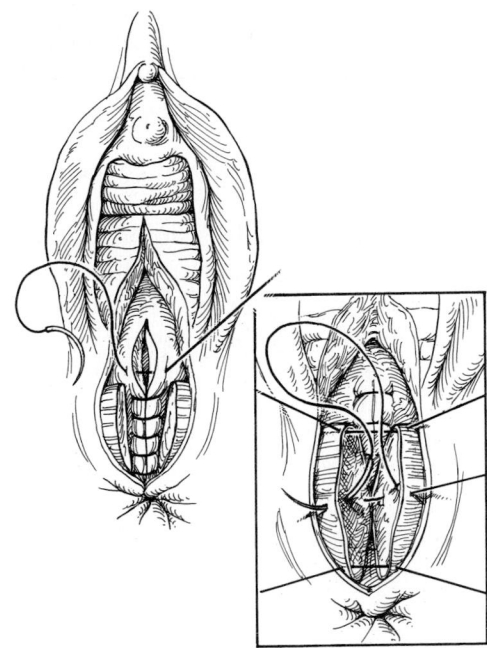

3. Then, holding the Allis clamps in one hand, place four interrupted 2-0 or 3-0 sutures into the fascial wall of the rectal sphincter. Place one below, one behind, and one above the torn muscle, and then, releasing the Allis and Gelpi clamps, place one in front of the muscle. This will bring the donut-shaped muscle back together.

4. Repair the remaining laceration as one would a second-degree episiotomy.

Follow-Up

1. Routine follow-up includes warm sitz baths two to four times a day and local anesthetic gels if needed. Nonsteroidal analgesia will relieve pain.

2. Infection can occur, as evidenced by foul odor and discharge. Treatment includes antibiotics, sitz baths, and possibly removal of suture material.

B | Bibliography

Graham ID, Graham DF: Episiotomy counts: trends and prevalence in Canada 1981/82 and 1993/94. Birth 1997;24:141–147.

Hagymasy L, Gaal J: A comparative study of vertical and horizontal deliveries in the presence and with the assistance of the woman's partner. J Psychosom Obstet Gynecol 1998;19:98–103.

Kaczorowski J, Levitt C, Hanvey L, et al: A national survey of use of obstetric procedures and technologies in Canadian hospitals. Birth 1998;25:11–18.

Labrecque M, Baillargeon L, Dallaire M, et al: Association between median episiotomy and severe perineal lacerations in primiparous women. CMAJ 1997;156:797–802.

Sultan AH, Kamm MA, Hudson CN, et al: Anal-sphincter disruption during vaginal delivery. N Engl J Med 1993;328:1906–1911.

129 Breast-Feeding

Rebecca Williams

Breast milk is the recommended food for infants. Although physician involvement is primarily through advocacy and counseling, conditions do arise that require medical treatment. Listed below are the steps involved in breast-feeding promotion and support.

Physician Promotion of Breast-Feeding

Because women who decide to breast-feed before or early in pregnancy are far more likely to succeed, breast-feeding promotion ideally should precede pregnancy. This process of counseling and support occurs best in offices and hospitals that are breast-feeding friendly.

Breast-Feeding–Friendly Office
1. Distribute educational materials.
2. Provide private space for breast-feeding.
3. Avoid formula promotion.
4. Educate office staff about breast-feeding concerns.

Annual Exams
1. Discuss breast-feeding with women contemplating pregnancy.
2. Emphasize benefits to the infant:
   a. Decreased episodes of diarrhea, pneumonia, meningitis, otitis media
   b. Fewer office visits and hospitalizations
   c. Fewer food allergies
   d. Decreased incidence of some cancers
3. Advise of benefits to the mother:
   a. Decreased fertility while nursing
   b. Faster return to prepregnancy weight
   c. Convenient and economical
   d. Enhanced bonding with infant

Prenatal Visits
1. Discuss infant feeding decisions at the first prenatal visit.
2. Emphasize benefits.
3. Explore reasons behind the decision to bottle-feed.

Social Support and Prenatal Instruction
1. Identify a support person with breast-feeding experience.
2. Consider referral to the local chapter of the La Leche League.
3. At term, review the basic processes of positioning and latch-on.
   a. Latch-on: attachment of the baby to the nipple. The infant's mouth should be as far back on the areola as possible with lips turned outward.
   b. Positioning: Cradle, side-lying, and football positions all involve the infant facing the breast with the neck straight. The football position is very useful after cesarean section.
4. Anticipate and address common problems.
5. Consider referral to a prenatal breast-feeding class.

Hospital Care
Advocate a "baby friendly" hospital. The UNICEF/WHO 10-step guidelines are based on proven methods of hospital based breast-feeding support.
1. Develop a written hospital policy on breast-feeding and communicate the policy to staff.
2. Train all health care staff to implement this policy.
3. Inform all pregnant women about the benefits and management of breast-feeding.
4. Help mothers initiate breast-feeding within 30 minutes of birth.
5. Show mothers how to breast-feed and maintain lactation if separated from their infants.
6. Give newborns no food or drink other than breast milk unless medically indicated.
7. Practice rooming-in.
8. Encourage breast-feeding on demand.
9. Give no pacifiers.
10. Foster the establishment of breast-feeding support groups.

Physician Support of Breast-Feeding

Most women who stop breast-feeding prematurely do so in the first 10 days of lactation. Two common problems account for most cases: breast or nipple pain and fears about inadequate milk supply. Physicians can support breast-feeding by providing anticipatory guidance and proper treatment for the conditions.

Breast and Nipple Pain

Etiology

1. Improper positioning and latch-on cause nipple trauma.
2. Infrequent early breast-feeding causes lymphatic swelling, engorgement.
3. Bacteria (generally staphylococci or streptococci) invade the traumatized nipple, causing mastitis.
4. Inadequately treated mastitis leads to breast abscess.
5. *Candida* infection causes breast and nipple pain.

Diagnosis

1. Persistent nipple pain
   a. *Candida* infection: stabbing or burning pain. Nipple may appear normal or exhibit an erythematous satellite rash.
   b. Sore nipples: common in the first few days of lactation. Nipple appears macerated and may be fissured.
2. Breast pain
   a. Engorgement: day 2 to 3 of lactation with bilateral breast swelling and low-grade fever
   b. Mastitis: fever with unilateral breast pain and a wedge-shaped area of erythema. Early symptoms resemble the "flu."
   c. Breast abscess occurs with unresolved mastitis. Ultrasound with or without needle aspiration may be helpful to diagnose and guide treatment.

Treatment

1. Observe breast-feeding for proper technique.
2. Engorgement is treated with frequent feedings, compresses, and analgesics.
3. Initiate feedings on less affected breast.
4. Sore nipples: Allow nipples to air dry, apply purified lanolin for comfort.
5. *Candida*: Treat both mother and infant (even if asymptomatic) with topical and/or oral antifungal agents.
   a. Nystatin is the drug of choice for infants.
   b. Ketoconazole (Nizoral) cream applied topically at least qid for mothers
   c. Oral fluconazole (Diflucan), 100 mg daily, for mothers with recurrent infection
6. Mastitis: Continue breast-feeding, analgesics, antibiotics.

a. Cephalexin (Keflex), 500 mg PO every 6 hours for 10 to 14 days
b. Dicloxacillin (Dynapen), 500 mg PO every 6 hours for 10 to 14 days
7. Abscess: Continued breast feeding or pumping; antibiotics; needle aspiration every 2 to 3 days or open drainage.
8. Recurrent mastitis: Treat as for mastitis and consider antibiotic suppression with erythromycin, 250 mg bid.

Prevention

1. Prenatal education
   a. Proper positioning and latch-on
   b. Importance of frequent (every 1 to 2 hours) early feedings
2. Early lactation support
   a. Confirmation of technique
   b. Encouragement
   c. Patient education
      (1) Pain persisting beyond the first few minutes of feeding is abnormal.
      (2) Fever or pain requires urgent evaluation (within 24 hours).

Fears About Inadequate Milk Supply

Treatment/Prevention

1. Patient/staff education on normal breast-feeding physiology
   a. Colostrum: produced for 3 to 5 days; high in calories, rich in immunoglobulins. Small amounts (3 to 5 ml per feed) provide sufficient nourishment for healthy newborns.
   b. Milk supply: produced on demand; the breast responds to suckling by increased production. Frequent early feedings produce sufficient supply in vast majority. Once established, feeding on demand will regulate supply.
2. Evaluating adequacy of feedings.
   a. The newborn that sucks well and cries loudly is adequately nourished.
   b. Urine and stool output increase daily, with stools gradually changing from green to yellow. After the fifth day of life, expect five voids and three yellow stools per day.
   c. Abandon measurement of weight before and after feeds. Hospital infant scales are not sufficiently accurate to measure weight changes associated with intake of a few milliliters of fluid.
   d. Measuring milk expressed by a breast pump underestimates intake from breast-feeding. Pumping may interfere with latch-on.

Follow-Up for Breast-Feeding Infants

1. Early office follow-up: 3 days for 24-hour discharge and 1 week for others
2. See infants frequently (at least weekly) until weight gain is adequate (30 gm/day).
3. Anticipatory guidance: jaundice, growth spurts, breast milk expression, return to work, and signs of illness.

Bibliography

Bear K, Tigges B: Management strategies for promoting successful breastfeeding. Nurse Pract 1993;18:52–58.

Cunningham A, Jelliffe D, Jelliffe E: Breast-feeding and health in the 1980s: a global epidemiologic review. J Pediatr 1991;118:659–666.

Lawrence R: The clinician's role in teaching proper infant feeding techniques. J Pediatr 1995;126:S112–S117.

Newman J: Breast-feeding: the problem of "not enough milk." Can Fam Physician 1986;32:571–574.

Saadeh R, Akre J: Ten steps to successful breast-feeding: a summary of the rationale and scientific evidence. J Birth 1996;23:154–160.

130 Preterm Labor

Tracey Lee Norton

Etiology

1. History of previous preterm labor
2. Dehydration
3. Chorioamnionitis, often associated with premature rupture of membranes (PROM)
4. Extrauterine infections
   a. Urinary tract infection: most common
   b. Vaginal infections: Trichomoniasis and bacterial vaginosis very common.
   c. Some association seen with severe respiratory infections.
5. Uterine structural defects
   a. Incompetent cervix
   b. Leiomyomata
   c. Septate uterus
6. Excessive uterine enlargement
   a. Hydramnios
   b. Multiple gestation
   c. Macrosomia
7. Placental abnormalities or insufficiency
   a. Abruptio placentae
   b. Placenta previa
   c. Marginal cord insertion
8. Maternal smoking
9. Substance abuse
10. Other serious maternal conditions
    a. Abdominal: surgery, cholecystitis, pancreatitis, peritonitis
    b. Trauma
    c. Diabetes
    d. Hypertension
11. Psychosocial stresses: socioeconomic, emotional, or occupational
12. Iatrogenic: induction of labor

Symptoms

1. Abdominal cramping: may or may not be associated with diarrhea
2. Backache: described as low and dull; may come and go, unaffected by position change
3. Increase in vaginal discharge: watery, blood tinged; passage of mucous plug
4. PROM
5. Menstrual-like cramping: May be constant or intermittent.
6. Pelvic pressure or ache
7. Uterine contractions every 10 minutes or closer: May be painless or only mildly uncomfortable.

Key Symptoms

- Uterine contractions
- Backache
- Abdominal cramping
- Increased or changes in vaginal discharge
- Menstrual cramping
- Fluid leakage
- Pelvic pressure

Clinical Findings

History

1. Obtain a detailed history of the patient's symptoms: onset of pain, intensity, duration, frequency, location.
2. Assess the presence, quality, and quantity of vaginal discharge with the focus on infection, amniotic fluid loss, and/or bleeding.
3. Review the dating criteria of the pregnancy.
   a. Reliable menstrual dates?
   b. Ultrasounds done early in the pregnancy?
   c. Review the prenatal record; do dates and uterine size and growth correlate?
4. Review maternal history for presence of risk factors or obstetric problems such as diabetes, hypertension, smoking, known fetal growth delay.
5. Complete review of systems to identify other maternal problems that affect evaluation and management. Include history of fever, dysuria, malaise, and flu-like symptoms or history of trauma.

Physical Examination

1. General physical examination to identify fever, hypertension, abdominal pain, trauma, or signs of infection

2. Cervical dilatation or effacement in a preterm patient is a warning sign.
   a. Nulliparous cervix less than 2 cm long or open early in pregnancy indicates increased risk.
   b. Multiparous cervix greater than 2 to 3 cm dilated at 28 weeks indicates increased risk.

3. Diagnosis of active preterm labor relies on the findings of abnormal uterine activity and ruptured membranes or cervical change (significant dilatation or effacement) with intact membranes.
   a. External electronic fetal monitoring is performed routinely for at least 30 minutes to identify the frequency and duration of uterine contractions.
   b. Uterine contractions: four in 20 minutes or eight in 60 minutes
   c. Greater than 2 cm dilatation or 75 per cent effacement in the presence of active contractions defines established preterm labor.

4. An experienced examiner should also palpate the uterus to assess the intensity of contractions as well as evaluate fetal size and presentation.

5. Subtle changes in cervical dilatation and effacement on serial examinations are important to diagnosis and to evaluation of management of preterm labor. When possible, serial examinations should be performed by the same examiner.

Ultrasound

1. Sonographic evidence for cervical change may be helpful by providing documentation of threatened preterm labor.

2. Gestational age
   a. When confronted with potential preterm labor/delivery, this is one of the most important determinations to be made.
   b. When the mother and fetus are deemed stable, obtain fetal biometric measurements.

3. Fetal weight is estimated from biometrics. Although error is inherent in the estimation of fetal weight by sonography, birth weight is the cornerstone for immediate neonatal prognosis, so determination of fetal weight is useful for predelivery counseling and preparation for delivery.

4. Data indicate that preterm labor and delivery may be associated with suboptimal fetal growth.

   a. At the lower limits of fetal viability (i.e., 22 to 26 weeks), sonography may underestimate fetal age, resulting in the declaration that a fetus is previable.
   b. At the other end of the prematurity spectrum (32 to 36 weeks), it is not uncommon to find fetal pulmonary maturity at amniocentesis, a case of suboptimal fetal growth presenting as preterm labor.

5. Fetal demise is a contraindication to tocolysis.

6. Multiple gestations result in preterm labor 12 times more often than singletons, and require great care be taken when applying parenteral tocolytic therapy.

7. Fetal malpresentation is a common finding in patients with preterm labor.
   a. The incidence of malpresentation is inversely related to gestational age.
   b. There is a known higher incidence of fetal malformation in the breech preterm infant.
   c. In this country, the breech-presenting fetus from 28 to 34 weeks facing inevitable delivery is delivered by cesarean section.

8. Fetal well-being
   a. Fetal tone, movement, amniotic fluid volume, and fetal breathing movements (fundamental parts of the biophysical profile), become manifest weeks prior to the classic heart reactivity.
   b. If these four criteria are present according to specific formulas, the clinician can be reassured of sufficient fetal oxygenation.

9. The presence of fetal breathing movements (FBMs) has been shown to be an indicator that pregnancy is not likely to be in true preterm labor.
   a. Castle and Turnbull have demonstrated that, if FBMs are not seen on real-time observation of the fetal chest over a 45-minute period, delivery is inevitable within the next 48 hours, and these patients should be considered for tocolysis.
   b. The application of FBMs to the management of preterm labor is unclear, but represents an exciting area of pertinent clinical investigation.

10. Other applications of sonography in the evaluation and management of preterm labor include
    a. Identification of fetal malformations
    b. Evaluation of polyhydramnios/oligohydramnios
    c. Placental, fundic, and uterine evaluation

Key Signs

- Early cervical dilatation or effacement

- Uterine contractions: four in 20 minutes or eight in 60 minutes

- Cervical change associated with uterine contractions

- Sonographic information on cervical/uterine condition, size, weight, well-being, presentation of fetus

Laboratory Tests

1. Complete blood count (CBC) to look for signs of infection or recent hemorrhage

2. Blood type and screen if cesarean section is being considered

3. Testing for infection
   a. Urinalysis and culture
   b. Cervical cultures for group B streptococcus, possibly chlamydia and gonorrhea
   c. Vaginal normal saline wet prep for *Trichomonas* or clue cells (evidence of bacterial vaginosis)

4. Test vaginal fluid for evidence of rupture of membranes
   a. Nitrazine-positive indicates rupture.
   b. Presence of ferning indicates rupture.

5. Amniocentesis can be considered to evaluate fetal lung maturity (FLM).
   a. Lecithin/sphingomyelin (L/S) ratio of more than 2.3 indicates probable lung maturity.
   b. The presence of phosphatidylglycerol with a mature L/S ratio prevents the development of hyaline membrane disease.

6. Amniocentesis can be used to look for intrauterine infection.
   a. Bacteria present on Gram's stain of the amniotic fluid is a better predictor of infection than the presence of white blood cells.
   b. Aerobic and anaerobic cultures.

Key Tests

- CBC: consider blood type and screen

- Urinalysis, culture and sensitivity

- Cervical culture for group B streptococcus

- Cervical culture or DNA probe for chlamydia and gonorrhea

- Normal saline wet preparation of vaginal fluid

- Ultrasound

- Amniocentesis: for evaluation of FLM and infection

Differential Diagnosis

1. Preterm labor is uterine contractions associated with documented cervical change occurring in a pregnancy between 22 and 36 weeks' gestation.

2. Increasing uterine activity without associated cervical change should be monitored because it can represent a clinical precursor to labor.

Treatment of Established Preterm Labor

1. Should the patient be transferred to a high-risk perinatal unit with a neonatal intensive care unit?
   a. Decision depends on condition of the mother, condition of the fetus, likelihood of rapid progression to delivery, the resources of the presenting hospital, and the availability of a trained perinatal transport team.
   b. The decision to transfer a patient must involve consultation with the receiving perinatologist.

2. Dehydration is known to lead to uterine irritability, so therapy of preterm labor begins with intravenous hydration. Ringer's lactate, 500 to 1000 ml, is infused over 1 hour, followed by infusion at a rate of 125 ml/hour.

3. As described under "Prevention," treat the underlying conditions that may be associated with or causal to the preterm labor.
   a. Antibiotic therapy should be begun for the diagnosis of urinary tract infection.
   b. Antibiotic therapy for group B streptococcus should be begun in the presence of PROM.
   c. Aggressive antibiotic therapy should be begun in the presence of the clinical diagnosis of chorioamnionitis.

Medication

1. A number of tocolytic therapies have been used to manage preterm labor (Table 130–1). However, there is still no clear-cut evidence that pharmacologic suppression of labor prolongs pregnancy beyond a couple of days.

2. It is usual for a patient with the diagnosis of preterm labor to begin tocolysis with a single medication, which is either added to or replaced by another if the original regimen is unsuccessful.

3. Adverse side effects, serious or even life-threatening to the mother, can occur, and this

TABLE 130-1. THERAPEUTIC AGENTS FOR PRETERM LABOR

AGENT	ACTION	DOSE	COMMENTS
Magnesium sulfate	Competes with Ca^{2+} for entry into cells	Initial 4 gm IV, then 1–4 gm/hr	Sweating, nausea and weakness. Follow levels. Respiratory arrest. Do not use with Ca^{2+} channel blockers.
Terbutaline	β-Adrenergic agent	IV: 0.01–0.025 mg/min SQ: 0.25 mg q1–4h PO: 2.5–5.0 mg q3–4h	Palpitations, tremor, headache, nausea. Fluid overload, pulmonary edema.
Ritodrine	β-Adrenergic agent	IV: 0.1–0.35 mg/min	Palpitations, tremor, headache, nausea. Fluid overload, pulmonary edema.
Indomethacin	Prostaglandin synthetase inhibitor	Initial 50 mg PO or 100 mg rectal suppository; then 25 mg q4h	Gastrointestinal upset/bleed. Headaches. Do not use after 34 weeks (premature constriction of ductus arteriosus).
Nifedipine	Ca^{2+} channel blocker	Initial 20–30 mg PO; then 10–20 mg PO q6h	Headaches. Peripheral edema. Constipation. Do not use with magnesium sulfate.

possibility must be considered in the decision to implement a given therapy.

4. Therapy tends to be more aggressive when the fetus is less mature, and generally is discontinued by 36 weeks' gestation.

5. When possible, a 24- to 48-hour delay in delivery allows the maternal dosing of steroids to enhance FLM.

   a. It has been concluded that steroids help reduce the incidence and the severity of infant respiratory distress syndrome (RDS).

   b. Intracerebral hemorrhage and necrotizing enterocolitis, the sequelae of RDS, also occur less frequently in infants whose mothers received steroids.

   c. The indications for steroid administration in preterm labor include

      (1) A fetus at 24 to 34 weeks' gestation

      (2) No maternal or fetal contraindications to the delay of delivery for 24 to 48 hours

      (3) No maternal contraindications to steroids

   d. Dosage regimens for steroid use

      (1) Betamethasone (Celestone), 12 mg IM, two doses 24 hours apart, *or*

      (2) Dexamethasone (Decadron), 6 mg IM, four doses 12 hours apart

   e. Dosing is repeated weekly through 34 weeks' gestation.

6. Once a patient has been evaluated and initial management begun, it should quickly be determined if she is a satisfactory candidate for to-colytic therapy. The following are selection criteria for beginning tocolysis:

   a. There are no contraindications to the chosen medication.

   b. There are no contraindications to prolonging the pregnancy.

   c. The fetus is healthy, not anomalous.

   d. The diagnosis of preterm labor is clearly established.

   e. The cervix is dilated less than 4 cm.

   f. The gestational age is between 24 and 34 weeks.

   g. There is not significant vaginal bleeding.

Diet

1. No special recommendations

2. Monitor fluid intake if on β-agonists.

Activity

1. Bed rest

2. If labor is stopped, recommend reduced activity and no strenuous activity.

Patient Education

1. Review the warning signs of preterm labor.

2. Insist on early reporting of symptoms of recurrence of preterm contractions.

3. Review the side effects of oral tocolytic therapy.

Prevention

Medication

1. Aggressive antibiotic treatment of cervical, vaginal, or urinary tract infection

a. Urinary tract infection: amoxicillin, 500 mg orally tid for 10 to 14 days. Cephalosporins possible second choice.

b. Group B streptococcus: Oral penicillin effective.

c. Trichomonas or bacterial vaginosis: metronidazole (Flagyl), 500 mg orally bid for 7 days (safe after 12 weeks' gestation). Amoxicillin, 500 mg tid for 7 days is an alternative.

d. Chlamydia: azithromycin (Zithromax), 1 gm orally, immediately

2. Prophylactic antibiotic treatment for patients with warning signs of preterm labor is controversial.

3. In patients with PROM, antibiotic therapy does delay the onset of preterm labor.

4. Prophylactic oral tocolytics are controversial in patients with warning signs because of the lack of proof of their efficacy and their side effect profile.

a. Terbutaline 2.5 mg orally q6h, increasing to 5 mg q6h as indicated. Alternative is ritodrine (Yutopar), 20 mg orally q6h.

b. Nifedipine (Procardia), 10 mg orally q6h; may be increased to 20 mg q6h. High incidence of side effects.

c. Magnesium gluconate, 1 gm q4–6h; magnesium oxide, 200 mg q3–4h.

Diet

1. No specific recommendations
2. Consider supplementation with 2 gm of elemental calcium per day.

Activity

1. Reduce workload.

a. Less than an 8-hour day and fewer than 5 days per week recommended for those at risk.

b. Reduce long hours of standing.

2. Bed rest recommended for increased warning signs, despite the absence of evidence to support effectiveness.

3. Coital abstinence recommended.

Patient Education

1. Patients should be taught to recognize the signs and symptoms of preterm labor.

2. Patients need to learn to report the occurrence of any symptoms immediately.

3. Providers must evaluate symptoms and not "write them off" as round ligament pain or Braxton Hicks contractions.

Key Treatment

- Tocolytics: magnesium sulfate, terbutaline and ritodrine, nifedipine
- Glucocorticoids: betamethasone or dexamethasone

Follow-Up

1. Early preterm labor

a. Weekly prenatal visits and cervical examinations beginning at 22 weeks for high-risk patients

(1) Assess cervical length and dilatation.

(2) Consider examination of all patients at 28 weeks regardless of risk status.

b. Sonogram every 4 weeks for high-risk patients beginning at 16 weeks

(1) Assess cervical length and dilatation.

(2) Assess fetal growth and well-being.

(3) Twice-weekly fluid volume assessments for women with PROM

c. Home uterine activity monitoring

(1) Controversial; frequent nursing contact may be of equal benefit.

(2) Some established efficacy for multiple gestations and polyhydramnios.

2. Established preterm labor

a. Weekly office visits for fetal assessment and cervical evaluation

b. Consider home monitoring, particularly for multiple gestation or patients with difficulty perceiving contractions.

Bibliography

American Academy of Family Physicians: Preterm Labor. In Advanced Life Support in Obstetrics Course Syllabus, 3rd ed, pp 61–70. Kansas City, MO, American Academy of Family Physicians, 1996.

American College of Obstetricians and Gynecologists: Preterm Labor (Technical Bulletin no 206). Washington, DC, American College of Obstetricians and Gynecologists, 1995.

Amon E, Petrie RH: Role of ultrasonography in the management of preterm labor. In Chervenak FA, Isaacson GC, Campbell S (eds): Ultrasonography in Obstetrics and Gynecology, Vol II, pp 1467–1478. Boston, Little, Brown & Co, 1993.

Castle BM, Turnbull AC: The presence or absence of fetal breathing movements predicts the outcome of preterm labour. Lancet 1983;2:471.

Premature rupture of membranes, preterm labor and preterm birth. In Beckman C, Ling F, Barzansky B, et al (eds): Gynecology and Obstetrics, 2nd ed, pp 123–127. Baltimore, Williams & Wilkins, 1995.

131 First Trimester Bleeding

Scott T. Henderson

Etiology

1. One fourth of all pregnant women experience vaginal bleeding in early pregnancy. In one half of these women spontaneous abortion will occur.

2. Various other causes, such as ectopic pregnancy, trophoblastic disease, and cervical and vaginal lesions, have been identified.

3. In a number of cases no apparent cause for the bleeding can be identified.

Symptoms

1. Vaginal bleeding: ranging from a scant pinkish or brownish discharge to massive hemorrhage

2. Pelvic or suprapubic pain

3. Uterine cramping

4. Gastrointestinal symptoms: abdominal pain and cramping, nausea and vomiting, and urge to defecate

5. Dizziness and syncope

6. Symptoms of pregnancy

Key Symptoms

- Vaginal bleeding
- Pelvic pain
- Abdominal pain
- Uterine cramping

Clinical Findings

Findings will vary depending on the cause of the bleeding.

1. Cervical dilatation (inevitable or incomplete abortion)

2. Rupture of membranes (inevitable abortion)

3. Passage of products of conception (incomplete abortion)

4. Soft and involuted uterus (ectopic)

5. Cervical motion tenderness (ectopic)

6. Abdominal tenderness (ectopic)

7. Adnexal/pelvic mass (ectopic)

8. Fever

9. Shock

Key Signs

- Cervical dilatation
- Passage of tissue
- Rupture of membranes
- Adnexal/pelvic mass

Laboratory Tests

1. Pelvic and/or transvaginal ultrasound (US): to determine the location of the pregnancy or products of conception and assess fetal viability

2. Culdocentesis: Assess for hemoperitoneum if the diagnosis of ectopic pregnancy is in question.

2. Complete blood count and differential

3. Blood type and Rh factor

4. Clotting studies and platelet count if history of coagulation disorder or if missed or septic abortion is present.

5. Qualitative serum β-human chorionic gonadotropin (β-hCG) level: Decreasing or abnormally low levels are predictive of problems.

6. Serum progesterone level: Levels less than 25 ng/ml may indicate ectopic or spontaneous abortion.

7. Type and cross-match

8. Vaginal wet prep and cultures for gonorrhea, chlamydia, and group B streptococcus

Key Tests

- Pelvic or transvaginal ultrasound
- Complete blood count
- Blood type and Rh factor
- Serum β-hCG

Differential Diagnosis

1. Spontaneous abortion

   a. Threatened: uterine bleeding in first half of pregnancy with or without contractions but without cervical dilatation or rupture of membranes

   b. Inevitable: rupture of membranes with cervical dilatation

(1) Incomplete: part of products expelled

(2) Complete: all of products expelled

c. Missed: conceptus dies but the products are retained in utero for 8 or more weeks.

2. Gestational trophoblastic disease: ranges from benign hydatidiform mole to invasive mole or gestational choriocarcinoma

3. Ectopic pregnancy: The fertilized ovum implants elsewhere than the endometrial cavity. Bleeding occurs in 50 to 94 per cent of patients.

4. Subchorionic bleeding: Can be due to excessive physical activity, gastrointestinal illness with vomiting or diarrhea, placenta previa, or the early stages of spontaneous abortion.

5. Lesions: including adenomas, uterine leiomyomas, cervical or uterine polyps, cervical erosions/ulcerations, and neoplasm

6. Genital trauma

7. Infections: vaginitis, cervicitis, or pelvic inflammatory disease

8. Implantation bleeding: slight bleeding occurring when the ovum burrows and implants into the uterus. Usually occurs near the time of the first missed menstrual period.

9. Incorrect menstrual dating: Bleeding may actually be a normal period.

10. Maternal disease: including coagulopathies, blood dysplasias, or leukemia

Treatment

The treatment of first trimester bleeding depends on the etiology. If life-threatening conditions, such as shock, are present, management must include appropriate advanced life-support measures.

1. Spontaneous abortion: If less than 6 to 8 weeks' gestation, the patient may be able to pass the tissue without medical or surgical intervention. An ultrasound may be necessary to assess for any residual tissue. If the bleeding is excessive or the pregnancy is past 8 weeks, the contents of the uterus need to be evacuated with a dilatation and curettage (D&C).

2. Gestational trophoblastic disease: Once diagnosed, the uterus must be evacuated immediately. D&C under general anesthesia is the preferred procedure. Oxytocin should be given during the procedure to help control bleeding. All patients should have β-hCG determinations followed for evidence of malignant disease.

3. Ectopic pregnancy: Surgical intervention by laparotomy or laparoscopy is required in the majority of cases. If an unruptured tubal pregnancy is less than 4 cm in diameter, it may be treated conservatively with methotrexate.

4. Subchorionic bleeds: No specific intervention is indicated, but activity should be limited and the patient put at pelvic rest. Additionally, bleeding should be followed up with an ultrasound examination in 4 to 8 weeks.

Medication

1. Drugs of choice

a. $Rh_o(D)$ immune globulin (RhoGAM): If patient is Rh negative, an intramuscular injection should be given within 72 hours of the fetomaternal hemorrhage. $Rh_o(D)$ immune globulin is supplied in two different unit doses, standard and microdose. Generally only a single injection is needed to provide protection. The microdose should be used only if the gestation is less than 12 weeks.

b. Oxytocin: intravenous (10 units at a rate of 20 to 100 mU/min) or intramuscular (10 units) route to control uterine bleeding following operative procedure such as D&C. To prepare an intravenous solution, add 10 to 40 units of oxytocin to 1000 ml of a nonhydrating diluent, resulting in a final solution concentration of 10 to 40 mU/ml.

2. Alternative drugs—ergots: Intramuscular or oral agents such as methylergonovine maleate (Methergine) may be used in place of oxytocin. Usual oral dosage is 0.2 or 0.4 mg two to four times daily, usually for 2 days. Intramuscular dosage is 0.2 mg (1 ml) and may be repeated in 2 to 4 hours if bleeding is severe.

Diet

Variable

Activity

1. Bed rest until resolution, if appropriate

2. Pelvic rest—no coitus, tampons, or douching

Patient Education

Inform the patient that there is an increased risk of abortion and fetal loss in subsequent pregnancies in women who experience first trimester bleeding.

Follow-Up

1. If the patient proceeds to have an abortion, the products of conception must be identified to confirm diagnosis.

2. If the patient goes on to have an abortion or if the ectopic pregnancy is managed conservatively, the β-hCG level must be followed until it returns to normal.

3. If the patient has gestational trophoblastic disease, the β-hCG levels should be followed for evidence of malignant disease.

4. Psychological support to the woman and her partner is necessary.

5. If the pregnancy is lost, the patient should be advised to use some form of birth control and not attempt another pregnancy until she has had at least two to three normal menstrual cycles.

6. If the patients continues to carry the pregnancy, there may be an increased risk of low birth weight, placenta previa, abruptio placentae, preterm delivery, and neonatal death. Close obstetric follow-up care is indicated.

 Bibliography

For more information on first trimester bleeding, see
Chamberlain G: Vaginal bleeding in early pregnancy—I. BMJ 1991;302:1141–1143.
Chamberlain G: Vaginal bleeding in early pregnancy—II. BMJ 1991;302:1195–1193.
Pernoll ML, Garmel SH: Early pregnancy risks. In DeCherney AH, Pernoll ML (ed): Current Obstetric and Gynecologic Diagnosis and Treatment, 8th ed, pp 306–330. Norwalk, CT, Appleton & Lange, 1994.
For more information on abortion, see
Abortion. In Cunningham FG, MacDonald PC, Gant NF, et al (eds): Williams' Obstetrics, 20th ed, pp 579–605. Stamford, CT, Appleton & Lange, 1997.
For more information on ectopic pregnancy, see
Ectopic pregnancy. In Cunningham FG, MacDonald PC, Gant NF, et al (eds): Williams' Obstetrics, 20th ed, pp 607–634. Stamford, CT, Appleton & Lange, 1997.

132 Third Trimester Bleeding

Peter R. Warrington

Bleeding from the genital area in later pregnancy (after fetal viability, 23 to 24 weeks) occurs in 2 to 5 per cent of all pregnancies. Most serious bleeding episodes arise from placental or uterine pathology, but multiple sources have been described. In reported series, up to 50 per cent of cases with third trimester bleeding *do not* have serious pathology.

Placenta Previa

Etiology
1. Prior uterine surgery
   a. Cesarean section: If placenta previa is present and patient has had prior cesarean section, there is an increased risk of placenta accreta.
   b. Dilatation and curettage, elective abortion
2. Risk increases with age of patient.
3. Risk increases with increasing parity.

Symptoms
1. Vaginal bleeding, frequently painless. There may be no history of trauma, or bleeding may occur after coitus or pelvic examination or with onset of contractions.
2. Crampy lower abdominal pain can occur with bleeding in up to 25 per cent of cases.

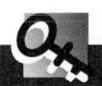

Key Symptom

Vaginal bleeding

Clinical Findings

> **WARNING**
>
> The initial history and physical examination will usually reveal the source of bleeding. However, although it depends on the level of expertise of the examiner, internal vaginal examination (digitally or by speculum) should be deferred in most cases until placenta previa has been ruled out.

1. Breech or transverse lie on abdominal examination is seen in about one third of cases. If vertex lie, vertex palpates well above pelvic brim.
2. Uterine contractions are present in up to 25 per cent of cases.
3. Uterine tenderness is seen in up to 10 per cent of cases as a result of coexisting abruption.
4. If blood loss is large enough, signs of hypovolemia can be present.
5. If hypovolemia is present, signs of fetal distress can be seen on heart monitor.
6. *If speculum examination is done*, bleeding from cervical os is noted.

Key Signs

- Vaginal bleeding
- Signs of hypovolemia
- Abnormal lie or nonengaged vertex
- Fetal distress

Laboratory Tests
1. Ultrasound of uterus: Area of cervix is viewed with patient's bladder full and then empty. Recently, vaginal probe ultrasound, carefully done, has been shown to resolve some questions when abdominal ultrasound is unclear (e.g., with posterior placenta previa). *Ultrasound examination has up to a 7 per cent false-negative rate.*
2. Complete blood count
3. Type and crossmatch at least 2 units of packed red blood cells.
4. Magnetic resonance imaging (MRI): Recent studies show that MRI can image cervix better and can be useful if ultrasound findings are unclear. Risk to the fetus is thought to be minimal, but adequate studies are not yet done.

Key Tests

- Ultrasound of uterus
- Complete blood count
- Type and crossmatch 2 units

Differential Diagnosis

1. Abruptio placentae: In up to 10 per cent of cases of placenta previa there is coexisting abruption.
2. Vasa praevia: If bleeding is from this source, signs of fetal distress will be seen on heart monitor after relatively little blood loss.
3. Ruptured uterus at site of cesarean section scar: If prior vertical uterine incision, one third of those that do rupture do so before labor. If prior horizontal uterine incision, rupture, if it occurs, is almost always with labor.
4. Bleeding from other genital site.

Treatment

1. Stabilize patient with volume replacement and transfusion as necessary. If bleeding is sufficient to endanger mother or fetus, delivery should be by immediate cesarean section regardless of gestational age.
2. If pregnancy is confidently known to be term, deliver by cesarean section.
3. If pregnancy is of unclear gestational age or less than 36 to 37 weeks and patient is stable, hospitalize at bed rest. Perform weekly amniocentesis and deliver when fetal lungs mature.
4. In certain circumstances, after initial hospitalization with stable patient, expectant management can be done on an outpatient basis.

Follow-Up

1. Postpartum hemorrhage is more common.
2. Risk of recurrence with subsequent pregnancy is 4 to 8 per cent.

Abruptio Placentae

Etiology

1. Maternal hypertension: In one study, almost 50 per cent of severe abruptions were in hypertensive patients.
2. Trauma
3. Cocaine use
4. Sudden uterine decompression (e.g., after rupture of membranes or after birth of first twin)
5. Severely small for gestational age
6. Prolonged rupture of membranes
7. Smoking

Symptoms

1. Vaginal bleeding

2. Abdominal or low back pain, crampy or continuous in nature
3. Decreased or absent perceived fetal movement

WARNING

Placental abruption, even severe, can occur silently without pain or bleeding.

 Key Symptoms

- Vaginal bleeding
- Decreased perceived fetal movement
- Abdominal or low back pain

Clinical Findings

1. Uterine tenderness
2. Bleeding from cervical os
3. Uterine contractions, frequently with uterine "irritability" (mild contractions of short duration with a frequency of 1 to 2 minutes)
4. Fetal distress on fetal heart monitor
5. Labor (uterine contractions with progressive cervical changes)
6. Fetal death
7. Shock: Can occur without excessive external blood loss as a result of occult collection of blood within the uterus.
8. Consumptive coagulopathy: When this accompanies abruption, there is almost always fetal demise.

 Key Signs

- Bleeding from cervix
- Uterine tenderness
- Uterine irritability
- Fetal distress

Laboratory Tests

1. Ultrasound of uterus
2. Complete blood count
3. Coagulation studies
4. Type and crossmatch at least 2 units packed red cells.

WARNING

A normal ultrasound does not rule out abruption.

Key Tests

- Ultrasound
- Uterine and fetal monitoring
- Type and crossmatch 2 units
- Coagulation studies
- Complete blood count

Differential Diagnosis

1. Placenta previa
2. Vasa praevia
3. Uterine rupture
4. Normal labor with "bloody show"
5. Bleeding from other genital site

Treatment

1. If the fetus is alive and abruption is mild in a term pregnancy, expeditious delivery should be accomplished by rupture of membranes, with oxytocin as needed.
2. With mild abruption and immature fetus, a judgment must be made as to whether intrauterine environment or intensive-care nursery is safer for fetus.
3. If abruption is more severe (fetal distress, maternal hypovolemia), delivery may need to be by cesarean section if vaginal birth is judged not to be imminent.
4. With abruption and fetal demise, one should expedite labor and perform cesarean section only when either labor is contraindicated or blood loss is excessive and labor is progressing too slowly.

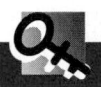

Key Treatment

- Delivery
- Volume and blood replacement

Follow-Up

1. Increased incidence of postpartum bleeding
2. Recurrence risk of 10 per cent for subsequent pregnancy

Vasa Praevia

Etiology

Velamentous insertion of umbilical cord with cord vessels surrounded only by membranes in front of presenting fetal part. It is more common with multiple gestations.

Symptoms

Vaginal bleeding onset with rupture of membranes.

Key Symptom

Vaginal bleeding onset with rupture of membranes

Clinical Findings

1. Bleeding from cervical os
2. Palpable vessels in membranes felt at internal os of cervix
3. Variable decelerations in fetal heart rate
4. Onset of persistent fetal distress with membrane rupture and bleeding

Key Signs

- Bleeding from cervical os
- Palpable vessels in membranes
- Onset of fetal distress with membrane rupture and bleeding

Laboratory Tests

1. Rapid test for fetal hemoglobin on blood from vagina (e.g., Apt test, Kleihauer-Bethke smear)
2. Recent articles suggest that vasa praevia can sometimes be visualized by abdominal or vaginal ultrasound.

Key Test

Rapid test for fetal hemoglobin

Differential Diagnosis

1. Placenta previa
2. Abruptio placentae
3. Uterine rupture
4. Bleeding from other genital site

Treatment

Rapid delivery, almost always by cesarean section

Bibliography

Clark SL: Placenta previa and abruptio placentae. In Creasy RK, Resnik R (eds): Maternal-Fetal Medicine: Principles and Practice, 4th ed, pp 616–631. Philadelphia, WB Saunders Company, 1999.

Crane S, Chun B, Acker D: Treatment of obstetric hemorrhagic emergencies. Curr Opin Obstet Gynecol 1993; 5:675–682.

Cunningham FG, MacDonald PC, Gant NF, et al (eds): Williams' Obstetrics, 20th ed, pp 745–760. East Norwalk, CT, Appleton & Lange, 1997.

Gabbe SG, Niebyl JR, Simpson JL (eds): Obstetrics: Normal and Problem Pregnancies, 3rd ed, pp 505–515. New York, Churchill Livingstone, 1996.

Lavery JP: Placenta previa. Clin Obstet Gynecol 1990;33: 414–421.

Lowe TW, Cunningham FG: Placental abruption. Clin Obstet Gynecol 1990;33:406–413.

Scott JR: Placenta previa and abruption. In Scott JR, Disia PG, Hammond LB, Spellacy WN (eds): Danforth's Obstetrics and Gynecology, 8th ed, pp 407–418. Philadelphia, Williams & Wilkins, 1999.

133 Postpartum Hemorrhage

Michael S. Wolkomir

Etiology

Early Postpartum Hemorrhage (Immediate to 24 Hours After Birth)

1. Uterine atony
   a. Rapid *or* prolonged labor
   b. Overdistended uterus (twins, macrosomia, polyhydramnios)
   c. High parity or history of previous atonic bleeding
   d. Induction or augmentation of labor
   e. Chorioamnionitis
2. Lower genital tract trauma
   a. Episiotomy (average loss = 200 ml)
   b. Vulvar lacerations and hematomas (generally secondary to uncontrolled delivery of head)
   c. Vaginal vault laceration and hematoma
      (1) Forceps can produce vault tears, especially over ischial spines.
      (2) Vacuum can cause avulsion of vaginal mucosa.
   d. Cervical laceration
      (1) Rapid first stage of labor
      (2) Pushing against undilated cervix; manual dilatation or vacuum before complete dilatation of cervix
      (3) Usually occurs at 3- and 9-o'clock positions.
      (4) Can extend beyond vault to broad ligament, producing life-threatening intra-abdominal bleeding.
   e. Other rare events
      (1) Uterine rupture: associated with previous uterine surgery, including classic cesarean section (vaginal births after cesarean section show no increased risk)
      (2) Uterine inversion: associated with mismanagement of third stage of labor

---

WARNING

Never attempt to separate the placenta by pulling on the cord without lifting the fundus away using the Brandt maneuver!!

---

3. Retained placenta or membranes (more common with previous cesarean section)
   a. Retained cotyledon or accessory lobe of placenta
   b. Abnormality of implantation (accreta, increta, percreta)
4. Coagulopathies (rare): Obstetric causes include pre-eclampsia, abruptio placentae, amniotic fluid embolism, and dead fetus syndrome.

Late Postpartum Hemorrhage (More Than 24 Hours)

1. Late recognition of *any* of the causes of early postpartum hemorrhage (PPH)
2. Failure of the placental bed to involute normally
3. Retained products of conception
4. Infection—chorioamnionitis
5. Consider especially coagulopathies.

Symptoms

1. Early PPH: May be none (physiologic adaptations include increase of 40 per cent or more blood volume, and patient may be supine).
2. Late PPH
   a. Nurse's or experienced mother's report of excessive lochia
   b. Dizziness or lightheadedness on standing, syncope

 Key Symptoms

- Early: mental status changes or frank shock
- Late: dizziness or syncope

Clinical Findings

Early PPH

1. Obvious vaginal bleeding in excess of your experience. Average blood loss is 500 ml. *Triple your "gut" estimate!*
2. Occult bleeding: Large amounts of blood can be lost slowly and easily hidden by drapes.

3. Classic symptoms of impending shock—tachypnea, tachycardia, hypotension, mental status changes—appear *late in the process.*

> **WARNING**
>
> **Pre-eclamptic mothers are exquisitely sensitive to blood loss (shock) and to its treatment (congestive heart failure and pulmonary edema).**

Late PPH

1. Orthostatic hypotension, tachycardia
2. Hemoglobin level fall of 1.5 gm = 1 unit of blood.
3. Low urine output (<30 ml/hour)
4. Signs of puerperal infection
5. Bleeding from other sites (e.g., venipuncture) suggests coagulopathy.

> **WARNING**
>
> **Signs of acute anemia without visible external bleeding, especially with expanding abdominal girth, may represent broad ligament hematoma and constitute a surgical emergency.**

Key Signs

- Early
  - Visible hemorrhage
  - Signs of shock
- Late
  - Orthostatic hypotension
  - Laboratory signs of anemia out of proportion to expected loss

Laboratory Tests

1. All mothers should have a preadmission hemoglobin and hematocrit for comparison.
2. At first sign of excessive bleeding
   a. Repeat complete blood count (CBC) with platelet count.
   b. Cross and type 4 units of packed red cells and keep 4 units on hand.
   c. Disseminated intravascular coagulation screen, including prothrombin time/partial thromboplastin time, fibrinogen, fibrin split products, and antithrombin III if available. (Do early before transfusions confuse the issue.)
   d. Qualitative clot retraction is easy to do but detects only platelet disorders.
3. For late PPH
   a. CBC with differential. Repeat as necessary to follow, at least daily.
   b. Cultures of lochia and blood as clinically indicated
   c. Coagulation screen as above
   d. Ultrasound may be useful in identifying retained products of conception or hematomas.

Key Laboratory Tests

- Early
  - Cross and type packed red cells in sufficient quantity
  - Coagulation screening
- Late
  - Infection work-up
  - Ultrasound of pelvis

Treatment

General Principles

PPH is a rapidly evolving emergency!

1. Get obstetric consultation and treat blood loss and shock *early.*
2. Treat for *atony* while looking for any other causes.
3. Start fluid replacement with two large-bore intravenous needles (18 or larger); lactated Ringer's, 1000-ml challenge, then 250 ml/hour. (Reduce rate in pre-eclamptics to prevent fluid overload.)
4. Administer oxygen, 2 to 6 L/minute.
5. Replace other components with reference to the patient's laboratory values. If this is not possible, consider 1 unit fresh frozen plasma for each 3 units of packed red blood cells.
6. Use intravenous analgesia if necessary to do an adequate pelvic examination.

Specific Causes

1. Atony: Vigorous bimanual massage, tamponade. Keep one hand in the vagina, the other on

the abdomen, and squeeze/massage the uterus between.

> **WARNING**
>
> Packing the uterus is *almost never* justified.

2. Birth trauma: *These tissues are friable. Avoid synthetic suture materials. Be gentle!*
   a. Vulvar trauma
      (1) Perineal laceration: Close like episiotomy if bleeding.
      (2) Periurethral: Place a catheter before starting to sew.
         (a) Interrupted or figure-of-eight sutures of 5-0 chromic *only if bleeding*
         (b) Clitoral region is very vascular. Be careful; use minimum suture.
      (3) Hematomas
         (a) If less than 3 cm and stable, observe, ice packs, and compression.
         (b) If more than 3 cm or enlarging, consider exploration and identification of specific bleeding sites. Can be oversewn with 3-0 or 4-0 chromic.
   b. Vault lacerations: *Good visualization is the key!* Use assistants for retraction.
      (1) If secondary to forceps, assume these are *bilateral!*
      (2) Look in hidden places (fornix, posterior vault).
      (3) Make sure you start sutures *above* the apex of laceration.
      (4) Close with one or two layers of figure-of-eight or running 3-0 chromic suture.
   c. Cervical laceration
      (1) Look at 3- and 9-o'clock positions.
      (2) Grasp upper and lower lip of cervix with ring forceps, and visualize apex of laceration.
      (3) Close with running lock suture of 3-0 chromic suture, beginning *above* the apex.
3. Retained placenta or membranes
   a. If undelivered by 30 minutes, infuse 10 International Units of pitocin in 20 ml of normal saline into umbilical vein.
   b. Manual exploration, removal: Sedation may be necessary.
      (1) Insert hand into uterus and sweep hypothenar ridge under the cleavage plane

of the placenta, sweep the uterine wall, and remove the products.
      (2) If plane does not develop, consider placenta accreta.
   c. Carefully inspect placenta for missing cotyledon or vessels coursing off membranes, indicating an accessory lobe.
   d. If not controlled, consider surgical evacuation.
      (1) Use suction curettage or large "banjo" curette.
      (2) Very gentle touch is necessary to prevent Asherman's syndrome or perforation.
   e. Cover with antibiotics for infection and pitocin for atony.
4. Rare traumatic events
   a. Uterine rupture: discovered on manual exploration. If bleeding, requires laparotomy.
   b. Uterine prolapse: requires *immediate* reinsertion. *Don't wait for a consultant!*
      (1) May require a tocolytic: Be prepared for massive bleeding and shock.
      (2) Leave placenta attached.
      (3) With one hand on the abdomen and the other in the vagina, revert the uterus like turning a sock inside out.
5. Coagulopathies (manage as described in Ch. 168, Bleeding Disorders)
6. Surgical management: In the event of failure of conservative management, several procedures are available. The purpose of these is to reduce the pulse pressure and allow hemostasis to occur.
   a. Ligation of hypogastric uterine or ovarian arteries
   b. Selective catheter embolization of the iliac or hypogastric arteries (still investigational)
   c. If all else fails, hysterectomy may be necessary.

Late PPH

1. Subinvolution is usually self-limited. Dilatation and curettage (D&C) is rarely indicated.
2. Intramuscular methylergonovine is a good therapy in the absence of hypertension.
3. Consider ultrasound to aid in the diagnosis of retained products before electing D&C.
4. Cover with antibiotics for endometritis, as described in Ch. 120, Endometritis.

Diet

After recovery, encourage balanced diet high in iron and protein to aid recovery.

Activity

1. Increase activity as tolerated.
2. Avoid intercourse until all healing has occurred (usually after the 6-week check).

Patient Education

1. Recurrence risk depends on the specific cause. The physician should review the current literature before discussing this with the patient.
2. Make sure patient is educated in the signs and symptoms of recurrent bleeding, acute anemia, and infection.

Key Treatment

Drugs of Choice

- Pitocin, 20 to 40 IU/L rapid IV infusion (IV bolus can cause circulatory collapse!). May also be given by IM or intramyometrial (IMM) injection.

- Methylergonovine, 0.2 mg IM or IMM—*not IV*

- Prostaglandin $F_{2\alpha}$ (Hemabate), very effective; 0.25 to 1 mg IM or IMM q 15–60 min prn to maximum of 12 mg.

- Dinoprostone, 20 mg per rectum q2h (avoid in hypotensive patients)

Follow-Up

1. Make sure the patient feels free to call if there are any problems.
2. Consider seeing her early. An ideal time is when seeing the baby for a 2-week check.

Bibliography

American College of Obstetricians and Gynecologists: Postpartum Hemorrhage (ACOG Education Bulletin no 243). Washington, DC, American College of Obstetricians and Gynecologists, 1998.

American College of Obstetricians and Gynecologists: Hemorrhagic Shock (ACOG Education Bulletin no 235). Washington, DC, American College of Obstetricians and Gynecologists, 1997.

Cunningham FG, et al: Obstetrical hemorrhage. In Cunningham FG, MacDonald PC, Gant NF, et al (eds): Wiliams' Obstetrics, 20th ed, pp 745–782. Stamford, CT, Appleton & Lange, 1997.

Etches D, Smith D: Post partum hemorrhage. In Advanced Life Support in Obstetrics, 3rd ed, pp 181–192. Kansas City, MO, American Academy of Family Physicians, 1996.

Watson P: Postpartum hemorrhage and shock. Clin Obstet Gynecol 1980;23:985.

134 Postpartum Depression

Mary Helen Morrow

Etiology

1. Postpartum depression (PPD) occurs in approximately 10 per cent of women. It can manifest as early as a few days after delivery or up to 1 year postpartum. There is little evidence to support a biologic basis for PPD.

2. Psychosocial: Women at increased risk are those who have experienced stressful life events, have a poor or absent social support system, or are going through marital conflict. Also at increased risk are first-time mothers, women who experienced complications during or after delivery, and women who perceive their infants as difficult.

3. History: Women who have a past history of depressive disorder, those who experienced antepartum depression, and the presence of the "postpartum blues" all increase the risk of developing PPD.

Symptoms

1. Postpartum blues occurs in 50 to 80 per cent of women. Symptoms include insomnia, tearfulness, irritability, fatigue, and mildly depressed affect. These symptoms are interwoven with periods of happiness. Symptoms start within 2 weeks of delivery and usually resolve within 2 weeks to 3 months.

2. PPD symptoms range from mild to severe and include uncontrollable crying, insomnia, exhaustion, nervousness and anxiety, poor concentration, overconcern for the baby, lack of interest in the baby, feelings of guilt or inadequacy, appetite and sleep disturbances, fear of harming self or baby, and actual suicide or infanticide attempts.

3. Postpartum psychosis is the most severe of the postpartum disorders. It occurs at a rate of 1 to 2 per 1000. Presenting symptoms include insomnia, agitation, bizarre feelings and behavior, delusions, and hallucinations.

Key Symptoms

- Excessive guilt/inadequacy
- Uncontrollable crying
- Loss of appetite
- Overconcern for baby
- Inappropriate fears of harm to baby
- Hopelessness
- Depressed mood
- Nervousness and anxiety
- Poor concentration
- Suicidal/homicidal ideation

Clinical Findings

1. The patient may present with somatic complaints ranging from fatigue to back pain to muscle and joint pains. Likewise, patients may not complain of their symptoms because they feel guilty for not being the ideal mother.

2. Women with PPD frequently describe their infants as demanding and difficult. This may be due to a difficult delivery (i.e., cesarean or multiple birth) or due to an irritable baby or one with poor motor control.

3. Women with PPD more often have poor social support systems. They may be unwed or having marital problems. They may be unemployed or have multiple other social stressors.

Key Signs

- Lack of and/or poor social support
- Within 6 months of delivery
- Feeling inadequate as a mother
- Difficulties with significant other
- Stressful childbirth
- Perception of infant as difficult

Laboratory Tests

1. It is necessary to rule out thyroid disease and assess for anemia as a cause of postpartum fatigue.

2. All prenatal patients should be screened for symptoms of depression early in their pregnancy and then re-evaluated during the preg-

nancy as needed. All women should be screened again postpartum.

3. Ideally postpartum evaluation should take place within 2 weeks of delivery. Follow-up screens should be performed as needed.

4. A variety of screening tools exist to evaluate for depression. The tool that is chosen should have good reliability and validity and be easy to use in clinical practice. General screening tools include the Beck Depression Inventory, the Hamilton Anxiety and Depression Scales, and the Zung Anxiety and Depression Self-Assessment Scale. Tools specific to PPD include the Postpartum Support Questionnaire and the Edinburgh Postnatal Depression Scale.

Key Tests

- Thyroid-stimulating hormone
- Edinburgh Postnatal Depression Scale
- Hemoglobin
- Beck Depression Inventory
- Screen EVERY prenatal and postnatal patient for depression.

Differential Diagnosis

1. Other postpartum mood disorders: postpartum blues and postpartum psychosis
2. Endocrine disorders: hypothyroidism, thyrotoxicosis, pituitary and adrenal disorders
3. Abusive home situation

WARNING

- **Diagnosis of postpartum psychosis warrants emergent hospitalization.**
- **Suicidal or infanticidal plan or intent demands immediate intervention.**

Treatment

1. Treatment varies with the type and severity of disease. If PPD is mild, it will sometimes resolve on its own. Moderate and severe cases need counseling and/or medication. Support groups can be very helpful to validate feelings, educate, and offer continuing support.
2. The treatment course is usually at least 6 to 12 months.
3. There is no question that some intervention is necessary and produces better long-term maternal-child interactions. In addition, chil-

dren whose mothers did not receive treatment for PPD were more likely to have impaired cognitive and emotional development.

4. Severe cases of postpartum depression may need to utilize electroconvulsive therapy (ECT). ECT has been used both during pregnancy and in PPD and has been shown to be both safe and effective even for breast-feeding mothers.

Medication

1. As with other depressive syndromes, the selective serotonin reuptake inhibitors (SSRIs) are now the drugs of first choice. Any SSRI or other antidepressant may be used for women who are not breast-feeding. Starting doses are the same and the drug dose is titrated upward until the desired response is achieved.

2. For breast-feeding mothers with PPD, the decision must be weighed carefully whether to institute pharmacotherapy. There are several drugs that have been shown to have undetectable levels of parent drug in infant serum (amitriptyline [Elavil], nortriptyline [Pamelor], desipramine [Norpramin], clomipramine [Anafranil], doxepin [Sinequan], and sertraline [Zoloft]).

3. Nondetectable levels of parent drug do not absolve the drug of possible long-term effects on the child. The longest studies to date are 5-year follow-ups. Risks and benefits must be weighed and discussed thoroughly with the parents and other involved health care providers. The options include counseling alone, the use of medications as listed above, and the possibility of weaning. All discussions and decisions should be documented in the medical record.

4. Serum levels should be monitored in infants less than 10 weeks of age. In infants greater than 10 weeks of age, serum levels should be checked when there are behavioral changes, sedation, or significant parental anxiety.

5. For women with antenatal depression, studies have indicated that the use of fluoxetine (Prozac) has not increased the rate of congenital abnormalities. Fluoxetine in pregnancy is Category B (probably safe). However, it is not safe for use by women who are breast-feeding. If women are given fluoxetine antenatally, it must be tapered over the weeks prior to delivery and another medication chosen for use postpartum.

6. Research is underway to evaluate the use of hormonal therapy. One small study using the estrogen patch demonstrated success in treating PPD.

Diet

There is no specific diet recommended for PPD. However, breast-feeding mothers require 2000 to 2200 calories/day to maintain their milk supply.

Activity

There were no specific recommendations in the literature reviewed regarding exercise.

Patient Education

1. Every prenatal patient should be extensively counseled regarding postpartum adjustment to the parental role. It is important to help parents set up reasonable expectations. This is especially important for those at risk for PPD. They should be educated about the postpartum mood disorders and be a partner in their detection.

2. Every primary care provider with access to new mothers and their families should screen for signs of PPD.

3. Encourage early reporting of any symptoms indicative of PPD.

4. There are national and international organizations offering education and support to both patients and health care providers. They are Depression After Delivery (phone: 1-215-295-3994; Internet: *www.infotrail.com/dad/dad.html*) and Postpartum Support International (*www . chss . iup . edu / anthropology / projects / depression/postpart.html*).

Key Treatment

Drugs to Choose From for Breast-Feeding Mothers

- Amitriptyline
- Nortriptyline
- Desipramine
- Clomipramine
- Doxepin
- Sertraline

Follow-Up

1. At the beginning of treatment, visits should occur at weekly or biweekly intervals to assess the effect of the medication or counseling. Once the patient is on the optimal dose of medication, the visits can gradually space to every other or every third month. This schedule coincides nicely with the well-child visit schedule.

2. Treatment should continue for at least 6 to 12 months.

3. Prophylactic treatment or increased vigilance should be instituted prior to any subsequent births to allow for early detection and treatment.

Bibliography

Cooper PJ, Murray L: Postnatal depression. BMJ 1998; 316:1884–1886.

Llewellyn AM, Stowe ZN, Nemeroff CB: Depression during pregnancy and the puerperium. J Clin Psychiatry 1997;58(Suppl 15):26–32.

Nonacs R, Cohen LS: Postpartum mood disorders: diagnosis and treatment. J Clin Psychiatry 1998;59(Suppl 2):34–40.

Pariser SF, Nasrallah HA: Postpartum mood disorders: clinical perspectives. J Womens Health 1997;6:421–434.

Susman JL: Postpartum depressive disorders: J Fam Pract 1996;43(Suppl 6):17S–24S.

Wisner KL, Perel JM, Findling RL: Am J Psychiatry 1996; 153:1132–1137.

Indications

1. Post-term pregnancy (gestation longer than 42 weeks' menstrual age)
2. Prelabor rupture of membranes at term
3. Pre-eclampsia
4. Maternal diabetes
5. Chronic hypertension
6. Chorioamnionitis
7. Placental abruption
8. Maternal renal disease
9. Isoimmunization
10. Fetal demise
11. Suspected placental insufficiency as manifested by intrauterine growth retardation, abnormal antenatal testing, oligohydramnios, or suspected meconium passage.

Labor induction is associated with elevated risk of cesarean section, forceps and vacuum-assisted delivery, reactions to drugs, maternal infection, and complications of premature delivery. Continuing a post-term pregnancy may be associated with increased risk of meconium aspiration syndrome, fetal demise, and maternal disseminated intravascular coagulation. Prolonging the duration of pregnancy complicated by pre-eclampsia is associated with increased risk of bleeding diatheses; maternal pulmonary, renal, hepatic, and neurologic injury; fetal demise; and intrauterine growth retardation.

Contraindications

There may be clinical situations in which elective cesarean delivery is preferable to labor induction. These include

1. Significant fetal heart rate abnormalities on antenatal testing indicating imminent fetal cardiac arrest
2. Known pelvic obstruction
3. Placenta previa

4. Active genital herpes
5. Breech presentation
6. Previous uterine surgery other than low transverse cesarean section. A previous low transverse cesarean section is not a contraindication to induction.

WARNING

Labor should not be induced in the case of a normal fetus with any uncertainty about fetal maturity. In such a case, amniotic fluid testing for fetal lung maturity is indicated. Labor induction should *NOT* be scheduled for the convenience of physician, patient, or hospital.

Preparation

1. Accurate assessment of gestational age
2. Capability to perform cesarean delivery, forceps delivery, and vacuum extraction
3. Capability to perform neonatal resuscitation
4. Capability to perform maternal resuscitation

Equipment

1. Electronic fetal monitoring
2. Intravenous access
3. Infusion pump(s)
4. Neonatal resuscitation equipment and supplies
5. Maternal resuscitation equipment and supplies

Anesthesia

Appropriate obstetric analgesia

Precautions

1. Fetal distress
2. Maternal hypertension
3. Maternal fluid and electrolyte imbalance
4. Uterine hyperstimulation

Technique

1. Oxytocin
   a. Significant practice variation exists for initial dose and the schedule and amount of incremental increase.
   b. Evidence suggests that "high-dose" (2.5-μg) regimens are more often associated with uterine hyperstimulation and ominous fetal heart rate changes than are "low-dose" (1.25-μg) regimens, and that "low-dose" regimens provide equivalent decreases in time to delivery.
   c. It is customary in the United States to mix 10 units of oxytoxin in 1000 ml of 5 per cent dextrose in water. Beginning infusion rates are often in the range of 0.5 mU/minute; incremental increases vary by amount and in-

terval. For example, some protocols call for increases every 15 minutes, others every 30 minutes.

2. Prostaglandins: Dinoprostone, misoprostol, and mifeprostone have been used alone and in combination with each other to achieve cervical ripening before oxytoxin induction with good success and a relatively low complication rate. Also in the literature are descriptions of successful inductions using these agents alone, without oxytoxin. Recommended dosages are

   a. Dinoprostone (Cervidil, Prepidil, Prostin E2), 10 mg in cervical canal

   b. Misoprostol (Cytotec), 25 to 50 μg orally every 3 to 6 hours

   c. Mifeprostone (RU 486), 200 mg on days 1 and 2 before oxytoxin induction on day 4

3. Saline infusion has been compared with misoprostol in women with unfavorable cervices in a randomized controlled trial, with equivalent time to delivery, complication rate, and cesarean section rate.

4. Amniotomy

   a. Risks include cord prolapse, infection, caput succedaneum, and umbilical cord compression during contractions. Saline amnioinfusion techniques have reduced risk for umbilical cord compression after amniotomy.

   b. Amniotomy alone, when compared to amniotomy with oxytoxin infusion started 1 hour later in women with a Bishop score of 6 or higher, was associated with shorter time until delivery but longer duration of latent labor, with comparable morbidity rates.

5. Digital separation of the chorionic membranes from the lower uterine segment (stripping the membranes), when done at 38 weeks, may be associated with a decreased instance of post-term pregnancy, but studies are not conclusive. No increase in significant perinatal morbidity has been reported, although some authors report more vaginal bleeding near term.

6. Nipple stimulation: No standard regimen has been well studied in clinical trials, and some clinicians express fear that uterine hyperstimulation is more common, although no increase in perinatal morbidity has been demonstrated. This method has been shown to shorten the time to effective contractions, and deserves further study.

Augmentation of Labor

1. Numerous protocols for the use of oxytoxin and amniotomy for augmentation of labor exist, and indications vary by and within institutions. An evidence-based recommendation is not currently available.

2. Many clinicians elect augmentation when cervical dilation does not follow Friedman's curve, but no evidence supports the use of medication or amniotomy when mother and baby are well.

3. Clinical evaluation for presence of malpresentation, true cephalopelvic disproportion, and maternal exhaustion must be performed carefully before oxytoxin is administered or amniotomy is performed in the face of progression of labor more slowly than the clinician expects.

Note

Induction of labor can decrease maternal and fetal morbidity, but data giving clinicians guidance as to which patients should be offered induction are currently insufficient for the construction of a comprehensive clinical guideline. Published research has focused on induction for post-term pregnancy, and research on induction methods for other indications is incomplete or has not been published. Current practices vary widely, and discussions with patients about whether and how to induce labor should feature quantitative differences in risk for various interventions, including watchful waiting, so that patients can assess and express their own preferences with respect to risks and choices for interventions and outcomes.

Bibliography

Crowley P: Elective induction of labour at 41+ weeks gestation. In Enkin MW, Keirse MJNC, Renfrew MJ, et al (eds): Pregnancy and Childbirth Module: Cochrane Database of Systematic Reviews (Update Software 1993; review no 04144, disk issue 2). Oxford, Cochrane Updates on Disk, 1993.

Hourvitz A, Alcalay M, Korach J, et al: A prospective study of high- versus low-dose oxytoxin for induction of labor. Acta Obstet Gynecol Scand 1996;75:636–641.

Ozgur K, Kizilates A, Uner M, et al: Induction of labor with intravaginal misoprostol versus intracervical dinoprostone. Arch Gynecol Obstet 1997;261:9–13.

Vengalil SR, Guinn DA, Olabi NF, et al: A randomized trial of misoprostol and extra-amniotic saline infusion for cervical ripening and labor induction. Obstet Gynecol 1998;91(5 Pt 1):774–779.

Wing DA, Ortiz-Omphroy G, Paul RH: A comparison of intermittent vaginal administration of misoprostol with continuous dinoprostone for cervical ripening and labor induction. Am J Obstet Gynecol 1997;177:612–618.

135 Pregnancy-Induced Hypertension

Gary R. Mennie

Description

The classic triad of findings in pre-eclampsia consists of hypertension, proteinuria, and edema, along with acute excessive weight gain developed during pregnancy after 20 weeks' gestation.

Etiology

1. The etiology of pregnancy-induced hypertension (PIH) or pre-eclampsia is not clearly understood; however, recent data support the presence of immunologic and genetic factors in the etiology of the disease.

2. The key event in the pathophysiology of pre-eclampsia is vasospasm, accompanied by activation of the coagulation system and endothelial injury and dysfunction, causing damage to vascular beds and end-organ damage.

3. Placental insufficiency on the fetal side secondary to vascular bed damage which leads to reduced placental perfusion.

4. Imbalance in the ratio of thromboxane A2 (potent vasoconstrictor) to prostacyclin I2 (potent vasodilator). Data suggest this imbalance may be responsible for the maternal hyperreactivity to angiotension II.

5. Because pre-eclampsia is more common in primigravidas and in woman with collagen vascular disease, an immunologic component has been suspected.

Symptoms

1. Headache and neurologic symptoms are the most obvious and most immediate threat to mother and fetus (i.e., intracerebral ischemia, hemorrhage, and edema).

2. Epigastric or right upper quadrant (RUQ) pain can be secondary to hepatic congestion, capsular swelling, or hepatic ischemia.

3. Visual disturbances may be secondary to retinal arteriolar spasm, cerebral ischemia, retinal hemorrhage, or papilledema.

4. Vaginal bleeding may be secondary to abruption, thrombocytopenia, or disseminated intravascular coagulation (DIC).

5. Oliguria results from decreased renal perfusion leading to decreased glomerular filtration rate and decreased uric acid clearance.

Key Symptoms

- Headache
- Visual disturbances
- Abdominal pain

Clinical Findings

1. Hypertension: defined as a blood pressure (BP) of 140/90 or greater or an increase in systolic BP of 30 mm Hg or diastolic BP of 15 mm Hg. Severe is considered a BP of 160/110 or greater (Table 135–1).

2. Edema: a clinically apparent edema or a rapid weight gain greater than 5 lb in a week. Edema is common in pregnancy; however, it is pathologic if it is rapid.

3. Proteinuria: is 0.3 gm/24 hours (>300 mg/24 hours) or concentration of 0.1 gm/L in at least two random urine samples collected 6 hours apart. It is severe if greater than 5 g/day.

4. Oliguria: less than 500 ml/24 hours.

Key Signs

- Systolic BP greater than 140 mm Hg or diastolic BP greater than 90 mm Hg
- Rapidly worsening edema
- Proteinuria

Clinical Course

Severe pre-eclampsia is marked by progression that may be gradual or rapid. These patients are at risk

TABLE 135–1. CRITERIA FOR SEVERE PRE-ECLAMPSIA*

BP greater than 160/110	Elevated serum creatinine
Proteinuria >5 gm/24 hr	Thrombocytopenia
Elevated liver enzymes	Cerebral or visual disturbances
Oliguria <500 ml/24 hr	RUQ or epigastric pain
Pulmonary edema	

*Developed by the American College of Obstetricians and Gynecologists.

for seizures, encephalopathy secondary to hypertension, pulmonary edema, acute renal failure, DIC, abruptio placentae, rupture liver, HELLP (hemolysis, elevated liver enzymes, and low platelet count) syndrome, fetal demise, and maternal demise.

Risk Factors

The risk factors include primigravida, familial incidence, extreme of age, lower socioeconomic status, multigestation, collagen disorders, first pregnancy with different father, diabetes mellitus, chronic hypertension, renal insufficiency, hydatid mole, fetal hydrops, polyhydramnios, and use of condoms. Epidemiologic reports indicate the prevalence of PIH was decreased in women who received heterologous blood or practiced oral sex, or when a long monogamous relationship preceded the pregnancy.

Laboratory Tests

1. Initial evaluation should include complete blood count (CBC), uric acid, liver functions, blood urea nitrogen and creatinine, urinalysis, and urine culture (Table 135–2). Remember that laboratory evaluation is more useful in the management of PIH patients than in the diagnosis of PIH.
2. Twenty-four-hour protein and creatinine clearance measurements should be done each trimester in patients with PIH or in patients at high risk.
3. Patients with hyperglycemia or wide BP swings: a 24-hour urine collection should be done for vanillylmandelic acid and metanephrines to rule out pheochromocytoma.
4. Remember, chronic renal disease may alter laboratory results.

Key Tests

- CBC
- Urinalysis
- Uric acid
- Aspartate transaminase
- Alanine transaminase
- Creatine

Differential Diagnosis

1. Chronic hypertension is the most likely cause in the first and second trimesters and persistent hypertension is most likely postpartum.
2. Transient hypertension of pregnancy is an increase in BP near term that resolves postpartum.

TABLE 135–2. LABORATORY VALUES THAT INDICATE PIH

Proteinuria >300 mg/24 hr or 1 gm/L	Thrombocyopenia
Uric acid >5.5 mg/dl mild, >9.5 mg/dl severe	Elevated PT
	Elevated FDP
CrCl <90 ml/min	Elevated liver function
Creatinine >1.0 mg/dl or BUN >16 mg/dl	
UA: granular cast, RBC cast, WBC cast, renal tubular cast	

Abbreviations: BUN, blood urea nitrogen; CrCl, creatinine clearance; FDP, fibrin degradation product; PT, prothrombin time; RBC, red blood cell; UA, urinalysis; WBC, white blood cell.

3. Chronic hypertension with superimposed PIH is marked by a rise in BP, development of proteinuria, increase in uric acid levels, and thrombocytopenia.

Treatment

1. Patients with mild chronic hypertension can be followed closely; those with moderate to severe hypertension need antihypertensive therapy. Patients with pre-eclampsia should be hospitalized, preferably in a tertiary care center. Those patients with severe pre-eclampsia or eclampsia need to be delivered as soon as possible.
2. The drug of choice for seizure prophylaxis is magnesium sulfate ($MgSO_4$).
   a. Give 4- to 6-gm IV loading dose over 15 to 20 minutes.
   b. Give 2 gm IV additional for second seizure.
   c. Give 2 to 3 gm/hour by IV infusion for maintenance.
   d. Magnesium levels are given in Table 135–3.
   e. Antidote is calcium gluconate, 1 gm IV over 3 minutes.
3. Methyldopa is given in divided dose to a maximum of 4 gm/day either IV or PO. It's the most extensively studied antihypertensive in pregnancy.
4. Hydralazine (Apresoline) is given 5 to 10 mg IV

TABLE 135–3. NORMAL, THERAPEUTIC, AND TOXIC $MgSO_4$ LEVELS

Normal	1.3–2.6 mg/dl
Therapeutic	4–8 mg/dl
Toxic	
Loss of patellar reflex	8–10 mg/dl
Somnolence	10–12 mg/dl
Respiratory depression	12–17 mg/dl
Paralysis	15–17 mg/dl
Cardiac arrest	30–35 mg/

every 20 to 30 minutes. This is the drug of choice to acutely lower BP. Side effects are headache, tachycardia, nausea, vomiting, tremors, and flushing, which are also symptoms of pre-eclampsia.

Alternative Medications

1. Diazoxide is given in 30-mg miniboluses every 2 to 5 minutes if hypertension is refractory to hydralazine. Miniboluses must be used to prevent uncontrolled hypotension.
2. β-Blockers are controversial. Labetalol has been used in several trials and is under consideration as a second-line choice. Concerns in using β-blockers include decreased uteroplacental flow, which can lead to a decreased fetal response to hypoxia.
3. Calcium channel blockers are promising. Nifedipine (Procardia) is under consideration but still lacks long-term studies. Nifedipine is given in doses of 30 to 120 mg/day divided into four doses or daily as an extended-release tablet. (*Remember*: Magnesium sulfate can potentiate the effect of calcium channel blockers, leading to hypotension.)
4. Nitroprusside should be avoided and used only as a last resort. It causes decreased uterine blood flow, plus the possibility of fetal cyanide toxicity. Keep the dose less than 4 μg/kg/minute.
5. Diuretics can be used in salt-sensitive patients when all other antihypertensives have failed. They decrease normal volume expansion in pregnancy.
6. Prazosin (Minipress) is used in pregnant patients with pheochromocytoma.
7. Angiotensin-converting enzyme inhibitors have no place in pregnancy and should never be used. They are associated with acute renal failure, neonatal anuria, oligohydramnios, intrauterine growth retardation (IUGR), and congenital abnormalities.

Diet

1. Recent trials indicate calcium supplementation, 1 to 2 gm/day, may sometimes prevent pre-eclampsia, but this was noted mainly in selective population with a relatively high incidence of pre-eclampsia (>8 to 10 per cent). Trials are now underway to evaluate its efficacy.
2. Protein, 80 to 100 mg/day.

Activity

Patients with pre-eclampsia or severe hypertension should be hospitalized and placed on bed rest.

Prevention

1. Patient education is the key. Patients should be educated on the signs and symptoms of pre-eclampsia and instructed to seek immediate medical attention if they develop.
2. Patients should be counseled on the potential side effects of the medications used to prevent hypertension and pre-eclampsia.
3. Patients should be counseled on avoiding excessive weight gain (>25 to 30 lb)
4. Recent studies indicate low-dose aspirin (60 mg/day), started in the 12th week of pregnancy, may sometimes prevent pre-eclampsia. Trials are now underway to evaluate its efficacy.

Key Treatment

- Delivery
- Methyldopa
- Hydralazine
- MgSO$_4$

Follow-Up

1. Patients with hypertension should be followed every 2 weeks in the first two trimesters and then weekly in the third trimester.
2. Monitoring with serial ultrasound for evidence of IUGR.
3. Nonstress tests weekly after the 26th week in severe hypertension and after the 34th week in mild hypertension.
4. Always recheck BP postpartum for evidence of chronic hypertension.

 ## Bibliography

American College of Obstetricians and Gynecologists: Hypertension in Pregnancy (ACOG Technical Bulletin no 219). Washington, DC, American College of Obstetricians and Gynecologists, 1996.

Hypertensive disorders in pregnancy. In Cunningham FG, MacDonald PC, Gant NF, et al (eds): Williams' Obstetrics, 19th ed, pp 763–803. Norwalk, CT, Appleton & Lange, 1993.

Magness RR, Gant NF: Control of vascular reactivity in pregnancy: the basis for therapeutic approaches to prevent pregnancy-induced hypertension. Semin Perinatol 1994;18:45–69.

Smith JF: The clinical management of eclampsia. Female Patient 1991;16:34–38.

Taylor RN: Immunobiology of pre-eclampsia. Am J Reprod Immunol 1997;37:79–86.

136 Gestational Hyperglycemia/Diabetes

Kimberle J. Vore

Etiology

1. Gestational diabetes mellitus (GDM) is hyperglycemia first recognized during pregnancy.

   a. Glucose intolerance resulting in postprandial hyperglycemia occurring later in pregnancy that is thought to be due to the influence of placental hormones causing insulin resistance; usually resolves after delivery

   b. Diabetes that existed prior to pregnancy but was unrecognized

2. Diabetes mellitus (DM) recognized as existing prior to pregnancy (see Ch. 174, Diabetes Mellitus, Type I; Ch. 175, Diabetes Mellitus, Type II).

Symptoms

1. GDM patients are usually asymptomatic.

2. Patients with pre-existing DM may have symptoms of hyperglycemia (polyuria, polydipsia, polyphagia).

3. Both types are prone to infections, especially urinary tract infections and vaginal candidiasis, and may have symptoms associated with these diseases—frequency, urgency, dysuria; vaginal itching and discharge.

Clinical Findings

1. Infants of diabetic mothers

   a. Hyperglycemia during pregnancy puts infants at increased risk of morbidity and mortality.

      (1) There is a threefold increase in congenital malformations if DM is uncontrolled in the first trimester.

      (2) Metabolic derangements can occur at birth, including hypoglycemia, hypocalcemia, hypomagnesemia, polycythemia, and hyperbilirubinemia.

      (3) Fetal macrosomia leading to possible birth trauma

      (4) Stillbirth

      (5) Increased risk of respiratory distress syndrome if born premature

   b. These infants inherit a predisposition to diabetes.

2. Pregestational diabetic mothers

   a. Increased incidence of pre-eclampsia–eclampsia

   b. Increased risk of operative delivery or traumatic vaginal delivery

   c. Greater incidence of polyhydramnios

   d. Greater risk of infections

3. Gestational diabetic mothers

   a. Up to 50 per cent of women diagnosed with GDM will have no identifiable risk factors.

   b. The risk factors listed under Key Signs are associated with GDM.

Key Signs

- Age older than 30 years

- Obesity

- Family history of DM

- Parity more than 5

- Glycosuria in current pregnancy

- Previous pregnancy with
  - GDM
  - Fetal macrosomia
  - Prematurity
  - Stillbirth

Laboratory Tests

1. Glucola screening is recommended for all women between weeks 24 and 28. A 50-gm oral glucose load is given without regard to meals. A venous plasma glucose drawn 1 hour after administration that is 140 mg/dl or greater indicates the need for 3-hour diagnostic oral glucose tolerance test.

2. The diagnostic test for GDM is a 100-gm oral glucose load administered after obtaining a fasting plasma glucose; then hourly plasma glucose tests are drawn for the next 3 hours, during which time the patient should not eat, drink, or smoke. In preparation for the test, the patient should have unrestricted diet and exercise for 2 to 3 days before test and then fast 8 to 12 hours (overnight). Two or more abnormal values indicate a positive test.

3. Once a diagnosis of GDM is made, periodic fasting and 2-hour postprandial plasma glucose

measurements are obtained to monitor treatment. Ideal levels are fasting blood glucose (FBG) levels below 105 mg/dl and 2-hour postprandial (pp) levels below 120 mg/dl.

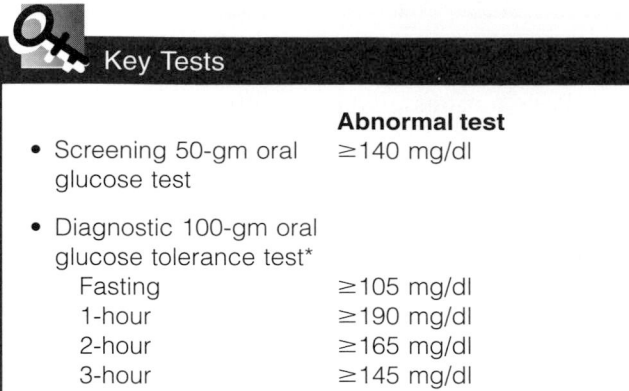

Key Tests

	Abnormal test
• Screening 50-gm oral glucose test	≥140 mg/dl
• Diagnostic 100-gm oral glucose tolerance test*	
Fasting	≥105 mg/dl
1-hour	≥190 mg/dl
2-hour	≥165 mg/dl
3-hour	≥145 mg/dl

*Requires two abnormal levels.
Based on criteria from National Diabetes Data Group.

Differential Diagnosis

Pre-existing DM should be diagnosed prior to pregnancy to allow for strict control of glucose before pregnancy.

Treatment

1. In patients with pre-existing DM, strict control of blood glucose needs to be maintained before and during pregnancy to prevent complications.

2. Ultrasound screening for congenital defects and to date pregnancy should be done at 16 to 18 weeks of gestation when mother has pre-existing DM.

3. Maintenance of glucose control (FBG <105 mg/dl and 2-hour pp <120 mg/dl) in patients with GDM is initially attempted through diet and exercise, but, when these levels are consistently elevated, insulin therapy is initiated.

4. Monitoring of fetal well-being with weekly nonstress testing is initiated at 32 weeks' gestation in patients requiring insulin.

5. Delivery is accomplished at or near term unless deterioration of fetal well-being indicates need for earlier delivery.

Medication

1. Human insulin is drug of choice to maintain glucose control.

2. Insulin requirements vary throughout pregnancy and require frequent monitoring and adjustment of insulin dosages.

3. Oral hypoglycemic agents should not be used during pregnancy because they cross the placenta, leading to possible fetal teratogenesis and prolonged serious neonatal hypoglycemia.

Diet

1. American Diabetes Association diet that provides 30 to 35 kcal/kg of ideal body weight on a daily basis

2. If the patient loses weight on this diet, calories may need to be increased.

Activity

Moderate aerobic exercise of 20 to 30 minutes three times a week will help to maintain normal glucose levels. Walking and swimming are ideal exercises.

Patient Education

1. All patients with glucose intolerance or overt diabetes need to visit a dietitian for dietary counseling.

2. If insulin is initiated during pregnancy, the patient will need instruction in self-administration of insulin and how to monitor blood glucose levels with a glucometer.

3. Preconception counseling about risks of congenital defects, risks during pregnancy, and need for strict glucose control should be done with all young diabetics considering pregnancy.

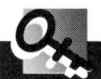

Key Treatment

Drug of Choice

Insulin

Follow-Up

1. Once the infant is delivered, the mother's blood glucose level should be monitored because insulin requirements for diabetics vary for several days, and gestation diabetics who required insulin during pregnancy often no longer need it.

2. Testing of patients with GDM at the 6-week postpartum examination is recommended. Fasting levels greater than 126 mg/dl or a 2-hour value greater than 200 mg/dl after a 75-gm oral glucose load indicate underlying diabetes. If initial testing is normal, yearly follow-up testing should be done because of high incidence of developing diabetes in women with GDM.

3. All women should be counseled in contraceptive use. Estrogen-progestin oral contraceptives and intrauterine devices should be avoided in women with overt diabetes.

 ## Bibliography

Carr DB, Gabbe S: Gestational diabetes: detection, management, and implications. Clin Diabetes 1998;16:4–11.

Endocrine disorders. In Cunningham FG, MacDonald PC, Gant NF, et al (eds): Williams Obstetrics, 20th ed, pp 1203–1221. Stamford, CT, Appleton & Lange, 1997.

Hollingsworth DR, Moor TR: Diabetes and pregnancy. In Creasy RK, Resnik R (eds): Maternal Fetal Medicine: Principles and Practice, 2nd ed, pp 925–988. Philadelphia, WB Saunders Company, 1989.

Langer O: Diabetes in pregnancy. In Cherry SH, Merkatz IR (eds): Complications of Pregnancy: Medical, Surgical, Gynecologic, Psychosocial, and Perinatal, 4th ed, pp 979–993. Baltimore, Williams & Wilkins, 1991.

O'Sullivan MJ, Skylar JS, Raimer KA: Diabetes and pregnancy. In Gleicher N (ed): Principles and Practice of Medical Therapy in Pregnancy, 2nd ed, pp 357–378. East Norwalk, CT, Appleton & Lange, 1992.

137 Epididymitis

Henry Martin-del-Campo

Etiology

Epididymitis is usually an infectious process. It normally occurs by spreading from an acute urinary tract infection or acute/chronic prostatitis followed by reflux of infective material down the vas deferens. Increasing bladder pressure from bladder neck obstruction can lead to reflux into the vas deferens, causing epididymitis. Structural abnormalities of the termination of the trigone and posterior urethra are the predisposing factors to retrograde epididymitis. Epididymitis may also occur with obstruction of the vas deferens following a vasectomy.

In heterosexual males less than 35 years of age, *Neisseria gonorrhoeae* and *Chlamydia trachomatis* are the most common pathogens. In the over-35-year age category, *Escherichia coli* and *Proteus mirabilis* are the most common pathogens. *Escherichia coli* is the most common pathogen in homosexual men. Other causes of acute epididymitis are anatomic and chemical causes.

1. Bacterial
   a. *Neisseria gonorrhoeae*
   b. *Treponema pallidum*
   c. *Escherichia coli*
   d. *Proteus mirabilis*
   e. *Chlamydia trachomatis*
   f. Uncommon organisms: *Salmonella*, *Haemophilus*, and tuberculosis
2. Atypical bacteria
   a. *Ureaplasma urealyticum*
3. Other infections
   a. Trichomoniasis
   b. Brucellosis
   c. Cryptococcosis
   d. Parasitic
   e. Viral (mumps)
4. Anatomic: epididymal torsion of appendix
5. Neoplastic
6. Trauma
7. Chemical: amiodarone (antiarrhythmic agent)

Symptoms

1. Tenderness or pain over the epididymis and/or testis
2. Dysuria
3. Urethral discharge
4. Fever
5. Scrotal swelling
6. Abdominal pain
7. Inguinal pain—may radiate to the flank
8. Scrotal pain, usually unilateral

Key Symptoms

- Scrotal pain
- Dysuria
- Abdominal pain
- Scrotal swelling
- Urethral discharge

Clinical Findings

Typically tenderness begins over the lower pole of the epididymis, or globus major, and progresses to include the entire epididymis. Radiation may occur into the spermatic cord and/or the inguinal region, and may include the lower quadrant of the abdomen on the affected side. Inflammation may progress to the body of the testis, where it may be difficult to distinguish between testicular and epididymal tenderness. The degree of pain varies from tenderness to excruciating pain.

1. Urethral discharge
2. Scrotal edema, with loss of rugae
3. Scrotal erythema
4. Increased scrotal temperature
5. Scrotal abscess formation
6. Vas deferens swelling and tenderness
7. Tenderness of testis, lower quadrant abdominal tenderness

Key Signs

- Prehn's sign: Elevation and support of the scrotum for approximately 1 hour usually can relieve the pain of epididymal orchitis (but not of torsion).

- Epididymal/testicular tenderness and edema

- Scrotal erythema, edema, and increased temperature

Laboratory/Radiologic Tests

1. Complete blood count may show an elevation of white cell count.
2. Urethral Gram's stain: intracellular gram-negative diplococci consistent with gonococcal urethritis
3. DNA probe (or culture) for *N. gonorrhoeae* or *C. trachomatis*
4. Urinalysis: can demonstrate white blood cells, blood, and bacteria. Midstream pyuria suggestive of epididymitis.
5. Urine: culture and sensitivities
6. Radionuclide scanning: may help differentiate between spermatic cord torsion versus epididymitis
7. Ultrasound: Color Doppler imaging (CDI) can be the modality of choice for the evaluation of the acute scrotum. CDI can assist in distinguishing between torsion and an inflammatory condition.

Differential Diagnosis

1. Epididymitis: bacterial.
2. Testicular appendage torsion: appendix epididymis or appendix testis. Blue dot sign seen through the skin of the scrotum.
3. Torsion of the spermatic cord

WARNING

Spermatic cord torsion is a serious emergency. This is a critical factor. Testicular infarction is the rule after 24 hours. Maximum salvage was noted when patients were operated on prior to 12 hours after onset of symptoms. It is believed that the anterior portion of each testis torques toward the midline; therefore, it should be rotated outward to achieve detorsion. Some experts believe anyone less than 15 years of age with the diagnosis of epididymitis requires surgical exploration to rule out spermatic cord torsion.

---

4. Intermittent testicular torsion
5. Incarcerated inguinal hernia
6. Testicular neoplasm
7. Traumatic testicular torsion (torsion following trauma)
8. Mumps orchitis

Complications

1. Failed treatment may lead to abscess formation.
2. Testicular atrophy
3. Infertility
4. Chronic pain

WARNING

Prostate palpation or massage prior to institution of antibiotics may cause increased reflux of infected material down the affected vas deferens. It may convert a unilateral process to a bilateral process.

Treatment

Supportive therapy consists of antibiotics, analgesics, bed rest, heat, and scrotal elevation. Infiltration of the spermatic cord with an anesthetic is an option for severe distress. Hot baths four times a day for 20 to 40 minutes are recommended. A hot, wet washcloth may be of benefit.

1. Nonsteroidal anti-inflammatory drugs and/or narcotics may be required for pain management.
2. Antibiotics: treatment options
   a. Gonococcal urethritis
      (1) Ceftriaxone (Rocephin), 250 mg IM once
      (2) Cefixime (Suprax), 400 mg PO once
      (3) Ofloxacin (Floxin), 400 mg once
      (4) Ciprofloxacin (Cipro), 500 mg PO once
      (5) Spectinomycin (Trobicin), 2 gm IM once
   b. *Chlamydia trachomatis*
      (1) Azithromycin (Zithromax), 1.0 gm PO once
      (2) Doxycycline (Vibramycin), 100 mg bid ×7 days
      (3) Ofloxacin (Floxin), 400 mg PO bid ×7 days
   c. Nongonococcal urethritis
      (1) Tetracycline, 500 mg qid ×10 days
      (2) Doxycycline, 100 mg bid ×10 days
      (3) Azithromycin, 1.0 gm PO once
      (4) Erythromycin, 500 mg qid ×7 days
      (5) Ofloxacin, 300 mg PO bid ×10 days
   d. Bacterial uropathogens: enterobacteria
      (1) Ciprofloxin, 500 mg PO bid ×10 to 14 days
      (2) Ofloxacin, 200 mg PO bid ×10 to 14 days
      (3) Ampicillin/sulbactam (Unasyn), 3 gm q6h IV
      (4) Cephalosporins: third generation, e.g., cefotaxime (Claforan) 2 gm q8h IV

(5) Piperacillin-tazobactam (Zosyn), 3.375 gm q6h IV

(6) Ticarcillin-clavulanate (Timentin), 3.1 gm q4–6h IV

Follow-Up

1. Verification of adequacy of treatment should take place within 2 to 6 weeks.
2. Consider syphilis and human immunodeficiency virus testing on individuals at risk.

 Bibliography

Brendan MR: Practical Strategies in Outpatient Medicine, 2nd ed, pp 1047–1078. Philadelphia, WB Saunders Company, 1991.

Gillenwater JY: Adult and Pediatric Urology, 3rd ed, vol 3, pp 2637–2655. St. Louis, Mosby–Year Book, 1996.

Herbener TE: Ultrasound in the assessment of the acute scrotum. J Clin Ultrasound 1996;24:405–421.

McDonald SW: Vasectomy reviews: sequelae in the human epididymis and ductus deferens. J Clin Anat 1996; 9:337–334.

The Sexually Transmitted Diseases (Section 10). In Rakel RE (ed): Conn's Current Therapy 1998, pp 731–739. Philadelphia, WB Saunders Company, 1998.

138 Varicocele

E. Robert Schwartz

Definition

An abnormal degree of venous dilatation in the pampiniform vascular plexus of the scrotum

Etiology

1. The exact causes of varicocele are not clearly known, but a possible cause is vascular dilatation caused by valvular incompetence in the internal spermatic veins.
2. Another possible cause is elevated hydrostatic pressure in the left renal vein, inferior vena cava, and internal spermatic veins. Because the left spermatic vein empties into the left renal vein, while the right spermatic vein empties into the inferior vena cava, varicoceles almost always occur on the left.
3. Varicocele also may be caused by the effect of mechanical pressure from the superior mesenteric artery.

Symptoms

1. The patient is often asymptomatic.
2. The patient may experience heaviness in the scrotum and/or rarely a dull ache.
3. There may be concern on the part of the patient about the physical findings associated with varicocele (i.e., many dilated and engorged veins in the scrotom).

Key Symptoms

- Asymptomatic
- Heaviness or dull ache

Clinical Findings

1. Patients should in general be examined while standing in order to accentuate the dilated veins.
2. The Valsalva maneuver or coughing may help identify the veins.
3. Greater than 90 per cent of varicoceles occur on the left.
4. On palpation, a varicocele often feels like a "bag of worms."

5. The dilated veins are found most often superior to the testis and above the epididymis and slightly posterior.
6. There is a grading system for varicocele:
   a. Grade I: palpable only while the patient performs a Valsalva maneuver
   b. Grade II: palpable on physical examination while standing
   c. Grade III: Visual inspection of the scrotum reveals varicocele.
7. There is a significant incidence of infertility associated with varicocele.

Key Signs

- Palpable veins in scrotum
- Greater incidence on the left than on the right

WARNING

With sudden appearance of a right-sided varicocele, rule out obstruction of right spermatic vein caused by retroperitoneal neoplasm.

Laboratory Tests

1. Noninvasive
   a. Ultrasound
   b. Labeled blood-pool scintigraphy
   c. Thermography
   d. Echo Doppler
2. Invasive: phlebography, internal spermatic vein

Key Tests

- Scrotal ultrasonography
- Spermatic venography ("gold standard")

Differential Diagnosis

1. Hernia
2. Epididymitis
3. Hydrocele
4. Spermatocele
5. Testicular tumor

Treatment

1. Surgical ligation
2. Laparoscopic varicocelectomy
3. Percutaneous varicocele occlusion
4. Guidewire-directed detachable balloon for embolization technique

Medication

None

Diet

None

Activity

1. If patient is asymptomatic, no restrictions are indicated.
2. If patient has scrotal heaviness or discomfort, an athletic supporter may be helpful.

Patient Education

1. Patient reassurance that varicocele is a common problem and that there is no evidence that it is a precursor to malignancy
2. If infertility is a cause of concern, explanation of the possible association with spermatogenesis and potential improvement of fertility with surgical correction
3. Clinical course of varicocele is unpredictable.

Key Treatment

- Surgical ligation
- Laparoscopic varicocelectomy
- Percutaneous varicocele occlusion
- Guidewire-directed detachable balloon for embolization technique

Follow-Up

1. In adolescents, there is strong evidence that close follow-up and early treatment may improve long-term fertility.
2. In asymptomatic patients without a history of infertility, no clear guidelines have been established. Yearly physical examination would seem prudent.
3. Good evidence exists that, for men with proven infertility, treatment is beneficial, but periodic physical examinations are necessary in order to diagnose recurrence and/or development of post-treatment complications.

 ## Bibliography

Jarow J, Assimos D, Pittaway D: Effectiveness of laparoscopic varicocelectomy. Urology 1993;42:544–547.

Laven JS, Haans LC, Mali WP, et al: Effects of varicocele treatment in adolescents: a randomized study. Fertil Steril 1992;58:756–762.

Morvay Z, Nagy E: The diagnosis and treatment of intratesticular varicocele. Cardiovasc Intervent Radiol 1998;21:76–78.

Skoog SJ, Roberts KP, Goldstein M, et al: The adolescent varicocele: what's new with an old problem in young patients? Pediatrics 1997;100:112–121.

Witt M, Lipshultz L: Varicocele: a progressive or static lesion? Urology 1993;42:541–543.

139 Hydrocele/Spermatocele

Grant C. Fowler

Etiology

1. The visceral lining of the testicle is known as the visceral tunica vaginalis. This layer is surrounded by the parietal tunica vaginalis. A hydrocele is a collection of peritoneal fluid in the potential space between these two layers.

    a. Communicating hydrocele: usually congenital, resulting from incomplete obliteration of the processus vaginalis. This communication allows fluid to descend from the peritoneal cavity and fill the potential space between the parietal and visceral vaginalis.

    b. Noncommunicating: imbalance between secretory and absorptive capacities of tunica vaginalis resulting from epididymitis, orchitis, filariasis (caused by lymphatic obstruction), germ cell testicular tumors, testicular trauma, renal transplantation with ligation of the spermatic cord, radiation therapy, or unknown etiology.

2. Spermatocele: Cause is not certain. It probably arises from cystic structures on the upper pole of the testis or weaknesses in the tubes of the epididymis.

Symptoms

Both are usually painless. Occasionally, either can be of sufficient size to cause pain and warrant surgical exploration or correction. Symptoms are usually described as a heaviness, often unilateral, in the scrotum or a pain in the inguinal area or lower back. Symptoms may also result from trauma with subsequent hemorrhage into a hydrocele. Pain may occur in association with epididymitis or if a hydrocele or spermatocele becomes infected. Rarely, torsion of a spermatocele has been described as causing symptoms.

Key Symptoms

- None

- "Heaviness" in the scrotum

Clinical Findings

1. Hydrocele

    a. Usually nontender scrotal mass or swelling that transilluminates. Often more prominent anteriorly, it may entirely surround the testis.

    b. Mass may be soft and cystic or large and tense. In a young boy with a communicating hydrocele, it may be small and soft in the morning, becoming larger and more tense at night.

    c. May be associated with a hernia. Auscultation of a hydrocele should not reveal bowel sounds. Hydroceles usually do not vary in size with respiration or Valsalva maneuver.

2. Spermatocele

    a. Very common, nontender, round scrotal masses that transilluminate. They may be freely movable. They are separate from and usually superior and posterior to the testis.

    b. May be solitary or multiple. Most are less than 1 cm in size. Spermatoceles do not vary in size with respiration or Valsalva maneuver.

Key Sign

Soft, nontender scrotal mass that transilluminates

Laboratory/Diagnostic Tests

1. Aspiration may result in infection requiring surgical repair and should be avoided if possible. However, aspiration of a hydrocele may be necessary for a thorough examination and usually results in clear, yellow fluid. Aspiration of a spermatocele often produces a thin, white, cloudy fluid with dead sperm on microscopic examination.

2. High-frequency (7.5 to 10 MHz) ultrasound should be performed if the diagnosis is uncertain or if the mass prevents thorough examination of the entire contents of the scrotum. This is especially important in a young male with a newly developed hydrocele and no apparent cause (to exclude tuberculosis or cancer).

Key Tests

- Aspiration of fluid
- Ultrasound

Differential Diagnosis

1. Varicocele
2. Hernia
3. Tumor

WARNING

- An intratesticular mass or a mass adherent to the testicle is cancer until proven otherwise.
- If a hydrocele develops spontaneously between the ages of 18 and 35, careful evaluation should be made to exclude cancer.

Treatment

1. Hydrocele
   a. In infants, spontaneous closure may occur. Surgical repair is indicated, however, if the presence of bowel is suspected. If a hydrocele persists beyond 1 year of age, spontaneous closure is unlikely
   b. Very tense, large hydroceles that might compromise circulation to the testicle or that are uncomfortable or perhaps cosmetically unsightly may need surgical repair. Infected hydroceles require surgical repair. Otherwise, active therapy is not required. An athletic supporter may relieve symptoms.

2. Spermatocele: same as item 1b above

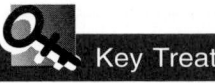

Key Treatment

Surgical repair

Bibliography

Disorders of the spermatic cord. In McAninch JW (ed): Smith's General Urology, 14th ed, pp 685–686. East Norwalk, CT, Appleton & Lange, 1995.

Goldstein M: Surgical management of male infertility and other scrotal disorders. In Walsh PC, Retik AB, Vaughan ED, et al (eds): Campbell's Urology, 7th ed, pp 1331–1377. Philadelphia, WB Saunders Company, 1998.

Junnila J, Lassen P: Testicular masses. Am Fam Physician 1998;57:685–692.

Pfenninger JL, Fowler GC, James RE: Selected disorders of the genitourinary system. In Taylor RB (ed): Family Medicine, Principles and Practice, 5th ed, pp 871–873. New York, Springer-Verlag, 1998.

Rozanski T, Bloom D, Colodny A: Surgery of the scrotum and testis in children. In Walsh PC, Retick AB, Vaughan ED, et al (eds): Campbell's Urology, 7th ed, pp 2193–2209. Philadelphia, WB Saunders Company, 1998.

140 Undescended Testicle

Timothy P. Daaleman

Etiology

1. Undescended testes (UDT), or cryptorchidism, is a frequent disorder of the male infant. The term "cryptorchidism" is taken from the Greek *kryptos* and *orchis*, which means "hidden testes."

2. The incidence of UDT is correlated with fetal maturity.
   a. In full-term male infants, the incidence of cryptorchidism is 3 per cent. This diminishes to 1 per cent at age 1 as a result of spontaneous descent.
   b. In preterm males who weigh more than 1500 gm, the incidence of UDT is 21 per cent, but it rises to 60 to 70 per cent among infants weighing less than 1500 gm.

3. Cryptorchidism has been demonstrated in up to 4 per cent of siblings and 6 per cent of fathers of cryptorchid children, which suggests a genetic influence.

4. UDT is seen more frequently in infant males with endocrine disorders, genetic abnormalities, or genitourinary anatomic anomalies.

5. There is no single unified cause of cryptorchidism. A mix of hormonal, neural, and mechanical factors that play a role in normal testicular descent has been implicated.

Symptoms

Cryptorchid males are asymptomatic.

Clinical Findings

1. The physical examination is critical in establishing the diagnosis and classification of UDT. The examination should be performed in a warm and nonthreatening environment and in a systematic manner.

2. For an optimal examination, the patient should be comfortably seated in a cross-legged position, which allows most retractile testes to descend spontaneously as a result of relaxation of the cremasteric muscles.

3. After warming his or her hands, the examiner should begin by evaluating the genitalia, with attention directed toward the scrotum. The overall size of the sac, as well as any discrepancies between the left and right sides, should be documented. In addition, any hernias, hydroceles, or evidence of hypospadias should be noted.

4. If an empty scrotum is found, liquid soap or KY jelly on the examiner's fingers is helpful prior to palpating along the inguinal canal. Begin at the inguinal ring and move medially toward the pubic bone. One helpful technique is to slide the second and third fingers over the canal while using the index finger of the opposite hand in a brushing motion preceding the sliding fingers. When a testis is palpated, an attempt should be made to manipulate it into the scrotum.

5. Undescended testes are generally classified as palpable or nonpalpable.
   a. In patients with nonpalpable testes, atrophy or agenesis should be considered. Most nonpalpable testes have an intra-abdominal location or an intracanalicular position that may be transient.
   b. Palpable testes may be either ectopic, retractile, or arrested in their normal descent.
      (1) Ectopic testes are usually perineal but may be located at the base of the penis, in the thigh or above the pubic bone, or in the opposite scrotal sac.
      (2) Testes may be retractile secondary to poor scrotal attachment or as a result of an overactive cremasteric reflex. Retractile testes are usually bilateral and are most commonly identified in preschool boys, although they may be present until puberty.
      (3) Testes that arrest along their normal descent generally reside superior to the external ring and superficial to the external oblique muscle.

Key Signs

- Nonpalpable testes
- Hydrocele
- Penile, pubic, inguinal, thigh, or perineal mass
- Hernia
- Asymmetric or empty scrotum
- Hypospadias

Laboratory Tests

1. When both testes are nonpalpable, baseline assays of luteinizing hormone (LH), follicle-stimulating hormone (FSH), and testosterone can be helpful in evaluating possible anorchidism. Elevated FSH and LH levels and a low baseline testosterone level suggest anorchidism. The presence or absence of testicular tissue also can be determined by human chorionic gonadotropin (hCG) stimulation (2000 IU/m² for 3 days). The lack of a several-fold rise in testosterone levels in hCG-stimulated males indicates an absence of functioning testicular tissue.

2. A variety of imaging techniques are useful in the diagnosis of cryptorchid testes.

   a. The use of ultrasound is an optimal diagnostic technique for testes along the inguinal canal, although there are limitations in its ability to identify intra-abdominal testes. Its low cost, noninvasiveness, and lack of radiation make it an attractive first-line technique.

   b. Computerized tomography (CT) and magnetic resonance imaging (MRI) are superior to sonography in localization and evaluation of the testes and cord structures. The risks associated with radiation exposure (CT) and the need for sedation in a pediatric population must be considered with these modalities.

   c. Selective gonadal venography is an infrequently used procedure because it is technically difficult, invasive, and radiation-exposing.

3. The use of laparoscopy continues to be a definitive modality in the localization and management of UDT. It allows direct visualization of the intra-abdominal testes. No other study is as sensitive or specific for localizing undescended testes.

Key Tests

- FSH, LH, and testosterone levels
- hCG stimulation test
- Ultrasound
- CT
- MRI
- Laparoscopy

Differential Diagnosis

Bilateral undescended testes are associated with a variety of endocrine disorders, genetic abnormalities, and anatomic variations.

1. Endocrine disorders: hypopituitarism, Kallmann's syndrome, testicular feminization disorder, anencephaly, 5α-reductase deficiency, congenital LH secretory failure

2. Genetic abnormalities: trisomy 13 and 18; Aarskog's, Laurence-Moon-Biedl, Freeman-Sheldon, prune belly, Prader-Willi, Cornelia de Lange's, Noonan's, Beckwith-Wiedemann, and Kleinfelter's syndromes

3. Anatomic variations: gastroschisis, omphalocele, exstrophy of the bladder, prune belly syndrome

Treatment

1. Consultation with a pediatric urologist or surgeon familiar with the diagnosis and treatment of cryptorchidism is advised.

2. Surgical treatment (orchidopexy and/or laparoscopy) is recommended after the age of 6 months and before 18 months of age for males with palpable or nonpalpable testes. Prepubertal males with retractile testes should be followed with yearly examinations. If the testis does not descend by puberty, orchidopexy is recommended.

3. Because of the increased risk of testicular cancer, postpubertal men younger than 32 years should be considered for orchiectomy. Men older than 32 years of age should be observed with frequent examinations.

4. The use of hormonal therapy (hCG, gonadotropin-releasing hormone, or both) has an uncertain place in the treatment of cryptorchidism. Although the efficacy of hormonal therapy has been questioned, this treatment can promote descent of retractile testes or enhance the success rates of subsequent surgical repair.

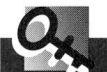

Key Treatment

Surgery: orchidopexy and/or laparoscopy

Follow-Up

1. The maintenance of fertility is the most important consideration in the cryptorchid male. Because there is histologic evidence of testicular germ cell damage by age 2, early identification and appropriate management of UDT are critical.

2. Testicular malignancies occur more frequently in cryptorchid males than in those with normal testicular position. In unilateral UDT, the contralateral, normally placed testicle has an in-

creased risk of having a malignancy. Early orchidopexy (prior to age 6) appears to diminish the chances of developing a malignancy.

3. In patients who have undergone surgical intervention and in those followed with hormonal or expectant management (retractile testes), the importance of annual physical examinations and monthly testicular self-examinations cannot be overstated.

Bibliography

Ellis DG: Undescended testes. In Ashcraft KW (ed): Pediatric Urology, pp 415–427. Philadelphia, WB Saunders Company, 1990.

Fonkalsrud EW: Current management of the undescended testis. Semin Pediatr Surg 1996;5:2–7.

Gandhi K, Maizels M: Management of the undescended testis. Compr Ther 1993;19:5–9.

Palmer JM: The undescended testicle. Endocrinol Metab Clin North Am 1991;20:231–240.

Rozanski TA, Bloom DA: The undescended testis: theory and management. Urol Clin North Am 1995;22:107–118.

141   Common Urinary Symptoms

SYMPTOM   HEMATURIA

Linda E. Tepper

Hematuria is a perplexing problem because of the numerous diagnostic possibilities and the invasive nature of the work-up. The presence of microscopic hematuria on screening urinalysis is common because 13 per cent of the general medical population manifests one erythrocyte per high-power field (HPF). However, only 2 per cent of these patients will have significant disease. Therefore, most physicians accept three erythrocytes per HPF as diagnostically significant hematuria.

Differential Diagnosis

1. Extrarenal causes
   a. Benign prostatic hypertrophy
   b. Infection of the bladder, urethra, or prostate
   c. Nephrolithiasis
   d. Neoplasm of the bladder, prostate, or ureter
   e. Endometriosis
   f. Meatal ulceration
   g. Vaginal bleeding
2. Glomerular renal diseases
   a. Poststreptococcal glomerulonephritis (GN)
   b. Berger's disease
   c. Henoch-Schönlein purpura
   d. Lupus erythematosus
   e. Vasculitis
   f. Goodpasture's syndrome
   g. Membranous GN
   h. Benign familial hematuria
   i. Proliferative GN
   j. Alport's syndrome
   k. Multiple myeloma
3. Nonglomerular renal diseases
   a. Hypertensive nephrosclerosis
   b. Drug-induced interstitial nephritis
   c. Papillary necrosis
   d. Polycystic kidney disease
   e. Renal infarct
   f. Medullary sponge kidney
   g. Obstructive or reflex nephropathy
   h. Tuberculosis
   i. Renal vein thrombosis
   j. Renal neoplasm
4. Other
   a. Coagulopathy
   b. Trauma from Foley catheter insertion
   c. Exercise such as running or bicycling
   d. False-positive results from food dyes and foods such as beets and blackberries, and myoglobin, hemolysis, and porphyrins
   e. Factitious sources
   f. Drugs such as phenytoin, rifampin, and sulfasalazine

History

1. Characterize the bleeding.
   a. Clots usually indicate lower urinary tract bleeding.
   b. Association with menses may suggest endometriosis.
   c. Relationship to exercise may indicate runner's hematuria.
   d. Association with flank pain may suggest infection, papillary necrosis, calculus, or obstruction, whereas painless bleeding is associated with cancer or GN.
   e. Association with hesitancy, frequency, or decreased force of stream is suggestive of prostatic hypertrophy.
2. Rule out systemic disease.
   a. Constitutional symptoms such as fatigue, weight loss, or anorexia may indicate cancer.
   b. Presence of rash, arthralgias, photosensitivity, Raynaud's phenomenon, or mouth ulcers may suggest GN secondary to collagen-vascular disease.
   c. Tendency toward bleeding may indicate a coagulopathy.

d. Hypertension (HTN) may indicate nephrosclerosis.

e. Atrial fibrillation or endocarditis may suggest emboli.

3. Rule out infection.

a. Symptoms of dysuria, fever, nausea, vomiting, urgency, or frequency may suggest urinary tract infection.

b. Pulmonary symptoms may suggest tuberculosis.

c. Complaints of vaginal or penile discharge may indicate presence of a sexually transmitted disease.

d. Recent upper respiratory tract infection may precede poststreptococcal GN, Berger's disease, or Henoch-Schönlein purpura.

e. Travel abroad may indicate schistosomiasis.

4. Screen for risk factors of urologic cancer, which include age greater than 50 years, tobacco use, pelvic irradiation, and use of analgesics or cyclophosphamide.

5. Screen for medication use.

a. Many drugs turn the urine red, such as rifampin, phenytoin, and pyridium.

b. Other drugs cause GN (e.g., penicillamine and gold) or cause interstitial nephritis (e.g., analgesics).

c. Anticoagulants often cause hematuria.

6. Screen for family history of sickle cell disease, polycystic kidney disease, Alport's syndrome, benign familial hematuria, or coagulopathy.

Clinical Findings

1. Vital signs: Check for fever, which may suggest infection, and HTN, which may be secondary to GN or may cause nephrosclerosis.

2. Cardiac: Auscultate for new heart murmur suggestive of endocarditis, or atrial fibrillation suggestive of emboli.

3. Back: Examine for costovertebral angle tenderness suggestive of infection.

4. Abdomen: Palpate to rule out any masses suggestive of cancer, enlarged kidneys suggestive of polycystic kidneys, or splenomegaly suggestive of endocarditis. Also, rule out tenderness consistent with infection, calculus, or papillary necrosis.

5. Genitourinary: Examine the urethral orifice and external genitalia for evidence of condylomata, ulceration, or stenosis. Examine the prostate to rule out the presence of hypertrophy, nodules, pain, and bogginess.

6. Extremities: Examine for edema suggestive of nephrotic syndrome or GN.

7. Skin: Examine for ecchymosis suggestive of coagulopathy, necrotizing lesions suggestive of vasculitis, and track marks suggestive of intravenous drug usage.

Tests

Because of the wide variety of causes of hematuria and the low frequency with which each diagnosis occurs, very large multicenter trials would be needed to compare the efficacy of all tests available and determine an algorithmic approach to hematuria. In the absence of such data, diagnostic approach should be guided by the history, physical examination, and urinalysis.

1. Microscopic urinalysis: Heavy proteinuria is evidence of glomerular disease and should be quantitated with a 24-hour urine protein measurement. Red blood cell (RBC) casts are again suggestive of glomerular disease. Pyuria suggests infection and should be followed by urine culture.

2. Phase-contrast microscopy: Dysmorphic (irregularly sized and shaped) erythrocytes may indicate glomerular bleeding. However, this test is limited by its specificity.

3. Screening laboratory tests: A baseline complete blood count, prothrombin time, partial thromboplastin time, and serum electrolytes should be performed. Again, other tests should be guided by the clinical picture. These might include antinuclear antibodies, antineutrophil cytoplasmic antibodies, complement level, anti–streptolysin O antibody, rapid plasma reagin test, urine protein electrophoresis, hemoglobin electrophoresis, tuberculin skin test, and prostate-specific antigen.

4. Urine cytology: Can detect lower urinary tract malignancies and should be obtained in patients older than age 50 and when suspicion of malignancy is high. False-positive results can occur with infection or nephrolithiasis.

5. Abdominal roentgenogram: Used to evaluate younger patients who have an increased incidence of nephrolithiasis. The results are limited by the proportion of calculi that are opaque and the presence of phleboliths.

6. Intravenous pyelogram (IVP): Provides good evaluation of anatomy and thus can detect silent stones, renal tumors, and hydronephrosis. It is less sensitive for bladder tumors.

7. Renal sonogram: Used if the patient is allergic to dye or if a cyst is suspected. It provides a good look at anatomy but is less sensitive than IVP for detecting ureteral stones or collecting system tumors.

8. Cytoscopy: Permits visualization of urethra, bladder, and ureteral orifices and is considered the gold standard for bladder cancer detection. However, in situ carcinomas and sessile or small tumors can be missed.

9. Renal biopsy: Done if glomerular bleeding is suggested by presence of HTN, RBC casts, dysmorphic RBCs, and proteinuria.

Management

Management depends on the diagnosis.

1. Medications that cause hematuria should be avoided.

2. Appropriate dietary recommendations should be made if the patient has HTN, renal failure, or a calculus.

3. If an infection is diagnosed, antibiotics should be instituted.

4. If bladder cancer is found, treatment with chemotherapy or surgery should be done.

5. If there is prostatic hypertrophy, α-adrenergic blockers, 5α-reductase inhibitors, or surgery may be instituted.

6. If nephrolithiasis is found, oral hydration, external wall lithotripsy, or surgery may be needed.

Follow-Up

In many patients, despite a thorough investigation, the cause remains obscure. Fortunately, studies of 5-year follow-up of patients who have undergone a previously negative work-up have shown that the future incidence of serious disease is low. One suggested protocol is

1. Those greater than age 50 or with risk factors for urologic cancer should have a urine cytology every 6 months and yearly cystoscopy and IVP for 3 years.

2. Those under age 50 who are asymptomatic and have no risk factors only require observation.

PEARLS

- Asymptomatic hematuria occurs commonly in the general medical population.

- In patients younger than age 50 with no risk factors for bladder cancer and normal physical examination, the incidence of serious disease is low, and work-up can be limited to abdominal roentgenogram, blood urea nitrogen, creatinine, and microscopic urinalysis.

- Patients older than age 50 require a full investigation because risk of serious disease is greater.

Bibliography

Ahmed Z, Lee J: Asymptomatic urinary abnormalities: hematuria and proteinuria. Med Clin North Am 1997; 81:641–652.

McCarthy JJ: Outpatient evaluation of hematuria. Postgrad Med 1997;101:125–128, 131.

Sultana R, Goodman CM, Byrne DJ, et al: Microscopic haematuria: urological investigation using a standard protocol. Br J Urol 1996;78:691–698.

Sutton JM: Evaluation of hematuria in adults. JAMA 1990;263:2475–2480.

Webb JA: Imaging in haematuria [editorial]. Clin Radiol 1997;52:167–171.

SYMPTOM PROTEINURIA

Joseph J. Lieber

The finding of protein by dipstick in a patient's urine is one of the key signs in nephrology. Proteinuria implies finding greater than 50 to 100 mg of protein in a 24-hour urine collection. Naturally, the amount of protein may vary, with greater quantities often implying more severe disease. Furthermore, the type of protein may vary as well. Always, a thorough history, physical examination, and key laboratory tests should be performed to help define the nature of the proteinuria, and its causes and possible treatments, if any.

Differential Diagnosis

1. *Glomerular* proteinuria is a manifestation of primary or secondary glomerular disease.

a. Usually composed of albumin with, at times, globulins and other proteins

b. When the amount of protein is greater than 3.5 gm in 24 hours, the patient has nephrotic-range proteinuria.

c. The specific glomerulopathies that cause proteinuria are quite varied and include minimal change disease, membranous nephropathy, diabetic nephropathy, focal sclerosis, amyloidosis, postinfectious glomerulonephritis, immunoglobulin A (IgA) nephropathy, and membranoproliferative glomerulopathy.

2. *Tubular* proteinuria normally is less than 1.5 gm in 24 hours

a. Composed mostly of β_2-microglobulin and Tamm-Horsfall protein

b. Caused by tubular cell damage with inability to resorb these proteins. This is usually seen with tubulointerstitial injury.

3. *Overflow* proteinuria is usually composed of light chain proteins and is caused by a plasma cell dyscrasia with the finding of a paraprotein in the urine.

a. Usual causes: multiple myeloma, amyloidosis, Waldenström's macroglobulinemia, and light chain nephropathy

b. Such patients may have secondary glomerular changes with glomerular proteinuria as well

c. Because the urine dipstick will detect only albumin, a large quantity of protein in a 24-hour sample with a trace dipstick reading should suggest a nonglomerular protein, often a light chain.

4. *Transient* proteinuria and orthostatic proteinuria are usually self-limited, although they may cause the patient some concern. Febrile illness, elevation in blood pressure, or exercise may lead to mild proteinuria that will usually remit in the near future. Other patients have persistent proteinuria, but the bulk of the protein is associated with ambulation. The prognosis is quite good.

Refer to Ch. 143, Acute Renal Failure; Ch. 144, Chronic Renal Failure; Ch. 145, Glomerulonephritis; Ch. 174, Diabetes Mellitus, Type I; and Ch. 175, Diabetes Mellitus, Type II.

History

1. A family history of kidney disease in the patient with proteinuria suggests a familial nephropathy.

2. A longstanding history of diabetes mellitus suggests diabetic nephropathy.

3. Recent pharyngitis, gross hematuria, arthritis, skin rash, or use of medications (including over-the-counter agents) should be questioned. Finding symptoms of a systemic disease, such as fever, weight loss, or myalgias, may suggest vasculitis or a secondary amyloid nephropathy. Furthermore, deep visceral infections, endocarditis, or hepatitis can have an associated glomerulopathy with proteinuria.

4. Careful assessment of risk factors for human immunodeficiency virus (HIV) is mandatory because HIV is associated with glomerular disease. In fact, abuse of illicit drugs such as heroin can cause a chronic glomerulopathy; "skin poppers" are at increased risk for amyloid.

5. Glomerular disease may rarely be a manifestation of an underlying solid tumor or hematologic malignancy; evidence for these should be considered in smokers and in patients with weight loss, diffuse symptoms, fevers, bleeding, and severe pain.

6. Many tubulointerstitial diseases are a result of toxins, abuse of analgesics, or exposure to industrial products. A good history will help determine if the patient is at risk for any of these. When asking about analgesic use, attempts to quantify doses are important because chronic injury is usually seen only with large amounts of these agents.

Clinical Findings

1. Assessment of blood pressure is crucial because hypertension may be a clue to fixed renal disease.

2. Edema and anasarca often imply more severe proteinuria, often in the nephrotic range.

3. A thorough eye examination to inspect for diabetic retinopathy is crucial. This will correlate with diabetic nephropathy. Other eye findings may include uveitis or episcleritis, which may suggest vasculitis.

4. A skin examination for a malar rash, erythema nodosum, or palpable purpura may again indicate a vasculitis or systemic lupus erythematosus. Amyloid may be associated with upper extremity purpura. Needle track marks are a clue to drug abuse.

5. Always assess for pericardial or pleural rubs that might be seen with lupus or, less likely, a systemic infection.

6. The findings of hepatomegaly and splenomegaly may be seen with amyloid, lymphoma, hepatitis, malignancy, or endocarditis. All of these may be associated with glomerular proteinuria.

7. The finding of active arthritis may be seen with lupus, vasculitis, and endocarditis. Clubbing may be a sign of neoplasia that could have an associated glomerulopathy.

8. Findings on ear, nose, and throat examination of ulcers, masses, and nodules may indicate Wegener's vasculitis.

9. Lymph nodes should be thoroughly palpated and followed to assess for lymphoma, metastatic cancer, or infection that may be associated with glomerular disease.

Tests

1. It is mandatory to quantify the proteinuria in a 24-hour sample to determine the degree of proteinuria. One might wish to quantify the proteinuria in a split collection, with the urine in one container obtained while the patient is ambulating and that in the other obtained while recumbent to confirm benign orthostatic proteinuria.

2. A urine protein electrophoresis and a urine sample for Bence Jones protein will determine the nature of the proteinuria. This should be done following a thorough microscopic examination of the urine. This may be crucial to help define the type of renal disease.

3. A renal sonogram assesses the size of the kidneys, determines chronicity of disease, and rules out obstruction. This will also be important if a renal biopsy is contemplated.

4. Serologic studies may include antinuclear antibodies (ANA), anti–glomerular basement membrane (anti-GBM), complement (C3 and C4), serum protein electrophoresis (SPEP), cryoglobulins, streptozyme, hepatitis profile, and anti–neutrophil cytoplasmic antibody (ANCA). These may be helpful, especially in patients with more severe glomerular proteinuria, azotemia, rash, evidence of a systemic disease, and arthritis.

   a. Complement levels are often helpful because usually only lupus nephritis, membranoproliferative glomerulonephritis (GN), post-streptococcal GN, and proliferative GN caused by endocarditis, hepatitis, or cryoglobulinemia lower complement levels.

   b. ANA testing may be helpful to diagnose lupus nephritis and some related conditions.

   c. An SPEP with a monoclonal spike is very suggestive of a plasma cell dyscrasia or amyloid.

   d. The anti-GBM and ANCA may be examined in patients with rapidly progressive azotemia and proteinuria, often associated with findings in the lungs, skin, and sinuses.

   e. Because many of these tests are expensive and may be diagnostic of less common entities, one should order only those tests that are of clinical value in that specific patient.

5. A renal biopsy may be indicated to specifically define the clinical entity. This is a relatively safe procedure and will give diagnostic as well as prognostic information. It is less crucial in patients with under 1 gm of proteinuria in 24 hours.

   a. Patients with greater amounts of proteinuria—especially in the nephrotic range—should undergo a biopsy unless the diagnosis is otherwise clear-cut.

   b. Patients with azotemia, normal-size kidneys, abnormal serologic studies, and severe proteinuria should also undergo biopsy.

   c. Patients with tubular proteinuria and orthostatic proteinuria are usually not helped by biopsy.

   d. If the renal sonogram reveals small kidneys, a biopsy is best deferred because this indicates chronic scarring and fibrosis.

Management

The management depends on the degree of proteinuria and its cause.

1. Patients with overflow proteinuria in whom the protein is a light chain should undergo a full assessment for myeloma and other plasma cell dyscrasias and be treated for the primary disease. Amyloidosis may be treated with regimens used to manage myeloma or the patient may be tried on colchicine.

2. Tubular proteinuria is usually not treated. The underlying nephropathies are usually not responsive to steroids or immunomodulating agents.

3. Transient proteinuria and benign orthostatic proteinuria are usually not treated.

4. Glomerulopathies with severe proteinuria should be treated based on pathologic and serologic findings.

   a. Steroids are usually the mainstay of therapy, with different lesions responding at varying degrees. Minimal change disease is quite steroid-responsive, whereas focal glomerulosclerosis is quite resistant. Cyclophosphamide (Cytoxan), azathioprine (Imuran), cyclosporine (Sandimmune), and chlorambucil (Leukeran) have been used as steroid-sparing agents and for their own immune effects. Lupus nephritis is often quite responsive to steroids and cyclophosphamide, as is Wegener's vasculitis and other vasculitides.

   b. General measures have been used to lessen the degree of proteinuria and attempt to preserve renal function.

      (1) Angiotensin-converting enzyme inhibitors will lower intraglomerular pressure and lessen protein excretion, especially in diabetic patients.

      (2) Nonsteroidal anti-inflammatory agents may be used to decrease proteinuria in

severe cases. These should be used with caution.

(3) Low doses of aspirin and other anti-platelet agents have been used with some glomerulopathies to help reduce sclerosis.

c. Restricted-protein diets may also lessen proteinuria. In patients with edema, sodium may need to be restricted as well. Patients with proteinuria and advanced renal insufficiency may need to limit their potassium intake.

d. It is crucial to recognize that stable patients with proteinuria need not always be treated. Such conditions as azotemia, nephrotic syndrome, and hypertension warrant aggressive therapy if such therapy exists. However, many of these regimens can cause considerable toxicity; this must be assessed when deciding on therapy. Patients are less likely to benefit from aggressive immunosuppressive therapy if signs and symptoms are mild.

e. Activity need not be restricted in patients with proteinuria.

PEARLS

- Diagnose proteinuria by dipstick. Always repeat the test at a later time if done during stress, fever, or exercise.

- Always quantify the degree of proteinuria and identify types of protein.

- Assess renal function and blood pressure, and examine the urine for formed elements.

- Search for clues of a systemic disease.

- Obtain appropriate serologies and sonography.

- Orthostatic proteinuria and transient proteinuria have a good prognosis. Consider renal biopsy if kidneys are normal size with severe proteinuria if diagnosis is not otherwise clear-cut. Azotemia and abnormal serologies may also add to the urgency of a biopsy.

B Bibliography

Carlson JA, Harrington JT: Laboratory evaluation of renal function. In Schrier RW, Gottschalk CW (eds): Diseases of the Kidney, 5th ed, vol 1, pp 380–392. Boston, Little, Brown, 1993.

Henry JB: Examination of urine. In Clinical Diagnosis and Management by Laboratory Methods, 18th ed, pp 413–415. Philadelphia, WB Saunders Company, 1991.

Lafayett RA, Perrone RD, Levey AS: Laboratory evaluation of renal function. In Schrier R, Gottschalk C (eds): Diseases of the Kidney, pp 330–342. Boston, Little, Brown, 1997.

Larson TS: Evaluation of proteinuria. Mayo Clin Proc 1994;69:1154–1158.

Mackenzie MS, Brenner BM: Current strategies for retarding progression of renal disease. Am J Kidney Dis 1998;31:161–170.

Rosenberg ME, Hostetter TH: Proteinuria. In Seldin D, Giebisch G (eds): The Kidney: Physiology and Pathophysiology, 2nd ed, vol 3, pp 3054–3055. New York, Raven Press, 1992.

SYMPTOM DYSURIA

Syed M. Ahmed

Dysuria refers to pain, difficulty, or a burning sensation during urination. Urinary tract infection (UTI) is the most common cause of dysuria. Although dysuria is very common in women, it is also a common symptom in men with UTI and urethritis. Because treatment varies based on etiology, the physician needs to explore possible underlying causes of dysuria.

Differential Diagnosis

1. UTI: more common in women. Patients can present with increased frequency. Urinalysis may be positive for nitrites, leukocyte esterase, pyuria, or hematuria.

2. Sexually transmitted disease (STD): In men with urethritis, symptoms include mild dysuria and clear-to-mucopurulent discharge. In women, dysuria, frequency, vaginal discharge, dyspareunia, and pelvic pain may be noted.

3. Vulvovaginitis: The most common complaint is of vaginal discharge with or without pruritis, offensive odor, and vulvar irritation. Vaginitis is the most common cause of dysuria in outpatient practice.

4. Atrophic vaginitis. In postmenopausal women, atrophic vaginitis may result in painful urination, burning, dyspareunia, and vaginal spotting.

5. Prostatitis/prostatocystitis: Patients may present with dysuria, frequency, urgency, or vague discomfort in lower abdomen, perineum, groin, or penis. In acute bacterial prostatitis, rectal ex-

amination may reveal a tender, hard, and irregular prostate.

6. Interstitial cystitis (IC). Patients with IC can present with dysuria, nocturia, urgency, or frequency. Although exact etiology is unknown, many authors suggest IC is a hypersensitive bladder condition based on abnormal urodynamics.

7. Female urethral syndrome: a "catch-all" diagnosis for a condition seen in a large number of women with dysuria, frequency, retropubic pressure, and often dyspareunia. Objective findings such as urinalysis or bacterial cultures are negative. Some authors suggest that infection of the microscopic female paraurethral gland is the cause of female urethral syndrome. Differential diagnosis also includes calculus, tumor, sexual abuse, and mechanical/chemical irritation.

History: Key Questions to Ask

1. When was the onset?

2. What is the duration?

3. Is it initial dysuria? Is it terminal dysuria? Or, is this dysuria throughout the micturition?

4. Is there frequency? Urgency? Hesitancy? Nocturia? Gross hematuria?

5. Is there any vaginal discharge? Itching?

6. Is there pain in abdomen? Groin? Perineum? Rectum? Testis? Penis?

7. Is there fever, chills, nausea or vomiting?

8. Is there any history of recurrence of genital or urinary infections?

9. Is there history of renal stone? Tumor? Prostatitis?

10. Are there new or multiple sexual partners? Sexual abuse?

11. Is a diaphragm or foam used as contraceptive?

12. What antibiotics were used in the past? Did they help? Any allergies?

Clinical Findings

1. Based on history, clinical examination should focus on revealing the cause of dysuria. Physicians need to keep the differential diagnoses in mind as they proceed toward physical examination and order the relevant tests.

2. Overall appearance: Look for any signs of systemic infections/toxicity.

3. Assess suprapubic or costovertebral angle tenderness.

4. Male genitourinary examination: Focus on urethral discharge, ulcers, erythema, tenderness of the testis, prostate, and rectum.

5. Vaginal examination: Focus on discharge, odor, atrophy, ulcers, erythema.

Tests

1. Dipstick urinalysis: A positive dipstick test is defined as one in which either nitrites or leukocyte esterase or both are present.

2. Urinalysis: It will assess nitrites, leukocyte esterase, pyuria, hematuria or proteinuria.

3. Urine culture and sensitivities: A reliably collected midstream urine culture is the mainstay in the diagnosis of UTI. Uncomplicated UTI in women may not require culture. Complicated UTI or UTI in men requires culture.

4. Vaginal discharge for wet mount and potassium hydroxide solution, if indicated.

5. STD tests for *Neisseria gonorrhoeae*, *Chlamydia trachomatis*, or herpes simplex if indicated.

6. Further tests may include urodynamics, cystoscopy, renal ultrasound, or intravenous urography to narrow the definitive diagnosis.

Management

1. UTI: The physician needs to determine if it is upper or lower tract and if it is a complicated or uncomplicated UTI. Outpatient or inpatient treatment is based on patient toxicity and patient ability to take oral medication. Three to 5 days of oral antibiotics is usually effective for acute bacterial uncomplicated UTI in women; 14 days or more of oral and parenteral treatment may be needed in complicated or upper UTI.

   a. Some of the oral antibiotics for UTI include

      (1) Sulfisoxazole, 120 mg/kg/day q6h

      (2) Trimethoprim-sulfamethoxazole (Bactrim DS), 160 mg/800 mg q12h

      (3) Nitrofurantoin (Macrobid, Macrodantin), 100 mg q6h

      (4) Ciprofloxacin (Cipro), 500 to 750 mg q12h

   b. Some of the parenteral antibiotics for UTI include

      (1) Ampicillin-sulbactam (Unasyn), 1.5 to 3.0 gm q6h

      (2) Ceftazidime (Fortaz), 1.0 to 2.0 gm q6–12h

      (3) Ticarcillin-clavulanate (Timentin), 3.1 gm q4–6h

   c. Pyridium, a urinary analgesic, may be prescribed for symptomatic relief.

2. STD: Treatment will be based on types of STD.

   a. Some choices for chlamydial urethritis or cervicitis are

(1) Doxycycline (Vibramycin), 100 mg PO bid ×7 days

(2) Azithromycin (Zithromax), 1 gm PO in a single dose

(3) Ofloxacin (Floxin), 300 mg PO qid ×7 days

b. Some choices for gonococcal infection include

(1) Ceftriaxone (Rocephin), 250 mg IM

(2) Cefpodoxime (Vantin), 200 mg PO

(3) Cefixime (Suprax), 500 mg PO

c. Follow the above by doxycycline, 100 mg bid ×7 days, or tetracycline, 500 mg qid ×7 days

3. Vulvovaginitis

a. For bacterial vaginosis some choices include

(1) Metronidazole (Flagyl), 500 mg PO bid ×7 days

(2) Clindamycin (Cleocin), 2% vaginal cream for 7 days

b. For candidal vaginitis, some choices include

(1) Fluconazole (Diflucan), 150 mg PO once

(2) Miconazole nitrate (Monistat), one suppository nightly

4. Atrophic vulvovaginitis: Some choices are

a. Premarin, 0.625 mg qd

b. Estrace, 1 mg qd

c. Estraderm patch, 0.05 mg applied to skin twice weekly

d. Intravaginal estrogen cream, 0.5 to 2 gm daily, depending on the severity of condition. Administration should be cyclic (e.g., 3 weeks on and 1 week off).

5. Prostatitis: Outpatient treatment for prostatitis includes at least 3 to 4 weeks' treatment with

a. Trimethoprim-sulfamethoxazole (Bactrim DS), 160 mg/800 mg 1 tablet bid

b. Ciprofloxacin (Cipro), 500 mg bid

c. Enoxacin (Penetrex), 400 mg bid

d. Norfloxacin (Noroxin), 400 mg bid

e. Ofloxacin (Floxin), 400 mg bid

f. Lomefloxacin (Maxaquin), 400 mg qd

6. Interstitial cystitis: There is no known curative therapy for IC. The Food and Drug Administration–approved oral therapy is pentosan polysulfate (Elmiron), 300 mg qd. Intravesical therapy includes hydrodistention of the bladder and use of dimethyl sulfoxide (DMSO; RIMSO-50).

Diet

1. Avoid over-the-counter decongestants and caffeine.

2. Cranberry or orange juice may help.

Patient Education

1. Maintenance of good hygiene is advised. Avoid perfumed soaps and toilet paper.

2. Use of condom for sexual intercourse needs to be encouraged.

3. Adequate fluid intake (e.g., 8 to 10 glasses of water) needs to be encouraged, along with frequent emptying of bladder.

4. Encourage evaluation and treatment of sexual partners of patients with STD.

Follow-Up

1. Follow-up depends on causes of dysuria. Uncomplicated lower UTI in women may need no follow-up if patient symptoms resolve. Complicated or recurrent UTI requires follow-up and further work-up.

2. For vulvovaginitis, follow-up and repeat examination is suggested if symptoms persist.

3. For prostatitis, do urinalysis and culture 30 days after initiating treatment.

PEARLS

- Dysuria is a symptom, not a disease.

- Explore risk factors (e.g., use of intrauterine device, diaphragm use, multiple sexual partners).

B **Bibliography**

Ahmed SM, Swedlund SK: Evaluation and treatment of urinary tract infections in children. Am Fam Physician 1998;57:1573–1580.

Hooten TM, Stamm WE: Diagnosis and treatment of uncomplicated urinary tract infection. Infect Dis Clin North Am 1997;11:551–581.

Kunin CM: Urinary Tract Infections: Detection, Prevention, and Management, 4th ed. Baltimore, Williams & Wilkins, 1997.

Kurowski K: The woman with dysuria. Am Fam Physician 1998;57:2155–2164.

Moul JN: Prostatitis: sorting out the different course. Postgrad Med 1993;94:191–194.

Oliguria is defined as the excretion of less than 400 ml of urine in 24 hours and is the result of a fall in the glomerular filtration rate. The etiology is classically divided into three pathophysiologic groupings: prerenal, renal, or postrenal causes. Anuria implies complete absence of urine flow and may be transient, intermittent, or permanent. Anuria, in contrast to oliguria, is usually the result of postrenal factors.

Differential Diagnosis

1. Prerenal (decreased renal blood flow)
   a. Hypotension
   b. Decreased blood volume
      (1) Gastrointestinal loss, burns, hemorrhage, excessive sweating, third spacing, diabetic ketoacidosis, addisonian crisis
      (2) Relative loss in blood volume: sepsis, liver failure, anaphylaxis, nephrotic syndrome
   c. Pump failure
      (1) Congestive heart failure (CHF), myocardial infarction (MI)
      (2) Pulmonary embolus
      (3) Mechanical ventilation
   d. Hypercalcemia
   e. Drugs
      (1) Angiotensin-converting enzyme inhibitors, nonsteroidal anti-inflammatory drugs
      (2) Anesthesia
      (3) Cyclosporine
      (4) Vasodilatory drugs
   f. Renal artery or vein occlusion
2. Renal
   a. Ischemia causing acute tubular necrosis (ATN) from prolonged prerenal events
      (1) Vasculitides: systemic lupus erythematosus, scleroderma, polyarteritis nodosa
      (2) Glomerulonephritis of any cause
      (3) Pregnancy
      (4) Malignant hypertension
   b. Toxins
      (1) Drugs: antibiotics, acyclovir, amphotericin, chemotherapeutic agents
      (2) Solvents: carbon tetrachloride, ethylene glycol
      (3) Heavy metals: mercury, cisplatin
      (4) Radiologic contrast
      (5) Endogenous toxins: myoglobin, hemoglobin, uric acid, calcium phosphate complexes
   c. Tumor
      (1) Multiple myeloma, lymphoma, leukemias
      (2) Tumor infiltration
   d. Interstitial nephritis
      (1) Infection: hantavirus, legionnaire's disease, hepatitis
      (2) Sarcoidosis
      (3) Allergic reactions to drugs
3. Postrenal (obstruction)
   a. Prostatic enlargement
   b. Intratubular obstruction: uric acid, calcium oxalate
   c. Intra- and extraluminal
      (1) Stone
      (2) Tumor
      (3) Fibrosis
      (4) Abscess
      (5) Clot

History

1. Medical conditions known to affect the kidney
   a. CHF, hypertension, diabetes
   b. Cancer
   c. Recent surgeries
   d. Fluid loss
2. Exposure to nephrotoxins
   a. Prescribed medications
   b. Recreational drug use, moonshine
   c. Occupational exposure
   d. Over-the-counter analgesic use
3. Recent skin rashes that may indicate collagen-vascular disease, embolic disease, or infection
4. Recent infections: streptococcal pharyngitis, tuberculosis
5. Urine excretion pattern (i.e., nocturia, polyuria); urine color (i.e., hematuria)
6. Review of systems may elicit symptoms not otherwise apparent: shortness of breath, joint pain, or hemoptysis

Physical Examination

1. Fluid status
   a. Daily intake and output
   b. Presence of peripheral edema
   c. Orthostatic blood pressure and pulse

d. Skin turgor

e. Dry or moist mucous membranes

f. Capillary refill: normal is less than 1.5 to 2.0 seconds

g. When in doubt, a central venous catheter or pulmonary artery catheter may need to be placed.

2. Cardiovascular

a. CHF

(1) Jugular venous distention

(2) Rales

b. Severe hypertension

(1) Malignant nephrosclerosis

(2) Glomerulonephritis

(3) Vasculitis

(4) Renal embolic disease

c. Murmurs

(1) Endocarditis

(2) CHF or MI

d. Friction rub

(1) Cardiac tamponade

(2) Indication for hemodialysis

3. Abdomen

a. Abdominal bruits: Obstruction of the renal arteries of any cause

b. Enlarged bladder suggests postrenal obstruction.

c. Ascites or enlarged liver implies a hepatic etiology.

4. Skin

a. Petechiae or purpura imply a collagen-vascular disease or a systemic inflammatory condition.

b. Livedo reticularis or skin hemorrhage denotes embolic disease, endocarditis, or vasculitides.

5. Neurologic

a. Uremic encephalopathy

b. Cranial nerve palsies indicate toxins or a vasculitis.

c. Altered or changing mental status suggest embolic disease or microangiopathy.

Tests

1. Urinalysis

a. Color

(1) "Dirty" brown is seen with ischemic or toxic ATN.

(2) Reddish color implies acute glomerulonephritis.

(3) Claret or pinkish urine suggests myoglobinuria.

b. Dipstick

(1) Hemoglobin is positive when myoglobin or hemoglobin is present.

(2) Proteinuria suggests a nephritic or a nephrotic condition.

c. Microscopy

(1) Granular casts and renal tubular cells are seen with ATN.

(2) Interstitial nephritis may demonstrate pyuria, white blood cell casts, and microhematuria.

(3) Eosinophilia present on Wright's or Hansel's stain indicates allergic interstitial nephritis.

(4) Crystals

(a) Uric acid crystals are usually seen with uric acid nephropathy.

(b) Calcium oxalate suggests ethylene glycol ingestion.

(c) Acetaminophen crystals may be present with toxicity with this drug.

2. Biochemical tests

a. Blood urea nitrogen/creatinine ratio greater than 20:1 indicates prerenal azotemia, whereas ratio of 20:1 or less is present with intrarenal disease.

b. Fractional excretion of sodium (FE_{Na}): In prerenal azotemia, the FE_{Na} is less than 1 per cent; it is greater than 1 per cent in ATN.

WARNING

Do not measure FE_{Na} after administration of loop diuretics, wait at least 24 hours.

$$FE_{Na} = \frac{(Urine\ [Na]/Plasma\ [Na])}{(Urine\ [Cr]/Plasma\ [Cr])} \times 100$$

3. Imaging

a. Renal ultrasound is valuable to assess kidney size. Normal-size kidneys suggest an acute cause, whereas shrunken kidneys imply a chronic disease. Ultrasound also gives valuable information concerning postrenal causes of oliguria. In addition, ultrasound may show evidence of intrarenal tumors or cystic structures indicative of polycystic kidney disease.

b. Doppler scans are useful in assessing renal blood flow (i.e., renal artery stenosis).

c. Angiography may be necessary to confirm renal artery occlusive disease.

d. Renal computerized tomography (CT) scans

are helpful to confirm masses or cystic structures noted on ultrasound. A CT scan may also be used to assess renal parenchymal disease.

  e. Renal biopsy is reserved for patients in whom the diagnosis of oliguria remains unknown despite an adequate work-up.

4. Other tests that may be useful depending on the clinical situation
  a. Spot urine for Na⁺, K⁺, creatinine, albumin, and eosinophils
  b. Pregnancy test
  c. Human immunodeficiency virus
  d. Antinuclear antibodies, erythrocyte sedimentation rate
  e. Complement tests: C3, C4, CH_{50}
  f. Antistreptolysin O titer
  g. Hepatitis profile
  h. Serum protein electrophoresis, serum immunoelectrophoresis, and urine protein electrophoresis
  i. Cryoglobulins

Management

1. A fluid challenge is useful in a patient who is depleted intravascularly, that is, a patient with trauma, dehydration, sepsis, pancreatitis, hypoalbuminemia, or low cardiac output states.
  a. A fluid bolus of 250 to 1000 ml should be adequate to gauge the response.
  b. A Swan-Ganz catheter may be indicated in volume-overloaded patients with decreased intravascular volume.
2. Diuretic therapy
  a. Loop diuretics are the preferred agents for use in oliguria. Thiazides are not useful beyond mild renal insufficiency.
    (1) Maximal effect occurs in doses of 160 to 200 mg of furosemide.

    (2) Hypovolemia or intravascular volume depletion may cause diuretic resistance.
  b. Add an oral thiazide if the response is inadequate. Dose between 50 and 100 mg once or twice a day.
  c. A vasopressor may need to be added to increase mean arterial pressure to 70 to 80 mm Hg.
  d. A continuous infusion of diuretic may increase urine output. Continuous infusions may keep more diuretic at its site of action longer than intermittent boluses. The initial rate of furosemide should be 10 mg/hour, titrated up to 30 to 50 mg/hour if needed.
  e. Albumin may be required to act as a carrier for the diuretic. The number of milligrams of furosemide per hour is multiplied by 12 and this number is added to 100 ml of 25% albumin. The combined infusion is then started at 8 ml/hour.
  f. Dopamine at 1 to 3 mg/kg/minute can be used to increase diuresis. If used in greater doses, its renal effect is lost.
  g. Hemodialysis is indicated if hyperkalemia, acidosis, pericarditis, encephalopathy, or volume overload unresponsive to diuretics develops.

B Bibliography

Brater DC: Drug therapy: diuretic therapy. N Engl J Med 1998;338:387–395.
DePriest J: Reversing oliguria in critically ill patients. Postgrad Med 1998;102:245–263.
Klahr S, Miller SB: Acute oliguria. N Engl J Med 1998; 338:671–675.
Thadhani R, Pascual M, Bonventre JV: Acute renal failure. N Engl J Med 1996;334:1448–1460.
Toto RD: Approach to the Patient with Acute Renal Failure. In Greenberg A (ed): Primer on Kidney Diseases, 2nd ed, pp 253–259. San Diego, Academic Press, 1998.

SYMPTOM PENILE DISCHARGE

John A. Andrilli

1. A common reason for doctor visit, especially for younger men
2. Usually caused by inflammation of the urethra, typically from infection with a sexually transmitted disease (STD)
3. Can have serious long-term complications if left untreated.
  a. Men can develop prostatitis, epididymitis, or urethral strictures.
  b. Transmission of infection to female sexual partners can lead to pelvic inflammatory disease and infertility.

Differential Diagnosis

1. Infectious: most common cause, nearly all sexually transmitted
  a. Gonococcal urethritis
    (1) Caused by *Neisseria gonorrhoeae*
    (2) *Twenty to 40 per cent have concomitant chlamydia infection*

b. Nongonoccal urethritis (NGU)

   (1) *Chlamydia trachomatis: most common of all causes* (23 to 55 per cent)

   (2) *Ureaplasma urealyticum* (25 to 35 per cent)

   (3) *Trichomonas vaginalis* (2 to 5 per cent)

   (4) *Mycoplasma hominis* and *Mycoplasma genitalium*

   (5) Herpes simplex virus and human papillomavirus: usually associated with typical external skin lesions

   (6) Other rarer causes: *Candida, Enterobacter*

   (7) Unknown cause in up to 20 to 30 per cent of NGU cases

c. Prostatitis: typically more painful and with occasionally bloody discharge

d. Epididymitis: Presents with associated testicular pain and swelling.

2. Noninfectious

a. Trauma/instrumentation: including straddle falls (bicycles, etc.), kick to groin, atypical sexual practices

b. Intraurethral growth or foreign body: warts, polyps, tumor

c. Reiter's syndrome: a reactive arthritis associated with human leukocyte antigen B-27 with symptoms of urethritis, conjunctivitis, and skin rashes; suspected to be an immunologic response to chlamydia or gastrointestinal infection

History

1. Urethral discharge: type and duration very variable, *sometimes only seen in morning prior to voiding*

a. Mucoid/purulent/yellow: Suggests gonococcal urethritis; usually evolves rapidly over 3 to 5 days after exposure.

b. Watery/clear: Suggests nongonococcal urethritis, especially chlamydia, usually mild or insidious in nature, developing over one to several weeks from exposure.

c. Bloody: trauma, prostatitis, condyloma, tumor

2. Dysuria

3. Suprapubic pain or meatal pressure/itching/swelling

4. Arthritis: seen in disseminated gonococcal infection or Reiter's syndrome from chlamydia

5. Pharyngitis/proctitis: Can be seen in gonococcal infection if oral/anal sex practiced.

6. Conjunctivitis/iritis/skin rash: seen in Reiter's syndrome

7. History of past STDs

8. History of unprotected sex, multiple sexual partners, or exposure to infected partner

9. History of recent gastrointestinal illness may suggest Reiter's syndrome.

10. *Up to 25 per cent of nongonococcal and 10 per cent of gonococcal infections may be asymptomatic.*

Clinical Findings

1. Urethral discharge: as described above; may need to milk penis to elicit.

2. Inguinal lymphadenopathy

3. Epididymal or prostatic tenderness

4. Joint swelling/rash/pharyngitis/conjunctivitis: suggests more severe or diffuse involvement rather than just localized urethritis

Diagnostic Tests

1. Gram's stain: Collect specimen with calcium alginate swab; sensitivity 95 to 98 per cent and specificity 95 per cent.

a. More than five white blood cells per high-power field needed for diagnostic stain.

b. Gonococcal: many white cells with gram-negative intracellular diplococci

c. NGU: white cells without intracellular bacteria

2. DNA probes: *now the diagnostic method of choice* in most cases because they can be performed on either urethral swab *or* urine specimens

a. Ligase chain reaction assay: greater than 90 per cent sensitivity and 100 per cent specificity

b. Polymerase chain reaction: greater than 95 per cent sensitivity and 100 per cent specificity

3. Antigen detection: chlamydia enzyme immunoassay from swab only, greater than 70 per cent sensitivity and greater than 99 per cent specificity

4. Culture: time consuming, less sensitive, therefore now usually performed only when resistance is suspected

5. Testing of pharyngeal and anal swab specimens should be performed if anal or oral intercourse was performed to increase chance of detection.

6. Wet prep: if persistent symptoms despite usual antibiotic treatment to assess for *Trichomonas*

7. Cystoscopy: Referral to urologist for cystoscopy usually required for bloody discharge unless

TABLE 141-1. CDC TREATMENT GUIDELINES FOR SEXUALLY TRANSMITTED DISEASES

ORGANISM	DRUG(S) OF CHOICE	ALTERNATIVE THERAPY
Gonorrhea (should treat for concomitant chlamydia)	Cefixime (Suprax), 400 mg PO once *or* Ceftriaxone (Recephin), 125 mg IM once *or* Ciprofloxacin (Cipro), 500 mg PO once *or* Ofloxacin (Floxin), 400 mg PO once	Spectinomycin (Trobicin), 2 gm IM once *or* Lomefloxacin (Maxaquin), 400 mg PO once *or* Norfloxacin (Noroxin), 800 mg PO once
Nongonococcal urethritis	Azithromycin (Zithromax), 1 gm PO once *or* Doxycycline 100 mg PO bid for 7 days	Erythromycin base, 500 mg PO qid for 7 days *or* Ofloxacin (Floxin), 300 mg PO bid for 7 days *or* Grepafloxacin (Raxar), 400 mg PO qd for 7 days
Trichomonas	Metronidazole (Flagyl), 2 gm PO once	Metronidazole (Flagyl), 500 mg PO bid for 7 days

Data from Centers for Disease Control and Prevention: 1998 Guidelines for treatment of sexually transmitted diseases. MMWR Morb Mortal Wkly Rep 1998;47(RR-1):1–111.

bleeding resolves rapidly and was caused by an obvious traumatic injury.

Management

Medication

1. Usually *treat immediately* based on history, appearance of discharge, and/or results of Gram's stain; use results of DNA probes for confirmation.
2. If etiology is unclear from history and no discharge is present at time of examination, treatment can be withheld until test results confirm etiology. Then treat accordingly.
3. *ALWAYS* treat for concomitant chlamydia infection in gonorrhea cases.
4. Specific treatment recommendations from the 1998 Centers for Disease Control and Prevention Treatment Guidelines for Sexually Transmitted Diseases are shown in Table 141–1.

Activity

1. Patient should avoid sexual activity until treatment is completed and symptoms are resolved (7 days is prudent).
2. Consider testing for syphilis and human immunodeficiency virus infection because patient is at risk for other STDs.
3. Patient must inform all sexual partners that they require evaluation and/or treatment.
4. Consider immunization for hepatitis A and B if clinically indicated.

Patient Education

1. Symptom relief usually occurs within 24 hours of treatment.
2. Explain importance of compliance with treatment to prevent transmission and complications.
3. Explain that you may be required to report case to the state/local health department.
4. Counsel on importance of safe sex practices, especially condom use.
5. No sexual contact with partners until they are tested/treated to prevent re-infection.

Follow-Up

1. No follow-up necessary unless symptoms persist or complications occur.
2. No need for post-treatment testing unless evidence of treatment failure present or noncompliance with therapy suspected.

PEARLS

- Need to maintain a high suspicion for urethritis even if discharge is scant or absent.
- Always treat for concomitant chlamydial infection when treating suspected or proven gonorrhea.
- DNA probes are currently the preferred tests to diagnose gonorrhea and chlamydia.

Bibliography

Carroll KC, Aldeen WE, Morrison M, et al: Evaluation of the Abbott LCx Ligase Chain Reaction Assay for detection of *Chlamydia trachomatis* and *Neisseria gonorrhoeae* in urine and genital swab specimens from a sexually transmitted disease clinic population. J Clin Microbiol 1998;36:1630–1633.

Centers for Disease Control and Prevention. 1998 Guidelines for treatment of sexually transmitted diseases. MMWR Morb Mortal Wkly Rep 1998;47(RR-1):1–111.

Krieger JN: Urethritis: etiology, diagnosis, treatment, and complications. In Gillenwater JY, Howards SS, Grayhack JT, et al (eds): Adult and Pediatric Urology, 3rd ed, pp 1879–1915. St. Louis, CV Mosby Company, 1996.

Krieger JN: Trichomoniasis in men: old issues and new data. Sex Transm Dis 1995;22:83–96.

Oriel JD: The history of non-gonococcal urethritis. Genitourin Med 1996;72:374–379.

SYMPTOM URINARY INCONTINENCE

Brian S. Murphy

Urinary incontinence is the involuntary loss of urine. This condition is estimated to affect some 10 million adults in the United States. The incidence of this problem increases with age, and it is believed to affect 50 to 70 per cent of nursing home residents. The annual cost of treating urinary incontinence is thought to exceed $10 billion. Incontinence is never a normal variant of aging.

Etiology

1. Urinary incontinence results from a derangement in the neuromuscular and psychologic axis that controls the storage of urine in the bladder. In the normal setting, filling of the bladder occurs with stretching of the bladder dome by β-adrenergic stimulation with concomitant constriction of the bladder neck and internal sphincter by α-adrenergic stimulation. Bladder capacity normally ranges between 300 and 600 ml of urine. For normal voiding to occur, bladder pressure must exceed the outlet resistance.

2. Voiding can occur in response to increased cholinergic tone, and involuntary bladder contractions are stimulated by the S2 through S4 reflex arc of the sacral micturition center. Relaxation of the internal and external sphincters is achieved through the simultaneous inhibition of both somatic and adrenergic impulses. Central control of urination is divided between the sensorimotor cortex of the frontal lobes, which have an inhibitory influence, and the brain stem, which facilitates micturition.

Clinical Findings

1. Urge incontinence
   a. The most common type seen in nursing home patients; also known as detrusor instability
   b. Etiology is rooted in a central nervous system defect caused either by multiple strokes, dementia, parkinsonism, or local irritation secondary to cystitis, tumors, or stones.
   c. Symptoms include loss of large amounts of urine (>50 ml), urgency, frequency, and nocturia.

2. Overflow incontinence
   a. Often caused by outlet obstruction, detrusor inadequacy, or impaired bladder sensation.
   b. Symptoms commonly include straining to urinate, incomplete emptying, frequent small voidings (10 to 50 ml), and hesitancy.
   c. Signs include a palpable bladder, prostate enlargement, difficult catheterization, and poor stream. Patients may also report nocturia.

3. Stress incontinence
   a. Occurs predominantly in women and is often the result of pelvic muscle laxity, neuropathy, or previous urologic surgery.
   b. Symptoms include loss of urine associated with coughing, laughing, or exercise.
   c. Loss of small urine volumes is a predominant sign along with daytime incontinence and the presence of atrophic vaginitis.

4. Functional incontinence
   a. Associated with the inability of a patient to reach the toilet because of environmental barriers or physical/psychological impairments.
   b. Drugs such as diuretics, sedatives/hypnotics, and alcohol have also been associated with this type of incontinence.

Tests

1. Urge incontinence results in urodynamics that reveal a normal postvoid residual but a small bladder capacity associated with uninhibited contractions.
2. Overflow incontinence has a urodynamic profile revealing a large postvoid residual (>150 ml), poor bladder contractions, and a bladder capacity greater than 500 ml.
3. Stress incontinence has a normal urodynamic profile.
4. Urinalysis and urine culture should be routine tests for all forms of incontinence.
5. Order cytology if malignancy is suspected.

Differential Diagnosis

One of the most important pieces of information to determine is whether the symptoms of incontinence are potentially reversible. This is where the history plays an important part of patient management.

TABLE 141-2. PHARMACOTHERAPY OF URINARY INCONTINENCE

INCONTINENCE TYPE	THERAPY

Urge (detrusor instability)	Estrogen replacement
	    Conjugated estrogens (Premarin), 0.625 mg
	Smooth muscle relaxants
	    Oxybutynin (Ditropan), 2.5–5.0 mg qd–tid
	    Dicyclomine (Bentyl), 20 mg qid
	    Flavoxate (Urispas), 100–200 mg tid–qid
	Anticholinergic agents
	    Imipramine (Tofranil), 10–50 mg qhs–tid
	    Propantheline (Pro-Banthine), 15 mg qid
	Muscarinic receptor antagonist
	    Tolterodine (Detrol), 2 mg bid
	Calcium antagonist
	    Nifedipine (Procardia), 10 mg tid

Overflow (atonic bladder)	Cholinergic agent
	    Bethanechol (Urecholine), 10–30 mg qd–tid
	α-Blockers
	    Prazosin (Minipress), 1–5 mg tid
	    Terazosin (Hytrin), 1–4 mg qhs

Outlet obstruction secondary to prostate enlargement	Finasteride (Proscar), 5 mg qid Terazosin (Hytrin), 1–4 mg qhs Doxazosin (Cardura), 1–6 mg qhs

Stress	Topical estrogen
	    Estrogen vaginal cream (Premarin), 2–4 gm qid for 1–2
	      wk, then 1 gm twice weekly
	α-Agonists
	    Phenylpropanolamine (Dimetapp), 25–50 mg tid–qid
	    Pseudoephedrine (Sudafed), 30–60 mg tid–qid
	Tricyclic antidepressants
	    Imipramine (Tofranil), 10–100 mg qhs
	    Doxepin (Sinequan), 25–100 mg qhs

1. Initial queries should focus on the timing of the incontinence (daytime or nocturia), including the onset, duration, frequency, possible precipitants, episodes of hematuria, and an estimation of the amount of urine lost.

2. Concurrent medications may serve as possible reversible precipitants of incontinence.

    a. The most common therapeutic agents associated with reversible incontinence are heavy alcohol use and diuretic therapy.

    b. Other agents leading to compromised urine retention are: psychotropic agents, narcotic analgesics, β-blockers, α-antagonists, and calcium channel blockers.

3. Co-morbid medical conditions associated with incontinence are a history of pelvic surgery, recurrent urinary tract infections, diabetes mellitus, depression, malignancies of the genitourinary system, neurologic disease, congestive heart failure, and multiparity.

Therapy

Urge Incontinence

1. Training regimens whereby the patient gradually lengthens the times between voiding

2. Medications (see Table 141–2 for dosages)

    a. Estrogen replacement therapy or progesterone cycling if a woman has an intact uterus

    b. Smooth muscle relaxants to act as smooth muscle depressants: oxybutynin, dicyclomine, and flavoxate

    c. Anticholinergic agents inhibit involuntary contractions of the detrusor muscle.

    d. Muscarinic receptor antagonist: tolterodine (Detrol) inhibits detrusor contractions.

    e. Calcium antagonists (nifedipine), which inhibit bladder contractions

Overflow Incontinence

1. Credé (external suprapubic compression) or Valsalva maneuver to enhance bladder emptying

2. Medications (see Table 141–2 for dosages)

    a. Hormonal therapy that suppresses androgen production to shrink a hyperplastic prostate (finasteride)

    b. Cholinergic agents to improve detrussor contractability (bethanechol)

    c. α-Blockers to reduce sphincter resistance (prazosin)

3. Surgery to help reduce the size of the prostate (transurethral resection of the prostate [TURP])

Stress Incontinence

1. Kegel exercises that strengthen the pelvic floor muscles. Includes teaching the patient to interrupt voiding. Exercises repeated three to four times per day with 10 to 20 repetitions per exercise.
2. Medications (see Table 141–2 for dosages)
   a. Topical estrogens to improve bladder outlet tone
   b. α-Agonists to increase smooth muscle tone at bladder outlet (phenylpropanolamine)
   c. Tricyclic antidepressants that increase outlet resistance but decrease detrusor contractility (imipramine)

3. Surgery may be an option in women who experience pelvic prolapse.

Bibliography

Burgio KL, Ives DG, Locher JL, et al: Treatment seeking for urinary incontinence in older adults. J Am Geriatr Soc 1994;42:208–212.
Busby-Whitehead J, Johnson T: Urinary incontinence. Clin Geriatr Med 1998;14:285–296.
Fourcroy JL: Urogynecology update: incontinence. Hosp Pract 1998;33:63–81.
Knapp PM: Identifying and treating urinary incontinence: the crucial role of the primary care physician. Postgrad Med 1998;103:279–294.
Sibley GN: Developments in our understanding of detrusor instability. Br J Urol 1997;80(Suppl 1):54–58.

SYMPTOM ENURESIS

Marc Ringel

Enuresis is involuntary voiding of urine. The term is usually reserved for children. (The condition is called urinary incontinence in adults.) Most children obtain bladder control between 2 and 4 years of age. By age 5, 20 per cent are still enuretic, gradually decreasing to an incidence of 1 per cent at 18 years. Boys with this problem predominate over girls 2:1 to 3:1. Although the prognosis for spontaneous "cure" is excellent, it can be a source of embarrassment for the child and of conflict within the family. There are quite effective treatments.

Differential Diagnosis

1. Idiopathic (familial, developmental)
2. Urinary tract infection
3. Polyuria secondary to excessive fluid intake
4. Sexual abuse
5. Fecal withholding, encopresis
6. Diabetes mellitus
7. Chronic renal failure
8. Diabetes insipidus
9. Renal tubular acidosis
10. Ectopic ureter
11. Sickle cell disease (dilute urine secondary to renal microinfarcts)

Enuresis is almost always developmental in etiology and self-limited. Unless there are reasons to suspect psychosocial disturbance or systemic illness, the work-up can routinely be quite brief.

History: Key Questions to Ask

1. Was either parent enuretic?
2. Is the enuresis at night (nocturnal) or during the day (diurnal) or both?
3. Has the child never been dry (primary enuresis), or have there previously been 6 months of dryness in a row (secondary enuresis)?
4. Does the child have diabetes, renal disease, sickle cell anemia, or other systemic illness?
5. Have growth and developmental milestones been normal?
6. Is there reason to suspect sexual abuse?
7. Have there been problems with constipation or encopresis (stool incontinence)?
8. How frequently does the child urinate? During the day? At night?
9. Does the child complain of urinary pain or urgency?
10. Is the incontinence sporadic, or is there constant dribbling?
11. What attempts have been made to treat the enuresis thus far?
12. Have family conflicts arisen as a result of this problem?
13. Has enuresis become a social embarrassment to the child? In what situations?

Questions about the social and familial context of enuresis are at least as important as the strictly medical aspects of the history. Family history is the best predictor of functional enuresis. If both parents were enuretic, for example, 77 per cent of their children will be. Factors that suggest an organic cause are daytime enuresis; secondary enuresis; other urinary symptoms (frequency, dysuria, urgency, etc.); history of systemic illness or developmental delays; and associated bowel problems.

Clinical Findings

1. Developmental delay
2. Tense family

3. Growth retardation
4. Genitourinary examination: perineal leak, hypospadias, meatal stenosis, labial adhesions, others
5. Distended bladder: urine withholding or neurogenic
6. Abnormal anal sphincter tone: evaluated non-invasively by presence of anal "wink" after perianal stroking
7. Distended colon: fecal withholding
8. Evidence of occult spina bifida: lumbosacral cleft, sinus, hair tuft, dimpling
9. Genital trauma, infection, and the like: sexual abuse

The office visit is as much an opportunity to observe parent-child interaction as to examine the child. Look for signs of serious systemic disease and for developmental delay.

Tests

1. Urinalysis
2. Bladder capacity (measure total urine volume in a single void after the child has held urine as long as possible)
3. Urinary tract imaging (intravenous pyelography, voiding cystourethrography, renal ultrasound)
4. Urine flow studies
5. Chemistry panel, complete blood count (to screen for systemic disease)
6. Developmental testing

For most cases of enuresis—particularly with a family history, nocturnal pattern, and unremarkable history and physical examination—a urinalysis to rule out urinary tract infection is all the laboratory work-up that need be done.

Treatment

1. First treat urinary tract infection, diabetes, encopresis, and any other physical contributor to this problem.
2. Nighttime wetness alarm (best ones fit in underpants)
3. Individual or family counseling
4. Hypnosis

Medication

1. Imipramine, 1–2 mg/kg at bedtime
2. Desmopressin (DDAVP) nasal spray, 2–4 sprays at bedtime
3. Placebo pills

Diet

1. Limit evening fluid intake.
2. High fiber (for stool withholders)

Activity

1. Behavior modification with "star chart" (stickers accumulated on a calendar for dry nights, resulting in an agreed-upon reward for achieving dryness goals)
2. Nighttime awakening and trips to the toilet (best if done by the child with own alarm clock). These activities may also be monitored on the "star chart."
3. Bladder stretching (holding urine as long as possible during the day)

Patient Education

1. Question about and educate parents on "normal" toilet training as part of routine health maintenance. Usually the child will let them know when he or she is ready.
2. Reassurance of parent and child that this is a problem that is almost always outgrown.
3. Discourage punitive attitudes by caregivers and self-blame by child.
4. Encourage giving child as much control as possible (e.g., pick out own stickers and calendar, set own alarm clock, change own sheets).

Simple reassurance, patience, and unintrusive behavioral interventions are all the treatment that is usually needed. Wetness alarms, used correctly, achieve dryness in up to 70 per cent of nocturnal enuretics, but usually take at least 3 weeks to begin showing results. Unless clearcut psychopathology is found, a psychological approach is rarely warranted. Use medications when all else has failed. Imipramine and DDAVP work well in the short term. Drugs are best used intermittently, to avoid embarrassment at a slumber party, for example. DDAVP has fewer side effects but is a lot more expensive. Relapse when either drug is discontinued is common. Enuresis is one of the few situations in which placebo pills may be effective.

Follow-Up

1. Frequent follow-up and reinforcement for the smallest success is crucial at the beginning of a behavioral regimen.
2. A long-term trusting relationship with a health care professional is most important to lasting success in treating this problem.

PEARLS

- Enuresis almost always resolves, with or without treatment.
- There is a strong familial component to this problem.

- Daytime wetness and other urinary symptoms, including frequency, urgency, and wetness, are more often attributable to underlying pathology than is nighttime wetness.

- Secondary enuresis is more likely to have an underlying cause than primary.

- A urinalysis is the only laboratory test that usually needs to be done in working up this problem.

- Behavioral methods are most effective.

- Unless there are strong social reasons to treat this problem, defer treatment until age 7, by which time 90 per cent of children will be dry.

- Use drug therapy to treat enuresis only if patient age, social situation, or previous treatment failures are factors.

- Always consider the possibility of sexual abuse, especially in secondary enuresis.

Bibliography

For more information on nocturnal enuresis, see
Tietjen DM, Husmann DA: Nocturnal enuresis: a guide to evaluation and treatment. Mayo Clin Proc 1996;71: 857–862.

For more information on management of secondary enuresis and behavioral management of nocturnal enuresis, see
Schmitt BD: Nocturnal enuresis. Pediatr Rev 1997;18: 183–191.

For more information on diurnal enuresis and the physical exam, see
Kelleher RE: Daytime and nighttime wetting in children: a review of management. J Soc Pediatr Nurs 1997;2: 73–82.

For more information on behavioral therapy of nocturnal enuresis, see
Moffatt ME: Nocturnal enuresis: a review of the efficacy of treatments and practical advice for clinicians. J Dev Behav Pediatr 1997;18:49–56.

For more information on complicated enuresis, see
Rushton HG: Wetting and functional voiding disorders. Urol Clin North Am 1995;22:75–93.

142 Hypercalciuria and Renal Calculi

P. George John

Hypercalciuria

Hypercalciuria is defined as urinary excretion of over 4 mg/kg/24 hours of calcium while on a regular diet (i.e., about 300 mg or more in men and 250 mg or more in women).

Etiology

Hypercalciuria With Hypercalcemia
(Table 142–1)

1. Hyperparathyroidism
   a. Found in 5 per cent of recurrent stone formers
   b. Suspect in patients who develop kidney stones in the fifth or sixth decade for the first time.
2. Granulomatous disease (e.g., sarcoidosis, tuberculosis). Hypercalcemia is due to elevated serum 1,25-dihydroxyvitamin D (1,25[OH]$_2$D).
3. Malignancies, including myeloma, lung cancer, and metastatic bone disease. The tumor cells may produce parathyroid hormone (PTH)–like hormone. Bone resorption may play a part also.
4. Prolonged immobilization: hypercalcemia caused by bone resorption
5. Milk alkali syndrome: taking too much calcium-containing antacids and milk, resulting in hypercalcemia
6. Metabolic diseases
   a. Hereditary hypophosphatemic rickets with hypercalciuria
   b. Hypophosphatasia

Hypercalciuria Without Hypercalcemia

1. Distal renal tubular acidosis: defect in hydrogen ion secretion in the distal tubule
2. Medullary sponge kidney.
3. Idiopathic hypercalciuria: About 60 per cent of renal stones and hypercalciuria is idiopathic.

Key Etiology

- Idiopathic hypercalciuria
- Systemic disease such as hyperparathyroidism (only 5 per cent)

Clinical Findings

1. The most common presenting symptom is nephrolithiasis.
2. Some patients, especially children, may have hematuria as a presenting symptom.

Key Finding

Renal stones

PEARLS

Suspect hypercalciuria:

- When the patient develops recurrent kidney stones

- When children present with unexplained hematuria

Laboratory Tests

1. Serum calcium, phosphate
2. Blood urea nitrogen (BUN), creatinine, electrolytes
3. A 24-hour urine collection for calcium, citrate, creatinine: Calcium excretion of 4 mg/kg/24 hours gives diagnosis of hypercalciuria.

Key Tests

- 24-Hour urine for calcium, citrate
- Creatine
- Serum calcium

WARNING

The 24-hour urine collection for calcium should be done only after the patient is on a regular diet and activity for a week.

TABLE 142–1. POSSIBLE MECHANISMS OF HYPERCALCIURIA

Primary Mechanism	Intestinal Calcium Absorption	Serum Calcium	Serum PTH	Urinary cAMP	Serum 1,24(OH)$_2$D	Net Bone Resorption	Serum PO$_4^{2-}$	Fasting Urine Ca/Creatinine	Urine Ca After Ca Load
Gluttony for Ca-rich food or abuse of Ca-containing antacids	Increased passive (fractional absorption of intake is low)	Normal (fasting) Increased after large Ca intake	Decreased or normal (high Ca)	Decreased	Decreased or normal	Decreased	Normal or high-normal (PTH suppression)	Normal (<0.34 mmol/mmol or <0.12 mg/mg)	Normal increment
Primary increased 1,25(OH)$_2$D synthesis (renal PO$_4^{2-}$ leak and hypophosphatemia, unknown central mechanism)	Increased active (fractional absorption of intake is high)	Normal (fasting) Increased after meals	Decreased or normal (high Ca, 1,25[OH]$_2$D)	Decreased	Increased	Normal (increased if diet Ca <10 mmol/day)	Normal Low if renal PO$_4^{2-}$ leak present	Normal or increased	Increased increment
Augmented intestinal Ca absorption independent of 1,25,(OH]$_2$D or enhanced sensitivity of gut to 1,25(OH)$_2$D	Increased	Normal (fasting) Increased after meals	Decreased or normal	Decreased	Normal	Normal or increased	Normal or high-normal	Normal or increased	Increased increment
Renal Ca "leak"—overt	Increased	Decreased or low-normal	Increased	Increased	Increased	Increased	Normal	Increased	Increased increment
Subtle renal Ca leak (acidosis, high protein diet, K depletion)	Normal	Normal	Normal	Normal	Normal	?Increased	Normal	High-normal	Normal increment
Primary hyperparathyroidism	Normal or increased	Increased	Increased	Increased	Increased or normal	Increased	Decreased	Increased (bone resorption)	Increased increment
Augmentation of net bone resorption independent of PTH or 1,25(OH)$_2$D	Normal or increased	Normal or increased	Normal or decreased	Normal or decreased	Normal or decreased	Increased	Normal or increased	Increased	Normal or increased increment

Abbreviations: Ca, calcium; 1,25(OH)$_2$D, 1,25-dihydroxyvitamin D; PO$_4^{2-}$, phosphate; PTH, parathyroid hormone.

Treatment

1. The purpose is to prevent kidney stones.
2. Treatment of hypercalciuria with hypercalcemia will depend on the cause.
   a. Hyperparathyroidism is best treated with surgery.
   b. Hypercalcemia due to granulomatous disease may be treated with steroids.
   c. Chloroquine 250 mg/day may reduce $1,25(OH)_2D$ level in granulomatous disease.
   d. Ketoconazole (Nizoral) 200 mg/day has been used with some success.
   e. Hypercalcemia of malignancy, including multiple myeloma, is treated with IV hydration with normal saline, corticosteroids, and chemotherapy.
3. Idiopathic hypercalciuria is treated with diet and drug therapy.
   a. Increased protein and sodium intake has been shown to increase the renal excretion of calcium.
   b. Dietary treatment includes restriction of protein to less than 60 gm/day, sodium restriction to 3 to 4 gm/day, and liberal intake of fluids.
   c. Dietary calcium should be restricted to 800 mg/day, which can be done by limiting intake of milk, cheese, or ice cream to one serving per day. More rigid restriction of calcium may lead to bone loss. In addition, very low dietary calcium intake may decrease the oxalate absorption and increase urinary oxalate, leading to stone formation (Table 142–2).

Key Diet

- Protein less than 60 gm/day
- Sodium 3 to 4 gm/day
- Liberal fluids

   d. Thiazide diuretics definitely reduce hypercalciuria by increasing the reabsorption of calcium in the distal tubule. There is also evidence that thiazide inhibits bone resorption. Thiazide may cause hypokalemia. Indapamide (Lozol) is also effective and may not cause hypokalemia.
4. Therapy for renal tubular acidosis is accomplished by alkalinization of urine with potassium citrate and liberal fluid intake.
5. Sodium cellulose phosphate, a calcium-binding resin, reduces calcium absorption when taken with meals. A controlled study showed that it is not superior to diet changes and increased fluid intake. Phosphate at the dose of 1500 mg of neutral potassium phosphate in three to six divided doses lowers the urinary calcium excretion, but efficacy needs to be proven by further study.

Key Treatment

Hydrochlorothiazide

Renal Calculi

Types of stones encountered are the following, in order of frequency (Table 142–3):

1. Calcium (oxalate, phosphate, or mixed)
2. Magnesium ammonium phosphate (struvite)
3. Uric acid
4. Cystine

TABLE 142–2. FACTORS INCREASING OR DECREASING URINARY CALCIUM EXCRETION BY CHANGING EITHER GLOMERULAR FILTRATION OR TUBULAR REABSORPTION OR CALCIUM

FACTORS INCREASING URINARY CALCIUM EXCRETION		FACTORS REDUCING URINARY CALCIUM EXCRETION	
Increased Filtered Calcium	**Reduced Tubular Reabsorption**	**Reduced Filtered Calcium**	**Increased Tubular Reabsorption**
• Dietary calcium intake	• Reduced PTH	• Hypocalcemia	• Increased PTH
• Hypercalcemia	• NaCl (volume expansion)	• Low glomerular filtration rate	• Alkali ingestion (HCO_3^-)
• Skeletal calcium mobilization	• Dietary protein intake		• Potassium
• Enhanced intestinal absorption	• Glucose, sucrose, ethanol		• Thiazide diuretics
	• Phosphate restriction		• Volume contraction
	• Magnesium		• PO_4^{2-} administration
	• Vitamin D deficiency		• Calcitonin
	• Loop diuretics		

TABLE 142–3. FREQUENCY OF DIFFERENT KIDNEY STONES

TYPE	FREQUENCY (%)
Calcium	70–80
Calcium oxalate	30–70
Calcium phosphate	36–70
Mixed	6–10
Magnesium ammonium phosphate (struvite)	6–20
Uric acid	6–17
Cystine	0.5–3
Miscellaneous	1–5

Incidence

1. Twelve per cent of the population will form kidney stones in their lifetime.
2. Men are affected two to three times as often as women.
3. Renal stones account for 7 to 10 of every 1000 hospitalizations.
4. Kidney stones are more common in hot, humid climates.
4. Peak age of onset is the third decade.

Etiology and Pathogenesis

1. Different factors that interact in the formation of stones are
   a. Supersaturation of urine
   b. Favorable conditions for crystallization
   c. Absence of crystal inhibitors
2. Supersaturation of urine not only depends on the solute load, but is also influenced by ionic strength and pH of the urine. The solutes of significance are calcium oxalate and uric acid. Calcium load is increased when there is hypercalciuria with or without hypercalcemia.

Hypercalciuria With Hypercalcemia

1. Hyperparathyroidism
2. Granulomatous diseases (e.g., sarcoidosis, tuberculosis, coccidioidomycosis)
3. Malignancies, including multiple myeloma, lung cancer, and metastatic bone disease
4. Hyperthyroidism
5. Prolonged immobilization
6. Milk alkali syndrome: ingestion of large amounts of calcium-containing antacids and milk
7. Hereditary hypophosphatemic rickets with hypercalciuria
   a. Hypophosphatasia
   b. Vitamin D overdosage
8. Systemic diseases cause only 5 per cent of kidney stones.

Hypercalciuria Without Hypercalcemia

1. Idiopathic hypercalciuria is found in 60 per cent of patients with nephrolithiasis.
2. Hyperuricosuria facilitates calcium oxalate crystallization.
3. Hypocitraturia resulting from primary metabolic defect, potassium depletion, or chronic diarrhea can facilitate kidney stone formation.
4. Renal tubular acidosis
5. Medullary sponge kidney
6. Kidney stone formation in the absence of hypocitraturia and hypercalciuria is due to absence of crystal inhibitors.

Uric Acid Stone

1. Uric acid stone formation (10 to 20 per cent of stones) is the result of hyperuricemia, which occurs in gouty diathesis or hematologic malignancy.
2. Hyperoxaluria can be a metabolic disorder or due to excess intake of oxalate-rich spinach, rhubarb, chocolate, peanuts, tea, strawberries, or wheat bran.

Cystine Stone

Cystine stone formation is due to a rare metabolic disorder.

Key Etiology

- Idiopathic hypercalciuria is the most common cause of renal calculi.
- Uric acid stone occurs in 10 to 20 per cent of cases.
- Absence of crystal inhibitors is a factor in small portion.
- Systemic disease such as hyperthyroidism occurs only in 5 per cent of cases.

PEARL

Think of hyperparathyroidism if the first episode of renal stone occurs after age 45 years in the absence of infection.

Symptoms

1. May be asymptomatic if the stone is in the calyces.
2. Severe unilateral colicky pain with nausea and vomiting is the typical symptom.

3. Stones in the renal pelvis and upper ureter cause flank and abdominal pain.

4. Stones in the middle of the ureter cause pain in the lower abdomen radiating to the inguinal region, labia, urethra, testes, or penis. Occasionally the pain may just be in the groin or testes.

5. Stones located in the intravesicle segment of the ureter may cause frequency and dysuria.

6. In some patients, especially children, the only symptom may be hematuria.

Key Symptom

Unilateral severe colicky pain in the lumbar region or lower abdomen radiating to groin, labia, testes or penis, very often with nausea and vomiting.

WARNING

Occasionally the patient may complain of pain in the groin or testes, without flank or abdominal pain. Rarely, the only symptom may be painless hematuria.

Laboratory Tests

1. History of colicky, unilateral pain.
2. Urinalysis: many red blood cells. Microscopy may show specific crystals.
3. Flat plate of abdomen: May show radiopaque stone (calcium stone).
4. Intravenous pyelogram (IVP) will show the size, location, and extent of obstruction.
5. Renal ultrasound is occasionally helpful.

Key Tests

- Urinalysis
- Microscopy for crystals
- Flat plate of abdomen
- IVP

Treatment (Table 142–4)

1. Pain control: IV Demerol and phenergan, parenteral anti-inflammatory agents such as ketorolac (Toradol), or indomethacin rectal suppository
2. Hydration
3. Elimination of the stone
4. Urologic procedures
   a. Extracorporeal shock wave lithotripsy (ESWL): relatively safe procedure. Complications include bruising, perinephrine hematoma, hematuria, renal colic from fragments of existing hypouria.
   b. Percutaneous nephrolithotomy: very useful for struvite stones
   c. Urethroscopy and removal of stone from below

Key Treatment

- Pain control
- Hydration
- Removal of stone

TABLE 142–4. SUGGESTED TREATMENT FOR DIFFERENT TYPES OF KIDNEY STONES

TYPE OF STONE	TREATMENT
All stones	High fluid intake
Calcium oxalate	Reduced sodium, protein, and calcium
Calcium phosphate	
Idiopathic hypercalciuria	Thiazide diuretics or indapamide
	Oral phosphate
	Sodium cellulose phosphate
Hypocitraturia	Potassium citrate
Renal tubular acidosis	Potassium citrate
Ileostomy/small intestinal malabsorption	Potassium citrate
Hyperoxaluria	
Dietary	Reduced oxalate intake
Enteric	Low-fat diet, calcium supplement, cholestyramine
Primary	Pyridoxine
Hyperuricosuria and uric acid stone	Allopurinol, potassium citrate
Cystine stones	Acetazolamide alkalinization, tiopronin, penicillamine
Struvite stones	Extracorporeal shock wave lithotripsy (ESWL), percutaneous nephrolithotomy, acetohydroxamic acid

Factors Influencing Management of Stones

1. Stone size: Stones smaller than 5 mm have 85 per cent chance of spontaneous passage.
2. Shape of stone: Smooth, round stone passes easier than spiculated stone.
3. Previous history of passage of stone increases the chance of spontaneous passage.

Indications for Urology Consult

1. Stone larger than 7 mm
2. Stone impacted for more than 24 hours
3. Evidence of significant obstruction
4. Evidence of infection

Indications for Antibiotics

1. Urine Gram's stain is positive.
2. The patient is febrile.
3. The patient has frequent urinary tract infections.

Key Decision for Urological Consultation

- Stones greater than 7 mm
- Stone impacted for more than 24 hours
- Evidence of significant obstruction
- Evidence of infection

Follow-Up

> **Important**
> All patients with kidney stones should be investigated for the etiology of kidney stones.

Because the recurrence rate is up to 50 per cent and there are associated morbidity and expenses, it is important to work up the cause of stones and treat the cause. Evaluation consists of the following:

1. Freshly voided urinalysis for pH, specific gravity, sediment (including crystals)
2. A 24-hour urine collection for calcium, citrate, oxalate, and urate; BUN; creatinine
3. Stone for analysis

> **WARNING**
> A 24-hour urine examination should be done only after the patient is on a normal diet and normal activities for a week.

Key Follow-Up Evaluation

- A 24-hour urine collection for calcium, citrate, uric acid, stone analysis
- Serum calcium, phosphorus

Diet

A diet high in protein and sodium causes hypercalciuria.

1. The protein intake should be less than 60 gm/day and sodium should be 3 to 4 gm/day.
2. Liberal fluid intake is recommended.
3. Restrict calcium intake to about 800 mg (less than 800 mg can cause osteopenia).
4. Dietary restriction of oxalate is necessary for patients with hyperoxaluria (avoid spinach, rhubarb, chocolate, peanuts, strawberries, tea, and wheat bran).
5. High doses of ascorbic acid should be avoided.
6. Pyridoxine may be beneficial in oxalate stones.

Key Diet

- Low sodium
- Low protein
- Restricted calcium
- Liberal fluid intake

Medication

1. If diet does not completely prevent stone formation, drug therapy is indicated.
2. Hypercalciuria may be treated with a thiazide diuretic or indapamide (Lozol). A calcium-binding resin, cellulose sodium phosphate (Calcibind), reduces calcium absorption when taken with meals. Neutral potassium phosphate 1500 mg in divided doses (K-Phos Neutral Tablets, 250 mg, two tablets three times daily), may reduce hypercalciuria.
3. Uric acid stones can be treated with alkalinization of urine with potassium citrate, increased fluid intake, and allopurinol. Low urinary citrate is treated with oral potassium citrate (Urocit-K), 10 to 20 mEq three times daily with meals.
4. Cystine stones are treated with increased fluid intake, reduced methionine-rich protein in diet, and alkalinization with potassium citrate to keep urine pH around 7.5. In addition, 250 mg of acetazolamide (Diamox) may be adminis-

tered at bedtime to inhibit proximal tubular bicarbonate absorption. If that does not work, penicillamine (Cuprimine), 250 to 500 ml may be given four times daily. This treatment is associated with several serious side effects, including agranulocytosis, thrombocytopenia, and glomerulonephritis. Tiopronin (Thiola) is better tolerated than penicillamine.

5. Infection stone (struvite stone) accounts for 10 per cent of kidney stones and are the most difficult to treat. Patients with neurologic bladder or paraplegia are prone to struvite stones. These stones resist pulverization with ESWL; may have to resort to percutaneous nephrolithotomy. Curative treatment requires elimination of all calculus material, followed by long-term antimicrobial agents. Urease inhibitors like acetohydroxamic acid (Lithostat) is a useful adjunct in the treatment even though they have significant side effects, including hemolytic anemia and deep venous thrombosis.

Bibliography

Asplin JR: Uric acid stone. Semin Nephrol 1996;16:412–424.

Cohen TD, Preminger GM: Struvite calculi. Semin Nephrol 1996;16:425–434.

Curhan GC, Willet WC, Rihm EG: A prospective study of dietary calcium and other nutrients and the risk of symptomatic kidney stones. N Engl J Med 1993;328:823–838.

Goldfarb S: Diet and nephrolithiasis. Annu Rev Med 1994;45:235–233.

Levy FL, Adams-Huet B: Ambulatory evaluation of nephrolithiasis: an update of 1980 protocol. Am J Med 1995;98:50–59.

Pacifici R: Idiopathic hypercalciuria and osteoporosis: distinct clinical manifestations of increased cytokine-induced bone resorption? [editorial]. J Clin Endocrinol Metab 1997;82:29–31.

Saklayen MG: Medical management of nephrolithiasis. Med Clin North Am 1997;81:785–799.

Schrier RW, Gottschalk CW: Diseases of the Kidney, 6th ed, pp 739–765. Boston, Little, Brown, 1997.

143 Acute Renal Failure

Cynthia L. Short

Definition

1. *Acute renal failure* (ARF): acute onset of complete or partial impairment in renal excretion of solute and/or fluid, resulting in a rise in serum creatinine of 0.5 to 2.0 mg/dl/day as well as urea nitrogen (*azotemia*). Because multiple factors can affect the rate of rise of blood urea nitrogen (BUN), such as a catabolic state, upper gastrointestinal (GI) bleed, increased protein intake, and steroid use, the rate of rise of BUN is not as indicative of the degree of renal failure as the rate of rise of serum creatinine.

> **Note**
> It is important to remember that the rate of rise of creatinine is only about 1.0 mg/dl/day even in the face of complete renal failure. Therefore, if the serum creatinine is 2.0 mg/dl today but was 1.0 mg/dl yesterday, the creatinine clearance is considered to be less than 10 ml/min. This is important in dosing drugs that are renally metabolized.

2. *Oliguric*: urine output less than 400 ml/day or less than 20 ml/hr
3. *Nonoliguric*: rising BUN and creatinine but maintenance of urine output (fluid removal without solute clearance)
4. *Anuric*: no urine output

Etiology

1. *Prerenal*: decreased renal perfusion
   a. Volume depletion (GI losses, insensible losses, blood loss, poor oral intake)
   b. Decreased effective circulating volume (sepsis, congestive heart failure, cirrhosis)
   c. Vasospasm (ischemia)
   d. Bilateral renal artery occlusion
2. *Renal*: direct damage to the renal parenchyma (interstitium)
   a. Acute tubular necrosis (ATN)
   b. Drug/toxin (aminoglycosides, amphotericin B, contrast dye, myoglobinuria/hemoglobinuria, acute interstitial nephritis secondary to medication, cholesterol emboli syndrome)

> **Note**
> After an angiogram, there are two major causes of renal failure: contrast nephropathy (onset within first 24 hours; rapid resolution) and cholesterol emboli (slower onset; other peripheral manifestations of emboli, such as livedo reticularis, purple toes, retinal changes, cerebrovascular accident; poor prognosis for renal recovery).

   c. *Intrinsic renal disease* (glomerular): rapidly progressive glomerulonephritis, a clinical syndrome of rapidly progressive renal failure, often associated with crescent formation on renal biopsy. Includes human immunodeficiency virus–associated nephropathy.
3. *Postrenal*: obstruction interrupting urine outflow and eventually leading to renal damage
   a. Bladder outlet (prostatic enlargement)
   b. Bilateral ureteral obstruction (stones)
   c. Bilateral renal vein occlusion

> **Note**
> In evaluating a patient for obstruction or vascular events, it is crucial to know if there are one or two kidneys present. Obstruction of one kidney has little or no effect on renal function if a second, normally functioning kidney is present. In the case of the single kidney, however, unilateral obstruction can lead to renal failure.

Symptoms

Most often *nonspecific*. The degree of symptomatology is often related to the rapidity of onset of renal failure.

1. Central nervous system: malaise, cognitive slowing, confusion, seizure, coma
2. GI: anorexia, nausea, vomiting, diarrhea, constipation, metallic taste
3. Cardiovascular: shortness of breath, dyspnea on exertion, pericarditis (chest pain), lower extremity and periorbital edema
4. Hematologic: easy bruising or bleeding (gingival), fatigue secondary to anemia
5. Genitourinary: decreased urine output, flank pain, hematuria, foamy urine

Key Tests

- Serum electrolytes, BUN, creatinine
- Urinalysis
- Renal ultrasound
- Complete blood count

Laboratory Tests

1. Electrolytes (BUN, creatinine, K^+, HCO_3^-)
2. Complete blood count (CBC): white blood cells (WBC), hematocrit (anemia caused by decreased erythropoietin production or hemoconcentration if dry)
3. Urinalysis: specific gravity, presence or absence of hematuria, proteinuria, granular, WBC count, red blood cell (RBC) casts
4. Urine electrolytes and fractional excretion of sodium (FENA) to elucidate renal versus prerenal in oliguric ARF

	PRERENAL	RENAL
Urine Na	<20	>40
$FENA = \dfrac{excreted\ Na}{filtered\ Na}$ $= \dfrac{U_{Na}}{P_{Na}} \times \dfrac{P_{Cr}}{U_{Cr}}$ $\times 100\%$	<1%	>15%

5. Creatinine kinase, urine myoglobin
6. Ultrasound: Especially helpful in ruling out obstruction, ruling out solitary kidney, checking renal size (patients with chronic renal failure often have smaller, shrunken kidneys).

Note

Ultrasound may not show evidence of hydronephrosis early on (within 24 to 48 hours) or in patients with retroperitoneal fibrosis, in whom the collecting system does not dilate.
Anterograde and/or retrograde pyelogram is the gold standard for ruling out obstruction and should be considered in all patients at high risk for obstruction.

---

7. Renal flow scan
8. Serologic tests: complement, antinuclear antibody, antistreptolysin O titer, anti–glomerular basement membrane titer, serum and urine protein electrophoresis, anti–neutrophilic cytoplasmic antibody
9. If creatinine is stable, 24-hour urine for creatinine clearance, total protein
10. Renal biopsy

Differential Diagnosis

1. Prerenal
   a. *Volume depletion*: Accurate volume assessment is essential in evaluating any patient with renal failure. This includes the estimation of both total-body volume and actual or effective intravascular volume (how much blood is actually perfusing the kidney). This is assessed by history, physical examination, laboratory values, and Swan-Ganz catheter readings if available.
      (1) Vital signs and orthostatic blood pressures, neck veins flat and at 45 degrees
      (2) Skin turgor
      (3) Intake and output, weight changes
   b. Decreased effective circulating volume
      (1) Sepsis
      (2) Poor cardiac output
      (3) Cirrhosis
      (4) Vasospasm (ischemia, cyclosporine, malignant hypertension, pre-eclampsia)
      (5) Bilateral renal artery stenosis or occlusion
2. Renal
   a. Nephritic (hypertension, hematuria, low-grade proteinuria, RBC casts, edema)
   b. Nephrotic (>3.5 gm of protein per 24-hour urine, hypoalbuminemia, edema, hypercholesterolemia)
   c. These are only broad classifications of renal disease, and there is often overlap between the two syndromes in a single patient. They can, however, guide the physician because some diseases (e.g., poststreptococcal glomerulonephrosis) tend to be more nephritic, whereas others (e.g., aggressive focal sclerosis) are more nephrotic.
3. Postrenal: obstruction
   a. Bladder outlet
      (1) Prostatic enlargement
      (2) Tumor
      (3) Neurogenic bladder
      (4) Clot
   b. Bilateral ureteral

(1) Stones

(2) Tumor

(3) Sloughed papillae (papillary necrosis)

(4) Retroperitoneal fibrosis

c. Bilateral renal vein thrombosis

Treatment

1. Maintain optimal intravascular volume.

   a. Diuretics (loop or thiazide/loop combination) if volume overloaded

   b. Volume expansion (normal saline, blood, albumin, etc.) if volume depleted

2. Optimize cardiac output.

3. Avoid further renal insults.

4. Treat hyperkalemia with resin binders and diuretics.

5. Treat underlying condition (e.g., antibiotics for sepsis, immunosuppressant agents for glomerulonephrosis, relieve obstruction).

6. Fluid restriction if euvolemic or volume overloaded (1 to 1.5 L/day)

7. Dialysis

   a. Intermittent hemodialysis

   b. Acute peritoneal dialysis

   c. Continuous replacement therapies: continuous venovenous hemofiltration (CVVH), continuous arteriovenous hemofiltration (CAVH). Treatment of choice in patients who are hemodynamically unstable and unable to tolerate standard hemodialysis.

Diet

1. Consider protein restriction for control of uremic symptoms, but remember to adjust to energy needs of catabolic patients.

2. Sodium restriction (2 to 4 gm/day)

3. Potassium restriction (2 to 3 gm/day)

Activity

As tolerated by the patient.

Patient Education

1. Allay fears regarding dialysis and outline limitations.

2. For most forms of ARF, the long-term prognosis is very difficult to predict at time of presentation, and the patient should be aware of this.

Key Treatment

- Maintain optimal intravascular volume.

- Optimize cardiac output.

Follow-Up

1. Resolving ATN: Increase in urine output usually seen before drop in serum creatinine. Post-ATN diuresis may occur, and it is important to avoid volume depletion.

2. Chronic dialysis or transplant

3. Termination of dialysis if the prognosis is poor and the patient/family agree

Bibliography

Demko TM, Diamond JR, Groff J: Obstructive nephropathy as a result of retroperitoneal fibrosis: a review of its pathogenesis and associations. J Am Soc Nephrol 1997;8:684–688.

Meyrier A, Hill GS, Simon P: Ischemic renal diseases: new insights into old entities. Kidney Int 1998;54:2–13.

Nolan CR, Anderson RJ: Hospital-acquired acute renal failure. J Am Soc Nephrol 1998;9:710–718.

Rahn KH, Heidenrach S, Bruckner A: How to assess glomerular function and damage in humans. J Hypertens 1999;17:309–317.

Thadani RI, Camargo CA Jr, Xavier RJ, et al: Atheroembolic renal failure after invasive procedures. Natural history based on 52 biopsy-proven cases. Medicine (Baltimore) 1995;74:350–358.

144 Chronic Renal Failure

Robert L. Benz

Etiology

1. Chronic renal failure (CRF) describes reduced kidney function that is characteristically prolonged (>3 months in duration), irreversible, and progressive in nature. These features differentiate it from acute renal failure (ARF). The presence of anemia and renal osteodystrophy favors the diagnosis of CRF, as does small kidney size.

2. Mild CRF may be referred to as "renal insufficiency," whereas "end-stage renal disease" (ESRD) refers to the development of symptoms or pathophysiologic alterations that require dialytic intervention or renal transplantation to preserve life.

3. The major categories leading to CRF include glomerulopathies (primary and secondary), hypertensive nephrosclerosis, chronic tubulointerstitial diseases, and obstructive uropathy. Diabetic nephropathy and hypertension represent the two leading causes of ESRD in the United States. Myeloma nephropathy may be diagnosed by finding light chains in the urine.

Symptoms

1. Symptoms of uremia typically develop when advanced CRF has been reached (creatinine clearance <30 ml/minute). The earliest symptom is often nocturia or polyuria resulting from loss of the concentrating mechanism.

2. Symptoms may be due to the anemia of CRF or neuromuscular sequelae (peripheral, autonomic, or central nervous system).

3. Other symptoms may stem from specific chemical disturbances related to phosphate, calcium, and parathyroid hormonal imbalance.

4. Bleeding-related symptoms may stem from platelet dysfunction or primary gastrointestinal problems that are increased in CRF patients, such as arteriovenous malformations.

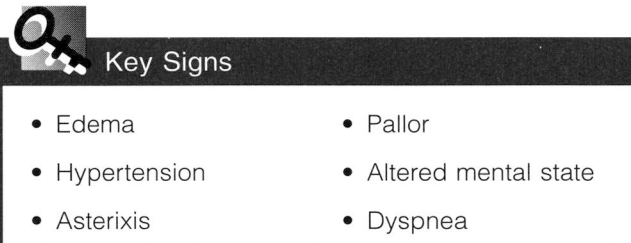

Key Symptoms

- Fatigue
- Nausea
- Anorexia
- Nocturia
- Pruritus
- Sleep disorders
- Confusion
- Dysgeusia

Clinical Findings

1. Clinical findings, like symptoms, do not usually manifest themselves until CRF is advanced (creatinine clearance <30 ml/minute).

2. Salt and water retention in CRF may be manifested by the following cardiovascular sequelae of volume overload: peripheral edema, new or worsening rise in blood pressure, ascites, congestive heart failure (CHF), pericardial effusion.

3. Neurologic manifestations may include

   a. Central nervous system: asterixis, confusion, lethargy, coma, or central sleep apnea

   b. Autonomic nervous system: orthostatic disturbances in blood pressure and pulse, gastroparesis

   c. Peripheral nervous system (typically sensory rather than motor): diminished vibratory sensation, hypoesthesia, diminished deep tendon reflexes, periodic limb movements in sleep, and restless legs syndrome

Key Signs

- Edema
- Hypertension
- Asterixis
- Pallor
- Altered mental state
- Dyspnea

Laboratory Tests

1. The necessary tests to diagnose CRF include markers of the retention of nitrogen waste products normally excreted by kidneys. In addition to tests that determine the level of kidney function directly are studies to detect sequelae of CRF that have occurred.

2. Tests

   a. Kidney status: serum creatinine and blood urea nitrogen (BUN), 24-hour urine for protein and creatinine clearance, renal ultrasound for renal size and to rule out obstruction, urinalysis

   b. Tests for metabolic, hematologic, and nutritional sequelae: calcium, phosphorus, albumin, hematocrit, bleeding time (if undergoing surgery), electrolytes, cholesterol, glucose (if diabetic), potassium, HCO_3^-, and parathyroid hormone

Key Tests

- BUN
- Creatinine
- Creatinine clearance
- Potassium
- Bicarbonate
- Hematocrit
- Urinalysis
- Ultrasound
- Calcium
- Phosphorus
- Serum albumin

Differential Diagnosis

1. The differential diagnosis for CRF is based on ruling out some degree of ARF superimposed on more modest underlying CRF.
2. Because ARF will typically resolve, whereas CRF will persist or progress, one should
   a. Check serial BUN and creatinine values over time.
   b. Try to correct any abnormalities that may be affecting renal function tests, such as medications, hypoperfusion, or obstruction.

Treatment

1. By definition, there is no treatment known to reproducibly correct CRF.
2. In general, the goal of therapy is to retard the rate of progression of CRF and limit the influence of its sequelae on the patient.

Medication

1. Treating the anemia of CRF can be achieved by ensuring adequate iron stores and then initiating recombinant human erythropoietin (rHu-EPO) subcutaneously.
2. Angiotensin-converting enzyme (ACE) inhibitors may preserve renal function by limiting hyperfiltration. Some fall in glomerular filtration rate may occur. Hyperkalemia must be watched for.
3. Control of renal osteodystrophy will require phosphate binders with meals (e.g., calcium acetate or $CaCO_3$) and active vitamin D (1,25-dihydroxycholecalciferol).
4. Diuretics may be necessary to control edema, potassium, and hypertension.
5. Bicarbonate replacement will neutralize associated metabolic acidosis.

6. Ultimately dialysis should be initiated when creatinine clearance is less than 10 ml/minute, or less than 15 ml/minute in diabetic patients. Transplantation is generally considered once the patient is on dialysis.

Diet

1. Anecdotal studies indicated that protein-restricted diets might retard CRF, but a recent multicenter study could not confirm this benefit.
2. It is best to ensure adequate nutrition and calories (35 kcal/kg/day).
3. Limit sodium and potassium to 2 gm daily while restricting phosphorus intake if phosphate levels are elevated.
4. Fluids should be restricted if edema, CHF, or hypertension is present.

Activity

Activity restrictions are few and mostly limited to trying to avoid exhausting activites that lead to hyperkalemia and acidosis.

Patient Education

1. Much education is necessary for the patient (and family), considering the serious nature of CRF and given its progressive course.
2. Once the patient reaches ESRD, dialytic intervention makes education that much more imperative.
3. Education generally requires a team that includes the nephrologist, nutritionist, social worker, dialysis nurse, and surgeon (once patient requires access to dialysis or transplantation).

Key Treatment

- Antihypertensives (especially loop diuretics)
- rHu-EPO
- ACE inhibitors
- Salt and potassium restriction
- Dialysis
- Transplantation

Follow-Up

1. Patients with CRF should be referred to nephrologists early on. The nephrologist and primary care physician should work together to closely monitor the patient's blood work, blood pressure, and progression.

2. As patients approach ESRD, frequent office visits and blood work will be necessary.

3. Counseling about eventual dialysis/transplantation is essential.

4. When creatinine clearance is less then 25 ml/minute or the serum creatinine is 3 to 4 mg/dl, the patient should have surgical consultation for access placement.

Bibliography

Brenner BM, Rector FC: The Kidney, pp 1997–2036. Philadelphia, WB Saunders Company, 1991.

Jacobson HR, Striker GE, Klahr S: The Principles and Practice of Nephrology, 2nd ed, pp 679–683. St. Louis, CV Mosby, 1995.

National Kidney Foundation: NKF-DOQI Clinical Practice Guidelines for Vascular Access, p 31. New York, National Kidney Foundation, 1997.

Schrier RW, Gottschalk CW: Diseases of the Kidney, 6th ed, pp 2581–2698. Boston, Little, Brown, 1997.

Suki WN, Massry SA: Therapy of Renal Diseases and Related Disorders, pp 649–738. Boston, Martinus Nijhoff, 1991.

145 Glomerulonephritis

Khalid Zafar

Etiology

The important glomerulonephritides are

1. Immunoglobulin A (IgA) nephropathy: Most common cause of glomerulonephritis.
2. Membranoproliferative glomerulonephritis (MPGN): Relatively uncommon in its idiopathic form but may be seen in a variety of systemic diseases:
   a. Hereditary complement-deficient states
   b. Hepatitis B and C
   c. Chronic visceral abscess
   d. Chronic lymphocytic leukemia
   e. Chronic transplant rejection
   f. Non-Hodgkin's lymphoma
   g. Malignant melanoma
   h. α_1-Antitrypsin deficiency
   i. Schistosomiasis
3. Rapidly progressive glomerulonephritis (RPGN): Characterized morphologically by crescent formation and clinically by progression to end-stage renal disease within weeks to months if left untreated. Three idiopathic forms are identified:
   a. Anti–glomerular basement membrane (GBM) disease, or Goodpasture's syndrome
   b. Antibody-negative RPGN
   c. Immune complex RPGN
4. Lupus nephritis
5. Postinfectious glomerulonephritis: Two diseases are often associated with glomerulonephritis:
   a. Poststreptococcal glomerulonephritis: May be seen 1 to 3 weeks after a streptococcal throat infection or 3 to 4 weeks after impetigo (skin infection).
   b. Bacterial endocarditis
6. Renal vascular diseases: Systemic vasculitis can cause glomerulonephritis:
   a. Polyarteritis, which includes classic polyarteritis nodosa, Churg-Strauss syndrome, and overlap syndrome
   b. Wegener's granulomatosis
   c. Hypersensitivity vasculitis, including Henoch-Schönlein purpura, essential mixed cryoglobulinemia, and serum sickness
7. Hereditary nephritis (Alport's syndrome): X-linked and associated with hearing loss and lenticular abnormalities
8. Fibrillary glomerulonephritis (immunotactoid glomerulopathy): Electron microscopy shows random fibrillar deposits in the mesangium.

Symptoms

1. Gross hematuria (tea-colored urine)
2. Facial and peripheral edema
3. Shortness of breath because of fluid overload
4. If renal failure is pronounced, the symptoms of uremia will predominate, including nausea, vomiting, loss of appetite, metallic taste, fatigue, and leg cramps.
5. Symptoms suggestive of individual diseases
   a. Sore throat or skin infection 2 to 4 weeks earlier: postinfectious glomerulonephritis
   b. Malar rash, Raynaud's phenomenon, alopecia, arthralgias: suggestive of systemic lupus erythematosus (SLE)
   c. Purpuric rash over the body: suggestive of vasculitis
   d. Fever: suggestive of endocarditis, vasculitis, and SLE
   e. Hemoptysis: suggestive of anti-GBM disease or Wegener's granulomatosis
   f. Rhinorrhea, sinus pain, cough, and upper respiratory tract symptoms: suggestive of Wegener's granulomatosis
   g. Deafness: Alport's syndrome

Key Symptoms

- Tea-colored urine
- Peripheral edema
- Shortness of breath

Clinical Findings

1. Evidence of fluid overload, including peripheral edema, jugular venous distention, and crackles on lung examination
2. Hypertension
3. Malar rash and oral mucosal ulcers in SLE

4. Palpable purpura in lower extremities in Henoch-Schönlein purpura

5. Cardiac murmurs, splinter hemorrhages, petechiae, Roth spots, Janeway lesions, and Osler nodes in endocarditis

6. Skin necrosis, especially in the distal portion of the body, in cryoglobinemia

Key Signs

- Peripheral edema
- Hypertension

Laboratory Tests

1. Urinalysis: showing evidence of hematuria, proteinuria, and red blood cell casts

2. Blood urea nitrogen (BUN) and creatinine to assess renal function

3. Serum electrolytes to rule out hyperkalemia and acidosis

4. Complete blood count (CBC) with differential

5. Erythrocyte sedimentation rate (ESR) and C-reactive protein

6. Antistreptolysin O titer

7. Complement levels, including C3, C4, and CH_{50}. Hypocomplementemia is seen in postinfectious glomerulonephritis, cryoglobulinemia, MPGN, and lupus nephritis.

8. Anti-GBM antibody

9. Antinuclear antibody (ANA)

10. Anti–double-stranded DNA antibody: positive in SLE

11. Serum cryoglobulins

12. Hepatitis serologies, including hepatitis B and C and liver function test

13. Anti–neutrophil cytoplasmic antibody (ANCA): positive in Wegener's and other vasculitides

14. Blood cultures: May be positive in endocarditis

15. Transthoracic or transesophageal echocardiogram to rule out valvular vegetation if endocarditis is suspected

16. Skin biopsy in case of a skin rash may be helpful

17. Chest radiograph to rule out pulmonary vascular congestion, and pulmonary hemorrhage in Goodpasture's syndrome

18. Kidney biopsy for definitive diagnosis

19. Nasopharyngeal mucosal biopsy or transbronchial or open lung biopsy if Wegener's granulomatosis is suspected

Key Tests

- Urinalysis
- Serum electrolytes
- BUN and creatinine

Differential Diagnosis

1. Acute interstitial nephritis: May present as acute renal failure with microscopic hematuria.

2. Urinary tract infection: May present with hematuria.

3. Lower genitourinary tract pathology: ureteral and bladder pathology, including stones, tumors, and trauma, may present with hematuria and renal insufficiency from obstruction.

4. Pigment nephropathy: Rhabdomyolysis can cause dark urine from myoglobinuria; also acute renal failure.

Treatment

Medication

1. No medication may be needed for poststreptococcal glomerulonephritis.

2. Steroids: Corticosteroids may be the mainstay of most of the glomerulonephritides. They are beneficial in
   a. Lupus nephritis
   b. MPGN
   c. RPGN
   d. Anti-GBM disease
   e. Vasculitis

3. Cyclophosphamide
   a. Mainstay therapy for Wegener's granulomatosis
   b. Lupus nephritis in conjunction with steroids
   c. Vasculitis in conjunction with steroids

4. Fish oil: Has shown some benefit with IgA nephropathy.

5. Antibiotics: Appropriate antibiotics are the only treatment needed for endocarditis-induced glomerulonephritis.

6. Diuretics: May be beneficial to treat the fluid overload.

7. Angiotensin-converting enzyme (ACE) inhibitors: In the absence of significant renal failure, ACE inhibitors are the preferred antihyperten-

sive to treat the hypertension because they diminish proteinuria by decreasing intrarenal hypertension.

8. Dialysis: May be required in patients with severe renal failure or volume overload.

9. Plasmapheresis: Indicated as a treatment tool for
   a. Anti-GBM disease
   b. Cryoglobulinemia
   c. RPGN

Diet

1. Low-sodium (2 gm) diet
2. Low-potassium and low-phosphorus diet in renal failure
3. Low-protein (0.6 to 0.7 gm/kg) diet

Activity

As tolerated

Patient Education

1. Patient should be instructed about the potential side effects of the medications, including steroids and cyclophosphamide.
2. Steroids can potentially cause
   a. Edema, weight loss, and cushingoid facies
   b. Osteoporosis
   c. Avascular necrosis of the hip
   d. Increased risk for infection; watch for sore throat, fever, dysuria, and the like.
   e. Abdominal striae
   f. Glucose intolerance and diabetes mellitus
   g. Hypertension
   h. Peptic ulcer
   i. Psychosis
3. Cyclophosphamide can potentially cause
   a. Bone marrow suppression—leukopenia
   b. Increased risk for cancer
   c. Increased risk for infection
   d. Infertility
   e. Hemorrhagic cystitis
4. Patients with renal failure should be educated about their diets, importance of close follow-up, and the potential need for dialysis. If necessary, they should be familiarized with the modalities of dialysis.

Key Treatment

- Steroids
- Cyclophosphamide
- Diuretics

Follow-Up

Close follow-up is necessary for most patients. Outpatient management includes

1. Immunosuppressive management: adjusting the dose of steroids and cyclophosphamide to keep the disease in remission
2. Monitoring of the parameters for disease activity, which may be different for individual diseases.
   a. In general, every follow-up visit should include:
      (1) Blood pressure
      (2) Weight
      (3) Serum BUN and creatinine
      (4) Serum electrolytes
      (5) CBC
      (6) Urinalysis
   b. In case of individual diseases, further laboratory testing is indicated:
      (1) ANA, anti–double-stranded DNA, complement levels, ESR, and C-reactive protein in lupus nephritis
      (2) Anti-GBM antibody in Goodpasture's syndrome
      (3) ANCA titers in vasculitis
      (4) Blood cultures, ESR, and echocardiogram for endocarditis
      (5) Aminoglycoside and vancomycin levels to avoid nephrotoxicity
3. Monitoring for side effects of medication clinically and on the basis of laboratory results
4. Adjusting antihypertensives and diuretics to keep patient normotensive and euvolemic

Bibliography

Appel GB, Silva FG, Pirani CL, et al: Renal involvement in systemic lupus erythematosus: a study of 56 patients emphasizing histologic classification. Medicine (Baltimore) 1976–1978;57:371.

Galla J: IgA nephropathy. Kidney Int 1995;47:377.

Gibson L: Cutaneous vasculitis: approach to diagnosis and systemic associations. Mayo Clin Proc 1990;65:221.

Rennke H: Secondary membranoproliferative glomerulonephritis. Kidney Int 1995;47:643.

Rose B: Pathophysiology of Renal Disease, 2nd ed, pp 254–262. New York, McGraw-Hill, 1987.

146 Pyelonephritis

Andy G. Pinson

Etiology

1. Acute pyelonephritis (APN) is an acute infection of the upper urinary tract. In the adult, chronic pyelonephritis does not generally develop unless there is a major underlying functional or anatomic abnormality.

2. APN usually occurs when colonic bacteria ascend through the urinary tract to invade the renal parenchyma.

3. The short length and the positioning of the female urethra in the vulvar area make it susceptible to contamination with bowel flora, and thus urinary tract infections (UTIs), including APN, are seen more frequently in women than in men.

4. Some women have an increased susceptibility to colonization by uropathogenic bacteria.

5. *Escherichia coli* is responsible for most episodes of APN, with other possible pathogens including *Proteus*, *Klebsiella*, *Staphylococcus saprophyticus*, and *Enterococcus*.

6. Some strains of bacteria possess virulence factors that make them more likely to cause APN.

Symptoms

1. Symptoms of APN usually include one or more of the following:
   a. Fever
   b. Chills
   c. Back or flank pain
   d. Nausea or vomiting

2. Symptoms of cystitis (dysuria, frequency, urgency) are often, but not always, present.

3. Based on localization tests, approximately 15 to over 50 per cent of patients with symptoms of cystitis also have evidence of occult infection of the upper urinary tract.

4. APN in the elderly may present atypically (altered mental status or vague abdominal pain being predominant).

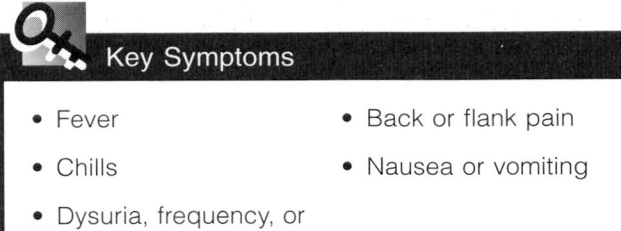

Key Symptoms

- Fever
- Chills
- Dysuria, frequency, or urgency
- Back or flank pain
- Nausea or vomiting

Clinical Findings

1. The presence of fever in the setting of symptoms of cystitis is suggestive of upper UTI.

2. Costovertebral angle tenderness is often present and may represent renal parenchymal inflammation.

3. A pelvic examination can help rule out other causes, such as pelvic inflammatory disease.

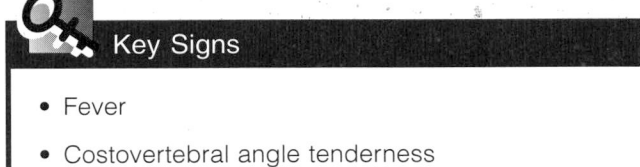

Key Signs

- Fever
- Costovertebral angle tenderness

Laboratory Tests

1. Clean-catch or in-and-out catheterization urinalysis
   a. Perform a urinalysis in all cases of suspected APN.
   b. In APN, an uncontaminated spun specimen should show five or more leukocytes per high-power field.
   c. A Gram's stain can be useful to help determine if gram-positive cocci are present (which can influence therapy).

2. Urine culture
   a. Should be obtained in all cases of suspected APN.
   b. A urine culture generally shows 100,000 or more colony-forming units per milliliter in APN, although lower colony counts are possible.

3. Blood cultures
   a. Should be obtained if the patient appears ill enough to warrant hospitalization.

b. There is no evidence that bacteremia predicts a worse prognosis or warrants longer therapy in an otherwise healthy individual with APN.

4. Bilateral ureteral catheterization and the bladder washout technique can be used to more definitively diagnose upper UTI, but these techniques are invasive and impractical for routine clinical use.

Key Tests

- Urinalysis
- Urine culture

Differential Diagnosis

1. Conditions that can be confused with APN include
   a. Pelvic inflammatory disease
   b. Acute appendicitis
   c. Acute cholecystitis
   d. Nephrolithiasis
2. A careful history, physical examination, and review of a spun urine specimen should help to rule out other diagnoses.
3. The absence of pyuria or an abnormal pelvic examination can be a clue that another diagnosis is present.

Treatment

1. The examining physician must determine if hospitalization is required or if outpatient therapy is possible.
2. Factors favoring hospitalization include
   a. Geriatric age group
   b. Underlying medical condition, such as diabetes or pregnancy
   c. Male gender (higher frequency of anatomic abnormality)
   d. Known genitourinary tract abnormality
   e. Inability to maintain oral hydration or take medications
   f. Severe illness (high fever, severe pain, or altered mentation)
3. Consider outpatient management for otherwise healthy young females who are reliable and who are tolerating oral intake.
4. Emergency room observation units can allow
   a. Hydration with intravenous fluids for 8 to 12 hours
   b. Administration of antiemetics
   c. Administration of one to two doses of parenteral antibiotics
   d. Reassessment of the patient by a physician to determine whether or not admission will be required

Medication

1. If hospitalization is required, numerous intravenous antibiotic regimens can be effective. Switch to an oral antibiotic (see item 2 below) after the patient has improved clinically.
   a. Ampicillin, 1 gm q6h, and gentamicin, 3 to 5 mg/kg/day or 1 mg/kg q8h, is the traditional regimen and still effective, especially if *Enterococcus* is suspected based on a Gram's stain of urine showing gram-positive cocci.
   b. Ceftriaxone (Rocephin), 1 to 2 gm q24h
   c. Other intravenous antibiotics with gram-negative coverage. Consider antibiotic sensitivity patterns of local pathogens.
2. For outpatient oral antibiotic therapy, choices include
   a. Fluoroquinolones such as ciprofloxacin (Cipro), 500 mg q12h, ofloxacin (Floxin), 200 to 300 mg q12h, levofloxacin (Levaquin), 250 mg qd, or norfloxacin (Noroxin), 400 mg q12h
   b. Trimethoprim-sulfamethoxazole (Bactrim DS), 160 mg/800 mg q12h: inexpensive and usually effective (an increase in the resistance of pyelonephritic strains to this antibiotic has been noted in recent years). A rash also sometimes develops.
   c. Cefixime (Suprax), 400 mg qd, or cefpodoxime proxetil (Vantin), 200 mg q12h
3. Total duration of antibiotic therapy: 10 days (in less ill patients) to 14 days (in more ill or pregnant patients).

Diet

Instruct patients to stay well hydrated.

Activity

Resume normal daily activities within a few days.

Patient Education

1. If outpatient therapy is chosen, the patient should be instructed to call or return for worsening symptoms.
2. Patients often improve markedly after 2 or 3 days of therapy but should be told to complete the entire antibiotic course.
3. Voiding after sexual intercourse can decrease the frequency of UTIs in some women.

Key Treatment (Inpatients)

Drugs of Choice	Alternative Drugs
• Ampicillin + gentamicin	• Other intravenous antibiotics with gram-negative coverge
• Ceftriaxone	

Key Treatment (Outpatients)

Drug of Choice	Alternative Drugs
• Fluoroquinolones	• Trimethoprim-sulfamethoxazole
	• Cefixime
	• Cefpodoxime

Follow-Up

1. For outpatients, a brief follow-up visit (or at least telephone follow-up) is recommended after 1 to 2 days to document clinical improvement.

2. Failure to improve or worsening symptoms after 48 to 72 hours may represent obstruction or abscess, so consider imaging studies such as an ultrasound or an intravenous pyelogram. If such a patient is being managed on oral antibiotics, consider hospitalization and intravenous antibiotics.

3. Routine post-treatment urine cultures in asymptomatic patients are no longer recommended.

4. If a woman has two recurrent episodes of APN, a urologic consultation or work-up (ultrasound or intravenous pyelogram and possibly cystoscopy) should be considered. In men, a single episode of pyelonephritis justifies a urologic work-up.

Bibliography

Hooton TM, Stamm WE: Diagnosis and treatment of uncomplicated urinary tract infection. Infect Dis Clin North Am 1997;11:551–581.

Meyrier A, Guibert J: Diagnosis and drug treatment of acute pyelonephritis. Drugs 1992;44:356–367.

Pinson AG, Philbrick JT, Lindbeck GH, Schorling JB: ED management of acute pyelonephritis in women: a cohort study. Am J Emerg Med 1994;12:271–278.

Pinson AG, Philbrick JT, Lindbeck GH, Schorling JB: Oral antibiotic therapy for acute pyelonephritis: a methodologic review of the literature. J Gen Intern Med 1992;7:544–553.

Sobel JD: Pathogenesis of urinary tract infection. Infect Dis Clin North Am 1997;11:531–549.

147 Acute Urinary Tract Infection in Adults

Steven K. Swedlund

Etiology

1. Urinary tract infections (UTIs) are largely a disease of sexually active females.
2. The female-to-male incidence ratio of UTI is 2:1 after the age of 60 years.
3. UTIs are the most common bacterial infection in the elderly, and are a common source of bacteremia.
4. Gram-negative coliforms are responsible for the majority of bacterial infections, with *Escherichia coli* predominating.

Symptoms

1. Dysuria is a very common symptom, often accompanied by frequency, nocturia, incontinence, and suprapubic pain.
2. Malodorous urine and gross hematuria may also be present.
3. Flank pain and fever are generally considered symptoms of UTI.
4. Elderly patients may also display a septic syndrome with altered mental status, tachycardia and tachypnea; an occasional patient may demonstrate hypothermia.
5. For some patients, gastrointestinal symptoms such as nausea, vomiting, and abdominal tenderness may falsely direct the clinician away from the urinary tract.

Key Symptoms

Lower Urinary Tract	Upper Urinary Tract
• Dysuria	• Flank pain
• Frequency	• Fever
• Nocturia	• Nausea and vomiting
• Suprapubic pain	• Mental changes (in the elderly)
• Hematuria	
• Malodorous urine	
• Incontinence	

Clinical Findings

1. For acute bacterial lower UTIs, the only positive physical finding may be suprapubic tenderness.

2. In addition, upper UTI may be associated with loin or flank tenderness, fever, tachypnea, tachycardia, and mental status changes (particularly in the elderly).

Key Signs

Lower UTI	Upper UTI
• Suprapubic tenderness	• Flank tenderness
	• Fever
	• Tachypnea
	• Tachycardia
	• Mental status change (elderly)
	• Vomiting

Laboratory Tests

1. Microscopic examination and culture of clean-catch midstream urine specimens are the primary laboratory tests for suspected UTI.
2. Pyuria is defined as 10 or more leukocytes/ml as measured on a fresh, uncentrifuged specimen of urine by microscopy in a hemocytometer chamber.
3. In the absence of a positive midstream urine culture (<100 uropathogens/ml), pyuria suggests infection by *Chlamydia trachomatis* or *Neisseria gonorrhoeae*, or tuberculosis.
4. Microscopic or gross hematuria may be observed in UTI but is nonspecific.
5. White cell casts noted on microscopy strongly suggest pyelonephritis in patients with symptoms of UTI.
6. Between 15 and 30 per cent of patients with acute pyelonephritis may be bacteremic with positive cultures. Elderly patients, diabetics, and individuals with urinary tract obstruction appear to have an increased risk of bacteremia.
7. Four biochemical screening tests for UTI have been devised: the glucose oxidase, catalase, nitrite reduction, and leukocyte esterase tests. Screening methods, in general, are insensitive at

bacterial counts less than 10^5 colony-forming units per milliliter.

Key Tests

- Urine microscopy

- Pyuria (>10 leukocytes/ml in uncentrifuged urine)

- White cell casts (indicate upper UTI)

- Leukocyte esterase test

- Clean-catch midstream urine culture

- Blood culture (in toxic or elderly patients with signs of upper UTI)

Differential Diagnosis

1. Acute bacterial lower UTIs in females may be mimicked by urethritis caused by *C. trachomatis*, *N. gonorrhoeae*, and herpes simplex virus.

2. Vaginitis from *Candida albicans* and *Trichomonas vaginalis* or bacterial vaginosis may also cause dysuria.

3. Acute upper UTI can be mimicked by diverticulitis, appendicitis, pneumonia, intestinal obstruction, and nephrolithiasis.

Treatment (Table 147–1)

1. Therapeutic standards have not been defined for many forms of acute bacterial UTIs. However, standards do exist for women with uncomplicated infections.

    a. For acute bacterial uncomplicated lower UTIs in females, 3 days of oral outpatient therapy is frequently effective.

    b. Treatment of uncomplicated bacterial upper UTIs in females and males includes 10 to 14 days of oral or parenteral antibiotics and may necessitate hospitalization.

2. For therapy of uncomplicated bacterial lower UTI in males, consider 7 days of therapy with an antibiotic that penetrates the prostate, e.g., a fluoroquinolone such as ciprofloxacin (Cipro), 250 mg q12h.

3. Factors that would designate a UTI as complicated include age greater than 65 years, indwelling catheter, recent genitourinary instrumentation, urinary calculi, renal impairment, prostatic involvement, diabetes mellitus, renal transplant, neutropenia, recent antibiotic therapy, recurrent UTI, pregnancy, steroid therapy, immunocompromising disease, and known structural or functional impairment.

TABLE 147–1. MEDICATION DOSAGES

Oral Regimens for Cystitis
- Trimethoprim-sulfamethoxazole (Bactrim DS, Septra DS), 160 mg/800 mg q12h
- Trimethoprim, 100 mg q12h
- Norfloxacin (Noroxin), 400 mg q12h
- Ciprofloxacin (Cipro), 100–250 mg q12h
- Levofloxacin (Levaquin), 250 mg q24h
- Ofloxacin (Floxin), 200 mg q12h
- Lomefloxacin (Maxaquin), 400 mg q24h
- Enoxacin (Penetrex), 400 mg q12h
- Sparfloxacin (Zagam), 400 mg day 1, then 200 mg q24h
- Cefixime (Suprax), 400 mg q24h
- Cefpodoxime proxetil (Vantin), 100 mg q12h
- Nitrofurantoin, 5–7mg/kg/d and give q6h (7 days)
- Macrocrystalline nitrofurantoin, 100 mg q12h (7 days)
- Cephalexin, 250–500 mg q6h
- Ampicillin, 250–500 mg q6h

Oral Regimens for Pyelonephritis
- Trimethoprim-sulfamethoxazole (Bactrim DS, Septra DS), 160 mg/800 mg q12h
- Ciprofloxacin (Cipro), 500 mg q12h
- Levofloxacin (Levaquin), 250 mg q12h
- Ofloxacin (Floxin), 200–300 mg q12h
- Norfloxacin (Noroxin), 400 mg q12h
- Enoxacin (Penetrex), 400 mg q12h
- Sparfloxacin (Zagam), 40 mg day 1, then 200 mg q12h
- Cefixime (Suprax), 400 mg q24h
- Cefpodoxime proxetil (Vantin), 200 mg q12h

Intravenous Regimens for Pyelonephritis
- Ceftriaxone, 1.0–2.0 gm q12h
- Gentamicin, 3 mg/kg/day q8h
- Ciprofloxacin (Cipro), 200–400 mg q12h
- Levofloxacin (Levoquin), 250 mg q24h
- Ofloxacin (Floxin), 200–400 mg q12h
- Trimethoprim-sulfamethoxazole (Bactrim, Septra), 160 mg/800 mg q12h

4. The presence of obstructing urinary calculi and acute bacterial upper UTI should be considered a surgical emergency and consultation obtained.

5. The clinician is limited in treating lower UTI in pregnant females because quinolones cannot be used during pregnancy nor can sulfonamides near the delivery date. Cephalexin is a reasonable first choice.

6. Antibiotic selection for all other complicated UTIs is dictated by the clinical situation. Duration of therapy is unknown in these situations. The clinician should consider treating for 14 days, and reculture to investigate for structural or functional impairment if there is recurrence.

Patient Education

1. Educate the patient to stay well hydrated.

2. In the female patient, discuss voiding after intercourse for prophylaxis.

3. Encourage patient to rest if toxic.

4. Discuss alternate contraception if recurrent UTI associated with use of diaphragm.

5. Consider chemoprophylaxis with recurrent lower UTI.

Key Treatment

Uncomplicated Lower UTI: Female (3 Days Oral Therapy)

Primary

- Trimethoprim-sulfamethoxazole

- Norfloxacin or other fluoroquinolone

Alternates

- Trimethoprim

- Nitrofurantoin or macrocrystalline nitrofurantoin (7 days)

Key Treatment

Uncomplicated Upper UTI: Female and Male (10 to 14 Days)

Primary

- Trimethoprim-sulfamethoxazole, *or*

- Ciprofloxacin, *or*

- Other quinolone

Parenteral

- Ampicillin and gentamicin, *or*

- Quinolone, *or*

- Third-generation cephalosporin

Follow-Up

1. Uncomplicated lower UTIs in females do not always require initial midstream culture, and do not require follow-up culture; consider urinalysis to document resolution of pyuria.

2. UTIs in men and complicated UTI require initial midstream culture, and also culture after completion of therapy.

3. UTIs in men require thorough genitourinary (GU) exam.

4. Recurrent and complicated UTIs in females require GU exam.

5. Utilize history and GU exam to tailor work-up to find functional or structural GU abnormality.

6. Simply assessing postvoid residual urine volume by catheterization may uncover functional bladder outlet obstruction.

7. Medical imaging techniques (ultrasonography, intravenous pyelography, computerized tomography, magnetic resonance imaging, nuclear scan) may assist in diagnosis of structural abnormalities such as calculi in the GU tract, renal abscess, bladder diverticula, fistulas, GU tumors, and congenital defects.

8. Urology consultation may also be indicated to evaluate for structural or functional GU deficit.

Bibliography

Gleckman RA: Urinary tract infection. Clin Geriatr Med 1992;8:793–803.

Hooten TM, Stamm WE: Diagnosis and treatment of uncomplicated urinary tract infection. Infect Dis Clin North Am 1997;11:551–573.

Morgan MG, McKenzie H: Controversies in the laboratory diagnosis of community acquired urinary tract infection. Eur J Clin Microbiol Infect Dis 1993;12:491–504.

Ronald AR, Nicolle LE: Infections of the upper urinary tract. In Schrier RW, Gottschalk CW (eds): Diseases of the Kidney, 5th ed, vol 1, pp 973–1027. Boston, Little, Brown, 1993.

Ronald AR, Nicolle LE, Harding GKM: Standards of therapy for urinary tract infections in adults. Infection 1992;20:S164–S167.

148 Acute Urinary Tract Infection in Children

Syed M. Ahmed

Etiology

1. Urinary tract infection (UTI) occurs in about 1 to 2 per cent of male children and about 5 per cent of female children.
2. In the neonatal age group there is a male predominance, whereas female predominance occurs afterward.
3. *Escherichia coli* is the most common infecting pathogen, accounting for 80 per cent of the cases.
4. Other pathogens include *Klebsiella pneumoniae*, *Proteus mirabilis*, *Pseudomonas aeruginosa*, *Enterobacter* species, *Staphylococcus aureus*, *Streptococcus viridans*, *Enterococcus* species, and *Candida albicans*.
5. Infection is usually caused by ascension of bacteria into the urinary tract, although in neonates the usual route of infection is presumed to be hematogenous.
6. Predisposing factors to the development of UTI include any condition that leads to urinary stasis (e.g., vesicoureteral reflux, obstructive uropathy, renal calculi, and voiding disorders).

Symptoms

1. Both history and physical examination are of limited value in detecting UTI in pediatric patients because symptoms are not specific and are seldom localized to the urinary tract.
2. Neonates with UTI may present with fever, vomiting, hypothermia, diarrhea, abdominal distention, lethargy, irritability, failure to thrive, convulsions, and bacteremia.
3. Older infants may have feeding problems, vomiting, fever, malodorous urine, and failure to thrive.
4. Older children can present with common symptoms of UTI, such as dysuria, frequency, hesitancy, enuresis, and suprapubic discomfort.
5. Children with pyelonephritis may present with flank pain, high fever, and toxic appearance.

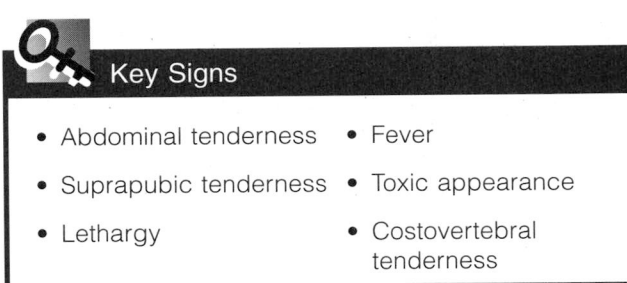

Key Symptoms

- Fever
- Vomiting
- Dysuria
- Frequency
- Flank pain
- Enuresis

Clinical Findings

1. Common signs include abdominal and suprapubic tenderness, pallor, lethargy, and palpable kidneys.
2. Patients with costovertebral tenderness and fever are usually assumed to have pyelonephritis until proven otherwise.
3. In case of a possible UTI, physical examination should exclude hypertension, abnormal genitalia, an abdominal mass, and neurologic deficits.

Key Signs

- Abdominal tenderness
- Suprapubic tenderness
- Lethargy
- Fever
- Toxic appearance
- Costovertebral tenderness

Laboratory Tests

1. A properly collected clean-catch midstream urine specimen is useful for diagnosis of UTI. In infants and children from whom it is difficult to obtain satisfactory clean-catch urine, suprapubic aspiration or bladder catheterization may be necessary.
2. "Dip and read" tests
   a. There are several different kinds of rapid, inexpensive tests available that determine the presence of leukocyte esterase and nitrite concentrations.
   b. False-negative and false-positive tests are common, occurring in 15 to 30 per cent of cases, and they are not sufficiently sensitive to determine the need for urine culture.
   c. Hematuria and proteinuria, assessed by dip-

stick, may occur with UTI but are not diagnostic.

3. Microscopic examination of urine

   a. Bacteria: The presence of one or more bacteria per oil-immersion field of uncentrifuged urine or greater than 10 organisms per oil-immersion field on a centrifuged unstained sediment correlates well with positive cultures.

   b. Pyuria: The presence of more than five white blood cells per high-power field in centrifuged urine has a high sensitivity for UTI. However, UTI can occur without pyuria.

   c. Gram's stain: The presence of one or more bacteria in an oil-immersion field of unspun urine correlates well with the finding of 10^5 colony-forming units or more bacteria per milliliter of urine.

   d. Urine culture: A reliably collected urine culture is the mainstay in the diagnosis of UTI.

      (1) More than 10^5 colonies from a midstream clean-catch urine, more than 10^3 colonies from an intermittent ("in-and-out") catheterization, and any number of colonies from a suprapubic bladder aspiration indicate UTI.

      (2) One positive culture associated with symptoms or two concurrent positive cultures in an asymptomatic child indicate UTI.

      (3) Most UTIs are caused by a single organism; the presence of two or more organisms usually suggests contamination.

      (4) A urine culture is not mandatory in adolescent females, particularly with a first episode. With recurrent episodes, episodes that fail therapy, in females with pyuria without bacteriuria, or in males, a culture is recommended.

Key Test

Positive urine culture is the definitive test.

Differential Diagnosis

1. In females, the differential diagnosis includes vulvovaginitis, gonococcal or chlamydial urethritis, acute urethral syndrome, and genital herpes infection. Local dermatitis from using contraceptive agents, foams, feminine hygiene products, soap, or other chemicals can present with UTI symptoms, such as dysuria.

2. In males, the differential diagnosis includes irritation from chemicals such as spermicidal foam, prostatitis, and gonococcal and nongonococcal urethritis. Physicians should consider torsion of testis and epididymitis when diagnosing a child with UTI.

Treatment

1. Outpatient treatment: The initial antibiotic therapy should be based on clinical severity, age, location of infection, presence of structural abnormalities, allergy to certain antibiotics, and cost of alternative antibiotics.

2. Reasonable choices for initial outpatient and inpatient antibiotic therapy are shown in Table 148–1. Based on the results of the urine culture and sensitivity, antibiotic therapy may require change.

3. The duration of treatment is controversial. There are studies reporting successful treatment of uncomplicated UTI with short-course therapy (e.g., a single dose of amoxicillin or a 3-day course of various antibiotics), although conventional therapy is for 7 to 10 days.

4. There is also controversy regarding the need for antibiotic treatment of asymptomatic bacteriuria, with reports showing no effects on the emergence of symptoms, kidney function, or kidney scars. Also, questions have been raised about whether treating organisms of low virulence can precipitate acute pyelonephritis by more virulent organisms. Some experts suggest treatment of asymptomatic bacteriuria if children are less than 5 years old or if they have a urinary tract structural abnormality.

TABLE 148–1. ANTIMICROBIAL DRUGS USED IN THE TREATMENT OF UTI IN CHILDREN

DRUG	DOSAGE
Oral therapy	
Amoxicillin	10–15 mg/kg/dose tid
Amoxicillin-clavulanate (Augmentin)	10–15 mg/kg/dose tid
Cephalexin (Keflex)	10–15 mg/kg/dose qid
Nitrofurantoin (avoid in newborns or patients with renal insufficiency)	1.25–1.75 mg/kg/dose qid
Sulfisoxazole (Gantrisin)	30–40 mg/kg/dose qid
Trimethoprim-sulfamethoxazole (Bactrim, Septra) (use cautiously during the first month of life because of risk of jaundice)	5 mg (trimethoprim)/kg/dose bid
Parenteral therapy	
Cefotaxime (Claforan)	50 mg/kg/dose q8h
Ceftriaxone (Rocephin)	50 mg/kg/dose q12–24h
Gentamicin	2.5 mg/kg/dose q8h (neonates q12h)

5. Hospitalization is suggested for symptomatic young infants (less than 3 months), children with clinical evidence of acute pyelonephritis, or children suspected of having upper UTI (toxic appearance, high fever, flank pain). An aminoglycoside in combination with ampicillin or a first-generation cephalosporin is the initial therapy of choice pending urine culture and sensitivity. A third-generation cephalosporin (ceftriaxone or cefotaxime) is also a safe choice, especially for neonates and patients with renal insufficiency. Intravenous therapy is continued until clinical signs (fever, pain, or signs of sepsis) resolve; then oral antibiotics should be taken for 2 to 3 weeks.

6. Ultrasonography is done to rule out obstruction. Although voiding cystourethrogram (VCUG) is usually deferred for 3 weeks to allow for resolution of changes, it can be done as soon as fever has resolved and the urine is sterile.

7. Prophylaxis is recommended for all children younger than age 5 with vesicoureteral reflux of certain grades or other structural urinary tract abnormalities and children with three documented UTIs in a year. With careful monitoring for side effects, prophylaxis can be obtained by a single nightly dose of nitrofurantoin (1 to 2 mg/kg/day) or trimethoprim-sulfamethoxazole (10 mg/kg/day) or sulfamethoxazole for 3 to 6 months or longer. Longer prophylaxis of several years is suggested in selected patients with persistent vesicoureteral reflux.

Patient Education

1. Avoidance or treatment of constipation is a recommended preventive measure against infection.

2. Good hygiene, including front-to-back wiping of the anus, especially in female children, is suggested.

3. The use of chemical irritants, bubble baths, and tight clothing should be avoided.

Key Treatment

Outpatient

• Antibiotics as in Table 148–1

Inpatient

• Aminoglycoside + ampicillin or a first-generation cephalosporin

Prophylaxis

• Trimethoprim-sulfamethoxazole or nitrofurantoin

Follow-Up

1. *Urine culture:* A urine culture should be done 3 to 7 days after completion of treatment to exclude relapse.

2. *Urologic evaluation*

   a. For children with systemic illness, any child less than 5 years of age, and any male children, after the first UTI, renal ultrasonography and cystography (VCUG or radionuclide cystogram [RCG]) are recommended. For female children over 5 years of age without systemic illness, medical imaging is not necessary with the first UTI but may be indicated with recurrent UTI.

   b. Fluoroscopic VCUG is recommended in males to rule out posterior urethral valves. Initial evaluation in females may be accomplished by RCG because obstruction within the urethra is rare. A RCG is a sensitive indicator of reflux. The VCUG can demonstrate obstruction, residual urine, reflux, or neuropathic bladder changes. Renal ultrasonography can demonstrate abnormalities of position or number, duplication, hydronephrosis, scarring, dysplasia, stones, or cysts. If both renal sonography and cystography are normal, no further evaluation is indicated.

   c. If reflux or morphologic changes are identified, further evaluation with renal cortical scintigraphy (RCS) or intravenous urography (IVU) is recommended, although RCS has become the standard for detection of pyelonephritis and renal scarring. RCS with dimercaptosuccinic acid (DMSA) offers the advantages of earlier detection of renal scars and acute inflammatory changes compared to IVU or ultrasound. DMSA scan is also useful in neonates and patients with poor renal function.

3. For children with recurrent infections and asymptomatic bacteriuria, a full work-up, including ultrasonography and cystography, is recommended.

4. *Urodynamics:* Urodynamic studies may prove useful for children with neurologic bladder or uninhibited bladder, especially if associated with reflux or hydronephrosis.

5. *Surgical intervention:* Vesicoureteral reflux, which is found in 30 to 50 per cent of children with UTI, is a risk factor for renal scarring. Grades I and II reflux can be treated with antimicrobial prophylaxis along with a strict voiding regimen; however, for grades III to V reflux, urologic consultation is recommended. Surgical

intervention may be indicated for severe reflux, although some recent studies reported no difference in breakthrough UTI, renal scarring, and renal functions when medical and surgical treatment were compared.

Bibliography

For more information on UTI in children younger than 5 years of age, see

Schlager TA, Lohr JA: Urinary tract infection in outpatient febrile infants and children younger than 5 years of age. Pediatr Ann 1993;22:8.

For current concepts on management of pediatric UTI, see

Hellerstein S: Evolving concepts in the evaluation of the child with a urinary tract infection [editorial]. J Pediatr 1994;124:513–519.

For evaluating the relation of vesicoureteral reflux and acute pyelonephritis, see

Ditchfield MR, De Campo JF, Cook DJ, et al: Vesicoureteral reflux: an accurate predictor of acute pyelonephritis in childhood urinary tract infection. Radiology 1994;190:413–415.

For overview of pediatric UTI, see

Ahmed SM, Swedlund SK: Evaluation and treatment of urinary tract infection in children. Am Fam Physician 1998;57:1573–1580.

Batisky D: Pediatric urinary tract infections. Pediatr Ann 1996;25:259–274.

Indications

1. Suspected urinary tract infection (UTI) or a need to exclude UTI as part of a septic work-up in an infant or toddler who is not yet toilet-trained or able to voluntarily void a clean-catch specimen.
    a. Bag specimens have unacceptably high false-positive rate secondary to perineal contamination.
    b. Generally used in children under 2 years of age.
    c. Fast: Takes less than 1 to 2 minutes to perform.
2. Lack of materials or trained personnel needed to perform urethral catheterization
3. Specimens obtained via catheterization with a 5-Fr feeding tube are also reliable for the above indications, but run the risk of introducing infection into the bladder

Contraindications

1. Bleeding disorders
2. Known or suspected genitourinary anatomic anomalies
3. Other gut anomalies
4. Abdominal organomegaly
5. Bowel distention (ileus, obstruction)
6. Skin infection at needle insertion site
7. Empty bladder (wet diaper within previous 30 to 60 minutes or marked dehydration)

Preparation

1. Explain procedure to parents or guardian.
2. Assemble all materials needed for procedure.
3. Check time of last known void and diaper for wetness.
4. Palpate and percuss abdomen for distended bladder.

Equipment

1. Povidone-iodine or other antiseptic surgical prep solution
2. 70% alcohol
3. Sterile 4 × 4 gauze pads
4. Sterile gloves
5. A 3- to 10-ml sterile syringe
6. A 1-inch, 22- or 23-gauge needle
7. Sterile urine specimen container
8. *Optional*: bedside ultrasound unit (recent work suggests that success rate is increased with the use of ultrasound guidance for the procedure, especially in neonates or premature infants)

Anesthesia

Not needed in infants because of the rapidity of procedure and only a single needle insertion is usually required. Local anesthetic is optional in older child, although the procedure is usually well tolerated without it.

Technique

1. Restrain patient in supine position, either frog-leg or with hips straight and thighs together.

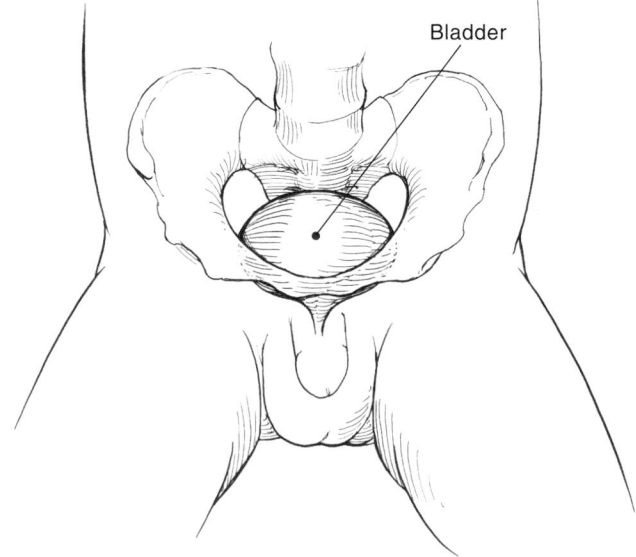

Bladder

2. Assistant prevents urination during procedure by application of gentle penile pinch in males, or gentle anterior pressure with fingertip in the rectum in females.

3. Cleanse the lower abdominal and suprapubic area with the antiseptic solution, and then alcohol.

4. Insert the needle through the skin 1 to 2 cm (about one fingerbreadth) above the symphysis pubis, in the midline. (*Note:* There is usually a transverse skin crease at this level as a landmark.) In neonates and infants, the syringe and needle should be held perpendicular to the table, or with the needle tip aimed slightly (10 degrees) toward the patient's head.

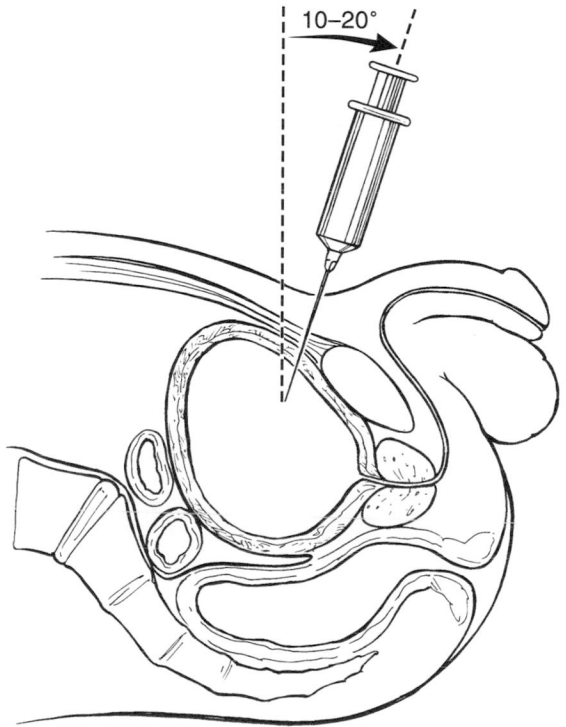

Most "dry taps" when urine is present in the bladder result from inserting too close to the symphysis or directing the needle toward the feet, thus passing below the bladder. Older children may require directing the needle slightly caudad.

5. Apply gentle suction with the plunger and advance the needle until urine is obtained or the hub reaches the skin (1 inch). If no urine is ob-

tained, withdraw the needle because multiple attempts usually are not warranted. Wait 30 to 45 minutes to allow bladder to fill before repeating, or consider alternative specimen collection such as catheterization. Consider ultrasound guidance for verification of urine and localization of bladder if multiple attempts are required.

6. After the needed amount of urine has been obtained, withdraw the needle and apply gentle pressure over the puncture site with a 4 × 4 pad and slight massage. Apply a small sterile dressing and clean off any remaining antiseptic solution residue.

7. Transfer urine into sterile specimen container and send for urinalysis and culture.

Follow-Up

No specific follow-up is needed other than observation for complications. Complications are rare (about 0.2 per cent in one large series), but may include

1. Hematuria (gross hematuria is rare and usually less than 24 hours, but brief microscopic hematuria is common)

2. Infection of skin or abdominal wall at the puncture site

3. Intestinal perforation (adverse sequelae are rare)

4. Bleeding at puncture site or abdominal wall hematoma

Bibliography

Custer JR: Appendix B: special procedures. In Hoekelman RA (ed): Primary Pediatric Care, 3rd ed, p 1806. St. Louis, Mosby–Year Book, 1997.

Hertz AL: Urinary tract infection. In Barkin RM (ed): Pediatric Emergency Medicine, 2nd ed, pp 1164–1168. St. Louis, Mosby–Year Book, 1997.

Kiernan SC, Pinckert TL, Keszler M: Ultrasound guidance of suprapubic bladder aspiration in neonates. J Pediatr 1993;123:789–791.

O'Grady DM: Procedures: suprapubic bladder aspiration. In Barone MA (ed): The Harriet Lane Handbook, 14th ed, pp. 76–77. St. Louis, Mosby–Year Book, 1996.

Pollack CV, Pollack ES, Andrew ME: Suprapubic bladder aspiration versus urethral catheterization in ill infants: success, efficiency, and complication rates. Ann Emerg Med 1994;23:225–230.

149 Nongonococcal Urethritis

Rose A. Recco

Etiology

Nongonococcal urethritis (NGU) is an inflammation of the urethra not caused by *Neisseria gonorrhoeae*. In the United States and many other developed countries, the incidence of NGU far exceeds that of gonococcal urethritis.

1. Common causes
   a. *Chlamydia trachomatis*
   b. *Ureaplasma urealyticum*
2. Infrequent causes: May be bacterial, viral, fungal, or parasitic.
   a. Bacterial: coliforms, genital mycoplasmas
   b. Viral: herpes simplex, condylomata acuminata
   c. Fungal: *Candida, Rhinosporidium*
   d. Parasitic: *Trichomonas vaginalis*, schistosomes
3. No cause found: No infectious etiology is found in as many as 20 to 30 per cent of cases.

Symptoms

The symptoms in NGU overlap with those of gonococcal urethritis but are generally considered milder, and the incubation period is longer than for gonococcal urethritis. NGU may be asymptomatic.

1. Urethral discharge: This is variable. It may be described as scant, profuse, clear, or colored brown, yellow, white, or green.
2. Dysuria or burning on urination
3. Itch in the urethra
4. Incubation period 1 to 5 weeks, peak 2 to 3 weeks

Key Symptoms

- Urethral discharge
- Dysuria
- Urethral itch

Clinical Findings

1. Typical findings
   a. Discharge: This may be spontaneous or expressed and may be mucoid or mucopurulent (i.e., thin cloudy fluid). (It is usually less florid than that with *N. gonorrhoeae*.)
   b. Crusting at meatus
   c. Redness around meatus
   d. Urethral tenderness
2. Unusual findings
   a. Conjunctivitis (*C. trachomatis*)
   b. Reiter's syndrome (*C. trachomatis*)
   c. Epididymitis (*C. trachomatis*)
   d. Regional lymphadenopathy and constitutional symptoms (herpes simplex virus)

WARNING

Differentiation of NGU from gonococcal and other forms of urethritis cannot be made on clinical findings alone.

Key Signs

- Mucopurulent discharge
- Meatal crusting and redness
- Urethral tenderness

Laboratory Tests

The diagnosis of NGU requires a determination of the presence of urethritis in the absence of urethral gonorrhea.

1. Determining the presence of urethritis
   a. Gram's stain of urethral discharge or endourethral swab (five or more polymorphonuclear leukocytes in five oil-immersion fields with no evidence of gram-negative diplococci).
   b. Examine urine sediment of the first 10 to 15 ml of urine (≥10 white blood cells per high-power field or positive leukocyte esterase test).
2. Establish the absence of urethral *N. gonorrhoeae* by Gram's stain and appropriate cultures.

3. Test for chlamydia
   a. Cultures: Isolation in cell culture is the "gold standard."
   b. Nonculture tests: These are primarily based on antigen detection or nucleic acid hybridization methods and may be used on urine and genital swabs.
4. Culture for *U. urealyticum* and other pathogens.

Key Test

Culture is the definitive test.

Differential Diagnosis

The differential diagnosis of NGU includes gonococcal urethritis and noninfectious forms of urethritis.

1. Gonococcal urethritis: Smears and cultures needed for diagnosis.
2. Noninfectious urethritis
   a. Urethral foreign body or calculi: Foreign bodies occasionally may be palpated and may produce bloody discharge. Calculi may produce large amounts of crystals in urine that may be visible on urine sediment. Pain is usually intermittent.
   b. A manifestation of systemic diseases
      (1) Stevens-Johnson syndrome
      (2) Wegener's granulomatosis
      (3) Tumors
   c. Chemical irrigation of the urethra, as with bath products, shampoos. History of use of such products is essential to the diagnosis.
   d. Congenital anomalies

Urethral Syndrome in Women

1. Women with dysuria, frequency, and nocturia in the absence of classic bacterial infection of the lower urinary tract are said to have acute urethral syndrome.
2. Causes may be similar to those in men (i.e., *Escherichia coli*, *N. gonorrhoeae*, *C. trachomatis*, and *U. urealyticum*).
3. *Chlamydia trachomatis* is often found in women with dysuria, frequency, and pyuria. In addition, urinary tract symptoms are reported by half of women with *C. trachomatis* isolated from the urethra. Hence, in some instances, the urethral syndrome may be the clinical counterpart of NGU in women.

Treatment

After the exclusion or treatment of gonococcal urethritis, the treatment of NGU is aimed at *C. trachomatis* and *U. urealyticum*. Any one of the following medications is appropriate.

1. Drugs of choice
   a. Doxycycline, 100 mg orally bid for 7 days
   b. Tetracycline, 500 mg orally qid for 7 days
   c. Azithromycin (Zithromax), 1 gm orally, single dose
2. Other choices
   a. Ofloxacin (Floxin), 300 mg orally bid for 7 days
   b. Erythromycin, 500 mg orally qid for 7 days
   c. Amoxicillin, 500 mg orally tid for 10 days
   d. Clindamycin, 450 mg orally qid for 10 days
   e. Sulfisoxazole, 500 mg orally qid for 10 days

Activity

Patients undergoing treatment for NGU should refrain from sexual intercourse until after treatment.

Patient Education

1. Because NGU is sexually transmitted and may be asymptomatic, patients should be cautioned to avoid promiscuity, use barrier contraceptives, and refer sex partners within the preceding 60 days for treatment.
2. *Chlamydia trachomatis* and *U. urealyticum* rarely cause serious physical consequences or infertility in males. In contrast, women with *C. trachomatis* genital infection may face infertility as a result of tubal occlusion, ectopic pregnancy, and chronic pelvic pain. Infection at term may be transmitted to the infant, causing conjunctivitis and pneumonitis.

Key Treatment

- A tetracycline or azithromycin
- Other choices depend on clinical situations (see text).
- Single-dose regimens improve compliance.

Follow-Up

Evaluation for cure is difficult because NGU may resolve without treatment and urethritis may persist despite microbiologic cure of *C. trachomatis* and *U. urealyticum*.

1. Patients symptomatic after completion of therapy
   a. Rule out inflammation.
   b. A patient should not be re-treated unless definite signs or laboratory evidence of urethral inflammation is present.
2. Persistent or recurrent urethritis
   a. Antibiotics should not be initiated unless signs of urethritis are present.
   b. Regimens for persistent symptoms or repeated occurrences after treatment have not yet been identified.
   c. Patients in this category may be re-treated with the initial regimen if they were noncompliant or re-exposed to an untreated sex partner.

d. Intraurethral swab culture and wet mount for *T. vaginalis* should be done.
e. Urologic evaluation is often not helpful in finding etiology.
f. Compliant patients in whom re-exposure is excluded may be treated with either metronidazole, 2 gm orally in a single dose, plus erythromycin base, 500 mg orally qid for 7 days, *or* erythromycin ethylsuccinate, 800 mg orally qid for 7 days.

Bibliography

Centers for Disease Control and Prevention: 1998 Guidelines for treatment of sexually transmitted diseases. MMWR Morb Mortal Wkly Rep 1998;47(RR-1):49–59.

Drugs for sexually transmitted diseases. Med Lett 1994;36(913):1–6.

Jones RB: Chlamydial diseases. In Mandell GL, Bennett JE, Dolin R (eds): Principles and Practices of Infectious Diseases, 4th ed, pp 1676–1701. New York, Churchill Livingstone, 1995.

McCormack WM, Rein MF: Urethritis. In Mandell GL, Bennett JE, Dolin R (eds): Principles and Practices of Infectious Diseases, 4th ed, pp 1063–1074. New York, Churchill Livingstone, 1995.

Stamm WE: Toward control of sexually transmitted chlamydial infectious. Ann Intern Med 1993;119:432–434.

150 Prostatitis

Michael O. Kirkpatrick

Etiology

Prostatitis is one of the most common and important causes of urinary tract infection (UTI) in adult males. *Acute prostatitis* is fairly uncommon yet potentially serious in nature. *Chronic prostatitis* is more common and may cause persistent and frustrating symptoms. Both require proper recognition and appropriate therapy. Both acute and chronic prostatitis originate from ascending urethral infection, reflux of infected urine, rectal infection extension, or hematogenous spread. The most common causative agents include

1. Gram-negative bacilli (*Escherichia coli*)
2. Enterococci
3. *Chlamydia*
4. *Ureaplasma* (this may be a causative agent in "nonbacterial prostatitis")

Symptoms

1. *Acute bacterial prostatitis*
   a. Constitutional: fever, chills, malaise, myalgias
   b. Local: decreased urine flow, dysuria, perineal and back pain, nocturia, urinary outlet flow obstruction
2. *Chronic prostatitis*: Exhibits a variable clinical presentation. The most common symptoms are associated with urinary outflow obstruction/infection and include
   a. Dysuria
   b. Decreased flow
   c. Hesitancy
   d. Dribbling
   e. Low-grade fever (possibly)
3. *Nonbacterial prostatitis*
   a. Characterized by a clinical presentation similar to chronic prostatitis, yet has no evidence of UTI despite the presence of leukocytes in prostatic secretions. Cultures of both urine and prostatic secretions yield no growth.
   b. *Prostadynia*, otherwise known as prostatosis, is also clinically similar to chronic prostatitis yet shows no inflammatory cells in prostatic secretions.

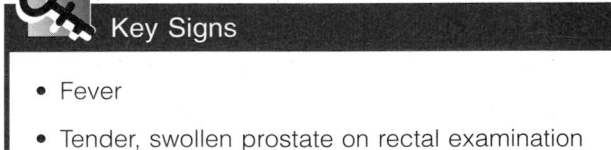

Key Symptoms

- Fever
- Dysuria
- Perineal/back pain
- Decreased flow

Clinical Findings

Gentle rectal examination (do not massage the gland) reveals a swollen, exquisitely tender, and boggy prostate gland, and often bladder distention is noted on abdominal examination.

Key Signs

- Fever
- Tender, swollen prostate on rectal examination

Laboratory Tests

1. Expressed prostatic secretions should be examined when diagnosis is in doubt, and bacterial cultures should be obtained when necessary.
2. Care should be taken in patients suspected of having acute bacterial prostatitis because of the possibility of bacteremia.
3. Older patients with negative cultures should be evaluated for neoplastic disease, and cystoscopy and possible prostatic biopsy should be considered, especially if laboratory data such as an elevated prostate specific-antigen level are present.
4. In order to accurately isolate the organism causing a chronic prostatic infection, a fractional urine specimen, along with expressed prostatic secretions, can be of benefit.

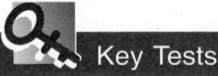

Key Tests

- Urinalysis
- Expressed prostatic secretions
- Urine and blood cultures if needed

Differential Diagnosis

The differential diagnosis of acute prostatitis is straightforward and readily evident with the findings of fever, dysuria, and tender prostate. Chronic prostatitis, on the other hand, may be more difficult to diagnose, and the differential should include

1. Benign prostatic hyperplasia
2. Prostatic carcinoma
3. Urethral stricture
4. Bladder carcinoma
5. Neurogenic bladder
6. Interstitial cystitis

Treatment

Treatment of acute prostatitis, with its diffuse, intense inflammation, allows for many antibiotics to be used.

1. If a patient is hospitalized, intravenous antibiotics may be used initially. Protocols include
    a. Ampicillin/aminoglycosides (gentamicin or tobramycin)
    b. Intravenous cephalosporin with aminoglycoside
2. Once a patient is converted to an oral antibiotic, or if an oral agent is instituted initially, the following regimens may be used:
    a. Trimethoprim-sulfamethoxazole (Bactrim DS), 160 mg/800 mg (double strength) twice a day, is the preferred regimen.
    b. Ampicillin, 500 mg four times a day
    c. Tetracycline, 500 mg four times a day
    d. Doxycycline (Vibramycin), 100 mg twice a day
    e. Carbenicillin (Geocillin), 1 gm four times a day
    f. Ciprofloxacin (Cipro), 500 mg twice a day. Some studies indicate that fluoroquinolones may have better cure rates in chronic prostatitis.
    g. Levofloxacin (Levaquin), 500 mg once daily.
3. All the preceding should be continued for at least 3 to 4 weeks to ensure resolution, and some authors suggest suppression therapy to last approximately 3 months. Regimens include but are not limited to
    a. Trimethoprim-sulfamethoxazole, 160 mg/180 mg once a day
    b. Ciprofloxacin, 500 mg once a day
    c. Doxycycline, 100 mg once a day

Diet

Diet may be altered to help patients avoid irritative urinary outlet symptoms.

1. Caffeine should be avoided, and over-the-counter decongestants should be discontinued.
2. Spicy foods should be avoided only if they cause an exacerbation of symptoms.

Activity

1. Activity usually is not restricted, and patients are encouraged to have a normal level of sexual activity.
2. If a patient has difficulty voiding, warm sitz baths may be of benefit.

Patient Education

1. Patient education includes a full discussion of the particular type of prostatitis and the understanding that prostatitis is *not* the equal of loss of sexual ability.
2. Patients also should be counseled that prostatitis is not the equal of prostate cancer.
3. Side effects of all medications used also should be discussed.

Key Treatment

Antibiotic regimens and possible suppression therapy

Follow-Up

1. Patients with acute prostatitis should be re-evaluated 48 to 72 hours after the initial evaluation or after discharge from the hospital.
2. Subsequent follow-up evaluations would then be in 2 to 3 weeks and then 1 month after discontinuing antibiotics.
3. Follow-up of other types of prostatitis should be individualized to each patient. If symptoms persist, referral to a urologist may be warranted.

Bibliography

Cox CE, Childs SJ: Treatment of chronic bacterial prostatitis with temafloxacin. Am J Med 1991;91:1345–1393.

de la Rosette JJ, Hubrentse MR, Meuleman EJ, et al: Diagnosis and treatment of 409 patients with prostatitis syndromes. Urology 1993;97:301–307.

Gleich P: Prostatitis: a state-of-the-art review of diagnosis and therapy. Consultant 1998;Feb:345–355.

Meares EM Jr: Prostatitis. Med Clin North Am 1991;75: 405–425.

Schwager EJ: Treatment of bacterial prostatitis. Am Fam Physician 1991;44:2137–2141.

Weidner W, Schiefer HG, Brahler E, et al: Refractory chronic bacterial prostatitis: a re-evaluation of ciprofloxacin treatment after a median follow-up of 30 months. J Urol 1991;146:350–352.

151 Benign Prostatic Hyperplasia

Neil K. Hall

Etiology

1. Exact cause is unknown.
2. Probably is prostate response to androgen hormones over time.
   a. Does not occur in the absence of testes or androgen.
   b. Begins in most men in their forties and tends to become symptomatic in their sixties.
3. Fat in diet also may play a role.

Symptoms

1. Obstructive symptoms from pressure on urethra from surrounding prostate tissue impeding urine flow
   a. "Dynamic" component caused by α-adrenergic tone in muscle fibers in prostate gland and capsule and in bladder neck, contraction of muscle fibers causing increased pressure on urethra.
   b. "Static" component caused by glandular mass impinging on urethra.
2. Irritative symptoms mostly from involuntary bladder muscle contractions and possibly bladder wall hypersensitivity.

Key Symptoms

Irritative	Obstructive
• Frequency	• Hesitancy
• Dysuria	• Straining
• Urgency	• Starting and stopping
• Nocturia	• Dribbling
• Incontinence	• Retention

Clinical Findings

1. Prostate examination
   a. May be enlarged, but size may appear normal despite symptoms, because rectal examination detects enlargement of peripheral zone of prostate, but symptoms come from periurethral zone, which is not palpable.
   b. Consistency usually rubbery and surface smooth. Nodules and areas of increased firmness must be considered possibly malignant.
2. Enlarged bladder may be palpable in severe obstruction.

Key Signs

- Enlarged prostate
- Palpable bladder

Laboratory Tests

1. Urinalysis
   a. Pyuria suggests infection.
   b. Hematuria may be a sign of malignancy.
2. Urine culture to rule out urinary tract infection (UTI) if there are irritative symptoms or positive urinalysis
3. Blood urea nitrogen and creatinine determinations to look for renal insufficiency
4. Prostate-specific antigen (PSA)
   a. Recommended by some to screen for malignancy.
   b. Values above 10 ng/ml suggest prostate cancer.
5. If retention suspected, abdominal ultrasound
   a. To detect hydronephrosis and other abnormalities of the upper urinary tract
   b. To check postvoid residual in bladder
6. Intravenous pyelogram not generally recommended, because ultrasound is much safer and gives adequate information in most cases.
7. Transrectal ultrasound
   a. If palpable nodule or elevated PSA
   b. Used by some urologists to estimate prostate size

Key Tests

• Urinalysis	• PSA
• Urine culture if irritative symptoms	• Blood urea nitrogen, creatinine

Differential Diagnosis

1. Prostatitis, acute or chronic
   a. May cause irritative and obstructive symptoms.
   b. Usually has a softer, more boggy gland, which may be tender, particularly if acute inflammation.
   c. Positive urine culture common, except in nonbacterial prostatitis.
2. Prostate cancer suggested by some signs.
   a. Hard nodule or area on examination
   b. Hematuria, microscopic or gross
   c. Elevated PSA

WARNING

Hematuria must always be followed up, even in the presence of urine infection, because of the possibility of underlying malignancy.

Treatment

1. Mild symptoms
   a. If not bothering patient greatly, consider no treatment, because many patients get better spontaneously over time.
   b. Avoid medicines that can worsen symptoms.
      (1) Decongestants and other sympathomimetics act on α-receptors to increase prostate muscle tone, increasing dynamic obstruction.
      (2) Anticholinergics, such as antihistamines, bowel antispasmodics, tricyclic antidepressants, and antipsychotics, decrease bladder muscle contraction, increasing retention.
2. Mild to moderate symptoms
   a. α-Blockers relax muscle fibers in the prostate gland and capsule and in the internal urethral sphincter, thus facilitating emptying.
      (1) Terazosin (Hytrin) starting at 1 mg at bedtime (first dose may give dizziness or syncope if not taken at bedtime), increasing up to 10 mg at bedtime as needed and tolerated
      (2) Doxazosin (Cardura), 4 to 8 mg daily, also may be used.
      (3) Tamsulosin (Flomax), 0.4 to 0.8 mg daily, has less hypotension as a side effect.
   b. Hormonal manipulation
      (1) Finasteride (Proscar), 5 mg daily, is well tolerated and effective but takes several months for maximum effect.
      (2) Other hormonal manipulations (estrogens, antiandrogens, gonadotropin-releasing hormone analogues) can be used, but only if finasteride is not tolerated because of adverse effects.
   c. May use hormonal and α-blocker treatment together.
   d. Avoid medicines that increase obstructive symptoms (noted above).
3. Severe or intolerable symptoms
   a. Surgery usually is required if significant urinary retention exists. Be sure to remove all drugs that might be contributing to retention before recommending surgery.
   b. Type of surgical procedure used is quite variable.
      (1) Transurethral resection of the prostate is most common, very effective, has few side effects, but may need to be repeated years later.
      (2) Open prostatectomy may be appropriate, especially for large glands; higher risk, but less need for repeat surgery.
      (3) Transurethral incision of the prostate is good for small glands. Fewer complications.
      (4) Other transurethral treatments include laser, electrovaporization, microwave thermotherapy, and needle ablation using radio waves.
   c. Urethral stents occasionally used for patients not candidates for surgery, but not yet approved therapy.
   d. Chronic catheter placement should be avoided because of risk of UTI and sepsis.

Diet

No dietary modification is usually needed.
1. Avoid caffeine and any foods that the patient finds exacerbate symptoms.
2. Despite possible role of dietary fat in etiology, effect of reducing fat is unknown.

Activity

No changes required.

Patient Education

1. Avoid drugs that can exacerbate symptoms or increase retention.
   a. Over-the-counter cold and allergy remedies
   b. Sedatives and over-the-counter sleeping pills
   c. Alcohol

2. Report any blood in the urine, UTI symptoms, and worsening of retention symptoms.

Follow-Up

1. If α-blockers used, check sitting and standing blood pressures weekly while titrating dose.

2. Evaluate symptoms and side effects every 6 months or so when treated with medications.

3. Annual rectal examination, as generally recommended for regular cancer screening (even open prostatectomy does not eliminate prostate cancer risk), with annual PSA recommended by most

4. Annual urinalysis

Bibliography

Alexander W: New guidelines—and many options—for BPH. Patient Care 1994; June 15:18–27. (*Note that this is a summary of* Agency for Health Care Policy and Research: Benign Prostatic Hyperplasia: Diagnosis and Treatment. [Clinical Practice Guideline No. 8. AHCPR publication no 94-0582]. Rockville, MD, Agency for Health Care Policy and Research, 1994. Free copy available: 1-800-358-9295; Also available on the Internet at *www.ahcpr.gov.*)

Hollander JB, Diokno AC: Prostatism: benign prostatic hyperplasia. Urol Clin North Am 1996;23:75–86.

Oesterling JE: Benign prostatic hyperplasia: medical and minimally invasive treatment options. N Engl J Med 1995;332:99–109.

Tammela T: Benign prostatic hyperplasia: practical treatment guidelines. Drugs Aging 1997;10:349–366.

152 Prostate Cancer

Timothy J. Wilt

Etiology and Epidemiology

1. Unknown etiology
2. Most common nonskin malignancy (incidence = 200,000 per year)
3. Second most common cause of cancer mortality in men (40,000 per year)
4. High prevalence of autopsy-detected asymptomatic cancer (30 to 40 per cent in men ≥ 50)
5. Mean age at diagnosis = 70
6. Ten-year disease-specific survival for localized disease is 80 to 90 per cent.
7. Risk factors: family history, age, black race, possibly dietary fat
8. Generally slow growing. Poorly differentiated tumors may grow rapidly. (See Table 152–1 for staging.)

Early Detection

1. Not demonstrated to reduce prostate cancer mortality and morbidity

TABLE 152–1. TNM STAGING SYSTEM FOR PROSTATE CANCER

STAGE	DESCRIPTION
T1a	Incidentally detected tumor, ≤5% of resected tissue
T1b	Incidentally detected tumor, ≥5% of resected tissue
T1c	Impalpable tumor, detected by needle biopsy (usually because of elevated prostate-specific antigen level)
T2a	Tumor confined to prostate, <50% of lobe involved
T2b	Tumor confined to prostate, >50% of lobe involved but not both lobes
T2c	Tumor confined to prostate, involves both lobes
T3a	Unilateral extension through prostate capsule
T3b	Bilateral extension through prostate capsule
T3c	Tumor invades seminal vesicle(s)
T4a	Tumor invades bladder neck, external sphincter, or rectum
T4b	Tumor invades levator muscles and/or fixed to pelvic wall
N1	Metastasis to lymph node, ≤2 cm in greatest diameter
N2	Metastasis to lymph node, >2 cm but ≤5 cm in greatest diameter
N3	Metastasis to lymph node(s), >5 cm in greatest diameter

From Thompson IM, Teague JL: Genitourinary tumors. In Rakel RE (ed): Conn's Current Therapy, p 680. Philadelphia, WB Saunders Company, 1994, with permission.

2. American Cancer Society, American Urological Association, U.S. Preventive Services Task Force, National Cancer Institute, and the American College of Physicians all state that routine testing with digital rectal examination (DRE) and prostate-specific antigen (PSA) without informed discussion is inappropriate. Men should understand the potential risks and benefits of screening and treatment for prostate cancer.

Symptoms

1. Usually asymptomatic: Detected by DRE, PSA testing, or incidentally during transurethral resection of the prostate (TURP) for symptoms caused by benign prostatic hypertrophy (BPH).
2. Local symptoms: Men with lower urinary tract symptoms consistent with BPH are not at increased risk for prostate cancer. Symptoms caused by urinary tract obstruction from prostate cancer may have more rapid onset than those resulting from benign causes and include nocturia, urgency, frequency, hesitancy.
3. Regional symptoms: Lower extremity edema, hematuria
4. Systemic symptoms: Back pain caused by spinal metastasis, weakness, weight loss

Key Symptoms

- Asymptomatic
- Rapid onset of urinary obstruction
- Back pain

Clinical Findings

1. DRE: prostatic nodule, induration, enlargement, or asymmetry. Can be normal.
2. May rarely present with hydronephrosis, adenopathy, back pain caused by bony metastasis, or biopsy revealing "adenocarcinoma of unknown primary."

Key Sign

Abnormal prostate on DRE

Laboratory Tests

1. PSA: Greater than 4 ng/ml abnormal (can be elevated in BPH or prostatitis). Normal PSA in approximately 40 per cent of prostate cancer cases. Less than 50 per cent of men with PSA greater than 10 ng/ml have pathologically localized prostate cancer.
2. Percentage of "free PSA"
3. Prostatic acid phosphatase: May be useful to evaluate for nonlocalized disease.
4. Bone scans: generally not indicated in patient with PSA less than 10 ng/ml and no bone pain
5. Transrectal ultrasound: Evaluate hypoechoic areas of prostate for biopsy.
6. Transrectal biopsy or aspiration: Biopsy required for diagnosis.

Key Tests

- PSA test widely utilized for early detection but not demonstrated to reduce prostate cancer mortality or morbidity.
- Biopsy or fine-needle aspiration of prostate are the only definitive tests.

Differential Diagnosis

Benign urologic diseases (prostatitis or BPH)

Treatment

1. Clinically localized prostate cancer
   a. Watchful waiting: palliative therapy for symptomatic/metastatic progression
   b. Radical prostatectomy: reserved for patients with life expectancy greater than 10 years
   c. Radiation therapy
   d. Brachytherapy: insertion of radioactive "seeds" into prostate
   e. Cryotherapy: New procedure; no long-term results available
   f. Options a through d appear to provide equivalent long-term survival and are all acceptable treatment options. Recommended therapy should include potential treatment risks, benefits, co-morbidities, and patient preferences. Randomized controlled trials are ongoing and necessary to determine preferred treatment option.
2. Regional or metastatic prostate cancer: Therapy is palliative.
   a. Mechanical interventions
      (1) TURP/transurethral incision of the prostate (TUIP)
      (2) Stents
   b. Hormonal therapy (Table 152–2)
      (1) Surgical orchiectomy
      (2) Medical orchiectomy: diethylstilbestrol, antiandrogens, luteinizing hormone–releasing hormone (LHRH) analogues.
      (3) Maximum androgen blockade: combination LHRH analogue or surgical orchiectomy and antiandrogen. Does not increase survival compared with either medical or surgical orchiectomy alone and may reduce quality of life.
   c. Radiation therapy
   d. Chemotherapy

TABLE 152–2. OPTIONS FOR HORMONAL TREATMENT OF PROSTATE CANCER

TREATMENT	ADVANTAGES	DISADVANTAGES
Bilateral orchiectomy	Inexpensive 100% compliance Minimal morbidity	Hot flashes Psychological effect Decreased libido/erections
Estrogens (oral)	Inexpensive	Higher risk of cardiovascular/thromboembolic complications Gynecomastia Hot flashes Decreased libido/erections
Luteinizing hormone–releasing hormone (LHRH) agonists	Convenient (q 3 mo dosing)	Very expensive Flare phenomenon Decreased libido/erections
Antiandrogens	Maintenance of potency	Very expensive Elevated testosterone
Combined androgen blockade	Possibly slight improvement in survival	Extremely expensive Combines complications of antiandrogen and either LHRH agonist or orchiectomy

Adapted from Thompson IM, Teague JL: Genitourinary tumors. In Rakel RE (ed): Conn's Current Therapy, p 680. Philadelphia, WB Saunders Company, 1994, with permission.

Key Treatment

Clinically localized disease

- Watchful waiting

- Radical prostatectomy

- Radiation (Brachytherapy or external beam)

Follow-Up

1. At 3- to 6-month intervals with DRE and PSA

2. Bone scan; if suspicious for bone metastasis

3. Hemoglobin, liver function tests if suspicious for metastatic disease

4. Evaluate for complications of treatment, including impotence, incontinence, bowel injury, hot flashes, breast tenderness, edema.

Bibliography

American College of Physicians: Screening for prostate cancer. Ann Intern Med 1997;126:480–484.

Catalona WJ, Partin AW, Slawing KM, et al: Use of the percentage of free prostate-specific antigen to enhance differentiation of prostate cancer from benign prostatic disease. JAMA 1998;279:1542–1547.

Chodak GW, Thisted RA, Gerber GS, et al: Results of conservative management of clinically localized prostate cancer. N Engl J Med 1994;330:242–248.

Fleming C, Wasson JH, Albertsen PC, et al: A decision analysis of alternative treatment strategies for clinically localized prostate cancer. JAMA 1993;269:2650–2658.

Middleton RG, Thompson IM, Austenfeld MS, et al: Prostate Cancer Clinical Guidelines Panel summary report on the management of clinically localized prostate cancer. J Urol 1995;154:2144–2148.

Pienta KJ, Esper PS: Risk factors for prostate cancer. Ann Intern Med 1993;118:793–803.

Wasson JH, Cushman CC, Bruskewitz RC, et al: A structured literature review of treatment for localized prostate cancer. Arch Fam Med 1993;2:487–493.

Wilt TJ: Prostate cancer screening: practice what the evidence preaches. Am J Med 1998;104:602–604.

Wilt TJ, Brawer MB: The Prostate Cancer Intervention Versus Observation Trial: a randomized trial comparing radical prostatectomy versus expectant management for the treatment of clinically localized prostate cancer. Oncology 1997;11:1133–1139.

153 Kidney Cancer

Deanna J. Wathington

Etiology

1. Renal cell carcinoma: Accounts for approximately 85 per cent of all primary malignant renal tumors.

   a. Typically proximal renal tubular in origin (adenocarcinoma)

   b. Balanced reciprocal translocation on short arm of chromosome 3; associated with both hereditary and sporadic forms of renal cell carcinoma

   c. Von Hippel–Lindau syndrome: also with change on short arm of chromosome 3

   d. Risk factors

      (1) Tobacco use/abuse consistently correlated with both epidemiologic case-control and case-cohort studies.

      (2) Products containing phenacetin also have shown correlation to renal cell carcinoma.

      (3) Various other factors (including exposure to cadmium, asbestos, and petroleum products; leather tanning; obesity; and diuretic use) have been associated with increased incidence but require further study.

2. Wilms' tumor: Accounts for 5 per cent of all childhood cancers. Chromosomal abnormalities are associated with both familial and sporadic forms.

Symptoms

1. Renal cell carcinoma more often diagnosed as an incidental finding on routine physical examination and/or imaging studies for an unrelated problem.

2. Can remain asymptomatic until late in progression of tumor; one third of patients have metastasis at the time of diagnosis.

3. In only 10 to 15 per cent of cases is the class triad of pain, hematuria, and a flank mass found; these patients often have advanced disease.

4. Weight loss, night sweats, and fever may be noted in the male patient.

5. Pain and hematuria are the most frequently presenting symptoms.

Key Symptoms

- Usually asymptomatic
- Pain and hematuria in 10 to 15 per cent

Clinical Findings

1. Microscopic hematuria

2. Hypertension may occur, usually secondary to increased renin release, segmental renal artery occlusion, or paraneoplastic syndromes.

3. Paraneoplastic syndrome

4. Stauffer's syndrome: nonmetastatic hepatic dysfunction with increased alkaline phosphatase, prolonged prothrombin time, white blood cell loss, fever, and areas of hepatic necrosis

5. Hypercalcemia in up to 10 per cent

6. Increased erythropoietin production leading to polycythemia

Key Sign

Microscopic hematuria

Tests

1. Computerized tomography (CT) scan is the radiologic procedure of choice for clinical staging and is obtained for any lesion on ultrasound that is not a simple cyst by strict criteria.

2. Renal ultrasound provides a method of distinguishing cystic versus complex versus solid masses.

3. Magnetic resonance imaging (MRI) and angiography prove useful for clarification of vascular involvement, such as invasion of the renal vein or inferior vena cava. These newer radiograph studies are increasing recognition of small renal masses and contributing to diagnosis at earlier stages.

4. To determine extent of metastatic disease, technetium-99m bone scan and CT can be utilized.

Key Tests

- CT scan
- Renal ultrasound
- MRI
- Hemoglobin, hematocrit
- Urinalysis
- Hepatic function panel
- Calcium

Differential Diagnosis

1. Angiomyolipoma
2. Oncocytoma
3. Other benign and malignant renal masses
4. Renal cyst
5. Previous renal infection or infarction
6. Xanthogranulomatous pyelonephritis
7. Granuloma
8. Congenital anomaly
9. Metastatic lesions to the kidney (most commonly these lesions occur secondary to lung or breast cancer).

Staging

See Table 153–1.

Treatment

1. Surgery
   a. Surgical excision continues to be the mainstay of treatment for primary renal cell carcinoma.
   b. Radical nephrectomy is the procedure of choice.
   c. Partial nephrectomy is being utilized with greater frequency in patients with small (<3-cm) renal cell masses that are limited to the kidney.
   d. Five-year survival rates associated with radical nephrectomy range from 60 to 82 per cent for T1 and T2 disease, to 50 per cent for T3 disease, to less than 20 per cent for metastatic disease.
2. Radiotherapy
   a. Radiotherapy has not yielded any successful or beneficial effect when used as primary treatment of renal cell carcinoma or as postoperative adjuvant therapy.
   b. Palliative radiotherapy has shown beneficial effects in the treatment of pain associated with metastasis.
   c. Role of radiotherapy in decreasing primary tumor size preoperatively or delaying local recurrence is under investigation.

TABLE 153–1. AMERICAN JOINT COMMITTEE ON CANCER STAGING CLASSIFICATION SYSTEM FOR RENAL CELL CARCINOMA (TNM CLINICAL CLASSIFICATION)

Primary Tumor (T)

TX	Primary tumor cannot be assessed
T0	No evidence of primary tumor
T1	Tumor 2.5 cm or less in greatest dimension limited to the kidney
T2	Tumor more than 2.5 cm in greatest dimension limited to the kidney
T3	Tumor extends into major veins or adrenal gland or perinephric tissue but not beyond Gerota's fascia
T3a	Tumor extends into adrenal gland or perinephric tissue but not beyond Gerota's fascia
T3b	Tumor grossly extends into renal vein or vena cava
T4	Tumor extends beyond Gerota's fascia

Regional Lymph Nodes (N)

NX	Regional nodes cannot be assessed
N0	No regional node metastasis
N1	Metastasis in a single node, 2 cm or less in greatest dimension
N2	Metastasis in a single node, more than 2 cm but not more than 5 cm in greatest dimension, or multiple nodes, none more than 5 cm in greatest dimension
N3	Metastasis in a node more than 5 cm in greatest dimension

Distant Metastasis (M)

MX	Presence of distant metastasis cannot be assessed
M0	No distant metastasis
M1	Distant metastasis

From Sokoloff M, deKernion J, Figlin R, et al: Current management of renal cell carcinoma. CA Cancer J Clin 1996;46:284–302, with permission.

3. Chemotherapy
   a. Most common agents include vinblastine and floxuridine.
   b. Neither single-agent therapy nor combination therapy has proven efficacious. Responses to these therapies have been limited.
4. Hormonal therapy remains investigational, as do retinoic acid studies.
5. Immunotherapy
   a. In the treatment of metastatic disease, systemic interleukin-2 is now clinically approved; however, the survival period has not been increased with this treatment.
   b. Combination therapy involving interleukin-2, interferon, and 5-fluorouracil appears to increase the response rate.
   c. The role of lymphokine-activated killer cells and tumor infiltration lymphocyte therapy in renal cell tumor regression is still investigational.

Patient Education

1. Smoking cessation
2. Family history

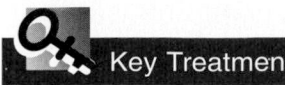

Key Treatment

Surgical excision

Follow-Up

1. After radial nephrectomy
   a. Physical examinations, laboratory studies, and chest radiographs every 6 months for 2 years, then annually
   b. CT scans every 12 months for 2 years and every 24 months after that
2. After partial nephrectomy
   a. Physical examination and laboratory studies at 3 months postoperatively
   b. Abdominal CT scans at 1, 6, 12, 18, and 24 months, then annually

 Bibliography

Belldegrun A, deKernion JB: Renal tumors. In Walsh PC, Retik AB, Vaughan ED, et al (eds): Campbell's Urology, 7th ed, vol 3, pp 2283–2326. Philadelphia, WB Saunders Company, 1998.

Figlin R, Gitlitz B, Franklin J, et al: Interleukin-2 based immunotherapy for the treatment of metastatic renal cell carcinoma: an analysis of 203 consecutively treated patients. Cancer J Sci Am 1997;3(Suppl 1):92S–97S.

Marshal F, Stewart A, Menck H: The national cancer database. Cancer 1997;80:2167–2174.

Motzer R, Russo P, Nanus D, et al: Renal cell carcinoma. Curr Prob Cancer 1997;21:185–232.

Sokoloff M, deKernion J, Figlin R, et al: Current management of renal cell carcinoma. CA Cancer J Clin 1996;46:284–302.

154 Bladder Cancer

David L. Hall

Etiology

1. Approximately 50,000 cases of bladder cancer are diagnosed annually, and it accounts for approximately 3 per cent of all cancer deaths in the United States. It is the second most common cancer of the genitourinary tract.
2. Among males, it is the fourth most common cause of cancer after lung, colorectal, and prostate cancer. It is the second most prevalent malignancy in middle-aged and elderly men.
3. Among females, it is the eighth most common form of cancer.
4. Occurs most often after the fifth decade of life; median age of diagnosis is 65 to 70 years of age.
5. Two to three times more common in men, and is more common in industrialized nations and urban areas.
6. About two times more common in Caucasian males than in African American males.
7. About 1.5 times more common in Caucasian females than in African American females.
8. Risk factors
   a. Occupational exposures: Account for one fourth to one third of all cases of bladder cancer. Primarily related to aromatic amines, which are used in synthesis of dyes used in textiles, printing, plastic, rubber, and cable industries. Those at risk include auto workers, painters, truck drivers, machinists, textile and paper manufacturers.
   b. Cigarette use: Accounts for about one third of all cases, including 50 per cent of cases in men. Fourfold higher incidence of bladder cancer among smokers versus nonsmokers; risk correlates with the number of cigarettes smoked and the number of years the individual has smoked.
   c. Analgesics: Increased incidence of bladder cancer seen in patients who ingest large amounts of analgesics containing phenacetin.
   d. Long-term use of cyclophosphamide
   e. Recurrent nephrolithiasis
   f. Recurrent UTIs; particularly associated with *Schistosoma haematobium* infections. This is a common infection in the Middle East; 10 to 40 per cent of malignant tumors in Egypt are associated with *Schistosoma*.
   g. Increased risk with chronic cystitis in presence of indwelling catheters
   h. Females treated with pelvic irradiation for cancer of cervix have two- to fourfold increased risk.
   i. Reports indicate 7 to 35 per cent of bladder cancers contaminated by human papillomavirus (HPV) DNA, but HPV role is unclear.
   j. Caffiene: Has been implicated in some studies; others show no increased risk.
   k. Artificial sweeteners and excessive alcohol use have been proposed as risk factors, but this is controversial.
   l. Endogenous tryptophan metabolites: Some studies have shown increased urinary tryptophan metabolite levels in bladder cancer patients; however, current studies suggest that tryptophan metabolites are not a factor in bladder cancer. The role of endogenous metabolites in bladder cancer is controversial.
   m. No epidemiology evidence exists for hereditary cause in most cases, but familial clusters have been reported.

Symptoms

1. Hematuria (especially painless hematuria): seen in 75 per cent of patients. May be intermittent.
2. Signs of bladder irritability
   a. Dysuria (in 25 per cent of patients)
   b. Urinary frequency (in 25 per cent of patients)
   c. Urgency (in 25 per cent of patients)
3. Ureteral obstruction and pelvic pain seen in a minority of patients.
4. Patients may occasionally present with symptoms of advanced disease, such as weight loss, lower extremity edema, and abdominal or bone pain.

Key Symptoms

- Painless hematuria—may be intermittent.
- Signs of bladder irritability

Clinical Findings

1. Physical examination is often unremarkable.
2. Hematuria on urinalysis
3. Urinary cytology, cystoscopy with biopsies needed for diagnosis. Saline bladder washes more accurate than voided samples.
4. Cell types
   a. Transitional cell cancer (about 90 per cent of cases)
   b. Squamous cell cancer (about 5 per cent of cases): Often associated with history of chronic infection, vesical calculi, or chronic catheter use. Accounts for about 60 per cent of bladder cancer in Egypt, parts of Africa, and Middle East where *Schistosoma* is a common source of infection.
   c. Mixed cell cancer (about 5 per cent of cases)
   d. Adenocarcinoma: very rare. May be preceded by cystitis and metaplasia.
   e. Transitional cell has best prognosis.

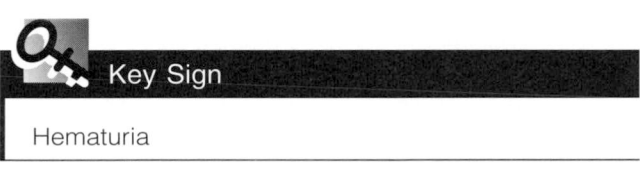

Key Sign

Hematuria

Laboratory Tests and Additional Studies

1. Urine cytology
2. Cystoscopy with multiple biopsies
3. Intravenous pyelography (IVP): Unilateral or bilateral ureteral obstruction, hydronephrosis, filling defects, or lack of bladder distensibility suggest cancer.
4. Serum chemistries, chest radiograph, and computerized tomography (CT) scan of abdomen and pelvis needed for staging.
5. In general, magnetic resonance imaging is not more helpful than CT for staging.
6. Bone scan may be helpful as baseline, but seldom reveals metastatic disease in patients with normal alkaline phosphatase.

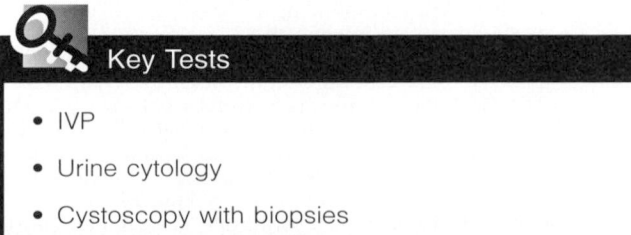

Key Tests

- IVP
- Urine cytology
- Cystoscopy with biopsies

Differential Diagnosis

1. Renal pelvic tumors
   a. Also presents with painless gross hematuria
   b. Pain and/or ureteral obstruction can occur but is rare.
   c. Diagnosis by IVP, which may show obstructed or nonvisualized kidney, or filling defects in visualized kidney.
   d. Cystoscopy will generally establish nature and location of tumor.
2. Nephrolithiasis
   a. Hematuria often present but rarely painless.
   b. Signs of bladder irritability can also occur.
   c. IVP usually confirms diagnosis.
3. Urinary tract infection: Diagnosis based on presence of pyuria and by positive urine culture.

Treatment

1. Depends on stage.
2. Staging: Based on Jewett-Strong-Marshall classification of 1952 or tumor-node-metastasis system (see Table 154–1).
3. Superficial (CIS, stage O and A)
   a. Endoscopic resection
   b. Fifty to 70 per cent of patients have superficial recurrences within 3 years of initial diagnosis.
   c. Recurrences sometimes treated with intravesical therapy such as doxorubicin, mitomycin, interferons, or bacillus Calmette-Guérin.
   d. Laser surgery: Has been used to treat some superficial bladder tumors and also in high-risk patients with muscle invasive tumors; has not been adopted for general use.
   e. Hydrostatic pressure treatment, in which the bladder is filled with saline under pressure, or a balloon is inserted in the bladder and inflated, was introduced in the early

TABLE 154–1. BLADDER CANCER STAGING SYSTEMS*

Tumor Involvement	J-S-M	TNM
Does not invade mucosa	—	CIS
Invades mucosa only	O	Ta
Invades submucosa	A	T1
Invades muscularis	B1	T2
Extends almost entire muscularis	B2	T3a
Extends into perivesical fat	C	T3b
Extends to prostate	D1	T4a
Extends to uterus or vagina	D1	T4b
Positive nodes below aortic bifurcation	D1	TxN+MO−
Positive nodes below aortic bifurcation or bone or soft tissue involvement	D2	TxN+M+

*J-S-M, Jewett-Strong-Marshall classification; TNM, tumor-node-metastasis system.

1970s. This treatment resulted in necrosis of bladder tumors. A major complication was bladder perforation, and the procedure has largely been abandoned.

 f. About 12 per cent develop invasive or metastatic disease.

4. Invasive disease (stage B1, B2; stage C; stage T2, T3a, or T3b)

 a. Radical or simple cystectomy most common treatment. Radical cystectomy in males usually accompanied by removal of prostate and seminal vesicles. In females, radical cystectomy usually accompanied by removal of uterus, fallopian tubes, ovaries, and part of vaginal vault.

 b. Radiation

 c. Cystectomy with preoperative radiation may be used, but studies have shown little added benefit of radiation therapy prior to surgery.

 d. Chemotherapy and radiation

 e. Five-year survival rate is 40 to 50 per cent regardless of mode of therapy.

 f. Surgical techniques to improve quality of life in patients with radical cystectomy include Kock's pouch, Indiana pouch, or Mainz pouch. All these procedures intended to allow urinary diversion by utilizing portions of small bowel as bladder reservoir.

5. Metastatic disease (stage D2, TxN+M+)

 a. Chemotherapy: cisplatin, methotrexate, doxorubicin, cyclophosphamide, vinblastine, or combination therapy

 b. Erythropoietin sometimes given to ameliorate myelosuppression, which is often seen in patients undergoing chemotherapy.

 c. Thirty to 70 per cent of patients show initial response to therapy, but effects rarely last more than 6 months.

 d. Most patients with metastatic disease die within 2 years.

6. Chemoprevention

 a. Vitamins A and E tested in study involving over 29,000, 50- to 59-year-old Finnish male smokers. Neither agent alone or in combination had any effect on development of bladder cancer.

 b. Vitamin B_6 (pyridoxine) was tested in randomized trials of patients with resected superficial tumors. The patients received either 20 mg of B_6 or placebo. No difference in recurrence rates was seen.

 c. One study showed high-dose multivitamins (40,000 units vitamin A, 100 mg vitamin B_6, 20,000 mg vitamin C, 400 units vitamin E, and 90 mg zinc) to be beneficial in preventing recurrence. However, this study has been questioned because of small size (65 patients) and mixed histologies and tumor histories of patients.

Key Treatment

- Superficial disease: endoscopic resection
- Invasive disease: cystectomy and/or radiation
- Metastatic disease: chemotherapy

Follow-Up

1. Superficial disease: Cystoscopy every 3 months for 2 years, then every 6 months for 2 years, then once a year.

2. Invasive and metastatic disease: Follow-up varies with invasiveness of disease and type of treatment used.

Screening

1. Urine cytology screening has been done in workers exposed to industrial carcinogens, but this is not cost effective for the general population.

2. Dipstick urinalysis for hematuria was utilized as a screening test in one study.

 a. Advantages: Test was inexpensive and compliance of subjects was good (2356 out of possible 3152 subjects responded).

 b. Disadvantages: Sensitivity of dipstick urinalysis as a screening test is unknown. Also, specificity of hematuria as a primary screening test was low.

Bibliography

Carroll PR: Urothelial carcinoma cancers of the bladder, ureter, and renal pelvis. In Tanagho EA, McAninch JW (eds): Smith's General Urology, 14th ed, pp 353–363. Norwalk, CT, Appleton & Lange, 1995.

Catalona WJ, Messing EM: Urothelial tumors of the urinary tract. In Walsh PC, Retik AB (eds): Campbell's Urology, 7th ed, vol 3, pp 2329–2410. Philadelphia, WB Saunders Company, 1998.

Droller MJ: Cancer of genitourinary system. In Niederhuber JE (ed): Current Therapy in Oncology, pp 458–461. St. Louis, Mosby–Year Book, 1993.

Scher HI, Motzer RJ: Bladder and renal cell cancer. In Fauci AS, Braunwald E, Isselbacker K, et al (eds): Harrison's Principles of Internal Medicine, 14th ed, vol 1, pp 592–594. New York, McGraw-Hill, 1998.

Shipley WU, Kaufman DS, Griffin PP, et al: Radiochemotherapy for invasive carcinoma of the bladder. In Ackerman R, Dielh V (eds): Malignancies of the Genitourinary Tract, pp 207–216. Berlin, Springer-Verlag, 1993.

Steineck G, Cordon-Cardo C: Bladder cancer. In Schrier RW, Gottschalk CW (eds): Diseases of the Kidney, 6th ed, vol 1, pp 803–821. Boston, Little, Brown, 1997.

Indications

1. Nonmedical
   a. Parental preference
   b. Religious tradition
2. Medical
   a. Prevention of conditions requiring circumcision later in life; phimosis, paraphimosis, balanitis
   b. Some studies have shown a decrease in urinary tract infections, penile cancer, and sexually transmitted diseases in circumcised males.

Contraindications

1. Congenital anomaly of the genitourinary system that might be repaired by using the foreskin: hypospadias, megalourethra, webbed penis
2. Other major anomaly that may require major surgery
3. Any signs or symptoms indicating an unstable medical condition or bleeding disorder
4. Premature birth: Circumcision is delayed until discharge.

Preparation

1. Avoid feeding the infant for 1 hour prior to the procedure to avoid emesis.
2. Perform dorsal penile nerve block (see "Anesthesia").
3. Swaddle the infant's arms and torso with a blanket.
4. Immobilize infant's arms on circumcision board.
5. Scrub the surgical field with povidone-iodine or other antiseptic solution.
6. Drape infant with fenestrated drape.
7. Inspect equipment tray to ensure that all necessary instruments are in working order.

Equipment

1. Gomco clamp with approximately sized cone; 1.1 or 1.3 size cones are usually a good fit for term infants.
2. Curved mosquito hemostats (2)
3. Straight hemostat (1)
4. Blunt-tipped probe (1)
5. Tissue scissors
6. Sterile safety pin
7. Scalpel with No. 10 blade
8. 4 × 4 sterile gauze (4)
9. Warm sterile water
10. Petroleum jelly gauze dressing

Anesthesia

Dorsal Penile Nerve Block

1. Have an assistant restrain the infant with the knees flexed and the hips externally rotated and cleanse the injection site with a topical antiseptic.
2. Draw 0.8 ml of lidocaine without epinephrine into a 1.0-ml tuberculin syringe.
3. Identify by palpation the symphysis pubis and corpora cavernosa at the penile root.
4. Stabilize the penis with one hand and position the needle at the 10 o'clock position, 0.5 to 1.0 cm distal to the point where the penile root passes under the pubic arch.
5. Pierce the skin and fascia with the needle at an acute angle, directly slightly posteromedially. The depth of injection should be about 2 to 5 mm.
6. The needle tip should be freely mobile. Aspirate to avoid intravascular injection.
7. Slowly inject 0.4 ml of lidocaine.
8. Repeat the injection at the 2 o'clock position.
9. Allow 3 to 5 minutes to take effect.
10. Anesthesia effectiveness is between ring block and EMLA (eutectic mixture of local anesthetics).

EMLA

1. Apply EMLA cream to the distal half of the penis.
2. Cover with semipermeable dressing for 90 minutes.
3. Effective method of anesthesia but less effective than ring block or dorsal penile nerve block.

Ring Block

1. Lidocaine 1% infiltrated circumferentially halfway along the shaft of the penis.
2. Found to be the most effective method of anesthesia by a randomized controlled trial.

Precautions

Remember that circumcision is usually an elective procedure and so should not be performed if there is concern regarding a possible contraindication.

Technique

1. Inspect the external anatomy of the penis to identify landmarks, specifically the slight bulge in the foreskin caused by the underlying edge of the corona.

2. Grasp the rim of the foreskin at the 10 o'clock and 2 o'clock positions with the curved mosquito hemostats.

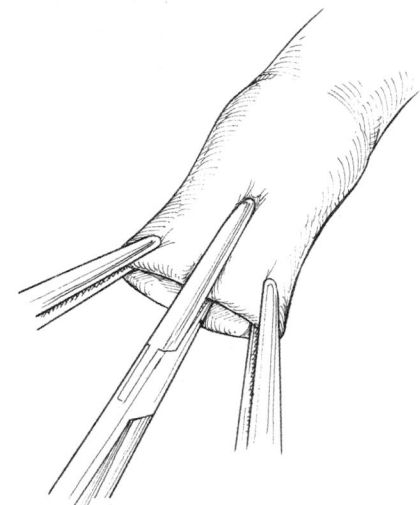

3. Insert the blunt-tipped probe just under the foreskin at the 12 o'clock position up to the corona. Sweep the probe over the glans penis, freeing the prepuce from the glans. Insert the straight hemostat in the closed position, open it and gently withdraw. This procedure assists in breaking down adhesions between the glans and the prepuce.

4. Make a crush line for the dorsal slit by inserting one blade of the straight hemostat under the foreskin at the 12 o'clock position to within a few millimeters of the corona. Close the hemostat and remove after a few seconds (see above figure).

5. Cut the dorsal slit along the crush line with the scissors. Make sure that the incision is confined to the crushed tissue.

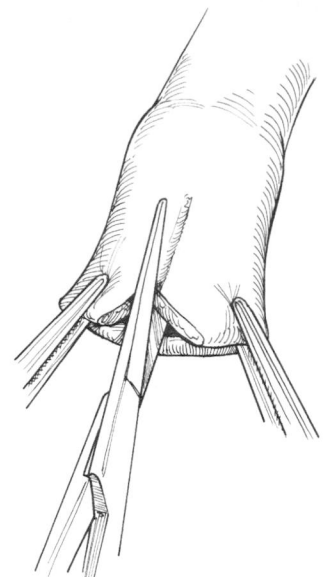

6. Inspect the glans to make sure that the urethral meatus is in the normal position. If you detect hypospadias that was hidden by the foreskin, stop the procedure and consult a pediatric urologist.

7. Retract the foreskin to expose the entire glans to the sulcus just proximal to the corona. Take down any adhesions with the blunt probe or by brushing with the 4 × 4 gauze. Be gentle while freeing adhesions on the inferior aspect of the glans because this is a common site of excessive bleeding.

8. Insert the cone of the Gomco clamp over the glans.

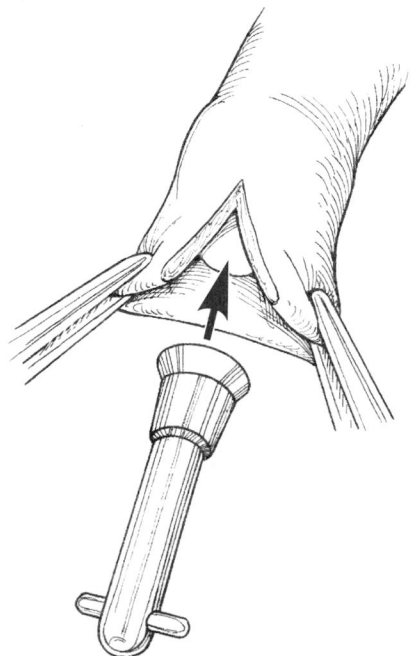

9. Draw the foreskin back over the cone, approximate the two edges of the dorsal slit and secure with the sterile safety pin. Remove the hemostats.

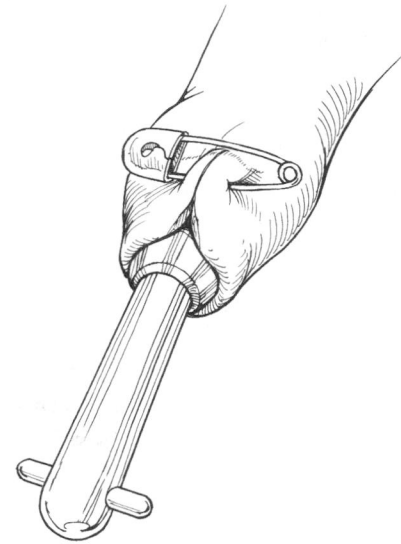

10. Twist the safety pin 90 degrees so that it is parallel to the shaft of the cone, then insert both through the hole in the base plate.

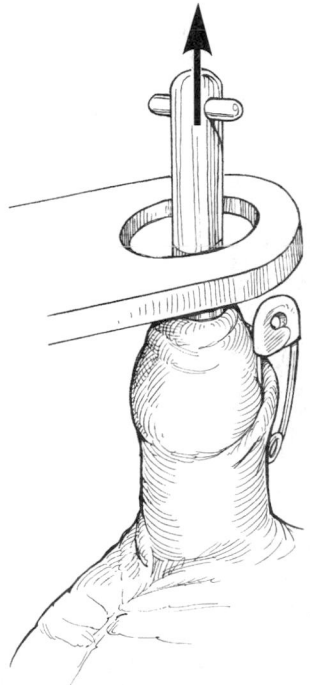

The curved hemostat may also be used to approximate edges of the dorsal slit and guide the prepuce through the base plate.

11. The top plate is hooked under the arms of the cone and slipped into place on the base plate. Inspect to be sure that a symmetrical rim of foreskin now lies above the base plate and that the entire length of the dorsal slit is visible above the base plate.

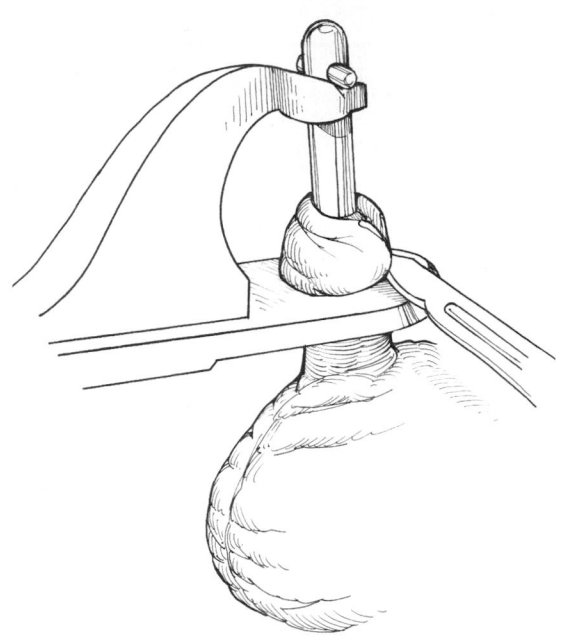

12. Attach the nut to the bolt on the base plate and tighten firmly. Trim off the foreskin just above the base plate, holding the scalpel nearly parallel to the base plate. Many authorities recommend that the clamp be left in place for 5 minutes to allow for hemostasis.

13. Unfasten the nut and remove the upper and lower plates. Gently brush the skin line off the cone with a 4 × 4 gauze.

14. Dress the area with petroleum jelly dressing. Extra gauze can be placed in the infant's diaper to supply additional compression.

Follow-Up

1. The infant should be observed for an hour to ensure that hemostasis has been achieved.

2. The parents should be instructed on how to gently clean the glans with water and to apply petroleum jelly to prevent adherence to the diaper.

3. Complications are rare but include hemorrhage, infection, urinary retention, urethrocutaneous fistula, foreskin adhesions, chordee, meatitis, and meatal ulcer.

4. Parents should be informed that in 1 to 2 days the healing glans will be covered with a yellowish membrane. This should not be confused with infection, which presents with redness and swelling of the glans. A fever, of course, may be a sign of serious infection and warrants immediate attention.

Bibliography

Fontaine P: Technique of neonatal circumcision. Personal communication, 1994.

Fontaine P, Toffler W: Dorsal penile nerve block for newborn circumcision. Am Fam Physician 1991;43:1327–1333.

Lander J, Brady-Fryer B, Metcalf JB, et al: Comparison of ring block, dorsal penile nerve block, and topical anesthesia for neonatal circumcision: a randomized controlled trial. JAMA 1997;278:2157–2162.

Schoen EJ, Anderson G, Bohon C, et al: Report of the Task Force on Circumcision. Am Acad Pediatr News 1989;5:7–8.

Circumcision is one of the oldest surgical procedures known; it has been practiced as long as recorded history. While both the Gomco clamp and the Plastibell are used on newborn infants, the Plastibell can also be used to circumcise children up to 10 years of age.

Indications

Although there is no absolute medical indication for routine circumcision of the newborn, the procedure is performed on 80 to 95 per cent of newborns in the United States.

1. Promotes good penile hygiene (possible without circumcision)
2. Social custom or religious tradition
3. Prevention of
   a. Phimosis: inability to retract the foreskin
   b. Paraphimosis: entrapment of the foreskin behind the corona
   c. Balanitis: inflammation of the glans penis
   d. Posthitis: inflammation of the foreskin
   e. Carcinoma of the penis (rare)

Contraindications

1. Genitourinary anomaly such as hypospadias, epispadias, congenital megalourethra, webbed penis
2. Sick or premature infant
3. Bleeding disorder
4. Imperforate anus, myelomeningocele

Preparation

1. Physical examination to rule out congenital abnormality

2. Sterile technique, including gloves, drapes, instruments, and liberal use of povidone-iodine or other antiseptic solution

Equipment

1. Plastibell and ligature: sizes 1.1, 1.2, 1.3 (most common), 1.5, 1.7 cm
2. Small curved mosquito clamp (2)
3. Small straight mosquito clamp
4. Blunt malleable probe
5. Straight tissue scissors
6. Scalpel (No. 11 or No. 15 blade or small curved scissors)
7. A 1-ml syringe with a 25- or 27-gauge needle
8. 1% lidocaine without epinephrine

Anesthesia

1. Ring block: Using a 1.0-inch 25- or 27-gauge needle, inject 0.8 ml of 1% lidocaine *without* epinephrine subcutaneously around the base of the penis, halfway along the shaft. A greater volume is injected dorsally in the midline than in other areas of the ring.
2. Dorsal penile nerve block: Inject 0.3 to 0.4 ml of 1% lidocaine *without* epinephrine subcutaneously at the base of the penile shaft at the 10 o'clock and 2 o'clock positions, 1 cm distal to the pubic bone. Avoid injecting deeper than the subcutaneous tissue.
3. With either technique, the total volume of lidocaine should should not exceed 0.8 ml. Allow 3 minutes for the anesthesia to take effect.

Precautions

Avoid performing a circumcision if there is any anatomic abnormality of the penis.

Technique

1. Grasp the distal edge of the foreskin at 10 o'clock and 2 o'clock with small curved clamps, being sure to catch both mucosa and skin. Pull gently while using the blunt probe to break any adhesions between the foreskin and the glans, taking care to avoid injury to the frenulum at 6 o'clock.

2. Place the small straight clamp between the two curved clamps at 12 o'clock.

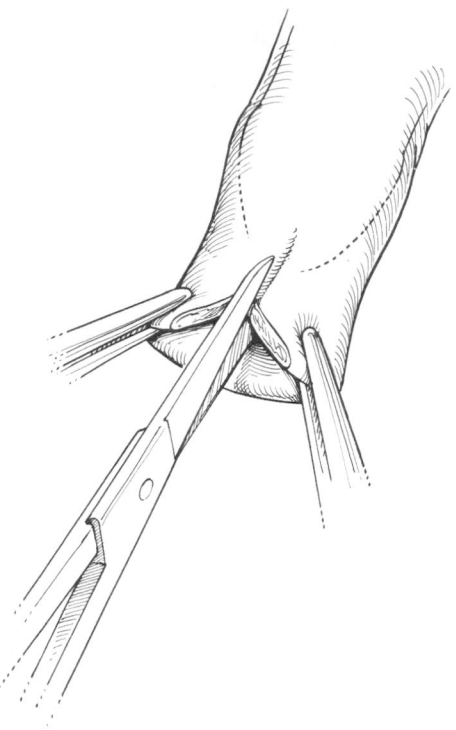

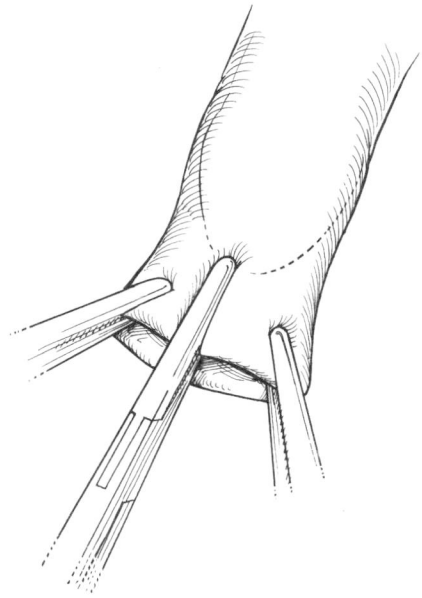

The length of the foreskin to be crushed should be approximately the same as the width of the glans. Making sure the clamp is not in the urethra, close it to achieve crush hemostasis and leave for approximately 10 seconds; then remove and use the scissors to cut down the center of the crushed area, making a dorsal slit.

Do not cut beyond the crushed area to avoid bleeding. If the slit is too short it can always be extended, but it is difficult to retrieve one that is made too long.

> **Note**
> The dorsal slit for the Plastibell technique is shorter than for the Gomco so that the foreskin can hold the Plastibell in place while the ligature is tied.

3. Using the two curved clamps, retract the foreskin proximally to expose the corona and sulcus. Under direct visualization, use the blunt probe to remove any remaining adhesions, again avoiding injury to the frenulum.

4. Select the proper size of Plastibell. The base should reach the corona without undue pressure on the glans and should not be so large that it extends beyond the corona, allowing the entire glans to slip through. If the bell is too small, it may injure the glans; if too large, it may slip over the corona onto the shaft. The apex of the dorsal slit should be distal to the bell's groove. The slit will usually be longer than shown in the next two illustrations. There should be approximately 1.0 cm between the sulcus and the groove of the bell where the ligature will be tied. A hemostat may be used to close the slit in order to hold the bell in place while tying the ligature.

5. Place the ligature around the base of the glans using a loose knot to hold it in place. With light pressure on the handle of the Plastibell, position the ligature in the bell's groove and inspect to ensure proper alignment and symmetry so that an even amount of foreskin is included around the entire circumference. Once appropriate positioning is confirmed, draw the ligature *tight* and tie with a surgeon's knot. Use the scissors to cut off excess ligature.

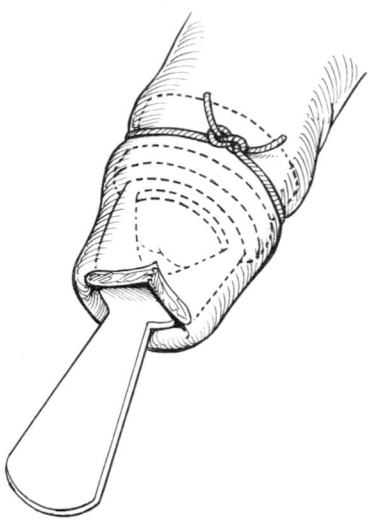

The tight ligature provides adequate hemostasis almost immediately.

6. Use the scalpel or small curved scissors to trim off the foreskin, with the outer ridge of the bell as a cutting guide.

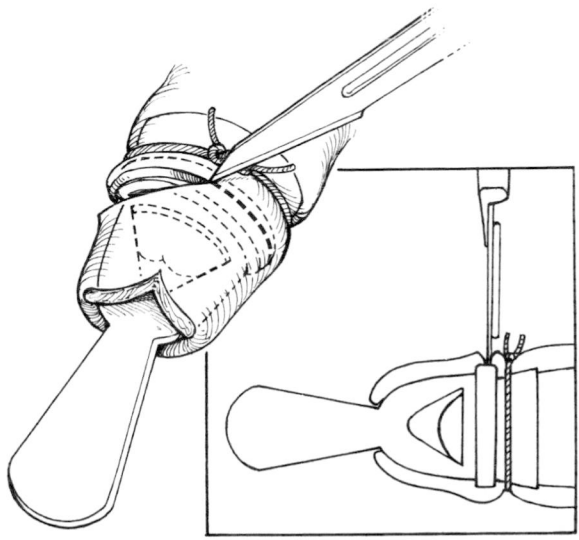

Maintaining slight traction on the foreskin while cutting will reduce the amount of remaining necrotic tissue, leaving a 1- to 2-mm cuff distal to the ligature.

7. Remove the handle by using a gauze pad to grasp the bell in one hand and use the other hand to break off the plastic handle.

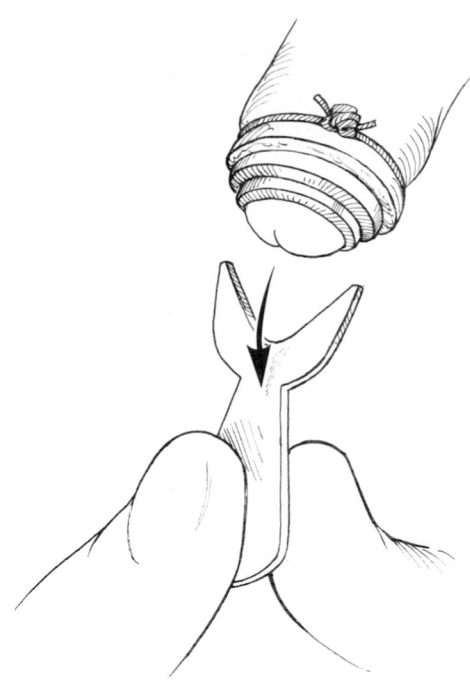

The handle is discarded. No dressing is necessary.

Follow-Up

1. Give the parents the follow-up instructions (*Now That Your Baby Has Been Circumcised*) that come with the Plastibell. This will avoid unnecessary concern and telephone calls before the next office visit. The bell will separate in 5 to 8 days, leaving a clean, healed line of incision. Remove the bell if it does not come off within 10 days.

2. Parents should confirm voiding over the next 24 hours and be instructed to keep the area clean by washing gently when bathing to avoid infection.

3. Complications
   a. Bleeding is much more common with the Gomco clamp and occurs with the Plastibell only if the ligature is tied too loosely or if the wrong size bell is used.
   b. Edema of the glans can occur if the bell is too small or if it is too large and migrates proximally, causing paraphimosis.
   c. Other complications are rare and consist of urinary retention, ulceration of the meatus, foreskin adhesions, necrotizing fasciitis, and urethrocutaneous fistulas. A rare but potentially serious complication of dorsal penile nerve block is methemoglobinemia, which can be induced by a variety of local anesthetics.

B Bibliography

American Academy of Pediatrics Task Force on Circumcision, Task Force Chairperson–Lannon CM: Circumcision policy statement. Pediatrics 1999;103:686–693.

Fontaine P, Dittberner D, Scheltema KE: The safety of dorsal penile nerve block for neonatal circumcision. J Fam Pract 1994;39:243–248.

Izzidien Al-Samarrai AY, Mofti AB, Crankson SJ, et al: A review of the Plastibell device in neonatal circumcision in 2000 instances. Surg Gynecol Obstet 1988;197:341–343.

Lander J, Brady-Fryer B, Metcalfe JB, et al: Comparison of ring block, dorsal penile nerve block, and topical anesthesia for neonatal circumcision: a randomized controlled trial. JAMA 1997;278:2157–2162.

Sorenson SM, Sorenson MR: Circumcision with the Plastibell device: a long-term follow-up. Int Urol Nephrol 1988;20:159–166.

Sprinkle RH: Care of the newborn. In Rakel RE (ed): Textbook of Family Practice, 5th ed, pp 589–591. Philadelphia, WB Saunders Company, 1995.

Indications

1. Neonatal circumcision reduces the incidence of urinary tract infection in the first year of life from 1 per cent to 0.1 per cent. Circumcision may reduce the incidence of some sexually transmitted diseases. The incidence of penile cancer after circumcision is near zero. Some religious groups practice ritual circumcision. However, most neonatal circumcisions are done for parental preference.
2. Beyond the neonatal period, circumcision is indicated for phimosis and paraphimosis.
3. The Mogen technique is faster and has less blood loss than the Gomco and Plastibell techniques. It anatomically places the angle of excision parallel to the corona. However, inadvertent partial amputation of the glans is possible if the surgeon does not give attention to a number of critical steps.

Contraindications

Bleeding disorders and structural abnormalities of the penis such as hypospadias are contraindications.

Preparation

1. An informed consent process must be followed with the parents.
2. Give the neonate nothing by mouth for 2 hours before the procedure.
3. Inspect the penis for any structural abnormalities.
4. A few swallows of glucose water given immediately before the procedure has been shown to reduce crying and distress.
5. Restrain the neonate on a Circumstraint or other such device. Leaving the arms unrestrained seems to reduce distress.
6. Dorsal penile nerve block (see "Anesthesia") is done before sterile prep to allow time for it to become effective.
7. The penis is prepped with an iodine solution such as povidone-iodine and draped with a sterile drape. Sterile gloves are worn.

Equipment

1. A 1-ml tuberculin syringe, 1/2-inch 30-gauge needle, 1 mEq/ml sodium bicarbonate solution, and 1% plain lidocaine solution are needed for dorsal penile nerve block.
2. Most circumcisions are done in hospital settings where a standard circumcision instrument tray

is used. This tray should contain a sterile drape with 1-inch fenestration, sterile 2 × 2 gauze pads, the Mogen clamp (neonatal, not adult, size), two delicate mosquito hemostats, a blunt probe, and a No. 10 blade scalpel. A 1-inch-wide petroleum jelly gauze strip is used for a dressing.

3. In addition, it is prudent to have Surgicel and 5-0 chromic suture on a taper-point needle available for bleeding complications.

Anesthesia

Neonates clearly feel pain. There is no excuse for doing a circumcision without adequate anesthesia. Dorsal penile nerve block is the technique of choice.

1. Draw up 0.1 ml of bicarbonate, then fill the syringe to 1.0 ml with 1% plain lidocaine.

WARNING

Do not use epinephrine-containing solutions because penile ischemia could result.

Neutralizing the lidocaine takes the sting out of injection. Exchange needles for a 30-gauge to minimize injection pain and ecchymoses.

2. Prep the dorsal root of the penis with an alcohol swab. Enter the skin at the 12 o'clock position dorsally, and advance between the skin and corpora to the 1 o'clock position. Inject 0.5 ml. Withdraw the needle, but leave the tip inside the skin. Advance to the 11 o'clock position and inject the remaining 0.5 ml.
3. Adequate anesthesia is usually obtained within 3 minutes—about the length of time needed to prep, glove, drape, and arrange instruments.

Precautions

1. Mogen clamps come in neonatal and adult sizes. *For a neonatal circumcision, the opening of the slot in the clamp must not exceed 2.5 mm.* Larger gaps can trap the glans, leading to inadvertent partial amputation of the glans.
2. It is critical to *free the foreskin fully* to allow the glans to slide back out of the way of the Mogen clamp. *Applying the Mogen clamp side-to-side, or during traction on the foreskin, is inviting partial amputation of the glans.*

Technique

1. First, free the foreskin off the glans. Grasp about 2 mm of the dorsal edge of the foreskin at the 12 o'clock position with a hemostat. While holding this hemostat in the nondominant hand, apply gentle traction along the axis of the penile shaft. Bluntly enter the plane between the dorsal foreskin and the glans with the closed second hemostat, starting just underneath the first hemostat. Holding the handles horizontally, advance the closed tips dorsally to the corona, *at all times tenting the foreskin up to prevent entry into the urethral meatus.* Once the tips are at the corona, open the hemostat. Use rotating, sweeping motions to free the foreskin off the glans

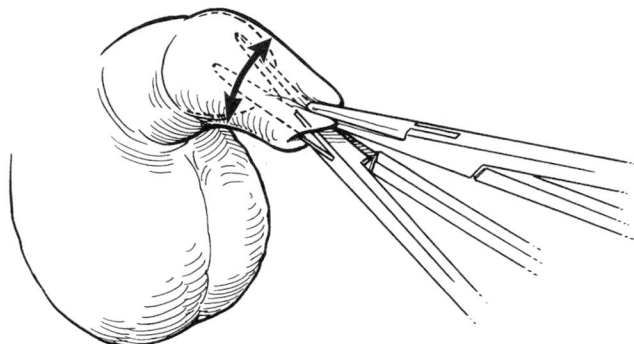

but *do not free between the 5 and 7 o'clock positions* where the urethral meatus and the frenulum containing the artery to the foreskin are located. Remove the dissecting hemostat from the cleavage plane.

2. Place a dorsal hemostat to hold the skin and mucosal surfaces of the foreskin together and to define the level of excision. Examine the penis carefully to find the ventral raphe. It is frequently rotated somewhat and not at the 6 o'clock position as might be expected. Determine if the true 12 o'clock position is to the left or right of the first hemostat's grasp. Open the second hemostat with handles held vertically. Enter the cleavage plane at the true 12 o'clock position with the bottom blade. While tenting the foreskin upward, advance until the tip is 5 mm short of the corona without traction.

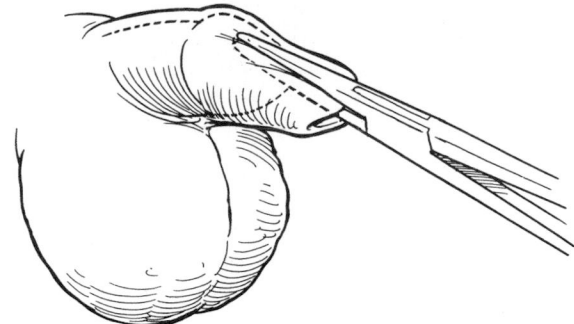

This should exactly follow the dorsal midline. Close and lock the hemostat. Remove the first hemostat.

3. The freed glans must be pushed back out of the way of the Mogen clamp's jaws to prevent inadvertent partial amputation of the glans. Hold the dorsal hemostat in the nondominant hand with handles vertically, wrapping the third, fourth, and fifth fingers around the hinge area. *Relax any traction on the hemostat.* Pinch the foreskin side-to-side underneath the hemostat blades using the thumb and index finger. This will push the freed glans back toward the root of the penis and out of the way. *Do not change this grasp until the Mogen clamp is fully placed.*

4. Open the Mogen clamp. Hold it in the dominant hand with the concave side toward the glans and the slot opening pointing downward. Carefully advance the slot across the foreskin from dorsal to ventral, starting at the tip of the grasping hemostat.

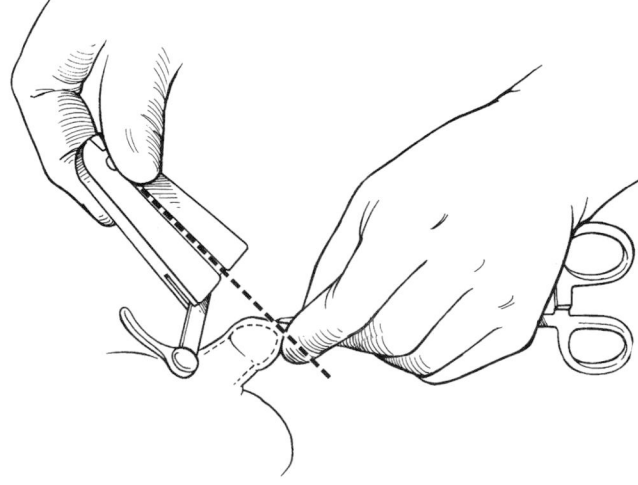

Angle the placement to follow the contour of the corona, taking less foreskin ventrally than dorsally. Slide the clamp as far across the foreskin as it will go. The nondominant hands' pinching grasp may now be dropped.

5. Check to be sure that the glans is not trapped before locking the Mogen clamp. Palpate the glans inside the shaft skin on the concave side of the clamp. Wiggle it up and down and side-to-side to *be sure that it is free of the clamp.*

6. Lock the Mogen clamp by pulling the locking bar across the slot opening, and closing the cam fully. Leave the clamp closed for 60 seconds.

7. While the Mogen clamp is locked, use the convex belly of the No. 10 scalpel blade to cut the foreskin away flush with the flat surface of the clamp.

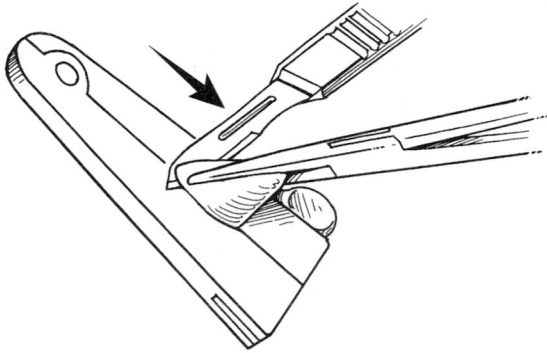

8. Unlock the Mogen clamp and remove it. The penis has an odd appearance now because the penile shaft skin is crushed together, concealing the glans.

9. Liberate the glans by grasping the penile shaft skin at the 3 and 9 o'clock positions and pushing down toward the root of the penis.

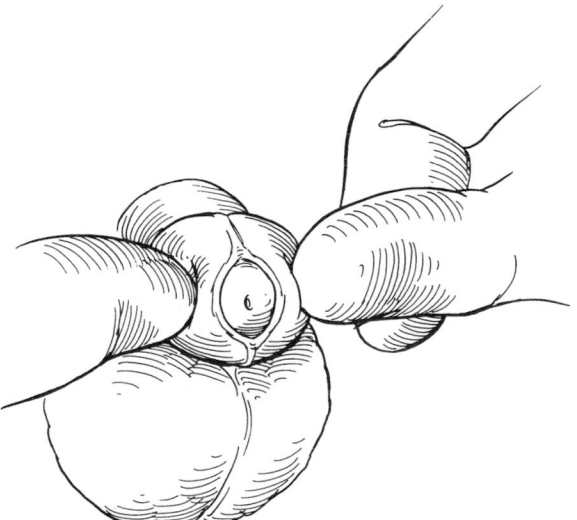

Pulling the remaining crush line apart while holding at the same positions will prevent paraphimosis. It is common to have some mucosa still adherent to the corona in some areas. The blunt probe is used to free these areas. To prevent bleeding, *avoid the meatal and frenulum areas.*

10. Wrap a petroleum jelly gauze dressing around the glans.

Follow-Up

1. Acetaminophen is given to minimize postoperative pain.

2. The petroleum jelly gauze dressing is left on until it becomes soiled by stool. Thereafter, a smear of petroleum jelly is placed in the front of each new diaper to prevent the healing glans from sticking to the diaper.

3. Tell parents to expect some yellowish exudate on the glans during a 4- to 7-day healing time. At each diaper change during this time, the shaft skin should be retracted away from the corona to prevent adhesions from forming between them. Petroleum jelly should be applied behind the corona to further prevent this.

Bibliography

Haouari N, Wood C, Griffiths G, et al: The analgesic effect of sucrose in full term infants: a randomized controlled trial. BMJ 1995;310:1498–1500.

Kaweblum YA, Press S, Kogan L, et al: Circumcision using the Mogen clamp. Clin Pediatr 1984;23:679–682.

Lenhart JG, Lenhart NM, Reid A, et al: Local anesthesia for circumcision: which technique is most effective? J Am Board Fam Pract 1997;10:13–19.

Reynolds RD: Use of the Mogen clamp for neonatal circumcision. Am Fam Physician 1996;54:177–182.

Wisniewski PM: Mogen circumcision utilizing transillumination. Female Patient 1992;17:29–32.

155 Anemia Work-up

Dominick Memoli

Etiology

1. Definition: reduction below normal of the number of erythrocytes, quantity of hemoglobin, or volume of packed red blood cells (RBCs) in the blood
2. Mechanism: Results from one or more combinations of three basic factors: blood loss, decreased RBC production, or increased RBC destruction (hemolysis).

Classification

The anemias can be broadly categorized into three major classifications according to the size, or mean corpuscular volume (MCV), of the erythrocytes.

1. Microcytosis (decreased MCV)
   a. Iron deficiency anemia
   b. α- or β-Thalassemias: inherited disorder, Asian and African varieties
   c. Anemia of chronic diseases: chronic inflammation or infection
   d. Sideroblastic anemias: acquired (antituberculosis drugs, lead) or congenital
2. Normocytosis (normal MCV)
   a. Normal variant: diagnosis of exclusion
   b. Anemia of chronic disease (see above)
   c. Acute hemorrhage
   d. Endocrinopathies: for example, myxedema, Addison's disease, eunuchoidism, panhypopituitarism
   e. Human immunodeficiency syndrome–related anemia
   f. Dilutional: overhydration of patients or rehydration of a dehydrated patient
   g. Sports anemia (runner's, etc.): multifactorial —hemolysis, plasma volume expansion, gastrointestinal blood loss
   h. Mixed anemias: the presence of two or more causes for anemia, such as iron deficiency anemia and vitamin B_{12}/folate deficiency
   i. Myelophthistic anemias: replacement of the normal marrow cells by leukemic, myeloma, or metastatic cancer cells or by myelofibrosis. Peripheral smear shows a leukoerythroblastic picture with teardrop RBCs, nucleated RBCs, and immature granulocytes (white blood cells). Thrombocytopenia and leukopenia also may be present.
   j. Liver disease, such as hepatitis or cirrhosis; marked variability of RBC size and shape as well as color
   k. Uremia: history of renal dysfunction; burr and spur RBCs on peripheral smear
   l. Hemoglobinopathies: for example, sickle cell anemia, hemoglobin C disease
3. Macrocytosis (increased MCV)
   a. Pure red cell aplasia: drug-induced (gold salts, diphenylhydantoin), underlying malignancies (thymoma, lymphoma), viruses (parvovirus B19)
   b. Alcoholism: unrelated to liver disease or B_{12}/folate deficiency. Bone marrow reveals vacuolization of erythroid precursors.
   c. Aplastic anemia: bone marrow failure resulting from a variety of causes, such as drugs (chloramphenicol), radiation, viral infections, hereditary (Fanconi's anemia). Characterized by stem cell destruction or suppression leading to pancytopenia in the peripheral smear. Paroxysmal nocturnal hemoglobinuria (PNH) is an uncommon cause of aplastic anemia characterized by a defect in the RBC membrane that increases sensitivity to hemolysis by complement. Sucrose hemolysis and Ham's acid tests are positive.
   d. Myelodysplastic syndromes: anemia of the elderly characterized by peripheral blood cytopenias, bone marrow abnormalities with or without an excess of marrow blasts, and hypercellularity; megaloblastoid changes in the erythroid precursors; B_{12}/folate levels normal (see Bibliography).
   e. Megaloblastic anemias: B_{12} or folate deficiency, hypersegmented neutrophils on peripheral smears, pancytopenia if deficiency severe
   f. Hemolytic anemias: variety of disorders characterized by reticulocytosis, erythroid hyperplasia in the marrow, increased levels

of serum bilirubin, hemoglobinemia, hemoglobinuria, hemosiderinuria, decreased serum haptoglobin, and increased serum lactate dehydrogenase. The direct Coombs' test may or may not be positive depending on the type of hemolytic anemia. The hemolytic anemias may be divided into the following:

(1) Extrinsic
   (a) Antibody-mediated: immunohemolytic anemias (drug-induced)
   (b) Microangiopathic hemolytic anemias: thrombotic thrombocytopenic purpura, disseminated intravascular coagulation, hemolytic-uremic syndrome
   (c) Toxins, malaria
(2) Intrinsic
   (a) RBC membrane defects: hereditary spherocytosis or elliptocytosis, PNH
   (b) Hemoglobinopathies: sickle cell disease, thalassemias
   (c) Enzymopathies: glucose-6-phosphate dehydrogenase (G6PD) deficiency, pyruvate kinase deficiency

Symptoms
1. Result from tissue hypoxia.
2. Severe anemia can produce weakness, headaches, dizziness, and fatigue.
3. If the anemia developed slowly, the patient may be asymptomatic.

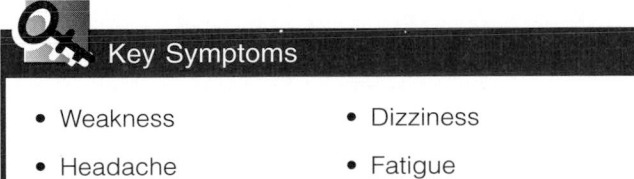

Key Symptoms

- Weakness
- Headache
- Dizziness
- Fatigue

Clinical Findings
1. On physical examination, orthostatic hypotension, tachycardia, and tachypnea may be present.
2. Jaundice and hepatosplenomegaly may be present (i.e., hemolytic anemias).
3. Neurologic manifestations, such as loss of vibratory or positional sensation, may be seen in B_{12} deficiency.
4. Evidence of underlying disease as cause for the anemia

Key Signs

- Orthostatic hypotension, tachycardia, and tachypnea on physical examination
- Jaundice and hepatosplenomegaly
- Neurologic manifestations

Laboratory Tests
1. Microcytic anemia: serum iron, total iron-binding capacity (TIBC), and serum ferritin; transferrin saturation; hemoglobin electrophoresis to identify thalassemias. Less commonly, free erythrocyte protoporphyrin (FEP) can be used to differentiate iron deficiency anemia from other causes of microcytic anemia (FEP) in increased MCV. Check feces for occult blood (see Table 155-1 for key tests and findings).
2. Normocytic anemia: evidence of underlying disease states with symptoms and signs of same, such as specific tests for a particular endocrinopathy based on clinical findings. Hemoglobin electrophoresis to identify hemoglobinopathies.
3. Macrocytic anemia: serum B_{12} and folate levels, thyroid function tests. For hemolytic anemias, see under "Etiology."
4. General: complete blood count with differential and platelet count, reticulocyte count, peripheral smear, and bone marrow biopsy and/or aspirate in most cases
5. Most anemias can be diagnosed by history, clinical findings, and physical examination; for example, pica for clay (geophagia) or ice (pagophagia) is a very common manifestation in iron deficiency anemia.
6. The RBC distribution width (RDW), like the MCV, indicates variations in RBC size. When the RDW is high, it is consistent with a marked variation in RBC size. Along with the MCV, the RDW can help to differentiate one anemia from another. For example, a low MCV and normal RDW favors thalassemia minor, whereas a low MCV and high RDW favors iron deficiency anemia.

Treatment
1. General: blood transfusion support in patients (particularly the elderly) who are symptomatic from their anemia, that is, orthostatic, short of breath, having anginal-type chest pain
2. Microcytic anemia: iron supplementation in iron deficiency anemia, blood transfusions in chronic diseases or thalassemias (watch for iron overload)

TABLE 155–1. KEY TESTS AND FINDINGS

	Serum Iron	TIBC	Serum Ferritin	Peripheral Smear	Hemoglobin Electrophoresis	Bone Marrow	Other
Iron deficiency anemia	Decreased	Increased	Decreased	Hypochromia	Normal	Erythroid hyperplasia No stainable iron	Increased free erythrocyte protoporphyrin (FEP) History of blood loss
α-Thalassemia	Increased	Normal or increased	Normal or increased	Basophilic stippling, target cells, nucleated RBCs, normochromia	Normal	Erythroid hyperplasia Increased stainable iron	Diagnosis of exclusion Asian type: more severe African type: less severe
β-Thalassemia	As above	As above	As above	As above	Increased hemoglobin A_2: Minor: 3–7% Major: 7–90%	As above	Mediterranean ethnic groups Minor: mild symptoms and hemolysis Major: more severe; iron overload FEP increased
Sideroblastic anemias	Increased	Normal or decreased	Increased	Dimorphism: microcytic and normocytic RBCs, basophilic stippling	Normal	Erythroid hyperplasia Increased stainable iron Increased number of ringed sideroblasts, vacuolated RBCs	
Anemia of chronic diseases	Decreased	Decreased	Increased	Hypochromia or normochromia	Normal	Increased stainable iron	Underlying chronic inflammation, malignancy

3. Normocytic anemia: treatment of the underlying disease. In the case of uremic patients, administration of erythropoietin usually beneficial; transfusion support in the hemoglobinopathies.

4. Macrocytic anemia: removal of toxic agents (drugs, alcohol, chemotherapeutic agents); in the megaloblastic anemias, the administration of B_{12} and/or folate will correct the anemia. In the extrinsic hemolytic anemias, the anemia resolves with treatment of the underlying disease; in the intrinsic type, avoidance of inciting drugs in G6PD or pyruvate kinase deficiency and splenectomy in hereditary spherocytosis or elliptocytosis are necessary.

Key Treatment

- Blood transfusion (general)

- Iron supplementation (microcytic)

- Treat underlying disease (normocytic).

- Removal of toxic agent (macrocytic)

Bibliography

Bennett JM: The classification of the acute leukemias: Cytochemical and morphologic considerations. In Wiernick PH, Caniellos GP, Kyle RA, et al (eds): Neoplastic Diseases of the Blood, vol 1, pp 201–217. New York, Churchill Livingstone, 1985.

Lee RG: Iron deficiency and iron deficiency anemia. In Wintrobe's Clinical Hematology, 9th ed, vol 1, pp 745–839, 885–910. Philadelphia, Lea & Febiger, 1993.

Steinberg MH, Adams JG: Laboratory detection of hemoglobinopathies and thalassemias. In Hoffman R, Benz EJ, Shattil SJ, et al (eds): Hematology, 2nd ed, pp 2241–2249. New York, Churchill Livingstone, 1995.

Williams WJ, Bentler E, Earsley AJ, et al (eds): Hematology, 4th ed. New York, McGraw-Hill, 1990.

156 Iron Deficiency Anemia

Mark Blumenthal

1. Anemia is a decrease in the red blood cell mass. Colloquially, anemia is defined as a reduction of hemoglobin or a decreased concentration of hemoglobin in the blood (hematocrit).

2. Because anemia is a condition rather than a disease, an underlying cause must be determined when anemia is identified.

3. Iron deficiency is the most common form of nutritional deficiency, and iron deficiency anemia is the most common cause of anemia worldwide.

4. Iron holds a pivotal role in many metabolic processes. In the form of hemoglobin, iron carries oxygen to the tissues from the lungs. As myoglobin, iron facilitates oxygen use and storage in the muscles, and, in the form of cytochromes, it is a transport medium for electrons within the cells. Iron also performs an integral role in enzyme reactions in various tissues.

5. Iron deficiency anemia can interfere with these physiologic functions, leading to both morbidity and mortality, and therefore must be accurately diagnosed and treated.

Etiology

1. In premature infants, iron deficiency anemia may result from lower iron stores than those in term infants, lower erythropoietin production compared to term infants, and frequent blood sampling in the neonatal nursery.

2. The iron stores of full-term infants can meet an infant's iron requirements until 4 to 6 months of age. However, a rapid growth rate accompanying inadequate intake of dietary iron places children less than 24 months of age at the highest risk of any age group for iron deficiency anemia.

3. Inappropriately low dietary iron intake frequently causes iron deficiency anemia in late infancy and early childhood.

    a. Introducing children to whole cow's milk before age 1 year, and children consuming greater than 24 oz daily after 1 year of age, incurs high risk. Cow's milk contains little iron, may replace foods with greater higher iron content and bioavailability, and often causes occult gastrointestinal bleeding.

    b. Iron-fortified formulas and iron-fortified cereals help protect against iron deficiency anemia.

4. During adolescence, iron requirements increase as a result of rapid growth, but stabilize among boys after the peak pubertal growth spurt.

    a. Among girls and women of childbearing years, menstrual blood loss is an important contributor to iron deficiency anemia.

    b. Intrauterine devices may also predispose women to menorrhagia, whereas the use of oral contraceptives reduces menorrhagia risk.

5. Only about 25 per cent of adolescent girls and women of childbearing age meet the Recommended Dietary Allowance of iron through diet.

6. The prevalence of iron deficiency anemia increases dramatically among pregnant women.

    a. Blood volume expands by approximately 35 per cent, and iron demands during the second and third trimesters increase threefold to approximately 5.0 mg iron/day.

    b. Women at high risk for iron deficiency anemia when not pregnant are also less likely to supplement their diets with iron during pregnancy.

7. Iron-deficiency anemia is relatively uncommon among adult men and postmenopausal women in the United States. No more than 2 per cent of men age 20 years or lower and 2 per cent of women age 50 years or older have iron deficiency anemia. Most men and women age 50 years or older meet the Recommended Dietary Allowance of iron through diet.

8. Among adult men and postmenopausal women who have iron deficiency anemia, nearly two thirds demonstrate clinical evidence of gastrointestinal bleeding. For the remainder of adults, the principal causes of anemia are chronic diseases and inflammatory conditions. Astute clinicians should not assume insufficient dietary intake to be the primary cause of iron deficiency anemia in low-risk adults.

Symptoms

1. In an asymptomatic patient, it is common to ultimately diagnose significant iron depletion, even with mild to moderate anemia.

a. In cases of chronic, slow blood loss, the body adapts to the increasing anemia, and patients can often tolerate extremely low concentrations of hemoglobin (e.g., <7 gm/dl) with remarkably few symptoms.

b. The symptoms accompanying iron deficiency depend on how rapidly the anemia develops.

2. As a rule, the only symptoms of iron deficiency anemia are those of the anemia itself, which may include easy fatigability, tachycardia, tachypnea on exertion, and palpitations. More unusual symptoms include headaches, tinnitus, and taste disturbance.

3. Many iron-deficient patients develop *pica*, an unusual craving for specific foods (dirt, clay, ice cubes, etc.) that may or may not contain iron.

Key Symptoms	
• Easy fatigability	• Tachypnea on exertion
• Tachycardia	• Palpitations

Clinical Findings

1. Many signs of iron deficiency anemia may be due to the underlying disease rather than the anemia itself.

2. Patients with pre-existing vascular disease can experience exacerbation of angina, claudication, or cerebral ischemia from compromise in oxygenation.

3. Gastrointestinal signs such as indigestion, nausea, and bowel irregularity may occur as a result of shunting of blood from the splanchnic bed.

4. Severe iron deficiency causes atrophy of the skin in about one third of patients, and nail changes such as koilonychia (spoon-shaped nails) result in brittle, flattened nails. Patients may also complain of angular stomatitis, in which painful cracks appear at the angle of the mouth, sometimes accompanied by glossitis.

5. Advanced iron deficiency may cause dysphagia because of the formation of esophageal webs (Plummer-Vinson syndrome), which are typically diagnosed on upper gastrointestinal endoscopy.

Key Signs	
• Angina	
• Indigestion	
• Skin or conjunctival pallor	

Laboratory Tests

1. Historically, complete blood count (CBC) with peripheral smear, ferritin, serum iron level, total iron-binding capacity (TIBC), transferrin saturation, and a reticulocyte count have been combined to form an "anemia panel."

2. Serum ferritin (<12 μg/L) or absent bone marrow iron stores (as demonstrated on bone marrow iron smears) are pathognomonic for iron deficiency anemia.

3. CBC with peripheral smear and serum ferritin level should be the first studies conducted when the clinician suspects iron deficiency anemia. Serum ferritin radioimmunoassay results may be elevated by underlying inflammatory or liver disease. Therefore, a normal (>15 μg/L) or high ferritin level does not entirely rule out iron deficiency.

4. The remaining studies in the anemia panel provide proxy measures for iron deficiency anemia.

a. The mean corpuscular volume (MCV) may appear completely normal in early iron deficiency anemia, in patients with liver disease, or in combined iron and vitamin B_{12} or folate deficiencies. Once hemoglobin levels fall below about 9 gm/dl (90 gm/L), microcytosis (MCV <78 μm^3 [78 fl]), poikilocytosis, and hypochromia become more prominent in the peripheral smear.

b. Low serum iron, in the presence of normal or elevated ferritin, may occur in acute and chronic inflammation, malignancy, and infection, as well as iron deficiency anemia.

c. TIBC is usually elevated (>300 μg/dl) in iron deficiency anemia, but may be low in inflammation, infection, or malignancy. TIBC may be normal in sideroblastic anemia, α-thalassemia trait, β-thalassemia, or other hemoglobinopathies.

d. Transferrin saturation levels below 15 per cent are consistent with but not diagnostic of iron deficiency anemia. In anemia of chronic disease, both iron and iron-binding capacity are also low, but with a transferrin saturation below 15 per cent but greater than 9 per cent.

5. Bone marrow iron stain remains the gold standard test for iron stores.

a. The assessment of iron stores as hemosiderin found within the reticuloendothelial cells usually rules out iron deficiency anemia if adequate iron storage areas are present in the aspirated material.

b. Although hemosiderin can be seen in unstained marrow particles, iron stains with potassium ferrocyanide are more accurate.

  c. The presence of any storage iron virtually rules out the diagnosis of iron deficiency anemia, unless the patient has been recently treated with iron supplementation or transfusion.

Key Tests

- CBC with peripheral smear
- Serum ferritin
- Bone marrow biopsy

Differential Diagnosis

1. Iron deficiency anemia accounts for the majority of hypochromic microcytic anemias. If ferritin is normal or high, the remainder of the anemia panel, including bone marrow examination if necessary, must be invoked.
2. Chronic diseases and inflammatory conditions
   a. If serum iron and TIBC are both decreased, one must look for the underlying chronic disease.
   b. If serum iron levels are normal or increased and TIBC is normal, hemoglobin electrophoresis may help diagnose β-thalassemia or another hemoglobinopathy.
      (1) Normal electrophoresis mandates examination of the bone marrow to exclude sideroblastic anemia or α-thalassemia trait.
      (2) Acquired sideroblastic anemia may result from lead intoxication, isoniazid, pyrazinamide, chronic ethanol consumption, chloramphenicol, and various chemotherapeutic agents.

Treatment

Effective management of iron deficiency anemia relies on both appropriate management of the underlying cause and iron replacement therapy.

Oral Therapy

1. In the pediatric population, 3 to 6 mg/kg of elemental iron drops, administered in divided doses between meals, may correct the peripheral anemia in as little as 4 weeks.
   a. Serial CBCs and reticulocyte counts should be used to follow the initial progress of iron repletion.
   b. To fully replete lost marrow iron stores, 4 to 6 months of oral therapy may be required.

Ferritin levels will then be greater than 15 μg/L.

2. In adults, oral therapy with ferrous sulfate, ferrous gluconate, or ferrous fumarate, sufficient to provide 200 mg of elemental iron daily, will fully replete lost iron stores in 4 to 6 months.
   a. The patient typically begins with 1 tablet daily, increasing intake by 1 tablet weekly until reaching the full 3-tablet regimen.
   b. The iron supplement must be taken between meals to maximize absorption. Taking ferrous sulfate with vitamin C–containing products and meats can improve absorption.
   c. A standard regimen includes 300 to 325 mg ferrous sulfate taken three times daily.
   d. Gastrointestinal side effects, including nausea, constipation, diarrhea, and abdominal cramping, occur in 20 to 25 per cent of patients. These side effects may be reduced by taking the tablets after meals, although this slows absorption and prolongs therapy.
3. Response to oral iron therapy may be noted within 7 to 10 days by a rise in the reticulocyte response and rising hematocrit. When following patients, it is reasonable to check a blood count 3 or 4 weeks after initiating therapy.
   a. Failure of response to iron therapy is usually due to noncompliance, although occasional patients may absorb iron poorly or have ongoing blood loss.
   b. Malabsorption is rarely a cause for treatment failure, except in patients who have undergone partial gastrectomy or those with malabsorption syndromes.

Parenteral Therapy

1. Indications for parenteral iron therapy include intolerance to oral iron, refractoriness to oral iron (poor absorption), gastrointestinal disease (usually inflammatory bowel disease) precluding the use of oral iron, and continued blood loss that cannot be corrected.

WARNING

Because of the possibility of severe and even fatal hypersensitivity reactions, parenteral iron therapy should be used only in cases of clinically significant documented iron deficiency after every reasonable attempt has been made to use oral therapy.

---

2. The total dose of parenteral iron dextran (Imferon) required equals the hemoglobin (Hb) def-

icit plus the amount needed to replete iron stores.

Hemoglobin deficit (mg) = (normal Hb

   − patient's Hb [gm/dl])

   × weight (kg) × 2.2

The total dose is typically 1.5 to 2 gm.

3. Iron dextran (Imferon) is dispensed as 50 mg elemental iron per milliliter and can be given intramuscularly or intravenously. Intravenous infusion has become the preferred route because intramuscular injections are slowly absorbed, with only 70 per cent bioavailability, cause local pain, and produce skin staining that may last for years.

4. Iron dextran is generally given undiluted at a slow, gradual rate not to exceed 50 mg (1 ml)/minute. Individual doses of 2 ml or less may be given on a daily basis until the calculated total amount required has been reached.

   a. A test dose of a 0.5-ml solution is given first, with epinephrine at the bedside, because of the risk of anaphylaxis, which occurs in less than 1 per cent of patients receiving the drug.

   b. Other side effects, which may occur within 4 to 6 days after the infusion, include arthralgias, fever, myalgias, hypotension, headache, abdominal pain, gastrointestinal distress, lymphadenopathy, urticaria, and pleural effusion.

5. Although the manufacturer does not recommend dilution of iron dextran injection or administration of the drug in single IV doses larger than 100 mg, numerous reports have been made in which the total dose of iron dextran was administered as a single dose either by direct IV administration or as an IV infusion.

   a. In the total-dose infusion technique, the total calculated dose of iron dextran is diluted in 250 to 1000 ml of 0.9% sodium chloride injection.

   b. The test dose of 25 mg of iron should be administered slowly over 5 minutes. If no reaction occurs, the remainder of the dose may be infused over 1 to 6 hours. After the infusion is completed, the vein is often flushed with 0.9% sodium chloride injection.

Diet

1. Foods containing large amounts of iron include liver, red meat, and legumes.
2. Vitamin C–rich foods may enhance iron uptake.
3. Substances that can reduce absorption include bran, eggs, milk, tea, coffee, calcium-rich antacids, and drugs such as cimetidine.

Activity

Activity should be tailored to the patient's physical well-being and underlying pathophysiology.

Key Treatment

Ferrous sulfate, 300 to 325 mg PO tid for 4 to 6 months

Follow-Up

1. Hemoglobin concentration should normalize by the end of 2 months of therapy.
2. By 4 to 6 months of therapy, iron stores should be replete, and ferritin levels will register greater than 15 μg/L.

Bibliography

Centers for Disease Control and Prevention: Recommendations to prevent and control iron deficiency in the United States. MMWR Morb Mortal Wkly Rep 1998; 47(RR-3).

Frewin R, Henson A, Provan D: ABC of clinical haematology: iron deficiency anaemia. BMJ 1997;314:360.

Guyatt GH, Oxman AD, Ali M, et al: Laboratory diagnosis of iron-deficiency anemia: an overview. J Gen Intern Med 1992;7:145–153.

Massey A: Microcytic anemia: differential diagnosis and management of iron deficiency anemia. Med Clin North Am 1992;76:549–566.

Shine J: Microcytic anemia. Am Fam Physician 1997;55: 2455–2462.

157 Megaloblastic Anemia

Wayne A. Bottner

Etiology

1. All megaloblastic states share a common pathophysiologic mechanism, interference with DNA synthesis.
2. Folic acid plays a crucial role in purine and pyrimidine synthesis. Cobalamin (vitamin B_{12}) is required for the proper metabolism of folate. Deficiency of either can ultimately lead to defective DNA metabolism and megaloblastosis.
3. Drugs may induce megaloblastosis by directly interfering with DNA synthesis (hydroxyurea) or by interfering with folate metabolism (methotrexate).

Symptoms

Three areas of involvement

1. Hematologic: anemia with resulting fatigue, pallor, intolerance of exertion
2. Epithelial (less common): atrophy of mucosal surfaces most commonly manifested by tongue or mouth pain
3. Neurologic (cobalamin deficiency only): paresthesias, weakness, gait disturbance, personality change, intellectual decline

Key Symptoms

- Fatigue, pallor, mouth/tongue pain
- Cobalamin deficiency only
  –Paresthesias, gait disturbance, weakness, intellectual/personality change

Clinical Findings

1. Signs reflect areas of involvement
   a. Patients may be profoundly anemic at presentation.
   b. Pallor and mild hyperbilirubinemia can impart a characteristic "lemon yellow" hue to the skin in severely anemic patients.
   c. Tongue may be smooth as a result of papillary atrophy.
   d. Folate-deficient patients may show signs of malnutrition.
2. Fortification of cereal products with folate may

lead to the masking of the hematologic manifestations of cobalamin deficiency in some patients.

WARNING

Patients with cobalamin deficiency may have no hematologic abnormalities and present with neurologic signs only.

Key Signs

- Pallor (lemon yellow)
- Smooth tongue
- Malnutrition (folate-deficient only)
- Cobalamin-deficient only
  –Diminished proprioception and vibratory sense
  –Spasticity
  –Dementia

Laboratory Tests

1. Identification of true tissue deficiency of cobalamin or folate is crucial for precise diagnosis and selection of appropriate therapy.
2. Evaluation should be carried out in two steps
   a. Establish deficiency of cobalamin or folate (or both).
   b. Determine underlying cause.
3. Serum levels alone may not accurately reflect conditions at the tissue level.
4. Peripheral blood findings are similar regardless of cause.
   a. Any or all cell lines may be affected.
      (1) Hypoproliferative anemia
      (2) Leukopenia and thrombocytopenia may be severe.
   b. High mean corpuscular volume (MCV; may be masked by coexisting iron deficiency), with oval macrocytes on smear
   c. Hypersegmented neutrophils
5. Hypercellular bone marrow reflects ineffective

erythropoiesis. Presence of megaloblasts is pathognomonic.

6. Elevation of lactate dehydrogenase (LDH) level may be striking.

7. Bilirubin usually is mildly high.

8. *Proving cobalamin deficiency and its cause*

   a. Serum cobalamin level has a relatively low sensitivity and specificity for tissue deficiency.

   (1) Serum or urine methylmalonic acid levels have been shown to be more sensitive than cobalamin levels. Availability may limit use.

   (2) Holotranscobalamin II level can also detect early cobalamin deficiency and may become the screening test of choice because of ease of performance. Availability may limit use.

   b. The Schilling test should only be used to determine the cause of cobalamin deficiency, not to prove its existence. Incomplete urine collection or renal functional impairment can affect the results.

   c. Anti–intrinsic factor antibodies have a high specificity for pernicious anemia, but only a 50 to 60 per cent sensitivity.

9. *Proving folate deficiency*: Serum folate rises and falls rapidly in response to fluctuations in dietary intake. Red blood cell folate is a better reflector of tissue levels.

Key Tests

- MCV
- Reticulocyte count
- Blood smear
- LDH
- Bilirubin
- Serum B$_{12}$ level
- Serum/red blood cell folate
- Methylmalonic acid
- Holotranscobalamin II
- Schilling test

Differential Diagnosis

1. Cobalamin deficiency

   a. Dietary: vegans

   b. Autoimmune: pernicious anemia

   c. Postsurgical: gastrectomy or ileal resection

   d. Inflammatory: Crohn's disease

   e. Infectious: bacterial overgrowth/parasitic

   f. Atrophic gastritis: elderly (normal Schilling test)

2. Folate deficiency

   a. Dietary: alcoholics/elderly

   b. Malabsorptive: sprue

   c. Drug: anticonvulsant

   d. Increased utilization: pregnancy/hemolysis

3. Chemotherapy: methotrexate/hydroxyurea/alkylating agents/cytarabine

4. Hereditary

Treatment

1. Cobalamin deficiency

   a. Until recently, intramuscular B$_{12}$ was considered the only effective treatment for all except vegans with dietary deficiency.

   b. Cyanocobalamin (vitamin B$_{12}$) used most often: 100 μg intramuscularly daily for 1 week, weekly for 1 month, then monthly or at more frequent intervals if deemed necessary.

   c. A recent randomized trial suggests that oral therapy may be as effective as IM cobalamin in patients with proven cobalamin deficiency.

   d. An intranasal cobalamin preparation (Nascobal), is also available.

2. Folate deficiency

   a. Oral folic acid will adequately treat all except those with malabsorption.

   b. An oral or parenteral dose of 1 mg daily is sufficient.

WARNING

Folic acid will correct the hematologic but *NOT* the neurologic manifestations of cobalamin deficiency. Accurate diagnosis is essential to prevent the erroneous use of folic acid in cobalamin-deficient patients.

Diet

1. Meat-based and vegetarian diets are generally rich in both cobalamin and folate.

2. Vegans should supplement their diet with oral cobalamin.

Patient Education

1. Emphasis on the importance of lifelong therapy will help to prevent relapse in those whose cause is not reversible.

2. Many patients can be taught to administer cobalamin at home to reduce cost and unnecessary clinic visits.

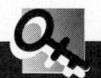

Key Treatment

Cobalamin Deficiency	Folate Deficiency
• Parenteral cyanocobalamin	• Oral folic acid

Follow-Up

1. Early follow-up is important to document response to therapy and rule out coexisting conditions (e.g., iron deficiency) that may interfere with response.

2. Periodic follow-up in patients on lifelong therapy may help to prevent relapse.

3. Pernicious anemia is associated with the development of gastric cancer. The ideal schedule for follow-up and the importance of early detection have not been established.

Bibliography

Babior BM, Stossel TP: DNA replications and hematopoiesis: Megaloblastic anemias. In Babior BM, Stossel TP: Hematology: A Pathophysiological Approach, 2nd ed, pp 73–91. New York, Churchill Livingstone, 1990.

Beck WS: Diagnosis of megaloblastic anemia. Annu Rev Med 1991;42:311–322.

Carmel R: Clinical aspects of megaloblastic anemia. In Bick RL (ed): Hematology: Clinical and Laboratory Practice, vol 1, pp 437–457. St Louis, CV Mosby Company, 1993.

Kuzminski A, Del Giacco EJ, Allen RH: Effective treatment of cobalamin deficiency with oral cobalamin. Blood 1998;92:1191–1198.

Savage DG, Lindenbaum J, Stabler SP, Allen RH: Sensitivity of serum methylmalonic acid and total homocysteine determinations for diagnosing cobalamin and folate deficiencies. Am J Med 1994;96:239–246.

158 Hemolytic Anemia

Aliasghar Mohyuddin

Premature destruction of circulating red blood cells (average life of 90 to 120 days) is called hemolysis. The resulting anemia is termed *hemolytic anemia.*

Etiology

Hemolysis can be intravascular or extravascular (spleen/liver). Extravascular hemolysis is more common. Hemolytic anemia can be divided into two broad categories.

1. Acquired
   a. Splenomegaly (with associated hypersplenism)
   b. Immune hemolytic anemia: hemolytic disease of the newborn; transfusion reactions
   c. Autoimmune/alloimmune (warm-reactive antibodies and cold-reactive antibodies)
      (1) Warm-reactive antibodies associated with neoplasms, collagen-vascular diseases (e.g., systemic lupus erythematosus), medication induced (e.g., penicillin, α-methyldopa, and quinidine); accounts for approximately 10 per cent of warm reactive antibody–induced reactions, idiopathic
      (2) Cold-reactive antibodies associated with mycoplasma infections (positive in ~90 per cent), Epstein-Barr virus, lymphoproliferative disorders, paroxysmal cold hemoglobinuria, idiopathic
   d. Hemolysis caused by trauma in circulation
      (1) Macroangiopathic: e.g., prosthetic heart valves (aortic)
      (2) Microangiopathic
         (a) Hemolytic-uremic syndrome
         (b) Thrombotic thrombocytopenic purpura
         (c) Disseminated intravascular coagulation
         (d) Graft rejection
   e. Direct toxic effect: malaria, babesiosis, toxoplasmosis, clostridial infections, typhoid fever
   f. Chemical/drug induced: sulfonamides, nitrofurantoin, phenacetin, salicylates, phenols, lead, copper, propylthiouracil, spider/snake venom
   g. Physical injury: burns, hypophosphatemia, march hemoglobinuria (e.g., prolonged physical exertion such as marching)
   h. Paroxysmal nocturnal hemoglobinuria (Hams's test)
   i. Spur cell anemia
   j. Vitamin E deficiencies in newborns
2. Hereditary
   a. Membrane defects
      (1) Hereditary spherocytosis
      (2) Hereditary elliptocytosis
      (3) Pyropoikilocytosis
      (4) Spherocytic elliptocytosis
      (5) Stomatocytic elliptocytosis
      (6) Hereditary stomatocytosis
      (7) Lecithin-cholesterol acyltransferase deficiency
      (8) High-phosphatidylcholine hemolytic anemia
      (9) Rh_{null} disease.
   b. Glycolytic enzyme defects: pyruvate kinase (~95 per cent of all defects), glucose phosphate isomerase deficiency, aldolase deficiency
   c. Abnormality of red blood cell nucleotide metabolism
   d. Deficiencies of enzymes in the pentose phosphate pathway and in glutathione metabolism (e.g., glucose-6-phosphate dehydrogenase [G6PD], glutathione synthetase/reductase)
   e. Thalassemias (e.g., α- and β-thalassemias)
   f. Hemoglobinopathies (e.g., sickle cell and autosomal dominant inherited unstable hemoglobins)

Symptoms

Patients with moderate to severe hemolysis develop noticeable fatigue, weakness, dyspnea on exertion, nausea, vomiting.

Moderate to Severe Hemolysis

- Fatigue

- Dyspnea on exertion

- Weakness

Clinical Findings

1. Anemia ± jaundice (acholuric and absence of pruritus) ± splenomegaly (present in chronic hemolysis)
2. Chronic leg ulcers (in chronic hemolysis)
3. Bony abnormalities (if hemolysis present in growth phase)
4. Cholelithiasis (in chronic hemolysis)
5. Flow murmurs (in moderate to severe hemolysis)

- Anemia

- ± Jaundice

- ± Splenomegaly

- Flow murmurs (moderate to severe, acute hemolysis)

- Chronic leg ulcers (chronic hemolysis)

- Cholelithiasis (chronic hemolysis)

- Bony abnormalities (hemolysis present in growth phase)

Laboratory Findings and Tests

1. Increase in unconjugated bilirubin
2. Low or absent haptoglobin (particularly in intravascular hemolysis)
3. Low or absent hemopexin (particularly in intravascular hemolysis)
4. Increase in lactate dehydrogenase (LDH), especially LDH-2
5. Increase in endogenous carbon monoxide production
6. Decrease in glycosylated hemoglobin (average 3.9 per cent in hemolysis)
7. Erythroid hyperplasia
8. Polychromatophilia
9. Reticulocytosis
10. Hemosiderinuria
11. Increase in urine and fecal urobilinogen
12. Peripheral smear
    a. *Spherocytes*: hereditary spherocytosis (osmotic fragility test), immunohemolytic anemia induced by warm antibodies
    b. *Acanthocytes*: abetalipoproteinemia, spur cell anemia, anorexia nervosa, vitamin E deficiency
    c. *Stomatocytes*: hereditary stomatocytosis
    d. *Target cells*: thalassemias, hemoglobin C disease, sickle cell disease, postsplenectomy, lecithin-cholesterol acyltransferase deficiency
    e. *Elliptocytes*: hereditary elliptocytosis, thalassemias, myelodysplastic/megaloblastic processes
    f. *Schistocytes/helmet cells*: disseminated intravascular coagulation, thrombotic thrombocytopenic purpura, hemolytic-uremic syndrome, cardiac valve hemolysis, burns, liver/renal disease, G6PD deficiency, pulmonary emboli

- Fractionated bilirubin

- Haptoglobin

- LDH

- Reticulocyte count

- Peripheral smear

Differential Diagnosis

1. Hemorrhage (into body cavities with marrow response)
2. Recovery from iron, folate B12 deficiencies
3. Recovery from marrow suppression (e.g., alcohol cessation)
4. Infiltrative marrow disorders
5. Myoglobinuria
6. Ineffective erythropoiesis

Treatment

Establish correct etiology.

1. Treat correctable causes (e.g., infection, drug exposure).
2. Observe for spontaneous recovery, as in usually self-limited G6PD deficiency.
3. Treat shock (cautious blood transfusion in severe hemolysis).
4. Exchange transfusion

5. Steroid therapy: 1 to 1.5 mg/kg/day prednisone equivalents (especially in warm antibody–induced hemolysis)

6. Splenectomy: in steroid-recalcitrant patients; best response in hereditary spherocytosis/elliptocytosis, some response in enzymatic deficiencies and unstable hemoglobins

7. Cytotoxic drugs: cyclophosphamide, azathioprine, 6-mercaptopurine (reserved for steroid resistant and nonsplenectomy candidates)

8. Other medications: danazol, intravenous immune globulin, cyclosporine

9. Folate replacement in chronic hemolysis (to prevent megaloblastic crisis)

Diet

1. Folate replacement in nutritionally replete diets and chronic hemolysis

2. Avoid exposure to fava beans (*Vicia fava*) in known G6PD patients.

Activity

As tolerated

Patient Education

Diet and medication education in G6PD patients (e.g., antimalarials, sulfonamides, nitrofurantoin)

Key Treatment

- Establish correct etiology

- Treat underlying cause (e.g., infection, drug-induced)

- Observe in some cases for spontaneous recovery (e.g., G6PD)

- Steroids, splenectomy, cytotoxic drugs

Follow-Up

Symptomatically

Bibliography

Beutler E: Hemolytic anemia due to infections with micro-organisms. In Beutler E, Lichtman MA, Coller BS, Kipps TJ (eds): Williams' Hematology, 5th ed, pp 674–676. New York, McGraw-Hill, 1995.

Domen RE: An overview of immune hemolytic anemias. Clev Clin J Med 1998;65:89–99.

Lee GR: Hemolytic disorders. In Pine JW Jr (ed): Wintrobe's Clinical Hematology, 10th ed, vol 1, pp 1109–1131. Baltimore, Williams & Wilkins, 1999.

Tabbara IA: Hemolytic anemias: diagnosis and management. Med Clin North Am 1992;76:649–668.

Zail S: Hereditary defects of the red cell membrane. In Harmening DM (ed): Clinical Hematology and Fundamentals of Hemostasis, 3rd ed, pp 146–163. Philadelphia, FA Davis Company, 1992.

159 Sickle Cell Disease

Mark S. Johnson

Etiology

1. In sickle cell disease the patient is homozygous for hemoglobin (Hb) S.

2. Hb S differs from Hb A in that valine replaces glutamic acid at the sixth position of the β chain.

3. Hb S is related to shortened red cell life because of hemolysis and both microvascular and macrovascular occlusion. The chronic hemolysis results in anemia and jaundice. Deoxygenation causes Hb S to polymerize; the red blood cell becomes stiff and adopts different shapes, such as the "sickle" shape from which the disorder derives its name. Such cells cannot traverse small blood vessels and capillaries, causing sludging. This increases the viscosity of the blood, which also inhibits flow. These findings are then related to the multiorgan damage that occurs in these patients.

4. The gene that is responsible for Hb S is present in approximately 8 per cent of African Americans. Sickle cell disease is present in about 1 out of every 375 African Americans.

5. Sickle cell disease is sometimes confused with Hb SC, where the patient is double heterozygous for Hb S and Hb C. Hb C has lysine in the place of glutamic acid at the sixth position of the β chain. Hb SC tends to be less severe than Hb SS.

6. Sickle cell trait: the mildest form of Hb S occurs when a patient has Hb A and Hb S. Sickling may occur under extreme conditions. Also, painless hematuria has been reported. Hb S can also be combined with one of the thalassemias.

7. Patients with persistent high levels of Hb F tend to have milder disease.

8. The life expectancy of sickle cell patients has improved. Recent advances in the care of sickle cell disease suggest that further decreases in morbidity and mortality can be made.

Symptoms

1. The constellation of symptoms associated with sickle cell disease are commonly known as a crisis. These problems are associated with pain and increasing anemia, and can be life-threatening.

2. The pain crisis is characterized by escalating pain, most often in the joints, muscles, or abdomen. This pain is more severe than that which is chronically experienced.

3. In children, acute chest syndrome is the second leading cause for hospitalization. In the adult population, acute chest syndrome is a leading cause of death.

    a. Patients present with fever, cough, dyspnea, and pulmonary infiltrates. It is difficult to differentiate between this and pneumonia, so it is necessary to start antibiotics early.

    b. These patients need to be monitored very closely because they can progress to respiratory failure rapidly.

    c. On a chronic basis, pulmonary infarcts can result in decreased pulmonary capacity and even pulmonary hypertension.

Key Symptoms

- Pain: joints, muscle, abdomen, chest
- Fever, cough, dyspnea

Clinical Findings

1. Crises

    a. *Aplastic crisis*: failure of red blood synthesis. Pain is associated with a dropping hematocrit and a reticulocyte count less than 10 per cent.

        (1) Often occurs coincident with surgery or an infection.

        (2) Can also result from folic acid deficiency.

    b. *Hemolytic crisis*: anemia associated with increasing hemolysis. The bilirubin is increased and the patient is jaundiced.

    c. *Sequestration crisis*: Acute increase in splenic trapping of red blood cells results in worsening of anemia to a hemoglobin of 2 gm/dl.

        (1) Potential for shock

        (2) Thrombocytopenia may be present

        (3) Second leading cause of death in children with sickle cell disease

(4) Fifty per cent of patients who survive a sequestration crisis will have another.

2. Pediatric

a. Infection: the leading cause of death in children with sickle cell disease. This is decreased by approximately 80 per cent with the use of prophylactic antibiotics. There is a special concern about encapsulated bacteria such as streptococcus, haemophilus, meningococcus, and salmonella. The functional asplenia that occurs contributes to this risk.

b. Cerebrovascular events: Stroke may be prevented by transfusion if the patient is assessed to be high risk by ultrasound evaluation of the circle of Willis.

c. Delayed growth and late onset of puberty: There is some evidence that this is related at least in part to nutritional status.

d. Gallstones: related to high bilirubin level from constant hemolysis

e. Splenomegaly

(1) Spleen size should be assessed at each visit and parents should be taught how to palpate the spleen when there is a concern about splenic sequestration.

(2) By adulthood the spleen is scarred down; if splenomegaly persists in an adult, the diagnosis should be confirmed, because splenomegaly in adults is common with hemoglobin SC.

3. Adult

a. Cardiomegaly: a consequence of chronic anemia

b. Retinopathy: more common in Hb SC than Hb SS. Both patients should have annual ophthalmology examinations.

c. Chronic renal insufficiency: May result from papillary necrosis. These patients may have difficulty concentrating urine. Renal and liver infarcts may occur

d. Gallstones

e. Priapism: may be recurrent and can occur in children

f. Orthopedic problems: It is important to try to differentiate between "regular" sickle cell pain and more serious problems such as bone infarcts or aseptic necrosis of the femoral or humeral head. Also, osteomyelitis occurs with increased frequency compared to the non–sickle cell population.

g. Sickle cell patients are at high risk for chronic leg ulcers.

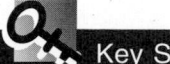

Key Signs

- Anemia
- Splenomegaly
- Gallstones
- Priapism

Laboratory Tests

1. Electrophoresis specific for Hb S and Hb A

2. Prenatal screening required in most states. Can be done on genetic material obtained from amniocentesis or fetoscopy. If prenatal screening not done, do electrophoresis at 2 months of age in high-risk groups (blacks and those from the Middle East or Mediterranean region).

3. Avoid screening tests based on solubility because of false negatives (especially in infants) and the lack of specificity needed for genetic counseling.

4. Prenatal testing can be done on genetic material obtained from amniocentesis or fetoscopy.

5. Peripheral blood smear shows sickling.

6. Hallmark of sickle cell disease is anemia.
   a. Hematocrit 20 to 30
   b. Reticulocyte count 10 to 20 per cent

7. Hyperbilirubinemia secondary to hemolysis

8. White blood cell count increased even in absence of infection.

9. Serum iron normal.

10. Watch for iron overload in patients receiving multiple blood transfusions.

11. Hepatitis C screening should be considered in patients who have received multiple transfusions.

Note

Hb S alters the results of Hb A_{1c} testing, decreasing the utility of this test in sickle cell patients who have diabetes mellitus.

Key Tests

- Complete blood count
- Blood smear
- Reticulocyte count
- Hemoglobin electrophoresis
- Serum bilirubin

Treatment

1. Frequent monitoring of symptoms and growth parameters; assessment of nutritional status (including protein intake); examination of heart, lungs, spleen, and feet; and measurement of hematocrit and reticulocyte count

2. Penicillin prophylaxis is the mainstay of management of children with sickle cell disease.
   a. Penicillin V, 125 mg PO bid from 3 months to 3 years of age
   b. Dose is increased to 250 mg PO bid until age 5.
   c. If the patient has not had any serious infections or a splenectomy and is receiving comprehensive care, prophylaxis can be stopped at age 5. The parents are cautioned to seek medical attention for any febrile illness.
   d. Erythromycin can be used in the penicillin-allergic child.
   e. As the incidence of penicillin-resistant *Streptococcus pneumoniae* increases, other antibiotics may be required.

3. Children with sickle cell disease should receive the usual recommended immunizations.
   a. Closely monitor postvaccination fever because it may in fact be sepsis.
   b. Additional immunizations are recommended:
      (1) Influenza vaccine annually
      (2) Pneumococcal vaccine at age 2 with a booster between the ages of 3 and 5
      (3) A single quadrivalent meningococcal vaccine after the age of 2

4. Pregnancy carries a higher maternal and perinatal risk compared to the general population. Women of childbearing age should be counseled of the risks. Oral progesterone-only contraception pills or depot medroxyprogesterone are preferred over estrogen-containing pills because of the increased risk of thrombosis.

5. Pain
   a. Create a pain management plan for each patient.
   b. Patients should have a supply of oral medications, either a nonsteroidal anti-inflammatory drug or a codeine-based narcotic, for home use.
   c. Instruct parents or other caregivers on the proper usage of pain medication in children.
   d. There is a tendency to underdose pain, which leads to other problems not the least of which is creating anxiety and preventing trust.
   e. Severe pain: parenteral medication or a fentanyl patch, with IV fluids (hydration reduces viscosity and sludging).
   f. Use oxygen judiciously; it can cause bone marrow suppression.
   g. Intractable pain: short course of oral steroids

6. Indications for transfusion
   a. Severe anemia
   b. Before surgery or arteriography
   c. Priapism
   d. Acute chest syndrome
   e. Stroke or transient ischemic attack (acutely or preventive to decrease reoccurrence)
   f. Chronic leg ulcers
   g. Pregnancy

7. Nutrition and exercise
   a. There is increasing evidence that sickle cell patients have higher nutritional requirements because of higher basal metabolic rates and protein turnover. This may be related in part to the growth delay that is often present.
      (1) Folic acid supplementation must be started early and continue throughout life.
      (2) Consider other vitamins, zinc, and magnesium.
   b. It is thought that sickle cell patients adopt a less rigorous lifestyle to adapt to their nutritional status. Patients must be cautioned about vigorous exercise because of the increased risk resulting from dehydration and increased oxygen demand.
   c. Patients must avoid unpressurized environments such as small planes and helicopters.

8. Hydroxyurea
   a. Hydroxyurea can stimulate Hb F production, which reduces polymerization. Research trials in both children and adults with severe sickle cell disease demonstrate an increase in Hb F and a reduction of symptoms.
   b. Hydroxyurea must be used with caution because of its potential hematologic and reproductive side effects.
   c. Erythropoietin may be used alone or in combination with hydroxyurea to stimulate Hb F.
   d. Iron may need to be given with erythropoietin, even if iron stores are normal.

9. Bone marrow transplantation (BMT): Internationally, over 100 BMTs for sickle cell disease have been performed, most of them in Europe. The overall survival rate is reported to be 90 to 95 per cent.

10. The next level of treatment for the future lies in genetic engineering.

Key Treatment

- Penicillin prophylaxis in children

- Pneumococcal, influenza, and meningococcal vaccines plus standard immunizations

- Analgesics

- Folic acid

- Blood transfusions

Follow-Up

1. Monitor pain medication

2. Patient education

3. Monitor for psychosocial concerns

4. Genetic counseling

Bibliography

Bunn HF: Pathogenesis and treatment of sickle cell disease. N Engl J Med 1997;337:762–769.

Charache S, Johnson CS (eds): Sickle cell disease. Hematol Oncol Clin North Am 1996;10.

Committee on Genetics, American Academy of Pediatrics: Health supervision for children with sickle cell disease and their families. Pediatrics 1996;98:467–472.

Davies SC, Roberts IAG: Bone marrow transplant for sickle cell disease—an update. Arch Dis Child 1996; 75:3–6.

Lane PA: Sickle cell disease. Pediatr Clin North Am 1996; 43:639–659.

160 Thalassemia Syndromes

Vipul N. Mankad

1. Definition: Thalassemias are inherited disorders characterized by hypochromic microcytic anemia caused by decreased synthesis of one of the globin chains.

2. Historical aspects: In 1925, Cooley described a group of children with severe anemia, striking skeletal and facial abnormalities and splenomegaly, bizarre morphology of red blood cells, and circulating nucleated red cells. The term *Cooley's anemia* is frequently used to describe this condition. Early observation that these children were of Italian or Greek ancestry led to the term *thalassemia* (*thalassa* = sea).

3. Malarial hypothesis: Although severe forms of the disease (e.g., homozygous β-thalassemia) were invariably fatal in the first 2 years of life and therefore could not contribute to propagation of the gene, autosomal recessive thalassemia genes were maintained in certain populations because of the protection conferred against malaria in individuals with the trait.

4. Geographic distribution and public health significance: Various forms of thalassemia are prevalent in Italy, Greece, Arabian peninsula, Turkey, Iran, India, Southeast Asia (including Thailand, Cambodia, and southern China), and in U.S. populations with ancestry from those areas; also in Africans and African Americans. The α-thalassemias are more common than the β-thalassemias. However, because the more severe forms of α-thalassemias lead to intrauterine death and do not pose a major public health problem, it is the β-thalassemias and hemoglobin E, a structural variant that produces a phenotype of thalassemia and which in combination with β-thalassemia can produce a severe form of anemia, that present a major international public health challenge.

Pathophysiology

The adult hemoglobin (Hb A) molecule is a tetramer of two α-globin and two β-globin polypeptide chains. When the synthesis of α- or β-globin chain is decreased as a result of one of the variety of mutations in the globin genes, imbalance in the synthesis of globin chains occurs. Excess globin chains precipitate in the red blood cells, aggregate into protein inclusions (Heinz bodies), and cause membrane changes resulting in hemolysis. Profound deficiency in synthesis of α- or β-globin chains results in marked reduction in synthesis of hemoglobin A and ineffective erythropoiesis.

Genetics

1. There are many mutations that account for β-thalassemia syndromes.

    a. Thalassemia major (Cooley's anemia), or "homozygous" β-thalassemia, is a clinically severe disease caused by the presence of two identical or dissimilar mutations causing decreased β-globin chain synthesis. The hypochromic anemia in these patients is so severe that dependency on blood transfusions is established at an early age because the hemoglobin levels decrease below 4 gm/dl.

    b. Thalassemia intermedia is characterized as a moderate disorder, usually caused by two β-thal mutations, not associated with transfusion dependence. These patients have hemoglobin levels over 7 gm/dl and have splenomegaly.

    c. Thalassemia minor is due to the presence of a single β-thal mutation and is characterized by microcytosis, hypochromia, and mild anemia; therefore, it is often misdiagnosed as iron deficiency anemia.

2. The α-globin synthesis is under control of two pairs of α-globin genes (total of four genes). The four α-thalassemias are

    a. α-Thalassemia-2 trait, or asymptomatic, silent carrier state

    b. α-Thalassemia-1 trait, resulting from deletion or malfunctioning of two α-globin genes and associated with mild, microcytic hypochromic anemia

        (1) The α-thalassemia-1 trait (i.e., deletion of two α-globin genes) can occur as a result of either removal of both loci from the same chromosome (*cis* deletion) or removal of one locus each from two chromosomes (*trans* deletion).

        (2) *Cis* deletion is found in Asian and Mediterranean populations, and therefore hydrops fetalis, deletion of four α-globin

genes, or homozygous occurrence of *cis* deletions is found in these populations.

   (3) African American populations are likely to have the *trans* deletion type of α-thalassemia-1 trait and therefore are not as likely to have hydrops fetalis as are Asian and Mediterranean people.

  c. Three loci of α-globin genes affected, as in hemoglobin H disease (a tetramer of β-globin chains): associated with moderately severe hemolytic anemia; usually not requiring chronic transfusions

  d. All four loci deleted or nonfunctional, which causes formation of Bart's hemoglobin (tetramer of γ-globin chains) and hydrops fetalis

3. Hemoglobin E (Hb E) syndromes

  a. Populations from Cambodia, Thailand, and Vietnam, including immigrants from these regions living in the United States, have high prevalence of hemoglobin E mutation. In this mutant, lysine replaces glutamic acid at the 26th position of the β-globin chain. The mutation in this "cryptic" RNA-splicing region causes a structurally abnormal hemoglobin, which is not translated appropriately.

  b. Heterozygous Hb E trait resembles a very mild β-thalassemia trait. Homozygous Hb E patients have more marked red cell abnormalities but are asymptomatic. Compound heterozygotes of Hb E and β-thalassemia produce hemolytic anemia similar to β-thalassemia intermedia or major (i.e., transfusion dependent).

  c. Hb E syndromes are important because they are so common in Southeast Asian populations.

Symptoms and Clinical Findings

1. Hematologic

  a. The child is not anemic at birth because fetal hemoglobin containing γ-globin chains predominates normally. Within the first few months of life, severe microcytic hypochromic anemia develops when β-globin chains fail to replace γ-globin chains. The hemoglobin level is usually 3 to 4 gm/dl. Fetal hemoglobin predominates (10 to 90 per cent) on electrophoresis. Hemoglobin A_2 level may be elevated.

  b. Serum bilirubin, aspartate transaminase, and alanine transaminase are frequently increased.

  c. Low levels of serum zinc and biochemical evidence of folic acid deficiency are found.

Increased iron level (serum ferritin) is found as a result of transfusional iron overload and/or increased absorption of iron from the gastrointestinal tract.

2. Skeletal abnormalities

  a. Hypertrophy and expansion of erythroid marrow results in skeletal deformities.

  b. The skull radiograph shows classic hair-on-end appearance as a result of bony trabeculae and widened diploic spaces. The maxilla is markedly overgrown, resulting in malocclusion of teeth. These changes cause the typical facial appearance called *Cooley's anemia facies*.

  c. Marked osteoporosis and cortical thinning may predispose to pathologic fractures of long bones and vertebrae, which may cause cord compression.

3. Hepatic changes: The liver is enlarged as a result of extramedullary hematopoiesis, cirrhosis and nodular regeneration, and iron deposition. Gallstones are present in more than 15 per cent of patients over age 15.

4. Cardiopulmonary abnormalities

  a. Cardiac dilatation and congestive cardiac failure secondary to severe anemia would be expected in untransfused thalassemia major patients. Blood transfusion therapy prevents this complication, but, in patients who are not on intensive chelation therapy, myocardial hemosiderosis occurs by the second decade.

  b. Increased P-R interval, first-degree heart block, and premature atrial or ventricular contractions and depression of ST segment are noted.

  c. Echocardiography provides a noninvasive assessment of cardiac function.

  d. Sterile pericarditis, friction rub, and pericardial effusion are not uncommon.

  e. Pulmonary problems are few, but restrictive or obstructive defects may be found.

5. Other organs

  a. The kidneys are frequently enlarged.

  b. Massive splenomegaly is unusual in transfused thalassemia major patients. However, splenectomy may help in lengthening the interval between transfusion therapy.

  c. Growth retardation, delayed or absent adolescent growth spurt, delayed menarche, oligomenorrhea or amenorrhea, poor development of secondary sexual characteristics, and hypogonadism are common.

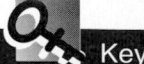

Key Symptoms

- Pallor
- Fatigue
- Dark urine

Key Signs

- Anemia, jaundice
- Hepatosplenomegaly
- Cooley's anemia facies
- Cardiac failure/dilation

Key Tests

- Complete blood count, reticulocyte count, and peripheral blood smear
- Hemoglobin electrophoresis
- Globin biosynthetic studies
- Assessment of iron overload

Laboratory Tests

1. Assessment of iron overload
   a. Serum iron, transferrin, transferrin saturation, and transferrin receptor concentration do not measure body iron stores quantitatively. Plasma or serum ferritin levels indirectly measure body iron stores. However, interpretation of ferritin values is confounded by ascorbate deficiency, fever, acute infection, chronic inflammation, acute and chronic hepatic damage, hemolysis, and ineffective erythropoiesis. Therefore, other indirect measurements, such as 24-hour deferoxamine-induced urinary iron excretion, imaging of tissue iron using computerized tomography, nuclear resonance scattering from mangenese-56, and magnetic resonance imaging, are often used to assess iron overload.
   b. Direct measurement of hepatic iron concentration is the most quantitative, specific, and sensitive method of determining iron burden in patients with thalassemia major. Although this procedure requires liver biopsy, some authors recommend measurement of hepatic iron concentration before initiating iron chelation treatment and for monitoring. Magnetic susceptometry using superconducting quantum interference device (SQUID) has been suggested but is generally not available.
2. Cardiac function and anterior pituitary reserve are assessed as indicators of organ function.

Treatment

Improved blood transfusion support and iron chelation therapy have transformed thalassemia major from a fatal disease to a chronic disease with prolonged survival and near-normal quality of life. Bone marrow transplantation is available to some patients, and future prospects of gene therapy have improved. In addition, agents such as 5-azacytidine, hydroxyurea, recombinant human erythropoietin, and various butyrate analogues are being investigated in β-thalassemia major to reactivate fetal hemoglobin. Aggressive programs of prenatal screening and diagnosis can reduce the frequency of birth of patients with thalassemia major. However, these benefits have not accrued to patients in poor, less industrialized countries.

1. Blood transfusion and iron chelation
   a. Patients transfused to levels of hemoglobin adequate to suppress endogenous hematopoiesis (i.e., never permitted to fall below 9.5 gm/dl) do not develop skeletal malformations and cardiomegaly. Higher baseline level of hemoglobin (e.g., Hb 11 gm/dl) would be more physiologic but would cause a greater iron overload. Ten milliliters per kilogram of packed leukocyte-poor red cells (achieved by using leukocyte filters) should be transfused every 2 to 3 weeks at a rate not to exceed 4 ml/kg/hour. Diuretics may be necessary for patients with potential cardiac decompensation. When requirements of blood exceed 200 ml/kg/year, splenectomy may be performed to reduce the transfusion needs. Such patients should receive a pneumococcal vaccine and be watched for serious infections. Because of risk of serious infections, splenectomy is not recommended before 5 years.
   b. Iron chelation is achieved by subcutaneous administration of deferoxamine at a dose of 25 to 40 mg/kg with a limit of 2 gm during 8 hours daily. Initiation and monitoring of dose should be guided by assessment of iron

stores as described above. Higher intravenous doses can be given for selected patients.

c. Toxicity of and compliance with iron chelation therapy: High-frequency hearing loss, retinal abnormalities, metaphysical and spinal abnormalities, and reduced growth are among toxicities of deferoxamine therapy. However, benefits of extended survival free of iron-induced complications and improved quality of life outweigh toxicities, which should be closely monitored. Compliance with monitored deferoxamine treatment is less than 70 per cent.

d. Oral chelators: Many compounds have been screened as oral iron chelators. From these, 1,2-dimethyl-3-hydroxypyrid-4-one (L_1, Deferiprone) has entered long-term trials in thalassemia patients.

2. Bone marrow transplantation and gene therapy

a. The ultimate therapy would be to remove patients' bone marrow cells, replace the abnormal gene or insert a normal β-globin gene, and reinfuse the marrow. Currently, this is not possible. However, several outstanding investigators around the world are attempting to achieve a genetic cure.

b. Bone marrow transplantation from a histocompatible donor is an alternative. Best results are achieved in patients who are young and are in good clinical condition. Lucarelli's group in Pesaro demonstrated that hepatomegaly and portal fibrosis were the two most important risk factors. The event-free survival varied from 94 per cent in class I patients (neither complication) to 80 per cent for class II (one risk factor) and 61 per cent for class III (both risk factors). The decision rests on weighing the risks described above and the benefits of cure with good quality of life.

Bibliography

Hoffbrand AV: Oral iron chelation. Semin Hematol 1996; 33:1–8.

Lucarelli G, Galimberti M, Polchi P, et al: Bone marrow transplantation in patients with thalassemia. N Engl J Med 1990;322:417–421.

Olivieri NF: Reactivation of fetal hemoglobin in patients with beta thalassemia. Semin Hematol 1996;33:24–42.

Olivieri NF, Brittenham GM: Iron-chelating therapy and the treatment of thalassemia. Blood 1997;89:739–761.

Weatherall DJ, Clegg JB: Thalassemia—a global public health problem. Nat Med 1996;2:847–849.

161 Neutropenia

Russell P. Gollard

Etiology

1. Neutropenia is the most frequent cause of leukopenia. Neutropenia is termed severe if there are fewer than 500 neutrophils (polymorphonuclear leukocytes and band leukocytes) per microliter, moderate if there are between 500 and 1000 neutrophils/μl, and mild if there are 1000 to 2000 cells/μl.

2. Neutropenia may arise from either decreased production, increased destruction, or peripheral margination.

3. Virtually all cytotoxic drugs (chemotherapeutic agents) cause a profound transient neutropenia 10 to 14 days after therapy.

   a. Noncytotoxic drugs such as antibiotics (chloramphenicol, penicillin, and sulfa drugs), antiviral drugs (zidovudine, gancyclovir), phenothiazines, some diuretics, antihydroid drugs, anti-inflammatory agents (gold salts, phenylbutazone), and histamine$_2$-blocking agents (ranitidine), and numerous other prescription drugs and toxic chemicals (benzene) can cause frank neutropenia or aplastic states of which neutropenia is a part.

   b. Drugs such as aminopyrine, α-methyldopa, phenylbutazone, mercurial diuretics, and some phenothiazines can cause peripheral destruction.

4. Hematologic diseases such as aplastic anemia, leukemia (lymphoid and myeloid), lymphomas (Hodgkin's and non-Hodgkin's), metastatic solid tumors, myelodysplasia, and myelofibrosis can cause neutropenia. In addition, genetic syndromes such as congenital hypoplastic neutropenia (Kostmann's syndrome) and cyclic neutropenia are known causes of neutropenia.

5. Chronic idiopathic neutropenia is characterized by a mild neutropenia of unknown cause. Patients with subpopulations of suppressor T lymphocytes that suppress granulopoiesis through a humoral factor have been described. These syndromes are more common in African Americans and may have a genetic basis. Vitamin B$_{12}$ and folate deficiencies are well-established causes of neutropenia, particularly in alcoholics. Neutropenia also may occur in individuals with eating disorders (bulimia, anorexia nervosa).

6. The infectious causes of neutropenia are many and include human immunodeficiency virus infection, bunyaviruses, arboviruses, phleboviruses, measles, infectious mononucleosis, viral hepatitis, and cytomegalovirus. Neutropenia caused by an acute viral infection is often accompanied by thrombocytopenia and/or transaminitis. Other infectious causes include tuberculosis, typhoid fever, brucellosis, tularemia, malaria, histoplasmosis, and leishmaniasis.

7. Neutrophils may be destroyed peripherally in individuals with Felty's syndrome or systemic lupus erythematosus (SLE).

   a. Antineutrophil antibodies also cause peripheral destruction, and, in cirrhotic individuals or those with Gaucher's disease, neutrophils may be trapped in the spleen.

   b. An overwhelming bacterial infection (sepsis syndrome), hemodialysis, and cardiopulmonary bypass all can cause peripheral margination.

Symptoms

1. Mild and moderate neutropenias may be clinically asymptomatic. When the neutrophil count falls below 1000 cells/μl, there is a progressively increasing susceptibility to infections with bacterial and fungal pathogens. Infections are uncommon in patients with absolute neutrophil counts greater than 500.

2. Infections are usually symptomatic, even while common localizing signs of inflammation may be absent.

3. Common pathogens include gram-negative bacilli, *Staphylococcus aureus*, *Staphylococcus epidermidis*, *Candida* species, and *Aspergillus* species.

4. The most likely source of bacteremia in a neutropenic patient with a fever and without an indwelling line is endogenous flora of the mouth and gut.

Key Symptoms

- Fever
- Odynophagia
- Painful defecation
- Respiratory distress
- Inflammation
- Lethargy
- Skin lesions

WARNING

Fever in a neutropenic patient is a medical emergency and generally requires hospital admission.

Clinical Findings

1. Findings frequently depend on the duration and severity of neutropenia.
2. Severely neutropenic patients frequently have oral thrush (postchemotherapy neutropenia and prolonged neutropenia) and perianal erythema or perirectal abscesses.
3. In addition, these patients frequently are found to have dullness to percussion and auscultation on lung examination. Hepatomegaly and splenomegaly also can be seen. Frequent findings in long-term neutropenic individuals include multiple poorly healed skin abscesses.
4. Patients may present with any combination of signs of the sepsis syndrome, including fever, tachycardia, cool clammy skin, hyperventilation, and postural hypotension.

Key Signs

- Fever
- Lymphadenopathy
- Oral thrush
- Skin abscesses
- Tachycardia
- Postural hypotension

WARNING

Digital rectal examinations are strongly contraindicated in neutropenic patients.

Laboratory Tests

1. The peripheral smear is important. A left-shifted differential (>10 per cent bands), toxic granulation, and the presence of Dohle bodies indicate a high likelihood of infection or a marrow in the recovery phase after a toxic insult. A paucity of immature forms, in contrast, suggests a toxic process. A low white count coupled with significant bandemia (and sometimes thrombocytopenia) suggests the sepsis syndrome.
2. Serial determinations of the complete blood count (CBC) for 4 to 6 weeks may be most useful in documenting the course of a mild neutropenia rather than other more invasive, expensive, or esoteric tests. (The normal range of white blood cells in African Americans and Yemenite Jews is somewhat less than average, and neutropenias in these populations are defined as less than 1.5×10^9 cells/L.)
3. The bone marrow is the gold standard for assessment of neutrophil production.
   a. Marrow infiltration (myelophthisis) may be seen in hematologic neoplasms (leukemia, lymphoma) and metastatic solid tumors or in certain infectious processes (presence of granulomas, organisms).
   b. When neutropenia is caused by a toxic insult, near-absence of immature forms, or "maturation arrest," will be seen.
   c. When neutrophils are destroyed peripherally or marginated (autoimmune processes, sepsis), immature granulocytes are abundant.
4. Macrocytosis (mean corpuscular volume > 100 fl) and nuclear-cytoplasm dyssynchrony suggest vitamin B_{12} and/or folate deficiency. Chronically ill individuals and alcoholics are particularly at risk, but patients receiving chemotherapy or suffering from myelodysplasia also can develop macrocytosis. Strict vegetarians need B_{12} supplementation. Vitamin B_{12} (normally 250 to 1100 pg/ml) may be drawn to assess stores in such individuals. Vitamin B_{12} deficiency may be masked by prior administration of this drug.
5. The anti-granulocyte antibody may be positive in autoimmune disorders and in such disorders as Felty's syndrome and SLE.
6. Chromosomal studies can be useful in differentiating myelodysplasia from drug- or toxin-induced suppression.
7. Blood cultures are mandatory in patients with neutropenia and fevers. Urine, sputum, or other body fluid cultures are suggested in clinically indicated patients.

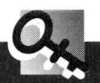

Key Tests

- CBC
- Bone marrow aspiration and biopsy
- Folate, B$_{12}$ levels
- Anti-granulocyte antibody
- Chromosome studies
- Body fluid cultures in febrile patients

Differential Diagnosis

1. Decreased production: drug or toxic effect, infection, hematologic neoplasm, metastatic disease, miscellaneous (chronic idiopathic neutropenia, cyclic neutropenia)
2. Peripheral destruction/margination: drug effect, autoimmune phenomena, splenic sequestration, sepsis, cardiopulmonary bypass, hemodialysis

Treatment

1. First, determine the underlying pathogenesis (drug, toxin, infection, neoplasm, vitamin deficiency). All possible drugs should be stopped immediately.
2. Folate is available in many forms and in deficiency states should be administered intraorally daily. Vitamin B$_{12}$ can be administered intramuscularly in deficient states, 1000 μg daily for 5 to 10 days and then 1000 μg monthly. New oral and nasal preparations are also available for patients not afflicted with pernicious anemia.
3. Granulocyte colony-stimulating factor (G-CSF; filgrastim [Neupogen]) and granulocyte-macrophage colony-stimulating factor (GM-CSF; sargramostim [Leukine, Prokine]) are commercially available genetically engineered cytokines useful in the treatment of severe neutropenia, especially in the postchemotherapy nadir period. Because of their expense and potential side effects or toxicities, it is suggested that they be given only under supervision of a hematologist or oncologist, at least initially. G-CSF and GM-CSF are given daily subcutaneously at a dosage of 5 mg/kg and 250 mg/m^2, respectively. G-GSF or GM-CSF should never be given concomitantly during the administration of chemotherapy or 24 hours thereafter, nor should either drug be given in patients with acute leukemia before induction chemotherapy.

4. Febrile neutropenia is a medical emergency and demands hospitalization, culturing of body fluids, and intravenous antibiotics. Prophylactic antibiotic therapy is a controversial issue, and therapy should always be individualized.

Diet

A low-bacteria diet is necessary in patients with prolonged neutropenia.

Activity

Patients should avoid individuals with known communicable diseases in the home and in the workplace. Most hospitals have infection control departments and have specific requirements for the care of neutropenic patients.

Key Treatment

- Folate
- Vitamin B$_{12}$
- G-CSF and GM-CSF
- Thiamine

Bibliography

For more information on the use of colony-stimulating factors in patients with neutropenic fever, see
Beveridge RA, Miller JA: Impact of colony stimulating factors on the practice of oncology. Oncology 1993; 7(Suppl):43–48.

For a general overview of leukopenia, see
Coates TD, Bachner R: Leukocytosis and leukopenia. In Hoffman R, Bent EJ, Shattil SJ, et al (eds): Hematology, 2nd ed, pp 769–784. New York, Churchill Livingstone, 1995.
Dale D: Neutropenia. In Beutler E, Lichtman MA, Coller BS, et al (eds): Williams' Hematology, 5th ed, pp 815–824. New York, McGraw-Hill, 1995.
Holland SM, Gallin JI: Disorders of granulocytes and monocytes. In Fauci A, Braunwald E, Isselhacher KJ, et al (eds): Harrison's Principles of Internal Medicine, 14th ed, pp 351–359. New York, McGraw-Hill, 1998.

For a detailed look at the treatment of infections in immunocompromised patients, see
Pizzo PA, Meyers J, Freifeld AG, et al: Infections in the cancer patient. In DeVita VT Jr, Hellman S, Rosenberg SA (eds): Cancer: Principles and Practice of Oncology, 5th ed, pp 2569–2704. Philadelphia, JB Lippincott Company, 1998.

For a general overview of neutropenia, with special emphasis on drug-related causes, see
Rapaport SI: Introduction to Hematology, 2nd ed, pp 409–412, 426–429. Philadelphia, JB Lippincott Company, 1987.

For more information on low-bacteria diets, see
Remington JS, Schimpff SC: Please don't eat the salads. N Engl J Med 1981;304:433–435.

162 Thrombocytopenia

Hal S. Shimazu

Platelets provide the first line of defense against bleeding, forming a platelet adhesive plug in traumatized capillaries and small arterioles. Thrombocytopenia is one of the most common acquired causes of abnormal bleeding. Normal platelet count is between 150,000 and 450,000/mm^3, with a 7- to 10-day platelet lifespan in the peripheral circulation. Twenty to 30 per cent of platelets are sequestered in the spleen.

Etiology

Thrombocytopenia (platelet count <150,000/mm^3) may be caused by (1) decreased platelet production, (2) increased platelet destruction, or (3) hypersplenic sequestration (see Table 162–1).

TABLE 162–1. ETIOLOGY OF THROMBOCYTOPENIA

Decreased Platelet Production
- Aplastic anemia
- Bone marrow replacement: myelophthisic process (e.g., leukemia, lymphoma, and tumor metastasis), granulomatous disease, myelofibrosis, multiple myeloma, lipid histiocytosis (e.g., Gaucher's disease)
- Ineffective thrombopoiesis: vitamin B$_{12}$, folate or iron deficiencies, myelodysplastic syndromes
- Acute viral infections: rubella, cytomegalovirus, Epstein-Barr virus (EBV), human immunodeficiency virus (HIV), hepatitis
- Drugs/physical agents: sulfas, thiazides, estrogen/diethylstilbestrol, alcohol, cocaine, phenylbutazone, cytotoxins, X-radiation, biologic response modulators (e.g., interferon and interleukin)
- Congenital: TAR syndrome (thrombocytopenia with absent radii), Fanconi's anemia, Wiskott-Aldrich syndrome, May-Hegglin anomaly

Increased Platelet Destruction
- Immune destruction
  - –Autoimmune: idiopathic thrombocytopenic purpura, secondary causes (e.g., systemic lupus erythematosus, lymphoma, chronic lymphocytic leukemia, Evan's syndrome with coexistant Coombs'-positive anemia)
  - –Drugs: over 150 drugs implicated (see Table 162–2)
  - –Infectious: acute EBV, HIV, viral hepatitis, bacterial septicemia, malaria, ?varicella
  - –Alloimmune: neonatal, post-transfusion purpura
- Nonimmune destruction
  - –Disseminated intravascular coagulation
  - –Thrombotic microangiopathies: thrombotic thrombocytopenic purpura, hemolytic-uremic syndrome, malignant hypertension, toxemia of pregnancy, pregnancy-related HELLP syndrome (hemolysis, elevated liver enzymes, low platelet count)
  - –Miscellaneous: dilution from massive transfusions, prosthetic intravascular devices, extracorporeal circulation (e.g., cardiopulmonary bypass and hemodialysis), giant cavernous hemangiomas

Hypersplenic Sequestration

1. Decreased platelet production
   a. Congenital syndromes are rare.
   b. The most common acquired defects are aplastic anemia, myelofibrosis, or malignant bone marrow infiltration, which also affects other cell lines.
   c. Other causes that can be more specific to defective thrombopoiesis include toxins (alcohol and cocaine), acute viral infections (including acute viral hepatitis and also human immunodeficiency virus [HIV], which more commonly causes immune thrombocytopenia), drugs (most commonly thiazides, estrogens, and cytotoxic agents), and nutritional deficiencies (vitamin B$_{12}$, folate, iron).

2. Increased platelet destruction: the most common cause of thrombocytopenia and mediated by immune and nonimmune means
   a. Immune thrombocytopenia: includes autoimmune, drug-induced antibodies, and alloantibodies
      (1) Immunoglobulin (Ig) G–mediated (rarely IgA, IgM) primary autoimmune thrombocytopenia (also known as idiopathic thrombocytopenic purpura [ITP]) is a diagnosis of exclusion. ITP presents differently in children and adults. In children ITP is acute; symptomatic, most often presenting at 2 to 4 years of age with equal sex distribution; commonly postviral; and self-limited, with spontaneous resolution in 80 per cent usually within a few weeks but up to 6 to 12 months. In adults, ITP is usually more insidious and chronic, typically affecting young women, with only 5 per cent spontaneous recovery.
      (2) Secondary autoimmune thrombocytopenias occur most commonly with systemic lupus erythematosus (20 per cent eventual risk) and lymphomas.
      (3) Over 150 drugs are implicated in immune thrombocytopenia, with quinine (remember tonic water), quinidine, and cimetidine most commonly responsible (see Table 162–2). Two mechanisms are described: a drug-platelet hapten or,

TABLE 162-2. COMMON DRUGS IMPLICATED IN IMMUNE THROMBOCYTOPENIA

Antibiotics	Penicillins, cephalosporins, sulfonamides, ciprofloxacin, rifampin, vancomycin, gentamicin, trimethoprim
Antihistamines	Histamine$_2$ antagonists, chlorpheniramine
Antihypertensives	Captopril, methyldopa
Cardiac	Digoxin, quinidine, procainamide, amiodarone, lidocaine, dipyridamole
Diuretics	Furosemide, thiazides, spironolactone
Neuropsychiatric	Tricyclic antidepressants, carbamazepine, phenytoin, valproic acid
Rheumatologic	Aspirin, nonsteroidal anti-inflammatory drugs, gold, chloroquine
Miscellaneous	Quinine, acetaminophen, heroin, heparin, iodinated contrast agents, insecticides

more commonly, the platelet as an "innocent bystander." Of special note, heparin-associated thrombocytopenia (HAT) occurs in up to 10 per cent of patients on IV heparin (subcutaneous less common). The much more common type I HAT is usually mild, asymptomatic, and probably not immune related. The less common but devastating type II HAT represents an immune-mediated process of platelet aggregation and activation leading to intravascular arterial and venous thrombosis with a severe consumptive thrombocytopenia.

(4) Among the infections that cause immune thrombocytopenia, HIV can affect 10 per cent of asymptomatic carriers and 30 per cent of acquired immunodeficiency syndrome patients and should be ruled out in the presence of risk factors. There is strong evidence that viral hepatitis (A, B, and C) can cause immune thrombocytopenia.

(5) Alloimmune post-transfusion purpura is rare but potentially severe, with the host (typically a multiparous female negative for the P1^{A1} platelet antigen) being sensitized to the P1^{A1} antigen from transfused blood products and developing a paradoxical destruction of the host's own platelets (unclear mechanism), leading to severe thrombocytopenia about 1 week post-transfusion. Neonatal alloimmune thrombocytopenia is based on the same P1^{A1} antigen, with an antigen-positive fetus sensitizing an antigen-negative mother.

b. Nonimmune thrombocytopenia

(1) Disseminated intravascular coagulation (DIC) can present in a myriad of serious clinical settings and is associated with excessive thrombin production, triggered coagulation cascade, and widespread microvascular thrombosis (see Ch. 171, Disseminated Intravascular Coagulation).

(2) Thrombotic thrombocytopenic purpura (TTP) and hemolytic-uremic syndrome (HUS) are serious disorders resulting from platelet consumption by platelet microvascular thrombosis without activation of the coagulation cascade; hence prothrombin time (PT), partial thromboplastin time (PTT), and fibrin split products (FSP) are normal. TTP (rare) and HUS (common cause of acute renal failure in children) share features including thrombocytopenia, microangiopathic anemia, and renal abnormalities (more severe in HUS), with central nervous system abnormalities prominent in TTP and less common in HUS.

3. Hypersplenic sequestration: Mild to moderate thrombocytopenia can result from splenomegaly from any cause, but most commonly alcoholic cirrhotic portal hypertension.

Symptoms

1. Bleeding from thrombocytopenia is typically into superficial sites, with easy bruisability, epistaxis, menorrhagia, mucosal bleeding, petechiae, and ecchymoses as common manifestations. In general, symptoms are as follows with various platelet counts.

   a. 100,000 to 150,000/mm^3: asymptomatic

   b. 50,000 to 100,000/mm^3: easy bruisability and bleeding post-traumatically

   c. 20,000 to 50,000/mm^3: at risk for serious, excessive post-traumatic bleeding

   d. <20,000/mm^3: at risk for spontaneous bleeding, including intracranial (infrequent but a major cause of mortality)

2. Historical queries should include prior platelet counts, past bleeding episodes (including surgical), family history of bleeding disorders, nutritional history (e.g., vegetarian), medications, alcohol, recreational drugs, high-risk sexual activity, and blood transfusions. Explore symptoms suggestive of hematologic, hepatic, immunologic, connective tissue, and infectious diseases.

Clinical Findings

1. Petechiae are the characteristic lesions occurring on skin and mucous membranes, especially in areas of increased capillary pressure or trauma (e.g., lower legs, face after coughing, buccal mucosa with chewing).
2. Physical examination should search for signs of lymphoma, hepatic disease, connective tissue disease, and infectious disease, with special focus for lymphadenopathy and hepatosplenomegaly.

Laboratory Tests

1. Complete blood count (CBC) and peripheral blood smear
   a. Essential to rule out "pseudothrombocytopenia" caused by the blood collection tube anticoagulant EDTA causing platelet clumping and an artificially low automated platelet count. Finger stick blood smear or an alternative anticoagulant, such as heparin or citrate, can confirm.
   b. Abnormalities of other cell lines suggest a marrow/production etiology, whereas isolated thrombocytopenia suggests peripheral destruction.
   c. Fragmented red blood cells (schistocytes) indicate a microangiopathic etiology.
   d. Elevated mean platelet volume (MPV) indicates increased thrombopoiesis as a result of increased platelet peripheral destruction or increased sequestration.
2. PT, PTT, and FSP are indicated in the ill, hospitalized, or postsurgical patient: abnormal in DIC and normal in TTP and HUS.
3. Bone marrow aspiration/biopsy is usually not necessary for isolated thrombocytopenia but is important to clarify platelet production problems when suspected with the presence of other cell line abnormalities.

4. Anti-platelet antibodies' usefulness is limited because of high false-positive and false-negative rates.
5. Other tests as indicated by history and physical findings (e.g., HIV antibodies, hepatosplenic imaging, viral serologies, rheumatologic serologies, serum protein electrophoresis)

Differential Diagnosis

1. Petechiae are characteristic of severe thrombocytopenia (although also seen in the rare occasions of microvascular pathology/dysfunction); otherwise easy bruisability and bleeding are nonspecific, representing any bleeding disorder.
2. ITP is a diagnosis of exclusion: An unremarkable history and physical with an isolated thrombocytopenia nearly rules out the differential of secondary causes.

Treatment

1. Platelet transfusion is indicated for serious bleeding or anticipated major surgery (6 units of random donor platelets [a "six pack"] increases the platelet count by 50,000/mm^3 in a 70-kg adult) and is the mainstay of therapy. A practical prophylactic transfusion guideline is to maintain platelet counts greater than 100,000/mm^3 for high-risk surgery; greater than 50,000/mm^3 for minor surgery, trauma, or presence of major bleeding; greater than 20,000/mm^3 in presence of minor bleeding; and greater than 5000 to 10,000/mm^3 if asymptomatic. Transfusions are generally contraindicated in post-transfusion purpura, TTP/HUS, and HAT.
2. Aminocaproic acid (antifibrinolytic agent) is effective for chronic mucosal bleeding: IV loading, then orally.
3. Decreased platelet production: Address underlying cause (e.g., offending drug, nutritional deficiency) and give transfusions as indicated.
4. Increased platelet destruction
   a. ITP and secondary autoimmune thrombocytopenia
      (1) First address possible primary disorders. Prednisone (1 to 2 mg/kg/day) is indicated for platelet counts less than 50,000/mm^3 with significant bleeding/bleeding risk or platelet counts less than

20,000/mm³. Response is usually within 1 to 3 weeks (80 per cent response rate), then taper to lowest effective dose to maintain 50,000/mm³.

(2) If ineffective or unacceptably high prednisone maintenance doses are needed, then splenectomy (80 per cent effective) is indicated (preoperative pneumococcal and *Haemophilus influenzae* vaccines are indicated).

(3) If splenectomy fails, danazol and immunosuppressive agents have been used with some success.

(4) Transfusions are limited to life-threatening bleeding because the platelet count increases for only a few hours.

(5) In childhood ITP, patients with platelet counts greater than 30,000/mm³ generally require no treatment. Those with platelet counts less than 20,000/mm³ with significant mucosal bleeding or less than 10,000/mm³ with minor purpura should receive IV IgG or steroids. Splenectomy is rarely needed.

b. Drug-induced thrombocytopenia: Discontinue suspected drug. If severe bleeding, a short course of prednisone may help. Platelet transfusions carry the same limitations and indications as in ITP.

c. Alloimune thrombocytopenia: Neonatal alloimmune thrombocytopenia is transient, benefiting from IV IgG and platelet transfusions (P1^A1-negative mother is most convenient donor) as indicated. Treatment of choice for post-transfusion purpura is IV IgG or plasmapheresis. Prednisone may help. Platelet transfusions are contraindicated.

d. Nonimmune thrombocytopenia

(1) DIC: see Ch. 171, Disseminated Intravascular Coagulation.

(2) TTP requires emergency plasmapheresis with fresh frozen plasma exchange. Steroids are typically used, although the roles of steroids as well as aspirin and dipyridamole are not clear. Platelet transfusions are generally contraindicated.

(3) HUS in adults is treated as for TTP plus renal support; in children, renal support is the primary therapy.

5. Hypersplenic sequestration: Usually mild to moderate thrombocytopenia, hence treatment is rarely necessary.

Patient Education

Precautions include contact sports, aspirin, nonsteroidal anti-inflammatory drugs, *Gingko biloba*, alcohol, IM injections, and pregnancy.

Key Treatment

- Address primary disorder or offending drug/toxin.
- No treatment usually necessary if asymptomatic.
- Platelet transfusions therapeutically/prophylactically
- Prednisone, splenectomy as indicated for autoimmune thrombocytopenia

Follow-Up

This is dictated by the severity of the thrombocytopenia and the nature of the underlying disorder, whether acute, chronic with exacerbations, or self-limited with possible recurrences.

Bibliography

George JN, Woolf SH, Raskol GE, et al: Idiopathic thrombocytopenic purpura: a practice guideline developed by explicit methods for the American Society of Hematology. Blood 1996;88:3–40.

Goldstein KH, Abramson N: Efficient diagnosis of thrombocytopenia. Am Fam Physician 1996;53:915–920.

Pulkrabek SM: Platelet antibodies. Clin Lab Med: Blood Banking 1996;16:817–834.

Rutherford CJ, Frenkel EP: Thrombocytopenia issues in diagnosis and therapy. Med Clin North Am 1994;78:555–575.

Schrier SL, Leung LLK: Disorders of hemostasis and coagulation. Sci Am Med 1997;5(Hematology VI):13–28.

163 Leukemia

Marc J. Chernoff

Leukemia is characterized by abnormal differentiation and proliferation of the lymphopoietic and hematopoietic stem cells. This disorder of normal cellular development and progression leads to accumulation of leukemic cells that respond poorly to normal regulatory cellular mechanisms, expand at the expense of normal lymphoid and myeloid cell lines, and infiltrate organs causing dysfunction.

Classification

For purposes of identification, prognosis, and treatment, the leukemias are divided into both acute and chronic forms.

Acute Leukemia

1. Acute myeloid leukemia (AML; acute nonlymphocytic leukemia, ANLL). This class is further divided into
   a. AML-M1
   b. AML-M2
   c. AML-M3 (acute promyelocytic)
   d. AML-M4 (acute myelomonocytic)
   e. AML-M5 (acute monocytic)
   f. AML-M6 (erythroleukemia)
   g. AML-M7 (megakaryocytic)
2. Acute lymphocytic leukemia (ALL). This class is further divided into
   a. ALL-L1
   b. ALL-L2
   c. ALL-L3 (Burkitt type)
3. Acute mixed lineage leukemia (AMLL)
4. Acute undifferentiated leukemia (AUL)

Chronic Leukemia

1. Chronic myelogenous leukemia (CML)
2. Chronic lymphocytic leukemia (CLL)
3. CLL variants
   a. Hairy cell leukemia
   b. T-cell chronic lymphocytic leukemia
   c. T-cell leukemia lymphoma
   d. Prolymphocytic leukemia

Etiology

The exact causes of leukemia are unknown, but there are associations with the following:

1. Hereditary factors, as in high-risk families

2. Congenital disorders
   a. Down's syndrome
   b. Bloom's syndrome
   c. Fanconi's anemia
   d. Kleinfelter's syndrome
   e. Ataxia-telangiectasia
   f. Osteogenesis imperfecta
   g. Wiskott-Aldrich syndrome
3. Underlying hematologic disorders
   a. Chronic myeloproliferative disorders (CML, agnogenic myeloid metaplasia, polycythemia vera, primary thrombocythemia)
   b. Preleukemic states/myelodysplastic syndromes
4. Irradiation
5. Chemical exposures (benzene, toluene)
6. Multiagent cytotoxic chemotherapy. Acute leukemia, predominantly myeloid, is a complication in patients treated with alkylators or immunosuppressive therapy in
   a. Hodgkin's lymphoma (especially those treated with MOPP)
   b. Non-Hodgkin's lymphoma
   c. Breast, ovary, lung, gastrointestinal tract, brain, ALL, myeloma
   d. Rheumatoid arthritis, Wegener's granulomatosis, histiocytosis X, polycythemia vera, Behçet's syndrome, Crohn's disease

Key Symptoms

- Fatigue, weakness

- Weight loss

- Bleeding: skin, gums, mucous membranes, genitourinary or gastrointestinal tract

- Infection: skin, throat, sinus, gums, respiratory or urinary tract

- Headache, nausea, vomiting, blurred vision, cranial nerve involvement

- Bone pain

- Abdominal distention and anorexia

- Lymphadenopathy
- Oliguria
- Obstipation
- Mental status alterations

Clinical Findings

1. The findings on examination also will parallel many of the symptoms.
2. A number of "unusual" presentations of leukemia may occur:
   a. Hyperleukocytosis
   b. Disseminated intravascular coagulopathy (DIC)
   c. Granulocytic sarcoma: tumors composed of myeloid cells, chloromas
   d. Central nervous system leukemia
   e. Leukemia cutis: leukemic skin infiltrates
   f. Sweet's syndrome: fever, neutrophilia, and painful, erythematous skin lesions
   g. Pyoderma gangrenosum: ulcerating, painful skin lesions
   h. Acute leukemia diagnosed during pregnancy

Key Signs

- Pallor, lethargy, and weakness
- Weight loss
- Purpura, petechiae, gingival hypertrophy or oozing, hematuria, melena
- Fever, chills, tissue infiltrates, pyoderma gangrenosum
- Papilledema, cranial nerve palsies, meningeal signs
- Bone tenderness
- Hepatosplenomegaly and abdominal tenderness
- Lymphadenopathy

Laboratory and Other Tests

1. Tests that may be useful
   a. Leukocyte alkaline phosphatase: decreased in CML
   b. Vitamin B_{12}: elevated in CML
   c. Urine and serum lysozyme (muramidase): seen in some forms of AML
   d. Serum protein electrophoresis: hypogammaglobulinemia seen in CLL
   e. Coombs' test: hemolytic anemias associated with leukemia

   f. Transfusion evaluation studies
   g. Human leukocyte antigen typing for potential bone marrow transplant candidates
   h. Human immunodeficiency virus (HIV) screen
2. Appropriate radiographic tests
   a. Chest radiograph
   b. Abdominal series
   c. Computerized tomographic scan
   d. Bone scan
   e. Sinus films
   f. Magnetic resonance imaging: especially in cases of suspected cord compression, dural, epidural, or meningeal involvement
3. Biopsy of infiltrated organs
4. Review the peripheral smear because there may be clues to help categorize the type of leukemia.
   a. Auer rods
   b. Hairy cells
   c. Smudge cells
   d. Platelet morphology
   e. Rouleaux formation
   f. Red cell morphology

Key Tests

- Complete blood count with differential
- Platelet count
- Electrolytes, including calcium, magnesium, PO_4, uric acid
- Liver function profile and renal function profile
- Coagulation studies: prothrombin time, International Normalized Ratio (INR), partial thromboplastin time; also a DIC panel: fibrinogen and fibrin split products
- Blood cultures when appropriate: aerobic, anaerobic, viral, fungal
- Bone marrow aspirate and core biopsy: histochemical, cytochemical, and immunologic staining and phenotyping, flow cytometry, and karyotypic analysis
- Analysis of the cerebrospinal fluid: cytology, cultures, and routine studies

Differential Diagnosis

1. Other considerations in the differential diagnosis include
   a. Distinction between marrow failure from

AML/ALL and other entities such as aplastic anemia

b. Marrow infiltration with nonhematopoietic tumors that may mimic clinical or laboratory features of ALL

   (1) In children, neuroblastoma or rhabdomyosarcoma

   (2) In adolescents and adults, Ewing's sarcoma or small cell lung carcinoma

c. When there is the presence of lymphadenopathy and/or splenomegaly, the following also should be considered:

   (1) Infectious causes: viral, bacterial, chlamydia, protozoan, mycotic, rickettsial, mycobacterial, HIV

   (2) Autoimmune causes: rheumatoid arthritis, lupus, dermatomyositis, mixed connective tissue disease, and Sjögren's syndrome

   (3) Iatrogenic hypersensitivity: serum sickness, drug hypersensitivity

   (4) Potentially malignant entities: angioimmunoblastic lymphadenopathy and Castleman's disease (angiofollicular lymph node hyperplasia)

   (5) Hodgkin's or non-Hodgkin's lymphoma

Treatment/Chemotherapy

Acute

1. AML: Treatment is divided into induction, consolidative, and maintenance therapy.

   a. Induction therapy consists of daunorubicin (Cerubidine) for 3 days and cytarabine (Cytosar) for 7 days, the so-called 7+3 regimen.

   b. Idarubicin (Idamycin), a synthetic anthracycline analogue, is also a potentially efficacious substitute for daunorubicin.

   c. High-dose cytarabine (ara-C) (HiDAC) is commonly used in patients with relapsed, refractory, or therapy-related AML.

   d. High-dose ara-C, 1 to 3 gm/m^2 of body surface area twice daily, is the preferred regimen for consolidation and maintenance therapy, and bone marrow transplant is usually reserved for "salvage" therapy.

   e. Treatment of the M3 subtype of AML is initiated by using all-*trans* retinoic acid, and further consolidation and maintenance with traditional agents.

2. ALL

   a. The most often used drugs in the induction of ALL are prednisone, vincristine (Oncovin), an anthracycline (e.g., daunorubicin), and asparaginase (Elspar).

   b. Consolidation therapy consists of regimens including agents such as VM26 (teniposide [Vumon]), VP16 (etoposide [VePesid]), HiDAC; combination therapy with VM26 and ara-C is promising.

   c. Maintenance therapy consists of mercaptopurine (Purinethol) and methotrexate.

   d. CNS prophylaxis: cranial irradiation; intrathecal methotrexate; administration of methotrexate, ara-C, and hydrocortisone via intraventricular reservoir; or high-dose systemic chemotherapy

Chronic

1. CML, chronic phase

   a. Busulfan (Myleran) and hydroxyurea (Hydrea) are agents of choice.

   b. Bone marrow transplant is also used in this phase.

2. CLL

   a. The major therapeutic modalities for CLL include chemotherapy and radiation therapy; splenectomy is also done.

   b. Commonly used agents are

   (1) Chlorambucil (Leukeran)

   (2) Cyclophosphamide (Cytoxan)

   (3) Fludarabine (Fludara)

   (4) 2-Chlorodeoxyadenosine (cladribine [Leustatin])

   (5) Deoxycoformycin (Nipent)

3. Hairy cell leukemia: promising results with 2-chlorodeoxyadenosine with or without interferon-alfa-2b (Intron A)

Bibliography

Burnett AK: Tailoring the treatment of AML. Curr Opin Hematol 1999;6:247–252.

Caligaris-Cappio F, Hamblin TJ: B-cell chronic lymphocytic leukemia: A bird of a different feather. J Clin Oncol 1999;17:399–408.

Faderl S, Talpaz M, Estrov Z, et al: Chronic myelogenous leukemia: biology and therapy. Ann Intern Med 1999; 131:207–219.

Melnick ST: Acute lymphoblastic leukemia. Clin Lab Med 1999;19:169–186.

Schumacher H: Acute Leukemia. Baltimore, Williams & Wilkins, 1998.

Tallman MS, Peterson LC, Hakimian D, et al: Treatment of hairy cell leukemia current views. Semin Hematol 1999;36:155–163.

Indications

1. Evaluate cytopenias (single or multiple cell line).
2. Determine marrow iron stores.
3. Evaluate leukocytosis: Consider flow cytometric and cytogenetic studies.
4. Diagnose suspected leukemias: Consider flow cytometric and cytogenetic studies.
5. Diagnose suspected myelodysplastic syndromes: Consider cytogenetic studies.
6. Diagnose suspected myeloproliferative disorders: Consider cytogenetic studies.
7. Diagnose suspected dysproteinemias.
8. Stage lymphomas/solid tumors.
9. Evaluate fever of unknown origin: Consider bacterial, fungal, acid-fast bacilli culture.
10. Assess result of therapy for leukemia or lymphoma.

Contraindications

1. Overlying skin infection
2. Local osteomyelitis
3. Major coagulopathy, including severe inherited factor deficiency, active disseminated intravascular coagulation, profound liver disease, or therapeutic anticoagulation with prothrombin/partial thromboplastin times above or at upper limits of therapeutic range
4. Thrombocytopenia, no matter how severe, is *not* a contraindication.
5. Prior therapeutic irradiation may result in a "dry tap" and nondiagnostic biopsy if procedure is performed in the same area.

Preparation

1. Obtain informed consent.
2. Obtain a complete blood count with differential on the day of the procedure.
3. Arrange for an assistant from the hematology section of the clinical laboratory to be present. The assistant should be able to prepare several bone marrow smears from a portion of the aspirate and to utilize the remainder to prepare a bone marrow clot (for fixation and histologic evaluation).

Equipment

1. Chux
2. Sterile drape
3. Povidone-iodine (Betadine) swabs (three)
4. Sterile 4×4 gauze (several packages)
5. Sterile gloves
6. Lidocaine (Xylocaine) 2% with epinephrine: Inquire regarding history of allergic reaction.
7. Sterile disposable needles: 25 gauge, ⅝ inch; 22 gauge, 1½ inch; 18-gauge
8. Sterile disposable Luer-tip syringes: 3, 6, and 12 ml
9. Sterile No. 11 blade (handle not needed)
10. Sterile Jamshidi needle: 11 gauge for most routine use; 8 and 13 gauge also available. A spare needle is recommended in case the original becomes contaminated prior to the end of the procedure.
11. Adhesive bandage
12. Sandbag: required only for prolonged tamponade of oozing site

Anesthesia

1. Premedicate (*after* obtaining informed consent) with intravenous midazolam (versed) (or alternative benzodiazepine) and meperidine (or alternative narcotic) in dosages appropriate for age, body size, and coexisting medical conditions (e.g., chronic pulmonary disease). Inquire regarding history of allergic reaction.
2. Raise skin bleb with Xylocaine-epinephrine solution (start with 25-gauge needle/6-ml syringe). Infiltrate through skin bleb, distributing remaining several milliliters of local anesthetic partly into subcutaneous tissues but *primarily* into periosteal surface (switch to 22-gauge needle). Inject several sites on periosteal surface, covering an area of at least 1 cm in diameter. (In obese patients, a spinal needle may be required for this step.)

Precautions

1. The posterosuperior iliac spine (PSIS) is the preferred site for both aspiration and biopsy.
2. The sternum (second or third intercostal space) and tibia (upper third) are alternative sites for aspiration. These sites are for experienced operators only. *Never attempt bone marrow biopsy at these sites.*

Technique

1. Position patient in lateral decubitus position with knees drawn up partly to the chest. Use left lateral decubitus position if target is right PSIS (for right-hand-dominant operator) or vice versa (for left-hand-dominant operator) (see figure below).

2. Administer intravenous premedication as discussed above.

3. Place a Chux underneath dependent buttock (to catch Betadine, blood)

4. Locate the PSIS by palpation. If this is difficult, follow the iliac crest anteriorly to posteriorly, searching for the large prominence on the medial border, several centimeters below the top of the crest.

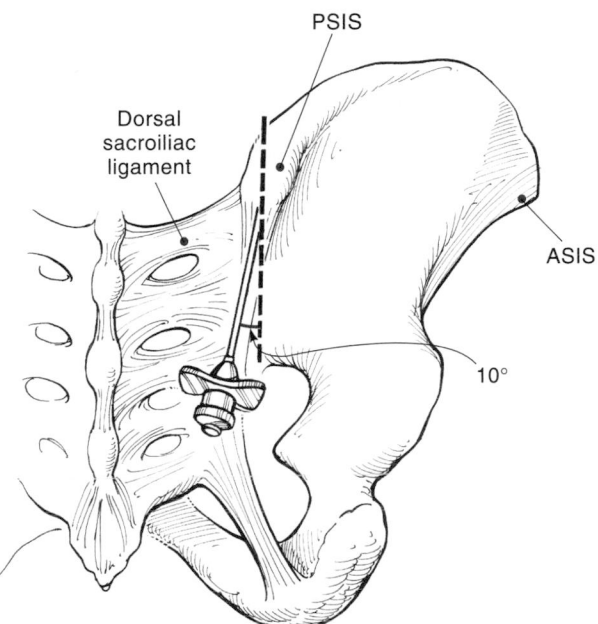

5. Use a marker (e.g., the nonwriting end of an office-type pen) to make an impression over the PSIS.

6. Prep the skin using Betadine over a wide area (diameter of at least 6 inches) centered on the PSIS. Drape the patient so that the anterosuperior iliac spine (ASIS) can be palpated through the sterile drape.

7. Administer local anesthetic as discussed above.

8. Make an incision at the previously marked site into the subcutaneous tissues with the No. 11 blade using a stabbing motion (see above).

9. While waiting for the anesthetic to take effect, examine the Jamshidi needle, ascertaining that it is complete with needle, stylette, screw cap, and probe.

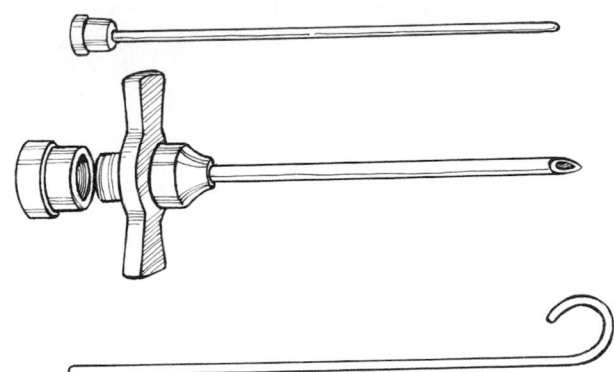

10. Grasp the handle of the reassembled Jamshidi needle with the dominant hand (the needle itself fitting between the third and fourth digits). Insert the needle into the incision site, and use the first and second digits of the nondominant hand to guide the needle down to the periosteum of the PSIS.

11. While stabilizing the needle at the skin using the first and second digits of the nondominant hand, introduce the needle into the PSIS using firm pressure and a rotatory motion with back-and-forth arcs of 180 degrees. Avoid the natural tendency for the needle to slide medially into the dorsal sacroiliac ligament by angling (pointing) the needle approximately 10 degrees *superior to the horizontal plane*, or toward the ASIS. The pressure required is variable depending on the mineralization of the iliac bone.

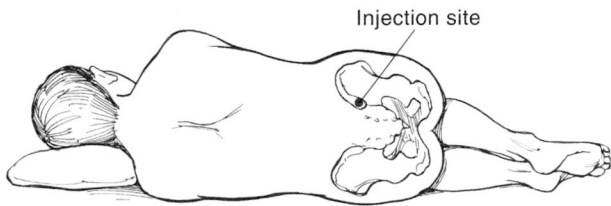

12. Check for solid placement of the needle by moving it parallel to the plane of the bed. The patient's entire pelvis should move with the needle. A "give" may be appreciated when the marrow cavity is entered, but this sensation is variable.

13. Verify that your assistant is ready to receive the aspirate specimen. If so, unscrew the needle cap and remove the stylette (but keep these sterile). Take a 12-ml syringe, aspirate and expel air through it once, and attach it firmly to the Jamshidi needle.

14. Warn the patient that this next step may be painful. Rapidly pull the plunger of the syringe back nearly all the way. Allow *no more* than

0.5 ml of marrow to enter the syringe. Immediately release all negative pressure on the plunger, detach the syringe, and hand it to the assistant. *This step should be accomplished as rapidly as possible (preferably within 3 seconds) to prevent clotting.* Place the stylette partly into the needle to decrease external bleeding.

15. Wait to see if the assistant finds bone marrow spicules in the specimen. If so, the aspiration is completed. If not, reinsert the stylette, reattach the screw cap, and withdraw the entire needle back to the subcutaneous tissue level. Repeat steps 11 through 14 at an adjacent periosteal site.

16. After the aspiration has been completed successfully, one may obtain (if indicated) additional marrow for culture and/or cytogenetics. A specimen of 10 ml of marrow (inoculated at the bedside into standard blood culture bottles) is recommended for culture; a specimen of 2 ml (collected in a heparinized syringe) is required for cytogenetics.

17. Failure of marrow to enter the syringe after step 14 (i.e., a dry tap) indicates either that the needle is not yet in the marrow cavity or that a pathologic condition (e.g., myelofibrosis, marrow replacement by tumor) is present. Advance the needle using the same rotatory motion about 1 to 2 cm and try aspirating again.

18. After completing the aspiration or establishing the presence of a dry tap, proceed to bone marrow biopsy. Withdraw the Jamshidi needle to the subcutaneous level, and replace the stylette and screw cap. Reintroduce the needle at a periosteal site 1 cm removed from where the aspirate was done by repeating steps 11 and 12 above. Remove the screw cap and stylette. Fold a 4×4 gauze over the proximal end, and advance the needle in its existing direction using the same grip, pressure, and hand motion described previously. Use the first and second digits of the nondominant hand at the skin line to ascertain that the needle has been advanced for another 2 to 3 cm.

19. When the needle has been advanced, it should contain a core specimen. Rotate the needle at least 360 degrees in each direction several times. Tilt the needle to the side in each of four quadrants to help break off the core specimen from surrounding bone. Withdraw the needle *in a controlled manner* while wobbling it from side to side. The core specimen may or may not be visible in the tip of the needle.

20. Use the probe to push the specimen from the *distal* to the *proximal* end of the needle (i.e., "backward"). If aspiration was successful, the biopsy specimen may be dropped directly into a fixative solution. If aspiration was not successful, the biopsy should first be placed on glass slides, where it may be rolled to obtain a cell touch prep, which is useful for evaluating cellular morphology and also can be used for cytochemical stains.

21. Fold the 4×4 gauze and tape firmly over the procedure site using the adhesive bandage. If there is much oozing, compress this area by hand for 10 minutes, and ask the patient to lie with the PSIS on the sandbag thereafter.

22. Properly dispose of all needles and sharp equipment. Write a procedure note.

Follow-Up

1. No special patient follow-up is normally required other than as dictated by the underlying disease. Acetaminophen should suffice for postprocedure pain.

2. Rare complications of the procedure include retroperitoneal hemorrhage and fracture of the iliac bone (for the PSIS) as well as perforation into the mediastinum and sternomanubrial separation (for the sternum).

Bibliography

Douglas DD, Risdell RJ: Bone marrow biopsy technic: artifact induced by aspiration. Am J Clin Pathol 1984; 82:92–94.

Hyun BH, Stevenson AJ, Hanau CA: Fundamentals of bone marrow examination. Hematol Oncol Clin North Am 1994;8:651–663.

Mainwaring CJ, Wong C, Lush RJ, et al: The role of midazolam-induced sedation in bone marrow aspiration/trephine biopsies. Clin Lab Haematol 1996;18: 285–288.

Perkins S: Examination of the blood and bone marrow. In Lee GR, Foerster J, Lukens J, et al (eds): Wintrobe's Clinical Hematology, 10th ed, vol 1, pp 9–35. Baltimore, Williams & Wilkins, 1999.

Wolff SN, Katzenstein A, Phillips GL, et al: Aspiration does not influence interpretation of bone marrow biopsy cellularity. Am J Clin Pathol 1983;80:60–62.

164 Polycythemia

Richard T. Silver

Definition

Polycythemia is defined as an increase in the volume of circulating red blood cells (RBCs) per kilogram of body weight or, equivalently, an increase in the RBC mass. This is expressed as an absolute increase in the number of red cells, usually but not always accompanied by corresponding increases in the hemoglobin and hematocrit. Increased RBC mass can be determined by using the widely available chromium-51–tagged RBC mass study.

Pathogenesis

An increase in RBC mass can occur as a primary disease of unknown cause, polycythemia vera, a myeloproliferative disease caused by aberrant stem cell growth, or as secondary manifestation of other illnesses (see below).

Symptoms

1. Pruritus: In polycythemia vera, this often increases in intensity after a tub bath and less often after showering
2. Burning, with throbbing pain in the legs, feet, or hands accompanied by a mottled redness. In polycythemia vera, especially when accompanied by increase in the platelet count.
3. Joint pain: Gout accompanies polycythemia vera in 10 per cent of cases.
4. Blood loss: The most common source of major hemorrhage is the upper gastrointestinal tract, because peptic ulcer occurs in about 10 per cent of patients with polycythemia vera.

Key Symptoms

- Easy fatigue
- Dizziness
- Visual disturbances
- Weakness
- Tinnitus
- Headaches
- Shortness of breath
- Bone pain
- Pounding in the ears

Clinical Findings

1. Injected or red conjunctivae
2. May show evidence of thrombosis or hemorrhage.

3. Liver palpable in about 50 per cent of patients
4. Spleen palpable in more than 75 per cent

Key Signs

- Splenomegaly
- Hepatomegaly

Diagnosis

1. Order chromium-51 RBC mass study to demonstrate an absolute increase in RBC mass
2. Proceed as in Table 164–1.

Differential Diagnosis

1. A clinical classification of the polycythemias is shown in Table 164–2.
2. Causes of secondary polycythemia can be classified for clinical use as those related to oxygen delivery that does not meet tissue needs and

TABLE 164–1. EVALUATION OF THE PATIENT WITH POLYCYTHEMIA

- History
- Physical examination, including neurologic and pelvic examinations
- Complete blood count, reticulocyte count, platelet count, and manual differentiation
- Urinalysis
- RBC volume: Should be >25 per cent above mean normal predicted value based on the International Council for Standardization in Haematology.
- Serum erythropoietin level
  –Low or absent in polycythemia vera
  –High in erythpoietin-secreting tumors
  –Unreliable in emphysema and chronic pulmonary conditions
- Serum vitamin B_{12} and vitamin B_{12}–binding capacity: usually increased
- Leukocyte alkaline phosphatase determination: usually increased in polycythemia vera
- Hemoglobin electrophoresis: An increase in red cell mass without concomitant rises in white blood cell and platelet counts may suggest polycythemia secondary to a hemoglobinopathy.
- Serum uric acid and potassium determinations
- Plasma cortisol determination: to exclude Cushing's syndrome
- Arterial oxygen tension and saturation determinations: A low level may suggest cardiopulmonary disease.
- Bone marrow biopsy with stains for iron, reticulin, and collagen
- Chest radiograph

TABLE 164–2. CLINICAL CLASSIFICATION OF POLYCYTHEMIA

1.0 *Secondary polycythemias*
   1.1 Related to inadequate oxygen delivery to tissues with respect to need
      1.11 Due to decreased arterial oxygen tension (low O_2 saturation)
         1.111 With physiologic or anatomic cardiopulmonary abnormalities:
- abnormalities of lungs, chest bellows, or ventilatory control mechanisms
- right-to-left vascular shunts

         1.112 Without physiologic or anatomic cardiopulmonary abnormalities
- low oxygen tension (e.g., high altitudes)
- impaired oxygen-carrying capacity of hemoglobin

      1.12 Due to decreased blood flow—congestive heart failure
   1.2 Unrelated to inadequate oxygen delivery, or need, and associated with high *erythropoietin level* and found with benign or malignant lesions of:
- kidney—cysts, hydronephrosis, adenoma, hypernephroma, sarcoma
- cerebellum—hemangioblastoma
- uterus—myoma
- liver—hepatoma, hamartoma
- other—adrenal (pheochromocytoma)

2.0 *Polycythemia vera*: Low erythropoietin level, usually normal O_2 saturation

TABLE 164–3. POLYCYTHEMIA VERA STUDY GROUP CRITERIA FOR THE DIAGNOSIS OF POLYCYTHEMIA VERA

*A_1 Increased red blood cell mass Male: ≥36 ml/kg Female: ≥32 ml/kg	B_1 Platelets ≥600,000 cells/μl
A_2 Arterial oxygen ≥92%	B_2 White blood cell count ≥12,000/μl in absence of fever
A_3 Splenomegaly	B_3 Elevated serum vitamin B_{12} (>900 pg/ml) or elevated unsaturated vitamin B_{12}-binding capacity (>2200 pg/ml)
	B_4 Elevated leukocyte alkaline phosphatase (>100) (no fever or infection)

*According to the International Council for Standardization in Haematology, the criteria now recommended are more than 25 per cent of the mean normal predicted value.

those not related to oxygen deprivation that are usually accompanied by increased serum erythropoietin levels.

3. Benign or malignant lesions of the kidney, cerebellum, uterus, liver, and other organs may give rise to a picture of polycythemia. Because these conditions are characterized by high erythropoietin levels, the determination of serum erythropoietin is of considerable value from a differential standpoint.

4. After demonstration of an increased RBC mass, determine whether the illness is a secondary manifestation of other illnesses or part of the disease complex polycythemia vera.

5. The diagnosis of polycythemia vera is often an exclusionary diagnosis.

   a. The criteria used for many years for diagnosing polycythemia vera were those of the P. Vera Study Group (Table 164–3). The diagnosis is acceptable if one of the two following combinations is present:

      (1) $A_1 + A_2 + A_3$,

      or, in the absence of splenomegaly,

      (2) $A_1 + A_2$ + any two items from category B

   b. The widespread availability of testing for serum erythropoietin levels has made the diagnosis easier. Serum erythropoietin levels should be low in all cases of polycythemia vera. A more simple modification for the diagnosis of polycythemia vera with or without splenomegaly is $A_1 + A_2$ + a low serum erythropoietin level (<25 μl).

   c. Other diagnostic criteria have also been proposed, especially those pertaining to panhypercellularity of the bone marrow and abnormal marrow karyotypes.

 Key Tests

- Complete blood count
- Platelet count
- Serum erythropoietin
- O_2 saturation

Treatment

1. It is most important to reduce the hematocrit to levels between 40 and 43 per cent with *phlebotomy* every week or biweekly if tolerated. Careful attention must be paid to possible platelet count rise.

2. Some form of myelosuppression usually must be employed. The most commonly used drug for this purpose is *hydroxyurea*, which may be given at a dose ranging between 500 and 1500 mg daily.

   a. Over the long term, hydroxyurea may be leukemogenic in approximately 10 per cent of cases.

b. It does not prevent progression of the disease to myelofibrosis.

c. *Interferon*, especially in young patients, may also be used, beginning with a dose of 1.0 MU SC three times a week, escalating to 3.0 MU three times a week with upward or downward adjustments as necessary. Interferon is of particular value because it has antierythropoietic and antimegakaryocytic activity.

4. Low-dose *aspirin* (81 mg daily) should be used to suppress platelet aggregation.

5. For younger patients who will not accept interferon, phlebotomy and anagrelide may be used.

6. For elderly patients, radioactive phosphorus can be considered.

Key Treatment

- Phlebotomy
- Hydroxyurea
- Interferon
- Aspirin

Bibliography

Najean Y, Rain JD: Treatment of polycythemia vera: the use of hydroxyurea and pipobroman in 292 patients under the age of 65 years. Blood 1997;90:3370.

Silver RT: Interferon alfa: effects of long-term treatment for polycythemia vera. Semin Hematol 1997;34:40.

Silver RT: Polycythemia vera and other polycythemia syndromes. In Conn RB, Borer WZ, Snyder JW (eds): Current Diagnosis, 9th ed, p 505. Philadelphia, WB Saunders Company, 1997.

Thiele J, Kvasnicka HM, Werden C, et al: Idiopathic primary osteo-myelofibrosis: a clinico-pathologic study on 208 patients with special emphasis on evolution of disease features, differentiation from essential thrombocythemia and variables of prognostic impact. Leuk Lymphoma 1996;22:303.

Weinfeld A, Swolin B, Westin J: Acute leukaemia after hydroxyurea therapy in polycythemia vera and allied disorders: prospective study of efficacy and leukaemogenicity with therapeutic implications. Eur J Haematol 1994;52:134.

165 Lymphadenopathy

Jeffrey T. Kirchner

Etiology

1. Lymph node enlargement occurs as a result of infection, inflammation, or malignancy.
   a. In the face of infection or an inflammatory process, there is an increase in the number of lymphocytes and macrophages in response to an antigenic challenge.
   b. In the case of primary malignancy, the lymph node enlarges as a result of in situ proliferation of malignant lymphocytes.
   c. With metastatic disease, there is infiltration of the node by malignant cells.
2. Small, nonpathogenic lymph nodes in the neck, groin, or axilla are normally palpable in some adults and children. Patients under age 30 will have a benign etiology in about 80 per cent of cases, whereas only 40 per cent of patients over age 50 will have a benign cause for their lymphadenopathy.

Symptoms

1. Lymph node enlargement may be transient, recurring, or chronic. It may develop as part of a systemic illness or syndrome, or may be noted in the presence or absence of nonspecific symptoms.
2. The presence of symptoms often depends on the etiology. These may include
   a. Fever
   b. Cough
   c. Fatigue
   d. Weight loss
   e. Night sweats
   f. Arthralgias
   g. Sore throat
3. Key questions
   a. How long has the node been present?
   b. Has it changed in size?
   c. Is it painful?

Key Symptoms

- Fever
- Fatigue
- Weight loss

Clinical Findings

Adenopathy may be localized or generalized (three or more locations). Nodes greater than 1 cm are considered enlarged and those larger than 3 cm suggest neoplastic disease. Palpable supraclavicular nodes are of clinical importance and often indicate a malignant process. Splenomegaly should also be assessed for because its presence suggests a systemic illness.

1. Infection: Nodes are tender and mobile; overlying skin may be inflamed or erythematous.
2. Malignancy: Nodes are stone-hard, fixed, and matted.
3. Inflammation: Nodes are tender and mobile.
4. Lymphoma: Nodes are firm, rubbery, nontender.

Laboratory Tests

1. These are variable and depend on the suspected etiology of the lymphadenopathy as determined by patient history and clinical presentation.
   a. Infection: complete blood count, purified protein derivative, erythrocyte sedimentation rate, C-reactive protein, human immunodeficiency virus antibody, hepatic transaminases, alkaline phosphatase, bacteriologic cultures; serology for Epstein-Barr virus, cytomegalovirus, *Toxoplasma gondii*, and *Bartonella henselae*.
   b. Inflammation: antinuclear antibody, rheumatoid factor, angiotensin-converting enzyme, chest radiograph
   c. Malignancy: excisional node biopsy. Tissue should be submitted for histologic studies, microbiologic culture, special staining for bacteria, mycobacterium, and fungi; consider special stains such as periodic acid–Schiff (Whipple's disease) or congo red (amyloid). Fine-needle aspiration is of low yield and thus not recommended.
2. Additional diagnostic studies may include bone marrow biopsy or liver biopsy. Ultrasonography, computerized tomography, and magnetic resonance imaging can assess for intra-abdominal, retroperitoneal, or hilar adenopathy.

TABLE 165–1. DIFFERENTIAL DIAGNOSIS OF LYMPHADENOPATHY BASED ON LOCATION

Generalized

Infections	Hypersensitivity reactions	Metabolic disease	Neoplasia
Mononucleosis	Serum sickness	Hyperthyroidism	Leukemia
HIV/AIDS	Vasculitis (RA, SLE)	Lipidoses	Hodgkin's disease
Toxoplasmosis	Drug reaction (phenytoin, hydralazine)		Non-Hodgkin's disease
Secondary syphilis	Graft-versus-host disease		

Localized

Anterior auricular	Viral conjunctivitis, rubella, scalp infection
Submandibular or cervical (unilateral)	Buccal infection, pharyngitis, thyroid malignancy, nasopharyngeal tumor, Kawasaki's disease
Cervical (bilateral)	Mononucleosis, pharyngitis, toxoplasmosis, sarcoidosis
Supraclavicular (left)	Renal, intra-abdominal, testicular, or ovarian malignancy
Supraclavicular (right)	Pulmonary, esophageal, or mediastinal malignancy
Axillary	Upper extremity infection, breast infection or malignancy
Epitrochlear	Hand infection, syphilis
Inguinal	Syphilis, genital herpes simplex, chancroid, local infection, lower extremity infection
Any region	Hodgkin's disease, non-Hodgkin's disease, cat-scratch disease, leukemia, metastatic cancer, sarcoidosis, granulomatous infection
Hilar region (bilateral)	Sarcoidosis, lymphoma, bronchogenic carcinoma, tuberculosis, fungal infections (histoplasmosis, coccidioidomycosis, cryptococcosis)
Hilar region (unilateral)	Sarcoidosis, lymphoma, tuberculosis, bronchogenic carcinoma

Abbreviations: HIV/AIDS, human immunodeficiency virus/acquired immunodeficiency syndrome; RA, rheumatoid arthritis; SLE, systemic lupus erythematosus.

Key Test

Biopsy is the gold standard for establishing a diagnosis

Differential Diagnosis

The differential diagnosis is extensive; thus it is helpful to determine clinically if the adenopathy is generalized, regional, or isolated (see Table 165–1). Patient age, sex, occupation, pet exposure, sexual history, and medication use should be considered.

Treatment

1. In the majority of patients, treatment will be self-limited and involve observation over days to weeks until the lymph node(s) have returned to normal size.
2. If a definitive diagnosis has been established, treatment will be directed at the underlying infection, inflammatory process, or malignancy.
3. In the absence of a definitive diagnosis and subsequent treatment, close follow-up is recommended.

Key Treatment

Empiric antibiotics or corticosteroids are not indicated.

Follow-Up

1. If the history and physical suggest a benign cause, follow-up at 2- to 4-week intervals is appropriate. Most authorities recommend biopsy of any node that is 3 cm or greater in size or that has persisted for more than 4 weeks without a diagnosis by noninvasive methods.
2. The reported yield on lymph node biopsies is variable but often as low as 50 per cent. In patients with a nondiagnostic biopsy, about 25 per cent eventually developed a disease related to the lymph node enlargement, and as many as 17 per cent may have lymphoma.

Bibliography

Henry PH, Longo DL: Enlargement of lymph nodes and spleen. In Fauci AS, Braunwald E, Isselhacher KJ, et al (eds): Harrison's Principles of Internal Medicine, 14th ed, 345. New York, McGraw-Hill, 1997.

Phatak PD, Janas JS, Sham RL, et al: Disorders that resemble lymphomas. Am J Hematol 1997;56:63–68.

Simon HB: Evaluation of lymphadenopathy. In Goroll AH, May A, Mulley AG (eds): Primary Care Medicine: Office Evaluation and Management of the Adult Patient, 3rd ed, pp 54–58. Philadelphia, JB Lippincott Company, 1995.

Slap GB, Connor JL, Wigton RS, et al: Validation of a model to identify young patients for lymph node biopsy. JAMA 1986;255:2768.

Williamson HA Jr: Lymphadenopathy in a family practice. J Fam Pract 1985;20:449.

166 Lymphoma

Barry R. Meisenberg

Etiology and Epidemiology

1. The non-Hodgkin's lymphomas (NHLs) are a diverse group of diseases that have in common malignant transformation of lymphocytes or lymphocyte precursors. Despite their common lineage, these diseases are quite heterogeneous with respect to their immunology, biology, natural history, and response to treatment.

2. Over 40,000 NHLs occur annually, equally split between aggressive and indolent forms. The average age of patients is in the early 40s. Ten to 20 per cent of NHLs arise outside the lymph nodes or spleen from lymphoid tissue in other organs. Predisposing conditions that have been associated with lymphomas include

   a. Immune suppression related to inherited or acquired conditions (especially the acquired immunodeficiency syndrome [AIDS])

   b. Viruses such as Epstein-Barr virus and HTLV-1

   c. Toxins such as herbicides or radiation

3. Most patients with NHL, however, do not have any recognized risk factor or predisposing condition.

Histologic Classification

Histologic classification is very complex, and competing systems exist. The International Working Class Formulation has attempted to bring some order to classification. In this system, NHL can be loosely grouped into three classes (Table 166–1).

Clinical Findings

1. Seventy-five per cent of patients present with palpable peripheral lymphadenopathy.

2. Most patients are asymptomatic, although 20 to 30 per cent have fevers, night sweats, or unexplained weight loss, the so-called B symptoms.

3. Other findings depend upon the location of the lymphoma.

Key Symptoms

B Symptoms Associated with NHL

- Fever >101.5°F

- Night sweats

- Unexplained weight loss of more than 10 per cent of total body weight

Key Signs

- Nodes may enlarge and decrease apparently spontaneously over several months.

- Involved lymph nodes are typically nontender and movable, and feel firm but not rock hard to the touch.

Laboratory Tests

1. Laboratory studies are used to confirm the diagnosis of lymphoma and aid in staging, which in turn helps make treatment decisions. Useful laboratory tests include

   a. Complete blood count with sedimentation rate (erythrocyte sedimentation rate may be useful in following the clinical course)

   b. A chemistry panel including lactate dehydrogenase (LDH) (the LDH is often a useful marker for disease activity and correlates with tumor bulk)

   c. Radiographic studies (computerized tomography scans of the chest and abdomen to aid in staging)

   d. Bone marrow biopsy for staging

   e. Additional studies as indicated

2. The most important test is an adequate surgical biopsy specimen, which should be reviewed by

---

TABLE 166–1. NHL GROUPING, INTERNATIONAL WORKING CLASS FORMULATION

Low Grade	Intermediate Grade
Small lymphocytic	Follicular large cell
Follicular small cleaved cell	Diffuse cleaved cell
Follicular mixed small and large cell	Diffuse mixed small and large cell
	Diffuse large cell
High Grade	
Large cell immunoblastic	
Lymphoblastic	
Small noncleaved cell	

an experienced pathologist. A needle aspiration of a suspicious lymph node does not allow determination of the nodal architecture and is not acceptable for initial diagnosis of a suspicious lesion. Needle aspiration may be useful in patients with known lymphoma who develop a recurrence but should not be performed to exclude lymphoma in a suspicious node.

Key Tests

- Surgical biopsy is the only definitive test.

- Do not rely on needle aspiration for diagnosis.

- Biopsy the largest lymph node that is accessible to avoid misdiagnosis.

Differential Diagnosis

1. Differential diagnosis of lymphadenopathy is extensive (see Ch. 165, Lymphadenopathy). Clinical judgment is required in determining whether a patient is at high risk for another diagnosis. For example:

   a. Isolated cervical adenopathy in a chronic smoker could be due to nasopharyngeal carcinoma.

   b. Isolated unilateral axillary adenopathy in a middle-aged or older woman suggests breast cancer.

Staging of Lymphoma

1. Staging of lymphoma follows the Ann Arbor Classification (Table 166–2).

2. Eighty per cent of indolent lymphomas present as stage IV disease (usually bone marrow involvement), whereas the more aggressive intermediate- or high-grade lymphomas are sometimes confined to one or more lymph node areas.

TABLE 166–2. STAGING OF LYMPHOMA, ANN ARBOR CLASSIFICATION*

Stage I:	Single lymph node region; for single, extralymphatic organ (1E)
Stage II:	Two or more lymph node regions on the same side of the diaphragm
Stage III:	Lymph node regions on both sides of the diaphragm
Stage IV:	Diffuse involvement of extralymphatic organs not affected by direct spread, such as lung, bone marrow, liver

*If B symptoms are present (see "Key Symptoms"), the classification changes to IB, IIB, IIIB, or IVB.

Treatment

1. The treatment of lymphoma is determined primarily by the histologic type as well as other factors, such as the age and underlying condition of the patient. Treatment relies primarily on chemotherapy with or without radiation therapy. The timing of treatment, treatment regimens, and therapeutic goals vary with the individual lymphoma type.

Key Treatment

Low-Grade Lymphoma

- Patients are older and often have stage IV disease.

- Indolent natural history with a 6- to 10-year average survival

- Chemotherapy leads to remission but not cure.

- Indications for treatment: symptomatic or bulky adenopathy, constitutional symptoms related to lymphoma, dangerous compressions of other vital structures by bulky nodes

2. Low-grade lymphoma is usually treated with one or more chemotherapy drugs such as cyclophosphamide (Cytoxan) or chlorambucil (Leukeran) along with prednisone. Vincristine (Oncovin) may be added. Remissions may be partial or complete and last several years, but adenopathy almost always returns. Additional treatment can be given but becomes progressively less successful.

3. Maintaining full-dose intensity is important. Patients who cannot receive full doses because of age or underlying disease have a poorer prognosis.

Key Treatment

Intermediate-Grade and High-Grade Lymphomas

- More aggressive biologically but with the potential for cure with aggressive chemotherapy.

- Standard treatment is combination CHOP (cyclophosphamide [Cytoxan], doxorubicin [Adriamycin], vincristine [Oncovin], and prednisone) given for six cycles.

- Durable complete remissions occur in 30 to 50 per cent.

- Important prognostic factors include age, bulk of disease, and histologic subtype.

- Lymphoblastic lymphoma is often treated like acute lymphocytic leukemia (see Ch. 163, Leukemia).

- Small noncleaved lymphoma is treated with high-dose cyclophosphamide in addition to methotrexate.

Bibliography

For information on the classification of lymphomas, see
Harris NL, Jaffe ES, Stein H, et al: A revised European-American classification of lymphoid neoplasma: a proposal from the International Lymphoma Study Group. Blood 1994;84:1361–1392.

For more information on the staging of non-Hodgkin's lymphomas, see
Moormeier JA, Williams SF, Golomb HM: The staging of non-Hodgkin's lymphomas. Semin Oncol 1990;17:43–50.

For more information on the treatment of lymphomas, see
Horning SJ: Treatment approaches to the low-grade lymphomas. Blood 1994;83:881–884.
Shipp MA: Prognostic factors in aggressive non Hodgkin's lymphoma: who has "high risk" disease? Blood 1994;83:1165–1173.

For information regarding the special considerations of lymphoma in patients with AIDS, see
Demario MD, Liebowitz ON: Lymphomas in the immunocompromised patient. Semin Oncol 1998;25:492–502.

167 Hodgkin's Disease

Kathryn Reilly

Etiology and Epidemiology

1. The age-specific incidence curve of Hodgkin's disease is bimodal.

   a. In the United States and other developed countries, the first peak occurs in adolescents and young adults (ages 15 to 24), most commonly female and of higher socioeconomic status. The second peak occurs in the fifth and sixth decades, primarily in males.

   b. In less developed areas of the world the first peak occurs between ages 5 and 9, mostly in boys. The second peak occurs in the fifth or sixth decade. These patients have a poorer prognosis because of predominance of mixed cellularity or lymphocyte-depletion disease and presence of more advanced disease at diagnosis.

2. Human immunodeficiency virus infection is associated with a high incidence of Hodgkin's disease, which is disseminated at diagnosis in at least three fourths of cases and associated with systemic symptoms in 70 per cent.

3. Epstein-Barr viral genome has been found in Reed-Sternberg cells, the malignant cell of Hodgkin's disease. However, because infection with this virus is almost universal, one or more cofactors are presumed to be needed to permit development of the disease, possibly involving an X-linked gene and/or human lymphocyte antigen typing.

Symptoms

1. Superficial lymph node enlargement in more than 70 per cent

2. Neck or supraclavicular in 50 per cent

3. Majority have no symptoms beyond lymphadenopathy.

4. Twenty-five to 30 per cent have constitutional symptoms.

   a. Low-grade fevers and night sweats

   b. Weight loss of more than 10 per cent over 6 months or less

   c. Generalized pruritus that may be associated with a skin rash

   d. Fatigue, weakness, and malaise

5. Pel-Epstein fevers: high fluctuating fevers associated with drenching night sweats that persist for several weeks and then disappear

6. Rare symptoms include

   a. Painful lymph nodes after ingesting alcoholic beverages (2 to 5 per cent)

   b. Cough, chest pain, shortness of breath, or hypertrophic osteoarthropathy

   c. Bone pain

   d. Obstruction of the superior vena cava

   e. Sudden spinal cord compression

   f. Headache or visual changes in intracranial Hodgkin's disease

   g. Abdominal pain, bowel disturbances, and ascites

Key Symptoms

- Painless lymphadenopathy
- Pruritis
- Weight loss
- Fevers

Clinical Findings

Nodes are firm, freely movable, and nontender.

Key Sign

Rubbery, large lymph nodes

Laboratory Tests

1. Biopsy from involved lymph nodes or other tissues is essential to diagnosis. Needle aspiration or needle biopsies do not contain enough tissue and are not adequate for diagnosis.

2. Criteria for diagnosis and classification of Hodgkin's disease are based on the Rye classification. Presence of the Reed-Sternberg cell is central to the diagnosis, but these cells are occasionally found in other conditions such as infectious mononucleosis and non-Hodgkin's lymphoma. Thus additional cellular and archi-

tectural features of Hodgkin's disease must be present in the tissue.

3. Chest radiograph demonstrates mediastinal adenopathy in 60 per cent. Chest computerized tomography (CT) should be obtained in patients with apparent thoracic disease to accurately define extent of disease. CT of the abdomen and pelvis is valuable for assessment of disease in the liver and abdominal lymph nodes, but it is not useful for evaluation of the spleen and involvement of nonenlarged nodes.

4. Blood studies include complete blood count, liver and renal function studies, and erythrocyte sedimentation rate, although none except the sedimentation rate has been shown to provide information about the extent of disease or organ involvement.

5. Bone marrow biopsy is needed unless disease is clearly stage IV.

6. Bipedal lymphangiogram demonstrates para-aortic and iliac lymph node enlargement and is more sensitive than CT. However, the accuracy of lymphangiogram is dependent on the experience of the radiologist.

7. Gallium scan is useful to follow response to treatment and to monitor for relapse. However, not all Hodgkin's disease absorbs gallium, so the scan must be done at the time of initial evaluation.

8. Staging laparotomy with splenectomy is standard for all patients except those with stage IV disease. The clinical stage of one third of patients is changed up or down after this procedure. Laparoscopy has been suggested as a less invasive procedure with shorter recovery time. Some authorities believe that staging laparotomy should be abandoned and that all patients should be treated with chemotherapy.

Key Tests

- Lymph node biopsy
- Chest radiograph
- CT of chest, abdomen, and pelvis
- Bone marrow biopsy

Staging After Biopsy Diagnosis

Appropriate treatment of Hodgkin's disease requires accurate staging. The Ann Arbor system is used to classify the extent of disease.

1. Stage I is disease involving one lymph node area.

2. Stage II disease involves two lymph node areas on the same side of the diaphragm.

3. Stage III disease involves lymph node areas on both sides of the diaphragm.

4. Stage IV is disseminated disease with bone marrow or liver involvement.

5. Patients with significant weight loss, night sweats, or fever are designated stage B; if none of these symptoms are present, the patient is designated as stage A.

Differential Diagnosis

1. Infections such as bacterial or viral pharyngitis, mononucleosis, cat-scratch disease, or toxoplasmosis

2. Other malignancies such as non-Hodgkin lymphoma or nasopharyngeal or thyroid cancer and, in older patients, carcinomas of the lung

3. Histoplasmosis can cause hilar adenopathy and is usually asymptomatic.

4. Drug reactions (especially phenytoin) can cause lymphadenopathy.

Treatment

1. Localized disease (stages IA and IIA) is treated with radiation therapy in most situations.

2. Patients with large mediastinal involvement have a greater risk of relapse with radiation and so are treated with radiation plus chemotherapy, even if they are in these early stages.

3. Patients with more extensive involvement (stages IIB and IIIA) can be treated with radiation alone, although their disease-free survival is less than those with early stages (70 vs. >80 per cent).

4. Combination chemotherapy is the treatment for advanced disease (stages IIIB and IV) and is frequently used for stages IIB and IIIA because of evidence for improved disease-free survival after chemotherapy.

5. MOPP (mechlorethamine, vincristine, procarbazine, and prednisone) has been used since the early 1970s. ABVD (doxorubicin, bleomycin, vincristine, and dacarbazine) is used either as an initial agent or as salvage therapy after relapse.

6. Treatment of elderly patients has not been optimally defined. However, it is known that suboptimal treatment in younger patients leads to poorer long-term outcomes. Current recommendations are that treatment for the elderly be based on the recommendations for younger patients, with modifications for specific risk profiles.

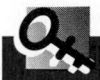

Key Treatment

Treatment depends on the stage of patient's disease.

Follow-Up

1. Relapse is usually treated with a different combination than that used to achieve remission. Poor prognostic variables include stage IV disease at diagnosis, B symptoms at relapse, or remission lasting less than 12 months.

2. Prognosis is dependent on numerous variables, including the age of the patient, stage at diagnosis, and histologic type, with lymphocyte depletion and mixed cellularity having poorer results. Bulky disease at diagnosis is also a poor prognostic sign.

3. Second malignancies are becoming more common as survival times have lengthened. The mean actuarial risk after 15 years is 17.6 per cent, with 13.2 per cent being solid malignancies.

   a. Acute nonlymphocytic leukemia and non-Hodgkin's lymphoma are the most common, and increase in frequency until 10 years after treatment, when the incidence plateaus.

   b. Solid tumors occur within the sites of radiation therapy (breast [RR 4], thyroid, lung, and basal cell cancers are the most common). The incidence of these tumors rises beginning 10 years after therapy.

4. Risk for cardiac disease is increased with radiation to the mediastinum (RR 3.1). Blocking to limit cardiac exposure does not eliminate this risk.

5. Thyroid dysfunction and gonadal dysfunction are both common.

Bibliography

Baccarani U, Carroll BJ, Hiatt JJ, et al: Comparison of laparoscopic and open staging in Hodgkin's disease. Arch Surg 1998;133:517–522.

Golumb H: Management of early-stage Hodgkin's disease: a continuing evolution. Semin Oncol 1998;25:476–482.

Greil R: Prognosis and management strategies of lymphatic neoplasias in the elderly. Oncology 1998;55:265–275.

Levine A: Hodgkin's disease in the setting of human immunodeficiency virus infection. J Natl Cancer Inst 1998;23:37–41.

Stiller CA: What causes Hodgkin's disease in children? [Review]. Eur J Cancer 1998;34:523–528.

168 Bleeding Disorders

Mary T. Brophy

Etiology

The approach to evaluating a bleeding patient is to first distinguish if the symptom is the result of an anatomic problem or a systemic hemostatic defect. Once a systemic bleeding disorder is suspected, the clinical evaluation should be directed toward differentiating congenital from acquired and coagulation from platelet-type disorders.

Congenital Defects

1. Coagulation factor deficiencies: reported for all factors, but the most common are
   a. Factor VIII (hemophilia A)
   b. Factor IX (hemophilia B or Christmas disease)
   c. Factor XI
2. Platelet disorders
   a. Quantitative disorders: rare, often accompanied by other congenital abnormalities
   b. Qualitative disorders: Glanzmann's thrombasthenia, granule deficiencies
   c. Both quantitative and qualitative disorders: Bernard-Soulier syndrome
3. Von Willebrand's disease (vWD): qualitative platelet and quantitative factor VIII defect
4. Fibrinolytic disorders: rare deficiencies in inhibitors of fibrinolysis

Acquired Defects

1. Coagulation disorders
   a. Vitamin K deficiency
   b. Medications: most common are heparin and warfarin
   c. Associated with underlying disorders: liver disease, dysproteinemia, amyloid
   d. Consumptive disorders
      (1) Diffuse: disseminated intravascular coagulation (DIC)
      (2) Localized: large hemangiomas, dissecting aneurysm
   e. Acquired specific inhibitors: most common are factor VIII and von Willebrand's factor
2. Platelet disorders
   a. Quantitative disorders
      (1) Immune destruction: immune thrombocytopenic purpura, drug-related, human immunodeficiency virus
      (2) Consumptive disorders: DIC, thrombotic thrombocytopenic purpura (TTP), hemolytic-uremic syndrome (HUS), large hemangiomas, dissecting aneurysm
      (3) Decreased production: secondary to medications, alcohol, toxins, virus, nutritional deficiencies, or bone marrow replacement
   b. Qualitative disorders
      (1) Medications: most common are aspirin, nonsteroidal anti-inflammatory drugs (NSAIDs)
      (2) Renal disease: uremia
      (3) Dysproteinemia: inhibition of platelet-platelet interaction
   c. Both quantitative and qualitative disorders
      (1) Myeloproliferative and myelodysplastic syndromes
      (2) Autoimmune: systemic lupus erythematosus
      (3) Cardipulmonary bypass
3. Fibrinolytic disorders
   a. Thrombolytic therapy
   b. Secondary to DIC

Symptoms

1. Coagulation disorders
   a. Bleeding is delayed after trauma or surgery.
   b. Severity is usually proportional to the degree of deficiency of the coagulation factor.
   c. Spontaneous bleeding in severe coagulopathies (less than 1 per cent activity)
2. Platelet disorders
   a. Bleeding is immediate after trauma or surgery.
   b. Severity of bleeding correlates with degree of platelet dysfunction.
   c. Spontaneous bleeding with platelet counts less than 10,000/μl

- Anatomic bleeding is usually a single bleeding episode from a single site.

- Bleeding that is spontaneous, more severe than expected, or from multiple sites suggests a systemic bleeding disorder.

Clinical Findings

1. Coagulation disorders
   a. Hematomas: visceral, intramuscular, retroperitoneal
   b. Hemarthroses are common.
   c. Mucous membrane bleeding with trauma
2. Platelet disorders
   a. Petechiae: skin, conjunctival, oral mucosal membranes
   b. Mucocutaneous bleeding: epistaxis, ecchymosis, gingival, gastrointestinal, genitourinary
   c. Spontaneous mucosal bleeding

- Coagulation disorders present with soft tissue and joint bleeds.

- Platelet disorders present with mucocutaneous bleeding.

Laboratory Tests

1. All patients with a bleeding disorder should have
   a. Complete blood count (CBC) with platelet count and blood smear evaluation
   b. Prothrombin time
   c. Activated partial thromboplastin time
2. The results of these tests, along with the history and clinical circumstances of the bleeding, will direct specific diagnostic testing (see Table 168–1).

WARNING

Results of laboratory test alone can be misleading. The importance of a clinical history of bleeding cannot be overemphasized. Mild hemostatic disorders may have normal screening tests. Screening tests can be abnormal with no bleeding diathesis.

- CBC

- Platelet count

- Prothrombin time

- Activated partial thromboplastin time

TABLE 168–1. DIFFERENTIAL DIAGNOSIS AND ADDITIONAL TESTING RECOMMENDED FOLLOWING SCREENING TESTS FOR PATIENTS WITH SUSPECTED IMPAIRED HEMOSTASIS

SCREENING TEST RESULTS	DIFFERENTIAL DIAGNOSIS	ADDITIONAL TESTING
nl Plt count, PT, and aPTT	Qualitative Plt disorders Mild vWD Fibrinolytic disorders	BT, ristocetin cofactor activity Plt aggregation studies Urea clot lysis time Factor XIII assay
↓ Plt count, nl PT and aPTT	Quantitative Plt disorders	Blood smear confirmation
↑ PT, nl plt count and aPTT	Vitamin K deficiency Early liver disease Coumarin effect ↓ Factor VII	Repeat PT after vitamin K administration
↑ aPTT, nl Plt count and PT	vWD ↓ Factors VIII, IX or XI Heparin effect	Ristocetin cofactor activity Mixing studies with incubation Factor levels (VIII, IX, XI) Thrombin and reptilase times
↑ PT and aPTT, nl Plt count	Hypo- or dysfibrinogenemia ↓ Factors V, X or II Liver disease	Fibrinogen level, TT, FDP Mixing studies with incubation Factor levels (V, X, II)
↑ PT and aPTT, ↓ Plt count	DIC, liver disease	Fibrinogen level, TT, FDP Mixing studies with incubation Factor VIII and V assay (nl in liver, ↓ in DIC)

Abbreviations: aPTT, activated partial thromboplastin time; BT, bleeding time; FDP, fibrin(ogen) degradation products assay; nl, normal; Plt, platelet; TT, thrombin time; vWD, von Willebrand's disease.

Differential Diagnosis

1. Primary vascular disorders
2. Connective tissue disorders

Treatment

1. Bleeds that are life-threatening or in critical locations require immediate correction of the hemostatic defect.
   a. Coagulation factor deficiencies are treated with IV administration of the required factor in the form of blood products or recombinant coagulation proteins.
   b. Quantitative platelet disorders (with the exception of TTP/HUS) and most qualitative platelet disorders (with the exception of uremia and dysproteinemia) are treated with platelet transfusion.
   c. Most fibrinolytic disorders respond to antifibrinolytic therapy.
2. Uncomplicated bleeds in noncritical area or minor traumatic injury can often be treated with topical hemostatics or hemostatic drugs.
   a. Antifibrinolytic amino acids for hemophilia, vWD, thrombocytopenia
   b. Desmopressin (DDAVP) for mild hemophilia A, type I vWD, qualitative platelet dysfunction secondary to granule deficiencies, uremia, myelodysplasia, and medications
3. Prophylactic therapy
   a. Patients with severe recurrent spontaneous bleeding from coagulation defects
   b. Platelet transfusion should not be given prophylactically because of the development of alloantibodies.
4. In acquired disorders, treatment of the underlying condition often improves the hemostatic defect.

Activity

Patients with bleeding diathesis should refrain from activity that could result in traumatic bleeds.

Patient Education

1. Medical alert bracelet should be worn by all patients with details about the type of bleeding diathesis.
2. Patients should be made aware that many commonly used medications, such as aspirin and NSAIDs, can exacerbate the bleeding problem and should be avoided.
3. Invasive procedures should not be done without consultation with the physician.

Key Treatment

The severity and location of the bleed determines the aggressiveness of therapy.

Follow-Up

Clinical monitoring is necessary to ensure that the bleeding has completely stopped. It may take several days before it is clear that adequate hemostasis has been achieved. In certain situations, laboratory monitoring is needed in order to ensure adequate levels of hemostatic factors.

Bibliography

Bowie EJW, Owen CA: Clinical and laboratory diagnosis of hemorrhagic disorders. In Ratnoff OD, Fores CD (eds): Disorders of Hemostasis, 3rd ed, pp 53–78. Philadelphia, WB Saunders Company, 1996.

Mannucci PM: Hemostatic drugs. N Engl J Med 1998; 339:245–253.

Rodgers GM, Bithell TC: The diagnostic approach to the bleeding disorders. In Lee GR, Foerster J, Lukens J, et al (eds): Wintrobe's Clinical Hematology, 10th ed, vol 2, pp 1557–1578. Baltimore, Williams & Wilkins, 1999.

Williams WJ: Classification and clinical manifestations of disorders of hemostasis. In Beutler E, Lichtan MA, Coller BS, et al (eds): William's Hematology, 5th ed, pp 1276–1281. New York, McGraw-Hill, 1995.

169 Use of Blood Products

Marion H. Sims

Indications for Transfusion

1. Red blood cells (RBCs)

   a. Acute anemia (blood loss): Previously healthy patients can tolerate the loss of 30 per cent of total blood volume (indicated by tachycardia and orthostatic hypotension without further signs of shock) without the need for transfusion.

      (1) Hemoglobin (Hgb) greater than 10 gm/dl: Rarely requires transfusion.

      (2) Hgb less than 6 gm/dl: Usually requires transfusion.

      (3) Hgb 6 to 10 gm/dl: Transfuse according to clinical scenario (tachycardia or hypotension unresponsive to volume correction, underlying cardiac, pulmonary, or cerebrovascular disease).

   b. Chronic anemias

      (1) Pharmacologic treatment (e.g., vitamin B_{12}, folic acid, erythropoietin, iron) should be used first if indicated.

      (2) Specific transfusion strategies are followed for sickle cell disease and thalassemia.

      (3) Transfuse only when necessary to minimize the symptoms and risks of anemia (usually at Hgb 5 to 8 gm/dl).

   c. Neonates

      (1) Hgb less than 7 gm/dl or hematocrit (Hct) less than 20 per cent: Requires transfusion.

      (2) Hgb 8 to 12 gm/dl or Hct 25 to 35 per cent: Transfusion requirements depend on various clinical conditions (e.g., tachycardia, tachypnea, the presence of respiratory distress syndrome or congenital heart disease).

   d. Obstetric patients: Transfusion guidelines for pregnant and postpartum patients are the same as for nonpregnant patients.

2. Granulocytes

   a. Profound neutropenia (<100 granulocytes/μl) with worsening sepsis or cellulitis despite appropriate antibiotic therapy

   b. *Note:* granulocytes are rarely transfused. Myeloid growth factors (granulocyte and granulocyte-macrophage colony-stimulating factors) are indicated in most cases of profound neutropenia needing intervention.

3. Platelets

   a. Decreased platelet production (acute leukemia, aplastic anemia, etc.)

      (1) Platelet count less than 5000 to 10,000/μl: Transfusion required.

      (2) Platelet count 10,000 to 50,000/μl: Transfuse for signs of bleeding resulting from thrombocytopenia (confluent petechiae, wound oozing, gastrointestinal hemorrhage, headaches, increasing retinal hemorrhage).

      (3) Prophylactically transfuse to counts of greater than 20,000/μl before minor procedures and greater than 50,000/μl before major procedures.

   b. Increased platelet destruction (immune thrombocytopenias, disseminated intravascular coagulation [DIC], etc.)

      (1) Transfuse if the platelet count is less than 20,000 to 50,000/μl and unexpected, excessive bleeding is present.

      (2) During/after cardiopulmonary bypass surgery, transfuse for counts of less than 100,000/μl with excessive bleeding or chest tube drainage.

   c. Platelet dysfunction

      (1) Congenital platelet defects: Weigh the risk of alloimmunization against the benefit of transfusion.

      (2) Aquired platelet dysfunction: Consider teatment with desmopressin instead of transfusion.

4. Fresh frozen plasma (FFP)

   a. Coagulopathy (congenital or aquired) with active bleeding or prior to invasive procedures, confirmed by one of the following: prothrombin time (PT) 1.5 times the midpoint of normal range, activated partial thromboplastin time (PTT) 1.5 times the high normal range, or coagulation factor assay less than 25 per cent activity

   b. Massive blood transfusion: transfusion of more than one total blood volume/24 hours

(5000 ml in a 70-kg adult) or 50 per cent of blood volume in 3 hours, with coagulopathy and continued bleeding

   c. Reversal of warfarin effect: presence of active bleeding or prior to emergency surgery/procedure with PT greater than 18 seconds or International Normalized Ratio greater than 1.6

   d. Treatment of congenital or acquired coagulation factor deficiency: FFP can be used when a specific concentrate is not available.

   e. Plasma exchange therapy: selected cases of thrombotic thrombocytopenic purpura or hemolytic-uremic syndrome

5. Cryoprecipitate

   a. Hypofibrinogenemia: DIC is the most common cause. If the clinical situation dictates rapid replacement of fibrinogen, cryoprecipitate transfusion is the treatment of choice.

   b. Coagulation factor deficiency: von Willebrand's disease and hemophilia A when factor concentrates are not available

Preparation for Transfusion

1. Informed consent: discussion about the reason for transfusion, the component to be transfused, expected benefits, risks, alternatives, and consequences of foregoing transfusion.

2. Compatibility testing: Routine testing ensures compatibility between recipient's and donor's blood. A, B, Rh, and D antigens are specifically tested for and recipient serum is screened for antibodies to other commonly occurring antigens. This testing takes about 1 hour.

3. Intravenous access: The catheter should be 18 gauge or larger.

4. Premedication: Antipyretics and/or antihistamines are not recommended because early recognition of adverse reaction may be hindered.

5. Autologous transfusions: Patients can donate blood for up to 35 days prior to elective surgery. Donate one unit per week (maximum = 1 unit/72 hours) and start oral iron therapy.

Equipment

1. In-line filter for microaggregates: This is routinely used except when transfusing donor-matched platelets.

2. Bedside filter for leukocytes: Not as effective as prestorage filtration for producing leukocyte-reduced blood.

3. In-line blood warmer: Used to prevent hypothermia with large-volume transfusions or to prevent cardiac arrhythmias in rapid transfusions through central venous catheters.

Precautions

1. Confirmation of proper identification: Clerical error in identifying pretransfusion blood sample or matching blood unit to be transfused to the proper patient is the most common cause of fatal transfusion reaction.

2. Consider the need for leukocyte-reduced blood component. Indications include

   a. A history of two previous febrile reactions to transfusion

   b. To prevent platelet refractoriness: Exposure to leukocytes bearing human leukocyte antigens (HLAs) can lead to platelet alloimmunization.

   c. To prevent cytomegalovirus (CMV) exposure: Important in neonatal, immunocompromised, and CMV-negative pregnant recipients. Leukocyte reduction is as effective as using a CMV-seronegative product.

Dosing

1. RBCs

   a. One unit (180 to 200 ml of RBCs plus plasma and additives for total volume of 260 to 320 ml) should raise the Hgb by 1 gm/dl and the Hct by 3 per cent in a 70-kg adult.

   b. In complete marrow failure, 1 unit of RBCs will be lost per week as a result of RBC aging.

2. Granulocytes

   a. One unit is equivalent to 10 per cent of the body's daily granulocyte production.

   b. Transfusions are given daily (because of the granulocyte's brief lifespan) and should be continued until the count remains greater than 500 granulocytes/μl.

   c. Irradiated granulocytes from HLA-matched donors are preferred.

3. Platelets

   a. One unit (about 50 ml; 1 platelet pheresis unit = 6 random donor units) will raise the recipient's count by 5000 to 10,000/μl and last 3 to 5 days.

   b. The plasma in 5 units of platelets provide the equivalent of 1 unit of FFP.

4. FFP: Two units (200 to 250 ml/unit with 1 unit of factor activity/ml) are the usual starting dose (or 1 plasmapheresis unit, 400 to 600 ml). If the PT is less than 22 seconds or the PTT less than 70 seconds, 1 unit may be sufficient. Up to 10 to 15 ml/kg may be needed in some patients.

5. Cryoprecipitate

   a. One unit has the volume of 9 to 16 ml and

contains 100 units of factor VIII:C, 80 units of von Willebrand's factor, 250 mg of fibrinogen, and 50 units of factor XII and is dosed as 1 unit/5 kg body weight for hypofibrinogenemia.

 b. A standard dose of 10 units should increase fibrinogen by 70 mg/dl in a 70-kg adult.

 c. Von Willebrand's disease: The usual dose is 1 unit of cryoprecipitate/10 kg/day.

 d. Hemophilia A: Each unit will raise the recipient's factor VIII activity level 2 per cent.

Follow-Up

1. RBC transfusion

 a. In massive blood transfusions: Monitor Hgb, platelet count, PT/PTT, fibrinogen level, and fibrinogen degradation products after 4 units. After 10 units, repeat these tests and test Ca^{2+}/Mg^{2+} levels, pH, and lactate.

 b. In less acute situations: The expected increase in Hgb/Hct can be observed within 1 hour of transfusion, and most recipients feel the benefit of the transfusion within 18 hours as 2,3-diphosphoglycerate is restored in the transfused cells.

 c. In patients requiring chronic transfusions, the chief complications requiring monitoring are alloimmunization and iron overload.

2. Platelet transfusion: A platelet count should be checked 10 to 30 minutes after transfusion.

 a. If the count rises by the expected increment, daily monitoring is adequate.

 b. An inadequate response to transfusion could be the result of multiple factors (infection, DIC, splenomegaly) but usually is due to recipient antibodies. This requires HLA-matched platelets for future transfusions.

3. FFP transfusion: PT/PTT should be checked at completion of transfusion. If the PT is greater than 18 seconds or the PTT is greater than 60 seconds, more FFP is usually needed. The PTT is typically the best indicator of treatment efficacy and need for repeat transfusions.

4. Cryoprecipitate transfusion

 a. Fibrinogen has a half-life of 3 to 5 days, but in DIC there is increased fibrinogenolysis. Concentrations should be followed daily or more often if clinically indicated.

 b. Management of von Willebrand's disease and hemophilia A requires hematology consultation.

Bibliography

Fresh-Frozen Plasma, Cryoprecipitate, and Platelets Administration Practice Guidelines Development Task Force of the College of American Pathologists: Practice parameter for the use of fresh-frozen plasma, cryoprecipitate, and platelets. JAMA 1994;271:777–781.

Sazama K: Practical issues in informed consent for transfusion. Am J Clin Pathol 1997;107(4 Suppl 1):72S–74S.

Simon TL, Alverson DC, AuBuchon J, et al, for the Red Blood Cell Administration Practice Guideline Development Task Force of the College of American Pathologists: Practice parameter for the use of red blood cell transfusions. Arch Pathol Lab Med 1998;122:130–138.

Walker RH: Mathematical calculations in transfusion medicine. Clin Lab Med 1996;16:895–906.

Westphal RG: Handbook of Transfusion Medicine, 3rd ed. Washington, DC, The American National Red Cross, 1996.

170 Adverse Reactions to Blood Transfusions

David H. Yawn

Immediate Immunologic Transfusion Reactions

1. Acute intravascular hemolysis (ABO-incompatible red cells or plasma)
   a. Caused by naturally occurring complement-fixing immunoglobulin (Ig) M and IgG antibodies to group A and B red cells
   b. Fever, pain at infusion site, hypotension, acute renal failure, hemoglobinemia, hemoglobinuria
   c. Occurs in less than 1 in 250,000 transfusions
   d. Prevented by transfusing ABO-compatible red cells and plasma

> ### WARNING
>
> **Clerical errors (misidentification of patient or crossmatch sample) cause most fatal hemolytic reactions.**

2. Urticarial reactions
   a. Patient sensitized to plasma proteins and/or other antigens
   b. Rapid onset of hives after or during transfusion
   c. 1 to 3 per cent of all transfusions
   d. Prevented by the use of washed red cells or by premedication with antihistamines
3. Anaphylaxis
   a. Anti-IgA in IgA-deficient recipients (rarely caused by antibodies to human leukocyte antigens [HLA] or platelet antigens)
   b. Sudden hypotension and respiratory distress during transfusion
   c. Expected in less than 1 in 1000 transfusions
   d. Prevented by recognition of IgA-deficient patients or by use of washed red cells or provision of blood components from IgG-deficient donors
4. Febrile nonhemolytic reactions
   a. Passive transfer of donor leukocytes to patients who have produced leukoagglutinins
   b. Rapid onset of fever and chills, rarely pulmonary distress
   c. 1 to 3 per cent of transfusions; more common in multiply transfused or multiparous recipients
   d. Prevented by use of leukocyte-depleted red cells, whole blood, and platelets
5. Adverse reactions caused by platelet alloantibodies
   a. HLA- or platelet antigen–specific antibodies (such as anti–PLA-1) in the recipient
   b. Fever, pulmonary edema, and failure to achieve increments after platelet transfusions. Antibodies to PLA-1 (a high-frequency platelet antigen): petechiae, associated with purpura and severe thrombocytopenia within days after transfusion (posttransfusion purpura).
   c. High frequency of platelet alloantibodies in multiply transfused recipients. Present in some multiparous women.
   d. Prevention of alloimmunization (primarily caused by the stimulating effect of HLA antigens on transfused leukocytes) by the use of leukocyte depletion filters for all cellular blood components
6. Transfusion-related acute lung injury
   a. Etiology uncertain. Volume overload and/or immunologic factors, leukoagglutinins in donor plasma, and complement activation.
   b. High-protein noncardiogenic pulmonary edema
   c. Rare but life-threatening, occurs in approximately 1 in 5000 transfusions.
   d. Avoid donors with plasma leukoagglutinins; use leukocyte depletion filters or washed red cells.

Immediate Nonimmunologic Reactions

1. Volume overload
   a. Rapid infusion of excess volume
   b. Right and left ventricular heart failure, pulmonary and peripheral edema
   c. Very common, frequently unrecognized
   d. Careful attention to cardiovascular function and volume status of the patient during transfusion therapy; diuretics for selected patients

2. Citrate toxicity
   a. Sudden lowering of ionized calcium
   b. Hypotension and cardiac dysfunction
   c. Rare except during rapid and massive blood transfusion (adult: 12 or more units of blood per hour)
   d. Treated with intravenous calcium gluconate or calcium chloride; washed red cells for neonates or small recipients
3. Air embolism
   a. Accidental infusion of air contained in blood component bags
   b. Loss of consciousness, vascular collapse, rapid heart rate, chest tightness, pain, and dyspnea
   c. An extremely rare complication (current risk greatest with intraoperative blood salvage systems)
   d. Prevention by awareness
   e. Treatment: Place the patient on the left side in a head-down, feet-up position (reduction of pumping of air in the right ventricle into the pulmonary arteries).
4. Potassium overload
   a. Elevated potassium in older or irradiated packed cells or whole blood
   b. Hyperkalemia in massively transfused or small patients, especially neonates and small children
   c. Very rare unless patient has pre-existing renal dysfunction or acidosis
   d. Prevented by the use of washed red cell components, especially important for neonates and small transfusion recipients

Delayed Transfusion Complications
1. Delayed immune hemolysis
   a. Sensitization to red cell antigens (especially Rh, Kidd, Duffy, MNS antigens) as a result of remote pregnancies or transfusions. Anamnestic production of non-complement-fixing IgG antibodies a few days after a recent blood transfusion. Extravascular removal of antibody-coated cells.
   b. Anemia, fever, arthralgia, mild hyperbilirubinemia. Positive direct antiglobulin test. Renal dysfunction usually mild (rarely severe).
   c. 1 in 1000 transfusions (previously transfused or multiparous recipients)
   d. Patient education. Wallet card identifying the offending antibodies. Transfusion from donors lacking the red cell antigen(s) to which the patient is sensitized.

2. Graft-versus-host disease
   a. Proliferation of transfused HLA-incompatible lymphocytes; immune-suppressed recipients or immune-competent recipients who receive blood components from relatives.
   b. Dermatitis, gastrointestinal and liver dysfunction, and immune suppression; high mortality rate
   c. Occurs in less than 1 in 1000 transfusions.
   d. Irradiate (at least 2500 rads) all blood components donated by family members or if transfusing immune-suppressed patients; absolutely required for bone marrow transplant recipients.
3. Transfusion-related immune suppression
   a. Mechanism unknown
   b. Increased risk for bacterial infections and cancer progression
   c. Common, subclinical, frequently unrecognized; occurs to some extent with every transfusion.
   d. Prevention by reducing homologous blood exposure; increase use of autologous blood components
4. Iron overload (transfusion hemosiderosis)
   a. There is 1 mg of iron in 1 ml of red cells.
   b. Chronically transfused patients at great risk with deposition of iron in liver, heart, lungs, and marrow.
   c. Common in chronically transfused patients
   d. Minimize unnecessary transfusion. Iron chelation therapy. Reduce transfusions with recombinant erythropoietin therapy.

Infections Transmitted by Transfusion
1. Deadly viruses
   a. Failure to recognize asymptomatic donors infected with human immunodeficiency viruses (HIV 1 or 2), human T-cell lymphotrophic viruses (HTLV-I or -II), hepatitis viruses, cytomegalovirus (CMV), and others
   b. Clinical features related to virus transmitted. Long latency period common with HIV and HTLV-I viruses. CMV not important unless recipient is immune suppressed.
   c. Risk per component transfused: HIV, <1 in 600,000; hepatitis B, 1 in 63,000; hepatitis C, 1 in 103,000; HTLV I/II, 1 in 641,000; CMV, 50 to 100 per cent of donors infected
   d. Reduce risk with careful donor screening and serologic testing. Nucleic acid testing for hepatitis C and HIV in all blood donors will soon reduce the transfusion transmission of these viruses. Leukocyte filters to remove

strictly cell-associated viruses (HTLV-I/II and CMV). Donors negative for antibodies to CMV less likely to transmit CMV. (Immune-compromised patients and premature neonates are candidates for CMV-seronegative donors and leukocyte-reduced blood components.)

2. Transmission of bacteria and endotoxins
   a. Unrecognized bacteremia in the donor or bacterial contamination during processing. Cryophilic organisms (*Escherichia coli* and *Pseudomonas*) associated with refrigerated blood components. *Yersinia, Serratia*, and *Salmonella* implicated with room temperature–stored blood components (platelets). Platelet contamination is a growing problem.

WARNING

Bacterial contamination of platelets is now the most common cause of transfusion-related fatality.

---

   b. High mortality rate: fever, shock, and disseminated intravascular coagulation
   c. One in 500,000 units of red blood cells may have bacterial contamination. One in 12,000 units of platelets may cause transfusion related sepsis. As viral transmission risk decreases, the risk of bacterial contamination becomes relatively more important.
   d. Prevention with correct cleaning of the donor phlebotomy skin area, good manufacturing practices, deferring donors with febrile ill-nesses, and the use of leukocyte-depleted blood components.

3. Parasitic agents
   a. Donors infected with parasites (e.g., malaria or trypanosome causing Chagas' disease)
   b. Clinical problems of the specific parasitic infection
   c. Rare in United States. Chagas' disease endemic in Central and South America. Increased risk of Chagas' disease by transfusion is a current growing concern in the United States.
   d. Prevention by donor screening and development of appropriate serologic tests

Bibliography

Blumberg N, Heal JM: Transfusion-associated immunomodulation. In Anderson KC, Ness PM (eds): Scientific Basis of Transfusion in Medicine, pp 580–598. Philadelphia, WB Saunders Company, 1994.

Dodd RY: Adverse consequences of blood transfusion: quantitative risk estimates. In Nance ST (ed): Blood Supply: Risks, Perceptions, and Prospects for the Future, pp 1–24. Bethesda, MD, American Association of Blood Banks, 1994.

Goodnough LT, Brecher ME, Kanter MH, et al: Transfusion medicine, first of two parts, blood transfusion. N Engl J Med 1999;340:438–447.

Lundberg GD (ed): Practice parameter for the use of fresh frozen plasma, cryoprecipitate, and platelets. JAMA 1994;271:777–781.

McCullough J: The nation's changing blood supply system. JAMA 1993;269:2239–2245.

Mollison PL, Engelfriet CP, Contreras M: Blood Transfusion in Clinical Medicine, 9th ed, pp 677–709. Oxford, Blackwell Scientific Publications, 1993.

Schreiber GB, Busch MP, Kleinman SH, et al: The risk of transfusion transmitted viral infections. N Engl J Med 1996;334:1685–1690.

171 Disseminated Intravascular Coagulation

Timothy P. Daaleman

Etiology

1. Disseminated intravascular coagulation (DIC) is an acquired thromboembolic disorder that virtually always occurs in the presence of a concomitant disease or clinical state.

2. DIC results from the activation of the coagulation and fibrinolytic systems and can be an acute or chronic event.

   a. Acute DIC is an uncompensated hemorrhagic and thrombotic disorder that involves both laboratory and clinical evidence of pathology.

   b. Chronic DIC is a compensated hematologic state with mild, protracted, or often subclinical disease manifested by laboratory abnormalities.

3. The causes of DIC are listed in Table 171–1.

Symptoms

1. Bleeding is the predominant clinical symptom.

2. Other symptoms (fever, tachycardia) are nonspecific and not diagnostically helpful.

3. Patients display the signs and symptoms of the concomitant primary disease rather than those of DIC.

Key Symptom

Bleeding

Clinical Findings

1. In the appropriate clinical settings, the following signs should warn the clinician of the possibility of acute DIC:

   a. Petechiae

   b. Ecchymoses

   c. Hemorrhagic bullae

   d. Wound-site bleeding

   e. Gangrene

   f. Gingival bleeding

   g. Vascular access site oozing

   h. Purpura

   i. Acral cyanosis

   j. Hematuria

   k. Epistaxis

   l. Purpura fulminans

2. Patients with chronic DIC present with bleeding that is problematic (i.e., epistaxis, gingival

TABLE 171–1.   CAUSES OF DISSEMINATED INTRAVASCULAR COAGULATION

Obstetric
Amniotic fluid embolism
Abruptio placentae
Eclampsia
Uterine rupture
Retained dead fetus
Septic or missed abortion

Tissue Injury
Trauma (head or crush injury)
Burns
Extensive surgery
Hypo- or hyperthermia
Anoxia/asphyxia
Ischemia/infarction

Immunologic
Anaphylaxis
Hemolytic transfusion reaction
Adverse drug reaction
Autoimmune vasculitis

Pulmonary
Adult respiratory distress syndrome (ARDS)
Pulmonary embolism
Pulmonary infarction

Infectious
Gram-negative/positive/anaerobic
Mycobacterial
Viral (cytomegalovirus, varicella zoster virus, hepatitis)
Rickettsial (Rocky Mountain spotted fever)
Fungal (*Aspergillus*, *Candida*, *Histoplasma*)
Protozoal (malaria)

Malignancy
Leukemia
Solid tumors

Cardiovascular
Giant hemangioma
Aortic aneurysm
Aortic balloon pump
Acute myocardial infarction
Vascular surgery
Peripheral vascular disease

Miscellaneous
Acute or chronic liver disease
Envenomation
Fat embolism
Amyloidosis

bleeding) but not life-threatening, in addition to diffuse thromboses.

Key Signs

- Petechiae
- Ecchymoses
- Hemorrhagic bullae
- Wound-site bleeding
- Gangrene
- Gingival bleeding
- Vascular access site oozing
- Purpura
- Acral cyanosis
- Hematuria
- Epistaxis
- Purpura fulminans
- Thromboses (chronic)

Laboratory Tests

1. There is no consensus regarding laboratory criteria that confirm a diagnosis of DIC. All laboratory values must be interpreted in the appropriate clinical setting.
2. The following laboratory tests support the diagnosis of DIC:
   a. Thrombocytopenia (generally less than 60,000/μl)
   b. Prolonged prothrombin time (PT) and/or partial thromboplastin time (PTT)
   c. Elevated fibrin(ogen) degradation products (FDPs)
   d. Low or falling fibrinogen levels
   e. Schistocytosis (fragmented red blood cells) on peripheral smear
   f. Elevated D dimer
   g. Microangiopathic anemia

Key Tests

- Complete blood count with peripheral smear
- Fibrinogen level
- FDPs
- PT and PTT
- Single-tube clot retraction and clotting time

Differential Diagnosis

Several diseases resemble DIC; however, they can be ruled out on clinical grounds.

1. Vitamin K deficiency
2. Renal failure
3. Dysfibrinogenemias
4. Systemic lupus erythematosus
5. Thrombotic thrombocytopenic purpura
6. Liver disease
7. Sickle cell crisis
8. Sepsis

Treatment

1. In acute DIC, identifying and treating the underlying disease process remain the cornerstones of treatment.
   a. Aggressive treatment of the primary disease (i.e., antibiotics, evacuate uterus) in addition to appropriate supportive measures to correct or prevent shock, hypoxemia, and acidosis often will be sufficient.
   b. The use of blood products should be guided by the clinical picture.
      (1) Fresh frozen plasma (FFP) provides volume replacement and clotting factors. The dosage of FFP is 10 to 15 ml/kg. The clinician should look to achieve a prothrombin time within 2 to 3 seconds of control.
      (2) Cryoprecipitate should be reserved for hypofibrinogen states. The dosage is 0.2 bag/kg (a 70-kg patient requires 12 to 15 bags).
      (3) Platelet transfusion is appropriate if the platelet count is less than 10,000 to 20,000/μl or if major bleeding is present with a count less than 50,000/μl.
   c. There is no clear consensus regarding the use of heparin in acute DIC. Heparin is probably indicated in the following clinical situations: amniotic fluid embolism, aortic aneurysm, evidence of thrombosis (in sepsis or malignancy), and severe transfusion reaction.
      (1) Heparin is contraindicated in patients with central nervous system injury or fulminant liver failure, and in most obstetric accidents.
      (2) Two dosing regimens are 80 to 100 units/kg subcutaneously every 4 to 6 hours or 5 to 10 units/kg by continuous intravenous drip. Improvement should be noted by decreasing FDPs and increasing fibrinogen levels.
2. Treatment of the underlying disease process is the initial therapy in chronic DIC.
   a. Anticoagulant therapy with low-dose subcutaneous heparin may be indicated.
   b. Combination antiplatelet agents also have been useful:

(1) Acetylsalicylic acid, 600 mg bid with 30 ml liquid antacid, plus dipyridamole, 50 mg qid

(2) Sulfinpyrazone, 200 mg bid with 30 ml liquid antacid, plus dipyridamole, 50 mg qid

Bibliography

Bick RL: Disseminated intravascular coagulation and related syndromes. In Bick RL (ed): Hematology: Clinical and Laboratory Practice, vol 2, pp 1463–1499. St. Louis, CV Mosby Company, 1993.

Gilbert JA, Scalzi RP: Disseminated intravascular coagulation. Emerg Med Clin North Am 1993;11:465–480.

Giles AR: Disseminated intravascular coagulation. In Bloom AL, Forbes CD, Thomas DP, et al (eds): Haemostasis and Thrombosis, 3rd ed, vol 2, pp 969–986. Edinburgh, Churchill Livingstone, 1994.

Marder VJ, Feinstein DI, Francis CW, et al: Consumptive thrombohemorrhagic disorders. In Colman RW, Hirsh J, Marder VJ, et al (eds): Hemostasis and Thrombosis: Basic Principles and Clinical Practice, 3rd ed, pp 1023–1063. Philadelphia, JB Lippincott Company, 1994.

Williams EC, Mosher DF: Disseminated intravascular coagulation. In Hoffman R, Benz EJ Jr, Shattil SJ, et al (eds): Hematology: Basic Principles and Practice, 2nd ed, pp 1758–1769. New York, Churchill Livingstone, 1995.

172 Hemochromatosis

David R. Little

Etiology

Hemochromatosis (HC) is the accumulation of excess iron in many organs, leading to cell damage and functional insufficiency. HC is the most common autosomal recessive disorder among whites, and is especially prevalent among individuals of northern European descent. Clinically apparent disease occurs only in homozygotes, and it is five times more frequent in males than in females.

1. Hereditary HC: Results from excessive intestinal absorption of iron.
2. Secondary iron overload: Results from disorders of ineffective erythropoiesis, or excessive iron intake.

Symptoms

Many cases are asymptomatic. The classic triad of "bronze diabetes"—diabetes mellitus, skin pigmentation, and hepatomegaly—presents in less than 10 per cent of cases. Other symptoms include

1. Abdominal pain: often in the right upper quadrant, caused by liver enlargement
2. Weakness and fatigue
3. Joint pain: caused by inflammatory arthritis
4. Skin pigmentation
5. Impotence and loss of libido: caused by testicular dysfunction and/or hypogonadism

Key Symptoms

- Often asymptomatic
- Abdominal pain
- Joint pain

Clinical Findings

1. Typical findings
   a. Liver involvement: abdominal pain, hepatomegaly, elevated transaminases
   b. Diabetes mellitus
   c. Bronze skin discoloration
   d. Inflammatory arthritis
   e. Increased susceptibility to infection

2. Late findings
   a. Liver fibrosis/cirrhosis
   b. Dilated cardiomyopathy and congestive heart failure
   c. Increased risk for hepatocellular carcinoma

Key Signs

- Hepatomegaly
- Diabetes mellitus
- Bronze skin discoloration

Laboratory Findings

1. Transferrin saturation percentage
   a. This value is calculated by the formula: Serum iron ÷ Total iron-binding capacity
   b. Values above 62 per cent are strongly suggestive of hemochromatosis.

2. Serum ferritin
   a. Reflects total body iron stores
   b. Normal range: 15 to 20 μg/L
   c. Ferritin levels are nonspecific and may be mildly elevated in a variety of conditions. Patients with hemochromatosis typically have ferritin levels above 400 μg/L.

3. Liver biopsy
   a. Liver biopsy will confirm the diagnosis and rule out other causes of liver disease.
   b. Biopsy will quantify the hepatic iron concentration, providing valuable prognostic information. When HC is accompanied by cirrhosis or a high hepatic iron content, the patient is at a higher risk for end-stage complications, including hepatocellular carcinoma.
   c. If biopsy is contraindicated, magnetic resonance imaging may provide helpful but less precise diagnostic and prognostic information.

Differential Diagnosis

The diagnosis of HC may be delayed or missed if the clinician does not maintain a high index of suspicion. HC must be included in the differential diagnosis of many undifferentiated complaints such as fatigue and/or weakness, abdominal pain, arthralgias, impotence, and congestive heart failure. Other conditions that must be distinguished from HC include

1. Causes of iron overload
   a. Disorders of ineffective erythropoiesis
      (1) β-Thalassemia
      (2) Sideroblastic anemia
      (3) Pyruvate kinase deficiency
   b. Excessive oral intake from medicinal iron
   c. Parenteral iron administration
      (1) Transfusions
      (2) Intramuscular injections
      (3) Hemodialysis
2. Causes of liver disease
   a. Alcoholic liver disease
   b. Chronic viral hepatitis
3. Causes of joint disease
   a. Calcium pyrophosphate deposition disease
   b. Gout
   c. Septic arthritis (especially among diabetic patients)

Treatment

1. Phlebotomy
   a. Acute phase
      (1) Removal of 1 unit of whole blood weekly or twice weekly
      (2) Continue this protocol until serum ferritin level drops below 50 μg/L.
      (3) This process may require 100 or more phlebotomy treatments.
   b. Maintenance phase
      (1) Regular phlebotomy every 3 to 4 months should prevent reaccumulation of iron.
      (2) Transferrin saturation and ferritin should be measured yearly.
      (3) The goal of treatment is to maintain ferritin below 200 μg/L.

2. Additional treatment options
   a. Deferoxamine (Desferal)
      (1) An IV iron chelator given twice weekly at 10 mg/kg/dose
      (2) Recommended only when rapid iron mobilization is necessary, such as in the instance of cardiac arrhythmias or congestive heart failure
      (3) May be used if phlebotomy is contraindicated.
   b. Deferiprone
      (1) An orally active iron chelator
      (2) Effective in some forms of iron overload, such as thalassemia, where phlebotomy is not an option
      (3) Associated with a high incidence of agranulocytosis

Follow-Up

The prognosis for patients with hemochromatosis is most closely related to the presence of cirrhosis. Early detection of hemochromatosis and aggressive iron mobilization will reduce the risk of cirrhosis and improve life expectancy.

1. Maintenance phlebotomy protocol (described above)
2. Monitoring for complications
   a. Hepatocellular carcinoma occurs in patients with HC and cirrhosis at a rate 219 times higher than in the general population. Consider periodic monitoring of α-fetoprotein levels and ultrasound examination of the liver in patients at risk
   b. Monitor clinically for additional complications, including cardiomyopathy, diabetes, and cirrhosis.
3. Screening
   a. The preferred screening test is the transferrin saturation percentage.
   b. Screening is currently recommended for individuals at risk (see Table 172–1). Some authorities recommend routine screening for all adults, or for all patients with diabetes.
   c. A genetic test has recently been discovered, but it is not currently recommended as a screening instrument until further population-based research is available.

TABLE 172–1. RISK FACTORS FOR HEMOCHROMATOSIS

Family history of iron overload disease
Clinical manifestations of iron overload
    Severe fatigue
    Impotence
    Hypogonadism
    Amenorrhea
    Cardiomyopathy
    Diabetes mellitus
    Liver disease
    Arthritis
Abnormalities found during routine health examination

Bibliography

Burke W, Thompson E, Khoury MJ, et al: Hereditary hemochromatosis: gene discovery and its implications for population-based screening. JAMA 1998;280:172–178.

Gandon Y, Guyader D, Heautot JF, et al: Hemochromatosis: diagnosis and quantification of liver iron with gradient-echo MR imaging. Radiology 1994;193:533–538.

Little DR: Hemochromatosis: diagnosis and management. Am Fam Physician 1996;53:2623–2628.

McDonnell SM, Witte D: Hereditary hemochromatosis: preventing chronic effects of this underdiagnosed disorder. Postgrad Med 1997;102:83–94.

Witte DL, Crosby WH, Edwards CQ, et al, for the Practice Guideline Development Task Force of the College of American Pathologists: Hereditary hemochromatosis. Clin Chim Acta 1996;245:139–200.

173   Common Endocrine Symptoms

SYMPTOM   HIRSUTISM

Laura Novak

Hirsutism is an excessive male pattern hair growth resulting from increased androgenic (male) hormone effect. It is often accompanied by amenorrhea, acne, and obesity (also caused by androgens). Although efforts are made to determine the source of the androgens (adrenal, ovarian, or both), and to rule out serious disease (which is rare), many women with hirsutism will have no laboratory abnormalities and are considered to be converting androgens peripherally. Even those women with diagnosable syndromes are treated with modification of their underlying imbalances rather than curative procedures. Therefore, it is important to approach this symptom holistically with concern for the woman's social, cosmetic, and self-esteem issues as well as her medical diagnosis.

Differential Diagnosis

1. Idiopathic/familial: usually caused by increased sensitivity of hair follicles to circulating androgens; more common in Mediterranean families

2. Polycystic ovarian disease: some combination of amenorrhea, hirsutism, obesity, infertility and bilateral cystic ovaries. May also be associated with increased insulin resistance.

3. Persistent anovulation: Consider hypothyroidism or prolactinemia.

4. Late-onset congenital adrenal hyperplasia (CAH): a deficiency in adrenal enzymes leading to increased androgens; presents with earlier onset, more rapid course. (*Note*: This can be passed on to offspring as severe, early-onset CAH.)

5. Exogenous testosterone: anabolic steroids (athletes), testosterone (Estratest), or dehydroepiandrosterone (over-the-counter "antiaging" pill)

6. Excess testosterone: If extreme, consider ovarian tumor.

7. Excess adrenal androgens: If extreme, consider adrenal tumor (rare).

8. Cushing's syndrome: truncal obesity, hypertension, striae, weakness, (rare).

History

1. Age at onset and rapidity of onset

2. Severity: May be disguised by hair removal.

3. Virilization: more severe male changes—balding, low voice, clitoromegaly. Presence implies more serious disease.

4. Menstrual and fertility history

5. Presence of galactorrhea or thyroid symptoms

6. Exogenous androgens

7. Family history

Clinical Findings

1. Coarse, dark hair growth in beard, mustache, chest, abdomen, thighs

2. Often accompanied by irregular menses, infertility, acne, and obesity

3. Possible virilization

4. Possible acanthosis nigrans (gray-brown discoloration of the axilla, groin, and vulva): seen with insulin resistance

Tests

The first three tests should be done on all patients. The other tests are used selectively.

1. Total serum testosterone
   a. Level greater than *80* ng/dl implies ovarian source
   b. Level greater than 200 ng/dl mandates tumor work-up (imaging study)

2. Serum dehydroepiandrosterone sulfate (DHEAS)
   a. Level greater than *350* μg/dl implies adrenal source
   b. Level greater than *700* μg/dl mandates tumor work-up (imaging study)
   c. There is wide variation of normal levels, and some people believe this is not a cost-effective test.

3. Serum 17-hydroxyprogesterone (17-OHP): Elevation indicates late-onset CAH. If greater

than 200 ng/dl, do adrenocorticotropic hormone (ACTH; Cortrosyn) test to confirm diagnosis (give ACTH, 0.25 mg IV, and check 17-OPH at 0 and 1 hours [use nomogram for normals]).

4. Low-dose dexamethasone test (*not dexamethasone suppression test*): If DHEAS is greater than *350* but less than 700 μg/dl, give 0.5 mg dexamethasone qid ×5 days and recheck DHEAS and testosterone. If levels decrease, the source is adrenal and low-dose dexamethasone will be an effective treatment.

5. Serum thyroid-stimulating hormone and prolactin if anovulatory

6. Pelvic ultrasound and luteinizing hormone/follicle-stimulating hormone (LH/FSH) ratio (>2 abnormal) may confirm polycystic ovarian disease.

Management

The goal of hirsutism management is to decrease circulating androgens (through decreased production, increased clearance, or changing the LH/FSH ratio). This usually results in markedly decreased further hair growth but will only partially eliminate already present hair. Therefore, cosmetic therapy is usually needed concomitantly.

1. Hormonal therapy
   a. Oral contraceptives: All brands of oral contraceptives will decrease circulating androgens, regulate periods, and (usually) decrease acne.
   b. Other hormones, such as medroxyprogesterone (Depo-Provera) or conjugated estrogens/medroxyprogesterone (Prempro, Premphase), can be effective.
   c. Ovarian suppression via Lupron or Danazole may be useful.

2. Dexamethasone, 0.5 mg qd, if indicated (see above)

3. Cosmetic therapy: bleaching, plucking, shaving, electrolysis (by licensed operator), laser therapy.

4. Weight loss: Will decrease insulin resistance and androgen production

5. Antiandrogen drugs: Often block peripheral binding.
   a. Usually need oral contraceptives because of side effect of dysfunctional uterine bleeding.
   b. Overall, these medications will decrease hair size and distribution by about 25 per cent

c. Reserve for difficult cases or use with a consultant: spironolactone, cyproterone, flutamide, ketoconazole, finasteride (experimentally; never in fertile women).

6. Fertility therapy: Patients with anovulation may be treated with ovulation inducers when desired. Metformin helps fertility in those with insulin resistance.

7. Insulin resistance: Promote ideal weight, exercise, risk reduction, and consider metformin (Glucophage).

Patient Education

1. Treatment is often slow (1 to 2 years) and partial, so the patient should have limited expectations.

2. Most hair removal products sold in magazines and on television are not effective.

3. Successful therapy may improve fertility, so contraception may be needed after therapy.

4. Shaving will not increase hair size or number, but will cause stubble.

PEARLS

- Cosmetic therapy is a necessary adjunct to medical therapy.

- Therapy is often partial and slow, so pictures or the Ferriman-Gallwey scale may be needed to see progress.

- Women with insulin resistance are at increased risk for diabetes and heart disease.

Bibliography

Andrew DE, Gagliardi C, Emmi AM: Hirsutism. In Decherney AH, Pernoll ML (eds): Current Obstetrics and Gynecology. Diagnosis and Treatment, 8th ed, pp 1016–1025. Norwalk, CT, Appleton & Lange, 1994.

Franks S: Polycystic ovarian disease. N Engl J Med 1995; 333:853–868.

Rosenfield RL: Current concepts of polycystic ovary syndrome. Baillieres Clin Obstet Gynecol 1997;11:307–333.

Hirsutism. In Speroff L, Glass R, Kase N (eds): Clinical Gynecologic Endocrinology and Infertility, 5th ed, pp 483–509. Baltimore, Williams & Wilkins, 1994.

Young R, Sinclair R: Hirsutes I: diagnosis. Aust J Dermatol 1998;39:24–28.

1. Gynecomastia is the enlargement of the male breast as a result of physiologic and pathologic changes in the estrogen-to-androgen hormone ratio.

2. Histologic changes of new-onset gynecomastia are characterized by a proliferation of glandular epithelium as well as hyperplasia and edema of stroma and connective tissue. In longstanding gynecomastia, fibrosis and hyalinization are the predominant tissue changes.

3. Physiologic male breast development of puberty is the most common type of gynecomastia, occurring in 65 per cent of all pubescent males. It usually resolves without any intervention. Gynecomastia in the older age groups is commonly associated with pathologic illness such as liver disease, renal failure, hyperthyroidism, gonadal failure, or various endocrine-secreting tumors. In both young and older age groups, several drugs have been recognized as causes of gynecomastia either by increasing estrogen levels and effects on tissue or by decreasing testosterone levels.

Differential Diagnosis

1. Childhood and adolescent male breast development
   a. Physiologic changes of the newborn or pubertal changes of the adolescent
   b. Medications
   c. Hypogonadal conditions
   d. Genetic disorders: Klinefelter's syndrome
2. Adult male breast development
   a. Medications
   b. Gonadal failure
   c. Chronic illnesses: liver disease, renal failure, hyperthyroidism, severe malnutrition
   d. Tumors: testicular, adrenal, bronchial, pancreatic, gastric, hepatic, and adrenal
3. Obesity
4. Hypertrophy of the pectoralis major
5. Carcinoma of the male breast
6. Neurofibromas

Drugs Associated With Gynecomastia

Estrogen, digitalis, cimetidine, ketoconazole, metoclopramide, finasteride, spironolactone, methyldopa, calcium channel blockers, isoniazid, metronidazole, omeprazole, reserpine, angiotensin-converting enzyme inhibitors, tricyclic antidepressants, phenothiazines, nadolol, diazepam, phenytoin, heroin, marijuana, alcohol, amphetamines, chemotherapy agents (alkylating drugs, cisplatin)

History

1. Age at time of onset
2. Duration of symptoms
3. Presence or absence of breast tenderness
4. History of chest wall trauma
5. Symptoms of testicular failure: loss of libido, impotence
6. Medication usage
7. History of illicit drugs
8. History of excessive alcohol
9. Symptoms of liver failure, renal insufficiency, hyperthyroidism
10. History of severe nutritional deficits
11. Symptoms of pituitary tumor growth: visual field defects or severe headaches

Clinical Findings

1. Breast mass centrally located beneath the nipple; most commonly bilateral but can be asymmetric and rarely unilateral
2. Mass that has a firm yet rubbery texture
3. Evaluate for
   a. Mobile mass
   b. Mass tenderness
4. Hypogonadism: small testes and absence of secondary sexual characteristics
5. Testicular examination for masses and size
6. Abdominal examination for adrenal tumors
7. Cushing's syndrome: suggestive of adrenal hyperactivity
8. Signs of hepatic failure: jaundice, ascites, spider angiomata
9. Thyrotoxicosis: hyperactive reflexes, tachycardia, exophthalmos, tender enlarged thyroid
10. Signs of renal insufficiency: peripheral edema, noncardiac pulmonary edema
11. Signs of Klinefelter's syndrome: tall, slim, underweight male; smaller than usual phallus and

testicular size; mental impairment variable from mental retardation to learning disabilities

---

PEARLS

- Benign breast mass are usually centrally located, bilateral, and mobile with a rubbery texture.

- Malignant masses are usually unilateral, eccentrically located, and immobile with a hard texture. Any nipple retraction or drainage strongly suggest a malignant process.

Diagnostic Tests

1. Because most cases of gynecomastia are caused by self-limiting benign physiologic changes, laboratory test are often unnecessary.
2. Baseline laboratory panel for: hepatic, renal, and thyroid functions
3. Hormonal measurements: testosterone, estradiol, luteinizing hormone
4. Quantitative human chorionic gonadotropin levels
5. Chest radiographs if pulmonary lesions suspected
6. Testicular ultrasound to evaluate for masses
7. Computerized tomography of abdomen to look for adrenal tumor
8. Breast tissue biopsy
9. Mammography
10. Chromosomal analysis if Klinefelter's syndrome suspected

Management

1. Observation and reassurance of the patient
2. Removal of the offending drug or agents
3. Treatment of underlying disease
4. Surgical excision: mastectomy, liposuction
5. Medications: usually most effective in new-onset gynecomastia; antiestrogen drugs (tamoxifen), aromatase inhibitor (testolactone), testosterone for hypogonadal states
6. Prophylactic radiation of breast tissue for those prostate cancer patients receiving hormones
7. Patient education
   a. Reassurance that most cases resolve without need for further intervention
   b. Reassurance that benign gynecomastia will not cause loss of virility and is not associated with feminization

Follow-Up

1. Recheck every 3 to 6 months for resolution of benign gynecomastia.
2. Follow laboratory test as indicated for specific underlying illnesses.
3. Survey for tumor regression or recurrence.

Bibliography

Frantz AG, Wilson JD: Endocrine disorders of the breast. In Wilson JD, Foster DW, Kronenburg HM, et al (eds): Williams' Textbook of Endocrinology, 9th ed, pp 885–892. Philadelphia, WB Saunders Company, 1998.

Glass AR: Gynecomastia. Endocrinol Metabol Clin North Am 1994;23:825–837.

Madani S, Tolia V: Gynecomastia with metoclopramide use in pediatric patients. J Clin Gastroenterol 1997;24:79–81.

Mahoney CP: Adolescent gynecomastia: differential diagnosis and management. Pediatr Clin North Am 1990;37:1389–1404.

Neuman JF: Evaluation and treatment of gynecomastia. Am Fam Physician 1997;55:1835–1844.

Wilson JD: Endocrine disorders of the breast. In Fauci AS, Braunwald E, Isselbacher KJ, et al (eds): Harrison's Principles of Internal Medicine, 14th ed, pp 2117–2118. Philadelphia, WB Saunders Company, 1998.

SYMPTOM **GOITER**

Isaac Kleinman

1. A goiter is any visible or palpable thyroid gland. (It may not be visible or palpable if located substernally.) It may be diffuse or nodular, toxic or nontoxic, endemic or sporadic, malignant or nonmalignant, congenital (rare) or acquired. The normal gland weighs about 20 gm.
2. Clinical goiter affects 200 million persons worldwide (7 per cent of the world population [World Health Organization, 1958]; 3 to 4 per cent of the United States population [Framingham Study]; and 15 per cent of the German population). Iodine deficiency is the most common cause worldwide (especially in Germany, Fiji, New Guinea, and the Himalayas). Thyroiditis is the most common cause in the United States. By postmortem examination in the United States, goiters or nodules are found in 50 per cent of the population.

Types

Congenital

1. Type I: associated with defects in iodine transport

2. Type II: associated with defects in organification of iodine

3. Type III: associated with defects in dehalogenase

4. Type IV: associated with defects in thyroglobulin synthesis

Acquired

1. Benign
   a. Nontoxic
      (1) Endemic (colloid) goiter: most common type of goiter; associated with puberty, menopause, and pregnancy. In addition to iodine deficiency, it may be caused by goitrogens such as turnips, aminosalicylic acid, and lithium: goitrogens block thyroxine formation, which leads to increased thyroid-stimulating hormone (TSH) secretion from the pituitary, which in turn induces gland hyperplasia. (This does not explain nodularity, a circumstance in which only parts of the gland undergo hyperplasia.) Colloid goiter patients may be euthyroid or hyperthyroid.
      (2) Hashimoto's thyroiditis (autoimmune thyroiditis)
         (a) Chronic; characterized by lymphocytic infiltrates
         (b) Most common cause of primary hypothyroidism
         (c) Frequently associated with autoimmune disorders and other endocrine disorders
         (d) Painless and nontender
   b. Toxic
      (1) Granulomatous thyroiditis (subacute, giant cell)
         (a) Acute, inflammatory type
         (b) Sudden onset
         (c) Fever
         (d) Neck pain
         (e) Tenderness
      (2) Silent thyroiditis
         (a) Mainly postpartum women
         (b) Nontender; transient hyperthyroid phase followed by a limited period of hypothyroidism
         (c) Probably autoimmune

2. Malignant
   a. Papillary: most common (50 to 70 per cent); female-to-male ratio 2.5 to 1; lymphatic spread
   b. Follicular: 15 per cent; hematogenous spread
   c. Mixed
   d. Medullary: May be associated with other endocrine disorders; metastasizes via lymphatics to cervical and mediastinal nodes, to lungs, and to bone; may be associated with ectopic production of other hormones; produces excessive calcitonin, which can lower calcium and phosphorus.

Differential Diagnosis of Anterior Neck Masses

1. Cystic hygroma (will usually transilluminate)
2. Thyroglossal duct cyst (may transilluminate)
3. Malignancy, metastatic
4. Lymphadenopathy and lymphoma
5. Goiter, toxic and nontoxic, benign and malignant

History may reveal symptoms of hypo- or hyperthyroidism or other endocrinopathies. Note mechanical symptoms and history of irradiation. Inquire about goitrogens.

Environmental Goitrogens

- Iodine deficiency
- Iodine process
- Radiation
- Chemicals: sulfonylureas, thiocyanate, lithium, propylthiouracil, resorcinol, cobalt, aminoglutethimide, fluoride, calcium, cassava, soya beans, turnips (contain thiouracil-like antithyroid substances)

Symptoms

Although most goiters are asymptomatic and present as a simple swelling in the neck, they themselves may produce symptoms that are mechanical or hormonal.

Mechanical

1. Dysphasia, dyspnea, sensation of constriction in chest or throat
2. Hoarseness, increased phlegm in the throat
3. Symptoms of superior vena caval obstruction (substernal goiter); positive Pemberton's sign (see below)

Hormonal

1. Hyperthyroidism
   a. Cardiac rhythm irregularities, tremor, nervousness, heat intolerance
   b. Tachycardia, increased appetite, frequent bowel movements, increased pulse pressure

c. Muscle weakness, eye signs (proptosis, lid lag, lid retraction, stare, conjunctival injection)

d. Weight loss

e. Thyroid storm (confusion, psychosis, coma, cardiovascular collapse)

2. Hypothyroidism

a. Hair loss, periorbital puffiness, drooping eyelids

b. Dry skin, macroglossia, bradycardia, menstrual disturbances

c. Mental sluggishness, myxedema coma (rare), change in personality, psychosis (rare)

Clinical Findings

Physical examination should first define the extent and character of the enlargement: diffuse or nodular, firm or soft, symmetric or asymmetric, associated lymphadenopathy. Check for Pemberton's sign (increased heart rate, usually with distention of the cervical veins, when the arms are abducted). Assess metabolic status and levels of thyroid hormone; look for associated endocrine changes or autoimmune disorders. General findings may include

1. Thyroid enlargement and/or nodularity

2. Tenderness (thyroiditis)

3. Symptoms and/or signs of thyrotoxicosis (see above)

4. Cardiac irregularity

5. Congestive heart failure

6. Muscle wasting and weakness

7. Displacement of trachea or esophagus

8. Superior vena caval obstruction (substernal goiter)

9. Symptoms and/or signs of hypothyroidism (see above)

Findings Suggestive of Malignancy

1. Young age

2. Male

3. Solitary nodule (multinodular goiters are 99 per cent benign)

4. Cold nodules on scan (20 per cent are malignant; "hot" nodules are rarely malignant)

5. History of radiation to head or neck

6. Stippled calcification on radiograph

7. Recent or rapid enlargement

8. Stony, hard consistency

9. Nodule with adjacent lymphadenopathy

10. Nodule with ipsilateral vocal cord paralysis

Tests

Laboratory tests are done to assess metabolic status and thyroid hormone levels and to search for associated endocrine disorders.

1. Triiodothyronine (T_3), thyroxine (T_4), TSH, reverse T_3, free T_4, thyrotropin-releasing hormone test, ^{131}I uptake, and thyroid-binding globulin: to assess thyroid function

2. Thyroid scans: to search for metastases (often not visible on radiograph)

3. Radiography, magnetic resonance imaging: to evaluate large tumors, substernal tumors

4. Calcitonin assay: in suspected medullary cancer

5. Ultrasound: to document size and follow growth or shrinkage; to determine if mass is solid or cystic; to document unilateral agenesis of a thyroid lobe

6. Laryngoscopy: to evaluate hoarseness (possible laryngeal nerve paralysis)

7. Needle biopsy: one of the most useful tests; potentially the most direct approach to diagnosis, short of open surgery.

a. There are four categories of biopsy reports:

(1) Cancer: In the case of medullary cancer, patients should be evaluated for other endocrinopathies, especially pheochromocytoma.

(2) Suspicious: occurs in 20 per cent of biopsies, usually follicular or Hürthle cell tumors. Twenty per cent of "suspicious" specimens ultimately prove to be malignant.

(3) Benign

(4) Inadequate specimen

b. Needle biopsy is not recommended in patients with a history of neck irradiation because 40 per cent of previously irradiated patients will have cancer in some other area of the gland than the nodule undergoing biopsy. Open biopsy should be used if biopsy is indicated in these patients.

Management

1. None required in asymptomatic euthyroid goiter. Iodine deficiency should be corrected and goitrogens discontinued if found. Surgical removal may be desirable for cosmetic reasons.

2. ^{131}I therapy: for thyrotoxicosis, especially in poor surgical risks

3. Surgery: indications

a. Suspicion of malignancy (cold nodules, follicular neoplasia, signs of invasion such as tracheal traction, lateral distortion or hoarseness, rapid growth, rock-hard gland)

b. Compressive symptoms

c. Cosmesis

d. Presence of autonomously functioning thyroid tissue

4. Medical

a. Nontoxic goiter: Two thirds of diffuse goiters and small nodular goiters will decrease in size on 150 to 200 μg/day levothyroxine. Change in size can be followed and documented by ultrasonography. Hashimoto's thyroiditis, pubescent goiter, and nontoxic goiter in younger patients respond best.

b. Toxic goiter: Propylthiouracil, 100 to 150 mg every 8 hours orally to start, or methimazole, 10 to 15 mg every 8 hours to start, are the mainstays of treatment. They work by impairing organification of iodine. When control of symptoms is achieved, the dose is reduced to the lowest level that maintains it (usually 100 to 150 mg/day of propylthiouracil or 10 to 15 mg of methimazole in divided doses bid or tid).

Classification of Goiter

- Stage 0A: no goiter

- Stage 0B: detectable by palpation but not visible even with the neck fully extended

- Stage I: palpable and visible only with the neck fully extended

- Stage II: visible with the neck in normal position

- Stage III: large goiter visible at a distance

PEARLS

- Thyroid disease in the elderly may be occult. Clues include cardiac irregularity, unexplained cardiac hypertrophy, occult congestive failure, and change in mental status.

- Thyroid hormone promotes bone mineral loss in postmenopausal women who are not receiving estrogen replacement therapy and may increase estrogen requirements.

- Avoid radiation treatment and hypothyroid status if possible during pregnancy.

- Avoid radiation treatment in the young patient.

Bibliography

Biassoni P, Ravera G, Bertocchi J, et al: Influence of dietary habits on thyroid status of a nomadic people, the Bororo shepherds, roaming a central African region affected by severe iodine deficiency. Eur J Endocrinol 1998;138:681–685.

Brunt M, Wells SA Jr: Advances in the diagnosis and treatment of medullary thyroid carcinoma. Surg Clin North Am 1987;67:263–277.

Chopra IJ: Hypothyroidism. In Rakel RE (ed): Conn's Current Therapy, pp 644–649. Philadelphia, WB Saunders Company, 1998.

Foley TP Jr: Goiter in adolescents. Endocrinol Metab Clin North Am 1993;22:593–606.

Roher H-D, Goretzki PE: Management of goiter and thyroid nodules in an area of endemic goiter. Surg Clin North Am 1987;67:233–249.

Schneider D, Barett-Conner E, Morton DJ: Thyroid hormone use and bone mineral density in elderly women. JAMA 1994;271:1245–1249.

174 Diabetes Mellitus, Type I   *O. David Dellinger, III*

Etiology

1. Type I diabetes mellitus is the result of the destruction of beta cells in the islets of Langerhans in the pancreas by either mechanical or chemical means or an autoimmune process.
2. The autoimmune destruction of beta cells involves a complex interaction between both genetic and nongenetic factors, with a concordance rate of between 20 and 50 per cent in monozygotic twins.
3. Several different immune events, including exposure to a variety of viruses, exposure to certain food components such as cow's milk, and maternal-fetal blood group incompatibility, have been associated with type I diabetes.

Symptoms

1. Increased blood glucose levels cause an osmotic diuresis (polyuria), leading to dehydration, possibly with orthostasis, and increased thirst (polydypsia).
2. Because the insulin-sensitive tissues cannot take up and utilize the glucose in the blood, those tissues begin to starve, producing increased hunger (polyphagia) and weight loss.
3. As blood glucose levels increase, blurred vision and paresthesias may develop.
4. As tissue starvation progresses, ketoacidosis ensues, with nausea and vomiting, and may lead to severe abdominal pain (which may mimic an acute abdomen). Vascular collapse, coma, and death will occur if left untreated.
5. Symptoms may develop gradually or quite suddenly.

Key Symptoms

- Polyuria
- Polydypsia
- Polyphagia
- Weight loss
- Orthostasis
- Blurred vision
- Abdominal pain
- Nausea and vomiting

Clinical Findings

1. Physical examination may be normal.
2. Body habitus is usually normal to wasted with signs of recent weight loss.

3. Usually younger patients (teens), but may be any age.
4. Signs of dehydration may be present.
5. Kussmaul respirations and an acetone smell will be noticeable if ketoacidosis is present.

Key Signs

- Examination may be normal
- Usually young and thin
- Evidence of recent weight loss
- Orthostatic hypotension
- Signs of dehydration
- Kussmaul respirations, acetone smell

Laboratory Tests

1. A fasting blood sugar greater than 126 mg/dl, any blood sugar greater than 200 mg/dl with symptoms, or a blood sugar greater than 200 mg/dl 2 hours after a 75-gm glucose load on two occasions is diagnostic.
2. An elevated glycosylated hemoglobin (or hemoglobin A_{1c}) is virtually diagnostic of diabetes mellitus, but normal values do not exclude the diagnosis.
3. The urine of untreated type I diabetics will show glucose and usually ketones.
4. C-peptide levels and serum insulin levels are low in untreated type I diabetes.
5. Islet cell antibodies are usually positive in autoimmune type I diabetes, but positive islet cell antibodies are not diagnostic or predictive of type I diabetes.

Key Tests

- Fasting blood sugar greater than 126 mg/dl
- Random blood sugar greater than 200 mg/dl with symptoms
- Blood sugar greater than 200 mg/dl 2 hours after 75-gm glucose load
- Elevated hemoglobin A_{1c}
- Glucosuria
- Ketonuria
- Low serum peptide C
- Low serum insulin

Differential Diagnosis

1. The only other consideration is type II diabetes mellitus.
2. Type II diabetics tend to be older, heavier, tend not to have ketosis, and often have signs of high insulin levels or other signs of insulin resistance.

Treatment

Medication

1. Some insulin must be provided every day, even if the patient is fasting.
2. The goal is to provide only as much insulin as the body needs in order to maintain blood sugars as close to normal as possible at all times.
3. The goal of insulin administration is to anticipate a rise in blood sugar and provide adequate insulin to control it, rather than "chasing" elevated blood sugars.
4. Many different insulin types are available or under development, and differ in their onset and duration of action (Table 174–1).
5. Conventional therapy for stable patients consists of two injections a day of a combination of an intermediate- (NPH) and short-acting (Regular) insulin.
   a. Initially, a daily insulin requirement of 0.5 to 1.0 unit/kg/day is assumed.
   b. Initially, two thirds of the total daily insulin dose is given before breakfast, and one third before the evening meal.
   c. The breakfast dose of insulin is two thirds intermediate-acting insulin and one third short-acting insulin.
   d. The evening dose is one half short-acting, and one half intermediate-acting insulin.
   e. The patient's blood sugar should be monitored before each meal and at bedtime.
   f. Insulin therapy for the following day can be fine tuned realizing that
      (1) The short-acting AM insulin affects the blood sugar before lunch.
      (2) The intermediate-acting AM insulin affects the blood sugar before supper.
      (3) The short-acting PM insulin affects the blood sugar at bedtime.
      (4) The intermediate-acting PM insulin affects the prebreakfast blood sugar.
   g. Insulin dosages are then adjusted based on the prior day's results.
6. Intensive therapy consists of at least four shots of insulin per day.
   a. If three meals a day are eaten, about one fourth of the total daily insulin is given in a short-acting form before each meal, with some adjustment for the size of the meal, the anticipated rise in blood sugar, and the blood sugar before the meal.
   b. The other one fourth is given as a long- or intermediate-acting dose before bedtime to maintain a basal insulin level throughout the night.
   c. Again, adjustments in insulin doses are based on the prior day's results.
7. Another alternative is to use an insulin pump.
   a. The pump requires an implanted delivery line and the use of an external reservoir.
   b. The pump uses short-acting insulin and is programmed to deliver about one fourth of the total daily insulin requirement continuously over 24 hours.
   c. Before each meal, the user presses a button that causes the release of a bolus of insulin.
8. The long-term advantage of each of these methods is controversial, and treatment should be individualized.
9. Future therapies may include nasal formulations of insulin, implantable pumps with glucose sensors, or islet cell transplantation.

Key Treatment

- Insulin, 0.5 to 1.0 units/kg/day initially
- Two thirds of total dose before breakfast, one third before supper
- Seventy per cent NPH/30 per cent Regular insulin in the AM, 50 per cent NPH/50 per cent Regular insulin in the PM

TABLE 174–1. TYPES OF INSULIN

	ONSET	PEAK EFFECT (hr)	DURATION (hr)
Lispro	Immediate	1–3	2–4
Regular	20 min	2–4	6–8
NPH/Lente	Slow	6–12	18–24
Ultralente/HOE 901	Slow	8–24	24+

- Adjust doses based on patterned blood sugars over 1 to 3 days

- Avoid "chasing" high blood sugars

- Never give *no* insulin in a 24-hour period

Diet

1. Total calories should be between about 30 and 45 kcal/kg depending on sex (males needing more), age (less with increasing age), and level of activity.

2. In general, total calories should be slightly low rather than high.

3. Protein should minimally be 0.9 gm/kg/day, but not more than about one third of total calories.

4. Fat should account for 30 per cent or less of calories, with mostly polyunsaturated fats and less than 300 mg of cholesterol per day; more recently, alternative diets with as much as 50 per cent of calories from monounsaturated fats have shown some benefit.

5. The balance of calories should consist mostly of complex carbohydrates.

Activity

1. A minimum of 20 to 30 minutes of aerobic exercise at least three times per week.

2. Because heart disease is more prevalent in diabetics, cardiovascular fitness should be assessed before initiation of an exercise program.

3. Pre-exercise blood sugar should be checked and an appropriate carbohydrate load given, realizing that exercise may lower blood sugar levels dramatically.

4. Avoid dehydration, and do not exercise if blood sugars are unusually high or low.

5. Carry "rescue" sugar, such as honey, in case of a sudden fall in blood sugar.

Patient Education

1. Patients need a basic understanding of the disease process and its control.

2. Blood glucose self-monitoring is essential for good control and should also be taught, along with proper insulin administration.

3. Recognition of the symptoms of both hypoglycemia and hyperglycemia are essential, as well as an understanding of their immediate treatment.

4. Feet should be inspected daily, and good-quality shoes always worn.

5. The need to increase insulin doses by up to 50 per cent during illness, with frequent blood sugar monitoring, should be discussed.

6. Finally, the need to seek professional help should blood sugars remain elevated, or if urine ketones are greater than trace positive, or for sustained nausea, vomiting, or abdominal pain, or any persistent, unusual symptom, should be emphasized.

Follow-Up

1. Assess control and understanding by asking about any high or low blood sugars and any measures taken to correct them.

2. Check the patient's blood sugar log and look for patterns of highs or lows.

3. Discuss diet, exercise, and overall well-being.

4. Check hemoglobin A_{1c} at least twice a year.

5. Blood pressure checks every visit

6. Eye exams at least once a year beginning at least within 5 years of diagnosis

7. Foot exams, including testing for early neuropathy (light touch) on every visit

8. Screening for microalbuminuria yearly

9. Cholesterol screening at least by age 30, then every year with aggressive therapy

10. Screen for associated autoimmune disease, such as Addison's disease, as appropriate.

Bibliography

Baker JR Jr: Autoimmune endocrine disease. JAMA 1997;278:1931–1937.

Bloomgarden ZT: International Diabetes Federation meeting, 1997, and Metropolitan Diabetes Society of New York meeting, November 1997. Diabetes Care 1998;21:658–665.

Holleman F, Hoekstra JB: Insulin Lispro. N Engl J Med 1997;337:176–183.

Purnell JQ, Hokanson JE, Marcovina SM, et al: Effect of excessive weight gain with intensive therapy of type I diabetes on lipid levels and blood pressure: results from the DCCT: Diabetes Control and Complications Trial. JAMA 1998;280:140–146.

Swift PGF: Optimization of insulin treatment in children. Ann Med 1997;29:419–424.

175 Diabetes Mellitus, Type II

Bruce E. Wilson

Etiology

1. Type II diabetes mellitus (DM II) is a heterogeneous group of clinical phenotypes that result in hyperglycemia that is generally not ketosis prone. This type of diabetes mellitus accounts for the vast majority of all cases of diabetes mellitus. Insulin resistance is central to the development of DM II. Other components of the pathogenesis of DM II include an insulin secretory defect; relative, but not absolute, insulin deficiency; and hepatic glucose overproduction. About 80 per cent of these individuals are obese, which worsens the underlying insulin resistance.

2. Heredity plays a significant role in the pathogenesis of DM II; there is a greater than 90 per cent concordance between monozygotic twins. It is unusual to identify an individual with DM II without a family history of diabetes mellitus. Certain ethnic groups have a higher likelihood of DM II (see below). DM II generally occurs in adults but may present in young people. There is an autosomal dominant type of non-insulin-requiring diabetes mellitus that presents in the preadult years.

Symptoms

DM II often has an insidious onset. Unfortunately, many people have DM II without any knowledge. Obviously, this increases the likelihood of future diabetic complications. It has been estimated that up to 50 per cent of the population with DM II are unaware that the disorder is present.

Key Symptoms

- Polyuria, polydipsia, thirst
- Fatigue
- Blurring of the vision
- Paresthesias or pain in the extremities
- Impotence
- Chronic cutaneous infections or genital candidiasis

Clinical Findings

1. Patients may present with classical symptoms of polyuria and thirst, but many individuals present with fatigue and vague symptoms that are not always associated with DM II. Therefore, it is important to know which subpopulations should be screened most stringently for DM II.

2. Patients, especially older individuals in nursing homes, may present in a classical nonketotic hyperosmolar state. In states of extreme physiologic stress, patients can present with ketoacidosis.

3. The majority of patients with DM II have central obesity. Oftentimes, there is associated hypertriglyceridemia, low levels of high-density lipoprotein (HDL) cholesterol, or hypertension. It is not uncommon for all of these disorders to be present in an individual with DM II.

4. Unfortunately, a subgroup of persons with DM II present with established complications of DM II: macrovascular disease (coronary artery disease or peripheral vascular disease), microvascular disease (retinopathy or nephropathy), or severe neuropathic pain syndromes.

Key Signs

- Obesity
- Family history of DM II
- History of gestational diabetes mellitus or delivery of neonates greater than 9 pounds
- History of impaired glucose tolerance or impaired fasting glucose
- African American, Pacific Islander, Hispanic American, Asian American, Native American ethnicity
- HDL cholesterol less than 35 mg/dl; triglyceride level greater than 250 mg/dl
- Hypertension
- History of polycystic ovarian syndrome or androgenic characteristics in a female
- Any established complication of diabetes mellitus

Laboratory Tests

The diagnosis of DM II may be made three ways: (1) demonstration of a fasting plasma glucose of greater than 126 mg/dl; (2) 2-hour glucose level of greater than 200 mg/dl during a 2-hour oral glucose tolerance test after ingestion of 75 gm glucose; or (3) demonstrating a casual glucose of greater than 200 mg/dl with symptoms of hyperglycemia. Any of these must be corroborated on a subsequent day with any of the other two criteria. A fasting glucose of greater than 110 mg/dl is considered impaired fasting glucose and identifies individuals at higher risk of future diabetes mellitus and/or cardiovascular disease.

1. *Glycosylated hemoglobin (Hb A_{1c})*: This remains the best estimate of glycemic control over the prior 2 to 3 months. Generally, diabetologists follow the Hb A_{1c} with a goal of 7 per cent, indicating an average serum glucose level of 150 mg/dl. Maintaining a Hb A_{1c} of 7 per cent or less decreases the likelihood of complications of diabetes mellitus.

2. *Urinary microalbumin*: If a patient with DM II has increased excretion of microalbumin in the urine, this indicates early nephropathy. Microalbuminuria is defined as a 24-hour urinary excretion of 30 to 300 mg albumin or 30 to 300 μg albumin/mg creatinine on a spot collection. Patients with microalbuminuria should be treated with an angiotensin-converting enzyme (ACE) inhibitor (with or without hypertension) or an angiotensin receptor–blocking agent. If there is greater than 300 mg albumin excretion in 24 hours, albuminuria is present and the patient should be seen by a nephrologist and/or diabetologist. Glycemic control and hypertension control are essential in these patients to avoid progression of the nephropathy.

3. *Serum lipid levels*: A patient with DM II has equivalent risk of coronary heart disease as the patient with a prior myocardial infarction. Low-density lipoprotein (LDL) cholesterol should be less than 100 mg/dl, with more stringent goals (75 to 90 mg/dl) a possible advantage. Ideally, serum triglycerides should be maintained at less than 200 mg/dl. Treatment of hypercholesterolemia should begin with restriction of dietary fats, but, if pharmacologic therapy is necessary to reach the goal, a 3-hydroxy-3-methylglutaryl coenzyme A (HMG CoA) reductase inhibitor is recommended, such as simvastatin. Pharmacologic treatment of isolated hypertriglyceridemia with gemfibrozil or fenofibrate is recommended if triglycerides are greater than 400 mg/dl.

Key Test

Fasting plasma glucose greater than 126 mg/dl on two separate occasions.

Differential Diagnosis

1. Drug toxicity: Many pharmacologic agents interfere with insulin secretion, such as β-adrenergic blocking agents, thiazides, and phenytoin. Estrogens, nicotinic acid, and glucocorticoids may induce insulin resistance.

2. Endocrine and metabolic disorders: Endocrine disorders such as hypercortisolemia (Cushing's syndrome), glucagonoma, pheochromocytoma, and acromegaly may induce diabetes mellitus. Diabetes mellitus may also be associated with hemochromatosis.

3. Chronic pancreatic disease or pancreatectomy.

4. DM II may be associated with myotonic dystrophy, ataxia-telangiectasia, leprechaunism, or genetic abnormalities in the insulin or proinsulin peptides.

5. Diabetes mellitus type I, in remission.

Treatment

The treatment of DM II has changed dramatically over the last few years, with more treatment options currently available. The goal of treatment of DM II is to maintain near-normal glycemic control, with a Hb A_{1c} of less than 7 per cent. In addition, it is necessary to modify all other risk factors for atherosclerotic cardiovascular disease, such as lipid levels, smoking, hypertension, and obesity.

Diet and Exercise

These remain the cornerstone of therapy for DM II. It is rare that a patient can have adequate therapy of DM II without adequate dietary modification and exercise. One must strive to eliminate processed sugar and saturated fat from the diet. An exercise program should suit the individual patient. It is extremely important to have some type of aerobic activity at least three to four times weekly for greater than 30 minutes. More exercise generally aids glycemic control and weight loss.

Medication

At this time, there are multiple oral medications for diabetes mellitus. Patients with DM II can be treated with a combination of oral agents or triple therapy to avoid insulin therapy.

1. Sulfonylurea drugs
   a. Commonly used for DM II and may be the agent of choice for the lean patient with DM II

b. Reduce glucose by enhancing insulin secretion

c. Common examples: glipizide and glyburide.

d. The latest sulfonylurea, glimepiride (Amaryl), may be the sulfonylurea of choice because of its favorable effects on the cardiovascular system; also, it does not appear to induce hypoglycemia as often as other sulfonylureas. Glimepiride, available as 1-, 2-, and 4-mg tablets, is prescribed once daily, 1 to 8 mg.

2. Metformin (Glucophage)

a. Reduces hepatic glucose production and is likely the agent of choice for patients with obesity or dyslipidemia associated with DM II.

b. Available as 500- and 850-mg tablets and is commonly prescribed in dosages of 500 to 2550 mg/day in divided doses.

c. Should not be used in patients with renal insufficiency or serum creatinine greater than 1.5 mg/dl in males or 1.4 mg/dl in females; also, it should be used with caution in patients with a history of congestive heart failure.

3. Troglitazone (Rezulin)

a. This thiazolidinedione reduces glucose levels by increasing insulin sensitivity by binding to nuclear receptors.

b. Should not be used in patients with hepatic dysfunction and may induce liver function abnormalities in about 2 per cent of patients.

c. Available as 200- and 400-mg tablets; the usual dosage is 200 to 600 mg/day in a single dose taken with food

d. Troglitazone can be used with insulin, metformin, or sulfonylurea drugs.

e. Rosiglitazone (Avandia) and pioglitazone are potentially less toxic thiazolidinedione agents.

4. Acarbose (Precose)

a. α-Glucosidase inhibitor; decreases absorption of glucose from the gut and is especially useful in patients with postprandial hyperglycemia.

b. Available as 50- and 100-mg tablets; taken with meals in doses of 25 to 100 mg

c. Side effects include flatulence, nausea, and diarrhea. Occasionally, a patient may experience reversible elevations in hepatic transaminases.

5. Repaglanide (Prandin)

a. This agent of the meglitinide class of glucose-lowering agents stimulates insulin secretion from pancreatic beta cells by a mechanism separate from that of sulfonylurea drugs.

b. Available as 0.5-, 1-, and 2-mg tablets; taken within 30 minutes before a meal in dosages of 0.5 to 4.0 mg.

c. Should be used with caution in patients with renal or hepatic impairment.

6. Insulin

a. Can be used in combination therapy with any of the oral antidiabetic agents often as a single or twice-daily injection of NPH insulin (see Ch. 174, Diabetes Mellitus, Type I).

b. Insulin lispro (Humalog) is an analogue of insulin that is injected directly before meals because it has peak serum levels within 1.5 hours in most patients. This can be utilized as adjunctive therapy in many patients not adequately controlled with oral agents.

c. Primary therapy in patients with severe hepatic or renal insufficiency, congestive heart failure, or inadequate endogenous insulin production.

d. Intensive insulin therapy in patients with DM II often results in significant weight gain.

7. Other

a. All patients with hyperlipidemia should receive dietary education and medical therapy, if necessary, to obtain goal levels of LDL cholesterol and triglycerides (see above).

b. Patients with DM II should receive aspirin, 81 to 325 mg daily, unless there is a specific contraindication.

c. Individuals with DM II should have a diet replete in vitamins or take multivitamins with vitamin E daily.

Patient Education

1. *Home blood glucose monitoring* is an essential tool for all patients with diabetes mellitus and has been shown to improve glycemic control. The benefits of glycemic control need to be stressed to all patients with DM II. However, very tight glycemic control (e.g., Hb A_{1c} <7 per cent) may induce significant morbidity in elderly, blind, or otherwise debilitated patients by inducing recurrent hypoglycemia.

2. *Foot and skin care*: Maintenance of skin integrity in the lower extremities is important for those patients with neuropathy and/or peripheral vascular disease to avoid the development of limb-threatening infections.

3. *Intercurrent illnesses* may induce elevations in glucose levels. All diabetic individuals must understand that intercurrent illness may lead to unresponsive hyperglycemia and necessitate temporary insulin therapy if treated with oral agents alone. Adequate fluid intake and frequent glucose monitoring is needed in these situations.

4. *Diet and exercise*: All persons with DM II should have dietary consultation and diabetes education to understand completely the benefits of dietary modification, exercise, and weight loss.

Key Treatment

Drugs of Choice	Alternative Drugs	
• Glimepiride	• Insulin	• Rosiglitazone
• Metformin	• Repaglanide	• Troglitazone
	• Acarbose	

Follow-Up

1. Annual *full* history and physical examination, including, but not limited to, weight and blood pressure, extremity examination, cardiovascular examination, and funduscopic examination. Review all goals, adequacy of current treatment programs, and diet/exercise program. An electrocardiogram should be obtained in all adults at baseline.

2. Persons with DM II should seek follow-up every 3 months with Hb A_{1c} measurement.

3. Tests for microalbuminuria should be ordered annually, with 24-hour urine studies for quantitative protein and creatinine clearance if there is evidence of renal insufficiency or significant albuminuria.

4. Hypertension should be aggressively treated with a goal of maintaining the blood pressure less than 130/85 to avoid the development of both micro- and macrovascular disease; treatment with an ACE inhibitor is preferred.

5. A fasting lipid profile should be evaluated annually and more frequently if a dyslipidemia is present (see above).

6. Annual ophthalmologic examination if there is evidence of retinopathy or microalbuminuria.

Bibliography

American Diabetes Association: Clinical practice recommendations 1998. Diabetes Care 1998;21(Suppl 1).

Estacio RO, Jeffers BW, Hiatt WR: The effect of nisoldipine as compared with enalapril on cardiovascular outcomes in patients with non-insulin-dependent diabetes and hypertension. N Engl J Med 1998;338:645–652.

Gilmer TP, O'Connor PJ, Manning WG, et al: The cost to health plans of poor glycemic control. Diabetes Care 1997;20:1847–1853.

Imura H: A novel antidiabetic drug, troglitazone—reason for hope and concern [editorial]. N Engl J Med 1998; 338:908–909.

Nestler JE, Jakubowicz DJ, Evans WS, et al: Effects of metformin on spontaneous and clomiphene-induced ovulation in the polycystic ovary syndrome. N Engl J Med 1998;338:1876–1880.

Pyorala K, Olsson AG, Pederson TR: Cholesterol lowering with simvastatin improves prognosis of diabetic patients with coronary heart disease: a subgroup analysis of the Scandinavian Simvastatin Survival Study (4S). Diabetes Care 1997;20:614–620.

Vegh A, Papp JG: Haemodynamic and other effects of sulphonylurea drugs on the heart. Diabetes Res Clin Pract 1996;31(Suppl):43S–53S.

Wei M, Gaskill SP, Haffner SM, et al: Effects of diabetes and level of glycemia on all-cause and cardiovascular mortality: the San Antonio Heart Study. Diabetes Care 1998;21:1167–1172.

176 Ketoacidosis

Robert B. Hash

Etiology

1. Ketoacidosis (KA) refers to the metabolic derangement wherein there is overproduction and accumulation of ketoacids (acetoacetate and β-hydroxybuterate) in the blood. This results in a metabolic acidosis, usually with a widened anion gap. KA is caused by a complete or relative deficiency of insulin in relation to anti-insulin hormones. The result is an inability to utilize glucose at the cellular level, glucose overproduction by the liver, and production of acetone and ketoacids. KA is usually caused by one of two conditions: diabetes or alcohol consumption.

2. Diabetic ketoacidosis (DKA) is not strictly defined but includes the presence of metabolic acidosis with a glucose greater than 250 mg/dl and serum ketones present. The principal causes of DKA are

   a. New onset of type I diabetes mellitus (~25 per cent of cases)

   b. Infection in a type I diabetic (~30 per cent of cases)

   c. Inappropriate therapy or noncompliance in a type I diabetic

   d. Myocardial infarction in a type I diabetic

   e. Pregnancy (known diabetic or pregnancy-induced diabetes)

   f. Trauma or severe physiologic stress in a type I diabetic.

> **Note**
> Any of the above can infrequently precipitate DKA in a type II diabetic.

3. Alcoholic ketoacidosis (AKA) is less well defined but is generally recognized to be a widened anion gap metabolic acidosis with ketonemia in the clinical setting of recent heavy alcohol consumption with acute cessation of drinking followed by vomiting, dehydration, and starvation.

Symptoms

1. Initially, polydypsia and polyuria (DKA)
2. Nausea and anorexia
3. Vomiting
4. Abdominal pain
5. Dyspnea
6. Weakness
7. Dizziness
8. Fatigue

Key Symptoms

- Nausea
- Vomiting
- Abdominal pain

Clinical Findings

1. Tachypnea (Kussmaul respirations)
2. Dehydration findings
3. Tachycardia
4. Acetone odor
5. Confusion (if osmolality >320)
6. Abdominal tenderness
7. Hypotension (late sign in severe disease)
8. Evidence of malnutrition and alcoholism (AKA)

Key Signs

- Tachycardia
- Tachypnea
- Dehydration
- Acetone odor on breath

Laboratory Tests

1. Glucose: Blood glucose elevated to greater than 250 mg/dl in DKA. Usually low or normal in AKA.

2. Ketones: Serum ketones are present at 1:2 dilution or higher. It is important to recognize that β-hydroxybuterate is preferentially produced in KA relative to acetoacetate and acetone but is not detected by nitroprusside reagent methods. This may result in a falsely negative nitroprusside test. As KA improves

with therapy, β-hydroxyburerate is converted to acetoacetate and acetone, causing a paradoxical increase in ketones with treatment.

3. Potassium: Virtually all patients with KA are total body potassium deficient. However, the initial serum potassium may be low, normal, or high.

4. Chloride: Usually low, as reflected in anion gap measurement. May be elevated if measured after chloride-containing fluids have been given in large amounts (i.e., after fluid therapy).

5. Bicarbonate: Usually low but may be near-normal if frequent vomiting, volume contraction.

6. Sodium: Measured Na^+ usually falsely low in DKA. Can be corrected as follows:

Correct Na = measured Na

$$+ \left[1.6 \times \left(\frac{\text{glucose (in mg/dl)} - 100}{100} \right) \right]$$

7. Arterial blood gases: pH less than 7.35, CO_2 decreased to compensate, pO_2 usually normal. Multiple acid-base disorders usually superimposed in AKA.

8. Complete blood count: White cell count usually elevated, but does not necessarily imply infection.

9. Anion gap

Anion gap = measured $Na^+ - (Cl^- + HCO_3^-)$

= 12 ($\pm$4)

Usually widened in ketoacidosis; may be normal after NaCl fluids.

10. Blood urea nitrogen: usually elevated as a result of volume depletion

11. Creatinine: usually falsely high because of interference with automated measurement

12. Amylase: Often elevated in DKA, but does not necessarily indicate pancreatitis.

13. Electrocardiogram (ECG), cardiac enzymes, computerized tomography of the head, blood cultures, toxicology studies: as indicated by history and clinical findings and suspicions

 Key Tests

- Glucose
- Electrolytes
- Serum ketones
- Arterial blood gases

Remember

Multiple acid-base problems are usually superimposed in AKA.

Differential Diagnosis

1. Ketoacidosis
   a. DKA
   b. AKA
   c. Prolonged starvation (mild acidosis)
   d. Inborn errors of metabolism (rare)
2. Widened anion gap acidosis
   a. Ketoacidosis
   b. Lactic acidosis
   c. Toxins
      (1) Methanol
      (2) Ethylene glycol
      (3) Formaldehyde
      (4) Paraldehyde
      (5) Cyanide
      (6) Toluene
   d. Medications
      (1) Salicylates
      (2) Iron
      (3) Isoniazid
   e. Uremia

Treatment

DKA

1. Always manage ABC's first: ensure patent airway and adequate ventilation, evaluate and treat circulatory collapse (shock).

2. Fluid replacement
   a. Give 1 to 2 L normal saline in first hour (may require more if shock is present, or less if disease is mild or co-morbidities such as cardiomyopathy are present), then 250 to 500 ml/hour of normal saline for 4 hours, then one-half normal saline at a rate of 100 to 250 ml/hour until rehydrated and oral intake re-established.
   b. Change to 5% dextrose fluids when blood glucose level drops below 250 mg/dl.

3. Insulin
   a. Initial dose of 10 units of Regular insulin as intravenous (IV) bolus. Thereafter administer continuous infusion of Regular insulin at a rate of 0.1 units/kg/hour. If an adequate response is not achieved, double the rate of infusion. If glucose is falling too rapidly, halve the dose. Optimal glucose response is a fall of 50 to 100 mg/dl/hour.

b. Change to subcutaneous therapy when ketosis is resolved and the patient is eating.

4. Potassium: All patients with DKA are total body potassium deficient. Remember that treatment of DKA will lower serum potassium.

   a. If the initial potassium level is less than 3 mEq/L, give 40 mEq of KCl IV infusion over 1 hour.

   b. If initial potassium level is 3 to 5 mEq/L, give 20 to 30 mEq KCl as continuous infusion over first hour. Thereafter give 20 to 30 mEq KCl with each liter of IV fluids.

   c. If potassium level is greater than 5 mEq/L, monitor potassium level and urine output closely and anticipate replacement needs.

   d. If potassium level is greater than 7 mEq/L or there are ECG changes of hyperkalemia (other than peaked T waves), treat for hyperkalemia.

5. Add glucose as 5% dextrose fluid when blood glucose falls below 250 mg/dl. Increase to 10% dextrose fluids if needed after insulin dose adjustment. *Remember*: Goal of treatment is to reverse ketogenesis, not achieve normoglycemia.

6. Bicarbonate: Usually not recommended unless there is severe acidosis (pH < 7.0), lactic acidosis, or hyperkalemia requiring treatment.

7. Phosphate: Replacement indicated only if serum phosphate level is less than 1 mg/dl.

8. Monitor urine output. Urine output should be at least 0.5 to 1 ml/kg/hour.

9. Treat precipitating factors.

10. Diet: Nothing by mouth until nausea, vomiting, abdominal pain, and ketonemia resolved. Begin on appropriate American Diabetic Association diet.

11. Activity: Bed rest initially until well hydrated and normal mental status. Activity may progress as tolerated thereafter.

12. Patient education: Review medication and dietary compliance, medication schedule, signs and symptoms of illness, sick day therapy, home glucose monitoring for DKA.

AKA

Treatment for AKA is similar to that for DKA with the following differences:

1. Fluid replacement: After initial fluid resuscitation with 1 to 2 L normal saline, 5% dextrose is added to all fluids.

2. Insulin: Insulin therapy is rarely required for AKA.

3. Thiamine: Administer 100 mg intravenously prior to glucose administration.

4. Magnesium: Administer 1 to 2 gm magnesium sulfate per liter of IV fluids after initial fluid resuscitation unless initial magnesium level is elevated. Watch for adequate urine output.

WARNING

- **Inadequate fluid replacement is a common treatment error in DKA.**

- **Therapy for KA will precipitate hypokalemia. Watch potassium level closely and maintain adequate potassium replacement.**

- **Thiamine should precede glucose in the treatment of AKA to prevent the precipitation of encephalopathy.**

 Key Treatment

- Intravenous fluid resuscitation

- Regular insulin for DKA

- Glucose infusion for AKA

- Potassium replacement

- Thiamine for AKA

- Evaluate and treat for precipitating factors.

Follow-Up

1. For DKA, patients should be evaluated in 1 to 2 weeks unless illness or predetermined glucose level abnormalities occur.

2. Patients with AKA should receive evaluation in 1 to 2 weeks, and should be offered counseling and treatment for alcoholism.

 ### Bibliography

Adams SL: Alcoholic ketoacidosis. Emerg Med Clin North Am 1990;8:749–760.

Fleckman AM: Diabetic ketoacidosis. Endocrinol Metab Clin North Am 1993;22:181–207.

Fulop M: Alcoholic ketoacidosis. Endocrinol Metab Clin North Am 1993;22:209–219.

Karam JH: Pancreatic hormones and diabetes mellitus. In Greenspan FS, Gordon JS (eds): Basic and Clinical Endocrinology, 5th ed, pp 595–663. Stamford, CT, Appleton & Lange, 1997.

Kitabchi AE, Wall BM: Diabetic ketoacidosis. Med Clin North Am 1995;79:9–37.

177 Hypothyroidism

Ronald S. Watts

Etiology

Hypothyroidism is a clinical disease characterized by decreased thyroid gland production of free thyroxin (T_4). The disease may be a primary thyroid disorder or a central pituitary disorder. Central hypothyroidism is due to a decrease in secretion of thyrotropin (thyroid-stimulating hormone [TSH]) from the pituitary (secondary hypothyroidism) or to a decrease in thyrotropin-releasing hormone (TRH) secretion or transport to the pituitary (tertiary hypothyroidism). Primary hypothyroidism is more common in women between the ages of 40 and 60 years.

Primary Hypothyroidism (Thyroprivic Hypothyroidism)

1. Autoimmune thyroid disease: most common cause of primary hypothyroidism
   a. Hashimoto's thyroiditis: chronic lymphocytic thyroiditis is most common cause of goitrous or atrophic hypothyroidism
   b. Idiopathic hypothyroidism: TSH receptor–blocking antibodies
   c. Graves' disease remission: without prior radioiodine (^{131}I) therapy or surgery
   d. Polyglandular failure: rare syndrome of adrenal failure, type I diabetes mellitus, pernicious anemia, hypoparathyroidism, ovarian failure, and hypophysitis
2. Postablative hypothyroidism
   a. Following radioactive iodine (^{131}I) treatment for Graves' disease or thyroid carcinoma
   b. Following external irradiation to neck for lymphoma
   c. Following thyroidectomy for treatment of Graves' disease or thyroid carcinoma
3. Thyroiditis: subacute, silent, or postpartum; may have transient or permanent hypothyroidism
4. Drugs
   a. Antithyroid drugs: propylthiouracil and methimazole; may cause goiter and/or hypothyroidism
   b. Iodine excess: goiter and/or hypothyroidism
      (1) Underlying thyroid disease and chronic use of iodine-containing cough medicine or amiodarone
      (2) Iodine goiter without hypothyroidism endemic in areas where seaweed (kelp) is consumed in large quantities.
      (3) Iodine administration to pregnant mothers commonly causes goiter and hypothyroidism at birth, and possibly death from neonatal asphyxia.
   c. Lithium: Chronic administration can cause goiters and/or hypothyroidism.
5. Rare causes of hypothyroidism
   a. Sporadic cretinism: developmental defect of the thyroid causing severe hypothyroidism in infancy, resulting in retardation of mental and physical development
   b. Iodine deficiency: worldwide problem, but rare in North America
      (1) Endemic goiter: Some may develop hypothyroidism if iodine deficiency is severe, but most are euthyroid.
      (2) Endemic cretinism: Both parents usually have endemic goiters and developmental disorder in addition to the clinical signs of cretinism. Thyroid is goitrous or atrophic.
   c. Genetic defects in hormone biosynthesis
      (1) Goiters are present at birth or appear later in life.
      (2) Iodide transport defect, organification defect, iodotyrosine coupling defect, iodotyrosine dehalogenase defect, and abnormal secretion of iodoproteins
   d. Infiltrative disorders: scleroderma, amyloidosis, hemochromatosis, sarcoidosis, Riedel's thyroiditis

Central Hypothyroidism (Trophoprivic Hypothyroidism)

1. TSH deficiency, secondary hypothyroidism
   a. Rarely occurs alone without other pituitary hormone deficiency (panhypopituitarism). There is also deficiency of growth hormone, gonadotropins (luteinizing hormone, follicle-stimulating hormone), adrenocorticotropic hormone (ACTH), or vasopressin.
   b. Pituitary macroadenomas, Sheehan's syndrome, craniopharyngiomas, infiltrative disorders of the pituitary, hypophysitis, or after severe head trauma with basal skull fracture

2. TRH deficiency: Tertiary hypothyroidism caused by hypothalamic disease is rare.

Symptoms

1. Clinical symptoms are listed below; subclinical disease is asymptomatic.

2. History of symptoms in multiple organ systems: general fatigue, lethargy, cold intolerance, *mild weight gain*, dry rough skin, hair loss, brittle nails, puffy face, memory or concentration problems, personality disturbances, weakness, muscle stiffness or cramps, arthralgia, nausea, constipation, decreased exercise tolerance, decreased libido, decreased fertility, and menstrual abnormalities.

3. Severity of symptoms may be related to duration of onset of hypothyroidism; a rapid onset of hypothyroidism is associated with more symptoms than is gradual onset.

4. Many of the symptoms are common complaints, which are not specific by themselves but together make up a constellation of symptoms and signs of clinical hypothyroidism.

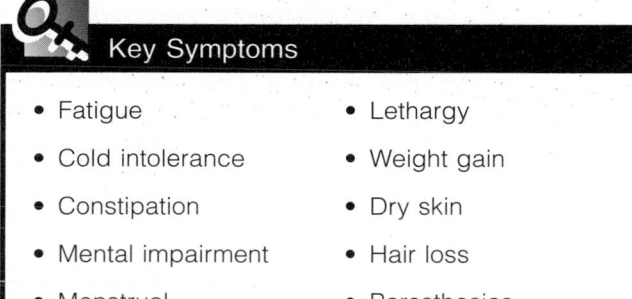

Key Symptoms

- Fatigue
- Cold intolerance
- Constipation
- Mental impairment
- Menstrual abnormalities
- Lethargy
- Weight gain
- Dry skin
- Hair loss
- Paresthesias

Clinical Findings

1. Physical examination may reveal typical puffy facies; periorbital edema; dry, coarse, thick skin and hair; brittle nails; hypersomnolence; slow speech; bradykinesia; hoarseness; large tongue; bradycardia; mild diastolic hypertension; psychological disorders; cerebellar ataxia; carpal tunnel syndrome; hyporeflexia; delayed relaxation phase of reflexes; or seizures.

2. Thyroid may be nonpalpable (atrophic) or goitrous. Goiter may be smooth or nodular.

3. Myxedema is characterized by clinical signs of pallor; carotenemia; nonpitting edema of hands, face, and ankles; secondary to dermal infiltration with mucopolysaccharides. The patient may also have ascites, pleural effusion, and pericardial effusion.

4. Myxedema coma is severe hypothyroidism presenting with altered mental status (lethargic to comatose), hypothermia, bradycardia, hypoventilation, hypoglycemia, adrenal insufficiency, and usually a precipitating factor such as noncompliance with levothyroxine, infection, or stress.

Key Signs

- Bradycardia
- Bradykinesia
- Hyporeflexia
- Muscle weakness
- Dry, coarse, thick skin
- Nonpitting edema (myxedema)
- Delayed relaxation phase of reflexes
- Goiter

Laboratory Tests

1. Laboratory tests consistent with primary hypothyroidism confirm clinical suspicion.

   a. Low free T_4 by radioimmunoassay (RIA) and elevated TSH

   b. Low total T_4, triiodothyronine (T_3) resin uptake, and free thyroxine index (FTI)

   c. Free T_3 by RIA usually normal, or may be mildly decreased in primary hypothyroidism; not necessary to measure free T_3 in evaluation of primary hypothyroidism.

   d. Transient TSH elevation common during recovery from subacute or silent thyroiditis.

   e. Transient TSH elevation common during recovery from postpartum thyroiditis, but greater risk of eventual hypothyroidism because of underlying autoimmune thyroiditis.

   f. High titer of antimicrosomal antibody usually indicates permanent hypothyroidism.

2. Low free T_4 and free T_3 by RIA and low, normal, or mildly elevated TSH

   a. Central hypothyroidism: TSH is usually very low or normal; rarely mildly elevated.

   b. Nonthyroidal illness (sick euthyroid syndrome): marked decrease in free T_3 in nonthyroidal illness, "low T_3 syndrome"; TSH usually normal, or mildly increased. Reverse T_3 will be increased in nonthyroidal illness.

3. Normal free T_4 and mildly increased TSH (5 to 15 μU/ml)

   a. Subclinical hypothyroidism

   b. Recovery from subacute, silent, or postpartum thyroiditis

   c. Recovery from nonthyroidal illness

4. Thyroid antibodies
   a. Antimicrosomal antibody: thyroid peroxidase antibody inhibiting the enzyme activity
      (1) Diagnostic for Hashimoto's thyroiditis when present in high titers (>1:400)
      (2) Degree of elevation correlates with clinical hypothyroidism.
      (3) Antibody titers tend to fall when hypothyroidism is present for a long time.
   b. Antithyroglobulin antibody not as specific for Hashimoto's thyroiditis, but also increased.
   c. If no antibodies are detected at time of diagnosis, it is idiopathic hypothyroidism, which may still be a form of autoimmune thyroiditis.
   d. It is not always necessary to check for antibodies if it is not going to make a difference in a decision to treat or not.
5. Other laboratory abnormalities: elevated creatinine kinase, normochromic normocytic anemia, hyperlipoproteinemia, hyponatremia, hyperprolactinemia, hyperlipoproteinemia, and abnormal electrocardiogram with nonspecific ST and T wave abnormalities, or low voltage of QRS complexes
6. Radioactive iodine scan and uptake are not necessary in the evaluation of hypothyroidism; indicated only in the evaluation of a single nodule or to confirm multinodular goiter.
7. Euthyroid hypothyroxinemia: low total T_4, increased T_3 resin uptake, normal or mildly decreased FTI, and normal TSH as a result of decreased thyroid-binding globulin. Free T_4 and TSH are usually normal because these patients are euthyroid.

Key Tests

- Thyrotropin (TSH)
- Free T_4 or FTI
- Antimicrosomal antibody

Differential Diagnosis

1. Nonthyroidal illness is often associated with decreased free T_3 and/or decreased free T_4 without clinical hypothyroidism. Usually the TSH is normal or could be mildly increased during recovery from nonthyroidal illness.
2. Euthyroid hypothyroxinemia: euthyroid with decreased T_4 as a result of decreased thyroid-binding globulin concentration caused by ne-

phrotic syndrome, exogenous testosterone, or high-dose steroids. Also, total T_4 may be decreased by drugs that inhibit T_4 binding, such as phenytoin, phenobarbital, and salicylates.

Treatment

Medication

1. Levothyroxine (e.g., Synthroid): synthetic preparation of T_4
   a. Dose: 1.6 to 1.8 μg/kg of ideal body weight. Healthy patients can be started on a full replacement dose. Patients who are elderly or have coronary artery disease need to start on 25 μg by mouth daily (or 12.5 μg daily) and increase gradually by 25 μg daily (or 12.5 μg daily) every 4 to 6 weeks. If angina occurs during levothyroxine replacement, the dose should be decreased and cardiac evaluation and treatment done before continuing to increase the levothyroxine.
   b. Lower dose could be given in the treatment of subclinical hypothyroidism (0.5 to 1.0 μg/kg).
   c. If diagnosis of hypothyroidism is uncertain in a patient already on levothyroxine, the dose can be reduced by half and the free T_4 and TSH reassessed in 6 to 8 weeks. If the TSH is increasing, resume the previous dose. If the TSH is normal, discontinue the levothyroxine and check the TSH again in 6 to 8 weeks for any increase.
   d. The goal of TSH replacement in primary hypothyroidism is to normalize, not suppress, the TSH. Suppressed TSH causes decreased bone mineral density over several years.
   e. The replacement goal in central hypothyroidism is to normalize the free T_4 because TSH is not reliable.
   f. TSH suppression is indicated only for those with a history of thyroid carcinoma, nontoxic simple goiter, or benign thyroid nodule.
   g. Drugs that commonly interfere with absorption include cholestyramine and ferrous sulfate.
2. Treatment of myxedema coma: ventilatory support if indicated, treatment of hypothermia, and intravenous levothyroxine, 300 to 500 μg daily to restore thyroxine concentrations to normal quickly.

Key Treatment

Levothyroxine

Follow-Up

1. After therapy has been initiated with levothyroxine, the laboratory should check levothyroxine levels in 6 to 8 weeks to determine whether adjustment of the levothyroxine dose is necessary. Increasing the levothyroxine dose more often than at 6- to 8-week intervals will probably lead to overreplacement.

2. Once a stable dose of levothyroxine has been obtained, the TSH level in primary hypothyroidism or the free T_4 level in central hypothyroidism can be checked biannually or annually.

Bibliography

For more information on subclinical hypothyroidism, see
Ayala A, Wartofsky L: Minimally symptomatic (subclinical) hypothyroidism. Endocrinologist 1997;7:44–50.

For more information on thyroid disease, see
Behnia M, Gharib H: Primary care diagnosis of thyroid disease. Hosp Pract 1996;31:121–134.

For more information on treatment of hypothyroidism, see
Singer PA, Cooper DS, Levy EG, et al: Treatment guidelines for patients with hyperthyroidism and hypothyroidism. JAMA 1995;273:808–812.

For more information on myxedema coma, see
Jordan RM: Myxedema coma: pathophysiology, therapy, and factors affecting prognosis. Med Clin North Am 1995;79:185–194.

178 Hyperthyroidism

Ronald S. Watts

Etiology

Thyrotoxicosis is defined as elevated concentration of free thyroxine (T_4) and/or free triiodothyronine (T_3). Thyrotoxicosis may be due to hyperthyroidism, which is an increase in thyroid hormone synthesis and release, but thyrotoxicosis may also be due to increased T_4 and/or T_3 concentrations without hyperthyroidism (increase in thyroid hormone synthesis). It is more common in young women.

Thyrotoxicosis and Hyperthyroidism: Increased Thyroid Radioactive Iodine Uptake (RAIU)

1. Graves' disease: most common cause of thyrotoxicosis
2. Toxic multinodular goiter (MNG): multiple autonomous functioning thyroid nodules
3. Toxic adenoma (Plummer's disease): solitary large autonomous functioning thyroid nodule
4. Hashitoxicosis: coexistent Hashimoto's thyroiditis and Graves' disease
5. Pituitary (thyrotroph) adenoma: thyrotropin (thyroid-stimulating hormone [TSH])–secreting adenoma
6. Selective pituitary resistance to thyroxine: hypersecretion of TSH without adenoma
7. Trophoblastic tumor: human chorionic gonadotropin (hCG)–secreting tumor
8. Exogenous iodine excess: only cause of hyperthyroidism with low RAIU—caused by iodine-containing drugs, such as cough medicine, amiodarone, contrast agents, or kelp (seaweed)

Thyrotoxicosis Not Caused by Hyperthyroidism: Decreased Thyroid RAIU

1. Subacute thyroiditis: inflammatory response causing increase in thyroxine release
2. Silent thyroiditis: inflammatory response causing increase in thyroxine release
3. Postpartum thyroiditis: inflammatory response 2 to 6 months postpartum
4. Surreptitious exogenous thyroid hormone use: typically the health care professional
5. Struma ovarii: ectopic thyroid tissue
6. Functioning metastatic thyroid cancer: ectopic thyroid tissue

Pathogenesis of Common Causes of Thyrotoxicosis

1. Graves' disease: Thyroid-stimulating immunoglobulins (TSI) bind TSH receptors, stimulating T_4 synthesis.
2. Subacute thyroiditis: Antecedent viral infection causes a subsequent inflammatory infiltrate of neutrophils, lymphocytes, histiocytes, and multinucleated giant cells.
3. Silent thyroiditis: May be a variant of lymphocytic thyroiditis; focal or diffuse acute lymphocytic infiltration that appears like chronic lymphocytic thyroiditis
4. Postpartum thyroiditis: underlying chronic autoimmune thyroiditis
5. Toxic adenoma and toxic MNG: gradual growth of autonomous functioning nodule(s)
6. Exogenous iodine excess: Causes hyperthyroidism with underlying subclinical thyroid disease, but the thyroid RAIU will be low instead of high.

Symptoms

Symptoms of common causes of thyrotoxicosis

1. Graves' disease: symptoms of ophthalmopathy, such as dry eyes, excessive tearing, proptosis, diplopia, impaired visual acuity, or field defects
2. Subacute thyroiditis: Preceded by 1 to 2 weeks by a viral syndrome and presents with thyroid or neck pain, which may radiate to jaw or ear.
3. Silent and postpartum thyroiditis: mildly symptomatic or asymptomatic
4. Toxic MNG and toxic adenoma: insidious onset, few symptoms, and more common in the elderly

Key Symptoms

- Hyperactivity
- Nervousness
- Irritability
- Palpitations
- Heat intolerance
- Sweating

- Increased appetite
- Fatigue
- Weight loss
- Weakness
- Frequent defecation
- Menstrual abnormalities

Clinical Findings

1. Thyrotoxicosis usually causes clinical disease, but can present with subclinical disease.
   a. General: hyperactivity, nervousness, anxiety, and warm, moist, smooth skin
   b. Eyes: lid retraction, lid lag, and stare
   c. Thyroid: firm smooth or nodular goiter present in most causes of thyrotoxicosis
   d. Cardiac: sinus tachycardia, paroxysmal supraventricular tachycardia, atrial fibrillation, hyperactive precordium, systolic flow murmurs, congestive heart failure, and angina
   e. Neurologic: fine tremor of hands, tongue, or closed eyelids, hyperreflexia, proximal muscle weakness, myopathy, emotional lability, and psychiatric manifestations
2. Clinical signs in specific causes of thyrotoxicosis
   a. Graves' disease: Degree of thyrotoxicosis varies from mild to severe.
      (1) Diffuse firm thyroid enlargement that may have bruit
      (2) Infiltrative ophthalmopathy
         (a) Bilateral proptosis, defined as exophthalmometer measurements exceeding 20 mm
         (b) Lid retraction, corneal ulcers, keratitis, conjunctivitis, periorbital edema
         (c) Diplopia with upward and lateral extremes of gaze, or may be constant.
         (d) Papilledema, or impairment of vision as a result of involvement of optic nerve
      (3) Rarely, localized myxedema, or thyroid acropachy (thickening of extremity)
      (4) Coexistent Hashimoto's thyroiditis with a lobular thyroid consistency
      (5) Thyroid storm: severe thyrotoxicosis with hyperpyrexia, tachyarrhythmias, shock, and acute metabolic encephalopathy. Look for precipitating factor such as infection, noncompliance with antithyroid drugs, trauma, iodine, or parturition.
   b. Subacute thyroiditis: Thyroid pain and tenderness the predominant problem in a firm goiter, mild to moderate in size, and mild thyrotoxicosis.
   c. Silent and postpartum thyroiditis: painless with mild thyrotoxicosis or subclinical disease
   d. Toxic multinodular goiter and toxic adenoma
      (1) Usually appears in elderly with prior history of goiter for several years.
      (2) In elderly, may have only cardiac signs or weight loss.
      (3) May occur in young patients with progressively enlarging goiter.
      (4) Toxic adenoma, usually more than 3.0 cm
   e. Surreptitious exogenous T_4 or T_3 use: Suspect whenever thyrotoxicosis is present without a goiter. The only cause of low thyroglobulin concentration in thyrotoxicosis.

Key Signs

- Restlessness
- Tachycardia or arrhythmia
- Systolic hypertension
- Hyperreflexia
- Tremor
- Stare
- Eyelid retraction
- Goiter
- Muscle weakness
- Warm, moist, smooth skin

Laboratory Tests

1. Thyroid function tests consistent with chemical thyrotoxicosis confirm clinical suspicion.
   a. Elevated free T_4 and/or T_3 concentrations by radioimmunoassay (RIA)
   b. Elevated total T_4, T_3 resin uptake, and free thyroxine index (FTI)
   c. Suppressed TSH (<0.1 μU/ml) utilizing a sensitive TSH assay. Exception: TSH is not suppressed in TSH-secreting pituitary adenoma or pituitary resistance to T_4.
   d. Serum thyroglobulin is suppressed only in surreptitious T_4 or T_3 use.
2. Other tests
   a. Erythrocyte sedimentation rate increased in subacute or silent thyroiditis
   b. TSI and TSH receptor antibodies confirm Graves' disease, and low titer may predict remission with antithyroid drug treatment.
   c. Antimicrosomal antibodies: high titer in postpartum thyroiditis and hashitoxicosis

d. Molar ratio of alpha subunit to TSH greater than 1.0 only in pituitary TSH-secreting adenoma

e. May have hypercalcemia, anemia, hypokalemia, osteoporosis

3. RAIU is required in all evaluations of thyrotoxicosis.

a. Increased thyroid RAIU in hyperthyroidism

(1) Graves' disease, hashitoxicosis, toxic MNG, and toxic adenoma

(2) Pituitary (TSH-secreting) adenoma, selective pituitary resistance to T_4, and trophoblastic (hCG-secreting) tumor are all rare causes of hyperthyroidism.

WARNING

If TSH is not suppressed (>0.1 μU/ml) and RAIU is increased, evaluate the pituitary by computerized tomography or magnetic resonance imaging for either TSH-secreting pituitary adenoma or selective pituitary resistance to T_4 if imaging of the pituitary is normal.

---

b. Decreased thyroid RAIU in other causes of thyrotoxicosis

(1) Thyroiditis: subacute, silent, and postpartum

(2) Exogenous thyroid hormone use and exogenous iodine excess

(3) Struma ovarii and functioning metastatic thyroid cancer: rare

c. Thyroid radioiodine scan is not always necessary in evaluating thyrotoxicosis.

(1) Diffuse homogeneous uptake confirms Graves' disease but is probably unnecessary in a patient with a diffusely enlarged goiter on examination.

(2) Useful test if there is a concern about a palpable thyroid nodule(s) in a thyrotoxic patient; may reveal heterogeneous uptake (toxic multinodular goiter), or a single hot nodule (toxic adenoma), or a cold nodule (coexistent neoplasm).

4. Euthyroid hyperthyroxinemia: elevated total T_4, decreased T_3 resin uptake, normal or mildly elevated FTI, or normal to mildly increased free T_4 by RIA; commonly caused by increase in thyroid-binding globulin or, rarely, to nonthyroid illness, generalized resistance to thyroid hormone

Key Tests

- Free T_4 or FIT, total T_3

- Thyrotropin (TSH)

- Thyroid RAIU

- Thyroid radioiodine scan—necessary only if palpable nodule(s)

Differential Diagnosis

1. Laboratory tests confirm chemical thyrotoxicosis. The specific cause of thyrotoxicosis may be determined clinically and by the thyroid RAIU (explained above).

2. If euthyroid findings exclude thyrotoxicosis, consider disorders associated with hypermetabolism, such as anxiety disorder, diabetes mellitus, pheochromocytoma, myeloproliferative disorder, cirrhosis, and chronic obstructive pulmonary disease.

3. Euthyroid hyperthyroxinemia: euthyroid with increased T_4 as a result of increase in thyroid-binding globulin concentration commonly caused by estrogens or hepatitis; rarely due to nonthyroidal illness, familial dysalbuminemia (increased albumin-binding T_4), or increased T_4 binding to thyroid-binding prealbumin and anti-T_4 antibodies

Treatment

Medication

1. β-Blockers

a. Mechanism: decrease the β-adrenergic–mediated effects of thyrotoxicosis, and decrease the peripheral conversion of T_4 to T_3

b. Drugs: propranolol, 10 to 80 mg by mouth qid; atenolol, 50 to 100 mg by mouth daily; nadolol; or metoprolol

c. Indication: all forms of thyrotoxicosis; titrate dose according to heart rate

d. Side effects: bronchospasm, bradycardia, decreased cardiac output, depression

2. Antithyroid drugs: propylthiouracil (PTU) and methimazole (MMI) (Tapazole)

a. Mechanism: both PTU and MMI inhibit T_4 synthesis. Only PTU inhibits peripheral conversion of T_4 to T_3. Possible immunosuppressive effect.

b. Dose: PTU, 50 to 300 mg by mouth every 6 to 8 hours; or MMI, 5 to 20 mg by mouth every 12 hours

(1) Treatment is usually required for 1 to 2 years for a possible remission to occur.

(2) If not in remission by 2 years, should consider ^{131}I or surgery.

(3) Remission is more likely if goiter is small or decreasing in size, or if mild thyrotoxicosis is controlled with minimal dose of antithyroid drugs.

(4) Recurrence after remission is possible.

c. Indications: hyperthyroidism (increased RAIU)

(1) Drugs of choice for treating pregnant Graves' patient or children

(2) Before and/or after radioiodine (^{131}I) therapy to help control severe hyperthyroidism

d. Contraindicated in low RAIU thyrotoxicosis

e. Side effects

(1) Common (<5 per cent): rash, transient leukopenia, and drug fever

(2) Rare (<0.5 per cent): agranulocytosis, aplastic anemia, thrombocytopenia, lupus-like syndrome, hepatitis, cholestasis, gastrointestinal symptoms, abnormal taste, and arthralgia

f. Check neutrophil count and liver enzymes before and periodically during therapy.

WARNING

Patients should be instructed, if temperature is greater than 101° F, to discontinue antithyroid drugs until neutrophil count is checked to exclude agranulocytosis.

---

3. Anti-inflammatory and immunosuppressive drugs

a. Acetylsalicylic acid (ASA) in moderate doses, or nonsteroidal anti-inflammatory drugs (NSAIDs) indicated for treatment of subacute silent thyroiditis. If no improvement, switch to steroids.

b. Steroids

(1) Prednisone, 40 to 60 mg by mouth daily, tapered over 4 weeks for subacute thyroiditis

(2) Decreased T$_4$ secretion and T$_4$-to-T$_3$ peripheral conversion in severe hyperthyroidism

(3) Temporary therapy for severe Graves' ophthalmopathy until surgery or irradiation

4. Radioactive iodine-131 (^{131}I): therapy of choice for Graves' disease

a. Mechanism: Inflammation and radiation destroy the thyroid gland.

b. Indication: hyperthyroidism (increased RAIU); contraindicated if RAIU is low

c. Contraindication: pregnancy—must check serum hCG before treatment.

d. Dose: One treatment of 10 to 20 mCi of ^{131}I is effective in 75 per cent of patients, and 10 to 20 per cent of patients will require more than one treatment with ^{131}I.

e. In toxic MNG or toxic adenoma, more than 20 mCi of ^{131}I usually required.

f. Side effects: pain in neck, radiation thyroiditis, and increase in T$_4$ release

g. Very safe without increased risk of cancer or gonad chromosomal abnormalities

h. Hypothyroidism is expected, and free T$_4$ and TSH levels should be monitored after therapy.

5. Iodine-containing compounds: potassium iodide (SSKI), Lugol's solution, ipodate sodium

a. Mechanism: acutely decrease T$_4$ release and decrease T$_4$-to-T$_3$ peripheral conversion

b. Indication: adjunctive therapy after ^{131}I treatment, preparation for surgery, or management of severe hyperthyroidism or "thyroid storm"

c. Contraindication: pregnancy—must check serum hCG before treating.

d. Dose: SSKI or Lugol's solution, 3 to 5 drops qid by mouth or IV

e. Comments: Begin only after one dose of antithyroid drug has already been given to block T$_4$ synthesis. One treatment will decrease RAIU and prevent effective treatment with radioactive ^{131}I for several months.

6. Therapy of thyroid storm: fluid resuscitation, treatment of hyperpyrexia, high dose of β-blockers, high dose of antithyroid drugs, "cold" iodides (SSKI, Lugol's solution, or ipodate), and high-dose (stress) steroids

Surgery

1. Indications

a. Severe thyrotoxicosis during pregnancy when antithyroid drugs have been unsuccessful

b. Suspicion of malignancy: palpable thyroid nodule, lymphadenopathy, hoarseness, and rapid growth of goiter

c. Toxic adenoma or toxic MNG in a good surgical candidate

2. Preparation: Patient should be rendered euthyroid with an antithyroid drug and "cold" iodide (SSKI, or Lugol's solution) before surgery.

3. Procedure: Near-total thyroidectomy should be done only by an experienced surgeon.

4. Complications: recurrent laryngeal nerve damage, hypocalcemia, bleeding, infection, and expected hypothyroidism

Key Treatment

- β-Blockers: propranolol, nadolol, or metoprolol

- Antithyroid drugs: PTU and MMI

- Anti-inflammatory and immunosuppressive drugs: only indicated for thyroiditis—ASA, NSAIDs, steroids

- ^{131}I

Follow-Up

1. Hypothyroidism

   a. Expected after treatment of Graves' disease with surgery, ^{131}I, or antithyroid drugs

   b. Recovery from thyroiditis (subacute, silent, or postpartum) may cause transient hypothyroidism, but most patients eventually become euthyroid. Thyroxine therapy should be withheld unless the patient has many symptoms of hypothyroidism or TSH elevation persists for a long time. If treatment is started for symptoms, titrate dose according to symptoms and not to completely normalize the TSH.

2. Recurrent thyrotoxicosis possible with Graves' disease or thyroiditis.

3. Thyroxine replacement: levothyroxine, approximately 1.6 to 1.8 μg/kg by mouth daily to normalize TSH

Bibliography

For more information on radioactive iodine treatment, see
Kaplan MM, Meier DA, Dworkin HJ: Treatment of hyperthyroidism with radioactive iodine. Endocrinol Metab Clin North Am 1998;27:205–223.

For more information on current treatment of hyperthyroidism, see
Gittoes NJ, Franklyn JA: Hyperthyroidism: current treatment guidelines. Drugs 1998;55:543–553.

For more information on antithyroid drug treatment of hyperthyroidism, see
Vitti R, Rago P, Chiovato L, et al: Clinical features of patients with Graves' disease undergoing remission after antithyroid drug treatment. Thyroid 1997;7:369–375.

For more information on subclinical hyperthyroidism, see
Haden S, Marqusee E, Utiger R: Subclinical hyperthyroidism. Endocrinologist 1996;6:322–327.

179 Thyroid Nodule; Thyroid Carcinoma

Harold V. Werner

Etiology

1. Thyroid nodules are very common (50 per cent prevalence by autopsy or ultrasound), but fewer than 1 in 10 are palpable; about 5 per cent of palpable nodules harbor malignancy but very few cause death. Do not do scans or ultrasound studies to *screen* for cancer because of extremely high false-positive rate.

2. Very little is known of specific causes of nodules.

3. Presence of palpable nodules, however, is influenced by

   a. Age

      (1) Prevalence of nodules increases linearly with age.

      (2) Palpable nodules are present in more than 5 per cent of people over 60 years of age.

      (3) Multinodular goiters start to appear ages 30 to 50; malignancy potential of a dominant nodule probably equals that of a solitary nodule.

      (4) Nodule in a child less than 14 years old has high malignancy potential.

   b. Sex

      (1) Five to six times more nodules in women, thus most cancers are in women.

      (2) Malignant potential, however, probably is higher in nodules in men.

   c. History of neck irradiation

      (1) Ascertain by history or records that significant (more than 50 rads) irradiation did occur.

      (2) Twenty-seven per cent of all irradiated patients get nodules (16.5 per cent by examination, 11 per cent more by scan).

      (3) One third of nodules are malignant by histology, but not more aggressive.

   d. Family or personal history suggesting multiple endocrine neoplasia type II, including hypercalcemia (hyperparathyroidism), hypertension (pheochromocytoma), and medullary carcinoma of thyroid

Symptoms

1. Often the patient or a family member discovers the nodule accidentally, or it is found incidentally by computerized tomography scan or ultrasound ("incidentaloma").

2. Ascertain at once that there are no obstructive symptoms (e.g., inspiratory stridor). Then the only goal is to exclude malignancy of the thyroid nodule safely and at lowest cost, usually by fine-needle aspiration (FNA) cytology.

3. No symptom or combination of symptoms can positively identify malignancy or eliminate malignancy. Nevertheless, surgery is recommended if any *one* of the following is present:

   a. Rapidly enlarging solid nodule

   b. Unexplained hoarseness and vocal cord paralysis by laryngoscopy

   c. Nodule discovered at less than age 14

Key Symptom

None or unexplained hoarseness

Clinical Findings

1. At other times the nodule is found by the physician palpating during screening physical examination or in response to pain, mass, or tenderness in the neck.

2. Again, no signs on physical examination can identify malignancy, but surgery is recommended if any *one* of the following is found:

   a. Hard nodule

   b. Nodule or thyroid "fixed" to adjacent tissues

   c. Ipsilateral neck lymph node enlargement(s)

Key Signs

- Palpation of a hard thyroid nodule
- Ipsilateral lymph node enlargement

Laboratory Tests

1. Rarely, unexplained metastases to lung (chest

film) or to bone (scan) lead to a single palpable thyroid nodule; surgery is recommended.

2. Obtain thyroid function tests in all patients with a nodule.

   a. If subclinical hyperthyroidism is present (low thyroid-stimulating hormone [TSH], normal free thyroxine [T_4]), give levothyroxine (L-T_4) for 4 weeks at a dose of 0.025 mg/day more than usual replacement dose for that age of patient.

   b. If subclinical *or* overt (very low TSH, high free T_4) hyperthyroidism is present, do a radioactive thyroid scan, preferably radioiodine scan. If the nodule is "hot," then follow by clinical examination.

3. Only a small minority of nodules are those at high risk (already to surgery as above) or those with a "hot" nodule. All the rest have FNA done in the office.

   a. The person doing the aspiration must be experienced and *currently* performing a significant number monthly. The cytopathologist (not a general pathologist) reading the biopsy should also *currently* be doing a significant number monthly. Major false negatives occur if *either* of these criteria is not met.

   b. If the FNA is read as "malignant" or "suspicious" or "indeterminant," surgery is performed.

   c. If the FNA is read as "benign," the patient is followed (see below).

   d. If the FNA is "inadequate sample" or "nondiagnostic," it is repeated until an adequate sample is obtained, using ultrasound-guided FNA if necessary.

Key Tests

- Werner's maneuver is done first to find the nodule and then to define its characteristics.

- FNA is performed on most nodules (contraindicated if patient anticoagulated). It is not a definitive test but a very important adjunct to management.

Differential Diagnosis

Modern diagnosis of thyroid cancer depends very much on confident palpation of the thyroid to identify a nodule in the first place.

1. Is the neck mass truly thyroid gland?

   a. Locate the notch of the thyroid cartilage, then the lower border of the thyroid carti-

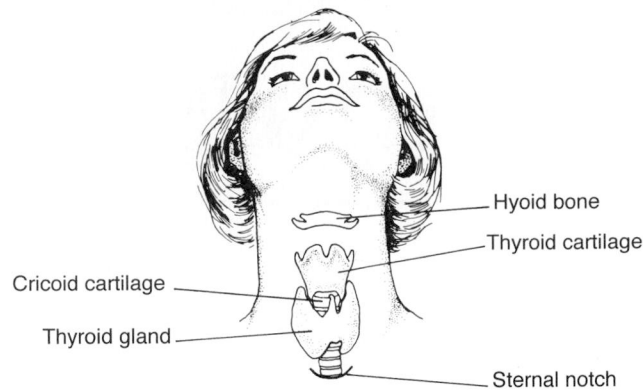

Figure 179–1 Landmarks for the anatomic location of the thyroid gland. (From Wartofsky L: The thyroid gland: introduction. In Becker KL [ed]: Principles and Practice of Endocrinology and Metabolism, p 264. Philadelphia, JB Lippincott Company, 1990; reprinted with permission.)

lage, and the cricoid cartilage immediately below it (see Fig. 179–1).

   b. The thyroid gland almost always will be between the cricoid and the sternal notch.

   c. From behind the patient, move the third and fourth digits downward, both hands at the same time, sensing for the upper edges of each lobe. Have the patient swallow. The thyroid gland will move upward under the examiner's fingers. If the nodule or mass moves upward with swallowing, it is likely thyroid-related. If it does not rise with swallowing, it probably is not a thyroid nodule.

   d. If the nodule is in the thyroid, palpate each lobe in turn using Werner's maneuver. Stand behind the seated patient. With the patient's head slightly flexed forward, to palpate the left lobe, the patient turns his or her head 15 to 20 degrees to the left to relax the left sternocleidomastoid muscle. The physician slides the right hand under the muscle and palpates the left lobe. Next retract the relaxed muscle with the fingers of the left hand and again palpate the left lobe with the right hand. Do the reverse for a nodule in the right lobe.

2. If the mass (nodule) is in the thyroid, then perform FNA and proceed as outlined above.

3. Rarely the neck mass is not thyroid.

   a. If it is midline, it may be

      (1) Thyroglossal duct cyst

         (a) One- to 2-cm remnant of pyramidal lobe, thus located above isthmus

         (b) Usually adjacent and inferior to hyoid bone

         (c) May rise on swallowing too, but it

also rises with maximal tongue protrusion.

(2) Epidermoid cyst

  (a) Usually nontender

  (b) Located in submental, infrahyoid region

b. If mass is not midline, think

  (1) Laryngocele

    (a) Expands with Valsalva maneuver but is not pulsatile (Valsalva may cause a vascular anomaly to enlarge but it is pulsatile).

    (b) May be bilateral (Dizzie Gillespie)

    (c) May be seen with chronic obstructive pulmonary disease.

  (2) Branchial cleft cyst

    (a) One to 2 cm in size

    (b) Located along anterior aspect of sternocleidomastoid muscle

4. Nonthyroid neck masses in adult: "80 per cent rule"

  a. Eighty per cent are neoplastic, 80 per cent of these are malignant, and 80 per cent of these are metastatic to the neck.

  b. Eighty per cent of primary tumors arise above the clavicles and are metastatic to neck nodes.

Treatment

1. If the FNA either is "malignant" or "benign," the issue is clear.

2. If either patient is high-risk or FNA is "suspicious" or "indeterminant" or "malignant," surgery is indicated. Only the extent of surgery is controversial.

  a. Near-total thyroidectomy probably is indicated in all except less than 1-cm differentiated carcinoma or minimally invasive follicular carcinoma. Get the best surgeon!

  b. In differentiated cancers, occult multifocal cancer occurs in 30 per cent and occult lymph node metastases are found in 50 per cent. Extensive surgery still is not needed, and only involved lymph nodes found at surgery need be removed before ablation treatment.

  c. Lymph node spread, however, is a more serious prognostic finding in anaplastic, lymphoma, medullary, or less differentiated papillary or follicular cancers. Expect more aggressive behavior in these, so treat vigorously, including radiotherapy.

  d. Dictating more aggressive postsurgery abla-

tion therapy are age less than 30 or more than 60; invasion outside thyroid capsule; nodule size more than 4 cm; male; intraglandular invasion of follicular cancer; tall cell variant of papillary; markedly multicentric cancer.

e. Postsurgical ^{131}I ablation therapy in all except solitary, less than 1 cm papillary or minimally invasive follicular cancer. Patient may desire ablation therapy even for these latter cancers, so offer it to them because there is some evidence of benefit.

  (1) TSH should be more than 30 μU/ml before using ^{131}I. Thus always stop L-T$_4$ therapy (0.1 mg/day) 6 weeks before ^{131}I, then give levotriiodothyronine (L-T$_3$) maintenance dose (Cytomel, 25 μg tid) the next 4 weeks; for last 2 weeks before ^{131}I, stop L-T$_3$ and have the patient eat a low-iodine diet.

  (2) In "low-risk" patients, use low-dose (30 mCi) ^{131}I. If needed, a second low dose is given 6 months later. If whole-body ^{131}I scan and serum thyroglobulin levels determine further ablation is needed, 100 mCi is given. Above preparation to get TSH more than 30 μU/ml always is done before ^{131}I ablation.

  (3) In "high-risk" (see above) patients, use the same procedure except treat with 100 mCi ^{131}I initially, and repeat same dose if needed (in 6 months).

3. If the nodule is "benign" by FNA, medical therapy or careful follow-up is done.

  a. Until recently all nodules would have been treated with suppressive doses of L-T$_4$ either to decrease the size or stop further growth of the nodule.

  b. Suppressive therapy either should not be done or the length of time a therapeutic trial is done should be limited strictly because

    (1) Double-blind, placebo-controlled study showed no effect in reducing size of nodules over 6 months' suppression (but may be subgroup with good response).

    (2) Suppressive doses of L-T$_4$ accelerate osteoporosis.

  c. How the patient is followed depends on the clinical context. If the nodule is an "incidentaloma" or "hot," follow by palpation every 3 to 6 months and then yearly. If the patient has a history of childhood irradiation, also follow with serial ultrasound studies and L-T$_4$ suppression of TSH. Keep the TSH more than 0.05 μU/ml.

4. If surgery is refused in a patient with "suspicious" FNA and no risk factors (e.g., woman 30 to 60 years and small nodule), try thyroid hormone suppression (keep TSH suppressed but not <0.05 μU/ml) and repeat FNA in 6 months. Alternatively, the nodule could be followed by serial ultrasonography at 6 and 12 months, with excision should the nodule enlarge.

Key Treatment

- If nodule is "high risk" or FNA is "malignant" or "suspicious," surgery is indicated.

- If FNA is "benign," medical therapy is indicated.

Follow-Up

1. In a patient with a "benign" nodule by FNA, thorough palpation of the thyroid (including Werner's maneuver), as well as regional lymph nodes is performed carefully at *all* future examinations. Appearance of *any* of the above high-risk findings (e.g., rapid growth, nodule hardens, obstructive symptoms) dictates immediate surgery.

2. Patients having thyroid cancer already operated are ablated with ^{131}I until total-body ^{131}I scan and serum thyroglobulin are both negative (tested 6 months and 12 months later).

3. Total-body ^{131}I scans are then done about every 5 years in "low-risk" patients and every 2 years in "high-risk" patients, or more frequently if se-

rum thyroglobulin levels increase. The latter are done every 6 months at first after ablative therapy and later every 1 to 2 years.

Bibliography

For more information on FNA, see
Gharib H: FNAB of thyroid nodules. Mayo Clin Proc 1994;69:44–49.

For more information on risk factors for malignancy in nodules, see
Hamming JF, Goslings BM, van Steenis GJ, et al: Value of FNAB in patients with nodular thyroid disease divided into groups of suspicion or malignant neoplasms on clinical grounds. Arch Intern Med 1990;150:113–116.

For more information on suppression by levothyroxine, see
Gharib H, James EM, Charboneau JW, et al: Suppression therapy with levothyroxine for solitary thyroid nodules. N Engl J Med 1987;317:70–75.
La Rosa GL, Lupo L, Giuffrida D, et al: Levothyroxine and iodine are both effective for treating benign solitary solid cold nodules of the thyroid. Ann Intern Med 1995;122:1–8.

For more information on levothyroxine and osteoporosis risk, see
Paul TL, Kerrigan J, Marie Kelly A, et al: Long-term L-thyroxine therapy is associated with decreased hip bone density in premenopausal women. JAMA 1988; 259:3137–3141.

For more information on management of thyroid nodules after neck irradiation, see
Schneider AB, Bekerman C, Leland J, et al: Thyroid nodules in the follow-up of irradiated individuals: comparison of thyroid ultrasound with scanning and palpation. J Clin Endocrinol Metab 1997;82:4020–4027.

For more information on "incidentalomas," see
Tan GH, Gharib H: Thyroid incidentalomas: management approaches to nonpalpable nodules discovered incidentally on thyroid imaging. Ann Intern Med 1997; 126:226–231.

180 Thyroiditis

Terry F. Davies

1. Thyroiditis implies inflammation within the thyroid gland, and such lymphocytic infiltrates may be infective, destructive, or benign.

2. The four most important clinical pointers to help diagnose the different types of thyroiditis are pain, diffuse gland enlargement, serum thyroid-stimulating hormone (TSH) levels, and the presence of thyroid autoantibodies.

   a. Pain within the thyroid depends upon the speed with which the gland swells, causing increased pressure within the thyroid capsule. Hence, a slowly progressive thyroid gland enlargement is rarely painful.

   b. Similarly, an intense infiltrate will feel firm, particularly if much time has passed and additional fibrosis has begun.

   c. Serum TSH remains the most vital diagnostic test for thyroid failure, rising significantly even before thyroid hormone levels can be detected as falling.

   d. Thyroid autoantibodies to thyroglobulin and thyroid peroxidase also remain the primary indicator of autoimmune involvement in the disease, although low levels are found in many normal individuals.

3. The different forms of thyroiditis are shown in Table 180–1.

Autoimmune Thyroiditis

Etiology

1. This is the most common form of thyroid failure. The cause is unknown but is considered to be a combination of genetic susceptibility and environmental triggers.

TABLE 180–1. TYPES OF THYROIDITIS

Type	Etiology	Treatment
Acute	Bacterial	High-dose broad-spectrum antibiotics
Subacute	Viral	Pain: aspirin/prednisone Hyperthyroid phase: propranolol Hypothyroid phase: low-dose T_4
Chronic	Autoimmune	T_4 replacement
Postpartum	Autoimmune	Hyperthyroid phase: propranolol Hypothyroid phase: low-dose T_4

2. Up to 20 per cent of the general population have easily detectable titers of antibodies to thyroid peroxidase (TPO) and thyroglobulin (Tg). However, only about 1 per cent of the population develop autoimmune thyroid failure, indicating that other, more important, risk factors also need to be present (e.g., T-cell abnormalities and appropriate human leukocyte antigens [HLAs]).

3. Patients with thyroid autoantibodies and a mildly raised TSH progress to clinical thyroid failure at a rate of approximately 3 to 5 per cent per year; hence the term *subclinical* or *mild thyroid failure* has been applied to such a disease state.

4. Autoimmune thyroiditis has been divided into types 1, 2, and 3 (Table 180–2). Type 1 refers to patients at risk for developing thyroid failure; such individuals may or may not have a goiter on examination by hand or, preferably, by ultrasound. Type 2 patients have thyroid failure as defined by markedly increased TSH levels. The goitrous type 2 patient is the type of patient described originally by Hashimoto, although we tend to call all forms of autoimmune thyroid failure "Hashimoto's disease." Type 3 refers to the thyroiditis that accompanies Graves' disease.

Symptoms

1. The classical symptoms and signs of thyroid failure may or may not be present depending upon the severity of the disorder. Although many patients have no specific symptoms, tiredness and weight gain are common.

2. Patients may present with, or without, an obvious goiter that is painless and slowly enlarging. These goitrous and atrophic varieties of the disease may represent two distinct varieties of the disease on the basis of HLA typing and natural history (e.g., the early goitrous variety may show periods of remission).

3. A large gland with Hashimoto's disease may, occasionally, cause pressure effects on the trachea or even a recurrent laryngeal nerve, which may be best relieved by a careful surgeon. Postoperative precautions must be taken to prevent

TABLE 180–2. CLASSIFICATION OF AUTOIMMUNE THYROIDITIS

Type 1 Autoimmune Thyroiditis:
Type 1A	Goitrous
Type 1B	Non-goitrous
	Status:
	Euthyroid with normal TSH level. Autoantibodies to hTg and hTPO present.

Type 2 Autoimmune Thyroiditis:
Type 2A	Goitrous (classical Hashimoto's disease)
Type 2B	Non-goitrous (primary myxedema, atrophic thyroiditis)
	Status:
	Persistent hypothyroidism with increased TSH levels. Autoantibodies to hTg and hTPO usually present. Some of Type 2B are associated with blocking type TSH receptor autoantibodies.
Type 2C	Transient aggravation of thyroiditis
	Status:
	May start as transient destructive thyrotoxicosis (increased serum thyroid hormones with low thyroidal radioactive iodine uptake). This is often followed by transient hypothyroidism. However, some patients show transient hypothyroidism without the preceding destructive thyrotoxicosis. Autoantibodies to hTg and hTPO usually present. Example, postpartum thyroiditis.

Type 3 Autoimmune Thyroiditis:
Type 3A	Hyperthyroid Graves' disease
Type 3B	Euthyroid Graves' disease
	Status:
	Hyperthyroid or euthyroid with suppressed TSH. Diagnostic autoantibodies to the TSH receptor of the stimulating variety are present. Autoantibodies to hTg and hTPO are also usually detected.
Type 3C	Hypothyroid Graves' disease
	Status:
	Orbitopathy with hypothyroidism. Diagnostic autoantibodies to the TSH receptor of the blocking or stimulating variety may be detected. Autoantibodies to hTg and hTPO are usually present.

From Davies TF, Amino N: A new classification for human autoimmune thyroid disease. Thyroid 1993;3:331–333, with permission.

tracheal collapse where there has been pressure atrophy of the supporting tracheal cartilage.

4. Occasionally, patients with autoimmune thyroiditis may present first with hyperthyroidism, a condition sometimes referred to as "hashitoxicosis." Acute autoimmune-mediated apoptosis of thyroid epithelial cells leads to an outpouring of thyroid hormone from the gland as colloid is released from within and without the cells. This transient hyperthyroidism may also be caused by local thyroid stimulators, such as prostaglandins from damaged cells, acting upon the remaining functional follicular cells.

Key Symptoms

- Low energy
- Weight gain
- Painless goiter

Clinical Signs

1. Most patients are women. Classical signs of weight gain, dry skin, hair loss, and loss of facial expression are rarely seen these days be-

cause of early diagnosis. Mild forms of these signs, however, are very common.

2. A diffuse firm goiter may or may not be present.

Key Signs

Firm, painless goiter, often visible

Laboratory Tests

1. In the definitive presentation, serum TSH is increased and free thyroxine (T_4) is decreased. TSH values above normal but less than 10 μU/ml should be confirmed. The measurement of triiodothyronine (T_3) is of no value in the diagnosis of thyroid failure.

2. Antibodies to thyroglobulin and thyroid peroxidase (microsomal antigen) are present, usually in high levels.

3. If the patient presents with destructive thyroiditis, serum T_3 and T_4 are increased, as is serum thyroglobulin, resulting in suppression of serum TSH.

Differential Diagnosis

1. Goiter: The thyroid in autoimmune thyroiditis has a classical firm feeling on examination. Sim-

ple goiters, including colloid goiters, are usually soft on examination. Iodine-deficiency goiters are often accompanied by thyroiditis and may also feel firm before the onset of multinodularity.

2. Thyroid cancer/lymphoma: Areas of the thyroid gland with Hashimoto's disease may feel extremely firm and nodular, raising the suspicion of neoplasia. In such patients, thyroid biopsy may be unhelpful because many of the aspirated lymphocytes may appear atypical, and normal thyroid epithelial cells can have the characteristics of papillary carcinoma. Hence, once a biopsy has been performed, there may be little alternative to a hemithyroidectomy if such a cytology reading is obtained. The presence of thyroid failure and high levels of thyroid autoantibodies should help avoid this situation, but thyroid cancer may be more frequent in autoimmune thyroid disease, just as thyroid lymphomas are occasionally seen.

3. Depression: Thyroid failure is often mistaken for depression and vice versa. The clinician must be astute in evaluating both these conditions.

4. Destructive thyroiditis: This condition may be difficult to distinguish from the onset of hyperthyroid Graves' disease, although it is usually milder in presentation and the presence of a firm goiter may be an indicator.

Treatment

1. Mild disease
   a. Patients with serum TSH level only just above the normal range (4 to 10 μU/ml) and with normal free T_4 and free T_3 levels have been referred to as suffering from "subclinical" or "mild" thyroid failure. The need for treatment of such patients has been questioned. There are good epidemiologic data on the poor consequences of patients with TSH greater than 10 μU/ml and normal free T_4 in regard to lipid profile and cardiac function, but few data for the more borderline category of patients.
   b. As mentioned earlier, the risk of worsening thyroid failure in such patients is 3 to 5 per cent per year only if they have thyroid autoantibodies. Hence, the presence of these autoantibodies in such patients may justify T_4 treatment to be instigated if there are clinical symptoms that require attention. Other patients may choose to be observed to determine progression of the disease.

2. Thyroid failure
   a. Patients who have symptoms consistent with

thyroid failure and whose thyroid function studies indicate reduced free T_4 concentrations combined with increased TSH levels should unquestionably be prescribed thyroid hormone replacement therapy ($\sim$1.5 to 2.0 μg/kg T_4 daily).
   b. It is inappropriate to prescribe thyroid hormones on the basis of suspicion alone; there must always be clearly documented evidence of thyroid failure.

3. Patient documentation: Because thyroid hormone replacement is lifelong, every patient should be provided with clear documentation of their need for thyroid hormone. One of the most common clinical problems is the lack of evidence for a patient already taking thyroid hormone replacement.

4. Thyroid replacement
   a. The dose of thyroid hormone prescribed in the long term is decided by titrating the patient's TSH with the daily dose of T_4.
   b. Most patients should be replaced with sufficient T_4 to normalize their TSH levels, preferably without decreasing their TSH below the normal range.
   c. A suppressed TSH indicates excessive thyroid hormone and entertains the possible long-term effects of such therapy on bone structure, particularly in postmenopausal women, and cardiac dysrhythmias.

5. Elderly patients: CAUTION should be exercised in the treatment of elderly patients and those with coronary artery disease. These patients should be replaced with small initial doses of thyroxine (25 μg daily) and monitored carefully for dysrhythmias and an influence on concurrent drug therapy. It may not be necessary to reduce the TSH levels of such patients to within the normal range, allowing them to remain in the 5- to 8-μU/ml range (normal <4).

6. Adrenal insufficiency: CAUTION should be exercised in patients suspected of adrenal insufficiency. Thyroid hormone replacement can precipitate an adrenal crisis by increasing metabolic demands.

7. Destructive autoimmune hyperthyroidism
   a. If symptomatic, treatment is with β-adrenergic blockade (e.g., propranolol, 20 to 40 mg qid).
   b. The condition may be difficult to distinguish from the onset of hyperthyroid Graves' disease, although it is usually milder in presentation and the presence of a firm goiter may be indicative of thyroiditis.
   c. These patients may rapidly become hypothy-

roid if antithyroid drugs are inappropriately used, and their underlying autoimmune thyroiditis will soon be revealed after drug withdrawal.

Key Treatment

Thyroxine replacement to normalize serum TSH

Follow-Up

1. Once a patient is appropriately replaced with T_4, then annual reviews are necessary for the checking of serum TSH levels.
2. Any change in the dose of T_4 prescribed should be followed by a delay of 4 to 6 weeks before repeating the TSH to allow for the slow equilibration to take place.

Postpartum Thyroiditis

Etiology

1. Levels of thyroid antibodies fall during pregnancy. Autoimmune thyroid disease, most obviously Graves' disease, characteristically improves during this time.
2. An associated switch from aggressive T cells to suppressive types of T cells, which is thought to be secondary to the presence of a variety of placental factors that favor immunosuppression during gestation, has also been observed to account for this phenomenon.
3. After delivery, thyroid antibody levels rebound to levels often greater than seen before pregnancy and then gradually return to normal. This time of rebound, 3 to 9 months postpartum, may be associated with a variety of postpartum thyroid syndromes, usually transient, in up to 8 per cent of women.
4. The most common form of the disorder is postpartum autoimmune thyroiditis, which essentially is a variant of Hashimoto's disease in a transient form.

Symptoms

1. Hyperthyroid phase: Thyrotoxic symptoms such as anxiety, palpitations, and weight loss may be a consequence of widespread thyroid cell destruction in early postpartum thyroiditis (PPT) just as it may be seen in autoimmune thyroiditis (see above). Evidence suggests that this form of presentation may be more common in the postpartum period than the early phase of classical autoimmune thyroiditis.

2. Hypothyroid phase: When PPT is mild, there may be no symptoms, but transient lethargy, depression, and weight gain or a failure to lose weight are common.

Key Symptoms

- Anxiety in hyperthyroid phase
- Postpartum depression in hypothyroid phase

Signs

1. A small, firm goiter may appear.
2. The thyroid is usually painless.

Key Sign

Small, firm, painless goiter

Laboratory Tests

1. Serum TSH is the guide to diagnosis. Although it may be suppressed in the early hyperthyroid phase, the TSH rises as thyroid failure ensues. Free T_3 is increased in the hyperthyroid phase and free T_4 falls as the thyroid fails. Sometimes the rise in TSH is delayed after a period of hyperthyroidism, and a falling free T_4 may be the first indication of failure.
2. Almost all patients show positive thyroid antibodies (especially anti-TPO), often at levels higher than before or during pregnancy.
3. Serum thyroglobulin is usually greatly increased in thyroiditis and may be a helpful distinguishing feature. Thyroglobulin can only be measured in patients without serum anti-thyroglobulin.
4. Thyroid biopsies in such cases have shown profuse mononuclear cell infiltration with follicular destruction, as seen in classical Hashimoto's disease. They are not necessary for diagnosis.
5. Radioiodine uptake is suppressed in thyroiditis. It is not needed for diagnosis, especially when patients are likely to be breast-feeding.

Key Tests

- TSH for hyperthyroidism and hypothyroidism
- Thyroid antibodies for diagnosis

Differential Diagnosis

1. Hyperthyroid phase
   a. This condition has to be distinguished from the onset of true Graves' disease, usually by the natural evolution of the condition. The onset of Graves' eye disease may also be diagnostic.
   b. An increased 24-hour radioiodine uptake in Graves' disease may be helpful (if the patient is not breast-feeding) but is rarely needed.
   c. The detection of thyroid-stimulating antibodies to the TSH receptor is also diagnostic of Graves' disease.
2. Hypothyroid phase: Genuine postpartum depression is the major differential in many patients at a time of great stress. Thyroid function testing provides the answer.

Treatment

1. Most episodes of PPT are transient, and rapid recovery can be expected over a 2- to 4-month period. Symptoms of thyroid failure and low thyroid function tests should be treated with thyroxine replacement therapy (50 to 150 μg daily) and the T_4 and TSH monitored.
2. Because only replacement therapy is prescribed, the problem of drugs in breast-feeding mothers does not arise.
3. As thyroid autoantibody levels fall, thyroid cell regeneration will be possible, and T_4 replacement should be reduced and withdrawn.
4. Antithyroid drugs will be unhelpful in the hyperthyroid phase because of their long delay in action and the transient nature of the condition. This phase may be very mild and even diagnosed only by biochemical changes. If significantly symptomatic, the appropriate treatment is β-adrenergic blockage (e.g., propranolol, 20 to 40 mg qid) prior to the onset of thyroid failure.

Key Treatment

- β-Adrenergic blockade for hyperthyroid symptoms
- Thyroid hormone replacement if symptomatic thyroid failure

Follow-Up

1. It is uncertain what percentage of such patients obtain full recovery.
2. Many patients no longer require T_4 supplementation but have evidence of continuing thyroid-

itis on the basis of high levels of thyroid auto-antibodies, and may even have a relapse following their next pregnancy.
3. In other patients, full recovery clearly does not ensue, as shown by continuing high TSH levels indicating the onset of classical Hashimoto's disease. Such patients will require long-term T_4 replacement.

Subacute (de Quervain's) Thyroiditis

Etiology

1. This uncommon disorder has been associated with evidence for a variety of viral infections, but no single agent has been described. The natural history and pathology are consistent with a viral type of infection.
2. It is possible that many individuals experience a mild form of the disease, but only with the onset of pain do they present to their physician. Indeed, a painless form of subacute thyroiditis has been recognized, although much less commonly, presumably with a lower grade of inflammation.
3. As with all forms of thyroiditis, there may be a hyperthyroid phase as the gland is lysed and a hypothyroid phase once the cells are destroyed.

Symptoms

1. General malaise and fever are common.
2. Severe pain and tenderness in the area of the thyroid gland, usually bilaterally
3. Symptoms of hyperthyroidism (anxiety and palpitations) may be present early in the disease even in patients with the rarer painless form.

Key Symptoms

- Malaise and fever
- Pain in the neck

Clinical Findings

1. The important clinical finding is that of extreme thyroid tenderness, often so severe that the patient will not allow the physician to palpate.
2. When palpated, the thyroid gland is smooth, firm, and very tender.
3. The thyroid pain and tenderness may sometimes be unilateral and move in progression from one side to the other.

Key Sign

Tender thyroid gland

Laboratory Tests

1. There is a diagnostic increase in the sedimentation rate in these patients (often >100 mm/hour).
2. Serum thyroglobulin levels are also very elevated.
3. Thyroid function tests may show a suppressed TSH early in the course of the disease and a rising TSH as the thyroid cells are destroyed.
4. Radioiodine uptake is often less than 1 to 2 per cent at 24 hours because of the thyroid cell destruction.
5. Thyroid autoantibody levels may be transiently present during subacute thyroiditis.

Key Tests

- Sedimentation rate
- Suppressed radioiodine uptake at 24 hours

Treatment

1. Most patients require no more than aspirin therapy to relieve the neck tenderness.
2. Severe tenderness may be devastating and, in this situation, prednisone, 30 to 40 mg daily over a 5- to 10-day period and gradually reducing the dose over the subsequent 2 weeks, is highly effective. The sedimentation rate is the appropriate guide to the necessity for steroid support.
3. Massive destruction of thyroid tissue leads to an outpouring of thyroid hormone, which may cause symptoms of hyperthyroidism. Some patients may require β-adrenergic blockade in the form of propranolol, 20 to 40 mg qid.
4. T_4 supplementation may be required in the hypothyroid phase depending on both the symptoms and the serum T_4/TSH results.
5. T_4 supplements may be continued for 6 to 8 weeks. It is important to realize, however, that thyroid cell regeneration may be enhanced by increased serum TSH levels in this and all other forms of thyroid destruction, and that T_4 supplementation should not be excessive (50 to 100 μg daily) unless the symptoms become gross.
6. Gradual withdrawal should lead to the return of normal thyroid function.

Key Treatment

- Pain relief: aspirin and steroids
- Rest the thyroid gland with T_4 replacement.

Follow-Up

1. Many patients retain an autoimmune diathesis after the disease, as evidenced by thyroid autoantibodies.
2. Serum thyroglobulin may be a useful marker to assess the degree of thyroiditis during thyroid hormone supplementation (in the absence of anti-Tg).
3. Some patients seem to have a chronic form of this disorder with continuing pain and discomfort. Putting the thyroid gland "to sleep" with full T_4 replacement is often effective in such patients.

Suppurative Thyroiditis

1. Septicemia and local infections from the chest and cervical lymph nodes may spread to the thyroid gland itself and cause an acute suppurative thyroiditis.
2. The gland may be enlarged and acutely tender, with systemic symptoms of fever, tachycardia, and malaise. Thrombophlebitis of the external jugular veins may complicate the presentation.
3. The diagnosis is usually obvious, and treatment involves appropriate high-dose antibiotics combined with incision and drainage when indicated. T_4 replacement may be necessary if there is much destruction of the gland, but full recovery usually ensues.

Reidel's Thyroiditis

1. This previously well-recognized chronic form of fibrous replacement of the thyroid is now rarely seen clinically. Although its etiology is uncertain, an association with Hashimoto's disease has been recognized and an autoimmune reaction to fibrous tissue may be involved.
2. There may be fibrosis of associated nonthyroid tissues, including the retroperitoneum.
3. The only effective treatment reported in addition to T_4 replacement is surgical correction of any resulting obstruction.

Bibliography

Davies TF, Amino N: A new classification for human autoimmune thyroid disease. Thyroid 1993;3:331–333.

Larson PR, Hay I, Davies TF: The thyroid gland. In Wilson JD, Foster DW, Larsen PR, et al (eds): Williams' Textbook of Endocrinology, 9th ed, pp 389–516. Philadelphia, WB Saunders Company, 1998.

Singer PA, Cooper DS, Levy E, et al: Treatment guidelines for patients with hyperthyroidism and hypothyroidism. JAMA 1995;273:808–812.

Tomer Y, Davies TF: The genetic susceptibility to Graves' disease. Baillieres Clin Endocrinol Metab 1998;11: 431–450.

Vanderpump MPJ, Tunbridge WMG, French JM, et al: The incidence of thyroid disorders in the community: a twenty-year follow-up of the Whickham survey. Clin Endocrinol 1995;43:55–68.

Wejda B, Hintze G, Katschinski B, et al: Hip fractures and the thyroid: a case-control study. J Intern Med 1995;237:241–247.

181 Cushing's Syndrome/Disease

Andrew J. Norton

Etiology

1. Endocrinologic syndrome of persistent inappropriate hypercortisolemia
2. Two etiologic categories determined by presence or absence of the stimulatory hormone adrenocorticotropic hormone (ACTH) at the time of measured hypercortisolemia
   a. ACTH-dependent
      (1) Pituitary neoplasm (Cushing's disease): 65 per cent of total
      (2) Nonpituitary neoplasm (ectopic): 15 per cent of total
      (3) Hypothalamic or ectopic corticotropin-releasing hormone–producing tumors: rare
   b. ACTH-independent
      (1) Adrenal neoplasm (adenoma or carcinoma): 15 per cent of total
      (2) Nodular adrenal hyperplasia: 5 per cent of total
         (a) Primary pigmented nodular adrenal disease
         (b) Macronodular adrenal hyperplasia
      (3) Iatrogenic: common
      (4) Factitious: uncommon
3. ACTH-dependent Cushing's syndrome is most commonly associated with a pituitary adenoma secreting ACTH (classic Cushing's disease).
   a. Female/male ratio 8:1
   b. Usual onset age 20 to 40 years
4. Ectopic ACTH-dependent Cushing's syndrome
   a. Most commonly caused by tumors of the amine precursor uptake and decarboxylation (APUD) system
      (1) Small cell carcinoma of the lung
      (2) Medullary carcinoma of the thyroid
      (3) Carcinoid
         (a) Bronchial
         (b) Thymic
      (4) Pheochromocytoma
      (5) Islet cell tumors
   b. Female/male ratio 1:1

Symptoms

1. General
   a. Weight gain—usually central (truncal)
   b. Weakness/fatigue
2. Dermatologic
   a. Easy bruisability
   b. Excessive hair growth in women
   c. Poor wound healing
3. Neuropsychiatric
   a. Depression
   b. Insomnia
4. Gonadal
   a. Menstrual disturbances/amenorrhea
   b. Impotence
   c. Decreased libido
5. Musculoskeletal
   a. Back pain
   b. Muscular weakness
6. Metabolic
   a. Polyuria
   b. Ureteral colic

Key Symptoms

- Weakness/fatigue
- Weight gain
- Dermatologic changes
- Depression
- Gonadal dysfunction

Clinical Findings

1. General
   a. Obesity and fat redistribution
      (1) Central obesity, particularly facial rounding and supraclavicular fullness
      (2) Generalized weight gain may occur.
   b. Hypertension
2. Dermatologic
   a. Hirsutism, particularly increased facial lanugo hair growth
   b. Acne and facial plethora
   c. Wide-based purple striae on the abdomen

d. Skin/subcutaneous thinning with ecchymosis

e. Superficial fungal infections

3. Neuropsychiatric: depression

4. Musculoskeletal

   a. Osteopenia/osteoporosis with pathologic fractures (vertebral, rib)

   b. Proximal muscle weakness

5. Metabolic

   a. Impaired glucose tolerance or diabetes mellitus

   b. Kidney stone formation

Key Signs

- Central obesity with supraclavicular fullness
- Facial rounding with plethora
- Hypertension
- Proximal muscular weakness
- Hirsutism and acne
- Glucose intolerance

Laboratory Tests

1. Basic laboratory studies are usually normal.

2. Leukocytosis, lymphopenia, polycythemia, hyperglycemia, and hypokalemia may be seen. Hypokalemia is commonly found (60 per cent) in ectopic ACTH production but is unusual in pituitary Cushing's syndrome (10 per cent).

3. Dexamethasone suppression test

   a. Screening test for Cushing's syndrome

   b. Give 1 mg dexamethasone orally in the late evening (2300 hours) with early morning serum cortisol determination in nonstressed ambulatory individual.

   c. Normal values less than 3 μg/dl

   d. False-positive results with physiologic stress, renal failure, estrogen and anticonvulsant drug therapy, and endogenous depression

4. Urine free cortisol

   a. Best test for confirmation and when initial clinical suspicion is high

   b. 24-hour urine collection for free cortisol and creatinine

   c. False-positive result uncommonly seen in physiologic stress, alcoholism, endogenous depression, and exogenous steroid use

   d. False-negative result seen in intermittent cortisol secretion syndromes (uncommon)

Key Tests

- Overnight dexamethasone suppression test
- A 24-hour urine free cortisol determination

Differential Diagnosis

1. Diagnostic confirmation of Cushing's syndrome and determination of its cause should be done with the collaboration of an experienced endocrinologist.

2. Determine plasma ACTH level by immunoradiometric assay (IRMA) technique to distinguish ACTH-dependent from ACTH-independent Cushing's syndrome.

3. If ACTH-dependent (>10 pg/ml)

   a. High-dose overnight dexamethasone suppression test

     (1) Give 8 mg dexamethasone in the late evening (2300 hours) with early morning cortisol.

     (2) In pituitary ACTH-dependent Cushing's syndrome, the morning cortisol is usually less than 50 per cent of baseline. In ectopic ACTH or ACTH-independent Cushing's syndrome, the cortisol level usually does not suppress.

   b. Magnetic resonance imaging of the pituitary

   c. Referral for bilateral inferior petrosal sinus sampling for ACTH to definitively ascertain the source of ACTH production (pituitary or ectopic)

4. If ACTH independent (<5 pg/ml), abdominal computerized tomographic scan for adrenal neoplasm

Treatment

1. Surgery

   a. Transsphenoidal pituitary microsurgery is the treatment of choice for pituitary ACTH-secreting adenoma and should be done by an experienced neurosurgeon.

   b. Adrenalectomy (unilateral or bilateral) for adrenal adenoma or hyperplasia and for persistent or recurrent pituitary Cushing's syndrome after pituitary microsurgery

2. Radiotherapy is adjunctive therapy for pituitary Cushing's syndrome.

3. Medical management of Cushing's syndrome employs drugs that inhibit adrenal hormone biosynthesis. Drugs used include

   a. Ketoconazole (Nizoral)

b. Metyrapone (Metopirone)

c. Aminoglutethimide (Cytadren)

d. Mitotane (Lysodren)

 ## Bibliography

For general information, see
Orth DN: Cushing's syndrome. N Engl J Med 1995;323: 791–803.

For more detailed information, see
Nieman N, Cutler GB: Endocrinology, 3d ed, pp 1741–1769. Philadelphia, WB Saunders Company, 1995.

For a review of the diagnostic work-up, see
Meier CA: Clinical and biochemical evaluation of Cushing's syndrome. Endocrinol Metab Clin North Am 1997;26:741.

For a review of ectopic ACTH syndromes, see
Findling JW, Raff H: Ectopic ACTH. In Mazzaferri EL, Samaan NA (eds): Endocrine Tumors, pp 554–566. Cambridge, England, Blackwell Scientific Publications, 1993.

182 Adrenal Insufficiency

James K. Rone

Etiology

Primary Adrenal Insufficiency (PAI; Lesion of the Adrenal Glands)

1. Autoimmune adrenalitis (component of autoimmune polyglandular syndromes)
2. Infections (recovery possible with early treatment)
   a. Tuberculous
   b. Fungal: histoplasmosis, paracoccidioidomycosis, blastomycosis, coccidioidomycosis
   c. Acquired immunodeficiency syndrome–related: cytomegalovirus, *Mycobacterium avium*, cryptococcus, cytokines
3. Bilateral adrenal hemorrhage
   a. Sepsis-induced (Waterhouse-Friderichsen syndrome)
   b. Associated with severe illness and physiologic stress—resulting in massive adrenal perfusion—plus coagulopathy, thromboembolic disease, or postsurgical states (especially primary anti-phospholipid antibody syndrome and heparin-induced thrombocytopenia)
4. Drugs
   a. Steroidogenesis inhibitors (ketoconazole, etomidate, adrenolytic agents)
   b. Inducers of steroid catabolism (rifampin, phenytoin, phenobarbital, levothyroxine)
5. Adrenoleukodystropy/adrenomyeloneuropathy
6. Systemic amyloidosis
7. Metastatic cancer or primary adrenal lymphoma
8. Other: sarcoidosis, hemochromatosis, bilateral adrenalectomy, congenital

Secondary Adrenal Insufficiency (SAI; Central Lesion)

1. Hypothalamic-pituitary-adrenal (HPA) axis suppression
   a. Exogenous glucocorticoids or adrenocorticotropic hormone (ACTH), inhaled steroids, megestrol acetate
   b. Endogenous Cushing's syndrome
2. Pituitary/hypothalamic lesion resulting in ACTH deficiency (rare)
   a. Tumors: pituitary adenoma, craniopharyngioma, metastatic
   b. Surgery/irradiation/trauma
   c. Lymphocytic hypophysitis
   d. Sarcoidosis
   e. Eosinophilic granulomatosis
   f. Infection: *Nocardia*, actinomycosis, tuberculosis
   g. Infarction (Sheehan's syndrome)
   h. Isolated ACTH or corticotropin-releasing hormone deficiency

Symptoms

1. The clinical presentation of adrenal insufficiency (AI) is variable.
   a. *Acute AI* (addisonian crisis) is a medical emergency presenting with fluid- and pressor-resistant shock. *Chronic AI* is an insidious disorder characterized by nonspecific "neurotic" complaints that may go undiagnosed for long periods.
   b. In *PAI* all adrenocortical hormones are lost (glucocorticoids, mineralocorticoids, androgens). *SAI* affects glucocorticoids and androgens, while the renin-angiotensin-aldosterone axis remains intact.
2. Symptoms
   a. Fatigue and weakness
   b. Anorexia/revulsion to food
   c. Nausea and vomiting
   d. Other gastrointestinal complaints: abdominal pain, constipation, diarrhea
   e. Psychiatric symptoms: depression, apathy, confusion, psychosis, paranoia
   f. Amenorrhea and decreased libido in women
   g. Salt craving as a result of mineralocorticoid loss (PAI only)
   h. Postural dizziness or syncope (more marked in PAI)
   i. Diffuse musculoskeletal pain
   j. Hypoglycemic symptoms
   k. Reduced insulin requirement in a type I diabetic

Clinical Findings

1. Weight loss
2. Hyperpigmentation (PAI only) over sun-exposed skin, palmar creases, nipples, lips, buccal mucosa, gingival margin, scars, areas of chronic mild trauma (elbows, knees, knuckles, under belts/bra straps)
3. Hypotension resulting from decreased cardiac contractility, decreased vascular resistance, catecholamine insensitivity (glucocorticoid loss), and volume contraction (mineralocorticoid loss)
4. Spontaneous resolution of hypertension
5. Decreased axillary and pubic hair in women (loss of primary androgen source)
6. Vitiligo (suggests autoimmune etiology)

Laboratory Tests

1. General findings
   a. Hyponatremia
      (1) Mineralocorticoid deficiency promotes urinary sodium loss.
      (2) Glucocorticoid deficiency promotes free water retention as a result of direct renal effect and antidiuretic hormone excess (loss of inhibition, decreased contractility, nausea, hypovolemia).
   b. Hyperkalemia (PAI only) resulting from mineralocorticoid deficiency, hypovolemia, and acidosis
   c. Hypercalcemia: typically mild but may be life-threatening
   d. Normocytic normochromic anemia, neutropenia, eosinophilia, lymphocytosis
   e. Hyperchloremic metabolic acidosis (PAI)
   f. Prerenal azotemia
   g. Fasting hypoglycemia
2. Screening and diagnostic testing

a. Basal serum cortisol levels vary widely in normal subjects but can be helpful. At a minimum, draw a cortisol prior to treating suspected acute AI. Therapy must not be delayed waiting for results.
   (1) *Random cortisol* during severe physiologic stress, such as shock (normal, ≥ 18 μg/dl; definite AI, <5 μg/dl; presumptive AI, 5 to 13 μg/dl)
   (2) *Morning cortisol* (0600 and 0800; normal, ≥ 20 μg/dl; definite AI, ≤ 3 μg/dl)
b. ACTH stimulation tests
   (1) Procedure
      (a) *Standard dose*: Inject 250 μg ACTH (Cortrosyn) intravenously or intramuscularly, and measure serum cortisol at 30 and 60 minutes (normal, ≥ 18 μg/dl at any point, although 30-minute result most indicative).
      (b) *Low dose*: Inject 1 μg ACTH and measure cortisol at same intervals; same normal values; more sensitive than the standard-dose test for partial SAI.
   (2) Standard-dose stimulation is the diagnostic test of choice in most settings.
   (3) Can be run in suspected acute AI if dexamethasone, which does not interfere with cortisol measurement, is used for initial treatment. Therapy must never be delayed.
   (4) Evaluates the entire HPA axis and will detect most PAI and SAI. Low sensitivity in mild or recent-onset SAI. In such cases a low dose test or insulin tolerance test is needed.
c. Insulin tolerance test (ITT)
   (1) Procedure: Induce symptomatic hypoglycemia (glucose <40 mg/dl) with regular insulin, 0.10 to 0.15 units/kg body weight IV bolus. Once hypoglycemia occurs, draw a serum glucose and cortisol at 0, 30, 60, and 90 minutes (treat the hypoglycemia). A peak cortisol greater than 18 μg/dl is normal.
   (2) Physician must be present. Fatal hypoglycemia may occur. Testing is contraindicated in elderly, cardiovascular, or seizure patients.
   (3) The ITT is the gold standard assessment of the HPA axis but is rarely needed. It offers no advantage over ACTH stimulation—and significantly more dis-

comfort and risk—except when partial or early ACTH deprivation is suspected.

3. Localization (PAI vs. SAI)

   a. Serum ACTH

     (1) Markedly elevated (always >100 pg/ml) in PAI

     (2) Low or inappropriately normal (8 to 75 pg/ml) in SAI

     (3) Should be drawn with the initial cortisol level in the evaluation of AI.

   b. Aldosterone response to ACTH stimulation (levels <4 ng/ml suggest PAI)

4. Other testing: If the etiology of AI is not obvious, consider chest radiography, purified protein derivative testing for tuberculosis, and adrenal computerized tomography (PAI) or pituitary magnetic resonance imaging (SAI). In PAI, consider screening for associated autoimmune diseases (especially hypothyroidism and diabetes).

Key Tests

- ACTH stimulation test
- Serum ACTH

Differential Diagnosis

1. Consider *acute AI* in all cases of unexplained hypotension or shock, especially if associated conditions are present or the patient has been on glucocorticoid therapy in the past year. May mimic acute abdomen, sepsis, and hypovolemic shock.

2. *Chronic AI* should be considered in any patient with chronic fatigue, especially if associated with weight loss, gastrointestinal symptoms, or hyperpigmentation. The differential diagnosis is broad and may include

   a. Major depression

   b. Mild thyrotoxicosis, especially in the elderly ("apathetic hyperthyroidism")

   c. Gastrointestinal malignancy

   d. Chronic infection

   e. Insulinoma: hypoglycemia associated with *increased* appetite and weight *gain*

   f. Other hyperpigmented conditions: racial, pregnancy, hemochromatosis, heavy metal toxicity, Peutz-Jegher's syndrome

   g. Paraneoplastic ectopic ACTH secretion may present with weight loss, fatigue, hyperpigmentation, and elevated ACTH levels, but these patients also have hypertension, hyper-

glycemia, hypercortisolemia, and hypokalemic metabolic alkalosis.

Treatment

Medication

1. Acute adrenal insufficiency

   a. Hydrocortisone (HC), 100 mg IV every 6 to 8 hours and rapidly taper, typically to 100 to 150 mg total on the second day, 50 to 75 mg the third day, and maintenance starting the fourth day. Taper patients with other serious illnesses more slowly.

   b. Alternatives include equipotent doses of methylprednisolone or dexamethasone, although HC is preferred because of greater mineralocorticoid action. Dexamethasone is often used for the first dose while ACTH stimulation testing is accomplished.

   c. Mineralocorticoid effect from high-dose HC is adequate. Supplement in PAI once dose drops below 100 mg/day.

   d. Give boluses of normal saline with 5% dextrose to correct volume depletion, hyponatremia, and hypoglycemia.

   e. Search for and treat precipitating events.

2. Chronic therapy

   a. Use a short-acting oral glucocorticoid in the lowest effective dose. Avoid dexamethasone because clearance rates vary and the long half-life may increase adverse effects.

   b. HC (or cortisone acetate, which is converted to HC) is preferred. Some authorities recommend prednisone with its slightly longer half life and lower cost.

     (1) HC dose: 12 to 15 mg/m^2 orally daily

     (2) Usually two thirds of the total dose in the morning and one third in late afternoon (typically 20 and 10 mg, respectively, or 25 and 12.5 mg of cortisone acetate)

     (3) To prevent subtle overreplacement, taper initial dose until evidence of deficiency appears (fatigue, gastrointestinal symptoms, hyponatremia), then increase slightly.

     (4) Single daily dosing (HC, 20 or 25 mg every morning) may improve compliance and lessen side effects.

     (5) For poor symptom control, consider three divided doses (HC, 10 mg tid), or prednisone, 3 to 4 mg/m^2 daily (4 to 5 mg on arising and 1 to 2.5 mg at 3 PM).

   c. Mineralocorticoid replacement (only PAI): fludrocortisone (Florinef), 0.05 mg every other day to 0.2 mg daily, typically 0.1 mg/day. Higher doses needed if a glucocorticoid other than HC is used.

d. Stress coverage

(1) Minor stress (fever >100° F, vomiting, diarrhea): double maintenance glucocorticoid replacement. Parenteral therapy needed if patient unable to tolerate oral intake.

(2) Major stress (severe trauma, illness, or surgery): as for acute AI

Diet

High sodium intake beneficial in PAI.

Activity

As tolerated

Patient Education

1. Patients and families must understand the need for stress coverage and how to make dosage adjustments when a physician is not available.

2. Patients should wear identification jewelry, such as a Medic Alert bracelet.

3. Patients should have in their possession and know how to use parenteral glucocorticoids in case of emergency (especially if traveling in remote areas).

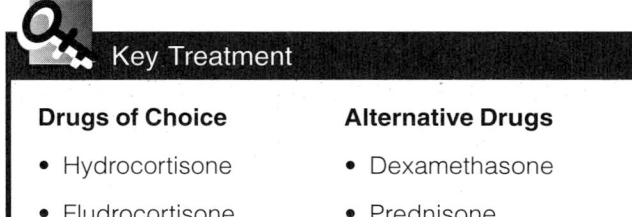

Key Treatment

Drugs of Choice	Alternative Drugs
• Hydrocortisone	• Dexamethasone
• Fludrocortisone	• Prednisone

Follow-Up

1. Monitoring glucocorticoid replacement

a. Follow clinical findings (appetite, well-being, body weight) and serum sodium. Urine free cortisol should be maintained in the normal range. ACTH and cortisol levels are not helpful.

b. Signs of Cushing's syndrome suggest over-replacement.

c. Measure bone mineral density periodically.

2. Monitoring mineralocorticoid replacement

a. Titrate serum potassium and renin levels to the upper normal range.

b. Monitor blood pressure. Dangerous hypertension may occur, especially when recumbent.

Bibliography

Carey RM: The changing clinical spectrum of adrenal insufficiency. Ann Intern Med 1997;127:1103–1105.

Chodosh LA, Daniels GH: Addison's disease. Endocrinologist 1993;3:166–181.

Grinspoon SK, Biller BMK: Laboratory assessment of adrenal insufficiency. J Clin Endocrinol Metab 1994;79:923–931.

Oelkers W: Adrenal insufficiency. N Engl J Med 1996;335:1206–1212.

Tordjman K, Jaffe A, Grazas N, et al: The role of the low dose (1 μg) adrenocorticotropin test in the evaluation of patients with pituitary diseases. J Clin Endocrinol Metab 1995;80:1301–1305.

183 Pheochromocytoma

Victor R. Lavis

Etiology

The etiology of pheochromocytoma is unknown. It occurs frequently in association with mutations of the *ret* proto-oncogene, which cause multiple endocrine neoplasia type II (MEN II), or of the *VHLD* tumor suppressor gene, which cause von Hippel–Lindau disease (VHLD), but the molecular pathogenesis has not been elucidated.

Symptoms

1. The classical symptoms are paroxysms of headache, sweating, palpitations, pallor, and anxiety. These reflect activation of the sympathetic nervous system.
2. Other common symptoms are tremulousness, nausea, chest or abdominal pain, and weakness.
3. Chest pain can be related to hypertension, sympathetic drive of the heart, or cardiomyopathy. Dyspnea on exertion may indicate cardiomyopathy or myocardial ischemia.
4. Weight loss is common and reflects hypermetabolism; in addition, there may be urinary loss of calories owing to uncontrolled diabetes mellitus.

Key Symptoms

- Headaches
- Palpitations
- Sweating

Ninety-five per cent of patients with pheochromocytoma will have at least one of the above three key symptoms. A hypertensive patient with none of the above is extremely unlikely to have a pheochromocytoma.

Clinical Findings

1. Hypertension, sustained or paroxysmal, may be extreme. Hypertensive crisis and pulmonary edema may occur.
2. Postural hypotension is very common.
3. Inappropriate tachycardia or reflex bradycardia are also very common.
4. Other common findings are pallor, tremulousness, and hyperglycemia.

5. Findings of associated diseases
   a. MEN II
      (1) Pheochromocytomas are located in the adrenals, and are almost always bilateral.
      (2) All forms of MEN II include medullary carcinoma of the thyroid.
      (3) Hypercalcemia owing to parathyroid hyperplasia (in MEN IIa)
      (4) Marfanoid habitus, mucosal neuromas, and thickened corneal nerves (in MEN IIb)
   b. VHLD
      (1) Retinal angiomas
      (2) Hemangiomas of cerebellum and spinal cord
      (3) Renal or pancreatic cysts or tumors
   c. Neurofibromatosis
      (1) Neurofibromas
      (2) Café-au-lait spots
   d. Tuberous sclerosis
      (1) Seizures
      (2) Skin lesions (adenoma sebaceum)
      (3) Mental retardation
6. Pheochromocytoma may present as an incidentally discovered adrenal nodule.

WARNING

Before attempting angiography, needle aspiration, or surgery on a patient with an adrenal mass, one should exclude pheochromocytoma.

Key Findings

- Paroxysmal hypertension accompanied by headache, pallor, and cold sweat; often with anxiety, palpitations, chest pain, and nausea
- Sustained hypertension is quite common.
- Postural hypotension
- Tachycardia

Laboratory Tests

1. The standard diagnostic tests are determinations of vanillylmandelic acid (VMA), metanephrine and normetanephrine, and epinephrine and norepinephrine in a 24-hour urine specimen. To validate the completeness of collection, urinary creatinine should also be measured. The patient should not have taken any adrenergic blocking drug, methyldopa, methocarbamol, tricyclic antidepressant, L-DOPA, monoamine oxidase inhibitor, or radiocontrast dye for the preceding 2 weeks, and should not have ingested any guaifenesin, vanilla, chocolate, bananas, nuts, coffee, tea, or citrus fruits for several days before collection of the urine. See Chapter 6 of Manger and Gifford (1996) for an extensive list of medicines that can interfere with these tests.

2. Measurement of plasma catecholamines (epinephrine and norepinephrine) can be helpful. For this test to be valid, the blood pressure should be elevated at the time of the test. The patient should be euglycemic, euthyroid, and euvolemic; should not be hypoxic, acidotic, in heart failure, or under stress; and must have been supine for at least 20 minutes before the blood is drawn. Ideally, the patient should be put at rest, an indwelling venous catheter inserted, and the blood drawn 30 or more minutes later.

3. Elevation of plasma or urinary epinephrine in a patient with pheochromocytoma indicates that the tumor is located in an adrenal gland or the organ of Zuckerkandl.

4. Clonidine suppression test: In the 3 hours following oral administration of clonidine, 0.3 mg/70 kg of body weight, plasma free catecholamines and blood pressure normally fall, but rise or stay the same in patients with pheochromocytoma.

5. Imaging procedures for localization
   a. Computerized tomography (CT) of the abdomen is simple and reliable, especially for patients with MEN, who are known to have adrenal pheochromocytomas.
   b. On magnetic resonance imaging (MRI), pheochromocytomas characteristically show high signal intensity on T_2-weighted images.
   c. [131]I-*meta*-Iodobenzylguanidine (MIBG) scan is especially useful for detection of extra-adrenal pheochromocytomas and metastases.

Key Tests

Diagnosis

- A 24-hour urine for VMA, metanephrines, and catecholamines

- Plasma catecholamines

- Clonidine suppression test

Localization

- CT scan of abdomen and pelvis

- MRI of abdomen and pelvis

- MIBG scan

WARNINGS

- **The clonidine suppression test should be carefully supervised because profound sedation and hypotension may occur in persons without pheochromocytoma.**

- **Provocative tests such as administration of glucagon are potentially dangerous and very seldom necessary. They should be performed only in specialized centers.**

- **Imaging procedures such as CT and MRI are of no use for the *diagnosis* of pheochromocytoma and may yield misleading results. They should be employed only for localization, *after* the diagnosis has been well established by means of appropriate biochemical studies of urine and blood.**

Differential Diagnosis

1. Panic attacks; anxiety states
2. Nontherapeutic drugs
   a. Cocaine
   b. Alcohol
   c. Amphetamines
3. Therapeutic drugs
   a. Congeners of catecholamines (e.g., phenylpropanolamine)
   b. Ingestion of tyramine-containing foods, in patient taking monoamine oxidase inhibitors
4. Withdrawal from clonidine
5. Menopausal flushes
6. Thyrotoxicosis
7. Paroxysmal tachyarrhythmias
8. Migraine

9. Acute hypoglycemia
10. Carcinoid tumor and mastocytosis: usually associated with flushing and hypotension
11. Autonomic hyperreflexia
12. Angina pectoris
13. Subarachnoid hemorrhage and other intracranial lesions

Treatment

Whenever possible, pheochromocytomas should be removed surgically, or at least debulked if complete resection is not feasible. It is very important to prepare the patient for operation with adrenergic blockade and volume replenishment, in order to avoid intraoperative hypertensive crises and arrhythmias, as well as postoperative hypotension.

Medication

1. First, one should control hypertension with α-adrenergic blockade.
   a. Traditionally, phenoxybenzamine (Dibenzyline) has been employed, starting at a dose of 10 mg twice daily.
   b. α_1-Adrenergic antagonists (e.g., prazosin [Minipress], doxazosin [Cardura], terazosin [Hytrin]), or labetalol (Trandate, Normodyne) also may be used.
   c. Expect some postural hypotension because vasodilatation occurs.
   d. Allow the patient free access to sodium.
   e. Titrate the dosage of α-blocker upward over several days to the maximum level tolerated with liberal intake of sodium.
2. *After* establishment of α-adrenergic blockade, β-adrenergic blockers such as metoprolol (Lopressor) may be added for control of tachycardia.
3. For patients with unresectable or metastatic disease, α-methyl-*p*-tyrosine, an inhibitor of catecholamine biosynthesis, may be employed.

WARNING

- If pheochromocytoma is suspected, do not begin treatment with β-adrenergic blocking drugs, which may precipitate hypertensive crisis. One must first establish α-adrenergic blockage.

- Substantial α-adrenergic blockade should be established prior to surgery, in order to avoid severe postoperative hypotension.

Diet

As noted above, it is important to liberalize sodium intake along with administration of adrenergic blocking drugs, in order to replete intravascular volume.

Follow-Up

1. Following resection of a pheochromocytoma, 24-hour urinary excretion of VMA, metanephrines, and catecholamines should be checked a few weeks postoperatively, and then annually for several years.
2. In MEN II, pheochromocytomas are bilateral. Therefore, patients with MEN II must be kept under surveillance after resection of one adrenal.
3. Patients with pheochromocytoma should be screened for MEN II and VHLD.
   a. Genetic screening for MEN II is commercially available, but genetic analysis for VHLD is still a research procedure.
   b. The lesions of VHLD may be detected by dilated funduscopic examination and computerized imaging of the brain, kidneys, and pancreas.
   c. If a patient has either of these syndromes, first-degree relatives should be screened.

Bibliography

Bravo EL, Gifford RW, Manger WM: Adrenal medullary tumors: pheochromocytoma. In Mazzaferri EL, Samaan NA (eds): Endocrine Tumors, pp 426–447. Boston, Blackwell Scientific Publications, 1993.

Keiser HR: Pheochromocytoma and other diseases of the sympathetic nervous system. In Becker KL (ed): Principles and Practice of Endocrinology and Metabolism, 2nd ed, pp 762–770. Philadelphia, JB Lippincott Company, 1995.

Keiser HR: Pheochromocytoma and related tumors. In DeGroot LJ (ed): Endocrinology, 3rd ed, vol 2, pp 1853–1877. Philadelphia, WB Saunders Company, 1995.

Manger WM, Gifford RW: Clinical and Experimental Pheochromocytoma, 2nd ed. Cambridge, MA, Blackwell Science, 1996.

Maurea S, Cuocolo A, Reynolds JC, et al: Iodine-131-metaiodobenzylguanidine scintigraphy in preoperative and postoperative evaluation of paragangliomas: comparison with CT and MRI. J Nucl Med 1993;34:173–179.

184 Hyperprolactinemia

Frederick C. Stone, Jr.

Etiology

Hyperprolactinemia is commonly a disease of adult life, with many physiologic and pathologic causes.

1. Physiologic causes
   a. Stress and exercise
   b. Food intake, especially arginine
   c. Pregnancy
   d. Breast-feeding, breast stimulation and suckling
2. Pathologic causes
   a. Prolactinomas
   b. Medications: phenothiazines, butyrophenones, metoclopramide, tricyclic antidepressants, verapamil, monoamine oxidase inhibitors, α-methyldopa, reserpine
   c. Tumors and infiltrative processes (e.g., sarcoidosis, hemochromatosis, tuberculosis)
   d. Hypothyroidism
   e. Renal disease
   f. Cirrhosis of the liver
   g. Adrenal insufficiency
   h. Chest wall injury/stimulation of intercostal nerve
   i. Idiopathic

Signs and Symptoms

1. Symptoms are generally more apparent in women. Oligomenorrhea, secondary amenorrhea, hirsutism, decreased libido, infertility, osteoporosis, and galactorrhea are common.
2. Postmenopausal women may have the above symptoms. They do not have the usual vasomotor symptoms of hot flashes expected with menopause because of low follicle-stimulating hormone and luteinizing hormone levels.
3. Common symptoms in men include decreased libido, erectile dysfunction, gynecomastia, and galactorrhea. Infertility resulting from decreased sperm count is less common.
4. Psychological symptoms can include anxiety, depression, and altered personality.
5. Tumor mass effects may result in chronic headaches, visual field defects, or hypopituitarism as a result of compression of the pituitary stalk.

Two thirds of patients with a visual field defect will have classical bitemporal hemianopsia. Cranial nerve palsies, seizures, or hydrocephalus can occur.

Key Symptoms

- Oligomenorrhea, amenorrhea
- Decreased libido
- Galactorrhea
- Infertility
- Erectile dysfunction (men)
- Headaches
- Visual field defects
- Anxiety
- Depression

Clinical Findings

1. Generally, the history will provide more clues to the diagnosis of hyperprolactinemia than the physical examination. A milky discharge may be expressible on breast examination. A visual field defect may be picked up; if present, it is usually bitemporal hemianopsia.
2. Findings consistent with a concomitant underlying process may be present.

Key Signs

- Galactorrhea
- Visual field defects

Laboratory and Other Diagnostic Tests

1. Confirm a laboratory determination of elevated prolactin level with repeated measurements. Keep this in mind, particularly if the elevation is minimal. Stress and exercise can elevate the prolactin level. Try to do testing in late morning or early afternoon, and at least 1 hour after a meal.
2. Laboratory evaluation
   a. Thyroid-stimulating hormone (TSH), renal function, liver enzymes, and a pregnancy test will exclude causes except hypothalamic-pituitary disease.

b. Adrenocorticotropic hormone, growth hormone, or urinary free cortisol might be ordered, depending upon particular history and physical examination findings and other laboratory results.

3. Computerized tomography (CT) or magnetic resonance imaging (MRI) of the pituitary should be done if history or physical examination suggests a neurologic cause or was completely unrevealing. These scans will pick up prolactinomas, infiltrative disorders, and other tumors. Note that the limit of resolution of CT/MRI for a prolactinoma is 2 to 3 mm. Complications of missing such a minute lesion are very small with close follow-up (see below). Also order a scan in a woman with a prolactin level of 20 to 30 ng/ml to assess for a pseudoprolactinoma or nonsecreting tumor.

4. Visual field examination with Goldmann perimetry: Check visual fields if scan shows tumor to be less than 2 mm from the optic chiasm or if there is suprasellar extension.

Key Tests

- Blood urea nitrogen, creatinine, liver enzymes, TSH, pregnancy
- CT/MRI scan of pituitary
- Visual fields testing

Treatment

Treatment of hyperprolactinemia is guided in part by size of the prolactinoma (if present) and how bothersome symptoms of hyperprolactinemia are for the patient. Treatment options are medication, surgery, and radiation. Surgery tends to be reserved for patients not responding to medical therapy or intolerant of it. Radiation therapy is a complement to medical or surgical therapy. Growth of adenomas treated with radiation is rare, but hypopituitarism can occur.

1. Microadenomas (<10 mm diameter)

   a. Generally these have little propensity to grow over many years.

   b. Treat medically if symptoms are bothersome or if amenorrhea is present, because this can lead to premature osteoporosis.

   c. Microadenomas respond well to dopamine agonist therapy (see below).

   d. Surgery is an option, although not as effective as once thought.

2. Macroadenomas (>10 mm diameter)

   a. Macroadenomas have already demonstrated their tendency to increase in size. Tumor size and prolactin level correlate, up to a point.

   b. These respond well to dopamine agonist therapy. Fall in prolactin level precedes tumor shrinkage. Responsiveness to medication is present in 90 per cent of cases, with half of the tumors shrinking more than 50 per cent in size. Responsiveness to medication is also present in about 90 per cent of cases with visual symptoms. This determines whether visual changes are permanent; if so, surgery is unlikely to be of much added benefit.

   c. Transsphenoidal surgery achieves good results, especially with tumors 1 to 2 cm in size and prolactin level greater than 200 ng/ml.

3. Pseudoprolactinomas: Tumor size is disproportionately big in relation to moderate levels of prolactin elevation. Less responsiveness is seen with dopamine agonist therapy than with prolactinomas.

4. Functional hyperprolactinemia: Treat if amenorrhea present because of risk of premature osteoporosis. Also treat if there is a desire for pregnancy.

Medication: Dopamine Agonists

1. *Bromocriptine* (Parlodel) has been the mainstay. Start with a low dose and titrate upward. Check prolactin level in 4 to 8 weeks.

   a. Pseudoprolactinomas have a poor response.

   b. Side effects include nausea, vomiting, abdominal cramps, vertigo, postural hypotension, headaches, drowsiness, and psychotic reactions, and are most likely initially and with increases in dose.

   c. Vaginal administration avoids the gastrointestinal side effects. Rectal administration is not absorbed.

2. *Cabergoline* (Dostinex) is the latest in the line of dopamine agonists. Side effects are less severe than those associated with bromocriptine. Cabergoline is long acting. Vaginal administration can be an effective alternative for patients who do not tolerate the oral route.

3. *Pergolide* (Permax) has fewer side effects than bromocriptine. Concerns about uterine neoplasms in rodents has deterred Food and Drug Administration approval for use in hyperprolactinemia.

4. *Quinagolide* has fewer side effects than bromocriptine and passes the blood-brain barrier more easily. About 50 per cent of adenomas resistant to bromocriptine will respond to quina-

golide. This is currently being used in Europe but is not yet approved for use in the United States.

Diet

There are no special diets recommended for patients with hyperprolactinemia.

Activity

There are no particular activities recommended or restricted in patients with hyperprolactinemia.

Patient Education

1. From a patient's perspective, the possibility or diagnosis of a "pituitary tumor" or "brain tumor" can produce many feelings of fear and anxiety. Careful explanations of the disease is essential, along with taking time to explore and address the concerns of the patient.

2. Symptoms to watch for and treatment options need to be clearly discussed.

Follow-Up

1. Follow prolactin levels and CT/MRI scans annually for 2 years. If stable and no new symptoms appear, then just prolactin levels can be followed.

2. Tapers in medication can be attempted slowly with close follow-up of prolactin levels and symptoms.

Key Treatment

- Periodic re-evaluation of prolactin level

- Periodic repeat of CT/MRI scan to reassess size of tumor

- Dopamine agonist medical therapy

- Surgery and radiation as second-line interventions

Bibliography

Conner P, Fried G: Hyperprolactinemia: etiology, diagnosis and treatment alternatives. Acta Obstet Gynecol Scand 1998;77:249–262.

Jeffcoate WJ, Pound N, Sturrock NDC, et al: Long-term follow-up of patients with hyperprolactinemia. Clin Endocrinol 1996;45:299–303.

Maor Y, Berezin M: Hyperprolactinemia in postmenopausal women. Fertil Steril 1997;67:693–696.

Molitch ME: Pathologic hyperprolactinemia. Endocrinol Metab Clin North Am 1992;21:877–901.

185 Hyperparathyroidism

S. Shekar Chakravarthi

Parathyroid hormone (PTH), secreted by the four parathyroid glands located behind the upper and lower poles of the thyroid gland, is important for maintaining calcium-phosphorus homeostasis. PTH release is stimulated by a fall in serum calcium or a rise in serum phosphate. PTH increases the calcium level by reducing urinary calcium excretion, stimulating bone resorption, and increasing the gastrointestinal absorption of calcium. It is also phosphaturic. In primary hyperparathyroidism, one or more adenomatous or hyperplastic parathyroid glands secrete excess PTH.

Etiology

1. Eighty per cent of primary hyperparathyroidism is due to a hyperfunctioning parathyroid adenoma. About 15 per cent of patients have parathyroid hyperplasia; various causes, including parathyroid malignancies or multiple parathyroid adenomas, account for the remaining few per cent.

2. Primary hyperparathyroidism occurs in a familial pattern in 10 to 15 per cent of cases. These patients may harbor multiple adenomas resulting from an autosomal dominant trait with variable penetrance. Classically, the multiple endocrine neoplasia (MEN) syndromes are divided into two major types.

    a. In MEN type I, the major associated abnormalities are adenomas of the pituitary and the pancreas.

    b. In MEN type IIA, parathyroid abnormalities may occur with medullary carcinoma of the thyroid and pheochromocytomas. In MEN type IIB, the additional findings include cutaneous neuromas and marfanoid habitus.

Symptoms

Although hyperparathyroidism is detected in asymptomatic patients by routine laboratory screening, patients may occasionally present with symptoms of hypercalcemia and kidney disease, specifically nephrolithiasis.

1. Symptoms of hyperparathyroidism are often subtle and may consist of fatigue, weakness, lethargy, and difficulty concentrating.

2. Vague gastrointestinal complaints such as nausea, abdominal discomfort, and constipation can occur (see Ch. 186, Hypercalcemia).

3. Bone symptoms such as pain, tenderness, arthralgia, gout, pseudogout, osteoporosis, and pathologic fractures may be seen.

Key Symptoms

- General: weakness, fatigue
- Musculoskeletal: bone pain, arthralgia
- Neurologic: confusion, depression
- Gastrointestinal: nausea, vomiting, constipation, ulcers
- Genitourinary: renal colic, polyuria

Clinical Findings

The physical examination in most patients with hyperparathyroidism (with the exception of MEN IIB) is unremarkable.

1. Possible findings are changes in muscle strength, altered mental status, bone tenderness, loosened teeth, and soft tissue calcification.

2. Sometimes patients with prolonged hypercalcemia have corneal calcifications, which are found on slit-lamp examination.

Key Signs

- Musculoskeletal: weakness, bony tenderness, joint effusion
- Neurologic: confusion, hyperreflexia, coma
- Gastrointestinal: tenderness, obstipation
- Cardiovascular: hypertension
- Ophthalmologic: corneal bands

Laboratory Tests

After confirming hypercalcemia, measuring the immunoreactive parathyroid hormone (iPTH) in a reliable laboratory is critical. An elevated fasting iPTH in the presence of hypercalcemia confirms hyperparathyroidism. Because an elevated calcium should suppress PTH secretion, a high-normal or mildly elevated level may indicate hyperparathyroidism in hypercalcemic patients.

1. Other biochemical abnormalities associated with hyperparathyroidism include a mild hyperchloremic acidosis and a low serum phosphorus. The chloride-to-phosphate ratio generally is greater than 33:1. Enhanced bone resorption can elevate the alkaline phosphatase level.

2. Routine radiographs are rarely helpful. Subperiosteal bone resorption of the digits and at the sternoclavicular joints may be evident. Additional findings include bone cysts, renal calcifications, pathologic fractures, and a rare "brown tumor."

3. Imaging procedures to localize the parathyroid glands are usually necessary only when hyperparathyroidism recurs and a reoperation is required. Ultrasound is cost-effective and accurate but lacks sensitivity. Other noninvasive imaging methods include computerized tomography, magnetic resonance imaging, and thallium scan.

4. In rare cases where the initial exploration was negative or hyperparathyroidism persists, arteriography and selective venous catheterization with iPTH measurements are needed to identify the parathyroid glands.

Key Tests

- Serum calcium and phosphorus
- Fasting iPTH

Differential Diagnosis

The differential diagnosis consists of other causes of hypercalcemia (see Ch. 186, Hypercalcemia). Hyperparathyroidism may be primary, secondary, or tertiary.

1. Primary hyperparathyroidism is the idiopathic, abnormally regulated secretion of PTH by the parathyroid gland(s). It is two to four times more common in women and increases in incidence over age 50.

2. Secondary hyperparathyroidism results from disease in another organ system, usually the kidneys. Renal failure is associated with a high phosphate and a low calcium and stimulates parathyroid hyperplasia.

3. Tertiary hyperparathyroidism occurs in renal failure, when PTH secretion becomes independent of the serum calcium.

4. Familial hypocalciuric hypercalcemia may be confused with primary hyperparathyroidism. Although PTH levels usually are normal, a limited number of patients show mild elevations, but the urinary calcium is extremely low.

Treatment

Management of primary hyperparathyroidism can be surgical or medical. In general, the higher the serum calcium level, the more likely patients will develop symptoms requiring surgical interventions.

1. Although surgery is curative, mild and uncomplicated asymptomatic cases of primary hyperparathyroidism may be followed medically.

   a. These patients should have a serum calcium less than 11.5 mg/dl and must be compliant with regular follow-up visits. Bone density should be normal, and there must be no evidence of renal insufficiency.

   b. Medical management also may be considered when contraindications to surgery exist and in some very frail elderly patients.

   c. Patients need semiannual checkups to follow blood pressure, serum calcium concentration, and bone mass.

   d. Patients should avoid dehydration, immobilization, and thiazide diuretics.

   e. Hypertension should be treated aggressively.

   f. Some clinicians use estrogen therapy for postmenopausal women.

2. Surgery is the treatment of choice.

   a. Exploration requires identification of all parathyroid glands. Single or multiple adenomas are removed. In four-gland hyperplasia, three glands are removed, and portions of the fourth are implanted in the forearm.

   b. An experienced surgeon is highly desirable because the normal glands are very small and may be aberrant in location. The initial surgical success rate is about 90 per cent.

   c. Complications include vocal cord paralysis, hypocalcemia, and hematoma formation.

Key Treatment

Surgery

Follow-Up

1. Perioperatively, patients need observation for hypocalcemia and tetany.
2. Flare-ups of gout, pseudogout, and decreased renal function may occur. Monitoring clinical symptoms and serum calcium is essential, and some patients may require calcium and vitamin D supplementation to avoid hypocalcemia and prevent bone demineralization.
3. In familial forms of hyperparathyroidism, family members require periodic monitoring. Genetic screening is now available for MEN syndromes.

Bibliography

al Zahrani A, Levine MA: Primary hyperparathyroidism. Lancet 1997;57:1233–1237.

Allerheiligen DA, Schoeber J, Housten RE, et al: Hyperparathyroidism. Am Fam Physician 1998;83:1795–1802.

Consensus development conference statement: Diagnosis and management of asymptomatic primary hyperparathyroidism. Ann Intern Med 1991;114:593–597.

Deftos LJ, Parthemore JG, Stabile BE: Management of primary hyperparathyroidism. Ann Rev Med 1994;44:19–26.

Petti G: Hyperparathyroidism. Otolaryngol Clin North Am 1990;23:339–355.

Ott SM: Calcimimetrics—new drugs with potential to control hyperparathyroidism. J Clin Endocrinol Metab 1998;83:1080–1082.

186 Hypercalcemia

Kurt Kurowski

Etiology

1. Common causes
   a. Primary hyperparathyroidism
   b. Malignant neoplasm
2. Less common causes
   a. Medications: thiazide diuretics, lithium, estrogens, antiestrogens
   b. Granulomatous diseases: sarcoid, tuberculosis, histoplasmosis, coccidioidomycosis
   c. Renal insufficiency
   d. Immobilization in patients with rapid bone turnover (e.g., growing children, Paget's disease of bone, bone metastases)
   e. Hyperthyroidism

WARNING

Hypercalcemia should not be attributed to Paget's disease of the bone unless the patient has also been immobilized.

---

3. Rare causes
   a. Vitamin D or A toxicity
   b. Parenteral nutrition
   c. Familial hypocalciuric hypercalcemia (aka familial benign hypercalcemia)
   d. Milk-alkali syndrome
   e. Other endocrine etiologies: adrenal insufficiency, pheochromocytoma, vasoactive intestinal polypeptide–secreting pancreatic islet cell tumors

Symptoms

The symptoms of hypercalcemia tend to correlate only with the degree of hypercalcemia present, irrespective of the etiology. Because the highest degrees of hypercalcemia are seen in patients with hyperparathyroidism or malignancy, these patients are most likely to have symptoms related to the hypercalcemia.

1. Neurologic: fatigue, impaired mentation, loss of recent memory, coma if severe
2. Gastrointestinal: constipation, anorexia, nausea, vomiting
3. Polyuria, polydipsia, nocturia, dry mouth
4. Weakness

Key Symptoms

- Impaired mentation
- Constipation
- Polyuria, polydipsia

Clinical Findings

1. Altered mental status: confusion, lethargy, coma
2. Calcifications: soft tissue, including skin; nephrolithiasis, nephrocalcinosis; chrondrocalcinosis; band keratopathy in the medial and lateral limbic regions of the cornea
3. Cardiovascular: hypertension, shortened Q-T interval on electrocardiogram
4. Gastrointestinal: pancreatitis, possible increase in peptic ulcer disease

---

WARNING

Patients are usually asymptomatic and without clinical findings unless their serum calcium exceeds 11.5 to 13.5 mg/dl.

Key Signs

- Altered mental status
- Soft tissue calcifications

Laboratory Tests

1. Confirm that the patient is hypercalcemic. A serum calcium level should be obtained and interpreted with knowledge of the serum albumin level. For each 1-gm/dl drop below 4 g/dl in serum albumin, the serum calcium level should be increased by 0.8 mg/dl.
2. If confirmed, begin the search for possible causes.
   a. A parathyroid hormone level: This is always drawn with a simultaneous measurement of serum calcium.

b. Urine calcium levels should be checked particularly in patients with a family history of hypercalcemia and normal parathyroid hormone levels. A 24-hour urine collection for calcium and creatinine allows identification of hypocalciuric and renal failure patients.

3. If parathyroid hormone is normal or suppressed, hypercalcemia persists despite discontinuation of potential exacerbating medications, and no obvious malignancy is present, continue investigation with the following:

   a. Serum 1,25-dihydroxyvitamin D level

   b. Serum parathyroid hormone–related peptide level (PTHrP)

   c. Thyroid-stimulating hormone

   d. Serum protein electrophoresis

4. Consider occult malignancy if parathyroid hormone–related peptide is elevated and 1,25-dihydroxyvitamin D levels are low. Some of the following may be appropriate in search of the primary malignancy, depending on individual patient characteristics and risk factors.

   a. Chest radiograph

   b. Mammography

   c. Urinalysis

   d. Ear, nose, and throat examination

   e. Prostate-specific antigen

   f. Endoscopic evaluation of gastrointestinal tract (especially esophagus)

   g. Computerized tomography scan of abdomen and pelvis

Key Test

Parathyroid hormone level with simultaneous serum calcium

Differential Diagnosis

1. Primary hyperparathyroidism: This diagnosis can be made when both serum calcium and parathyroid hormone levels are elevated and renal function is normal.

2. Hypercalcemia of malignancy: Carcinomas of the lung, breast, head, and neck and multiple myeloma and lymphomas are the most commonly associated malignancies. Renal, prostate, gastrointestinal (especially esophagus), and ovarian malignancies also account for some cases. Lytic bone metastases secondary to any primary are also associated with hypercalcemia.

3. Medication-induced

   a. Prescription medication: thiazide diuretics, lithium, estrogens or antiestrogens

   b. Vitamin D or A toxicity

   c. Large quantities of bicarbonate and milk ingestion

4. Granulomatous disease: Sarcoidosis accounts for most of these cases.

5. Endocrine etiologies exclusive of hyperparathyroidism: Hyperthyroidism is the most common of these.

6. Familial hypocalciuric hypercalcemia patients are asymptomatic and will remain so without treatment.

Treatment

Milder (serum calcium <11.2 mg/dl) asymptomatic or minimally symptomatic hypercalcemic patients do not require pharmacotherapy, but need to be evaluated for the underlying cause and need to be well hydrated and avoid immobilization.

1. Principal medications

   a. Normal saline intravenous solution for rehydration. Normal saline at 200 ml/hour with close monitoring of intake and output and evidence of congestive heart failure. This is reserved for patients with severe hypercalcemia (>13.5 mg/dl)

      (1) Thiazide diuretics are avoided.

      (2) Loop diuretics such as furosemide, 20 mg q6–12h, are also given only if there is clinical evidence of fluid overload.

   b. Pamidronate (Aredia) (a biphosphonate), 30 to 60 mg in a liter of normal saline, is infused over 24 hours (90 mg if the patient's calcium is >13.5 mg/dl). Etidronate (Didronel) is an alternative. Takes 3 to 6 days for the calcium level to decline, but the effect may be sustained for weeks.

   c. Calcitonin (Calcimar, Miacalcin), 4–8 IU/kg IM or SC q6–12h

      (1) Begins to lower calcium after just a few hours.

      (2) Will not usually completely normalize calcium, and its effects wane even with further doses after several days.

   d. Estrogen, 0.625 mg of conjugated estrogens (Premarin) PO qd; or 0.5 mg of estradiol (Estrace) PO qd; or 0.05 mg estradiol patch (Estraderm), applied to skin two times a week.

      (1) All of these estrogen preparations should be given with daily medroxyprogesterone (Provera) 2.5 mg PO qd, or cycled

with 5 mg of medroxyprogesterone qd if the patient has an intact uterus.

(2) This therapy is most appropriate for postmenopausal women (especially if osteoporosis is present) with mild hypercalcemia secondary to hyperparathyroidism who have no contraindications to the estrogen.

2. Less commonly used medications

a. Glucocorticoids (e.g., prednisone, 20 to 40 mg PO bid) initially. Reserved for treatment of hypercalcemia secondary to steroid responsive conditions such as multiple myeloma, lymphoma, sarcoidosis.

b. Plicamycin (Mithracin), 25 μg/kg/day in 1 L of 5% dextrose in water IV over 4 hours $\times$ 3 days.

(1) Less effective and not as well tolerated as pamidronate.

(2) Use limited to acute treatment of severe hypercalcemia unresponsive to principal medications.

c. Gallium nitrate (Ganite), 200 mg/m^2 in 1 L of 5% dextrose in water q24h $\times$5 days

(1) Reserved for severe, acute hypercalcemia.

(2) Nephrotoxicity limits use.

d. Phosphorus, 500 mg of elemental phosphorus PO bid

(1) Not usually used because calcium phosphate salts can deposit in soft tissues.

(2) Only used when there is a concomitant severely low phosphorus level (<2 mg/dl). Hyperphosphatemia must be avoided.

Diet

1. Adequate oral fluids to avoid dehydration
2. Dietary calcium intake restriction of 300 to 800 mg/day *only* if patient's hypercalcemia is associated with elevated serum levels of 1,25-dihydroxyvitamin D (vitamin D intoxication and some cases of primary hyperparathyroidism and granulomatous disease). All others should have moderate calcium intake of 800 to 1000 mg/day.

Activity

Mobilization and full activity are encouraged. Inactivity can promote hypercalcemia.

Patient Education

1. Patients need to avoid situations that could restrict their access to fluids or promote dehydration.
2. Patients need to know the potential symptoms of worsening hypercalcemia (lethargy, confusion, anorexia, nausea) and that they need urgent assessment when these develop.

Key Treatment

- Hydration and mobilization
- Pharmacotherapy based on severity, symptoms, and underlying cause

Follow-Up

Intensity and frequency of follow-up is based on the degree of hypercalcemia present, how symptomatic (if at all) the patient is, and the underlying etiology. Patients with hypercalcemia secondary to malignancy and primary hyperparathyroidism may develop severe elevations and need closer monitoring.

1. Severe hypercalcemia (>13.5 mg/dl) warrants follow-up serum calciums and clinical reassessment within hours of starting therapy.

2. Patients with moderate hypercalcemia (11.2 to 13.5 mg/dl) should have follow-up serum calcium levels approximately 1 week after starting biphosphonate therapy.

3. Patients with mild hypercalcemia from an established etiology may only need serum calcium levels every 6 months, with earlier checks if they become symptomatic.

Bibliography

Allerheiligen DA, Schoever J, Houston RE, et al: Hyperparathyroidism. Am Fam Physician 1998;57:1795–1802.

Bilezikian JP: Management of hypercalcemia. J Clin Endocrinol Metab 1993;77:1445–1449.

Locker FG, Silverberg SJ, Bielzikian JP: Optimal dietary calcium intake in primary hyperparathyroidism. Am J Med 1997;102:543–550.

Mundy GR, Guise TA: Hypercalcemia of malignancy. Am J Med 1997;103:134–145.

Sharma OP: Vitamin D, calcium and sarcoidosis. Chest 1996;109:535–539.

187 Hypocalcemia

Leland Graves, III

Etiology

1. Hypoalbuminemia is the most common cause of a low total serum calcium.

   a. In the circulation, calcium is present bound to protein (45 per cent), in the free ionized form (45 per cent), and complexed to anions (10 per cent).

   b. Free calcium ion is the form of calcium important for the neuromuscular, enzymatic, and secretory functions of calcium. If free ionized calcium is normal, the patient does not have a hypocalcemic disorder. Free ionized calcium can be measured directly; however, many clinical laboratories do not have this capability.

   c. Total serum calcium can be corrected for hypoalbuminemia by adding 0.8 mg/dl to the serum calcium for every decrease of 1 gm/dl in serum albumin.

   d. The percentage of calcium bound to albumin varies in the critically ill patient, particularly in extremes of pH and osmolality. In these situations the correction formula may not accurately reflect ionized calcium.

2. Decreased parathyroid hormone (PTH) activity resulting from decreased PTH secretion or peripheral resistance to PTH activity will result in hypocalcemia. Normally, PTH acts to raise serum calcium by increasing calcium resorption from bone, increasing calcitriol production, and increasing renal calcium reabsorption.

   a. Hypoparathyroidism (inadequate PTH secretion by the parathyroid glands) may result following surgical removal, autoimmune destruction (isolated or associated with other hormone resistance syndromes), or irradiation. Severe hypomagnesemia and, less commonly, infiltrative and genetic disorders may also cause hypoparathyroidism.

   b. Resistance to PTH action peripherally occurs with chronic renal failure, magnesium deficiency, vitamin D deficiency, and pseudohypoparathyroidism.

3. Vitamin D deficiency may be a consequence of inadequate intake and sun exposure, malabsorption, anticonvulsant therapy, hepatobiliary disease, and rarely vitamin D–resistant states.

4. Calcium sequestration (soft tissue deposition, increased bone deposition, or chelation) is a common cause of hypocalcemia in the critically ill patient.

   a. Acute pancreatitis may cause saponification of calcium by free fatty acids.

   b. Hyperphosphatemic disorders such as chronic renal failure, rhabdomyolysis, and tumor lysis syndrome may cause the calcium/phosphorus product to exceed 60. This predisposes calcium-phosphorus complex deposition in soft tissues.

   c. Citrate, present as the anticoagulant in transfused blood, may chelate calcium, resulting in hypocalcemia in patients requiring multiple blood transfusions.

   d. Increased influx of calcium into bone may occur following surgical correction of hyperparathyroidism ("hungry bone syndrome"). Osteoblastic metastasis may also result in hypocalcemia.

5. Sepsis syndrome may produce hypocalcemia; the mechanism is multifactorial.

6. Medications

   a. Anticalcemic agents used to treat Paget's disease or hypercalcemia, including bisphosphonates, calcitonin, plicamycin, and phosphate, may cause hypocalcemia.

   b. Antineoplastic agents such as doxorubicin, cytosine arabinoside, and cisplatin may cause hypocalcemia directly or by causing hypomagnesemia.

Note

Correct calcium for hypoalbuminemia:
Corrected serum calcium = 0.8 (4 − serum albumin) + serum calcium

---

Symptoms

1. Neuromuscular symptoms result from neuromuscular excitability induced by hypocalcemia. Symptoms are related to the degree and the rate of drop of ionized calcium. Mild symptoms include perioral numbness and paresthesia in the extremities. Symptoms progress with muscle cramping, carpopedal spasm, tetany, and laryngospasm.

2. Central nervous system manifestations include lethargy, depression, psychosis, hyperirritability, and seizures.

Key Symptoms

- Paresthesias
- Muscle cramp, carpopedal spasm
- Tetany, laryngospasm
- Lethargy, confusion, psychosis
- Seizures
- Symptoms of heart failure, hypotension, and bradycardia

Clinical Findings

1. Signs of neuromuscular excitability resulting from hypocalcemia may be present spontaneously or may be induced with maneuvers during the physical examination.

   a. Chvostek's sign is contraction of the facial muscles produced by tapping over the facial nerve just anterior to the ear. This may be present in hypocalcemia or hypomagnesemia but is also present in 10 per cent of normal individuals.

   b. Trousseau's sign is demonstrated by inflation of the blood pressure cuff to the level of the systolic blood pressure for 3 to 5 minutes. In hypocalcemia, ensuing mild ischemia induces neuromuscular excitability, and carpal spasm occurs.

2. Cardiovascular manifestations result from impaired contractility, vasodilatation, and conduction abnormalities. Hypocalcemia may present with hypotension, congestive heart failure, prolonged Q-T interval, and arrhythmia.

3. Chronic hypocalcemic conditions may be associated with the presence of subcapsular cataracts, dry skin, brittle nails, intracranial calcification, papilledema, and parkinsonian movement disorders.

Key Signs

- Chvostek's sign
- Trousseau's sign
- Prolonged Q-T interval
- Congestive heart failure
- Hypotension
- Tetany
- Seizure

Laboratory Tests

1. Free ionized calcium should be determined. Serum albumin can be used to calculate corrected serum calcium, or ionized calcium can be measured directly.

2. Laboratory tests should assess parathyroid function, renal function, magnesium, vitamin D levels, and possible causes of sequestration.

3. Cardiovascular effects and stability should be assessed by electrocardiography (ECG), and continuous monitoring may be indicated.

Key Tests

- Albumin
- Phosphorus
- PTH
- Vitamin D
- ECG
- Creatinine
- Magnesium

Differential Diagnosis

Hypomagnesemia may cause hypocalcemia or may produce many of the same clinical manifestations as hypocalcemia.

Treatment

1. Emergency management: Patients with symptomatic hypocalcemia should receive calcium replacement to a level at which the patient is no longer symptomatic or at risk of complications of hypocalcemia. Therapy for tetany, seizures, or cardiovascular manifestations of hypocalcemia should include

   a. Intravenous calcium gluconate 10%, 10 to 20 ml (93 mg elemental calcium/10-ml vial) infused over 10 minutes

   b. In situations of persistent hypocalcemia (e.g., postparathyroidectomy), a continuous infusion may be necessary and may be given at 10 to 15 mg/kg over 8 to 10 hours. This could be expected to raise the serum calcium by 2 to 3 mg/dl.

   c. Calcium should be monitored closely, every 4 to 6 hours. The calcium infusate should be as dilute as possible. Extravasation may cause soft tissue injury and necrosis.

WARNING

Phosphorus and bicarbonate are not compatible in the same IV line with calcium. Patients taking digitalis should be monitored closely if intravenous calcium is required because calcium potentiates digitalis toxicity.

---

2. Management of chronic hypocalcemia: Disorders such as hypoparathyroidism causing chronic hypocalcemia require a combination of oral calcium and vitamin D supplementation.

   a. Oral calcium supplementation should be started using 1 to 3 gm elemental calcium daily in a tid dose. Calcium carbonate is the least expensive and most widely used. If calcium carbonate is not tolerated, other forms of calcium, such as calcium lactate or calcium citrate, are available.

   b. Vitamin D is usually required in chronic hypocalcemic disorders such as hypoparathyroidism. Vitamin D is most frequently given in the form of ergocalciferol or calcitriol.

      (1) Ergocalciferol (vitamin D_2) should be given in an initial dose of 50,000 units (1.25 mg/capsule) daily. The onset of action is 2 to 4 weeks. If toxicity (hypercalcemia) occurs, the effects of ergocalciferol may persist for 2 to 8 weeks.

      (2) Calcitriol (1,25-dihydroxyvitamin D) is the active form of vitamin D. The onset of action is 1 to 3 days. If hypercalcemia occurs, the time to reverse toxicity is 3 to 10 days. Initial dosage is 0.25 to 0.5 μg daily, with the usual dose range 0.5 to 2.0 μg/day. Dosage may be increased as indicated at 2- to 4-week intervals.

      (3) Ergocalciferol is the least expensive preparation; however, the onset of action and the shorter half-life in cases of toxicity make calcitriol the agent of choice in many cases.

Follow-Up

The goal of therapy is to alleviate symptoms of hypocalcemia and avoid the toxicity of hypercalcemia and hypercalciuria.

1. Serum calcium should be restored to the low-normal range (8 to 8.5 mg/dl). At that time urinary calcium should be determined. If hypercalciuria (>250 mg/24 hours) is present, vitamin D dosage should be decreased.

2. If hypercalcemia develops, vitamin D and calcium should be discontinued and serum calcium monitored frequently until hypercalcemia resolves. In cases of symptomatic hypercalcemia, prednisone may be beneficial.

3. While calcium and vitamin D dosages are being adjusted, serum calcium should be monitored once or twice weekly. After maintenance dose has been reached, serum calcium and 24-hour urinary calcium should be monitored every 3 months.

Bibliography

Bringhurst FR, Demay MB, Kronenberg HM: Hormones and disorders of mineral metabolism. In Wilson JD, Foster DW, Kronenberg HM, et al (eds): Williams Textbook of Endocrinology, 9th ed, pp 1155–1209. Philadelphia, WB Saunders Company, 1998.

Popovtzer MM, Knochel JP, Kumar R: Disorders of calcium, phosphorus, vitamin D, and parathyroid hormone activity. In Schrier RW (ed): Renal and Electrolyte Disorders, 5th ed. Philadelphia, Lippincott-Raven, 1997.

Rude RK: Magnesium metabolism and deficiency. Endocrinol Metab Clin North Am 1993;22:377–395.

Tohme JF, Bilezikian JP: Hypocalcemic emergencies. Endocrinol Metab Clin North Am 1993;22:363–375.

Zaloga GP: Hypocalcemia in critically ill patients. Crit Care Med 1992;20:251–262.

188 Hypoglycemia

Harris C. Taylor

Etiology

1. Hypoglycemia is either *reactive* (within the first 5 hours after eating) or *fasting* (more than 5 hours after eating). Contrary to common belief, reactive hypoglycemia is infrequent. The typical office presentation of a young (often female) patient with postprandial "spells" and the self-diagnosis of hypoglycemia is infrequently confirmed by serum glucose measurement while symptomatic. These patients usually have pseudohypoglycemia, the cause of which is unclear. True postprandial hypoglycemia may be caused by
   a. Gastrointestinal surgery such as vagotomy and pyloroplasty, gastrectomy, or gastrojejunostomy
   b. Early diabetes mellitus (unusual)
   c. True idiopathic "functional" hypoglycemia (unusual)

2. Among true hypoglycemic patients, the large majority have the fasting type. However, even patients with insulinoma, a classic example of fasting hypoglycemia, may have symptoms postprandially. The following are the causes of fasting hypoglycemia in approximate declining order of frequency in emergency room and hospitalized patients. Keep in mind that underlying malnutrition or even missed meals, together with chronic liver and/or renal disease, accentuate the hypoglycemia.
   a. Drugs
      (1) Insulin and sulfonylureas (therapeutic or factitious use)
      (2) Alcohol, with or without another drug (impairs gluconeogenesis)
      (3) Propranolol (more often in patients on hemodialysis)
      (4) Salicylates (mostly in children)
      (5) Quinine (intravenously for cerebral malaria)
      (6) Pentamidine (usually in undernourished acquired immunodeficiency syndrome patients)
      (7) Disopyramide (Norpace) (usually in elderly nondiabetics with liver or renal disease)
   b. Renal insufficiency
   c. Substrate deficiency
      (1) Severe malnutrition (in the United States in nursing home patients)
      (2) In pregnancy, where it is usually asymptomatic
   d. Liver disease with hepatic failure or severe heart failure; cirrhosis, especially when accompanied by sepsis
   e. Septicemia
   f. Insulinoma
      (1) May be benign or malignant
      (2) Nesidioblastosis (diffuse growth of insulin-producing cells from pancreatic ductules), usually in children
   g. Hormone deficiency
      (1) Adrenal insufficiency, primary and secondary (more common in children).
      (2) Growth hormone deficiency
      (3) Thyroxine, catecholamine, and glucagon deficiency (unusual)
   h. Mesenchymal tumor, generally very large and located in the abdomen, pelvis, or thorax; also may be seen with adrenal, renal, and gastrointestinal carcinomas and hepatoma; detectable by physical examination, plain radiograph, or computerized tomographic scan. Insulin-like growth factor 2 may cause the hypoglycemia.
   i. Glycogen storage disease (rare and begins in childhood)
   j. Systemic carnitine deficiency (rare)
   k. Artifactual hypoglycemia may be seen in leukemia if red stopper tubes are used. Employ gray stopper tubes instead.
   l. Autoimmune insulin syndrome and anti-insulin receptor antibody

Symptoms

Plasma glucose values of less than 50 mg/dl usually, but not always, produce symptoms. Fasted young healthy women may have plasma glucose levels well under 50 mg/dl without symptoms. Conversely, poorly controlled diabetics may experience symptoms of hypoglycemia with serum glucose levels of 70 mg/dl and above. Symptoms are subdivided into adrenergic and neuroglycopenic.

1. Frequent adrenergic symptoms are anxiety, tremulousness, hunger, sweating, irritability, and palpitations.
2. Frequent neuroglycopenic symptoms are headache and visual, cognitive, and behavioral (aggressive and abusive) changes. Patients may, however, manifest more severe symptoms, including hemiparesis, aphasia, coma, and convulsions.

Key Symptoms

Adrenergic	Neuroglycopenic
• Anxiety, hunger	• Headache; behavioral, cognitive, and/or visual changes; fatigue
• Sweating, palpitations	
	• Seizures, coma

Clinical Findings

1. Adrenergic signs: tachycardia, diaphoresis, hypo- and hyperthermia
2. Neuroglycopenic signs: seizures (more often in children), coma, aphasia, hemiparesis, and extensor plantar reflexes

Key Signs

Adrenergic	Neuroglycopenic
• Tachycardia ± premature ventricular contractions	• Convulsions, aphasia
	• Coma, Babinski's sign
• Diaphoresis, hypothermia, or hyperthermia	

Laboratory Tests

1. Hypoglycemia may be arbitrarily defined as a laboratory (not a portable monitor) plasma or serum glucose of less than 50 mg/dl.
2. In a known diabetic who experiences hypoglycemia, clinical circumstances may suggest determining serum alcohol and cortisol level, liver function tests, blood urea nitrogen (BUN), and creatinine.
3. In a nondiabetic, when hypoglycemic, obtain preceding plus
   a. Total insulin with insulin antibodies and C-peptide. If insulin antibodies are present, obtain free insulin.

b. If total (free) insulin and C-peptide are inappropriately increased for the hypoglycemia (greater than 6 μU/ml insulin), obtain a sulfonylurea level. Remember, the usual commercial assay for sulfonylureas is not very reliable for second-generation drugs.
   c. If total insulin is increased, no insulin antibodies are present, and C-peptide is normal or low, obtain anti–insulin receptor antibodies.
4. If drugs, alcohol, liver or renal disease, malnutrition, sepsis, and previous gastrointestinal surgery are not identified as causes of hypoglycemia on first evaluation, endogenous hyperinsulinemia is more likely. If the initial hypoglycemic serum does not demonstrate inappropriately increased levels of insulin and C-peptide, perform a 72-hour fast. Occurrence of hypoglycemia with increased insulin and C-peptide levels in the absence of insulin antibodies and sulfonylureas makes the diagnosis of insulin-producing tumor. If anti-insulin antibodies are present, the autoimmune insulin syndrome or surreptitious injection of insulin must be ruled out.

Key Tests

(Initial hypoglycemic serum [preferred] or later 72-hour fast)

• Glucose, BUN, creatinine	• Insulin, C-peptide, and insulin antibodies
• Alcohol and cortisol level	• Sulfonylurea level if insulin increased
• Liver function tests	

WARNING

Five-hour glucose tolerance should not be used to diagnose hypoglycemia. Unless insulinoma is diagnosed biochemically or there is a high suspicion of a large mesenchymal tumor, computerized tomographic scanning of the pancreas and/or abdomen is not routinely indicated. Neither patient nor physician should use a portable glucose monitor to diagnose hypoglycemia in a nondiabetic individual.

Differential Diagnosis

1. Office patients (without past gastrointestinal surgery) presenting with the self-diagnosis of

hypoglycemia occurring several hours after meals usually are found to have pseudohypoglycemia. Other disorders to be considered in this setting where complaints are similar to the adrenergic symptoms of hypoglycemia are

   a. Generalized anxiety disorder

   b. Panic attacks

   c. Hyperventilation

   d. Pheochromocytoma

2. Neuroglycopenic symptoms of hypoglycemia usually, although not always, are encountered in inpatients or in the emergency room. Consider

   a. Seizure disorder

   b. Psychosis

   c. Drug or alcohol intoxication

   d. Transient ischemic attack or cerebrovascular accident

   e. Multiple causes of coma

Treatment

Therapy of hypoglycemia is divided into the acute phase (where treatment is the same independent of cause) and chronic phase (where therapy does depend on the underlying cause).

1. Acute therapy: 6 to 12 ounces of juice or non-diet soda if the patient is responsive. If unresponsive, give 50 ml of 50% glucose intravenously, followed by continuous drip of 10% to 20% dextrose in water until the patient is able to eat. Remember, any cause of hypoglycemia may produce prolonged and/or recurrent depression of the serum glucose level, and continued intravenous therapy and/or repeat boluses of 50% glucose may be required.

2. After treatment of the acute episode and availability of diagnostic tests, the underlying disorder can be treated.

   a. Patients with pseudohypoglycemia often do well on a six-feeding high-protein, low-carbohydrate diet.

   b. Alcohol must be discontinued if implicated.

   c. Sulfonylurea doses should be decreased and/or discontinued, and/or metformin (Glucophage), rosiglitazone (Avandia), or shorter-acting glipizide (Glucotrol) substituted for longer-acting glyburide (Micronase) and chlorpropamide (Diabinese).

   d. Decrease and adjust insulin doses; adjust diet; accept poorer control in diabetics with neuroglycopenia.

   e. If other drugs are at fault, consider substitutes.

   f. Patients with renal failure not on dialysis require increased amounts of carbohydrate in their diet and/or more frequent feedings; those on dialysis may benefit from a decrease in the dialysis glucose concentration.

   g. Patients with severe hepatic failure require continuous intravenous glucose administration until recovery has begun.

   h. Malnutrition requires implementation of adequate nourishment; nasogastric tube feeding or percutaneous enteral gastrostomy tube may be necessary.

   i. Cortisol replacement for adrenal insufficiency

   j. Insulinomas and mesenchymal tumors require endocrine consultation and expert surgical resection. Nonoperable insulinomas can be managed with diazoxide and thiazide.

Key Treatment

Drug of Choice

- Glucose

Alternative Drug

- Fructose

Other Treatment

- Discontinue or change doses of offending drugs

- Diet for pseudohypoglycemia, malnutrition, or renal failure

- Surgery for insulinoma or large mesenchymal tumor

Follow-Up

Observe for recurrence of original symptoms. If present, obtain serum glucose.

Bibliography

Comi RJ: Approach to acute hypoglycemia. Endocrinol Metab Clin North Am 1993;22:247–262.

Field JB (ed): Hypoglycemia. Endocrinol Metab Clin North Am 1989;18:1–252.

Marks V, Teale JD: Hypoglycemia in the adult. Baillieres Clin Endocrinol Metab 1993;7:705–730.

Palardy J, Havrankova J, Leparge R, et al: Blood glucose measurements during symptomatic episodes in patients with suspected postprandial hypoglycemia. N Engl J Med 1989;321:1421–1425.

Service FJ: Hypoglycemia. Endocrinol Metab Clin North Am 1997;26:937–955.

189 Hyperkalemia

John P. Speck

1. Hyperkalemia is often encountered in patients with disturbed renal function, among those taking medications that alter potassium homeostasis, and in those subjected to a massive influx of potassium. Hyperkalemia is often multifactorial, and its incidence increases with aging.

2. The kidneys play a pivotal role in potassium homeostasis. However, it takes hours for the kidneys to change urinary potassium excretion. The body's acute defense against rises in the serum potassium consists of insulin and probably catecholamine release. In response to acute rises in the plasma potassium, insulin is released, which then drives potassium as well as glucose into cells. Diabetics are at increased risk of developing hyperkalemia as a result of their impaired insulin release. Another probable defense mechanism against hyperkalemia involves the acute release of catecholamines. The overall effect of released norepinephrine and epinephrine is to relocate plasma potassium intracellularly.

3. In a slower but powerful way, the kidneys protect against hyperkalemia. Potassium is freely filtered by the glomerulus into the tubular fluid. In a complex manner, it is then completely reabsorbed, with the potassium appearing in the urine, having been actively secreted by the collecting tubule under the influence of aldosterone. The kidneys have a remarkable ability to vary potassium excretion into the urine from less than 5 to 100 mEq/L. Factors that favor potassium excretion include increased plasma aldosterone, increased tubular sodium flow, diuretics, and bicarbonate appearing in the urine.

Etiology

Table 189–1 summarizes the causes of hyperkalemia.

1. Pseudohyperkalemia: This is a fairly frequent occurrence and results from
   a. Excessively long tourniquet application before phlebotomy, causing potassium egress from muscle cells distal to the tourniquet
   b. Hemolysis, during or after phlebotomy: For hemolysis to raise serum potassium more than 0.5 mEq/L above the baseline, gross hemolysis should be evident to the naked eye.
   c. Thrombocytosis and/or leukocytosis: If the platelet count is more than 1 million or the white cell count is over 100,000, the normal process of clot formation and retraction causes lysis of some of the platelets or white blood cells with attendant release of their rich intracellular potassium into the serum. If this condition is suspected, one should obtain a plasma potassium determination: the blood is drawn into an anticoagulated tube and spun down. Normal serum potassium is only 0.1 to 0.2 mEq/L more than plasma potassium. If the plasma potassium is normal in the face of an elevated serum potassium, the diagnosis is made and no treatment is needed.

2. Massive influx of potassium into the plasma
   a. There can be release of the high intracellular potassium into the plasma from tissue destruction, such as hemolysis or rhabdomyolysis, or from resorption of a hematoma.
   b. Exuberant oral intake of high-potassium foods (such as citrus fruits and potassium salt substitutes), and intravenous potassium supplements can cause hyperkalemia, espe-

TABLE 189–1. CAUSES OF HYPERKALEMIA

Pseudohyperkalemia

Massive Potassium Influx Into the Plasma
Oral or intravenous potassium salts
Dietary indiscretions
Salt substitutes
Hemolysis
Rhabdomyolysis

Redistribution From Within Cells Into Plasma
Medications (digoxin toxicity, succinylcholine, β-blockers, α-agonists, arginine, and lysine)
Hyperosmolar states
Hyperkalemic periodic paralysis
Normal anion gap metabolic acidosis

Inadequate Renal Potassium Excretion
Adrenal disorders (hyporenin hypoaldosteronism, Addison's disease)
Tubular secretory defects (systemic lupus erythematosus, obstructive uropathy, sickle cell disease, renal transplant)
Renal failure
Medications (potassium-sparing diuretics, nonsteroidal anti-inflammatory drugs, angiotensin-converting enzyme inhibitors, cyclosporin A)
Diminished effective circulating plasma volume

cially if other causes of hyperkalemia are present.

3. Redistribution of potassium from within cells into the plasma

   a. Multiple medications can cause at least mild hyperkalemia by inhibiting potassium movement into cells. These include digoxin (at toxic levels), succinylcholine, β-blockers, α-agonists, arginine, and lysine (often used in hyperalimentation).

   b. Hyperosmolar states, as from hyperglycemia, can cause hyperkalemia, probably as a result of intracellular flux of water into the plasma, which drags potassium with it.

   c. Normal anion gap (but not large anion gap) metabolic acidosis causes intracellular potassium to translocate into the plasma. A drop in pH of 0.1 here raises the serum potassium up to 0.6 mEq/L. Large anion gap metabolic acidosis from organic acidoses such as lactic acidosis or ketoacidosis and respiratory acidosis has little effect on the plasma potassium.

   d. A rare disorder, periodic paralysis, can cause hyper- and/or hypokalemia.

4. Inadequate renal potassium excretion

   a. Adrenal disorders such as Addison's disease and hyporenin hypoaldosteronism (renal tubular acidosis) can cause hyperkalemia via diminished aldosterone-mediated tubular potassium secretion.

   b. Hyporenin hypoaldosteronism is a fairly common cause of hyperkalemia. It occurs in middle-aged to elderly patients who have mild to moderate renal insufficiency that is not of itself severe enough to cause hyperkalemia. Half are diabetic. Glucocorticoid function is normal, and most patients have low-normal or low plasma renin and aldosterone levels. If efforts are made to stimulate plasma renin and aldosterone release (as by salt deprivation or furosemide administration), the plasma renin and aldosterone levels are definitely low. Some of these patients have normal renin studies but low aldosterone levels.

   c. When renal failure has progressed to a creatinine clearance of less than 5 ml/minute, renal potassium excretion is inadequate and hyperkalemia often occurs.

   d. Medications such as potassium-sparing diuretics (spironolactone, triamterene, amiloride) may cause hyperkalemia. Nonsteroidal anti-inflammatory drugs (NSAIDs), heparin, and angiotensin-converting enzyme inhibitors each may cause at least some degree of hyperkalemia by blocking aldosterone release.

   e. Diminished effective plasma volume, which causes diminished sodium delivery to the distal tubule, can cause mild hyperkalemia.

Diagnosis

1. A finding of hyperkalemia should be confirmed with at least one other measurement of serum potassium, with particular attention to nontraumatic phlebotomy and proper blood handling.

2. Hyperkalemia is often multifactorial, with several mild disorders combining to cause severe hyperkalemia. An example would be the patient with mild chronic renal failure who is taking an NSAID and a potassium salt substitute. The diagnosis of pseudohyperkalemia is outlined above. Adrenal insufficiency can be diagnosed by doing a cosyntropin stimulation test. Hyporenin hypoaldosteronism should be suspected by the finding of otherwise unexplained hyperkalemia in a middle-aged patient with mild renal failure. Baseline and stimulated plasma renin and aldosterone levels are confirmatory tests.

3. In chronic hyperkalemia, the transtubular potassium gradient (TTKG) may be useful. It is defined as $(U_K/S_K) \times (S_{osm}/U_{osm})$, where U_K and U_{osm} are the urine potassium and osmolar concentration done on a spot sample and S_K and S_{osm} are the serum potassium and osmolar concentration. It helps differentiate hyperkalemia caused by potassium influx from that caused by diminished renal potassium excretion. A TTKG greater than 6 implies potassium influx (from excess intake or cell death). Conversely, a TTKG less than 6 implies impaired renal potassium excretion (e.g., from hyporenin hypoaldosteronism). To use the TTKG, the serum potassium needs to be greater than 6 and the urine osmolality greater than the serum osmolality.

Symptoms and Clinical Findings

The signs and symptoms of hyperkalemia are muscle weakness and perioral paresthesias. These findings are inconsistently present and are not to be relied upon.

Key Signs and Symptoms

- Muscle weakness (inconsistently present)
- Perioral paresthesias (inconsistently present)

Tests

The life-threatening danger of hyperkalemia arises from its depolarizing effect on the myocardium. With progressive rises in the plasma potassium, there is peaking of the T waves on the electrocardiogram (ECG), especially in the precordial leads (inverted T waves become shorter), prolongation of the PR interval, and loss of the P wave. The Q-T interval does not become prolonged. As hyperkalemia worsens, the QRS complex widens and then degenerates into a sine wave and the patient arrests (Fig. 189–1). Prior to cardiac arrest, these ECG changes can be reversed within minutes or seconds by prompt efforts to stabilize the myocardium and lower the plasma potassium.

Key Test

Electrocardiogram (ECG)

Treatment

1. If the serum potassium is less than 6.5 mEq/L and either no ECG changes are present or there is at most T wave peaking, treatment can usually consist of prompt efforts to identify and correct the cause of hyperkalemia. For example, if the patient is taking potassium salts or NSAIDs, these medications should be stopped and the serum potassium rechecked.

2. If the patient has hyperkalemia from advanced renal failure, tubular defects, or hyporenin hypoaldosteronism, loop diuretics may augment potassium excretion. Additionally, in hyporenin hypoaldosteronism, fludrocortisone (Florinef) may be used, starting at a dose of 0.1 mg daily. Loop diuretics may cause dehydration and Flor-

inef can worsen hypertension and edema. A sodium-potassium exchange resin, sodium polystyrene sulfonate (Kayexalate), mixed with 1 ml 70% sorbitol per gram Kayexalate, may also be used. A starting dose of 15 gm Kayexalate orally on alternate days is reasonable.

WARNING

If serum potassium is 8 mEq/L or greater *or* if ECG changes beyond peaked T waves are present, emergency therapy is needed.

---

3. Emergency therapy

   a. An intravenous line must be placed immediately with continuous ECG monitoring; 10 to 30 ml of a 10% solution of calcium gluconate should be given immediately by IV push. This does not change the plasma potassium level but transiently stabilizes myocardial cells. Calcium begins to work within minutes but lasts for only a half hour.

   b. As soon as calcium has been given, the IV line should be cleared and IV glucose and insulin and/or sodium bicarbonate should be given: 200 to 500 ml of 10% dextrose with 1 ampul of sodium bicarbonate should be infused over 30 minutes with regular insulin, 10 units intravenously or subcutaneously, given concurrently. This combination may be repeated several times. The glucose/insulin and bicarbonate both cause potassium to move from the plasma into cells. (Sodium bicarbonate is ineffective in treating hyperkalemia in end-stage renal disease.) Plasma potassium begins to drop in 30 minutes. The effect lasts several hours.

   c. More long-lasting lowering can be achieved with Kayexalate, 25 to 50 gm given with sorbitol (see above), administered as an oral solution or as a 1-hour retention enema. It takes hours to begin to work, and peak effect is seen at 4 hours.

   d. Hemodialysis lowers plasma potassium efficiently; peritoneal dialysis removes potassium slowly.

   e. β_2-Adrenergic agonists inconsistently lower plasma potassium and are not recommended.

4. When there is suspicion of continuing influx of potassium into the plasma (from ongoing tissue necrosis), treatment of hyperkalemia must be extremely aggressive.

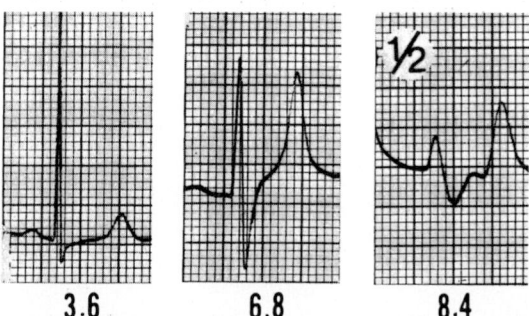

3.6 6.8 8.4

Figure 189–1 ECG changes with hyperkalemia. When serum potassium (K⁺) is 6.8, there is prolongation of the PR and QRS intervals. When K⁺ is 8.4, the P wave is difficult to identify and QRS is further widened. (From Braunwald E [ed]: Heart Disease: A Textbook of Cardiovascular Medicine, 3rd ed, p 236. Philadelphia, WB Saunders Company, 1984, with permission.)

Bibliography

DeFronzo RA: Hyperkalemia and hyporeninemic hypoaldosteronism. Kidney Int 1980;17:118.

Grem AS: Disorders of potassium homeostasis. Pediatr Clin North Am 1990;37:419.

Kamel K, Ethier JH, Richardson RA: Urine electrolytes and osmolality: when and how to use them. Am J Nephrol 1990;10:89.

Kupin WL, Marins RG: The hyperkalemia of renal failure: pathophysiology, diagnosis, and therapy. Contrib Nephrol 1993;102:1.

Michael MF: Hyperkalemia in the elderly. Am J Kidney Dis 1990;16:296.

190 Hypokalemia

Kevin C. Oeffinger

Etiology

1. Definition
   a. Serum potassium less than 3.5 mEq/L
      (1) Mild hypokalemia: 3.0 to 3.4 mEq/L
      (2) Moderate: 2.5 to 2.9 mEq/L
      (3) Severe: 2.4 mEq/L or less
   b. Total body potassium: 50 to 55 mEq/kg body weight
   c. Extracellular fluid: 3.5 to 5.0 mEq/L
   d. Intracellular fluid: 140 to 150 mEq/L
2. Potassium homeostasis
   a. Normal dietary intake averages between 50 and 100 mEq/day.
   b. Ninety per cent of the potassium is absorbed.
   c. Excreted predominantly in the urine (60 to 90 per cent) and the feces (8 to 10 per cent); negligible loss in sweat unless quite profuse
3. Prevalence of hypokalemia
   a. Can be found in about 2 per cent of the normal healthy adult population.
   b. About 20 per cent of hospitalized patients are hypokalemic.
4. Causes
   a. Dietary
      (1) Inadequate intake of potassium is very unusual, even in alcoholics.
      (2) When dietary intake is inadequate, there are generally multiple other factors that affect the potassium homeostasis, compounding the hypokalemia.
      (3) Clay ingestion decreases the absorption of potassium and can lead to hypokalemia.
   b. Renal
      (1) Loss of potassium by way of renal excretion is the most common cause of hypokalemia.
      (2) Potassium is normally excreted in the distal tubule and the collecting duct, mediated by the Na^+/K^+-ATPase pump.
      (3) When an increased sodium load is delivered to the distal nephron, such as in the use of diuretics, sodium reabsorption occurs with an increased loss of potassium.

   (4) Aldosterone stimulates potassium excretion. Release of aldosterone is stimulated by decreased glomerular blood flow (volume contraction, congestive heart failure, nephrotic syndrome, or cirrhosis). Aldosterone levels may also increase as a result of secretion from an adrenal adenoma/hyperplasia or secondarily from renovascular hypertension or a renin-secreting tumor.
   (5) Absorption rates of chloride and sodium can affect potassium excretion. When magnesium depletion occurs, the reabsorption of chloride is slowed, resulting in an increased loss of potassium. Increased rate of sodium reabsorption, which occurs with Liddle's syndrome or mineralocorticoid excess, increases the rate of potassium excretion.
   c. Gastrointestinal
      (1) Can result from diarrhea, laxative or cathartic use, enemas, or villous adenomas.
      (2) Vomiting results in little loss of potassium through emesis, but rather causes hypokalemia by the increased secretion of aldosterone secondary to volume depletion.
   d. Cellular shifts: Shift of potassium into the intracellular fluid may occur with secretion of aldosterone or administration of insulin or β_2-agonists or presence of alkalosis.
5. Pseudohypokalemia: May rarely occur when the blood sample contains a large number of white blood cells (generally over 50,000/mm^3) and sits at room temperature for a prolonged period of time.

Symptoms

1. Most patients with hypokalemia are asymptomatic.
2. Progressive loss of potassium can result in muscle cramps, myalgias, and weakness; generally affects the lower extremity and proximal muscles. As the involvement of muscle groups increases, rhabdomyolysis may occur.
3. May experience an ileus secondary to diminished activity in the intestinal smooth muscle;

manifested by abdominal distention, nausea, and vomiting.

4. Most profound effect can be on the cardiac muscle and conducting system, manifested by increased palpitations or symptoms of an arrhythmia.

5. Familial hypokalemic periodic paralysis, a rare disorder where the Na^+/K^+-ATPase activity is markedly increased secondary to different stimuli, can result in quadriplegia and progress to respiratory failure.

6. Chronic hypokalemia: nocturia, polydipsia, and polyuria

Key Symptoms

Skeletal Muscle (Proximal/Lower Extremities)

- Muscle cramps
- Myalgias
- Weakness
- Fasciculations
- Rarely: paralysis, respiratory failure, rhabdomyolysis

Smooth Muscle (Gastrointestinal)

- Nausea/vomiting
- Constipation
- Obstipation

Cardiac Muscle/Conduction System

- Palpitations
- Symptoms of arrhythmias

Clinical Findings

1. Referable to the symptoms noted above: demonstrable weakness, diminished bowel sounds, and audible ectopy

2. Electrocardiogram (ECG) may show ST segment depression/flattening, T-wave inversion, development of a U wave.

3. Severity of hypokalemia does not correlate well with changes seen on the ECG.

4. Monitoring of the heart may show increased ectopy and arrhythmias.

5. Cardiac manifestations, especially ventricular arrhythmias, are more likely in the face of a myocardial infarction or digitalis therapy/toxicity.

Key Signs

Skeletal Muscle Signs

- Increased creatine phosphokinase in severe hypokalemia

Gastrointestinal Signs

- Diminished bowels sounds
- Radiographic evidence of an ileus

Cardiac Signs

- ECG changes
  - ST depression
  - ST flattening
  - T wave inversion
  - U wave
- Arrhythmias

Laboratory Tests

1. History and physical will generally provide answer for hypokalemia.

2. If the etiology of hypokalemia is not obvious from the history and physical examination, check sodium, chloride, bicarbonate, glucose, magnesium, blood urea nitrogen, and urine potassium.

3. If surreptitious diuretic use is suspected, the urine chloride and urine potassium will be elevated.

4. If laxative or cathartic abuse is suspected, the stool potassium will be increased and melanosis coli will often be seen on flexible sigmoidoscopy.

Differential Diagnosis

1. Increased urinary potassium (>20 to 25 mEq/L)
   a. Normotensive
      (1) Acidosis: diabetic ketoacidosis, renal tubular acidosis (RTA) type I or II, ileostomy, ureterosigmoidostomy
      (2) Alkalosis: diuretics, Bartter's syndrome, magnesium depletion (alcoholism, cisplatin)
   b. Elevated blood pressure
      (1) Decreased renin: primary hyperaldosteronism, Cushing's syndrome, Liddle's syndrome, licorice, congenital adrenal hyperplasia
      (2) Increased renin: malignant hypertension, renovascular disease, renin-producing tumor

2. Decreased urinary potassium (<20 mEq/L)
   a. Gastrointestinal loss: diarrhea, laxatives, enemas, cathartics, villous adenoma

b. Cellular shifts: alkalosis, insulin, β_2-agonists, familial periodic paralysis

3. Miscellaneous
   a. Clay ingestion
   b. Secondary hyperaldosteronism: congestive heart failure, cirrhosis, nephrotic syndrome

Treatment

Treat the underlying cause.

1. Severe hypokalemia (<2.4 mEq/L)
   a. Generally represents a potassium deficit of about 600 mEq.
   b. Replacement route and rate are dictated by concurrent medical problems. In a patient with an acute myocardial infarction or digitalis toxicity, where the threshold for arrhythmia is lowered, potassium should be replaced intravenously.
   c. Be careful not to overcorrect; monitor serum potassium every 1 to 2 hours.
   d. Use potassium chloride at a rate of 30 mEq/hour.
   e. In an emergency, the rate can be increased to 40 mEq/hour if given through a central venous catheter.
   f. Administer intravenously in small volumes, such as 50 to 100 ml of 5% dextrose in water (D_5W), over short intervals, such as 1 to 2 hours.
   g. Rates above 30 mEq/hour tend to be irritating to the peripheral vein.
   h. Use cardiac monitor during replacement for severe hypokalemia, or if there is any evidence of cardiac irritability.
   i. Estimate total deficit, administer slowly after the serum potassium level is greater than 3.0 mEq/L.
   j. Slower rate of replacement (10 to 15 mEq/hour) should be used in patients with heart block, acidosis, type IV RTA, or recent use of nonsteroidal anti-inflammatory drugs (NSAIDs) or β_2-blockers.

2. Moderate hypokalemia (2.4 to 2.9 mEq/L)
   a. Replace in a slower fashion unless there is a concurrent arrhythmia.
   b. Intravenous or oral route
   c. If intravenous route is chosen, rates of 10 to 20 mEq/hour are adequate.
   d. If the patient does not have evidence of cardiac arrhythmia or irritability, cardiac monitoring is not necessary for rates of 20 mEq/hour or less.
   e. Monitor serum potassium as needed to avoid overcorrection.

f. If the potassium does not respond to replacement therapy, check a magnesium level. In patients with magnesium depletion, hypokalemia will be difficult to correct until the magnesium level is corrected.

3. Mild hypokalemia (3.0 to 3.4 mEq/L)
   a. Replace with oral potassium.
   b. Oral potassium can cause irritation of the gastric mucosa.
   c. Use potassium citrate for replacement in patients with hypokalemia secondary to RTA or ureterosigmoidostomy.

 Key Treatment

Severe (<2.4 mEq/L)
- IV K^+ 30 to 40 mEq/hour
- D_5W, 60 mEq/100 ml over 2 hours
- Cardiac monitor
- Check K^+ every 1 to 2 hours
- Slower rate for patients with heart block, acidosis, type IV RTA, or concurrent use of NSAIDs or β_2-agonists

Moderate (2.5 to 2.0 mEq/L)
- Oral or IV K^+ 10 to 15 mEq/hour
- Check K^+ every 12 to 24 hours
- Correct the underlying cause

Mild (3.0 to 3.4 mEq/L)
- Oral K^+
- Potassium citrate for hypokalemia secondary to RTA or ureterosigmoidostomy
- Correct the underlying cause

Follow-Up

Recheck potassium until normalized and cause is corrected. In patients with an untreatable cause, chronic replacement with periodic monitoring of the potassium level is necessary.

 Bibliography

Freedman BI, Burkart JM: Hypokalemia. Crit Care Clin 1991;7:143–153.

Kamel KS, Quaggin S, Scheich A, et al: Disorders of potassium homeostasis: an approach based on pathophysiology. Am J Kidney Dis 1994;24:597–613.

Mandal AK: Hypokalemia and hyperkalemia. Med Clin North Am 1997;81:611–639.

Rodriguez-Soriano J: Potassium homeostasis and its disturbances in children. Pediatr Nephrol 1995;9:364–374.

Zull DN: Disorders of potassium metabolism. Endocr Metab Emerg 1989;7:771–794.

191 Hypernatremia

Michael N. Doupé

Etiology

1. The primary cause of hypernatremia (serum sodium >145 mEq/L) is *impaired water intake*, usually secondary to
   a. Defect in thirst sensation and/or
   b. Restricted access to water
2. Usually occurs in setting of increased water losses.
   a. Pure water loss: fever, hyperventilation, diabetes insipidus
   b. Hypotonic fluid loss: burns, diarrhea, diuretic therapy, osmotic diuresis
3. Geriatric patients are at increased risk because
   a. Thirst sensation declines with age.
   b. Renal concentration ability lost with aging.
4. Hospitalized patients also at increased risk secondary to
   a. Altered sensorium, sedation, intubation, and/or nothing-by-mouth status
   b. Iatrogenic administration of inappropriate intravenous or enteral fluids (usually not enough free water)

Categories

Disease states of hypernatremia may be divided into three categories.

1. Extrarenal water loss
   a. Insensible losses
      (1) Skin: sweat with fever, heat exposure, exercise, and burns
      (2) Respiratory: tachypnea, mechanical ventilation
   b. Gastrointestinal losses
      (1) Diarrhea (e.g., infectious, inflammatory bowel disease, malabsorption)
      (2) Vomiting, nasogastric suctioning, biliary and pancreatic drainage
2. Renal water loss
   a. Osmotic diuresis
      (1) Glucose (e.g., nonketotic hyperosmolar hyperglycemia, diabetic ketoacidosis)
      (2) Urea (e.g., enteral tube feedings)
      (3) Mannitol (e.g., cerebral edema)
   b. Central (hypothalamic) diabetes insipidus (inadequate antidiuretic hormone [ADH])
      (1) Head trauma
      (2) Postneurosurgical: hypophysectomy
      (3) Brain neoplasm: primary or metastatic
      (4) Granulomatous diseases (e.g., sarcoidosis)
      (5) Meningitis/encephalitis
      (6) Cerebrovascular (e.g., aneurysm, stroke, Sheehan's syndrome)
      (7) Idiopathic
   c. Acquired nephrogenic diabetes insipidus (inadequate response to ADH)
      (1) Electrolyte disorder: hypercalcemia, severe hypokalemia
      (2) Drugs: lithium, demeclocycline
      (3) Recovery phase of acute renal failure
      (4) Tubulointerstitial kidney diseases (e.g., multiple myeloma, polycystic kidney disease, sickle cell nephropathy)
      (5) Postobstructive uropathy
3. Iatrogenic
   a. Administration of hypertonic sodium (e.g., $NaHCO_3$ in cardiac arrests, 3% hypertonic saline)
   b. Improper diluting of concentrated infant formula

Symptoms

The signs and symptoms of hypernatremia are nonspecific and relate to cellular dehydration, especially in the brain. As the brain "shrinks," traction on dural veins and venous sinuses can lead to intracranial hemorrhage, particularly in children.

Key Symptoms

- Irritability, lethargy
- Confusion, coma

Clinical Findings

1. Patients with hypotonic fluid losses (e.g., diarrhea) present with signs of hypovolemia. In contrast, patients with pure water losses (e.g., diabetes insipidus) lose water from both

intracellular and extracellular compartments, and may not produce signs of volume depletion unless losses are extreme.

2. Infants and toddlers present with tachycardia, decreased skin turgor, sunken eyes and anterior fontanelle, dry mucous membranes, lack of tears, hypotonia, and diminished social interaction.

3. Adults present with depressed or altered sensorium and, often, signs of hypovolemia (e.g., "relative" hypotension, orthostatic hypotension, tachycardia, and dry mucous membranes). Seizures may occur in all age groups.

Key Signs

- Depressed sensorium
- Evidence of hypovolemia (orthostatic hypotension, tachycardia)

Laboratory Tests

The most commonly useful laboratory tests are

1. Serum electrolytes (sodium, potassium, chloride, and bicarbonate) will confirm hypernatremia. Hypokalemia or acid-base disorders reflect co-morbid conditions requiring evaluation and treatment.

2. Complete blood count with differential: A leukopenia or leukocytosis may reflect an infection or sepsis, not uncommonly found in the geriatric nursing home patients with a urinary tract infection or pneumonia.

3. Serum glucose to rule out hyperglycemia

4. Blood urea nitrogen (BUN) and creatine to evaluate renal function

5. Serum osmolality (normal range 280 to 295 mmol/kg) may be measured or calculated:

$$2(Na) + \frac{glucose}{18} + \frac{BUN}{2.8}$$

6. Urine osmolality will aid in differential diagnosis of hypernatremia.

Key Tests

- Serum sodium
- Urine osmolality

Differential Diagnosis: Key Questions to Ask

1. Is there a reason for water loss or sodium gain?
   a. Increased insensible losses (fever, tachypnea, sweat losses)?
   b. Diarrhea or vomiting?
   c. Renal water loss (>3 L/24 hours of dilute urine)?
   d. Iatrogenic administration of hypertonic sodium solutions?

2. Is there a reason for inadequate water intake?
   a. Impaired thirst?
   b. Altered mental status?
   c. No access to water?
   d. Primary neurologic disorder (stroke, meningitis, tumor)?

3. Is polyuria present (urine volume >3 L/24 hours)?
   a. Urine osmolality 300 mOsm/L or greater (osmotic diuresis, e.g., saline, glucose)? With diuretics, osmotic diuresis, or salt wasting, the urine tends to be isotonic.
   b. Urine osmolality less than 150 mOsm/L (diabetes insipidus)? Vasopressin (ADH) test will distinguish central from nephrogenic.

Treatment

1. The mortality rate from hypernatremia is reported to be 40 to 55 per cent, but the majority of deaths are related to the underlying disease process. However, delayed or inappropriate treatment is associated with an increase in deaths.

2. In chronic hypernatremia (>48 hours), there has been time for brain adaptation with an accumulation of organic solutes (idiopathic osmoles). This puts the patient at risk for cerebral edema if the hypernatremia is corrected too rapidly.

3. When symptomatic hypovolemia is present, the first priority is rapid expansion of the extracellular fluid volume with 0.9% saline or lactated Ringer's solution.

4. Once volume status is restored, calculation of the free water deficit should be performed.

$$H_2O \text{ deficit} = \text{Total body water}$$
$$\times \left[\frac{Na^+ \text{ (measured)} - Na^+ \text{ (desired)}}{Na^+ \text{ (desired)}} \right]$$

5. A safe rate of correction of hypernatremia is to decrease the serum sodium concentration no faster than 0.5 to 1.0 mEq/L/hour. Approximately half the water deficit can be given in the first 24 hours, with the rest administered over the next 48 hours.

6. Saline 0.45% replaces both H_2O and sodium (each liter delivers about 500 ml free water).

7. Dextrose 5% in water (D_5W) is most efficient in correcting hypernatremia (each liter delivers 1 L of free water), but should be avoided in hyperglycemia and may lead to cerebral intracellular lactic acidosis.

8. Frequent rechecking of serum sodium should be done to monitor therapy.

9. Remember that free water may be given via oral, nasogastric tube, or intravenous routes.

Key Treatment

- If volume depletion present, give 0.9% saline initially.

- Calculate water deficit, then give hypotonic fluids.

- Avoid a drop in serum sodium greater than 1 mEq/hour.

- Monitor serum sodium frequently during therapy.

Follow-Up

1. Recognition and treatment of the underlying disorder associated with hypernatremia is most important.

2. In both children and adults, survivors of severe hypernatremia have a 10 to 15 per cent likelihood of permanent neurologic deficits.

3. Whenever access to water is an issue, whether in a home residence or nursing home, education of the primary caregiver and nursing staff may be quite valuable in preventing future recurrences.

EXAMPLE

A 76-year-old woman, a nursing home resident, is found to have a serum [Na^+] of 168 mEq/L while being evaluated for altered mental status. She weighs 60 kg. Blood pressure is 94/60 and pulse is 125. To restore volume, a liter of 0.9% saline is given over 1 hour. The water deficit is then calculated:

$$(0.5 \times 60) \times [168 - 140/140] = 6.0 \text{ L}.$$

Approximately half of the deficit (3.0 L) should be given over 24 hours, with the rest given over 48 hours. Assume maintenance fluid requirement of 1.0 L/24 hours. A total of 4.0 L (3.0 L + 1.0 L) free water is to be given as 0.45% saline at 330 ml/hour (total of 8.0 L in 24 hours) or D_5W at 165 ml/hour (total of 4.0 L). The downward correction rate of [Na^+] is 0.58 mEq/hour.

 ## Bibliography

Ayus JC, Arieff AI: Abnormalities of water metabolism in the elderly. Semin Nephrol 1996;16:277–288.

Beck LH: Changes in renal function with aging. Clin Geriatr Med 1998;14:199–209.

Falevsky PM, Bhagrath R, Greenberg A: Hypernatremia in hospitalized patients. Ann Intern Med 1996;124: 197.

Fried LF, Palevsky PM: Hyponatremia and hypernatremia. Med Clin North Am 1997;81:585–609.

Preston RA: Hypernatremia. In Acid-Base, Fluids, and Electrolytes Made Ridiculously Simple, pp 65–76. Miami, Med Master, Inc, 1997.

192 Hyponatremia

Jon V. Martell

Definition

Hyponatremia is a measured serum sodium less than 135 mmol/L.

Etiology

Hyponatremia results from disturbances of osmotic regulation. Regardless of the underlying pathophysiology, hyponatremia is always caused by one of the following conditions:

1. Laboratory error or artifact (pseudohyponatremia)
2. Large amounts of osmotic substances in the serum
3. Intake of massive amounts of dilute fluids, either IV or oral, in persons with normal volume status
4. Hypovolemic release of antidiuretic hormone (ADH) with intake of free water, either IV or oral, in persons with volume depletion
5. ADH released inappropriately (syndrome of inappropriate ADH secretion [SIADH]).
   a. Medications: Antidepressants, neuroleptics, chemotherapy, narcotics, carbamazepine
   b. Central nervous system (CNS) disorders: trauma, tumors, infections, advanced atrophy
   c. Lung diseases: pneumonia, abscess, tuberculosis
   d. Malignancy: bronchogenic carcinoma, genitourinary cancers, pancreatic, lymphoma
   e. Hypothyroidism

Symptoms

The symptoms of hyponatremia are nonspecific. Symptoms are more severe if the hyponatremia develops rapidly or is profound.

Key Symptoms

- Weakness
- Cramps
- Lassitude
- Anorexia

Clinical Findings

Clinical findings rarely offer clues to the presence of hyponatremia but are critical to determining the cause. Patients should be assessed for the following:

1. Volume status: dehydrated, overloaded, or normal
2. Edematous states: congestive heart failure (CHF), kidney or liver disease
3. Lungs: infections or severe pulmonary disease
4. CNS lesions: trauma, focal neurologic deficits
5. Malignancies

Key Signs

- Mental status changes: disorientation, delirium
- Seizures

Laboratory Tests

The following laboratory tests are helpful to determine a cause and in the initiation and monitoring of therapy.

1. Serum sodium
   a. Mild hyponatremia: 130 to 134 mEq/L
   b. Moderate hyponatremia: 120 to 129 mEq/L
   c. Severe hyponatremia: 110 to 119 mEq/L
   d. Critical hyponatremia: less than 110 mEq/L
2. Serum osmolality
   a. Normal: 280 to 295 mOsm/kg
   b. Hypo-osmolar: less than 280 mOsm/kg
   c. Hyperosmolar: greater than 295 mOsm/kg
3. Urine sodium
   a. Salt wasting: greater than 30 mmol/L
   b. Dehydration: less than 20 mmol/L
4. Urine osmolality
   a. ADH turned on: greater than 150 mOsm/kg
   b. ADH turned off: less than 150 mOsm/kg

Key Tests

- Serum and urine sodium
- Serum and urine osmolality

Differential Diagnosis

1. Hypovolemic
   a. Dehydration (urine Na$^+$ <20 mmol/L): diarrhea, other loss
   b. Salt wasting (urine Na$^+$ >30 mmol/L): diuretics, nephritis, renal tubular acidosis, Addison's disease
2. Euvolemic
   a. ADH off, iso-osmolar (urine osmolality <150 mOsm/kg, serum osmolality 280 to 295 mOsm/kg): lab error, or paraproteinemia, or high triglycerides
   b. ADH off, hyperosmolar (urine osmolality <150 mOsm/kg, serum osmolality >295 mOsm/kg): hyperglycemia or mannitol, IV contrast
   c. ADH on, hypo-osmolar (urine osmolality >150 mOsm/kg, serum osmolality <280 mOsm/kg): SIADH
3. Hypervolemic
   a. ADH off (urine osmolality <150 mOsm/kg): acute renal injury
   b. ADH on (urine osmolality >150 mOsm/kg): CHF, liver disease, nephrotic syndrome

Treatment

WARNING

Overly aggressive treatment of severe hyponatremia may lead to central pontine myelinolysis, which can cause severe neurologic damage and death. Hypoxia increases the risk.

Critical Hyponatremia or Severe Hyponatremia With Seizure or Coma

Goal: Increase serum sodium by 10 mmol/L or to 120 mmol/L, whichever is less, in the first 6 hours.

1. Admit to intensive care unit and monitor closely.
2. Avoid hypoxia; use oxygen liberally as indicated.
3. Serum sodium determinations every 1 to 2 hours
4. Furosemide, 40 mg (0.5 mg/kg) IV, to establish a diuresis of 200 to 400 ml/hour
5. Saline 3% at 150 ml/hour (2 ml/kg/hour).
6. Adjust IV rate and furosemide based on clinical situation and laboratory results.

7. When goal is met, continue treatment as for severe hyponatremia.

Severe Hyponatremia

Goal: Increase serum sodium to 125 mmol/L with an average rise in serum sodium no more than 0.5 mmol/L/hour.

1. Close monitoring until clinically stable
2. Serum sodium determinations every 4 hours
3. If patient is hypovolemic, replace volume with normal saline and skip items 4 and 5.
4. Establish a diuresis with furosemide, 20 to 40 mg IV.
5. Replace urine output with normal saline IV.
6. When goal is met, proceed with treatment as for moderate hyponatremia.

Moderate Hyponatremia

1. Hypovolemic
   a. Replace volume with 0.9% saline solution.
   b. Identify and treat cause of volume loss or identify and treat salt wasting syndromes.
2. Euvolemic
   a. Fluid restriction: 1500 to 2000 ml/day.
   b. Evaluation of polydipsia, if indicated
   c. Identify cause of SIADH and treat appropriately. Consider demeclocycline, 600 to 1200 mg/day.
3. Hypervolemic
   a. Fluid restriction: 1500 to 2000 ml/day.
   b. Identify underlying cause and treat appropriately.

Mild Hyponatremia

Mild hyponatremia does not usually require specific treatment. Underlying causes should be identified and treated if possible.

Bibliography

Cluitmans FH, Meinders AE: Management of severe hyponatremia: rapid or slow correction? Am J Med 1990; 88:161–166.
DeVita MV, Michelis MF: Perturbations in sodium balance. Clin Lab Med 1993:13:135–148.
Laureno R, Karp BI: Myelinolysis after correction of hyponatremia. Ann Intern Med 1997;126:57–62.
Robertson G, Berl T: Pathophysiology of water metabolism. In Brenner BM (ed): The Kidney, 5th ed, vol 1, pp 899–913. Philadelphia, WB Saunders Company, 1996.
Sterns RH: Severe symptomatic hyponatremia: treatment and outcome. Ann Intern Med 1987;107:656–664.

193 Fluid Balance

Diane S. Voss

1. The fluid balance or volume status of a patient is dictated by the *total body sodium content*. The vast majority of total body sodium (85 to 90 per cent) is in the extracellular space. Sodium is thus the principal osmotic ion in the extracellular space. Solutes are actively moved between compartments by ion pumps. Water passively follows ions and equilibrates among all body compartments (Fig. 193–1). Total body sodium content is regulated primarily by absorption, reabsorption, and release via the renal and gastrointestinal (GI) systems.

2. There is no formula to accurately estimate the total body sodium. The clinical assessment (history and physical examination) is the most accurate way to evaluate sodium content.

3. A common mistake is to attempt to derive the fluid status from the serum sodium concentration on the electrolyte panel. This is like trying to estimate how full a cup of coffee is by checking if it is weak (dilute) or strong (concentrated). The serum sodium concentration indicates only the ratio of salt to water. It gives no information about total body sodium content. Total body salt and total body water are regulated independently.

Volume Depletion (Extracellular Volume Depletion)

Etiology

1. Vascular: acute hemorrhage
2. Skin: profuse diaphoresis, large burns, extensive dermatitis
3. Interstitial fluid shifts ("third space"): crush injury, pancreatitis, peritonitis, bowel obstruction, bowel necrosis, rhabdomyolysis, noncardiac pulmonary edema
4. GI: vomiting, nasogastric suction, GI fistulas, diarrhea
5. Renal
   a. Solute diuresis: diuretics, urea, ketones, glucosuria, sodium chloride, bicarbonaturia (renal tubular acidosis), hypoaldosteronism (adrenal insufficiency, interstitial nephritis)
   b. Water diuresis: diabetes insipidus, ethanol, mannitol, postobstructive diuresis
6. Increased vascular capacitance: septic shock, autonomic dysfunction, medications

---

WARNING

Rule out causes of decreasing cardiac output, such as congestive heart failure, cardiac tamponade, or tension pneumothorax.

Clinical Findings

1. Total body sodium depletion is detected clinically by history and physical examination findings of extracellular volume contraction (Table 193–1).

2. Because true fluid depletion and poor cardiac output may share many presenting characteristics but are treated very differently, it is imperative to differentiate these by a careful clinical evaluation. If the clinical assessment is equivocal, consider invasive hemodynamic evaluation.

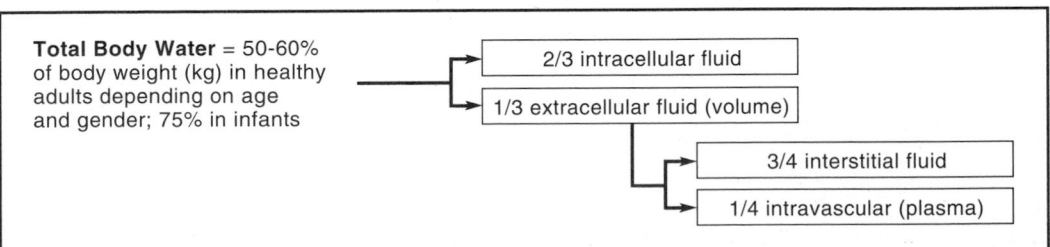

Figure 193–1 Body fluid compartments.

TABLE 193–1.   CLINICAL EVALUATION AND KEY FINDINGS OF VOLUME DEPLETION

SEVERITY	KEY SYMPTOMS	KEY SIGNS	KEY LABORATORY FINDINGS
Mild (<5%), 1–2 L*	Thirst, fatigue	Dry mucosa; concentrated urine	Urine osm >500, ↑ urine sp gr Hemoconcentration (↑ Hct, ↑ protein)

Moderate
(5–10%), 2–4 L*
	Anorexia, nausea, cramps, cry sans tears, no axillary sweat, near-syncope	↑ Resting heart rate, ↓ urine output, ↓ weight, flat neck veins
		Orthostatic changes:
		  ↑ HR >20
		  ↓ BP sys >20
		  ↓ BP dias >10
		Associated with symptoms
			↑ BUN, BUN/creatinine ratio >20, hyperuricemia, ↑ phosphate, ↑ systemic vascular resistance

Severe (>10%), 1–6 L*	Lethargy, confusion	Sunken eyes, hypotension, hypothermia	↑ Creatinine
Moribund (>20%), 8 L*	Cool extremities	Vasoconstriction, shock, coma	

Abbreviations: BP dias, diastolic blood pressure; BP sys, systolic blood pressure; BUN, blood urea nitrogen; Hct, hematocrit; HR, heart rate; osm, osmolality; sp gr, specific gravity; ↓, decreased; ↑, increased.

*In a 70-kg person.

Key Findings

Tachycardia, orthostatic changes, urine electrolytes, osmolality, and specific gravity are the most reliable signs of volume depletion. The sensitivity of such parameters may vary depending on the rate of fluid loss, age, and renal and cardiac function.

Differential Diagnosis

If the history and physical examination are not conclusive, the following steps may help define the etiology of volume depletion.

1. Check serial hematocrits to rule out blood loss if there is a history of trauma or acute bleeding. Initial measurements may be falsely high if water has not had a chance to re-equilibrate.

2. Check urinary Na^+ and pH as well as serum K^+ and HCO_3^-, and follow the algorithm in Figure 193–2.

3. Patients with metabolic alkalosis have obligatory sodium loss resulting from bicarbonaturia. High urinary sodium in this setting will be misleading in the face of nonrenal hypovolemia. Therefore, if the urinary pH exceeds 7, measure the urinary Cl^- in Figure 193–2 instead of uri-

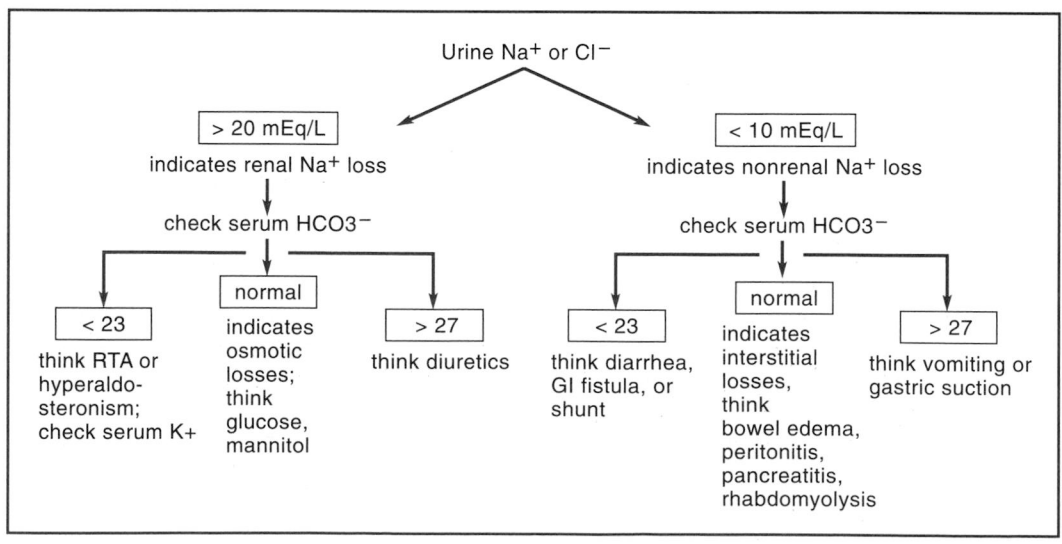

Figure 193–2 Differential diagnosis of extracellular volume depletion. RTA, renal tubular acidosis.

nary Na^+. Laboratory values for Cl^- are the same as those for Na^+.

4. From a clinical standpoint, volume status and electrolyte loss can be predicted based on the type of fluid being lost, and replacement needs anticipated (Table 193–2).

Treatment

1. Restore the intravascular volume. Give sodium (normal saline or an osmotic equivalent such as lactated Ringer's) as rapidly as possible until the patient is hemodynamically stable.

2. Administer packed red blood cells or other plasma expanders to replace blood loss.

3. Stop or reverse medications that may contribute to the problem (diuretics, antihypertensives, sedatives). Remember to remove transdermal medications (clonidine and nitrate patches).

4. Reassess the volume status of the patient every 1 to 8 hours depending on presentation and the underlying pathologic process. Adjust therapeutic plan as indicated by response to therapy (vital signs, symptoms, examination and laboratory data).

5. The ratio of total body sodium and water can then be therapeutically adjusted as indicated by the type of fluid being lost and the serum sodium concentration when the patient is hemodynamically stable. Remember to monitor electrolytes and replace as anticipated and needed.

6. Mild volume depletion in the stable patient may be replaced orally with 2 to 4 L of water/day and (in patients without renal or cardiac failure) a 10- to 20-gm sodium diet, or with approximately isotonic oral fluids.

7. Evaluate and treat the underlying cause of the volume depletion when the patient is hemodynamically stable. *Volume depletion is a consequence, not a primary pathologic process.*

WARNING

The most common mistakes are:

• Inadequate rate and volume of saline replacement (undertreating the situation)

• Neglecting to re-evaluate the patient's status and laboratory findings frequently enough

• Failure to anticipate changes in fluid and electrolyte status

---

Volume (Total Body Sodium) Overload

Etiology

1. Sodium retention
   a. Renal failure: acute and chronic
   b. Hormonal: hyperaldosteronism, syndrome of inappropriate antidiuretic hormone, Cushing's syndrome (these are generally not associated with edema)

2. Decreased effective circulating volume
   a. Decreased cardiac output: acute myocardial infarction, cardiomyopathy, hypertensive emergency, cor pulmonale
   b. Cirrhosis
   c. Nephrotic syndrome

WARNING

Rule out underlying infection as a cause of decompensation.

---

3. Iatrogenic excess intake: intravascular fluid, total parenteral nutrition, medication (e.g., sodium-containing penicillins)

TABLE 193–2. ESTIMATED ELECTROLYTE LOSSES/LITER OF COMMON BODY FLUIDS AND RECOMMENDED IV FLUID REPLACEMENT

| | ELECTROLYTE LOSSES (mEq/L) | | | | RECOMMENDED |
FLUID LOST	Na^+	K^+	Cl^-	HCO_3^-	REPLACEMENT
Urine	10–60	20–40	90	—	½ NS + 20 mEq KCl
Gastric	40–110*	10	120	—	NS
Small bowel	130	10	110	30	NS
Colon	120	30	90	50	½ NS + KCl + NaHCO₃‡
Skin: insensible	10	—	—	—	D_5W
Skin: active loss	20–70†	—	—	—	½ NS

Abbreviations: NS = normal saline; D_5W = 5% dextrose in water.
*Low at low pH, high at high pH.
†Burns, extensive dermatitis, profuse sweating.
‡Each ampul of $NaHCO_3$ has 45 mEq of Na^+.

TABLE 193-3.   CLINICAL EVALUATION AND KEY FINDINGS OF FLUID OVERLOAD

Symptoms	Signs	Laboratory Tests
Fatigue	Tachypnea	Chest radiograph
Extremity swelling	Tachycardia	BUN/creatinine
↑ girth	Crackles	Urine specific gravity
Exertional dyspnea	S₃	Fractional excretion of Na⁺ or Cl⁻
Paroxysmal nocturnal dyspnea	↑ weight	Hemodynamic monitoring
Resting dyspnea	Dependent edema	Echocardiogram
Early satiety	Jugular venous distention	Abdominal ultrasonography
	Hepatojugular reflux	
	Tender hepatomegaly	
	Ascites	
	Pleural effusion	
	Subungual edema	

Clinical Findings

See Table 193–3.

Key Finding

Weight gain is the most sensitive and consistent sign of fluid overload. Weight should be obtained daily to assess the response to therapy. Edema and other clinical signs are often not evident until there is an excess of 2 to 4 L of fluid (300 to 600 mEq of sodium and its requisite free water). In the outpatient setting, it is often helpful to ask the patients with chronic CHF or renal disease to weigh themselves regularly and report any change over 3 to 5 lb.

Differential Diagnosis

Rule out the diagnoses of pericardial tamponade, venous lymphatic obstruction, venous thrombosis, and idiopathic lymphedema (Table 193–4).

Treatment

1. Sodium restriction (regardless of serum sodium): acutely as little as 1 gm/day. Realistically it is difficult to consume less than 2 gm/day long term.

2. Water restriction: less than 1.5 L/day (orally and intravenously combined)

3. Diuresis (*except pericardial tamponade or right ventricular infarction*): Generally, cor pulmonale can be aggressively treated with loop diuretics. Unless the patient has pulmonary edema, volume overload can be treated less aggressively (0.5 to 1 kg/day) to avoid intravascular volume depletion. In patients with ascites but no peripheral edema, the diuretic dose must be adjusted to provide a more gentle diuresis of about 0.25 kg/day. Spironolactone is the diuretic of choice because it does not need to be filtered by the kidney to exert its effect. The use of diuretics should be re-evaluated in patients with a rising creatinine level.

TABLE 193-4.   DIFFERENTIAL DIAGNOSIS OF VOLUME OVERLOAD: KEY FINDINGS

Disease	Key Symptoms	Key Signs	Key Laboratory Findings
Nephrotic syndrome	Anasarca	Periorbital edema	Urine protein >3.5 gm/day, ↓ serum albumin, ↑ cholesterol, normal BUN, creatinine
Renal failure	Nausea, vomiting; anorexia	Uremic fetor	↑↑ BUN, creatinine
Hyperaldosteronism	Few symptoms	Hypertension	↓ Serum K⁺
Cirrhosis	↑ Abdominal girth	Spider angiomas, palmar erythema, gynecomastia, asterixis, ascites, no jugular venous distention	↑ Bilirubin
Left ventricular failure	Dyspnea, paroxysmal nocturnal dyspnea, orthopnea	Rales, S₃, ↑ pulse and respiratory rate	Pulmonary edema on chest film, ↑ PCWP*
Right ventricular failure	Dependent edema with clear lungs	Jugular venous distention, hepatojugular reflex, hepatic congestion	↑ Central venous pressure

*PCWP, pulmonary capillary wedge pressure.

> **WARNING**
>
> **Avoid inducing intravascular volume depletion in the edematous patient.**

4. Discontinue drugs that may interfere with renal sodium excretion or cardiac performance, such as nonsteroidal anti-inflammatory drugs and negative inotropes.

5. Mechanical removal of fluid if indicated (paracentesis, thoracentesis, hemodialysis) may provide temporary relief for the patient and diagnostic information.

6. Treatment of pulmonary edema and the associated symptoms and hypoxia may be augmented with nitrates or morphine in the acute setting to reduce vascular pressure.

7. Bed rest, the safest diuretic, may be helpful in mobilizing fluid in the patient with decreased effective circulating volume.

8. Treat the underlying problem when the patient is hemodynamically stable. *Fluid overload is a consequence, not a primary pathologic process.* See the appropriate chapters for the evaluation of cirrhosis, chronic heart failure, and nephrosis.

 Key Treatment

- Sodium restriction
- Water restriction
- Diuresis

 ## Bibliography

Abraham WT: Renal sodium excretion, edematous disorders, and diuretic use. In Schrier RW (ed): Renal and Electrolyte Disorders, 5th ed, pp 72–129. Philadelphia, Lippincott-Raven, 1997.

Lafayette RA: Hyponatremia and hypernatremia. In Harrington JT (ed): Consultation in Internal Medicine, 2nd ed, pp 237–251. St. Louis, CV Mosby Company, 1997.

Muther RS: Clinical disorders of sodium balance. In Muther RS, Barry JM, Bennett WM (eds): Manual of Nephrology, pp 187–209. Philadelphia, BC Decker, 1990.

Pemberton B: Treatment of water, electrolyte, and acid-base disorders in the surgical patient. New York, McGraw-Hill, 1994.

Singer GG: Fluid and electrolyte management. In Carey CF, Lee HH, Woeltje KF (eds): The Washington Manual of Medical Therapeutics, 29th ed, pp 39–48. Philadelphia, Lippincott-Raven, 1998.

194   Common Nutritional Symptoms

SYMPTOM   LOSS OF APPETITE

John B. Coombs

1. Just as the body's control of appetite is multifactorial and intertwined, so are both the internal and external factors that influence appetite. With loss of appetite, the physician's recognition of which of the basic phases of appetite are affected will assist in the efficient identification of the most likely cause. These phases include the desire to eat, hunger, satiety, prospective anticipation, and the pleasure of eating.

2. Loss of appetite is most often temporary and of no medical concern. Given that, in the public's mind, a robust appetite is closely associated with well-being, if loss persists for more than 10 to 14 days, the patient and/or the family become anxious, most often fearing cancer or a serious illness. An organized, efficient approach by the physician toward persistent loss of appetite avoids unnecessary testing and expense and, perhaps of greatest importance, helps to put the patient's mind at ease. The presence or absence of objective weight loss is pivotal when considering the source of loss of appetite. In the absence of weight loss, a physiologic or iatrogenic cause is most likely, with a change in mood next in line. Given weight loss and loss of appetite, somatic/organic illness or more severe forms of those conditions leading to loss of appetite without weight loss factor more prominently into the differential diagnosis.

Differential Diagnosis

All the listed conditions may be seen either with or without associated weight loss.

1. Loss of appetite most often without weight loss
   a. Physiologic causes: those causes associated with normal fluctuations within the life cycle
      (1) The "picky eater" of childhood (most often presenting at age 15 to 36 months)
      (2) Adolescent poor eating habits
      (3) Anorexia in the elderly: decreased taste, smell, vision; decreased "feeding drive"
      (4) Pregnancy
      (5) Food aversion
   b. Iatrogenic causes
      (1) Drug effect: antidepressants, smoking, excessive alcohol, chemotherapy, digoxin, nonsteroidal anti-inflammatory drugs
      (2) Food faddism/self-imposed dietary habits
      (3) Poor attention to oral health
   c. Changes in mood
      (1) Depression/melancholia
      (2) Stress, fear, anxiety
   d. Other
      (1) Exercise-induced: brief suppression with delayed onset of eating
      (2) High altitude exposure
2. Loss of appetite most often with weight loss
   a. Preceding conditions with more pronounced presentations
   b. Somatic illness
      (1) Cancer, malignancy
      (2) Psychiatric conditions: anorexia nervosa, severe depression, psychosis (Stunkard, 1997)
      (3) Gastrointestinal disturbances: chronic liver disease, lactose intolerance, esophageal dysfunction, gallstones, gastroparesis
      (4) Diabetes mellitus
      (5) Infection, human immunodeficiency virus/acquired immunodeficiency syndrome (HIV/AIDS)
      (6) Renal dysfunction/failure

Appetite varies in all of us at different stages of the life cycle. The physician's first consideration should be directed toward these cyclic changes. Likewise, many drugs affect taste sensation (potassium preparations, antibiotics), mouth moisture (antidepressants), suppression of appetite (antineoplastics), and

TABLE 194–1. HOW VARIOUS CONDITIONS AFFECT SELECTED PHASES OF APPETITE

| | PHASE OF APPETITE | | |
CONDITION	Hunger/Desire to Eat	Satiety	Pleasure of Eating
Physiologic (elderly	↓ or normal	↑	↓
Depression	↓	↑	↓
Somatic illness	↓	Normal	Normal

sense of smell (antihistamines and bronchodilators) —all of which can change appetite.

In the presence of otherwise unexplained weight loss, somatic illness should strongly be considered. Most often, attention to a complete history (including the dietary and psychosocial components) and physical examination allows the physician to focus concern. Historical attention to the phase of appetite that is or is not affected sharpens the physician's diagnostic acumen (Table 194–1).

History: Key Questions to Ask

1. Dietary history
   a. Desire to eat?
   b. Hunger?
   c. Satiety?
   d. Prospective anticipation?
   e. Pleasure of eating?

Note

In compiling the dietary history, a food diary kept for a 24-hour or 72-hour time period by the patient or personal care helper that takes into account the listed information is a useful and essential tool (see Fig. 194–1).

---

2. Psychosocial history
   a. Does patient live alone? Eat alone?
   b. Have there been recent sad events/changes in lifestyle?
   c. Are there adequate resources (money, time to shop) to support good nutrition?
   d. Has the patient noticed a change in sleeping habits?
3. Weight loss

   a. Has the patient noticed a loss of weight?
   b. If so, how has this been recognized?
   c. Has this occurred before?
4. System review: A complete review of systems, especially in light of weight loss, allows the examiner to focus on particular somatic/system-specific complaints.

The duration of symptoms, nature of onset, and associated changes/symptoms are crucial in directing one's investigation. Likewise, in the absence of findings and persistence of symptoms, follow-up history in 4 to 6 weeks or if the patient/family notices change is the proper approach.

Clinical Findings

1. Anthropometric measurements
   a. Is there weight loss? Evidence of malnutrition? Standardized measures of body composition and size, such as body mass index (BMI) or growth charts, is essential.
   b. Skinfold measurement may be of use in determining nutritional status.
   c. Trended measurements are essential to map progress or future relative change.
2. General appearance: Sad? Anxious? Well-nourished? Well-kept? Chronically ill? Well cared for (in the case of children)?
3. Sensory dysfunction: signs of conditions that might interfere with sensory input (taste, smell, vision) or oral health (mouth lesions, poor dentition, jaw dysfunction)
4. Focal signs on physical examination: associated findings with specific organic disease conditions.

Type/How Much	What Kind	Time	Where	Alone or With Whom	Activity	Mood

Figure 194–1 Sample food diary.

Measuring height and weight and applying the BMI nomogran (Bray) is essential in assessing nutritional status and, over time, the impact of weight loss/gain as well as effect of therapeutic intervention. The finding of an abdominal mass, an enlarged liver, or an abnormal psychometric screen influences the physician's concern for the presence of organic disease.

Tests

1. The use of tests in the absence of specific findings on history or physical examination is not recommended. As an example, less than 1 per cent of tests in children with apparent poor appetite and failure to thrive proved to be of diagnostic value when ordered without some degree of suspicion created by history or physical examination.

2. With persistent weight loss and no specific findings, the physician should consider:
   a. Complete blood count, chemistry profile (liver, renal, and thyroid function), and urinalysis
   b. Chest radiograph

3. A number of psychometric tests and measures of eating behavior have been developed. Measurements found in the Eating Inventory or Eating Attributes (EAT) may be useful to the practitioner seeking objective measures to establish or reinforce diagnosis (Stunkard), 1997).

Management

Following establishment of a working diagnosis, management should be directed toward the root cause. All therapeutic management plans should include provisions for patient education, dietary alteration (if indicated), and ongoing surveillance and follow-up.

1. Physiologic cause
   a. In the absence of weight loss, explanation alone followed by surveillance for weight loss and new symptoms/signs is recommended.
   b. Given documented weight loss or poor nutritional status, dietary change or nutritional supplementation discussed below should be followed.
   c. In the elderly, nutritional supplementation in the undernourished has been shown to be beneficial, whereas, of the many drugs available to enhance appetite, none are ideal for use in the elderly at this time. Often this may require the consultative expertise of a registered dietitian.

2. Somatic/organic cause

a. Therapy directed toward the root condition and education/nutritional intervention as outlined below in the presence of weight loss or malnutrition.
b. If medications are causative, either change of dose, medication type, or patient education as to source followed by an ongoing trial is indicated.

3. In pronounced conditions, such as the anorexia/cachexia phase of cancer or infection (HIV/AIDS), even forced caloric intake may not resolve associated anorexia, wasting, weight loss, and impaired immune function. In these situations, the use of pharmacologic agents (discussed below) to stimulate appetite is recommended.

Diet

1. Dry mouth: Add liquid (gravy/sauces) or butter/margarine to meals; casseroles are more acceptable.

2. Early satiety: Small, frequent meals—emphasis on a breakfast rich in calories and protein

3. Altered taste and smell: Experiment with seasonings; enhance or minimize food odors. Serve food at room temperature; eliminate offensive foods.

4. Nausea: Bland foods; eat when less nauseated; coordinate meals with an antiemetic.

5. Malnutrition: Supplemental nutritional products may be required.

Patient Education

1. Explain working diagnosis (key points); allay fear by explaining what the condition is not; anticipate individual concerns.

2. Create a therapeutic alliance. Lay out a therapeutic course and approach to ongoing surveillance. "Red flags" prompting early return also should be provided to the patient and/or family.

3. At follow-up, reassess and then reinforce or adjust the outlined approach.

Obviously, treatment of a symptom such as loss of appetite relies on addressing the underlying cause. When loss of weight or malnutrition exists, good nutritional principles should be applied to remedy the identified condition. Most often, loss of appetite can be addressed by a simple adjustment of diet, good patient education, and sound, timely surveillance. When it is the harbinger of a more serious condition, loss of appetite should be managed aggressively with the assistance of a registered dietitian and the modalities of dietary adjustment, nutritional support, and ongoing evaluation so as to maintain or restore good nutritional health.

Pharmacologic Intervention

When clinical depression is identified in association with loss of appetite and/or weight loss, the addition of tricyclic antidepressants is useful. In the management of anorexia/cachexia syndrome associated with cancer or disseminated infection (e.g., HIV/AIDS), the use of progestogens (megestrol acetate), corticosteroids (prednisone), metoclopramide, or tetrahydrocannabinol (dronabinol) may provide therapeutic benefit (Puccio and Nathanson, 1997).

PEARLS

- Loss of appetite: think of
  - Life cycle–associated change
  - Drug related
  - Mood related

- Loss of appetite with weight loss

- Look carefully and sequentially, if needed, for focal historical or physical clues.

- Limited laboratory, image, or psychometric screening indicated unless associated symptom or sign directed.

Bibliography

Chapman KM, Nelson RA: Loss of appetite: managing unwanted weight loss in the older patient. Geriatrics 1994;49:54–59.

King NA, Burley VI, Blundell JE: Exercise-induced suppression of appetite: effects on food intake and implications for energy balance. Eur J Clin Nutr 1994;48:715–724.

Morley JE: Anorexia of aging: physiologic and pathologic. Am J Clin Nutr 1997;66:750–773.

Puccio M, Nathanson L: The cancer-cachexia syndrome. Semin Oncol 1997;24:277–287.

Stunkard A: Eating disorders: the last 25 years. Appetite 1997;29:181–190.

Von Roenn I, Knopf K: Anorexia/cachexia in patients with HIV: lessons for the oncologist. Oncology 1996;10:1049–1056.

SYMPTOM WEIGHT LOSS

Lawrence G. Smith

Weight loss is a common presenting complaint to primary care physicians. This complaint frequently triggers extensive medical work-ups in search of organic causes of the weight loss. These work-ups often prove unrewarding. Key to the understanding and successful management of weight loss is the fact that severe underlying organic illnesses rarely present with only weight loss. However, significant involuntary weight loss, especially in the elderly, is a marker for increased mortality.

Differential Diagnosis

1. Psychiatric conditions are especially common causes of weight loss, particularly in outpatients, accounting for over 20 per cent of patients.
2. Malignancy accounts for an additional 20 per cent of patients with involuntary weight loss.
3. A gastrointestinal (GI) disease accounts for approximately 10 per cent.
4. An additional 10 per cent have a variety of disorders, such as drug reactions, endocrine problems such as hyperthyroidism and diabetes, and other severe systemic illnesses.
5. Twenty-five per cent of all patients presenting with weight loss have no medical cause discovered, even after extensive evaluation. Adverse social conditions and dementia should be considered, especially in the elderly.

Major Causes of Weight Loss (in Order of Frequency)

1. Psychiatric disease
2. Malignancy
3. GI disease
4. Severe systemic illness
5. Hyperthyroidism
6. Medication side effect

History

1. Essential to this evaluation is the assessment of the extent of actual weight loss. Over half of all patients complaining of weight loss to primary care physicians do not have that weight loss verified. Thus verification of weight loss is essential before any evaluation takes place.

2. One must be certain that the patient has not engaged in voluntary weight loss and simply does not offer that as an explanation. One should look for clues, such as lack of concern over weight loss or distorted body image, that may signify a primary eating disorder such as anorexia nervosa.

3. A dietary history and assessment of appetite, as well as a careful review of systems, must be carried out, searching in detail for systemic illness, especially malignancy and GI disorders.

4. Most important, throughout the history taking, the physician must be attuned to the presence of psychiatric disorders, specifically depression.

5. One key concept to remember while taking the history is that weight loss with increased appetite causes one to think of diagnoses such as hyperthyroidism, malabsorption, diabetes, and certain hypermetabolic states associated with malignancy, whereas weight loss with associated anorexia would draw one's attention toward depression and other systemic illnesses and GI disorders that would decrease appetite. Classifying weight loss early in history taking as belonging to one of these two broad categories is extremely helpful.

6. Questions concerning the social state of the patient and his or her ability to carry out activities of daily living must be asked. This is specifically important with elderly patients, whose ability to purchase or prepare food may be important in the etiology of the weight loss. Weight loss resulting from a combination of depression and social situation is particularly common when there has been a recent change in the social support structure of the patient, such as the death or institutionalization of a spouse. These are particularly vulnerable periods when the ensuing weight loss may be the only sign that brings the patient to the attention of the health care system.

Clinical Findings

1. Physical signs of significant weight loss

   a. Weight loss should not be considered significant unless there has been a 5 per cent loss of body weight over 6 months, without significant voluntary reduction in the caloric in-take or the institution of diuretic therapy for an edematous state.

   b. Clues to significant weight loss would be changes in clothing size, general appearance of the patient, and testimony from observers, such as family members.

2. Following verification of significant weight loss, the remainder of the physical examination should focus on the presence or absence of overt psychiatric disorders, as well as severe systemic disease.

3. It is most important to note that a systemic illness rarely presents without other signs and symptoms at the time that significant weight loss exists.

Tests

There is much controversy regarding the extent of medical evaluation for weight loss. It seems clear from the medical literature that extensive evaluations, including computerized tomographic scans, without specific symptoms to guide the evaluation are not fruitful. A suggested initial screen for weight loss would be

1. Complete blood count
2. SMA12
3. Urinalysis
4. Chest radiograph
5. Stool for occult blood
6. The evaluation of upper and lower GI tract: only if signs or symptoms are present
7. Thyroid testing: only if signs and symptoms are suggestive, or in elderly patients, in whom apathetic hyperthyroidism may exist

Testing directed at confirming a specific diagnosis because other clues are present in the history or physical examination should be done when appropriate. When no diagnosis is evident, long-term follow-up with appropriate evaluation, depending on subsequent pattern of illness, should be planned.

Management

1. The management of involuntary weight loss focuses on the underlying problem. If there is a primary eating disorder, referral to an appropriate specialized center needs to be made because these conditions can become life threatening.

2. Otherwise, a focus on the presence or absence of other psychiatric conditions, underlying severe systemic disease, GI disorders, or hormonal disorders is needed.

3. Specific attempts at forced feeding without correction of the underlying problem have been universally unsuccessful.

PEARLS

- Weight loss should be verified before an extensive evaluation is performed.

- Psychiatric conditions dominate the outpatient setting.

- Systemic diseases, such as malignancy, rarely present only with weight loss.

- Extensive evaluations without the presence of signs or symptoms rarely produce a diagnosis.

- Involuntary weight loss in the elderly is a predictor of increased mortality.

Bibliography

Chapman KM, Nelson RA: Loss of appetite: managing unwanted weight loss in the older patient. Geriatrics 1994;49:54–59.

Garfinkel PE, Garner DM, Kaplan AS, et al: Differential diagnosis of emotional disorders that cause weight loss. Can Med Assoc J 1983;129:939–945.

Rabinovitz M, et al: Unintentional weight loss: a retrospective analysis of 154 cases. Arch Intern Med 1986;146:186–187.

Thompson MP, Morris LK: Unexplained weight loss in the ambulatory elderly. J Am Geriatr Soc 1991;39:497–500.

Wallace JI, et al: Involuntary weight loss in older outpatients: incidence and clinical significance. J Am Geriatr Soc 1995;43:329–337.

195 Nutritional Assessment in Clinical Practice

Hilary I. Hertan

Malnutrition occurs when nutritional requirements are not met by dietary intake. This is discovered by means of a nutritional assessment, which includes clinical and dietary history, physical examination, body composition analysis, biochemical tests, and evaluation of immune competence.

Etiology

1. Dietary: frequency, types, consistency of meals; changes in diet
2. Gastrointestinal and other disease states: ulcers, malabsorption, bowel obstruction, inflammatory bowel disease, liver and pancreatic disease, malignancy, diabetes, renal failure
3. Other conditions: surgery, trauma, burns, pregnancy, lactation, infections, acquired immunodeficiency syndrome, neurologic disorders
4. Drugs: antibiotics, analgesics, chemotherapy
5. Socioeconomic factors: marital status, age, poverty
6. Habits: alcohol, smoking, drug abuse, food fads

 Key Symptoms

- Weight loss: extent and rate are important
- Anorexia
- Nausea
- Vomiting
- Diarrhea
- Steatorrhea
- Constipation
- Dysphagia
- Early satiety
- Fatigue

Clinical Findings

1. In protein-calorie deficiency
   a. Muscle and fat wasting
   b. Edema
   c. Liver and parotid enlargement
2. In vitamin and mineral deficiency
   a. Poor dentition
   b. Glossitis
   c. Stomatitis
3. In zinc deficiency: dermatitis
4. In B_{12}, iron, and folate deficiency: pallor resulting from anemia

 Key Signs

- Muscle and fat wasting
- Peripheral edema
- Stomatitis, glossitis
- Hair loss
- Dermatitis
- Neurologic abnormalities
- Growth retardation

Laboratory Tests

Protein and calorie deficiency is more common than individual vitamin or mineral deficiency.

1. Body composition analysis; anthropometric measurements: estimate fat and protein stores
   a. Body weight
      (1) Body weight compared with usual weight
         (a) Body weight 85 to 95 per cent usual weight: mild malnutrition
         (b) Body weight 75 to 85 per cent usual weight: moderate malnutrition
         (c) Body weight less than 75 per cent usual weight: severe malnutrition
      (2) Percentage of ideal body weight (IBW): based on Metropolitan Life tables (which list ideal weights for a given sex, height, and body frame)
         (a) IBW 80 to 90 per cent: mild malnutrition
         (b) IBW 70 to 80 per cent: moderate malnutrition
         (c) IBW less than 70 per cent: severe malnutrition
   b. Fat stores: 20 per cent of body weight for a healthy male adult; measured by multiple skinfold thickness based on assumption that 50 per cent of body fat is subcutaneous
   c. Triceps skinfold (TSF): most commonly used; measured midway between acromial and olecranon processes of upper arm in millimeters. When compared with age- and sex-specific standards, the following relationships between TSF percentile and nutritional status are accepted:

(1) TSF 35 to 45 per cent of predicted: mild malnutrition

(2) TSF 25 to 35 per cent of predicted: moderate malnutrition

(3) TSF less than 35 per cent of predicted: severe malnutrition

d. Muscle mass represents 4 to 6 kg of the body's 10 to 12 kg of protein. It is the main protein source in starvation and stress.

e. Mid-arm circumference (MAC) and mid-arm muscle circumference (MAMC): estimate somatic protein mass; measured at same level as TSF in centimeters with a tape measure and compared with normal values for given sex and age. The following relationships between the percentile of MAC and MAMC and nutritional status are accepted:

(1) MAC/MAMC 35th to 45th percentile: mild malnutrition

(2) MAC/MAMC 25th to 35th percentile: moderate malnutrition

(3) MAC/MAMC less than 25th percentile: severe malnutrition.

MAMC is derived from the TSF and the MAC by the following equation

$$MAMC = MAC - (0.314 \times TSF)$$

Problems with using these parameters include interobserver variation and uneven muscle and fat distribution; these measurements are helpful in following a patient's progress over weeks to months.

2. Biochemical measurements
   a. Somatic protein mass
      (1) The 24-hour urinary creatinine: Creatine from muscle is metabolized to creatinine, which cannot be utilized and is excreted. This is a good reflection of muscle mass.
      (2) Creatinine-height index (CHI): determined by comparing patient's 24-hour creatinine excretion with expected creatinine excretion for adults of the same sex and height. Decreased CHI indicates somatic protein depletion.
         (a) CHI 60 to 80 per cent predicted: moderate protein loss
         (b) CHI less than 60 per cent predicted: severe protein loss
   b. Visceral protein mass: measurement of circulating transport proteins synthesized in the liver; decreased in malnutrition, catabolism, and liver disease
      (1) Albumin: the major protein synthesized

by the liver. Decreased levels indicate decreased intake, or stress. Half-life is 18 to 20 days. Drops rapidly in catabolic states such as severe acute pancreatitis. Falsely low in overhydration and elevated in dehydration. Albumin parallels visceral protein depletion.

(a) Albumin greater than 3.5 gm/dl: normal

(b) Albumin 2.8 to 3.5 gm/dl: mild depletion

(c) Albumin 2.1 to 2.8 gm/dl: moderate depletion

(d) Albumin less than 2.1 gm/dl: severe depletion

(2) Transferrin: reflects acute changes in protein stores. Half-life is 8 days. Falsely elevated by iron deficiency. Transferrin is related to the total iron-binding capacity (TIBC) as follows:

$$Transferrin = 0.8 \times TIBC - 43$$

Tranferrin parallels protein stores:

(a) Transferrin greater than 200 mg/dl: normal

(b) Transferrin 150 to 200 mg/dl: mild protein deficiency

(c) Transferrin 100 to 150 mg/dl: moderate protein deficiency

(d) Transferrin less than 100 mg/dl: severe protein deficiency

3. Immune competence: Malnutrition affects cellular and humoral immunity.
   a. Total lymphocyte count (TLC): a gross assessment of immune competence; predicts postoperative sepsis. Affected by radiation, chemotherapy, drugs, infections.

   $$TLC = Total\ white\ blood\ count \times \%\ Lymphocytes$$

   TLC relates to malnutrition as follows:
   (1) TLC greater than 2000: normal
   (2) TLC less than 2000: mild malnutrition
   (3) TLC less than 1200: moderate malnutrition
   (4) TLC less than 800: severe malnutrition

   b. T-cell function: delayed hypersensitivity: Common skin test antigens (tuberculin, *Candida*) are administered intradermally on patient's forearm. Induration greater than 5 mm at 48 hours is a positive skin test. If none of three skin tests is positive, patient is anergic, which is associated with increased morbidity and mortality. Altered results can

TABLE 195–1. PARAMETERS FOR NUTRITION ASSESSMENT

MEASUREMENT	DEGREE OF MALNUTRITION		
	Mild	Moderate	Severe
Anthropometric			
Ideal body wt	80–90%	70–80%	<70%
Usual wt	85–95%	75–85%	<75%
TSF (percentile)	35th–45th	25th–35th	<25th
MAC, MAMC (percentile)	35th–45th	25th–35th	<25th
Biochemical			
Serum albumin	2.8–3.5 gm/dl	2.1–2.8 gm/dl	<2.1 gm/dl
Transferrin	150–200 mg/dl	100–150 mg/dl	<100 mg/dl
Total lymphocyte count	1200–2000	800–1200	<800
Creatinine-height index		60–80%	<60%

be seen in infections, cirrhosis, uremia, trauma, and immunosuppressive medication without malnutrition.

In summary, anthropometric measurements and laboratory tests are readily available and provide the necessary tools to assess nutritional status. The most useful tests are body weight compared with usual weight, TLC, and albumin level (Table 195–1).

Treatment

1. Calculate caloric requirements: Harris-Benedict equation determines basal energy expenditure (BEE) (in kilocalories/day)

   Males: 66 + (13.8 × weight)
   + (5 × height) − (6.8 × age)

   Females: 655 + (9.6 × weight)
   + (1.8 × height) − (4.7 × age)

   (Weight in kilograms, height in centimeters, age in years) BEE is multiplied by a stress factor and an activity factor to determine total caloric need (in kilocalories/day).

   Total caloric need = BEE × stress factor
   × activity factor

   a. Stress factors
      (1) Mild stress: 1.3
      (2) Trauma, sepsis: 1.5
   b. Activity factors
      (1) In bed: 1.3
      (2) Ambulatory: 1.3
2. Calculate protein requirements (grams/day)
   a. Normal person: weight (kg) × 0.8 gm/kg
   b. Mild to moderate stress: weight (kg) × 1.0 gm/kg
   c. Severe stress: weight (kg) × 1.5 gm/kg

Based on these data, adequate protein and calories are administered in the form of regular food, enteral feedings, or parenteral feedings. Different preparations have different protein concentration and caloric density.

Bibliography

Jeejeebhoy KN: Clinical and Functional Assessments. In Shils ME, Olson SA, Shike M (eds): Nutrition in Health and Disease, pp 805–811. Philadelphia, Lea & Febiger, 1994.

Lukakski HC: Methods for the assessment of human body composition: traditional and new. Am J Clin Nutr 1987;46:537–556.

Mullen JL, Smith LE: Nutritional assessment and indications for nutritional support. Surg Clin North Am 1991;71:449–457.

Rolandelli RH, Ulrich JR: Nutritional support of the frail elderly surgical patient. Surg Clin North Am 1994;74:79–92.

Wright RA, Heymsfield S: Nutritional Assessment. Boston, Blackwell, 1984.

196 Obesity

Donald F. Kirby

Etiology and Epidemiology

1. *Definition*: Obesity is defined as being 20 per cent or more above the ideal body weight (IBW).

   a. Determination of excess body fat may include anthropometric techniques (pinch methods), bioelectrical impedance, near-infrared interactance and, currently the gold standard, underwater weighing.

   b. Body mass index (BMI) is often used clinically to define and classify obesity (Table 196–1). BMI is calculated by dividing the body weight in kilograms by the square of the height in meters (kg/m^2). (See calculated table in Appendix, p 915.)

2. *Epidemiology*: At least one third of men and two thirds of women are 20 per cent or more over their IBW. African American and Hispanic females have the highest rates of obesity.

   a. As the level of obesity rises, obesity is an independent risk factor for increased mortality.

   b. Associated with many diseases (Table 196–2)

3. Causes

   a. Common causes (multiple causes may be interacting)

      (1) Excessive intake of calories

      (2) Decreased energy expenditure: affected by age and muscle mass

      (3) Genetics: Accounts for about 40 per cent of tendency to be overweight.

      (4) Environment: Accounts for about 60 per cent.

      (5) Drugs and medications: alcohol, sulfonylureas, insulin, estrogen, contraceptive pills, corticosteroids, phenothiazines, tricyclic antidepressants, others

   b. Less common causes (not an exhaustive list)

      (1) Genetic disorders: Prader-Willi syndrome, Laurence-Moon-Biedl syndrome, others

      (2) Hypothalamic disorders: trauma, inflammation, infiltration, and tumors

      (3) Other endocrine disorders: pituitary gland, hypothyroidism, parathyroid or adrenal gland dysfunction, testicular and ovarian causes

Symptoms

1. Depending upon the degree of obesity, symptoms may vary from none to severely disabling, mainly as a result of the diseases associated with obesity (Table 196–2). The history should focus on the presenting complaint, but the impact of obesity should be considered.

2. Common symptoms include weakness, dyspnea, joint pain, headaches, depression, and excessive somnolence.

3. History taking should include issues about achieving a more healthy weight and discussion of any previous attempts to lose weight.

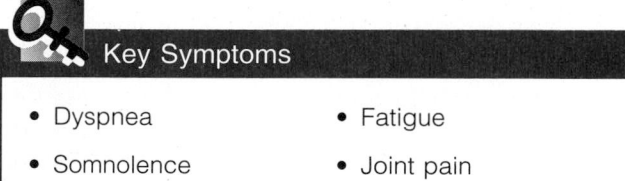

Key Symptoms

- Dyspnea
- Somnolence
- Fatigue
- Joint pain

TABLE 196–1.   HEALTH RISK ASSOCIATED WITH BMI

BMI RANGES	COMMENTS
19–<25	Desirable weight ranges
25–<27	Borderline overweight
27–<30	Moderate risk associated with this range; higher risk with the presence of co-morbid conditions
30–<40	High risk in this range; presence of co-morbid conditions further increase risk
≥40	Extremely high risk for increased morbidity and mortality

TABLE 196–2. MEDICAL RISKS ASSOCIATED WITH OBESITY

Asthma	Chronic venous disease	Coronary artery disease
Dermatologic diseases	Diabetes mellitus	Fatty liver
Gallbladder disease	Gastroesophageal reflux	Gout
Hyperlipidemias	Hypertension	Job prejudice
Osteoarthritis	Psychological disorders	Restrictive lung disease
Sleep apnea	Thromboembolic disease	

Increased cancer rates for breast, colon, endometrial, and prostate cancers

Clinical Findings

1. Distribution of excess fat is clinically important. Truncal obesity (upper body and central body fat; apple shape or beer belly) is more highly associated with symptoms (previously listed) compared to lower body obesity (peripheral fat; pear shape, large buttocks and thighs).

2. Physical examination may reveal a number of co-morbid conditions such as hypertension, congestive heart failure, peripheral edema, pulmonary wheezing and/or rales, dermatologic disorders, and joint disease.

3. Two endocrine disorders, Cushing's disease and hypothyroidism, may have physical signs that warrant further evaluation. Patients with Cushing's disease may have hirsutism, purple striae, proximal myopathy, central obesity, and buffalo hump. Patients with hypothyroidism may have dry skin, hoarseness, and bradycardia.

4. Many genetic disorders may be associated with hypogonadism and mental retardation.

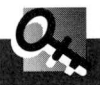

Key Signs

- BMI of 27 kg/m² or higher
- Hypertension

Laboratory Tests

1. A thorough history and physical examination will generally help guide whether laboratory tests or radiologic imaging tests are indicated, but these are not needed to make a diagnosis of obesity. The genetic disorders are often diagnosed in childhood.

2. A routine panel of serum chemistry tests, complete blood count, serum magnesium, lipid profile, and a screening test for hypothyroidism (i.e., thyroid-stimulating hormone level) are generally recommended prior to initiating a weight loss program. Obtaining an electrocardiogram is also prudent to look for gross changes or risk for arrhythmic events predicted by the Q-Tc interval.

3. Other tests may be indicated from sequelae of the obesity and its effect on end-organ function.

Key Tests

- Blood glucose
- Key electrolytes (potassium, phosphorus, and magnesium)
- Electrocardiogram
- Lipid profile
- Liver enzymes

Differential Diagnosis

1. Most patients will have obesity from a combination of dietary excess and insufficient exercise, making the diagnosis straightforward.

2. Patients who have recent onset of fairly rapid weight gain should be evaluated for a hypothalamic or endocrine disorder.

Treatment

1. The hallmarks of obesity treatment include lifestyle changes that are lifelong—a healthful diet and increased exercise. These are difficult practices to maintain over time, and this explains why most patients regain their weight. Behavior modification techniques may also be beneficial to help patients understand and hopefully change their behavior.

2. For other patients, use of medications may be a helpful adjunct. Unfortunately, these medications are not without risk, as witnessed by the 1997 removal of fenfluramine and dexfenfluramine from the U.S. market. Although primary pulmonary hypertension was a known but infrequent complication of these drugs, it was not until fenfluramine was combined with phentermine (Fen/Phen) that the question of heart valve damage emerged.

3. A more drastic treatment approach to obesity involves surgery. With careful selection of patients, this can be a very successful option.

Diet

1. Dietary therapy should be emphasized to any patient who wishes to lose weight. A balanced, low-calorie diet should be designed, optimally with a registered dietitian skilled in weight loss planning. This can be very helpful to patients who also have co-morbid risk factors such as diabetes or hypertension.
2. Very-low-calorie diets (VLCDs) provide about 800 kcal/day with 60 to 90 gm of protein and all the essential vitamins and minerals. This type of diet should be reserved for those patients who are 30 per cent or more above IBW and where more conservative approaches have failed. VLCDs are usually prescribed for varying periods of time (12 to 16 weeks), and should include patient education on food and behavior modification as well as exercise. Medical screening and follow-up with the laboratory tests previously mentioned should be performed. Contraindications to VLCD include pregnancy, lactation, unstable angina or cardiac arrhythmia, type I diabetes, and gout. Monitoring for "key" electrolyte depletion (K^+, phosphorus, and Mg^{2+}) and prolongation of Q-Tc interval is important with this type of diet.

Exercise

1. Increasing physical activity is a key element to improving cardiovascular fitness and expending calories. It can help maintain weight loss, but is generally not sufficient by itself to produce sustained weight loss.
2. For morbidly obese patients, consultation with an exercise physiologist or physical therapist might assist with creative ways to help patients exercise as well as decreasing their risk of injury.

Behavior Modification

Effecting lifestyle changes in eating and exercise are keys to successful weight loss and its maintenance. Groups such as Weight Watchers may be useful to some patients, whereas others may benefit from more intensive therapy (individual or group), with a trained counselor, psychologist, or psychiatrist.

Medications

It is the American way to want a "quick fix" for a chronic problem such as obesity. Medication therapy can have a positive supportive effect in some patients. Use of medications should be monitored by physicians as part of a program that includes diet, exercise, and behavior modification. There are currently several prescription options as well as many herbal remedies (Table 196–3).

1. Herbal products are not regulated and their purity and dosage may not be uniform even among the same lot. *Ma huang* is chemically related to ephedrine and can dangerously raise blood pressure in susceptible patients. *St. John's wort* has been used in Europe as a natural treatment for depression. It has been used in this country for depression and weight loss, but controlled trials are not available.
2. Phentermine, a sympathomimetic amine, has been available in this country for over 20 years. It is a useful adjunct for many patients, but does not appear to be as effective as when it was previously combined with fenfluramine (Fen/Phen) as an "off-label" usage and prescribed for prolonged periods. Fenfluramine (Pondimin)

TABLE 196–3. WEIGHT LOSS MEDICATIONS BY CLASS OF ACTION

GENERIC NAME	TRADE NAME EXAMPLE	COMMENTS
Noradrenergic		
Phenylpropanolamine	Dexatrim	Over-the-counter (OTC)
Ma huang (*Ephedra sinica*)		Herbal OTC
Diethylpropion*	Tenuate	C-IV
Phentermine*	Fastin, Ionamin	C-IV
Dextroamphetamine†	Dexedrine	C-II
Methamphetamine†	Desoxyn	C-II
Serotonergic		
Fenfluramine	Pondimin	Removed from market in 1997
D-Fenfluramine	Redux	Removed from market in 1997
Fluoxetine	Prozac	Not approved for this indication
St. John's wort (*Hypericum*)		Herbal OTC
Serotonin-Noradrenalin Reuptake Inhibitor		
Sibutramine*	Meridia	C-IV
Gastric and Pancreatic Lipase Inhibitor		
Orlistat	Xenical	

*Controlled substance-Schedule IV.
†Amphetamines are strongly discouraged for use in weight loss management.

and dexfenfluramine (Redux) were taken off the market in 1997.

3. Meridia (sibutramine) is a serotonin and noradrenaline reuptake inhibitor that was released in 1998. Its place in the treatment of obesity is still being defined; it is associated with an increase in blood pressure. Other medications for weight loss are still being evaluated.

Surgery

1. Patients who weigh more than twice their IBW or are 100 lb or more above their IBW may be candidates for surgery. Although some individuals believe that this option is a drastic way to deal with obesity, it can be very successful for selected individuals.

2. Gastric bypass is generally associated with a loss of two thirds of the excess body weight, by forcing patients to change their eating patterns. However, because this is a very obese population, surgery carries a risk of morbidity and mortality.

3. Exercise and behavior modification are still important to obtain the best results.

4. The amount of weight loss achieved with surgery can significantly ameliorate sleep apnea, hypertension, diabetes, hyperlipidemia, and osteoarthritis.

Key Treatment

- Diet
- Medication
- Exercise
- Surgery
- Behavior modification

Follow-Up

1. Because obesity is a chronic disease and achieving optimal weight loss can take a long time, many patients lose interest and regain weight. Calorie control and exercise are commitments that must be lifelong; therefore, reasonable expectations for weight loss should be promoted.

2. The role of medications for this disease is still unsettled, but they can be useful in carefully chosen patients.

3. Surgery is an option that is associated with a high degree of success but has a defined morbidity and mortality.

Bibliography

Connolly HM, Crary JL, McGoon MD, et al: Valvular heart disease associated with fenfluramine-phentermine. N Engl J Med 1997;337:581–588.

Kirby DF: Obesity. In Rakel RE (ed): Conn's Current Therapy 1996, pp 549–554. Philadelphia, WB Saunders Company, 1996.

Kirby DF, DeLegge MH: Nutritional assessment. the high and low tech tour. In Kirby DF, Dudrick SJ (eds): Practical Handbook of Nutrition in Clinical Practice, pp 1–18. Boca Raton, FL, CRC Press, 1994.

Pi-Sunyer FX: Medical hazards of obesity. Ann Intern Med 1993;119:655–670.

Technology Assessment Conference Panel: Methods of voluntary weight loss and control: Technology Assessment Conference Statement. Ann Intern Med 1993; 119(7 Pt 2):764–770.

Selected Body Mass Index (BMI*) Calculations

BMI Height	25	26	27	28	29	30	→	35	40	45	50
						Weight (in pounds)					
4'10"	119	124	129	134	138	143		167	191	215	240
4'11"	124	128	133	138	143	148		173	198	220	245
5'0"	128	133	138	143	148	153		179	204	230	255
5'1"	132	137	143	148	153	158		185	211	237	264
5'2"	136	142	147	153	158	164		191	218	245	273
5'3"	141	146	152	158	163	169		197	225	253	282
5'4"	145	151	157	163	169	174		203	233	262	290
5'5"	150	156	162	168	174	180		210	240	270	300
5'6"	155	161	167	173	179	185		216	247	278	309
5'7"	159	166	172	178	185	191		223	255	287	319
5'8"	164	171	177	184	190	197		230	263	295	328
5'9"	169	176	182	189	196	203		237	270	304	338
5'10"	174	181	188	195	202	209		243	278	312	348
5'11"	179	186	193	200	207	215		250	286	322	358
6'0"	184	191	199	206	213	221		258	294	331	368
6'1"	189	197	204	212	219	227		265	303	340	378
6'2"	194	202	210	218	225	233		272	311	350	389
6'3"	200	208	216	224	232	240		279	319	359	399
6'4"	205	213	221	230	238	246		287	328	369	410

*BMI is calculated by body weight (in kg) divided by height (in m^2). A BMI of 27 kg/m^2 or higher with co-morbid risk factors correlates with a higher risk to health. A BMI of 30 kg/m^2 or higher is an independent risk factor for increased morbidity and mortality from excess weight.

197 Malnutrition

Diana S. Dark

1. Undernutrition is widespread in the developing countries of the world. It is estimated that 400 million persons worldwide suffer from serious nutritional deficiencies. Although severe malnutrition is not widespread in the United States, it does exist. In this country, cases of severe undernutrition are the result of ignorance, extreme poverty, neglect, mental illness, or unusual environmental conditions.

2. Malnutrition is a condition in which there is an actual nutritional deficiency or potential alteration in the dietary or nutritional requirements, which may lead to an abnormality in body mass or composition. Although this definition includes both obesity and undernutrition, this chapter will focus on protein-energy malnutrition (PEM).

3. Major forms of PEM are
   a. Marasmus: deficiency primarily of energy-providing foods
   b. Kwashiorkor: characterized by protein deficiency
   c. Marasmic kwashiorkor: deficiencies of both energy and protein

4. The patient may also have a deficiency of a specific nutrient. Isolated vitamin and mineral deficiencies can occur even in the face of apparent good nutrition.

Etiology

1. PEM occurs when there is/are
   a. Insufficient energy or protein available to meet metabolic demands
   b. Increased metabolic demands as a result of disease
   c. Increased nutrient losses

2. Protein deficiency may also arise in the face of adequate protein intake if the dietary protein is of poor quality.

3. Protein nutrition is also influenced by the intake of energy relative to the intake of protein, because the efficient utilization of dietary protein requires energy from nonprotein calories.

Symptoms

1. Body weight is the most commonly used indicator of caloric status. A decrease of more than 10 per cent of the usual body weight, particularly when the rate of loss is greater than 3 to 6 per cent per month, is a good indicator of PEM.

2. The patient may complain of listlessness, loss of energy, and fatigue.

Key Symptoms

- Weight loss
- Fatigue and loss of energy

Clinical Findings

1. Reduction in subcutaneous fat together with weight loss constitute the most obvious and constant physical features of PEM in adults.

2. Significant reduction in fat mass can be overlooked unless quantitative criteria are assessed.

3. Decreased muscle mass can be recognized on physical examination, although mild malnutrition is usually underestimated.

4. Changes in hair, skin, eyes, lips, teeth, and tongue are common.

5. Many organ systems may be affected, including the cardiovascular system, gastrointestinal system, and nervous system, particularly if malnutrition is severe.

Key Signs

- Weight loss, evidence of pronounced wasting of subcutaneous fat
- Dry, wire-like, easily plucked hair
- Scaling skin, dependent edema, pallor
- Cheilosis, glossitis

Tests

Laboratory Tests

Biochemical tests: No single biochemical indicator is diagnostic. The combined use of several indicators provides a much better measure of status.

1. Measures of plasma protein compartment
   a. Measurement of serum albumin is usually done routinely. However, the validity of serum albumin as a reflection of the status of the visceral protein compartment is poor in the setting of acute or critical illness. The long half-life of albumin (20 days), the fact that it is distributed extensively in the extravascular as well as intravascular compartment, and the fact that its synthesis is influenced by the presence of circulating inflammatory mediators and by liver function all limit its value as a measure of nutrition.
   b. Serum proteins with shorter half-lives, such as transferrin, prealbumin, and retinol-binding protein, are better indicators than albumin in this circumstance.
2. Measures of immune system integrity: anergy
   a. Malnutrition is associated with depressed immune competence manifested by decreased lymphocyte count. Total lymphocyte count can be affected by an acute stress response or by the presence of a large wound.
   b. Additionally, skin testing to common recall antigens (mumps, *Candida*) may be done, and the presence of one positive test indicates intact immunity. However, a wide variety of medical treatments and metabolic abnormalities (e.g., trauma, sepsis, malignancy, and edema) can interfere with the skin reactions.

Other Tests

1. Anthropometric measurements (body size and composition)
   a. Height, weight, and skinfold thickness are measurements frequently used.
   b. Skinfold thickness measurements provide information about fatness and leanness. The width of the fat layer that lies directly beneath the skin is measured in various places on the body by means of a caliper. Skinfold thickness measurements obtained are then compared with averages for persons of the same age and sex.
2. A thorough diet history can signal the possibility of malnutrition, can serve as a check on the findings of the physical examination and laboratory tests, and can provide a basis for making changes in food habits should this be necessary.

Key Tests

- Measurement of serum proteins, including serum albumin, prealbumin, and transferrin
- Measurement of total lymphocyte count or measure of delayed hypersensitivity
- Anthropometric measurements
- Diet history

Treatment

1. The etiology of malnutrition should be vigorously pursued to rule out other disease processes such as pancreatic insufficiency, malabsorption, malignancy, or acquired immunodeficiency syndrome. There also may be socioeconomic factors that should be discussed with the patient. In the face of terminal disease, the patient may prefer to withhold supplemental nutrition.
2. Nutritional assessment should be done to estimate the protein and energy needs of the patient.
   a. Basal energy expenditure (BEE) represents the resting basal metabolic rate. It is dependent on the size of lean tissue mass and is influenced by metabolic demands, fever, ambient temperature, and activity. Although there are more than 150 formulas for estimating energy expenditure, the most widely used is the Harris-Benedict equation (see Ch. 195, Nutritional Assessment, and Ch. 199, Parenteral Nutrition). Indirect calorimetry also can be used but is labor-intensive, requires expensive equipment, and may be inaccurate unless a steady state is reached. The BEE obtained is then usually increased by the addition of a stress/activity factor, depending on severity of illness and patient activity.
   b. Protein needs should be estimated, depending on severity of illness. The majority of calories will be delivered by carbohydrates and fats, both of which are required for adequate nutritional support.
3. Alteration of diet or oral supplementation is always the preferable method for correcting dietary inadequacies.
4. If oral intake is inadequate, and oral supplementation not feasible, the patient may need nutritional supplementation either enterally or parenterally.

Enteral Nutrition

1. Enteral nutrition has significant advantages over parenteral nutrition. Feeding the patient with an enteral formulation is the simplest, least expensive, least invasive, and most physiologic means for supplementation.

2. Feedings can be done by way of a nasally introduced soft-bore tube into either the stomach or the small bowel.

3. For patients who will need supplementation long term, a semipermanent enteral feeding tube can be placed percutaneously using endoscopic guidance (percutaneous endoscopic gastrostomy) or surgically (gastrostomy tube, jejunostomy tube).

4. There are a number of enteral formulations available for use. Specialty formulas are available for a number of disease states, including diabetes, severe renal disease, and severe hepatic disease.

Parenteral Nutrition

Total parenteral nutrition (TPN) may be delivered by either peripheral or central intravenous access.

1. Peripheral nutrition uses a lipid-based solution with lower osmolality. It is designed for short-term use (≤ 10 days) because of potential difficulty with continued peripheral access; fluid volume required to deliver adequate calories is usually higher than with central TPN.

2. Central TPN requires central intravenous access. The solution can be concentrated if fluid restriction is necessary and can be given long term, even on an outpatient basis if semipermanent access is placed. The solution can be tailored to the patient's specific needs and either delivered continuously or cycled to be delivered only during the night. There is a significant risk of line sepsis, particularly in a hospital setting.

Patient Education

Both the patient and the family need to be instructed as to the importance of proper nutrition.

Key Treatment

- Oral supplementation is preferred.

- If oral intake is not adequate, enteral alimentation should be used.

- Parenteral nutrition can be given either peripherally or via a central line.

Follow-Up

1. Follow-up should include determination of nitrogen balance. It is a measure of the extent of protein utilization. Daily nitrogen intake is measured and nitrogen excretion is calculated using a 24-hour urine urea nitrogen collection, with additional insensible loss estimated.

2. Plasma proteins (prealbumin, albumin, transferrin) should be followed to document improvement in nutritional status and ensure adequacy of nutritional support.

3. Routine tests of hepatic and renal function should also be followed, as well as other tests such as hematocrit, serum chemistries, and electrolytes, in order to avert complications related to nutritional supplementation.

Patients will need long-term follow-up to ensure that nutrition remains adequate and that nutritional state continues to improve. Periodic weights and nutritional assessment are needed to prevent malnutrition from recurring or worsening.

Bibliography

Cahill GF: Starvation in man. N Engl J Med 1970;282: 668–675.

Mahan LK, Arlin MT: Krause's Food, Nutrition and Diet Therapy, 9th ed. Philadelphia, WB Saunders Company, 1996.

Souba WW: Nutritional Support. N Engl J Med 1998; 336:41–48.

Spiekerman AM: Proteins used in nutritional assessment. Clin Lab Med 1993;13:353–369.

198 Bulimia and Anorexia Nervosa

Dawn M. Grinenko

Etiology

1. Anorexia nervosa and bulimia nervosa are believed to be primarily psychiatric in origin, although both have significant medical sequelae.
2. The mean age of onset for anorexia nervosa is 13.5 years, with a bimodal distribution, occurring in early adolescence associated with puberty and in later adolescence associated with college. Bulimia typically occurs in later adolescence through adulthood.
3. The etiology of eating disorders is unknown but is believed to be multifactorial.
   a. Biologic: hypothalamic, opiate receptor theories
   b. Psychological: deficits in the individual's self-identity/autonomy
   c. Familial: interactions that discourage development of independence and autonomy (enmeshment, overprotectiveness, rigidity, a lack of conflict resolution)
   d. Sociocultural: societal emphasis on diet and thinness

Symptoms

1. Presenting symptoms in anorexia nervosa are nonspecific and include weight loss, amenorrhea, abdominal pain, bloating, vomiting, constipation, cold intolerance, and dizziness.
2. Common behavioral symptoms include increased exercise, obsessive behavior, and sleep disturbance. Denial is typical.
3. Bulimics usually present with more symptoms of depression and a sense of loss of control, despair, or anxiety. Common complaints include fatigue, swelling, bloating, diarrhea, polyuria, and weakness. Bulimics tend to have more insight into the possibility that they have an eating disorder.
4. Patients with anorexia nervosa may present with some bulimic behaviors, especially self-induced vomiting.

Key Symptoms

Anorexia Nervosa	Bulimia Nervosa
• Weight loss	• Bloating
• Amenorrhea	• Swelling
• Constipation	• Depression
• Cold intolerance	• Fatigue
• Hyperactivity	• Diarrhea

Clinical Findings

1. Anorexia nervosa often presents with severe weight loss with emaciation. The patients often wear baggy clothing to conceal their body habitus.
2. Other physical findings in anorexia nervosa include
   a. Bradycardia, hypotension
   b. Hypothermia
   c. Bradypnea
   d. Yellow, dry-appearing skin, increased lanugo, hair loss
   e. Edema of the lower extremities
   f. Active, restless, fidgety
3. Physical findings in bulimia nervosa include normal or slightly increased weight, parotid gland swelling, dental enamel erosion from gastric acid, and excoriation or bruising of the pharynx or the dorsum of the hand from mechanical induction of vomiting.
4. Ominous findings in either disorder include those of metabolic derangement such as
   a. Dehydration evidenced by orthostasis
   b. Hypokalemia manifested through muscle cramping or cardiac arrhythmias
   c. Metabolic acidosis or alkalosis presenting with syncope or seizures
   d. Lethargy in an anorexic heralds physiologic decompensation.

TABLE 198–1. LABORATORY TESTS IN EATING DISORDERS

LABORATORY TEST	PURPOSE
• Electrolytes	• Exclude ↓ K, phosphorus, acidosis, alkalosis
• Urinalysis	• Evaluate diuretic use
• Thyroid function tests	• Exclude thyrotoxicosis; in anorexia ↓ T_3, ↑ rT_3, nl T_4, and TSH
• Cholesterol	• Usually normal or elevated in acute anorexia
• Carotene	• Exclude malabsorption; ↑ in anorexia
• Erythrocyte sedimentation rate	• Exclude inflammatory bowel disease; ↓ in anorexia
• Albumin, total protein	• Usually normal in anorexia
• Exercise tolerance testing	• Helpful in convincing patients of severity of disease
• Gastric emptying study	• Excludes achalasia, but often abnormal in anorexia

Abbreviations: ↓, decreased; ↑, increased; nl, normal; rT_3, reverse triiodothyronine; T_3, triiodothyronine; T_1, thyroxine; TSH, thyroid-stimulating hormone.

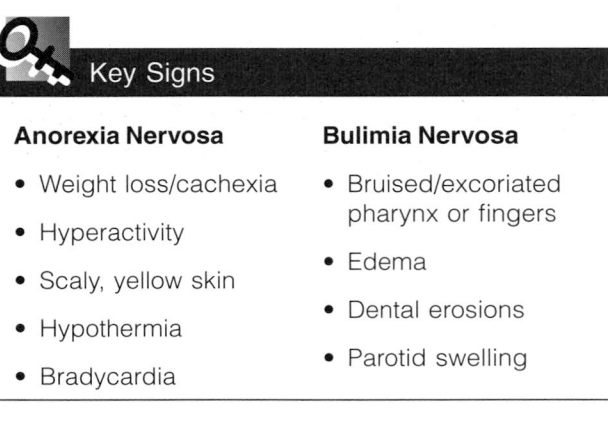

Key Signs

Anorexia Nervosa	Bulimia Nervosa
• Weight loss/cachexia	• Bruised/excoriated pharynx or fingers
• Hyperactivity	• Edema
• Scaly, yellow skin	• Dental erosions
• Hypothermia	• Parotid swelling
• Bradycardia	

Laboratory Tests

1. In general, laboratory and radiographic evaluations are more useful in excluding organic disorders and medical complications than in making the diagnosis of an eating disorder (Table 198–1).

2. Useful laboratory tests may include

   a. Electrolytes, including phosphorus, calcium, and magnesium

   b. Urinalysis, including urine electrolytes

   c. Complete blood count

   d. Thyroid function tests

   e. Electrocardiogram

   f. Cholesterol

   g. Carotene

   h. Erythrocyte sedimentation rate

   i. Albumin, total protein, prealbumin

   j. Exercise tolerance test

   k. Gastric emptying study/upper gastrointestinal radiography

3. Diagnostic testing should be used prudently because unnecessary testing may augment, encourage, or exacerbate the patient's denial.

Diagnostic Criteria

1. Anorexia nervosa

   a. Morbid fear of gaining weight

   b. Refusal to maintain minimal normal weight for age and height (Fig. 198–1)

   c. Disturbance in body image with denial of seriousness of low weight

   d. Amenorrhea of at least 3 months' duration

2. Bulimia nervosa

   a. Recurrent episodes of binge eating characterized by consuming a larger amount of food than most people would consume in a discrete time period

   b. Fear of inability to stop eating during a binge episode

   c. Recurrent inappropriate compensatory behavior (regular self-induced vomiting and laxative or diuretic use)

   d. Minimum of two binge episodes per week for 3 months

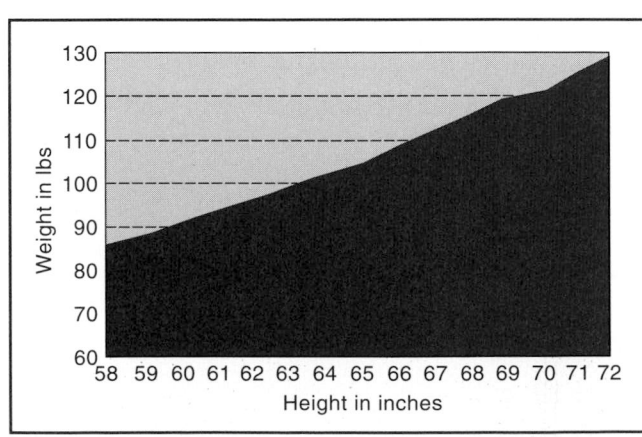

Figure 198–1 Weight criteria for anorexia nervosa (15 per cent below ideal body weight for height).

e. Self-esteem unduly influenced by body shape and weight

Differential Diagnosis

1. Gastrointestinal disorders are the most frequently encountered organic disorders to consider in the differential diagnosis.
   a. Inflammatory bowel disease (regional enteritis, ulcerative colitis)
   b. Acid peptic disease
   c. Malabsorption syndromes (sprue, protein-losing enteropathy)
   d. Hepatitis
   e. Irritable bowel syndrome
2. Chronic infection with intestinal parasites, tuberculosis, Epstein-Barr virus, and human immunodeficiency virus should be considered.
3. Psychiatric disorders to consider in the diagnosis include schizophrenia and major depressive disorders. The main difference between major depression and the eating disorders is that appetite is suppressed in depression but normal or increased in eating disorders.
4. Endocrine disorders to consider include
   a. Thyrotoxicosis
   b. Insulin-dependent diabetes mellitus
   c. Addison's disease
5. Malignancy may present with weight loss, but usually the history and examination are not consistent with an eating disorder.
6. Very rare conditions to consider include
   a. Diencephalic (hypothalamic) tumors
   b. Cystic fibrosis variants
   c. Juvenile rheumatoid arthritis
   d. Systemic lupus erythematosus

Treatment

1. Establish the seriousness of the condition with the patient and the family.
2. Evaluate and replenish metabolic and nutritional deficits.
   a. In hypokalemic alkalosis, correct hypomagnesemia along with potassium supplementation.
   b. When refeeding, be aware of the possibility of hypophosphatemia.
   c. When supporting nutritional plans, the goal should be to increase the caloric intake by 200 kcal/day, with care to limit weight gain to no more than a half-pound or 200 gm/day.
3. Coordinate treatment team activities. Team members should include the patient, family, primary care physician, psychiatrist, and, optimally, a nutritionist, psychotherapist, and physical therapist. Behavior modification is a crucial component of treatment.
4. Criteria for acute hospitalization
   a. Severe bradycardia or dysrhythmia
   b. Hypotension or hypovolemia
   c. Marked emaciation/severe caloric restriction (<500 kcal/day)
   d. Hypokalemia
   e. Neurologic deficits/listlessness in anorexia
   f. Inability to gain weight with outpatient regimen
   g. Adverse home environment
5. Provide patient and family education

Key Treatment

- Establish seriousness of condition with patient and family.
- Evaluate and replenish metabolic and nutritional deficits.
- Behavior modification is a critical component of treatment.

Follow-Up

1. Communication with treatment team members, especially psychiatric members, is crucial for both disorders.
2. The mortality rate in anorexia nervosa is 2 to 8 per cent and is attributable to starvation and suicide.
   a. Thirty to 40 per cent recover
   b. Twenty-five to 30 per cent improve
   c. Fifteen to 20 per cent are chronically affected and do not improve
   d. Two to 8 per cent die
3. Frequently encountered problems in anorexics after treatment include a change to bulimic behavior patterns, irritable bowel syndrome, peptic ulcer disease, and constipation.
4. In bulimia nervosa, roughly 50 per cent may be cured through appropriate intervention. Again suicide contributes significantly to morbidity.
5. The primary care physician should remain involved in a sensitive, supportive role even if the greater part of treatment is provided by a psychiatrist.

Bibliography

American Psychiatric Association: Diagnostic and Statistical Manual of Mental Disorders, 4th ed, pp 539–550. Washington, DC, American Psychiatric Press, 1994.

Commerci G: Eating disorders in adolescents. Pediatr Ann 1992;21:707–774.

Commerci G: Medical complications of anorexia nervosa and bulimia nervosa. Med Clin North Am 1990;74:1293–1310.

Fisher M, Golden NH, Katzman DK, et al: Eating disorders in adolescents: a background paper. J Adolesc Health 1995;16:420–437.

McClain CJ, Humphries LL, Hill KK, Nickl NJ: Gastrointestinal and nutritional aspects of eating disorders. J Am Coll Nutr 1993;12:466–474.

Powers PS: Anorexia nervosa: evaluation and treatment. Compr Ther 1990;16:24–34.

199 Parenteral Nutrition

David J. Cooper

Etiology

1. *Definition*: Malnutrition results from depletion of essential nutrients secondary to inadequate intake or abnormalities in digestion, absorption, metabolism, or excretion.
2. *Epidemiology*: It has been reported that malnutrition could be identified in 30 to 50 per cent of hospitalized patients.
3. *Risk factors*: Malnutrition can occur over long periods of time, such as chronic disease states, or suddenly, in response to stress (e.g., infection, fever, catabolic illness) or injury. This leads to depletion of the body's energy reserve and total-body proteins, so-called *protein-energy (protein-calorie) malnutrition*.

Symptoms

1. Most patients do not present with symptoms or a chief complaint except decreased energy reserve and easy fatigability. This accounts for the large number of hospitalized patients who are never diagnosed with malnutrition.
2. It is the secondary symptoms of malnutrition that alert most clinicians to its presence. Left untreated, patients develop depressed immune function, a higher likelihood of infection, and decreased wound healing.

Key Symptom

None except for a complaint of decreased energy and fatigue

Clinical Findings

1. Weight loss is the most useful indicator of risk for malnutrition. The largest determinant of basal metabolic rate or energy reserve is lean body mass. Decreases in this body compartment lead to malnutrition and inadequate nutritional reserves to combat acute stress or injury.
   a. The most commonly accepted value is a 10 per cent weight loss from either usual body weight or "pre-illness" weight or over a short time period (3 months).
   b. If patients are more than 15 per cent below ideal body weight, they are also at risk for malnutrition with decreased lean body mass and energy stores.
2. Although not specific for malnutrition, there is a decrease in immune function with anergy to common skin antigen tests. A normal response is restored with repletion of nutrients.
3. Methods of analyzing body composition involving anthropometric measurements such as triceps skinfold and mid-arm circumference have fallen from favor because of their low sensitivity, low specificity, and examiner-dependent variability. Bioimpedance devices may be more reliable.

Key Signs

Primary Signs	Secondary Signs
• Ten per cent weight loss (most reliable)	• Infection
	• Depressed immunity
• Fifteen per cent below ideal body weight	• Decreased wound healing

Laboratory Tests

1. The most useful indicator for malnutrition is serum albumin, because it reflects hepatic protein synthesis and the body's protein stores.
   a. The serum albumin level, however, can be falsely lower in fluid overload states and in sepsis as a result of redistribution of serum proteins.
   b. In addition, the half-life of albumin is approximately 2 weeks; therefore, levels obtained on hospitalization may reflect protein stores from 2 weeks before.
2. Prealbumin or transferrin have shorter half-lives; however, they are more expensive to follow and can rise as acute-phase reactants.
3. Decreased nutrient intake leads to a selective lymphopenia and ultimately to anemia.
4. Other tests available but used less frequently are 24-hour urinary creatinine determination with calculation of the creatinine/height index, 24-hour urine for nitrogen balance, and total-body nitrogen isotope studies.

- Serum albumin (most useful)

- Lymphocyte count and complete blood count

- Anergy to common skin antigens

Differential Diagnosis

A previously healthy individual can show signs of nutritional deficits with semistarvation or reduced caloric intake after 2 weeks. During the first 48 to 72 hours of starvation, an individual with normal reserves suffers only water and glycogen losses. This normal response to decreased nutrient intake should be distinguished from that of the hospitalized patient, who may be catabolic secondary to disease or nutritional stresses that require nutritional support.

WARNING

After 7 days of minimal or no nutrient intake, almost all hospitalized patients require nutritional support—sooner if they are nutritionally stressed with fever, infection, or catabolic disease or are elderly with reduced lean body mass.

Treatment

1. Total parenteral nutrition (TPN) is widely prescribed in the hospital setting and even in the home. As much care and deliberation should go into deciding on and prescribing TPN as for other interventions such as dialysis or chemotherapy.

2. Only patients with either a nonfunctioning (e.g., malabsorption) or inaccessible (e.g., esophageal carcinoma, coagulopathy) gastrointestinal tract in whom use of a feeding tube is not possible should be considered for TPN.

   a. If the patient meets the definition of protein-energy malnutrition, is a candidate for TPN, and requires nutritional support secondary to nutritional stress, then the patient's daily caloric needs must be calculated and nutrients prescribed.

   b. Calculating daily caloric needs

      (1) **Method One:** Calculate patient's basal energy expenditure (BEE) using the Harris-Benedict equation, which takes into account height (H, in centimeters), weight (W, in kilograms), age (A, in years), and sex:

Women: BEE = 655.10 + 9.56W + 1.85H − 4.68A

Men: BEE = 66.47 + 13.75W + 5.00H − 6.76A

Then multiply BEE times a stress factor (0.85 for mild starvation to 1.55 for severe infection or trauma) and then times an activity factor (1.25 if patient is ambulatory or 1.0 if paralyzed or on a ventilator). Result will be in kilocalories (kcal).

      (2) **Method Two**—"Rough rule of thumb": Multiply 30 kcal times the patient's weight in kilograms (try to use ideal body weight or average of actual and ideal if large discrepancy). This will deliver sufficient calories in 90 per cent of hospitalized patients and possibly overfeed 10 per cent.

3. TPN prescription: After the daily caloric requirements are determined by either method one or method two, individual nutrients are prescribed as follows:

   a. Protein requirements: 0.8 to 1.0 gm/kg/day in normal adults and 1.5 gm/kg if nutritionally stressed.

   b. Carbohydrate requirements: 2.0 to 5.0 mg/kg/minute. Use 3.5 mg/kg/minute and adjust down for brittle diabetic or carbon dioxide retainer and upward for severely catabolic, such as a burn patient.

   c. Only protein and carbohydrates are required. Intralipids are used to "fill in calories" to meet daily needs and to prevent fatty acid deficiency.

   d. Add electrolytes: sodium, potassium, chloride, phosphorus, calcium, magnesium, and acetate (as needed for electron neutrality).

   e. Add 10 ml of multivitamins and 3 ml of trace elements per day in TPN.

   f. Add 1 unit of heparin per 1 ml of TPN to prevent thrombus formation at catheter tip.

   g. Insulin and other TPN-compatible drugs can be added as needed.

4. Calculating nutrient calories and volume (Table 199–1)

   a. Protein (the amino acid mix) is 4 cal/gm and currently available in an 8.5%, 10%, or 15% solution.

   b. Carbohydrate or dextrose is 3.4 cal/gm (glucose is 4 cal/gm), and a 70% (D70) solution is used.

TABLE 199–1. CALCULATION OF TPN

Example: A 5-foot 10-inch, 70-kg man is admitted to the hospital for exacerbation of Crohn's disease and has not eaten in 7 days. He is febrile and thought to be catabolic; TPN is requested.

CALCULATION

Step 1: Total daily caloric needs equal 70 (kg) $\times$ 30 (kcal/day) = 2100 kcal/day

Step 2: Calculate required nutrients:
  a. Calculate required *protein* calories: 70 kg $\times$ 1.5 gm/kg = 105 grams; then 105 gm/day $\times$ 4 kcal = 420 protein kcal/day
  b. Calculate required *carbohydrate* calories: 70 kg $\times$ 3.5 mg/kg $\times$ 1440 minutes/day divided by 1000 mg/gm = 353 gm/day; then 353 gm/day $\times$ 3.4 kcal/gm = 1200 kcal/day
  c. Calculate remaining caloric needs and provide lipid calories: 2100 kcal/day $-$ 420 protein kcal/day $-$ 1200 carbohydrate kcal/day = 480 kcal/day
  d. *Intralipids* are 2 kcal/ml, so 240 ml (480 divided by 2) of 20% intralipid will be added to the TPN.

Step 3: Calculate volume and rate of TPN:
  a. Protein: using an 8.5% amino acid solution will require 105 gm/day divided by 0.085 gm/ml = 1235 ml/day
  b. Carbohydrate: using a 70% dextrose solution will require 353 gm/day divided by 0.70 gm/ml = 504 ml/day
  c. 1235 ml of amino acids + 504 ml of carbohydrate + 240 ml of intralipid = 1979 ml/day (abc). The rate would be 1979 ml/day divided by 24 hours/day = 82 ml/hr.

Step 4: Add electrolytes, 10 ml of multivitamins, and 3 ml of trace elements as well as 2000 units of heparin (1 unit/ml) to TPN.

---

c. The intralipid is a 20% solution and contains 2 cal/ml.

WARNING

The TPN formulation must be adjusted in certain disease states. Protein should be reduced in liver or renal failure, as well as potassium, phosphorus, magnesium, and fluid concentration. Salt and fluid concentration should be restricted in congestive heart failure and carbohydrates reduced in diabetes or chronic obstructive pulmonary disease. TPN is highly osmolar and must be administered via a central line.

Follow-Up

1. Initially, daily electrolytes must be followed and strict fluid intake and output monitored. Platelet counts must be followed to rule out thrombocytopenia secondary to heparin or the need to restrict lipids (lipids may interfere with platelet quantity and function). When fluid and electrolytes are stabilized, can reduce to twice-weekly blood tests.

2. Must watch for signs of catheter sepsis or wound infection.

3. Patient's weight should be followed at least weekly. A 24-hour urinary nitrogen balance should be obtained weekly to assess sufficient protein calories.

4. Gastrointestinal activities should be monitored for bowel sounds and function. Oral intake should be resumed as soon as possible with calorie counts to guide cessation of TPN.

5. Patients who require TPN for prolonged periods of time should be assessed and counseled for home TPN.

Bibliography

For more information on nutritional support, see
ASPEN Board of Directors: Guidelines for the use of parenteral and enteral nutrition in adult and pediatric patients. JPEN 1993;17:1SA–26SA.
Birmigham CL: Total parenteral nutrition in the critically ill patient. Lancet 1999;353:1116–1117.
Heyland DK, MacDonald S, Keefe L, et al: Total parenteral nutrition in the critically ill patient: a meta-analysis. JAMA 1998;280:2013–2019.
Wilmore DW, van Woert JH: Enteral and parenteral nutrition in hospital patients. In Rubenstein E, Federman D (eds): Scientific American, sec 4, chap 14, pp 1–21. New York, Library of Congress, 1992.

For more information on complications of TPN, see
Meadows N: Monitoring and complications of parenteral nutrition. Nutrition 1998;14:806–808.

For more information on home TPN, see
Tjellesen L: Assessment of nutritional status in patients on home parenteral nutrition. Nutrition 1999;15:54.

200 Common Bone Symptoms

SYMPTOM **BONE PAIN AND SWELLING** *Karl E. Miller*

Bone pain and/or swelling can be a presenting symptom of a wide range of medical conditions, from a simple contusion to a pathologic fracture. The pain is usually self-limited and responds to conservative therapy. In cases that do not respond or have no history of trauma or overuse, an evaluation of the rarer causes must be performed.

Differential Diagnosis
1. Trauma
2. Overuse syndromes
   a. Stress fractures
   b. Anterior compartment syndrome—shin splints
3. Primary or secondary neoplasias
4. Padget's disease
5. Osteomyelitis

History: Key Questions to Ask
1. Character of pain
2. Onset and course
3. Duration
4. Intensity of pain
5. What exacerbates the pain/swelling
6. What relieves the pain/swelling
7. Mechanism of any injury, abrupt versus subtle onset
8. Change in training intensity
9. Skin changes over painful/swollen area
10. Fever, chills, night sweats, weight loss
11. Medical history of cancer or other medical illnesses

Most bone pain/swelling is self-limiting and lasts for a few days. The pain can range from a dull ache to a severe, stabbing sensation. The key to establishing the diagnosis is the presence or absence of trauma. Without a history of trauma, the next important area to explore is overuse syndromes. With a dramatic increase in the intensity and/or duration of training, the incidence of overuse syndromes in-creases dramatically. The most common overuse syndrome is anterior compartment syndrome, which presents as pain on the lateral side of the tibia, usually the middle to lower portion. The pain may not be present during the activity but usually occurs after exercise. The other overuse syndrome is stress fractures that involve the tibia and fibula. Presenting complaints can range from a persistent low-grade pain to severe pain. If an individual who trains has bone pain in the lower extremity, stress fracture must be considered. If there is no history of trauma or overuse of the bone, the rarer causes of bone pain/swelling need to be considered, such as primary or metastatic cancer of the bone, osteomyelitis, or Padget's disease.

Clinical Findings
1. Tenderness over the painful area
2. Swelling may or may not be present.
3. Skin color changes may or may not be present.
4. The joint above and below the painful area need to be evaluated.
5. Neurovascular examination below the painful/swollen area

Trauma over a bone can result in pain and/or swelling. It is important to evaluate the joint above and below the injured area in order to ensure the trauma did not injure either joint. Skin changes are uncommon, but, if the area over the bone is red and warm to touch, an infectious process needs to be considered. In anterior compartment syndrome, the swelling can become severe enough to compress the vascular supply. In the case of severe bone pain with no evidence of trauma, a general physical examination should be performed.

Tests
1. Bone radiographs (anteroposterior and lateral) of the painful area and the joint above and below the area
2. Bone scan
3. Laboratory studies as indicated

Bone radiographs can determine if there is evidence of a fracture, neoplasia, osteomyelitis, or Padget's disease. The minimal views needed to evaluate the bone are lateral and anterior-posterior views. In trauma, the joint above and below the injury should also receive radiographic evaluation. Bone scans can identify stress fractures, neoplasias, and osteomyelitis. Laboratory studies such as a sedimentation rate and a white blood cell count with a differential are indicated if osteomyelitis is suspected.

Management

1. Pain relief with rest, ice, elevation, immobilization when indicated, and medications
2. Exercise for muscle strengthening once the pain has resolved. Physical therapy may be needed in cases that do not respond to simple exercise programs.
3. Surgery if fractured and unstable

Medication

1. Analgesics such as acetaminophen, aspirin, nonsteroidal anti-inflammatory drugs (NSAIDs), and narcotics
2. Osteomyelitis: appropriate antibiotics
3. Primary or metastatic cancer: chemotherapy and/or radiation therapy

Activity

1. Rest involved bone. May need traction in unstable fracture.
2. Cold therapy for the first 48 to 72 hours in acute injuries
3. Activity can be increased as pain decreases and exercise initiated when pain free.

Patient Education

1. If related to trauma, reassure that the process is usually self-limiting.
2. In the case of overuse syndromes, instruction about appropriate training techniques, intensity, equipment, and surfaces during exercise or activity.

When dealing with benign processes such as trauma and overuse syndromes, the appropriate treatment consists of pain relief, rest, and NSAIDs. Patients should not return to activity until they are pain free. It is important in overuse syndromes to establish the appropriate intensity, time, and equipment in order to reduce the strain on the affected bone. In some cases that do not respond to the first-line therapies, physical therapy treatments aimed at stretching and strengthening muscle groups around the involved bone can improve patients' response. In the case of osteomyelitis, treatment is directed at the causative bacteria. In cases where the bone pain or swelling is related to cancer, the appropriate treatment consists of chemotherapy or radiation therapy depending on the tumor type.

Follow-Up

1. In the case of trauma and overuse syndromes, follow up in 2 to 4 weeks to assess response to therapy.
2. In fractures, follow-up would be based on the bone that is fractured and the severity of the fracture.
3. In cancer, follow-up would be based on the type of cancer and the treatment modality used.
4. In osteomyelitis, follow-up depends on the response to antibiotic therapy.

PEARLS

- Most bone pain or swelling is self-limiting and lasts for a few days.
- It is important to evaluate the joint above and below the area when bone pain is related to trauma.

Bibliography

Ballas MT, Tytko J, Mannarino F: Commonly missed orthopedic problems. Am Fam Physician 1998;15:267–274.

Buckwalter JA, Brandser EA: Metastatic disease of the skeleton. Am Fam Physician 1997;55:1761–1768.

Buckwalter JA, Brandser EA: Stress and insufficiency fractures. Am Fam Physician 1997;56:175–182.

Jaovisidha S, Subhadrabandhu T, Siriwongpairat P, et al: An integrated approach to the evaluation of osseous tumors. Orthop Clin North Am 1998;29:19–39.

Payne R: Mechanism and management of bone pain. Cancer 1997;80(8 Suppl):1608–1613.

201 Osteoporosis

Kenneth K. Steinweg

Etiology and Epidemiology

1. Osteoporosis is defined as a disease characterized by low bone mass and microarchitectural deterioration of bone tissue leading to enhanced bone fragility and a consequent increase in fracture incidence. Osteoporosis is measured in relationship to peak bone mass density, usually reached between the ages of 25 and 35. The World Health Organization uses standard deviations from peak bone mass to define bone loss and classify risk. For each standard deviation below peak bone mass, the risk of fracture doubles (Table 201–1).

2. Bone mass usually begins to decline after the age of 35, and in women accelerates during the postmenopausal years to as much as 3 to 7 per cent per year for up to 7 years. Later in life, bone loss slows to 1 to 2 per cent a year in both men and women.

   a. For women in the immediate postmenopausal years, the bone loss is thought to be related to increased resorption resulting from increased interleukin and cytokine activity caused by the loss of estrogen.

   b. Bone loss associated with age is thought to be related to calcium deficiency, causing subtle secondary hyperparathyroidism. Additionally, aging skin and decreased exposure to sunlight result in low vitamin D levels, with resulting poor absorption of calcium. Most older adults do not ingest adequate amounts of vitamin D and calcium in their diet, aggravating this situation.

3. Osteoporosis is epidemic in the United States and affects approximately 25 million people, the vast majority of them women. By age 70, more than 30 per cent of women have osteoporosis. In blacks osteoporosis is rare; whites and Asians have a higher incidence of osteoporosis. The costs are comparable to those of congestive heart failure and are estimated to be $14 billion per year.

Symptoms

1. Osteoporosis is a silent disease that remains asymptomatic for decades.

2. Common presentations are fractures of the vertebral column, hips, and forearms. These conditions cause extensive disability and increased mortality.

Key Symptoms

- Osteoporosis is asymptomatic during its early and intermediate stages.

- A common presentation is sudden compression fractures of the spine with minimal trauma (bending, lifting, coughing).

- Fractures of the forearm (Colles' fracture) or hip fractures associated with falls are also common indications of osteoporosis.

Clinical Findings

1. Classical presentations of patients with the late stages of osteoporosis are most commonly those with vertebral compression fractures and to a lesser degree forearm and hip fractures. Not all compression fractures are acutely symptomatic, and they may not come to the attention of medical providers. Only about half of vertebral compression fractures present to the clinician with acute pain, and therefore a high index of suspicion is indicated in examining patients with back pain and disability. Minimal trauma such as coughing or bending can precipitate a fracture, most typically in the lower thoracic or upper lumbar vertebrae.

2. Loss of height and kyphosis may be important clinical signs. The curvature of the thoracic

TABLE 201–1. WORLD HEALTH ORGANIZATION CLASSIFICATION OF BONE MINERAL DENSITY

CATEGORY	BMD T-SCORE (SD FROM PEAK BONE MASS)
Normal	> -1
Osteopenia	≤ -1 but > -2.5
Osteoporosis	≤ -2.5
Severe osteoporosis	≤ -2.5 + fragility fracture

From World Health Organization: Assessment of Fracture Risk and Its Application to Screening for Postmenopausal Osteoporosis (Technical Report Series no 843). Geneva, World Health Organization, 1994, with permission.

spine characteristic of this condition is called dowager's hump.

3. Falls associated with fractures of the forearm or hip are another common presentation of osteoporosis.

4. Radiographs of the chest and other areas of the body when done for other indications may accidentally detect osteoporosis, osteopenia, or compression fractures. Such evidence of loss of bone density should prompt a thorough evaluation.

Key Signs

- Sudden onset of acute back pain
- Kyphoscoliosis (dowager's hump)
- Rapid loss of height
- Incidental finding on radiographs

Laboratory Tests

1. Bone mineral density (BMD), or bone mass measurement, is considered the gold standard in the diagnosis of osteoporosis. Although radiographs will often reveal evidence of osteoporosis or osteopenia, a precise measurement is best obtained using dual-energy absorptiometry (DXA).

2. Because it is preferable to identify this condition during the asymptomatic phase, screening often involves the use of risk factors and BMD testing (Table 201–2). However, risk factors are often not very accurate in predicting this condition because genetic factors play a large role (up to 80 per cent) in the incidence of osteoporosis. BMD can be used to establish the diagnosis and severity of the disease and to monitor therapy. It is also accurate in risk assessment in asymp-

tomatic patients. Currently mass screening for osteoporosis is not recommended. Recommended indications for testing are listed in Table 201–3.

3. The Food and Drug Administration has recently approved quantitative ultrasound devices for measuring bone mineral density at the calcaneus. The use of these devices in screening, diagnosis, and treatment follow-up are uncertain at this time.

4. Once osteoporosis is confirmed, appropriate laboratory evaluation should be performed to establish the etiology.

Key Tests

- Complete blood count
- Urinalysis
- Serum calcium, phosphorus
- Alkaline phosphatase
- Liver function tests
- Thyroid panel
- Serum creatinine, blood urea nitrogen
- Testosterone (men only)
- 25-Hydroxyvitamin D (if suspected malabsorption or malnutrition)

Adapted from Navas LR, Lyles KW: Osteoporosis. In Duthie EH, Katz PR (eds): Practice of Geriatrics, 3rd ed, pp 217–227. Philadelphia, WB Saunders Company, 1998, with permission.

Differential Diagnosis

1. Osteoporosis can be classified as either primary or secondary (Table 201–4). Most forms of osteoporosis are primary, that is, not associated with other diseases.

   a. The vast majority of osteoporosis cases are

TABLE 201–2. RISK FACTORS FOR OSTEOPOROSIS

MODIFIABLE	NONMODIFIABLE
Alcohol	Age
Smoking	Gender
Nutrition	Early menopause
Exercise	Genetics (family history)
Medications	Race/ethnic background

From World Health Organization: Assessment of Fracture Risk and Its Application to Screening for Postmenopausal Osteoporosis (Technical Report Series no 843). Geneva, World Health Organization, 1994, with permission.

TABLE 201–3. NATIONAL OSTEOPOROSIS FOUNDATION GUIDELINES FOR BMD MEASUREMENT

- Estrogen deficiency (when treatment decisions would be based on the results)
- Osteopenia (on radiograph)
- Long-term glucocorticoid therapy (longer than 3 months)
- Asymptomatic primary hyperparathyroidism
- Low-trauma fractures
- Monitoring treatment of osteoporosis

From Jonston CC, Melton LJ, Lindsay R, et al: Clinical indications for bone mass measurements: a report from the Scientific Advisory Board of the National Osteoporosis Foundation. J Bone Miner Res 1989;4(Suppl 2):1–28, with permission.

TABLE 201–4. CLASSIFICATION OF PRIMARY AND SECONDARY OSTEOPOROSIS

Primary Osteoporosis
Involutional
  Type I, postmenopausal
  Type II, age-related
Idiopathic (juvenile and adult)

Secondary Osteoporosis
Drugs: alcoholism, anticonvulsants, glucocorticoids, heparin,
  methotrexate, excess thyroid hormone
Endocrine: Cushing's syndrome, hyperparathyroidism,
  hyperthyroidism, hypogonadism
Gastrointestinal: chronic liver disease, gastrectomy,
  inflammatory bowel disease, malnutrition
Renal: renal failure

Adapted from Navas LR, Lyles KW: Osteoporosis. In Duthie EH, Kate PR (eds): Practice of Geriatrics, 3rd ed, pp 217–227. Philadelphia, WB Saunders Company 1998, with permission.

type I, or postmenopausal osteoporosis. This type becomes clinically evident 15 to 20 years after menopause in women.

  b. Type II, or age-associated osteoporosis, occurs in both men and women over 70 years of age. The female-to-male ratio is 2:1 to 3:1.

2. Secondary osteoporosis is relatively uncommon in women, but is thought to comprise almost half of the cases of osteoporosis in men. Secondary causes of osteoporosis in men include hypogonadism, postgastrectomy status, glucocorticoid use, and alcoholism.

3. All patients should have an appropriate evaluation for treatable conditions.

Treatment

Successful intervention requires early identification of people at risk in the asymptomatic period and appropriate intervention when the condition is diagnosed. The goal of therapy is to prevent further bone loss and increase bone density to prevent fractures.

Activity

Exercise is an important component in osteoporosis prevention and treatment. Reduced physical activity results in declining bone mass. Exercise promotes higher levels of BMD.

Diet

Adequate calcium and vitamin D are necessary for maintenance of healthy bone. Current recommendations are for 1500 mg/day of elemental calcium for postmenopausal women and men over age 65. Vitamin D requirements are between 400 and 800 IU/day. Calcium and vitamin D supplements have demonstrated increases or maintenance of bone density in pre- and postmenopausal women.

Medication

There are expanding pharmacological options in treating primary osteoporosis.

1. Estrogen replacement therapy is an important option for women for both prevention and treatment of this condition. In women with osteoporosis, estrogen therapy has been proven to improve BMD and reduce fractures. There are a variety of strengths and delivery methods. Depending on the presence of a uterus, some women will need progesterone therapy to decrease the incidence of endometrial hyperplasia and endometrial cancer. Therapy with estrogens has a number of complications, including uterine bleeding, breast swelling and tenderness, and weight gain.

2. Bisphosphonates inhibit the action of osteoclasts and decrease bone resorption. Alendronate (Fosamax) is approved for both prevention and treatment of osteoporosis in men and women. This drug improves bone mineral density in the spine and the hip. It is associated with a 48 per cent reduction in vertebral fracture rate in susceptible women.

3. Raloxifene (Evista), a member of a new category of medications known as selective estrogen receptor modulators (SERMs), has been approved for osteoporosis prevention in women. SERMs produce tissue-specific estrogen-like effects on bone and lipids without influencing the uterus or breast. This medication prevents bone loss associated with the postmenopausal period.

4. Calcitonin (Calcimar) is approved only for the treatment of postmenopausal osteoporosis, not prevention. It slows bone resorption. It only has efficacy in the spine and not the hip. It is available as a nasal spray (Miacalcin) of 200 IU/spray, with one spray given each day.

Key Prevention and Treatment Therapies

- Exercise
- Calcium and vitamin D
- Pharmacologic options

Prevention	**Treatment**
• Estrogen	• Estrogen
• Alendronate (bisphosphonate)	• Alendronate
	• Calcitonin
• Raloxifene (SERM)	

Follow-Up

Appropriate follow-up is dictated to a certain degree by the extent of the disease, treatment modalities chosen, and the patient's age. Presently it is recommended that bone mineral density testing be done at least 12 to 18 months apart because of the slow changes in bone density and the error tolerance of the measurements.

Bibliography

Black D, Cummings S, Karpf D, et al: Randomized trial of effect of alendronate on risk of fracture in women with existing vertebral fractures. Lancet 1996;348:1535–1541.

Dawson-Hughes B, Harris SS, Krall EA, et al: Effect of calcium and vitamin D supplementation on bone density in men and women 65 years of age and older. N Engl J Med 1997;337:670–676.

Navas LR, Lyles KW: Osteoporosis. In Duthie EH, Katz PR (eds): Practice of Geriatrics, 3rd ed, pp 217–227. Philadelphia, WB Saunders Company, 1998.

Prestwood KM, Kenny AM: Osteoporosis: pathogenesis, diagnosis, and treatment in older adults. Clin Geriatr Med 1998;14:577–599.

World Health Organization: Assessment of Fracture Risk and Its Application to Screening for Postmenopausal Osteoporosis. (Technical Report Serial no 843). Geneva, World Health Organization, 1994.

202 Paget's Disease of Bone

Mark E. Hroncich

Etiology

1. Paget's disease is caused by hyperactivity of multinucleated osteoclasts with intact bone formation. The resultant lamellar bone is formed in a disordered mosaic pattern. The cause of the osteoclast activation is unknown.

2. Paget's disease may be caused by a slow virus.
   a. Paramyxovirus-like particles have been found in pagetic bones by structural studies and immunohistochemistry.
   b. The long latency period is similar to that of other slow virus diseases.
   c. Polymerase chain reaction techniques do not confirm a viral presence.

3. There is a hereditary component of Paget's disease.
   a. Twelve per cent of cases have a family history of the disease.
   b. Paget's disease is very common in England, the United States, Australia, New Zealand, and Western Europe.
   c. HLA-DQw1 antigen is common.

4. An immune cause or effect of Paget's disease is possible, because a low CD4/CD8 ratio is present.

Symptoms

1. Eighty to 90 per cent of Paget's disease is asymptomatic. It is incidentally discovered as an elevated alkaline phosphatase or an abnormal radiograph.

2. Paget's disease has multiple osseous manifestations.
   a. Painful bones are present, worse on weight bearing. The following bones are affected in decreasing order of frequency:
      (1) Pelvis
      (2) Lumbar spine
      (3) Femur
      (4) Skull
      (5) Other bones
   b. Bone deformities
   c. Loss of height
   d. Deafness (cranial nerve entrapment)
   e. Visual loss (cranial nerve entrapment)
   f. Headache (skull involvement)
   g. Increased hat size (cranial thickening)

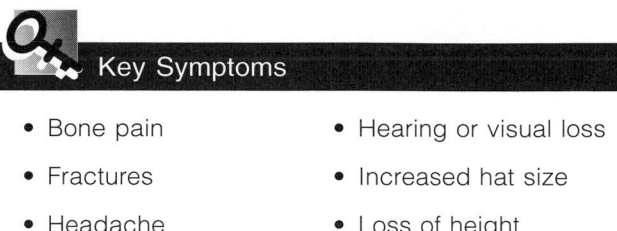

Key Symptoms

- Bone pain
- Fractures
- Headache
- Hearing or visual loss
- Increased hat size
- Loss of height

Clinical Findings

1. Warmth over affected bones as a result of the increased blood supply that is present.
2. The weight-bearing bones become bowed with a genu varum pattern.
3. Fractures are common.
4. Skull thickening is common. The most severe form of this is platybasia. Patients present with paraparesis. The cranium compresses the spinal cord, brain stem, and its blood supply.
5. Cranial nerves I, II, V, VII, and VIII can become compressed.
   a. Deafness
   b. Blindness
6. Spinal cord compression
7. Radiculopathies
8. High-output congestive heart failure
9. Bruit over affected areas
10. Osteosarcomas (<1 per cent), fibrosarcomas, benign giant cell tumors

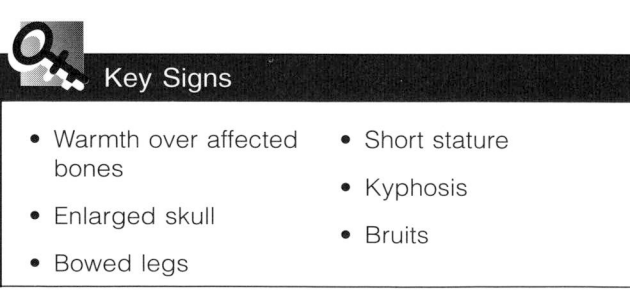

Key Signs

- Warmth over affected bones
- Enlarged skull
- Bowed legs
- Short stature
- Kyphosis
- Bruits

Laboratory Tests

1. A universal feature of Paget's disease is an elevation of serum alkaline phosphatase and urinary hydroxyproline. These tests are useful for

diagnosing the disease as well as following treatment responses.

a. Laboratory tests that increase with disease activity
   (1) Alkaline phosphatase
   (2) Urinary hydroxyproline
   (3) Osteocalcin
   (4) β_2-Microglobulin
   (5) Calcium (only if immobilized)
b. Laboratory test that decreases with disease activity: 24,25-$(OH)_2$ vitamin D_3 level
c. Laboratory tests that do not change with Paget's disease
   (1) Calcium (ambulatory)
   (2) Phosphorus
   (3) Parathyroid hormone
   (4) 25-OH vitamin D_3
   (5) 1,25-$(OH)_2$ vitamin D_3

2. Radiologic studies are extremely helpful in the diagnosis and treatment of Paget's disease. Plain roentgenograms show a characteristic fluffy appearance with expansion and cortical thickening. Lytic lesions also occur. The characteristic lesions of Paget's disease advance in untreated bones at a rate of 1 cm/year. The nuclear medicine bone scan is very sensitive at detecting pagetic lesions and may help determine prognosis. Magnetic resonance imaging (MRI) is useful in diagnosing nerve entrapments.

3. Biopsy of pagetic bone shows a very characteristic pattern of giant multinucleated osteoclasts. These are on a background of disorganized lamellar bone called a "mosaic pattern."

Key Tests

- Alkaline phosphatase
- Urinary hydroxyproline
- Plain roentgenograms
- Bone scan

Differential Diagnosis

1. The combination of elevated urinary hydroxyproline and serum alkaline phosphatase, along with the characteristic radiographic appearance, is usually sufficient to diagnose the disease.

2. Prostate cancer can give a similar radiologic appearance but can be detected with an elevated prostate-specific antigen. Both diseases are common, and occasionally, a bone biopsy may be necessary to distinguish between the two or confirm the presence of both. Myeloma also can give a similar radiologic appearance, as can other metastatic tumors. Osteogenic sarcoma and benign giant cell tumors rarely occur in pagetic bones and are detected on MRI scans. Definitive diagnosis requires biopsy.

3. Degenerative disease and Paget's disease frequently coexist. Both diseases affect the same populations. It can be difficult to determine the source of a patient's pain. A therapeutic trial of anti-Paget therapy can be very helpful in this situation.

Treatment

Many patients require no treatment. Nonsteroidal anti-inflammatory drugs are frequently enough for pain control. Reasons to use specific anti-Paget therapy would be

1. Neurologic complications
2. Impending fractures or bone surgery
3. Hypercalcemia
4. Hypercalciuria

Medication

1. Calcitonin
   a. Salmon calcitonin (Calcimar) is effective for acute disease and much stronger than the human form. Side effects include nausea, flushing, and allergic reactions. The response is short lived. Nasal preparations are sometimes used. Relapses are common. The dosage is 50 to 100 IU subcutaneously or intramuscularly daily or every other day.
   b. Human calcitonin (Cibacalcin) is reserved for use in patients allergic to salmon calcitonin. The dosage is 0.5 mg subcutaneously three times weekly.

2. Bisphosphonates
   a. Alendronate (Fosamax) is effective in Paget's disease. A dose of 40 mg/day is given orally for 6 months. Patients are then monitored for recurrence on an every-6-months basis. Patients may have long remissions. The major side effects at this dose were upper gastrointestinal tract–related problems and musculoskeletal pains.
   b. Etidronate (Didronel) is also approved for the treatment of Paget's disease. The drug causes long remissions of the disease but may cause abnormal bone mineralization and cannot be given continuously. The dosage is 5 mg/kg daily for no greater than 6 months continuously.
   c. Pamidronate (Aredia) is a new bisphosphonate that is given in an intravenous form. Its side effects are an elevated temperature and

lymphopenia. It does not cause abnormal mineralization. A solution of 30 mg in 500 ml of normal saline is infused over 4 hours.

3. Plicamycin (Mithracin) works well for Paget's disease. It is usually reserved for refractory cases because it causes significant bone marrow toxicity.

4. Gallium nitrate (Ganite) is administered in the nuclear medicine department. The agent works quickly to destroy osteoclast function but is only used in refractory cases.

Diet

There is no specific dietary therapy for Paget's disease.

Activity

Exercise that avoids undue stress to affected bones is encouraged.

Patient Education

The Paget Foundation (1-800-23-PAGET) is an excellent source of information and support for patients.

Key Treatment	
Drugs of Choice	**Alternative Drugs**
• Salmon calcitonin	• Pamidronate
• Disodium etidronate	• Plicamycin
• Alendronate	• Gallium nitrate
	• New investigational bisphosphonates

Follow-Up

1. A minimum of annual physical examination and alkaline phosphatase level is recommended.
2. Disease activity can be followed with urinary hydroxyproline levels.
3. There is no satisfactory system of tumor surveillance.

Bibliography

Bone HG, Kleerekoper M: Clinical review 39: Paget's disease of bone. J Clin Endocrinol Metab 1992;75:1179–1182.

Gallacher SJ: Paget's disease of bone. Curr Opin Rheumatol 1993;5:351–356.

Nunziata V, Giannattasio R, DiGiovanni G, et al: Vitamin D status in Paget's bone disease. Clin Orthop 1993;293:366–371.

Siris ES: Paget's disease of bone. In Favus MJ (ed): Primer on the Metabolic Bone Diseases and Disorders of Mineral Metabolism, 3rd ed, pp 409–419. Philadelphia, Lippincott-Raven, 1996.

Siris ES, Weinstein RS, Althan R, et al: Comparative study of alendronate versus etidronate for the treatment of Paget's disease of bone. J Clin Endocrinol Metab 1996;81:961–967.

203 Osteomyelitis

Thomas B. Golemon

Etiology

1. Osteomyelitis occurs by hematogenous spread of bacteria (20 per cent), contiguous contact of bone with an infected wound (45 per cent), and in association with peripheral vascular disease (35 per cent).
2. Hematogenous spread
   a. Infants and children: metaphyses of long bones. *Staphylococcus aureus* most common isolate; group B streptococcus and *Escherichia coli* common in the age group 12 months and under. For the age group 1 to 16 years, *Staphylococcus*, *Streptococcus*, and *Haemophilus influenzae* are most common. *Salmonella* species are seen with sickle cell disease.
   b. In adults, hematogenous spread less common. Occurs in vertebrae; *S. aureus* or aerobic gram-negative rods. Immunosuppressed: tuberculosis, *Monilia* or *Cryptococcus*.
3. Contiguous spread
   a. Origins include contaminated wounds, postoperative infections, and open fractures.
   b. For dental, foot, intra-abdominal, sinuses, human bites, and decubiti: polymicrobial and anerobic coverage required.
4. Associated peripheral vascular disease
   a. Diabetes and atherosclerotic disease predispose. Bacteriology diverse, *S. aureus* and *Staphylococcus epidermidis* are leaders. Various streptococci, gram-negative rods, and *Pseudomonas* species are seen.
   b. Unrecognized trauma, fissures, chronic ulcers are portals of entry.

Symptoms

1. Pain: varies in severity depending on age and mechanism of infection
   a. Hematogenous spread in children: half with vague pain for 1 to 3 months; may refuse to walk or bear weight. Can mimic septic joint. In adults, dull, constant pain over vertebral body with focal pain on percussion. Paravertebral spasm and ache common.
   b. Contiguous spread: Sensory neuropathy will diminish symptoms.
2. Fever: variable
   a. Hematogenous spread in pediatric patients: 50 per cent present with abrupt fever and lethargy, as with classic septicemia. Other children and most adults have low-grade or absent fevers.
   b. Contiguous spread: often without fever
3. Chronically draining sinuses

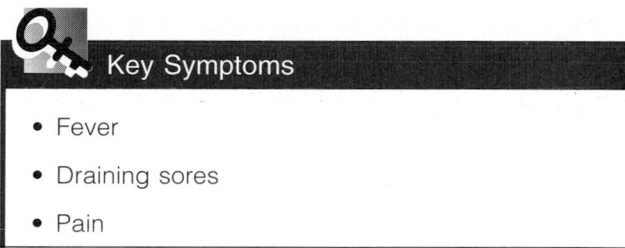

Key Symptoms

- Fever
- Draining sores
- Pain

Clinical Findings

1. Local pain and tenderness
2. Erythema (may be minimal or absent)
3. Draining sinuses connecting skin to infected bone
4. Fever, especially with hematogenous disease
5. Chronic skin ulcers in setting of vascular disease

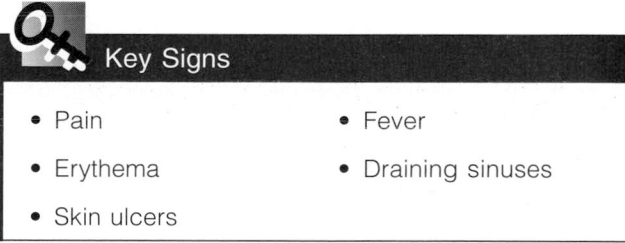

Key Signs

- Pain
- Erythema
- Skin ulcers
- Fever
- Draining sinuses

Laboratory Tests

1. Blood and bone cultures (percutaneous or at surgery); cultures of sinus tracts unreliable (exception: *S. aureus*).
2. White blood cell count (WBC): greater than 15,000 (most reliable in children)
3. Erythrocyte sedimentation rate (ESR): often 50 to 100 mm/hour; C-reactive protein (CRP) increased (may be followed for treatment response).
4. Imaging tests
   a. Radiographs: Should always be obtained; periosteal elevation or cortical erosion oc-

curring 10 to 20 days after onset specific but not sensitive.

b. Computerized tomography (CT): relatively high sensitivity and specificity

c. Magnetic resonance imaging (MRI): highest sensitivity, good specificity; allows differentiation from soft tissue infection; most accurate but most expensive.

d. Radionuclide studies: technetium, gallium, and indium; good sensitivity but less specific than CT; cost less but often require more than one scan type.

5. Doppler studies: important in peripheral vascular disease to determine vascular adequacy

Key Tests

- Blood cultures
- Bone cultures
- WBC count
- ESR, CRP
- Plain radiographs
- MRI or CT scans
- Doppler studies
- Radionuclide imaging

Differential Diagnosis

1. Hematogenous spread—children
   a. Septicemia
   b. Meningitis
   c. Septic arthritis
2. Hematogenous spread—adults (uncommon)
   a. Arthritis of spine
   b. Back strain and/or spasm
   c. Compression fracture of spine
   d. Metastatic or primary tumor of vertebral body
3. Contiguous spread
   a. Cellulitis
   b. Chronic skin ulcer/decubitus

Treatment

1. Intravenous antibiotics: 4 to 6 weeks, followed in many cases by oral antibiotics for another 2 months. Follow ESR and CRP. Time course individualized with other components of therapy. Home intravenous therapy ideal in this disease.
2. Surgical débridement with obliteration of dead space
3. Partial amputation or suppressive antibiotics; best choice in critically or terminally ill
4. Balloon angioplasty may be helpful prior to surgery.

Medication

1. *Staphylococcus aureus*: A penicillinase-resistant penicillin (oxacillin [Prostaphilin], nafcillin [Nafcil], methicillin [Staphcillin], cloxacillin [Tegopen]) is drug of choice. Alternative: first-generation cephalosporins. Vancomycin (Vancocin) for methicillin-resistant staphylococci. Add rifampin (Rifadin) in chronic staphylococcal infections.
2. *Haemophilus influenzae*: Use cefuroxime (Ceftin) or a third-generation cephalosporin.
3. *Pseudomonas*: May use ticarcillin–clavulanic acid (Timentin), a third-generation cephalosporin, or a quinolone. Fluoroquinolones also active against most gram-negative organisms; may offer less costly alternative to intravenous drugs but have not yet attained the same level of confidence. Watch use in pediatric age groups (cartilage).

Diet

Usually unchanged; may need higher protein content.

Activity

1. As tolerated. Individualize for pain and postoperative needs.
2. Home treatment: Offers greater freedom in rehabilitation phase.

Patient Education

1. Must understand need for long-term antibiotic therapy for compliance.
2. Home therapy: Requires teaching on care of intravenous access lines.

Follow-Up

1. Home therapy: nursing visits for care of intravenous lines and/or wounds and compliance on antibiotic regimen
2. Physician visits (home or office): biweekly, weekly, or bimonthly, as required by severity and availability of physician extenders.

 Bibliography

Bamberger DM: Osteomyelitis. Postgrad Med 1993;94: 177–183.

Boutin R, Brossmann J, Sartoris D, et al: Update on imaging of orthopedic infections. Orthop Clin North Am 1998;29:41–66.

Mackowiak PA, Jones SR, Smith JW: Diagnostic value of sinus-tract cultures in chronic osteomyelitis. JAMA 1978;239:2772–2775.

Sanford JP, Gilbert DN, Moellering RC Jr, et al: The Sanford Guide to Antimicrobial Therapy. Dallas, Antimicrobial Therapy Inc, 1997.

204 Common Immune Symptoms

Multiple systemic illnesses can be responsible for recurrent infections. This chapter reviews the evaluation and treatment of the patient who presents with multiple episodes of an infectious disease.

Differential Diagnosis

Before embarking on a work-up to determine the presence of a primary immunodeficiency syndrome, it is important to consider the more common etiologies of "recurrent" infections. These include inadequate treatment of a persistent infection, medications that can cause immunosuppression, other diseases that may mimic an infectious process, and underlying illnesses that may predispose to infectious diseases.

1. Pyelonephritis, prostatitis, chronic sinusitis, and subacute bacterial endocarditis, among others, may require a protracted course of antibiotics for a cure. These patients may present with what looks like a new episode of infection that actually is a reactivation of a previously existing infection.

2. Medications, including steroids and other immunosuppressants, such as chemotherapy agents, may predispose to recurrent infections. Common drugs that can induce a neutropenia include trimethoprim-sulfamethoxazole, propylthiouracil, ticlopidine, angiotensin-converting enzyme inhibitors, nonsteroidal anti-inflammatory drugs, acetaminophen, diuretics, and many others.

3. Many illnesses can mimic an infectious disease. Some of these include
   a. Urinary tract infection: Can be mimicked by interstitial cystitis or suprapubic mass (urinary frequency, urgency, with or without terminal hematuria, no pyuria, sterile cultures).
   b. Pneumonia: Can be mimicked by pulmonary infiltration with eosinophilia, Wegener's granulomatosis, hypersensitivity pneumonitis.
   c. Bacteremia/sepsis: can be mimicked by causes of fever of unknown origin, including chronic lymphocytic leukemia and other malignancies, especially lymphomas and leukemia; connective tissue diseases; drug fever; thyrotoxicosis; salicylate overdose (especially in elderly).

4. Underlying diseases that may predispose to recurrent infections include diabetes, renal failure, malnutrition, IV drug abuse, cirrhosis, malignancy, alcohol use, and collagen-vascular diseases. Diabetes, renal failure, cirrhosis, and alcohol abuse can cause decreased neutrophil phagocytosis. Malignancy is associated with decreased immunoglobulin levels.

5. Recurrent sinusitis, pneumonia, urinary tract infections, and the like can result from structural lesions and obstruction by tumor, Wegener's granulomatosis, or an inhaled foreign body. Foreign bodies in the nose may cause recurrent sinus disease. Cystic fibrosis may cause recurrent pneumonia.

6. Polyglandular autoimmune syndromes can present with multiple endocrinopathies and recurrent mucocutaneous candidiasis.

Primary Immunodeficiency Syndromes

Once the common causes of recurrent infections have been ruled out, a primary immunodeficiency syndrome should be considered. The primary immunodeficiency syndromes can be categorized by the component of the immune system involved. These include defects in antibody production, defects in T-cell function, and defects in the complement system. The list below is not exhaustive; many other primary immunodeficiency syndromes occur. Prenatal diagnostic procedures are available for many of the illnesses below and should be considered in the kindred of appropriate patients.

Antibody Deficiencies
1. Immunoglobulin A (IgA) deficiency
   a. Defined as a serum IgA of less than 5 mg/dl with normal serum immunoglobulin G (IgG) and immunoglobulin M (IgM) levels

b. Presents in childhood; the most common primary immunodeficiency syndrome, occurring in about 1:500 individuals.

c. Most patients are asymptomatic, but individuals may have recurrent sinusitis, otitis, and other airway infections.

d. Several medications can cause an IgA deficiency, including phenytoin, carbamazepine sulfasalazine, gold, D-penicillamine, and others. These drugs may be environmental triggers in patients predisposed to this illness.

e. Patients with an IgA deficiency may have an anaphylactic reaction when given blood products, including transfusions and IV IgG, which contains trace amounts of IgA. IgG should not be administered to these patients unless it is from an IgA-deficient donor. Additionally, they should only receive red cells that have been washed five times or that are from an IgA-deficient donor.

f. May progress to combined variable immunodeficiency.

2. IgG deficiency

a. Generally presents in childhood.

b. IgG is composed of several subclasses: IgG_1, IgG_2, IgG_3, IgG_4. A deficiency of any subclass may predispose to infectious complications, especially recurrent bacterial and viral respiratory infections.

c. Many normal individuals may have low values of a subclass, especially of IgG_4. Thus it is important to perform a functional assay. Draw serum for an immunoglobulin electrophoresis, administer diphtheria-tetanus vaccine, *Haemophilus influenzae* vaccine, and/or 23-valent pneumococcal vaccine. Check for postimmunization antibody levels 2 to 3 weeks after immunization. If these rise appropriately, the diagnosis of IgG deficiency is ruled out.

3. Common variable immunodeficiency disease (CVID)

a. Patients have low serum levels of IgG, IgM, and IgA.

b. Presents in the third or fourth decade in a previously healthy individual.

c. Symptoms include recurrent respiratory tract infections or recurrent sinusitis in a previously healthy individual, especially from encapsulated organisms such as *Pneumococcus* and *Haemophilus*. As the disease progresses, patients may develop chronic diarrhea, recurrent herpes zoster, recurrent herpes simplex, and opportunistic infections, including *Pneumocystis* pneumonia.

d. Twenty-five per cent have splenomegaly; autoimmune disorders are common.

e. Patients also have an increased incidence of gastric cancer and lymphoma.

f. The same drugs that trigger IgA deficiency may also trigger CVID.

4. X-linked (Bruton) agammaglobulinemia

a. Serum has low levels of IgG and no detectable IgM and IgA. Transient neutropenia may be seen.

b. Occurs in males; manifestations begin between 9th and 12th month of life when transplacentally acquired IgG is depleted.

c. Patients present with recurrent otitis media, sinusitis, pneumonia, and pyoderma. The main organisms causing infection include *H. influenzae*, *S. pneumoniae*, and *Mycoplasma*. Patients may incur local tissue destruction, especially in the lungs, leading to bronchiectasis.

d. May present with large joint arthritis (generally from *Mycoplasma* or *Ureaplasma*), chronic diarrhea, weight loss, and a protein-losing enteropathy.

5. Hyper-IgM syndrome

a. Serum levels of IgA and immunoglobulin E (IgE) are undetectable, with low levels of IgG. IgM and immunoglobulin D may be in the high-normal range or quite elevated.

b. Seventy per cent of cases are X-linked.

c. Presentation is with pyogenic infections, similar to those found in individuals with X-linked agammaglobulinemia.

Cellular Defects

1. Hyper-IgE syndrome (Job's syndrome)

a. Main defect is poor chemotaxis.

b. Patients present with severe eczema, recurrent episodes of pyoderma (so-called cold abscesses), mucocutaneous candidiasis, and recurrent pulmonary infections with abscess formation and bronchiectasias.

c. Normal neutrophils exposed to serum from patients with hyper-IgE syndrome function properly, so that the defect seems to be in the neutrophils rather than as a result of elevated IgE.

2. Severe combined immunodeficiency

a. Sixty per cent of cases are X-linked.

b. Patients have lymphopenia and the absence of cellular immunity.

c. Onset is by 3 months of age with recurrent thrush or candidal diaper rash. Patients may have a persistent cough from *Pneumocystis* pneumonia and may have a morbilliform rash soon after birth, indicating a graft-versus-host reaction from transplacentally acquired maternal lymphocytes.

d. Death can occur rapidly from any type of infection, including viral and bacterial causes. Treatment is emergent bone marrow transplant.

3. Wiskott-Aldrich syndrome

a. Serum studies show elevated IgA and IgE levels with normal levels of IgG and low levels of IgM. T-cell response to mitogenic effects of antibodies to CD3 is poor or absent, and the number of T cells drops as the number of B cells increases.

b. X-linked recessive; onset early in life

c. The complex of thrombocytopenia with small platelets and recurrent infections is pathognomonic of this syndrome.

d. Patients present with recurrent diarrhea, severe eczema, and pyogenic and opportunistic infections.

4. DiGeorge syndrome

a. Characterized by typical facial features and cardiac, thymus, and parathyroid abnormalities along with poor response of T cells to mitogens or even absence of T cells in the peripheral blood. The number of T cells and their response to mitogens is variable, however.

b. Patients may have hypocalcemia as a result of parathyroid disease, and the thymus may be absent.

c. Mucocutaneous candidiasis is a frequent presenting symptom.

Complement Disorders

1. These are rare and may manifest as recurrent meningococcemia and gonococcemia.

2. Chronic granulomatous disease

a. Defect in the ability of phagocytes to produce hydrogen peroxide. Thus ingested organisms are not killed. About 50 per cent are X-linked.

b. Generally presents in childhood with recurrent infection with catalase-positive organisms such as *Staphylococcus aureus* and *Escherichia coli*.

TABLE 204–1.   MANAGEMENT OF PRIMARY IMMUNODEFICIENCIES

DISEASE	DEFECT	LABORATORY FINDINGS	AGE AT CLINICAL PRESENTATION	TREATMENT
IgA deficiency	Antibody	Low IgA; normal IgG and IgM	Variable; may be clinically normal	None generally needed
X-linked agammaglobulinemia	Antibody	Low IgG; undetectable IgM and IgA	9–12 months	Intravenous immune globulin: (400 mg/kg for 3 wk); increase to 600 mg/kg if needed
IgG deficiency	Antibody	Low IgG or subclass of IgG after antigenic stimulation	Variable; may be clinically asymptomatic	As above but efficacy not well established
Common variable immunodeficiency	Antibody	Low IgG, IgA, IgM	3rd or 4th decade	As above
X-linked hyper-IgM syndrome	Antibody, cellular (variable neutropenia)	Elevated IgM; IgA and IgE undetectable; low levels of IgG	Young childhood to young adulthood	As above
Hyper-IgE syndrome (Job's syndrome)	Cellular	Elevated IgE; poor chemotaxis	Infancy or early childhood	Aggressive antibiotic treatment and abscess drainage
DiGeorge's syndrome	Cellular	Low T-cell levels; variable response to mitogens; cardiac and facial abnormalities (hypertelorism, micrognathia, low-set ears); hypocalcemia	Neonatal tetany from hypocalcemia	Fetal thymus transplant; thymic hormones
Chronic granulomatous disease	Cellular	Abnormal NBT test	Childhood	Bone marrow transplant
Wiskott-Aldrich syndrome	Cellular	Thrombocytopenia; small platelets; elevated IgA, IgE; normal IgG; low IgM	Variable; early in life	Bone marrow transplant
Severe combined immunodeficiency	Cellular	Marked lymphopenia	By 3 months	Bone marrow transplant

c. Patients have multiple draining wounds, especially from lymph nodes.

d. Diagnosis is by the nitroblue tetrazolium (NBT) test. Neutrophils ingest NBT. This should be reduced to a blue color if hydrogen peroxide is being generated. The absence of blue granules in the neutrophil is classical for this illness.

Diagnosis

1. Because primary immunodeficiency syndromes can mimic human immunodeficiency virus/acquired immunodeficiency syndrome (HIV/AIDS) in their presentation, it is important to rule out HIV/AIDS as a cause of immunodeficiency, either by history or by laboratory testing.

2. Perform a complete blood count followed by a quantitative immunoglobulin electrophoresis. This will help to categorize the diagnosis if it is abnormal.

3. If the immunoglobulin electrophoresis is normal, perform a CH50. The CH50 is a measure of complement activation and will be low if there is a complement defect.

4. If the CH50 is normal, a test of the T-cell line should be done. T cells can be measured directly by most laboratories using an antibody test that will differentiate between T3, T4, and T8 cells. T-cell function can be assessed by the presence or absence of delayed hypersensitivity using an "anergy panel" (e.g., skin tests to *Candida*).

Neutrophil function is difficult to quantitate and can usually only be done by special laboratories.

Management

The management of this heterogeneous group of disorders is complex, and a detailed discussion is beyond the scope of this manual. However, general guidelines are provided in Table 204–1. Immunoglobulin deficiencies are amenable to treatment by a primary care physician. Specialized testing and bone marrow or thymus transplant may be required for those patients with cellular defects.

WARNING

Patients with immune deficiency disorders should not have live virus vaccines!

 Bibliography

Behrman RE (ed): Nelson Textbook of Pediatrics, 15th ed. Philadelphia, WB Saunders Company, 1996.

Buckley RH: Breakthroughs in the understanding and therapy of primary immunodeficiency. Pediatr Clin North Am 1994;41:665–690.

Markert ML, Hummell DS, Rosenblatt HM: Complete DiGeorge syndrome: persistence of profound immunodeficiency. Pediatrics 1998;132:15–21.

Ochs HD, Smith CIE: X-linked agammaglobulinemia: a clinical and molecular analysis. Medicine 1996;75:287–299.

Rosen FS, Cooper M, et al: Medical progress: the primary immunodeficiencies. N Engl J Med 1995;333:431–440.

205 Asymptomatic HIV Infection

Nancy O. Tatum

Etiology

1. Human immunodeficiency virus (HIV), a human retrovirus, has been known since 1983 to be the etiologic agent for acquired immunodeficiency syndrome (AIDS).
2. By coding for the enzyme reverse transcriptase, this virus inserts itself into the cellular genome and causes persistent and latent infection.
3. Although the virus may be found in all body fluids, only blood, semen, and vaginal secretions have been implicated in transmission.
4. Although there are no overt symptoms during the asymptomatic phase, the virus continues to replicate, infects more host cells, and progressively destroys cellular immunity.
5. There are three known routes of transmission.
   a. Sexual transmission (anal, oral, or vaginal intercourse)
   b. Blood or blood products (transfusions, infected needles)
   c. Perinatal transmission (in utero, at delivery, or via breast-feeding)
6. In the United States there are more than 640,000 cases of AIDS and an estimated 1.5 million people infected with HIV who are asymptomatic.
7. The World Health Organization estimates that over 10 million people worldwide are HIV infected.
8. Whereas homosexual men and IV drug users account for the majority of HIV/AIDS cases in the United States, AIDS is expected to be a predominantly heterosexual disease by the end of the 1990s.

Symptoms and Clinical Findings

1. Asymptomatic HIV patients must have had no previous signs or symptoms attributable to HIV infection.
2. History may be suggestive of an acute mononucleosis or influenza-like syndrome with or without aseptic meningitis.

Laboratory Tests

1. A positive enzyme-linked immunosorbent assay (ELISA) test followed by a positive Western blot test confirms HIV infection.
2. After confirmation of HIV-seropositive status, CD4 and CD8 lymphocyte subsets and HIV-1 RNA (viral load copies/milliliter) are used to stage HIV infection.
3. Other initial laboratory evaluations should include complete blood count, comprehensive chemistry panel, rapid plasma reagin, hepatitis B profile, *Toxoplasma gondii* and cytomegalovirus titers, tuberculin skin test, and β-human chorionic gonadotropin (women).

Key Tests

- ELISA for HIV antibodies
- Western blot test
- CD4 and CD8 lymphocyte counts
- HIV-1 RNA

Differential Diagnosis

1. The acute primary infection phase of HIV may be confused with mononucleosis, influenza, or a number of acute self-limited viral illnesses that have associated fever, myalgias, sore throat, and generalized skin rash.
2. Only a high index of suspicion of HIV exposure would suggest HIV infection; clinical findings in the asymptomatic stage are completely lacking.

Treatment

1. Treatment for asymptomatic patients is directed toward controlling viral replication and preventing opportunistic infections, and
   a. Should be considered for all HIV patients who have detectable HIV-1 RNA if the patient requests treatment and is committed to lifelong adherence to therapy.
   b. Is recommended for all HIV patients with CD4 cell counts below 500/mm^3 or HIV-1 RNA levels greater than 5000 to 10,000 copies/ml regardless of CD4 cell count.
   c. May be deferred for patients with low HIV-1 RNA levels and high CD4 counts (with reevaluation every 3 to 6 months).
2. Decision to treat asymptomatic patients must be balanced between

a. Benefits of early intervention

b. Cost and availability of treatment options

c. Complexity and side effects of treatment regimens

d. Potential for developing drug-resistant viral strains if adherence is not strictly maintained.

3. Initial treatment regimens should be aggressive and include combinations of nucleoside reverse transcriptase inhibitors (NRTI), protease inhibitors (PI), and non-nucleoside reverse transcriptase inhibitors (NNRTI).

a. NRTI-1, and NRTI-2, and PI (recommended)

b. NRTI-1, and NRTI-2, and NNRTI (alternative)

4. Prophylaxis for opportunistic infections should be considered when CD4 cell counts fall below 200 (*Pneumocystis carinii*) or below 100 (*Cryptococcus, Toxoplasma, Mycobacterium avium*, esophageal candidiasis).

Diet

1. Patients with asymptomatic HIV infection should follow good general nutrition principles, choosing foods from all major food groups daily. Multivitamin supplementation is recommended.

2. Care must be taken to prevent possible exposures to potentially deadly gastrointestinal pathogens (particularly *Campylobacter*, *Listeria*, and *Salmonella*). Avoid nonpasteurized milk products and rare or undercooked meats.

Activity

1. Regular aerobic exercise, in moderation only, is encouraged because of its beneficial effects on immune function.

2. Extreme exercise regimens (e.g., marathon racing) may damage the immune system and are generally discouraged.

Patient Education

1. Education of patients with HIV and those people at risk for HIV exposure has proved to be the only effective means of prevention.

2. Patients should be cautioned to use "safer sex" practices.

3. Consistent use of latex condoms, preferably with nonoxynol-9, a viricidal spermacide, is recommended to prevent sexual transmission of HIV. Petroleum-based lubricants should be avoided because they increase the risk of condom rupture.

4. Sexual partner notification of risk of HIV exposure is essential to prevent transmission.

Key Treatment (Asymptomatic)

- HIV-1 RNA viral load greater than 5000 to 10,000 copies/ml: *recommend* aggressive treatment.

- HIV-1 RNA viral load detectable, less than 5000 copies/ml: *consider* aggressive treatment.

- HIV-1 RNA viral load low and CD4 cell high: may *defer* treatment with close follow-up. *Note*: aggressive treatment consists of two NRTIs and one PI.

Follow-Up

1. Follow-up intervals depend on changes in clinical and laboratory parameters.

a. For high CD4 cell counts and low or undetectable viral loads, patients should be reevaluated every 6 to 12 months.

b. For patients with low CD4 cell counts and high viral loads, follow-up should be every 3 months.

2. For patients with rapidly declining CD4 counts, rapidly rising viral loads, or the onset of symptoms (e.g., persistent generalized lymphadenopathy, oral candidiasis, herpes zoster), more frequent follow-up is indicated.

3. Recommended routine immunizations include tetanus-diphtheria, measles-mumps-rubella (MMR), *Haemophilus influenzae*, type B conjugated vaccine, pneumococcal, influenza, hepatitis B vaccine, and enhanced inactivated poliovirus vaccine. Avoid live attenuated vaccines except MMR. More frequent boosters are often indicated.

4. Visits for psychosocial evaluation may also be indicated because of the incidence of family dysfunction, depression, and suicide associated with HIV infection.

Bibliography

Carpenter CCJ, Fischl MA, Hammer SM, et al: Antiretroviral therapy for HIV infection in 1997; updated recommendations of the International AIDS Society–USA Panel. JAMA 1997;277:1962–1969.

Fauci AS: Multifactorial nature of human immunodeficiency virus disease: implications for therapy. Science 1993;262:1011–1018.

Ho DD: Viral counts count in HIV infection. Science 1996;272:1124–1125.

Mellors JW, Kingsley LA, Rinaldo CR, et al: Quantitation of HIV-1 RNA in plasma predicts outcome after seroconversion. Ann Intern Med 1995;122:573–579.

O'Brien WA, Hartigan PM, Martin D, et al: Changes in plasma HIV-1 RNA and CD4+ lymphocytes and the risk of progression to AIDS. N Engl J Med 1996;334:426–431.

206 Early Symptomatic HIV Infection

Linda L. Krishna

Etiology

1. Human immunodeficiency virus (HIV) is spread via contact with parenteral/bodily fluids.
2. HIV binds to CD4 protein receptors on T-helper lymphocytes as well as monocytes, macrophages, and other cells.
3. With disease progression, CD4 lymphocyte counts decrease. Below 200 cells/μl, there is increased risk of opportunistic infections. Also, immune complexes may lead to renal disease, vasculitis, myalgias, arthralgias, and thrombocytopenias.
4. Early symptomatic HIV infection usually occurs when CD4 counts begin to decrease and CD4/CD8 ratio inverts.

Symptoms

1. Weight loss
2. Night sweats
3. Fever/chills
4. Fatigue/malaise
5. Lymphadenopathy
6. Changes in cognition
7. Personality change
8. Cough, shortness of breath
9. Myalgia/arthralgia
10. Paresthesias
11. Oral lesions/ulcers
12. Abdominal discomfort
13. Diarrhea
14. Vesicular skin lesions
15. Skin rashes

Key Symptoms

- Weight loss
- Fever, chills, sweats
- Diarrhea
- Lymphadenopathy
- Oral ulcers/lesions
- Skin rashes/lesions
- Fatigue/malaise
- Myalgias/arthralgias

Clinical Findings

1. Generalized wasting
2. Hairy leukoplakia
3. Oral candidiasis
4. Periodontal disease
5. Oral herpes
6. Aphthous ulcers
7. Cotton wool spots
8. Lymphadenopathy
9. Hepatosplenomegaly
10. Herpes zoster
11. Tinea infections
12. Seborrheic dermatitis
13. Folliculitis/acne
14. Rashes
15. Myopathy
16. Neuropathy
17. Genital lesions
18. Ataxia
19. Decreased cognition
20. Depression

Key Signs

- Generalized wasting
- Hairy leukoplakia
- Oral candidiasis
- Lymphadenopathy
- Skin rashes
- Tinea infections
- Decreased cognition
- Myopathy
- Neuropathy

Laboratory Tests

1. HIV diagnosis: Seroconversion is nearly always within 3 to 6 months of HIV exposure.
   a. HIV enzyme-linked immunosorbent assay (ELISA)
   b. Western blot for confirmation
2. Follow up with periodic CD4 counts and HIV-1 RNA quantitative viral load
3. Complete blood count (CBC) with differential
4. Chemistry panel (SMA-20)
5. Stool studies, if indicated (ovum and parasites, routine culture, fecal leukocytes, *Clostridium difficile* toxin, colon biopsy if other tests are negative)

6. Purified protein derivative (PPD) with control and baseline chest radiograph
7. Pap smears and sexually transmitted disease screening
8. Serologic tests for syphilis: rapid plasma reagin (RPR) or Venereal Disease Research Laboratory (VDRL)
9. Biopsies of uncertain skin and mucous membrane lesions
10. Sputum for culture, acid-fast, *Pneumocystis carinii* smear, if indicated
11. Iron studies, B_{12}, folate
12. Cerebrospinal fluid studies if indicated
13. Antinuclear antibodies, sedimentation rate
14. *Toxoplasma gondii* immunoglobulin G antibodies (IgGAb)
15. Hepatitis B surface antigen

 Key Tests

- ELISA/Western blot
- CD4 count
- HIV-1 RNA viral load
- CBC with differential
- Stool studies
- *Toxoplasma gondii* antibodies

Differential Diagnosis

1. Lymphoma
2. Leukemia
3. Other cancers
4. Tuberculosis
5. Malabsorption syndromes
6. Fungal/viral infections
7. Pneumonias
8. Mononucleosis
9. Systemic lupus erythematosus/rheumatologic disorders
10. Subacute bacterial endocarditis

Treatment

Medication

1. Antiretroviral medications: indicated for HIV-1 RNA plasma loads of 5000 to 10,000 copies/ml or CD4 counts less than $500/\mu l$, or for evidence of primary HIV infection, central nervous system disease, or acquired immunodeficiency syndrome–defining illness
   a. Initial regimen recommended by National Institutes of Health is two nucleoside analogue reverse transcriptase inhibitors plus one protease inhibitor or one non-nucleoside reverse transcriptase inhibitor.
      (1) Nucleoside analogue reverse transcriptase inhibitors
         (a) Zidovudine (AZT, Retrovir): 200 mg tid or 300 mg bid. Can cause anemia, nausea, insomnia.
         (b) Didanosine (ddI, Videx): 200 mg bid (if <60 kg, 125 mg bid). Can cause neuropathy, pancreatitis.
         (c) Lamivudine (3TC, Epivir): 150 mg bid (if <50 kg, 2 mg/kg bid). Can cause restlessness, insomnia.
         (d) Stavudine (d4T, Zerit): 40 mg bid (if <60 kg, 30 mg bid). Can cause neuropathy.
         (e) Zalcitabine (ddC, Hivid): 0.75 mg tid. Can cause neuropathy, oral ulcers, rash.
      (2) Non-nucleoside reverse transcriptase inhibitors
         (a) Delavirdine (Rescriptor): 400 mg tid. Can cause rash.
         (b) Nevirapine (Viramune): 200 mg bid. Can cause rash.
      (3) Protease inhibitors
         (a) Indinavir (Crixivan): 800 mg every 8 hours. Can cause nephrolithiasis, hyperbilirubinemia.
         (b) Nelfinavir (Viracept): 750 mg tid. Can cause diarrhea, rash.
         (c) Ritonavir (Norvir): 600 mg bid. Can cause nausea, vomiting, diarrhea, anorexia.
         (d) Saquinavir (Fortase, Invirase): 600 mg tid (hard gelcap) or 1200 mg tid (soft gelcap) Can cause nausea, diarrhea.
   b. Alternate therapy if failure to initial regimen occurs; use two different nucleoside analogues plus different protease inhibitor or non-nucleoside reverse transcriptase inhibitor.
2. *Pneumocystis carinii* pneumonia (PCP) prophylaxis: for CD4 count less than 200 cells/μl, HIV-related thrush, unexplained fever for 2 weeks, or previous PCP infection.
   a. Trimethoprim-sulfamethoxazole (TMP-SMZ) (Bactrim, Septra): one DS tablet/day, *or*
   b. Dapsone: 100 mg/day, *or*
   c. Aerosolized pentamidine: 300 mg monthly
3. *Toxoplasma gondii* prophylaxis: for CD4 count near 100 cells/μl or seropositive for IgGAb

a. TMP-SMZ: one DS tablet/day, *or*

b. Dapsone, 50 mg/day, plus pyrimethamine, 50 mg/week, plus leucovorin calcium, 25 mg/week

4. *Mycobacterium tuberculosis* prophylaxis: for PPD greater than 5 mm, prior untreated positive PPD, or active tuberculosis exposure

   a. Isoniazid, 300 mg/day plus pyridoxine HCl, 50 mg/day, for 12 months, *or*

   b. Rifampin: 600 mg/day for 12 months

5. *Mycobacterium avium* complex prophylaxis: for CD4 count less than 50 cells/μl

   a. Clarithromycin (Biaxin): 500 mg bid, *or*

   b. Azithromycin (Zithromax): 1200 mg a week, *or*

   c. Rifabutin (Mycobutin): 300 mg/day

6. *Candida albicans* (oral)

   a. Ketoconazole (Nizoral): 400 mg/day for 14 days, then 200 mg/day for 7 consecutive days a month

   b. Fluconazole (Diflucan): 100 to 200 mg/day for 14 days, then 100 to 200 mg/week

7. Diarrhea: symptomatic treatment

   a. Imodium, 4 mg orally, then 2 mg orally every 6 hours or prn

   b. Lomotil, 2.5 to 5 mg orally 3 to 6 times per day, then tid or prn

   c. Paregoric (0.4 mg morphine/ml), 5 to 10 ml orally every day qid or prn

   d. Octreotide (Sandostatin), 100 μg subcutaneously tid, then increase for a maximum of 500 μg subcutaneously qid

8. Weight loss

   a. Megestrol (Megace), 80 mg orally tid (maximum 800 mg orally daily)

   b. Dronabinol (tetrahydrocannabinol, Marinol), 2.5 mg orally bid before meals

Vaccines

1. Pneumococcal
2. Yearly influenza
3. Hepatitis series (if seronegative and at risk)
4. Tetanus-diphtheria every 10 years
5. Hepatitis A (if at risk)

Diet

High protein, calories, vitamins, minerals, with small, frequent meals and generous fluids.

Activity

As tolerated. Increased physical activity has not been shown to increase HIV progression.

Patient Education

1. Explain natural course of HIV and manifestations.
2. Explain safe sex/abstinence and encourage patient to inform appropriate others to be tested for HIV.
3. Educate/assist with housing, financial assistance, counseling.
4. Inform patient of the state's HIV reporting requirements.
5. Educate about oral/skin care, laboratory tests and follow-up, medication side-effects and specific instructions, and strict medication compliance to decrease viral resistance.

Key Treatment

Recommended Nucleoside Analogue Combinations

- Zidovudine + didanosine
- Zidovudine + zalcitabine
- Zidovudine + lamivudine
- Didanosine + stavudine
- Stavudine + lamivudine
- Use one of above combinations with a protease inhibitor or a non-nucleoside reverse transcriptase inhibitor

Alternative Drugs

- Two different nucleoside analogue combinations *and*
- One different protease inhibitor or non-nucleoside reverse transcriptase inhibitor

---

Follow-Up

1. CD4 count: every 6 months for CD4 greater than 600 cells/μl, every 3 months for CD4 count greater than 200 and less than 600, every 3 months for CD4 less than 200 to assess antiretroviral therapy's effect
2. HIV-1 RNA viral load every 3 to 4 months. More frequent for change in medications
3. High risk: regular PPD, chest radiograph
4. VDRL or RPR every year or less if indicated. If patient had previous syphilis, follow up with nontreponemal serologies at 1, 2, 3, 6, 9, and 12 months after treatment and annually afterward.

5. Regular oral, funduscopic, dental, physical, and pelvic examinations.

Bibliography

Early HIV Infection Guideline Panel (Wafaa El-Sadr, et al): Managing early HIV infection. Am Fam Physician 1994;49:801–814.

Goldschmidt RH, Dong BJ: Treatment of AIDS, and HIV-related conditions. J Am Board Fam Pract 1994;7(2): 155–175.

Maenza J, Flexner C: Combination antiretroviral therapy for HIV infection. Am Fam Physician 1998;57:2789–2798.

Myers RA: Outpatient management of HIV-infected adults. Postgrad Med 1998;103:219–228.

Polsky B: Human immunodeficiency virus infection and its complications. In Rakel RE (ed): Conn's Current Therapy 1998, pp 43–55. Philadelphia, WB Saunders Company, 1998.

207 Late Symptomatic HIV Infection

Philip C. Johnson

Etiology

1. *Definition*: CD4 cell count less than 300/mm³
2. Progressive destruction of CD4 cells by human immunodeficiency virus (HIV) infection places the person at risk for
   a. Opportunistic infection and routine infections
   b. Malignancies (e.g., Kaposi's sarcoma, B cell lymphoma)
   c. Sequelae related to immune imbalance
      (1) Drug allergies and sinusitis
      (2) Wasting syndrome

Symptoms

1. Depend on reactivation of previous infectious diseases or exposures to new infections.
2. Fever invariably seen with infectious diseases.
3. Other symptoms depend on the organ systems affected.
4. Headache: May be associated with fever.
5. Seizures
6. Blindness and blurred vision
7. Dyspnea
8. Diarrhea
9. Weight loss
   a. Febrile illnesses
   b. Odynophagia and dysphagia
   c. *Mycobacterium avium* complex
      (1) Presents with abdominal complaints and fever.
      (2) CD4 count less than 100/mm³.

Key Symptoms

- Headache
- Seizures
- Blindness and blurred vision
- Dyspnea
- Diarrhea
- Weight loss

Clinical Findings

1. Tachypnea
   a. Best early indication of a pulmonary process
   b. May be seen in septic shock.
   c. Pulse oximetry not useful because most patients maintain adequate oxygen saturation by increasing their respiratory rate; check arterial blood gas.
2. Oral lesions
   a. Candidiasis: reddened satellite lesions or cottage cheese–like plaques
   b. Herpes simplex: shallow-based ulcers
3. Retinitis and papilledema
4. Dullness on chest percussion
   a. Pleural effusions unlikely in *Pneumocystis carinii* pneumonia (PCP).
   b. Can be seen with other pulmonary processes.
5. Hepatomegaly, splenomegaly, and lymphadenopathy
6. Cranial nerve palsies

Key Signs

- Tachypnea
- Retinitis and papilledema
- Dullness on chest percussion
- Hepatomegaly, splenomegaly, and lymphadenopathy
- Cranial nerve palsies

Laboratory Tests

1. CD4 cell count is main indicator, but it can vary widely.
2. Tests for specific diseases
   a. Aphthous ulcers: Exclude herpes simplex and cytomegalovirus (CMV)
   b. Candidiasis: smear and culture in difficult cases
   c. *Coccidioides immitis*
      (1) Culture
      (2) Spherule found in bronchial secretions or sputum
      (3) Serology is useful.
      (4) Skin testing invariably negative.
   d. Community-acquired pneumonia

(1) Lobular infiltrate on chest radiograph

(2) Gram's stain with bacterial organisms

(3) Resident oral flora influenced by antibiotics

e. Cryptococcal meningitis

(1) Cryptococcal antigen in serum or cerebrospinal fluid (CSF) positive in 97 per cent.

(2) India ink test of CSF positive in 75 per cent.

(3) Fungal culture

f. CMV

(1) Viral culture with determination of CMV early antigen

(2) CMV immunoglobulin M (IgM) serology

(3) Pathology: frequently negative

g. Diarrhea

(1) Fecal leukocytes indicate diffuse colonic inflammation.

(2) Bacterial, acid-fast bacilli (AFB) culture

(3) Parasite examination, including *Cryptosporidium parvum*

(4) *Clostridium difficile* toxin assay

h. Kaposi's sarcoma of the lung: Bronchoscopy

i. *Mycobacterium avium* complex

(1) Lysis centrifugation blood culture

(2) Bone marrow culture and smear

(3) Stool culture

j. PCP pneumonia

(1) Interstitial infiltrates on chest roentgenogram

(2) Elevated lactate dehydrogenase (LDH)

(3) Increased A-a gradient on arterial blood gas analysis

(4) Sputum or pulmonary secretions show organism after Giemsa staining.

(5) Atypical presentations for people taking aerosolized pentamidine prophylaxis

k. Progressive disseminated histoplasmosis

(1) *Histoplasma capsulatum* antigen by radioimmunoassay (RIA) of urine or serum

(2) Lysis centrifugation blood culture

(3) Bone marrow examination or peripheral smear shows yeast.

(4) Biopsy of skin lesions

(5) Elevated LDH, ferritin

l. Progressive multifocal leukoencephalopathy

(1) Fluffy or diffuse non–contrast-enhancing subcortical white matter lesions on

computerized tomography (CT) of brain

(2) Brain biopsy

(3) No treatment, and so empiric treatment of toxoplasmosis is usually tried first.

m. Toxoplasmosis

(1) Multiple spherical ring-enhancing lesions with mass effect on CT of brain

(2) *Toxoplasma* serology helpful if there is a seroconversion.

(3) *Toxoplasma* IgM-positive

(4) Response to empiric therapy establishes the diagnosis. It usually takes 2 weeks.

n. Tuberculosis

(1) AFB smear and culture

(2) Knowledge about purified protein derivative (PPD) status or exposures

(3) Diagnosis of tuberculosis meningitis is difficult—CSF sugar normal or low, CSF protein modest increase, lymphocytic pleocytosis.

Key Tests

- CD4 cell count
- HIV RNA by polymerase chain reaction (viral load)
- Fecal leukocytes
- Chest radiograph
- Cryptococcal antigen
- Lumbar puncture with opening pressure
- Lysis centrifugation blood culture
- Fiberoptic bronchoscopy
- *Histoplasma capsulatum* antigen by RIA
- Automated chemistry
- Arterial blood gases
- CT of brain

Differential Diagnosis

1. Side effects from medications

2. Other infectious disease processes or multiple infections

   a. Cryptococcal meningitis

   (1) Cranial nerve palsies

   (2) Nuchal rigidity

   (3) Headache that improves after spinal tap and relief of increased intracranial pressure

   (4) Blurred vision and papilledema

   b. Toxoplasmosis

   c. Progressive multifocal leukoencephalopathy

d. B cell lymphoma
e. Tuberculosis
f. CMV retinitis
g. PCP
h. Progressive disseminated histoplasmosis
i. *Coccidioides immitis*
j. Kaposi's sarcoma of the lung
k. Community-acquired pneumonia
l. Mucocutaneous candidiasis
m. Oral herpes
n. Aphthous ulcers
o. Malabsorption
p. Hepatitis B or C
q. *Mycobacterium avium* complex
r. Syphilis

Treatment

Primary Therapy for HIV

1. Most people have already started therapy by this time.
2. Treatment for HIV requires three-drug regimens, including one choice each from the protease inhibitor and the nucleoside reverse transcriptase inhibitor options listed below. Drugs are listed in random, not priority order.
   a. Protease inhibitors
      (1) Indinavir
      (2) Nelfinavir
      (3) Ritonavir
      (4) Saquinavir soft gel capsule
      (5) Ritonavir and saquinavir
      (6) Agenerase
   b. Nucleoside reverse transcriptase inhibitors
      (1) Zidovudine and didanosine
      (2) Stavudine and didanosine (potent)
      (3) Zidovudine and zalcitabine
      (4) Zidovudine and lamivudine (potent)
      (5) Stavudine and lamivudine (potent)
3. Alternative: Efavirenz, a non-nucleoside reverse transcriptase inhibitor + two nucleoside reverse transcriptase inhibitors (2b above)
4. Not generally recommended
   a. Two nucleoside reverse transcriptase inhibitors
   b. Saquinavir hard gel capsule and two nucleoside reverse transcriptase inhibitors
5. Not recommended
   a. Monotherapy
   b. Stavudine and zidovudine
   c. Zalcitabine and didanosine

d. Zalcitabine and stavudine
e. Zalcitabine and lamivudine

Prophylaxis

1. Candidiasis
   a. Clotrimazole (Mycelex) troches tid
   b. Nystatin swish and swallow tid
   c. Ketoconazole (Nizoral), 200 mg orally daily, on an empty stomach with citrus juice
2. Herpes simplex: acyclovir (Zovirax), 200 mg orally tid
3. Influenza: yearly vaccination
4. *Mycobacterium avium* complex: Rifabutin (Mycobutin), 300 mg orally daily when CD4 count less than 100/mm^3
5. PCP
   a. Use when CD4 count less than 200/mm^3 or CD4 cells less than 20 per cent.
   b. Trimethoprim-sulfamethoxazole (TMP-SMX) (Bactrim, Septra), one double-strength tablet orally every Monday, Wednesday, and Friday
   c. Dapsone, 100 mg every Monday, Wednesday, and Friday
   d. Aerosolized pentamidine, 300 mg via Respirgard nebulizer
6. Pneumococcal pneumonia: vaccination once in a lifetime
7. Tuberculosis: isoniazid, 300 mg orally daily for 1 year of PPD-positive or at high risk
8. Varicella zoster: acyclovir, 800 mg bid

Treatment of Opportunistic Infections

1. Aphthous ulcers
   a. Symptomatic therapy
   b. Trial therapy for CMV if lesions severe
2. Candidiasis
   a. Clotrimazole (Mycelex) troches, q4h
   b. Ketoconazole (Nizoral), 200 mg orally daily, taken on empty stomach with citrus juice
   c. Fluconazole (Diflucan), 200 mg orally daily (most expensive option)
3. *Coccidioides immitis*
   a. Amphotericin B, 2.5-g total dose
   b. Suppression therapy with fluconazole, 400 mg orally daily
4. Community-acquired pneumonia: Cefotaxime (Claforan), 2 gm intravenously q8h, plus erythromycin, 500 mg intravenously q6h
5. Cryptococcal meningitis
   a. Amphotericin B, 0.7 mg/kg intravenously for 14 days, then fluconazole, 400 mg

orally daily for suppression; if flucytosine used with amphotericin B, 100 mg/kg q6h.

b. Control of intracranial pressure is vital to prevent complications.

(1) Measure opening pressure initially.

(2) If more than 18 cm H_2O, remove enough CSF to decrease pressure.

(3) Retap with symptoms of headache, meningismus, or cranial nerve palsies.

(4) Some patients require a lumboperitoneal shunt.

(5) Increased intracranial pressure can occur after successful treatment is started.

(6) Risk of herniation even with very high pressures is extremely small.

6. CMV

a. Ganciclovir (Cytovene), 5.0 mg/kg intravenously q12h for 2 weeks, then 6.0 mg/kg intravenously daily for 5 days each week

b. Foscarnet (Foscavir), 60 mg/kg intravenously (infuse over 2 hours) q8h for 2 to 3 weeks, then 90 to 120 mg/kg intravenously daily

7. Diarrhea

a. Trial of ciprofloxacin (Cipro), 500 mg orally q12h for 5 days, and metronidazole (Flagyl), 250 mg orally q8h for 7 days unless specific pathogen is known

b. Symptomatic treatment with loperamide, 2 mg orally q4h as needed, in the absence of dysentery

8. Kaposi's sarcoma of the lung

a. Liposomal daunorubicin

b. Do not give next dose until white cell count exceeds 4000/mm³.

9. *Mycobacterium avium* complex

a. All regimens have clarithromycin, 500 to 1000 mg orally q12h (azithromycin is a second-line agent).

b. In addition, one or more of the following drugs

(1) Ciprofloxacin, 500 mg orally q12h

(2) Rifabutin, 300 mg orally daily

(3) Ethambutol, 15 mg/kg orally daily

(4) Amikacin (Amikin), 7.5 mg/kg intravenously daily

10. PCP

a. TMP-SMX (Bactrim, Septra), two double-strength tablets q6h for 21 days, or TMP-SMX IV (equivalent of TMP 5 mg/kg daily intravenously q6h) for 21 days

b. Atovaquone (Mepron), 750 mg orally q8h

(1) Take with food; food increases absorption.

(2) Mild cases only

c. Dapsone, 100 mg orally daily, and trimethoprim, 5 mg/kg orally q6h for 21 days

d. Pentamidine isethionate

(1) Four mg/kg intravenously daily

(2) Aerosolized 600 mg via Respirgard nebulizer daily for 14 days

e. Prednisone, 40 mg orally q12h (or equivalent) for 5 days; then 40 mg orally daily for 5 days, then 20 mg orally daily for remainder of PCP therapy if:

(1) PCP documented

(2) pO_2 under 60 mm Hg on room air

11. Progressive disseminated histoplasmosis

a. Amphotericin, 0.7 mg/kg IV daily until stable, then itraconazole, 200 mg orally q12h

b. Itraconazole (Sporanox), 200 mg orally q12h if patient is stable

12. Progressive multifocal leukoencephalopathy

a. Empiric treatment for toxoplasmosis usually tried for 2 weeks

b. High-dose zidovudine and cytarabine (experimental treatment)

13. Toxoplasmosis

a. Pyrimethamine, 50 to 75 mg orally daily, and clindamycin, 450 mg orally q8h (or 600 mg intravenously q6h), plus folinic acid, 10 mg orally daily

b. Sulfisoxazole can be added if patient is allergic to pyrimethamine or clindamycin.

c. Steroids are needed if there is brain edema on CT.

14. Tuberculosis: combination therapy

a. Isoniazid, 300 mg orally daily, with pyridoxine, 25 mg orally daily

b. Rifampin, 600 mg orally daily; rifabutin if on protease inhibitors

c. Pyrazinamide, 15 to 25 mg/kg/day

d. Ethambutol, 15 mg/kg/day

e. Can simplify regimen when susceptibility is known.

Follow-Up

1. All infections and malignancies are likely to be chronic and recurrent at this stage.

2. Resistance to treatment develops.

Bibliography

Bartlett JG: Antiretroviral therapy in HIV-infected patients: update. Infect Dis Clin Pract 1994;3:340–344.

Carpenter CC, Fische MA, Hammer SM, et al: Antiretroviral therapy for HIV infection in 1998: updated recommendations of the International AIDS Society–USA Panel. JAMA 1998;280:78–86.

Cohen PT, Sande MA, Volberding PA (eds): The AIDS Knowledge Base, 3rd ed. Philadelphia, Lippincott Williams & Wilkins, 1999. (also available at *http://hivinsite.ucsf.edu*)

Hammer SM, Kessler HA, Saag MS: Issues in combination antiretroviral therapy: a review. JAIDS 1994;7(Suppl 2):524–537.

Sande MA, Gilbert DN, Moellering RC: The Sanford Guide to HIV/AIDS Therapy. Hyde Park, VT, Antimicrobial Therapy, Inc, 1999.

208 Drug Allergy

Stephen F. Kemp

Etiology

1. The risk of an allergic reaction for most drugs is 1 to 3 per cent. Between 15 and 30 per cent of hospitalized patients experience adverse drug reactions (up to 0.3 per cent may be fatal) and 0.2 to 29.3 per cent of outpatients require hospitalizations for adverse drug reactions.

2. Any drug or biologic agent potentially can cause an adverse reaction.

   a. At least 80 per cent of adverse drug reactions are type A reactions, which are common and predictable. These reactions include

      (1) *Overdosage or toxicity*: an exaggerated but characteristic effect from an excessive dose

      (2) *Side effects*: excessive expressions of known pharmacologic effects of a drug that can occur at recommended dosages

      (3) *Drug interactions*: can occur when a patient takes two or more medications.

   b. Type B adverse drug reactions are uncommon, unpredictable, and occur only in particularly susceptible patients. These reactions include

      (1) *Intolerance*: an undesirable outcome that occurs at a subtherapeutic dosage

      (2) *Idiosyncratic reaction*: an uncharacteristic response to the administration of a drug

   c. *Allergic reaction* or *hypersensitivity*: These reactions occur in small numbers of patients (6 to 10 per cent of adverse drug reactions), and they require previous exposure to the same or a chemically related drug. They develop rapidly after re-exposure and produce clinical syndromes commonly associated with immunologic reactions.

3. Allergic reactions associated with specific drugs

   a. β-Lactam antibiotics are responsible for most allergic drug reactions.

   b. Sulfonamides most commonly cause maculopapular eruptions, but urticaria, erythema multiforme, and potentially life-threatening mucocutaneous reactions, such as Stevens-Johnson syndrome (SJS) and toxic epidermal necrolysis (TEN), may occasionally occur. Clinical cross-reactivity with structurally similar compounds is rare.

   c. "Red man syndrome" is a dose-dependent reaction to vancomycin that is characterized by generalized erythema, pruritus, and a diffuse burning sensation. Vancomycin directly stimulates cutaneous mast cells to release histamine and other mediators, and a decrease in the rate of vancomycin infusion will reduce or prevent symptoms for most affected patients.

   d. Aspirin and other nonsteroidal anti-inflammatory drugs (NSAIDs) may cause nonimmunologic drug reactions such as gastrointestinal irritation/bleeding, renal insufficiency, and hepatotoxicity. Immunologic drug reactions include urticaria/angioedema, respiratory sensitivity, and anaphylaxis. Excessive leukotriene production is the most commonly proposed mechanism. Aspirin desensitization and/or treatment with a leukotriene-modifying agent may reduce respiratory sensitivity.

   e. Angiotensin-converting enzyme (ACE) inhibitors may produce syndromes of cough or angioedema via inhibition of bradykinin and substance P metabolism. Life-threatening angioedema may potentially occur any time during treatment. ACE inhibitors should not be given to patients with any history of angioedema. Anaphylaxis associated with ACE inhibitors has also been reported.

   f. β-Blockers may cause bronchospasm in patients with underlying bronchial hyperreactivity. Patients at risk for anaphylaxis should not take β-blockers because these agents competitively inhibit epinephrine.

   g. Anticonvulsants are frequent causes of maculopapular eruptions and serum sickness, and they have also been associated with hepatic necrosis, aplastic anemia, and the anticonvulsant hypersensitivity syndrome.

   h. Local anesthetic reactions usually result from vasovagal syncope, anxiety, overdosage, accidental intravenous injection, or systemic effects of the epinephrine contained in many preparations. Immunologic reactions to local anesthetics are exceedingly rare.

i. Radiocontrast media (RCM), opiates, and thiamine cause mast cell histamine release by non–immunoglobulin E (IgE)-mediated mechanisms. Repeat reactions to RCM occur in 15 to 30 per cent of patients who again receive RCM without premedication.

j. Hemolytic anemia and drug-induced lupus may result from autoantibodies formed in response to drugs such as methyldopa or penicillamine. Drug cessation usually provides rapid relief of symptoms.

Symptoms and Clinical Findings

The patient history and the nature of the reaction frequently will suggest the culprit drug and the likelihood of a recurrence upon subsequent administration. Most allergic reactions have cutaneous manifestations with or without other immunologic features.

1. Urticaria/angioedema: an IgE-mediated mechanism predicts recurrence upon subsequent administration. Mast cell degranulation in the superficial dermis and deep dermis produces urticaria and angioedema, respectively.

2. Maculopapular and morbilliform eruptions: These are the most common drug-induced cutaneous reactions. These eruptions are symmetric, frequently confluent macules and papules that typically spare the palms and soles. β-Lactam antibiotics, sulfonamides, anticonvulsants, NSAIDs, and allopurinol are particularly common causes. These eruptions may occur in 50 to 80 per cent of patients with concomitant viral infections or leukemia. Progression to SJS or TEN is rare.

3. Phototoxic or photoallergic dermatitis: These are toxic or immunologically mediated eruptions, respectively, and both require activation by light.

4. Allergic contact dermatitis: This is the most common example of drug-induced delayed hypersensitivity. It is an eczematous eruption caused by a medication applied topically to the skin. Sensitization usually requires 5 to 7 days of drug exposure, but subsequent application of the drug may elicit dermatitis within 24 hours.

5. SJS and TEN: Potentially lethal mucocutaneous reactions for which drugs are associated with 50 per cent of cases; sulfonamides, NSAIDs, allopurinol, and anticonvulsants account for two thirds of these drug-associated cases. Viral infections, such as herpes, may also be responsible.

6. Serum sickness: This syndrome, which is due to immune complex (immunoglobulin G) tissue deposition, may develop 1 to 3 weeks after drug or heterologous serum administration. It is most frequently associated with fever, arthralgias, urticaria, and malaise.

Key Signs and Symptoms

- Urticaria/angioedema
- Maculopapular/ morbilliform eruptions
- Eczematous eruption
- Anaphylaxis
- Generalized pruritus
- Fever
- Hepatic/renal insufficiency
- Anemia
- Arthralgias
- Oral or other mucosal ulceration

Diagnostic Testing

1. Published protocols are available for the diagnosis and management of a number of drugs and biologic agents. General goals are to stop the reaction and simultaneously identify both the culprit drug and a therapeutic alternative. The most recently administered drug is usually implicated, but any drug administered within 3 weeks of the reaction should be considered.

2. Allergy skin testing: Detection of drug-specific IgE antibody enables the prediction of subsequent IgE-mediated drug reactions to some drugs and biologic agents. Skin testing is not useful for detecting allergic reactions caused by haptens. Routine penicillin skin testing can facilitate the safe use of penicillin in up to 90 per cent of patients with a previous history of penicillin allergy.

3. Drug-specific IgE must be clinically relevant to be useful. For example, IgE anti-insulin antibodies are common in patients who receive insulin, but allergic reactions to insulin are rare.

4. Patch testing may identify the cause of contact dermatitis.

5. Patients with purported drug allergy have usually experienced type A reactions for which dose modification or drug substitution may be adequate intervention. A small test dose may be administered for reassurance if a serious reaction after re-administration appears unlikely and if therapeutic alternatives are unavailable. These challenges should only be administered in a setting where drug reactions can be treated promptly and adequately.

- Drug cessation or dosage adjustment (type A reactions)
- Complete blood count, chemistries, serum drug levels (where indicated)
- Drug-specific allergy skin tests
- Patch testing (delayed-type skin hypersensitivity)
- Provocative dose challenge

Treatment

1. Treatment of adverse drug reactions
   a. Withdrawal of the drug may be the only treatment required.
   b. Anaphylaxis is an acute, life-threatening immunologic reaction that develops rapidly and includes generalized erythema, urticaria, angioedema, bronchospasm, laryngeal edema, hyperperistalsis, hypotension, or cardiac arrhythmias, alone or in combination.
      (1) The key to treatment of anaphylaxis is the early and appropriate use of 1:1000 epinephrine, 0.3 to 0.5 ml (0.01 ml/kg) SC or IM, repeated every 15 minutes as necessary.
      (2) Supplemental therapy may include oral or intravenous antihistamines (e.g., diphenhydramine, 1 to 2 mg/kg, up to 50 mg) and a short-acting corticosteroid (e.g., methylprednisolone, 1 to 2 mg/kg IV). Antihistamines and corticosteroids have limited effects on acute anaphylaxis but may prevent prolonged episodes or late-phase reactions that occur in some patients 6 to 18 hours after the initial episode.
      (3) Nebulized β-agonists may be useful for bronchospasm initially unresponsive to epinephrine.
   c. Morbilliform rashes or serum sickness may require 1 to 2 weeks of symptomatic treatment with antihistamines and/or systemic corticosteroids.
   d. Early use of corticosteroids in SJS may prevent visceral involvement. TEN is treated supportively, and prognosis depends on the amount of skin loss and visceral involvement.
   e. Maculopapular rashes often resolve spontaneously. However, any suggestion of SJS/TEN or anaphylaxis requires prompt treatment and immediate discontinuation of the offending drug.

2. Prevention of adverse drug reactions
   a. An alternative, chemically unrelated drug should be used if safe re-introduction of the culprit drug is impossible.
   b. Premedication may reduce the risk of subsequent *non*–IgE-mediated reactions. For example, the most common protocol for RCM premedication is prednisone, 50 mg administered 13 hours, 7 hours, and 1 hour before RCM; diphenhydramine, 1 mg/kg 1 hour before RCM; ephedrine, 25 mg orally 1 hour before RCM (contraindicated by hypertension or angina); and use of a lower osmolarity RCM.
   c. Short-term desensitization to antimicrobials, allopurinol, NSAIDs, and polypeptides (e.g., insulin) is frequently successful. If drug therapy is interrupted, however, allergic manifestations will appear again and anaphylaxis may potentially occur. Desensitization should be attempted only under the supervision of an experienced allergist-immunologist.
   d. Leukotriene-modifying agents may reduce respiratory sensitivity to NSAIDs.

- Discontinue offending drug.
- Epinephrine for anaphylaxis
- Antihistamines and/or corticosteroids for protracted anaphylaxis, serum sickness, or dermatitis
- Premedication for selected non–IgE-mediated reactions
- Short-term desensitization
- Leukotriene-modifying agent for NSAID respiratory sensitivity
- Therapeutic alternative (if necessary)
- Patient education
- Avoid unnecessary medication.

Follow-Up

1. Patients with adverse drug reactions should receive education in risk reduction.
2. Unnecessary medications should always be avoided.

3. Patients with a history of life-threatening reactions should wear a medical warning bracelet or neck chain and carry epinephrine syringes for self-administration.

4. The Food and Drug Administration (FDA) maintains a surveillance system for adverse drug reactions. Physicians who observe an adverse drug reaction should contact either the pharmaceutical manufacturer or the FDA. The FDA MedWatch telephone number is 1-800-FDA-1088.

Bibliography

deShazo RD, Kemp SF: Allergic reactions to drugs and biologic agents. JAMA 1997;278:1895–1906.

DeSwarte RD, Patterson R: Drug allergy. In Patterson R, Grammer LC, Greenberger PA (eds): Allergic Diseases: Diagnosis and Management, 5th ed, pp 317–412. Philadelphia, Lippincott-Raven, 1997.

Lazarou J, Pomeranz BH, Corey PN: Incidence of adverse drug reactions in hospitalized patients: a meta-analysis of prospective studies. JAMA 1998;279:1200–1205.

Patterson R, DeSwarte RD, Greenberger PA, et al: Drug Allergy and Protocols for Management of Drug Allergies, 2nd ed, pp 1–27. Providence, RI, OceanSide Publications, 1995.

Rawlins MD, Thompson W: Mechanisms of adverse drug reactions. In Davies DM (ed): Textbook of Adverse Drug Reactions, pp 18–45. New York, Oxford University Press, 1991.

209 Food Allergy

W. Anderson Nish

General

1. Adverse food reaction: any untoward reaction after the ingestion of a food
   a. "Food intolerances" account for most reactions and are not immunologically mediated.
   b. "Food allergies" refer to those reactions that are immunologically mediated.
2. Estimated incidence of food allergy is 4 per cent in children and 1 per cent in adults, although studies vary, and up to 40 per cent of adults report adverse food reactions.
3. The role of food allergy in some patients
   a. Established: atopic dermatitis, anaphylaxis, chronic urticaria, food protein gastroenteropathy, eosinophilic gastroenteritis
   b. Uncertain: migraine, chronic asthma or rhinitis, irritable bowel syndrome, inflammatory bowel disease, serous otitis media
   c. Unlikely or uncommon: attention-deficit disorder, behavior problems

Etiology

1. Children: cow's milk, egg, soy, peanut, wheat
2. Adults: peanut, true nuts, fish, shellfish
3. Oral allergy syndrome: fresh fruits, vegetables
4. Food-associated exercise-induced anaphylaxis: wheat, celery, shellfish
5. Increased incidence of food allergy in young children and atopic individuals
6. Latex allergy has been associated with allergy to avocado, potato, banana, tomato, chestnut, kiwi, and possibly other foods.
7. Airborne food particles from cooking, particularly shrimp, fish, and wheat, can induce allergic reactions.

Symptoms

1. Oral allergy syndrome: pruritus, tingling, and edema of oral mucosa, lips, tongue, and pharynx
2. Generalized reactions
   a. Cutaneous: pruritus, urticaria/angioedema, increased eczema
   b. Respiratory: shortness of breath, chest tightness, cough, hoarseness, rhinitis
   c. Gastrointestinal: cramping, diarrhea, nausea, emesis
   d. General: syncope, feeling of impending doom
   e. Genitourinary: uterine cramping, incontinence
3. History should include suspected food(s), amount eaten, time between ingestion and symptoms, any symptoms at other times with that food, and if other factors such as exercise are necessary for a reaction.

Key Symptoms

- Pruritus
- Increased eczema
- Shortness of breath
- Diarrhea
- Urticaria/angioedema
- Chest tightness
- Abdominal cramping

Clinical Findings

1. Cutaneous: urticaria/angioedema, eczematous lesions, flushing
2. Respiratory: wheezing, rhinorrhea, stridor
3. Cardiovascular: hypotension, tachycardia
4. Ocular: conjunctivitis

Key Signs

- Urticaria/angioedema
- Wheezing
- Hypotension
- Flushing
- Oropharyngeal edema
- Tachycardia

Laboratory Tests

1. Elimination diet followed by reintroduction, for chronic symptoms only
2. Prick skin tests with appropriate extracts
   a. Sensitive for immunoglobulin E (IgE)–mediated allergy
   b. Not specific; must be correlated with history
   c. Fresh fruits or raw vegetables may need to

956 • XIII Diseases of the Immune System

be used for testing if skin test negative with standard extract.

3. Radioallergosorbent testing (RAST)
   a. Also detects IgE antibody
   b. Less sensitive than skin testing
   c. Consider if cannot skin test because of medicines or concern about anaphylaxis in a very food-sensitive patient or one with extensive skin disease.
4. Double-blind, placebo-controlled food challenge
   a. Gold standard for confirming food allergy
   b. Must be done under carefully controlled conditions.
5. No role for leukocytotoxic testing, provocation/neutralization, antigen-antibody complexes, or immunoglobulin G for food allergy.

Key Tests

- Prick skin tests
- Double-blind, placebo-controlled food challenge

Differential Diagnosis

1. Reactions to food additives
   a. Monosodium glutamate: Chinese restaurant syndrome (in some cases may be caused by histamine in foods)
   b. Sulfites: may trigger asthma
2. Food toxicity
   a. Bacterial: *Salmonella, Shigella, Escherichia coli*
   b. Toxins: *Vibrio*, botulism, ciguatera, scombroid
3. Pharmacologic effects
   a. Alcohol: vasodilatation and flushing
   b. Tyramine in wine and cheese: headache
4. Enzyme deficiencies
   a. Disaccharidase deficiency: lactose intolerance
   b. Galactosemia
5. Gastrointestinal disease
   a. Gastroesophageal reflux
   b. Inflammatory bowel disease
6. Functional/psychological

Treatment

1. The only appropriate treatment for food allergy at present is avoidance.

2. There is no current role for food immunotherapy.

Medication

1. Patients with suspected or proven food anaphylaxis must be given an epinephrine kit.
2. Proper instruction for use of epinephrine kit is essential.
   a. Patient must have it available at all times.
   b. Patient and caregivers/family members must know how to use it.
   c. Administer for reaction that is initially severe or with any progressive symptoms; then seek care at an emergency room.

Diet

1. Elimination diet trial for chronic symptoms
2. Strict avoidance of foods causing anaphylaxis
3. For food allergy prophylaxis, breast-feeding and/or use of hypoallergenic formulas during the first 6 months of life combined with delaying introduction of the most allergenic foods may at least delay the onset of food allergy in atopy-prone infants.

Patient Education

1. Instruct in proactive avoidance of food(s) causing allergy.
2. Instruct about special caution at day care, school, parties, and restaurants.
3. Explain ubiquitous nature of some allergens, such as peanuts.
4. Patients with exercise-induced anaphylaxis should not eat implicated foods for at least 4 to 6 hours prior to exercise.
5. Medic Alert bracelet stating food allergy

Key Treatment

- Food avoidance
- Epinephrine kit

Follow-Up

1. Periodic follow-up to reinforce education and renew epinephrine kit if necessary
2. Particularly in children, cow's milk, soy, and egg may be tolerated after a period of time.
3. Allergy to peanuts, true nuts, fish, and shellfish is likely to persist.
4. Follow growth of patients on a restricted diet.
5. Egg-allergic patients need further evaluation prior to receiving measles-mumps-rubella, influenza, or yellow fever vaccines.

Bibliography

For more specific information on food allergy, see
Sampson HA: Food allergy. JAMA 1997;278:1888–1894.

For more information on the relation of food allergy to atopic dermatitis, see
Burks AW, James JM, Hiegel A, et al: Atopic dermatitis and food hypersensitivity reactions. J Pediatr 1998; 132:132–136.

For more information on food allergy in children, see
Anderson JA: Milk, eggs and peanuts: food allergies in children. Am Fam Physician 1997;56:1365–1374.

For more information on the association of allergy to latex and to foods, see
Beezhold DH, Sussman GL, Liss GM, et al: Latex allergy can induce clinical reactions to specific foods. Clin Exp Allergy 1996;26:416–422.

For more information on reactions to food additives, see
Weber RW: Food additives and allergy. Ann Allergy 1993; 70:183–190.

210 Anaphylaxis

James K. Buck, II

Etiology

1. Anaphylaxis is a clinical syndrome of systemic allergic response to any of a number of potential inciting agents. Through one of several initial pathways, these agents cause the release of mediators from mast cells and basophils throughout the body. These mediators include histamine, platelet-activating factor, leukotriene (LT) C_4, LTD_4, and LTE_4 (slow-reacting substance of anaphylaxis), and others. They act on blood vessels, airways, and other tissues and are responsible for the physiologic effects that comprise the syndrome.

2. Virtually any substance from a number of types might induce anaphylaxis in a given susceptible individual. An exhaustive list of inciting agents is beyond the scope of this text. Some of the more common causes of anaphylaxis are
   a. Antibiotics
      (1) Penicillins
      (2) Cephalosporins
      (3) Sulfonamides
      (4) Ciprofloxacin
      (5) Vancomycin
      (6) Amphotericin B
   b. Other drugs and therapeutic agents
      (1) Insulin
      (2) Protamine
      (3) Allergen extracts
      (4) Vaccines
      (5) Opiates
      (6) Radiocontrast media
      (7) Aspirin and nonsteroidal anti-inflammatory drugs
      (8) Streptokinase
   c. Foods and food additives
      (1) Nuts
      (2) Fish
      (3) Shellfish
      (4) Legumes
      (5) Egg whites
      (6) Dairy products (especially milk)
      (7) Fruits and berries
      (8) Metabisulfites
   d. Blood products
      (1) Whole blood
      (2) Plasma
      (3) Immunoglobulin
      (4) Cryoprecipitate
   e. Venoms
      (1) Fire ant venom
      (2) Hymenoptera venom (beesting)
      (3) Snake venom
   f. Miscellaneous
      (1) Latex
      (2) Exercise
   g. Idiopathic

Symptoms

1. Anaphylactic reactions are generally rapid, and initial symptoms are typically noticed seconds to minutes after exposure. The vast majority of these reactions occur within 1 hour of antigen exposure.

2. Individual patients' symptoms may vary widely in scope and severity. A given patient may present with any subset or combination of the following:
   a. General: Warmth, flushing, and generalized pruritus (as well as nasal, palatal, and ocular pruritus in particular) may be seen. Other general complaints may include a feeling of faintness and a sense of impending doom.
   b. Respiratory: Initial symptoms may include sneezing, cough, rhinorrhea, hoarseness, or "a lump in the throat" and may progress quickly to shortness of breath and dyspnea.
   c. Cardiovascular: Palpitations or a sensation of faintness may be present.
   d. Gastrointestinal: Symptoms may include a peculiar taste (possibly metallic), dysphagia, nausea, bloating, and/or abdominal cramping.

3. Pulmonary and/or cardiovascular symptoms and signs are the most potentially troublesome because pulmonary complications account for the large majority of anaphylactic deaths, followed by cardiovascular complications.

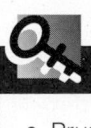

Key Symptoms

- Pruritus
- Lump in throat
- Hoarseness
- Shortness of breath
- Cough
- Sneezing
- Abdominal cramping
- Nausea
- Palpitations
- Faintness

Clinical Findings

1. Clinical signs also may vary widely from patient to patient. In the patient with profound anaphylactic shock, there may be few or no distinguishing clinical features present.

2. Possible clinical findings include

   a. Dermatologic: Classical skin manifestations include *urticaria*, usually pruritic and more prominent on the trunk and proximal limbs, and *angioedema*, usually seen as periorbital and circumoral edema. Generalized flushing also may be seen.

   b. Respiratory: Early signs may include sneezing, cough, and/or rhinorrhea. These may progress rapidly to include wheezing, stridor, tachypnea, use of accessory muscles, and cyanosis, possibly leading to complete asphyxia.

   c. Cardiovascular: Patients may manifest hypotension, shock, syncope, tachycardia, conduction defects, and dysrhythmias. Myocardial infarction may complicate anaphylaxis or its treatment in some patients.

   d. Gastrointestinal: Signs may include vomiting, diarrhea, and/or bloating.

Key Signs

- Urticaria
- Angioedema
- Flushing
- Rhinorrhea
- Wheezing
- Tachypnea
- Stridor
- Hypotension
- Shock
- Syncope
- Tachycardia
- Vomiting

Laboratory Tests

1. The diagnosis of anaphylaxis is a clinical one, and laboratory studies are generally not helpful in making the diagnosis acutely.

2. General laboratory studies (electrocardiogram, arterial blood gases) are helpful in some patients in the acute setting for evaluating specific complications such as hypoxemia, cardiac dysrhythmias, and acid-base disruptions and in monitoring the response of these complications to therapeutic measures.

Differential Diagnosis

1. In a patient who has collapsed or cannot give a history and who may lack urticaria or angioedema, the differential diagnosis may be extensive. One should consider

   a. Other conditions associated with sudden loss of consciousness (e.g., acute myocardial infarction, arrhythmias, seizure disorders, vasovagal syncope)

   b. Other conditions manifesting acute respiratory compromise (e.g., epiglottitis, status asthmaticus, foreign body aspiration, pulmonary embolus)

   c. Other conditions with similar skin or respiratory findings (e.g., carcinoid syndrome, hereditary angioedema, mastocytosis)

2. Vasovagal syncope may be the most common similar syndrome but usually may be differentiated by the presence of bradycardia (as opposed to tachycardia in anaphylaxis) with diaphoresis and maintenance of blood pressure, as well as pale appearance (as opposed to generalized flushing) and lack of pruritus or true respiratory difficulty.

Treatment

1. The treatment of acute anaphylaxis must begin with prompt evaluation and recognition, because complications and death may occur within minutes. As in other medical emergencies, the initial management is aimed at establishing an effective airway and circulatory system.

2. General measures include establishing intravenous access and the administering of intravenous fluids (i.e., saline) and supplemental oxygen (by cannula, mask, or endotracheal tube, if necessary). Cardiac monitoring should be instituted.

Medication

1. *Epinephrine* is the initial drug of choice in treating acute anaphylactic reactions.

   a. Epinephrine is routinely administered as a subcutaneous or intramuscular injection of 0.01 ml/kg of aqueous epinephrine 1:1000 (maximum adult dose 0.3 to 0.5 ml). The dose may be repeated approximately every 5 to 10 minutes if symptoms persist or recur.

b. For patients in profound circulatory collapse, continuous intravenous infusion of epinephrine may be necessary but should be used with extreme caution. An epinephrine drip may be started with 2 ml of 1:1000 solution added to 500 ml of saline at a rate of 2 to 20 μg/minute.

2. Both H_1 and H_2 antihistamines are recommended for treatment of anaphylaxis.

a. A suggested regimen would include diphenhydramine, 25 to 50 mg intravenously or intramuscularly, and ranitidine (Zantac), 50 mg intravenously. In the absence of hypotension, the use of an H_2 antihistamine is optional.

b. Patients generally should be maintained on H_1 antihistamines orally every 6 hours for 48 hours after the initial attack to help protect against rebound and/or relapse.

3. Corticosteroids are too slow in onset of action to be efficacious in acute episodes of anaphylaxis; it is recommended that they be used early, primarily to prevent late-phase reactions or recurrences. Higher doses (i.e., hydrocortisone, 5 mg/kg intravenously) are given initially and are often followed by a quickly tapered oral regimen.

4. Other medications to consider in specific circumstances are

a. Aerosolized β agonists (i.e., albuterol) to further combat bronchospasm (also may consider aminophylline)

b. Atropine or isoproterenol for refractory bradycardia

c. Dopamine or levarterenol for refractory hypotension (give adequate intravenous fluids for volume expansion first).

d. Glucagon may be useful in patients on β-blocking drugs (which may make them refractory to epinephrine treatment).

Diet

1. The patient should be kept to nothing by mouth until the acute episode is under control.

2. No other dietary restrictions apply, unless one or more foods are suspected as causative agents (in which case they should be avoided).

Activity

1. Patients with moderate systemic anaphylactic reactions should be monitored for at least 8 to 12 hours prior to discharge.

2. Those with severe, life-threatening reactions should be admitted to a hospital for continued evaluation and treatment.

3. There are no other specific limitations on activity once the acute event has been stabilized.

Patient Education

1. The patient should be counseled on the nature of his or her illness and the steps to take to avoid the offending agent(s) if possible.

2. Patients should be prescribed an emergency epinephrine kit (Ana-Kit, EpiPen) and instructed in its use in case of recurrent anaphylactic episodes.

Key Treatment

Drugs of Choice	Alternative Drugs
• Epinephrine 1:1000, 0.01 ml/kg SC or IM (see text)	• None (to epinephrine)
• Diphenhydramine, 25 to 50 mg IV or IM	• Hydroxyzine and others
• Ranitidine 50 mg IV or IM	• Cimetidine and others
• Hydrocortisone 5 mg/kg IV	• Methylprednisolone and others

Follow-Up

All patients who experience significant anaphylactic reactions should be referred to a specialist in allergy and immunology for further evaluation, testing, counseling, and/or preventive therapy as specifically indicated.

Bibliography

Atkinson TP, Kaliner MA: Anaphylaxis. Med Clin North Am 1992;76:841–855.

Lieberman P: The use of antihistamines in the prevention and treatment of anaphylaxis and anaphylactoid reactions. J Allergy Clin Immunol 1990;86:684–686.

Marquardt DL, Wasserman SI: Anaphylaxis. In Middleton E, Reed CE, Ellis EF (eds): Allergy Principles and Practice, 4th ed, vol 2, pp 1525–1536. St Louis, Mosby–Year Book, 1993.

Reisman RE, Lieberman P (eds): Anaphylaxis and anaphylactoid reactions. Immunol Allergy Clin North Am 1992;12:501–690.

Saryan JA, O'Laughlin JM: Anaphylaxis in children. Pediatr Ann 1992;21:590–598.

Winbery SL, Lieberman PL: Anaphylaxis. Immunol Allergy Clin North Am 1995;15:447–475.

211 Common Musculoskeletal Symptoms

SYMPTOM **NECK PAIN** *Kevin M. McKown*

Neck pain is a very common problem in adults. Prior incidences of 35 per cent or more and prevalences of 10 per cent have been reported. The pain is usually self-limited, with 70 per cent of episodes resolving within 1 month. Once unusual and potentially serious causes of neck pain are excluded, treatment is conservative in almost all instances.

Differential Diagnosis

1. Cervical spondylosis
2. Neck strain/sprain
3. Radiculopathy
4. Cervical myelopathy
5. Trauma
6. Chronic pain syndrome
7. Rheumatoid arthritis (RA)
8. Torticollis
9. Neoplasm
10. Vertebral osteomyelitis
11. Referred pain—especially from the shoulder, diaphragm, apical lung, heart, and aorta
    a. Temporomandibular joint pain
    b. Bursitis, tendinitis, or arthritis of the shoulder
    c. Reflex sympathetic dystrophy
    d. Thoracic outlet syndrome
    e. Bronchogenic carcinoma
    f. Coronary artery disease
    g. Aortic dissection
    h. Peptic ulcer disease
    i. Pancreatitis
    j. Cholecystitis
12. Ankylosing spondylitis (AS) or other spondyloarthropathies
13. Giant cell arteritis, polymyalgia rheumatica
14. Paget's disease
15. Fibromyalgia
16. Meningitis

In most patients, a definite cause of neck pain cannot (and need not) be established, and the pain is attributed to neck strain or cervical spondylosis. Cervical spondylosis describes degenerative changes in disks, ligaments, and joints of the cervical vertebral column (which are ubiquitous with aging). Psychologic factors are important predictors of chronic, unexplained neck pain. History and physical examination will identify other causes of neck pain.

> Refer to Ch. 203, Osteomyelitis; Ch. 216, Temporomandibular Joint Syndrome; Ch. 217, Osteoarthritis; Ch. 218, Rheumatoid Arthritis; Ch. 221, Myofascial Syndromes (Fibromyalgia and Myofascial Trigger Points); and Ch. 315, Reflex Sympathetic Dystrophy.

History: Key Questions to Ask

1. Duration, onset, and course of pain?
2. Trauma?
3. Radiation of pain?
4. Character of pain and any radiation?
5. Better or worse with certain activities, movements?
6. Relieved by rest?
7. Numbness or weakness?
8. Loss of bowel or bladder control?
9. Fever, weight loss, other active problems?
10. Cancer, other past medical history?

Most neck pain lasts days to a few weeks, is nonradiating, and is influenced by movement and position. Cervical spondylosis pain may radiate short distances in a fairly constant, achy, nondermatomal fashion. Radiculopathy pain is intermittent, sharp, and dermatomal and can be associated with numbness and weakness. Pain improved by activity suggests a spondyloarthropathy. Pain *not* relieved by rest or that is progressive suggests infection or neoplasm. Bowel or bladder dysfunction or lower extremity numbness, weakness, or ataxia suggests myelopathy. Systemic complaints and past history may suggest infection, neoplasm, or referred pain. Patients with RA are prone to instability. Patients with AS are prone to fracture with trivial trauma. Psychosocial factors may be important in chronic cervical spondylosis pain.

Clinical Findings

1. Tenderness, loss of motion of neck, shoulders
2. Numbness or weakness of upper or lower extremities
3. Hypo- or hyperreflexia
4. General physical examination if *any* suspicious history

Neck pain *without* neck tenderness, loss of neck motion, or pain with neck motion suggests a referred cause. Nuchal rigidity suggests meningitis. Polyradiculopathy suggests neoplasm, infection, or widespread spondylosis. Lower extremity ataxia, hyperreflexia, or hypertonicity suggests myelopathy. A general physical examination should be done with any suggestion of an unusual source of neck pain.

WARNING

Never force a neck when evaluating range of motion.

Tests

1. Cervical radiographs (anteroposterior and lateral)
2. Magnetic resonance imaging (MRI) or computerized tomography (CT)
3. Bone scan
4. Electromyography/nerve conduction velocity studies (EMG/NCVs)
5. Laboratory studies as indicated

Cervical radiographs can demonstrate evidence of neoplasm, osteomyelitis, fracture, or traumatic subluxation. In trauma or RA, add odontoid view. Gentle flexion-extension views may show instability in RA. Radiographs may be omitted in young patients with a straightforward, nontraumatic history and examination. Bone scans can demonstrate early osteomyelitis or neoplasm. MRI is superior to CT for soft tissue imaging; both are used for preoperative imaging. They should not be obtained routinely—many asymptomatic individuals have disk degeneration, herniated disks, or foraminal stenosis by MRI. EMG/NCV may be helpful preoperatively or in differentiating neurologic problems.

Management

1. Pain relief with relative rest, medications, physical modalities
2. Exercises: once there is improvement in pain
3. Surgery: occasionally indicated

Medication

1. Analgesics: acetaminophen, aspirin, nonsteroidal anti-inflammatory drugs, mild narcotics
2. "Muscle relaxants": benzodiazepines, cyclobenzaprine, methocarbamol

Activity

1. Relative rest. May use cervical pillow, soft cervical collar, traction.
2. Physical modalities, such as hot, cold, and ultrasound, may give relief.
3. Isometric exercises: once pain lessens

Patient Education

1. Reassurance as to self-limited nature of problem
2. Instruction on proper body positioning during daily activities

No treatment has been shown to alter the natural history of mechanical neck pain. Management is directed at patient comfort and the hope of secondary prevention by improving posture and muscle strength. Manipulation by skilled physicians should be used cautiously, if at all; neurologic catastrophes can result. Trigger point and epidural injections may give additional relief in skilled hands. Surgery is indicated for myelopathic symptoms; instability with neurologic abnormalities or severe pain, and severe radicular pain from a definable lesion not resolving after weeks to months of conservative therapy.

Follow-Up

1. Return in 2 to 4 weeks to reassess clinically for improvement.
2. Encourage patients to call for systemic or neurologic symptoms or unremitting pain.

PEARLS

- Unremitting pain suggests neoplasm, infection.
- Cervical myelopathy presents with lower extremity corticospinal tract signs.

B ## Bibliography

Barnsley L: Neck pain. In Klippel JM, Dieppe PA (eds): Rheumatology, 2nd ed, pp 4.4.1–4.4.11. London, Mosby International, 1998.

Bland JH: Disorders of the Cervical Spine, 2nd ed. Philadelphia: WB Saunders Company, 1994.

Ellenberg MR, Monet JC, Treanor WJ: Cervical radiculopathy. Arch Phys Med Rehabil 1994;75:342–352.

Nakano KK: Neck pain. In Kelley WN et al (eds): Textbook of Rheumatology, 5th ed, pp 394–412. Philadelphia, WB Saunders Company, 1997.

Thorn RP, Curd JG: A systemic approach to disorders of the cervical spine. Hosp Pract 1993;28:49–58.

SYMPTOM WHIPLASH

David C. Agerter

Many milder injuries of the cervical spine, such as those resulting from whiplash mechanisms, represent partial ligamentous tears or sprains. These patients characteristically have nonfocal neck pain without neurologic changes. Radiographs are normal and symptoms usually resolve spontaneously. *Whiplash of the neck* remains a controversial term; the symptoms are often vaguely described and the mechanisms of injuries are not fully understood. Many authorities would argue that the use of *whiplash* is best mentioned for historical purposes only. However, the term is so well ingrained among practitioners that it still is currently used. It would be best to describe the method of injury in terms of deceleration or acceleration forces. This would more accurately describe the mechanics of the force being hyperflexion or hyperextension.

Etiology

The cervical spine and head may be subjected to six general types of injuries:

1. *Pure flexion injury*: May result in posterior ligamentous injury with possible stable wedge fracture of a vertebral body.
2. *Flexion injury with rotation*: May cause posterior ligaments to rupture.
3. *Hyperextension injuries*: May cause vertebral fracturing. Hyperextension loading may cause rupturing of the disk and involvement of the anterior longitudinal ligament. If sufficient force is applied, spinal cord paralysis may result.
4. *Hyperextension with rotation*: May be associated with fractures and dislocations.
5. *Vertical compression*: Often seen with diving accidents. The vertical load shatters vertebral endplates and forces the nucleus of the disk into the vertebral body, causing it to explode.
6. *Lateral flexion injuries*: May be associated with brachial plexus injuries, with or without compression fracture. These often occur in playing football.

Differential Diagnosis

Whenever there is a head injury, one must always rule out any associated cervical spine involvement.

1. Myofascial sprain: an injury of tearing of the muscle ligamentous components of the neck

2. Herniated disk (also so-called slipped disk): The nucleus pulposus is extruded through a tear in the annulus fibrosis, with resultant nerve root irritation or compression.
3. Spinal stenosis: a narrowing of the cervical spinal canal that may predispose the patient to spinal cord or nerve injury with relatively minor trauma
4. Cervical instability: Occurs when ligamentous injury has occurred. It may or may not be associated with cervical fractures.
5. Fractures: There is injury to the bony components of the spine, usually resulting in compression of vertebral bodies. These may be classified as stable, where the integrity of the spine is still preserved, or unstable, where excess movement between adjacent osseous elements is occurring.

History

Whenever a patient has a suspected "whiplash" injury or neck pain, it is important to obtain the following information:

1. What was the exact mechanism of injury (in the patient's own words)?
2. If the injury is a result of a motor vehicle accident, was the patient wearing a seatbelt?
3. Has the patient had any previous injury to the head or neck? Previous injuries to the cervical (C) spine predispose the patient to a new injury that is likely to be more disabling.
4. What factors aggravate or alleviate the pain? Are there any associated symptoms to include involvement of upper extremities?
5. Do Valsalva's maneuvers accentuate the neck pain?

Clinical Findings

1. All patients who present to the family physician's office with chief complaint of "whiplash" are immobilized.
2. Obtain a lateral C-spine film to be certain there is no evidence of an underlying unstable fracture.
3. Check for cervical range of motion; then palpate for evidence of paraspinous muscle spasm and localized tenderness that may be present.

TABLE 211–1. NEUROLOGIC DEFICITS WITH CERVICAL OR NERVE ROOT INJURIES (FROM FRACTURES, DISK RUPTURES, ETC.)

DISK SPACE	NERVE ROOT AFFECTED	DISTRIBUTION OF MOTOR DEFICIT	SENSORY ABNORMALITIES (USUALLY NUMBNESS)	REFLEX ABNORMALITIES
C4	C5	Deltoid	Lateral aspect of shoulder	None
C5–6	C6	Biceps	Thumb	Biceps
C6–7	C7	Triceps	Middle finger	Triceps

4. Check for neurologic deficits, including weakness and reflex changes (Table 211–1).

Tests

1. Although most C-spine radiographs are normal, it is important to obtain these in patients with acute trauma to the C-spine. In order to properly evaluate the C-spine, the following views should be obtained:
   a. Odontoid view
   b. Anteroposterior view
   c. Lateral view
   d. Right/left oblique views
2. It is extremely important to be certain that all seven cervical vertebrae are visualized. Often C7 is not well delineated. It is then important to depress the shoulders by gentle but firm downward traction of the arms. If this is not possible, a so-called swimmer's view may be obtained. This view is done when the patient lies in a prone and oblique position with the higher tube-side arm above the head and the lower table-side arm beside the body.
3. Magnetic resonance imaging, computerized tomography, or myelography should be used in only those patients who do not respond to the usual treatment, or who have definite suspected spinal cord injury or nerve root compressions.

Treatment

1. Hospitalization is rarely indicated in the absence of a fracture-dislocation.
2. Antispasmodics or muscle relaxants may be helpful, but should be used for short periods of time only, such as 5 to 7 days. Analgesics such as nonsteroidal anti-inflammatory agents may be of benefit.
3. A soft collar that is properly fitted and correctly used is of significant benefit for many patients. The flexed position for the collar is advocated because this position separates the facets and opens the foramina. A soft collar is preferable to a more rigid collar. Duration for wearing a collar will vary widely. Most authorities recommend brief splinting and early mobilization. Brief splinting implies approximately 7 to 10 days. The collar should also be worn during sleep.
4. Once the patient's pain is markedly reduced, gentle range-of-motion exercises should be begun. Heat applied before exercising may be of benefit.
5. The use of cervical traction is not uniformly accepted at this time. It is often used based on the physician's personal preference. It may best be reserved for the patient who does not show good improvement within 2 to 3 weeks after the initial injury.
6. It has been clearly documented in the medical literature that whiplash injuries are often slow to resolve because of impending litigation.

PEARLS

• Suspect C-spine injury in all cases of head injuries.

• Always visualize C7.

• Early mobilization is the key to avoiding long-term disability for most patients.

Bibliography

Bring G, Westman G: Chronic posttraumatic syndrome after whiplash injury. Scand J Primary Health Care 1992;9:135–141.

Bucholz RW: Orthopaedic Decision Making, 2nd ed. St. Louis, CV Mosby Company, 1996.

Carroll PG: Acute neck strain—the value of judicious early mobilization. Aust Fam Physician 1992;21:275–276.

Torg JS, Ramsey-Emrhein JA: Cervical spine and brachial plexus injuries: return-to-play recommendations. Sportsmedicine 1997;25:60–88.

Torg JS, Thibault L, Sennett B, et al: The pathomechanics and pathophysiology of cervical spinal cord injury. Clin Orthop 1995;321:259–269.

Wilson FC, Lin PP: General Orthopaedics. New York, McGraw-Hill, 1997.

Patients of all ages are affected by both acute and chronic shoulder pathology. Many causes of shoulder pain are resistant to treatment and require patience on the part of both physician and patient. The judicious use of surgery is helpful in selected cases. Timely diagnosis and initiation of appropriate care afford the best chance of a favorable outcome for those afflicted with shoulder pain.

Differential Diagnosis

A history of prior trauma will focus the initial differential diagnosis.

1. Prior trauma
   a. Rotator cuff tear: more common in the elderly
   b. Dislocation: 90 per cent are anterior dislocations
   c. Fractures: clavicle, humerus, rarely scapula
   d. Acromioclavicular joint or sternoclavicular joint injury
2. No prior trauma
   a. Rotator cuff inflammation
   b. Bursitis: subacromial, subdeltoid
   c. Adhesive capsulitis: frozen shoulder
   d. Biceps tendinitis or rupture
   e. Arthritis: glenohumeral, acromioclavicular, sternoclavicular
   f. Glenohumeral instability
   g. Neurologic disorders: cervical spine, brachial plexus
   h. Neoplastic process: primary or metastatic
   i. Infection

> Refer to Ch. 213, Bursitis; Ch. 214, Tendinitis and Tendinosis; Ch. 217, Osteoarthritis; Ch. 218, Rheumatoid Arthritis; Ch. 221, Myofascial Syndromes (Fibromyalgia and Myofascial Trigger Points); and Ch. 237, Shoulder Dislocations.

History

1. Prior trauma: Increases likelihood of fracture, acute rotator cuff tear, clavicle injury, or dislocation.
2. Age: Adhesive capsulitis, bursitis, and tendinitis common in elderly.
3. Work-related activities: Patients in occupations requiring repetitive movement of the arms are at high risk for bursitis and rotator cuff tendinitis (e.g., carpenters, painters, assembly-line workers).
4. Recreational activities: Overhand-throwing athletes and swimmers are at high risk for rotator cuff impingement and tears as well as glenohumeral instability and labrum tears (e.g., pitcher, quarterback, tennis and volleyball players).
5. Night pain: Pain caused by bursitis and rotator cuff inflammation is often worse at night.
6. Sensation of slipping or instability of the head of the humerus: suggestive of prior dislocation
7. Crepitations or popping with movement: common with calcific tendinitis.
8. Weakness of distal extremity: suggests cervical spine or axillary nerve injuries
9. Constitutional symptoms may suggest infectious or neoplastic process.

Clinical Findings

1. Inspection: The shoulder should be carefully inspected for any signs of swelling, warmth, or deformity. Atrophy of the muscles of the shoulder—in particular the deltoid, which overlies the head of the humerus—points toward a neurologic injury. A depression above the humeral head (sulcus sign) is suggestive of glenohumeral instability and ligamentous laxity.
2. Palpation: The clavicle, acromioclavicular joint, and sternoclavicular joint are palpated. Deformities of these structures or pain with palpation points to an underlying injury. Anterior shoulder pain is found in a recently dislocated shoulder. The axilla and supraclavicular area are examined for lymphadenopathy.
3. Range-of-motion (ROM) testing: Decreased ROM is often the first indication of underlying rotator cuff difficulties, adhesive capsulitis, or bursitis. Limits to abduction and internal or external rotation should be searched for carefully.
   a. Passive ROM limitations: indicative of adhesive capsulitis
   b. Active ROM limitations: indicative of rotator cuff inflammation
   c. Method of testing
      (1) Abduction: Patient standing and elbow fully extended. Arm is raised out from side. Normal is zero degrees (arm at side) to 180 degrees (arm straight up).
      (2) Flexion: Patient standing and elbow fully extended. Arm is raised forward. Normal is zero degrees (arm at side) to 180 degrees (arm straight up).
      (3) Rotation: Patient supine, arm abducted

90 degrees, elbow flexed 90 degrees, and forearm perpendicular to table surface (reference position). Normal internal and external rotation is approximately 90 degrees from reference position.

4. Resistive testing: Patient's arm is placed in position to isolate each of the tendons of the rotator cuff. Inflammation of the rotator cuff will produce pain and/or weakness when patient raises arm against examiner's resistance.
   a. Supraspinatus: abduction; usually first tendon to be affected
      (1) Patient standing
      (2) Arm abducted to approximately 80 to 90 degrees and 20 to 30 degrees anterior of coronal plane
      (3) Elbow fully extended
      (4) Arm internally rotated and the thumb pointed to the floor
      (5) Arm pushed upward against the examiner
   b. Subscapularis: internal rotation; best isolated using lift-off test
      (1) Dorsum of hand placed on ipsilateral buttock
      (2) Patient instructed to lift hand away from buttock against examiner resistance
   c. Teres minor and infraspinatus: external rotation
      (1) Elbow flexed to 90 degrees and held at patient's side
      (2) Arm rotated externally against examiner resistance
      (3) Important that patient does not lift elbow away from side while rotating arm
   d. Biceps: resisted flexion of elbow
5. Apprehension testing
   a. Evaluates glenohumeral instability
   b. Positive in patients with anterior dislocations, glenohumeral subluxation, and glenoid labrum tear
   c. Method of testing
      (1) Patient supine with arm abducted 90 degrees, elbow flexed to 90 degrees, and arm externally rotated until limit of rotation or patient feels discomfort
      (2) Upper arm is pulled forward (anteriorly). If instability present, the discomfort is worsened with this anterior pressure (positive apprehension sign).
6. Impingement testing: Forces rotator cuff against coracoacromial ligament, worsening pain if in-

flammation, tear, or rotator cuff abnormality is present. Testing done with patient supine.
   a. Impingement I: With the elbow fully extended and arm internally rotated, the arm is flexed forward (toward the patient's head) and held close to the patient's head.
   b. Impingement II: Upper arm held perpendicular to table, elbow flexed to 90 degrees, arm rotated internally until limit of rotation or pain produced
   c. Impingement III: Elbow extended, arm brought across front of patient's chest
7. Neurologic testing: Evaluates for cervical or axillary nerve injury.
   a. Biceps (C5, C6) and triceps (C6, C7, C8) deep tendon reflexes
   b. Light touch of arm and hand. Careful attention should be paid to area overlying deltoid muscle because hypoesthesia in this area can be early indicator of underlying neurologic abnormality.
   c. Grip strength and intrinsic muscle strength of hand

Tests

1. Plain film radiographs: useful to evaluate for following:
   a. Fractures of clavicle, humerus, or, rarely, scapula
   b. Calcification of rotator cuff tendons (indicates chronic inflammation)
   c. Widening or calcifications of acromioclavicular or sternoclavicular joint
   d. Lytic or sclerotic bone lesions
   e. Dislocation of humerus
2. Magnetic resonance imaging (MRI)
   a. Useful for the detection of both inflammation and tear of the rotator cuff
   b. Detection of partial and full thickness tears enhanced with the use of MRI arthrography
   c. MRI arthrography also useful for detection of glenohumeral abnormalities
3. Computerized tomography (CT) arthrography: most useful for detection of glenoid labrum tear
4. Nerve conduction studies (EMG): to evaluate for nerve root injuries
5. CT or MRI of cervical spine if indicated by EMG

Management

1. Fractures
   a. Clavicle: Careful observation or figure-of-eight splint; surgery is rarely indicated.

b. Humerus: Sling and swath initially, and begin physical therapy as soon as possible; prolonged immobilization should be avoided.

c. Scapula: physical therapy for ROM and strengthening as soon as pain subsides

2. Rotator cuff inflammation and tears, subacromial bursitis

a. Nonsteroidal anti-inflammatories and aggressive physical therapy to increase ROM and strength; immobilization should be avoided.

b. Injection of the subacromial bursa with corticosteroids is a helpful adjunct to physical therapy when therapy is limited because of severe pain but should never replace an aggressive rehabilitation program.

c. Arthroscopic surgery for rotator cuff tears if not helped by therapy or injections: should not be first-line treatment.

3. Dislocations

a. Patients under age 20 have a very high risk of recurrence and should be evaluated by an orthopedic surgeon following the initial injury.

b. Patients over 40 have low risk of subsequent dislocation and should begin physical therapy as soon as symptoms permit.

c. Choice of surgery versus physical therapy for patients between 20 and 40 depends on frequency of subsequent dislocations and/or the physical activity of the patient.

4. Acromioclavicular and sternoclavicular inflammation and injury

a. Symptomatic treatment for pain

b. Corticosteroid injection for persistent pain

c. Resection of distal clavicle for recalcitrant pain of acromioclavicular joint

5. Cervical nerve root or axillary nerve abnormalities: surgical decompression if indicated

6. Lytic bone lesions: Search for underlying cause.

 Bibliography

Flatow EL: The rotator cuff, Part 1. Orthop Clin North Am 1997;28:1–78.

Flatow EL: The rotator cuff, Part 2. Orthop Clin North Am 1997;28:205–224.

Fongemie AE, Buss DD, Rolnick JR: Management of shoulder impingement syndrome and rotator cuff tears. Am Fam Physician 1998;57:667–684.

Kneeland JB: Update in musculoskeletal imaging. Radiol Clin North Am 1997;35:77–116.

Matsen FA, Lippitt SB, Sidles JA, et al: Practical Evaluation and Management of the Shoulder. Philadelphia, WB Saunders Company, 1994.

Indications

Surgical procedures in the distribution of nerves blocked, such as paronychia, wound repair, nail removal, or foreign body removal

Contraindications

1. Hypersensitivity to local anesthetic. Reactions are usually to epinephrine or preservatives. Hypersensitivity to the amide-type local (e.g., lidocaine, bupivacaine) anesthetics is rare.

2. Injection through areas of infection may spread infection to deeper structures. Often the nerve may be blocked successfully at a site more proximal to the infection.

Equipment

1. Local anesthetic solution
2. Antiseptic solution
3. Syringe with 23- to 27-gauge 1½-inch needle

Precautions

1. *Do not exceed toxic dose of local anesthetic (e.g., 4.5 mg/kg for lidocaine, 7 mg/kg for lidocaine with epinephrine, and 3 mg/kg for bupivacaine).*

2. No epinephrine in areas of terminal circulation (e.g., fingers, toes, nose, ear, penis)

3. Severe pain during the injection suggests that the needle bevel lies within the nerve bundle, and the injection should be halted and the needle repositioned slightly.

WARNING

Aspirate before injecting large doses of local anesthetic in the vicinity of blood vessels.

Technique

Wrist Block

1. Review the three nerves supplying the hand, and determine the nerves that supply the surgical field.

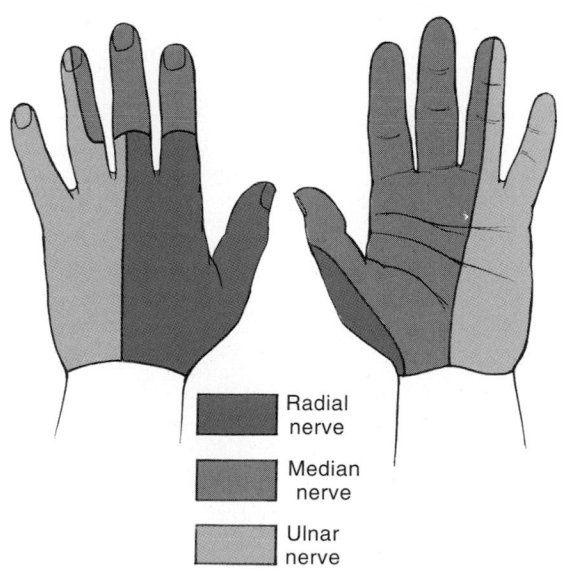

Radial nerve

Median nerve

Ulnar nerve

2. The ulnar nerve is most easily located and blocked in the ulnar notch at the elbow. The needle is placed in the ulnar notch, and 3 to 5

ml of local anesthetic is injected. If a paresthesia is elicited, 1 to 2 ml will be sufficient.

3. The median nerve is located between the palmaris longus tendon and the flexor carpi radialis tendon at the level of the proximal volar crease of the wrist. The needle is introduced, and 3 to 5 ml of local anesthetic is infiltrated into the space between the tendons.

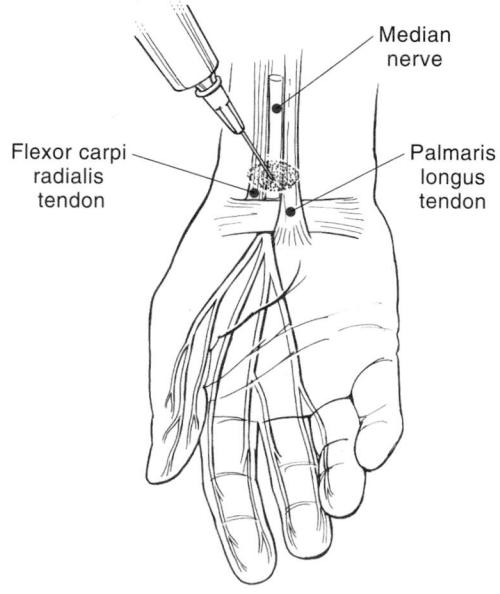

Median nerve

Flexor carpi radialis tendon

Palmaris longus tendon

If a paresthesia is elicited, then 2 ml of solution is injected at that location.

4. The radial nerve is represented by several sub-cutaneous branches at the level of the wrist. These supply the dorsal aspect of the hand on the radial side. The location of these branches is variable and is blocked with a continuous subcutaneous cuff of local anesthetic.

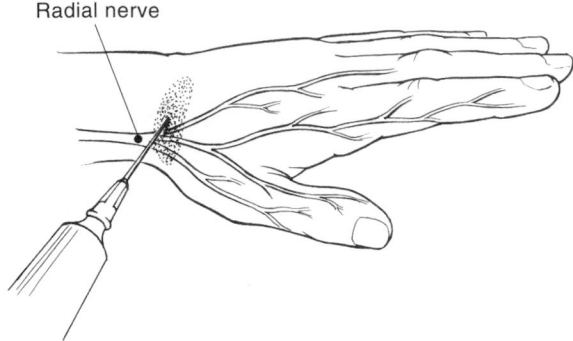

Radial nerve

5. It is crucial to allow 10 to 15 minutes for the anesthetic to diffuse and the block to become complete. This time can be spent preparing the skin, draping, and organizing the instruments.

Digital Block

1. The principal nerves innervating the digit lie on either side of the phalanx toward the palmar (plantar) surface located at the 5 and 7 o'clock positions as seen in cross section.

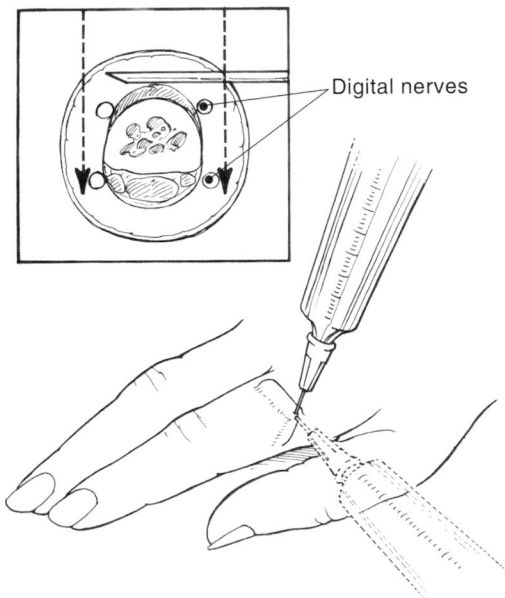

Digital nerves

The dorsal aspect of the digit is innervated by smaller dorsal branches at 10 and 2 o'clock.

2. A fine-gauge (25- to 27-gauge) needle is introduced at the base of the proximal phalanx at a point dorsal and lateral. The needle is advanced until the point lies at the estimated position of the palmar digital nerve, and 1.0 ml of local anesthetic is injected.

3. The needle is withdrawn to just beneath the skin while injecting a subcutaneous wheal of local anesthetic.

4. The needle is redirected 90 degrees, and a subcutaneous wheal is placed across the dorsum of the digit (see illustration above).

5. The needle can be introduced on the opposite side of the digit through this dorsal wheal, sparing the patient the pain of a second needle stick. The block is completed by injecting 1.0 ml at the location of the remaining palmar digital nerve and placing a subcutaneous wheal along the lateral aspect.

6. The total volume injected should not exceed 4 ml, because large volumes can compress the digital vessels and produce ischemia. For the same reason, vasoconstrictors (epinephrine) should never be used.

7. It is crucial to allow 5 to 10 minutes for the anesthetic to diffuse and the block to become complete. This time can be spent preparing the skin, draping, and organizing the instruments.

B **Bibliography**

Adriani J: Labat's Regional Anesthesia, 4th ed, pp 524–526. St. Louis, Warren H. Green, 1985.
Brown DL: Atlas of Regional Anesthesia, 2nd ed. Philadelphia, WB Saunders Company, 1998.
Ferrera PC, Chandler R: Anesthesia in the emergency setting: I. Hand and foot injuries. Am Fam Physician 1994;50:569–573.
Moore DC: Regional Block, 4th ed, pp 189–230. Springfield, IL, Charles C Thomas, 1979.
Valvano MN, Leffler F: Comparison of bupivacaine and lidocaine/bupivacaine for local anesthesia/digital nerve block. Ann Emerg Med 1996;27:490–492.

Elbow injuries are among the most challenging that face the primary care physician. The central positioning of the elbow in the upper extremity predisposes to overuse microtrauma, as well as referred pain from the neck, shoulder, and wrist.

> Refer to Ch. 213, Bursitis; Ch. 214, Tendinitis; Ch. 215, Epicondylitis; Ch. 221, Myofascial Syndromes (Fibromyalgia and Myofascial Trigger Points); and Ch. 230, Carpal Tunnel Syndrome and Other Nerve Entrapments.

Differential Diagnosis

Overuse Injuries

1. Anterior
   a. Biceps tendinitis
   b. Pronator teres syndrome: median nerve entrapment
2. Posterior
   a. Triceps tendinitis
   b. Olecranon impingement syndrome
   c. Olecranon bursitis
3. Lateral
   a. Tennis elbow: lateral epicondylitis
   b. Posterior interosseous nerve entrapment
   c. Radial tunnel syndrome
4. Medial
   a. Golfer's elbow: medial epicondylitis
   b. Ulnar collateral ligament strain
   c. Cubital tunnel syndrome: ulnar nerve entrapment

Traumatic Injuries

1. Fractures
2. Dislocations
3. Compartment syndromes

Unique Pediatric Injuries

1. Anterior: forearm "splints"
2. Posterior: olecranon apophysitis
3. Medial: medial epicondylar stress lesion
4. Lateral: osteochondritis dissecans of the capitellum

Overuse injuries represent the predominant form of musculoskeletal injury seen by physicians. Tennis elbow is the most common overuse injury involving the elbow, occurring nearly twice as often as medial epicondylitis. Little League elbow occurs frequently in young throwing athletes and involves a constellation of injuries, including a medial apophyseal stress lesion, lateral osteochondritis dissecans of the capitellum, and olecranon apophysitis.

History

1. The character of the pain should be clearly established.
   a. Onset: traumatic versus overuse
   b. Quality
      (1) Aching pain: tendon overuse
      (2) Burning pain and tingling: nerve entrapment
   c. Frequency and duration
   d. Activities that exacerbate or relieve the pain
2. History of injury
   a. Prior elbow fracture or dislocation
   b. Prior elbow overuse injury
   c. History of cervical radiculopathy or carpal tunnel syndrome
3. Occupational and sports history
   a. Racquet and throwing sports predispose to overuse injuries.
   b. Occupations requiring repetitive wrist motion predispose to injury (e.g., carpenters, typists, auto mechanics).

The history is the key to a good pathoanatomic diagnosis. The physician's inquiry should search to identify a recent period of transition, such as a vigorous tennis weekend, a new racquet, increased typing, or the start of Little League baseball.

Clinical Findings

1. A careful examination includes inspection, palpation, range-of-motion testing, special tests, and neuromuscular testing of the entire upper extremity.
2. Normal carrying angles measure 5 degrees of valgus in males and 10 to 15 degrees in females.
3. Passive limitation of extension: mechanical blockade or a muscular flexion contracture. Pain with forced extension: olecranon impingement syndrome
4. Palpation should include all four quadrants through a full range of motion.
   a. The point of maximal tenderness for tennis elbow is at the insertion of the wrist extensors at the lateral epicondyle.
   b. The point of maximal tenderness for golfer's elbow is at the flexor origin at the medial epicondyle.

c. A Tinel's test should be performed at the cubital tunnel, where the ulnar nerve crosses the elbow.

5. Both varus and valgus instability should be assessed at 0 and 30 degrees of elbow flexion and compared with the other extremity.

6. Resisted dorsiflexion, palmar flexion, pronation, and supination should be performed to identify musculoskeletal dysfunction.

Pain with resisted dorsiflexion with the elbow in full extension suggests a better prognosis than with the elbow in 90 degrees of flexion. Classical signs of Little League elbow include tenderness over the medial epicondyle and pain with resisted flexion and/or pronation. Findings that suggest more advanced involvement include tenderness over the lateral condyle, swelling, and a limitation of elbow motion.

Tests

1. Standard radiographs include anteroposterior and lateral views. Special views include oblique, axial, radial head, and stress views.

2. Computerized tomographic arthrography and magnetic resonance imaging can be used to evaluate for loose bodies, soft tissue mechanical blockade, and osteochondritis.

3. Electromyography and nerve conduction velocity studies can be used to evaluate for ulnar nerve dysfunction, median nerve entrapment with the pronator syndrome, and posterior interosseous nerve entrapment.

In the young patient with open growth plates, radiographs of both elbows should be ordered. Fat pad signs are frequently helpful in diagnosing subtle fractures. Posterior fat pads are always considered abnormal and suggestive of elbow fracture. Anterior fat pads are frequently present normally. When a fracture is present, the anterior fat pad can elevate, indicating the classical "sail sign."

Management

1. Pathoanatomic diagnosis: Successful treatment begins with an accurate diagnosis.

2. Control of inflammation
   a. Medication
      (1) A 7- to 10-day course of a nonsteroidal anti-inflammatory drug, such as Naproxen, 375 mg twice a day for 7 days, frequently helps to control pain and inflammation.
      (2) Corticosteroid injections: Short-term relief, but corticosteroid can cause tissue degeneration.
   b. Modalities: High-voltage pulsed galvanic stimulation, iontophoresis, and phonophoresis can all be of assistance in managing elbow overuse pain.
   c. Protection: Elbow immobilization is used only in select cases because stiffness and atrophy are not infrequent complications. Protection is most effectively provided by appropriate activity modification.

3. Promotion of healing: The promotion of healing only occurs through rehabilitative exercise and cardiovascular conditioning.
   a. Exercise progresses from isometrics to isotonics, with emphasis on wrist flexors and extensors.
   b. The entire upper extremity should be rehabilitated, including the shoulder and scapular stabilizers.
   c. Home isoflex (surgical tubing) exercises are very effective.

4. Control abuse
   a. Control of force loads: re-education of proper sports and/or occupational technique and control of intensity and duration of activity
   b. Counterforce bracing: helpful in rehabilitation and in early return to sport
   c. Proper equipment is important to avoid overuse injury.

5. Patient education
   a. Ongoing maintenance rehabilitation is necessary to avoid recurrent injury.
   b. Progression should be gradual.
   c. Patients should never play or participate through the pain.
   d. Premedicating with pain medication before athletic or occupational activity should be avoided.

Rest from abusive activity should be relative and not complete. Surgery for elbow overuse injuries is indicated only after failure of a quality rehabilitative program (3 to 6 months), persistent pain at rest or with activities of daily living, and an unacceptable quality of life.

PEARLS

- When tennis elbow fails to improve, posterior interosseous nerve entrapment should be ruled out.

- The patient with an elbow overuse injury frequently has associated rotator cuff tendinitis.

- Cervical radiculopathy and carpal tunnel syndrome not uncommonly produce referred pain patterns involving the elbow.

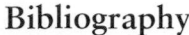

Bibliography

Behr CT, Altchek DW: The elbow. Clin Sports Med 1997; 16:681–704.

Foley AE: Tennis elbow. Am Fam Physician 1993;48: 281–288.

Morrey BF, Regan WD: Tendinopathies about the elbow. In De Lee JC, Drez D (eds): Orthopaedic Sports Med-

icine: Principles and Practice, pp 860–881. Philadelphia, WB Saunders Company, 1994.

Nirshl RP: Elbow tendinosis/tennis elbow. Clin Sports Med 1992;11:851–870.

O'Connor FG, Ollivierre CO, Nirchl RP: Elbow and forearm injuries. In Lillegard WA, Butcher JD, Rucker KS (eds): Handbook of Sports Medicine, 2nd ed, pp 141–157. Boston, Butterworth Heinemann, 1999.

SYMPTOM WRIST AND HAND PAIN

Kenneth M. Bielak

The hand and wrist are important mediators with our environment, responsible for touch, manipulation, and interaction. Any disorder that detracts from or destroys that interaction has a monumental impact on our ability to manually communicate with our environment effectively. In a fall, the hand and wrist are typically the first or trailing part of the body to impact the ground by trying to break the fall. In everyday common use, our hands are needed for typing, writing, and molding materials for our benefit, but usually at a cost of more chronic problems of fatigue and soreness. This chapter provides a breadth of disorders to consider in narrowing the focus to an accurate assessment and beginning appropriate rehabilitation.

Differential Diagnosis

The differential diagnosis is extensive. It can be helpful to isolate by anatomic site, historic features, and temporal relationships to narrow the differential to a more workable size.

1. Tendinitis (see also Ch. 214, Tendinitis and Tendinosis)
   a. Extensor tenosynovitis of the six dorsal compartments of the wrist
      (1) de Quervain's tenosynovitis (abductor pollicis longus and extensor pollicis brevis): positive Finkelstein's test (pain with ulnar and radial deviation); rule out arthritis, scaphoid fracture, Wartenberg's or intersection syndrome.
      (2) Intersection syndrome: inflammation at the intersection of the first and second dorsal compartment (extensor carpi radialis longus and brevis); edema and pain with flexion and extension
      (3) Extensor pollicis longus
      (4) The four extensor digitorum communis tendons and the extensor indicis propius (EIP) tendon
      (5) Extensor digiti minimi
      (6) Extensor carpi ulnaris

   b. Flexor tenosynovitis
      (1) Flexor carpi radialis
      (2) Flexor carpi ulnaris
2. Sprains
   a. Carpal bone ligaments
   b. Triangular fibrocartilage complex (TFCC): ulnar wrist
   c. Wrist sprain
   d. Collateral ligament tears involving proximal interphalangeal (PIP) joints
3. Nerve entrapments
   a. Carpal tunnel syndrome: median nerve
   b. Inflammation of the dorsal sensory branch of the radial nerve
4. Fractures and dislocations (see also Ch. 239, Finger Dislocations; Ch. 241, Wrist Fractures; Ch. 242, Finger Fractures)
   a. Wrist fracture
      (1) Colles': apex volar
      (2) Smith's: apex dorsal
      (3) Barton's: anterior fracture/dislocation of the radial head with articular involvement
      (4) Fracture of radius and ulna
   b. Carpal bone fracture
      (1) Fracture of scaphoid: proximal/middle portions, with adverse sequelae resulting from poor blood supply
      (2) Fracture of hook of hamate
   c. Metacarpal fractures: head, neck, shaft, or base
      (1) Boxer's: typically third or fourth metacarpal
      (2) Bennett's: volar lip fracture of first carpometacarpal bone of the thumb
      (3) Rolando's: intra-articular fracture/dislocation of the first carpometacarpal bone
   d. Phalangeal fractures
      (1) Tuft fracture: distal phalanges

(2) Flexor or extensor tendon avulsion fracture
  e. Dislocations and disassociations
    (1) Carpal bone dislocation
    (2) Scapholunate dissociation
    (3) PIP joint dislocation
5. Arthritic and connective tissue disorders
  a. Localized systemic problems of scleroderma, polymyalgia rheumatica, osteoarthritis, rheumatoid arthritis
  b. Reflex sympathetic dystrophy
6. Avascular necrosis
  a. Avascular necrosis of the capitate
  b. Kienbock's disease: avascular necrosis of the lunate
7. Cysts and masses
  a. Trigger finger: typically nodular mass at first annular pulley with triggering noted on flexion. Rule out infection, laceration, foreign body, subluxation, or connective tissue disease.
  b. Ganglion

History: Key Questions to Ask

1. What was the mechanism of injury? An acute event (such as fall, or hit by an object) or one that occurred over time (chronic overuse)?
2. What activities or motions aggravate it? Relieve it?
3. Is the pain located on the dorsal or volar aspect of the wrist or hand?
4. Is there a noise such as grinding, popping, snapping, or clicking associated with the pain?
5. Was any swelling noted either acutely or over time?
6. What has been done to date for treatment? Response to date?

It is important to establish as complete an understanding as possible of the acute event or the nature of a chronic condition from repetitive overuse. By understanding the type of occupation or sport that requires a forceful grip coupled with ulnar deviation or repetitive use of the thumb (such as racquet sports, fly fishing, golfing, knitting; laboratory technicians, filing clerks, mail sorters), the examiner can focus on the likely anatomic areas involved. Noises such as popping, clicking, or grinding can help isolate bony, tendon, or arthritic pathology. Paresthesias (numbness, tingling, or electrical signals) point toward nerve involvement, such as entrapment.

Clinical Findings
1. Direct observation

  a. Skin changes: erythema, edema, abrasions, and ecchymosis
  b. Deformity: dislocation, fracture (closed or open)
2. Direct palpation: crepitus (bony, ligaments or tendons)
3. Palpation of bony and ligamentous landmarks can aid in localizing the source of discomfort. Landmarks should include
  a. Distal forearm bones of the radius and ulna, styloid process
  b. Carpal bones: trapezium, trapezoid, capitate, hamate, triquetrum, pisiform, lunate, and navicular or scaphoid
  c. Snuffbox: scaphoid
  d. Radioulnar joint
  e. TFCC: ulnar wrist
  f. Base of metacarpals
  g. Metacarpophalangeal joints
  h. PIPs
  i. Distal interphalangeal joints
4. Muscle testing
5. Ligament and joint testing: flexibility (laxity, loss of motion). Range of motion, both active and passive, should be assessed in all planes of function, including ulnar and radial deviation, pronation and supination of the wrist.
6. Muscular changes: atrophy, loss of strength
7. Neurovascular findings: loss of sensation, loss of strength, capillary refill/pulses

Comparison to the contralateral side affords a basis of normality to assess appearance, strength, motion, flexibility, and function. The neurovascular examination is essential to rule out serious disorders of the nerves and blood vessels, which would require immediate consultation. It is helpful to follow the dermatomes outline by the distribution of the ulnar, radial, and medial nerves.

Tests
1. Range of motion of the wrist
  a. Flexion: normal is 80 degrees
  b. Extension: normal is 70 degrees
  c. Ulnar deviation: normal is 50 degrees
  d. Radial deviation: normal is 20 degrees
2. Allen test: After patient holds a firm grip, the examiner occludes the radial and ulnar artery as the patient releases the grip and examiner observes the filling pattern to the hand as either the radial or ulnar artery occlusion is released. Vascular disruption will show delayed filling on the disrupted side.
3. Finkelstein's test: Ulnar deviation of the wrist

with the thumb in extreme adduction tucked under the flexed fingers typically ignites the pain of tenosynovitis of the first dorsal compartment (de Quervain's).

4. Watson's test (scapholunate instability): Place thumb on scaphoid tuberosity with wrist in ulnar deviation, then deviate wrist radially. The scaphoid moves dorsally in a positive test.

5. TFCC test: The wrist is dorsiflexed with ulnar deviation, then rotated. Clicking suggests compromise to the TFCC.

6. Tinel's test: Any tapping along the peripheral nerves may elicit an electrical or tingling sensation, suggesting nerve impingement; seen commonly when checking for carpal tunnel syndrome by tapping at the volar wrist area overlying the median nerve.

7. Phalen's test: Extreme volar flexion of the wrist for more than 40 to 60 seconds may reproduce paresthesias of median nerve entrapment of carpal tunnel syndrome.

8. Plain radiographs
   a. Minimum two views at right angles
   b. Oblique and comparison views of the contralateral extremity when clinical suspicion is high and with immature growth plates of children and adolescents
   c. Specialized views: ulnar deviated anteroposteriorly for scaphoid view; carpal tunnel view to rule out hamate fracture

9. Aspiration of joint fluid for analysis is especially useful to rule out septic joint, investigate for crystals or inflammation.

10. Magnetic resonance imaging (MRI)
    a. Soft tissue disorders of intrinsic ligaments
    b. Chronic occult complaints with restricted motion
    c. Avascular necrosis
    d. Occult fractures
    e. Osteomyelitis
    f. Failed carpal tunnel surgery
    g. Establish originating site of ganglion

11. Computerized tomography scans
    a. Highlight subtle bony involvement, especially in chronic or complicated conditions
    b. Occult fractures

12. Electromyography/nerve conduction velocity tests: documentation of peripheral nerve entrapment or injury

13. Technetium-99m bone scan: rule out stress fractures; skeletal surveys; limited utility

14. Arthrography: intrinsic ligament injury, such as TFCC tear; the standard MRI may soon overtake

For any suspicion of fracture or ligamentous disruption, plain radiographs are the most economical and utilitarian investigations to establish a diagnosis. More sophisticated investigations are useful in the chronic or suspected occult fractures. Serial radiographs are useful to follow up initial repair of fractures or to rule out occult fractures with persistent symptoms. A high index of suspicion should prompt conservative treatment in the face of negative radiographs until serial radiographs show conclusively that no occult fracture exists. For systemic and inflammatory conditions, appropriate history, examination, and screening laboratory investigations are indicated.

Management

1. Management of acute initial injury should follow the acronym of PRICEMM:
   a. *Protect*: splinting is the safest and most effective
   b. *Rest*
   c. *Ice*: to minimize further swelling
   d. *Compression*: if swelling is noted
   e. *Elevation*: to eliminate further swelling
   f. *Medications*: for example, nonsteroidal anti-inflammatory drugs (NSAIDs)
   g. *Modalities*: ultrasound, phono-/iontophoresis, galvanic stimulation

2. For acute fractures, a splint is effective in immobilizing the affected joint while allowing access to decrease swelling. Cast immobilization is desired when swelling has subsided and operator skill level allows effective use of this technique.

3. Early consideration for physical and occupational therapy, especially in conjunction with evaluations by hand specialists

4. For sprains and tendinitis after adequate control of the acute process, work on stretching, range of motion, strengthening of muscle function, then endurance (generally in this order).

Medication

NSAIDs of choice, based on cost, effectiveness, and fewest gastrointestinal side effects, especially for the high-risk patient

Diet

1. No restrictions for most disorders
2. Avoidance of purine-rich diets for gouty arthritis

3. Special diet restrictions for rheumatoid arthritis (antioxidants and vegetarian diets are two examples)

4. Adequate calcium and vitamin D intake to promote bone healing in fractures; consideration for vitamin B$_6$ daily supplements with carpal tunnel syndrome.

Activity

1. Relative rest is essential.

2. Any activity that provokes or prolongs discomfort is to be avoided.

3. In general, fractures require 6 to 8 weeks of immobilization and some added time to increase strength and endurance; other injuries may take longer.

Patient Education

1. Clear understanding of provocative activities and subsequent avoidance

2. Consideration for biomechanical evaluation to improve efficiency and eliminate chronic problems for the occupational overuse syndromes

Follow-Up

Serial follow-up is necessary to ensure adequate healing response and to consider whether initial assessment is accurate enough for management to effect complete resolution.

B Bibliography

Barry NN, McGuire JL: Overuse syndromes in adult athletes. Rheum Dis Clin North Am 1996;22:515–530.

Mastey RD, Weiss APC, Akelman E: Primary care of hand and wrist athletic injuries. Clin Sports Med 1997; 16:705–723.

Riley SA: Wrist pain in adult athletes. Postgrad Med 1995;98:147–154.

Schreibman KL, Freeland A, Gilula LA, et al: Imaging of the hand and wrist. Orthop Clin North Am 1997;28: P537–P582.

Tiedeman JJ, Ferlic TP: Hand and wrist injuries. In Mellion MB, Walsh WM, Shelton GL (eds): The Team Physician's Handbook, 2nd ed, pp 474–490. Philadelphia, Hanley and Belfus, Inc, 1997.

SYMPTOM BACK PAIN   *Sarah S. Kramer*

The syndrome of low back pain (LBP) is ubiquitous, afflicting up to 90 per cent of people over their life spans. Most LBP resolves with conservative management, but physicians are commonly vexed in their management of these patients because the pathophysiology of LBP is poorly understood. The cause of pain may evolve during the course of illness or be multifactorial. Pain from the spine is poorly localized, and pain from visceral structures of the chest, abdomen, or pelvis may refer dorsally. The management of LBP is complicated by patients' common misconceptions (e.g., "slipped disk," "pinched nerve") and imprecise terminology. This discussion focuses on musculoskeletal pain syndromes of the back.

Differential Diagnosis

1. Myofascial: muscle strain, insertion tendinitis, enthesopathies (most common)

2. Diskogenic: herniated nucleus pulposis (HNP) or degenerative disk disease

3. Osteoarthritis, including facet joints

4. Spondylolisthesis (spondylolysis controversial as a cause of pain)

5. Spinal stenosis: congenital or acquired

6. Fractures: traumatic or pathologic

7. Inflammatory or rheumatologic diseases (e.g., Reiter's sacroiliitis)

8. Infiltrative diseases: infection, malignancy, Paget's disease

The likelihood of diagnosis is age-related. Disk disease and myofascial pain are responsible for almost all LBP in adults age 50 and younger, with spondylolysis and inflammatory diseases occurring less commonly. Spinal stenosis, malignancies, and Paget's disease should be considered in adults over age 50, although they are still less common than the first two etiologies.

Refer to Ch. 202, Paget's Disease of Bone; Ch. 217, Osteoarthritis; and Ch. 221, Myofascial Syndromes (Fibromyalgia and Myofascial Trigger Points)

History

1. Pain descriptors: acuity of onset, duration, location, and radiation of pain; precipitating factors; positional variance (flexion vs. extension); history of LBP

2. Occupational history: especially presence of heavy lifting, repetitive twisting, and operating heavy equipment (4- to 6-Hz vibration)

3. Neurologic symptoms, including pain, numbness, or paresthesia in either radicular or myofascial referral patterns, motor weakness (e.g.,

footdrop) neurogenic claudication, and pelvic visceral dysfunction

4. Psychosocial factors, including job dissatisfaction, perception of disability, and secondary gain (e.g., workers' compensation, litigation, avoidance of responsibilities)

As with any disease, the history is of paramount importance in the diagnosis of LBP and also commonly directs therapy. Positive motor symptoms mandate further examination and diagnostic testing. However, the psychosocial history is most predictive of eventual outcome.

Clinical Findings

1. Neurologic examination: gait abnormalities (try toe walking, heel walking), muscle strength, tendon reflexes, and perianal sensation

2. Posture, range of motion, hamstring flexibility

3. Point tenderness: spine, muscles, tendon insertions, sacroiliac joints

4. Pelvic stress tests: Patrick's or Faber's maneuver

Perianal sensory loss with pelvic floor dysfunction or loss of anal tone implies cauda equina syndrome, which is rare but requires urgent surgical referral. Straight-leg lift testing is widely used but has poor predictive value. Posture is often very revealing, with acute HNP patients preferring to stand and myofascial pain patients preferring to sit or recline.

Tests

1. Plain radiographs can reveal fractures, lytic lesions, spondylolysis, and degeneration and, with the neurologic examination, will exclude most serious causes of LBP. Recommended in all trauma patients, adolescents, and adults over 50 years.

2. Bone scans reveal inflammatory and infiltrative processes, occult fractures, and active spondylolysis. Highly sensitive for ruling out serious pathology.

3. Computerized tomography and magnetic resonance imaging (MRI) are usually reserved for patients who may require surgery. T_2-weighted MRIs give myelogram-like information.

4. Myelogram: not recommended unless MRI is not available

5. Electromyelography tests peripheral nerve function

6. Blood tests: Erythrocyte sedimentation rate screens for inflammation and chronic infection; other serologic tests can screen for specific rheumatologic disorders.

Most patients with LBP are managed clinically. Testing should be reserved for trauma, patients with known cancer, those with abnormal neurologic examinations or systemic illness, or those with symptoms that worsen or do not improve despite 6 weeks of appropriate therapy. Symptoms and functional disability generally correlate poorly with objective tests.

Management

Medications

1. Nonsteroidal anti-inflammatory drugs (e.g., ibuprofen)

2. Tricyclic antidepressants (TCAs) or related compounds for chronic pain. Newer anticonvulsants, such as gabapentin (Neurontin), are gaining in popularity as alternatives to TCAs.

3. Other analgesic agents (e.g., acetaminophen)

4. Oral or intrathecal steroids for HNP (recent studies have shown these to not result in improved outcomes)

5. Oral narcotics are *not* recommended except in postoperative or trauma patients. In routine LBP, they are associated with poorer outcomes.

6. Muscle "relaxers" such as methocarbamol are probably of no benefit. Benzodiazepine use delays recovery.

Physical Modalities

1. Ice, heat, ultrasound

2. Osteopathic or chiropractic manipulation

3. Lumbosacral corset or thoracolumbosacral orthosis: diskogenic pain, spinal stenosis, spondylolisthesis, sacroiliac pain

4. See also Ch. 221, Myofascial Syndromes (Fibromyalgia and Myofascial Trigger Points).

Activity

1. Relative rest, with early return to normal activities

2. Aerobic exercise

3. Trunk muscle exercises (see Procedure on Low Back Pain Exercises)

4. Bed rest is to be avoided in the absence of a truly unstable lesion.

Diet

1. Weight loss

2. Tobacco cessation

Patient Education

1. Reassurance: avoid overdiagnosis, overtesting. Correct misconceptions about spinal anatomy and physiology, natural history of disease.

2. Modified workplace ergonomics is marginally effective in reducing new back injury.

3. Education in biomechanical stresses of disks (back school) has been widely used but not validated by well-designed trials.

4. Resolution of psychosocial stressors

5. Lifelong fitness

Patients should be encouraged to plan an active role in their rehabilitation. Passive modalities such as traction and massage are not only ineffective but encourage inactivity.

Follow-Up

1. Should be oriented to promotion of early return to activity.

2. Consider referral to physical therapy or chiropractic care early in course if not improving.

3. Surgical consultation: any patient with progressive neurologic findings or cauda equina syndrome. Consider in patients whose pain had not improved within 6 weeks.

PEARLS

- Observation of the patient's gait, posture, and affect often yields the diagnosis.

- In the absence of hard neurologic findings, there is usually more danger in too much rest than in too much exercise.

- Scrupulously avoid narcotics and benzodiazepines in nonsurgical LBP.

- Attention to psychosocial factors rather than biomechanical ones has better outcomes.

Bibliography

Borenstein D: Epidemiology, etiology, diagnostic evaluation, and treatment of low back pain. Curr Opin Rheumatol 1995;7:141–146.

Burton AK, Erg E: Back injury and work loss: biomechanical and psychosocial influences. Spine 1997;22:2575–2580.

Hartigan C, Miller L, Liewehr SC: Rehabilitation of acute and subacute low back and neck pain in the work-injured patient. Orthop Clin North Am 1996;27:841–860.

Twomey L, Taylor J: Exercise and spinal manipulation in the treatment of low back pain. Spine 1995;20:651–659.

Waddell G, Feder G, Lewis M: Systematic reviews of bed rest and advice to stay active for acute low back pain. Br J Gen Pract 1997;47:647–652.

Goals in Prescribing Exercises for Low Back Pain Patients

1. Decrease pain
2. Increase endurance and fitness
3. Increase strength
4. Improve posture
5. Decrease mechanical stress
6. Stretch contracted muscles
7. Improve mobility
8. Decrease the number and severity of future back problems

Types of Exercises Used in the Therapy of Low Back Pain Patients

1. Aerobic fitness with low-impact activities
2. Mobility and strengthening exercises
3. Lumbar flexion exercises (Willliams)
4. Lumbar extension exercises (McKenzie method)

There are no good data to favor the utility of one method over the other (flexion vs. extension). However, the literature is suggestive to favor the extension program in pain of discogenic origin. It also appears that the extension program is not especially helpful in chronic low back pain.

Indications

1. Acute low back pain after some response to conservative therapy
2. Low back pain associated with postural factors
3. Fibrositis or fibromyalgia syndrome
4. As part of a general rehabilitation and flexibility program
5. Chronic low back pain

Contraindications

1. Signs of systemic illness, such as fever, weight loss, malaise
2. Acute trauma
3. The young and the elderly who have not had sufficient work-up
4. Cauda equina syndrome: This is the only surgical emergency in acute low back pain of musculoskeletal origin.
5. Radiculopathy and muscle atrophy without adequate work-up

Preparation

1. Patient's pain should have partially responded to rest (no more than 4 days), nonsteroidal anti-inflammatory drugs, and/or muscle relaxants.
2. Patient should be in athletic or nonbinding clothes.
3. Physical therapist or physician should instruct the patient and check progress.

Equipment

Exercise pad on the floor or examining table and pillow

Precautions

1. Flexion exercises should not be done if
   a. There is acute disk prolapse.
   b. The exercise is to begin immediately after a prolonged bed rest, because hyperhydrated disks are susceptible to injury.
   c. Back pain is postural as a result of flexion or lateral trunk list.
2. Extension exercises may cause an increase in symptoms in patients who
   a. Have acute disk prolapse
   b. Have had multiple back surgeries
   c. Have limited range of motion as a result of paraspinous scarring
   d. Have spinal stenosis
   e. Have facet syndrome

Technique

Mobility and Strengthening Exercises

Do in sets of 5 to tolerance.

1. Low back stretch
   a. Lie supine on the floor with the legs extended.
   b. With the right hand, pull the left leg over the right leg.
   c. Shoulders should remain on the floor; turn the head to the left.
   d. Pull up the left thigh to stretch the lower back and buttocks.
   e. Repeat from the other side.
2. Full spinal stretch
   a. Lie supine flat on the floor with the knees bent.

b. Place hands on the back of the thighs and bring the thighs to the abdomen.

c. Curl the head up toward the knees; uncurl; repeat.

3. Heel cord stretch

a. Stand facing a solid wall.

b. Place one foot about 18 inches from the wall and the other behind about 8 to 12 inches.

c. Keep the rear foot flat and place hands shoulder-high against the wall.

d. Bend the forward leg and move the chest toward the wall and feel the stretch in the calf; change the anterior and posterior feet, and repeat.

4. Hamstring stretching

a. Sit with one leg flexed and one leg straight.

b. Reach toward the toes and stretch gently.

c. Change the position of the legs so that the opposite hamstring is stretched.

5. Hip flexor stretching

a. Lie supine with one leg straight and one flexed.

b. Take the flexed thigh and pull toward the chest.

c. Prevent the extended leg from elevating; repeat by changing legs.

6. Back rotation

a. Lie supine with both knees flexed.

b. Keep shoulders flat and swing the knees from side to side to tolerance.

Flexion Exercises (Williams Exercises)

All flexion exercises should begin with the pelvic tilt as illustrated to decrease lumbar lordosis. The lower back should be flat against the floor. Repeat in sets of 5 to tolerance.

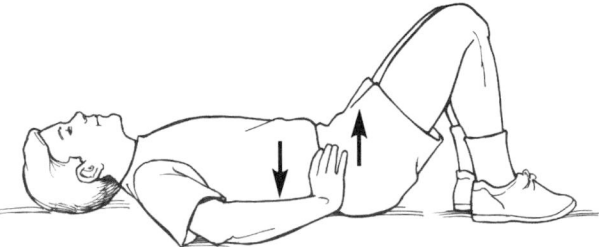

1. Knee to chest

a. Begin by lying on the back with the knees flexed.

b. Place the hands on the knees and pull to chest.

c. Alternative method: can do one leg at a time.

d. Raising head slightly will stretch neck and other paraspinal muscles.

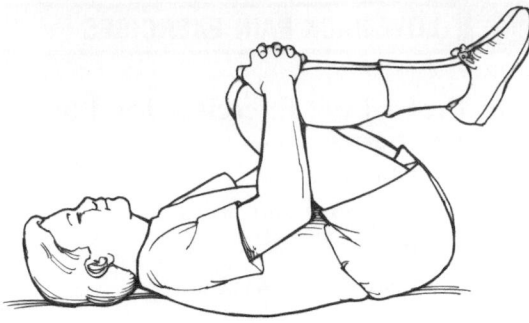

2. Curl-up: strengthens the abdominal muscles

a. Lie supine with knees flexed and feet on floor.

b. Place hands on chest; pelvic tilt.

c. Bring head and shoulders off the floor and hold for count of three.

d. Relax by uncurling.

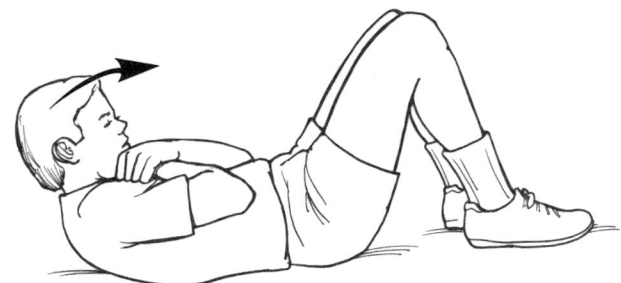

Extension Exercises (McKenzie Technique)

Repeat each exercise in sets of 5 to tolerance.

1. Lying exercises

a. Lie prone, face to one side, arms to side, relax. Pain should lessen or move toward the lower back.

b. Lie prone and then place forearms under shoulders and lift the chest off the floor; hold and then repeat.

c. Lie prone, place hands under shoulders, and push up, lifting chest; straighten elbows to tolerance; eventually get elbows straight and chest and part of the abdomen off the floor.

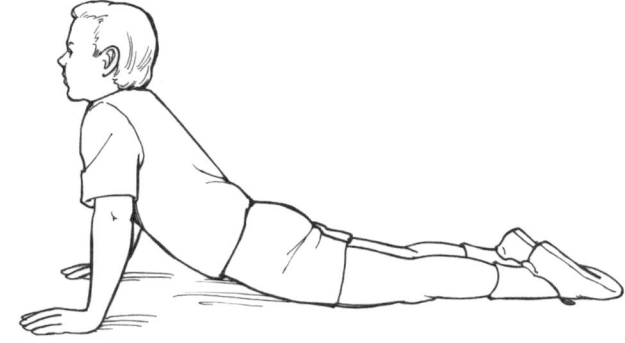

2. Extension in standing

a. Stand with feet apart, hands on hips with

fingers toward the small of the back or hands clasped in small of the back.

b. Bend the trunk backward at the waist as far as possible, keeping the knees straight.

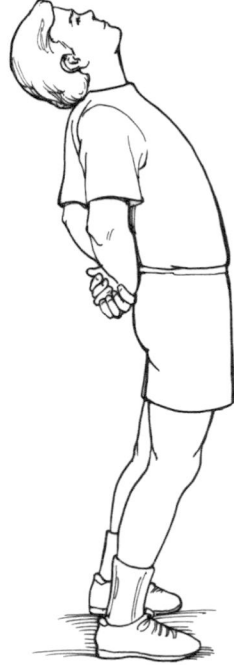

c. Repeat after holding a second or two, trying to extend a little farther each time.

Follow-Up

1. Because many people with acute and chronic low back pain are in poor physical condition,

a prudent program of major muscle group strengthening and cardiorespiratory fitness should be begun when the patient's acute pain is improved.

2. If the McKenzie method exercises are used, flexion exercises should be instituted after the acute pain is resolved. This should help to prevent recurrence of the symptoms. Both sets of exercises should be done on most days of the week.

3. The flexion and extension exercises can be used in chronic back pain to help maintain flexibility and to strengthen and balance the muscles used in maintaining and erect posture. These exercises are also useful in the long-term conservative management of some herniated disks without progressive neurologic signs.

Bibliography

Agency for Health Care Policy and Research: Acute Low Back Problems in Adults: AHCPR Clinical Practice Guidelines, pp 53–57. Washington, DC, Agency for Health Care Policy and Research, 1994.

Borenstein DG, Wiesel SW: Low Back Pain: Medical Diagnosis and Comprehensive Management, 2nd ed, pp 614–624. Philadelphia, WB Saunders Company, 1995.

Cole AJ, Herring SA: The Low Back Pain Handbook, pp 125–140. Philadelphia, Hanley and Belfus, 1997.

McKenzie R: Treat Your Own Back, 4th ed, pp 40–49. London, Spinal Publications, 1991.

Nwuga G, Nwuga V: Relative therapeutic efficacy of the Williams and McKenzie protocols in back pain management. Physiother Pract 1985;1:99–104.

SYMPTOM HIP PAIN

Thurayya Arayssi

The hip joint serves a crucial function in locomotion and weight bearing. It may be subject to extreme stresses or trauma, and diseases that affect it may cause severe disability. Much of this disability is secondary to the pain associated with these processes.

Of all the symptoms of hip disease, hip pain is the most common. Although often manifest as groin pain, it may also be felt in the thigh or buttocks; moreover, pain felt about the proximal femur or more superior pelvis is often also described by patients as "hip pain." The structures that underlie these complaints must also be considered in the diagnosis and management of hip pain.

Hip pain in children and adolescents presents a diagnostic dilemma that may be distinct from that encountered in adults. At the same time, diseases of the hip that begin in childhood may lead to pain and disability in adulthood.

Differential Diagnosis

Groin, Anterior Thigh, and Medial Thigh Pain

1. Osteoarthritis (OA)
2. Transient synovitis
3. Hip fracture
4. Rheumatoid arthritis (RA)
5. Idiopathic avascular necrosis
6. Polymyalgia rheumatica (PMR)
7. Septic arthritis/osteomyelitis
8. Ankylosing spondylitis (AS)
9. Pigmented villonodular synovitis
10. Referred pain (e.g., from testicular torsion)
11. Adductor/quadriceps muscle strain
12. Iliopectineal or iliopsoas bursitis
13. Snapping hip

With specific relation to children and adolescents

14. Slipped upper femoral epiphysis
15. Juvenile RA
16. Perthes' disease
17. Sickle cell disease
18. Hemophilia
19. Acute leukemia

Lateral Hip and Thigh Pain

1. Trochanteric bursitis
2. Fascia lata syndrome
3. Abductor, gluteus muscle strain

Posterior Hip and Thigh Pain

1. Radiculopathy
2. Tumors
3. Diskitis
4. Spondylolisthesis
5. Ischial bursitis
6. Sacroiliitis

The most common cause of hip pain in adults is degenerative joint disease or OA. Other rheumatic conditions, such as PMR and RA, as well as bursitis, fractures, and avascular necrosis, make up the majority of the remaining etiologies. More rarely, conditions such as AS, pigmented villonodular synovitis, and septic arthritis are found to be the cause. Referred pain from structures outside the hip joint itself must also be considered. Lumbar spinal problems and disorders of the pelvic cavity may refer pain to the hip.

In children, acute septic arthritis and osteomyelitis of the proximal femur/greater trochanter must be given more attention in the differential diagnosis. Other causes of acute hip pain include traumatic injuries, the sequelae of acute systemic illnesses, and the entity known as "irritable hip." Conditions that lead to more chronic hip pain in children include chronic slipped upper femoral epiphysis and Perthes' disease, both of which may lead to OA in adulthood.

History: Key Questions to Ask

1. Where is the pain located? ("Point with one finger to the area where you are having pain.")
2. Does the pain move or radiate from its primary location?
3. What were you doing when the pain came on? Was there any trauma?
4. Did the pain come on suddenly or more gradually?
5. What things make the pain better or worse (specifically with regard to activity)?
6. Is there pain in any other distinct location or joint?

7. Is there stiffness in the joint (i.e., pain with movement) in the morning? If so, how long does it last?
8. Do your medications include steroid drugs? How do you use alcohol?
9. Do you have a fever or feel feverish?

The effect of activity on the hip pain is particularly important. For example, hip stiffness may improve with activity in RA but will worsen with OA. Also, bilateral pain that comes on with walking and is relieved by rest may point more specifically to vascular or neurogenic claudications. As outlined above, the location of the pain may be important in eliciting the correct diagnosis and treatment plan. Associated trauma or injury also helps to narrow the differential diagnosis. More general questions regarding systemic symptoms and medication/substance use may bring diagnoses such as infection and avascular necrosis, respectively, to the fore.

Clinical Findings

1. Gait abnormalities, including adductor lurch, antalgic gait, and Trendelenburg gait (pelvis on side opposite the affected side drops during the stance phase)
2. Muscle atrophy in quadriceps denotes severe disease in the hip joint.
3. Positive Trendelenburg sign (non–weight-bearing side of pelvis drops when the patient is asked to stand on the affected leg/hip) is suggestive of hip abductor weakness.
4. The presence of ecchymosis or abrasions is suggestive of trauma.
5. Tenderness to palpation along the lateral aspect of the hip and the greater trochanter points toward trochanteric bursitis.
6. Abnormalities in range-of-motion testing, mainly limitation of abduction and internal rotation, are common with intra-articular hip disease.
7. Pain on hip extension suggests sacroiliac pain, lumbar spine disease, or articular hip pain.
8. Sensory and motor neurologic examination abnormalities are suggestive of radiculopathy.

Tests

1. Radiographic examination is done of both hips with weight-bearing films.
2. Magnetic resonance imaging of both hips if plain films are nonrevealing
3. Complete blood count, sedimentation rate, and serum uric acid level are essential to differentiate inflammatory from noninflammatory causes of hip pain.

4. Aspiration of the hip joint for Gram's stain and culture if septic arthritis is a concern

The interpretation of the above tests should be done in the context of the history and physical examination. Special attention should be paid to findings on x-ray film that do not always correlate with pathology; for example, the presence of osteophytes in a patient with hip pain does not necessarily mean that the patient has OA as a cause of the symptoms.

Management

Management includes the use of medications, surgery, physical therapy, and patient education to relieve pain and maintain function.

Pharmacologic Therapy

1. Nonsteroidal anti-inflammatory medications can be helpful in reducing hip pain of noninfectious etiology. The choice of the medication depends on the response of the patient.
2. Acetaminophen can reduce pain if used on a regular basis.
3. Depot corticosteroids injected locally can be helpful in treating trochanteric bursitis.
4. Low-dose tricyclic antidepressants may be useful for chronic hip pain.
5. Topical medications such as capsaicin may provide some relief.
6. Short-term use of narcotics may be necessary for severe acute pain.

Nonpharmacologic Therapy

1. Local heat and ultrasound therapy can reduce symptoms secondary to bursitis and muscular strain.
2. Physical therapy referral is advised to maintain range of motion and strengthen target muscle groups when pain is adequately controlled.
3. Weight loss is recommended.
4. Femoral osteotomy or hip replacement surgery may be indicated for specific causes of articular hip pain unresponsive to more conservative therapy.

Important

The treatment of hip pain caused by infection (osteomyelitis or septic arthritis) deviates from the general scheme outlined above. In this case, prompt antibiotic therapy based on culture data is essential to the prevention of irreversible joint destruction. Surgical débridement and drainage may also be indicated.

Activity

1. Activity and weight bearing are restricted in the acute phase.
2. Graduated increase in activity and weight bearing is soon recommended.
3. Assistive devices such as cane or crutches can be helpful to unload the affected hip.

Patient Education

Education for weight loss is recommended in obese patients, especially those with OA of the hip.

PEARLS

- OA is the most common cause of hip pain in adults over 50 years of age.

- If infection is suspected, prompt diagnosis and antibiotic treatment, preferably based on specific culture data, are essential.

- Palpation over the proximal lateral thigh and/or greater trochanter that reproduces or exacerbates the patient's pain is highly suggestive of trochanteric bursitis.

- Findings on plain radiographs consistent with OA do not necessarily rule out other etiologies for hip pain.

Bibliography

Boyd RJ: Evaluation of hip pain. In Goroll AH, May LA, Mulley AG Jr (eds): Primary Care Medicine, 3rd ed, pp 762–765. Philadelphia, JB Lippincott Company, 1995.

Dillingham MF, Barry NN, Lannin JV: Hip and knee pain. In Kelley WN, Harris ED, Ruddy S, et al (eds): Textbook of Rheumatology, 5th ed, pp 457–470. Philadelphia, WB Saunders Company, 1997.

Hill RA, Fixsen JA: Investigation and management of the painful hip in childhood. Br J Hosp Med 1994;51:270–274.

Schon L, Zuckerman JD: Hip pain in the elderly: evaluation and diagnosis. Geriatrics 1988;43:48–62.

Types of Regional Anesthetic Blocks

1. Specific nerve block (peripheral block): placed to anesthetize a specific area by blocking a specific nerve
   a. *Advantage*: no distortion of surgical area
   b. *Disadvantage*: requires precise knowledge of anatomy
2. Infiltrative nerve block: Anesthetic is injected in area of procedure.
   a. *Advantage*: Simplicity
   b. *Disadvantages*
      (1) Larger amounts of anesthetic agent usually needed
      (2) Possible tissue distention and distortion of surgical field
      (3) Tissue distention may interfere with vascular supply
      (4) Painful
      (5) Multiple injections may be needed.

Indications for Regional Anesthesia

1. Local and regional anesthesia makes office procedures possible.
2. Patient has medical condition that increases risk for general anesthesia.
3. Postoperative anesthesia

Precautions

1. Vascular insufficiency to extremity
2. Peripheral neuropathies
3. Allergy to local anesthetic
4. Skin infections near site of injection
5. Maximum dose of lidocaine over 90 minutes
   a. With epinephrine, 7 mg/kg
   b. Without epinephrine, 4.5 mg/kg
   c. 1% solution = 10 mg/ml

Complications From Local Anesthesia

1. Central nervous system
   a. Stimulation: seizures, restlessness, disorientation
   b. Depression: unconsciousness, lethargy, dysphasia
2. Cardiovascular
   a. Anaphylactic shock
   b. Bradycardia
   c. Hypotension
   d. Arrhythmia

Preparation for Complications

1. Intubation equipment

2. Electrocardiographic monitoring capabilities
3. Defibrillator
4. Intravenous equipment available
5. Drugs available
   a. Ephedrine to treat hypotension
   b. Atropine to treat bradycardia

Specific Nerve Blocks to Lower Extremity

Common Peroneal Nerve at the Knee

1. Anatomy: Exits the popliteal fossa laterally, passing posterior to the head of the fibula, coursing lateral to the neck of the fibula, entering the head of the peroneus longus muscle, and dividing into the superficial and deep peroneal nerves.

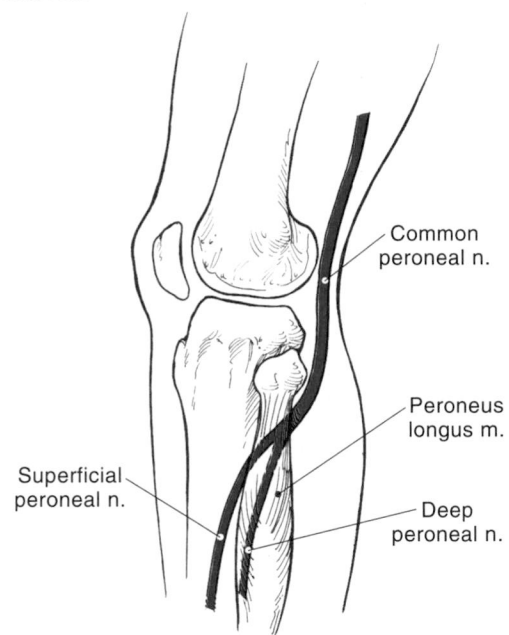

2. Area of anesthesia: lateral calf, ankle, and dorsal foot
3. **Technique**
   a. Identify landmarks: head and neck of fibula.
   b. Prepare skin with antiseptic.
   c. Raise skin wheal 2 cm posterior to head of fibula.
   d. Advance needle, attempt aspiration, inject 5 ml of local anesthetic posterior to head of fibula.

Tibial Nerve at Ankle

1. Anatomy: At the ankle, the tibial nerve passes medially between the Achilles tendon and the flexor digitorum longus tendon posterior to the medial malleolus.

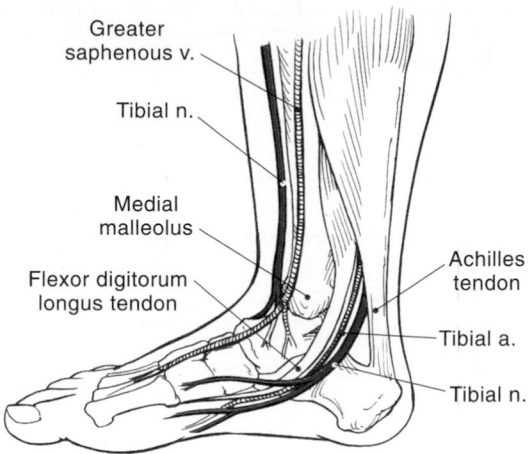

Greater saphenous v.
Tibial n.
Medial malleolus
Flexor digitorum longus tendon
Achilles tendon
Tibial a.
Tibial n.

2. Area of anesthesia: plantar surface of the foot

3. **Technique**

   a. Identify landmarks: palpation of posterior tibial artery posterior to medial malleolus.

   b. Inject 2 to 3 ml of anesthetic just posterior to artery at depth of 1 to 2 cm.

   c. To avoid vascular injection, always aspirate, because the posterior tibial vein is between the artery and nerve.

Sural Nerve

1. Anatomy: Passes 1 to 1.5 cm posterior to the lateral malleolus.

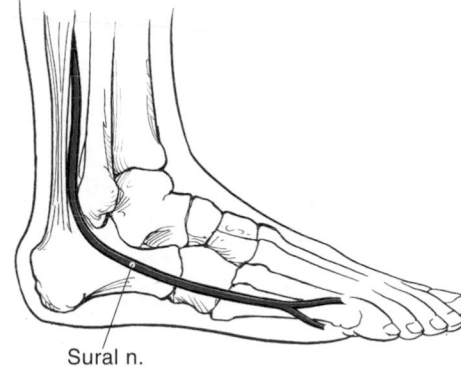

Sural n.

2. Area of anesthesia: lateral fifth metatarsal area

3. **Technique (two options)**

   a. Specific block

      (1) Identify landmark: lateral malleolus.

      (2) Infiltrate subcutaneous tissue 0.5 to 2 cm posterior to lateral malleolus with 3 to 5 ml of anesthetic.

   b. Infiltrative block: 5 to 6 cm proximal to lateral malleolus, inject subcutaneous tissue from lateral edge of tibia to Achilles tendon.

Saphenous Nerve

1. Anatomy: courses in the superficial fascia in the distal anterior medial foreleg, just medial to the greater saphenous vein and lateral to the medial malleolus.

2. Area of anesthesia: distal anterior medial foreleg, including medial malleolus area

3. **Technique (two options)**

   a. Specific block

      (1) Identify landmark: medial malleolus.

      (2) Palpate nerve just anterior and lateral to medial malleolus at ankle. Inject 1 to 2 ml of anesthetic medial to greater saphenous vein.

   b. Infiltrative block: 5 to 6 cm proximal to malleolus, inject subcutaneous tissue from medial edge of tibia to medial edge of Achilles.

Digital Block

1. Anatomy: Each toe has four sensory nerves, two running medially and two laterally along the dorsal and planter surface. The nerves are *subcutaneous*, close to the dermis.

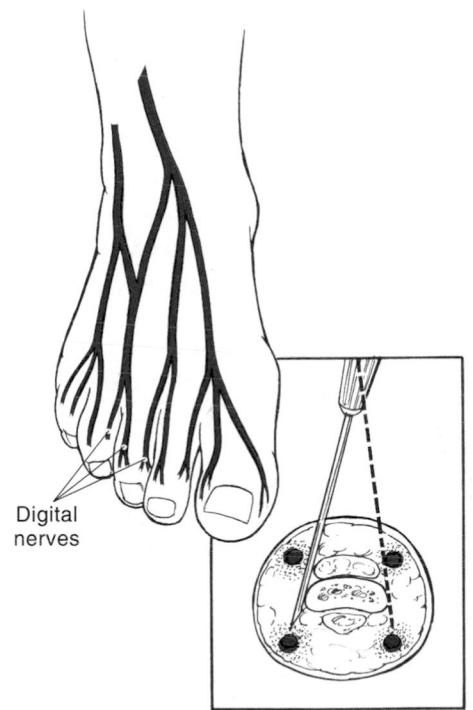

Digital nerves

2. **Technique:** Two wheals of anesthetic agent are injected on the lateral-dorsal and medial-dorsal surfaces in the proximal digit. The needle is then advanced dorsally to the dermis on the planter surface. Then 1 ml of local anesthetic is injected both laterally and medially.

 Bibliography

Brown DL: Regional Anesthesia and Analgesia. Philadelphia, WB Saunders Company, 1996.

Clemente CD: Anatomy: A Regional Atlas of the Human Body. Baltimore, Williams & Wilkins, 1997.

Lutter LD: Atlas of Adult Foot and Ankle Surgery. St. Louis, CV Mosby Company, 1997.

Myerson M: Current Therapy in Foot and Ankle Surgery. St. Louis, BC Decker, 1993.

Williams PL: Gray's Anatomy: The Anatomical Basis of Medicine and Surgery, 38th ed. New York, Churchill Livingstone, 1995.

SYMPTOM KNEE PAIN

Craig C. Young

Knee pain is a common complaint. The etiology of the pain varies with age, illness, and mechanism of injury. Correct diagnosis of the cause will determine the appropriate treatment of the patient.

Differential Diagnosis

Acute Knee Pain: Traumatic Injury

1. Very common cause: medial collateral ligament sprain
2. Common causes
   a. Anterior cruciate ligament (ACL) sprain
   b. Medial meniscus tear
   c. Subluxed or dislocated patella
   d. Contusions
   e. Traumatic bursitis
3. Uncommon causes
   a. Lateral collateral ligament sprain, fracture, traumatic patellofemoral pain syndrome (PFPS), posterior cruciate ligament (PCL) sprain
   b. Muscle strain: includes quadriceps, hamstrings, gastrocnemius, soleus
4. Rare cause: muscle rupture—includes plantaris, quadriceps, hamstrings

Acute Knee Pain: Nontraumatic Injury

1. Common causes
   a. Arthritis
   b. Gout
   c. Calcium pyrophosphate dihydrate (CPPD) crystal deposition disease
   d. Referred pain
      (1) In adults, includes herniated disk, muscle strain, and hip injury.
      (2) In children, hip pathology commonly refers pain to the knee.
2. Uncommon causes: septic knee, ruptured Baker's cyst
3. Rare cause: popliteal aneurysm rupture

Chronic Knee Pain

1. Very common causes
   a. Arthritis
   b. PFPS

2. Common causes
   a. Patellar tendinitis, "jumper's knee"
   b. Iliotibial band syndrome, "runner's knee"
   c. Meniscal tears
   d. Pes anserine bursitis
   e. Osgood-Schlatter disease (common in adolescents)
   f. Quadriceps tendinitis
3. Uncommon causes
   a. Baker's cyst, plica syndrome, recurrent patellar subluxation
   b. Loose bodies, "joint mice": chondral fracture, osteochondral fracture, osteochondritis dissecans (OCD)
4. Rare causes: osteochondritis dissecans, neoplasm, popliteal aneurysm

> Refer to Ch. 213, Bursitis; Ch. 214, Tendinitis and Tendinosis; Ch. 217, Osteoarthritis; Ch. 218, Rheumatoid Arthritis; Ch. 229, Osteochondritis (Osgood-Schlatter Disease); and Ch. 233, Runner's Injuries.

History

1. Onset of injury
   a. Sudden versus gradual onset
   b. Associated change in training pattern, intensity, or activities
   c. Ability to continue activities after injury
2. Mechanism of injury
   a. Varus or valgus contact: ligament sprains, patellar subluxation, meniscal tear, fracture
   b. Direct blow: patellofemoral joint injuries, PCL sprain, fracture
   c. Hyperextension injury: ACL sprain, PCL sprain, posterior capsule injuries
   d. Deceleration injury: ACL sprain
   e. Rotational injury: meniscal injury, ligament injuries, osteochondral fracture, patellar dislocation or subluxation
   f. Dashboard injury: fracture, ligament and capsular injuries
   g. Other important factors: weight-bearing

or non–weight-bearing; direct or indirect force

3. Pop or snap: May indicate rupture of ligament, tendon, or muscle or a fracture.
4. Swelling: how quickly the swelling occurred; bloody effusion immediately after injury indicates a high probability of ACL rupture.
5. Pain: location, radiation pattern, and type
   a. Sharp, stabbing pain more likely to be associated with mechanical problems.
   b. Dull, aching pain more likely to be associated with degenerative and overuse problems.
6. Buckling: Does the knee give way?
   a. Which activities cause it to give way: changing directions, pivoting, walking, or running?
   b. Buckling is associated with ACL injury.
7. Pseudobuckling: a feeling of giving way but without actual giving way of knee; associated with ACL injury, PFPS, arthritis
8. Locking: knee getting caught in specific positions; associated with meniscal injury, loose bodies, OCD, patellar dislocation
9. Pseudolocking: knee feels like it catches without actually locking; associated with PFPS, arthritis, patellar subluxation
10. Other important factors: stiffness, level of function, previous injury

Clinical Findings
1. Observation
   a. Effusions, quadriceps atrophy, standing position, gait
   b. Anatomic malalignment
      (1) Anatomic variances are frequently associated with overuse injuries.
      (2) Common malalignments: Q-angle, patellar position, tibial torsion
2. Palpation: effusion, patellar facets, tendons, joint line
3. Range of motion (ROM): passive, active, resisted, patellar tracking
4. Ligament stability
   a. Lachman's test: Evaluates ACL integrity.
   b. Varus and valgus stress testing: Evaluates collateral ligament integrity.
   c. Posterior drawer test: Evaluates PCL integrity.
   d. Sag test: Evaluates PCL integrity.
5. Grind test: Evaluates PFPS.
6. Apprehension test: Evaluates patella subluxation and dislocation.

7. McMurray's test (circumduction tests): Evaluates meniscus.
8. Functional tests: walking (forward and backward), squatting, bounce squat, stairs, running, figure-of-eights, jumping

Tests
1. Joint aspiration
   a. Bloody effusion: traumatic injury (especially ACL sprain), Charcot joint, tumor, sickle cell joint. Fat droplets indicate intra-articular fracture.
   b. Purulent effusion: septic joint (bacterial, tuberculosis, fungal) is more than 80,000 white blood cells (WBCs)/mm^3, 90 per cent polymorphonuclear leukocytes (PMNs), very low glucose
   c. Inflammatory effusion: rheumatoid arthritis, gout, CPPD, viral arthritis is 1000 to 50,000 WBCs/mm^3, 30 to 50 per cent lymphocytes, 50 to 70 per cent PMNs
   d. Crystal examination: Gout—rods or needles, negatively birefringent (yellow); CPPD—rods, rectangles, or rhomboids, weakly positively birefringent (blue)
2. Radiographs: Use to evaluate possible fractures and injuries that are not responding to treatment. Standard series: anteroposterior weight-bearing (to evaluate joint space), lateral, notch, Merchant's (or other tangential/skyline view).
3. Magnetic resonance imaging: especially useful for evaluation of ligaments, menisci, bone bruises
4. Computerized tomography: especially good for evaluation of OCD and other bony pathology
5. Bone scan: useful for evaluation of overuse injuries, infection, and tumors
6. Arthrography: useful for evaluation of menisci and plica

Management
1. Arthritis: See Ch. 217, Osteoarthritis; and Ch. 218, Rheumatoid Arthritis.
2. Acute treatment (goals: control pain, minimize swelling, minimize tissue damage): protection, rest, ice, compression, elevation
3. Short-term treatment (goals: control pain, maintain ROM): protection, relative rest, ice, painless ROM, nonsteroidal anti-inflammatory drugs (NSAIDs)
4. Intermediate-term treatment (goals: prepare for return to normal activities): wean off NSAIDs, strengthening (start with isometric strengthening; advance to eccentric and concentric

strengthening), stretching, cardiovascular conditioning, functional drills, full ROM exercises

5. Long-term treatment (goals: prevention of future injury): strengthening and stretching

> ## PEARLS
>
> - Bags of poly-wrapped frozen corn kernels make a good reusable substitute for crushed ice.
>
> - Artificial ice substitutes are colder than ice and thus place the body at greater risk for frostbite. Always wrap artificial ice in towels before placing against skin.

Bibliography

For more information on physical assessment, see
Magee D: Orthopedic Physical Assessment, 3rd ed, pp 506–598. Philadelphia, WB Saunders Company, 1997.
For more information on imaging, see
Gray SD, Kaplan PA, Dussault RG: Imaging of the knee: current status. Orthop Clin North Am 1997;28:643–648.
For more information on assessment and treatment of pediatric knee injuries, see
Davids JR: Pediatric knee: clinical assessment and common disorders. Pediatr Clin North Am 1996;43:1067–1090.
For more information on assessment and treatment of athletic knee injuries, see
Fadale PD, Hulstyn MJ: Common athletic knee injuries. Clin Sports Med 1997;16:479–499.
For more information on assessment and treatment of occupational knee injuries, see
Westrich GH, Hass SB, Bono JV: Occupational knee injuries. Orthop Clin North Am 1996;27:805–814.

SYMPTOM ANKLE AND FOOT PAIN

James R. Barrett

A Gallup poll showed that three fourths of Americans over the age of 18 complained that their feet hurt. Amazingly, nearly two thirds thought that their feet were supposed to hurt. Foot and ankle pain are common problems that are often seen by primary care physicians. Although rarely life-threatening, these complaints do cause significant discomfort and disability because of the importance of ambulation for work and pleasure. For this reason, it is important for the primary care physician to have a working knowledge of the most common causes of ankle and foot pain.

Ankle Pain

Differential Diagnosis (in Order of Likelihood)

1. Ankle sprain, including syndesmotic sprains
2. Fracture, including stress fractures: tibia, fibula, talus, calcaneus, fifth metatarsal
3. Peroneal tendonitis/subluxation/dislocation
4. Arthritides: rheumatoid, degenerative joint disease (DJD), gout, pseudogout, ankylosing spondylitis, Reiter's syndrome, psoriatic
5. Anterior/posterior impingement
6. Complex regional pain syndrome (CRPS) (new term for reflex sympathetic dystrophy)
7. Osteochondritis dissecans

> Refer to Ch. 217, Osteoarthritis; Ch. 218, Rheumatoid Arthritis; Ch. 233, Runner's Injuries; Ch. 243, Ankle Fractures; and Ch. 244, Foot Fractures.

History: Key Questions to Ask

1. Description of the pain: exact location, quality, timing, relieving or aggravating features, referral to other areas, associated symptoms
   a. Acute-onset pain with no trauma? Early morning stiffness? (arthritis)
   b. Pain with extreme dorsi-/plantar flexion? (anterior/posterior impingement)
   c. Pain out of proportion to injury? Vasomotor disturbances and/or edema? (CRPS)
2. Mechanism of injury (if injured)?
3. Previous foot or ankle injury?
4. Occupational or athletic history
5. Family history of arthritis, cancer, hypertension, or cardiovascular disease?
6. Can the patient ambulate?
7. Swelling or ecchymosis?
8. Mechanical symptoms: popping or snapping noticed? (peroneal tendon dysfunction); locking or instability of ankle? (osteochondritis dissecans)

Clinical Findings

1. Skin appearance, including swelling, ecchymosis, erythema, mottled appearance
2. Range of motion (ROM)
3. Palpable tenderness over bones, ligaments, and tendons
4. Neurovascular examination
5. Anterior drawer/talar tilt/compression test of tibia and fibula

Tests

1. Radiographs of ankle (anteroposterior, lateral, and oblique) if fracture suspected; consider radiograph of *entire* tibia/fibula (especially medial sprains) or foot (fifth metatarsal tenderness).
2. Bone scan for suspected stress fracture
3. Tomography or computerized tomography for suspected osteochondral lesion
4. Magnetic resonance imaging for soft tissue pathology or osteochondral lesion

Treatment

1. Acute treatment based on *RICED* mnemonic:
   a. *R*est from pain-producing activities
   b. *I*ce for 20 minutes several times a day while area is swollen
   c. *C*ompression with padding and a wrap
   d. *E*levation above level of heart to reduce edema
   e. Nonsteroidal anti-inflammatory *D*rugs for pain and inflammation if not contraindicated
2. Physical therapy (PT) aimed at improving motion, strength, flexibility, and proprioception. Non–weight-bearing exercises early until protected weight bearing is tolerated (pain as a guideline) and inflammatory phase subsides.
3. Peroneal tendon dysfunction: peroneal tendon stretching, medial heel wedge, ankle brace, PT, occasionally surgery
4. CRPS: pain relief with anti-inflammatories or mild narcotics, early ROM, PT, occasional referral to anesthesia for sympathetic blocks

Heel Pain

Differential Diagnosis (in Order of Likelihood)

1. Inferior
   a. Plantar fasciitis or fascial rupture
   b. Arthritides: rheumatoid, DJD, gout, pseudogout, ankylosing spondylitis, Reiter's syndrome, psoriatic
   c. Calcaneal fracture
   d. Nerve entrapment
   e. Lumbar radiculopathy (S1)
2. Posterior
   a. Achilles tendinitis (calcaneal apophysitis [Sever's disease] in children) or rupture
   b. Haglund's deformity ("pump bump")
   c. Bursitis
3. Medial
   a. Posterior tibial tendinitis
   b. Tarsal tunnel syndrome

c. Nerve entrapment

History: Key Questions to Ask

1. Description of the pain (see "Ankle Pain")
   a. Pain when first step down after sleeping or sitting? (plantar fasciitis)
   b. Pain activity-related? History of increased activity? (tendonitis or stress fracture)
   c. Burning or tingling sensation/pain at night? (neurologic origin)
2. Occupational or athletic history
3. History of low back pain or injury? (radiculopathy)

Clinical Findings

1. Palpable tenderness over bone, tendon, plantar fascia, soft tissue
2. Pain with
   a. Medial and lateral compression of calcaneus? (stress fracture)
   b. Active inversion? (posterior tibialis tendinitis)
   c. Percussion? (fracture)
3. Lumbar back examination, including straight-leg raise (S1 radiculopathy)
4. Positive Tinel's sign (tarsal tunnel syndrome)
5. Palpable gap in Achilles tendon; positive Thompson test: squeeze calf—no plantar flexion noted (Achilles tendon rupture)
6. Foot type: cavus or pronated (associated with plantar fasciitis)

Tests

1. Radiograph: calcaneus
2. Laboratory: erythrocyte sedimentation rate, human leukocyte antigen B27, rheumatoid factor if arthritis is suspected
3. Electromyography/nerve conduction velocity (EMG/NCV) for neurologic abnormalities

Treatment

1. RICED (see "Ankle Pain")
2. Supportive footwear with a firm heel counter and arch support, lace-up shoes
3. Plantar fasciitis: heel pad or wedge, stretching exercises for plantar fascia, PT, low dye taping, orthotics, steroid injection, night splints, surgery
4. Posterior tibialis tendinitis: medial arch support or wedge, PT
5. Haglund's deformity, Achilles tendinitis, bursitis: 1/4-inch heel wedge, calf stretching, PT, surgery

6. Achilles tendon rupture: surgical consultation (debated in literature whether casting or primary repair results in better outcome)

Forefoot Pain

Differential Diagnosis (in Order of Likelihood)

1. First metatarsal pain
   a. Bunion/hallux valgus
   b. Hallux limitus/rigidus
   c. Sesamoiditis
   d. Arthritides: rheumatoid, DJD, gout, pseudogout, ankylosing spondylitis, Reiter's syndrome, psoriatic
   e. Diabetic neuropathy
   f. Infection
2. Forefoot pain (metatarsalgia)
   a. Interdigital neuroma
   b. Sprain
   c. Calluses/warts
   d. Stress fracture
   e. Nerve entrapment: posterior tibial
   f. Diabetic neuropathy
   g. Infection

History: Key Questions to Ask

1. Description of the pain (see "Ankle Pain")
   a. Pain better with shoe off? Better with massage of foot? Burning or sharp pain with weight-bearing? "Electric shock?" (neuroma)
   b. Numbness or tingling into the toes? (neurologic origin)
   c. Great toe pain when toeing off? On tiptoes? (hallux rigidus or sesamoiditis)
   d. Atraumatic hot, swollen first toe? Gnawing or throbbing pain? (gout/infection)
   e. Stocking distribution to pain? (diabetic neuropathy)
   f. Pain only with activity? During standing or weight-bearing? (stress fracture)
2. Frequent use of high-heeled shoes with narrow toe box?

Clinical Findings

1. Evaluation of footwear: Does it fit correctly? Wear pattern? Wide or narrow toe box? Is heel counter firm? Height of heel?
2. Palpable tenderness: on metatarsal head, metatarsal body, between metatarsal heads, at ball of foot, over sesamoids?
3. Warmth/swelling

4. Foot type
5. Decreased plantar/dorsiflexion at first metatarsophalangeal joint (hallux rigidus/limitus)
6. Any visual deformities of the foot; protuberance medially or laterally (bunion)
7. Hyperesthesia in web space (neurologic origin)
8. Palpable mass on plantar aspect; positive Mulder's sign—pain on compressing forefoot from side to side while squeezing the tissue between metatarsal heads with fingertip (neuroma)

Tests

1. Radiograph of foot
2. Joint aspiration if gout, pseudogout, or joint infection suspected
3. EMG/NCV for suspected neurologic problem

Treatment

1. RICED (see "Ankle Pain")
2. Avoid constrictive footwear—use wide toe box, low heel, and supportive arch.
3. Neuroma: metatarsal pad, corticosteroid injection, PT, surgery
4. Hallux limitus/rigidus: padding to shift weight laterally, hard-soled shoe, joint injection with steroid/anesthetic, surgery
5. Hallux valgus: Trim hyperkeratotic area, bunion shield/pad medial side, orthotics, surgery for severe deformity or pain unresponsive to conservative measures.
6. Sesamoiditis: crescent-shaped pad, stiff-soled shoe, orthotics, PT, rarely surgery
7. Calluses: Remove hyperkeratotic area with scapel or pumice stone, insoles or orthotics to relieve friction.
8. Warts: keratolytic agent (trichloroacetic acid, salicylic acid), cryosurgery, electrodesiccation

---

PEARLS

- Urgent referral to orthopedic surgeon if acute neurovascular impairment

- Referral or consultation for displaced ankle fracture, Jones' fracture, peroneal tendon dislocation, or osteochondritis dissecans

- Warts can be distinguished from calluses by interruption of skin lines, blood vessels in the core, and tenderness on squeezing.

- Stress fractures are common in the foot and frequently do not show up on radiographs; have a high index of suspicion for them.

Bibliography

Birrer R, DellaCorte M, Grisafi P: Common Foot Problems in Primary Care. Philadelphia, Hanley & Belfus, 1998.

Calliet R: Foot and Ankle Pain. Philadelphia, FA Davis Company, 1997.

Garrick J, Webb D: Sports Injuries: Diagnosis and Management, pp 279–320. Philadelphia, WB Saunders Company, 1990.

Kwong P (ed): Foot and Ankle Injuries. Clin Sports Med 1994;13:683–952. Philadelphia, WB Saunders Company, 1994.

McBryde AM Jr: Disorders of the ankle and foot. In Grana WA, Kalenak A (eds): Clin Sports Med. Philadelphia, WB Saunders Company, 1991; pp 466–489.

212 Ankle Sprain

Ben L. Glaspey

Etiology

1. Inversion and plantar flexion: injury to lateral ligaments (anterior and posterior talofibular, calcaneofibular). Anterior talofibular usually injured first.
2. Eversion: injury to medial ligaments (deltoid, anteroinferior tibiofibular, interosseous membrane)

Symptoms

1. Aid in determining grade or severity of sprain. Classified as grades 1, 2, and 3 (Table 212–1).
2. One or more of the following should be present: pain, inability to bear weight (especially with grades 2 and 3), swelling (immediate with grades 2 and 3, hours later with grade 1), decreased range of motion (ROM).

Clinical Findings

1. In conjunction with symptoms, used to determine grade or severity of injury
2. One or more of the following should be present: swelling, ecchymosis, point tenderness over ligament or insertion point, diffuse tenderness, laxity when ligaments stressed (only with grades 2 and 3).

> **WARNING**
>
> Severe ankle sprains (especially grade 3) can be associated with either fractures of adjacent bones or sprains in other areas (e.g., knee). As with all significant orthopedic injuries, palpate adjacent joints and bones to screen for associated injuries.

Laboratory Tests

1. Ottawa Ankle Rules: Determine necessity of ankle and foot radiographs (see Fig. 212–1 legend for guidelines). *Note:* A 28 per cent decrease in numbers of radiographs ordered (foot and ankle) with no "significant" fractures missed.
2. Stress radiographs or arthrograms: Differentiate grades 2 and 3 by widening of the ankle mortise. Grade 3 injury shows widening of anterior tibial tubercle–fibula interval more than 5 mm.
3. If septic joint or inflammatory arthritis is suspected, do arthrocentesis, joint fluid analysis.

Differential Diagnosis

1. Fracture of the lateral malleolus, medial malleolus, dome of talus, tarsal navicular, or proximal fifth metatarsal. *Note:* Proximal fifth metatarsal fractures are often missed because the area is not palpated.
2. Growth plate injury: In children, the ligaments and joint capsules are two to five times stronger than the physis; therefore, growth plate injuries are more common than sprains.
3. Syndesmosis sprains (i.e., sprains of the tibiofibular ligament)
4. Arthritis (e.g., gout, septic joint): Onset may coincide with or be triggered by trauma.
5. Myositis ossificans: extraskeletal ossification that can be confused with sarcoma

> **PEARL**
>
> Myositis ossificans usually involves the diaphysis; pain and mass decrease with time, and radiographs demonstrate an intact underlying cortex. This is a contraindication to early mobilization.

6. Compartment syndrome of the leg

TABLE 212–1.   CLASSIFICATION OF LIGAMENT INJURIES

Grade	Amount of Tear	Able to Continue Activity?	Swelling	Laxity
1	<25%	Yes	Hours later	None
2	25–75%	No	Within minutes	Mild (firm end point)
3	75%–complete	No	Within minutes	Yes (soft end point, "clink")

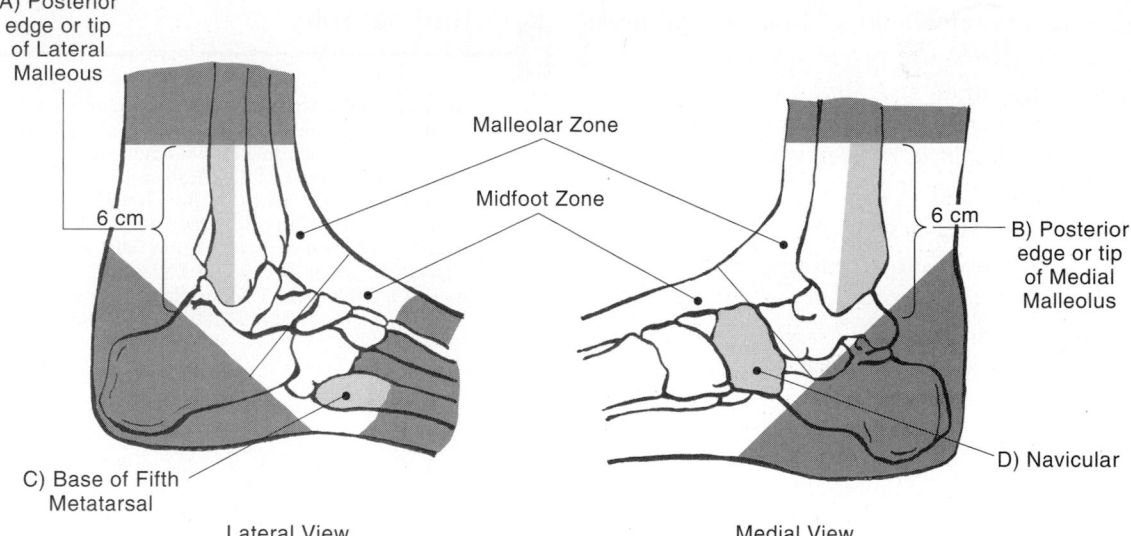

A) Posterior edge or tip of Lateral Malleous

Malleolar Zone

Midfoot Zone

6 cm

6 cm

B) Posterior edge or tip of Medial Malleolus

C) Base of Fifth Metatarsal

D) Navicular

Lateral View

Medial View

Figure 212–1 Ottawa Ankle Rules. An ankle radiologic series needed with malleolar pain and tenderness at A, B, C, or D, or inability to bear weight both immediately and in emergency department. (Modified from Stiell IG, Greenberg GH, McKnight RD, et al: Decision rules for the use of radiography in acute ankle injuries: refinement and prospective validation. JAMA 1994;271:827–832. Used with permission.)

Treatment

PRINCE

1. *Protection:* Use compression wrap first (see below), then follow with air stirrups or other form of ankle support.

2. *Rest:* crutches until painless weight-bearing. Begin ROM exercises when swelling stops. Exception is myositis ossificans—refer.

3. *Ice:* first 24 to 48 hours. Apply ice bag for 10 to 20 minutes every 1 to 2 hours during the day. Then contrast baths when swelling stops until swelling resolves. For example, perform ROM exercises for 4 minutes in warm water followed by 1 minute in cold, repeated 4 times. Trace alphabet in large letters with big toe.

4. *Nonsteroidal anti-inflammatory drugs (NSAIDs):* Use around the clock, *not* as needed (prn), for first couple of days.

5. *Compression:* Proper use of the compression wrap is paramount for preserving ROM and strength. Place pair of felt horseshoes or donuts around medial and lateral malleoli and hold in place with elastic bandage or stockinette. Keep in place for first 24 to 36 hours.

6. *Elevation:* ideally, above the heart for 24 to 48 hours

Medication

1. NSAIDs: Ibuprofen is inexpensive and effective. Use every 6 hours around the clock for 24 to 48 hours and then prn. Take with food!

2. Narcotic analgesics in conjunction for more severe sprains

---

Key Treatment

PRINCE

- *P*rotection
- *R*est
- *I*ce
- *N*SAIDs
- *C*ompression
- *E*levation

Follow-Up

1. Ankle rehabilitation

   a. Passive ROM exercises early: flexion/extension with towel under ball of foot, toe circles, heel walk, toe walk. May use water exercises in pool.

   b. Athletes: Progress through stages and advance when activity no longer hurts.

      (1) Stages: walk, run in straight line, run in wide circles, run in figure-of-eight

      (2) Rule of thumb: Football player can practice when he can run tight (20-yard-long) figure-of-eight with little or no pain.

      (3) Return to previous stage if pain or disability increases.

   c. Persistent ankle pain 6 or more weeks after injury may be caused by insufficient rehabilitation, impingement syndrome, talar dome fracture, or syndesmosis injury. Clinical pearl for talar dome fracture: episodes of brief, spontaneous lancinating pain, like an "ice pick," during rehabilitation.

d. Chronic unstable ankles: 3-mm lateral heel and sole wedge to prevent inversion

e. Follow-up office visit in 3 to 4 weeks with repeat radiographs, bone scan or magnetic resonance imaging for persistent pain.

2. Avoid reinjury

a. Tape ankle after first injury.

b. Braces for chronic or recurrent sprains (lace-up, air splints). Consider underlying cause of recurrent sprains.

c. High-top, lace-up shoes/sneakers

Bibliography

Bassewitz HL, Shapiro MS: Persistent pain after ankle sprain. Physician Sportsmed 1997;25:58–68.

Garrick JG, Schelkun PH: Managing ankle sprains. Physician Sportsmed 1997;25:56–68.

Meisterling RC, Johnson RJ: Recurrent lateral ankle sprains. Physician Sportsmed 1993;21:123–132.

Shea MP, Manoli A: Recognizing talar dome lesions. Physician Sportsmed 1993;21:109–121.

Stiell IG, McKnight RD: Implementation of the Ottawa Ankle Rules. JAMA 1994;271:827–832.

213 Bursitis

Lawrence D. Powell

Etiology

1. Anatomy: There are over 150 bursae in the human body. They function to reduce friction between fascial planes. The subacromial, iliopectineal, ischiogluteal, semimembranous, gastrocnemius, and suprapatellar bursae communicate with the adjacent joint. Most other bursae, like the prepatellar, are freestanding. Types of bursae:

   a. Constant: formed during embryonic development. The epithelium lined with synovial cells secrete a lubricating fluid.

   b. Adventitial: form later in life from myxomatous degeneration of fibrous tissue (i.e., bunion, bunionette, or head of fifth metatarsal). They do not have an endothelial lining and therefore do not secrete synovial fluid.

2. Pathophysiology: Tissue injury stimulates the inflammatory cascade. The bursae fill with fluid and enlarge. If the condition is not treated, fibrous bands, loose bodies of scar tissue, and thickening may develop.

3. Cause

   a. Microtrauma: cumulative trauma that leads to chronic thickening. There may be associated mechanical causes such as soft tissue injury to adjacent structures, as in supraspinatus tendinitis. Chronic inflammation can predispose to calcific bursitis.

   b. Macrotrauma: secondary to a single event, such as a direct blow. There is often hemorrhage into the bursa, common in superficial bursae such as the prepatellar or olecranon.

   c. Septic: Infection is usually secondary to breakdown in the skin defenses (i.e., laceration, ulceration, or cellulitis) and the transcutaneous spread of pathogens. Iatrogenic puncture wounds, gout, hemodialysis, and atopic dermatitis are other risk factors. *Staphylococcus aureus* is the major pathogen. Hematogenous spread is possible. Septic bursitis can be associated with septic arthritis as a result of communication between the joint space and the bursa.

> **Note**
>
> *Common Pathogens*
> - *Staphylococcus aureus* (90 per cent)
> - Group A streptococci and *Staphylococcus epidermidis* (9 per cent)
>
> *Rare*
> - *Candida*
> - *Mycobacterium tuberculosis* and *marinum*
> - *Propionibacterium acnes*
> - *Haemophilus influenzae*
> - *Bacillus subtilis*
> - *Escherichia coli*
> - *Pseudomonas*

---

   d. Crystalline-induced: Apatite crystals are most common; these include calcium pyrophosphate, hydroxyapatite, and fluoroapatite. Monosodium urate, calcium oxalate, and cholesterol crystals are other causes. Gout and pseudogout are associated disorders that can cause crystalline-induced bursitis.

   e. Systemic disease: Bursitis is seen with rheumatoid arthritis and spondyloarthropathies. Syphilis, hypothyroidism, and systemic scleroderma are less commonly associated with bursitis.

Symptoms

1. Pain: Onset is acute if traumatic and insidious if overuse is the cause. It is characterized as aching in quality, well localized, and constant. The severity is subjective. Activity aggravates it, especially against resistance. It is relieved with rest.

2. Swelling: usually present but may not be apparent in bursa located deep or under thick subcutaneous tissue

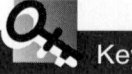

Key Symptom

Localized pain exacerbated by activity

Clinical Findings

1. There is usually localized tenderness to palpation.
2. Swelling is usually present, except in bursae not located superficially.
3. Passive range of motion is usually normal, but active range of motion may be limited by pain.
4. Erythema may be present, especially in septic bursitis.
5. Disuse atrophy and weakness may indicate a chronic bursitis.

Key Signs

Localized tenderness and swelling

Common Sites

1. Subacromial/subdeltoid: located below acromion. Pain is worse with overhead maneuvers and lying on affected shoulder. Tenderness can be demonstrated below the acromion, near the supraspinatus tendon, or along the supraspinatus muscle. Neer's and Hawkin's impingement signs and supraspinatus challenge test are positive.
2. Subscapular: located on the superomedial, superolateral, and inferomedial border of the scapula. Usually presents with a "snapping scapula."
3. Olecranon ("miner's elbow"): located superficially near the olecranon process of the ulnar. Presents with tender, swollen, red area on the back of elbow. In septic bursitis the person may be febrile.
4. Iliopectineal/iliopsoas: located between pectineus and psoas muscle over lesser trochanter. Presents with groin pain exacerbated by hyperextension, adduction, and internal rotation of hip against resistance. Position of comfort is hip in flexion and external rotation.
5. Ischiogluteal ("weaver's bottom"): located over ischial tuberosity. Presents with pain with sitting and walking. Pain worse with passive flexion or hip extension against resistance. Pain may radiate because bursa overlies sciatic and posterior femoral cutaneous nerve.
6. Greater trochanter: located over greater trochanter. Seen commonly in overweight, middle-aged women. Presents with lateral hip pain worse with hip abduction and external rotation against resistance, and when lying on affected side.

7. Medial collateral ligament: located on anterior attachment of medial collateral ligament on the tibia. Usually follows external rotation twisting knee injury. Presents with medial knee pain inferior to joint, worse with knee extension.
8. Pes anserine: located where sartorius, semitendinosus, gracilis tendons insert on the tibia. Pain over medial anterior tibia below knee. Associated with obesity, jogging, or frequent knee bending, and with sports such as basketball, soccer, or racket sports. Pain worse with active knee flexion.
9. Prepatellar ("housemaid's knee," "coal-miner's knee"): located over patella. Presents as swelling anterior to patella. Because of superficial location, frequently associated with traumatic and/or septic bursitis.
10. Calcaneal: Two bursae are located near the insertion of the Achilles tendon. The superficial bursa is located just anterior to Achilles tendon. Bursitis at this site is associated with ill-fitting shoes. The retrocalcaneal bursa is located posterior to the Achilles tendon. Bursitis at this site is associated with prominent posterosuperior angle of the calcaneus (Haglund's deformity). Both of these conditions can co-exist with Achilles tendinitis. Presents with posterolateral and posteromedial heel pain and swelling. Pain is worse with passive dorsiflexion.

Laboratory Tests

1. Usually requires no tests
2. Culture and Gram's stain are obtained from bursal aspirate if infection is suspected. Normal bursal fluid has a clear to turbid appearance with a low white cell count and a predominance of monocytes. If septic, the fluid aspirate is purulent in appearance, the culture is positive, and the white cell count is elevated with a predominance of polymorphonuclear leukocytes. The Gram's stain is unreliable.

Note

- **Normal:** White blood cell count less than 2000/mm^3
- **Inflammatory:** White blood cell count 2000 to 50,000/mm^3
- **Infectious:** White blood cell count greater than 50,000/mm^3

---

3. Fibrocartilaginous bodies (rice bodies) suggestive of rheumatoid arthritis and other spondyloarthropathies

4. Bone scan may be useful to rule out other causes of pain.

Differential Diagnosis

1. Consider local soft tissue injury, tendinitis, ligament sprain, muscle strain, meniscal injury, and synovitis.
2. Other infectious processes, such as abscess and septic arthritis, should also be considered.
3. Bone pathology, such as degenerative joint disease, fracture, and osteomyelitis, should be ruled out.
4. Referred pain from vertebral disk disease and spinal nerve root radiculopathy are possibilities.
5. Systemic diseases, such as gout, pseudogout, Reiter's syndrome, or rheumatoid arthritis, can cause similar symptoms.
6. Other conditions, such as femoral aneurysms, metastatic tumors, lymphadenopathy, hernia, and vascular malformations, could be causative.

Treatment

1. Nonoperative management
   a. Active rest such as swimming, cycling, or pool running
   b. Topical ice, ice massage, or ice bath
   c. Compression wrap to reduce acute swelling or fluid reaccumulation after intrabursal aspiration
   d. Physical therapy modalities such as iontophoresis or phonophoresis. Stretching and strengthening exercises also are of benefit.
   e. Oral nonsteroidal anti-inflammatory drugs such as
      (1) Ibuprofen, 200 to 400 mg tid or qid
      (2) Naproxen sodium (Aleve), 200 mg bid or tid
   f. Steroid injections for refractory symptoms
      (1) Betamethasone acetate (Celestone Soluspan), 6 mg/ml, 0.5 to 1 ml with 2 to 4 ml lidocaine
      (2) Triamcinolone acetonide (Kenalog), 20 mg/ml or 40 mg/ml, 0.5 to 1 ml with 2 to 4 ml lidocaine

      (3) Complications of steroid injection are skin depigmentation, subcutaneous atrophy, and crystal-induced postinjection flare.
2. Septic bursitis
   a. Empiric oral therapy with β-lactamase–resistant antibiotic for 4 weeks
      (1) Dicloxacillin, 500 mg PO qid
      (2) Keflex, 500 mg PO qid
   b. Parenteral therapy and surgical drainage may be required for severe cases.
3. Operative procedures, such as bursectomy, partial tendon release, or surgical removal of bony defects, are rarely needed.

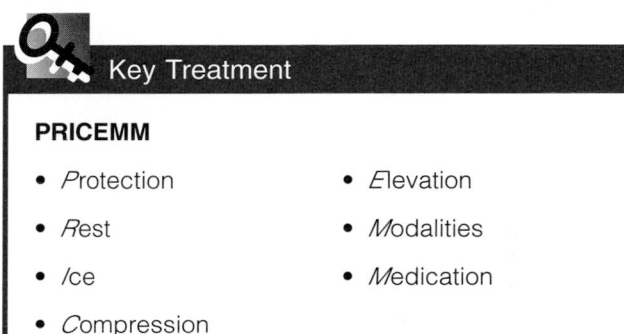

Key Treatment

PRICEMM

- *P*rotection
- *R*est
- *I*ce
- *C*ompression
- *E*levation
- *M*odalities
- *M*edication

Follow-Up

1. Evaluate response to nonoperative treatment.
2. Consider orthopedic consultation if poor response to conservative treatment or if fluid reaccumulates after aspiration while on antibiotic therapy.

Bibliography

Butcher JD, Salzman MC, Lillegard WA: Lower extremity bursitis. Am J Fam Pract 1996;53:2317–2324.
Dillingham MF, Barry NN, Lannin JV: Hip and knee pain. In Kelly WN, Ruddy S, Harris ED, et al (eds): Textbook of Rheumatology, 5th ed, vol 1, pp 457–478. Philadelphia, WB Saunders Company, 1997.
Larsson L, Baum J: The syndromes of bursitis. Bull Rheum Dis 1986;36:1–8.
Salzman KL, Lillegard WA, Butcher MC: Upper extremity bursitis. Am J Fam Pract 1997;56:1797–1806.
Zimmerman B 3rd, Mikolich DJ, Ho G Jr: Septic bursitis. Semin Arthritis Rheum 1995;24:391–410.

214 Tendinitis and Tendinosis

Daniel T. Davison

Definitions

1. Tendon injuries often occur by traumatic means or, more usually, by overuse during sporting activity, work, or day-to-day activities.
2. Certain inflammatory arthropathies may present as tendinitis:
   a. Rheumatoid arthritis
   b. Systemic lupus erythematosus
3. Macrotrauma: traumatic tendinitis
   a. An acute traumatic injury resulting from an excessive compressive force (contusion) or sudden overstretching (strain)
   b. Macrotrauma is an event, not a process.
4. Microtrauma: overuse, overload
   a. An injury that occurs to a particular anatomic structure that cannot adapt to the cumulative stress of a repetitively applied force
   b. Overuse is a process, not an event; repetitive microtrauma accumulates over time and results in local tissue injury.
   c. Tendon injuries are likely the most common overuse conditions encountered in sports.
   d. Tendons most susceptible to overload are "those that undergo large loads in an eccentric or stretching mode in which the tendon is storing and releasing energy" (Tietz and Garrett, 1997).
   e. The risk of overuse tendon injury is related to the amount of activity and age.
   f. The basic pathologic process identified within the overloaded tendon is degenerative rather than inflammatory, and thus the term *tendinosis* is more applicable than *tendinitis*.

Etiology

Traumatic Tendinitis

1. Strains
   a. Result from excessive tensile forces on the musculotendinous junction, causing overstretching and tearing.
   b. Contributing factors: lack of sufficient flexibility, inadequate warm-up, local corticosteroid injection, fatigue, deconditioning, recent injury

2. Contusion
   a. Result from high-velocity compressive forces.
   b. The more contracted the muscle at the time of injury, the more severe is the injury.

Tendinosis

1. Age: Older individuals are more susceptible to tendon overload.
2. Excessive pressure on the tendon: acromial clavicular arthritis causing rotator cuff tendinosis
3. Friction between soft tissue planes: iliotibial band tendinosis resulting from the iliotibial band rubbing over the lateral femoral condyle
4. Tissue overload, as in patellar or Achilles tendinosis
5. The sheath of tendons that overlies a joint may be a bursa, which becomes irritated from friction of the tendon as it moves under a rigid arch, as in subacromial bursitis secondary to shoulder impingement syndrome.
6. Bursitis may result as a secondary effect of the proximity of the bursa to the irritated tendon, as in retrocalcaneal bursitis secondary to Achilles tendinosis.
7. Extrinsic risk factors
   a. Athletic training/work errors: The amount, intensity, and frequency of the activity (work, exercise) are major factors in the evolution of overuse: too much, too fast, too soon, too often; too long.
   b. Play/work surface: hard (concrete vs. asphalt), soft (dirt vs. grass), canted (track vs. road)
   c. Alteration in athletic training/work routine
      (1) Interval training, hill running
      (2) A normally sedentary individual who suddenly performs physical work
   d. Improper technique
   e. Inappropriate/deteriorated equipment/footwear: Overuse injury risk increases when runners accumulate more than 500 miles on their running shoes.
   f. The biomechanics of the sport or activity involved usually dictates the body part/tissue at risk.

8. Intrinsic risk factors
   a. Anatomic malalignment: excessive femoral neck anteversion, foot pronation/supination, tibial torsion, genu varum (bow legs), genu valgum (knock knees).
   b. Leg-length discrepancy
   c. Muscle imbalance: very important in all levels of activity
   d. Muscle weakness: more important in lesser trained individuals
   e. Flexibility/inflexibility
   f. Excessive joint laxity: Chronically unstable shoulder joint is a cause of rotator cuff tendinosis (the rotator cuff is a dynamic stabilizer of the shoulder).
   g. Associated disease states: rheumatoid arthritis
   h. Previous injury *not* treated properly
   i. Growth process/the growth spurt: Longitudinal bone growth leads to relative muscle-tendon tightness and inflexibility.

Symptoms

Traumatic Tendinitis

1. Mechanism of injury: An accurate description of the injury mechanism frequently leads to the correct diagnosis.
2. Recent injury: One of the more common causes of a reinjury is a previous injury that was misdiagnosed or was diagnosed properly but improperly treated.
3. An audible "pop" or "snap" indicates significant muscle-tendon tearing.
4. Patients frequently report they thought they were struck by a stick or were kicked.
5. Initially, if the tearing is mild to moderate, there may be very little pain and disability, and patients report they could return to the activity.
6. Swelling, pain, and disability progress over several hours and are maximal the day following the injury.
7. Referred/radicular pain
   a. Hamstring pain from lumbar disk herniation
   b. Shoulder pain from carpal tunnel syndrome

Tendinosis

1. The degree of pain in overuse injuries provides a prognostic measure.
2. Grading of overuse injuries
   a. Grade 1: Symptoms are present for less than 2 weeks.
      (1) "Soreness" after aggravating activity

(2) Pain resolves quickly, usually within hours.
(3) No functional impairment
   b. Grade 2: Symptoms persist for 2 to 3 weeks (true overuse).
      (1) Pain during the latter phase of the aggravating activity
      (2) Pain persists after the activity is completed.
      (3) No functional impairment
   c. Grade 3: Symptoms present for 3 to 4 weeks.
      (1) Pain during most of the aggravating activity that continues after the activity is completed but will subside with rest
      (2) Performance is impaired.
   d. Grade 4: Symptoms are present for more than 4 weeks.
      (1) Pain is continuous, present before, during, and after the aggravating activity.
      (2) Performance is definitely affected and frequently prevented by the injury.
      (3) Activities of daily living frequently impaired.

Clinical Findings (Table 214–1)

Traumatic Tendinitis and Tendinosis

1. Always compare affected side with its opposite.
2. Skin: warmth/coolness
3. Always assess circulatory, motor, and sensory status.
   a. Weakness without reproduction of pain indicates a nerve injury.
   b. A compartment syndrome may occur in virtually any extremity injury, and one should always consider it.

Strains/Contusions

1. In general, early on, the pain from a traumatic muscle-tendon injury is increased by active resisted motion testing.
2. Grading of traumatic muscle-tendon injuries
   a. A mild or first-degree strain is a "pulled muscle"; it is an overstretching of the muscle-tendon unit with no palpable defect and mild inflammatory changes.
   b. A moderate or second-degree strain consists of a more significant disruption (10 to 90 per cent tearing) of the musculotendinous unit, resulting in a palpable defect with surrounding intact tissue and more significant inflammatory changes.
   c. A severe or third-degree strain is a complete rupture of the muscle-tendon unit resulting

TABLE 214–1. TENDON INJURIES

Injury	Etiology/Mechanisms	Symptoms	Signs
Traumatic Tendinitis			
Acute Achilles tendon strain	Rapid, unexpected plantar flexion as in stepping into a hole Following longstanding Achilles tendinitis	"Feeling like someone kicked my Achilles"	Defect palpable 3–6 cm proximal to calcaneus Positive Thompson's sign (lack of plantar response with passive calf squeeze)
Adolescent Overuse Tendinitis			
Patellar apophysitis (Osgood-Schlatter disease)	Rapid growth Traction apophysitis of patellar tendon	Usual age 10–15 years Painful prominence of tibial tubercle	Pain with palpation of tibial tubercle Tight hamstrings and quadriceps
Calcaneal apophysitis (Sever's disease)	Rapid growth Traction apophysitis of Achilles tendon	Usual age 10–11 years Pain in heel typically following sports	Focal pain with palpation of calcaneal apophysis Tight calf muscles
Overuse Tendinitis/Tendinosis			
Rotator cuff tendinitis (RCT)	Activities that require repetitive overhead motion	Several-week history of shoulder pain, usually anterior, lateral; exacerbated by activity	Positive supraspinatus sign Positive infraspinatus sign
RCT secondary to impingement	Narrowing of subacromial space (i.e., acromioclavicular joint arthritis)	As with RCT	As with RCT Positive Neer's sign (the shoulder is passively forward flexed and internally rotated) Positive Hawkin's sign (pain with active resistance of the shoulder placed at 90 degrees of forward flexion and internally rotated)
RCT secondary to shoulder instability	Hypermobility of the shoulder leading to instability	As with RCT "Feeling that my shoulder slips out of joint"	Positive apprehension sign Painful click with resisted internal and external rotation, indicative of glenoid labral tear

in a large, palpable defect with a proximal contracted ball of torn tissue; should be referred to an orthopedist.

    d. When soft tissue swelling is severe, be wary of a developing compartment syndrome.

Tendinosis

1. Palpation of the involved portion of the tendon will frequently elicit a tender, palpable nodule and reproduces the patient's pain.

2. Resisted active contraction of the involved tendon generally reproduces the patient's pain.

Traction Apophysitis—"Tendinitis of Adolescence"

1. An apophysis is a growth cartilage site to which tendon(s) attach.

    a. Inflammation and pain develops in these sites as a result of growth and the resultant muscle-tendon tightness.

    b. Traction apophysitis is actually an avulsion fracture of the apophysis at the tendon attachment.

2. Sever's disease (os calcis apophysitis): pain in the Achilles tendon attachment at the calcaneus growth plate (apophysis)

3. Osgood-Schlatter disease (tibial apophysitis)

    a. Pain in the tibial tubercle growth plate at the patellar tendon attachment

    b. Associated with tight hamstrings

4. Anterior superior iliac spine/iliac crest apophysitis: apophyseal avulsion fracture at the origin of the sartorius and rectus femoris muscles

Differential Diagnosis/Complications

1. Vascular: compartment syndrome

    a. Suspect in traumatic tendinitis/myositis resulting from blunt trauma.

    b. Suspect in cases of tendinosis in which pain occurs early in the activity.

2. Neurologic

    a. Radicular pain may mimic tendinosis pain.

    b. Peripheral neuropathies may present with proximal symptoms and mimic tendinosis pain: carpal tunnel syndrome may present as shoulder/rotator cuff tendinosis.

3. Collagen-vascular disorders may cause tendinitis or be complicated with acute tendon rupture.

4. Steroid abuse: Suspect steroid abuse in cases of tendon rupture at unusual sites, as in patellar tendon rupture.

5. Myositis ossificans: an abnormal formation of cartilage or bone following an acutely strained or contused muscle

6. Coagulation disorders: Numerous bruises in an individual, especially after mild trauma, should cause one to suspect an underlying coagulation disorder (i.e., hemophilia).

7. Stress fracture

Tests

1. Radiographs: should be done to assess for a stress fracture risk and to rule out soft tissue calcifications.
   a. Radiographs for suspected stress fractures may be "normal" for 6 to 8 weeks or more.
   b. Soft tissue radiographs should be obtained when myositis ossificans is suspected and repeated in 2 to 4 weeks to prove the diagnosis.

2. Bone scan: gold standard for stress fracture diagnosis

3. Rheumatologic conditions should be screened with an erythrocyte sedimentation rate and further collagen-vascular tests if warranted.

4. Coagulation laboratory tests: bleeding time, factor VIII assay.

5. Compartment pressures: usually diagnostic in an acute compartment syndrome; however, normal pressures may be found even following exercise in chronic compartment syndrome.

Treatment

Traumatic Tendinitis

1. PRICE: *p*rotect; relative *r*est; *i*ce; *c*ompression; *e*levation

2. Jones dressing: two alternating layers of cast padding and Ace wrap applied from distal to proximal

3. Nonsteroidal anti-inflammatory drugs (NSAIDs): short course for pain relief

4. Early mobilization: painless range of motion

5. Strengthening exercises as swelling subsides and range of motion improves

6. Aerobic conditioning as tolerated using pain as limit

7. Return to activity when pain-free, equal range of motion, and able to complete functional testing (i.e., running and cutting 100 yards following lower extremity injury rehabilitation)

Tendinosis

1. Grade 1: ice; reduce/adjust training regimen.

2. Grade 2: ice; reduce training program 25 to 50 per cent; NSAIDs for 7 to 10 days; specific flexibility and strengthening exercises; progress to kinetic chain exercises.

3. Grade 3: same as grade 2 except
   a. Rest from aggravating activity until able to perform pain-free.
   b. May perform nonaggravating aerobic exercises (i.e., bicycling generally permissible with running-induced injuries).
   c. NSAIDs for 10 to 14 days
   d. Cross friction massage to irritated tissue every other day: especially helpful in tendinosis of the elbow, shoulder, knee, and Achilles
   e. Physical therapy modalities for pain relief: phonophoresis with 10% hydrocortisone, interferential current, micro-current
   f. Cortisone injection: Consider local cortisone injection if significant symptoms persist.
   g. Correct functional biomechanical deficit.

4. Grade 4: Same as grade 3 except rest from aggravating activity until pain-free for 1 to 2 weeks

Follow-Up

Traumatic Tendinitis

1. Re-evaluate grade 2 and 3 injuries within 7 to 10 days.

2. Refer grade 3 injuries to an orthopedist.

3. Evaluate adolescent patients before return to activity, especially adolescent athletes.

4. NSAIDs should not be continued to permit return to activity, especially in adolescents.

Tendinosis

1. Re-evaluate grades 2, 3, and 4 injuries every 2 to 4 weeks.

2. Consider a local cortisone injection in difficult cases.

3. Follow-up all grade 3 and 4 injuries prior to return to activity.

4. Discontinue NSAIDs prior to return to activity.

5. Consider referring injuries that do not improve in 2 to 3 months.

Bibliography

Griffin JR, Stanish WD: Overuse tendinitis and rehabilitation. Can Fam Physician 1993;39:1762–1769.

Kibler WB, Chandler TJ: Principles of rehabilitation after chronic tendon injuries. Clin Sports Med 1992;11: 661–671.

Kibler WB, Livingston B: Shoulder rehabilitation: clinical application, evaluation, and rehabilitation protocols. Instr Course Lect 1997;46:43–51.

Teitz CC, Garrett WE: Tendon problems in athletic individuals. Instr Course Lect 1997;46:569–582.

Young JL, Laskowski ER: Thigh injuries in athletes. Mayo Clin Proc 1993;68:1099–1106.

215 Epicondylitis

Aaron Rubin

Etiology

1. Definition
   a. Lateral epicondylitis (tennis elbow)
      (1) Pain near the lateral muscle mass of the elbow. The wrist extensors originate at the lateral elbow. Condition may be due to tendinitis or, in more chronic cases, tendinosis.
      (2) Most commonly involved are the origin of the extensor carpi radialis brevis, followed by the extensor digitorum communis and the extensor carpi radialis longus.
   b. Medial epicondylitis (medial tennis elbow, golfer's elbow)
      (1) Pain near the medial muscle mass of the elbow. The wrist flexors and forearm pronators originate at the medial epicondyle.
      (2) Most often involved are the pronator teres, flexor carpi radialis, and palmaris longus, but the flexor carpi ulnaris and flexor sublimis may also be involved.
2. Cause
   a. Overuse: repetitive eccentric extensor muscle overload for lateral epicondylitis and eccentric flexor/pronator overload for medial epicondylitis. *Eccentric* means contraction of a muscle while an applied force is causing it to lengthen.
   b. In the younger group the cause is sports-related injury; in the much larger group of older individuals, the cause is workplace overuse injury.
   c. Typical characteristics
      (1) Patients 30 to 50 years old
      (2) High-repetition activity
      (3) Symptoms for 3 to 6 weeks (usually chronic condition when reported)
      (4) In tennis, consider improper grip size, improper string tension, practice longer than 2 hours per day, improper backhand technique (snapping wrist). More advanced players may get medial epicondylitis from repeated flexion during serve or imparting topspin on forehand strokes.
      (5) In golf, consider evaluating proper swing mechanics.

Symptoms

1. Lateral epicondylitis
   a. Pain over lateral elbow, worsened with activities that cause resisted extension of wrist. This may include lifting objects with wrists in extension.
   b. Often able to lift only with elbow flexed and adducted and forearm supinated
2. Medial epicondylitis: pain over medial epicondyle, worsened by resisted wrist flexion or forearm pronation

Key Symptoms

Lateral Epicondylitis

- Pain over lateral elbow and muscle mass
- Worsens with use of wrist extensors

Medial Epicondylitis

- Pain over medial elbow and muscle mass
- Worsens with use of wrist flexors and forearm pronators

Clinical Findings

History should include questions about recent and remote injuries to elbow, upper extremity, and neck. One should also question regarding type of work, sport, and other activity, eliciting information about repetitious motions and biomechanics of activities.

1. Lateral epicondylitis
   a. Tender over lateral epicondyle and conjoined tendon of the common extensors
      (1) Tenderness more posterior suggests posterior interosseous nerve entrapment (see "Differential Diagnosis")
      (2) Lack of tenderness with paresthesia suggests cervical radiculopathy.

b. May note diminished grip strength when tested.

c. Increased pain with resisted extension at wrist as well as third finger metacarpophalangeal joint

d. Motion loss of 10 degrees compared with unaffected side is noted with more chronic process.

2. Medial epicondylitis

a. Tenderness at the medial epicondyle

(1) Tenderness more anterior or pain with application of valgus stress suggests collateral ligament injury.

(2) Tenderness over cubital tunnel (posterior to medial epicondyle) and positive Tinel's sign are suggestive of ulnar nerve entrapment.

b. Motion may be decreased with chronic problem.

Key Signs

Lateral Epicondylitis

- Tenderness over lateral epicondyle and lateral proximal muscle mass

- Increased tenderness with resisted extension of wrist

Medial Epicondylitis

- Tenderness at the medial epicondyle and medial proximal muscle mass

- Increased tenderness with resisted flexion

Laboratory Tests

Radiographs are necessary in cases of trauma and to narrow differential. Look for calcifications or exostosis in extensor or flexor area, although they are of little known prognostic significance.

Differential Diagnosis

1. Lateral elbow pain

a. Radial nerve irritation

(1) Radial tunnel syndrome with paresthesia, a positive Tinel's over the nerve, tenderness to palpation 4 cm distal to the lateral epicondyle, pain with resisted supination with elbow extended, weakness of full finger extension

(2) Posterior interosseous nerve (deep branch of radial nerve) can become entrapped within the supinator muscle,

producing small finger extensor weakness.

b. Radial head fracture

c. Lateral epicondyle avulsion fracture

d. Radiculopathy of C6 nerve root

2. Medial elbow pain

a. Medial collateral ligament injury

b. Valgus extension overload

c. Ulnar nerve entrapment

d. T1 nerve root radiculopathy

3. Medial or lateral pain

a. Rheumatoid, gouty, or degenerative arthritis

b. Loose bodies

c. Referred pain from shoulder arthritis, carpal tunnel syndrome, angina pectoris

d. Joint space infection

e. Primary or metastatic tumor

Refer to Procedure on Joint Aspiration and Injection (after Ch. 218)

Treatment

1. Acute phase

a. Relative rest: Eliminate the activity that causes pain. May return to activity (e.g., golf or tennis) when symptoms have decreased, generally in 1 to 2 weeks.

b. Continue passive then active range of motion through pain-free range.

c. Cryotherapy: Cold reduces swelling, edema, and pain. Ice bag should be placed over area for 20 minutes three times a day or ice massage applied to area for 5 minutes three times a day. No excessive use of area should occur soon after icing. Cryotherapy is contraindicated in patients with Raynaud's disease and similar cold-induced disease. Relative contraindications include history of frostbite, cold hypersensitivity, peripheral vascular disease, impaired sensation, and fragile skin.

d. Counterforce (tennis elbow) brace

e. Wrist splint in 20-degree extension may be used. It relieves tension on the extensor mass in lateral epicondylitis and prevents pronation in medial epicondylitis.

f. Ultrasound may increase rate of tissue healing, reduce interstitial edema, and increase elasticity of tendons. It is generally recommended for 2 to 4 minutes three times per week. Caution is advised in possible infected joint, over open growth plates, and during pregnancy.

g. High-voltage galvanic stimulation may increase healing rate.

h. Nonsteroidal anti-inflammatory drugs (NSAIDs) (see below)

i. Consider injection with corticosteroids (see below).

2. Improvement phase

a. Normal range of motion is present with no pain. There may be some discomfort at extremes of range.

b. Continue stretching wrist in extension and flexion.

c. Begin active resistance exercise, initially isometrically, then with light weights (a hammer works very well) or surgical tubing. Begin with elbow flexed then progress elbow extension until the following are done with the elbow fully extended:

(1) Wrist flexion

(2) Wrist extension

(3) Radial and ulnar deviation

(4) Forearm pronation and supination

3. Return-to-sport/activity phase

a. Continued work on strength

(1) Isometric and higher resistance exercise to build strength

(2) High-repetition exercise to build endurance

(3) Sports-specific activity

b. Gradual return to sports activity with close attention to causative factors

Medication

1. NSAIDs: may be helpful for lateral and medial epicondylitis. Be cautious about side effects. Patient should undergo one or two courses, 2 to 3 weeks each.

2. Local medications

a. Lateral epicondyle

(1) Careful injection of corticosteroid with local anesthetic deep in area of lateral epicondyle has been helpful in reducing pain and inflammation in area and found superior to anesthetic alone.

(2) Injection with local anesthetic prior to steroid helps to localize the area for the steroid injection.

(3) Side effects include tendon weakening and rupture if injected directly into tendon (but this is generally not a major problem in this area), flair-up of pain for several days (which may be reduced by application of cryotherapy), local dimpling or discoloration of skin (occurs in too-superficial injection).

(4) Technique

(a) Prepare syringe with anesthetic (1% lidocaine plain [without epinephrine]). This may be mixed with 0.25% bupivacaine for longer lasting results. Mix or prepare separate syringe with triamcinolone suspension, 20 mg/ml, or triamcinolone, 25 mg/ml (or physician's corticosteroid of choice), with small-gauge needle. A second syringe may be used with local anesthetic for local infiltration of the skin.

(b) Area is prepped.

(c) Area of tenderness is palpated and sprayed with Fluori-Methane spray or ethyl chloride spray, then injected with local anesthetic followed by deeper injection with the steroid/anesthetic combination. Injection should be deep to the extensor carpi radialis brevis tendon, approximately 2 to 5 mm anterior and distal to the lateral epicondyle. Injection may be repeated three times over several months.

(5) Controversy exists about return to activity. Some recommend 2 to 3 weeks off strenuous activity. Studies have shown that full tendon strength has returned by this time. One should certainly wait until local anesthetic has worn off.

b. Medial epicondyle: Same preparation as above may be used—with extreme caution because of proximity of ulnar nerve.

c. Phonophoresis (use of ultrasound) with fluocinonide (Lidex) gel 0.05% for 2 to 5 minutes two to three times per week for 3 weeks is an alternative method of treatment with corticosteroid. Efficacy is uncertain.

Activity

1. The athlete should be closely observed for recurrence of symptoms and given early treatment and activity modification as well as appropriate coaching changes to prevent problems.

2. The worker should avoid repetitive overuse. Modification of length of time, position, and equipment should be considered. The worker should be instructed in a rehabilitation program.

Key Treatment

- Relative rest
- Pain-free range of motion exercises
- Cold applications
- NSAIDs
- Countertraction brace (tennis elbow)

ACKNOWLEDGMENT: Special thanks to David Anderson, M.D., for assistance in preparing this chapter.

Bibliography

Amundson M: Golf. In Mellion MB, Walsh WM, Shelton GL (eds): The Team Physician's Handbook, pp 806–815. Philadelphia, Hanley & Belfus, 1997.

Foley AE: Tennis elbow. Am Fam Physician 1993;48: 281–288.

Gelman H: Tennis elbow (lateral epicondylitis). Orthop Clin North Am 1992;23:75–82.

Johnson TR: Elbow and forearm. In Snider RK (ed): Essentials of Musculoskeletal Care, pp 139–143. Rosemont, IL, American Academy of Orthopedic Surgeons, 1997.

Nicola TL: Tennis. In Mellion MB, Walsh WM, Shelton GL (eds): The Team Physician's Handbook, pp 816–827. Philadelphia, Hanley & Belfus, 1997.

Nirschl RP: Elbow tendinosis/tennis elbow. Clin Sports Med 1992;11:851–870.

216 Temporomandibular Joint Syndrome

T. K. Cumarasamy

Etiology

1. The term *temporomandibular joint (TMJ) syndrome* may be used to describe the following collection of symptoms of temporomandibular disorders, given in general temporal order of appearance:
   a. Pain in and around the TMJs: Occurs early.
   b. Tenderness/spasm of the muscles of mastication and head and neck: Occurs early with or without joint pain and limited jaw movement.
   c. Joint noises: Occur late.
   d. Limited mandibular movement: Occurs later, usually with joint noises
2. When the first two symptoms mentioned are the only or predominant ones the term *myofascial pain dysfunction (MPD) syndrome* has been used, indicating fatigue or spasm of the muscles of mastication and of the head and neck. This primarily comes from muscle overuse or tension. Prolonged muscle dysfunction can contribute to intra-articular dysfunction. The term *TMJ syndrome* generally refers to the presence of all of the above symptoms of joint and muscle dysfunction arising from malfunction or pathology. Malfunction is seen more frequently than pathology, because risk factors favor malfunction.
3. Persistent malfunction of the TMJ gradually causes derangement of the intra-articular disk, resulting in displacement, deformity, and eventually perforation of the disk, concurrent meniscitis, synovitis, capsulitis, and in later stages bone-to-bone contact, all of which cause pain, tenderness, or spasm in the related regional muscles, noises in the joint as a result of disk derangement, and limited mandibular movement.
4. Epidemiology
   a. May be seen in all after the first decade of life but more commonly in white women in the second to fourth decades.
   b. The TMJ syndrome with clinically detectable signs may be present in over 50 per cent of the population, but only about half may be aware of the problem and only about another half of that number need treatment.
   c. Patients who have signs but are symptom-free when TMJ dysfunction is discovered during routine examinations should be evaluated for the presence of risk factors, which are frequently subtle.
5. Risk factors that predispose the TMJs to traumatic injury and thus malfunction include
   a. Fatigue and spasm of regional muscles (MPD syndrome) caused by
      (1) Stress and tension for various reasons
      (2) Parafunctional habits (bruxism, clenching of teeth, excessive gum chewing) with or without stress
   b. Malocclusion of teeth, as well as missing teeth and malfitting dentures
   c. Excessive and prolonged opening of the mouth
   d. Maxillary/mandibular malalignment
   Whereas major trauma is easily recognized, minute trauma to the intra-articular structures because of malalignment is not and thus escapes the attention of the patient and physician until the cumulative effect has caused irreversible damage and associated symptoms.
6. Pathologic causes of TMJ dysfunction include
   a. Inflammatory and degenerative joint diseases (rheumatoid arthritis, degenerative joint disease, gout)
   b. Infectious arthritis
   c. Tumors of the joint structures and surrounding areas
   d. Developmental joint anomalies

Symptoms

1. Joint and regional pain: dull to sharp pain aggravated by jaw movement with possible radiation to the ear, eye, head, and face, and tenderness in the muscles of mastication and of the head and neck. Patients may thus complain of earache, headache, facial pain, neck pain, anxiety, and stress.
2. Joint sounds: clicking, grinding, and grating sounds audible to the patient and, if loud enough, also to those in close proximity to the patient. Patients may have already started to avoid opening wide to bite into a hamburger or

apple, started to cut food into smaller than usual pieces, and also changed to a softer texture.

3. Limited jaw movement/stiffness: Occurs as a result of inflammation and displacement of the disk. Patients may find the jaw locking during the opening or closing movement, resulting in decreased opening, deviated movements, and having to do wiggling actions to unlock.

Key Symtoms

- Joint pain
- Joint noises
- Joint stiffness
- Limited jaw movement

Clinical Findings

1. A normal to very tense patient
2. Tender muscles of mastication and of the head and neck with or without spasm: Palpate regional muscles.
3. Joint sounds such as clicking, grinding, or grating: Auscultate over joint with stethoscope during movement.
4. Limitation or deviation in opening and closing movements of the jaw (normal interincisal opening for adults is 40 to 50 mm, and dental midline lateral deviation is 8 to 10 mm)
5. The presence of risk factors mentioned above. Unless quite obvious, these risk factors will require a TMJ specialist to detect as well as eliminate.

Key Signs

- Joint tenderness
- Altered jaw movement
- Joint sounds
- Muscle tenderness/ spasm

Diagnostic Tests

1. TMJ radiographs: Consist of panoramic, reversed Towne's, and transcranial views and can be used as a screening measure. Bony changes can be seen in advanced cases.
2. Computerized tomography (CT) scans may be used to identify bony changes over plain radiographs or plain tomograms. Early changes can be seen better with CT scans.
3. Magnetic resonance imaging (MRI) scans are very good to see soft tissue pathology in the disk, synovium, and capsule.

4. TMJ arthrography will demonstrate disk deformity, abnormal motion, and perforation. Although MRI scans show more detail in the soft tissue changes, arthrography is a popular technique to evaluate joint dynamics.
5. Arthroscopy of the TMJ is done for both diagnostic and therapeutic reasons.
6. Injection of local anesthetic solution into the joint or trigger points in the muscles confirms the source of pain.

Key Tests

- Plain TMJ radiograph
- Arthrography
- CT/MRI
- Arthroscopy

Differential Diagnosis

Otitis media, neuralgia, sinusitis, arthritis (rheumatoid, degenerative joint disease, gout, psoriatic, septic), tooth pain, parotid gland pathology, tumors of the brain, tumors of the head and neck, and muscular and neurologic conditions all can cause pain and/or limitation of jaw movement.

Treatment

1. Initially
   a. Mandibular rest, softer diet, and local application of heat with use of nonsteroidal anti-inflammatory drugs (NSAIDs; e.g., ibuprofen, naproxen) control symptoms. Anxiolytics and muscle relaxants may be of value in individual cases.
   b. Use of intra-articular or systemic steroids is not common now. Narcotic analgesics should almost always be avoided because of the protracted nature of the condition.
   c. The preceding conservative management for 2 to 4 weeks may provide relief for an extended period of time.
2. Later
   a. Referral to a *TMJ specialist* is prudent after remission of symptoms for further investigation of risk factors.
   b. Behavior modification to eliminate stress and parafunctional habits as needed includes use of occlusal bite guards, occlusal repositioning appliances, biofeedback, hypnosis, and psychological counseling, usually performed by the TMJ specialist and his or her team.
3. Surgery: Advanced internal derangement of the joints requires surgical management, usually carried out by the oral and maxillofacial surgeon with view to improve symptoms. Arthro-

scopic surgery is now widely performed in appropriate situations.

Key Treatment

Initially	Later
• NSAIDs	• Surgery
• Soft diet	
• Local heat	
• Stop habits/change behavior	

Follow-Up

During acute symptoms, a biweekly follow-up helps to reassure the patient and reinforce conservative measures. Because long periods of remission from symptoms do occur, the patient may neglect to undertake further evaluation. Patients should thus be motivated to see the TMJ specialist earlier in the disease rather than later.

Bibliography

Dolwick MF, Sanders B: TMJ Internal Derangements and Arthrosis. St. Louis, CV Mosby Company, 1985.

Okeson JP, de Kanter RJ: Temporomandibular disorders in medical practice. J Fam Pract 1996; 43:347–356.

Parameters of care for oral and maxillofacial surgery. Oral Maxillofac Surg 1995;53(Suppl 5).

Peterson LJ: Principles of Oral and Maxillofacial Surgery. Philadelphia, JB Lippincott Company, 1992.

Sarnat BG, Laskin DM: The Temporomandibular Joint: A biological Basis for Clinical Practice. Philadelphia, WB Saunders Company, 1992.

217 Osteoarthritis

David H. Neustadt

Etiology

1. Osteoarthritis (OA) is the most common form of arthritis and one of the oldest known diseases, but the etiology is not fully known. Two major forms predominate:
   a. Primary (idiopathic): considered genetic in origin (e.g., Heberden's and Bouchard's nodes)
   b. Secondary to trauma or overuse, congenital joint abnormality, developmental defects, and biomechanical failure usually associated with excess load (obesity) and increasing age
2. Key etiologic risk factors and contributing causes of OA
   a. Hereditary factors: gene mutation
   b. Trauma
   c. Aging: typically greater than 60 years
   d. Altered cartilage biomechanics
   e. Inflammatory component

Symptoms

Many patients with clinical evidence of OA may be asymptomatic.

Key Symptoms

Insidious Onset and Inexorable Course

- Pain in affected joints—especially knee and hip on weight-bearing

- Soreness and stiffness in neck or back in patients with OA of cervical spine and lumbar spine

- Progressive disability in advanced disease associated with considerable underlying joint damage

Clinical Findings

Physical features of OA are variable, and depend on sites of involvement.

Key Signs

Hands

- "Lumpy-bumpy" (wavy) digits with knobby appearance (large Heberden's nodes, Bouchard's nodules)

- Tender "squared-off" trapeziometacarpals (thumb bases)

Knees

- Pain on motion with limitation of motion

- Local tenderness and crepitus (creaking)

- Occasional synovitis (small effusions)

Hips

- Positive Patrick's test (fabere sign)

- Limited range of motion in significant hip involvement

Feet

- Enlarged bunion joint with hallux valgus when first metatarsophalangeal joint is affected

---

WARNING

Inflammatory (cystic erosive) OA may resemble rheumatoid arthritis, when the proximal interphalangeal (PIP) joints (Bouchard's nodules) are involved, but metacarpophalangeals (MCPs), with the exception of the first carpometacarpal (CMC), are usually spared.

Laboratory Tests

There are no typical laboratory abnormalities or specific markers.

Key Tests

- Erythrocyte sedimentation rate (ESR), C-reactive protein, and hemograms are usually normal

- Synovial fluid, when obtained, is typically viscous noninflammatory, with white blood cell (WBC) count less than 1800/mm^3 and a normal differential count, predominantly mononuclear cells rather than the polymorphonuclear (PMN) leukocytosis found in rheumatoid arthritis (RA).

Imaging Procedures

Radiographic evidence of OA is present in 85 per cent of persons after 65 years of age. Typical evidence of OA includes narrowing of the joint space, osteophyte (spur) formation, subchondral bony sclerosis (eburnation), and (subchondral) cystic erosions in inflammatory OA. Computerized tomography and magnetic resonance imaging are rarely indicated.

Differential Diagnosis (Table 217–1)

OA was confused with RA until the turn of the twentieth century. Differential considerations include

1. RA, psoriatic, and other forms of spondyloarthropathy
2. Calcium pyrophosphate deposition disease, pseudogout
3. Diffuse idiopathic skeletal hyperostosis (DISH)
4. Neuropathic (Charcot's) joint disorder (relatively painless)
5. Ochronosis (alkaptonuria), a rare metabolic disorder
6. Fibromyalgia: soft tissue "rheumatism" without joint involvement

Treatment

There is no cure for OA; thus the major goals of treatment are

1. To control pain and reduce stiffness
2. To maintain functional capacity and prevent disabling features
3. To maintain or improve quality of life

Nonpharmacologic Measures: The First Step

1. Patient education and lifestyle modifications
2. Reduce joint loading and impact
3. Weight reduction program
4. Physical modalities (therapy) with emphasis on range of motion, stretching, and isometric muscle strengthening exercises (e.g., isometric quadriceps drill)
5. Use of adaptive equipment (e.g., elevated toilet seat) and walking aids (e.g., canes and crutches)
6. Regular application of moist hot packs or warm soaks to painful area

Pharmacotherapy: The Next Step

1. After the institution of the basic management program, the next step is the judicious addition of nonopioid analgesics, nonsteroidal anti-inflammatory drugs (NSAIDs), and intra-articular (IA) therapy.
2. Guidelines for management strategies with drug therapy
   a. Acetaminophen, 1 gm, three to four doses daily
   b. Nonacetylated salicylates (e.g., salsalate and trisalicylate), 1 to 1.5 gm bid
   c. NSAIDs (numerous agents available)
   d. IA steroid therapy: May be given up to three or four times/year
   e. IA hyaluronate for OA of the knee: Three to five injections at 1-week intervals depending on preparation selected.

WARNING

Acetaminophen should be used with caution in patients with pre-existing renal or liver conditions (rare interaction with Coumadin [warfarin] if international normalized ratio >4).

TABLE 217–1. DIFFERENTIAL DIAGNOSIS

	RA	OA
Sites commonly involved	Wrists, MCPs, PIPs, elbows, knees	Distal interphalangeal joints, CMC, knees, hips, spine
Morning stiffness	>45 min (prolonged)	<15 min (brief)
Joint findings	Synovitis (soft tissue swelling [STS])	Bony enlargement (occasional synovitis)
Extra-articular features	Fatigue, weight loss, pulmonary	Absent
Laboratory findings		No specific abnormalities
Subcutaneous rheumatoid nodules	In 30% of patients	Absent
Synovial fluid	"Watery," turbid (opaque) fluid with >70% PMN	Viscous, clear fluid, <2000 WBCs with <35% PMN
Radiographic	Erosive destruction	Narrowing joint space with osteophyte formation

Other Forms of Therapy

If patient is resistant to conventional medical treatment, do

1. Joint lavage (needle tidal irrigation)
2. Arthroscopic débridement and/or synovectomy
3. Osteotomy to correct malalignment of the knee
4. Arthrodesis (fusion) for unstable joints
5. Total joint replacement: salvage procedure

Investigational Therapy

1. Disease-modifying drugs
   a. Tetracycline derivatives (doxycycline, minocycline) to inhibit degradative enzymes (e.g., collagenase)
   b. Hydroxychloroquine (study in progress)
   c. Nitric oxide inhibitors (experimental)
2. Pulsed electromagnetic fields (device under study)
3. Chondrocyte transplantation (limited to focal surface defects)
4. Gene therapy (methods under exploration)

New Developments

1. Two isoforms of cyclo-oxygenase (COX) have been recognized.
   a. COX-1: constitutive in gastrointestinal tract, kidney, and platelets. Responsible for "housekeeping" functions, the cause of unwanted side effects.
   b. COX-2: inducible at inflammatory sites in synovia and cartilage

---

WARNING

Increased risk of NSAID-related side effects from inhibition of COX-1 (chiefly gastrointestinal, renal, and hematologic) is associated with high dosage, long duration of therapy, and advanced age.

---

2. Selective COX-2 inhibitors (celecoxib [Celebrex], rofecoxib [Vioxx]) are highly effective for the management of OA, and tolerability and safety profiles appear to be superior to available COX-1 NSAIDs.

Key Treatment

Mild OA

- Nonpharmacologic measures

  +

- Acetaminophen or nonacetylated salicylate (weak COX inhibitor)

Moderate OA

- Add nonopioid analgesics (propoxyphene, tramadol) and/or NSAIDs

  +

- IA hyaluronate and/or IA steroids

Severe OA

- Add opioids if resistant

- Consider surgical procedures: arthroscopy, osteotomy with realignment, total joint replacement

Bibliography

Hochberg MC, Altman RD, Brandt KD, et al: Guidelines for the medical management of OA. Part 1: OA of the hip. Arthritis Rheum 1995;38:1535–1540.

Hochberg MC, Altman RD, Brandt KD, et al: Guidelines for the medical management of OA. Part 2: OA of the knee. Arthritis Rheum 1995;38:1541–1546.

Moskowitz RW: Osteoarthritis—symptoms and signs. In Moskowitz RW, Howell DS, Goldberg VN, et al (eds): Osteoarthritis: Diagnosis/Medical Surgical Management, pp 255–261. Philadelphia, WB Saunders Company, 1993.

Neustadt DH: Intra-articular steroid therapy. In Moskowitz RW, Howell DS, Goldberg VM, et al (eds): Osteoarthritis: Diagnosis and Medical/Surgical Management, 2nd ed, pp 493–510. Philadelphia, WB Saunders Company, 1992.

Neustadt DH: Osteoarthritis. In Rakel RE (ed): Conn's Current Therapy, 50th anniv ed, pp 995–999. Philadelphia, WB Saunders Company, 1998.

218 Rheumatoid Arthritis

Raymond H. Feierabend, Jr.

Etiology

1. Chronic inflammatory disease of uncertain etiology
2. Genetic predisposition appears to be important.
3. Cellular and immune mechanisms result in destructive inflammatory process, primarily involving the synovium.
4. Inciting factor suspected to be infectious, although no specific agent has been identified.

Symptoms

1. Course
   a. Affects women two to three times more commonly than men
   b. Highly variable
   c. Begins insidiously in most cases but may be abrupt in onset (10 per cent of cases).
   d. Usually progressive but often with exacerbations and remissions (incomplete)
2. Musculoskeletal symptoms
   a. Multiple painful and tender joints; typically symmetrical distribution
      (1) Proximal interphalangeal (PIP), metacarpophalangeal (MCP), and wrist joints typically involved.
      (2) Metatarsophalangeal (MTP), ankle, knee, and elbow joints and cervical spine also commonly involved.
      (3) Hip, shoulder, and temporomandibular joints are less commonly involved.
      (4) Distal interphalangeal joints and thoracic and lumbar spine are typically spared.
   b. Characteristic morning stiffness lasting more than 1 hour, improving with activity
3. Constitutional symptoms
   a. Malaise
   b. Easy fatigability
   c. Muscle weakness
   d. Anorexia
   e. Weight loss
   f. Low-grade fever
4. Symptoms may be associated with extra-articular manifestations, including pleural effusions, pulmonary nodules, pulmonary fibrosis, pericarditis, cardiac rheumatoid nodules, vasculitis, compression neuropathies, mononeuritis multiplex, Sjögren's syndrome, scleritis, and episcleritis.

Key Symptoms

- Morning stiffness
- Painful, swollen joints
- Malaise, easy fatigue, weakness
- Symmetric joint involvement
- PIPs, MCPs, wrists
- MTPs, ankles, knees

Clinical Findings

1. Musculoskeletal
   a. Swelling (typically "boggy" to feel), warmth, tenderness, and decreased range of motion of affected joints; typical fusiform-shaped swelling of PIP joints
   b. Effusions of larger affected joints
   c. Effects of joint destruction, including subluxations, dislocations, and ankylosis
2. Rheumatoid nodules (up to 50 per cent of patients): subcutaneous nodules over extensor surfaces and juxta-articular regions
3. Signs associated with extra-articular manifestations noted above

Key Signs

- Symmetric joint findings
  - Tenderness
  - Warmth
  - Boggy swelling
  - Effusion
  - Decreased motion
- Rheumatoid nodules
- Joint deformities

Laboratory Tests

1. Blood
   a. Rheumatoid factor: single most useful test
      (1) Helps to confirm the diagnosis if positive in a patient with history and clinical findings consistent with rheumatoid ar-

thritis (RA). Positive in about 80 per cent of RA patients.

    (2) Does not establish the diagnosis if clinical findings are not present. False-positive results occur in other systemic diseases and in about 1 per cent of normal population (especially older women).

    (3) Does not exclude the diagnosis if negative.

        (a) Negative in up to 20 per cent of RA patients

        (b) Often negative during the first several months of clinical disease

  b. Anemia of chronic disease commonly present.

  c. Erythrocyte sedimentation rate typically elevated. Nonspecific but may be helpful in monitoring severity of disease.

  d. Antinuclear antibodies positive with high titers in up to 30 per cent of RA patients, usually with diffuse immunofluorescence pattern.

  e. Hypergammaglobulinemia with polyclonal gammopathy often present.

2. Synovial fluid: inflammatory; white blood cell count 2000 to 50,000/mm^3 (usually 10,000 to 30,000/mm^3)

3. Radiologic

  a. Periarticular soft tissue swelling

  b. Juxta-articular osteoporosis

  c. Juxta-articular erosions characteristic in RA

  d. Joint space narrowing

Key Signs

- Rheumatoid factor
- Sedimentation rate
- Joint fluid analysis
- Radiographs, especially of hands

Differential Diagnosis

1. Osteoarthritis
2. Spondyloarthropathies
  a. Ankylosing spondylitis
  b. Psoriatic arthritis
  c. Reiter's syndrome
  d. Colitic arthritis
3. Systemic lupus erythematosus
4. Systemic sclerosis
5. Lyme disease

6. Crystal-induced arthritis
  a. Gout
  b. Pseudogout

Treatment

1. No curative therapy
2. Integrated approach is necessary, including patient education, physical and occupational therapy, pharmacotherapy, and surgery.
3. Pharmacotherapy is rapidly changing; must be individualized.

Medication

1. Nonsteroidal anti-inflammatory drugs (NSAIDs)
  a. Useful as sole or initial agents in mild disease and as adjunctive therapy when other agents are needed
  b. Aspirin most economical.
  c. Other NSAIDs
2. Corticosteroids
  a. Limited role because of serious toxicity
  b. Intra-articular injection useful for acutely inflamed joints.
  c. Low-dose oral therapy may have some role.
3. Slow-acting drugs, some of which may modify the disease course
  a. Gold salts: Parenteral preparations much more effective than oral, but less well tolerated.
  b. Methotrexate: Generally effective and well tolerated, but serious toxicity may occur, including hepatic fibrosis and hypersensitivity pneumonitis.
  c. Penicillamine, hydroxychloroquine, and sulfasalazine may be useful in selected patients; preferred agents according to some rheumatologists.

Surgery

Useful in patients with more severe disease with joint erosions/destruction

1. Synovectomy
2. Joint fusion
3. Arthroplasty

Diet

No specific role other than maintenance of overall good nutrition

Activity

1. Balance between rest and activity is essential.
  a. Adequate physical rest; up to 10 hours of bed rest per 24 hours
  b. Prolonged immobilization may be counterproductive.

2. Physical therapy is of major importance. Regular exercise program to include
   a. Aerobic exercise to maintain overall physical conditioning
   b. Passive and active range-of-motion exercises to prevent contractures and maintain function
   c. Isometric and isotonic exercises to develop and maintain muscle strength
   d. Immobilization of specific joints with splinting may be useful.
   e. Heat modalities such as hot packs and paraffin baths

Patient Education
Essential for the patient's overall well-being

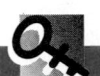

Key Treatment

Medications	**Physical Therapy Modalities**
• Aspirin and other NSAIDs	• Heat
• Gold salts	• Splinting
• Methotrexate	• Exercises
Surgery for More Advanced Disease	

Follow-Up
Regular re-evaluation and appropriate alteration of management are essential.

Bibliography

Bhardwaj N, Paget SA: Rheumatoid arthritis. In Paget SA, Fields TR (eds): Rheumatic Disorders, pp 19–78. Boston, Andover Medical Publishers, 1992.

Borenstein DG, Silver G, Jenkins E: Approach to initial medical treatment of rheumatoid arthritis. Arch Fam Med 1993;2:545–551.

Cash JM, Klippel JH: Second-line drug therapy for rheumatoid arthritis. N Engl J Med 1994;330:1368–1375.

Goronzy JJ, Weyland CM: Rheumatoid arthritis: Epidemiology, pathology, and pathogenesis; Anderson RJ: Rheumatoid arthritis: Clinical and laboratory features; Paget SA: Rheumatoid arthritis: Treatment. In Klippel JH (ed): Primer on the Rheumatic Diseases, 11th ed, pp 155–174. Atlanta, Arthritis Foundation, 1997.

Pincus T: A pragmatic approach to cost-effective use of laboratory tests and imaging procedures in patients with musculoskeletal symptoms. Prim Care 1993;20: 795–814.

Indications

1. Pain relief
   a. Aspiration of tense hemarthrosis or joint effusion
   b. Injection of bursitis, tendonitis, arthritis
2. Diagnostic
   a. Nontraumatic history
      (1) Septic arthritis
      (2) Crystal-induced arthritis
      (3) Rheumatic arthritis
   b. Traumatic or activity-related
      (1) Intra-articular fracture
      (2) Ligamentous tear
      (3) Synovial/capsular tear

Contraindications

1. Absolute
   a. Localized abscess or cellulitis at injection site
   b. Active herpes simplex virus or tuberculosis infections
   c. Previous hypersensitivity to injectable anesthetic
2. Relative
   a. Bleeding diatheses
   b. Anticoagulant therapy
   c. Bacteremia
   d. Partial tendon rupture at injection site
   e. Joint prothesis

Preparation

1. Obtain informed consent.
2. Ensure proper, comfortable patient position.
3. Identify landmarks; mark site of insertion with a scratch, sterile marking pen, or skin indentation.
4. Wide-field skin cleaning/sterilization with povidone-iodine
5. Assemble materials while solution is drying on skin.
6. Apply sterile drape.
7. Always use sterile gloves; mask and gown optional

Equipment

1. Povidone-iodine (Betadine) solution, alcohol wipes
2. Sterile 4×4 gauze
3. Sterile gloves, drape; mask and gown optional
4. Needles for aspirations: 18 and 20 gauge
5. Needles for injections: 22 and 25 gauge
6. Syringes: 6 ml, two 12 ml, two 35 ml
7. Lidocaine 1% (single dose vials are ideal)
8. Injectable corticosteroids
9. Sterile dressings and Ace wrap(s)
10. Purple-top (EDTA-containing) and red-top tubes
11. Appropriate culture medium
12. Glass microscope slides/cover slips

Anesthesia

Local anesthesia (aspirations only)

1. Lidocaine 1% with 25- to 30-gauge needle
2. Apply localized skin wheal, then redirect toward joint.
3. Apply liberal amount at joint capsule: this area is the most pain-sensitive.
4. Continuously aspirate while directing the needle.

Precautions

1. When using anesthetic agents, have IV diazepam ready if seizures occur.
2. Appropriate clotting factors should be given to patients with bleeding diatheses prior to arthrocentesis.
3. When redirecting needle, always withdraw to subcutaneous tissue prior to redirecting.
4. Avoid removing needle completely from skin and reinjecting.
5. Localized cutaneous atrophy can be avoided by not allowing injectable steroids to leak out into near-surface (<5 mm) tissues.
6. Postprocedural compression/ice will reduce subcutaneous swelling/pain.
7. Practice sterile technique (postprocedural infection rate 1:10,000). Always use unopened vials of injectable solutions or single-dose vials.
8. Avoid tendons to avoid tendon damage.
9. Postinjection steroid "flares" (pain developing 6 to 12 hours postinjection) can be relieved with nonsteroidal anti-inflammatory drugs and ice.

Remember
Joint fluid will flow easily when the joint capsule is penetrated.

Technique

Shoulder

1. Injection for subacromial bursitis:
   a. Patient position: sitting, with arm at side, humeral head detracted distally as far as possible
   b. Locate: Palpate superiorly along spine of scapula to posterolateral portion of the acromion (acromial angle), superior to humeral head.
   c. Insert 4-cm, 25-gauge needle 1 cm below acromial angle. Direct anteromedially, staying close to inferior border of acromion; insert approximately 2.5 cm. Avoid rotator cuff tendon inferiorly.

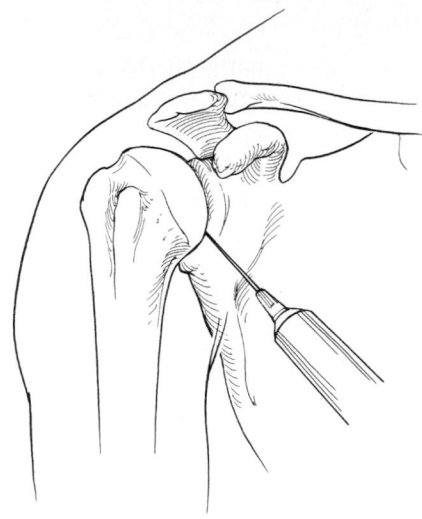

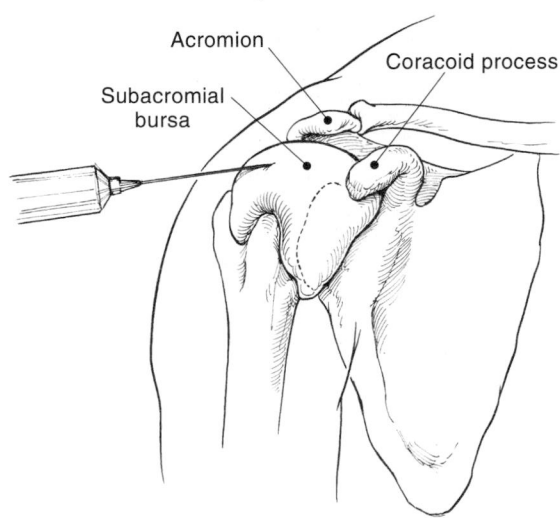

   d. Inject 8 to 12 ml of anesthetic and corticosteroid mixture. Following injection, move the joint through full range of motion to distribute mixture. To avoid potential tendon damage, the patient should avoid strenuous activity for 2 to 7 days.

2. Glenohumeral joint aspiration
   a. Patient position: sitting forward with arm in lap
   b. Locate inferolateral border of coracoid process, the anterolateral border of the acromion, and the medial border of the humeral head.
   c. Insert 4-cm, 22-gauge needle in space between inferolateral border of coracoid and humeral head. Direct posteriorly toward glenoid rim. Aspirate fluid for studies.

Elbow

1. Injection for lateral epicondylitis:
   a. Patient position: sitting with shoulder abducted to allow for the forearm to rest on a side table; elbow flexed 90 degrees with hand pronated.
   b. Locate point of maximum tenderness near lateral epicondyle. The patient may extend wrist with a clenched fist to increase localized tenderness.
   c. Insert 1-cm, 25-gauge needle into point of maximum tenderness, parallel to the tendon direction

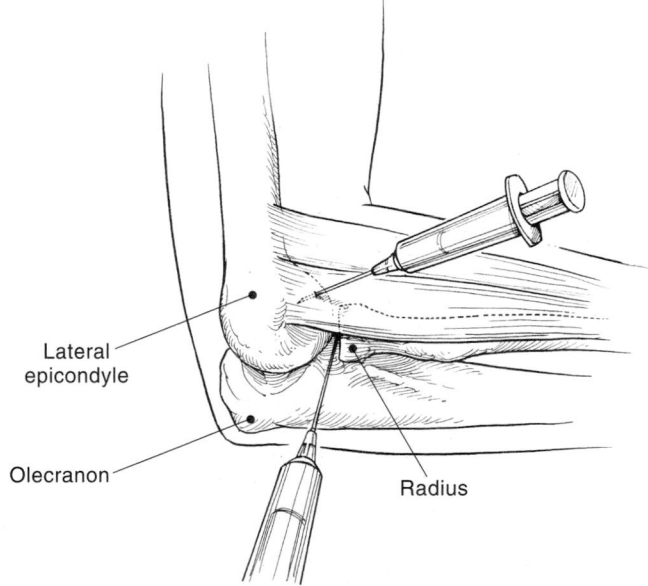

   d. Inject 3 to 5 ml of anesthetic and corticosteroid mixture, bathing the tendon sheath.

> **WARNING**
> **Avoid insertion of needle directly into tendon.**

2. Radiohumeral joint aspiration
   a. Patient position: same as above
   b. Locate space between distal lateral epicondyle and proximal tip of olecranon process of radial head.
   c. Insert 4-cm, 22-gauge needle at 90-degree angle to skin. Direct medially. Aspirate fluid for studies.

Knee

Aspiration of joint fluid: lateral approach

1. Patient position: Supine, with leg extended
2. Locate space between the superolateral border of the patella and the lateral femoral epicondyle.
3. Insert 4-cm, 20-gauge needle (for septic joint, use 18 gauge), parallel to floor, in space 1 cm lateral to patella border. Direct toward undersurface of patella; with the quads relaxed, the patella may be lifted to ease insertion.

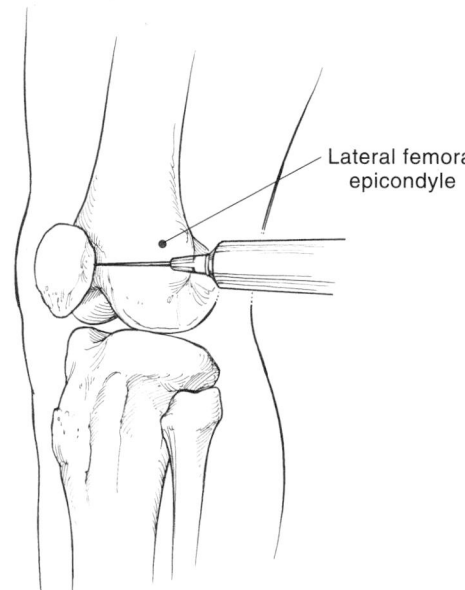

Lateral femoral epicondyle

The knee is capable of having 50 to 100 ml of interarticular fluid: have three 35-ml syringes ready to aspirate joint fluid/effusion.

Ankle

Aspiration of tibiotalar joint

1. Patient position: supine with leg fully extended, foot partially plantar flexed
2. Locate the joint line 1 cm superior to the line joining the inferior borders of the malleoli, and bordered medially by the tibialis anterior tendon. Also locate the points where the anterior tibial artery and extensor hallicus longus tendon cross the joint line.

3. Insert 4-cm, 22-gauge needle anywhere along the joint line, avoiding the artery and tendons. Direct the needle superiorly 2 to 3 cm into joint space. Aspirate fluid for analysis.

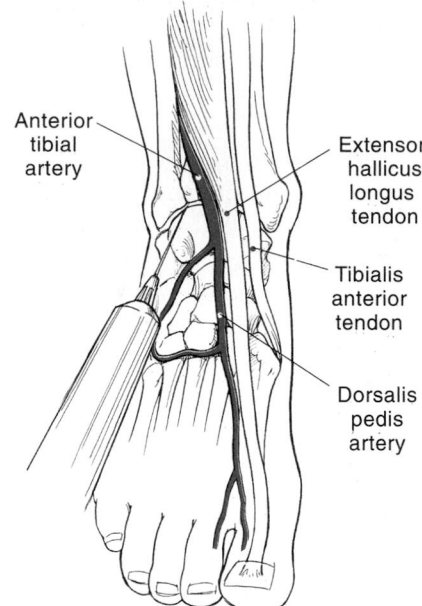

Anterior tibial artery

Extensor hallicus longus tendon

Tibialis anterior tendon

Dorsalis pedis artery

Joint Aspirate Studies

1. Cell count and differential (EDTA tube)
2. Gram's stain, culture and sensitivity
3. Crystal analysis under polarized light
   a. Urate: needle-shaped, negative birefringence
   b. Calcium pyrophosphate: rhomboid-shaped, positive birefringence
4. Glucose: compare to serum glucose
5. String test: Normal fluid, when gently pushed from a syringe, will form a 5- to 10-cm "string." With infection, the string will be shorter.

Bibliography

Bach BR, Bush-Joseph C: Subacromial space injections: a tool for evaluating shoulder pain. Physician Sports Med 1992;20:93–97.

Benjamin GC: Arthrocentesis. In Roberts JR, Hedges JR (eds): Clinical Procedures in Emergency Medicine, 3rd ed, pp 919–932. Philadelphia, WB Saunders Company, 1998.

Pfenninger JL: Injections of joints and soft tissue (Part I) and (Part II). Am Fam Physician 1991;44:1196–1202 and 44:1690–1701.

Saunders S, Cameron G: Injection Techniques in Orthopaedic and Sports Medicine. Philadelphia, WB Saunders Company, 1997.

Williams JR: Elbow. In Carr AJ, Harnden A (eds): Orthopaedics in Primary Care, pp 19–31. Oxford, Butterworth-Heinemann, 1997.

Williams KD: Infectious Arthritis. In Canale ST (ed): Campbell's Operative Orthopaedics, 9th ed, vol 1, pp 601–625. St. Louis, Mosby, 1998.

219 Gout

Thomas P. Harder

Gout is best known as an acutely painful recurrent inflammatory arthritis that only sometimes becomes chronic and disabling. The precursor to gout is hyperuricemia. *Hyperuricemia* is defined as a uric acid level 2 standard deviations above the mean of a random population or as the supersaturation of uric acid in the plasma (≥ 7 mg/dl). Four stages characterize the natural history of gout: asymptomatic hyperuricemia, acute gouty arthritis, intercritical gout, and chronic tophaceous gout.

Etiology

1. Monosodium urate crystal deposits in connective tissue lead to gout.
2. Polymorphonuclear cells initiate the inflammatory response when they ingest the crystals.
3. Hyperuricemia is the most important risk factor for gout, resulting from
   a. Undersecretion by the kidneys (80 to 90 per cent of patients with gout) *and/or*
   b. Metabolic overproduction (10 to 15 per cent of patients with gout)
4. Additional risk factors for gout and hyperuricemia
   a. Male gender (most common inflammatory joint disorder in men over age 40)
   b. Alcohol abuse
   c. Obesity
   d. Age: at highest risk are middle-aged men and postmenopausal women
   e. Family history of gout
   g. Drugs: includes diuretics, salicylates (low-dose), and cyclosporine
   h. Other: renal insufficiency, hypertension, hematologic malignancy, lead poisoning
5. Provocative factors that can trigger an acute attack
   a. Repetitive joint trauma
   b. Surgical stress
   c. Drugs (especially the initiation of antihyperuricemics)
   d. Binge on alcohol or "rich" foods

Symptoms

1. Stage I: Asymptomatic hyperuricemia—no symptoms

2. Stage II: Acute gouty arthritis
   a. Attacks are often sudden, occurring at night in a lower extremity joint.
   b. Joint symptoms: Within hours of slight discomfort the joint becomes
      (1) Excruciatingly painful, sensitive even to light touch
      (2) Throbbing
      (3) Swollen
      (4) Hot
   c. Systemic symptoms include anorexia, malaise, headache, and mild chills.
3. Stage III: Intercritical gout: defines the asymptotic intervals between attacks
4. Stage IV: Chronic tophaceous gout: Recurrent attacks may damage joints or lead to the deposition of tophi. Tophi are deposits of urate in connective tissue.
   a. Joint damage leads to chronic pain, stiffness, and loss of function.
   b. Tophi become symptomatic if they ulcerate and become infected or if they enlarge and subsequently restrict movement.

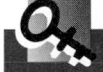

Key Symptom

Acute severe throbbing joint pain

Clinical Findings

1. Stage I: Asymptomatic hyperuricemia—no signs
2. Stage II: Acute gouty arthritis
   a. Affected sites show signs of inflammation:
      (1) Warmth
      (2) Redness
      (3) Swelling
      (4) Tenderness
   b. Acute attacks are usually monarticular:
      (1) Podagra (acute arthritis of first metatarsophalangeal joint) is most common.
      (2) Less common initially involved joints include, in decreasing frequency, the in-

step, ankles, heels, knees, wrists, fingers, and elbows.

   c. Skin may peel as inflammation subsides.

   d. Fever is more likely if polyarticular.

3. Stage III: Intercritical gout—generally no signs

4. Stage IV: Chronic tophaceous gout: defined by tophi and disabling arthritis. Tophi are firm and movable; overlying skin can be thin and red. Tophi form first in cooler body parts such as the pinnae, the olecranon tips, and the distal joints in the hands and feet.

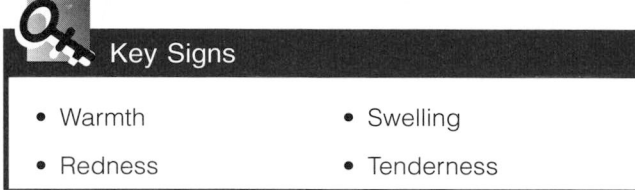

Key Signs

- Warmth
- Redness
- Swelling
- Tenderness

Laboratory Tests

1. Synovial fluid or tophaceous aspiration is the gold standard.

   a. Aspirate is usually turbid.

   b. Polarized microscopy reveals classic intracellular needle-shaped crystals that are strongly negatively birefringent (yellow when parallel to the long axis; blue when perpendicular).

   c. Wet mount may reveal pathognomonic crystals.

   d. White blood cell (WBC) count is typically 10,000 to 30,000/μl.

   e. Gram's stain and culture (crystals do not rule out septic arthritis)

2. Serum uric acid is usually elevated but can be within normal limits (30 per cent of acute attacks).

3. Radiographs

   a. Early stages: effusions and soft-tissue swelling

   b. Chronic stages

     (1) Tophi appear as cloud-like increases in density; may be calcified.

     (2) Gouty erosions have a punched-out appearance with overhanging edges, usually located in juxta-articular bone.

   c. Latest stages: demineralization and loss of articular structures

4. The 24-hour excretion of uric acid has therapeutic implications (see "Treatment").

5. Peripheral WBC count is usually normal; occasionally elevated to 15,000/μl.

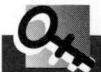

Key Tests

- Serum uric acid
- Synovial fluid analysis

Differential Diagnosis

1. Differential diagnosis for acute gouty arthritis

   a. Infection: septic arthritis or cellulitis

   b. Rheumatoid arthritis

   c. Calcium pyrophosphate dihydrate deposition disease (CPPD), called "pseudogout"

   d. Bursitis (usually prepatellar or olecranon)

   e. Acute trauma

   f. B27-associated diseases (includes Reiter's syndrome and reactive arthritis)

   g. Other: lipid crystal and intra-articular steroid-induced inflammation

2. Differential diagnosis for a tophus

   a. Rheumatoid nodule

   b. Benign nodule

   c. Other: neoplasm, granuloma annulare, xanthomatosis, leprosy, sarcoidosis

Treatment

Medication

Goals are to terminate the acute attack, prevent recurrent attacks, and normalize the hyperuricemia.

1. *Terminate the acute attack*: Treat immediately. Medications include nonsteroidal anti-inflammatory drugs (NSAIDs), colchicine, and corticosteroids.

   a. NSAIDs: initial drugs of choice (most NSAIDs are effective in full doses)

     (1) Indomethacin, 50 to 75 mg orally, and then 50 mg orally every 8 hours; or naproxen, 750 mg orally, and then 250 mg orally every 8 hours

     (2) After attack resolves, taper over 48 hours.

     (3) Side effects: gastrointestinal (GI) bleed, GI ulcer, nausea, rash, fluid retention, and, in less than 1 per cent, either renal or hepatic impairment

   b. Colchicine: oral or intravenous (effective if given within 48 hours of onset)

     (1) *Oral*: 0.5 to 0.6 mg every hour until attack resolves or toxicity develops; use limited by side effects of nausea, vomiting, diarrhea, and abdominal pain; do not exceed total of 5 to 6 mg.

(2) *Intravenous*: 1 to 2 mg in 20 ml of normal saline infused slowly over 20 minutes. Rarely used because of low benefit/toxicity ratio; if used, do not give additional oral or intravenous colchicine for 7 days.

c. Corticosteroids: oral, intramuscular, intra-articular, or adrenocorticotropic hormone (ACTH) preparations

(1) *Oral or intramuscular*: Prednisone, 30 mg orally bid, tapered quickly over 5 to 7 days; or triamcinolone acetonide, 60 mg intramuscularly, may be effective.

(2) *Intra-articular injection or ACTH subcutaneously or intramuscularly*: Both are options in patients with contraindications or resistance to other medications.

2. *Prevent recurrent attacks*

a. Avoid prophylaxis until after second or third acute attack.

b. Medication options for prophylaxis include

(1) Colchicine, 0.5 to 2.0 mg orally daily, adjusted not to cause diarrhea

(2) NSAIDs: One example is indomethacin, 25 mg orally bid.

c. Consider concomitant therapy for hyperuricemia.

d. May discontinue if attack-free for 6 to 12 months.

e. Treat risk factors and review medications for drugs that cause hyperuricemia, notably salicylates and diuretics.

3. *Normalize the hyperuricemia*

a. Patients with asymptomatic hyperuricemia

(1) First treat risk factors and attempt to correct the underlying cause.

(2) If that does not work, consider medical therapy for either

(a) Patients with a serum uric acid greater than 12 mg/dl *or*

(b) Patients who excrete more than 1100 mg uric acid per 24 hours.

b. Antihyperuricemic therapy is indicated in patients with gout and progressive tophi, joint erosions, or uric acid kidney stones.

c. Medication options to lower uric acid; remember to start at least 48 hours after acute attack has resolved.

(1) Uricosuric agent: Drug of choice in "undersecreter" who is less than 60 years old, has good renal function, and has no history of kidney stones. These agents require intake of large amounts of fluid.

(a) Before using uricosuric, measure 24-hour uric acid excretion: 330 to 600 mg per 24 hours is normal.

(b) Probenecid (Benemid), is the uricosuric of choice; start with 500 mg orally bid; maximum daily dose is 1500 mg orally bid. Probenecid is a safe drug; side effects include skin rash and GI upset.

(2) Allopurinol (Zyloprim), to decrease uric acid production: With allopurinol, there is no need to check 24-hour uric acid excretion. Side effects can be severe: GI upset, headache, rash, marrow suppression, fever, liver or kidney failure, vasculitis, alopecia, lymphadenopathy. Start with 300 mg orally once daily; up to 600 or 800 mg daily is occasionally necessary. In patients with renal insufficiency start at doses of 100 mg or 200 mg once daily. Initiation of uric acid lowering therapy can precipitate acute gouty arthritis. Give an NSAID or colchicine as prophylaxis for the first week or two of allopurinol therapy.

(3) Adjust medications on response after 2 to 6 months. The goal is to reduce serum uric acid to 6 mg/dl or less.

Diet

Instruct patients to modify dietary and alcohol-use patterns. Purine restriction is difficult to follow and of uncertain benefit. Weight loss may be very beneficial.

Activity

Restrictions apply to patients with chronic arthritis; encourage activities that limit stress on the joints.

Patient Education

1. Teach patients that gout is a "symptom" of the disease hyperuricemia.

2. Teach patients the causes of gout and hyperuricemia.

3. Teach patients the indications for and the side effects of their medications.

Key Treatment

- NSAIDs
- Colchicine
- Corticosteroids

Follow-Up

1. Follow up in 1 to 2 weeks after acute attack to review therapy, laboratory results, and medication side effects and to plan antihyperuricemic therapy.
2. See patient again in 4 to 6 weeks to adjust medications and to review treatment goals.
3. Eventually, the well-managed patient can be followed yearly.

Bibliography

Emmerson BT: The management of gout. N Engl J Med 1996;334:445–451.

George TM, Mandell BF: Individualizing the treatment of gout. Cleveland Clin J Med 1996;63:150–155.

Joseph J, McGrath H: Gout or 'pseudogout': how to differentiate crystal-induced arthropathies. Geriatrics 1995;50:33–39.

Kelley WN, Schumacher HR Jr: Gout. In Kelley WN, Harris ED, Ruddy S, et al (eds): Textbook of Rheumatology, 4th ed, vol 2, pp 1291–1336. Philadelphia, WB Saunders Company, 1993.

Tiliakous NA: Gout. In Hurst JW (ed in chief): Medicine for the Practicing Physician, 3rd ed, pp 202–206. Boston, Butterworth-Heinemann, 1992.

220 Costochondritis

Russell D. White

Etiology and Epidemiology
1. Etiology is unknown
2. Defined as inflammation of the costochondral or costosternal junction
3. Female/male ratio is 3:1.
4. Incidence increased with age greater than 40 years.

Symptoms
1. Greater than 90 per cent experience multiple sites of involvement.
2. Left side is more commonly involved than right: left third costochondral junction is most frequently involved.
3. Pain in the parasternal area
4. Aggravated by twisting, deep inspiration, and overhead reaching
5. Must differentiate from Tietze's syndrome and exclude angina.

Key Symptom
Pain aggravated by twisting, deep inspiration, overhead reaching

Signs
1. Multiple areas of pain to palpation over anterior chest wall
2. Localized tenderness to palpation over costochondral/costosternal junctions that reproduces symptoms
3. No visible swelling
4. May find erythema of overlying skin.

Key Sign
Localized tenderness at costochondral or costosternal junctions

Tests
1. Chest radiograph: Rule out other disease states.
2. Electrocardiogram: Rule out ischemic heart disease.
3. Complete blood count (CBC)/erythrocyte sedimentation rate: May rule out other causes but usually of little value.
4. Cardiac enzymes: Rule out acute myocardial infarction.
5. Ultrasound: best test to define Tietze's syndrome
6. Other radiographic tests
   a. Computerized tomography: not useful
   b. Technetium bone scan: useful in confirming septic arthritis
   c. Gallium scanning: useful in evaluating soft-tissue inflammation or monitoring response to treatment

Key Tests
- Chest x-ray
- ECG
- Erythrocyte sedimentation rate

Differential Diagnosis
1. Angina pectoris: confusing because it may co-exist and both are aggravated by activity
2. Contusion
3. Muscle spasm/strain
4. Rib fracture
5. Cervical/thoracic osteoarthritis
6. Pleuritis
7. Costochondral cartilage separation
8. Slipping rib syndrome
9. Septic arthritis
10. Herpes zoster
11. Scoliosis (mechanical abnormality)
12. Ankylosing spondylitis
13. Tietze's syndrome: Rare syndrome characterized by isolated swelling/pain of second and third costal junctions in patients under age 40.
14. Chondrosarcoma
15. Rheumatoid arthritis
16. Reiter's syndrome
17. Xiphoidalgia

18. Neoplasm (breast, prostate, plasma cell cytoma)
19. Sternalis syndrome

Treatment

Treated by nonsteroidal anti-inflammatory drugs (NSAIDs) and topical moist heat.

1. Medical
   a. Analgesics (acetaminophen) in mild cases
   b. Salicylates or NSAIDs such as ibuprofen (Motrin), naproxen (Naprosyn), indomethacin (Indocin), or diclofenac (Cataflam)
   c. Local injection with lidocaine/corticosteroid (2 ml 1% lidocaine and 20 mg methylprednisolone)
   d. Topical moist heat
2. Surgical: resection of inflamed cartilage in painful, refractory cases

Activity

1. Avoid activity that aggravates condition.
2. Stretching exercises after resolution of acute pain

Patient Education

Inform patient that process is *self-limited* (1 to 3 months), although some cases may last longer.

Key Treatment

- NSAIDs
- Topical moist heat

Bibliography

Aeschlimann A, Kahn MF: Tietze's syndrome: a critical review. Clin Exp Rheumatol 1990;8:407–412.

Gilliland BC: Tietze's syndrome and costochondritis. In Fauci AS, Braunwald E, Isselbacher KJ, et al (eds): Harrison's Principles of Internal Medicine, 14th ed, p 1958. New York, McGraw-Hill, 1998.

Massie JD, Sebes JI, Cowles SJ: Bone scintigraphy and costochondritis. J Thorac Imaging 1993;8:137–142.

Semble EL, Wise CM: Chest pain: a rheumatologist's perspective. South Med J 1988;81:64–68.

Wolf E, Stern S: Costosternal syndrome: its frequency and importance in differential diagnosis of coronary heart disease. Arch Intern Med 1976;136:189–191.

221 Myofascial Syndromes (Fibromyalgia and Myofascial Trigger Points)

Jimmy H. Hara

Etiology

1. *Fibromyalgia* (or *fibrositis*) is a chronic rheumatologic syndrome seen in 4 to 11 per cent of the population, more common in women. Etiology is unknown.

2. *Myofascial trigger points* are seen in up to 50 per cent of the normal healthy population, equally common in men and women, representing tender foci of muscle hyperirritability with specific reference zone pain radiation caused by muscular strain. Muscular strain is often a product of

   a. Mechanical stresses, such as structural asymmetry (leg-length discrepancy, pelvic asymmetry, short humerus), poor posture, or prolonged immobilization

   b. Nutritional deficiency (especially B and C vitamins)

   c. Metabolic/endocrine inadequacies (especially thyroid)

   d. Emotional stress/distress and sleep disturbance

Symptoms

1. In fibromyalgia, patients complain of "total body" pain and fatigue, sleep disturbance, and various psychophysiologic symptoms (especially irritable bowel).

2. Patients suffering from myofascial trigger points (or tension myalgia) complain of pain and dysfunction specific to the affected muscle(s).

   a. The pain of a specific myofascial trigger point is in the distribution of the reference zone pain pattern (areas where pain radiates when pressure is applied to the trigger points) for that specific muscle. Frequently, multiple myofascial trigger points occur in the same patient.

   b. Some myofascial trigger points (such as the sternomastoid) have associated autonomic epiphenomena (such as lacrimation and rhinorrhea).

3. Commonly encountered myofascial trigger points and their specific reference zone pain patterns include

   a. The upper trapezius trigger located along the superior margin of the trapezius and referring up the neck, behind the ear, and over the ear to the angle of the jaw

   b. The levator scapular trigger at the superomedial angle of the scapula and referring up the neck, laterally across the shoulder, and down the back

   c. The posterior cervical trigger located a few centimeters below the nuchal ridge and referring up to the occiput

 Key Symptoms

Fibromyalgia	Myofascial Trigger Points
• Total-body pain	• Pain in reference zone pattern
• Sleep disturbance	• Dysfunction of affected muscle
• Psychophysiologic symptoms	• Autonomic epiphenomena possible

Clinical Findings

1. In fibromyalgia, a patient must have 11 of 18 tender points (Fig. 221–1) on digital examination (with 4 kg/cm^2 of pressure).

   a. Eight of the tender points (four pairs) are those of tendinitis or bursitis: lateral epicondylitis, anserine bursitis, supraspinatus impingement tendinitis, and trochanteric bursitis.

   b. Two of the tender points are those of costochondritis.

   c. Eight of the tender points are true myofascial trigger point pairs (upper and middle trapezius, posterior cervical, and quadratus lumborum).

2. Myofascial trigger points are identified by the finding of the trigger point specific for the affected muscle, which reproduces the reference

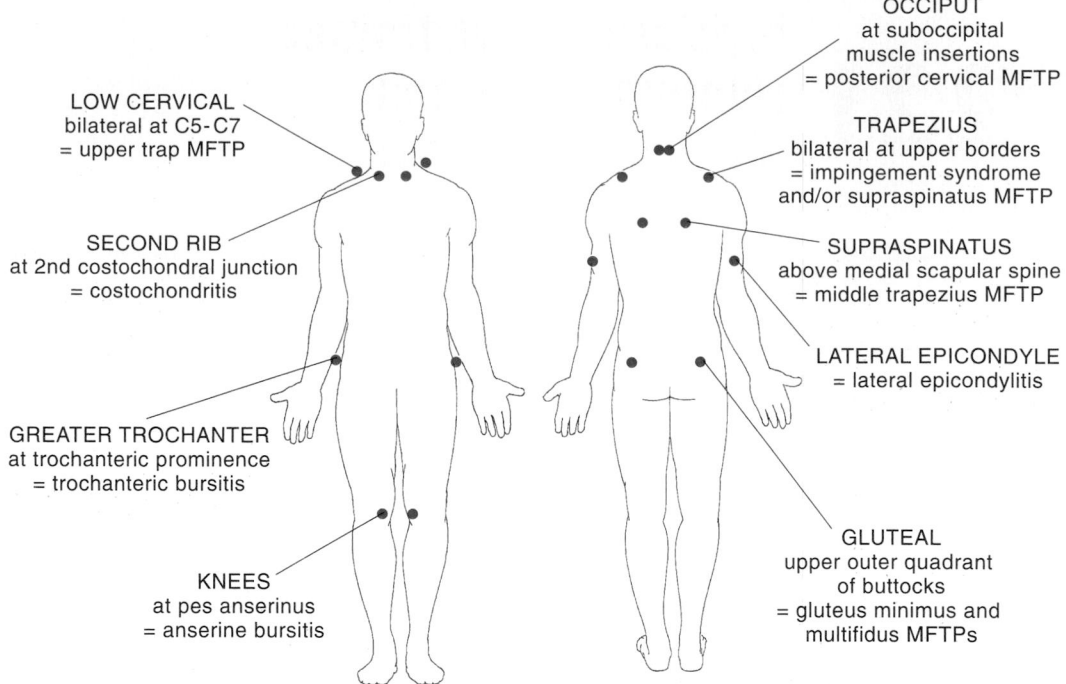

Figure 221–1 Myofascial trigger points. Occipital/suboccipital corresponds to posterior cervical myofascial trigger point (MFTP). Low cervical corresponds to the upper trapezius myofascial trigger point. Trapezius corresponds to the supraspinatus peritendinitis/impingement syndrome tender point. Supraspinatus corresponds to the middle trapezius myofascial trigger point. Lateral epicondyle corresponds to lateral epicondylitis tendinosis/enthesitis. Gluteal corresponds to gluteus minimus and multifidus myofascial triggers. Second rib corresponds to costochondritis tender points. Knees correspond to tender points of the anserine bursitis.

zone pain pattern when palpated with firm digital pressure.

Key Signs

- Tender points in fibromyalgia
- True trigger points in myofascial syndrome

Laboratory Tests

1. There are no specific diagnostic laboratory tests recommended (complete blood count and erythrocyte sedimentation rate are typically normal).
2. Specialized immunologic testing may reveal an increased CD4/CD8 level (helper/suppressor ratio) in fibromyalgia.
3. Sleep electroencephalogram may reveal an alpha/delta pattern.

Differential Diagnosis

1. The differential diagnosis of fibromyalgia includes depression, metabolic imbalance, hypothyroidism, polymyalgia rheumatica, and polymyositis.
2. The differential diagnosis of specific myofascial trigger point syndromes includes any cause of

pain or dysfunction in the involved anatomic site.

Treatment

1. Pharmacotherapy for fibromyalgia includes low-dose selective serotonin reuptake inhibitor (SSRI) antidepressants (fluoxetine [Prozac], sertraline [Zoloft], paroxetine [Paxil]); low-dose heterocyclic antidepressants (trazodone [Desyrel], bupropion [Wellbutrin], venlafaxine [Effexor]; and cyclobenzaprine [Flexeril]). Clonazepam (Klonopin) or zolpidem (Ambien) may help sleep; tramadol (Ultram) or gabapentin (Neurontin) may help pain.
2. Tendinitis, bursitis, and costochondritis tender points may be injected with Xylocaine and steroid.
3. Anesthetic injection of trigger points with 0.5% procaine (patient should experience pain/warmth in reference zone pain pattern as anesthetic is infused)
4. Stretch and intermittent cold therapy (vapocoolant stretch and spray) may be applied to specific myofascial trigger point muscle.
5. Other stretching modalities may be applied, such as the Lewit technique, strain-counterstrain, or proprioceptive neuromuscular facilitation.

6. Ischemic compression may be applied for approximately 3 minutes to extinguish trigger point pain. Shiatsu and acupressure may be effective as ischemic compression techniques.
7. Patients with higher levels of dysfunction may benefit from multidisciplinary group programs utilizing cognitive-behavioral techniques, physical therapy, and pharmacotherapy.

Diet

1. Basic nutritionally sound diet.
2. Ensure adequate water-soluble vitamins.

Activity

1. Advise exercise as tolerated.
2. Focus on adequate stretching of involved muscles.

Patient Education

1. Explain chronic nature of fibromyalgia.
2. Prevent precipitating factors if identified (poor body mechanics, compensations for body asymmetry, poor diet).
3. Encourage stretching of involved muscles.

Key Treatment

For Fibromyalgia	For Trigger Points
• Low-dose SSRI or heterocyclic antidepressant	• Injection with procaine
	• Stretching modalities
• Injection with Xylocaine/steroid	• Ischemic compression

Follow-Up

1. Fibromyalgia patients require periodic follow-ups to treat symptomatic tender points and titrate drugs.
2. Patients with chronic and recurrent myofascial trigger points may need periodic revisits for injections or stretch and intermittent cold therapy.
3. Patients with acute or episodic myofascial trigger point syndromes do not typically require follow-up.

Bibliography

Bennett RM: Multidisciplinary group programs to treat fibromyalgia patients. Rheum Dis Clin North Am 1996;22:351–367.

Hara JH: Fibromyalgia. In Taylor RB (ed): Manual of Family Practice, pp 544–545. New York, Little, Brown, 1996.

McCain, GA: Treatment of fibromyalgia and myofascial pain syndrome. In Rachlin ES (ed): Myofascial Pain and Fibromyalgia, pp 31–44. St Louis, Mosby–Year Book, 1994.

Wallace JB: Making Sense of Fibromyalgia, pp 1–210. New York, Oxford University Press, 1999.

Yunus MB: Fibromyalgia syndrome and myofascial pain syndrome: Clinical features, laboratory tests, diagnosis, and pathophysiologic mechanisms. In Rachlin ES (ed): Myofascial Pain and Fibromyalgia, pp 3–29. St. Louis, Mosby–Year Book, 1994.

222 Rhabdomyolysis

Bobbi B. Adcock

Etiology

The term *rhabdomyolysis* is derived from the Greek meaning "striped muscle dissolution." Rhabdomyolysis is injury of skeletal muscle causing muscle cell lysis because of disruption of the calcium transport system. Myocyte contents (e.g., creatine, myoglobin, aldolase, potassium, lactate dehydrogenase) are released into the plasma. Diagnosis of rhabdomyolysis may be difficult; therefore, clinicians must maintain a high index of suspicion. Causes of rhabdomyolysis with examples include

1. Muscle injury (common): compression, heat exhaustion, extreme physical exertion, seizures, electrical burns, trauma
2. Drugs: salicylates, clofibrate, lovastatin, phenothiazines, corticosteroids, phenytoin
3. Toxins: alcohol (common), cocaine, venom (snakes, hornets), carbon monoxide
4. Metabolic abnormalities: hypokalemia, hypophosphatemia, hypomagnesemia, hyponatremia, hypernatremia, diabetic ketoacidosis
5. Infections: influenza, *Legionella*, gram-negative sepsis, *Salmonella*
6. Hereditary causes: McArdle's disease, carnitine palmitoyltransferase deficiency, Duchenne's muscular dystrophy, malignant hyperthermia
7. Ischemia: sickle cell anemia, vascular insufficiency, vasculitis
8. Multifactorial
9. Idiopathic

Symptoms

Symptoms can be subtle and may include
1. Muscle pain, stiffness, and spasm
2. Dark urine: often the first clue
3. Weakness
4. Malaise
5. Nausea
6. Confusion

Key Symptoms

- Muscle pain
- Weakness
- Dark urine

Clinical Findings

1. Muscle swelling and tenderness
2. Fever
3. Decreased range of motion

Key Sign

Muscle swelling and tenderness

Laboratory Tests

1. Urinalysis: The urine dipstick (orthotoluidine test) will be positive for blood, but the microscopic evaluation will show no red blood cells.
2. Serum creatine kinase (CK) is the most sensitive indicator of rhabdomyolysis. CK is usually at least five times the normal level and can be greater than 100,000 IU/L.
3. Myoglobin

   a. Urine myoglobin via radioimmunoassay is diagnostic for rhabdomyolysis. Once the renal threshold for myoglobin (21 mg/dl plasma) is reached, myoglobin is cleared at 75 per cent of the glomerular filtration rate.

   b. Serum myoglobin is not a good indicator of clinical disease because of rapid renal clearance. However, if there is marked muscle breakdown, the serum myoglobin level may be high. Myoglobin is not detectable until the serum level is greater than 1.5 mg/dl, which equals dissolution of 100 gm of skeletal muscle.

4. Electrolytes/metabolites

   a. Hypernatremia secondary to dehydration because of third spacing

   b. Hyperkalemia secondary to its release into the interstitial fluid and circulation

   c. Hyperuricemia secondary to enhanced release of purine precursors

   d. Lactic acidosis secondary to glycogen depletion and anaerobic metabolism

Differential Diagnosis

1. Dark brown urine: hemoglobinuria, porphyria, urobilinogen, medications (nitrofurantoin, primaquine, metronidazole)
2. Myalgia: polymyositis, dermatomyositis, rheumatoid arthritis, fibrositis, polymyalgia rheumatica, tendinitis, infection, medications (steroids, diuretics).

Treatment

Medication

1. Intravenous fluids at 2.5 ml/kg/hour must be given to maintain adequate urine output (goal of >2 ml/kg/hour) to prevent acute tubular necrosis. Four to 6 L of normal saline may be needed in the first 24 hours.
2. Bicarbonate causes alkalinization of urine, which prevents nephrotoxic effects of myoglobin. Maintenance of the urine pH greater than 6 prevents disassociation of myoglobin into ferrihemate and globin. Bicarbonate should be used cautiously because it can cause hypocalcemia.
3. Mannitol, an osmotic diuretic and renal vasodilator, dilutes the concentration of myoglobin and decreases nephrotoxicity. It can be given as a single dose of 0.25 to 1.0 gm/kg IV over 30 minutes. If needed, furosemide 40 to 120 mg can be given IV over 10 minutes, but it can acidify the urine.
4. Treatment should be continued until the urine dipstick is negative for blood, creatinine is normal, and other laboratory evidence of rhabdomyolysis is negative.
5. Monitor for complications:
    a. *Acute renal failure* may develop secondary to acute tubular necrosis because of the decreased glomerular filtration rate and tubular obstruction, primarily by myoglobin. Dialysis may be indicated.
    b. *Metabolic complications* can include hyperkalemia, hypokalemia, hypercalcemia, hypocalcemia, hyperuricemia, hyperphosphatemia, and hypoalbuminemia. Cardiac monitoring is necessary because of potential for arrhythmias. Hyperkalemia can be treated with glucose and insulin, kayexalate, or calcium chloride, but the latter can cause other metabolic abnormalities. Intravenous fluids will usually correct hypercalcemia, hypocalcemia, and hyperphosphatemia.
    c. *Compartment syndrome* is caused by increased compartmental pressure and ischemia, which cause neuromuscular and circulatory compromise. Manifestations include edema, pain, paresthesias, and diminished pulses. A fasciotomy is usually performed when the compartment pressure is 30 to 45 mm Hg.
    d. *Disseminated intravascular coagulopathy* (DIC) is caused by the apparent release of thromboplastin and plasminogen activator from damaged muscle. Treatment involves management of the cause of DIC, and resolution of DIC typically occurs spontaneously after several days. If bleeding occurs, treatment is fresh frozen plasma.
    e. *Miscellaneous:* cardiomyopathy, respiratory failure

Diet

Increased fluids

Activity

Rest

Patient Education

1. Encourage adequate hydration, carbohydrate intake, and rest.
2. Discourage exhaustive exercise.
3. Limit activities during extremely high temperatures and humidity.

Follow-Up

The patient should follow up if there are recurrent signs or symptoms.

Bibliography

Better OS, Stein JH: Early management of shock and prophylaxis of acute renal failure in traumatic rhabdomyolysis. N Engl J Med 1990;322:825–829.

Curry SC, Chang D, Conner D: Drug- and toxin-induced rhabdomyolysis. Ann Emerg Med 1989;18:1068–1084.

Poels PJE, Gabreels FJM: Rhabdomyolysis: a review of the literature. Clin Neurol Neurosurg 1993;95:175–192.

Reilly KM, Salluzzo R: Rhabdomyolysis and its complications. Resid Staff Physician 1990;36:45–52.

Slater MS, Mullins RJ: Rhabdomyolysis and myoglobinuric renal failure in trauma and surgical patients: a review. J Am Coll Surg 1998;186:693–716.

223 Restless Legs Syndrome

Brian S. Murphy

Etiology

1. Restless legs syndrome (RLS) affects 10 to 15 per cent of the population, and 40 per cent of those afflicted recall the onset of symptoms before age 20.
2. RLS is defined as an unpleasant sensation in the legs that occurs at rest and is relieved by movement.
3. Most cases are idiopathic.
4. Physiologic causes have been implicated, including iron deficiency anemia, folate and B_{12} deficiency, hypothyroidism, chronic renal failure, second or third trimester of pregnancy, rheumatoid arthritis, and diabetes mellitus.
5. Drugs, such as β-blockers, caffeine, lithium, antihistamines, and tricyclic antidepressants, have also been associated with RLS.
6. It is not uncommon to find a positive family history of RLS.
7. On a cellular level, the etiology of RLS is postulated to involve a disturbance of inhibitory subcortical pathways allowing for the expression of a normally suppressed neural generator at the level of the spinal cord.

Symptoms

1. The diagnosis of RLS is clinically based on the patient's history.
2. Paresthesias, if present, are usually located in the calves and are often bilateral and symmetric in intensity. The unpleasant sensations of RLS are noted to be deep inside the leg and are often described by patients as creeping or crawling in nature. This sensation is often associated with a compelling motor restlessness.
3. The course of RLS can be intermittent, with long asymptomatic periods between attacks.
4. Symptoms can develop at any age, and a family history suggests an autosomal dominant pattern of inheritance.
5. Walking has been reported to relieve the symptoms; flexing or massaging the legs can also bring relief.
6. Symptoms usually develop at night and are often associated by sleep disturbances. More than 80 per cent of patients with RLS also experience periodic movements of sleep (PMS) that are characterized by stereotypic flexion movements of the legs during non–rapid-eye-movement sleep.

Key Symptoms

- Restlessness at night
- Paresthesias
- Creeping or crawling feeling in legs

Differential Diagnosis

1. Syndromes such as fibromyalgia, paresthesias, and nocturnal leg cramps can be distinguished from RLS on the basis of the patient's history.
2. Akathisia, often neuroleptic induced, is often present throughout the day and occurs both at rest and with activity.

Treatment

1. Secondary causes of RLS should be evaluated and removed. This includes reducing or eliminating caffeine-containing drinks, alcohol, and tobacco products.
2. Treatment of any underlying medical problem is also effective in relieving symptoms of RLS. This would include iron supplementation in patients with iron deficiency anemia and folate supplements in pregnant women.

Medication

1. Dopaminergic agents
   a. Carbidopa-levodopa (Sinemet CR) has been shown to control or diminish the symptoms of RLS in several randomized controlled trials. The usual dosage is half a 25/100-mg tablet before bed, with patients able to titrate the dose up to a full tablet if needed.
   b. Although levodopa has been shown to be effective for up to 5 years of therapy, a complicating factor of therapy is the development of daytime paresthesias and restlessness, which are termed *restless leg augmentation* (RLA). RLA has been associated with the pretreatment of restless legs symptoms before 6 PM and a daily dosage of levodopa exceeding 200 mg.

2. Dopamine agonists
   a. Bromocriptine (Parlodel) has been shown to be an effective treatment in a small double-blind crossover study with the daily dosage ranging between 5 and 15 mg.
   b. Pergolide (Permax), a long-acting dopamine agonist, has also been used to treat RLS, but it is rarely used as a first-line agent because of side effects such as nausea, insomnia, and light-headedness. Pergolide has been shown to be effective in the treatment of patients who experience RLA. Treatment regimens usually start with 0.05 mg prior to sleep, with the dose increased by 0.05 mg every 2 nights until symptoms are controlled or until a maximum dose of 0.6 to 0.8 mg is attained.
3. Carbamazepine: A double-blind trial of 174 patients revealed that carbamazepine (Tegretol) relieved symptoms of RLS, but this medication was noted to cause side effects in 40 per cent of the treated group. Further clinical studies have shown that this medication lacks significant efficacy, and its use has been curtailed in the treatment of RLS.
4. Benzodiazepines
   a. Benzodiazepines often decrease arousal from sleep but do not affect limb movements in RLS. Clonazepam (Klonopin) has been most studied and is administered in doses of 0.5 to 2.0 mg. Other drugs in this class used in treating RLS include triazolam (Halcion), 0.125 to 0.25 mg; and temazepam (Restoril), 7.5 to 30 mg.
   b. Because many patients with RLS may be elderly, a significant concern with using benzodiazepines is the increased risk of falls as a result of sedating side effects. These same side effects can complicate the course of patients with sleep apnea and may produce daytime somnolence in patients.
   c. These medications have been shown to be useful in conjunction with levodopa or dopamine agonist therapy.
5. Opioids
   a. Opioid agents are usually reserved for treatment when other modalities have failed, and those that act on the mu receptor have been shown to be effective at relieving the symptoms of RLS.
   b. In cases of mild symptoms, codeine and propoxyphene (Darvon) are useful in initial dosages of 30 mg and 65 mg, respectively. If these are not effective, higher potency agents such as oxycodone, at an average dose of 10 to 15 mg each day, have improved the symptoms of RLS.
6. Clonidine
   a. Clonidine (Catapres) has been showed to be effective in controlling the symptoms of RLS in patients with the uremic or idiopathic types. Dosages range from 0.1 to 0.9 mg in divided doses.
   b. Side effects associated with clonidine include lightheadedness and dry mouth.

Key Treatment

- For mild symptoms: intermittent use of a benzodiazepine (clonazepam) or low-potency opioid (codeine) when symptoms become exacerbated

- Continuous and disruptive of sleep: carbidopa-levodopa

- If side effects pre-empt the use of carbidopa-levodopa or if the treatment becomes ineffective, switch to pergolide.

- If daytime augmentation develops when using pergolide or if side effects make the drug prohibitive, use higher potency opioids or a benzodiazepine plus levodopa.

Bibliography

Kreuger BR: Restless legs syndrome and periodic movements of sleep. Mayo Clin Proc 1990;65:999–1006.

O'Keefe ST: Restless legs syndrome—a review. Arch Intern Med 1996;156:243–248.

O'Keefe ST, Gavin K, Lavan JN: Iron status and restless legs syndrome in the elderly. Age Ageing 1994;23:200–203.

O'Keefe ST, Noel J, Lavan JN: Restless legs syndrome in the elderly. Postgrad Med J 1993;69:701–703.

Silber MH: Restless legs syndrome. Mayo Clin Proc 1997;72:261–264.

224 Systemic Lupus Erythematosus

Monica O. Watts

Etiology

1. The cause of systemic lupus erythematosus (SLE) is unknown.

2. The disease affects women more than men at a ratio of 9:1. If affects 1 in 250 black women and 1 in 1000 white women.

3. The disease is usually chronic and is often relapsing. It can also lead to a rapid death in a small percentage of those affected.

Symptoms

The symptoms of SLE can vary widely. A patient will certainly not present with all the symptoms at once but during the course of the disease most will occur.

1. Arthralgia is often the most common presenting complaint.

2. Other common symptoms may include fever, malaise, oral ulcers, photosensitivity, weight loss, and anorexia.

3. The malar or "butterfly" rash that is often associated with SLE is usually seen in only one half of patients. There may often be other cutaneous lesions, including splinter hemorrhages, periungual erythema, alopecia, and discoid lupus.

4. Abdominal pains, photophobia, transient blindness, and blurred vision are also frequent complaints.

5. An estimated 20 per cent of SLE patients present with symptoms of Raynaud's phenomenon.

6. Often patients present with signs of cognitive impairment, such as memory loss or trouble thinking clearly.

Clinical Findings

1. On clinical examination, patients with SLE often have an increased pulse rate. The increase in rate strongly correlates with flares of the disease.

2. Other findings may include hypertension, cardiac arrhythmias, and accelerated atherosclerosis.

3. SLE can affect the lungs and pleura, manifesting as pleurisy, pleural effusion, and pneumonia.

4. The majority of SLE patients also have renal involvement in the form of lupus nephritis; in black patients, up to 75 per cent have been found to be affected. Lupus nephritis can be mild, as in the form of mesangial glomerulonephritis and focal proliferative glomerulonephritis, or it can be severe, as in the form of diffuse proliferative glomerulonephritis. Renal biopsy can help determine the severity of disease.

5. Hematologic disturbances can include anemia of chronic disease, iron deficiency anemia, hemolytic anemia, thrombocytopenia, and leukopenia.

6. Neurologic findings include psychosis, seizures, organic brain syndrome, stroke, and transverse myelopathy. Many SLE patients also present with depression.

7. Osteoporosis, osteonecrosis, and fibromyalgia are common musculoskeletal problems.

Key Signs

A patient must have 4 or more of the following 11 criteria to be classified as having SLE:

- Malar rash
- Discoid rash
- Photosensitivity
- Oral ulcers
- Arthritis
- Serositis
- Renal disease

Key Symptoms

- Arthralgia
- Alopecia
- Discoid lesions
- Fever
- Malar rash
- Oral ulcers
- Photosensitivity
- Weight loss

- Neurologic disease

- Hematologic disorders

- Immunologic abnormalities

- Positive antinuclear antibodies (ANA)

Adapted from Tan EM, Cohen AS, Fries JF, et al: The 1982 revised criteria for the classification of systemic lupus erythematosus. Arthritis Rheum 1982;25:1271–1277; reprinted with permission.

Laboratory Findings

1. Laboratory tests should include complete blood cell count, chemistry panel, and urinalysis. As mentioned earlier anemia, leukopenia, and thrombocytopenia are frequent laboratory abnormalities. There may also be proteinuria and hematuria.

2. ANA test is positive in almost all SLE patients, but it is not specific to SLE. Antibodies to double-stranded DNA (dsDNA) and antibodies to Sm are more specific but are not present in 40 to 70 per cent of patients.

3. False-positive test for syphilis occurs in about 25 per cent of SLE patients.

4. Lupus anticoagulant and anti-cardiolipin antibodies may also be present in 7 and 25 per cent, respectively.

5. Complement levels are often decreased. Levels of C3 are the most useful to follow as an indicator of active disease.

Key Tests

- ANA

- Anti-dsDNA

- Anti-Sm

- Complement levels (especially C3)

- False-positive test for syphilis

Differential Diagnosis

1. Several drugs have been known to cause a condition similar to lupus. These include sulfa drugs, hydralazine, procainamide, and isoniazid. In drug-induced lupus, the ratio of affected men to affected women is 1:1. There are also no antibodies to dsDNA and complement levels are normal.

2. SLE should be differentiated from primary antiphospholipid antibody syndrome. This syndrome consists of thrombosis, recurrent or late pregnancy loss, and thrombocytopenia. The patient may have anti-phospholipid antibodies but

no other specific features of SLE. Patients with active SLE usually have a loss early in the pregnancy.

3. The differential diagnosis of SLE also includes scleroderma, vasculitis, and rheumatoid arthritis.

Treatment

Because SLE can vary widely in the severity of the disease, treatment is reserved for symptomatic patients regardless of positive serologic test.

1. Minor joint pains are the most common complaint, and nonsteroidal anti-inflammatory drugs (NSAIDs) are used for this. When the joint pain is not responding to NSAIDs, antimalarial drugs such as hydroxychloroquine (Plaquenil), are used.

2. Corticosteroids are used when patients have polyarthralgias that do not respond to NSAIDs or antimalarials. Hemolytic anemia, thrombocytopenia, myocarditis and lupus nephritis are also treated with corticosteroids. Severe flare-up can be treated with intravenous methylprednisolone sodium succinate (Solu-Medrol), 1000 mg daily for 3 days. For maintenance, the smallest dose of corticosteroids necessary to control symptoms should be used, preferably less than 10 mg/day.

3. Immunosuppressive drugs such as methotrexate or azathioprine (Imuran), are reserved for conditions that are resistant to all other therapies.

4. Medical treatment for SLE can also include estrogen, calcitonin, and bisphosphonates to prevent osteoporosis associated with long-term steroid use and menopause.

Diet

1. For the patient with SLE, the diet should be low in cholesterol. This is to lower the incidence of premature atherosclerosis, which is one of the long-term causes of mortality. Patients with SLE have higher levels of homocysteine, a risk factor for atherosclerosis.

2. The diet should also include the daily recommended allowance of vitamin D and calcium to help maintain bone mass and prevent osteoporosis.

Patient Education

1. Patient education should stress the importance of taking medications as prescribed and keeping follow-up appointments. Because the medications used to treat SLE can have serious side effects, frequent monitoring is necessary so that the lowest doses needed to control the disease can be used.

2. The patient should be informed that the complications of SLE may be silent, and regular evaluations may be the only way to detect them early.

3. Smoking cessation is also important.

Key Treatment

- NSAIDs

- Antimalarials: hydroxychloroquine

- Corticosteroids: Solu-Medrol, prednisone

- Immunosuppressive drugs: methotrexate, azathioprine

Follow-Up

1. Follow-up should include laboratory monitoring of renal and hematologic abnormalities. Cognitive changes can also be monitored at that time.

2. Follow-up should also include ophthalmologic examination every 6 months to screen for retinal changes from hydroxychloroquine. It is also necessary to check for steroid-induced cataracts and glaucoma.

3. Bone density measurements are important because of the increased risk of osteoporosis.

4. Pneumococcal and flu vaccines are also recommended.

Bibliography

Hellmann DB: Systemic lupus erythematosus. In Tierney LM (ed): Current Diagnosis and Treatment, 35th ed, vol 1, pp 742–745. Norwalk, CT, Appleton & Lange, 1996.

Karlson EW, Daltroy LH, Lew RA, et al: The relationship of socioeconomic status, race and modifiable risk factors to outcomes in patients with systemic lupus erythematosus. Arthritis Rheum 1997;40:47–55.

Petri M: Treatment of systemic lupus erythematosus: an update. Am Fam Physician 1998;57:2753–2760.

Roberts WN: Keys to managing systemic lupus erythematosus. Hosp Practice 1997;32:113–126.

Tan EM, Cohen AS, Fries JF, et al: The 1982 revised criteria for the classification of systemic lupus erythematosus. Arthritis Rheum 1982;25:1271–1277.

225 Scleroderma (Systemic Sclerosis)

Carlos M. Swanger

Etiology

1. The cause of systemic sclerosis is unknown.
2. Theories of pathogenesis
   a. Genetic predisposition: haplotype HLA A1, B8, DR3
   b. Connective tissue: excessive deposition of tissue matrix proteins, primarily collagen
   c. Vascular: microvascular and endothelial injury
   d. Immunologic: the association of specific antinuclear antibodies, the presence of mononuclear cell infiltrates, and evidence for antimaternal graft-versus-host reactions in some women developing systemic sclerosis after their childbearing years

Symptoms

1. Raynaud's phenomenon: episodic digital ischemia
   a. Presents as pallor followed by cyanosis and rubor. Pallor is the most reliable component of this triad.
   b. Syndrome occurs in 90 to 98 per cent of patients with systemic sclerosis; it is the first symptom in 70 per cent of cases.
2. Skin
   a. Skin thickening
      (1) Often begins with hands
      (2) Development of taut facial skin that may lead to restriction of mouth opening
      (3) Areas of hyper- or hypopigmentation
   b. Edema
      (1) Swelling mainly of hands
      (2) May also be present on trunk, proximal arms, and face.
3. Musculoskeletal
   a. Morning stiffness and arthralgias. Arthritis occurs as the initial symptom in up to 66 per cent of patients.
   b. Limitation of joint function and movement
   c. Muscle weakness secondary to disuse atrophy and/or myositis
4. Gastrointestinal
   a. Intermittent heartburn and regurgitation secondary to esophageal involvement
   b. Dysphagia and odynophagia
   c. Early satiety
   d. Telangiectasias may cause symptoms of both upper and lower gastrointestinal bleeding.
   e. Persistent vomiting from functional gastric outlet obstruction
   f. Acute and chronic diarrhea
   g. Symptoms associated with small bowel obstruction
5. Pulmonary
   a. Worsening dyspnea on exertion
   b. Nonproductive cough
   c. Less commonly, there may be chest pain, pleurisy, or productive cough.
6. Cardiac
   a. Palpitations from atrial or ventricular arrhythmias
   b. Congestive heart failure manifest as dyspnea or edema
   c. Chest pain—such as that associated with pericarditis
7. Renal: symptoms associated with severe hypertension
   a. Headaches
   b. Visual disturbances
   c. Symptoms of acute left ventricular failure
8. Other
   a. Sicca syndrome: dry eyes, dry mouth
   b. Numbness, paresthesias, and weakness associated with entrapment neuropathies and facial nerve palsies

Key Symptoms

- Raynaud's phenomenon
- Edema
- Skin thickening
- Arthralgias/arthritis
- "Heartburn"
- Dysphagia/odynophagia
- Hematemesis, melena
- Dyspnea, nonproductive cough
- Headaches
- Visual disturbances
- Sicca syndrome

Clinical Findings

1. Vascular: Nailfold capillary microscopy shows a dropout of capillary loops. This has also been found to be a strong predictor of the subsequent development of systemic sclerosis among patients with Raynaud's phenomenon.
2. Skin and musculoskeletal
   a. Shiny and taut appearance
   b. Skin thickening—involving forearms, hands, and face in limited scleroderma (LSS)
   c. Skin thickening extends proximally in diffuse scleroderma (DSS).
   d. Palpable tendinous friction rubs: wrists, ankles, knees
   e. Subcutaneous calcinosis of fingers and distal extensor surfaces occurs in 40 per cent of patients with LSS.
3. Gastrointestinal: There is impaired function of the lower esophageal sphincter and impaired peristalsis of the lower two thirds of the esophagus.
4. Pulmonary
   a. Reduced lung volumes and diffusing capacity lead to hypoxemia.
   b. Pulmonary hypertension, more common in LSS, leads to signs of right ventricular overload and failure.
5. Renal: scleroderma renal crisis
   a. Signs of malignant hypertension and rapidly progressive renal insufficiency, which may be accompanied by microangiopathic hemolytic anemia
   b. Often associated with rapid progression of skin involvement
6. Cardiac
   a. Atrial, nodal, and ventricular arrhythmias
   b. Signs of left ventricular failure

Key Signs

- Skin thickening
- Microscopic nailfold capillary dropout
- Accelerated/malignant hypertension
- Tendinous friction rubs
- Subcutaneous calcinosis
- Inspiratory rales
- Signs of pulmonary hypertension
- Arrhythmias
- Left ventricular gallops

Laboratory Tests

Antinuclear antibodies: present in 90 per cent of patients

1. Scl-70 (topoisomerase I): sensitivity approximately 75 per cent and specificity 99 per cent for diffuse scleroderma
2. Centromere/kinetochore
   a. More commonly seen in LSS: Sensitivity is between 50 and 96 per cent in various studies.
   b. Present in less than 10 per cent of individuals with DSS

Key Tests

- Antinuclear antibodies
- Anti-Scl-70
- Anticentromere

Differential Diagnosis

1. Disorders characterized by or associated with skin thickening on the fingers and hands
   a. Acrodermatitis chronica atrophicans
   b. Adult celiac disease
   c. Vibration disease
   d. Bleomycin-induced scleroderma
   e. Reflex sympathetic dystrophy
   f. Amyloidosis
   g. Vinyl chloride disease
   h. Mycosis fungoides
   i. Digital sclerosis of diabetes mellitus
2. Disorders characterized by or associated with generalized skin thickening but typically sparing the fingers and hands
   a. Scleroderma adultorum of Buschke
   b. Scleromyxedema
   c. Eosinophilic fasciitis
   d. Eosinophilic-myalgia syndrome
   e. Generalized subcutaneous morphea
   f. Human adjuvant disease
   g. Amyloidosis
   h. Porphyria cutanea tarda
   i. Graft-versus-host disease
   j. Pentazocine-induced disease
3. Disorders characterized by asymmetric skin change
   a. Morphea
   b. Linear scleroderma
   c. *Coup de sabre*

4. Disorders characterized by similar internal organ involvement
   a. Primary pulmonary hypertension
   b. Primary biliary cirrhosis
   c. Intestinal pseudo-obstruction
   d. Idiopathic pulmonary fibrosis
   e. Infiltrative cardiomyopathy
   f. Collagenous colitis
5. Disorders characterized by Raynaud's phenomenon

Treatment

Medication

1. D-Penicillamine
   a. May lead to improvement of cutaneous manifestations.
   b. Decreases incidence of new visceral involvement.
   c. Initial dose is 250 mg/day, with the goal being 750 to 1500 mg/day.
2. Corticosteroids
   a. Do not slow disease progression.
   b. Can be helpful in inflammatory myositis, arthralgias/myalgias, and some cases of interstitial lung disease.
   c. Can precipitate normotensive renal crisis at doses of 30 or more mg/day of prednisone or the equivalent.
3. Calcium channel blockers
   a. May produce subjective relief of Raynaud's phenomenon.
   b. Available doses of long-acting calcium channel blockers include nifedipine (Adalat, Procardia), 30 to 90 mg qd; diltiazem (Cardizem), 120 to 300 mg/day; isradipine (DynaCirc CR), 5 to 20 mg/day; amlodipine (Norvasc), 2.5 to 10 mg/day; and nicardipine (Cardene), 60 to 120 mg/day.
4. Angiotensin-converting enzyme inhibitors
   a. Control hypertension.
   b. May slow progression of renal insufficiency.
   c. Captopril (Capoten) in doses up to 50 mg tid and enalapril (Vasotec) in doses up to 20 mg bid are the agents of choice for renal crisis.
5. Nonsteroidal anti-inflammatory drugs may be of benefit for arthralgias and myalgias.
6. Histamine$_2$ blockers: ranitidine (Zantac), up to 150 mg qid.
7. Proton pump inhibitors (PPIs): omeprazole (Prilosec), 20 to 40 mg qd; metoclopramide (Reglan), 5 to 10 mg qid; or
8. Prokinetic agents: cisapride (Propulsid), 10 to 20 mg qid
9. Other/experimental: immunosuppressive agents, iloprost, pentoxifylline, apheresis, photophoresis, and psoralen ultraviolet A-range (PUVA) therapy

Patient Education

1. Avoid cold temperatures; wear layered clothing.
2. Abstain from smoking.
3. Use skin lubrication.
4. Use range-of-motion exercises.
5. Elevate head of bed.
6. Avoid large meals.
7. Avoid tight clothing, especially about the abdomen.
8. Frequent blood pressure monitoring.

Bibliography

Artlett CM, Smith JB, Jimencz SA, et al: Identification of fetal DNA and cells in skin lesions from women with systemic sclerosis. N Engl J Med 1998;338:1186–1191.

Black HR: Scleroderma—clinical aspects. J Intern Med 1993;234:115–118.

Fritzler MJ: Autoantibodies in scleroderma. J Dermatol 1993;20:257–268.

Medsger TA: Treatment of systemic sclerosis. Ann Rheum Dis 1991;50:877–886.

Seibold JR: Scleroderma. In Kelly WN, Edwards ED, Ruddy S, et al (eds): Textbook of Rheumatology, 5th ed, vol 2, pp 1133–1162. Philadelphia, WB Saunders Company, 1997.

Silver RM: Clinical aspects of systemic sclerosis (scleroderma). Ann Rheum Dis 1991;50:854–861.

226 Polymyositis and Dermatomyositis

John Meyerhoff

Etiology

1. Rare idiopathic disease with an incidence of less than 1 in 100,000
   a. One peak in childhood
   b. Second peak in forties
   c. More common in women
2. Occurs as part of other rheumatologic diseases:
   a. Rheumatoid arthritis
   b. Systemic lupus erythematosus
   c. Scleroderma
3. Controversy exists as to whether or not there is an association with malignancy.

Symptoms

1. Muscle weakness
   a. Reported by 70 to 90 per cent of patients
   b. More frequent in proximal muscles and lower extremities
   c. Patients without polymyositis may use "weakness" to describe other symptoms.
      (1) Pain or stiffness in muscles or joints
      (2) Fatigue
      (3) Malaise
2. Muscle pain
   a. Reported frequency varies widely (25 to 73 per cent).
   b. Generally not very severe
   c. Absent often enough that polymyositis is often listed as a cause of painless weakness
3. Joint pain
   a. Occurs in approximately 25 per cent of idiopathic cases.
   b. More frequent in cases associated with other rheumatologic diseases
   c. Generally not as severe as seen in rheumatoid arthritis
4. Rash
   a. Blue/purple discoloration on upper eyelids (heliotrope rash)
   b. Scaly violaceous rash on knuckles (Gottron's papules)
   c. Defines the disease as dermatomyositis.

Key Symptoms

- Muscle weakness
- Muscle pain
- Rash (in dermatomyositis)

Clinical Findings

1. Muscle weakness
   a. Present in 92 to 100 per cent of patients
   b. Usually more proximal than distal and more often affects lower than upper extremity
2. Muscle tenderness occurs in 40 to 50 per cent of patients.
3. Rash consistent with dermatomyositis in 40 per cent of patients.
4. Systemic involvement may also occur.
   a. Not due to muscle involvement
      (1) Generalized: fatigue, fever, weight loss
      (2) Joints: arthralgias and arthritis
      (3) Pulmonary: interstitial fibrosis
      (4) Cardiac: tachyarrhythmias and conduction abnormalities
   b. Due to muscle involvement
      (1) Oropharyngeal: uncoordinated swelling and aspiration
      (2) Gastrointestinal: dysphagia, delayed gastric emptying, reduced motility
      (3) Cardiac: cardiomyopathy and cor pulmonale

Key Signs

- Muscle weakness
- Muscle tenderness
- Rash (in dermatomyositis)

Diagnostic Studies

1. Creatine phosphokinase (CPK) elevated in 64 to 96 per cent.
   a. "Normal" is higher in African Americans > Hispanics > Whites.

b. Normal values for black women about the same as for white men.
2. Muscle biopsy
   a. Abnormal in 90 per cent
   b. Allows diagnosis of subgroups of polymyositis/dermatomyositis (PM/DM) and other diseases:
      (1) Inclusion body myositis (IBM)
      (2) Parasitic diseases
3. Abnormal electromyography in 90 per cent
   a. Not necessary if biopsy is abnormal
   b. Use in patients with normal CPK to confirm muscle involvement before biopsy.
4. Autoantibodies
   a. Antinuclear antibodies present in 50 to 90 per cent of patients.
      (1) Do not indicate lupus by their presence.
      (2) Should lead one to consider an overlap syndrome if findings of lupus or scleroderma exist.
   b. Specific myositis antibodies (MSAs)
      (1) Usually anti-tRNA synthetase antibodies
      (2) Most associated with presence of interstitial lung disease and arthritis.
      (3) Anti-histidyl-tRNA (Jo-1) most common (50 per cent of cases) and is associated with Raynaud's phenomenon.

Key Tests

- CPK
- Muscle biopsy

Differential Diagnosis
1. Neurologic diseases
   a. Muscular dystrophies
   b. Neuromuscular diseases
   c. Glycogen and lipid storage disorders
   d. Neuropathies
2. Endocrine disorders
   a. Hypo- and hyperthyroidism
   b. Hypo- and hyperparathyroidism
   c. Hypo- and hyperadrenalism
3. Acute rhabodomyolysis
4. Drugs and toxins (see Table 226–1)
5. Infectious agents (see Table 226–2)

Treatment
1. Rule out and treat other diseases.
   a. Stop potentially toxic drugs.

TABLE 226–1. DRUGS AND TOXINS PRODUCING PM/DM-LIKE EFFECTS

Chloroquine	Ethanol	Penicillin
Cimetidine	Heroin	Phenytoin
Clofibrate	Hydralazine	Procainamide
Colchicine	Ipecac	Rifampin
Corticosteroids	Levadopa	Simvastatin
Danazol	Lovastatin	Sulfonamides
Emetine	Penicillamine	Vincristine
		Zidovudine

b. Treat infections.
c. Look for endocrine disorders.
d. Make sure patients are up to date with recommended routine cancer screening.
2. Corticosteroids remain mainstay of treatment.
   a. PM/DM as reported from community hospitals may be more steroid responsive.
   b. Starting dose of prednisone around 60 mg/day.
      (1) Usually given as single daily dose in university settings
      (2) Every-other-day dosing effective in 40 per cent of cases in community hosptials.
      (3) Split dose may be helpful if response slows.
   c. Responders show following responses:
      (1) Fifty per cent reduction in CPK in 1 month
      (2) Normalization of CPK in 3 to 4 months
      (3) Improvement in muscle strength in 3 to 4 months
   d. Taper as tolerated once CPK has normalized.
      (1) No universally accepted regimen
      (2) CPK usually a good guide to speed of taper.
   e. "Steroid failure" can be defined as lack of improvement in 4 months.

TABLE 226–2. INFECTIOUS AGENTS PRODUCING PM/DM-LIKE EFFECTS

BACTERIA	PARASITES	VIRUSES
Borrelia	Cysticercus	Adenovirus
Mycobacterium	Sarcocystis	Coxsackievirus
Rickettsia	Toxoplasma	Echovirus
	Trichinella	Epstein-Barr virus
	Trypanosoma	Hepatitis B virus
		Human immunodeficiency virus
		Influenza
		Mumps
		Rubella
		Varicella-zoster

f. Osteoporosis prophylaxis with calcium and vitamin D is necessary.

3. Steroids less effective in patients with MSAs and even less effective in IBM.

4. Treatment of steroid failure
   a. Methotrexate and azathioprine (Imuran)
      (1) May be best agents to add to regimen, together or separately.
      (2) May be appropriate to start at onset in patients with MSAs and IBM.
   b. Cyclosporine (Sandimmune), intravenous immune globulin (Gamimune N), and cyclophosphamide (Cytoxan) have all been used.

5. Intensity of exercise to improve muscle strength depends on amount of weakness.
   a. Range of motion exercises if patient too weak to lift against gravity
   b. Isometric exercises preferred intially.
   c. Vigorous isotonic exercises as strength improves

Key Treatment

- Corticosteroids
- Exercise

Follow-Up

1. Taper steroids as tolerated.
2. Watch for complications of therapy.
3. Minimize aspiration in patients with dysphagia.
   a. Elevate head of bed.
   b. Speech therapy consultation
4. Prepare patients, particularly those with MSAs and IBM, for a long course of therapy.

Bibliography

Black HR, Quallich H, Gareleck CB: Racial differences in serum creatine kinase levels. Am J Med 1986;81:479–487.

Bohan A, Peter JB, Bowman RL, et al: A computer assisted analysis of 153 patients with polymyositis and dermatomyositis. Medicine 1977;56:255–286.

Maoz CR, Langevitz P, Livneh A, et al: High incidence of malignancies in patients with dermatomyositis and polymyositis: an 11-year analysis. Semin Arthritis Rheum 1998;27:319–324.

Mastaglia FL, Phillips BA, Zilko PJ: Immunglobulin therapy in inflammatory myopathies. J Neurol Neurosurg Psychiatry 1998;65:107–110.

Villalba L, Hicks JE, Adams EM, et al: Treatment of refractory myositis: a randomized crossover study of two new cytotoxic regimens. Arthritis Rheum 1998;41:392–399.

227 Polymyalgia Rheumatica

John Meyerhoff

Etiology

The etiology of polymyalgia rheumatica (PMR) is unknown. Many theories have been suggested, but none has held up. Although it is clearly inflammatory, joint and muscle biopsies are negative in PMR patients.

Symptoms

1. Onset of symptoms over age 50
2. Bilateral shoulder pain
3. Stiffness (or gelling) in the proximal shoulder (more often than hip girdles) with inactivity, usually longer than 1 hour in the morning
4. May be felt to be "just getting old" by patients
5. Often associated with mild weight loss and/or depression
6. May be associated with symptoms of temporal arteritis (see Ch. 228, Temporal Arteritis).

Key Symptoms

- Shoulder pain
- Morning stiffness
- Depression
- Weight loss

Clinical Findings

1. Pain on range of motion of the shoulder joints
2. True weakness not present, but patients frequently report pain in the shoulder muscles on muscle strength testing.
3. Muscle tenderness, in distinction to joint tenderness, is common in PMR but is rare in other rheumatologic diseases involving the shoulder.
4. Osteoarthritis frequently found in these patients; inflammatory arthritis rarely.
5. Findings of temporal arteritis also may be seen (see Ch. 228, Temporal Arteritis).

Key Sign

Pain in the shoulder with range-of-motion testing, muscle strength testing, and palpation of the muscles

Laboratory Tests

1. Anemia of chronic disease often present if symptoms have been present long enough.
2. Erythrocyte sedimentation rate (ESR) is frequently very elevated.
3. PMR can occur with a normal hemoglobin and a normal ESR, and neither should be used to rule out the disease.
4. Muscle enzymes (creatine phosphokinase [CPK] or aldolase) must be normal.
5. Muscle, joint, and other biopsies (other than temporal artery) are uniformly normal and should not be done.
6. Bone scans may be abnormal but are not helpful.

Key Tests

- Complete blood count
- ESR
- CPK

Differential Diagnosis

1. Painful muscle syndromes are most likely to be confused with PMR.
   a. Fibromyalgia is more diffusive and associated with tiredness (nonrestorative sleep) and pain in the morning more than stiffness. May be associated with tender points that are not found in PMR and occurs below age 50.
   b. Myalgias caused by viral infections may be similar but rarely last more than 4 weeks.
2. Joint disease may be confused with PMR.
   a. Rheumatoid arthritis (RA) often will give morning stiffness greater than 1 hour in duration, pain on motion of the shoulders, anemia, and an elevated ESR. RA usually does not give tenderness of the shoulder muscles, and PMR does not usually give a peripheral arthritis.
   b. Osteoarthritis may give morning stiffness, but it usually rarely lasts more than 10 to 15 minutes. These patients also may have pain

on motion of the shoulders, but they also usually do not have muscle tenderness either. Anemia is rare, and ESR should be normal.

3. Bursitis and tendinitis of the shoulder gives pain on motion and tenderness and occasionally morning stiffness, but it is rarely symmetric.

4. Polymyositis will give true muscle weakness and is usually painless, and affects distal as well as proximal muscles.

5. Neoplastic disease may present similarly to PMR, and patients with known primary neoplastic disease, lack of response to corticosteroids, or symptoms suggestive of neoplasia should be screened carefully for primary or secondary neoplasia.

6. Depression may present with the muscle pain, morning stiffness, and fatigue. These patients should not have anemia or an elevated ESR and often will appear depressed.

Treatment

Medication

1. Corticosteroids are the treatment of choice.
   a. Response is dramatic, with improvement overnight and almost complete resolution within 48 hours.
   b. Failure to respond dramatically is usually due to one of the following:
      (1) Incorrect diagnosis, particularly depression or neoplasia-related
      (2) Underlying or coexisting condition such as bursitis, tendinitis, osteoarthritis, or RA, which will improve more slowly
   c. Low doses of prednisone with rapid taper to replacement doses are often effective in many patients as follows: 15 mg/day for 3 to 5 days, 10 mg/day for 1 to 2 weeks, 5 mg/day for 12 months, then taper by 1 mg/day per month afterward.
   d. If patients have a flare, symptoms are easily controlled by resuming previous dose (or 5 mg/day if on less) for 1 to 2 weeks with taper afterward.
   e. Patients may have recurrent, consistent flares of PMR or coexisting osteoarthritis as prednisone is tapered below 5 mg/day and may need to be kept on 1 to 4 mg/day of prednisone for a prolonged period of time.
   f. Consider rheumatologic consultation for use of an alternative schedule in patients in whom prednisone cannot be tapered or for the use of other drugs such as steroid-sparing agents in patients who are having steroid side effects and whose dosage cannot be tapered.

2. Nonsteroidal anti-inflammatory drugs are rarely effective.

Patient Education

1. Patients should be instructed in the signs and symptoms of temporal arteritis (see Ch. 228, Temporal Arteritis) and should be told to take 60 mg prednisone immediately if they develop any of these findings and then to call their physician.

2. Patients should be instructed in the treatment and follow-up schedule because they will be seeing their doctor for an asymptomatic condition.

Key Treatment

- Low-dose prednisone
- Regular follow-up
- Surveillance for temporal arteritis

Follow-Up

1. Patients should keep in touch over the first several weeks to ensure that they have the expected response to steroids.

2. The initial follow-up visit should be scheduled at 4 to 6 weeks after the initial visit, and further visits at 2- to 4-month intervals for the first year depending on the patient's compliance.

3. At each visit, patients should be asked about symptoms of PMR and GCA, with emphasis on what they should do if they develop symptoms of GCA.

4. Visits should be every 1 to 2 months as prednisone is being tapered from 5 mg.

Bibliography

Bird HA, Esselinckx W, Dixon AS, et al: An evaluation or criteria for polymyalgia rheumatica. Ann Rheum Dis 1979;38:434–439.

Ellis ME, Ralston S: The ESR in the diagnosis and management of the polymyalgia rheumatica/giant cell arteritis syndrome. Ann Rheum Dis 1983;42:168–170.

Hellmann DB: Immunopathogenesis, diagnosis, and treatment of giant cell arteritis, temporal arteritis, polymyalgia rheumatica, and Takayasu's arteritis. Curr Opin Rheumatol 1993;5:25–32.

Kyle V, Hazelman BL: The clinical and laboratory course of polymyalgia rheumatica/giant cell arteritis after the first two months. Ann Rheum Dis 1993;52:847–850.

Meyerhoff J: Rapid tapering of initial prednisone dose in polymyalgia rheumatica. Arthritis Rheum 1998;41: 261S.

228 Temporal Arteritis

Michael Lewko

Etiology

1. Temporal arteritis (TA), or giant cell arteritis, is a disease of the elderly, rarely found in those under age 50. It is more common in females and is not as rare in blacks, Hispanics, and Asians as once thought.
2. TA: vasculitis of unknown etiology
   a. Possible pathogenic factors: genetic, infectious, immunologic
   b. May be etiologically related to polymyalgia rheumatica (PMR).
   c. Recently, it has been discovered that the majority (60 to 70 per cent) of TA and PMR patients express the HLA-DR4 allele.
3. TA affects medium- to large-sized arteries with internal elastic lamina.
   a. Preferential sites of involvement: branches of internal and external carotid arteries, particularly temporal artery
   b. Typically inflammation consists of primarily macrophages and CD4+ T lymphocytes of Th1 type; infiltrative granuloma, usually with giant cells; and disruption of the internal elastic membrane.

Symptoms

1. Onset may be abrupt or insidious.
2. Classic symptoms: headache, jaw claudication, visual changes, PMR
3. Loss of vision is the most serious complication, frequently preceded by diplopia or amaurosis fugax.
4. Atypical presentations: fever of unknown origin, weight loss, failure to thrive in elderly

Key Symptoms

- New headache
- Jaw claudication
- Visual symptoms
- Proximal myalgias/arthralgias
- Weight loss
- Malaise
- Fever
- Cough
- Claudication of the extremities

Clinical Findings

1. Localized temporal artery tenderness, decreased pulsation, induration, or even scalp necrosis. Temporal arteries are normal in one third of patients.
   a. Ophthalmologic findings: ophthalmoplegia, visual loss
   b. Funduscopic abnormalities
      (1) Pallor and swelling of optic disks (early)
      (2) Optic atrophy (late)
2. Systemic manifestations usually result from ischemia of affected arteries or inflammation related to giant cell arteritis.
   a. Bruits in head and neck
   b. Absent upper extremity pulses
   c. Neurologic deficits: mononeuritis, progressive dementia, delirium, stroke, transient ischemic attacks
   d. Inflammatory signs: synovitis, pericarditis, breast masses

Key Signs

- Temporal artery tenderness or decreased pulsation
- Ophthalmoplegia
- Visual field cuts
- Ptosis
- Retinal or optic disk ischemia
- Neurologic deficits
- Bruits, head and neck
- Diminished or absent pulses in upper extremities

Laboratory Findings

1. Erythrocyte sedimentation rate (ESR) by Westergren method
   a. Almost always increased
   b. Usually greater than or equal to 50 mm/hour
   c. May be normal in 15 per cent of patients.

2. Diagnostic temporal artery biopsy is recommended in patients with suspected TA. A negative biopsy does not always rule it out.
3. To increase the biopsy yield
   a. Biopsy segment should be 3 to 6 cm long.
   b. Biopsy should be bilateral if frozen sections of initial biopsy are negative (at 1- to 2-mm intervals).
   c. Pathologists should evaluate in detail multiple sections of biopsied segment.
   d. Upon initiation of steroid therapy, in general biopsy should be obtained within 7 days.
4. Other laboratory findings include
   a. Elevated C-reactive protein (frequently >10 mg/dl)
   b. Normocytic, normochromic anemia
   c. Abnormal liver function test: elevated alkaline phosphatase (elevated three- to fivefold)
   d. Elevated globulin fraction in serum electrophoresis
   e. Elevated von Willebrand factor

Key Tests

- ESR
- Temporal artery biopsy

Differential Diagnosis

1. Temporal arteritis is distinguishable from other forms of vasculitis by differences in organ involvement, histopathology, clinical manifestations, age, and affected population.
2. The differential diagnosis consists of Takayasu's arteritis, Wegener's granulomatosis, polyarteritis nodosa, hypersensitivity, and vasculitis.
3. Other possibilities include arteriosclerotic disease, malignancy, infection, primary amyloidosis, other causes of fever, headache, blindness, arthralgias, and myalgias.

WARNING

The most common dreaded complication is vision loss resulting from untimely diagnosis and inadequate treatment.

Treatment

1. The treatment for temporal arteritis is high-dose corticosteroids.
   a. Prednisone, 40 to 60 mg/day in two to four divided doses *or*
   b. Equivalent dosage of another corticosteroid (Medrol) *or*

c. Intravenous pulse Solu-Medrol in patients with recent blindness, less than 24 to 36 hours
2. High-dose corticosteroids should be initiated promptly when the suspicion is high and when visual symptoms are present.
   a. Only high-dose corticosteroids will prevent blindness
   b. Alternate-day regimens are not effective in the initial treatment
   c. The decision to continue treatment or initiate treatment will depend on the results of the temporal artery biopsy, the clinical presentation, and laboratory tests.
3. Clinical response to treatment is usually
   a. Rapid and dramatic—within 3 to 7 days
   b. The ESR normalizes in 2 to 4 weeks.
   c. Reversal of blindness is rare.

Medication

1. Treatment with prednisone
   a. Initial dose is 40 to 60 mg/day in two to four divided doses.
   b. Consolidate total dose to one single morning dose once response has occurred.
   c. Initiate reduction of daily dose when symptoms have resolved and the ESR has normalized.
2. Reduction of prednisone is
   a. Empirical
   b. Gauged by symptoms and ESR
   c. Gradual to prevent exacerbations
3. An approach to reduction
   a. Reduce the dose by 10 per cent every 2 to 4 weeks down to a total dose of 15 to 30 mg, and maintain at this dose for several months.
   b. Follow this by 2.5-mg decrements every 2 to 4 weeks down to a total dose of 5 to 7.5 mg, and maintain at this dose for several months.
   c. Follow by 1-mg decrements every 1 to 3 months until discontinued.
   d. In general, treatment is necessary up to 1 to 2 years or sometimes longer, up to 5 years or more.
4. Corticosteroid toxicity is common and should be anticipated in older patients. It may result in
   a. Cushingoid features
   b. Osteopenia
   c. Hypertension
   d. Impaired wound healing
   e. Fractures
   f. Proximal myopathy

g. Cataracts

h. Glucose intolerance

i. Easy bruisability

j. Depression

k. Insomnia

5. Prevention of corticosteroid-induced toxicity

   a. Monitor blood pressure, glucose, and calcium.

   b. Add calcium, 1 to 1.5 gm, with vitamin D, 400 to 800 IU daily, to diet.

   c. Switching to alternate-day steroids is not recommended.

   d. Addition of steroid-sparing agents, methotrexate, dapsone, or azathioprine (Imuran) may be appropriate.

   e. Do not treat the ESR; adjust corticosteroid dose mainly on the basis of symptoms.

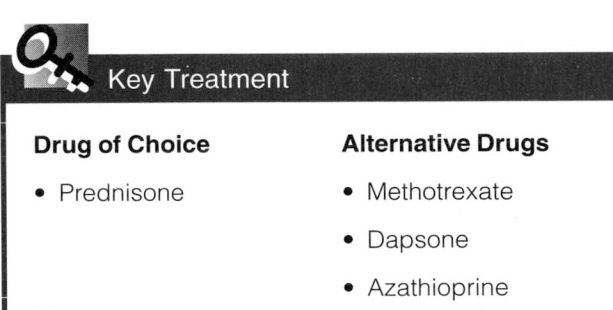

Key Treatment

Drug of Choice	Alternative Drugs
• Prednisone	• Methotrexate
	• Dapsone
	• Azathioprine

Follow-Up

1. Prognosis of treatment is good.

2. Risk of death from TA appears to be increased within first 4 months of treatment.

3. Death occurs from vascular complications such as stroke, myocardial infarction, ruptured aneurysm, or dissecting aneurysm.

4. After 4 months, there is no difference in survival from rest of the age-matched general population.

5. Blindness rarely occurs during treatment.

6. In most cases, remission is maintained after withdrawal of therapy.

Bibliography

Buchbinder R, Detsky AS: Management of suspected giant cell arteritis: a decision analysis. J Rheumatol 1992; 19:1220–1228.

Goodwin SJ: Progress in gerontology: polymyalgia and temporal arteritis. J Am Geriatr Soc 1992;40:515–525.

Nesher G, Sonnenblick M: Steroid sparing medications in temporal arteritis: report of three cases and review of 174 reported patients. Clin Rheumatol 1994;8:84–92.

Nescher G, Sonnenblick M, Friedlander Y, et al: Analysis of steroid related complications and mortality in temporal arteritis: a 15 year survival of 43 patients. J Rheumatol 1994;21:1283–1286.

Nordborg E, Nordborg C, Malmvall BE, et al: Giant cell arteritis. Rheum Dis Clin North Am 1995;21:1013–1026.

Wind BE: Temporal arteritis: aggressive treatment prevents visual complications. Postgrad Med 1992;91: 337–338, 341–342.

229 Osgood-Schlatter Disease

Victoria S. Kaprielian

Etiology

1. Rather than a true disease, Osgood-Schlatter is a clinical syndrome that may include a number of different precise etiologies. All involve inflammation at the insertion of the patellar tendon to the apophysis at the tibial tubercle in a growing adolescent (Fig. 229–1); thus it is sometimes referred to as a traction apophysitis. Potential etiologic factors include

   a. Relative inflexibility as a result of growth of musculotendinous structures lagging behind that of bones, leading to increased traction forces at the tendon insertion site.

   b. Repetitive microtrauma causing multiple minute avulsion fractures

   c. Osteochondral stress fracture of the apophysis

   d. Heterotopic bone formation in the tendon near its insertion

2. Because this is a problem of a growth point, it occurs only before achievement of full skeletal height, typically between the ages of 10 and 15 years

3. It occurs more commonly in males, though the incidence is increasing in females, perhaps as a result of increased sports participation.

Symptoms

1. Anterior knee pain, usually insidious in onset; increased with activities requiring forceful contraction of the quadriceps (e.g., running, jumping, climbing stairs), decreased with rest

2. Swelling and tenderness below the knee, often making kneeling painful

3. Often bilateral; may be greater on one side than the other

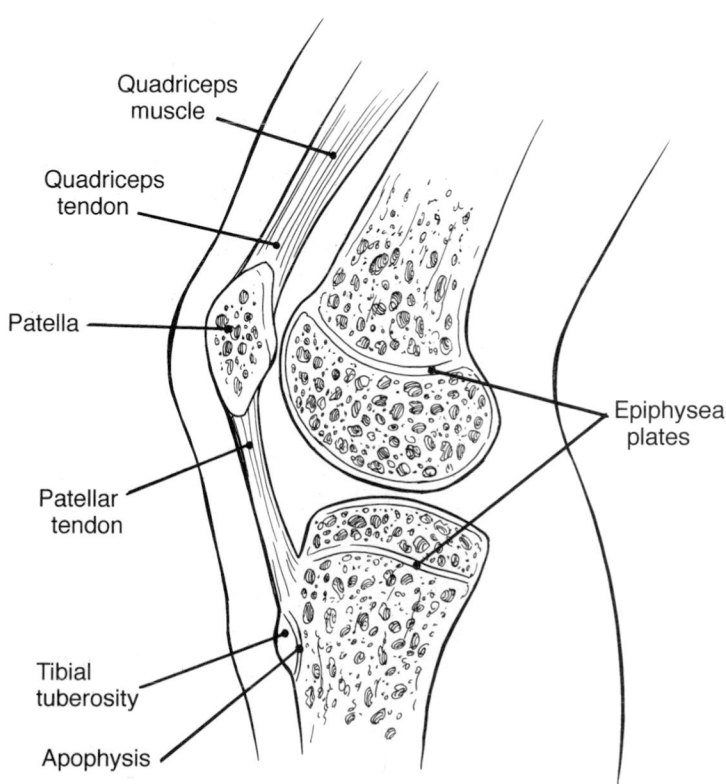

Figure 229–1 Anatomy of Osgood-Schlatter disease.

- Pain and swelling anteriorly just below the knee
- Pain increased with sports activities, decreased with rest

Clinical Findings

1. Point tenderness of the tibial tubercle
2. Soft tissue swelling over the tibial tubercle, sometimes with increased warmth
3. Pain elicited by resisted extension of the knee (especially in flexed position)
4. Examination of the knee joint itself is normal.

Tender, swollen tibial tubercle(s) with otherwise normal knee examination

Tests

In cases where symptoms are unilateral or poorly responsive to conservative measures, radiographs may be worthwhile to rule out other pathologic lesions such as tumors or osteomyelitis. There are no specific radiographic findings for Osgood-Schlatter disease. Lateral views of the knee may show an enlarged, irregular, fragmented tibial tuberosity with overlying soft tissue swelling. These findings are normal, however, and not diagnostic.

- Diagnosis is made by history and physical examination.
- Radiographs may be used to rule out other problems.

Differential Diagnosis

1. Common problems to consider (pain and tenderness localized to slightly different sites)
   a. Sindig-Larsen-Johansson syndrome: apophysitis at the inferior pole of the patella
   b. Patellofemoral syndrome: inflammation of the patellofemoral joint as a result of poor tracking
   c. Patellar tendonitis: inflammation of the tendon itself; more common after skeletal maturity
   d. Pes anserinus bursitis: inflammation at tendinous insertion point inferomedial on the tibia
2. Less common, more severe conditions to be ruled out as appropriate (usually unilateral)
   a. Stress fracture
   b. Partial avulsion of the quadriceps tendon
   c. Tumor
   d. Osteomyelitis
   e. Complete avulsion of the tibial tubercle
   f. Referred hip pain (e.g., slipped capital femoral epiphysis, Legg-Calvé-Perthes disease)

Treatment

1. Simple conservative therapy is generally successful.
   a. Medication: nonsteroidal anti-inflammatory agents to reduce acute inflammation
   b. Activity: relative rest—decreasing frequency and intensity of activities requiring forceful knee extension (running, jumping, kicking)
   c. Patient education: Explanation of the cause, treatment, and anticipated course of the condition is essential to reassure the patient and parents. It is vital that they have sufficient understanding to make educated decisions regarding sports activities.
   d. Ice after activities reduces recurring inflammation.
   e. Stretching of the quadriceps and hamstring muscle groups to decrease traction on the affected insertion point
   f. Gradual strengthening of the knee extensor mechanism, after acute symptoms relieved
2. Specific equipment may be helpful in certain cases.
   a. Knee pads are recommended for kneeling and activities that may lead to direct trauma to the tibial tubercle.
   b. Neoprene sleeves with patellar cutouts provide some compression and protection, and may be preferred by some patients.
   c. Patellar tendon straps may be helpful in patients who are unwilling or unable to eliminate activities that exacerbate symptoms.
   d. Knee immobilizer and/or crutches may be necessary in resistant cases.

Key Treatment

- Rest
- Ice
- Anti-inflammatory medication
- Stretching

WARNING

Steroid injection is not recommended because this increases risk of tendon rupture.

Follow-Up

Definitive cure is accomplished with achievement of skeletal maturity and closure of the growth plate. In those rare cases where pain persists after skeletal maturity and does not respond to conservative measures, surgical removal of bony ossicle(s) in the patellar tendon may be considered. Some residual prominence of the tibial tubercle is common, and may be of cosmetic concern, especially to female patients.

Bibliography

Dunn JF: Osgood-Schlatter disease. Am Fam Physician 1990;41:173–176.

Kaeding CC, Whitehead R: Musculoskeletal injuries in adolescents. Primary Care 1998;25:211–223.

Peck DM: Apophyseal injuries in the young athlete. Am Fam Physician 1995;51:1891–1895.

Snider RK (ed): Osgood-Schlatter disease/Sindig-Larson-Johansson syndrome. Essentials of Musculoskeletal Care, pp 624–625. Rosemont, IL: American Academy of Orthopedic Surgeons, 1997.

Tachdjian MO: Clinical Pediatric Orthopedics: The Art of Diagnosis and Principles of Management, pp 107–108. Stamford, CT, Appleton & Lange, 1997.

230 Carpal Tunnel Syndrome and Other Nerve Entrapments

Kevin R. Nelson

Carpal Tunnel Syndrome

Etiology

1. The carpal tunnel is bounded by the volar transverse ligament and dorsally by the carpal bones. Coursing through the carpal tunnel are the flexor tendons of the digits and the median nerve. The carpal tunnel is physically confined in a large proportion of otherwise normal individuals. Symptoms of carpal tunnel syndrome (CTS) are produced by increased pressure within the tunnel, leading to nerve ischemia, demyelination, and perhaps axonal injury.

2. Medical conditions associated with CTS include diabetes, pregnancy, rheumatoid arthritis, hypothyroidism, chronic renal failure, multiple myeloma, amyloidosis, and acromegaly.

3. A generalized peripheral neuropathy of any cause often predisposes to CTS and other nerve entrapments.

4. Occupations requiring repetitive wrist movements, the use of vibrating tools, or sustained hand positions involve a higher incidence of CTS.

5. Local infections, fractures, tenosynovitis, aberrant anatomy, or masses of the wrist also may lead to CTS.

6. A congenitally narrow canal increases the risk of nerve compression, particularly in later life when degenerative changes further compromise the space or with the aggravating factors described above.

Symptoms

1. The earliest symptom is typically intermittent hand paresthesias or pain, often awaking the patient at night.

2. Digital sensory disturbances may impair fine motor tasks.

3. Pain occurs in the wrist and hand and may radiate up the arm.

4. Symptoms are provoked by repetitive motion and sustained hand positions (e.g., driving).

5. Relief is sometimes obtained by shaking or moving the wrist.

Key Symptoms

- Nocturnal hand paresthesias or pain
- Median sensory disturbance
- Wrist or hand pain

6. Patients may complain of poor grip and often drop objects.

7. Symptoms typically involve the dominant hand and may be bilateral.

Clinical Findings

1. Sensory loss (especially two-point discrimination) occurs in the median nerve distribution (digits I, II, III, and sometimes IV).

2. Weakness of thumb abduction is usually found only after sensory symptoms are well developed.

3. Thenar atrophy occurs late in the course.

4. Flexing the wrist for 1 minute (Phalen's maneuver) or tapping over the median nerve at the wrist (Tinel's sign) may provoke symptoms in the hand. Tinel's sign may be found in normal persons, and positive results should be interpreted with caution.

Key Signs

- Sensory loss in the first three digits
- Thenar wasting
- Phalen's or Tinel's sign

Laboratory Tests

1. Nerve conduction studies (NCS) demonstrate slowed median nerve conduction through the wrist. This will usually be recorded from the sensory fibers first.

   a. NCS have a high degree of diagnostic sensitivity and specificity. Best laboratory method of establishing the diagnosis of CTS.

   b. NCS also will detect underlying generalized neuropathies.

c. In mild or acute CTS, the NCS may be normal.

2. Obtain wrist radiographs in patients suspected of having fractures and joint disease.

3. Laboratory studies to evaluate associated diseases (as indicated)

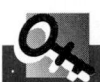

Key Test

NCS is the most definitive test.

Differential Diagnosis

1. C6 and C7 radiculopathies may present with sensory symptoms within the median nerve territory. Neck pain or pain radiating down the arm, weakness in the muscles proximal to the wrist, and reflex loss may be present.

2. Tenosynovitis and osteoarthritis produce wrist pain worsened by movement.

3. A generalized neuropathy (e.g., diabetic) can predispose to isolated nerve compressions.

4. Proximal median nerve injury (e.g., at elbow)

5. Brachial plexus lesion

6. Rarely transient ischemic attack

Treatment

1. Medical

   a. Avoid activities that flex and extend the wrist.

   b. Splint the wrist in the neutral position. The splint should be worn at night as well as during the day, particularly if the symptoms are nocturnal.

   c. Scheduled nonsteroidal anti-inflammatory agents (NSAIDs) for several weeks

   d. Oral steroids for 7 to 10 days should be considered for patients with severe symptoms.

   e. Steroid injections into canal may provide temporary or longstanding relief. This should be performed by experienced physicians.

   (1) Complications include local infection, inflammation, and permanent nerve injury.

   (2) Multiple injections risk damaging the flexor tendons and predispose them to later rupture.

   f. Thiazide diuretics may be effective for CTS associated with pregnancy, if treatment is needed.

2. Indications for surgical decompression

   a. Symptoms that are sufficient to interfere with work or daily life and are unresponsive to conservative therapy

   b. Persistent or progressive neurologic deficits, particularly motor weakness

   c. Acute CTS with severe pain and weakness (e.g., hemorrhage) may require immediate decompression.

Key Treatment

- NSAIDs
- Surgical release
- Wrist splinting
- Avoid provocative activity.

Follow-Up

1. Most patients with mild disease do well with conservative treatment. Improvement may take several weeks or months.

2. If a 3- to 6-month trial of medical therapy fails, consider surgery.

3. Patients may report marked improvement shortly after surgical decompression. Continued improvement may be evident over several months.

4. Patients with recurrent symptoms after surgery should be considered for re-exploration. Repeat NCS may be helpful in this instance.

Ulnar Nerve Compression at the Elbow

Etiology

1. Excessive forearm flexion/extension and leaning on the elbow can traumatize the nerve over time. Persons with a shallow condylar groove or a dislocating ulnar nerve are vulnerable to nerve injury.

2. Patients at risk are those who are comatose, anesthetized, or at prolonged bed rest.

3. Elbow fractures (acute or remote), degenerative or rheumatoid arthritis, or masses near the elbow may entrap the nerve.

4. In many patients, no antecedent cause is found. In some, the nerve is compressed by fibrous tissue in the condylar groove or the cubital tunnel (aponeurosis of the flexor digitorum sublimus muscle).

Key Symptoms

- Progressive hand weakness
- Numbness in an ulnar distribution

Clinical Findings

1. Sensory deficits are usually found within the ulnar distribution (digits, IV, V) distal to the wrist crease. Sensory loss that splits the ring finger is typical of an ulnar nerve injury and is uncommon with a radiculopathy.
2. Weakness is often prominent and is found in finger abduction, thumb adduction, and other intrinsic hand muscles.
3. Atrophy may be seen in the hypothenar area, over the first web space, and in the dorsum of the hand.
4. "Claw hand" deformity is produced by hypertension of the metacarpophalangeal joints and flexion at the interphalangeal joints of the fourth and fifth digits. This arises from unopposed action of muscles innervated by the median and radial nerves.
5. Pain may be present at the elbow or more diffusely in the arm.
6. Tapping the ulnar nerve at the elbow may elicit paresthesias in the hand (Tinel's sign). The specificity of this sign is poor.

Key Signs

- Ulnar sensory disturbance
- Shallow condylar groove
- Claw hand
- Atrophy of intrinsic hand muscles

Key Tests

- NCS and electromyography
- Elbow radiographs

Differential Diagnosis

1. C8/T1 radiculopathy
2. Lower trunk brachial plexopathy
3. Early motor neuron disease (amyotrophic lateral sclerosis)
4. Ulnar entrapment at the wrist or hand

Treatment

1. Avoid activities that can compress the nerve.
2. Protect the nerve with an elbow pad.
3. Scheduled NSAIDs
4. In patients with an elbow mass, a dislocating nerve, or structural deformities of the elbow, surgical transposition should be considered early.

Follow-Up

1. Patients should be given a trial of medical treatment (usually 2 to 3 months)
2. Consider surgery in patients with severe or progressive weakness that is resistant to therapy.

Peroneal Nerve Compression at the Fibular Head

Etiology

Causes include habitual leg crossing, frequent squatting, positioning during anesthesia or coma, weight loss, leg casts, and masses in the knees. The nerve is also subject to injury from fibular fractures, knee dislocations, and blunt injury.

Key Symptom

Footdrop (tripping)

Clinical Findings

1. Weakness of ankle and toe dorsiflexion. Often foot eversion is preserved.
2. When walking, the patient lifts the foot high for the toes to clear the ground as the leg swings forward. The leg is then brought abruptly down, slapping the foot (steppage gait).
3. Sensory loss occurs in the peroneal nerve distribution.

Key Signs

- Weak ankle dorsiflexion
- Steppage gait

Key Tests

NCS and electromyography are the definitive tests

Differential Diagnosis

1. L5 radiculopathy
2. Lumbosacral plexopathy
3. Sciatic neuropathy
4. Central nervous system cause for footdrop (e.g., stroke)

Treatment
1. Avoid activities that can compress the nerve (see above).
2. Shoes with support above the ankle or an ankle-foot orthosis may assist the patient's gait and reduce tripping.
3. Rarely, acute swelling of the anterior tibial muscle from trauma will compress the nerve (compartment syndrome). This should be emergently surgically decompressed.

Follow-Up
1. The prognosis for pressure palsies is generally good. Time of recovery varies from days to months among patients.
2. Surgical exploration of the peroneal nerve at the fibular head might be considered if weakness persists.

Bibliography

American Association of Electrodiagnostic Medicine, American Academy of Neurology, American Academy of Physical Medicine and Rehabilitation: Practice parameters for electrodiagnostic studies in carpal tunnel syndrome: summary statement. Muscle Nerve 1993;16:1390–1391.

Chang MH, Chiang HT, Lee SS, et al: Oral drug choice in carpal tunnel syndrome. Neurology 1998;51:390–393.

Jablecki CK, Andary MT, So YT, et al: Literature review of the usefulness of nerve conduction studies and electromyography for the evaluation of patients with carpal tunnel syndrome. Muscle Nerve 1993;16:1392–1414.

Katz RT: Carpal tunnel syndrome: a practical review. Am Fam Physician 1994;49:1371–1379.

Rosenbaum RB, Ochoa JL: Carpal Tunnel Syndrome and Other Disorders of the Median Nerve. Boston, Butterworth-Heinemann, 1993.

Stewart JD: Focal Peripheral Neuropathies, 2nd ed. New York, Raven Press, 1993.

231 Thoracic Outlet Syndrome

Toni M. Cutson

Definition and Demographics

1. The thoracic outlet is demarcated by the first rib, the upper mediastinum medially, and the fifth cervical nerve cephalad. It contains the brachial plexus and subclavian and axillary veins and arteries.
2. Compression of the structures result in symptoms/signs of thoracic outlet syndrome (TOS).
3. Incidence: 0.3 to 0.7 per cent; 4:1 women to men
4. Average age of occurrence: 35 years (25 to 40 years)
5. Sixty to 70 per cent report precedent trauma; many cannot remember specific injury.

Types

1. Neurogenic type constitutes the majority of cases (80 to 90 per cent)
   a. Nerve compression leads to intraneural edema and pressure, resulting in Schwann cell denervation and fibrosis. Ante- and retrograde axonal transport abnormalities occur.
   b. "Double crush" injury: High-level compression renders distal nerve more susceptible to pressure injury (e.g., carpal or cubital tunnel).
   c. High-level TOS is at C1 to C7; lower (most common) is at C8 to T1; may overlap.
2. Vascular type constitutes about 10 to 20 per cent of cases.
   a. Venous compression results in vascular congestion and possible thrombosis. Compression is usually due to soft tissue abnormalities (e.g., thick subclavian muscle).
   b. Arterial compression results in ischemia, claudication, poststenotic aneurysm with thrombus, and possible embolism/necrosis. Arterial compression usually due to bony abnormalities.

Etiology

1. Potential anatomic areas of compromise
   a. Interscalene triangle: bordered by the anterior scalene, middle scalene, first rib. The interscalene triangle area opening may be narrowed by the following:
      (1) Variations of insertion of anterior scalene on the first rib (e.g., broad insertion, crossing with middle scalene muscle insertion)
      (2) Intermingled scalene muscle fibers impinging upon neurovascular structures
      (3) Fibrous bands (congenital or secondary to trauma)
      (4) Cervical rib (incidence, 0.5 per cent; 50 to 80 per cent bilateral)
      (5) Prominent C7 transverse process
   b. Costoclavicular space may be narrowed by the following:
      (1) Healed fractures/callus formation
      (2) Hypertrophied subclavius muscle
      (3) Downward displacement of shoulder (poor posture/trauma)
   c. Retropectoralis minor muscle
2. Congenital
   a. Abnormal placement/insertion of muscles (scalenes on first ribs)
   b. Fibromuscular bands
3. Acquired
   a. Trauma: inflammation to scar to spasm and contracture
   b. Anterior scalene stretch injury may induce increase in type II (tonic) fibers, resulting in tight and rigid muscles increasing compression.
   c. Muscular imbalance: poor posture with stooped shoulders, head-forward position; sleeping with arm over head. Leads to muscle tightness and shortening, decreasing the outlet space and increasing compression.
4. Osseous etiology constitutes 30 per cent of TOS cases.

Symptoms

1. Neuropathic: pain, weakness, heaviness, easy limb fatigability, paresthesias
   a. Upper (C5 to C7): Symptom distribution includes side of neck and face, upper back, external side of arm in the radial distribution; weak shoulder girdle, biceps, triceps.
   b. Lower (C8 to T1): Symptom distribution in-

cludes upper anterior chest and upper back, medial arm in the median distribution.

   c. Unusual symptoms include difficulty breathing and swallowing, stuffiness in the ear. Although these symptoms may be due to TOS, they should lead to consideration of neurotic symptoms and psychiatric referral.

2. Vascular

   a. Venous

     (1) Symptoms: edema, cyanosis, pain and heaviness. Subsequent thrombosis (Paget-Schroetter syndrome) may cause passive ischemia.

     (2) Risks: postphlebitc syndrome with chronic edema, lymphedema, disuse

   b. Arterial (relatively rare)

     (1) Symptoms: ischemia, claudication, color change, weakness

     (2) Risks: thromboembolism, necrosis

Key Symptoms

- Neurologic: weakness, pain, heaviness and fatigue, paresthesias possibly involving side of face or anterior chest, difficulty swallowing

- Vascular: edema, cyanosis, pain (congestive ischemia), claudication

Clinical Findings

1. General signs: Raynaud's phenomenon or color changes, decreased ipsilateral pulse, tenderness in supra- and infraclavicular spaces

2. Later signs may include muscle atrophy.

3. Vascular signs include edema, venous distention, cyanosis, embolism/necrosis.

Key Signs

- Color change of extremity (Raynaud's phenomenon)

- Swelling

- Venous distention

- Diminished pulse

- Tenderness in the supra- /infraclavicular area

Tests

1. There is no definitive test for the neurogenic (and most common) type. Diagnosis is dependent upon patient history, examination, and re-

production of symptoms in the absence of other pathology.

2. Radiography may disclose a suspected bony abnormality (e.g., cervical rib).

3. Vascular-type TOS may be tested with angiography or duplex ultrasound.

4. Clinical provocative tests (each performed for 2 minutes; positive test = reproduction of symptoms)

   a. Adson's test: Pulse decreases as patient inhales with head extended and turned to affected side.

   b. Neck tilt: Tilt the head away from the affected side.

   c. Costoclavicular compression: Examiner presses down on the patient's shoulder.

   d. Wright's test: Patient sits/stands with shoulders in hyperabduction and externally rotated. Positive test = decrease in pulse on affected side with symptoms.

   e. EAST (*elevated arm stress test*)/Roos test: Arms are held in the "surrender" position, patient opens and closes fists for 3 minutes.

5. Electromyography/somatosensory tests are not specific and not recommended.

Key Tests

- *There is no definitive test.*

- Vascular: angiography, duplex ultrasound

- Radiography: May disclose bony abnormality (e.g., cervical rib).

- Clinical tests: Maneuvers designed to diminish the thoracic outlet are considered positive if symptoms or signs are induced.

Differential Diagnosis

1. Other compressive neuropathies (e.g., carpal tunnel, cubital tunnel)

2. Cervical disease with nerve compression

   a. Test with Spurling's manuever: With patient's head turned and slightly flexed to the affected side, examiner applies compression to the head. Positive test = parethesias/shooting pain into arm indicating cervical root compression.

   b. Consider magnetic resonance imaging.

3. Reflex sympathetic dystrophy

4. Apical lung disease (especially with vascular symptoms, e.g., Pancoast's tumor): chest ra-

diograph with lordotic views to rule out apical disease

5. Inflammatory shoulder conditions: rotator cuff tendinitis, arthritis

6. Myofasciitis of upper back

Treatment

1. Nonsurgical treatment reserved for mild/moderate neurogenic type; consider physical/occupational therapy

    a. Posture-improving exercises: proper alignment of axial structures

    b. Shoulder stretching/strengthening exercises (e.g., chin tucks/cervical retractions, shoulder shrugs, circles, lateral neck stretches)

    c. Nonpharmacologic pain treatments transcutaneous electrical nerve stimulation (TENS), heat, massage

    d. Environmental adaptations (e.g., avoidance of overhead work, repetitive arm movements)

2. Surgical referral recommended for severe neurologic or vascular types.

    a. Surgical approaches

        (1) Scalenectomy (supraclavicular approach) preferred for upper-type TOS

        (2) First and/or cervical rib resection preferred for the lower types of TOS

            (a) Transaxillary: primary approach

            (b) Posterior thoracotomy: reserved for recurrence

            (c) Supraclavicular approach: increased surgical time and risks phrenic nerve paralysis

    b. Efficacy: 90 per cent complete or partial relief of symptoms of neurogenic TOS; 2.2 to 5 per cent recurrence within 6 months

    c. Venous thrombosis (rare; <5 per cent of cases) is treated with urokinase/streptokinase followed by anticoagulation for 3 to 4 months. Surgical resection of the first rib and scalenectomy can then be performed.

Key Treatment

- Nonsurgical
    - Posture exercises, shoulder strengthening
    - Pain control: massage, TENS
    - Environmental/work restrictions (e.g., restrict using arms overhead)

- Surgical
    - Cervical or first rib resection
    - Scalenectomy
    - Combination

Bibliography

Atasoy E: Thoracic outlet compression syndrome. Orthop Clin North Am 1996;27:265–303.

Nichols AW: The thoracic outlet syndrome in athletes. J Am Board Fam Pract 1996;9:346–355.

Novack CB: Conservative management of thoracic outlet syndrome. Semin Thorac Cardiovasc Surg 1996;8: 201–207.

Roos DB: Thoracic outlet syndromes: update 1987. Am J Surg 1987;154:568–573.

Roos DB: TOS: historical perspectives and anatomic considerations. Semin Thorac Cardiovasc Surg 1996;8: 183–189.

232 Swimmer's Injuries

Shaun Berry

"Swimmer's shoulder" is a term used to describe the most common musculoskeletal complaint among swimmers. Up to 66 per cent of competitive swimmers have a history of pain that interferes with training.

Etiology

1. "Swimmer's shoulder," like any other overuse injury, is multifactorial in its etiology. It is most commonly caused by subacromial impingement syndrome, resulting from compression of the tissues of the subacromial space between the head of the humerus, the coracoacromial arch, and the anterior acromion. The subacromial bursa, the tendon of the long head of the biceps, and the supraspinatus tendon are the structures inflamed by subacromial impingement. These tissues are in an impingement position with each repetitive arm stroke while swimming.

2. Contributing factors include rotator cuff fatigue, multidirectional glenohumeral instability, and imbalance in rotator cuff muscle strength.

3. Additional investigation into etiology should include stroke technique, overtraining, and past history of shoulder injury. Freestyle (crawl) and butterfly strokes are the most common strokes associated with shoulder pain.

4. Adolescents may also suffer as a result of exacerbation by less developed shoulder musculature, increased glenohumeral laxity, and bone immaturity.

Symptoms

1. Anterior or anterolateral shoulder pain during or after swimming:
   a. Pain while swimming is common during the adduction and internal rotation of the underwater pull-through of freestyle, or during the extreme abduction of the above-water recovery phase.
   b. A snapping sensation in the shoulder is commonly noted during either the pull-through or recovery phase.

2. Less commonly pain may be localized to the posterior or lateral shoulder.

3. Commonly a chronic problem lasting longer than one year.

Key Symptom

Anterior shoulder pain during or after swimming

Clinical Findings

1. Impingement test: The Hawkins test is performed by flexing the patient's shoulder forward to 90 degrees, then passively internally rotating the shoulder. Reproduction of pain is a positive test and sensitive for diagnosing subacromial impingement.

2. Apprehension test: Abduct the patient's arm to 90 degrees, then passively externally rotate the arm while pushing the humeral head anteriorly with the thumb. Apprehension, resistance, or pain are positive results for possible glenohumeral instability.

3. Drawer test: An additional test for glenohumeral instability. Hold the acromion process with one hand and with the other grasp the proximal humerus, and test the anterior-posterior translation of the glenohumeral joint. Inferior instability is assessed by the sulcus test, with downward traction on the arm in neutral position.

4. Palpation of the supraspinatus tendon and the long head of the biceps tendon will aid in diagnosis of tendinitis.

Key Signs

- Positive impingement test
- Positive apprehension test

Laboratory Tests

1. Plain radiographs should include an anteroposterior view, an axillary view, and an outlet view. Calcific tendinitis or underlying degenerative joint disease may aid in diagnosis.

2. Magnetic resonance imaging or arthrography may aid in diagnosis of a rotator cuff tear.

Key Test

Plain radiograph

Differential Diagnosis

1. Rotator cuff tear
2. Bicipital tendinitis
3. Labral damage
4. Subluxation
5. Stress fracture of proximal humeral physis (in youths)
6. Apophyseal injury (in youths)

Treatment

1. Physical therapy to strengthen the rotator cuff, especially the external rotators, and improve glenohumeral stability
2. Medications
   a. Subacromial steroid injections should be reserved for those who fail conservative treatments.
   b. Nonsteroidal anti-inflammatory drugs should be prescribed when appropriate for their beneficial analgesic and anti-inflammatory actions.

Activity

1. A period of rest or activity below the threshold of pain should be recommended. During rest other activities, such as training with a kickboard during swim practices, should be encouraged to avoid deconditioning.
2. Preseason conditioning programs including strengthening of the external rotators
3. Investigate stroke techniques closely with coaches and trainers.
4. Avoid swimming with hand paddles because this may exacerbate symptoms.
5. Frequent icing of shoulder, especially after practices

Patient Education

1. Swimmers should be aware of this condition and its chronicity.
2. Emphasize proper preseason conditioning and stretching before and after practices.
3. Swimmers, parents, and coaches must be alert to the risks of overtraining.

 ## Bibliography

Bak K, Magnusson S: Shoulder strength and range of motion in symptomatic and pain free swimmers. Am J Sports Med 1997;25:454–459.

Koehler S, Thorson D: Swimmer's shoulder: targeting treatment. Physician Sportsmed 1996;24:39–50.

McMaster W, Roberts A, Stoddard T: A correlation between shoulder laxity and interfering pain in competitive swimmers. Am J Sports Med 1998;26:83–86.

Russ D: In-season management of shoulder pain in a collegiate swimmer: a team approach. J Orthop Sports Phys Ther 1998;27:371–376.

Rupp S, Berninger K, Hopf T: Shoulder problems in high level swimmers—impingement, anterior instability, muscular imbalance? Int J Sports Med 1995;6:557–562.

233 Runner's Injuries

David M. Barclay, III

Iliotibial Band Syndrome

Etiology

Iliotibial band (ITB) syndrome is caused by repetitive rubbing of the band against the lateral epicondyle of the femur.

1. Intrinsic causes
   a. Tight gluteus maximus and tensor fascia lata
   b. Leg-length differences: ITB syndrome develops in the shorter leg
   c. Increased forefoot varus
   d. Increased knee, Q angles
2. Extrinsic causes
   a. High weekly training miles or increasing weekly mileage too quickly
   b. Downhill running
   c. Running on crowned roads, which produces a functional leg-length difference
   d. Excessive pronation

Symptoms

Pain over the lateral femoral condyle that is made worse with long runs, running up or down hills, or ascending or descending stairs

Key Symptom

Pain over lateral femoral condyle

Clinical Findings

1. Pain with palpation over the lateral aspect of the knee
2. Pain with flexion and adduction of the hip
3. Pain with flexion and extension of the knee (worse at 30 degrees of flexion)

Key Sign

Pain with palpation over lateral femoral condyle

Laboratory Tests

1. Imaging studies are of little use unless a complete tendon rupture is suspected, which may appear as a soft-tissue density on a plain film, or meniscus injury is suspected, in which case magnetic resonance imaging (MRI) is indicated.
2. Significantly thicker bands on MRI scans than in controls without symptoms

Key Test

- Imaging studies may be useful to rule out other disorders

Differential Diagnosis

1. Patellofemoral pain syndrome
2. Early degenerative joint disease
3. Lateral meniscus injury
4. Superior tibiofibular joint sprain

Treatment

1. Nonsteroidal anti-inflammatory drugs (NSAIDs) for 1 or 2 weeks
2. Ice massage to painful area after running and several times a day
3. Phonophoresis alone or in combination with corticosteroids
4. Temporary use of a knee immobilizer for 2 to 3 days in severe cases
5. A comprehensive stretching program for the ITB and the proximal hip musculature
6. Exercises to strengthen the lateral stabilizers of the hip musculature, especially the gluteus medius

Tibial Stress Syndrome (Shin Splints)

Etiology

Tibial stress syndrome refers to a spectrum of pathology ranging from tenderness and swelling of the pretibial or posttibial muscle groups to the more severe tibial stress reaction or fracture.

1. Intrinsic causes
   a. Reduced ankle dorsiflexion secondary to tightness in the gastrocnemius-soleus musculature
   b. Hindfoot and forefoot varus with compensatory hyperpronation

2. Extrinsic causes
   a. Increasing training mileage too quickly
   b. A sudden increase in running speed
   c. Running on hard surfaces too often
   d. Running in worn-out running shoes

Symptoms
Dull pain over the medial distal two thirds of the tibia. During the acute phase, pain may disappear shortly into a run and return several hours later. As the condition progresses pain is constant and present even with walking.

Key Symptom

Pain over the distal two thirds of the tibia

Clinical Findings
1. Tenderness over the posterior medial edge of the tibia, most commonly the distal third.
2. Pain with dorsiflexion and plantar flexion of the foot

Key Sign

Tenderness over the distal two thirds of the tibia

Laboratory Tests
1. Plain radiographs are only indicated if a fracture line is detected.
2. MRI has been shown to be superior to isotope bone scanning to evaluate the four degrees of tibial stress injuries.

Key Test

Radiographs if a fracture line is detected

Differential Diagnosis
1. Tibial stress reaction, an inflammation of the periosteum
2. Tibial stress fracture

Treatment
1. Decrease running until pain is relatively improved.
2. Ice massage to painful area after running and several times a day
3. NSAIDs during acute phase

4. Running on soft, flat surfaces
5. Cross-training
6. Phonophoresis alone or in combination with corticosteroids
7. Consider orthotics to correct hyperpronation.

Achilles Tendinitis

Etiology
Foot pronation exerts an internal rotational force on the tibia, whereas knee extension exerts an external rotational force. If the foot remains excessively pronated during normal knee extension, the Achilles tendon is exposed to the extreme force created by these contradictory forces.

1. Intrinsic causes
   a. Hyperpronation of the foot
   b. Tight gastrocnemius and soleus muscles
2. Extrinsic causes
   a. High weekly training miles or increasing weekly mileage too quickly
   b. A sudden increase in running speed
   c. Running in worn-out running shoes

Symptoms
The Achilles tendon is tender just proximal to the calcaneus. Tenderness is worse with hill running.

Key Symptom

Tenderness just proximal to the calcaneus

Clinical Findings
1. Pain with palpation of the tendon
2. In the early stages, the foot loosens during the beginning of a run.
3. In the advanced stages, pain increases throughout the run and is often present with walking.
4. With more severe tendinitis, the tendon sheath becomes thickened, erythematous, and inflamed.
5. In chronic cases of tendinosis, nodules may be palpated in the body of the tendon.

Key Sign

Pain with palpation of the tendon

Laboratory Tests

Plain radiographs are of little use. MRI can differentiate paratendinous adhesions and swelling from actual tendon degeneration and partial tears.

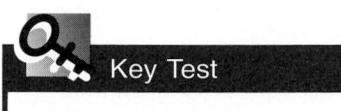

Key Test

MRI

Differential Diagnosis

1. Superficial tendo Achillis bursitis
2. Sever's disease, a traction apophysitis at the insertion of the tendon into the calcaneous, seen in adolescents
3. Posterior impingement syndrome
4. Calcaneus stress fracture

Treatment

1. NSAIDs for 1 or 2 weeks
2. Ice massage to painful area after running and several times a day
3. Phonophoresis alone or in combination with corticosteroids (iontophoresis)
4. Consider whirlpool treatments, posterior splinting, and heel lifts.
5. No hill running
6. Strengthen tendon and associated muscle groups with toe raises in a pain-free range of motion.

Patellofemoral Pain Syndrome

Etiology

Patellofemoral pain syndrome is the most common sports-related injury to the knee. Maltracking of the patella in the femoral trochlea leads to high contact pressures and anterior knee pain.

1. Intrinsic causes
   a. Femoral neck anteversion leads to a medially directed femoral trochlea and lateral positioning of the patella.
   b. Compensatory external tibial torsion pulls the patella laterally.
   c. Flatfoot deformity and pronation with hindfoot valgus further displace the patella.
   d. Atrophy of the vastus medialis oblique muscle allows unchecked lateral displacement of the patella.
   e. Tight iliotibial band
   f. All of the above changes are reflected in an increased Q angle.

2. Extrinsic causes
   a. High weekly training miles or increasing weekly mileage too quickly
   b. Increased patellofemoral loading from prolonged sitting with knees flexed (theater sign)
   c. Ascending or descending stairs or hills and hiking

Symptoms

1. Dull, aching anterior knee pain of insidious onset
2. Occasional sharp pain when ascending or descending stairs or hills
3. Pain after sitting for prolonged periods
4. Pain is worse with activity and relieved by rest.

Key Symptom

Dull, aching anterior knee pain

Clinical Findings

1. Apprehension with lateral displacement of the patella (apprehension sign)
2. Compression of the patella on the femoral condyles produces pain.
3. Contraction of the quadriceps muscles while grasping both sides of the patella produces pain.
4. Pain on the posterior surface of the patella
5. Q angle exceeds 16 degrees.

Key Sign

Apprehension sign

Laboratory Tests

Radiographs are indicated if there is no response to conservative therapy after 6 weeks. Unrelated diagnoses such as bone tumors, degenerative joint disease, and accessory ossification centers can be identified with plain films.

Key Test

• Radiograph only if there is no response to conservative therapy

Differential Diagnosis

1. Meniscus injury
2. Plica syndrome

3. Inflammatory or degenerative arthritis

4. Tumors of the joint

5. Patellar tendinitis

6. Osteochondritis dissecans

Treatment

1. NSAIDs are rarely useful unless there is an effusion present.

2. Stretching and strengthening exercises directed toward the hamstrings and gastrocnemius-soleus, and, particularly, ITB stretching

3. Correct hyperpronation with orthotics.

4. Consider a Neoprene knee sleeve as a transitional measure in the rehabilitation process in patients unable to perform strengthening exercises pain-free.

5. A dynamic patellar stabilization orthosis may benefit patients with a hypermobile patella or recurrent patellar subluxation.

Bibliography

Ballas MT, Tytko J, Cookson D: Common overuse running injuries: diagnosis and management. Am Fam Physician 1997;55:2473–2480.

Fadale P, Hulstym M: Common athletic injuries. Clin Sports Med 1997;16:493–499.

Fredericson M: Common injuries in runners: diagnosis, rehabilitation and prevention. Sports Med 1996;21:49–72.

Fredericson M: Diagnosing tibial stress injuries in athletes. West J Med 1995;162:150.

234 Knee Injuries

John Midtling

Overuse Injuries

Patellofemoral Pain Syndrome

See Ch. 235, Patellofemoral Pain Syndrome.

Patellar Tendinitis

Etiology
1. Overuse injury secondary to excessive jumping or running
2. Repetitive force leads to microscopic tears and inflammation of patellar tendon.
3. Dorsiflexor weakness secondary to ankle injury

Symptoms
1. Pain at patellar tendon at attachment to inferior pole of patella
2. Infrapatellar pain worse after exercise.

Key Symptom

Pain over inferior pole of patella worse after exercise

Clinical Findings
1. Tenderness at insertion of patellar tendon into inferior pole of patella
2. Vastus medialis oblique weakness with extensor dysfunction
3. Weak ankle dorsiflexors

Key Sign

Tenderness over inferior pole of patella

Tests
1. Radiograph of knee shows irregularity at inferior pole of patella and possibly patella alta.
2. Magnetic resonance imaging (MRI) shows degenerative changes in patellar tendon.

Key Test

Radiograph of knee

Differential Diagnosis
1. Tumor
2. Osteoarthritis
3. Osgood-Schlatter disease

Treatment
1. Rehabilitation with quadriceps strengthening
2. Strengthening of ankle dorsiflexors
3. Nonsteroidal anti-inflammatory drugs (NSAIDs)
4. Phonophoresis, iontophoresis with corticosteroids, ultrasound

Key Treatment

- Rehabilitation strengthening
- NSAIDs
- Physical modalities

Apophysitis (Osgood-Schlatter Disease)

See Ch. 229, Osteochondritis (Osgood-Schlatter Disease).

Iliotibial Band Syndrome

Etiology
1. Chronic inflammation over lateral side of knee where iliotibial band moves over lateral femoral epicondyle
2. Overuse secondary to running
3. Running on irregular surface
4. Varus malalignment, unequal leg lengths, foot pronation

Symptoms
1. Lateral knee pain with activity
2. Occasional popping

Key Symptom

Lateral knee pain with activity

Clinical Findings
1. Tenderness over lateral femoral epicondyle
2. Tight iliotibial band
3. Positive Ober's test

Key Sign

Tenderness over lateral femoral epicondyle

Differential Diagnosis
1. Popliteus tendinitis
2. Vastus lateralis tendinitis
3. Lateral meniscal injury
4. Plica

Treatment
1. Iliotibial band stretching exercises
2. Lateral strengthening
3. Rest
4. NSAIDs
5. Ultrasound, phonophores, iontophoresis
6. Injection
7. Orthotics

Key Treatment

- Iliotibial band stretching
- Rest
- Physical modalities

Ligamentous Injuries

Medial Collateral Ligament

Etiology
1. Valgus stress to knee with external rotation
2. Lateral blow

Symptoms
1. Pain on medial side of knee
2. Knee gives way into valgus
3. May hear pop

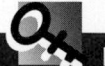
Key Symptom

Pain on medial side of knee with valgus stress

Clinical Findings
1. Knee in 30 degrees of flexion: medial laxity with valgus stress
2. Medial swelling
3. Ligament extends from adductor tubercle to anteromedial tibia, inserting at level of tibial tuberosity, providing medial stabilizing structure.

Key Sign

Medial laxity with knee in flexion and valgus stress

Tests
1. Radiograph of knee looking for fracture of distal femur or proximal tibia, epiphyseal fractures in adolescents
2. Abduction stress radiograph of knee
3. MRI

Key Tests

- Radiograph of knee
- MRI

Differential Diagnosis
1. Epiphyseal fracture at distal femur or proximal tibia
2. Medial meniscal tear

Treatment
1. Rest, ice, compression, elevation during acute phase
2. Functional rehabilitation
3. Grade III (complete) usually require surgical repair.

Key Treatment

- Rehabilitation
- Surgical intervention for grade III

Lateral Collateral Ligament

Etiology
1. Varus or twisting injury
2. May be noncontact.
3. Posterolateral ligaments may be injured by hyperextension mechanism.

Symptoms
1. Pain over lateral ligament complex
2. Knee gives way on twisting, cutting, or pivoting

Key Symptom

Pain over lateral ligament complex

Clinical Findings
1. With knee in 30 degrees of flexion: lateral laxity with varus stress
2. Ligament extends from lateral femoral epicondyle to head of fibula.
3. Frequently associated with cruciate ligament and peroneal nerve injuries

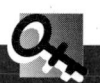

Key Sign

Lateral laxity with knee in flexion and varus stress

Tests
1. Radiograph of knee looking for avulsion of fragment of proximal lateral tibia or avulsion fracture of proximal fibula
2. MRI

Key Tests

- Radiograph of knee
- MRI

Differential Diagnosis
1. Medial compartment osteoarthritis
2. Posterior cruciate ligament injury
3. Lateral meniscus tear
4. Knee dislocation
5. Peroneal nerve injury

Treatment
1. Rest, ice, compression, elevation during acute phase
2. Functional rehabilitation
3. Grade III (complete) usually require surgical repair.

Key Treatment

- Rehabilitation
- Surgical intervention for grade III

Anterior Cruciate Ligament

Etiology
1. Usually torn from femur or tibia or in midportion
2. Hyperextension, varus and internal rotation, or valgus and external rotation is cause.
3. May avulse tibial spine.
4. Must be noncontact injuries.

Symptoms
1. Large effusion: second-degree hemarthrosis
2. Knee gives way on twisting, pivoting, or cutting.
3. Autonomic symptoms
4. Popping or snapping sensation
5. Knee gives out and there is sense of instability.
6. Effusion
7. Pain in anterior knee or at posterolateral joint line

Key Symptom

Popping sensation and effusion at knee following hyperextension of the knee

Clinical Findings
1. Large hemarthrosis
2. Positive Lachman's test
3. Positive anterior drawer sign
4. Ligament extends from anterior central tibia to medial aspect of lateral femoral condyle, stabilizing and limiting anterior tibial displacement.

Key Signs

- Hemarthrosis
- Positive Lachman's test (knee in 15 degrees of flexion yields anterior translation of tibia beneath femur and lack of a firm end point)

Tests

1. Radiograph of knee looking for lateral capsular sign, avulsion of tibial spine, osteochondral fracture
2. MRI

Differential Diagnosis

1. Rule out other causes of hemarthrosis, such as osteochondral fracture.
2. Rule out ligamentous injury or meniscal tear.

Treatment

1. Acute treatment consists of rest, ice, compression, and elevation.
2. Grade III (complete) or instability requires surgical repair (usually delay 3 to 5 weeks).

Posterior Cruciate Ligament

Etiology

1. Valgus or varus stress in full extension
2. Direct blow to anterior proximal tibia
3. Usually a contact injury associated with trauma

Symptoms

1. Less swelling than with anterior cruciate ligament injury
2. Feeling of femur sliding anteriorly off tibia
3. Sense of instability and reluctance to fully extend knee

Clinical Findings

1. Abduction or adduction stress test positive in *full extension*.
2. Posterior drawer sign
3. Popliteal tenderness

4. Positive sag test
5. Ligament extends from posterior central tibia to lateral aspect of medial femoral condyle, limiting posterior tibial displacement.

Tests

1. Radiograph of knee looking for avulsion of tibial attachment
2. MRI

Differential Diagnosis

1. Differentiate from posterior lateral corner injury.
2. Meniscal tear

Treatment

1. Acute treatment consists of rest, ice, compression, and elevation.
2. Grades I and II may be treated with functional rehabilitation and protective bracing.
3. Grade III usually requires surgical repair.

Meniscal Injuries

Medial Meniscus

Etiology

1. Disruption of medial meniscus from single traumatic episode or degenerative process
2. Most tears are posterior horn tears.
3. Most important factor is whether the tear is in the peripheral vascular zone or central nonvascular zone (blood supply only to peripheral third of meniscus).

4. Mechanism is twisting or squatting with valgus tibial rotation while weight bearing in a partially flexed position.
5. Frequently associated with acute ligamentous injuries

Symptoms
1. Mild effusion
2. Medial joint line pain
3. Knee locks in full extension or locks as a result of fragments.
4. Slipping or catching of knee at joint line
5. Impingement
6. May feel snap or pop.
7. Difficulty squatting

Key Symptom

Medial joint line pain

Clinical Findings
1. Positive McMurray's test
2. Positive Apley compression test
3. Tender over medial joint line
4. Mild effusion

Key Sign

Positive McMurray's test with external rotation of tibia and movement from flexion to extension

Tests
1. Radiograph of knee looking for osteoarthritis
2. MRI

Key Tests

- Radiograph of knee
- MRI

Differential Diagnosis
1. Medial collateral ligament injury
2. Patellar problems
3. Synovial plicas
4. Loose bodies causing significant locking
5. Osteoarthritis

Treatment
1. Acute treatment consists of rest, ice, compression, and elevation.
2. Functional rehabilitation
3. Surgical intervention depending upon time constraints, type of injury, and symptomology

Key Treatment

- Rehabilitation
- Consideration of surgical intervention

Lateral Meniscus

Etiology
1. Disruption of lateral meniscus from single traumatic episode or degenerative process
2. Most important factor is whether peripheral vascular zone or central nonvascular zone is injured.
3. Mechanism is twisting or squatting with varus stress.
4. Less common than medial meniscal injuries
5. Often the result of rotation while in maximally flexed position (squatting)

Symptoms
1. Mild effusion
2. Lateral joint line pain
3. Knee locks in full extension or locks as a result of fragments.
4. May feel snap or pop.
5. Impingement

Key Symptom

Lateral joint line pain

Clinical Findings
1. Positive McMurray's test
2. Positive Apley compression test
3. Tender over lateral joint line
4. Mild effusion

Key Sign

Positive McMurray's test with internal rotation of tibia and movement from flexion to extension

Tests

1. Radiograph of knee looking for osteoarthritis
2. MRI

Key Tests

- Radiograph of knee
- MRI

Differential Diagnosis

1. Lateral collateral ligament injury
2. Loose bodies causing significant locking
3. Osteoarthritis
4. Popliteal tendinitis
5. Iliotibial band syndrome

Treatment

1. Acute treatment consists of rest, ice, compression, and elevation.
2. Functional rehabilitation
3. Surgical intervention depending upon time constraints, type of injury, and symptomatology

Key Treatment

- Rehabilitation
- Consideration of surgical intervention

Bibliography

Garrick JG: Knee injuries. In Garrick JG, Webb DR (eds): Sports Injuries: Diagnosis and Treatment, pp 197–255. Philadelphia, WB Saunders Company, 1990.

Garrick JG: Knee ligament injuries. In Sallis RE, Massimino F (eds): Essentials of Sports Medicine, pp 412–417. St. Louis, CV Mosby Company, 1997.

Garrick JG: Meniscal injuries. In Sallis RE, Massimino F (eds): Essentials of Sports Medicine, pp 418–420. St. Louis, CV Mosby Company, 1997.

Levandowski R: Knee injuries. In Birrer RB (ed): Sports Medicine for the Primary Care Physician, pp 506–530. Boca Raton, FL, CRC Press, 1994.

Richards DB, Kibler WB: Rehabilitation of the injured knee. In Sallis RE, Massimino F (eds): Essentials of Sports Medicine, pp 433–436. St. Louis, CV Mosby Company, 1997.

Wieting JM, McKeag DB: Anterior knee pain and overuse. In Sallis RE, Massimino F (eds): Essentials of Sports Medicine, pp 421–432. St. Louis, CV Mosby Company, 1997.

235 Patellofemoral Pain Syndrome

Mark W. Niedfeldt

Etiology

1. Definition
   a. Patellofemoral pain syndrome (PFPS) is a common source of knee symptoms and disability in the athlete and is the most common type of knee disorder encountered in clinical practice. It is often seen in girls and those participating in sports that involve running.
   b. Other names commonly referring to PFPS include anterior knee pain, chondromalacia patella, lateral hypercompression syndrome, excessive lateral pressure syndrome, patellofemoral arthralgia, and runner's knee. The term *chondromalacia patella*, commonly used in the past, should be avoided except in the very specific instance of chondral changes on the patella actually visualized by arthroscopy or various special imaging techniques. It should not be applied merely to patients with painful symptoms around the anterior knee.

2. Anatomy
   a. The patella is contained within the quadriceps mechanism as a sesamoid bone and functions to increase the mechanical advantage of the extensor muscles by transmitting force across the knee at a greater distance from the axis of rotation. The stability of the patella is a function of bony, ligamentous, and muscular components.
   b. The proximal two thirds of the posterior surface of the patella is V-shaped and can be divided into medial and lateral facets. These facets articulate with the distal femur in the region of the intercondylar notch and are covered with the thickest articular cartilage in the body.
   c. The four muscles of the quadriceps muscle group insert in a layered arrangement into the proximal patella at different angles, creating vectors of force on the patella. The vastus medialis and lateralis contribute to the medial and lateral retinacula, which in turn attach to the proximal tibia.

3. Biomechanics
   a. Significant patellofemoral contact does not occur until approximately 20 degrees of knee flexion, and at greater than 90 degrees of flexion the quadriceps tendons begin to contact the femoral trochlea articular surface.
   b. Peak pressure on the patellofemoral joint occurs at 45 degrees of knee flexion. Up to 10 times the normal body weight can be generated across the patellofemoral joint when the knee is extended against resistance forces. Even relatively slight degrees of malalignment may cause a significant concentration of loading forces, leading to anterior or peripatellar knee pain.

4. Risk factors: Malalignment of the patellofemoral articulation with resulting abnormal articular contact pressures may develop from a combination of factors. These risk factors include excessive femoral anteversion at the hip, genu valgum (knock knees), patella alta (high patella), hyperpronated foot, lateral placement of the tibial tubercle, loose retinacular ligaments, and weakness of the quadriceps muscles, particularly the oblique head of the vastus medialis (VMO). Activities that place the patient at risk include running and repetitive weight-bearing movements involving knee flexion.

Symptoms

1. Symptoms may occur gradually as a result of an overuse process or suddenly following a specific traumatic event. Both knees are affected in two thirds of cases.

2. The knee tends to feel stiff, with dull, achy pain located about the anterior aspect of the knee. The discomfort may be diffuse or localized to the medial or lateral patellofemoral joint and retinaculum.

3. Ascending or descending stairs, squatting, kneeling, and sitting with the knee flexed for a long period of time, as in a movie theater or when traveling in a car, aggravate the condition as a result of increased compressive forces within the patellofemoral joint. Symptoms gradually become more severe with increased activity or may wax and wane as activity levels change but tend to be relieved with rest.

4. The discomfort of PFPS is thought to be caused by abnormal pressure transmitted to nerve-rich subchrondral bone and inflamed synovium.

5. There is usually no history of swelling, although some patients may complain of mild recurrent puffiness.

6. Patients may notice crepitation in the knee prior to the onset of symptoms, and some individuals may have crepitation in an asymptomatic knee.

7. On occasion, patients may have some complaints of the knee giving way. This occurs as a result of muscular reflexes, and patients should not report a sensation of actual bony subluxation.

Key Symptoms

- Stiffness with dull, achy anterior or peripatellar pain

- Pain aggravated on stairs, with squatting or sitting with the knee flexed

- Worsened with increased activity and improved with rest

Clinical Findings

1. Palpation of the patella frequently reveals tenderness along the medial patellar facet. Crepitation of the patellofemoral joint may be noted with movement of the knee, but the presence of crepitation does not always correlate with pain and dysfunction. An effusion should not be present. Forced knee extension against resistance often creates pain.

2. Compression of the patella against the anterior aspect of the femur may cause crepitation or pain. This compression test is performed by holding the proximal pole of the patella firmly in place while the quadriceps muscles are contracted. Some patients may be unable to contract the quadriceps because of discomfort.

3. With the patient standing, look for excessive varus or valgus of the lower extremity and pes planus (flat feet), which can contribute to malalignment.

4. The Q angle measurement can be performed with the patient lying supine. While the quadriceps muscles are contracted, the angle from the anterior superior iliac spine to the tibial tuberosity is measured using the center of the patella for reference. The Q angle is considered increased if it is greater than 10 degrees in males and 15 degrees in females.

5. Flexibility in the hamstrings and gastrocnemius-soleus complex should also be assessed.

Key Signs

- Tenderness along the medial patellar facet

- Pain with forced knee extension

- Patellar compression reproduces pain.

Laboratory Tests

1. Routine radiographs are usually unremarkable. If taken, radiographs may show accessory ossification centers, degenerative joint disease, bone tumors, or osteochondritis dissecans.

   a. Patellar position may be assessed and patella alta or baja may be noted in the anteroposterior (AP) view. The inferior pole of the patella usually rests at the upper extreme edge of the intercondylar notch shadow.

   b. The lateral view may show traction changes on the patella and tibial tuberosity as well as osteochondritis dissecans.

   c. The axillary view, often known as a sunrise or Merchant's view, may show lateral patellar tilt, lateral displacement, or degenerative changes in the patellofemoral joint.

2. Further testing, including bone scans, computerized tomography, and magnetic resonance imaging, are generally unnecessary. Advanced testing may be warranted if another disease process is suspected based on physical examination and outcome of initial treatment.

Key Tests

- Radiographs usually normal.

- Radiographs should include AP, lateral, and axillary views.

- Further testing usually unnecessary.

Differential Diagnosis

1. Patellar tendinitis is demonstrated by tenderness of the patellar tendon at its attachment to the distal pole of the patella. Quadriceps tendinitis presents as tenderness at the proximal pole of the patella where the quadriceps tendon attaches.

2. Patellar instability may be evaluated by a positive apprehension test. As the patella is displaced laterally over the lateral femoral condyle, the patient experiences apprehension and discomfort. An effusion following an injury or a feeling of giving way in the knee may be in-

dicative of a patellar dislocation, ligamentous, or meniscal injury.

3. Osteochondritis dissecans is characterized by primary necrosis of subchrondral bone with subsequent involvement of the overlying articular cartilage. The knee is the most common site affected. It usually occurs in the second decade of life, and boys are affected three times more often than girls. Radiographs may reveal the lesion, usually on the lateral side of the medial femoral condyle.

Treatment

Nonsurgical treatment is the cornerstone of dealing with PFPS and is focused on stabilization of the patella in its articulation with the femoral trochlea.

Medication

1. Nonsteroidal anti-inflammatory drugs (NSAIDs) are often used for this condition.

2. These medications should be used as a short-term adjunct to rehabilitative exercise or for intermittent flaring of symptoms.

Activity

1. Most cases of PFPS are due to overuse. Relative rest and modification of activities, including eliminating the offending activity and substituting other activities, is required initially. Brisk walking, bicycling, or swimming may be substituted for other weight-bearing activities. A gradual return to activities is essential.

2. Rehabilitative exercises attempt to affect dynamically the malaligned forces that are at the root of the pain.

    a. Exercises involving isometric quadriceps strengthening targeting a portion of the VMO in full extension (i.e., straight-leg raises) are used.

    b. Another major component of rehabilitative exercise is flexibility, especially of the hamstrings, calf, quadriceps, and iliotibial band.

Other Treatments

1. Ice should be used for 15 to 20 minutes after activity.

2. Correction of biomechanical abnormalities should be performed. Patients with a correctable foot deformity such as pes planus may benefit from arch supports or orthotics to decrease the forces on the knee extensor mechanism.

3. Patellar taping (McConnell taping) has been used with success by therapists in some patients. This technique attempts to re-educate the muscles while providing external support for the patella.

4. Braces often use a passive lateral buttress or straps to support and realign the patella and also provide proprioception.

5. Surgical treatment can usually be avoided, but in a small group of patients surgical management will be required. Conservative treatment should be continued for at least 3 to 6 months prior to surgery. Procedures include lateral retinacular release, extensor mechanism reconstruction, and patellofemoral decompression procedures.

Key Treatments

- Relative rest and gradual return to activity
- NSAIDs
- Quadriceps strengthening (especially VMO)
- Hamstring and calf stretching
- Ice
- Correct biomechanical abnormalities.
- Patellar taping or bracing
- Surgery after 3 to 6 months of conservative treatment

Follow-Up

Although short-term success is achieved in 75 per cent of patients, many may have a return of symptoms during the following year. Patients often need to continue stretching and strengthening exercises beyond the acute phase, and whenever possible correction of underlying biomechanical abnormalities should be performed.

Bibliography

Arroll B, Ellis-Pegler E, Edwards A, et al: Patellofemoral pain syndrome: a critical review of the clinical trials on nonoperative therapy. Am J Sports Med 1997;25:207–212.

Bellemans J, Cauwenberghs F, Witwrow E, et al: Anteromedial tibial tubercle transfer in patients with chronic anterior knee pain and a subluxation-type patellar malalignment. Am J Sports Med 1997;25:375–381.

Cutbill JW, Ladly KO, Bray RC, et al: Anterior knee pain: a review. Clin J Sport Med 1997;7:40–45.

Davids JR: Pediatric knee: clinical assessment and common disorders. Pediatr Clin North Am 1996;43:1013–1033.

Timm KE: Randomized controlled trial of Protonics on patellar pain, position, and function. Med Sci Sports Exerc 1998;30:665–670.

236 Plantar Fasciitis

Kelley Withy

Etiology

1. Plantar fasciitis is the most common cause of localized heel pain and accounts for about 4 per cent of all running injuries.

2. The plantar fascia is a band of white fibers that originates at the medial tubercle of the calcaneus and fans out to insert onto the metatarsal heads. It provides support for the plantar aspect of the foot and the arch.

3. Plantar fasciitis is an overuse condition caused by repetitive traction and stretching of the plantar fascia, resulting in microtears of the fascia and periostitis at the attachment of the plantar fascia on the calcaneus.

4. The reparative inflammatory response causes thickening and stiffness of the fascia. Inflammation and sudden stretching of the stiff fascia cause pain.

5. Fifty per cent of patients with plantar fasciitis will develop heel spurs, which may be caused by periostitis, chronic tension on the bony attachment, and bone remodeling. Heel spurs also occur without fasciitis, can be asymptomatic, and require no treatment.

6. Anatomic factors can predispose to plantar fasciitis.

   a. Cavus deformities: high arch; excessive supination
   b. Pes planus (flat foot): excessive pronation
   c. Excessive tightness of the Achilles tendon
   d. Age-related loss of calcaneal fat pad

7. Obesity and lack of conditioning also predispose to plantar fasciitis.

8. Plantar fasciitis rarely occurs in children and adolescents.

9. Plantar fasciitis is rarely traumatic, but can be caused by sudden excessive loading and fascial rupture.

Symptoms

1. Patients present with pain on the plantar and medial aspects of their foot and heel.

   a. The pain is usually described as burning, aching, sharp, or piercing.
   b. Sometimes the pain is described as radiating anteriorly from the heel.
   c. Pain is most severe upon initial weight bearing following a period of non–weight bearing, because of sudden stretching of the stiff, inflamed, and thickened fascia.
   d. The pain decreases with stretching and activity, then recurs after or toward the end of a vigorous workout or during prolonged weight bearing. As the condition worsens, pain is not relieved with activity.

2. Plantar fasciitis usually has a gradual onset over a number of weeks.

3. Symptoms are usually unilateral, but may be bilateral in 15 to 30 per cent of cases.

Key Symptoms

Burning pain on the bottom of the foot and heel area, most severe with the first step of the day

Clinical Findings

1. Pain on palpation of the anterior and medial calcaneus, the plantar fascia, and sometimes the abductor hallucis muscle.

2. Pain may be duplicated or intensified by dorsiflexion of the foot or the great toe.

3. Affected area may have swelling, but no other skin changes are present.

4. Tightness of the Achilles tendon is seen in a majority of patients.

5. Mid-stance pronation (pes planus) or high rigid arch (cavus deformity) may be seen.

6. Unusual wear pattern on shoes: either medial heel wear (pes planus) or lateral heel wear (cavus deformity)

Key Signs

Point tenderness over the medial process of the calcaneal tuberosity (attachment of the plantar fascia onto the calcaneus)

Tests

1. A lateral foot radiograph can be done if there is suspicion of calcaneal fracture. Fifty per cent of radiographs will show heel spurs, which have no clinical significance.

2. A bone scan can help differentiate between calcaneal stress fracture and fasciitis.

Key Tests

No laboratory or radiology tests are recommended unless other causes are suspected or symptoms do not respond to treatment.

Differential Diagnosis

1. Other local conditions may cause similar symptoms of foot pain, but severe pain with the first step of the day is strongly indicative of plantar fasciitis.

   a. Calcaneal fracture: onset more acute, possible history of trauma, pain worsens with activity, positive heel squeeze test

   b. Nerve compression: medial calcaneal nerve entrapment or tarsal tunnel syndrome—pain worse at night, positive Tinel's sign (symptoms duplicated with nerve percussion)

   c. Sever's disease: calcaneal apophysitis seen in children and adolescents

   d. Posterior calcaneal spur and Haglund's deformity (painful bump at Achilles tendon insertion): Cause posterior heel pain.

   e. Local infection: usually presents with erythema and warmth

   f. Arterial insufficiency: Symptoms are worse with activity, pulses are diminished.

   g. Self-limited musculoskeletal causes: abductor hallucis spasm, medial plantar bursitis, heel contusion

2. Systemic causes should also be considered: rheumatoid arthritis, Reiter's syndrome, systemic lupus erythematosus, gout, ankylosing spondylitis, Paget's disease, cancer, and S1 radiculopathy.

Treatment

Patient education and lifestyle modification are the most successful treatment modalities for symptom relief and long-term prevention of plantar fasciitis pain.

Medication

Nonsteroidal anti-inflammatory medication regularly for a 2- to 4-week period (if no contraindications)

Activity

1. Ice after weight-bearing activity and when painful (at least four times a day for 20 minutes). Avoid hot soaks.

2. Limit injury-provoking activity or excessive weight bearing until symptoms resolve.

3. Stretching exercises: at least 10 repetitions three to five times a day

   a. Achilles tendon stretch

   b. Gastrocnemius and soleus muscle stretch

   c. Plantar fascia stretch

   d. To avoid morning pain, patient should dorsiflex and plantar-flex the affected foot 10 times before standing.

4. Strengthening exercises

   a. Intrinsic foot muscle strengthening: Repeatedly bunch towel with toes.

   b. Gastrocnemius strengthening: heel raises with weights or arc-of-motion exercises with rubber tubing or bicycle inner tube

5. Proper foot support

   a. Patient must always wear properly fitting shoes with good medial arch support, a close fitting heel, adequate room for the toes, and a soft sole. Lace-up running or walking shoes are recommended. Avoid slippers, flats, and barefoot walking. A prescription to wear running shoes at work may be helpful.

   b. Arch support: either over-the-counter shoe inserts or custom-made orthotics

   c. Heel cup or pads are helpful in the case of diminished fat pad or prolonged standing.

   d. Plantar taping, such as low-dye taping, to prevent excessive pronation

6. Transverse friction massage at the origin of the plantar fascia on the calcaneus

7. Posterior night splints: short-leg posterior splint in position of maximum dorsiflexion to be worn during sleep until symptoms resolve

8. Physical therapy (2 to 4 weeks) for stretching exercises, massage, ultrasound, and iontophoresis

9. Corticosteroid injection may be given up to three times, at least 6 weeks apart. There is a small risk of fascial weakening and rupture, loss of calcaneal fat pad, infection, bleeding, and allergic reaction.

Procedure

After spraying medial aspect of foot with ethyl chloride anesthetic spray, immediately inject 0.5 to 1 ml of medium- or long-acting steroid (betamethasone phosphate/acetate or methylprednisolone acetate) mixed with 1 to 2 ml of local anesthetic (1% lidocaine) using a 1.5-inch 22- to 25-gauge needle. Enter the skin through the medial foot 1.5 cm superior to the plantar aspect (sole) of the foot. Infiltrate the area around the attachment of the plantar fascia onto the calcaneus, where the pain is the greatest.

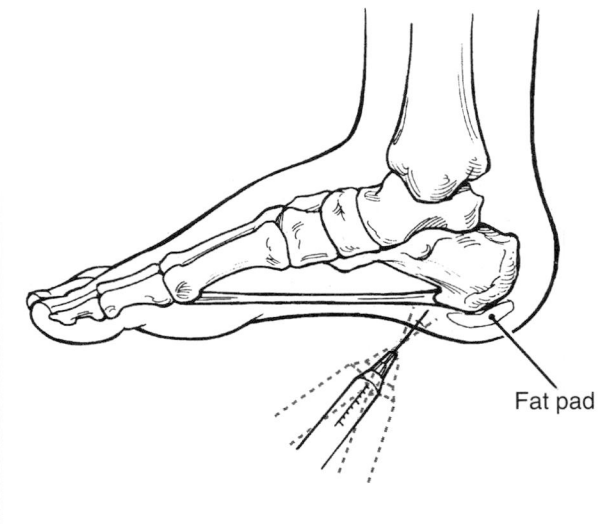

Fat pad

10. Cast immobilization with short-leg walking cast for 4 weeks

11. Surgical fasciotomy and spur removal are only recommended if all other modalities fail and symptoms are lifestyle-limiting for over 9 to 12 months.

Patient Education

1. Rest, ice, proper arch support and footwear
2. Avoid applying heat and going barefoot.

3. Utilize stretching and strengthening exercises as listed above.

Follow-Up

If diagnosed and treated early, most patients will improve significantly within 6 weeks using conservative measures. Ninety per cent of cases will resolve completely within 1 year. Symptoms may recur if weight-bearing activities are restarted prematurely or if the patient has not made lifestyle modifications such as appropriate footwear at all times, regular stretching, strengthening, icing, and rest as needed.

1. Patient should be seen after 2 to 3 weeks of rest, ice, stretching, proper footwear, nonsteroidal anti-inflammatory drugs, and over-the-counter orthotics.

2. If there is no improvement in 2 to 3 weeks, taping, physical therapy, and/or night splints can be utilized.

3. If there is still no improvement in 4 more weeks, casting, custom orthotics, and/or corticosteroid injection can be utilized.

4. If symptoms persist despite all treatment modalities, surgery can be considered as last resort after 9 to 12 months of pain and limitation of activities.

Bibliography

Ballas M, Tytko J, Cookson D: Common overuse running injuries: diagnosis and management. Am Fam Physician 1997;55:2473–2480.

Kalb R: Evaluation and treatment of foot and ankle pain. Hosp Pract 1998;33:127–132.

Ryan J: Use of posterior night splints in the treatment of plantar fasciitis. Am Fam Physician 1995;52:891–898.

Singh K, Angel J, Bentley G, et al: Fortnightly review: plantar fasciitis. BMJ 1997;315:172–175.

Wyngarden T: The painful foot, Part II: common rearfoot deformities. Am Fam Physician 1997;55:2207–2212.

237 Shoulder Dislocations

Joe E. Himes

Shoulder dislocations may be the result of acute trauma or chronic instability of the glenohumeral joint. Primary care physicians most commonly recognize the anterior shoulder dislocation but may not appreciate the more subtle details of its pathophysiology and treatment. On the contrary, posterior shoulder dislocations may be much more difficult to recognize. Posterior shoulder dislocations may present as a chronic process and pose special treatment challenges.

Etiology

1. Anterior shoulder dislocation: abduction, external rotation, and extension of arm
2. Posterior shoulder dislocation: adduction, internal rotation, and flexion of arm

Symptoms

1. Anterior and/or posterior shoulder pain
2. Periarticular muscle spasms
3. Possible neurovascular compromise to ipsilateral extremity

Key Symptoms

- Shoulder pain
- Limitation of glenohumeral motion

Clinical Findings

1. Anterior shoulder dislocation
   a. Inability to rotate arm
   b. Apprehension
   c. Fullness in anterior shoulder
2. Posterior shoulder dislocation
   a. Inability to rotate
   b. Inability to fully supinate hand with shoulder in forward flexion
   c. Findings subtle and may be missed on initial examination in 60 to 80 per cent of cases.

> **WARNING**
>
> **Always evaluate and document the neurovascular status of the entire extremity at the time of injury and after treatment. Compromised neurovascular status constitutes a true medical emergency.**

Laboratory Tests

Radiographic Evaluation

1. Purposes
   a. Identify fracture of humerus, clavicle, and glenoid fossa (Bankart lesion)
   b. Identify Hill-Sachs lesion of posterior humerus
   c. Confirm suspected dislocation
2. Recommended views
   a. True anteroposterior view of shoulder with internal and external humeral rotation
   b. True lateral view of scapula (scapular Y view)
   c. Axillary view
   d. Westpoint view (identify glenoid rim fractures, e.g., Bankart lesions)

Differential Diagnosis

1. Fracture of humerus, clavicle, glenoid fossa
2. Combined fracture-dislocation
3. Muscular contusion
4. Brachial plexopathy
5. Acromioclavicular separation

Treatment

1. Anterior shoulder dislocation
   a. Elevation and internal rotation of humerus while applying posterior pressure to anterior humeral head
   b. Stimson maneuver: Position patient prone, hanging affected arm off edge of table. Apply weights to arm to provide traction (Fig. 237–1). It is important that weights hang from arm. Patient holding weights interferes with shoulder relaxation. May enhance pa-

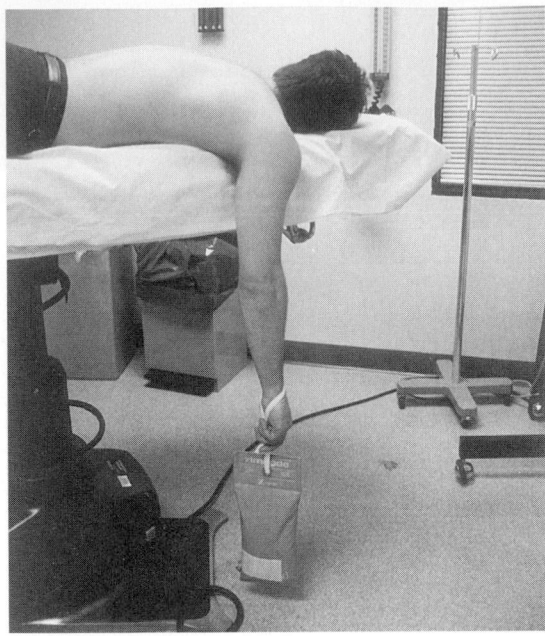

Figure 237–1 Stimson technique for relocation of anterior shoulder dislocation.

tient relaxation with muscle relaxants, analgesics, or anesthesia.

   c. Double-sheet method: Patient supine on treatment table. One sheet is held around the patient's torso by an assistant. A second sheet around the patient's upper arm provides lateral traction while the physician provides firm, but gentle, traction to the arm along the axial plane. "Arm lock" technique may be used in place of second sheet (Zahiri et al. 1997).

2. Posterior shoulder dislocation: With patient supine, apply lateral traction with internal rotation followed by external rotation.

WARNING

Those patients with neurologic and/or vascular compromise, those with open growth plates, and those presenting as first-time dislocators should be treated as true emergencies. These patients should receive radiologic evaluation prior to relocation attempts and orthopedic and vascular surgery consults should be considered early in treatment.

Surgery

1. Surgical reduction indicated if conservative approach to reduction unsuccessful.
2. Surgical stabilization following reduction if patient at high risk of recurrence

   a. Acute anterior shoulder dislocation recurrence
     (1) If patient younger than age 20, greater than 80 per cent
     (2) If patient older than 20, about 25 per cent (higher if more active)
   b. Acute posterior shoulder dislocation recurrence: less than 40 per cent, with younger patients more likely to suffer
   c. Chronic dislocators
     (1) Attempt to identify voluntary dislocators and educate them.
     (2) Much less likely to respond to conservative treatment

---

WARNING

Voluntary subluxors/dislocators are not considered suitable for surgical stabilization because they often continue subluxing/dislocating habits, thereby lengthening the repair in the early postoperative period.

Medication

1. Prereduction: Rapid identification and reduction can obviate need for muscle relaxants.
2. Reduction: intramuscular lidocaine at site, intravenous benzodiazepines or narcotics, and occasionally general anesthesia
3. Postreduction: Analgesics and anti-inflammatory medications can provide pain relief and minimize soft tissue swelling.

Activity

1. Following reduction of acute, first-time dislocations, arm is immobilized for 2 to 4 weeks, followed by sling for comfort, to a total of 6 weeks.
2. Chronic dislocations are likely to occur with less force and less soft tissue damage. Conservative therapy includes relocation with subsequent shoulder stabilization exercises.

Patient Education

1. Educate the patient regarding recurrent dislocations.
2. For patients active in sports, educate regarding proper strength, conditioning, technique.

Follow-Up

1. Follow-up radiographs to document:
   a. Successful relocation
   b. Bankart or Hill-Sachs lesions

2. Physical therapy
   a. Control pain and swelling.
   b. Restore range of motion.
   c. Restore strength and endurance.
   d. Relearn proprioceptive and functional reflexes.
3. Bracing
   a. Anterior shoulder dislocation: Limits abduction and external rotation of shoulder.
   b. Posterior shoulder dislocation: No effective bracing available.

 Bibliography

Allen AA, Warner JJP: Shoulder instability in the athlete. Orthop Clin North Am 1995;26:487–504.

Brown DD, Friedman RJ: Postoperative rehabilitation following total shoulder arthroplasty. Orthop Clin North Am 1998;29:535–547.

Hulstyn MJ, Fadale PD: Shoulder injuries to the athlete. Clin Sports Med 1997;16:663–679.

Matthews DE, Roberts T: Intraarticular lidocaine versus intravenous analgesic for reduction of acute anterior shoulder dislocations. Am J Sports Med 1995;23:54–58.

Zahiri CA, Zahiri H, Tehrany F: Anterior shoulder dislocation reduction technique—revisited. Orthopedics 1997;20:515–521.

238 Elbow Dislocations

Kim Edward LeBlanc

1. Accounts for approximately 20 per cent of all dislocations.
2. Most commonly seen between between the ages of 5 and 25 years
3. May have associated fractures and soft tissue injuries.
4. Most commonly (>80 per cent) are posterior or posterolateral dislocations.
5. Usual mechanism of injury: fall on outstretched arm with arm in extension and adduction
6. Radial head subluxation: commonly known as "nursemaid's elbow"; seen in young children usually between ages 2 and 3 years, resulting from abrupt axial and pronating force on radius
7. Note any previous injuries to elbow.

Symptoms

1. Moderate to severe pain, particularly with motion
2. Inability to flex and extend, with impaired ability to pronate and supinate
3. May be unable to determine exact source of pain with nursemaid's elbow, although palpation and passive motion will localize to elbow (palpate wrist and shoulder first).

Key Symptom

Severe elbow pain

Clinical Findings

1. Swelling may obscure bony landmarks.
2. Pain is severe, particularly with motion.
3. Elbow held in partial flexion, unable to extend.
4. Very prominent olecranon process with anteriorly displaced humerus
5. Usually an obvious deformity
6. Possible neurovascular compromise

Key Signs

- Elbow held in flexion
- Readily apparent swelling and deformity
- Assess for neurovascular compromise.

Diagnostic Tests

1. Anterolateral and posterior radiographs; may require comparison views.
2. Type of dislocation defined by radiographs: posterior, anterior, medial, lateral, or divergent.
3. Radius and ulna almost always dislocate together.
4. Dislocation may have associated fracture: coronoid process, epicondyle, or radial head.
5. Nursemaid's elbow usually does *not* require radiographic examination, particularly if symptoms resolve quickly postreduction.
6. Exclude supracondylar fractures in skeletally immature patients (refer to orthopedics).

Key Tests

- Obtain radiographs before and after reduction to rule out fracture.
- Comparison radiographic views, particularly in the skeletally immature patient
- Observe lateral film for fat pad sign (anterior displacement of antecubital fat pad secondary to bleeding about elbow): usually indicative of fracture.

Differential Diagnosis

1. Subluxation of elbow
2. Elbow sprain or contusion
3. Fracture about the elbow: supracondylar, radius, olecranon

Management

1. Reduction should be performed as soon as possible with minimal trauma.

2. Delayed reduction results in increased swelling and decreases ability to ensure anatomic alignment.

3. Open reduction rarely required for simple dislocation.

4. Displaced fracture should be surgically reduced.

5. Document neurovascular status both pre- and postreduction.

6. Reduction, if performed early, may not require anesthesia; regional or general anesthesia decreases force required for reduction.

7. Reduction accomplished by applying gentle, longitudinal firm traction to forearm with elbow flexed while countertraction applied to arm.

8. Palpable clunk and full range of motion indicates proper medial and lateral alignment.

9. Nursemaid's elbow: elbow held in one hand with thumb overlying radial head, reduction by slowly flexing elbow while rotating forearm from full pronation to full supination; palpable click usually felt at radiocapitellar joint (indicates reduction).

Postreduction Management

1. Place forearm in long-arm, well-padded splint with elbow at 90 degrees.

2. Frequent reassessment of neurovascular status imperative.

3. Obtain repeat radiographs 3 to 5 days following reduction.

4. Nursemaid's elbow: following reduction full range of motion should be noted. Splinting is unnecessary. No radiographs are required.

Follow-Up

1. Immobilize for 7 to 10 days (2 to 3 weeks for dislocations with instability).

2. Follow immobilization with program of active exercises.

3. Immobilization beyond 3 weeks increases risk of loss of motion and development of flexion contractures.

4. Outcome worsened if dislocation has associated fractures.

5. Complications may result in long-term or permanent disability and include neurovascular problems, recurrent instability, joint stiffness, myositis ossificans, heterotopic calcifications, and prolonged swelling.

6. Nursemaid's elbow should not be immobilized or restricted in any way.

Key Treatment

- Closed reduction with early mobilization exercises
- Frequent assessment of neurovascular status

Bibliography

In Browner BD, Jupiter JB, Levine AM, et al (eds): Skeletal Trauma, 2nd ed, vol 2, pp 1474–1480. Philadelphia, WB Saunders Company, 1998.

Griggs SM, Weiss APC: Bony injuries of the wrist, forearm, and elbow. Clin Sports Med 1996;15:373–400.

Mehlhoff TL, Bennett JB: Elbow injuries. In Mellion MB, Walsh, WM, Shelton GL (eds): The Team Physicians' Handbook, 2nd ed, pp 461–473. Philadelphia, Hanley & Belfus, Inc, 1997.

In Steinberg GG, Akins CM, Baran DT, et al (eds): Ramamurti's Orthopedics in Primary Care, 2nd ed, pp 75–85. Baltimore, Williams & Wilkins, 1992.

Timmerman LA, Andrews JR: Arthroscopic treatment of posttraumatic elbow pain and stiffness. Am J Sports Med 1994;22:230–235.

Distal Interphalangeal Joint

Etiology: Mechanism of Injury

1. Dislocation is usually the result of hyperextension—uncommon injury.
2. Ligament and tendon injuries are more common at distal interphalangeal (DIP) joint.

Symptoms

1. Pain, swelling, or inability to flex or extend at DIP joint
2. Complaint of obvious deformity: May have been reduced already.

Clinical Findings

1. Deformity of distal phalanx position
   a. Displaced dorsally or laterally—most common (see Fig. 239–1 for normal anatomy)
   b. Volar dislocations are rare.

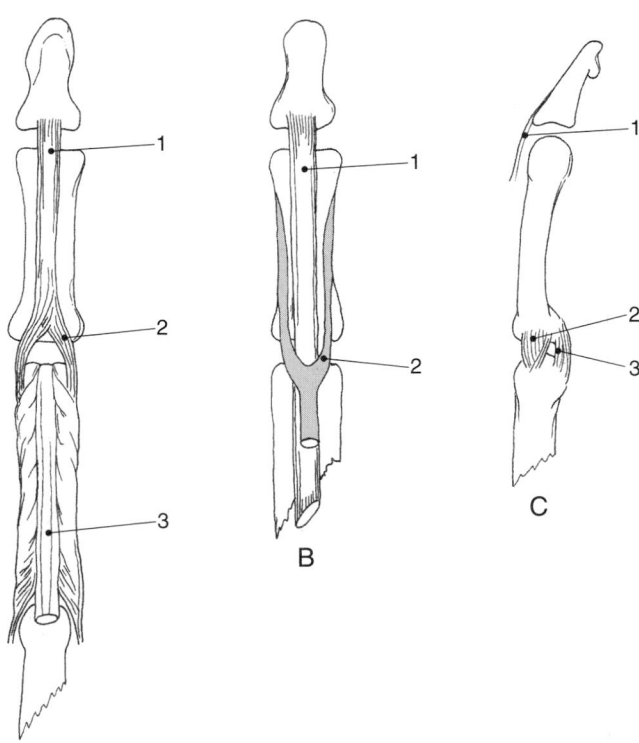

Figure 239–1 Normal anatomy. *A*, Dorsal (1) extensor tendon, (2) central slip, (3) extensor digitorum. *B*, Palmar (1) flexor digitorum profundus, (2) flexor digitorum superficialis. *C*, Lateral (1) extensor tendon, (2) collateral ligament, (3) volar plate.

2. *Careful* inspection for an open wound. Nail bed injuries should be repaired.

Radiographic Findings

1. Anteroposterior (AP) and lateral views of individual digits for clear view
2. Evaluate for avulsion fracture
3. Refer to hand surgeon if fracture greater than 25 per cent of articular surface

Associated Ligament Injuries (Compare Injured with Uninjured Side)

1. Collateral ligament sprains: Assess with varus and valgus stress in extension and 10 to 15 degrees of flexion.
2. Volar plate injuries: Assess with hyperextension stress at DIP.

Associated Tendon Injuries (Compare Injured with Uninjured Side)

1. Extensor tendon rupture ("baseball" or "mallet" finger)
   a. Result of forced flexion during active extension
   b. Assess active and resisted extension at DIP joint.
2. Flexor digitorum profundus tendon (FDP) rupture (Jersey finger)
   a. Result of forced hyperextension during active flexion
   b. Test for active and resisted flexion at DIP and with other digits held in extension to isolate FDP tendon.

Treatment

1. DIP dorsal dislocations/volar plate and collateral ligament injury
   a. Open dislocations should be referred to hand surgeon.
   b. Digital block should produce adequate anesthesia.
   c. Apply gentle traction in line with digit and pressure on dorsal aspect of distal phalanx until relocated.
   d. Evaluate for associated ligament/tendon injuries and repeat radiographs to rule out articular fracture after reduction.

e. Dorsal splint for 3 weeks with DIP in 10 to 15 degrees of flexion

2. Tendon injuries

a. Extensor tendon rupture with or without associated avulsion fracture: Splint DIP in full extension for 6 to 8 weeks.

b. FDP rupture: Splint in slight flexion and refer to hand surgeon; requires surgical repair within 7 to 10 days.

Activity/Follow-Up

1. DIP dorsal dislocations/volar plate and collateral ligament injury

a. Continue usual activities with splint for initial 3 weeks.

b. For sports, splint for additional 6 to 8 weeks.

2. Tendon injuries

a. Continue usual activity with splint for 6 to 8 weeks and then only for sports for additional 6 to 8 weeks.

b. FDP injury: per hand surgeon based on severity of injury

Proximal Interphalangeal Joint

Etiology/Mechanism of Injury

Dorsal dislocation resulting from axial loading and hyperextension

Symptoms

1. Pain and swelling at proximal interphalangeal (PIP) joint

2. Complaint of previous deformity: May have already been reduced.

Clinical Findings

1. Deformity of middle phalanx in relation to proximal phalanx

a. Dorsal dislocation most common: Involves volar plate tear.

b. Volar dislocation—rare injury: Disrupts extensor mechanism.

2. Location of tenderness suggests structures involved.

Radiographic Findings

AP and lateral views of individual digit for unobstructed view

1. Evaluate for articular surface or avulsion fracture.

2. If fracture greater than 25 per cent of articular surface, refer to hand surgeon.

Associated Ligament Injuries (Compare Injured with Uninjured Side)

1. Volar plate tear: Can occur alone or with dorsal dislocation.

a. Pain on volar surface of PIP joint

b. Laxity and pain with hyperextension of PIP

2. Collateral ligament injury (jammed or "stoved" finger)

a. May occur alone or with other injuries.

b. Detected by laxity with varus and valgus stress at PIP

Associated Tendon Injury: Central Slip Injury

1. Results from blunt trauma, lacerations, or forced hyperflexion.

2. Inability to extend at PIP actively or with resistance

3. Failure to treat leads to boutonnière deformity.

Treatment

1. Dorsal dislocations: Digital block may be used for anesthesia.

a. Relocate by accentuating deformity, applying *gentle* traction, and flexing finger to normal position.

b. Radiograph after reduction to rule out articular fracture.

c. Assess for associated injuries: Volar plate usually torn.

d. Splint PIP in 25 to 30 degrees of flexion for 2 to 3 weeks.

2. Volar plate tears splinted in 20 to 30 degrees of flexion for 2 to 3 weeks.

3. Collateral ligament injuries

a. Buddy tape in slight flexion until pain-free (about 4 to 6 weeks).

b. Complete tears may require surgical correction.

4. Central slip tears: Splint PIP in extension for 5 to 6 weeks.

Activity/Follow-Up

1. Encourage early motion with protection.

2. Dorsal dislocation: Buddy tape until pain-free motion.

3. Volar plate tears: Continue usual activities with splint for initial 2 to 3 weeks, then extension block splint until pain-free, and then buddy tape with sports activities for 2 to 3 more weeks.

4. Collateral ligament injury: Buddy tape until pain-free.

5. Central slip injury: Initial treatment for 5 to 6 weeks.
   a. Protective splint/buddy tape for additional 6 to 8 weeks
   b. Surgical repair for boutonnière deformity

Metacarpophalangeal Joint (Including Thumb)

Etiology/Mechanism of Injury
1. Dorsal dislocation results from forced hyperextension.
2. Second or fifth digit most commonly involved.
3. Lateral and volar dislocations much less common.

Symptoms
1. Pain and disability in flexion at metacarpophalangeal (MCP) joint
2. Deformity of proximal phalanx at MCP joint

Clinical Findings
1. Dorsal dislocation may be simple or complex.
   a. Simple dislocation presents with the proximal phalanx in 60 to 90 degrees of hyperextension on dorsum of metacarpal head; articular surfaces remain in contact.
   b. Complex dislocation shows only slight hyperextension and a characteristic dimple of palmar skin.
2. Lateral dislocation associated with collateral ligament injury
   a. Tenderness over involved collateral ligament
   b. Swelling in the space between the metacarpal heads
   c. Laxity with varus and valgus stress with MCP in full flexion
   d. Thumb requires specific evaluation (see "Thumb–Ulnar Collateral Ligament Injuries" below).

Radiologic Findings
1. Simple dorsal dislocations show articular surfaces in contact.
2. Complex dorsal dislocation: Pathognomonic sign is sesamoid within joint space.

Associated Ligament Injuries
1. Volar plate is torn from insertion on neck of metacarpal.
   a. Complex dislocation results from entrapment of volar plate between base of proximal phalanx and metacarpal head.

b. Simple dislocation can become complex when closed reduction is done incorrectly.
2. Collateral ligament injury with lateral dislocation

Associated Tendon Injury: Rupture of Extensor Hood
1. Results in tendon subluxation between metacarpal heads.
2. Decreased extension at MCP joint with weakness

Treatment
1. Simple dorsal dislocation: Traction may cause complex dislocation.
   a. Anesthesia: wrist or metacarpal block
   b. Wrist and interphalangeal joints flexed to relax tendons
   c. Proximal phalanx hyperextended to approximately 90 degrees—*no traction*
   d. Push base of proximal phalanx across articular surface.
   e. Flex gently to confirm positioning.
   f. Splint in 50 to 70 degrees of flexion for 7 to 10 days.
2. Complex dislocation: Refer to hand surgeon for open reduction.
3. Collateral ligament injury with lateral dislocation
   a. Without fracture: Splint in 50 to 70 degrees of flexion for 3 weeks.
   b. Unstable joint or avulsion fracture: Refer to hand surgeon.

Activity/Follow-Up
1. Simple and complex dislocations: early active motion with buddy tape until pain-free
2. Collateral ligament injury: Buddy tape for an additional 4 weeks.

Thumb–Ulnar Collateral Ligament Injuries

Etiology/Mechanism of Injury
1. Sudden valgus (abduction) stress with hyperextension
2. Commonly called "gamekeeper's" or "skier's" thumb.

Symptoms
1. Pain and swelling at MCP joint
2. Point of greatest pain localizes to ulnar aspect of MCP joint.

Clinical Findings

1. Tenderness at ulnar aspect of MCP joint
2. Assess degree of laxity: partial or complete tear
   a. Test in both flexion and extension.
   b. Compare injured and uninjured thumb.
3. Stener lesion develops when adductor aponeurosis lies between ends of torn ligament.

Radiographic Findings

Avulsion fracture of proximal phalanx or articular surface

Treatment

1. Partial tear: thumb spica cast for 3 to 6 weeks
2. Complete tear: operative repair; refer to hand surgeon.
3. Avulsion fractures
   a. Nondisplaced: thumb spica cast for 3 to 6 weeks
   b. Displaced greater than 5 mm or greater than 25 per cent articular surface: Refer.

Activity/Follow-Up

1. Partial tears and nondisplaced fractures: Continue usual activities with appropriate splint for 3 to 6 weeks, then activity as tolerated.
2. Operative repair: activities with cast for 4 weeks
   a. Removable splint for 2 to 3 weeks after casting
   b. Activity without splint *not* allowed until 10 to 12 weeks.

Bibliography

Aronowitz ER, Leddy JP: Closed tendon injuries of the hand and wrist in athletes. Clin Sports Med 1998;17: 449–467.

Duay GJ, Eaton RG: Dislocations and ligament injuries in the digits. In Green DP (ed): Operative Hand Surgery, 3rd ed, pp 767–791. New York, Churchill Livingstone, 1993.

Green DP, Strickland JW: Hand and wrist, section B: the hand. In DeLee JC, Drez D Jr (eds): Orthopedic Sports Medicine: Principles and Practice, vol 1, pp 945–983. Philadelphia, WB Saunders Company, 1994.

Langford SA, Whitaker JH, Toby EB: Thumb injuries in the athlete. Clin Sports Med 1998;17:553–566.

Palmer RE: Joint injuries of the hand in athletes. Clin Sports Med 1998;17:513–531.

240 Patellar Dislocations

Carl Winfield

Etiology

1. Mechanism of injury
   a. Lateral force vector associated with cutting maneuver
   b. Flexion and valgus positioning of the knee with forceful contraction of the quadriceps
   c. Direct trauma (rare) forcing patella out of trochlear groove
2. Risk factors
   a. Tight lateral structures
   b. Quadriceps dysplasia (weak vastus medialis obliques [VMO])
   c. Patella alta
   d. Increased Q angle
   e. Hypermobile patella
   f. More common in females
3. Pathology: tear of the medial patellofemoral ligament and VMO muscle complex from the femoral origin at the adductor tubercle (in the majority of patients)

Symptoms

1. Pain
2. Swelling
3. Inability to bear weight
4. Most spontaneously reduce when the knee is extended.

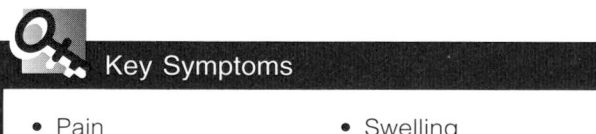

Key Symptoms

- Pain
- Swelling

Clinical Findings

1. Deformity: Patella located laterally, knee slightly flexed
2. Large effusion
3. Abnormal patellar tracking
4. Tenderness to palpation at medial retinacular structures and adductor tubercle
5. Patellar apprehension while pushing patella laterally

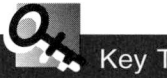

Key Signs

- Deformity
- Effusion
- Tenderness medial to patella

Tests

1. Radiographs to look for loose bodies and/or intra-articular fracture of articular surface of patella or lateral femoral condyle
2. Posteroanterior, lateral, and skyline or Merchant's views

Key Test

- Radiographs

Differential Diagnosis

1. Anterior cruciate ligament tear
2. Medial collateral ligament sprain
3. Patellar tendon rupture

Treatment

1. Prompt reduction via extension of the knee and gentle lateral pressure applied to the patella provides significant pain relief (DO NOT FORCE IF IT DOES NOT REDUCE EASILY).
2. RICE: *r*est, *i*ce, *c*ompression, and *e*levation
3. Immobilize in 10 degrees of flexion in knee immobilizer
4. Nonsteroidal anti-inflammatory drugs
5. Close follow-up
6. Orthopedic surgery referral
7. Arthroscopic removal of loose bodies if present
8. As far as definitive treatment to prevent recurrence, nonoperative versus operative approaches are controversial. No single operative procedure has obtained widespread approval.
9. Surgical procedures include extensor realignment procedures, lateral release.

10. Patellar stabilizing braces
11. Rehabilitation: Quadriceps/VMO retraining and strengthening
    a. Electrical stimulation
    b. Resistance exercise (isometric contractions early, then progressive resistance)
    c. Gradual return to activity with elimination of symptoms, normal strength, and range of motion

Key Treatment

- Extension with gentle lateral pressure—DO NOT FORCE

- Removal of loose bodies (arthroscopy)

Bibliography

Gaith WP, Pomphrey N, Merrill K: Functional treatment of patellar dislocation in an athletic population. Am J Sports Med 1996;24:785–791.

Garrick JG: Knee ligament injuries. In Sallis RE, Massimino F (eds): ACSM's Essentials of Sports Medicine, pp 412–417. St. Louis, Mosby–Year Book, Inc., 1997.

Maenpaa H, Lehto MOK: Patellar Dislocation: the long-term results of non-operative management in 100 patients. Am J Sports Med 1997;25:213–217.

Scuder GR: Surgical treatment for patellar instability. Orthop Clin North Am 1992;23:619–630.

Sallay PI, Poggi J, Speer KP, et al: Acute dislocation of the patella: A correlative pathoanatomic study. Am J Sports Med 1996;24:52–60.

241 Wrist Fractures

Reid B. Blackwelder

Etiology

1. One of the most common fractures
2. Usually occur as a result of a fall on an outstretched hand

Symptoms

1. Painful, swollen distal forearm and wrist and a history of a fall
2. Serious complications may be damage to an associated nerve, most commonly the median nerve; sensory deficits in the distribution of this nerve may be found.
3. As for any trauma, be aware of associated symptoms unrelated to the wrist injury that may be important to address, such as syncope, seizures, and so on.
4. A thorough history is essential in approaching a wrist injury.
   a. Ask about mechanism of injury, specifically about dorsi- or volar flexion, supination or pronation of forearm, point of contact, and activity (fall or blow).
   b. Ask about motor and sensory function.
   c. Document which hand is dominant.

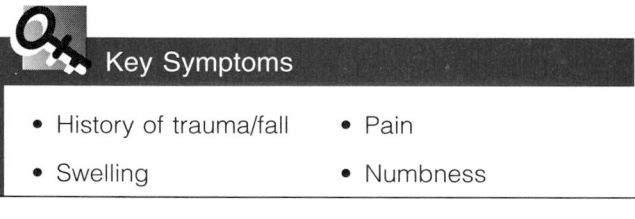

Key Symptoms

- History of trauma/fall
- Pain
- Swelling
- Numbness

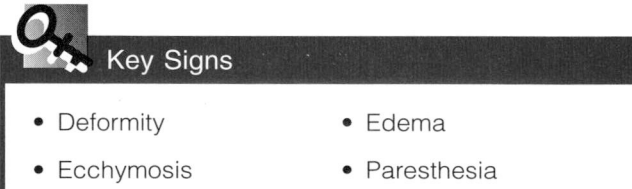

Key Signs

- Deformity
- Edema
- Ecchymosis
- Paresthesia

Anatomy

1. Knowledge of the anatomy of the wrist is essential; missed diagnoses can lead to difficult management problems and instability in the long run.
2. Wrist starts 3 cm proximal to the radiocarpal joint and extends to the carpometacarpal joints.

3. Bony components
   a. Distal end of the radius, the articular disk and the articulations with the proximal carpal row (scaphoid, lunate, and triquetral); this inherently unstable joint is strengthened by several groups of strong ligaments.
   b. Ulna has no direct bony articulations.
   c. Scaphoid, or navicular bone, serves a critical function as the stabilizer of the wrist complex during motion.
4. Muscular components
   a. No muscles originate or insert in the wrist.
   b. Extrinsic muscles arise on the forearm and insert at the base of the metacarpals, except for the flexor carpi ulnaris, which inserts on the pisiform; this arrangement causes motion to be translated across the rows of carpal bones and emphasizes the importance of the stability the scaphoid provides for the carpal bones.
5. Neurovascular components
   a. Radial and ulnar arteries cross the wrist to enter the palm, with superficial and deep branches forming arches.
   b. Ulnar nerve provides motor innervation to almost all the intrinsics and sensation to entire ulnar 1 1/2 fingers.
   c. Radial nerve does not supply any motor function to intrinsic muscles but does provide sensation to the dorsum of the hand and the dorsum of the radial 3 1/2 fingers and motor function to the extrinsic wrist and finger extensors.
   d. Median nerve travels in the carpal tunnel and supplies sensation to the palmar aspect and the dorsal fingertips of the radial 3 1/2 fingers and motor function to the thenar muscles.

Tests

1. Examination
   a. Completely expose the injured arm, and remove all rings, bracelets, and the like; often helpful to compare it with the uninjured side.
   b. Observe hand in relaxed position: Should see slight flexion, with normal curve of digits.

c. Inspect both dorsal and volar surfaces for deformity, laceration, swelling, and discoloration.

d. Palpate gently to try to localize the site of maximal pain. Pay particular attention to the anatomic "snuff box" located between the tendons of the extensor pollicus longus and the extensor pollicus brevis; pain in this area raises the possibility of a fracture of the scaphoid.

e. Assess vascular function by checking radial and ulnar pulses, performing Allen's test, and checking capillary refill. Be concerned about a pulsatile swelling, which may indicate an arterial injury.

f. Assess neurologic function by performing a complete sensory examination of the hand; deficits may be created by direct nerve damage, associated vascular injury, or compression.

(1) Checking light touch is not sufficient.

(2) Use a pin to test sensation to sharp and dull and a paper clip for two-point discrimination (>4 mm is suspicious for injury); check at each side of the finger pulp.

(3) Distribution of any sensory changes points to the nerve involved; as stated previously, median nerve injuries are the most common with wrist fractures.

(4) Realize the value of serial neurovascular checks, especially if a reduction is planned; signs of ischemia from compression may be slow to develop.

(5) Any symptoms suggesting nerve damage warrant immediate attention and, if not transient, referral to an orthopedist.

g. Assess motor function, including strength of muscle groups and range of motion of the wrist and fingers, specifically flexion, extension, and pronation-supination.

2. Radiographs

a. Radiographs are crucial in the evaluation of wrist injuries.

b. Obtain anteroposterior (AP; *some texts say PA*) and true lateral views with wrist in neutral position (no ulnar-radial deviation or palmar dorsiflexion of hand or wrist), and oblique views with 45 degrees each of supination and pronation.

c. May need scaphoid view if a carpal fracture is suspected.

Key Tests

- Complete vascular examination
- Complete neurologic examination
- Wrist radiographs

Differential Diagnosis

1. Colles' fracture

   a. The most common type, which presents with the classic "silver (dinner) fork" deformity

   b. Distal radius is fractured and displaced dorsally, often with shortening and radial deviation of the distal fragment; sometimes associated ulnar styloid or ulnar collateral ligament injury.

2. Smith's fracture (reverse Colles'): Results from fall with forearm supinated and hand extended, or after throwing a punch, or after sustaining a direct blow to the dorsum of the wrist with hand flexed and forearm pronated.

3. Barton's fracture: Involves an oblique dorsal rim fracture-dislocation through the articular surface of the distal radius.

4. Pediatric wrist fractures

   a. Epiphyseal fracture-separation (pediatric Colles')

      (1) Diagnosis may be difficult if nondisplaced; remember wrist sprains are uncommon in children because the ligamentous complexes are stronger than the epiphyseal plate.

      (2) Tenderness over epiphysis strongly suggests fracture.

   b. Torus fractures

      (1) Occur approximately 2.5 cm proximal to wrist.

      (2) No displacement occurs; radius "buckles."

5. Scaphoid fracture

   a. Most commonly encountered carpal bone fracture; must be considered in differential diagnosis of wrist fractures.

   b. Complication is avascular necrosis, although 90 per cent heal without complication.

   c. Clinical examination will reveal pain at the wrist but particularly in the anatomic snuffbox.

   d. Diagnosis is by clinical suspicion followed by scaphoid films 1 to 2 weeks after the injury if pain persists.

Treatment

Reduction of Fractures

1. General points
   a. If seen within a few hours, usually can reduce under local anesthesia (hematoma block).
   b. Reduction involves reversing the forces causing the injury.
   c. Always repeat a neurovascular examination after any reduction.
2. Colles' fracture
   a. Disimpact the distal fragment with longitudinal traction and thumb pressure to reduce the dorsal angulation.
   b. Provide ulnar deviation with thumb pressure to reduce the radial displacement.
   c. Apply upward pressure with wrist slightly flexed and ulnarly deviated to maintain reduction until a cast is placed, usually a sugar-tong splint for 3 to 7 days.
   d. Elevate with ice for 48 to 72 hours, with active motion of the fingers.
   e. Repeat radiograph within 7 to 10 days. Occasional loss of reduction may occur when the swelling subsides—may be acceptable in older patients.
   f. Immobilize with sugar-tong or short-arm cast for 6 weeks.
3. Smith's fracture
   a. If no involvement of the articular surface, may be treated as Colles', except the wrist is immobilized in supination.
   b. If the articular surface is involved, refer for treatment.
4. Barton's fracture: Refer in all cases because often requires open reduction and fixation.
5. Pediatric fractures
   a. Epiphyseal fracture-dislocation
      (1) With presence of tenderness, consider placing a short-arm cast or sugar-tong even if the radiographs are normal.
      (2) Repeat radiograph in 2 weeks. If callus, continue cast 2 more weeks; if none, can remove cast and sprain has been treated.
      (3) Important to discuss the possibility of growth plate injury with parents; risk of premature closure and shortening of the limb exists.
      (4) Consider referral to orthopedic surgeon; definitely refer for displacement with angulation.
   b. Torus fracture: Treat with short-arm cast for 3 to 4 weeks.

6. Scaphoid fracture—either documented or suspected
   a. Because fractures are often not initially seen on radiograph, may treat as fracture with immobilization for 2 weeks and repeat film; if study is still inconclusive and the clinical picture is still suspicious, get bone scan.
   b. Good reduction is necessary; put palmar-to-dorsal pressure on the distal fragment to reduce volar flexion.
   c. Place in short-arm spica thumb cast to the tip of the thumb; may require up to 12 to 24 weeks.
   d. Refer for greater than 1 mm displacement.

Medications

1. Unless contraindicated, nonsteroidal anti-inflammatory drugs are often helpful.
2. Appropriate analgesia is always beneficial—broken bones hurt!
3. Consider mild sedation prior to reduction of fractures.

Patient Education

1. Elevate wrist for 24 to 48 hours after treatment.
2. Ice may be applied, but keep cast dry; limit icing to 20 minutes an hour.
3. If sugar-tong placed, provide a sling.
4. Discuss signs and symptoms of ischemia and need to contact physician immediately if numbness, cyanosis, or severe pain occurs.

Key Treatment

- Definitive treatment depends on type of fracture.
- Initial treatment is reduction, if needed, or referral.
- Rest, ice, compression, elevation, nonsteroidal anti-inflammatory drugs (RICED)
- Splint/immobilize
- Repeat radiograph if reduced and splinted/casted.
- Analgesia

Follow-Up

1. See patient in 3 to 4 days to evaluate cast.
2. If necessary, radiographs may be taken with the cast on to check adequacy of reduction.
3. Once the appropriate time has passed, usually 6 weeks, remove the cast and repeat radiograph.
4. Initiate rehabilitation exercises for hand and wrist.

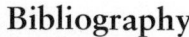

Bibliography

Bisschop P: The wrist, thumb and hand. In Ombrecht L, Bisschop P, ter Veer HJ, et al (eds): A System of Orthopaedic Medicine, pp 335–352. London, WB Saunders Company, 1995.

Breen TF: Wrist and hand. In Steinberg GG, Akins CM, Baran DT, et al (eds): Ramamurti's Orthopaedics in Primary Care, 2nd ed, pp 105–123. Baltimore, Williams & Wilkins, 1992.

Mercier LR: Practical Orthopedics, 3rd ed, pp 119–124. St. Louis, Mosby–Year Book, 1991.

Morgan RL, Linder MM: Common wrist injuries. Am Fam Physician 1997;55:857–868.

Tolo VT, Wood B: Pediatric Orthopaedics in Primary Care, pp 55–61. Baltimore, Williams & Wilkins, 1993.

242 Finger Fractures

Kenneth L. Taylor-Butler

1. Because finger function is crucial to so many activities of daily living, it is important to have a clear understanding of the anatomy of the finger and hand in order to develop a system for proper injury evaluation, treatment, and referral. In order to prevent long-term disability, the supporting ligaments and tendons of the metacarpophalangeal and proximal interphalangeal joints must be evaluated and treated quickly.

2. It is easy to assume that the inability to move a joint is a result of the pain and swelling of the injury. However, soft tissue injuries are a major source of instability with functional impairment. Therefore, the assumption that, as swelling dissipates, function will return is not always valid. Furthermore, fractures may be occult, with patients having performed "on-the-field" reduction of the finger, returning it to a normal appearance. For that reason the fate of the injured hand will be determined by the judgment of the physician who first sees the patient.

3. In evaluating the finger, it is important to understand first the normal biomechanics and second the mechanism of injury.

   a. The most frequently seen fractures in the body are those of the metacarpals and phalanges. Phalangeal fractures are commonly seen in ball sports.

   b. The etiology of finger fractures is often age dependent: sports are the leading cause among those 10 to 29 years of age, whereas falls predominate in those over 70 years of age.

   c. Common fractures, such as the mallet/baseball finger, can be diagnosed readily based on the disability and mechanism of injury. Unusual injuries such as the Jersey finger will require a high index of clinical suspicion in order to make the diagnosis.

   d. Because the distal hand is most readily exposed to trauma, it is understandable that the long finger is injured twice as often as the next most injured digit, the thumb.

Tests

1. Inspect for maximum tenderness and swelling.
2. Test neurologic function (two-point discrimination, strength).
3. Assess vascular status (capillary refill).
4. Evaluate individual joint range of motion.
5. Look for signs of instability: rotation or angulation.

PEARL

Because there is wide variability of laxity in individuals, always compare with the uninjured side. During stress testing, flex the joint at 30 degrees in order to reduce the stabilizing effects of the volar plate.

---

6. Perform stress testing of anatomic structures involved.
7. Three radiographic views (posteroanterior, lateral, and oblique) are necessary in order to completely evaluate any swollen digit.

Complications

1. Malunion: malrotation, volar or lateral angulation, shortening
2. Loss of motion
3. Infection
4. Post-traumatic arthritis

Clinical Findings

Is there articular surface disruption? Fractures that involve more than 25 per cent of the articular surface are considered unstable and require surgical intervention in order to prevent long-term disability with stiffness, deformity, and pain.

1. Rotation is disruption of the fracture around the center of the longitudinal axis of the digit. When alignment is correct, the tubercle of the scaphoid is the focus of all fingers (Fig. 242–1).
2. Angulation is disruption of the longitudinal axis of the digit with the fracture fragment falling out of alignment.

PEARLS

Referral to orthopedic service for operative repair is generally necessary for fractures that are irreducible, open, or unstable.

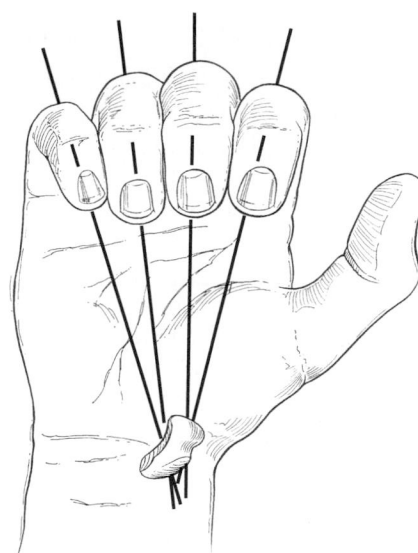

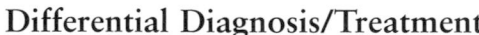

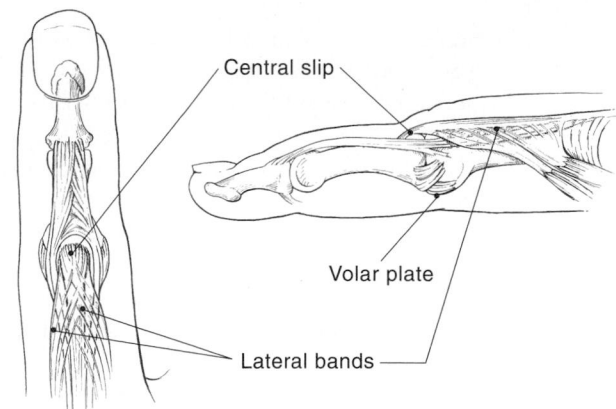

Figure 242–2 Injury to central clip with volar subluxation of lateral bands. (Copyright Joan M. Beck, Beck Visual Communications, Inc., Minneapolis, MN. Used with permission.)

Figure 242–1 With correct alignment, tubercle of the scaphoid is the focus of all fingers. (Copyright Joan M. Beck, Beck Visual Communications, Inc., Minneapolis, MN. Used with permission.)

Differential Diagnosis/Treatment

1. Fractures of the distal phalanx
   a. Extra-articular
      (1) Longitudinal, comminuted, transverse
      (2) Treatment
         (a) Splint the distal interphalangeal (DIP) joint for 4 weeks.
         (b) Treat soft tissue; evacuate hematoma.
   b. Intra-articular
      (1) Dorsal avulsion (mallet finger)
         (a) Hyperflexion at DIP joint. Extensor tendon may be stretched, ruptured, or avulsed from its attachment to the distal phalange.
         (b) Treatment: Immobilize in extension with dorsal splint for 4 weeks.
      (2) Flexor digitorum profundus avulsion (Jersey finger)
         (a) Hyperextension of the DIP joint while the flexor tendon is contracting
         (b) Treatment: Requires early referral to a hand surgeon because the tendon tends to retract into the palm.
2. Fractures of the middle and proximal phalanx
   a. Crush injuries with force perpendicular to the long axis of the digit
   b. Treatment
      (1) Stable (no angulation, rotation, or displacement): dynamic splinting (buddy taping); early range of motion

(2) Unstable; early surgical reduction with immobilization
3. Volar plate disruption: hyperextension of the proximal interphalangeal (PIP) joint, often with dislocation (Fig. 242–2).
   a. Swan neck deformity: distal disruption of the volar plate
   b. Pseudoboutonnière deformity: proximal disruption of the volar plate.
   c. Treatment: immobilization or dynamic splinting of the PIP joint for 4 weeks
4. Boutonnière deformity: injury to central slip (Fig. 242–2) with volar subluxation of lateral bands
   a. Direct dorsal trauma over the joint
   b. Forced flexion of the PIP joint
   c. The postinjury volar position of the lateral bands makes them extensors of the DIP joint.
   d. Treatment
      (1) Splint the PIP joint in extension for 4 to 6 weeks.
      (2) Dynamic splinting with range-of-motion exercises.

PEARLS

This injury can be categorized by examining the DIP joint. In a true boutonnière injury, the DIP joint will be hyperextended, whereas in the pseudoboutonnière injury the DIP joint will be in a normal position.

---

5. Thumb injuries
   a. Ulnar collateral ligament strain (gamekeeper's thumb): abduction stress with the metacarpophalangeal joint in extension

(1) Stener lesion: The adductor pollicis longus aponeurosis folds back on itself and becomes interposed between the ends of the ligament, preventing healing.

(2) Treatment: Because Stener lesion occurs frequently, it is recommended that gamekeeper's thumb injuries be treated surgically in order to prevent chronic instability.

b. Carpometacarpal joint of the thumb (Bennett's fracture)

(1) Fracture/subluxation at the base of the first metacarpal; occurs when the thumb metacarpal is axially loaded and partially flexed. The abductor pollicis longus is the deforming force pulling the metacarpal fragment radially, proximally, and dorsally.

(2) Treatment

(a) Nondisplaced: long-arm thumb spica cast for 3 weeks, followed by 3 weeks in a short-arm thumb spica cast

(b) Displaced: Internal fixation required.

(c) An active exercise program in order to obtain full range of motion in both nondisplaced and displaced treatment

Bibliography

Bowman SH, Simon RR: Metacarpal and phalangeal fractures. Emerg Med Clin North Am 1993;11:671–702.

DeJonge JJ, Kingma J: Phalangeal fractures of the hand. Br J Hand Surg 1994;198:168–170.

Hoffman DF, Schaffer TC: Management of common finger injuries. Am Fam Physician 1991;43:1594–1607.

Lo I, Richards RS: Combined central slip and volar plate injuries at the PIP joint. J Hand Surg [Br] 1995;20:390–391.

Mastey RD, Weiss APC: Primary care of hand and wrist athletic injuries. Clin Sports Med 1997;16:705–724.

Seno N, Hashizume H: Fractures of the base of the middle phalanx of the finger. J Bone Joint Surg [Br] 1997;79:758–763.

Stern PJ: Fractures of the metacarpals and phalanges. In Green DP (ed): Operative Hand Surgery, pp 695–758. New York, Churchill Livingstone, 1993.

243 Ankle Fractures

Allan V. Abbott

Etiology

1. Patients commonly remember the event, but cannot recall details of the mechanism of injury.

2. The most common mechanism of injury is inversion of the ankle with lateral ligament sprains and distal fibula fractures; however, a wide variety of injury mechanisms are possible with many resultant fractures.

3. Certain sports are associated with particular injuries: skiing is associated with fractures of the tibia or fibula, football with anteroinferior tibiofibular ligament injuries, basketball with ankle sprains, and dancing with tendinitis and stress fractures.

4. In elderly patients, ankle fractures may present as subacute problems and may reflect neglect by the patient or caregiver.

5. In cases of fractures resulting from seemingly minor trauma in older patients, an evaluation for osteoporosis is warranted.

Symptoms

1. When the patient recalls a "crack" or a "pop," a serious ligament rupture or fracture should be considered.

2. Inability to bear weight suggests a fracture.

Key Symptoms

- A history of a "crack" or "pop" suggests a fracture or ligament rupture.

- Severe pain and rapid swelling suggests a serious injury.

Clinical Findings

1. After the injury, rapid progression of swelling and severe pain suggest the presence of a fracture, hemarthrosis, or serious ligament rupture.

2. Examination starts with assessment of perfusion, deformity, ecchymosis, and edema.

3. Next, passive and active range of motion are tested.

4. Assessment of point tenderness may localize bone, ligament, or tendon injury, particularly when the examination is performed soon after the injury.

5. Assessment of ability to bear weight should proceed if (1) suspicion of serious fracture is low, (2) location of point tenderness does not indicate need for radiographs, or (3) radiographs have ruled out a fracture.

6. Obvious deformity or dislocation will require radiographs and urgent orthopedic consulation.

7. The anterior drawer test can also help determine ankle stability. An anterior shift of 8 to 10 mm compared to the opposite ankle suggests a tear of the anterior talofibular ligament. To perform this test, stabilize the distal tibia, grasp the heel with the dominant hand, and apply anterior force.

8. Determine if the fracture is open (compound). Even the smallest laceration or puncture site near a fracture should arouse suspicion of an open fracture.

Key Signs

- Inability to bear weight

- Deformity or neurovascular compromise

- Tenderness of bone over malleoli

- Joint instability

- Open fracture

Tests

1. Radiographs

   a. The "Ottawa Rules" are widely recognized as guidelines for identifying patients who need radiographs after ankle injury. These rules state that radiographs are required when

   (1) There is bone tenderness at the posterior edge of the distal 6 cm or tip of either malleolus.

   (2) The patient is unable to bear weight for at least four steps immediately after injury and at the time of evaluation.

b. The Ottawa Rules do not apply in cases of subacute or chronic injury.

2. Standard views include the anteroposterior (AP), lateral, and mortise views.

    a. *The AP view* identifies fractures of the malleoli, distal fibula and tibia, horizontal surface of the tibia (plafond), talus, and calcaneus. The AP view should include the entire fibula if there is lateral tenderness proximal to the lateral malleolus.

    b. *The lateral view* identifies the anterior and posterior tibial margins, talar neck, posterior talar process, and calcaneus. Any incongruity of the articular space between the talar dome and the distal tibia suggests instability.

    c. *The mortise view* (taken with the ankle in 15 to 25 degrees of internal rotation) allows evaluation of the congruity of the articular surface between the dome of the talus and the mortise. This joint space should be equal throughout the joint. The presence of any joint space abnormality suggests instability.

3. Plain films can miss subtle fractures or ligamentous injuries. When radiographs are negative, or when unexplained symptoms persist, other imaging or orthopedic consultation is appropriate.

    a. *Stress radiographs* with the ankle in inversion can confirm lateral ankle ligament disruption and instability (compare with the opposite ankle).

    b. A *bone scan* can detect soft tissue injuries such as syndesmotic disruption, and subtle stress fractures (as early as 1 to 2 days after the stress fracture) or osteochondral fractures.

    c. *Computerized tomography* scans image bones and soft tissue in a manner superior to plain films and can help in cases of subtle fractures and ligamentous injury.

    d. *Magnetic resonance imaging* provides clear imaging of soft tissue structures, ligaments, tendons, and muscles. It is becoming the preferred and definitive imaging method in sports medicine.

Key Tests

- Neurovascular examination
- AP, lateral, and mortise view radiographs

Differential Diagnosis

1. Ankle sprains: May require radiographic evaluation to determine the absence of fracture.

2. Syndesmosis sprains: sprains of the tibiofibular ligament

3. Arthritis: Onset may be triggered by trauma.

4. Growth plate injury in children

Treatment

1. The RICE (*rest, ice, compression, elevation*) acronym is appropriate for the initial treatment of the injured ankle. The ankle is splinted, elevated, and iced, and an elastic bandage is applied to minimize swelling.

2. Orthopedic consultation is required in all open, displaced, or potentially unstable fractures (Table 243–1).

    a. Dislocations or displaced fractures must be reduced rapidly, at least within 6 to 8 hours.

    b. The goal in displaced fractures is to achieve a nearly perfect reduction before even minor changes in the integrity of the ankle joint can have disastrous results.

3. A small avulsion chip fracture from the distal fibula can be treated like an ankle sprain.

4. Lateral malleolar fractures and minor ankle fractures with no displacement can be treated by a primary care physician.

    a. A posterior splint and elastic bandage will allow for increased swelling during the first few days after the fracture.

    b. A circumferential short leg cast can be applied after 5 to 10 days when the swelling has subsided.

    c. The patient should be non–weight-bearing for the first 2 to 3 weeks, and may then be allowed to bear weight if the fracture remains stable.

    d. The cast can be replaced after 4 to 6 weeks with a functional brace that allows some an-

TABLE 243–1. FRACTURES REQUIRING ORTHOPEDIC CONSULTATION

Unimalleolar fractures
Fibula fracture at or just proximal to the tibiotalar joint line
Lateral malleolar fracture with deltoid ligament rupture
Lateral malleolar fracture with widened medial clear space
Displaced lateral malleolar fracture
Displaced medial malleolar fracture
Medial malleolar fracture with lateral collateral ligament rupture
Unimalleolar fracture with syndesmotic diastasis
Displaced posterior malleolar fracture
Posterior malleolar fracture involving more than 25% of joint surface
All bimalleolar fractures
All trimalleolar fractures
All intra-articular fractures with step deformity
All open fractures
All pilon fractures

kle motion until the fracture is completely healed. Early joint mobilization improves subsequent return of normal joint function.

e. Physical therapy and rehabilitation exercises are important after removal of the cast, and until full function is regained.

f. Full sports activities should not be resumed for approximately 3 months.

Medication

1. Unless contraindicated, nonsteroidal anti-inflammatory drugs are often helpful. Ibuprofen is inexpensive and effective when given every 6 to 8 hours.

2. Pain relief with acetaminophen and codeine and similar medications is helpful, especially within the first few days after a fracture.

Activity

1. Ankle fractures should be elevated as much as possible to minimize swelling during the first 2 to 3 days after injury.

2. The patient should remain non–weight-bearing for the first 2 to 3 weeks after fracture, then may walk in a walking cast or boot.

Patient Education

1. Call the doctor immediately for increasing pain, numbness, or loss of function under the cast; these suggest that the ankle has swollen and that the cast is too tight.

2. The casted ankle should be elevated to a level above the heart for the first several days to reduce swelling.

3. Walking on the casted ankle should not occur until directed by the physician.

4. Do not get the cast wet.

5. Do not scratch the skin around the cast or poke things down inside the cast.

Key Treatment

- Initial RICE treatment includes rest (immobilization), ice, elevation, and light compression to minimize swelling.

- Treatment depends upon the type of fracture.

- Orthopedic consultation is required in all open, displaced, or potentially unstable fractures.

- Fracture-dislocations that threaten neurovascular function or soft tissue viability should receive consultation and reduction immediately.

- Minor stable fractures are immobilized and casted for 6 to 8 weeks.

Follow-Up (of Minor Stable Fractures)

1. The patient should return for re-examination in 24 to 48 hours after casting to ensure that the cast is not too tight.

2. The patient should return again at 1 week and 3 weeks for re-evaluation with radiographs to ensure maintenance of position.

3. At 3 weeks, the cast should be reapplied if it has loosened, or converted for weight bearing. A cast-boot can be applied for walking.

4. At 6 to 8 weeks the cast is removed, and the patient can begin careful ambulation if the examination and radiographs reveal adequate healing.

Bibliography

Cooper C: The crippling consequences of fractures and their impact on quality of life. Am J Med 1997;103: 12S–17S.

Dovan JR, McKeag DB: Ankle splinting, taping, and casting. In Pfenninger JL (ed): Procedures for Primary Care Physicians, pp 1003–1013. St. Louis, CV Mosby Company, 1994.

Geissler WB, Tsao AK, Hughes JL: Fractures and injuries of the ankle. In Rockwood CA, Green DP, Bucholz RW, et al (eds): Rockwood and Green's Fractures in Adults, 4th ed, pp 2201–2266. Philadelphia, JB Lippincott Company, 1996.

Rosen: Emergency Medicine: Concepts and Clinical Practice, 4th ed, pp 821–835. St. Louis, Mosby–Year Book, 1998.

Tropp H, Norlin R: Ankle performance after ankle fracture: a randomized study of early mobilization. Foot Ankle Int 1995;16:79–83.

Indications

1. Fractures of the extremities
2. Ligament sprains and tears
3. Overuse injuries

Contraindications

1. Unstable or irreducible fractures
2. Avoid circumferential casting for an acute injury with soft tissue swelling; splint instead.

Preparation

1. Size and position of cast or splint
   a. Each injury is unique (see Bibliography for sources discussing the types of cast/splint for a particular injury).
   b. Immobilize joint above and below the fracture.
   c. Immobilize forearm and hand injuries in position of function (wrist extension 30 degrees, hand like it is holding a half tennis ball).
   d. Keep foot in neutral or slight dorsiflexion for lower leg and foot injuries.
2. Determine type of material.
   a. Plaster: inexpensive and easy to form but falls apart when wet and may impede radiographic evaluation.
   b. Fiberglass: strong, lightweight, waterproof, and radiolucent. However, harder to mold and expensive.
   c. Thermoplastics: used for splints, expensive
   d. Be familiar with package insert of the material.
3. Select appropriate width of material.
   a. Circumferential casts
      (1) Five- to 6-inch rolls for the upper leg
      (2) Four- to 5-inch rolls for the lower leg
      (3) Two- to 4-inch rolls for the hand, wrist, and lower arm
   b. Splints are one-half the circumference of the extremity.
4. Remove jewelry from injured extremity (e.g., rings).

5. Assistant to control the extremity

Equipment

1. Casting or splint material
2. Sink with plaster trap
3. Soap and water
4. Stockinette
5. Thick cotton padding (Webril)
6. Heavy-duty scissors
7. Elastic wrap for splints
8. Gloves for handling material
9. Cast shoe, sling, or crutches

Anesthesia

Local or digital block with lidocaine (Xylocaine) for some closed reductions

Precautions

1. Avoid cast that is too tight and does not allow for soft tissue swelling.
2. Avoid pressure over bony prominences and superficial neurovascular bundles; pad liberally.
3. Cast or splint should not be too loose or poor stablization of joint or fracture will result.

WARNING

- **Be vigilant for any patient complaints in the first 24 to 48 hours after cast application:**
  - **Increasing pain, especially with passive movement of digits**
  - **Paralysis**
  - **Paresthesia**
  - **Pallor**
  - **Pulselessness**

- **To treat, bivalve the cast, cotton padding, and stockinette.**

- **If problem persists, suspect compartment syndrome, and obtain urgent orthopedic consultation.**

Technique

1. Measure the material needed over the patient's uninjured side.
2. For casting, stockinette should be 3 inches longer than needed on each end. Gently slide this over the injured extremity, and avoid bunching the material.
3. Wrap thick cotton padding (Webril) over the stockinette. Start distally and work proximally, overlapping the rolls 50 per cent. Apply extra padding over bony prominences and superficial neurovascular bundles.
4. When handling plaster or fiberglass, wear gloves. Hold the edge of the roll between the index finger and thumb so that the beginning of the roll is not lost as it is immersed in water. Immerse plaster roll in tepid water (77° to 95° F) until bubbles stop rising from the roll. Remove from water and gently compress the ends of the roll inward to remove excess water from the plaster.

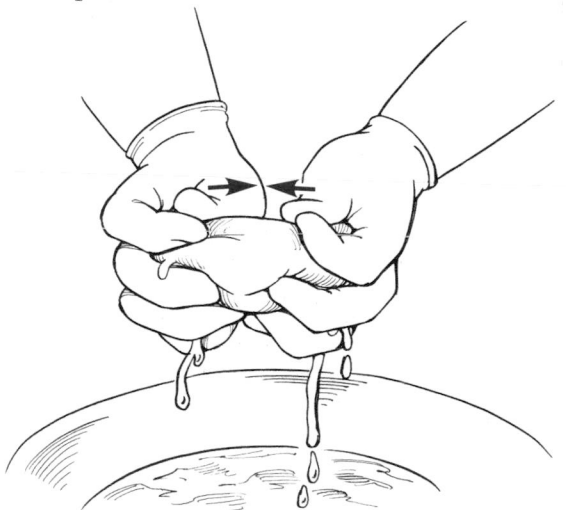

For fiberglass, immerse in cool water (68° F) and squeeze the roll several times. Remove and shake excess water off the fiberglass roll before application. Keep in mind, the warmer the water, the faster the material sets.

5. Follow the direction of the cotton padding to apply the rolls of casting material to the extremity, overlapping each roll by 50 per cent. Do not pull or stretch the material; simply lay it down. Tuck and smooth excess material with the palms.

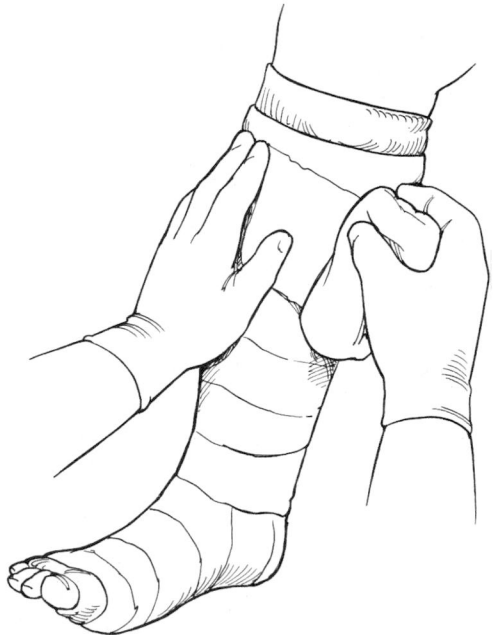

Use three to four layers of fiberglass or four to six layers of plaster to make the cast. Thicken weight-bearing areas and incorporate longitudinal splints into the cast to give extra support where needed, especially when using plaster.

6. Be careful not to indent plaster with the fingertips. Trim rough edges. Fold extra stockinette back over the ends of the cast, then apply the final layer of casting material. This will create smooth and comfortable cast edges.
7. Splinting requires 12 strips of plaster measured slightly longer than the injured extremity. Three to four strips of fiberglass achieve the same purpose. The splinting material is immersed in water, squeezed out in an accordion fashion, laid flat, and gently massaged into a uniform slab. Apply a cover of four layers of cotton padding on both sides of the splint, and wrap the padded splint on the extremity with elastic wrap.

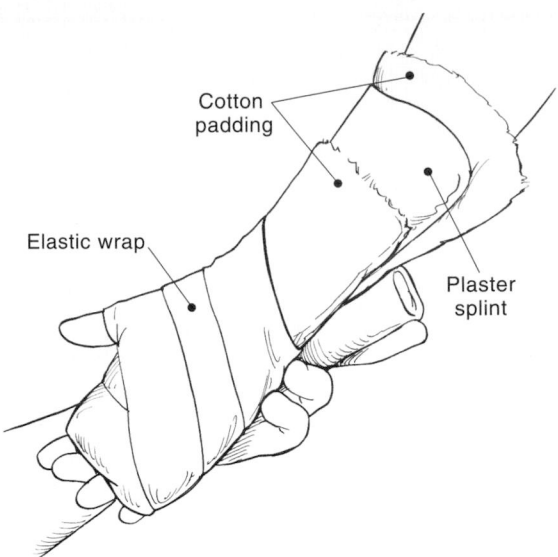

Cotton padding

Elastic wrap

Plaster splint

As an alternative, preformed splinting material may be used.

8. Plaster will set within 5 to 10 minutes and completely harden within 48 hours. Fiberglass also sets in 5 minutes and hardens for weight bearing in 20 minutes. Avoid manipulation of the cast after it has set.

9. Use a cast shoe to protect the lower extremity cast. A rubber walking platform can be incorporated into the bottom of the cast for weight-bearing patients.

Follow-Up

1. Repeat radiograph after casting a fracture that requires closed reduction

2. Care of the extremity

   a. Keep elevated for 24 to 48 hours.

   b. Move muscles and joints that are free.

   c. Watch for danger signs of compression.

   d. Avoid getting cast and padding wet (syn-thetic stockinette and padding required if fiberglass cast expected to get wet).

3. Re-evaluate patient in 1 to 2 weeks.

4. Cast removal

   a. Brace hand when using cast saw.

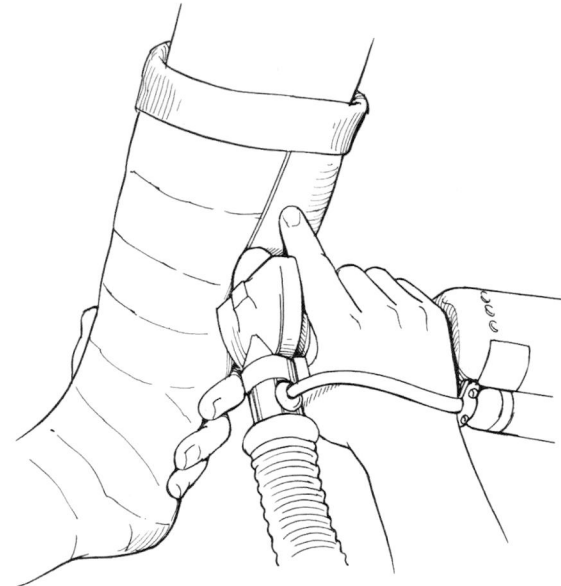

   b. Bivalve the cast, then use cast separator.

 Bibliography

Billotti JD, McKeag DB, Menkes JS: Fast splinting techniques for fractures. Patient Care 1993;148–180.

Connolly J: The Management of Fractures and Dislocations, 3rd ed, pp 115–120. Philadelphia, WB Saunders Company, 1981.

Dvorkin ML: Office Orthopaedics, pp 1–296. Norwalk, CT, Appleton & Lange, 1993.

Eathorne SW, McKeag DB: Cast immobilization. In Pfenninger JL, Fowler GC (eds): Procedures for Primary Care Physicians, pp 1014–1027. St. Louis, CV Mosby Company, 1994.

Snider RK, Bruch RF, Schwarter JF, et al: Splinting principles. In Snider RK (ed): Essentials of Musculoskeletal Care, pp 59–66. Rosemont, IL, American Academy of Orthopedic Surgeons, 1997.

244 Foot Fractures

Robert L. Hatch

Tarsal Fractures

There are two broad classes of tarsal fractures, with different etiologies and management.

Tarsal Avulsion Fractures

Etiology
Twisting injury (usually)

Symptoms
Localized pain following injury

Clinical Findings
Point tenderness at fracture site, mild to moderate swelling

Differential Diagnosis
1. Sprain (examination may be identical, but radiograph should be normal with a sprain)
2. Accessory ossicle or old fracture. Radiographically, these generally appear rounded, are well corticated on all sides, and are usually nontender. Acute avulsion fractures are more irregular, lack cortical thickening along the inside edge, and are point tender.

WARNING

Beware of chip fractures that involve articular surfaces (the dome of the talus is a common site). These injuries often lead to severe degenerative joint disease. Referral of such fractures is strongly recommended (management differs from below). Suspect a talar dome fracture when an ankle sprain is slow to heal.

Treatment and Follow-Up
1. Recommend consultation or referral if tender on both sides of foot (possible subluxation), if fragment displaced more than 2 mm, or if fragment larger than 5 mm.
2. Nondisplaced or minimally displaced (i.e., less than 2 mm)
   a. Following initial management (Tables 244–1 and 244–2), apply short-leg walking cast (SLWC) for 4 to 6 weeks. Some avulsions are best managed without casting.
   b. Special considerations
      (1) Consider referral if fragment becomes more distracted.
      (2) Healing may occur without development of obvious callus, so base further treatment decisions less on follow-up radio-

TABLE 244–1. INITIAL MANAGEMENT OF AN ACUTE FRACTURE

1. Rule out complications that require emergent referral/consultation: neurovascular injury, significant soft tissue injury, open fracture, and compartment syndrome.
2. Splint, ice, elevation, pain control. If must apply cast acutely (e.g., fracture unstable), strongly recommend splinting cast to avoid iatrogenic compartment syndrome.
3. Give instructions about warning signs of vascular compromise.

TABLE 244–2. FOLLOW-UP OF FOOT FRACTURES: GENERAL GUIDELINES

1. Apply cast when no further swelling is expected (preferably after most swelling has resolved, i.e., 2 to 5 days after injury).
2. Consider cast check in 12 to 24 hours to be sure cast is comfortable and to rule out iatrogenic compartment syndrome (especially if compliance with elevation questionable or high risk for more swelling).
3. If fracture is stable (i.e., unlikely to lose position), examine out of plaster in 3 to 6 weeks (varies by fracture).
   a. Discontinue cast if radiographic and clinical evidence of healing is present (i.e., callus seen on radiograph and resolution of all but minimal point tenderness at the fracture site).
   b. If not yet healed, replace cast and re-evaluate every 1 to 2 weeks until healed or until benefits of continued casting are outweighed by drawbacks (such as permanent decreased range of motion resulting from prolonged immobilization); consultation beneficial if unsure.
   c. After removal of cast, begin range-of-motion (ROM) exercises and gradual resumption of activity; re-evaluate 2 to 4 weeks after cast removal to assess progress, and consider referral to physical therapist if ROM/normal function slow to return.
4. If fracture unstable or potentially unstable, repeat radiographs *in plaster* (i.e., do not remove cast) before callus expected (i.e., 8 to 10 days after fracture for an adult). If fracture has lost position, refer it then while it is relatively easy to reposition. If position maintained, obtain later radiographs in plaster when possible.

graphs and more on symptoms such as pain and tenderness.

Fractures Through the Body of a Tarsal Bone

Etiology

High-energy blows (e.g., crush or a fall from a great height), twisting injuries

Symptoms

Swelling and pain, which may be marked

Clinical Findings

Swelling, tenderness, ecchymosis (later)

Differential Diagnosis

1. Dislocation (comparison view of other foot or reference to radiographic anatomy text may facilitate recognition of a dislocation, particularly in children)
2. Navicular fractures often mistaken for a sprain (similar mechanism of injury, fracture may only be seen on lateral view).

WARNING

Because of the mechanism of injury, patients with calcaneus fractures frequently have associated thoracic or lumbar spine fractures. Strongly consider radiographs of these regions.

Treatment

1. Consultation or referral recommended
   a. May require inpatient observation.
   b. Talus may develop avascular necrosis.
   c. If fracture extends to a joint surface, there is a high risk of future degenerative joint disease (DJD) even if position anatomic.
2. Some primary care physicians manage selected calcaneal fractures (if nondisplaced and no extension to joint surface) (see Eiff et al. 1998, pp 209–227, for discussion of management).

Metatarsal Fractures

Multiple Metatarsal Fractures

1. Compared with fractures of a single metatarsal (MT), these fractures
   a. Have a higher risk of associated dislocation or vascular compromise (which may be delayed, i.e., compartment syndrome)
   b. Often have significant displacement (may require fixation)

2. Consider referral unless experienced in the management of these fractures; management similar to that outlined below (first MT).

Avulsion Fracture of Proximal Fifth Metatarsal (Fracture of Styloid)

Probably the most common fracture of the lower extremity

Etiology

Inversion of ankle

Symptoms

Acute lateral foot pain following inversion injury

Clinical Findings

Local swelling and point tenderness

Radiographic Findings

Transverse or oblique lucency less than 1.5 cm from proximal tip of fifth MT

 Key Test

Palpate proximal fifth MT of all patients who sustain ankle inversion injuries to avoid missing this fracture.

Differential Diagnosis

1. Jones' fracture or diaphyseal stress fracture (see below)
2. Apophysis (growth center seen in older children and adolescents). Lucency of apophysis lies *parallel* to long axis of fifth MT; fracture usually transverse. If apophysis is tender
   a. Obtain comparison view of other foot to rule out avulsion of apophysis.
   b. Consider referring or treating like a Salter I fracture even if radiograph is normal.
3. Sesamoid bone (os peroneum or os vesalianum)

Treatment

1. Consider consultation or referral if displaced more than 2 to 3 mm (unusual).
2. If displacement is less than 2 to 3 mm,
   a. Generally require only a firm-soled, comfortable shoe for 4 to 8 weeks, plus initial ice and elevation.
   b. If patient is very symptomatic despite above, SLWC (for 2 weeks) may help.

Follow-Up

1. Follow up every 2 to 4 weeks until patient has resumed most normal activities.

2. Switch patient to normal shoes when symptoms allow.
3. Patient occasionally may need physical therapy (more likely if cast used).

Acute Fracture of Metaphyseal-Diaphyseal Junction (Jones' Fracture)

Etiology
Sudden force under distal fifth MT

Symptoms
Sudden pain following injury

Clinical Findings
Point tenderness over proximal fifth MT

Radiologic Findings
Transverse lucency through proximal diaphysis extending into the joint between the bases of the fourth and fifth metatarsals

Differential Diagnosis
1. Avulsion fracture
2. Apophysis
3. Diaphyseal stress fracture

Treatment and Follow-Up
1. Consider referral because delayed union or nonunion may occur.
2. Following usual acute care (see Tables 244–1 and 244–2) short-leg non–weight-bearing cast for 6 to 12 weeks until radiographic healing; re-evaluate every 2 to 3 weeks, and refer for possible internal fixation if no healing by 10 to 12 weeks.

Stress Fracture of the Fifth Metatarsal

Etiology
Chronic overloading (especially pivoting); usually occurs in young adult male athletes

Symptoms
Pain for weeks, often with sudden worsening

Clinical Findings
Point tenderness 3 to 4 cm from tip of styloid; swelling may be minimal.

Radiologic Findings
Radiographs often negative initially, but may show narrowing of medullary canal (earliest finding), periosteal reaction, or faint lucent line. Over time, the lucency may become widened (type II), and may go on to type III (nonunion with obliteration of the med-

ullary canal by callus). Early diagnosis may require bone scan.

Differential Diagnosis
1. Avulsion fracture of styloid
2. Acute fracture of diaphysis
3. Benign apophysis

> **WARNING**
>
> Stress fractures of the proximal fifth metatarsal have a high risk of delayed union or nonunion. Consider referral for early internal fixation, especially in young athletes.

Treatment and Follow-Up
1. Consider referral in all cases: Many patients (especially athletes) require early internal fixation. Conservative therapy (casting without internal fixation) is an option for patients with
   a. Type I (early) stress fractures (radiographs ranging from normal to a thin fracture line)
   b. Type II fractures (widened fracture line) in patients who are unable to undergo surgery or who prefer immobilization (which may be prolonged) to surgery.
2. Conservative therapy consists of
   a. Short-leg non–weight-bearing cast for 2 to 6 months
   b. Follow every 4 to 6 weeks.
   c. When clinical and radiographic evidence shows that healing is well underway, allow protected weight bearing in a short-leg cast for an additional 2 to 4 weeks.
   d. Thereafter, patient may *very gradually* resume former activities.

Proximal Metatarsal Fractures (Other Than Fifth)

High incidence of associated tarsometatarsal joint (Lisfranc) injuries, which may be subtle, disabling, and difficult to manage. Recommend referral of proximal fractures, especially if multiple.

Midshaft or Distal Fracture of a *Single* Metatarsal (Second to Fifth)

Etiology
1. Direct blow or twist with toes fixed
2. Common site of stress fractures, which usually occur after a sudden increase in activity (e.g., athletes and new military recruits, i.e., "march" fracture)

Symptoms

1. Forefoot pain, increased with weight bearing
2. With stress fracture, onset gradual.

Clinical Findings

1. Point tenderness, usually with swelling and ecchymosis
2. Pain with axial compression

Radiographic Findings

Fracture usually spiral or oblique, generally with little or no displacement (if adjacent metatarsals are intact, they "splint" the fracture). Consider referral if

1. Fracture involves a joint surface (high risk of future DJD even if anatomic position).
2. Significant angulation of metatarsal head (develop abnormal forefoot biomechanics and chronic keratosis if not corrected)

Key Test

A full foot series (anteroposterior, oblique, and lateral) is necessary to assess all potential metatarsal fractures. Because of overlying shadows on lateral view, it is necessary to carefully follow the cortex of each metatarsal to determine the position of the fracture. Undetected angulation can lead to significant long-term sequelae.

Treatment and Follow-Up

If displaced 2 mm or less and no significant angulation: usual initial care and follow-up (see Tables 244–1 and 244–2), using SLWC for 2 to 3 weeks, followed by early ambulation in well-padded shoe. Many patients can be managed without casting (i.e., with only firm, padded shoe and partial weight bearing as tolerated).

First Metatarsal

Etiology

Usually a high-energy crushing injury

> **WARNING**
>
> **Crush injuries (particularly of the foot) are prone to extensive soft tissue damage, which may be more problematic than the fracture itself. Consider early referral/consultation if suspected.**

Symptoms/Clinical Findings

Similar to those of midshaft or distal fracture of a single metatarsal (above)

Treatment

1. Vast majority should probably be referred.
    a. May require overnight observation of vascular status.
    b. Anatomic position more important because of its important weight-bearing function.
    c. Associated dislocation possible if fracture is proximal.
2. For selected patients with nondisplaced, stable fracture:
    a. Initial care as in Table 244–1 (special emphasis on immediate return if signs of vascular compromise develop)
    b. Follow up as in Table 244–2, including recheck at 12 to 24 hours and repeat films at 8 to 10 days to check position. Use a short-leg non–weight-bearing cast until healing, with re-evaluation every 2 weeks.

Toes

First Toe (Great Toe)

Etiology

Usually a direct blow (falling object or stubbing injury)

Symptoms

Pain (patient often presents days after injury)

Clinical Findings

1. Point tenderness
2. Swelling
3. Ecchymosis
4. Subungual hematoma (especially first toe)

Differential Diagnosis

1. Sprain
2. Contusion
3. Dislocation

Treatment and Follow-Up

1. Important weight-bearing function, so consider referral if displaced (especially proximal phalanx) or if intra-articular (especially MTP joint).
2. Nondisplaced
    a. Buddy tape (i.e., tape to adjacent toe with padding between them)
    b. Firm-soled shoe
    c. Crutches with partial weight bearing for 2 to 3 weeks
    d. If pain control not adequate, use SLWC with toe platform for 2 weeks, followed by above; see also Tables 244–1 and 244–2.

Lesser Toes

Etiology, symptoms, findings, and differential diagnosis as in first toe (great toe) above.

Treatment and Follow-Up
1. Rarely need referral unless open fracture is present.
2. Nondisplaced
   a. Buddy tape for comfort.
   b. Re-evaluate in 2 to 4 weeks.
   c. Rarely require follow-up radiographs; see also Tables 244–1 and 244–2.
3. Displaced
   a. Following local anesthesia (achieved with ice for 5 to 10 minutes or occasionally with digital block), reduce using gentle traction.
   b. Buddy tape to hold position.
   c. Same follow-up as for nondisplaced toe fracture

Bibliography

Eiff MP, Hatch RL, Calmbach WL: Fracture Management for Primary Care. Philadelphia, WB Saunders Company, 1998.

Holubec KD, Karlin JM, Scurran BL: Retrospective study of fifth metatarsal fractures. J Am Podiatr Med Assoc 1993;83:215–222.

Lawrence SJ, Botte MJ: Jones' fractures and related fractures of the proximal fifth metatarsal. Foot Ankle 1993;14:358–365.

Shea MP, Manoli A II: Recognizing talar dome lesions. Physician Sportsmed 1993;12:109–121.

245 Common Infectious Disease Symptoms

Body temperature is determined by the balance between heat production and heat loss. This balance is under control of the nervous system and regulated by neurons predominantly in the "preoptic region" of the hypothalamus to maintain a set body temperature. This process is so effective that an individual's body temperature rarely varies more than 1° C from baseline. Fever results from a resetting of the hypothalamus, so that heat production and loss are balanced to maintain a higher body temperature. The hypothalamus can be reset by:

1. Circulating substances (termed *pyrogens*): The most common mechanism that elicits fever is the elaboration of endogenous pyrogens by stimulated circulating monocytes and tissue macrophages.

2. Damage from hemorrhage, infarction, or compression

Because of individual and diurnal variations, there is no well-established discrete body temperature that defines fever. Simplifying the complex issues of clinical thermometry, an oral temperature greater than 38° C in an adult will be defined as a fever. Although some individuals without recognizable illnesses may have body temperatures above 38° C, this value will be sensitive enough to detect almost all of those patients with significant disorders that produce fever. Chills are a secondary symptom associated with fever, resulting from the need for muscular activity to increase heat production and raise body temperature to the level desired by the reset hypothalamus. Thus chills are most often seen while the body temperature is rising. Fever is a common presenting symptom, accounting for 2 to 6 per cent of unselected adults presenting to hospital emergency departments or ambulatory walk-in clinics.

Differential Diagnosis

1. Fever can be due to
   a. Infection: essentially all causes, whether bacterial, viral, or parasitic. The potential causes depend on the patient's age, under-lying host factors, and epidemiologic associations. For example, an acute undifferentiated fever in Southeast Asia is often due to malaria, whereas a similar presentation in rural areas of the mid-Atlantic United States during the spring and summer is possibly Rocky Mountain spotted fever.
   b. Immunologic disorders: associated with an inflammatory reaction, such as acute inflammatory arthritis, serum sickness, immune hemolytic anemia
   c. Neoplastic disorders: sometimes seen with solid tumors and often seen with reticuloendothelial tumors
   d. Vascular thrombosis or infarction: acute myocardial infarction, deep venous thrombosis, pulmonary emboli, cerebrovascular accidents
   e. Trauma: usually involves significant skeletal muscle injury from a crushing mechanism.
   f. Miscellaneous: acute gout, acute porphyria, acute adrenal insufficiency, hyperthyroidism, tonic-clonic seizures
   g. Drug-induced: Drugs most often reported include methyldopa, quinidine, procainamide, phenytoin, carbamazepine, penicillin, cephalothin, tetracycline, sulfonamide, isoniazid, bleomycin.

2. Acute bacterial infection is the etiology for which timely diagnosis and treatment is important. The initial diagnostic approach to evaluating an adult with an acute fever usually involves detecting a treatable infection (most often bacterial) or excluding such an infection to a reasonable degree of clinical certainty. Patients without a diagnosis on initial evaluation can usually be followed expectantly.

History

1. Fever: onset, duration, maximal value, chronologic pattern (although of little diagnostic value)

2. Secondary symptoms: chills, sweats, malaise, and myalgias

3. Localizing symptoms: Most otherwise healthy adults with the acute onset of fever also report localizing symptoms (e.g., sore throat, cough, dysuria) caused by the specific illness producing the fever.

4. Medical history: underlying disorders that reduce resistance or predispose to infection, especially diabetes, malignancy, acquired immunodeficiency syndrome, sickle cell anemia, alcoholism, intravenous drug use

5. Current medications: especially antipyretics or leftover antibiotics

6. Epidemiologic factors: others ill at home with fever, recent travel, unusual exposures

Clinical Findings

1. An oral temperature above 38° C should be considered a fever and should prompt a search for a definite cause. Because of age, diurnal variation, or antipyretic use, patients may report a history of fever but will not have an oral temperature above 38° C at presentation.

2. Secondary clinical findings: chills, sweats, and malaise

3. Tachypnea, tachycardia, or hypotension with fever may represent the systemic "septic" response and is associated with a 37 to 47 per cent incidence of bacteremia.

4. Observe general condition: Does patient appear acutely ill (or "toxic"), or to tolerate fever without obvious effects?

5. The following clinical findings suggest a focal disorder or infection:
   a. Altered mental status: lethargy, confusion, stupor, or coma
   b. Head and neck: inflamed tympanic membranes, pharyngeal erythema or exudate, sinus tenderness, nasal exudate or congestion, cervical adenopathy
   c. Chest: localized rales, rhonchi, or evidence of consolidation
   d. Heart: regurgitant valvular murmur
   e. Abdomen: focal tenderness, guarding, or rebound
   f. Genitourinary: flank or kidney tenderness, exudate from cervical os, cervical motion, or adnexal tenderness
   g. Rectum: focal anal tenderness or swelling, exudate
   h. Extremities; focal erythema, tenderness, or swelling; monoarticular joint effusion
   i. Skin: petechial, pustular, or other rashes

6. Using the combination of symptoms and clinical findings, the clinician can categorize the patient into a general syndrome. For example
   a. Upper respiratory infection: nasal congestion, earache, sore throat, postnasal drip
   b. Lower respiratory infection: cough, rales, evidence of consolidation
   c. Acute gastroenteritis: nausea, vomiting, diarrhea
   d. Urinary infection: dysuria, frequency, urgency, costovertebral angle or flank tenderness

Diagnostic Tests

1. Laboratory tests are most useful when the results will alter diagnosis, treatment, or disposition and are least useful (possibly not necessary) when results will not change decisions.

2. For otherwise healthy febrile adults with localizing symptoms or findings, specific laboratory tests are chosen based upon the clinical syndrome; there is little need for "shotgun" testing. Useful examples include
   a. Streptococcal screen for patients with exudative pharyngitis
   b. Urinalysis for patients with urinary symptoms
   c. Chest radiograph for patients with a productive cough

3. For febrile adults, ancillary tests—such as the white blood cell (WBC) count, urinalysis, chest radiograph, and blood culture—to detect occult bacterial infection are useful in
   a. Febrile adults without localizing symptoms or findings: up to a 30 per cent incidence of occult bacterial infection and 15 per cent incidence of bacteremia
   b. Febrile neutropenic patients
   c. Febrile adults with systemic immunodeficiencies

4. The WBC count has little utility when used indiscriminately, but has a modest predictive value for bacterial infection or bacteremia in
   a. Febrile adults without localizing symptoms or findings: WBC count greater than 15,000/mm^3 associated with approximately a 50 per cent incidence of bacterial infection and 30 per cent incidence of bacteremia.
   b. Febrile patients when the history suggests the possibility of neutropenia: neutrophil count less than 1000/mm^3

c. The febrile elderly patient: WBC count greater than 14,000/mm^3 associated with about a 50 per cent incidence of bacterial infection.

5. The white cell differential also has modest predictive value in detecting bacterial infection or bacteremia in

   a. Febrile adults without localizing symptoms or findings: Neutrophil band count greater than 1500/mm^3 associated with about a 50 per cent incidence of bacterial infection and 20 per cent incidence of bacteremia.

   b. The febrile elderly patient: Neutrophil band greater than 6 per cent associated with about 70 per cent incidence of bacterial infection.

6. Urinalysis is useful in

   a. Febrile adults with urinary symptoms: internal dysuria, frequency, urgency, flank or abdominal pain. Upper urinary tract infections in otherwise healthy adults are almost always associated with pyuria with WBC count greater than 5 per high-power field. The absence of pyuria essentially excludes this diagnosis, except in neutropenic patients.

   b. Febrile adults without localizing symptoms or findings: about 10 to 15 per cent incidence of occult urinary tract infection

   c. Elderly febrile patients

7. Urine culture: The large majority of otherwise healthy adults with pyelonephritis respond to empiric antibiotic selection, and so culture and determination of sensitivity, although commonly performed, do not influence treatment. Urine culture is recommended when bacteriologic diagnosis is important.

   a. Febrile neutropenic or immunocompromised patients

   b. Febrile patients with urinary tract obstruction

8. Chest radiographs: The clinical examination lacks accuracy in detecting pulmonary consolidation; the chest radiograph is the most accurate technique to detect pneumonia. Clinically occult infiltrates have been detected by chest radiography in 3 to 4 per cent of

   a. Febrile adults without localizing symptoms or signs

   b. Febrile neutropenic patients without pulmonary symptoms

   c. Febrile adults with a productive cough but no auscultatory abnormalities

9. Blood culture: Indiscriminate use of blood cultures has low utility. Blood cultures are recommended for

   a. Situations in which blood culture is the primary modality for diagnosis (e.g., bacterial endocarditis). Two populations are at special risk: febrile intravenous drug users and patients with prosthetic heart valves.

   b. Febrile adults without localizing symptoms or signs when the WBC count is greater than 15,000/mm^3 or the neutrophil band count is greater than 1500/mm^3 have about a 20 to 30 per cent incidence of bacteremia. Conversely, when the WBC count is less than 15,000/mm^3 and the neutrophil band count is 1500/mm^3, the incidence of bacterial infection is 3 per cent and the incidence of bacteremia is less than 1 per cent.

   c. Febrile elderly patients

   d. Febrile neutropenic or immunocompromised patients

10. Stool cultures: seldom contributory for evaluation of sporadic cases of gastroenteritis. A stool culture positive for enteric pathogens has a yield of 40 to 50 per cent in febrile adults evaluated for gastroenteritis.

Management

1. Specific antibiotic treatment is indicated when a clinical syndrome has a sufficient probability of being caused by bacteria. For example, exudative tonsillitis, fever, and cervical adenopathy in a 20-year-old has up to a 60 per cent likelihood of being due to streptococci, and treatment with penicillin is recommended.

2. Empiric antibiotic therapy is indicated when the clinical syndrome suggests the possibility of a serious, potentially fatal bacterial infection. For example, patients with acute meningitis or septic shock should receive empiric antibiotics before cultures and other ancillary tests are completed. Ideally, such treatment is initiated after appropriate cultures are obtained, but antibiotics should not be unduly delayed.

3. Broad-spectrum antibiotic therapy for undifferentiated febrile illnesses is to be avoided.

4. Antipyretic therapy is appropriate for patient comfort with

   a. Acetaminophen, 10 to 15 mg/kg orally every 4 hours

   b. Ibuprofen, 5 to 10 mg/kg orally every 6 hours

PEARLS

- The patient's general condition and how well the illness is being tolerated determine the need for hospitalization.

- Febrile adults with serious co-morbid conditions or underlying immunodeficiencies are usually admitted to the hospital for fear of serious complications developing rapidly because of delayed diagnosis or treatment.

- As with the febrile 5-month-old with a "negative septic work-up," febrile adults with a nondiagnostic evaluation upon initial contact should be seen again or contacted by phone in 24 hours.

Bibliography

Bossink AW, Groeneveld J, Hack CE, et al: Prediction of mortality in febrile medical patients: how useful are systemic inflammatory response syndrome and sepsis criteria? Chest 1998;113:1533–1541.

Gallagher EJ, Brooks F, Gennis P: Identification of serious illness in febrile adults. Am J Emerg Med 1994;12:129–133.

Mellors JW, Horwitz RI, Harvey MR, et al: A simple index to identify occult bacterial infection in adults with unexplained fever. Arch Intern Med 1987:147:666–671.

Trivalle C, Chassagne P, Bouaniche M, et al: Nosocomial febrile illness in the elderly: frequency, causes, and risk factors. Arch Intern Med 1998;158:1560–1565.

Van Dissel JT, Schijf V, Vogtlander N, et al: Implication of chills. Lancet 1998;352:374.

246 Fever of Unknown Origin
Cynthia M. Moore-Sledge

Definition

1. Most fevers of unknown origin (FUO) are due to the atypical presentation of common illnesses. Thorough evaluation, including history, physical examination, and selected tests, will reveal the etiology in most cases.

2. The criteria established by Petersdorf and Beeson in 1961 eliminated illnesses of shorter duration that were thought to be self-limited or more easily diagnosed. The criteria for adults are

   a. The illness is of more than 3 weeks' duration
   b. The temperature is documented to be higher than 38.3° C (101° F) on several occasions
   c. No diagnosis is made after 1 week of study in the hospital. Improved diagnostic technology, infectious disease training, and economic constraints have led to the alteration of this criterion to "no diagnosis after 1 week of intelligent and intensive evaluation." This allows inclusion of patients evaluated in the outpatient setting.

3. Pediatric patients with febrile illness lasting for more than 2 weeks with no diagnosis are considered by Dechovitz and Moffet to have FUO.

Etiology

1. More than 200 causes of FUO have been identified. The major categories are infection, neoplasms, rheumatologic disease, miscellaneous, and undiagnosed. These major categories have remained constant since Petersdorf and Beeson's investigation in the 1950s.

2. Most studies indicate that infections cause 30 to 40 per cent of cases; neoplasms, 20 to 30 per cent; rheumatologic diseases, 10 to 20 per cent; miscellaneous sources, 15 to 20 per cent; and undiagnosed sources, 5 to 15 per cent.

3. The most common cause of FUO in the pediatric, adult, and geriatric populations is infection.

4. The recent recognition of new causes of FUO, such as Lyme disease, *Bartonella* endocarditis, and Sweet's syndrome, has led to the development of a new classification system:

   a. Classic FUO
      (1) Fever of 38.3° C or higher for more than 3 weeks with no diagnosis after three outpatient visits or 3 days in the hospital
      (2) Causes include tuberculosis, mononucleosis syndrome, pelvic/abdominal abscess, osteomyelitis, fungal disease, neoplasm, infective endocarditis, granulomatous disease, and drug fever.

   b. Neutropenic FUO
      (1) Fever of 38.3° C or higher on several occasions in a patient with less than 500 neutrophils/mm^3 or expected to fall to that level in 1 to 2 days without identification of the cause in 3 days of hospitalization and at least 2 days of culture incubation.
      (2) Causes include *Candida*, *Aspergillus*, herpes simplex, and cytomegalovirus (CMV).

   c. Human immunodeficiency virus (HIV)–associated FUO
      (1) Fever of 38.3° C or higher of 4 weeks' duration in outpatient or 3 days' duration in inpatient setting in a patient with HIV
      (2) Causes include *Mycobacterium avium-intracellulare*, tuberculosis (TB), toxoplasmosis, CMV, *Cryptococcus*, histoplasmosis, non-Hodgkin's lymphoma, and drug fever.

   d. Nosocomial FUO
      (1) Fever of 38.3° C or higher for 3 days and infection not present or incubating at the time of admission, with a minimum of 3 days' admission and 2 days of culture incubation without diagnosis
      (2) Causes include infected IV lines, recurrent pulmonary embolisms, and drug fever.

Symptoms

1. The most common symptom in all patients is fever. Symptoms otherwise are nonspecific. The pattern of the fever has not been shown to reliably lead to a diagnosis.

2. Twenty to 30 per cent of elderly patients have a blunted or absent fever response. An increase of 2° C above baseline temperature is an indi-

cation of fever in this population. Altered mental function, decreased functional capacity, weight loss or failure to thrive, weakness, falls, and generalized pain may signal infection in the elderly.

3. Symptoms such as jaw claudication, joint pain, abdominal pain, and syncope may aid in narrowing the differential diagnosis of FUO.

Key Symptoms

- Fever

- Altered mental function

Clinical Findings

1. Fever must be documented to be genuine. Factitious fever may be suspected in a patient who appears healthy in spite of elevated temperature, has unusually high temperatures (>41° C), defervesces rapidly without diaphoresis, exhibits temperature-pulse disparity, lacks the usual diurnal variation, and may have signs of self-mutilation. Patients with habitual hyperthermia have exaggerated diurnal variation in temperature.

2. Patients on medication should have all medications stopped if possible. Drug-related fever should resolve within 48 hours of drug withdrawal.

3. A detailed history and carefully performed physical examination is imperative. These may need to be repeated during the evaluation to reveal information that may have been overlooked as well as signs that may develop with progression of the disease.

   a. Information regarding alcohol intake; medications; travel; occupational exposure; exposure to pets, chemicals, or plants; familial illnesses; previous illnesses; previous surgeries; previous TB skin test results; exposure to TB; rashes; and joint symptoms is to be included in the history.

   b. Diagnosis and appropriate use of ancillary tests may be directed by findings on a physical examination.

   c. Signs that may aid in diagnosis are periodontal disease (oral abscess), position-dependent diastolic murmur (atrial myxoma), malar rash (systemic lupus erythematosus [SLE]), retinitis (CMV or toxoplasmosis), Roth's spots (infective endocarditis), thrush (HIV), oral leukoplakia (HIV), thyromegaly (thyroiditis), bony tenderness (osteomyelitis),

right upper quadrant pain (liver abscess, hepatobiliary disease, hepatic lymphoma, hepatitis), and lymphadenopathy (lymphoma, lymphadenitis, mononucleosis syndrome).

Key Signs

- Documentation of fever

- Infection

Laboratory Tests

1. The diagnosis of FUO is rarely made with screening laboratory tests. Screening labs may direct further investigation. The yield of tests is increased if ordered based on "potentially diagnostic clues." The yield of tests is increased in patients with continuous fever, high erythrocyte sedimentation rate, and low hemoglobin. Anemia and abnormal liver function tests are common, nonspecific findings in patients with FUO.

2. First-stage or screening labs include complete blood count with differential, renal profile, hepatic profile, urinalysis, urine culture, blood culture, antinuclear antibody, anti–neutrophil cytoplasmic antibody, rheumatoid factor, chest radiograph, and abdominal ultrasound.

3. Second-stage tests may include computerized tomography (CT) scan of the abdomen or chest, echocardiography, small and large intestinal radiography, magnetic resonance imaging, serology (CMV, Epstein-Barr virus, *Mycoplasma pneumoniae*, *Brucella*, toxoplasmosis, *Borrelia*, *Chlamydia psittaci*, HIV, leptospirosis, *Coxiella burnetti*, respiratory syncytial virus, rubella, *Yersinia enterocolitica*), sinus radiographs, thyroid testing, scintigraphy, and cultures of sputum or other sites.

   a. Use of second-stage tests should be based upon findings of the history, physical examination, and screening laboratory tests.

   b. Scintigraphy or the use of radiolabeled white blood cells or immune globulin has revealed inflammatory and neoplastic lesions not revealed with CT.

4. Third-stage tests may include small intestine biopsy, skin biopsy, skin-muscle biopsy, liver biopsy, or laparoscopic examination. Lymph node biopsy in patients with generalized lymphadenopathy is more likely to aid in diagnosis than biopsy in patients with localized lymph node enlargement. Temporal artery biopsy may be

done early in the evaluation of patients over 55 years of age with no focal findings.

5. The history and physical should be repeated throughout the evaluation.

Key Tests

- Complete blood count
- Urinalysis
- Blood culture
- Erythrocyte sedimentation rate

Differential Diagnosis

Causes are categorized as infections, neoplasms, rheumatologic diseases, and miscellaneous causes.

1. Infection may include infective endocarditis, intra-abdominal abscess, urinary tract infection, osteomyelitis, and TB.
2. The most common neoplasms are renal cell carcinoma, Hodgkin's disease, and leukemia.
3. Rheumatologic diseases include Still's disease, SLE, and vasculitis.
4. Miscellaneous disorders include sarcoidosis, drug fever, factitious fever, recurrent pulmonary emboli, alcoholic hepatitis, and Mediterranean fever.

Treatment

1. Treatment is directed by the findings of the evaluation. Empiric therapy with corticosteroids or antibiotics should be withheld if possible. Debilitating fever should be treated with aspirin, acetaminophen, or nonsteroidal anti-inflammatory drugs (NSAIDs). Aspirin, NSAIDs, and antibiotics may cause fever.
2. Empiric therapy is begun to avoid (1) tachycardia in persons with cardiac compromise, (2) hyperventilation in patients with pulmonary compromise or dehydration, and (3) enceph-

alopathy in persons with neurologic disorders and children with a history of febrile seizures. Temperatures less than 41° C have been proven not to cause neurologic damage and do not require treatment.

3. Patients who are unstable or have rapidly progressive disease should be admitted. They may be considered for treatment with steroids or antibiotics. Steroids should be started only after infection is ruled out. Antibiotics should be used judiciously. Multiple antibiotic regimens should be avoided.

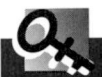

Key Treatment

Treatment should be withheld whenever possible until a diagnosis is made.

Follow-Up

1. Despite extensive evaluation, 9 to 25 per cent of patients with FUO remain undiagnosed.
2. Patients who remain stable generally have a good prognosis. These patients should be followed monthly.
3. Pediatric patients with prolonged periodic fever with no identified etiology may be at risk to develop neurologic abnormalities.

Bibliography

Avnow P, Flaherty J: Fever of unknown origin. Lancet 1997;350:575–580.

deKleign E, van Lier HJ, Van der M: Fever of unknown origin (FUO): II. Diagnostic procedures in a prospective multicenter study of 157. Medicine 1997;76:401–441.

Hirschman J: Fever of unknown origin in adults. Clin Infect Dis 1997;24:291–302.

Meller J, Ivancevic V, Conrad M, et al: Clinical value of immunoscintigraphy in patients with fever of unknown origin. J Nucl Med 1998;39:1248–1253.

Miller L, Sisson B, Tucker L, et al: Prolonged fevers of unknown origin in children: patterns of presentation and outcome. J Pediatr 1996;12:419–423.

247 Fungal Infections

S. Anthony Swaldi

Etiology

1. Fungi are ubiquitous in nature, and, in most settings, they pose no health threat. Invasive disease is usually prevented by a normal functioning immune response, normal bacterial flora, and intact mucosal barriers. Disruption of this balanced system, however, can lead to infection. Patients at highest risk for fungal infections are those with immunodeficiency caused by human immunodeficiency virus infection, hematologic malignancy, or cancer chemotherapy. Other predisposing conditions include diabetes mellitus, chronic or broad-spectrum antibiotics, and treatment with high-dose corticosteroids. Person-to-person spread generally does not occur.

2. Systemic diseases: Most begin as primary pulmonary infections, which disseminate to involve multiple organ systems.

   a. Aspergillosis (*Aspergillus fumigatus, A. flavus, A. niger*): Commonly found on decaying vegetation. Inhalation of spores leads to infection. Involvement of lungs, paranasal sinuses, skin, or gastrointestinal tract begins before dissemination. Neutropenic patients are at highest risk of death from systemic infection.

   b. Blastomycosis (*Blastomyces dermatitidis*): uncommon. Found in soil and rotting vegetation. Prevalent areas include states bordering the Mississippi and Ohio rivers. Inhalation is the principal route of infection.

   c. Candidiasis (*Candida albicans, C. tropicalis, C. parapsilosis, C. glabrata*): Human body is natural habitat. Most common species is *C. albicans*. Fungi found in mouth, stool, and vagina in small numbers. Premature neonates are particularly prone to infection. Chronic catheterization, antibiotic use, and immunosuppression are risk factors.

   d. Coccidioidomycosis (*Coccidioides immitis*): soil saprophyte endemic to arid regions of Southwest United States. Infection arises from inhalation of spores that are disrupted by dust storms or construction.

   e. Cryptococcosis (*Cryptococcus neoformans*): Enters host by inhalation. Wide geographic distribution. Found on fruit, soil, and especially pigeon dung. Cryptococcal meningitis is a common acquired immunodeficiency syndrome (AIDS)–defining illness.

   f. Histoplasmosis (*Histoplasma capsulatum*): acquired by inhalation. Endemic to Middle Atlantic and Central regions of the United States. Isolated in moist soil under trees and in caves. Grows best in association with bird and bat droppings.

   g. Mucormycosis (*Rhizopus, Rhizomucor*): Grows on decaying vegetation, dung, and food high in sugar, such as strawberries and breads. Diabetics are especially predisposed to infection of sinuses or lungs.

   h. Paracoccidioidomycosis (*Paracoccidioides brasiliensis*): deep fungal infection endemic to Mexico, Central America, and South America; resembles blastomycosis.

   i. Sporotrichosis (*Sporothrix schenckii*): worldwide soil saprophyte of plants. Fungi of thorny bushes, tree bark, and moss. Animals, fish, and insects may harbor *Sporothrix*. Infection begins after inoculation into subcutaneous tissue; lymphangitic spread follows. Systemic disease is rare.

Symptoms

1. Aspergillosis: hypersensitivity, cough, wheezing, hemoptysis, fever, facial pain, epistaxis

2. Blastomycosis: indolent onset, chronically progressive fever, cough, hemoptysis, pleuritic chest pain, arthralgia, myalgia

3. Candidiasis: fever, malaise, tachycardia, hypotension, altered mental states, blurred vision, scotoma

4. Coccidioidomycosis: 60 per cent asymptomatic; mild flu-like illness to severe pneumonia, fever, arthralgias, rash

5. Cryptococcosis: headache, nausea, confusion, blurred vision, fever, chest pain, cough

6. Histoplasmosis: asymptomatic or mild infection often with gradual onset, cough, weight loss, night sweats, fever, abdominal pain; symptoms may be chronic.

7. Mucormycosis: low-grade to high fever, nasal congestion, headache, diplopia, facial pain, bloody discharge, cough

8. Sporotrichosis: painless skin lesions, joint pain, cough; systemic involvement rare.

Clinical Findings

1. Aspergillosis
   a. Pulmonary: wheezes, rales, rhonchi; perihilar infiltrate; can lead to acute pneumonia with cavitation or aspergilloma ("fungus ball") formation.
   b. Other: sinusitis; otitis; keratitis; endocarditis; myocarditis

2. Blastomycosis
   a. Pulmonary: fibronodular upper lobe infiltrate, pleural thickening
   b. Skin: verrucous, pustular, or ulcerative lesions of skin and mucosal surface
   c. Other: joint effusion, prostate or epididymal lesions, meningitis, osteomyelitis

3. Candidiasis
   a. Systemic: endocarditis, arthritis, myositis, hepatosplenomegaly, brain abscess
   b. Oral (thrush): adherent white plaques on oral mucosa
   c. Skin: erythema, maceration, and pustules of intertriginous areas, scrotum, or perineum
   d. Other: esophagitis, balanitis, cystitis, endophthalmitis, vaginitis

4. Coccidioidomycosis
   a. Pulmonary: single lobe infiltrate, hilar adenopathy, pleural friction rub
   b. Skin: verrucous lesions, erythema nodosum

5. Cryptococcosis
   a. Meningoencephalitis: altered mental status, papilledema, cranial nerve palsies, hydrocephalus; nuchal rigidity rare.
   b. Pulmonary: circumscribed dense infiltrate, hilar adenopathy, pleural effusion
   c. Other: prostatitis, endophthalmitis, hepatitis, pericarditis, ulcerative skin lesions

6. Histoplasmosis
   a. Pulmonary (acute): perihilar adenopathy, patchy pneumonitis
   b. Disseminated (acute): Addison's disease, hepatosplenomegaly, anemia, thrombocytopenia
   c. Chronic disease: fibronodular infiltrates, emphysema, cor pulmonale, calcification

7. Mucormycosis
   a. Craniofacial: red necrotic turbinates, sinus opacification, proptosis, reduced ocular motion, blindness
   b. Pulmonary: necrotic cavitary pneumonia

8. Sporotrichosis
   a. Skin: painless erythematous papule at inoculation site, nodules or vesicles along lymph channels
   b. Other: inflammatory arthritis; systemic involvement rare.

Laboratory Tests

1. Aspergillosis: culture of endobronchial brushing or sputum, complete blood count (CBC) (eosinophilia), skin reactivity to *Aspergillus* antigen; blood culture rarely positive.
2. Blastomycosis: culture and smear
3. Candidiasis
   a. Systemic: biopsy or culture of blood, cerebrospinal fluid (CSF), joint fluid, or suspect catheter tip; serum *Candida* antigen
   b. Superficial: KOH wet smear for pseudohyphae; culture and/or biopsy occasionally necessary.
4. Coccidioidomycosis: wet smear, culture, serology, CBC, skin testing
5. Cryptococcosis: CSF for culture and smear (India ink), glucose (low), protein (elevated), cell count with differential (20 to 60 white blood cells/μl, lymphocytic predominance); sputum culture; biopsy
6. Histoplasmosis: culture, serology, skin testing (indicates exposure)
7. Mucormycosis: biopsy with smear and culture
8. Sporotrichosis: culture of pus, joint fluid, or sputum; skin biopsy

Differential Diagnosis

1. General systemic pulmonary: tuberculosis (TB); malignancy; lung abscess; viral, bacterial, or *Mycoplasma* pneumonia; chronic obstructive pulmonary disease; sarcoidosis; other opportunistic infections
2. Cryptococcal meningoencephalitis: TB, syphilis, progressive multifocal leukoencephalopathy, herpes simplex virus, toxoplasmosis, lymphoma, viral meningitis, AIDS dementia
3. Sporotrichosis: infection with *Nocardia asteroides, Mycobacterium marinum, Mycobacterium kansasii, Leishmania braziliensis*.

Treatment

Medication

1. Aspergillosis: amphotericin B (Fungizone), 1 to 1.5 mg/kg/day intravenously for 4 to 12 weeks; or itraconazole (Sporanox), 200 mg orally bid
2. Blastomycosis; itraconazole, 100 to 200 mg PO bid; or amphotericin B, 0.5 to 0.6 mg/kg/day

intravenously; alternative: ketoconazole (Nizoral), 400 to 800 mg/day orally

3. Candidiasis: amphotericin B, 0.5 to 1 mg/kg/day intravenously ± flucytosine (Ancobon), 100 to 150 mg/kg/day orally; alternative: fluconazole (Diflucan), 400 mg intravenously or orally daily. Remove infected devices. For cystitis: local irrigation with amphotericin B.

4. Coccidioidomycosis: fluconazole, 400 to 800 mg/day orally; or amphotericin B, 0.5 mg/kg/day intravenously

5. Cryptococcosis: amphotericin B ± flucytosine; alternative: fluconazole, 400 mg orally daily. Check CSF culture weekly.

6. Histoplasmosis: itraconazole, 200 mg orally bid; or amphotericin B, 0.5 to 0.6 mg/kg/day intravenously

7. Mucormycosis: amphotericin B, 1 to 1.5 mg/kg/day intravenously; débridement

8. Paracoccidioidomycosis: itraconazole, 100 mg/day orally; or amphotericin B, 0.4 to 0.5 mg/kg/day intravenously

9. Sporotrichosis: itraconazole, 100 to 200 mg/day orally; or potassium iodide (SSKI), 1 to 5 ml orally tid

Diet

1. Diabetics: American Diabetic Association diet to control serum glucose

2. Neutropenic patients: Avoid fresh fruits and vegetables (raw).

3. Other: *Lactobacillus*-containing dairy products may aid in restoring normal flora

Activity

1. Hospitalization required for severe systemic infections, meningitis, or fungemia

2. Neutropenic patients: reverse isolation; avoid flowers.

Patient Education

1. Avoidance of high-risk areas and activities (see "Etiology")

2. Importance of diabetic control

3. Importance of prophylactic antifungal when undergoing treatment with antibiotics or immunosuppressive agents

4. Protection from contact (i.e., wearing dust masks or gloves)

Follow-Up

1. In general, patients receiving amphotericin B will require weeks to months of therapy. Because of the high toxicity of this drug, monitoring SMA 7 and CBC twice weekly is recommended.

2. Follow cultures until sterile.

3. Monitor pulmonary function tests in patients with reactive airways (aspergillosis).

4. Follow with chest radiograph for clearing of lesions.

5. Follow with serologic titers every 2 weeks during therapy (coccidioidomycosis, candidiasis).

6. Monitor and maintain suppressive antifungal therapy in AIDS patients (cryptococcosis, histoplasmosis).

Bibliography

Abramowicz M: Systemic fungal drugs. Med Lett Drugs Ther 1994;36(916):16–18.

Fungal and algal infections. In Connor DH, Chandler FW, Schwartz DA, et al (eds): Pathology of Infectious Diseases, Part IV, pp 927–1120. Stamford, CT, Appleton & Lange, 1997.

Feigin RD, Cherry JD: Textbook of Pediatric Infectious Diseases, 4th ed, vol 1, pp 2337–2349. Philadelphia, WB Saunders Company, 1998.

Louria DB: Fungal pneumonias. In Gorbach SL, Bartlett JG, Blacklow NR (eds): Infectious Diseases, 2nd ed, pp 605–613. Philadelphia, WB Saunders Company, 1998.

Mycoses. In Mandell GL, Bennett JE, Dolin R (eds): Mandell, Douglas and Bennett's Principles and Practice of Infectious Diseases, 4th ed, Section G, pp 2288–2375. New York, Churchill Livingstone, 1995.

248 Bacteremia/Sepsis

Peter M. Reiser

Etiology

1. Septic shock is the most common cause of shock and a leading cause of mortality in most intensive care units.

2. Gram-negative organisms such as *Escherichia coli, Pseudomonas*, and *Klebsiella* are the most common causative agents in septic shock and associated mortality.

3. Gram-positive organisms as causative agents are increasing in frequency; some studies suggest they cause up to 40 per cent of septic shock cases.

4. In immunosuppressed or neutropenic patients, viremia/fungemia must be considered as a cause of septic shock. Rickettsia and malaria can cause a sepsis syndrome.

5. *Bacteremia* refers to the presence of viable bacteria in the blood; positive blood cultures may be found in up to 40 per cent of septic shock patients.

6. Sepsis is assumed to begin with bacteremia, release of bacterial cell wall products, or a nidus of infection that triggers cell-mediated activity via macrophages, neutrophils, lymphocytes, platelets, and endothelial cells interacting. These interactions result in cytokine mediators and other humoral factors being released.

7. Endotoxin, found in the blood of about 40 per cent of gram-negative septic shock patients, and exotoxins are important triggers of cell-mediated activity.

8. Tissue necrosis factor, interleukins, prostaglandins, complement, nitric oxide, and other mediators cause myocardial depression and peripheral vascular injury with circulatory failure, leading to maldistribution of blood flow, depressed contractility, decreased ejection fraction, and decreased systemic vascular resistance (SVR).

9. Arterial and venodilation, loss of endothelial integrity, and tissue hypoxemia lead to increased vascular capacitance and loss of fluid from the vascular space (i.e., relative hypovolemia).

WARNING

Gram-positive and gram-negative causes of sepsis cannot be differentiated from each other based on the clinical examination or hemodynamics alone.

Definitions (Society of Critical Care Medicine Consensus Conference)

1. *Sepsis* is the systemic response to infection and often occurs in the absence of bacteremia. Frequency has been increasing recently, with approximately 500,000 cases per year in the United States. About 40 per cent of these patients develop shock.

2. *Systemic inflammatory response syndrome* (SIRS) is the systemic response to a variety of insults, such as trauma, burns, or pancreatitis, where infection is not apparent. Eighteen per cent develop severe sepsis; 4 per cent develop septic shock.

3. *Septic shock* is sepsis with hypotension refractory to adequate fluid resuscitation together with evidence of organ hypoperfusion (lactic acidosis, oliguria, or altered mental status).

4. *Hypotension* is defined as systolic blood pressure (BP) less than 90 mm Hg, mean arterial pressure (MAP) less than 60 mm Hg, or a reduction in systolic BP greater than 40 mm Hg from the patient's normal systolic pressure.

Symptoms/Presumptive Source of Infection

1. Fevers with or without chills/rigors: primary bacteremia; consider a vascular catheter as a source.

2. Respiratory distress/cough: pneumonia/chest

3. Nausea, vomiting, diarrhea: abdominal

4. Dysuria/flank pain: genitourinary

5. Rash/cellulitis: skin/soft tissue

6. Headache, seizures, nuchal rigidity: central nervous system abscess or meningitis

- Fever
- Respiratory distress
- Abdominal complaints
- Dysuria
- Altered mental status

Clinical Findings

1. For sepsis or SIRS, two or more of the following should be present:
   a. Temperature greater than 38° C or less than 36° C
   b. Heart rate greater than 90 beats/minute
   c. Respiratory rate greater than 20 breaths/minute or partial pressure of CO_2 less than 32 mm Hg
   d. White blood cell (WBC) count greater than 12,000 or less than 4000/mm^3 *or* 10 per cent bands
2. For septic shock:
   a. Two or more of items a through d above *plus*
   b. Hypotension: systolic BP less than 90 mm Hg, MAP less than 60 mm Hg
   c. Organ hypoperfusion (oliguria <0.5 ml/kg/hour), lactic acidemia, or altered mental status
3. Source-specific findings: Increase respiratory rate, sputum production suggest pneumonia. Abdominal tenderness or pain suggests a gastrointestinal source.
4. Gram-negative and -positive septic shock can look identical clinically and hemodynamically. Many patients have warm extremities and strong pulses.

- Increased temperature, heart rate, or respiratory rate
- Decreased blood pressure and urine output

Laboratory Tests

1. All patients should have a complete blood cell count and blood cultures plus urine, sputum, or skin/wound sites cultured as indicated by history and physical examination.

2. Initial work-up requires an electrocardiogram, chest radiograph, and usually arterial blood gases. If clinically indicated, other studies such as lumbar puncture, computerized tomography (CT) of the head and sinuses, abdominal CT, renal ultrasound, or transesophageal cardiac ultrasound may be required to determine the source of infection.
3. Laboratory findings include
   a. Respiratory alkalosis—early
   b. Lactic acidosis (metabolic anion gap acidosis)—later on
   c. Thrombocytopenia, commonly without disseminated intravascular coagulopathy
   d. Increased WBC count, increased bands are usual; prognosis is worse with leukopenia.
   e. Hypoxemia
   f. Hyperglycemia not uncommon. Hypoglycemia may occur late in the clinical course.
   g. Hyperbilirubinemia and elevated liver enzymes
4. Echocardiogram: May show biventricular dilation, decreased ejection fraction in many patients in the first 3 to 4 days of septic shock.

- WBC count with differential
- Blood cultures

Differential Diagnosis

1. Other causes of shock: Hypovolemia, cardiogenic, or an extracardiac cause such as pulmonary embolus may coexist. Pulmonary artery catheterization and echocardiogram are useful to differentiate forms of shock.
2. Other causes of hypotension: Toxic shock syndrome, severe liver disease, anaphylactic reaction, adrenal insufficiency, vasodilator or sedative/hypnotic overdose are associated with decreased SVR and blood flow maldistribution.
3. Consider thyroid storm, heat stroke, systemic vasculitis, neuroleptic malignant syndrome, cocaine or organophosphate intoxication, drug withdrawal syndrome, bacterial endocarditis.
4. Extensive tissue injury (pancreatitis, burn) with SIRS

Treatment

1. Early recognition is crucial and requires a high index of suspicion as well as a complete his-

tory and physical examination to attempt to identify a source of infection. Pay attention to the "ABCs." Place a Foley catheter to monitor renal function; an arterial line for blood gases and BP monitoring is very desirable.

2. Early aggressive fluid resuscitation with 200 to 500 ml of isotonic saline or other volume expander in 10 to 15 minutes if hypoperfusion or hypotension. Several liters of fluid may be required in the first several hours of septic shock. With a low hemoglobin, blood is an excellent volume expander and also increases oxygen-carrying capacity.

3. A pulmonary artery flotation catheter is very useful to differentiate various forms of shock and manage fluids to optimize filling pressures and cardiac performance and decrease risk of fluid overload. The goal should be a wedge pressure between 12 and 18 mm Hg.

4. The hemodynamics of septic shock typically reveal increased cardiac output (if volume expanded) and decreased SVR with a low or normal wedge pressure.

5. Early, empiric broad-spectrum antibiotics directed at *all* potential sources of infection, which should always initially include coverage for *Staphylococcus aureus*, should be given as soon as possible and preferably after obtaining blood, urine, sputum, or other appropriate cultures.

6. Closed-space infections must be drained and devitalized tissue must be removed despite the patient not being totally stable hemodynamically. Acquired nosocomial infection may be another reason for deterioration after an initial response to therapy.

7. Refine initial antibiotic choices over the next 36 to 48 hours based on new data, culture and sensitivities, scans, or other information that points to a specific organism or source.

8. Antibiotic choices

   a. If no source of infection evident in a normal host, use: ceftriaxone (Rocephin), 2 gm IV q12h; cefotaxime (Claforan), 2 gm IV q6h; or piperacillin-tazobactam (Zosyn), 3.375 gm IV q6h. If resistant *S. aureus* are commonly found in this location, vancomycin must be included in initial regimen.

   b. In an immunocompromised host with no apparent source, use piperacillin (Pipracil), 3 gm IV q4h, and gentamicin (Garamycin), 1.5 mg/kg q8h; *or* ceftazidime (Ceptaz), 2 gm IV q8h, and vancomycin (Vancocin) 500 mg IV q6h. Amphotericin (Abelcet)

may be required if shock develops while on antibiotics or fungal infection is suspected.

   c. If an intra-abdominal process is suspected, use ampicillin (Unasyn), 2 gm IV q6h, and gentamicin, 1.5 mg/kg q8h, and metronidazole (Flagyl), 500 mg IV q8h.

   d. If urinary tract source suspected, consider ampicillin and gentamicin.

   e. Atypical pneumonia should include coverage for *Legionella* species.

9. Steroids, antiendotoxin, anti–tumor necrosis factor, and anti-interleukin therapies have not improved survival up to this point in time.

10. If hypotension persists despite volume resuscitation, vasopressors are required to bring the MAP above 60 mm Hg. Consider dopamine 2.0 to 20 μg/kg/minute initially. Norepinephrine (Levophed), 1 to 30 μg/minute or phenylephrine (Neo-Synephrine), 2 to 10 μg/kg/minute, can be used as alternatives. Consider the possibility of adrenal insufficiency.

11. Progressive respiratory distress, tachypnea, and hypoxemia with a partial pressure of O_2–to–inspired oxygen concentration ratio less than 200, associated with worsening infiltrates on chest radiograph and a wedge pressure less than 18 mm Hg, suggests acute respiratory distress syndrome (ARDS).

Key Treatment

- Broad-spectrum antibiotic coverage for gram-positive and gram-negative bacteria as early as possible

- Specific antibiotic choices depend on likely source of organisms (see text).

Prognosis

1. Overall mortality of septic shock is 40 to 90 per cent and seems to be decreasing recently. About 50 per cent of deaths are due to refractory hypotension within the first week. The vast majority of these deaths result from refractory vasodilation, not myocardial pump failure. The other half die from progressive multiorgan failure syndrome after the first week.

2. *Pseudomonas*, *S. aureus*, and fungi are especially associated with increased mortality. Risk factors for increased mortality are elderly, immunosuppressed, cirrhosis, asplenia, shock, diabetes, hypothermia, low neutrophil count, inappropriate antibiotics, and requirement for high-dose pressors. Sustained elevation of

interleukin-6 is associated with increased mortality. Acute lung injury is common, with about 20 per cent developing ARDS.

3. Proper nutritional support is crucial to outcome.

4. Prevention of septic shock is desirable. Hand washing between patients, use of aseptic technique for invasive procedures, monitoring catheters for infection, and use of vaccination in high-risk groups may be helpful.

Bibliography

Bone RC: The pathogenesis of sepsis. Ann Intern Med 1991;115:457–469.

Brun-Buisson C, Doyon F, Carlet J: Bacteremia and severe sepsis in adults. Am J Respir Crit Care Med 1996;154: 617–624.

Fein AM, Abraham E, Back R, et al: Sepsis and Multiorgan Failure. Baltimore, Williams & Wilkins, 1997.

Hall JB, Schmidt GA, Wood LH: Principles of Critical Care, 2nd ed. New York, McGraw-Hill, 1998.

Parillo JE: Pathogenic mechanism of septic shock. N Engl J Med 1993;328:1471–1477.

249 Toxic Shock Syndrome

Yangheng Fu

Etiology

1. Microbiology and host immunity
   a. The vast majority of cases of toxic shock syndrome (TSS) are mediated by toxic shock syndrome toxin-1 (TSST-1), produced exclusively by certain strains of *Staphylococcus aureus*. Colonizing toxigenic *S. aureus* in an individual without antibody to TSST-1 is the most important factor in developing TSS. More than 90 per cent of the general population have the antibody to TSST-1, which is protective in TSS.
   b. Twenty per cent of *S. aureus* strains produce TSST-1. One to 4 per cent of healthy individuals harbor TSST-1–producing strains of *S. aureus*. Any site of toxigenic *S. aureus* infection or colonization could be associated with TSS. The nares, axillae, vagina, pharynx, or damaged skin surfaces are the places for colonization. Rates of vaginal colonization during menstruation (with *S. aureus* producing TSST-1) are nearly 5 per cent.
   c. There was a dramatic increase in the incidence of TSS (16 cases per 100,000 women) in the early 1980s, mainly in association with the introduction of superabsorbent tampons (taken off the market since then). The incidence of menstrual TSS had declined to fewer than 3 cases per 100,000 women in 1990. In recent years, menstrual TSS accounts for two thirds of all cases. TSS-1 can be identified in greater than 90 per cent of menstrual TSS and 50 per cent of nonmenstrual cases, whereas other staphylococcal enterotoxins, such as B and C (mainly B), explain non–TSST-1-related cases.
2. Mechanisms of TSS
   a. *Staphylococcus aureus* does not need to invade tissue to cause TSS. Colonized *S. aureus* elaborate TSS-1, which is absorbed via endocytosis through epithelial cells coated with TSST-1 receptors.
   b. TSST-1 and other staphylococcal enterotoxins are superantigens because of their ability to activate large proportions of T cells. For example, TSST-1 is able to activate all T cells bearing the Vβ2 chain of the T-cell receptors, which account for 5 to 20 per cent of resting T cells (as compared with 0.01 per cent of T cells for conventional antigens). Those exponentially expanded T cells will further activate monocytes/macrophages. T cells and monocytes release excessive quantities of cytokines (such as tumor necrosis factor, γ-interferon, and interleukin-1, -2, -6, and -8), which cause fever, shock, capillary leak, and multiorgan failure.

Symptoms

1. Fever 38.9° C or higher
2. Vomiting
3. Diarrhea
4. Confusion
5. Dizziness
6. Headache
7. Severe myalgias
8. Sore throat

Key Symptoms

- Fever 38.9° C or higher
- Vomiting and diarrhea
- Myalgias

Clinical Findings

1. Rashes: Vast majority of patients develop sunburn-like erythroderma (macular but not papular) and subsequent desquamation (the latter is a relative specific sign, usually declares itself 1 to 2 weeks after the clinical presentation).
2. Vaginal, oropharyngeal, or conjunctival hyperemia; strawberry tongue in 50 per cent of cases
3. Hypotension (systolic blood pressure ≤90 mm Hg) or orthostatic changes occurs early in the course of disease.
4. Complications include rhabdomyolysis, renal failure, adult respiratory distress syndrome, toxic encephalopathy, aseptic meningitis, arrythmias, myocardial depression, disseminated intravascular coagulation.
5. Mortality in menstrual TSS is about 2 to 3 per cent, whereas that in nonmenstrual TSS is two

to three times higher. Influenza-associated TSS has a very high mortality rate in children (up to 90 per cent).

6. Recalcitrant erythematous desquamating syndrome is a form of TSS occurring more frequently in patients with acquired immunodeficiency syndrome.

7. Recurrent TSS, up to 5 episodes, has been reported.

Key Signs

- Rashes, mucosal hyperemia
- Hypotension
- Confusion

Laboratory Tests

1. Platelet count 100,000/mm³ or less
2. Culture-negative pyuria
3. Creatinine level at least twice the upper limit of normal
4. Fivefold increase in creatinine phosphokinase (CPK)
5. Bilirubin and transaminases at least twice the upper limit of normal
6. Hypoalbuminemia, severe hypocalcemia, hypophosphatemia, hypomagnesemia
7. Isolation of *S. aureus* from infected or colonized sites

Key Tests

- Platelet count
- Blood, vaginal, wound cultures
- Serum creatinine
- Serum calcium
- Bilirubin and transaminases
- Serum CPK

Diagnosis

1. The criteria for the diagnosis of TSS includes sudden onset of fever, hypotension, characteristic rashes with subsequent desquamation, and involvement of three or more organ systems (see lists from symptoms, clinical findings, and laboratory tests) and excludes other diseases resembling TSS. The absence of erythroderma and desquamation does not exclude the diag-

nosis because rash can be limited or evanescent. Clean wound or flu-like symptoms do not suggest an alternative diagnosis.

2. Blood cultures and cultures from vagina or wound should be obtained. Isolation of *S. aureus*–producing TSST-1 is suggestive but not diagnostic of TSS because there is a 1 to 4 per cent colonization rate in the healthy population and higher in hospitalized patients. Failure to identify *S. aureus* should not exclude the diagnosis because the true colonization sites may not be suspected.

3. The above strict case definition by the Centers for Disease Control and Prevention will certainly miss many less serious cases with the same pathogenesis. For example, neonatal TSS-like exanthematous disease occurs in the first week of life with fever, small erythematous rash, and thrombocytopenia. Desquamation, hypotension, or multiorgan failure have not been reported and disease is self-limited. Nearly 100 per cent of patients were carriers of methicillin-resistant *S. aureus*. TSST-1 seems responsible for this disease. Maternal antibody to TSST-1 or immaturity of the immune system in the newborn may explain why those patients do not develop full-blown TSS.

Differential Diagnosis

1. Streptococcal TSS (STSS)

   a. Exotoxin A or C from some strains of *Streptococcus pyogenes* are superantigens, which is why STSS is clinically indistinguishable from staphylococcal TSS. Identifying *S. pyogenes* from blood or other sterile site confirms the diagnosis.

   b. Bacteremia is rare in TSS but is present in up to 60 per cent of patients with STSS. Desquamation is less common in STSS, whereas cellulitis (80 per cent) and fasciitis (70 per cent) suggest STSS.

   c. Early recognition and thorough surgical intervention cannot be overemphasized, because mortality from STSS is up to 30 to 70 per cent.

   d. The presence of fever with unexplained severe musculoskeletal pain, marked left shift, and elevated CPK are the best early clues of the disease.

2. Kawasaki's syndrome (KS)

   a. Fever, rashes with subsequent desquamation in KS make it difficult to differentiate from TSS. Some data suggested KS could be a microbial superantigen-induced disease.

   b. The following features suggest KS: age less

than 5 years old, subacute onset, no hypotension, papular component of the rash, azotemia and thrombocytopenia (rarely).

3. Rocky Mountain spotted fever (RMSF) and meningococcemia can cause fever, hypotension and multiple organ failure. Histories of travel, exposure to ticks, and purpuric rashes suggest the diagnosis of RMSF. Lumbar puncture will confirm the diagnosis of meningitis. One caveat is that *S. aureus* septicemia can cause purpuric lesions mimicking those of RMSF and meningococcemia.

4. Other differential diagnoses include leptospirosis, septicemia, scarlet fever, staphylococcal scalded skin syndrome, drug eruptions, acute viral syndrome, and measles.

Treatment

1. Removal of foreign body and cleaning of focal wound are very important even when the wound looks normal (e.g., removal of tampon and irrigation of vaginal vault in menstrual TSS and opening any closed wound in nonmenstrual cases).

2. Fluid resuscitation (10 to 20 L) may be required in the first 24 hours; vasoactive agents may be necessary.

3. Monitoring and correcting electrolyte abnormality should not be overlooked.

Medication

1. Some authors advocate clindamycin (900 mg IV q8h) as the first-line drug because bacteria at stationary phase are not susceptible to agents that interfere with cell wall synthesis.

2. Methicillin resistance is uncommon because TSS usually develops in healthy individuals, but, when suspected, vancomycin should be used.

3. Two weeks of antistaphylococcal antibiotics is recommended. Addition of a broad-spectrum antibiotic is reasonable pending culture results or when the diagnosis is uncertain. Alternative drugs are nafcillin, cefazolin.

4. Intravenous immune globulin (IVIG) should be used in severe cases; it showed promise in a small case-control study of STSS and in anecdotal reports of TSS. IVIG can be given 400 mg/kg as a single dose over several hours. Antibody to TSST-1 in IVIG may partially account for its therapeutic effect, but immunomodulation may also play a role.

5. Corticosteroids have no proven role in TSS.

Key Treatment

- Remove foreign body
- Clean wound
- Fluid resuscitation
- Correct electrolyte abnormality
- Clindamycin
- IVIG

Follow-Up

1. Reversible alopecia and nail losses occur several months after acute illness. A late rash occurs several weeks after illness.

2. There may be persistent neuropsychological symptoms, such as fatigue, depression, and memory loss.

3. Two thirds of patients will not develop antibody to TSST-1 after first episode of TSS; they should refrain from using tampons or barrier contraceptives and use another catamenial product such as sanitary napkins or pads.

Bibliography

Centers for Disease Control and Prevention: Toxic-shock syndrome—United States. MMWR Morb Mortal Wkly Rep 1997;46(RR-22):492–495.

Lowy FD: *Staphylococcus aureus* infections. N Engl J Med 1998;339:520–532.

Parsonnet J: Nonmenstrual toxic shock syndrome: new insights into diagnosis, pathogenesis, and treatment. Curr Clin Top Infect Dis 1996;16:1–20.

Stevens DL: The toxic shock syndromes. Infect Dis Clin North Am 1996;10:727–746.

Takahashi N, Nishida H, Kato H, et al: Exanthematous disease induced by toxic shock syndrome 1 in the early neonatal period. Lancet 1998;351:1614–1619.

250 Infectious Diarrhea

Bradley W. Fenton

Sporadic, Endemic Diarrhea

Etiology

1. Most episodes of acute, endemic diarrhea (the sporadic type occurring in the United States) are self-limited, lasting less than 5 to 10 days. More than half are of viral origin. Fewer than 30 per cent involve a bacterial agent, and less than 5 to 10 per cent of all acute episodes are true dysenteries—the bloody, mucoid diarrhea associated with fever and caused by invasive organisms or their cytotoxic products. Therefore, antibiotic treatment should be considered in fewer than 1 in 10 cases of endemic diarrhea. Reassurance, symptomatic treatment, dietary changes, and occasionally rehydration are usually all that is required in the management of routine cases. Diarrhea lasting more than 10 to 14 days and that occurring in immune-impaired hosts (human immunodeficiency virus [HIV]-positive individuals and those with acquired immunodeficiency syndrome) requires a more comprehensive and aggressive initial evaluation.

   a. Common noninfectious causes of acute diarrhea

   (1) Drugs: laxatives, magnesium-containing antacids, antibiotics, colchicine, quinidine, digitalis

   (2) Lactose intolerance

   (3) Sucrose-containing dietetic foods, candies, and gum

   (4) Irritable bowel syndrome

   (5) Inflammatory bowel disease

   b. Bacterial agents in acute diarrhea

   (1) *Campylobacter* species

   (2) *Salmonella* species

   (3) *Shigella* species

   (4) *Clostridium difficile*

   (5) *Escherichia coli*: enterotoxigenic and enterohemorrhagic strains

   (6) *Aeromonas hydrophila*

   (7) *Plesiomonas shigelloides*

   (8) *Yersinia enterocolitica*

   (9) *Vibrio* species

   c. Viral pathogens

   (1) Rotavirus

   (2) Norwalk-like agents

   (3) Caliciviruses

   (4) Adenoviruses

2. Acute diarrhea lasting more than 10 to 14 days is more likely to be caused by

   a. Transient lactose intolerance secondary to a self-limited viral or bacterial diarrhea

   b. Protracted courses of usual pathogens (*Salmonella*, *Shigella*, *Campylobacter*)

   c. *Entamoeba histolytica*

   d. *Giardia lamblia*

   e. Bacterial overgrowth

Symptoms

1. Acute food poisonings caused by preformed toxins are brief, self-limited illnesses usually lasting less than 24 to 48 hours, and vomiting as well as diarrhea are prominent symptoms. Fever is not. *Staphylococcus aureus*, *Clostridium perfringens*, and *Bacillus cereus* are the most common agents. In these intoxications (to differentiate them from true infection), the secretory activity of the small bowel overcomes the absorptive capacity of the distal small bowel and proximal colon, resulting in diarrhea.

2. The abdominal discomfort characteristic of viral gastroenteritis and nondysenteric, toxin-mediated bacterial infection is usually diffuse or periumbilical cramping, reflecting small bowel involvement. Most of the dysenteric pathogens also initially produce toxins active in the small bowel, resulting in profuse watery diarrhea as a prelude to the small-volume dysentery of colonic involvement. The abdominal discomfort of infectious gastroenteritis is more likely to be relieved temporarily by a bowel movement than is a surgical or mechanical problem, which waxes and wanes irrespective of stool passage.

3. Small-volume diarrhea with frequent mucoid movements, suprapubic crampy pain, tenesmus, and rectal discomfort are characteristic of the true dysenteries caused most commonly in the United States by *Campylobacter*, *Shigella*, and *Salmonella* species. Fever and grossly bloody mucoid stools are characteristic of dysentery. Ten to 15 or more small stools a day is not uncommon.

4. Enterohemorrhagic *E. coli* (EHEC) serotype 0157:H7 is an increasingly recognized pathogen cultured from undercooked ground beef, unpasteurized drinks, and unwashed fruits and vegetables. It causes a characteristic syndrome beginning as abdominal pain and diarrhea for a few days, followed by grossly bloody, watery stools for 2 to 4 days, usually without associated fever. In the young and elderly, hemolytic-uremic syndrome may develop upon recovery from the diarrhea in 8 to 10 per cent of cases.

5. Signs and symptoms of volume depletion (thirst, oliguria, and orthostatic dizziness) are uncommon in usual cases but may be more prominent in very young or elderly patients and those with other significant medical problems who are taking medications such as diuretics and other antihypertensive agents.

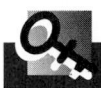

Key Symptoms

Viral Gastroenteritis	Bacterial Dysentery
• Vomiting	• ±Vomiting
• Fever	• Fever
• Profuse, watery diarrhea	• Bloody, mucoid loose stool
• Abdominal crampy pain (periumbilical or generalized)	• Suprapubic crampy pain (temporarily relieved by bowel movements)
• Myalgias	• Tenesmus
• Arthralgias	• Often begins as watery diarrhea
• Headache	

Clinical Findings

1. An office visit is not always necessary in the patient without complicating medical problems, significant volume depletion, or clear-cut dysenteric stools. Symptoms suggestive of abdominal obstruction or other surgical problems (severe pain, persistent vomiting, feculent vomitus, marked abdominal distention, or the cessation of flatus and bowel movements) warrant urgent evaluation.

2. A toxic appearance, scleral icterus, fever, and orthostatic signs should be noted on clinical examination. The presence of marked guarding, referred or rebound pain, a quiet abdomen, or high-pitched rushes suggesting obstruction may warrant an evaluation for an acute surgical abdomen with plain films and a surgical consultation.

3. In the female patient, when the clinical picture is unclear and lower abdominal symptoms are present, a pelvic examination should be performed.

4. Rectal examinations with occult blood testing should almost always be done in patients examined for acute abdominal pain and diarrhea. Testing negative for occult blood is helpful. However, occult or gross blood from concurrent hemorrhoids or fissures can confuse the picture.

5. Extraintestinal complications are listed in Table 250–1.

Key Signs

Findings Consistent With a Nonsurgical Abdomen

- Mild tenderness
- Soft abdomen
- Hyperactive bowel sounds
- Absence of peritoneal signs

Laboratory Tests

1. For those patients examined, all that is usually necessary as the initial laboratory work-up of acute diarrhea is stool testing for occult blood.

   a. Fecal white cell smears using methylene blue or Gram's stain are positive for white cells in approximately two thirds of invasive or dysenteric diarrheas.

      (1) A specimen of stool obtained from a rectal swab or freshly passed stool is thinly smeared on a glass slide and flooded with two or three drops of methylene blue and allowed to stain the white cell nuclei for three or four minutes.

      (2) The polymorphonuclear plus mononuclear cells (nuclei) per high-power field are counted. More than 25 are consistent with dysentery.

   b. Alternatively, a Gram's stain of a thin fecal

TABLE 250–1. EXTRAINTESTINAL COMPLICATIONS OF ACUTE DIARRHEAL ILLNESS

PATHOGEN	COMPLICATION
Escherichia coli 0157:H7	Hemolytic-uremic syndrome
Non-*Salmonella* species, *Y. enterocolitica*	Reactive arthritis
Campylobacter species	Guillain-Barré syndrome
Listeria monocytogenes	Meningitis/sepsis

smear can be just as satisfactory for counting cells.

2. In the United States, when a patient is acutely ill with diarrhea, cultures are not generally necessary or cost-effective unless the diarrhea lasts more than 7 to 10 days. In the absence of recent foreign travel to high-risk areas, ova and parasite determinations can be delayed for at least the first few weeks of an illness, and then three separate specimens should be evaluated by an experienced, reliable laboratory.

   a. Giardia antigen testing on fresh stool is available, sensitive, and inexpensive.

   b. A freshly passed specimen for *C. difficile* toxin assay (rather than culture) can be obtained in the appropriate setting.

   c. For HIV-positive patients, diarrhea persisting more than 5 to 7 days usually warrants a more comprehensive initial laboratory evaluation, including stool culture for enteric pathogens, ova and parasite determinations, and acid-fast smears that can identify mycobacteria, *Cyclospora*, *Isospora*, and cryptosporidia.

3. Sigmoidoscopy has no place in the routine office management of acute diarrhea in uncomplicated cases.

   a. One exception is diarrhea occurring within 2 months following antibiotic therapy, when antibiotic-associated pseudomembranous colitis can be diagnosed endoscopically by recognizing the characteristic whitish-yellow membranes.

   b. Sigmoidoscopy or colonoscopy is indicated in cases of persistent diarrhea in HIV-positive patients whose bacterial cultures, *C. difficile* toxin assays, and ova and parasites determinations have been unrevealing.

Key Test

Stool white cell smear

Differential Diagnosis

1. Figure 250–1 outlines a practical approach to the differential diagnosis for the patient presenting with acute diarrhea. Once surgical problems and other noninfectious etiologies have been considered and satisfactorily ruled out, the algorithm helps to direct diagnostic and therapeutic decisions.

2. More than 60 per cent of cases in the United States are due to a viral etiology. Norwalk and related viruses attack older children and adults, often causing outbreaks in the household or workplace. Rotaviruses are the most common cause of watery diarrhea in children and in adults in contact with children.

3. Twenty-five to 30 per cent of the cases of infectious diarrhea in patients older than 6 months are caused by the invasive enteropathogens *Campylobacter*, *Shigella*, and *Salmonella*. Less frequently, *Y. enterocolitica*, enterohemorrhagic *E. coli* (serotype 0157), *A. hydrophila*, and *Plesiomonas* species are isolated. *Vibrio* species are now causing isolated cases in individuals exposed to seafood from the Gulf Coast of the United States.

4. Although many epidemiologic associations (particularly foods) have been documented in texts and medical literature, such information is rarely useful clinically. The incubation period of agents causing acute infectious diarrhea ranges from a few hours to 2 weeks. Patients tend to associate their illness with foodstuffs eaten just before the onset of symptoms.

Management

1. Because the majority of cases of endemic diarrhea will not respond to antibiotic therapy, becoming adept at *treating symptoms* will provide more rapid comfort to patients and minimize absenteeism from work or school and decompensation of underlying medical problems.

   a. *Adsorbents* such as attapulgite (Kaopectate) will firm up stools but do not decrease total stool volume and so have little to offer from a practical standpoint. Currently they are the only agents available for use by pregnant women.

   b. Bismuth subsalicylate (Pepto-Bismol) is an *antisecretory agent* that also has antibacterial properties. It is useful for reducing the amount of watery diarrhea by about 50 per cent. Co-administration of salicylates should be avoided to prevent salicylism. A black tongue and dark stools usually develop.

   c. The *antiperistaltic agents*, which include codeine, paregoric, and the synthetic opioids loperamide HCl (Imodium) and diphenoxylate HCl with atropine sulfate (Lomotil), are the most active and useful for diminishing abdominal cramps as well as reducing the number of stools.

      (1) Anticholinergics (e.g., atropine) have no demonstrated role in the treatment of diarrhea and so the safety and side-effect profile makes loperamide currently the agent of first choice. Recent studies in

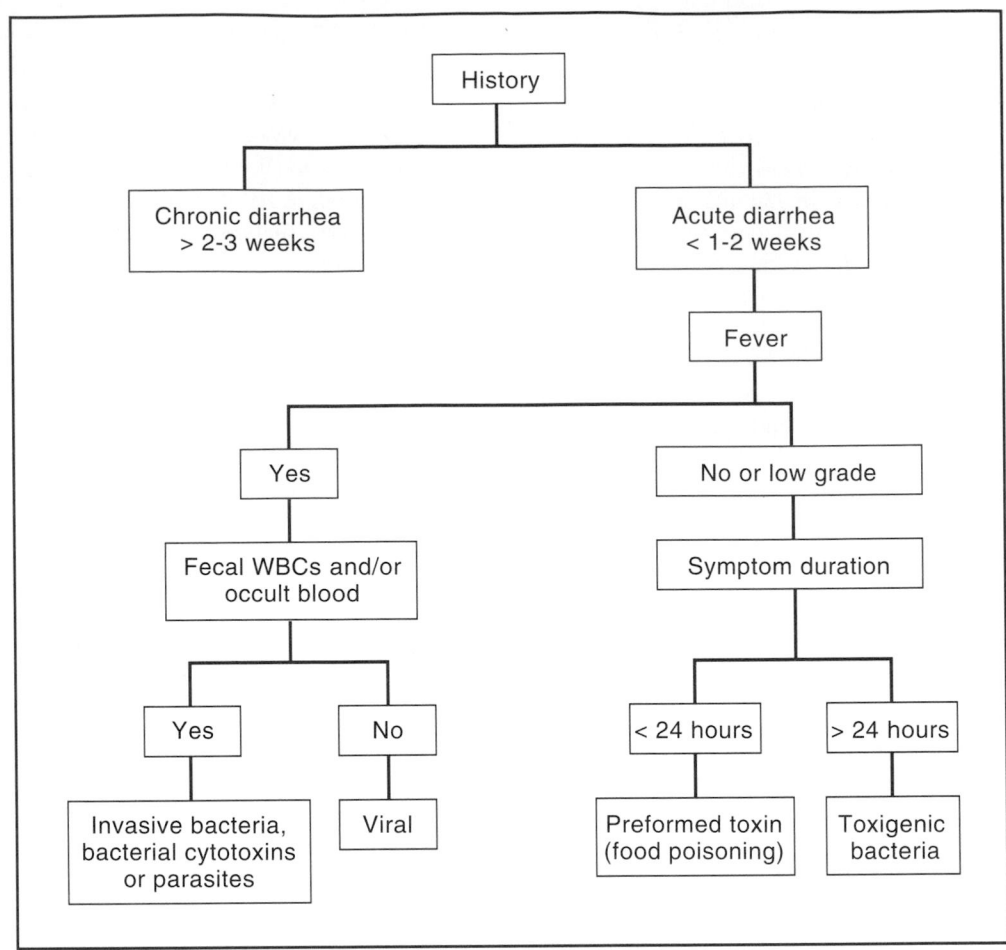

Figure 250–1 Diagnostic approach to acute diarrheal illnesses. WBCs, white blood cells. (Adapted from Blaser MJ: Current approach to acute diarrheal illnesses. Drug Ther 1983;13:114, with permission.)

travelers' diarrhea confirm the utility and safety of loperamide even in the presence of bacterial pathogens. Patients with low-grade fever (<101.5° F) and occult blood–positive stool that grew *Shigella* and *Campylobacter* responded well. *Salmonella* carriage may occasionally be prolonged by antiperistaltic agents, but clinical deterioration is rare.

   (2) These agents should be avoided in toxic-appearing patients with high fevers and grossly bloody stools lest they contribute to the development of a toxic megacolon.

2. The *antibiotics* of choice for empiric therapy in adult patients ill with fever and dysentery are the quinolones: ciprofloxacin HCl (Cipro), norfloxacin (Noroxin—unlabeled use), and ofloxacin (Floxin).

   a. Although antibiotic therapy for 3 days shortens clinical illness in *Campylobacter* and *Shigella* infections and shortens intestinal shedding and communicability in *Shigella* in-

fections, no therapy has a beneficial effect in nontyphoidal *Salmonella* enteritis, and antibiotics may prolong fecal carriage.

   b. *Salmonella typhi* infection (typhoid fever) should always be treated, as should patients with bacteremic *Salmonella* infections with nontyphoidal strains, which can occur in 5 per cent of those with gastroenteritis. Those at risk of bacteremic complications include individuals with lymphoproliferative disorders, sickle cell anemia, prosthetic heart valves, aortic aneurysms, and HIV infection.

   c. Because of resistance, ampicillin and trimethoprim-sulfamethoxazole are no longer predictably active against *Shigella* and *Salmonella* and are never effective for *Campylobacter*. If cultures and antibiotic sensitivities are available, they can be used to specifically direct therapy for a duration of no more than 3 to 5 days.

   d. Antibiotics have no benefit in hemorrhagic colitis caused by EHEC, and there is some concern that they may predispose to the development of the hemolytic-uremic syndrome.

3. In antibiotic-induced pseudomembranous colitis caused by *C. difficile* infection, discontinuing the offending antibiotic may be all that is necessary to treat mild episodes. Although bile-acid–binding resins such as cholestyramine (Questran—unlabeled use) and colestipol HCl (Colestid—unlabeled use) may be effective in binding toxin and improving mild cases, metronidazole (Flagyl; Protostat—unlabeled use) or oral vancomycin (Vancocin, Vancoled) is recommended in moderate to severe cases. Metronidazole is much less expensive and currently is the drug of choice. Relapse may occur in 10 to 20 per cent of cases. Retreat with metronidazole.

Diet

1. Avoiding lactose-containing foods (especially milk, cheese, and ice cream) may decrease bloating, flatulence, and diarrhea. Infectious diarrhea can lead to lactase depletion in the intestinal epithelium of the proximal small bowel, lasting for days to weeks.

2. Caffeine stimulates intestinal motility and should also be avoided initially. Coffee, chocolate, nonherbal teas, and caffeinated sodas are included.

3. Hydration with broth, clear juices (containing no pulp), herbal teas, and commercial electrolyte-glucose solutions (Gatorade) is recommended, especially with high fever and profuse diarrhea.

4. Low-residue, carbohydrate-rich foods are the mainstay of nutrition once vomiting has ceased: noodles, rice, boiled or baked potatoes, and breads.

5. As diarrhea ceases, cooked vegetables, broiled or baked poultry, and fish can be reintroduced.

6. Meats, raw fruit and vegetables, and lastly lactose-containing dairy foods are reintroduced as tolerated.

7. Temporarily stopping diuretics may also be necessary.

Activity

Fever, malaise, myalgias, and abdominal discomfort will generally limit the patient's activities, including work. Control of diarrhea and cramping with dietary measures and antiperistaltic agents will allow early return to usual daily activities once a patient is confident that immediate access to the bathroom is not necessary. Food handlers should be culture negative before returning to work after bacterial enteritis has been documented.

Patient Education

1. Avoidance of high-risk foods (unpasteurized drinks and dairy products, raw eggs, undercooked poultry and meats, and raw seafood), thorough cooking, proper refrigeration, and attention to cross-contamination (separate handling of raw and cooked foods) may prevent infectious diarrheal illness.

2. Reminding patients of the need for hand washing after bathroom use is important to minimize family and other point source outbreaks.

3. Educating patients about the use of over-the-counter antidiarrheal agents and dietary restrictions may allow them to manage mild, uncomplicated illnesses without physician involvement.

Key Treatment

Symptomatic Therapy

- Bismuth subsalicylate (Pepto-Bismol), 30 ml or two tabs q30min up to maximum of eight doses

- Loperamide HCl (Imodium), 4 mg initially; 2 mg after each loose stool, not to exceed 16 mg/day

Antibiotic Therapy—Empiric

- Ciprofloxacin HCl, 500 mg PO bid ×3 days

- Norfloxacin HCl, 400 mg PO bid ×3 days

- Ofloxacin, 300 mg PO bid ×3 days (Quinolones should not be given to prepubertal children or to pregnant or lactating women.)

***Clostridium difficile* Enterocolitis**

- Metronidazole, 500 mg PO tid for 7 to 14 days

- Vancomycin, 125 mg PO qid for 7 to 14 days

Travelers' Diarrhea

1. In contrast to sporadic, endemic diarrhea, for which antibiotics are usually not indicated, travelers' diarrhea, which occurs in 30 to 40 per cent of individuals visiting less industrialized destinations, is caused by treatable bacteria in more than 75 per cent of cases.

2. The most common pathogens include enterotoxigenic *E. coli* (Mexico, Central and South America) and *Campylobacter* and *Salmonella* species (India, the Far East, and Africa). Parasites (amebae and *Giardia* most commonly) are usually not a consideration during travel of less than 2 weeks' duration.

TABLE 250–2. EMPIRIC THERAPY FOR TRAVELERS' DIARRHEA

DRUG	THERAPY	INDICATIONS
Ciprofloxacin	500 mg twice daily for 1–3 days	Diarrhea resulting from travel to Mexico (coastal areas year round and interior areas during the winter) and developing areas of Africa, Southern Asia, and South America. These areas are known for high rates of *Campylobacter* isolates and other trimethoprim-resistant pathogens.
Ofloxacin	300 mg twice daily for 1–3 days	
Norfloxacin	400 mg twice daily for 1–3 days	
Trimethoprim-sulfamethoxazole	160/800 mg twice daily for 1–3 days	Diarrea resulting from travel in the interior of Mexico during the summer.
Loperamide	4 mg initially 2 mg after each stool	Antimotility agent of choice to use at the onset of symptoms. Withhold in cases of bloody stools or high fever.
Bismuth subsalicylate	30 ml every ½ hr for up to 8 hr	High-volume, watery diarrhea—use at the onset of symptoms. Bismuth subsalicylate may be used prophylactically.
Ibuprofen	200–600 mg three times daily	Use with bismuth subsalicylate.

3. Typically travelers' diarrhea presents as nausea, abdominal cramps, malaise, low-grade fever, and four to five loose bowel movements per day. Untreated, this usually benign illness resolves spontaneously in 90 per cent of individuals within 7 days. However, vacations and business travel usually warrant prompt treatment.

4. To minimize the occurrence of diarrhea, usual dietary recommendations include avoiding local water, including ice (drinking bottled, carbonated beverages, wine, and beer), fresh uncooked vegetables and salads, fruits that cannot be peeled, and foods that stand at room temperature (buffets). The Peace Corps adage "Peel it, boil it or forget it" makes sense, but even well-informed travelers make serious food choice mistakes frequently.

5. Because adverse drug effects are common (including photosensitivity reactions), selection of resistant bacteria is a growing worldwide problem, and the question of antibiotic choice for prevention failures is unanswered, the consensus of experts is not to recommend prophylactic antibiotics for travelers except in very exceptional cases. In some areas of the world (Mexico) bismuth subsalicylate (Pepto-Bismol), two tablets four times a day with meals, has been 60 per cent effective in preventing diarrhea. Patients unable to take aspirin should abstain. Tinnitus, dark stools, and a black tongue can occur. Bismuth subsalicylate should not be used for more than 2 to 3 weeks consecutively.

Management

1. Antimotility agents are the first line of therapy and, combined with fluoroquinolones, often lead to resolution of symptoms within 12 to 36 hours (Table 250–2). Evidence suggests that the first day's entire dose can be given at once with loperamide and the remaining 2 days' (four doses) medication withheld if there is prompt resolution of symptoms. High fever (>103° F), toxicity, and grossly bloody stools warrant prompt medical evaluation.

2. A written handout outlining use of loperamide and antibiotics as well as usual dietary measures is very useful for prospective travelers. Dietary restrictions as noted above for endemic diarrhea apply for travel-associated diarrhea.

Bibliography

Ericsson CD, DuPont HL: Travelers' diarrhea: approach to prevention and treatment. Clin Infect Dis 1993;16:616.

Goodman LJ, Trenholme GM, Kaplan RL, et al: Empiric antimicrobial therapy of domestically acquired acute diarrhea in urban adults. Arch Intern Med 1990;150:541.

Gorbach SL: Drugs for intestinal agonies. Infect Dis Clin Pract 1997;6:597.

Johnson S, Gerding DN: Clostridium difficile-associated diarrhea. Clin Infect Dis 1998;26:1027.

Slutsker L, Ries AA, Maldney K, et al: Escherichia coli 0157:H7 diarrhea in the United States: clinical and epidemiologic features. Ann Intern Med 1997;126:505.

Tamkin GW: An approach to diarrhea. Emerg Med 1998; June:16.

251 Cellulitis

Carol L. Ellis

Etiology

1. Cellulitis is an acute infection of the skin and subcutaneous tissues. It may arise from
   a. Entry of bacteria through a disruption in the integrity of the skin (i.e., a laceration, puncture wound, or fungal intertrigo)
   b. Extension from a contiguous focus (i.e., an abscess)
   c. Metastatic dissemination from bacteremia (e.g., pneumococcal cellulitis)
2. Cellulitis is a serious disease because of the propensity of infection to spread via the lymphatics and blood stream, which may result in bacteremia and sepsis.
3. Certain conditions appear to predispose to cellulitis. These include
   a. Local trauma or abrasions
   b. Underlying skin lesions such as ulcers, eczema, psoriasis, or tinea
   c. Tinea pedis or "athlete's foot"
   d. Diabetes or peripheral vascular disease
   e. Impaired lymphatic drainage, as may be seen after saphenous venectomy, mastectomy, or radical pelvic surgery
   f. Parenteral drug injection
4. Causative organisms
   a. Group A β-hemolytic *Streptococcus* and *Staphylococcus aureus* are responsible for the majority of cases. Streptococci of other groups (groups C, G, B) may occasionally be causal.
   b. In immunocompromised or granulocytopenic patients, gram-negative rods (e.g., *Serratia*, *Proteus*, *Enterobacter*) and fungi (*Cryptococcus neoformans*) may be the etiologic agents.
   c. In persons handling fish, meat, or poultry, *Erysipelothrix rhusiopathiae* may be the cause of a cellulitis that begins on the hands.
   d. *Aeromonas hydrophila*, a gram-negative bacillus found in lakes, rivers, and soil, may cause cellulitis by contaminating an open wound in fresh water; salt water wounds exposed to *Vibrio* (e.g., *V. vulnificus*, *V. alginolyticus*, *V. parahaemolyticus*) can progress to cellulitis, necrosis, and bacteremia.

Symptoms

1. Within several days of the inciting trauma, local tenderness, pain, swelling, and erythema develop, rapidly intensify, and spread.
2. Fever, chills, and malaise may be present.

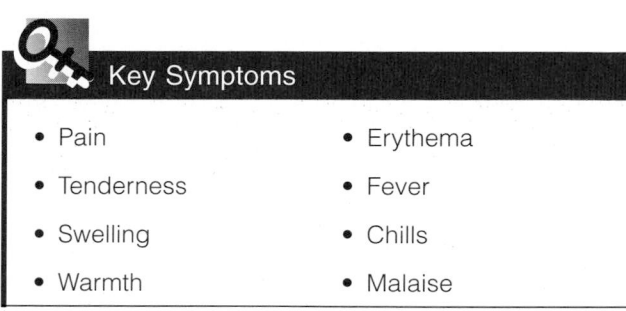

Key Symptoms

- Pain
- Tenderness
- Swelling
- Warmth
- Erythema
- Fever
- Chills
- Malaise

Clinical Findings

1. Erythema with indistinct margins, warmth and tenderness of the skin
2. Regional lymphadenopathy and lymphatic streaking are common.
3. Bullae, abscesses, and necrosis of the skin may occur.

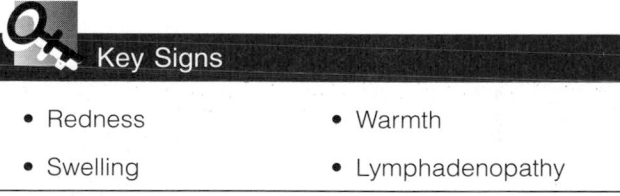

Key Signs

- Redness
- Swelling
- Warmth
- Lymphadenopathy

Laboratory Tests

1. Laboratory tests add little to the management of the typical patient; identification of the infecting organism is usually not obtained and may not be necessary.
2. Blood cultures and skin site cultures may prove helpful in guiding antibiotic therapy in patients who
   a. Fail to respond to standard therapy
   b. Have serious underlying medical problems
   c. Have ulcers or abscesses that could yield microorganisms

Differential Diagnosis

1. Erysipelas is superficial cellulitis involving skin but not soft tissue. It is characterized by bright

red color and a raised advancing border and caused by the same pathogens that produce other types of cellulitis.

2. It is important to differentiate cellulitis from skin infections that are rapidly progressive and cause tissue necrosis, such as necrotizing fasciitis or gas gangrene, where drainage and débridement will be required.

3. Cellulitis of the lower extremity in older patients is frequently complicated by deep vein thrombosis.

4. Diffuse inflammatory carcinoma of the breast and cutaneous neoplasms may look like cellulitis.

Treatment

Medication

Presumptive antibiotic therapy to cover streptococci and staphylococci is generally the appropriate choice.

1. Outpatient treatment
   a. A reasonable option if the cellulitis is limited and if the patient is not seriously ill and is without co-morbid conditions.
      (1) A penicillinase-resistant oral penicillin: dicloxacillin (Dynapen), 500 mg to 1 gm qid *or*
      (2) A first-generation cephalosporin: cephalexin (Keflex), 500 mg qid
   b. For penicillin-allergic patients: erythromycin, 500 mg qid
   c. For sicker patients: ceftriaxone (Rocephin), 1 gm intramuscularly daily for the first few days
   d. Duration of therapy: 10 to 14 days
2. Inpatient treatment
   a. When intravenous antibiotics are needed
      (1) Nafcillin (Nafcil, Unipen), 1 to 2 gm intravenously q4h
      (2) Cefazolin (Ancef), 2 gm intravenously q6h
   b. For immunocompromised patients
      (1) Ticarcillin-clavulanate (Timentin), 3.1 gm q6h
      (2) Cefoxitin (Mefoxin), 1 gm q6h

3. Atypical cellulitis
   a. *Erysipelothrix*: penicillin
   b. *Vibrio* species: aminoglycosides and tetracyclines
   c. *Aeromonas hydrophila*: aminoglycosides and chloramphenicol

Activity

1. Immobilization and elevation of an affected limb may be helpful initially.
2. Moist heat may serve to localize the infection.

Patient Education

The goal of education is to prevent recurrences. Use of support stockings, good skin hygiene, and foot care can reduce or eliminate recurrences.

Follow-Up

1. Follow-up is needed to ensure eradication of the infection.
2. Athlete's foot should be treated with oral antifungal agents. Coexistent tinea and bacterial infections of the foot may result in recurrent cellulitis.
3. Patients with predisposing factors should be evaluated to assess whether these conditions can be treated or improved (e.g., improve diabetic foot care). Patients without major predisposing conditions who have had recurrent bouts of cellulitis may benefit from prophylaxis with penicillin G (250 to 500 mg orally bid) or intramuscular benzathine penicillin G given every 2 weeks.

Bibliography

Baddour L: Primary skin infections in primary care: an update. Infect Med 1993;10:42–48.

Lindbeck G, Powers R: Cellulitis. Hosp Pract 1993; 28(Suppl 2):10–24.

Swartz M: Cellulitis and superficial infections. In Mandel G (ed): Principles and Practice of Infectious Disease, pp 796–807. New York, Churchill Livingstone, 1990.

Wang JH, Liu YC, Cheng DL, et al: Role of benzathine penicillin G in prophylaxis for recurrent streptococcal cellulitis of the lower legs. Clin Infect Dis 1997;25: 685–689.

Weekly CPC. N Engl J Med 1989;321:1029–1038.

252 Cat-Scratch Disease

Beck B. Soderberg

Etiology

1. Typically, a cat's scratch inoculates the skin with the zoonotic bacterium *Bartonella henselae*. After 3 to 10 days, a nontender, red-brown papule or pustule arises at the site of the scratch. This is followed by regional lymphadenopathy, which may persist for several days or 2 to 3 months. Flea feces, especially on younger cats, have been implicated as the primary bacterial reservoir and are transmitted to skin by not only scratching, but also by biting and licking.

2. Cat-scratch disease (CSD) has been divided into two groups. Typical CSD accounts for 90 per cent of presentations and is defined by uncomplicated signs and symptoms. Atypical CSD accounts for the remaining 10 per cent of cases, which have variable presentations. About 80 per cent of infected patients are less than 21 years old.

Symptoms

1. Regional lymph node enlargement, usually tender, is present in all cases of CSD.

2. Typical CSD
   a. Adenopathy only: 50 per cent
   b. Fever: 45 per cent
   c. Fatigue/malaise: 30 per cent
   d. Headache: 14 per cent
   e. Exanthem: 5 per cent

3. Atypical CSD
   a. Parinaud's oculoglandular syndrome: 6 per cent. A soft papule develops on the palpebra conjunctiva, often associated with preauricular adenopathy.
   b. Severe systemic disease: 2 per cent
   c. Central nervous system involvement: 1 to 2 per cent
      (1) Seizures, coma, and inflammatory syndromes
      (2) Symptoms usually clear completely.
   d. Osteolytic lesions, peripheral neuropathy or Bell's palsy, sepsis, erythema nodosum, arthralgias/arthritis, hematologic disorders, and abscess: less than 1 per cent

Key Symptoms

Regional lymph node enlargement, usually tender, is present in all cases of CSD.

Clinical Findings

1. A red-brown papule or pustule, commonly with crusting, at the site of a cat scratch and regional tender lymphadenopathy are the hallmarks of CSD.

2. Hepatosplenomegaly: 12 per cent
3. Conjunctivitis: 5 per cent
4. Parotid swelling: 2 per cent
5. Bacillary angiomatosis: numerous violaceous vasculoproliferative tumors; seen primarily in immunocompromised patients
6. Encephalopathy: less than 2 per cent

Key Signs

A red-brown papule or pustules, commonly with crusting, at the site of a cat scratch and regional tender lymphadenopathy are the hallmarks of CSD.

Laboratory Tests

1. The majority of infections are diagnosed clinically; however, for atypical disease or confirmation, serologic testing can be helpful.
   a. Immunofluorescent antibody (IFA) serology for *B. henselae* antibody
   b. Enzyme-linked immunosorbent assay (ELISA) for *B. henselae* immunoglobulin M (IgM) antibody
   c. Polymerase chain reaction for *B. henselae*–specific DNA sequences.

2. If suspicion remains high after negative testing, a lymph node biopsy for tissue staining and culture should be performed.

3. For atypical presentations, further work-up should be guided by clinical suspicion. Additional tests may include

a. Abdominal ultrasound or computerized tomography splenic/liver lesions or enlargement

b. Radiography or bone scan: lytic bone lesions

Key Tests

Typical CSD is primarily a clinical diagnosis, although IFA or ELISA for *B. henselae* IgM antibody will be helpful for confirmation.

Differential Diagnosis

1. Tender chronic lymphadenopathy: bacterial or viral lymphadenitis, syphilis, mononucleosis, *Mycobacterium* infection, lymphogranuloma venereum, tularemia, toxoplasmosis, sarcoidosis, connective tissue disease, lymphomas, chronic phenytoin therapy, necrotizing lymphadenitis, and angioimmunoblastic lymphadenopathy with dysproteinemia

2. Nontender chronic lymphadenopathy: *Sporothrix schenckii* infection, toxoplasmosis, *Mycobacterium* infections

3. In immunocompromised patients, the differential should also include Kaposi's sarcoma. This diagnosis requires biopsy of the suspicious lesion.

Treatment

1. In the immunocompetent patient, CSD is primarily self-limiting and does not require therapy. However, many studies show that antibiotic use can shorten disease duration. Effective therapy includes azithromycin (Zithromax), 500 mg orally once, then 250 mg daily for 4 days. Alternatives are rifampin (Rimactane), ciprofloxacin (Cipro), or intramuscular gentamicin (Garamycin), typically for 10 to 14 days, although the appropriate duration of therapy has not been well defined. These latter antibiotics should continue for at least 5 days after flu-like symptoms have resolved.

2. The immunocompromised patient should always receive antibiotic therapy for at least 6 weeks. Erythromycin, 500 mg four times daily, or doxycycline, 100 mg twice daily, are usually sufficient.

3. There are no specific dietary or physical restrictions.

Patient Education

1. Avoid cat scratches, especially from kittens less than 12 months of age.

2. Eradicate cat fleas, which are the primary reservoir for bacteria.

Key Treatment

Typical CSD does not usually require treatment, but azithromycin for 5 days can shorten duration of symptoms.

Follow-Up

1. Re-examine in 2 and 12 weeks to ensure clinical improvement and assess lymphadenopathy.

2. When untreated, the average duration of lymphadenopathy is 2 to 3 months although cases have been reported with persistence up to 2 years.

Bibliography

Bass JW, Freitas BC, Freitas AD, et al: Prospective randomized double blind placebo-controlled evaluation of azithromycin for treatment of cat-scratch disease. Pediatr Infect Dis J 1998;17:447–452.

Bass JW, Vincent JM, Person DA: The expanding spectrum of Bartonella infections: II. Cat-scratch disease. Pediatr Infect Dis J 1997;16:163–179.

Margileth AM: Antibiotic therapy for cat-scratch disease: clinical study of therapeutic outcome in 268 patients and a review of the literature. Pediatr Infect Dis J 1992;11:474–478.

Smith DL: Cat-scratch disease and related clinical syndromes. Am Fam Physician 1997;55:1783–1789.

Tompkins LS: Of cats, humans, and Bartonella [editorial]. N Engl J Med 1997;337:1916–1917.

253 Varicella Infections

Virginia E. Robertson

Etiology

1. Varicella zoster virus (VZV) of Herpesviridae family
2. VZV causes two distinct clinical presentations.
   a. The primary infection is *chickenpox*.
   b. Reactivation causes *herpes zoster* (shingles).
3. Transmission occurs through close contact with a VZV-infected person.
   a. Chickenpox may be acquired by
      (1) Inhalation of aerosolized respiratory droplets
      (2) Direct contact with open shingle lesions
      (3) Maternal-fetal transmission via placenta
   b. VZV becomes latent in dorsal root ganglia after primary infection, re-emerging as shingles when immune system surveillance wanes with age or other disease.

Chickenpox

Epidemiology

The primary infection is commonly a disease of childhood.

1. Equally distributed between genders and races
2. Endemic, with peaks during late winter and early spring
3. Secondary attack rates range between 60 and 90 per cent
4. Incubation is 14 to 15 days (range 10 to 20)
5. Infectious period begins 48 hours before onset of clinical symptoms and persists through the period of new lesion formation (3 to 5 days).

Symptoms

1. A prodrome of low-grade fever and general malaise may precede the defining rash by 1 to 2 days.
2. The classic rash begins as scattered small vesicles with erythematous bases, seen first on the trunk or face
   a. The lesions spread centrifugally to involve all skin surfaces and possibly mucous membranes (lips, vulva).
   b. The lesions are pruritic; many patients will scratch.

c. Intact and ruptured vesicles will be present simultaneously; scratching may yield excoriations and superficial skin infections.
3. Constitutional symptoms may occur, especially in older patients, or the patient may be otherwise asymptomatic.
   a. Mild anorexia, listlessness
   b. Low-grade fever, 100° to 103° F
   c. Myalgias or headaches
4. In an older or immunocompromised patient, symptoms present similarly, but expect an increased number of lesions, possible hemorrhagic bases, and more severe constitutional symptoms.

Key Symptoms

- Vesiculopapular rash
- Centrifugal spread of lesions
- Pruritus
- Mild constitutional symptoms

Clinical Findings

1. The classic description of the lesion is a "dewdrop on a rose petal," corresponding to a clear vesicle on erythematous base.
2. As rash spreads, multiple stages of lesions will be present simultaneously in a random, nonclustered pattern.
   a. New clear vesicles, 3 to 5 mm in diameter
   b. Older, cloudy-looking vesicles
   c. Recently ruptured or excoriated lesions
   d. Healing bases
3. Excoriations if scratching is prominent
4. Possible superinfected lesions
5. Evidence of constitutional symptoms
6. New lesions cease appearing within 3 to 5 days (range 3 to 7).
7. In utero infection yields various fetal malformations.

Laboratory Tests

1. Diagnosis usually rests on history of exposure, symptoms, and signs.
2. In difficult cases, possible serum studies include
   a. Acute and convalescent varicella serum titers
   b. Enzyme-linked immunosorbent assay, direct fluorescent antibody, or other radioassays
3. Direct skin studies may include
   a. Tzanck's smear of unroofed lesion to look for multinucleated giant cells (Wright's or Giemsa's stains)
   b. Tissue culture systems
   c. Skin biopsy
   d. Gram's stain/bacterial cultures of superinfected lesions

Differential Diagnosis

1. Atypical measles
2. Impetigo
3. Herpes simplex virus
4. Enteroviral infections, usually group A coxsackieviruses

Complications

1. In adolescent and older patients or those in an immunocompromised state (lymphoreticular cancer, human immunodeficiency virus [HIV]), complications are more common and may necessitate hospitalization and treatment.
2. Complications include
   a. Visceral VZV, especially pneumonia; also nephritis, myocarditis, arthritis
   b. Neurologic VZV or sequelae: meningitis, encephalitis, transverse myelitis, optic neuritis
   c. Superinfections of skin lesions, with cellulitis and, rarely, invasive group A *Streptococcus* or other life-threatening deep infections
   d. Hematologic complications: thrombotic thrombocytopenic purpura, purpura fulminans

> **WARNING**
>
> Reye's syndrome has been associated with aspirin use during varicella infection in children. No aspirin or aspirin-containing product should be used.

Treatment

Symptomatic therapy alone is needed by most patients.

1. Keeping lesions clean is crucial: Use mild soap for bathing, trim fingernails, and wash hands often.
2. Antipruritic measures include
   a. Lukewarm baths with colloidal oatmeal or baking soda
   b. Calamine, oatmeal, other topical anti-itch lotions
   c. Oral antihistamines may be useful.
      (1) Diphenhydramine: in children, 5 mg/kg/24 hours given q6h; in adults, 10 to 50 mg tid or qid
      (2) Hydroxyzine: in children, 2 mg/kg/24 hours given q6h; in adults, 25 to 100 mg tid or qid
3. Control fever with acetaminophen (see warning box above).
4. Antiviral therapy should be reserved for those who are at risk for more symptomatic or complicated chickenpox: immunocompromised individuals, older patients, and possibly secondary cases.
   a. In children 2 to 12 years old, acyclovir (Zovirax), 20 mg/kg qid for 5 days (max 800 mg/day), initiated within 24 hours
   b. In patients older than 12 years, give acyclovir 800 mg orally 5 times a day for 7 days.
   c. Consider intravenous acyclovir in immunocompromised patients.

Activity

Quarantine until all lesions heal to minimize transmission of varicella.

Patient Education

1. Reassurance of generally benign and limited course
2. Emphasize keeping lesions clean.
3. Inform family of expected secondary outbreaks and incubation period for susceptible individuals.

4. Recommend evaluation of pregnant or immunocompromised contacts if no prior history of VZV.
5. Warning signs of complications: change in mental status, dyspnea, signs of superinfection of lesions
6. Avoid use of aspirin.

Key Treatment

- Symptomatic therapy
- Acyclovir in selected populations

Prevention
1. Consider prophylaxis of susceptible high-risk individuals: Varicella zoster immune globulin (VZIG) is given up to 96 hours after exposure to prevent or reduce illness.
2. In hospital settings, or for hospital workers, isolation through the potential infectious period is recommended.
3. Varicella immunization (Varivax) is now recommended for susceptible people ages 12 months and older.
   a. Live, attenuated vaccine
   b. Dosages: 12 months to 12 years old: 0.5 ml SC once; 13 years and older: 0.5 ml SC followed by repeat dose in 4 to 8 weeks
   c. Contraindicated and reportable in first trimester of pregnancy
   d. A mild outbreak of varicella-like syndrome may appear after vaccination, typically with few lesions and low-grade fever.

Follow-Up
1. As needed if complications arise
2. Chickenpox is a reportable disease.

Shingles

Epidemiology
Shingles is seen primarily in the elderly or in the immunocompromised, especially those with HIV or lymphoreticular malignancies.
1. Incidence does not vary with gender or race.
2. Endemic without periods of epidemicity
3. May be seen in young children whose mothers had chickenpox during pregnancy (early reactivation).

Symptoms
1. Pain typically precedes any skin manifestations by several days.
   a. Pain is sharp or lancinating and often severe.
   b. Dermatomal distribution may or may not be recognized.
   c. Hyperesthesia of the area may be present.
2. The rash begins as erythematous maculopapules that become vesiculated in 12 to 24 hours; linear clustering is evident.
   a. Weeping and subsequent crusting occurs over 10 to 12 days.
   b. Resolution of the crusts, often with scarring, occurs within 2 to 3 weeks.
3. Pain during and after the rash is often remarkable.

Key Symptoms

- Erythematous vesicular rash
- Pain before, during, and after rash
- Dermatomal distribution

Clinical Findings
1. In the absence of the rash, pain and hyperesthesia may not be associated with specific clinical findings.
2. Defining rash: clear vesicles on an erythematous base clustered in a linear region along a unilateral dermatome and associated with pain. The appearance of the lesions may become
   a. Umbilicated and cloudy or frankly pustular
   b. Hemorrhagic
   c. Weeping
3. The rash characteristically stops at the midline.
4. Adjacent dermatomes may be involved.

Key Signs

- Erythematous vesicular rash
- Dermatomal distribution
- Unilateral, clustered lesions

Laboratory Tests
1. Diagnosis is usually made on clinical findings.
2. Direct skin tests may include
   a. Tzanck's smear of unroofed lesion to examine for multinucleated giant cells (Wright's or Giemsa's stain)
   b. Skin biopsy

Key Tests

- None usually required
- Consider Tzanck's smear or skin biopsy

Complications

1. These are more likely in some immunocompromised patients. Patients with HIV, however, do not appear to have more complications, although shingles is common.
2. Complications include
   a. Disseminated shingles
   b. Visceral VZV: pneumonia
   c. Multiple neurologic manifestations can occur.
      (1) Cranial nerve palsies
      (2) Motor weakness, transverse myelitis
      (3) Encephalitis, cerebral vasculitis
   d. Superinfections of lesions
   e. Persistent radicular pain after the rash heals, called *postherpetic neuralgia*

Differential Diagnosis

1. Before rash erupts, there may be a wide differential for the pain, given location, severity, and coincident symptoms.
2. The rash may resemble that of herpes simplex.

Treatment

For most patients, the major emphasis should be symptomatic relief and prevention of secondary skin infections.

1. Keeping lesions clean is critical, using appropriate measures such as soothing, cleansing soaks with Burow's solution.
2. Pain management depends on severity.
   a. Simple analgesics such as acetaminophen or ibuprofen
   b. Narcotic analgesics such as Demerol or dilaudid
   c. Radicular nerve blocks
   d. Transcutaneous electrical nerve stimulation (TENS)
   e. Consider consultation for managing pain
3. Antiviral agents will decrease time to healing and lessen risk of transmission if started within 48 hours of the onset of the rash.
   a. For mild to moderate cases
      (1) Famciclovir (Famvir), 500 mg PO tid for 7 days, or valacyclovir (Valtrex), 1 gm PO q8h for 7 days, has the added benefit

of decreasing likelihood of postherpetic neuralgia.
      (2) Acyclovir (Zovirax), 800 mg PO five times a day for 7 to 10 days
   b. For severe cases requiring hospitalization
      (1) Intravenous acyclovir, 10 to 12 mg/kg (1-hour infusion) q8h for 7 to 14 days; adjust for renal insufficiency.
      (2) Foscarnet sodium (Foscavir) if unresponsive to acyclovir (or if suspected resistance, especially in HIV patients)
4. Postherpetic neuralgia may be severe and linger over months.
   a. Tricyclic antidepressants
   b. Ongoing TENS
   c. Topical capsaicin cream

Activity

Quarantine until all lesions heal to minimize transmission of varicella.

Patient Education

1. Education and involvement of the patient in pain management issues, especially postherpetic neuralgia, is helpful.
2. Notification of possible transmission of varicella to susceptible contacts (will manifest in secondary cases as chickenpox)
3. Expect scarring.

Key Treatment

- Symptomatic care
- Acyclovir, famciclovir, or valacyclovir

Follow-Up

1. As needed, if complications arise
2. Ongoing pain management when appropriate
3. Consider VZIG prophylaxis of susceptible high-risk contacts.

Bibliography

Clements DA: Modified varicella-like syndrome. Infect Dis Clin North Am 1996;10:617–629.
Enders G, Miller E, Cradock-Watson J, et al: Consequences of varicella and herpes zoster in pregnancy:

prospective study of 1739 cases. Lancet 1994;343: 1548–1551.

Tyring S, Barbarash RA, Nahlik JE, et al: Famciclovir for the treatment of acute herpes zoster: effects on acute disease and postherpetic neuralgia. Ann Intern Med 1995;123:89–96.

White CJ: Varicella-zoster vaccine. Clin Infect Dis 1997; 24:753–763.

Whitley RJ: Varicella-zoster virus. In Mandell GL, Douglas RG, Bennett JE (eds): Principles and Practice of Infectious Diseases, 4th ed, pp 1345–1351. New York, Churchill Livingstone, 1995.

254 Rubella

Joseph V. Connelly

Etiology

1. Rubella (German measles) is caused by the rubella virus. Although it is usually a mild illness, it can cause devastating consequences to the fetus when it is acquired during pregnancy.

2. Humans are the only known host for the virus. There is no vector transmission.

3. Transmission is probably via respiratory droplets. Patients are most contagious when the rash is erupting, but viral shedding can occur from 10 days prior to 15 days after the onset of the rash.

4. Incubation period is 18 ± 3 days.

5. The disease is most commonly seen in the winter and spring.

Symptoms

1. Symptoms, if present at all, are usually mild.

2. Prodromal symptoms, when they occur, precede the rash by 1 to 5 days.

3. During the exanthem period there may be mild pruritus from the rash or a low-grade fever. Other symptoms usually disappear after the first day of the rash.

4. Children usually have a more mild illness.

Key Symptoms

- Eye pain
- Sore throat
- Headache
- Malaise
- Upper respiratory complaints

Clinical Findings

Postnatal (Acquired) Infection

1. Lymphadenopathy
   a. Begins 1 to 5 days before the rash.
   b. Along with generalized lymphadenopathy, suboccipital and postauricular nodes are characteristically involved.
   c. May be the only sign of infection.

2. Rash
   a. Appears first on face, then progresses down the body.
   b. Maculopapular. Lesions are discrete (not confluent); however, they sometimes coalesce on the trunk.
   c. Lasts 3 to 5 days.
   d. Sometimes desquamates during convalescence.

3. Occasionally an enanthem, consisting of petechial lesions on the soft palate, occurs at the same time as the exanthem.

4. Mild conjunctivitis

5. Fever
   a. Low-grade or absent
   b. Resolves by first day of rash.

6. Complications are rare but may include
   a. Arthritis and arthralgia: more common in adult women
   b. Thrombocytopenia or leukopenia
   c. Encephalitis (very rare)

Congenital Infection

1. The manifestations are most severe the earlier in pregnancy the illness occurs.

2. Fetal death, premature delivery, and many congenital abnormalities may result. These include
   a. Nerve deafness: 80 to 90 per cent frequency
   b. Growth retardation: 50 to 85 per cent
   c. Cataracts and/or retinopathy: 35 per cent each
   d. Patent ductus arteriosus: 30 per cent
   e. Pulmonary artery stenosis: 25 per cent
   f. Neurologic abnormalities including mental retardation, meningoencephalitis, and behavior disorders: 10 to 20 per cent each
   g. Hepatosplenomegaly: 10 to 20 per cent
   h. Bone lesions: 10 to 20 per cent
   i. Thrombocytopenic purpura: 5 to 10 per cent

3. Late-onset manifestations may include diabetes mellitus, thyroid disorders, hearing loss, central nervous system problems, and others.

Key Signs

Postnatal	Congenital
• Lymphadenopathy (suboccipital and postauricular)	• Deafness
	• Growth retardation
• Maculopapular rash	• Cataracts
• Exanthem	• Retinopathy
• Conjunctivitis	• Congenital heart disease
• Low-grade fever	• Mental retardation

Laboratory Tests

1. Laboratory testing is generally not useful or recommended in diagnosing the acute disease.
2. Viral isolation from nose, throat, urine, or other body fluid is the definitive test for acute or congenital infection.
3. Elevations in rubella immunoglobulin M (IgM) antibody can be measured, but false positives frequently occur.
4. Maternal and infant sera may be measured for IgM antibody. Its presence in the infant is highly suggestive of congenital infection.

Key Tests

- Usually not necessary for postnatal infection
- Virus isolation for congenital

Differential Diagnosis

1. Enteroviral infections
   a. Shorter incubation period (3 to 7 days)
   b. More common in younger children
   c. Frequently have a higher fever
   d. More common in summer and fall
2. Measles
   a. Frequently has a higher fever
   b. Rash is confluent
3. Scarlet fever
4. Infectious mononucleosis
5. Toxoplasmosis
6. Roseola
7. Erythema infectiosum
8. Drug reactions

Treatment

Symptomatic treatment is given for postnatal infection (e.g., starch baths for pruritus).

Medication

1. Acetaminophen for fever; aspirin for arthralgia
2. Some authors recommend immune globulin for the susceptible pregnant woman of less than 20 weeks' gestation who has been exposed within 72 hours.

Diet

No special diet is necessary.

Activity

1. Patients with rubella should not have contact with susceptible persons until 7 days after the onset of the rash.
2. Infants with congenital rubella should be isolated while in the hospital. They should avoid susceptible persons when at home.

Prevention

1. All adults born in 1957 or later should receive one dose of measles-mumps-rubella (MMR) vaccine unless
   a. They can provide proof of one dose of live vaccine having been given on or after their first birthday *or*
   b. They have documentation of physician-diagnosed disease *or*
   c. They have laboratory evidence of immunity.
2. Two doses of MMR vaccine for children:
   a. First dose at 12 to 15 months of age
   b. Second dose at age 4 to 6 years
   c. College students, military recruits, hospital workers, and those traveling to endemic areas who were born after 1957 should also receive two doses.
3. Contraindications to MMR vaccine:
   a. Previous anaphylactic reaction to this vaccine or its components
   b. Immunocompromised patients, including severely immunocompromised human immunodeficiency virus patients
   c. Moderate or severe acute illness
   d. Reception of blood products or immune globulin within past 11 months; consult *1997 Red Book* for direction.
   e. Pregnancy or possible pregnancy within 3 months
4. All cases should be reported to the appropriate authorities.

Bibliography

Centers for Disease Control and Prevention: Measles, Mumps, and Rubella—Vaccine Use and Strategies for Elimination of Measles, Rubella, and Congenital Rubella Syndrome and Control of Mumps: Recommendations of the Advisory Committee on Immunization Practices (ACIP). MMWR Morb Mortal Wkly Rep 1998;47 (No. RR-8).

Cherry J: Rubella Virus. In Feigin RD, Cherry JD (eds): Textbook of Pediatric Infectious Disease, 4th ed, pp 1922–1949. Philadelphia, WB Saunders Company, 1998.

Gershon A: Rubella Virus (German Measles). In Mandell GL, Douglas RG Jr, Bennett JE (eds): Principles and Practice of Infectious Diseases, 4th ed, pp 1459–1465. New York, Churchill Livingstone, 1995.

Maldonado Y: Rubella Virus. In Long SS, Pickering LK, Prober CG (eds): Principles and Practice of Pediatric Infectious Diseases, pp 1228–1237. New York, Churchill Livingstone, 1997.

Peter G, Hall C, Halsey N, et al (eds): Rubella. In 1997 Red Book: Report of the Committee on Infectious Diseases, 24th ed, pp 456–462. Elk Grove Village, IL, American Academy of Pediatrics, 1997.

255 Measles (Rubeola)

Ram Yogev

Etiology

The measles virus belongs to the Paramyxoviridae family and is the only human member of its genus *Morbillivirus*. The virus is spherical, and its envelope contains a single-stranded linear RNA genome that codes for six major proteins.

Symptoms

1. The incubation period is 8 to 12 days.
2. Early symptoms include fever and nonspecific upper respiratory inflammation (e.g., sneezing, congestion, coryza, and cough).

Key Symptoms

- Fever
- Coryza
- Conjunctivitis

Clinical Findings

1. Conjunctivitis without discharge (pus) appears shortly after the fever and the respiratory symptoms, accompanied by increased lacrimation, edema of the eyelids, and photophobia.
2. Koplik's spots (1-mm bluish white lesions on an erythematous base) can be seen only in the first couple of days of symptoms. They usually appear on the buccal mucosa opposite the lower molars and quickly coalesce into larger lesions.
3. The skin rash, erythematous maculopapular lesions that coalesce, usually appears 2 to 3 days after the onset of fever and respiratory symptoms. It first appears on the forehead and behind the ears and then spreads from the head to the feet. The rash begins to disappear in about 3 days in the same manner (from head down). Fine desquamation may occur during healing. The total duration of rash is about 7 days.
4. Pharyngitis, postauricular and/or suboccipital lymph node enlargement are common.
5. Less common findings include abdominal pain with or without vomiting or diarrhea, laryngitis, and croup.

Key Signs

- Koplik's spots
- Coalescing erythematous maculopapular rash
- Suboccipital and/or postauricular lymph node enlargement

Complications

1. Relatively common
   a. Otitis media
   b. Pneumonia: early in the disease—caused by measles virus; later—bacterial superinfection)
2. Less common
   a. Encephalitis
   b. Myocarditis, pericarditis
   c. Thrombocytopenic purpura
   d. Keratoconjunctivitis with corneal ulceration
   e. Reactivation of tuberculosis
   f. In pregnant women, increased abortion and premature labor rates
   g. Subacute sclerosing panencephalitis (SSPE) —years after the infection

> **WARNING**
> - **Vitamin A deficiency increases severity of disease and mortality.**
> - **In an immunocompromised host, the clinical presentation is frequently unusual (e.g., initial presentation is pneumonia with rash developing only later, seizures and encephalitis several months after clinical measles).**

Laboratory Tests

1. The diagnosis of measles is usually made from its clinically characteristic presentation.
2. Determining the presence of the virus
   a. Virus isolation in tissue culture from conjunctivae, nasal secretions, blood and urine

during febrile period is possible but technically difficult.

    b. Detection of measles antigen in tissue (e.g., exfoliative skin) by fluorescent antibody technique

    c. Detection of the measles genome with polymerase chain reaction

3. Serologic tests

    a. Enzyme-linked immunosorbent assay (ELISA)

    b. Single determination of immunoglobulin M antibody to measles 72 hours after appearance of rash

    c. Rise (at least fourfold) in neutralizing and/or hemagglutination inhibition (HI) antibodies in sequential serum samples 10 to 14 days apart

    d. In patients with SSPE measles, HI titers are extremely high both in serum and cerebrospinal fluid.

 Key Test

ELISA is the most sensitive and can be performed rapidly.

Differential Diagnosis

The differential diagnosis of measles includes all conditions with an erythematous maculopapular rash.

1. Viral etiologies

    a. Rubella

    b. Enteroviral infections

    c. Infectious mononucleosis

    d. Roseola infantum

    e. Erythema infectiosum

    f. Cytomegalovirus

2. Bacterial

    a. Scarlet fever

    b. Staphylococcal scalded skin syndrome

    c. Streptococcal or staphylococcal toxic shock syndrome

    d. *Mycoplasma pneumoniae* infection

    e. Meningococcemia

3. Other

    a. Kawasaki's disease

    b. Drug eruptions

    c. Toxic erythemas

    d. Sunburn

> ## PEARL
>
> Evaluation of the prodromal period, distribution of the rash, and presence of pathognomonic signs (e.g., Koplik's spots in measles) may be very helpful in the differential diagnosis.

Treatment

1. Only symptomatic treatment for uncomplicated disease

    a. Acetaminophen for headache and fever

    b. Fluids to prevent dehydration

    c. Bed rest in darkened room (for photophobia)

    d. Room humidification for cough, croup, or laryngitis

2. Vitamin A (100,000 IU for infants 6 to 12 months of age, 200,000 IU for infants older than 1 year of age) in selected circumstances, such as

    a. Patients 6 to 24 months of age with measles complications

    b. Patients with immunodeficiency

    c. Patients with malabsorption (e.g., cystic fibrosis, short bowel syndrome) or severe malnutrition

    d. Recent immigrants (e.g., adoptees) from countries with high mortality resulting from measles

If xerophthalmia, night blindness, or Bitot's spots (gray deposits adjacent to the cornea) are present, the dose of vitamin A should be repeated within 24 hours and 4 weeks later.

> ## WARNING
>
> - **Antibacterial agents *should not* be given routinely to prevent bacterial complications.**
>
> - **Ribavirin *should not* be used to treat measles pneumonitis in normal hosts. Its efficacy for pneumonia in immunocompromised patients is controversial.**

Prevention

1. Active immunization

    a. Two doses of live-virus measles vaccine (at 12 to 15 months of age and at 4 to 6 years) are recommended.

    b. In epidemic situations, the first dose can be given as early as 6 months of age; if the first dose was already given, revaccinate if at least 4 weeks after the first dose. Revaccinate at 12 months and 4 years.

c. Patients with known allergy to egg or neomycin (nonanaphylactic) can be vaccinated.

d. Patients with unknown vaccination status or vaccinated before 1 year of age should receive two doses of the vaccine.

e. Mild febrile illness (e.g., upper respiratory infection, otitis media) is not a contraindication for vaccination.

f. Immunocompromised patients (e.g., leukemia, malignancy) should not be vaccinated. Vaccination can be given 3 months after cessation of immunosuppressive therapy.

WARNING

If a patient has received an immune globulin (IG) preparation, measles vaccination should be postponed for variable periods of time depending on the IG dose (see *1997 Red Book*, p 353).

---

2. Passive immunization

a. To prevent measles in an immunocompetent child, intramuscular IG (0.25 ml/kg, maximum dose 15 ml) can be given within 6 days of exposure.

b. In immunocompromised patients, regardless of their measles vaccination status, 0.5 ml/kg (not to exceed 15 ml) of IG should be given. The only exception is patients who received intravenous IG up to 2 weeks before the exposure.

Follow-Up

Measles is a reportable disease and, if an outbreak is suspected and confirmed, measles vaccine should be given to all exposed persons without documented measles immunity.

 Bibliography

James JM, Burks AW, Roberson PK, et al: Safe administration of the measles vaccine to children allergic to eggs. N Engl J Med 1995;332:1262–1266.

Markowitz LE, Albrecht P, Rhodes P, et al: Changing levels of measles antibody titers in women and children in the United States: impact on response to vaccination. Pediatrics 1996;97:53–58.

Measles. In Peters G, Hall CB, Marcy SM, et al (eds): Red Book: Report of the Committee on Infectious Diseases, 24th ed, pp 344–357. Elk Grove Village, IL, American Academy of Pediatrics, 1997.

Stratton KR, Howe CJ, Johnston RB: Adverse events associated with childhood vaccines other than pertussis and rubella: summary of a report from the Institute of Medicine. JAMA 1994;271:1602–1605.

256 Infectious Mononucleosis

William R. Scheibel

Etiology/Epidemiology

1. Most frequently caused by Epstein-Barr virus (EBV)
   a. EBV is a double-stranded DNA virus from the herpesvirus family.
   b. Humans are the sole source, with transmission by intimate contact.
   c. EBV infects epithelial cells of oropharynx, cervix, and resting B lymphocytes, which disseminate throughout the body and proliferate until checked by activated T cells.
      (1) Transmission is usually by infected saliva and rarely by blood transfusions or bone marrow transplantation.
      (2) Viral excretion occurs for months, and asymptomatic carriage is common.
      (3) Transmission probably requires repeated and prolonged contact with infected oral secretions, yet few patients can identify a known contact.
   d. Incubation period is 3 to 7 weeks.
   e. Endemic in children in developing countries by age 5; infection delayed until adolescence and adulthood in developed or industrialized countries with high-quality sanitary conditions
   f. Reactivation of EBV can occur in transplant or immunocompromised patients only.
2. Infrequent causes (<10 per cent)
   a. Cytomegalovirus
   b. Human immunodeficiency virus
   c. *Toxoplasma gondii*
   d. Human herpesvirus type 6

Symptoms

1. Wide spectrum of disease from asymptomatic to fulminant infection and even death in immunocompromised patients
   a. Often unrecognized in infants and young children because it usually ranges from asymptomatic to a brief febrile illness.
   b. Overt illness most common in adolescents and young adults with triad of fever, sore throat, and lymphadenopathy.
2. Prodrome of malaise, fatigue, and persistent low-grade headache followed by severe sore throat
   a. Anorexia, myalgias, chills, nausea, abdominal discomfort, cough, or arthralgias may occur.
   b. Acute phase lasts 1 to 3 weeks, with most patients completely recovered by 6 to 8 weeks.

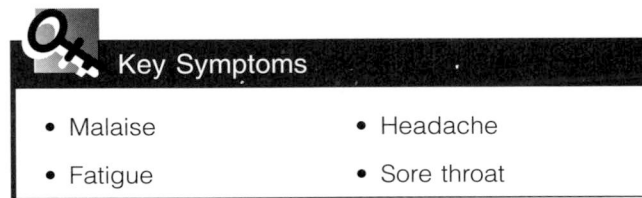

Key Symptoms

- Malaise
- Fatigue
- Headache
- Sore throat

Clinical Findings

1. Severe pharyngitis is the most prominent feature and can be exudative or accompanied by palatine petechiae.
2. Lymphadenopathy more characteristically involves the posterior cervical chain and the anterior cervical chain but can be generalized.
3. Splenomegaly is usually present by the second week.
4. Hepatomegaly, palatal exanthem, rash (usually transient, generalized, and maculopapular), jaundice, and periorbital swelling or palpebral edema may occur.
5. There is little support for EBV now as cause of chronic fatigue syndrome.
6. Complications
   a. Bacterial pharyngitis
   b. Splenic rupture
   c. Upper airway obstruction, pneumonitis
   d. Hematologic: hemolytic anemia, thrombocytopenia, or granulocytopenia
   e. Neurologic: seizures, meningoencephalitis, Bell's palsy, Guillain-Barré syndrome, psychosis, and Reye's syndrome
   f. Cardiac: myocarditis or pericarditis
   g. Dermatologic: rash after exposure to ampicillin
   h. Renal: glomerulonephritis
   i. Hepatic: jaundice

j. Malignant: Burkitt's lymphoma, nasopharyngeal carcinoma, or B lymphoma

Key Signs

- Lymphadenopathy
- Pharyngitis
- Fever
- Splenomegaly

Laboratory Tests

1. Mild hepatitis with two- to threefold increases of liver enzymes
2. Modest leukocytosis (up to 20,000/mm^3) during acute phase; lymphocytosis (>50 per cent) and atypical lymphocytes (>10 per cent)
3. Mild reduction of platelet count
4. Positive immunoglobulin (Ig)M heterophile antibodies (HA) in 90 per cent of patients by the third week of illness.
5. More specific serologic tests are useful when heterophile antibody is absent.
   a. IgM antibodies to EBV viral capsid antigen (anti-VCA) evolve quickly and persist only for weeks to months.
   b. IgG anti-VCA persist lifelong.
   c. IgA anti-VCA are useful in nasopharyngeal carcinoma.
   d. Antibodies to EBV early antigens (anti-EA) are of a diffuse or restricted pattern and appear 2 to 3 weeks after the onset of illness, then peak and gradually decline.
   e. Antibodies to EBV nuclear antigen (anti-EBNA) develop late and persist lifelong.
6. No EBV infection: negative serologic tests
7. Acute EBV infection: positive HA, IgM anti-VCA, IgG anti-VCA, and IgG anti-EA
8. Past EBV infection: positive IgG anti-VCA and anti-EBNA

Key Tests

- Absolute lymphocytosis (>50 per cent)
- Atypical lymphocytes (>10 per cent)
- Presence of heterophile antibodies

Differential Diagnosis

1. Bacterial disease
   a. Exudative pharyngitis with group A β-hemolytic streptococcus

b. Mycoplasma
   c. Bacteremia
2. Viral infection
   a. Cytomegalovirus, toxoplasmosis
   b. Respiratory viruses: influenza, parainfluenza, or adenovirus
   c. Viral hepatitis
   d. Rubella, mumps
   e. Human immunodeficiency virus, human herpesvirus type 6
3. Drug reaction
4. Hematologic malignancies: leukemia or lymphoma

Treatment

Medication

1. Uncomplicated acute infectious mononucleosis usually only requires supportive therapy.
   a. Warm salt water or anesthetic (lidocaine 2%, phenol 1.4%) gargles for pharyngitis
   b. Acetaminophen, 650 to 1000 mg every 4 hours, for fever or malaise
2. Antibiotic treatment of concomitant group A β-hemolytic Streptococcus pyogenes
   a. Penicillin or erythromycin for 10 days are first choices.
   b. Avoid amoxicillin or ampicillin because they usually produce a morbilliform rash in patients with mononucleosis.
3. Corticosteroids: prednisone, 40 to 80 mg/day and tapering over 5 to 14 days.
   a. May shorten duration of fever and pharyngitis in uncomplicated disease.
   b. There is concern that corticosteroids may adversely influence long-term immunity to EBV or increase the number of lymphocytes with EBV latent infection.
   c. Can reduce obstructive tonsillar enlargement and may improve autoimmune hemolytic anemia, thrombocytopenia, granulocytopenia, aplastic anemia, encephalitis, or myocarditis.
   d. No evidence corticosteroids improve splenomegaly or prevent rupture.
4. Acyclovir, ganciclovir, bromovinyldeoxyuridine, zidovudine, foscarnet, and human interferon inhibit replication of EBV in vitro.
   a. Acyclovir has little or no clinical benefit in uncomplicated infectious mononucleosis.
   b. Aforementioned agents are used in fulminant infections and immune deficient patients, but benefits may be only transient.

5. Vaccine development with a subunit or inactivated virus vaccine is ongoing.

Activity

1. Limited activity during acute phase, with gradual return to daily activities
2. Restrict strenuous activity to prevent precipitating splenic rupture.
3. No contact sports for 4 weeks, longer if spleen is still palpable or is enlarged on radiologic examination

Patient Education

1. Restricting intimate contact during the acute symptomatic phase may decrease transmission.
2. Isolation is unnecessary because EBV shedding continues after the acute illness.
3. Acute symptoms usually last 1 to 2 weeks, with resolution of fatigue over 2 to 4 weeks.

Key Treatment

- Uncomplicated acute infectious mononucleosis generally requires only supportive therapy.

- Penicillin or erythromycin is given for concomitant group A β-hemolytic *Streptococcus pyogenes*.

Bibliography

Bailey RE: Diagnosis and treatment of infectious mononucleosis. Am Fam Physician 1994;49:879–885.

Chetham MM, Roberts KB: Infectious mononucleosis in adolescents. Pediatr Ann 1991;20:206–213.

Hickey SM, Strasburger VC: What every pediatrician should know about infectious mononucleosis in adolescents. Pediatr Clin North Am 1997;44:1541–1556.

Maki DS, Reich RM: Infectious mononucleosis in the athlete. Am J Sports Med 1982;10:162–173.

Straus SE, Cohel JI, Tasato G, et al: NIH Conference. Epstein-Barr virus infections: biology, pathogenesis and management. Ann Intern Med 1993;118:45–58.

257 Chronic Fatigue Syndrome

William Fulcher

Chronic fatigue syndrome (CFS) is a debilitating illness of unknown etiology and accounts for approximately 2 to 5 per cent of the chronically fatigued patients seen in primary care practices. It is important to recognize so that physicians can offer affected patients current information on its etiology, treatment, and prognosis.

Etiology

CFS was initially thought to be caused by one of a number of viruses because of its frequent occurrence in "outbreaks" and its commonly reported sudden onset and "flu-like" symptoms; however, the etiology is still unknown. Current research is focusing on central nervous system and immune system abnormalities as potential causes.

Symptoms

1. Clinically evaluated, unexplained, persistent or relapsing chronic fatigue that is new in onset (not lifelong); is not the result of ongoing exertion; is not substantially alleviated by rest; and results in substantial reduction of previous levels of work, educational, social, or personal activities
2. Concurrent occurrence of four or more of the following symptoms for at least 6 months and not preceding the fatigue:
   a. Impairment in short-term memory or concentration
   b. Sore throat
   c. Tender cervical or axillary lymph nodes
   d. Muscle pain
   e. Multiple joint pains without joint swelling or tenderness
   f. Headaches of a new type, pattern, or severity
   g. Unrefreshing sleep
   h. Postexertional malaise

Exclusions

- Active medical conditions that explain the chronic fatigue state (see "Differential Diagnosis")
- Unresolved, previously diagnosed medical conditions accompanied by the symptom of fatigue
- Any past or current major depressive disorder, psychosis, dementia, anorexia nervosa, bulimia
- Alcohol or substance abuse within 2 years of the onset of the fatigue

3. Other commonly reported symptoms in CFS
   a. Anorexia
   b. Nausea
   c. Night sweats
   d. Increased pain perception
   e. Dizziness
   f. Altered temperature regulation

History

A complete and thorough history is the most important diagnostic procedure in patients with chronic fatigue. The physician should schedule an unhurried review of the following areas and allow the patient time to tell his or her "story":

1. Carefully review work, sleep, exercise, and social history.
2. Assess for current or premorbid psychiatric disorders.
3. Take a thorough "oral intake" history (medications, vitamins and supplements, alcohol, caffeine, nicotine, special diets).
4. Find out: What is the patient concerned about? What do they expect from your services?

Clinical Findings

There are no uniformly abnormal physical findings in patients with CFS. Some patients will have slightly tender lymph nodes (typically cervical) and areas of point tenderness in various muscle groups (*similar to those found in patients with fibromyalgia*). Some patients have signs of dysautonomia, such as orthostatic tachycardia or hypotension.

Key Signs

- Patients may look well or look depressed/tired
- Slightly tender cervical or axillary lymph nodes (some patients)
- Orthostatic hypotension (some patients)

Laboratory Tests

1. Complete blood count (CBC) with differential
2. Blood urea nitrogen (BUN), creatinine, electrolytes, glucose
3. Calcium, phosphorus, alanine transaminase (ALT), alkaline phosphatase
4. Total protein, albumin, globulin
5. Urinalysis
6. Erythrocyte sedimentation rate
7. Thyroid-stimulating hormone (TSH)
8. In special cases
   a. Antinuclear antibody
   b. Rheumatoid factor
   c. Lyme disease serology
   d. Hepatitis serology
   e. Human immunodeficiency virus antibody
   f. Tuberculosis skin test
   g. Serum cortisol
   h. Immunoglobulin levels

Key Tests

- CBC with differential
- BUN, creatinine, electrolytes, glucose
- Calcium, phosphorus, ALT, alkaline phosphatase
- Total protein, albumin, globulin
- Urinalysis
- Erythrocyte sedimentation rate
- TSH

Differential Diagnosis

1. Chronic infection: hepatitis, subacute bacterial endocarditis, tuberculosis, osteomyelitis
2. Hematologic disorders: anemias, polycythemia, hemoglobinopathies
3. Nutritional dysfunction: protein-calorie/vitamin deficiencies, obesity
4. Chronic exogenous intoxication: alcohol, heavy metals, gasoline, carbon monoxide
5. Chronic endogenous intoxication: uremia, liver failure
6. Endocrine disorders: diabetes, pituitary/adrenal dysfunction, thyroid disorders
7. Malignancies
8. Iatrogenic: drugs
9. Neuropsychiatric dysfunction: depression, chronic anxiety
10. Idiopathic: chronic fatigue syndrome

Treatment

Medication

There are no specific medications to treat CFS. CFS patients report extreme sensitivity to the effects of many drugs that affect the central nervous system; consequently, the primary physician should treat all underlying conditions with the least sedating medications possible.

1. Sleep disorder: Low-dose tricyclic antidepressants such as amitriptyline, 5 to 25 mg, or nortriptyline, 25 mg qhs
2. Depression: selective serotonin reuptake inhibitors such as sertraline, paroxitine, fluoxetine at usual starting doses but carefully watching for sensitivity to side effects; venlafaxine
3. Atopic disease/rhinitis: nonsedating antihistamines, intranasal steroids
4. Pain: nonsteroidal anti-inflammatory drugs (naproxen, ibuprofen), muscle relaxers (cyclobenzaprine)
5. Orthostasis: added salt diet, fludrocortisone (*not* a Food and Drug Administration–approved indication)

Diet

Well-balanced, low-fat prudent diet, plenty of water; avoid alcohol, caffeine, tobacco.

Activity

Several studies have recently shown that the perceived degree of fatigue is reduced in patients who perform regular aerobic activity/exercise at mild to moderate pace (i.e., walking). Physical therapy may be helpful in some patients.

Patient Education

Inform patients that they have a real illness that currently has no cure. Treatment should be focused on treating any identified conditions, such as fibromyalgia, depression, or allergies, and on preventing deconditioning. There are many resources and support groups that patients should be encouraged to contact.

Key Treatment

- Treat obvious disease states.
- Treat and manage stress and depression (consider referral to counselor)
- Adequate, efficient rest
- Well-balanced diet
- Drug, cigarette, and alcohol free if possible

- Regular mild- to moderate-intensity exercise
- Express concern but be optimistic/hopeful
- Schedule regular follow-up.

Follow-Up

Frequent follow-up initially to complete patient education and initiate therapy for any detected treatable diseases/syndromes, then every 3 to 4 months to monitor for new problems (initially, some patients may benefit from monthly visits). Maintain recommended health maintenance checkups.

Resources for Patients
CFIDS Asociation Inc.
PO Box 220398
Charlotte, NC 28222-0398
(phone: 1-800-442-3437)

Internet
CFS Network: *www.ncf.carleton.ca/ip/ social.services/cfseir/CFSEIR.HP.html*
CDC CFS homepage: *www.cdc.gov/ncidod/ diseases/cfs/cfshome.html*

Bibliography

Bates DW, Buchwald D, Lee J, et al: Clinical laboratory test findings in patients with chronic fatigue syndrome. Arch Intern Med 1995;155:97–103.

Bates DW, Schmitt W, Buchwald D, et al: Prevalence of fatigue and chronic fatigue syndrome in a primary care practice. Arch Intern Med 1993;153:2759–2765.

Fukuda K, Strauss SE, Hickie I, et al: The chronic fatigue syndrome: a comprehensive approach to its definition and study. Ann Intern Med 1994;121:953–959.

Komaroff AL, Buchwald DS. Chronic fatigue syndrome: an update. Annu Rev Med 1998;49:1–13.

Kroenke K, Wood DR, Mangelsdorff AD, et al: Chronic fatigue in primary care: prevalence, patient characterictics, and outcome. JAMA 1988;260:929–934.

258 Influenza

John G. Spangler

Etiology

1. Influenza A, B, and C are single-stranded RNA of Orthomyxoviridae family; classification based on hemagglutinin and neuraminidase antigens.
2. Frequent nuclear rearrangement (antigenic drift and antigenic shift) gives rise to epidemics and pandemics (especially with influenza A).
3. Influenza C is responsible for only mild respiratory illness.

Symptoms

1. Rapid onset of fever and headache
2. Respiratory symptoms such as sore throat, nasal stuffiness, and nonproductive cough (may become productive in setting of bacterial superinfection)
3. Muscle aches and extreme malaise lasting several days

Key Symptoms

• Fever	• Nonproductive cough
• Sore throat	• Muscle aches
• Nasal congestion	• Extreme malaise

Clinical Findings

Uncomplicated Influenza

1. Fever (frequently up to 103° F) for 3 to 5 days
2. Upper respiratory signs, including conjunctival injection, nasal discharge, pharyngeal erythema, and cough
3. Mild muscle tenderness to palpation
4. Paucity of pulmonary findings

Primary Influenza Viral Pneumonia

1. Severe, often fatal, disease frequently progressing to adult respiratory distress syndrome (ARDS)
2. Occurs predominantly in younger patients, patients with cardiovascular (especially rheumatic heart) disease, and pregnant women
3. Dyspnea, cyanosis, scant sputum production; occasional crackles

Secondary Bacterial Pneumonia

1. Bacterial superinfection of typical influenza in an elderly or chronically ill patient
2. Purulent sputum production, fever, pleuritic chest pain; localized rales or rhonchi with consolidation

Reye's Syndrome

1. Childhood complication of influenza with cerebral edema, fatty infiltration of the liver, and mental status changes; peak onset at 6 years of age
2. High association with aspirin use during respiratory viral diseases

Key Signs

Uncomplicated Influenza	Secondary Bacterial Pneumonia
• Fever	• Productive cough
• Myalgias	• Localized crackles or rhonchi
• Nonproductive cough	• Pleuritic chest pain
• Few pulmonary findings	**Reye's Syndrome**
Primary Viral Pneumonia	• Hepatomegaly (fatty liver)
• Severe dyspnea	• No jaundice
• Occasional rales	• Mental status changes
• Cyanosis	• Hypoglycemia
• Scant sputum	

Laboratory Tests

1. Viral culture of throat swab or sputum is definitive test, but takes 3 to 7 days.
2. Rapid test packs available for diagnosis in 10 minutes.
3. Serologic diagnosis requires a fourfold rise in complement-fixing antibody titers 2 to 4 weeks after acute illness.
4. Epidemiologic "diagnosis" can be presumed with 85 per cent certainty in setting of docu-

mented community outbreak of influenza with presence of fever, cough, and muscle aches.

5. Chest radiograph
   a. Primary viral pneumonia: patchy bilateral infiltrates, basilar streaking, or ARDS
   b. Secondary bacterial pneumonia: bilateral or unilateral lobar processes
6. Sputum Gram's stain and culture most helpful in secondary bacterial pneumonia, showing *Pneumococcus* and *Staphylococcus* in most cases; *Haemophilus influenzae* and gram-negative rods also common.

Key Tests

- Viral culture for definitive diagnosis
- Serology
- Chest film (in complicated influenza)
- Sputum microbiology (in secondary bacterial pneumonia)

Differential Diagnosis
1. Other respiratory viruses (e.g., adenovirus, measles, respiratory syncytial virus)
2. Primary bacterial pneumonias (e.g., *Mycoplasma*, *Pneumococcus*)
3. Rarely, pneumonic forms of *Rickettsia*, plague, or Hantavirus

Treatment

Uncomplicated Influenza
1. Bed rest, antipyretics, and cough suppressants
2. Amantadine (Symmetrel) and rimantadine (Flumadine), both 100 mg bid for approximately 5 days
   a. Can shorten course of influenza A if give within 48 hours of onset of symptoms.
   b. Renal impairment dosing adjustment needed (see Table 258–1).
3. Neuraminidase inhibitors: oseltamivir (Tamiflu), one 75 mg tablet twice daily for 5 days, and zanamivir (Relenza), two 5 mg inhalations twice daily for 5 days, reduce the duration of influenza A and B if given within 48 hours of onset of symptoms. Clinically significant drug interactions are unlikely and both are well tolerated, although oseltamivir has an increased rate of nausea compared to placebo, and zanamivir may cause bronchospasm in patients with underlying pulmonary disease.

Complicated Influenza
1. Primary viral pneumonia: intensive care hospitalization to maintain oxygenation
2. Secondary bacterial pneumonia: antibiotic treatment directed at most common organisms (see above)
3. Reye's syndrome: intensive care support to manage hypoglycemia, increased blood ammonia, and cerebral edema

Prevention
Influenza vaccine: Goal is to reduce the incidence of lower respiratory tract disease and its complications.
1. Inactivated, egg-grown, highly purified vaccine containing two influenza A subtypes and one influenza B subtype; updated annually
2. Contraindicated in anaphylactic egg allergy; patients with acute febrile illnesses should delay vaccination. Otherwise, side effects include local pain and swelling, and infrequently fever, malaise, and myalgias.
3. Target groups
   a. Persons 65 years old and older
   b. Long-term care facility residents
   c. All persons with cardiopulmonary disease (e.g., valvular heart disease, chronic obstructive lung disease), or chronic metabolic diseases (e.g., diabetes mellitus, sickle cell anemia, Addison's disease)
   d. Children on long-term aspirin (e.g., juvenile rheumatoid arthritis)
   e. Health care workers and others who may transmit influenza to high-risk individuals
   f. Pregnant women with medical conditions increasing their risk of severe influenza, or who will be in their third trimester during influenza season
   g. Immunocompromised individuals: large doses of corticosteroids, malignancies, chemotherapy, post–organ transplantation
   h. Patients with human immunodeficiency virus infection or acquired immunodeficiency syndrome
   i. Except in cases of egg allergy or previous hypersensitivity, the general population may receive vaccination, including children.
   j. Patients who are at risk for complicated influenza and who are unable to tolerate vaccine or who have not been vaccinated should be maintained on amantadine or rimantadine prophylaxis (100 mg bid) throughout the influenza season in their community (usually 5 to 6 weeks).

TABLE 258-1. AMANTADINE AND RIMANTADINE DOSAGE GUIDELINES

AGE, WEIGHT, AND/OR MEDICAL CONDITION	AMANTADINE DOSAGE		RIMANTADINE DOSAGE
Child <45 kg or <10 years old	5 mg/kg/d divided into 2 doses, not to exceed 150 mg/d total		5 mg/kg/d divided into 2 doses, not to exceed 150 mg/d total
Healthy adult or adolescent	100 mg twice per day		100 mg twice per day
Adult ≥65 years	≤100 mg once per day		Consider reduction to 100 mg once per day; if elderly nursing home patients, reduce dosage to 100 mg once per day
Renal impairment	**Creatinine Clearance (ml/min/1.73 m²)**	**Dosage**	100 mg once per day if creatinine clearance ≤10 ml/min
	30–50	200 mg on day 1 then 100 mg daily	
	15–29	200 mg on day 1 then 100 mg every other day	
	<15	200 mg every 7 days	
Severe liver dysfunction	No change		100 mg once per day

From Zimmerman RK, Ruben FL, Ahwesh ER: Influenza, influenza vaccine, oral amantadine/rimantadine. J Fam Pract 1997;45:107–122, with permission.

Patient Education

1. Influenza is self-limited in healthy individuals, but its potentially severe consequences must be stressed to elderly or chronically ill patients to ensure their annual vaccination.

2. Patients at risk for severe disease traveling abroad (May to September in Southern Hemisphere; October to April in North Hemisphere; year round in tropics) should be vaccinated.

3. Parents must not give aspirin to children during upper respiratory illnesses or chickenpox because of the risk of Reye's syndrome.

Key Treatment

Drug of Choice

- Amantadine or rimantadine (treat only influenza A)

Primary Viral Pneumonia

- Aggressive oxygen support

Secondary Bacterial Pneumonia

- Intravenous antibiotics

Reye's Syndrome

- Maintain euglycemia

- Monitor and treat cerebral edema

Follow-Up

Elderly or chronically ill patients require frequent monitoring for prolonged malaise, depression, or pulmonary complications.

Bibliography

For general reference on virology, epidemiology, and clinical aspects of influenza, see

Betts RF: Influenza virus. In Mandel GL, Bennett JE, Dolin R (eds): Principles and Practice of Infectious Diseases, 4th ed. New York, Churchill Livingstone, 1995, pp 1546–1567.

Zimmerman RK, Ruben FL, Ahwesh ER: Influenza, influenza vaccine, oral amantadine/rimantadine. J Fam Pract 1997;45:107–122.

For information regarding the use of amantadine and rimantadine, see

Nicholson KG: Use of antivirals in influenza in the elderly: prophylaxis and therapy. Gerontology 1996;45:280–289.

Wintermeyer SM, Nahata MC: Rimantadine: a clinical perspective. Ann Pharm 1995;29:299–310.

For influenza vaccine recommendations, see

Centers for Disease Control and Prevention: Prevention and control of influenza. MMWR Morb Mortal Wkly Rep 1997;46(RR-9):1–25.

For general information regarding Reye's syndrome, see

Quam DA: Recognizing a case of Reye's syndrome. Am Fam Physician 1994;50:1491–1496.

For information on the impact of influenza among the elderly, see

McBean AM, Babish JD, Warren JL: The impact and cost of influenza in the elderly. Arch Intern Med 1993;153:2105–2111.

259 Lyme Disease

Armando Jose Jarquin

Etiology

Lyme disease is caused by the spirochete *Borrelia burgdorferi*.

1. Most common vector-borne disease in the United States; approximately 12,000 cases per year
2. Transmitted to human by Ixodes ticks, which are part of the *Ixodes ricinus* complex.
3. White-footed mouse and white-tailed deer are the major animal reservoirs for *B. burgdorferi*.

Symptoms

Stage I: Early Localized Infection (1 to 4 Weeks After Bite)

1. Erythema migrans (found in 80 per cent of patients)
   a. Mostly asymptomatic; causes burning sensation, itching, or pain in 14 per cent of patients
   b. About 1 week after bite, lesion appears at the site, which is commonly in the groin or the axilla.
2. Flu-like symptoms (found in 50 per cent of patients): regional lymphadenopathy, fever, chills, malaise

Stage II: Early Disseminated Infection (1 to 4 Months)

1. Persistent malaise and fatigue (most common)
2. Migratory pain in joints, muscles, and tendons
3. Intermittent headaches and focal neurologic changes
4. Occasional palpitations or syncope

Stage III: Late Persistent Infections (4 Months to Years)

1. Prolonged arthritis and persistent arthralgias (60 per cent of patients)
2. Joint subluxations or tenderness below lesions of acrodermatitis
3. Various neurologic changes: ataxic gait, dementia, mood changes, paresthesias

Key Symptoms

- Stage I: fever, chills, malaise
- Stage II: headache, arthralgias, minor neurologic changes
- Stage III: severe fatigue and arthralgias, neurologic deficit

Clinical Findings

Stage I Manifestations

1. Erythema migrans: macule or papule enlarging to form annular lesion with red border and central clearing in trunk or extremities
2. Flu-like symptoms: fever, malaise, myalgia

Stage II Manifestations

1. Skin
   a. Worsening erythema migrans (5 to 40 cm in diameter)
   b. Secondary annular skin lesions: 17 per cent of patients
   c. Lymphocytoma (rare, only 1 per cent of patients): red and violet nodule occurring in earlobe or nipple; usually asymptomatic
2. Musculoskeletal
   a. Fatigue and malaise (most common)
   b. Migratory arthritis
   c. Panniculitis (rare)
3. Central nervous system: 10 to 20 per cent of patients
   a. Aseptic meningitis, encephalitis
   b. Bell's palsy, peripheral neuropathy
4. Cardiac: 4 to 10 per cent of patients
   a. First-degree atrioventricular (AV) block (PR segment <0.3 second)
   b. High-degree AV block
   c. Myocarditis or, in rare cases, pancarditis

Stage III Manifestations

1. Skin
   a. Acrodermatitis chronicum atrophicans (rare): bluish-red discoloration with edema

and central areas of atrophy, mostly on lower extremities

b. Scleroderma-like lesions: sclerotic or fibrotic plaques and subcutaneous nodules around knees and elbows

2. Musculoskeletal

   a. Prolonged arthritis: associated with human leukocyte antigens DR4 and DR2

   b. Synovitis, periostitis

   c. Severe fatigue

3. Central nervous system

   a. Subacute encephalopathy (most common): dementia, sleep disturbance, and mood changes

   b. Axonal polyneuropathy: distal paresthesias and radicular pain

   c. Leukoencephalitis (rare): ataxia, cognitive dysfunction, spastic paraparesis, and bladder dysfunction

Key Signs

- Stage I: malaise, expanding macule or papule with central clearing

- Stage II: headache, neuropathies, worsening erythema, palpitations

- Stage III: fatigue, dementia, ataxia, bluish-red lesions with atrophy

Laboratory Tests

1. Detection of specific antibodies to *B. burgdorferi*

   a. Indirect immunofluorescence assay

   b. Enzyme-linked immunosorbent assay (ELISA): In early disease, 50 per cent of patients are seronegative; in later stages, over 90 per cent are seropositive. Immunoblot (Western blot) analysis is used to confirm indeterminate or positive ELISA results.

2. Cultures

   a. Blood: About 30 per cent are positive.

   b. Cerebrospinal fluid: Less than 10 per cent are positive.

   c. Erythema migrans biopsy specimens: About 60 per cent are positive.

3. Special silver staining of chronic synovitis shows spirochetes in 33 per cent of patients.

Key Test

- ELISA is preferred, because it is more sensitive and specific.

- Immunoglobulin (Ig)M antibody appears first, at 2 to 4 weeks after skin lesions, peaks at 6 to 8 weeks, then declines after 4 to 6 months of illness. Persistent IgM suggests recurrent illness.

- IgG increases later, at 6 to 8 weeks of disease, peaks at 4 to 6 months, and remains high indefinitely.

Differential Diagnosis

1. Lyme disease as multisystemic disease

   a. Autoimmune diseases: fibromyalgia, systemic lupus erythematosus, rheumatoid arthritis

   b. Rocky Mountain spotted fever, rat-bite fever

   c. Chronic fatigue syndrome

   d. Secondary syphilis

2. Dermatologic manifestations

   a. Erythema migrans versus

      (1) Insect bites, drug eruptions

      (2) Erythema multiforme and tinea corporis

   b. Acrodermatitis chronica atrophicans versus

      (1) Venous insufficiency

      (2) Arterial insufficiency

      (3) Stasis dermatitis and scleroderma

   c. Lymphocytoma versus erythema nodosum, rheumatic nodules

3. Neurologic manifestations

   a. Bacterial and viral meningitis

   b. Multiple sclerosis

4. Cardiac manifestations: viral myocarditis

Treatment

Treatment should be given depending on the clinical findings of the disease.

Medication

1. Tetracycline, 500 mg orally qid; or doxycycline, 100 mg orally bid; or amoxicillin, 250 to 500 mg orally tid; or erythromycin, 250 mg orally qid; should be given for

   a. Erythema migrans (14 to 21 days)

   b. First-degree AV block (20 to 30 days)

   c. Arthritis (30 days)

   d. Acrodermatitis atrophicans (30 days)

   e. Bell's palsy (30 days)

2. Ceftriaxone (Rocephin), 2 gm intravenously

daily; or penicillin G, 20 million units in six divided doses per day intravenously; for

a. Neurologic disease other than Bell's palsy (14 to 28 days)
b. High-degree AV block (14 to 21 days)
c. Persistent arthritis (14 to 28 days)

Diet

Unless there is any particular objection, a regular diet should be given. Nasogastric tube feeding may be needed.

Activity

Activity should be undertaken as tolerated. Physical therapy may be needed for arthritis or any neurologic sequelae.

Patient Education

Patient and relatives should be well aware of the nature of this disease and complications.

Key Treatment

Drug of Choice	**Alternative Drugs**
• Tetracycline, 500 mg PO q6h for 10 to 30 days	• Amoxicillin or erythromycin
	• Nonsteroidal anti-inflammatory drugs should be given for symptoms.

Follow-Up

1. Should be individualized depending on the stage of the disease.
2. In noncomplicated cases, follow up as outpatient every week.
3. Complicated cases should be hospitalized and seen daily.

Bibliography

Fitzpatrick TB, Johnson RA, Polano MK, et al: Color Atlas and Synopsis of Clinical Dermatology, 2nd ed, pp 360–369. New York, McGraw-Hill, 1992.

Jacobs RA: Infectious diseases: spirochetal. In Tierney LM Jr, McPhee SJ, Papadakis MA (eds): Current Medical Diagnosis and Treatment, 38th annual rev, pp 1332–1352. East Norwalk, CT, Appleton & Lange, 1999.

Rahn DW, Felz MW: Lyme disease update. Postgrad Med 1998;103:51–70.

Steere AC: Lyme disease. N Engl J Med 1989;321:586–595.

Steere AC, Taylor E, McHugh GL, et al: The overdiagnosis of Lyme disease. JAMA 1993;269:1812–1816.

260 Salmonellosis

Lisa G. King

Etiology

1. *Salmonella* is a nonencapsulated, gram-negative bacillus.

2. *Salmonella* is transmitted by the fecal-oral route. Poultry, beef, eggs, and milk products are common sources. So are pet reptiles, chicks, and ducks.

3. Those most vulnerable are under 20 or over 70 years of age. Sickle cell disease and osteomyelitis predispose to infection.

Symptoms

Salmonella infection manifests itself in three clinical syndromes.

1. *Gastroenteritis* is the most common. "Food poisoning" may be salmonellosis. After an incubation period of up to 48 hours, these symptoms begin:

   a. An abrupt onset of nausea and vomiting

   b. Crampy abdominal pain

   c. Diarrhea ranging in severity from mild to dysenteric

   d. Self-limited fever

   Healthy adults are symptomatic for 2 to 5 days.

2. *Enteric fever (typhoid fever)* typically has a 1- to 2-week incubation period during which ingested bacteria penetrate the gut mucosa and travel via the lymphatics into the blood.

   a. The earliest symptoms are headache, malaise, chills, abdominal pain, and a fever that increases incrementally over a period of days.

   b. After about a week, the fever becomes sustained.

   c. Other manifestations may include constipation or mild diarrhea, anorexia, nausea, vomiting, epistaxis, rose spots, bronchitis, and altered mental status.

3. *Bacteremia and focal infections* may follow intestinal infection. The symptoms vary with the site of infection, which can be intravascular, skeletal, meningeal, splenic, hepatobiliary, urinary, or pulmonary. Most patients give a history of fever, chills, sweats, and weight loss.

Key Symptoms

***Salmonella* Gastroenteritis**

- Nausea

- Crampy abdominal pain

- Diarrhea

Enteric Fever

- Fever that increases in a stepwise manner over several days

- A flu-like syndrome

Clinical Findings

1. The gastroenteritis manifests mainly as periumbilical or right lower quadrant pain with watery stools that sometimes contain mucus or blood.

2. Enteric fever's primary signs are bradycardia relative to the degree of fever, a musty body odor, and right lower quadrant tenderness. Rose spots are evident on the trunk in over 50 per cent of patients. They appear as erythematous macules up to 0.5 cm in diameter that blanch with pressure.

3. For bacteremia with focal infections, the clinical findings are related to the site of infection.

Key Signs of Enteric Fever

- Prolonged fever

- Relative bradycardia

- Rose spots

Laboratory Tests

1. With gastroenteritis there is usually no leukocytosis, although there may be hemoconcentration. The stool smear will contain leukocytes. By the time a positive stool culture returns, the patient is typically recovering.

2. In enteric fever, blood cultures are usually positive for 1 to 3 weeks after symptoms begin. Cultures of stool, urine, and rose spots may in-

crease the diagnostic yield. Bone marrow cultures are the most sensitive; over 90 per cent are positive.

a. Nonspecific lab abnormalities include anemia, leukopenia to normopenia with relative bandemia, and thrombocytopenia. Bilirubin and aspartate transaminase may be elevated, and disseminated intravascular coagulation may occur. If the patient has diarrhea, the stool may show many leukocytes.

b. Two thirds of patients have a fourfold or greater elevation in the O or H antibody titers over 2 to 3 weeks. This is a positive Widal's test, but it is not diagnostic because of many false positives and false negatives.

3. Isolation of *Salmonella* from the blood or site of localized infection confirms the diagnosis in patients with bacteremia and focal infections.

Key Tests

Diagnosis is based on isolation of organisms from stool, blood, urine, bone marrow, rose spots, or tissue fluid.

Differential Diagnosis

1. For gastroenteritis consider *Escherichia coli*, *Campylobacter jejuni*, *Yersinia enterocolitica*, *Clostridium difficile*, *Shigella*, viruses, ulcerative colitis, and Crohn's disease.

2. In atypical cases enteric fever may resemble mononucleosis, rickettsiosis, brucellosis, leptospirosis, miliary tuberculosis, cytomegalovirus infection, malaria, viral hepatitis, or lymphoma.

Treatment

Medication

1. Gastroenteritis: Only those who are infants, elderly, immunocompromised, or at increased risk of focal infection should receive antibiotic therapy, because treatment does not alleviate symptoms and may prolong intestinal carriage.

   a. Drug of choice: amoxicillin or ampicillin for 3 to 5 days

   b. Alternative drugs: chloramphenicol or trimethoprim-sulfamethoxazole (Bactrim, Septra)

2. Enteric fever

   a. Drug of choice: chloramphenicol, 50 mg/kg/day intravenously or orally, in four divided doses for 2 to 4 weeks

b. Alternative drugs: amoxicillin, trimethoprim-sulfamethoxazole, fluoroquinolone or ceftriaxone (Rocephin)

3. Systemic infection: Antibiotic therapy must be accompanied by removal of infected tissue.

   a. Drugs of choice: parenteral chloramphenicol or third-generation cephalosporin

   b. Alternative drugs: trimethoprim-sulfamethoxazole or amoxicillin

Diet

The primary treatment of the gastroenteritis is oral fluids.

Patient Education

1. Education on proper hand washing and food preparation techniques can prevent the transmission of *Salmonella*.

2. Advise travelers to developing countries where enteric fever is endemic not to drink untreated water or eat ice, unpeeled fruit, or other uncooked foods. They may also wish to get the vaccine, which offers 70 per cent protection against serotypes of salmonellae that cause enteric fever.

Key Treatment

Salmonella Gastroenteritis

• Oral fluid replacement

Enteric Fever

Drug of Choice	*Alternative Drugs*
• Chloramphenicol	• Amoxicillin
	• Trimethoprim-sulfamethoxazole
	• Fluoroquinolones
	• Ceftriaxone

Follow-Up

1. Complications of enteric fever usually occur 2 to 4 weeks after the initial symptoms and can include intestinal ulcers with hemorrhage or perforation, cholecystitis, hepatitis, meningitis, pneumonia, arthritis, nephritis, myocarditis, osteomyelitis, parotitis, prostatitis, epididymitis, and orchitis.

2. About 10 per cent of patients with enteric fever experience a relapse after 4 to 5 weeks whether

or not the initial infection was treated. Relapses are treated in the same manner as a first episode.

3. Three per cent of patients who have had enteric fever and 0.5 per cent of patients exposed to other serotypes of *Salmonella* become chronic fecal carriers. True asymptomatic carriage is diagnosed when *Salmonella* are shed in the stool for a year or more. Chronic carriers are treated with 4 to 6 weeks of ampicillin or amoxicillin plus probenecid. Chronic carriers with gallstones may also require cholecystectomy.

 Bibliography

Butler T: Typhoid fever. In Bennett JC, Plum F (eds): Cecil Textbook of Medicine, 20th ed, pp 1641–1642. Philadelphia, WB Saunders Company, 1996.

Hornick R: Salmonella infections other than typhoid fever. In Bennett JC, Plum F (eds): Cecil Textbook of Medicine, 20th ed, pp 1643–1646. Philadelphia, WB Saunders Company, 1996.

Keusch GT: Salmonellosis. In Fauci AS, Braunwald E, Isselbacher KJ, et al (eds): Harrison's Principles of Internal Medicine, 14th ed, pp 950–956. New York, McGraw-Hill, 1998.

Miller SI, Hohmann EL, Pegues DA: Salmonella (including Salmonella Typhi). In Mandel GL, Bennett JE, Dolin R (eds): Principles and Practice of Infectious Diseases, 4th ed, pp 2013–2033. New York, Churchill Livingstone, 1995.

261 Malaria

Gary A. Goforth

Etiology

1. Parasitic agents (*Plasmodium falciparum, Plasmodium vivax, Pityrosporum ovale,* or *Plasmodium malariae*) infect humans, the host/reservoir, via the female *Anopheles* species mosquito vector.

2. Protective effect against *P. falciparum* infection if sickle cell disease or trait, glucose-6-phosphate dehydrogenase (G6PD) deficiency, or hereditary ovalocytosis. Resistant to *P. vivax* infection if Duffy-negative blood type.

Symptoms

1. Incubation period 9 to 40 days; average 12 days (*P. falciparum*), 13 days (*P. vivax*), 17 days (*P. ovale*), 28 days (*P. malariae*)

2. Initial symptoms: cold stage—rigors, chills; hot stage—fever, seizures; defervescent stage—diaphoresis

3. Periodicity of fever corresponds to release of merozoites from red blood cells in asexual cycle every 48 hours for *P. falciparum* (malignant tertian malaria), for *P. vivax* (benign tertian malaria), and for *P. ovale* and every 72 hours for *P. malariae* (quartan malaria).

4. Other common symptoms: nonproductive cough, myalgias, postural hypotension, diarrhea, persistent fatigue, marked lethargy (especially cerebral malaria)

Key Symptoms

- Periodic fever
- Diaphoresis
- Persistent fatigue
- Chills
- Diarrhea (often bloody)
- Lethargy/coma (cerebral malaria)

Clinical Findings

1. Common physical findings: mild jaundice, liver tenderness, hemolysis, splenomegaly (with chronic infection)

2. *P. falciparum* infection: Significant parasitemia common, with life-threatening complications including acute renal failure (blackwater fever), hemolytic anemia, pulmonary edema.

3. *P. malariae* infection: Nephrotic infection occasionally seen in chronic infections.

Key Signs

- Hemolytic anemia
- Liver tenderness
- Pulmonary edema
- Jaundice
- Splenomegaly (chronic infection)
- Renal failure

Laboratory Tests

1. Thick and thin blood smears standard for diagnosis. If malaria suspected but smear negative, repeat every 6 to 12 hours for 2 consecutive days. (Malaria is unlikely if smears remain negative.)

2. Other useful tests: complete blood count with peripheral smear (hemolytic anemia, leukopenia, thrombocytopenia); liver function tests (alanine transaminase [ALT], aspartate transaminase [AST], direct and indirect bilirubin elevated); albumin (decreased)

3. Quantitative buffy coat, DNA probe, and ribosomal RNA probes are under development as diagnostic tests.

Key Tests

- Thick and thin blood smears
- Liver function tests (ALT, AST, direct/indirect bilirubin)
- Complete blood count, peripheral smear

Differential Diagnosis

1. Severe *P. falciparum* infection: dysentery, acute gastroenteritis, viral syndrome, acute hepatitis, acute hemolytic anemia, meningitis, pneumonia, influenza, and other febrile illnesses in a tropical environment; cerebrovascular accident

2. Chronic infection: hyperreactive malarial syndrome, differential diagnosis of splenomegaly (infectious, inflammatory, hematologic neo-

plasms, nonmalignant hematologic disorders, congestive splenomegaly, infiltrative disorders, trauma)

Treatment

Medication—Drugs of Choice

1. P. malariae, P. vivax, P. ovale, or P. falciparum infection in areas with chloroquine sensitivity
   a. Oral therapy: chloroquine phosphate (Aralen)
      (1) Adults: 600 mg base (1 gm salt) followed by 300 mg base (500 mg salt) 6 hours later, then 300 mg base daily for 2 days.
      (2) Pediatric: 10 mg/kg base (max 600 mg base), followed by 5 mg/kg base 6 hours later, then 5 mg/kg base daily for 2 days.
   b. Parenteral therapy (if unable to tolerate oral therapy, parasitemia >5 per cent, or evidence of complications)
      (1) Adults: quinidine gluconate, 10 mg/kg salt in 500 ml of normal saline intravenously over 1 to 2 hours, then 0.02 mg/kg/minute continuous infusion until oral therapy can be started (maximum 72 hours). Central venous catheter to monitor fluid balance and cardiac monitoring necessary.
      (2) Pediatric: same as adults
2. P. falciparum infection acquired in areas with chloroquine resistance
   a. Oral therapy
      (1) Adult: quinine sulfate, 650 mg salt q8h for 3 to 7 days orally, plus tetracycline, 250 mg orally qid for 7 days, or pyrimethamine sulfadoxine (Fansidar), 3 tablets orally in single dose. If acquired in Thailand or the Amazon basin, 7-day course of quinine required.
      (2) Pediatric: quinine sulfate, 10 mg/kg salt q8h orally for 3 to 7 days, plus tetracycline, 5 mg/kg qid for 7 days, or pyrimethamine sulfadoxine (Fansidar) in single dose (<1 year, 1/4 tablet; 1 to 3 years, 1/2 tablet; 4 to 8 years, 1 tablet; 9 to 14 years, 2 tablets; >14 years, 3 tablets). The benefit of using tetracycline must be weighed against known adverse events in children under 8 years old.
   b. Parenteral therapy: See above under chloroquine-sensitive P. falciparum malaria.

Medication—Alternative Drugs

1. Mefloquine hydrochloride (Lariam), 15 mg/kg salt orally in single dose up to 1250 mg (adult and child)
   a. Treatment dose associated with dose-related increased incidence of neuropsychiatric side effects.
   b. Contraindicated for persons with known hypersensitivity or history of serious psychiatric or seizure disorder, children less than 15 kg, patients with cardiac conduction abnormalities, and during pregnancy.
2. Halofantrine (Halfan): adult dosage 6 tablets (250 mg salt each) orally, 2 tablets q6h × three doses; pediatric dosage 8 mg/kg salt orally q6h × three doses.
3. Pregnant patients: quinine (as above) plus clindamycin (Cleocin), 450 mg orally q8h × three days
4. Prevention: Use 1 week before arrival (1 to 2 days for doxycycline) and 4 weeks after leaving endemic area
   a. Chemoprophylaxis against all species except chloroquine-resistant P. falciparum: Chloroquine phosphate, 300 mg base (500 mg salt) or 5 mg/kg base (children) once weekly
   b. Chemoprophylaxis against chloroquine-resistant P. falciparum
      (1) Mefloquine, 228 mg base (250 mg salt) orally weekly; children 15 to 19 kg, 1/4 tablet; 20 to 30 kg, 1/2 tablet; 31 to 45 kg, 3/4 tablet; more than 45 kg, 1 tablet
      (2) Doxycycline, 100 mg orally daily (children >8 years, 2 mg/kg up to 100 mg/day)
   c. Prevention of P. vivax and P. ovale relapse (start after leaving endemic area): primaquine, 15 mg base (26.3 mg salt) or 0.3 mg/kg base (children) orally daily for 14 days, or 45 mg base (adults) or 0.9 mg/kg base (children) weekly for 8 weeks.

WARNING

Primaquine can cause hemolytic anemia in G6PD-deficient patients. Avoid during pregnancy.

Diet

No restrictions; oral fluids and feeding as tolerated in severe cases

Activity

Bed rest with febrile phase; gradual return to full activities when afebrile

Patient Education

Emphasize prevention of future disease to include chemoprophylaxis before and after travel to endemic area, use of personal protective measures against mosquito bites (DEET insect repellent, mosquito netting).

Key Treatment

Drugs of Choice	Alternative Drugs
• Chloroquine orally	• Mefloquine orally
• Tetracycline orally	• Halofantrine orally
• Quinine sulfate orally	• Pyrimethamine sulfadoxine orally
• Quinidine gluconate intravenously	• Quinine *plus* clindamycin

Follow-Up

1. Consult physician if treated for malaria while abroad or if febrile syndrome occurs after return.

2. Because of emerging *P. vivax* chloroquine resistance, recommend follow-up blood smear at 3 and 7 days after chloroquine treatment to assess parasite clearance. Treat as chloroquine-resistant *P. falciparum* if parasitemic within 3 weeks of treatment.

Bibliography

Barry M: Medical considerations for international travel with infants and older children. Infect Dis Clin North Am 1992;6:389–404.

Stanley J: Travel-related emergencies. Emerg Med Clin North Am 1997;15:113–149.

Strickland GT: Malaria. In Strickland GT (ed): Hunter's Tropical Medicine, 7th ed, pp 586–614. Philadelphia, WB Saunders Company, 1991.

Wyler D: Malaria chemoprophylaxis for the traveler. N Engl J Med 1993;329:31–37.

Zucker J, Campbell C: Malaria principles of prevention and treatment. Infect Dis Clin North Am 1993;7:547–567.

262 Typhoid Fever

Miriam T. Vincent

Etiology

1. Typhoid fever is a bacterial disease caused by *Salmonella typhi.*
2. *Salmonella* is a motile, gram-negative, nonencapsulated bacillus in the family of Enterobacteriaceae.
3. Transmission is by the fecal-oral route through contaminated water or food.

Symptoms (Table 262–1)

Typhoid fever is characterized by

1. Fever and chills, early (bacteremia)
2. Prolonged fever
3. Abdominal pain
4. Diarrhea
5. Delirium
6. Rose spots
7. Splenomegaly

Key Symptoms

- Persistent fever and chills
- Abdominal pain
- Diarrhea
- Headache

History, Signs, and Symptoms: When to Think Typhoid

- Travel to an endemic area, or food prepared by an individual from an endemic area
- Persistent and increasing fever, chills, headache
- Relative bradycardia
- Relative neutropenia

Clinical Findings (Table 262–1)

1. Early: fever, chills, headache (nonspecific), altered mental status, abdominal tenderness
2. Abdominal pain: right lower quadrant over terminal ileum
3. Prostration

4. Diarrhea ("pea-soup")
5. Rose spots: more than 50 per cent of body, most commonly on shoulders, thorax, and abdomen
6. Delirium, aphonia, or coma
7. Seizures (common in children)
8. Intestinal bleeding, intestinal perforation (5 per cent)
9. Inappropriate bradycardia at the height of fever
10. High spiking fevers in the absence of leukocytosis

Key Signs

- Fever
- Rose spots
- Delirium
- Relative bradycardia
- Relative neutropenia

Laboratory Tests

1. *Salmonella typhi* isolation from blood culture: positive in 90 per cent by week 1 to 3
2. Urine and stool cultures: less frequently positive than blood
3. Bone marrow culture (most sensitive)
4. Widal's test: agglutinating antibodies—O, somatic; F, flagellar; limited use, false-positive results in endemic areas
5. White blood cell count: normal or increased, with increased bands
6. Platelets are often decreased.
7. Elevation of aminotransferases and bilirubin

Key Tests

- Blood culture
- Stool and urine culture
- Bone marrow culture
- White blood cell count

TABLE 262-1. EVOLUTION OF SYMPTOMS AND SIGNS IN TYPHOID FEVER

TIME	SYMPTOMS	SIGNS	DISEASE
Week 1	Fever, chills, headache	Abdominal tenderness	Bacteremia
Week 2	Rash, diarrhea/constipation, delirium, exhaustion, abdominal pain	Rose spots, hepatomegaly, splenomegaly	Epidermal mononuclear vasculitis, Peyer's patch, ileal hyperplasia
Week 3	Complications: intestinal bleeds, perforation, shock	Melena, ileus, peritonitis, coma	Peyer's patch, ulceration or perforation
Week 4	Resolution, relapse, weight loss	Acute disease, cachexia	Cholecystitis, chronic carrier

Adapted from Butler T: Typhoid fever. In Bennett JC, Plum F (eds): Cecil Textbook of Medicine, 20th ed, p 1643. Philadelphia, WB Saunders Company, 1996, with permission.

Differential Diagnosis

1. Malaria
2. Hepatitis
3. Typhus
4. Amebic hepatic abscess
5. Shigellosis
6. Nontyhoid salmonellosis (*S. paratyphi* A, *S. paratyphi* B, *S. typhimurium*)
7. Septicemia
8. Influenza
9. Miliary tuberculosis
10. Meningococcemia
11. Bacterial endocarditis
12. Infectious mononucleosis
13. Septicemia: urinary tract, gastrointestinal tract, gallbladder

Treatment

Medication

1. Drugs of choice: ciprofloxacin (Cipro), 500 mg PO bid ×10 days (adults); ceftriaxone (Rocephin), 2 gm qd IV ×5 days
2. Alternative drugs: chloramphenicol, amoxicillin, trimethoprim-sulfamethoxazole (Bactrim), ampicillin

Patient Education

1. Education regarding proper hand washing and food preparation can prevent transmission.
2. Advise travelers going to nonindustrialized areas where typhoid fever is endemic to not eat ice, uncooked food, or unpeeled fruits or drink untreated water. Advise vaccines (variable efficacy: 60 to 80 per cent).

Follow-Up

1. Complications of typhoid fever (2 to 4 weeks after presentation) may include
   a. Intestinal ulcers with hemorrhage and perforation
   b. Cholecystitis
   c. Pneumonia
   d. Hepatitis
   e. Arthritis
   f. Nephritis
   g. Osteomyelitis
   h. Prostatitis
   i. Epididymitis
   j. Orchitis
   k. Meningitis
2. Ten per cent of patients will relapse regardless of treatment. Treatment is as per presentation. Three per cent of patients will become chronic fecal carriers (salmonella shed in the stool for >1 year).

B Bibliography

Butler T: Tyhoid fever. In Bennett JC, Plum F (eds): Cecil Textbook of Medicine, 20th ed, pp 1642–1644. Philadelphia, WB Saunders Company, 1996.

Hull A: Salmonellae. In Conn R, Borer WB, Synder J (eds): Conn's Current Diagnosis, 9th ed, pp 144–147. Philadelphia, WB Saunders Company, 1997.

Keusch GT: Salmonellosis. In Isselbacher KG, Braunwald E, Wilson JD, et al (eds): Harrison's Principles of Internal Medicine, 13th ed, pp 671–676. New York, McGraw-Hill, 1994.

Nirmal J, Milfred D: The use and misuse of new antibiotics: a perspective. Arch Intern Med 1995;155:569–577.

Oldach DW, Richard RE, Borza EN, et al: A mysterious death. N Engl J Med 1998;338:1764–1769.

263 Leprosy

Ronald E. Pust

Etiology and Epidemiology

1. Geographic: Although discovered by Hansen in Norway in 1873, the acid-fast bacillus *Mycobacterium leprae* now is transmitted mainly in developing nations. Leprosy is seen in immigrants from such countries and occasionally in U.S.-born persons from Hawaii and the Gulf Coast states. About 150 to 200 new cases are diagnosed in the United States each year, adding to the 5000 to 6000 previously diagnosed persons living in the United States.

2. Agent-host interaction: Three "basic science" facts about *M. leprae*, along with the spectrum of human immunologic response to it, determine clinical findings in leprosy:

   a. Slow growth, with a "doubling time" of 12 to 21 days

   b. Optimal growth at 82° F (28° C), favoring invasion of cooler body areas

   c. Affinity for nerves, especially in these cooler areas

3. Transmission from upper airways of untreated multibacillary cases results in secondary cases 2 to 8 or more years later in 5 to 7 per cent of close household contacts. Conversely, most new cases of leprosy have no obvious source case.

Symptoms

1. Leprosy should be considered in any person from an endemic area who has persistent unexplained findings in skin, upper airways, eyes, or peripheral nerves, especially in the limbs. All of these are cooler areas of the body.

2. These findings vary considerably, determined by the patient's placement on a five-type clinical continuum from multibacillary (lepromatous; LL) to paucibacillary (tuberculoid; TT) (see Table 263–1).

   a. Multibacillary patients have poor cell-mediated immune (CMI) responses specific to *M. leprae*. This is probably genetic but does not imply a broad-spectrum immune deficit.

   b. Paucibacillary patients have good CMI responses, yet this CMI response can cause early and severe damage to large nerves, especially in type I reactions (see below).

Clinical Findings

1. *Multibacillary (LL, BL, BB) leprosy*

   a. Often presents with multiple, infiltrated (raised), poorly marginated plaques or with nodules.

   b. Early in lepromatous disease, there may be only mild "stocking and glove" sensory loss. Often there is no motor nerve loss, even in advanced disease.

   c. Eye, ear, nose, and throat (EENT) lesions are common, including earlobe thickening, iritis or keratitis, and chronic nasal infiltration that may slowly progress to septal perforation.

2. *Borderline cases*, especially BB, show mixed features and are most susceptible to type I reactions, which can be an emergency.

3. *Paucibacillary (BT, TT) leprosy*

   a. Usually presents with only a few, well-marginated macules or plaques. These lesions nearly always show mild to profound anesthesia.

   b. Cutaneous or regional nerves are commonly enlarged, with associated sensory and often motor loss.

   c. If a motor nerve shows tenderness and acute loss of function, type I reaction should be suspected and steroids begun.

   d. The "pure neural" form of paucibacillary leprosy (i.e., without skin lesions) is rare in the United States.

4. The anesthesia in all types of leprosy, especially if progressive or untreated, leads to neuropathic injuries, ulcerations and the classic—but pre-

TABLE 263–1. COMPARISON OF CLINICAL ASPECTS OF MULTIBACILLARY AND PAUCIBACILLARY LEPROSY (HANSEN'S DISEASE)

Clinical Aspect	Multibacillary (Lepromatous)		Borderline	Paucibacillary (Tuberculoid)	
Ridley-Jopling type* Immunity (cell mediated, *M. leprae* specific)	LL Absent	BL Low	BB Moderate	BT High	TT Strong
Infectiousness (untreated)	Moderate		Slight	Minimal	None
Clinical features					
Skin lesions	Many, small, raised	Variable size, number		3–5, larger	1–2, flat, dry
Sensation, sweating	Slow "stocking-glove" loss		Varies	Moderate loss	Marked loss (early)
Nerve enlargement	None and/or late	Slow, variable			Marked and/or early
"Systemic" invasion (EENT, testes, bone)	Common (if untreated)	Variable, moderate		Rare	None
Clinical suspicion if:	Skin or EENT lesions (± peripheral anesthesia)			Anesthetic lesion or thickened nerve	
Diagnostic confirmation					
Skin Biopsy	AFB in subdermal histiocytes and nerves			Skin granulomas, nerve infiltrates; AFB rarely seen	
Bacillary index (on slit-skin smear)	5–6+	4–5+	2–4+	0–2+	0–1+
Reaction susceptibility					
Type I ("reversal")		←——————————————→			
Type II (ENL)	←——————————————→				
Potential dermatologic differentials include (consider neuropathy differential also)	Kaposi's sarcoma; neurofibromatosis; pityriasis; granuloma multiforme; leishmaniasis; lichen simplex or planus; drug eruption; keloids; syphilis (LL may have false-positive VDRL); etc.			Tinea corporis or versicolor; atopic or contact dermatitis; sarcoid; mycosis fungoides; psoriasis or other plaques; skin TB; SLE; etc	

Abbreviations: AFB, acid-fast bacilli; EENT, eye, ear, nose, throat; ENL, erythema nodosum leprosum; SLE, systemic lupus erythematosus; TB, tuberculosis; VDRL, Venereal Disease Research Laboratory [test].

*LL, lepromatous leprosy; BL, borderline lepromatous; BB, borderline; BT, borderline tuberculoid; TT, tuberculoid leprosy.

Adapted from Pust RE, Campos-Outcalt D: Leprosy in the United States: risks, recognition, regimens, resources. Postgrad Med 1985; 77:151–159, with permission.

---

ventable—deformities. Motor paralysis may contribute to further, sometimes severe, loss of limb function.

Key Signs

Acute Type I Reaction

- Tender swollen nerve(s) with acute loss of motor function—*treatment urgent*

- Anesthetic macules or plaques and/or stocking-glove hypesthesia

- Other typical persistent skin lesions (see Table 263–1)

- Enlarged or tender nerves

- Sensory or motor loss, especially in facial, ulnar, median, radial, peroneal, or posterior tibial nerves

- Ulcers and deformities resulting from damage to regions served by these anesthetic nerves

- Nasal or anterior eye damage, especially if other consistent findings

Type II Reaction: Erythema Nodosum Leprosum (ENL)

- Tender subdermal nodules, arising acutely, especially on extensor surfaces

Laboratory Tests

1. The 4-mm punch skin biopsy is the most useful diagnostic test in the United States. The specimen must be deep enough to include subdermal fat. Submitted in 10% formalin, it should be labeled to indicate the possibility of leprosy; this will also alert the pathologist to perform acid-fast bacilli (AFB) stains on the histologic specimen. Histopathologists experienced in leprosy, such as those at the U.S. Public Health Service (USPHS) Hansen's Disease Program, can classify the biopsy in one of the five Ridley-Jopling (LL to TT) categories, thus confirming the clinical picture and determining appropriate chemotherapy regimens.

2. Much like the direct sputum smear in tuberculosis, slit-skin smears stained for AFB may confirm the diagnosis of multibacillary leprosy and

quantify the bacterial load. In practice, however, nonleprologists are seldom prepared to do this test. Smears are not necessary to make the diagnosis in developed countries, where histopathology is readily available.

3. Numerous sophisticated diagnostic tests are proposed, including polymerase chain reaction, but so far none have proven as useful as clinical examination, punch biopsy, and slit-skin smears.

Key Tests

- Thorough EENT, skin, and limb examination is the best "test."

- Punch biopsy of skin lesion (mailed to USPHS Hansen's Disease Program)

- Slit-skin smears (not needed for initial diagnosis)

Differential Diagnosis

1. Skin
   a. The classic findings are virtually pathognomonic: Paucibacillary patients have skin lesions that are anesthetic; multibacillary cases have skin biopsies or smears showing AFB. In either type, nerve enlargement adds to the certainty of the diagnosis.
   b. Skin diseases that may be initially confused with leprosy include those in Table 263–1; however, none of these causes anesthesia.

2. Peripheral neuropathies
   a. Only peripheral nerves—never the central nervous system—are involved in leprosy.
   b. Leprosy and diabetes are the most common of the several causes of limb neuropathy in the world. However, in leprosy the clinician will virtually always find some of leprosy's other classic features.

3. EENT
   a. Perforation of the nasal septum can be found in congenital syphilis, Wegener's granulomatosis, or cocaine abusers.
   b. When chronic EENT changes suggest lepromatous leprosy, the clinician should examine the nerves and biopsy the skin.

Treatment

1. Regimens recommended in the United States since 1997 for chemotherapy of paucibacillary (TT and BT) and multibacillary (BB, BL, and LL) leprosy include rifampin, dapsone, and clofazimine.
   a. These same three drugs are the basis for the World Health Organization (WHO)–rec-

ommended regimens around the world. Although utilizing less frequent doses of rifampin, the WHO regimens are probably as effective as the U.S. regimens.
   b. Drug regimens of choice in the United States in 1999 are shown in Table 263–1 and in the Key Treatment box.

2. Treatment of *leprosy reactions* (see Key Treatment box)
   a. *Many patients first present to clinicians when they are in reaction.* All reactions except the most mild should be started on treatment with high-dose daily oral steroids.
   b. The only common "emergency" in leprosy is the acute motor neuropathy induced by a serious type I reaction. Prednisone will also control type II (ENL) reactions; thus it is not absolutely necessary for the nonleprologist to distinguish type I from type II in the emergency situation.
   c. An ENL reaction may persist for several months to a few years; in this situation thalidomide is also highly effective and avoids the complications of long-term steroids. Decisions about thalidomide use can be made later, in consultation with a physician authorized to prescribe it through the USPHS Hansen's Disease Program and/or Celgene Company, the U.S. manufacturer of thalidomide (Thalomid).

Key Treatment (Adult Doses)

Paucibacillary Leprosy (TT and BT)

- One year of daily rifampin (Rifadin), 600 mg, plus dapsone, 100 mg

Multibacillary Leprosy (BB, BL, LL)

- Two years of daily rifampin (Rifadin), 600 mg, plus dapsone, 100 mg, plus clofazimine (Lamprene), 50 mg

Acute Type I or II Leprosy Reactions

- Continue above regimen, consult with USPHS Hansen's Program, and *add* for

- Mildest reactions (no nerve pain or function loss or fever): hydroxychloroquine sulfate (Plaquenil) or nonsteroidal anti-inflammatory drugs

- All other reactions
  –Begin 60 to 80 mg prednisone daily; consider slow taper after 1 week.

  –Consider thalidomide (under proper precautions) for prolonged or recurrent type II (ENL) reactions.

Prognosis

1. With early diagnosis and recommended treatment, all forms of leprosy have an excellent prognosis. Skin lesions may become barely visible. Nerve and EENT damage is usually arrested but is rarely reversed by treatment. The clear exception is the full or partial recovery from acute motor neuropathy by prompt steroid treatment of type I reactions.

2. Physical therapists, orthotists, and podiatrists play crucial roles in tertiary prevention and in restoration of limb function.

3. Eye and ENT specialists contribute to the care of lepromatous complications.

Follow-Up

1. Leprosy patients should be seen every 1 to 3 months during their 1 to 2 years of chemotherapy, more often if in reaction. Intensity of long-term follow-up is determined by the complications of motor and sensory loss; this in turn requires patient education for prevention and treatment of secondary infections and limb or eye dysfunctions.

2. The USPHS Hansen's Disease Program is eager to be of assistance to any U.S. clinician. Their services include telephone clinical consultation about diagnosis and treatment, histopathology and slit-skin smear interpretation, provision of the recommended drugs (see Key Treatment box), professional and patient education, and, in some circumstances, acute hospitalization. The phone number is 1-504-642-7771 or toll-free 1-800-642-2477 in Carville or Baton Rouge, LA (U.S. central time zone). The American Leprosy Mission, 1 ALM Way, Greenville, SC 29601, is a nongovernmental international agency that also supplies clinical education materials in the United States.

3. Patients with leprosy who reside in the United States thus have available to them through these channels all of the resources needed for diagnosis, treatment, education, and follow-up.

Journals and Internet Sites Devoted to Leprosy

- *International Journal of Leprosy: http://www.allenpress.com/catalogue/index/lepr/index.html*

- *Leprosy Review* (British Leprosy Relief Association): *http://www.lepra.org.uk*

- American Leprosy Mission: *http://www.leprosy.org/*

- Netherlands Leprosy Relief Association (INFOLEP): *http://infolep.twinfo.nl/infolep*

Bibliography

Hastings RC (ed): Leprosy, 2nd ed. New York, Churchill Livingstone, 1994.

Leprosy. In Benenson AS (ed): Control of Communicable Disease Manual, 16th ed, pp 264–267. Washington, DC, American Public Health Association, 1995.

Pust RE, Campos-Outcalt D: Leprosy in the United States: risks, recognition, regimens, resources. Postgrad Med 1985;77:151–159.

Style A: Early diagnoses and treatment of leprosy in the US. Am Fam Physician 1995;52:172–178.

Yoder LJ, Guerra IE: Hansen's Disease: A Guide to Management in the United States. Greenville, SC, American Leprosy Mission, 1996.

264 Common Symptoms of Protozoan/Helminthic Diseases

Isaac Kleinman

1. The increase in travel and commerce between developed and undeveloped countries coupled with large-scale immigration has resulted in the importation of previously uncommon parasitic illness and increased the incidence of the familiar ones.

2. Parasitic diseases in humans are not trivial. They cause severe morbidity and economic loss worldwide and, indeed, are often lethal. An example is tinea soleum, or pork tapeworm infection, which in its trophozoite manifestation causes an estimated 50 million cases and 50,000 deaths worldwide as neurocysticercosis, which can be transmitted person to person. Moreover, the United States is currently experiencing large-scale immigration from Latin America, where this disease is endemic.

3. Malaria and amebiasis are potentially life threatening and must not be missed if suspected.

4. Some diseases, such as filariasis, paragonimiasis, and Chagas' disease, occur only after long or repeated exposure (like leprosy) and are rare in returned travelers. Many parasitic infections may not be evident for months or years after exposure.

Differential Diagnosis

The signs and symptoms of parasitic disease, except for the actual passage of a parasite, are varied and largely nonspecific; however, there are clues.

1. *History*

   a. Immigration or foreign travel (see Table 264–1). Question travelers carefully about areas visited, immunizations.

   b. Dietary habits: consumption of untreated water and undercooked food

   c. Exposures: tick bites, walking barefoot, wading, contact with sewage, contact with animals, day care

2. *Clinical findings*: Some constellations of clinical findings suggest parasitic disease. If the patient has

   a. Human immunodeficiency virus and the "wasting syndrome" (malabsorption, chronic watery diarrhea, and progressive weight-loss): cryptosporidiosis, *Isospora belli, Pneumocystis.*

   b. Fever and splenomegaly: trypanosomiasis, malaria, toxoplasmosis, acute schistosomiasis.

   c. Lymphadenopathy (submandibular and anterior cervical nodes): African trypanosomiasis (posterior cervical nodes), filariasis.

   d. Bronchopneumonia or pulmonary eosinophilic syndrome: *Strongyloides*, ascaris,

TABLE 264–1.   PROTOZOAN/HELMINTHIC DISEASES COMMON IN FOREIGN COUNTRIES

Africa	Malaria, trypanosomiasis, cutaneous leishmaniasis, intestinal parasites, schistosomiasis, filariasis, cutaneous myiasis, and tungiasis
Ethiopia	Strongyloidiasis, beef tapeworm and other intestinal parasites, *Schistosoma mansoni*, echinococcosis
Haiti	Malaria, intestinal parasites
Latin America and Mexico	Malaria, Chagas' disease, mucocutaneous and cutaneous leishmaniasis, cysticercosis, intestinal parasites, echinococcosis, cutaneous myiasis, and tungiasis
Mediterranean countries	Visceral and cutaneous leishmaniasis, intestinal parasites, echinococcosis
Middle Eastern countries	Cutaneous leishmaniasis, *Hymenolepis nana* and other intestinal parasites, echinococcosis, schistosomiasis
South Asia	Malaria, *H. nana* and other intestinal parasites, filariasis and tropical pulmonary eosinophilia
Southeast Asia	Melioidosis, malaria, liver flukes and other intestinal parasites, paragonimiasis, *Schistosoma mekongi* and *japonica*

Adapted from Wolfe MS: Diseases in immigrants. In Strickland GT (ed): Hunter's Tropical Medicine, 6th ed, pp 958–965. Philadelphia, WB Saunders Company, 1984, with permission.

hookworm, *Schistosoma*, paragonimiasis (crabs and crayfish), and echinococcus.

  e. Neurologic symptoms and fever: neurocysticercosis.

  f. Hepatic lesions or tenderness and fever (keep in mind that exposure may have occurred years before in these cases): amebiasis, echinococcus, liver fluke, biliary ascariasis.

3. *Physical findings*

  a. Myositis: Consider trichina, ascaris, hookworm, *Strongyloides, Toxocara*

  b. Diarrhea, flatulence: Consider protozoa, *Giardia, Entamoeba*, cryptosporidia, helminths, hookworm, *Strongyloides*, schistosomes, *Trichuris, Trichinella*.

    (1) About 50 per cent of all travelers to underdeveloped countries have symptoms during the first 2 weeks of travel.

    (2) The pathogens are not parasitic in the vast majority of cases. Chronicity should lead to suspicion of a parasite.

  c. Fever: Consider malaria, although fever can be seen in patients with trichina, trypanosomiasis, schistosomiasis, and amebiasis (liver abscess). High fever lasting for weeks suggests Chagas' disease.

  d. Abdominal pain: Suspect amebiasis (liver abscess), especially if the alkaline phosphatase is elevated.

  e. Headache or change in mental status: Consider malaria, but helminths and angiostrongylosis can also cause meningitis and encephalitis.

  f. Pneumonia and pulmonary eosinophilic syndrome: acute schistosomiasis, ascaris and hookworm migratory phases (ascaris and hookworm eggs are absent in stool at the time of this stage), *Strongyloides*, and paragonimiasis (crabs and crayfish) (see Table 264–2).

  g. Jaundice: malaria, drugs, cholangitis secondary to parasites in the biliary tree (liver flukes, ascaris).

  h. Skin lesions: cutaneous larva migrans ("creeping eruption"), cutaneous leishmaniasis, chronic ulcers (incubation period is several months), cutaneous myiasis (fly maggots).

4. *Laboratory findings*

  a. Hypochromic microcytic anemia: hookworm, *Ancylostoma duodenale, Necator americanus*

  b. Macrocytic anemia: Consider *Diphyllobothrium latum* (fish tapeworm).

TABLE 264–2. PULMONARY SYNDROMES

Loeffler's syndrome	Patchy migratory infiltrates, resolving over weeks; seen with helminthic parasites, especially ascaris
Chronic eosinophilic pneumonia	Dense peripheral infiltrates, fever; progressive; blood eosinophilia may be absent; acute presentation diagnosed by bronchoalveolar lavage; steroid responsive
Tropical pulmonary eosinophilia	Miliary lesions and fibrosis; heightened immune response causing one form of lymphatic filariasis; increased immunoglobulin E and antifilarial antibodies.

Modified from Weller PF: Eosinophilia in travelers. Med Clin North Am 1992;76:1423, with permission.

  c. Hemolytic anemia: malaria.

  d. Bone marrow infiltration: Chagas' disease.

  e. Eosinophilia: *Strongyloides*, cysticercosis, echinococcus, filaria, flukes, and certain drugs (see Table 264–3).

PEARL

The watchword in parasitic disease is persistence or chronicity. A sore that does not heal ought to make you think of parasitic infestation just as quickly as cancer.

---

5. Laboratory tests

  a. Tests to consider

    (1) Stool analysis

    (2) Duodenal drainage, string test

    (3) Serology: Available for a number of parasitic infections, including *Giardia*, filariasis, and amebiasis.

    (4) Rectal aspiration and mucosal biopsy (especially amebiasis and *Schistosoma*).

    (5) Lumbar puncture

TABLE 264–3. DRUGS PRODUCING EOSINOPHILIA

Semisynthetic penicillin, cephalosporin
Nitrofurantoin, sulfas, nonsteroidal anti-inflammatory agents
Dantrolene
Semisynthetic penicillin, tetracyclines
Allopurinol, phenytoin
Aspirin
β-Blockers
L-Tryptophan contaminant
Ampicillin, penicillins, cephalosporin

Adapted from Weller PF: Eosinophilia in travelers. Med Clin North Am 1992;76:1422, with permission.

(6) National Institutes of Health (NIH) smears

(7) Bone marrow aspiration (rarely required)

b. Laboratory tests are discussed in more detail under specific diagnoses elsewhere in this volume. Nevertheless, some comments are in order.

(1) The stool examination is the most important and frequently done test for parasitic disease.

(a) Formed stools should be examined and specimens of small portions taken both from the interior and from the surface to examine for *Schistosoma mansoni* organisms.

(b) The patient should have no barium, bismuth, mineral oil, antimicrobials, antacids, or stool softeners prior to testing.

(c) After the formed stools are obtained, give a saline cathartic such as Fleet Phospho-Soda or 15 gm of sodium sulfate to obtain three liquid stools. Enemas cannot be used because the ameba organism does not frequent the lower bowel.

(d) Take the liquid stool, tease out the mucus, and stain it in the usual manner.

(e) Stool specimens should be put in PVA preservative or refrigerated promptly after being obtained. Cysts of the ameba will last 14 to 20 days at 5° C but only 2 to 5 hours at 37° C.

(f) With one specimen you will find a positive stool in less than 50 per cent of known infested patients; the number of positives increases with the number of stools examined (usually requires three to six stools). Concentration should be employed on the stools as well.

(2) The NIH test (cellophane tape test) is best done in the perianal region within an hour of arising. Best results are obtained if the anal and perianal area is washed the night before to remove microscopic stool fragments and snug underpants are put on.

(3) In spinal fluid, eosinophils may be mistaken for neutrophils unless Wright's or Giemsa's stain is requested.

Treatment

Treatment is covered under specific diseases elsewhere in the text. In general, keep in mind the following points:

1. Acquired immunity in parasitic diseases is poor, as one might expect in the case of any successful parasite. Because of their low antigenicity, a number of protozoal diseases (malaria, toxoplasmosis, trypanosomiasis, Chagas' disease) and helminths (echinococcus, *Tenia*, *Strongyloides*, *Schistosoma*) may persist for a lifetime. Consequently, no vaccines are available.

2. Some treatment is surgical, such as the drainage of amebic hepatic abscess and the extraction of fly larvae from the skin in myiasis.

3. Mild diarrhea lasting more than 10 days in a returning traveler may first be treated empirically for *Giardia* before an extensive laboratory work-up is begun.

4. If diarrhea is large in volume, or there is weight loss or passage of blood or mucus, a complete work-up is indicated.

Preventive Measures

1. Maintain good personal hygiene. Keep fingers out of the mouth and wash hands frequently.

2. Wear shoes; avoid wading in fresh water.

3. Eat only well-cooked food and drink only properly treated water.

4. Maintain good nutrition.

5. Encourage and support good public health measures, including "pooper-scooper" laws to keep streets and yards free of animal droppings and vigorous enforcement of restaurant cleanliness laws.

6. Avoid insect exposure and take prophylactic measures where needed (malaria).

PEARLS

- Chronicity is the hallmark of parasitic infection.

- Fever in a traveler returning from a malarial area is due to malaria until proven otherwise.

- In comatose patients who have a travel history, do malarial smears.

- Request Giemsa's or Wright's stain on spinal fluid smears in suspected cases of parasitic central nervous system disease.

- With a sore that does not heal, think of parasitic infestation just as quickly as cancer.

- Remember, the most important public health measure ever devised is cooking of food.

Bibliography

Chappell CL, Okhytsen PC, Sterling CR, et al: Infectivity of Cryptosporidium parvum in healthy adults with pre-existing anti-C. parvum serum immunoglobulin G. Am J Trop Med Hyg 1999;60:157–164.

Christensen HA, de Vasquez AM, Petersen JL: Short report epidemiological studies on cutaneous leishmaniasis in eastern Panama. Am J Trop Med Hyg 1999;60:54–57.

Parija SC, Karki BM: Detection of circulating antigens in amoebic liver abscess by counter-current immunoelectrophoresis. J Med Microbiol 1999;48:99–101.

Strickland GT: Hunter's Tropical Medicine, 7th ed. Philadelphia, WB Saunders Company, 1991.

Symposium on Travel Medicine. Med Clin North Am 1992;76:1261–1497.

265 Pinworms

Valerie L. Hearns

Etiology

1. Pinworm infection (enterobiasis) is caused by the intestinal parasite *Enterobius vermicularis*. With U.S. prevalence of 20 to 42 million cases, it is thought to be the most common helminthic infection of humans. Children in the 5- to 10-year age group have the greatest rate of infestation. Children under 2 years of age are rarely affected. There is no association with poverty among children.

2. Transmission is via ingestion of eggs through the following methods:
   a. Direct infection from anal and perianal area by infected fingernails and soiled night clothes
   b. Contact with viable eggs on soiled bed linen and other contaminated objects
   c. Embryonic eggs in contaminated dust
   d. Larval migration from anal muscles into the sigmoid colon and rectum—retroinfection

Symptoms

Most cases of pinworms are asymptomatic.
1. The classic symptom is pruritis ani or perineal pruritis.
2. Abdominal pain
3. Conjunctivitis
4. Emesis
5. Hives
6. Insomnia
7. Anorexia

Key Symptom

Pruritis ani

Clinical Findings

1. Typical findings
   a. Direct observation of the mobile pinworms around the anus
   b. Restlessness at night
   c. Grinding of teeth
   d. Nose picking
   e. Vaginal and urethral inflammation
   f. Weight loss

2. Unusual findings
   a. Vaginal bleeding in pregnancy
   b. Eosinophilic colitis
   c. Salpingitis
   d. Appendiceal colic
   e. Acute urinary tract infections

Key Signs

- Scratching in the perianal region
- Restlessness at night

Laboratory Tests

Diagnosis is made on the identification of adult worms or eggs. This is accomplished by the *cellophane tape test*, which is best carried out in the mornings, shortly after waking and before bathing or defecation. The buttocks are spread and a strip of cellophane tape (sticky side downward) is pressed several times against the anus and perianal area. The strip is then adhered to a microscope slide and the worms and/or eggs should easily be visualized under ×100 magnification.

Key Test

Cellophane tape test with microscopic identification of eggs or worms

Treatment

1. Once a positive diagnosis is confirmed, a number of chemotherapeutic agents can be used for treatment. Mebendazole (Vermox) in a single dose of 100 mg is the treatment of choice. Because the drug is effective against the worms only (not the eggs), the dose should be repeated after 1 week.

2. The *Medical Letter* recommends pyrantel pamoate (Antiminth), 11 mg/kg in a single dose (up to 1 gm), as the drug of choice. It is necessary to repeat in 2 weeks.

3. Treat all family members simultaneously even if asymptomatic.

Patient Education

1. Hand washing (careful hand washing and finger scrubbing)
2. Keeping fingernails clipped short.
3. Good hygiene
4. Washing of bed linen daily
5. Cleanliness of living quarters

Key Treatment

- Mebendazole, 100-mg single dose; repeat in 1 week, *or*

- Pyrantel pamoate, 11 mg/kg (up to 1 gm); repeat in 2 weeks

Bibliography

Cook GC: Enterobius vermicularis infection. Gut 1994; 35:1159–1162.

Drugs for parasitic infections. Med Lett 1998;40(1017): 1–12.

Grencis RK, Hon S, Cooper ES, et al: Enterobius, Trichuris, Capillaria, and hookworm including Ancyclostoma caninum. Gastroenterol Clin North Am 1996;25: 579–597.

Hamblin J, Connor P: Pinworms in pregnancy. J Am Board Fam Pract 1995;8:321–324.

Schnell VL, Yandell R, Van Zandt S, et al: Enterobius vermicularis salpingitis: a distant episode from precipitating appendicitis. Obstet Gynecol 1992;80(3 Part 2): 553–555.

Zoorob RJ: Appendiceal colic caused by Enterobius vermicularis. J Am Board Fam Pract 1996;9:57–59.

266 Giardiasis

Mark A. Landis

Etiology

1. *Giardia intestinalis* causes infection through its cyst form and produces disease through its motile, trophozoite form. The trophozoite attaches itself to the villi in the small intestine.

2. Animals, particularly mammals, appear to serve as a reservoir for the disease. The disease is found in temperate and tropical regions throughout the world. It may be spread through water supply, direct transmission, swimming pools, genitorectal contact, and contaminated food.

3. *Giardia* is the most common human intestinal protozoal infection. Incubation period is 1 to 2 weeks.

4. There is a high prevalence (up to 81 per cent) of *Giardia* cysts in raw water supplies in the United States. The majority of U.S. cases come from overseas travelers. Children, travelers, and the immunocompromised are most at risk.

Symptoms

1. Infestation can be asymptomatic.

2. Symptoms can include self-limited to persistent diarrhea, abdominal discomfort, nausea, flatulence, lassitude, vomiting, steatorrhea, belching, cramps, and anorexia.

3. Low-grade fever and chills may be present in the early stages.

 Key Symptoms

- Persistent diarrhea
- Flatulence
- Abdominal cramps
- Nausea

Clinical Findings

1. Clinical findings include macrocytic anemia resulting from vitamin B_{12} or folate deficiency and weight loss.

2. The stool and/or breath may have a rotten egg (hydrogen sulfide) odor.

3. Children, in particular, may show signs of intestinal malabsorption and growth retardation.

 Key Signs

- Rotten egg odor to stool and/or breath
- Weight loss
- Macrocytic anemia
- Growth retardation (children)

Laboratory Tests

1. Stool for ova and parasites (O & P): three specimens over 2 weeks. This test may miss the diagnosis 15 to 50 per cent of the time because cysts are found in the stool only intermittently.

2. Fecal antigen detection (enzyme-linked immunosorbent assay [ELISA]) has a 92 to 96 per cent sensitivity and a 95 to 100 per cent specificity.

3. String test (enterotest)

4. Duodenal aspiration or endoscopic small bowel biopsy

5. Serology has limited value because it is only positive in the presence of mucosal damage and malabsorption.

Key Tests

- Stool for O & P
- Fecal antigen detection (ELISA)

Differential Diagnosis

Differential diagnosis includes irritable bowel syndrome, *Escherichia coli* traveler's diarrhea, malabsorption, pancreatic insufficiency, human immunodeficiency virus, enteropathy, ileocecal tuberculosis, disaccharidase deficiency, tropical sprue, and nontropical sprue. Other parasitic diarrheas, such as amebic dysentery, *Salmonella*, *Campylobacter*, and *Shigella*, may also be in the differential.

Treatment

Medication

1. Metronidazole (Flagyl)
   a. Adults: 250 mg tid for 7 to 10 days
   b. Children: 15 mg/kg/day in tid dosing for 7 to 10 days
2. Furazolidone (Furoxone)
   a. Adults: 100 mg qid for 7 to 10 days
   b. Children: 6 mg/kg/day divided qid for 7 to 10 days
3. Paromomycin (Humatin, Aminosidine): Less effective but nonabsorbed so *may* be useful during *pregnancy*.
4. Not available in the United States:
   a. Quinacrine (Atabrine)
      (1) Adults: 100 mg tid for 5 to 7 days
      (2) Children: 7 mg/kg/day in tid dosing for 5 to 7 days
   b. Tinidazole
      (1) Adults: 2-gm single-dose therapy; may be less effective than longer term therapy.
      (2) Children: 50 to 75 mg/kg single dose

Diet

Avoid reinfection by eliminating ingestion of potentially contaminated food and water.

Activity

Care must be taken to avoid spread of contamination, especially in areas with poor public sanitation facilities.

Patient Education

See "Diet" and "Activity." Instruct patient on method of transmission.

Key Treatment

- Metronidazole, 250 mg tid × 7 to 10 days
- Furazolidone, 100 mg qid × 7 to 10 days

Follow-Up

As needed.

Bibliography

Babb RR: Giardiasis: taming this pervasive parasitic infection. Postgrad Med 1995;98:155–158.

Farthing MJG: Giardiasis. Gastroenterol Clin North Am 1996;25:493–511.

Juckett G: Intestinal protozoa. Am Fam Physician 1996; 53:2507–2516.

Marshall MM, Naumovitz D, Ortega Y, et al: Waterborne protozoan pathogens. Clin Microbiol Rev 1997; 10:67–85.

Zaat JOM, Mank TA, Assendelft WJ, et al: A systematic review on the treatment of giardiasis. Trop Med Int Health 1997;2:63–82.

267 Amebiasis

Myrtho Montes

Etiology

1. Epidemiology

   a. Infection caused by *Entamoeba histolytica*, a protozoan that infects approximately 10 per cent of the world's population.

   b. *Entamoeba histolytica* is most prevalent in Central and South America, the sub-Saharan regions of Africa, the Indian subcontinent, and Indonesia.

   c. There is a 5 per cent incidence of infection in developed countries; confined mostly to certain high-risk groups such as recent travelers to or immigrants from endemic areas, institutionalized populations, and sexually active male homosexuals.

   d. Recent advances in diagnostic testing have helped identify two distinct species of *Entamoeba* that are morphologically indistinguishable, *E. dispar* and *E. histolytica*.

   e. *Entamoeba histolytica* is the only disease-producing member of *Entamoeba* genus. *E. dispar*, the more prevalent species worldwide, results in an asymptomatic carrier state and does not produce a serum antibody response.

   f. The principal hosts and reservoirs of *E. histolytica* are humans.

2. Pathophysiology

   a. *Entamoeba histolytica* exist in two forms: trophozoite and cyst.

   b. Cysts are the infective form and can remain viable for weeks or months in a moist environment.

   c. Infection is acquired by ingesting cyst form from contaminated water, fruit, or vegetables, or by direct fecal-oral contact.

   d. Cysts are resistant to usual concentrations of chlorine purification, but are destroyed by iodine, acetic acid, and temperatures of 68° C and above.

   e. Ingested cysts undergo excystation in the small bowel, releasing the motile feeding form of the organism, the trophozoite.

   f. Trophozoites cause symptomatic disease by invading the colonic mucosa. They can also ascend through the venous portal system to cause hepatic disease.

   g. Anti-amebic antibodies produced during acute infection are not effective in clearing the disease. They may protect against future episodes of invasive amebiasis.

Symptoms

1. Intestinal amebiasis

   a. Asymptomatic cyst passers

   b. Acute amebic colitis: 1- to 2-week history of abdominal pain, tenesmus, frequent loose and watery stools containing blood and mucus

   c. Fulminant amebic colitis: sudden-onset bloody diarrhea, fever, diffuse abdominal pain

   d. Chronic amebic colitis: recurrent episodes of bloody diarrhea over a period of years

   e. Ameboma: asymptomatic or tender abdominal mass

2. Extraintestinal amebiasis: Symptoms may develop weeks/months after leaving endemic area.

   a. Amebic liver abscess: acute presentation—fever and right upper quadrant abdominal pain; subacute presentation—weight loss, abdominal pain, anemia; lasting more than 2 weeks

   b. Pleuropulmonary amebiasis: cough, pleuritic chest pain, and shortness of breath. Sudden onset of respiratory distress and chest pain may indicate presence of empyema.

   c. Peritoneal amebiasis: fever, abdominal pain, distended rigid abdomen

   d. Pericardial amebiasis: fever, abdominal pain progressing to chest pain and symptoms of congestive heart failure

   e. Cerebral amebiasis: sudden onset of seizures, mental status change, or focal deficit

   f. Genitourinary amebiasis: painful genital ulcers

Key Symptoms

Amebic Colitis	Amebic Liver Abscess
• Diarrhea	• Fever
• Tenesmus	• Right upper quadrant pain
• Bloody stools	• Diarrhea
• Abdominal pain	• Weight loss
• Fever	

Clinical Findings

1. Intestinal disease

    a. Asymptomatic cyst passers

    b. Acute amebic colitis: abdominal tenderness, heme-positive stools

    c. Fulminant amebic colitis (toxic megacolon): rare presentation; fever, hypotension, abdominal tenderness, and signs of peritoneal irritation. Children, pregnant women, and patients who are malnourished or on corticosteroids may be at higher risk. Mortality greater than 50 per cent; usually requires surgical intervention.

    d. Chronic amebic colitis: weight loss, abdominal tenderness

    e. Ameboma: palpable extrahepatic tender abdominal mass

2. Extraintestinal disease: Amebic liver abscess is the most common complication of invasive amebiasis. Pleuropulmonary, peritoneal, and pericardial amebiasis are all complications of amebic liver abscess.

    a. Amebic liver abscess: Tender hepatomegaly found in 50 per cent of cases; fever is common (may present as fever of unknown origin); less than 30 per cent have diarrhea.

    b. Pleuropulmonary amebiasis: Most frequent (10 to 20 per cent) complication of amebic liver abscess. Fifty per cent of cases may have pleural effusion. Hepatobronchial fistula occurs rarely.

    c. Peritoneal amebiasis: Second most frequent (2 to 5 per cent) complication of amebic liver abscess. Caused by rupture of abscess into peritoneum.

    d. Pericardial amebiasis: Most serious complication of amebic liver abscess (mortality about 70 per cent). Caused by rupture of amebic liver abscess (mostly left lobe) into pericardium.

    e. Cerebral amebiasis: Rare, onset abrupt, can progress to death quickly if untreated.

    f. Genitourinary amebiasis: Rare; rectovaginal fistula or painful genital ulcers

Key Signs

Amebic Colitis	Amebic Liver Abscess
• Heme-positive stools (100 per cent)	• Abdominal tenderness (84 to 90 per cent)
• Abdominal tenderness (12 to 80 per cent)	• Fever (85 to 90 per cent)
• Fever greater than 38° C (10 per cent)	• Hepatomegaly (30 to 50 per cent)
	• Cough (10 to 30 per cent)
	• Jaundice (6 to 10 per cent)

Laboratory Tests (See Table 267–1)

1. Microscopy: Parasite can be identified in stool or biopsy specimen.

2. Serology: Serum anti-amebic antibodies can be found in some patients with invasive intestinal amebiasis and in almost all patients with amebic liver abscess. Indirect hemagglutination tests for anti-amebic antibody are highly sensitive, remain positive for years, and cannot differentiate acute from past infection. Agar gel diffu-

TABLE 267–1. APPROACH TO DIAGNOSIS

AMEBIC COLITIS	AMEBIC LIVER ABSCESS
1. Check stool for occult blood. If negative consider other diagnoses.	1. Obtain imaging study (ultrasound, computerized tomography, or magnetic resonance imaging).
2. Obtain three fresh stool specimens for ova and parasites, including permanent trichrome stain and/or antigen detection.	2. Obtain serum anti-amebic antibody. If negative, repeat in 7 d (consider empiric treatment if suspicion high).
3. Obtain serum anti-amebic antibody.	3. If unable to make a diagnosis using clinical profile, epidemiologic data, and serology when an abscess is noted on imaging studies, consider fine-needle aspiration.
4. If 2 and 3 are negative but suspicion is still high, obtain colonoscopy with scraping and biopsy of ulcer edge.	4. Do not aspirate abscess if there is suspicion of *Echinococcus*.

sion, enzyme-linked immunosorbent assay, and counterimmunoelectrophoresis may be more useful in differentiating acute disease from previous exposure.

3. Endoscopy: Colonoscopy may be preferable to sigmoidoscopy because disease may be localized to cecum or ascending colon. Diagnostic yield from biopsy and scrapings of ulcers is high.

4. Imaging studies: Should be done on all suspected cases of amebic liver abscess. Ultrasound, computerized tomography, and magnetic resonance imaging are equally sensitive.

5. New developments: Stool antigen detection tests are described as rapid and more specific than microscopy. Serum antigen detection test may prove helpful in diagnosis of amebic liver abscess. Polymerase chain reaction and DNA probes appear promising as future diagnostic tools.

Key Tests

Amebic Colitis	Amebic Liver Abscess
• Stool microscopy (Sn 60 per cent, Sp 50 per cent)	• Stool microscopy (Sn 8 to 44 per cent)
• Serology (Sn 90 to 100 per cent, Sp 80 per cent)	• Serology (Sn 90 to 100 percent, Sp 80 per cent)
• Stool antigen (Sn 80 per cent, Sp 93 per cent)	• Serum antigen (Sn 67 per cent, Sp 92 per cent)
• Serum antigen (Sn 57 per cent, Sp 92 per cent)	• Imaging study

Abbreviations: Sn, sensitivity; Sp, specificity.

Differential Diagnosis

1. Asymptomatic cyst passers: *Entamoeba dispar* cysts

2. Amebic colitis
   a. Infectious causes: *Shigella, Campylobacter, Salmonella, Vibrio*, and invasive *E. coli*; pseudomembranous colitis; cytomegalovirus colitis
   b. Noninfectious causes: inflammatory bowel disease, ischemic colitis, and diverticulitis

3. Ameboma: colon cancer

4. Amebic liver abscess: pyogenic abscess, echinococcal cyst, and hepatocellular carcinoma

Treatment

Treat only *E. histolytica*. Metronidazole (Flagyl) is not effective against *E. histolytica* cyst. Must give an intraluminal agent after treatment with metronidazole to eradicate cyst.

Medication

1. Asymptomatic cyst passers: Treat with an intraluminal agent to prevent invasive disease and transmission.

2. Amebic colitis: Treat with metronidazole followed by an intraluminal agent.

3. Hepatic abscess/extraintestinal amebiasis: Treat with metronidazole or another tissue agent followed by an intraluminal agent.

Diet

For travelers to endemic areas, avoid contaminated foods (unpeeled fruits and vegetables), use bottled water or purify water by boiling or iodination.

Activity

No limitations

Patient Education

1. Dispose of waste properly.

2. Avoid contaminated food and water (eat only cooked foods, peel fruits, boil water or use bottled water).

3. Avoid high-risk sexual activity.

Key Treatment

Intraluminal Agents	Tissue Agents
• Paronomycin (Humatin), 500 mg PO tid ×7 days	• Metronidazole (Flagyl), 750 mg PO tid ×5 to 10 days
• Iodoquinol (Yodoxin), 650 mg PO tid ×20 days	• Metronidazole, 500 mg IV q6h ×5 to 10 days
• Diloxanide furoate (Furamide), 500 mg PO tid ×10 days*	• Tinidazole (Fasigyn), 1 gm PO bid ×3 days†
	• Ornidazole (Tiberal), 500 mg PO bid ×5 days†

*Available through Centers for Disease Control and Prevention.
†Not available in United States.

Follow-Up

1. Follow-up stool examination after treatment is essential to ensure that cysts have been eradicated.

2. There is no chemoprophylaxis available to prevent amebiasis. Initial studies toward development of a vaccine appear promising.

Bibliography

Kimura K, Stoopen M, Reeder MM, et al: Amebiasis: modern diagnostic imaging with pathological and clinical correlation. Semin Roentgenol 1997;32:250–275.

Li E, Stanley SL: Protozoa amebiasis. Gastroenterol Clin North Am 1996;25:471–492.

Petri WA: Recent advances in amebiasis. Crit Rev Clin Lab Sci 1996;33:1–37.

Ravdin JI: Amebiasis. Clin Infect Dis 1995;20:1453–1466.

Reed SL: Entamoeba histolytica and other intestinal amoebae. In Gorbach SL, Bartlett JG, Blacklow NR (eds): Infectious Diseases, 2nd ed, pp 2393–2398. Philadelphia, WB Saunders Company, 1998.

268 Tapeworm Infections

Gregory Juckett

Broad or Fish Tapeworm (*Diphyllobothrium latum*)

Life Cycle
1. Common in fish-eating mammals (including humans), which serve as the final or definitive hosts
2. Host feces must enter water, where eggs hatch into a larval *coracidium* that then may be swallowed by a freshwater crustacean or copepod (the first intermediate host).
3. The copepod, now containing a procercoid larva, is in turn swallowed by a fish (the second intermediate host), in whose flesh the organism develops as a *pleurocercoid* or *sparganum*.
4. Larger fish become infected by *pleurocercoids* of any fish they swallow.
5. When raw infected fish is consumed by humans, these larvae survive digestion and grow rapidly into segmented adults.
6. The worms have a lifespan of many years and may reach 10 meters in length.

Epidemiology
1. Especially common in Scandinavia and the Baltic region, although it is also found in the northern Midwest and Alaska as well as parts of the Orient.
2. Raw or undercooked fish transmit the infection.
3. Fish-eating carnivores act as a reservoir for eggs, as does the discharge of untreated sewage into water.

Symptoms
1. Although mild infections may be asymptomatic, anorexia, nausea, abdominal discomfort, loose stools, and weight loss may occur.
2. An interesting megaloblastic anemia resembling pernicious anemia is well known in Finland; this worm competes effectively with its host for vitamin B_{12}.

Diagnosis
1. The appearance of characteristic proglottids (worm segments) in stools or the discovery of eggs leads to the diagnosis.
2. *Diphyllobothrium latum* proglottids are known to have a central rosette-shaped, egg-filled uterus.
3. The characteristic yellow eggs are 60 to 70 μm long with an operculum at one end and a small knob at the other.

Treatment
1. One regimen is currently approved for this (and most other) tapeworms in the United States: Praziquantel (Biltricide) 5 to 10 mg/kg taken once (adults and children).
   a. Side effects: usually well tolerated but malaise, headaches, dizziness, abdominal discomfort, and urticaria may occur as the tapeworm dies.
   b. Cure is not considered complete until stool ova and parasite testing is negative for 3 months. If found, the scolex, or "head," of the tapeworm should be examined after passage to aid in species identification.
2. Niclosamide, an alternate therapy, is no longer commercially available in the United States.

Prevention
Thorough cooking of fish is the most effective method of prevention, although freezing fish for 24 to 48 hours at $-10°$ C ($14°$ F) is also satisfactory.

Sparganosis

Life Cycle
1. *Spirometra mansonoides* and other tapeworms related to *D. latum* have a very similar life cycle involving copepods, numerous secondary intermediate hosts (amphibians, reptiles, birds, and mammals), and various final hosts that are carnivores (cats, racoons, etc.).
2. If humans ingest infected copepods in their drinking water, *pleurocercoids* or *spargana* may establish themselves in this abnormal intermediate host environment.

Epidemiology
1. Sparganosis is most common in the Orient, where it is contracted through copepods in drinking water or through Asian medical practices (split frog poultices, raw snake consump-

tion) that transfer the spargana to a human host.

2. Nonproliferating and less common, but much more serious, proliferating forms of the illness are known.

Symptoms

1. Swollen, tender cutaneous lesions or pustules develop that may mimic abscesses or even cancer if located in a region such as the breast.

2. Eye infections are common in Asia from frog poultices because the *sparganae* may migrate from such infected tissue.

Diagnosis

Incision of skin lesions may reveal the living wormlike *spargana* inside, but otherwise the diagnosis is often missed.

Treatment

Surgical removal usually suffices. Praziquantel may help in severe cases.

Prevention

1. Filtered or otherwise purified drinking water is the most important measure.

2. Contact with or ingestion of raw infected flesh should also be avoided.

Pork Tapeworm (*Taenia solium*) and Cysticercosis

Life Cycle

1. *Taenia solium* is a worldwide tapeworm for which the pig is the intermediate host and the human the final or definitive host.

2. Pigs consume the eggs deposited in human feces; hexacanth larvae then hatch in the intestine and develop into bladder worms or cysticerci in host tissue.

3. Humans contract the infection by consuming inadequately cooked infected (measly) pork.

4. The worm can live in its human host 25 years or more.

Epidemiology

1. Although not as common as the beef tapeworm, the pork tapeworm is far more dangerous because human autoinfection can take place either through the fecal-oral route or, rarely, by the migration of egg-laden proglottids to the stomach.

2. In such a situation, the bladder worms develop in human tissue (cysticercosis) rather than that of the pig, often with grave consequences. Thus humans may serve as either intermediate or final hosts.

3. Pork tapeworm infection is most common in Central and South America but may be found around the world.

Symptoms

1. *Adult tapeworm*: Infection often asymptomatic but may cause vague abdominal discomfort, nausea, malaise, or weight loss.

2. *Cysticercosis*

   a. Symptoms depend on where the cysticerci locate. Most commonly, this is in subcutaneous tissue where symptoms are minimal; however, the eye, brain, muscles, and internal organs may all be involved.

   b. Blindness or sudden onset of seizures may occur from eye or brain involvement; there is even the potential for fatal allergic reactions when a cysticercus dies.

Diagnosis

1. *Adult tapeworm*

   a. Active or passive migration of a proglottid from the anus usually results in a prompt diagnosis.

   b. The pork tapeworm proglottid has 7 to 13 lateral uterine branches as opposed to 15 to 20 in the beef tapeworm, but their eggs appear identical.

2. *Cysticercosis*

   a. Often calcified cysticerci are discovered incidentally on radiographs, on which they may appear as rice grains.

   b. The parasite also may appear on other imaging studies or, in the case of the eye, with direct visualization.

   c. Serologic tests have also been developed.

Treatment

1. *Adult tapeworm*: same as *D. latum*. Purging 2 hours after treatment reduces risk of egg release.

2. *Cysticercosis*

   a. Albendazole (Albenza), 15 mg/kg/day (maximum 800 mg/day) in two doses ×8 to 30 days, repeated as necessary, for adults and children. Usual adult dose: 400 mg bid. Side effects similar to those of mebendazole.

   b. Praziquantel (Biltricide) 50 mg/kg/day in three doses ×15 days. Contraindication exists in ocular cysticercosis because destruction of the parasite in the eye (or any sensitive neurologic structure) could cause further injury. Bioavailability is increased with cimetidine.

    c. Surgical excision when possible. Asymptomatic cysticercosis may not require treatment.

Prevention

1. Thorough cooking or freezing of pork kills cysticerci, although pickling and salting do not.
2. Proper disposal of human feces prevents swine infection.
3. Human cysticercosis may be prevented by prompt treatment of the adult worm and by taking measures to avoid fecal-oral contact.

Beef Tapeworm (*Taenia saginata*)

Life Cycle

1. *Taenia saginata* is an abundant cosmopolitan tapeworm, utilizing humans as the definitive host (harboring sexual stage) and cattle or another grazing animal as the intermediate (nonsexual phase) host.
2. Eggs are passed in human feces and can remain viable on pasture land for at least 4 months.
3. After eggs are consumed by cattle, cysticerci encyst in their muscle and, in turn, infect humans if they ingest this undercooked "measly" beef.
4. This tapeworm takes 10 to 12 weeks to mature in the intestines.

Epidemiology

1. *Taenia saginata* is one of the most common tapeworms in the world, with a high prevalence in South America, Africa, and some Muslim regions.
2. Fortunately, its cysticerci do not develop in people who happen to ingest eggs, and thus it is far less dangerous than the pork tapeworm.

Symptoms

1. Usually there are no symptoms; however, vague abdominal discomfort, decreased appetite, nausea, intestinal obstruction, and weight loss are reported.
2. Surprisingly, increased hunger is not very common.
3. Some symptoms, such as headache, dizziness, skin sensitivity, and even delirium, may be caused by the absorption of this and other tapeworm's excretions.

Diagnosis

1. Proglottids with 15 to 20 lateral uterine branches are passed in the stool with the eggs, or they may actively migrate out.

2. *Taenia saginata* eggs are more likely to be detected on anal swabs.

Treatment

Same as for *D. latum*

Prevention

1. Proper disposal of human feces and the thorough cooking of beef until it is no longer pink inside is very effective.
2. Cysticerci are killed at 56° C or by freezing for 1 week.

Unilocular Hydatid Disease (*Echinococcus granulosus*)

Life Cycle

1. *Echinococcus granulosus* is a tiny (3- to 6-mm) tapeworm of dogs (the definitive host), with sheep serving as the usual intermediate host.
2. Dogs are affected by consuming sheep organs that harbor infective cysts.
3. Sylvatic echinococcosis occurs in northern Canada and involves wolves and caribou.
4. Domestic sled dogs may become infected if they have access to caribou meat.

Epidemiology

1. Humans become abnormal intermediate hosts when they ingest the eggs (which are passed in dog feces).
2. The infection is common in sheep-rearing areas worldwide, especially if there is close contact between shepherds and their dogs.
3. The hydatid cyst, as the bladder stage is called, develops slowly with numerous brood capsules forming inside, each containing several larval protoscolices.
4. In some cases, up to 20 years may pass before symptoms appear, and the fluid-filled cyst can become huge if its growth is not restricted by its location.
5. A similar tapeworm, *Taenia* (*Multiceps*) *multiceps*, follows a similar life cycle and occasionally causes a central nervous system infection in humans called coenuriasis.

Symptoms

1. As in cysticercosis, symptoms depend on cyst location; however, these cysts are much larger.
2. Hydatids can cause spontaneous fractures if they grow in bone, biliary colic if in the liver, cough or hemoptysis in the lung, and neurologic symptoms mimicking brain tumor if in the brain.

3. Cyst rupture releases proteinaceous fluid, which may cause sudden, fatal anaphylaxis. Rupture also results in the development of multiple new hydatid cysts.

Diagnosis

1. "Cannonball"-shaped cysts may be noted on radiography or other imaging studies. At times, fremitus ("hydatid thrill") may be palpated over a large cyst.
2. Eosinophilia is present in only a minority of cases.
3. In the past, Casoni's test, an intradermal hydatid protein skin test, has been utilized, but it is now being replaced by enzyme-linked immunosorbent assay and other serologic tests.

Treatment

1. Surgical excision of the cyst requires predosing with steroids to prevent anaphylaxis in the event of accidental rupture. A partial cyst aspiration with replacement by hypertonic saline to kill the contents has also been recommended before removal.
2. Albendazole, 400 mg bid ×28 days repeated as necessary (pediatric: 15 mg/kg/day ×28 days). This medication causes cyst regression and is sometimes used in conjunction with surgery.

Prevention

Avoiding dog feces, the regular worming of dogs, and preventing canine consumption of infected sheep are all key interventions.

Alveolar Hydatid Disease (*Echinococcus multilocularis*)

Life Cycle

1. This is another small tapeworm with foxes (or occasionally dogs and cats) as definitive hosts and small rodents serving as intermediate hosts.
2. When hydatids within the rodent are consumed, the carnivore develops tapeworms.
3. The cycle repeats when rodents ingest the eggs passed in fox feces.

Epidemiology

1. Human infection is uncommon but is found in trappers or sled dog owners in the far north (including several states in the northern United States).
2. In these regions, pets feeding on infected mice could pass this infection to their owners through their feces.
3. Unlike the single cysts of unilocular hydatid disease, an aggregate of tiny alveolar cysts form in the host; these may infiltrate organs and even metastasize as cancer does.

Symptoms

1. The liver is usually involved and may become honeycombed to the point of cavitation.
2. Hepatomegaly and ascites are frequent manifestations of this chronic disease.

Diagnosis

1. Liver scanning suggests and liver biopsy confirms the diagnosis.
2. Even on gross examination, the affected organ is often thought to have been ravaged by a malignancy.

Treatment

1. Surgical excision is the only reliable option, but this infection must be caught while it is still operable.
2. Albendazole or mebendazole may help as long-term systemic therapy.

Prevention

1. Avoiding close contact with foxes or other host animals is necessary; in the case of pets, regular worming.
2. Washing wild berries before eating in endemic regions is recommended in case they are contaminated by fox feces.
3. This uncommon but dangerous sylvatic infection is difficult to eradicate because of the wild fox reservoir.

Dwarf Tapeworm (*Hymenolepis* [*Vampirolepis*] *nana*) and Rat Tapeworm (*Hymenolepis diminuta*)

Life Cycle

1. *Hymenolepis nana* is a tiny cosmopolitan tapeworm of mice and rats with an optional arthropod intermediate host (larval fleas or beetles); however, unlike all other known tapeworms, no intermediate host is required, and autoinfection is common.
2. Ingested eggs hatch in the duodenum, develop into tiny cysticercoids in the villi, then emerge within a week as adults in the small intestine.
3. *Hymenolepis diminuta* is a similar parasite of domestic rats with an obligate intermediate insect host that must be consumed (usually in grain) to cause human infection.

Epidemiology

1. This very common tapeworm infection of children is contracted by fecal-oral contact with infected rodent or human feces.
2. Infected grain beetles or fleas are an alternate source of infection with *H. nana* and the only one in the case of *H. diminuta*.

Symptoms

1. Usually asymptomatic, but heavy infections may cause abdominal discomfort, dizziness, pruritus, headaches, and weakness.
2. A host immune response may occur.

Diagnosis

1. *Hymenolepis nana* has ovoid eggs measuring 30 to 47 μm containing internal polar filaments on the inner membrane.
2. *Hymenolepis diminuta* eggs are larger (60 to 86 μm) and lack polar filaments.

Treatment

Similar in both infections: praziquantel, 25 mg/kg once (adult and pediatric)

Prevention

1. Rodent control and improved grain storage reduce numbers of both tapeworms.
2. Treatment of infected individuals and proper disposal of human feces may be even more important, especially with *H. nana*.

Dog Tapeworm (*Dipylidium caninum*)

Life Cycle

1. This common tapeworm of dogs and cats is worldwide in distribution; fleas and dog lice serve as intermediate hosts.
2. Larval fleas become infected by consuming eggs from the soil. Later, as adults, these fleas transmit the infection to pets when they are eaten.

Epidemiology

Children become infected infrequently but may harbor the adult tapeworm if they accidentally swallow fleas while playing with their pets.

Symptoms

Minimal, with mild anal itching (similar to pinworm)

Diagnosis

1. Active worm segments, bearing a striking resemblance to animated cucumber seeds, may pass from the rectum and are frequently mistaken for pinworms.
2. The distinctive egg clusters are encapsulated.

Treatment

Same as for *D. latum*.

Prevention

Flea eradication is the most practical method of control.

 Bibliography

Drugs for parasitic infections. Med Lett 1998;40(1017).

Marx MB: Parasites, pets, and people. Primary Care 1991;18:153–165.

Roberts LS, Janovy J Jr: Tapeworms. In Foundations of Parasitology, 5th ed, pp 325–353. Boston, Wm. C Brown, 1996.

Schantz PM, McAuley J: Current status of food-borne parasitic zoonoses in the United States. Southeast Asian J Trop Med Public Health 1991;22(Suppl):65–71.

Tanowitz HB, Wittner M: Cestode Infections. In Strickland GT (ed): Hunter's Tropical Medicine, 7th ed, pp 831–859. Philadelphia, WB Saunders Company, 1991.

269 Ascaris and Hookworm Infection

Mark Byler

Ascaris

Etiology

1. *Ascaris lumbricoides* (roundworm)
2. Distribution is worldwide. It is endemic in southeastern United States. Over 1 billion are infected worldwide.
3. Morphology
   a. Largest intestinal nematode: adult female, 20 to 35 cm; adult male, 15 to 20 cm; "pencil" size with tapered blunt ends.
   b. Color is white, cream, or pink.
4. Life cycle and transmission
   a. It lives primarily unattached in jejunum of host, where females lay up to 200,000 eggs per day. Eggs can survive for years in shaded soil at 25° C (77° F).
   b. Infection is spread by consumption of food or drink exposed to feces-contaminated soil. Eggs hatch in the intestine; the larvae then penetrate blood or lymph vessels and pass to the lungs, perforate the alveoli, and migrate up bronchial passages to the epiglottis and down the esophagus to the small intestine, where maturation occurs. Eggs appear in the stool 2 months after ingestion.

Symptoms/Clinical Findings

Both are dependent upon the parasite load. A few ascaris usually result in no symptoms.

1. Larval stage: During larval migration pneumonitis may develop with cough, fever, pulmonary infiltrate, and eosinophilia (Löffler's syndrome).
2. Adult stage: Adult worms cause no specific pathology except to compete for available ingested food. Symptoms during the adult stage depend primarily on two criteria:
   a. The number of adult worms in relation to the size of the host will determine symptoms. If the mass of worms is large enough, intestinal lumen obstruction may occur. In one series of acute abdominal emergencies in Cape Town, South Africa, 10 to 15 per cent were due to ascaris, with children having the peak incidence.

b. Adult worms are usually confined to the jejunum but may migrate. This migration may lead to obstruction of various ducts, resulting in appendicitis, pancreatitis, cholecystitis, or jaundice. Worms may also migrate up the esophagus to the eustachian tube and paranasal sinuses, emerging from the nose or mouth.

Key Symptoms

Larval Stage	Adult Stage
• Cough	• Usually none
• Pneumonitis	• Abdominal pain if obstruction present

Key Signs

Larval Stage	Adult Stage
• Fever	• Usually none
• Pulmonary infiltrates	• Malnutrition (weight loss)
	• Intestinal obstruction

Laboratory Tests/Diagnosis

1. Definitive diagnosis can only be made by three means:
   a. Identify eggs microscopically in feces (most common means).
   b. Identify adult worm in feces, emesis, nares, or at surgery.
   c. Identify larval worm in sputum or tissue sample.
2. Eosinophilia occurs only during the larva's tissue migration, *not* during the adult stage in the jejunum.

Treatment

See treatment for hookworm.

Hookworm

Etiology

1. Two species: *Ancylostoma duodenale* and *Necator americanus*

2. Distribution: subtropics and tropics. The two species overlap in many regions.

3. Morphology

    a. Pink or white in color

    b. Adult male, 8 to 11 mm; adult female, 10 to 13 mm

4. Life cycle and transmission: almost identical for the two species.

    a. Adults attach to mucosa of small intestine, where females lay 10,000 to 30,000 eggs per day. Once eggs are released into soil, a larva is hatched within 24 to 48 hours and can survive for months in warm, moist soil.

    b. On contact with unprotected human skin, the larva penetrates the epidermis, enters the venous system, and is carried to the lungs. There it penetrates the alveoli and migrates up the bronchial tree to the esophagus and back to the small intestine. Total elimination of the parasite takes 5 to 15 years if reinfection does not occur.

Symptoms/Clinical Findings

1. Larva stage: A dermatitis known as "ground itch" or "coolie itch" may occur at the site of larva penetration of the skin. During migration through the lung, the larvae seldom produce the severe reaction that can be seen with ascaris.

2. Adult stage: Findings depend on parasite load. There are primarily two pathologic features of infection:

    a. Anemia: The severity of the anemia is proportional to the content of iron in the diet, duration of infection, and parasite load. The anemia is classically hypochromic micro-

cytic. In diets low in vitamin B_{12} or folate, the anemia may be normocytic or macrocytic.

    b. Hypoproteinemia: Protein loss is usually in excess of the red blood cell loss. Protein loss is the consequence of plasma loss from ingestion by the worm and traumatized intestinal lumen. The resulting hypoproteinemia and hypoalbuminemia can lead to edema resembling kwashiorkor in children or congestive heart failure in adults.

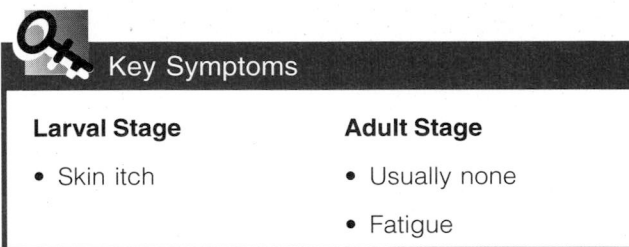

Key Symptoms

Larval Stage	Adult Stage
• Skin itch	• Usually none
	• Fatigue

Key Signs

Larval Stage	Adult Stage
• Rash in area of larval penetration	• Usually none
	• Malnutrition (weight loss)

Laboratory Tests

1. Hypochromic microcytic anemia

2. Hypoproteinemia and hypoalbuminemia

3. Eosinophilia, which is usually a mild elevation

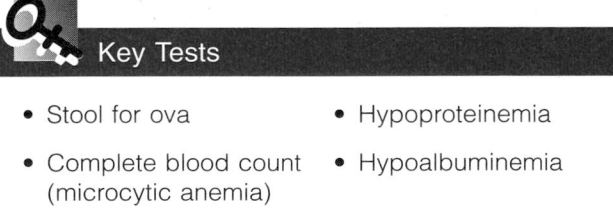

Key Tests

• Stool for ova	• Hypoproteinemia
• Complete blood count (microcytic anemia)	• Hypoalbuminemia

Diagnosis

Microscopic hookworm eggs found in the fecal sample are diagnostic.

Treatment for Ascaris and Hookworm

1. Treatment of choice is mebendazole (Vermox): pediatric and adult dosage, 100 mg bid ×3 days or 500 mg once

2. Alternative treatments

    a. Pyrantel pamoate (Antiminth): pediatric and adult dosage, 11 mg/kg once (maximum dose 1 gm)

b. Albendazole (Zentel): pediatric and adult dosage, 400 mg once

Key Treatment

Treatment of Choice	Alternative Treatment
• Mebendazole (Vermox)	• Pyrantel pamoate (Antiminth)
	• Albendazole (Zentel)

Bibliography

Drugs for parasitic infections. Med Lett Drugs Ther 1998;40(1017).

Jong EC, McMullen R: The Travel and Tropical Medicine Manual, 2nd ed. Philadelphia, WB Saunders Company, 1995.

Strickland GT (ed): Hunter's Tropical Medicine, 7th ed. Philadelphia, WB Saunders Company, 1991.

Warren S, Mahmound Adel AF (eds): Tropical and Geographical Medicine, 2nd ed. New York, McGraw-Hill, 1990.

Wilson ME: World Guide to Infections: Diseases, Distribution, Diagnosis. London, Oxford University Press, 1991.

270 Common Dermatologic Symptoms

SYMPTOM ITCHING

Terry S. Ruhl

Itching, or pruritus, is an unpleasant sensation that provokes the urge to scratch. Causes of itching range from the serious (lymphoma) to the simple (flea bites). Whatever the cause, itching can make life miserable and is worthy of careful evaluation and treatment.

Differential Diagnosis

The diagnostic possibilities for itching are daunting. Fortunately, most itching is caused by a primary dermatologic condition. The challenge is to focus on finding and treating common causes without forgetting that itching is occasionally the presenting symptom of serious systemic disease.

1. Dermatologic causes
   a. Xerosis (dry skin)
   b. Infections: dermatophytosis, folliculitis, *Candida*, varicella, human immunodeficiency virus (HIV)
   c. Infestations: scabies, lice, pinworms, other parasitic diseases
   d. Other: atopic dermatitis, contact dermatitis, urticaria, insect bites, seborrheic dermatitis, pityriasis rosea, psoriasis, stasis dermatitis, senile pruritus, dermatitis herpetiformis, lichen planus, pemphigus
2. Physical causes: sunburn, fiberglass, chemical irritants, overdrying, too-frequent bathing, pressure, low-intensity electrical stimulation, suction
3. Medication-related causes
   a. Allergy to drug
   b. Idiosyncratic drug reactions
   c. Pruritus-producing drugs: oral contraceptives and other hormones, opiates, barbiturates, aspirin, vitamin B complex, phenothiazines, tolbutamide, quinidine, and many others
4. Psychological: psychogenic itching, neurodermatitis, stress, depression
5. Pregnancy-related causes
   a. Nonspecific pruritus of pregnancy
   b. Intrahepatic cholestasis of pregnancy
   c. Pruritic urticarial papules and plaques of pregnancy (PUPPP)
6. Systemic causes
   a. Renal: uremia
   b. Obstructive biliary disease
   c. Hematologic: iron deficiency anemia, polycythemia vera, systemic mastocytosis
   d. Endocrine: hyperthyroidism, hypothyroidism, hypercalcemia, carcinoid
   e. Malignant: lymphoma, multiple myeloma, visceral malignancy
   f. Neurologic: multiple sclerosis, stroke, brain tumor or abscess, peripheral neuropathy

> Refer to Ch. 166, Lymphoma; Ch. 208, Drug Allergy; to Urticaria, elsewhere in this chapter (Ch. 257); Ch. 271, Atopic Dermatitis; Ch. 272, Seborrheic Dermatitis; Ch. 273, Contact Dermatitis; Ch. 282, Psoriasis; and Ch. 355, Insects and Spiders.

History: Key Questions to Ask

1. Where is the itching? (localized vs. generalized)
2. How severe is the itching? (interference with work, sleep, or daily activities)
3. When do you get the itching? (onset, duration, morning/night, time of year)
4. What makes the itching worse? (cold air, stress, sun, bathing, clothing)
5. What are you exposed to? (pets, allergens, soaps, irritants, medications including nonprescription, travel, occupational)
6. Is anyone else in your household itching?
7. What have you tried for the itching so far?
8. Do you have any other problems? (weight loss, fever, jaundice, fatigue, night sweats)

Clinical Findings

1. Nonspecific signs of scratching or rubbing
   a. Excoriations: linear arrays of erosions in areas within reach of fingernails
   b. Lichenification: thickening of skin with prominence of superficial markings
   c. Hyperpigmentation
2. Signs of skin disease (may be subtle)
   a. Rash suggestive of specific diagnosis
   b. Pattern of rash: localized versus generalized, fingernail-accessible
   c. Scaling, dryness, cracking: xerosis
   d. Erythema
   e. Urticaria (hives) or dermatographism (wheal after rubbing skin with blunt object)
   f. Interdigital lesions, linear or S-shaped burrows (scabies is often atypical)
   g. Lice or nits
3. Signs of underlying disease
   a. Jaundice
   b. Lymphadenopathy
   c. Thyromegaly
   d. Hepatosplenomegaly

Tests

Tests are usually not needed for the effective treatment of itching. A careful history and physical often reveal a cause. Often empiric treatment brings relief of symptoms even if the cause is not known. Tests should be reserved for those patients with significant itching, but without dermatologic disease, who have not responded to nonspecific treatment. Test selection should be guided by clinical judgment.

1. Complete blood count
2. Creatinine, blood urea nitrogen
3. Thyroid function tests
4. Calcium
5. Bilirubin
6. Urinalysis

Consider

7. Chest radiograph
8. Sedimentation rate
9. Serum protein electrophoresis
10. Liver function tests
11. Stool for occult blood
12. Electrolytes
13. Fasting glucose
14. Stool for ova and parasites
15. HIV test

Management

1. First treat any specific causes of itching (e.g., scabicides for scabies, dialysis for uremia).
2. Skin hydration measures are often the most effective treatment. Use them in addition to any other treatment selected.

Medication

1. Emollients (moisten skin)
   a. Use preparations without perfumes or additives. White petroleum jelly is effective and inexpensive.
   b. Use especially after washing and before bed.
   c. Avoid lotions and creams that may sensitize the skin
2. Creams with urea or lactic acid (hydration)
3. Camphor/menthol/phenol lotions (soothe by counterirritation)
4. Antihistamines (for histamine-related itching)
   a. Hydroxyzine (Atarax), chlorpheniramine, and other alkylamines are good choices.
   b. Nonsedating antihistamines are less effective because the sedation seems to be an important mechanism of action.
   c. Use of antihistamines for nonallergic itching is controversial and probably works through sedation.
5. Tricyclic antidepressants (histamine$_1$ blockade, sedation, and other mechanisms): Doxepin (Sinequan) is especially useful.
6. Hydrocortisone creams (use for specific indications)
7. Risks of systemic steroids must be considered if used for severe, intractable cases.
8. Specific treatments
   a. Phototherapy for itching caused by uremia
   b. Cholestyramine (Questran) for itching caused by cholestasis
9. Calamine lotion is very drying and should only be used on weeping wounds.
10. Topical anesthetics and antihistamines are often ineffective and sensitizing
11. A number of other therapies for itching have been suggested without definitive studies supporting their usefulness. Transcutaneous electrical nerve stimulation, acupuncture, EMLA cream, histamine$_2$ blockers, serotonin (5-HT$_3$) receptor antagonists, opiate antagonists, and capsaicin may eventually have a role in the treatment of itch.

Diet

1. Avoid spicy food, alcohol, hot foods, or hot liquids (vasodilatory).

2. Drink lots of fluids.

Activity

1. Use pressure with palm near pruritic area instead of scratching.
2. Apply cool washcloth or ice to area.
3. Trim fingernails short; keep them clean.
4. Hydration measures
   a. Minimize bathing, avoid hot baths.
   b. Pat dry instead of rubbing.
   c. Use bath oils (caution patients about slipping in bathtub).
   d. Use superfatted or nonalkaline soaps rather than drying soaps.
5. Avoid rough clothing (e.g., wool).
6. Double rinse clothes; add lotion to rinse cycle.
7. Change one sheet at a time to avoid static electricity.
8. Avoid the sun and sweating.

Patient Education

1. Because many of the interventions require changing longstanding habits, written instructions will help to increase compliance.
2. Increase humidity of the house.
3. Lower stress levels.
4. Have all pets evaluated for fleas and lice.

Follow-Up

1. Repeating a careful history and physical examination at follow-up visits may yield clues to the cause of the itching.

2. Consider scabies, HIV, and psychiatric causes for difficult cases.
3. Consider skin biopsy or dermatology referral.

PEARLS

- Most itching is caused by skin diseases, especially dry skin. Clues may be subtle, such as the fine scaling and cracking of xerosis (dry skin).

- If in doubt, treat dry skin. Even if it is not the cause of the itching, dry skin makes any itching worse.

- Reserve laboratory evaluation for patients who (1) have significant itching, (2) have no skin disorder, *and* (3) have not responded to empiric therapy.

Bibliography

Bernhard JD: Pruritus: Advances in treatment. Adv Dermatol 1991;6:57–71.
Denman ST: A review of pruritus. J Am Acad Dermatol 1986;14:375–392.
Fried RG: Evaluation and treatment of "psychogenic" pruritus and self-excoriation. J Am Acad Dermatol 1994;30:993–999.
Greco JG, Ende J: An office-based approach to the patient with pruritus. Hosp Pract 1992;27(5A):121–128.
Kam PCA, Tan KH: Pruritis—itching for a cause and relief? Anaesthesia 1996;51:1133–1138.

SYMPTOM URTICARIA AND ANGIOEDEMA

Constantine Saadeh

Urticaria (commonly known as hives) and angioedema are the result of a similar pathophysiologic defect: the release of histamine and other mediators.

1. Urticaria usually involves the epidermis and the upper portions of the dermis, whereas angioedema involves the deeper layers of the dermis and the subcutaneous tissue. The release of mediators leads to dilatation of the blood vessels with extravasation of fluid and edema in the interstitial region. Because urticarial lesions are superficial, the clinical appearance is that of swelling and redness, referred to as wheal and flare, respectively, whereas in angioedema the involvement is deeper; the skin may appear normal and only swelling is noted.

2. Angioedema usually occurs in association with urticaria. Approximately 20 per cent of the American population will experience at least one episode of acute urticaria during a lifetime. It usually subsides spontaneously. Acute urticarial episodes are transient and do not last more than 24 to 48 hours; chronic urticaria or angioedema occurs much less frequently, probably less than 10 per cent of cases.

Etiology and Differential Diagnosis

Urticaria and angioedema can be classified, based on the duration of the lesion, as acute or chronic. In chronic urticaria, a known etiologic agent can be identified in only about 20 per cent of cases.

1. If angioedema occurs in the absence of urticaria, suspect hereditary or, rarely, (acquired) C1 esterase inhibitor deficiency.

2. Acute urticaria usually subsides within 24 to 48 hours. The offending agent is probably an ingested substance such as a food item (peanut,

shellfish), drugs (penicillin, aspirin), or insect bite (*Hymenoptera* venom) and rarely aeroallergens.

3. Parasitic infestations can also be a cause of chronic urticaria.

4. Intravenous radiocontrast iodinated media can induce urticaria and/or anaphylaxis via direct stimulation of mast cells.

5. Recurrent acute urticaria can be induced by physical factors.

   a. Dermatographism (writing on the skin), which is probably the most common cause of physical urticaria: transient wheal and flare occurring within a few minutes of mechanical stroking of the skin. Dermatographism can be present by itself or can accompany other physical urticarial conditions listed below.

   b. Vibratory urticaria, which appears when vibration is the predominant motion, such as a shaking steering wheel.

   c. Solar urticaria is of six types and is related to sun exposure.

   d. Cold-induced urticaria is usually acquired and is noted within minutes after cold exposure.

   e. Pressure urticaria, which occurs at the site of pressure application, could be of two types: the immediate and the delayed, occurring within 5 to 10 minutes and 4 to 6 hours, respectively, following pressure application (e.g., wearing a tight belt). It is to be noted that the delayed reaction can be associated with other systemic symptoms such as fever and elevated sedimentation rate.

   f. Cholinergic urticaria is present after a hot shower or exercising in a humid environment. Typically, it appears around the neck area, and the lesions are smaller in size than the usual hives.

6. Chronic urticaria from autoimmune and malignant causes

   a. Essential mixed cryoglobulinemia (EMC) can present with urticaria, fever, elevated sedimentation rate with low complement levels (C3 and C4) and cryoglobulins.

   b. Similar urticarial rash can occur in association with other autoimmune diseases (lupus erythematosus and rheumatoid arthritis) and malignant conditions (Hodgkin's and non-Hodgkin's lymphomas).

7. If none of the above etiologies has been identified in a particular patient, the diagnosis of chronic *idiopathic* urticaria (CIU) is suspected. CIU, therefore, is defined by

   a. The absence of a known etiology of urticaria.

   b. Lesions appearing either continuously or several days during the week for at least 6 weeks.

8. Psychogenic factors and hyperthyroidism can worsen chronic urticarial lesions but by themselves cannot be the sole etiology.

   a. Histamine release could be related to immunoglobulin E (IgE)–dependent mechanism, as in food and in the physical urticarias. Direct release of histamine from the mast cell, independent of IgE, could also occur, as in the case of intravenous radio contrast dye and opiates.

   b. The activation of other mediators, as in the leukotriene pathway, could be important in aspirin-induced urticaria, although the true mechanism of this phenomenon is not fully understood.

Refer to Ch. 166, Lymphoma; Ch. 167, Hodgkin's Disease; Ch. 178, Hyperthyroidism; Ch. 208, Drug Allergy; Ch. 209, Food Allergy; Ch. 224, Systemic Lupus Erythematosus.

History

The diagnosis of urticaria/angioedema is usually obvious: the lesion is very typical, with a wheal and flare–type response in urticaria and a swelling in the normal-appearing area of the skin in angioedema. Investigation of the cause of the lesion depends on the history, such as the ingestion of certain food items, with peanuts and shellfish being the most commonly incriminated. The patient must have been eating the same type of food or have ingested the same drug earlier, based on an IgE-mediated reaction.

Physical Findings

Physical examination, such as a search for an underlying lymphoma and palpation of the thyroid gland, could identify subtle causes or exacerbating factors of urticaria/angioedema, respectively. The key findings of hereditary angioedema include

1. Attacks of angioedema of the extremities, eyelids, lips, larynx, or scrotal areas in early childhood, either spontaneously or in response to exercise or stress

2. The attacks usually last 48 to 72 hours in the absence of itching and urticaria.

Tests

1. Minimum laboratory investigation: a complete blood count to check for increased eosinophils

and anemia associated with chronic disease. Stool for ova and parasites in search for helminthic infections.

2. A urticarial eruption 5 minutes following stroking of the skin gently with a tongue depressor is characteristic of dermatographism, and placing a finger in a vortex tube with an immediate urticarial reaction suggests vibratory urticaria.

3. A positive satellite response to the subcutaneous application of methacholine is noted in one third of patients with cholinergic urticaria, whereas a giant hive appearing at the site 15 to 20 minutes following the application of ice cube is diagnostic of cold-induced urticaria.

4. Although a biopsy of an urticarial lesion is generally not necessary, there are two situations in which biopsy is helpful. In patients with EMC, lupus, and other autoimmune conditions, the biopsy will show leukocytoclastic vasculitis, whereas, in CIU, an increased number of mast cells that are degranulated and other inflammatory cells, such as T lymphocytes, macrophages, neutrophils, and eosinophils, usually in a perivascular location, is noted. An increased concentration of lymphocytes may predict poor response to antihistamines.

5. Recent data have shown that, in a subset of patients with CIU, an autoantibody directed against IgE or high-affinity IgE receptor was described. This suggests that CIU may be a form of an autoimmune process.

6. Other useful laboratory data include
   a. Erythrocyte sedimentation rate and anti–nucleic acid antibodies are elevated in EMC and lupus.
   b. Thyroid panel: CIU can be exacerbated by hyperthyroidism.
   c. Complement 4 (C4) is usually suppressed in hereditary angioedema, even between attacks, which makes this test very sensitive. If C4 is low, specific determination of a low C1 esterase inhibitor, either antigenically or functionally, will establish the diagnosis.

Management

1. Avoid the offending agent if known. Use epinephrine if a vital organ is involved, such as angioedema of the larynx. In most situations, however, the lesions will subside spontaneously within 24 to 48 hours.

2. If itching is persistent, antihistamines can be used, such as chlorpheniramine or hydroxyzine.

a. Hydroxyzine, classically, has been the drug of choice for chronic idiopathic urticaria and other forms of physical urticarias, and should be given in doses of 25 to 50 mg every 4 to 6 hours.

b. The major side effect of these antihistamines is sedation. Many patients can become tolerant to the sedative effect within a few days. For those who cannot, one can then resort to the new generation of antihistamines that are currently approved for the treatment of chronic urticaria/angioedema, including loratadine (Claritin), cetirizine (Zyrtex), and fexofendine (Allegra). Cetirizine is also effective in the management of delayed pressure urticaria.

3. In a patient with continued urticaria/angioedema despite the use of the newer antihistamines, a histamine$_2$ (H$_2$) blocker can be added: The combination of histamine$_1$ (H$_1$) and H$_2$ blockers has been shown to be effective in more than 60 per cent of the patients with this condition. Fortunately, most patients with CIU recover within weeks or months.

4. In the rare patient who continues to have problems despite the use of H$_1$ and H$_2$ blockers, referral to an allergist is necessary to try other agents, many of which are considered experimental, such as colchicine, dapsone, and methotrexate. Oral or parenteral steroids are usually effective but should be only used on a short-term basis (1 to 2 weeks) in resistant patients.

PEARLS

- Food is the most common cause of acute urticaria.

- Urticaria for more than 6 weeks with no known etiology is labeled chronic idiopathic urticaria.

- Hyperthyroidism can make chronic urticaria worse but is not a cause.

- Tonsillitis or cholecystitis are not causes of urticaria.

- Addition of an H$_2$ blocker to an H$_1$ blocker can induce remission in 60 to 80 per cent of patients with CIU.

- Hereditary angioedema does not itch and is not associated with urticaria.

- Eosinophilia with chronic urticaria suggests parasitic infestation.

Bibliography

Charlesworth EN: Urticaria and angioedema: a clinical spectrum. Ann Allergy Asthma Immunol 1996;76: 484–495; quiz 495–499.

Fox RW: Update on urticaria and angioedema (hives). Allergy Proc 1995;16:289–292.

Kaplan AP: Urticaria and angioedema. In Frank MM, Austin KF, Claman HN, et al (eds): Samter's Immunological Diseases, 5th ed, pp 1329–1343. Boston, Little, Brown, 1995.

Mahmood T: Physical urticarias. Am Fam Physician 1994;49:1411–1414.

Zuraw BL: Urticaria, angioedema, and autoimmunity. Clin Lab Med 1997;17:559–569.

SYMPTOM DRY SKIN

Anne Cawley

1. Dry skin (xerosis/asteatosis) is a problem that affects many people. Its pathophysiology remains unclear. The outermost layer of skin, the stratum corneum, consists of cells and intercellular lipids greater than 50 per cent of which are ceramides. Together these elements hold water in the skin. Skin lacking this hydration is dry. Aging skin is thought to contain fewer ceramides and so typically is drier than young skin.

2. Other factors that contribute to dry skin are

   a. General dehydration

   b. Exposure to sun

   c. Humidity less than 30 per cent (xerosis is uncommon at humidities >60 per cent); increased incidence of xerosis occurs in winter with its colder, drier ambient air and heated, drier indoor environs.

   d. Use of irritant soaps and detergents that disrupt the protective lipid barrier of the stratum corneum and increase water loss

Differential Diagnosis

1. Dermatologic

   a. Eczema—atopic, nummular

   b. Icthyosis vulgaris

2. Systemic conditions

   a. Hypothyroidism, human immunodeficiency virus infection, chronic renal failure/hepatic disease

   b. Occasionally underlying malignancies (e.g., leukemia, lymphoma), diabetes

   c. More rarely hypovitaminosis A

   d. Medications (e.g., fluconazole [Diflucan])

History: Key Questions to Ask

1. Is there a history of skin disease?

2. Behavioral aspects: bathing habits, use of moisturizers, exposure to heat and cold both inside and outside?

3. General health: symptoms or history suggestive of relevant systemic disease?

Clinical Findings

1. Common, mild

   a. Looks dry and scaly; feels rough

   b. Patient complains of itch.

   c. Loss of elasticity

   d. Erythema/accentuated skin creases

2. Chronic, severe: eczema and fissuring

3. Sites

   a. Usually extremities, especially anterior lower legs

   b. Trunk, hands, face

Diagnostic Tests

There are no specific diagnostic tests. Xerosis is a clinical diagnosis with the hallmarks of scaling and itching.

Management

Medication

1. Moisturizers/lubricants

   a. Enhance skin hydration. They hold added water in the skin and slow its evaporation. They also form a barrier, which slows water loss from the stratum corneum, enhances its elasticity, and prevents further irritation. They are best applied immediately after bathing when they can retain water absorbed through the skin from soaking.

   b. Various emollient forms

      (1) Ointments are mixtures of water in oil (e.g., petrolatum, Aquaphor, Lachydrin). They are occlusive and therefore very effective, but also very greasy and so variably tolerated by patients. Best used in acute or severe xerosis/asteatotic eczema.

      (2) Creams are mixtures of oil in water (e.g, Eucerin, Moisturel). They spread easily and are less greasy.

      (3) Lotions are mixtures of powder crystals dissolved in water and then held in suspension by surface-active agents (e.g., Lubriderm, KeriLotion).

(4) Creams and lotions are ideal for prevention of dry skin and treatment of mild conditions.

c. Various emollient ingredients

(1) Urea/lactic acid: Both serve as hydrating agents and should be used regularly, particularly during winter months. Lactic acid is available over the counter as 5% concentration and by prescription as 12%.

(2) Mineral oils, lanolin, and glycerin: Avoid lanolin in patients whose condition is exacerbated by contact with wool. Oils are helpful when added to bath water but will make the tub slippery, so are not recommended for elderly patients.

2. Topical steroids

a. Helpful in severe cases where eczema has developed and there is fissuring of the skin.

b. Best results if used in conjunction with an occlusive agent.

3. Oral antihistamines are occasionally helpful in the short term to relieve the symptom of itch and prevent further irritation or superinfection through scratching.

4. Oral antibiotics should be given to treat infection if it is present. Again, only necessary in cases where eczema has developed (e.g., dicloxacillin, erythromycin).

Diet

Diet has no exacerbating or relieving effects on xerosis.

Activity

1. Brief, tepid baths or showers serve to superhydrate the skin. Follow with patting dry rather than toweling and apply an emollient immediately to hold the added water. Do not bathe more than once a day. Use "mild" superfatted soaps and cleansers (e.g., Dove, Cetaphil) and *only* for the axillae, perineum, and feet.

2. Choose 100 per cent cotton clothing/linen thoroughly rinsed of detergents.

Patient Education

This should be aimed at preventing the occurrence of dry skin in the first instance as well as at managing the condition once it arises.

1. Short, tepid baths/showers no more than once daily—ideally every other day.

2. *All* soaps are drying to the skin. Limit their use to armpits and groin.

3. Regular use of moisturizers (i.e., at least daily) and always immediately after bathing.

4. Avoid woolen clothing next to the skin. Wool will not exacerbate xerosis but may cause itch.

5. Humid environment is helpful. Adjust heating to the lowest comfortable temperature. Consider humidifiers.

PEARLS

• Crisco (shortening): A cheap and effective emollient ointment

• Humidifier: The cheapest and quite effective model is a pot full of water by the heating outlet.

B ## Bibliography

Engelke M, Jensen J-M, Ekanayake-Mudiyanselage S, et al: Effects of xerosis and ageing on epidermal proliferation and differentiation. Br J Dermatol 1997;137:219–225.

Hardy MA: What can you do about your patient's dry skin? J Gerontol Nurs 1996;22(5):10–18.

Kumi J, Yuko H, Yutaka T, et al: Analysis of beta-glucocerebrosidase and ceramidase activities in atopic and aged dry skin. Acta Derm Venereol (Stockh) 1994;74:337–340.

Loden M: Biophysical properties of dry atopic and normal skin with special reference to effects of skin care products. Acta Derm Venereol Suppl 1995;192:1–48.

Shellow VR: Disturbances of skin hydration: dry skin and excessive sweating. In Goroll AH, May LA, Mulley AG (eds): Primary Care Medicine: Office Evaluation and Management of the Adult Patient, 3rd ed, pp 903–904. Philadelphia, JB Lippincott Company, 1995.

SYMPTOM **PURPURA**   *John J. Coon*

Purpura is a symptom noted in the skin and mucous membranes resulting from a number of different causes. The appearance is that of hemorrhagic spots of various sizes and shapes that characteristically do not blanch, as do telangiectasias, and may leave postinflammatory hyperpigmentation. Terms also used to describe these lesions include petechiae and ecchymoses. The disorder may be most readily divided into palpable and nonpalpable categories, although age and other factors may help in the differential diagnosis.

Differential Diagnosis

1. By age

a. Neonatal
  (1) Extramedullary erythropoiesis (blueberry muffin baby)
  (2) Coagulation defects
    (a) Protein C and S deficiency
    (b) Hemorrhagic disease of the newborn
    (c) Hereditary clotting deficiencies
  (3) Platelet abnormalities
    (a) Immune platelet destruction
      (i) Maternal autoimmune thrombocytopenia
      (ii) Drug-related immune thrombocytopenia
    (b) Primary platelet production/function defects
      (i) Wiscott-Aldrich syndrome
      (ii) Fanconi's anemia
      (iii) Congenital amegakaryocytic thrombocytopenia
      (iv) Other hereditary thrombocytopenias
    (c) Kasabach-Merritt syndrome
  (4) Infections
    (a) Congenital: toxoplasmosis, other (congenital syphilis and viruses), rubella, cytomegalovirus, and herpes simplex virus (TORCH)
    (b) Sepsis
    (c) Human immunodeficiency virus (HIV)
    (d) Parvovirus B19
  (5) Trauma
b. Children
  (1) Henoch-Schönlein (H-S) purpura
  (2) Acute hemorrhagic edema
  (3) Collagen-vascular diseases and systemic vasculitis
  (4) Pigmented purpura
  (5) Infection-associated purpura
    (a) Bacterial
    (b) Viral
    (c) Fungal
    (d) Parasites
  (6) Trauma/factitial purpura
  (7) Drug eruptions
c. Older
  (1) Drug effects/side effects
  (2) Toxins and venoms
  (3) Senile/trauma
  (4) Infections

  (5) Malignancies
2. By etiology
  a. Intravascular (usually nonpalpable). Alteration in platelet formation, destruction, or function
    (1) Drugs (aspirin, methyldopa)
    (2) Idiopathic thrombocytopenic purpura, thrombotic thrombocytopenic purpura
    (3) Disseminated intravascular coagulation
    (4) Infection (especially *Neisseria, Rickettsia, Staphylococcus*)
    (5) Splenic sequestration
    (6) Radiation therapy
    (7) Myelofibrosis
    (8) Myeloproliferative disorder
  b. Vascular (usually palpable)
    (1) Inflammatory vascular causes
      (a) Cutaneous vasculitis
      (b) Purely cutaneous vasculitis (secondary to medications)
      (c) H-S purpura
      (d) Polyarteritis nodosa
      (e) Granulomatous vasculitis (Wegener's granulomatosis, etc.)
      (f) Cutaneous vasculitis associated with collagen-vascular disease (systemic lupus erythematosus [SLE], rheumatoid arthritis [RA])
      (g) Giant cell arteritis
      (h) Mixed cryoglobulinemia
    (2) Noninflammatory causes
      (a) Trauma
      (b) Subacute bacterial endocarditis
      (c) Other embolic disease
      (d) Amyloidosis
  c. Extravascular and miscellaneous (may be palpable or nonpalpable)
    (1) Corticosteroids
    (2) Toxins and venoms
    (3) Senile purpura
    (4) Scurvy
    (5) Valsalva's maneuver
    (6) Pseudopurpura (Sweet's syndrome, cherry angiomas, angiokeratoma, Kaposi's sarcoma)

History: Key Questions to Ask
1. Drug ingestion
  a. Antibiotics
  b. Nonsteroidal anti-inflammatory drugs (NSAIDs)

c. Thiazides

d. Allopurinol

e. Phenytoin

2. Sexual history

   a. Gonorrhea

   b. HIV

3. Travel history: Rocky Mountain spotted fever

4. Insecticide exposure

5. Trauma history

6. Pulmonary symptoms

   a. Hemoptysis: Consider SLE, Wegener's granulomatosis.

   b. Asthma: Consider Churg-Strauss vasculitis (allergic angiitis and granulomatosis).

7. Associated malignancies

   a. Leukemia

   b. Lymphoma

   c. Multiple myeloma

   d. Colon carcinoma

8. Infections

   a. Group A β-hemolytic streptococcus

   b. *Staphylococcus aureus*

   c. *Rickettsia*

   d. *Neisseria*

   e. *Escherichia coli*

   f. Hepatitis B virus

   g. Coxsackievirus

   h. Enterovirus

   i. Echovirus

   j. Parvovirus B19

   k. HIV

Clinical Findings

Physical Examination

1. Elevated blood pressure: renal-associated vasculitis

2. Chest examination

   a. Evidence of infiltrates or effusions

   b. Murmurs

3. Abdominal examination

   a. Tenderness, guarding

   b. Heme-positive stools

     (1) H-S purpura

     (2) Bowel vasculitis

4. Spleen and lymph nodes

   a. Enlarged with malignancy

   b. Collagen-vascular disease

5. Genitalia

   a. Discharge (with gonococcus)

   b. Testicular tenderness (polyarteritis)

6. Musculoskeletal

   a. Tender, warm joints

   b. Pain with motion

7. Integument

   a. Palpable purpura

   b. Nodules

   c. Ulcers

   d. Livedo reicularis

Diagnostic Tests

1. Laboratory

   a. Complete blood count

   b. Erythrocyte sedimentation rate

   c. Blood culture

   d. Antinuclear antibody

   e. RA factor

   f. Urinalysis

   g. Blood urea nitrogen/creatinine

   h. Vitamin B_{12}, folate levels

   i. Liver function tests

   j. Prothrombin time, partial thromboplastin time, fibrinogen, D-dimer

   k. Capillary fragility

2. Biopsy

3. Other studies

   a. Chest radiograph

   b. Electrocardiogram

   c. Serum protein electrolytes

   d. Cryoglobulins

   e. Echocardiogram

   f. Bone marrow

Management

Treatment is best tailored to the specific etiology if this can be determined.

1. Corticosteroids: prednisone, 1 to 2 mg/kg for 4 to 6 weeks, then taper off

2. Pulse therapy with dexamethasone, 40 mg/day for 4 days out of 28 for six cycles

3. Treat underlying conditions/infections.

4. Stop drugs that are causative.

5. Antihistamines (type I and II) for allergic vasculitis or urticaria

6. NSAIDs

7. Danazol (Danocrine), 200 mg qid

8. Vincristine (Oncovin), 1 to 2 mg/week IV times four to six doses

9. Colchicine, 0.6 mg tid PO times 2 months

10. Dapsone, 75 mg PO daily times 2 months;

screen for glucose-6-phosphate dehydrogenase deficiency.

11. Cyclophosphamide (Cytoxan), 150 mg/day PO up to 8 weeks; adjust to mild neutropenia.

12. Azathioprine (Imuran), 150 mg/day PO up to 3 to 6 months; adjust to mild neutropenia.

13. Interferon alfa, 3 million U subcutaneously tiw times 4 weeks

14. Intravenous immune globulin (Gamimune N), (0.5 to 1.0 g/kg) as needed to prevent mucosal bleeding

15. Vinblastine (Velban), 5 to 10 mg IV every 1 to 4 weeks

16. Cyclosporine (Sandimmune), 1.25 to 2.5 mg/kg PO bid; follow creatinine and cyclosporine levels periodically.

17. Vitamins C and K if needed

18. Splenectomy in refractory cases

Follow-Up

Careful follow-up and monitoring is needed in all cases. Balance risk of treatment with severity of the condition. Referral to hematologist recommended for refractory cases or with use of unfamiliar or more toxic agents.

Bibliography

Baselga E, Drolet BA, Esterly NB, et al: Purpura in infants and children. Dermatology 1997;37:673–705.

George JN, Woolf SH, Raskob GE, et al: Diagnosis and treatment of idiopathic thrombocytopenic purpura: ASH ITP Practice Guideline Panel. Am Fam Physician 1996;54:2437–2447.

MacMillan R: Therapy for adults with refractory chronic immune thrombocytopenic purpura. Ann Intern Med 1997;126:307–314.

Stevens G, Adelman H, Wallach PM, et al: Palpable purpura: an algorithmic approach. Am Fam Physician 1995;52:1355–1362.

SYMPTOM ALOPECIA

Arnold Goldberg

1. The emotional and financial stress generated by hair loss makes it an extremely important symptom to evaluate, treat, supply accurate information on, and correctly refer.

2. Hair growth occurs in a repeating three-stage cycle: (1) anagen (active growth), 85 to 90 per cent of scalp hairs; (2) catagen (transitional), 3 per cent of scalp hairs; (3) telogen (resting), 10 to 15 per cent of scalp hairs.

3. Hairs on the top of the scalp, beard, axillary, and pubic areas are influenced by androgen hormones. The rest of the hairs are androgen independent.

Differential Diagnosis and Clinical Findings

The causes of hair loss can most easily be classified as generalized versus localized.

1. Generalized hair loss: a diffuse uniform loss, with many hairs left in the bald areas

   a. Telogen effluvium (TE)

      (1) Sudden nonscarring loss, 3 months after insult, of no more than 50 per cent of total scalp hair, which enters the telogen phase all at once and then sheds

      (2) Hair loss lasts for about 1 to 3 months, then hair spontaneously regrows. *Chronic TE* is a variant that lasts for months or years without any seasonal fluctuations or spontaneous recovery.

      (3) Causes of TE include severe illness, physical stress, hypo- and hyperthyroidism, childbirth, acute blood loss, high fever, and medications such as lithium, angiotensin-converting enzyme inhibitors, Coumadin, heparin, and propranolol.

   b. *Anagen effluvium (AE)*: Abrupt halt and sudden loss of hair follicles in their growth phase as a result of an insult such as chemotherapy, poisoning (i.e., arsenic and thallium), or radiation therapy, with recovery after the agent is stopped.

   c. Secondary syphilis causes "moth-eaten," patchy, generalized alopecia.

   d. Alopecia totalis (total scalp) and alopecia universalis (total body) both are likely to be chronic and resistant to treatment.

2. Localized hair loss: All or most of the hair is missing from the bald areas.

   a. Androgenic alopecia (AGA) in men

      (1) Physiologic reaction induced by androgen hormones in genetically predisposed men, starting after puberty

      (2) Specific polygenic hereditary patterns are a poor basis for predicting outcomes. Do not increase a patient's anxiety, because family history is only a general indication of the future.

      (3) Androgen-sensitive follicles on top of the head have their growth phase progressively shortened and the follicles miniaturize until the hair is shed and replaced

by a fine, light hair without scalp scarring.

    (4) Hair loss occurs in well-understood patterns: frontotemporal recession accompanied by midfrontal recession, then vertex hair loss with decreasing density over the top of the scalp.

b. AGA in women

    (1) Physiologic reaction induced by androgen hormones in genetically predisposed women, accelerating after menopause

    (2) A diffuse thinning in a mosaic pattern on the vertex of the scalp. Frontal hairline is usually retained.

    (3) Physical examination reveals a normal menstrual cycle with no abnormalities.

    (4) Adrenal androgenetic female pattern alopecia: central scalp alopecia in which serum adrenal androgens (dehydroepiandrosterone sulfate [DHEAS]) are elevated.

c. Alopecia areata (AA)

    (1) Asymptomatic disease with a rapid onset of total hair loss in a sharply defined 1- to 4-cm, usually round area on the scalp that is smooth and white or may have short stubs of hair

    (2) Wave of follicles prematurely enter telogen phase, and the shaft weakens, narrows, and breaks on reaching the surface.

    (3) Immunologically mediated

    (4) Hairs on the periphery of the lesion have a narrow base and normal upper shaft —the signature "exclamation point" hair with a peribulbar lymphocytic infiltrate.

    (5) Illnesses associated with AA include thyroid disease, Addison's disease, vitiligo, systemic lupus erythematosus (SLE), ulcerative colitis, and pernicious anemia.

    (6) Stress may play a role, but there is little hard evidence to support this.

    (7) Psychologically painful, affecting social comfort and self-esteem.

    (8) For information contact the National Alopecia Areata Foundation, P.O. Box 150760, San Rafael, CA 94915-0760.

d. Hirsutism: characteristic male pattern baldness or, when in women, a central scalp regression with retention of the frontotemporal hairline

e. Trichotillomania

    (1) Manual extraction of the hair, most common in young children, adolescents, and women; a recognized psychiatric symptom

    (2) Irregular angulated borders, incomplete balding with short, broken hairs in varying lengths, randomly distributed

f. Traction alopecia: Transient hair loss related to chronic tension on the hair by hair styles or equipment

g. Scarring forms of alopecia

    (1) Alopecia cutis congenita: prominent, permanent hair loss on the vertex

    (2) Epidermal nevi: hamartomas with circumscribed alopecia on the scalp

    (3) Facial hemiatrophy (Romberg's syndrome): frontal alopecia caused by localized scleroderma

    (4) Infectious agents

        (a) Tinea capitis

            (i) Various dermatophytes cause differing presentations.

            (ii) Commonly causes a patchy alopecia and fine, dry scaling without inflammation; usually found in children.

            (iii) Another type presents with a patchy alopecia, swelling, and purulent discharge known as a kerion.

        (b) Bacterial: folliculitis

        (c) Viral: herpes zoster

        (d) Protozoan: leishmaniasis

    (5) Neoplasms such as basal cell and squamous cell carcinoma, lymphomas, and metastatic tumors

    (6) Physical or chemical irritations resulting in numerous presentations

    (7) SLE: irregular macules or plaques that scar without hair

    (8) Lichen planus: may have accompanying bulla that scar without hair

    (9) Sarcoidosis: brown or violet papules or plaques that scar devoid of hair

    (10) Scleroderma: violet or tan macules developing firm scarring plaques

    (11) Pemphigoid: subepidermal blisters that scar devoid of hair

    (12) Graham-Little syndrome: progressive scarring alopecia of scalp, axillae, pubic area

    (13) Acne keloidalis: long-term pustular eruption localized to the occiput and

posterior neck that keloids devoid of hair

History: Key Questions to Ask

1. Is this a sudden or gradual loss?
2. Was there any psychological or physical stress within the last 3 months?
3. Are there any other systemic illnesses?
4. Were there any medications or physical or chemical exposure?
5. What is the family history of hair loss?

Tests

1. Hair pluck—trichogram
   a. Grasp 50 hairs at same height with rubber-tipped needle holder and, with a quick upward motion, extract hair. Cut excess hair 1 cm from roots, place on a wet microscope slide and examine under Z10 lens after staining with DACA (4-dimethyaminocinnamaldehyde), which stains anagen hair bulbs bright red.
   b. TE has 30 to 60 per cent telogen hairs with small unpigmented terminal ovoid bulbs, whereas AE shows the presence of 100 per cent telogen hairs.
2. Clip test: Grasp 30 hairs between the thumb and forefinger and cut hair at scalp. The hairs just above the fingers are cut and the remaining hairs examined on a wet microscope slide for their hair shaft diameters.
3. Hair pull: Grasp 60 hairs 3 cm above the auricle and pull; fewer than six club hairs should be extracted. Repeat the count on the opposite side of the head and in two other areas.
4. Daily counts
   a. Count and record in separate plastic bags for 14 days hairs lost in first morning combing, including those lost during washing. Normal loss is up to 100 hairs daily and 200 to 250 hairs on the day of shampooing. If hair is shampooed daily, the counts should be less than 100.
   b. Examine the bulbs to see if they are anagen or telogen.
5. Hair growth window (used to diagnose trichotillomania): Examine a 2×2-cm^2 occluded area after 1 week. Normal growth is 2.5 mm in 1 week and 1 cm in 1 month.
6. Fungal tests
   a. Wood's lamp for *Microsporum canis* and *M. audoinii*, giving a blue-green fluorescence
   b. Fungal cultures of plucked hairs
   c. KOH preparation looking for a "sack full of marbles" within and upon the hair shaft, visible under low power
7. Scalp biopsy: used for scarring alopecia or those cases in question
8. Part width: normal to slightly widened in TE; widened in AE
9. Hormone levels: In female patients with either female or male pattern alopecia, check serum DHEA-A, total serum testosterone (T), serum prolactin level, and testosterone-estradiol binding globulin (TeBG) for the T/TeBG ratio.

Management

1. Androgenic alopecia
   a. Minoxidil (Rogaine) 2% or 5% solution applied to dry scalp twice a day. Fewer than 5 per cent of patients have dense regrowth; 30 per cent have moderate regrowth in 8 to 12 months.
      (1) Need continued use to sustain hair.
      (2) Best in younger men with small areas of partial hair loss on the vertex; unreliable results in frontal temple areas
      (3) Thought to be effective in women, but some studies have not confirmed this.
      (4) Side effects are mild irritation, allergic contact dermatitis, photoallergic dermatitis, and hypertrichosis of the face, which is due to local contamination.
   b. Antiandrogens: Spironolactone and estrogenic oral contraceptive pills are of limited use in women. They just maintain present hair and have little effect on regrowth.
   c. Androgen blockade: 5-α-reductase inhibitor, finasteride (Propecia).
      (1) Blocks the conversion of testosterone to dihydrotestosterone, decreasing the serum and tissue dihydrotestosterone that is found in increased amounts in the miniaturized follicles of balding scalp.
      (2) Dose is 1 mg orally daily.
      (3) Three double-blind, randomized, placebo-controlled studies demonstrated hair growth out to 12 months, but the medication must be taken continuously.
      (4) Women who are pregnant should not take or handle the tablets because exposure may cause hypospadias in a developing male fetus. Exposure to semen of a man taking finasteride does not pose a risk to the pregnancy.
   d. Surgical methods: hair transplants, scalp reduction, flap formation, and hair weaves
2. Alopecia areata

a. Observation: Most patients with a few small areas can be reassured that the prognosis is excellent, as regrowth usually starts in 1 to 3 months.

b. Intralesional steroids
   (1) Deliver uniformly throughout the bald area, enough to blanch.
   (2) Use triamcinolone acetamide (Kenalog), 2.5 to 10 mg/ml.
   (3) Repeat at 4-week intervals.
   (4) Best for few small areas, not for progressive disease or for longer than 2 years
   (5) Side effects are transient atrophy, follicular atrophy, and pain. There is no hard evidence that this alters the course, and hair may be shed again.

c. Topical steroids
   (1) Have not been extensively evaluated but are frequently used.
   (2) Three months of bid applications with treatment of entire scalp if disease is widespread or actively flaring
   (3) Chronic treatment may be required to maintain hair growth.
   (4) Side effects are local folliculitis, acneiform facial lesions, and reversible hypertrichosis, without any systemic symptoms.

d. Systemic steroids: for rapidly progressive or extensive AA, although active hair loss does not always cease and loss may rapidly recur

e. Anthralin
   (1) Anthralin (Drithocreme) 0.5% applied overnight to entire scalp or 1% used as a short application (20 to 60 minutes); mean response was 3 months, with cosmetic response taking up to 60 weeks to achieve.
   (2) Side effects are pruritus and local irritation, which resolve if medication is stopped and restarted using shorter application times.

f. Topical minoxidil: See under Androgenic Alopecia treatment.

g. Oral minoxidil in severe AA: shown to have only an 18 per cent cosmetic effect.

h. Other therapies used with some variable success have been oral cyclosporine, oral inosiplex, topical nitrogen mustard, thymopentin, zinc, azathioprine, imipramine, and sulfones.
   (1) Psoralen and ultraviolet A (PUVA) therapy has not been shown to be superior to other treatment.
   (2) Treatment with topical diphenylcylopropenone shows some success, although is not curative.

i. Combination therapies
   (1) Topical 5% minoxidil with topical steroids applied 30 to 60 minutes later is superior to either drug used alone.
   (2) Minoxidil 5% with anthralin 0.5% cream applied at bedtime 1 or more hours after the second minoxidil application: Efficacy for long-term effect is not firmly established.

3. Tinea capitis
   a. Griseofulvin, 7 to 10 mg/kg/day, in daily or twice-daily dosing. Examine every 3 to 4 weeks, and, if KOH preps or cultures are positive, increase to 15 mg/kg/day.
   b. Continue for 2 weeks after cultures and KOH preps become negative (usually total duration 6 to 12 weeks), and monitor alanine transaminase every 3 weeks or if side effects occur.

4. Other infections, hirsutism, and systemic illnesses should respond to their specific therapy.

 Bibliography

Fiedler V, Alaiti S: Treatment of alopecia areata. Dermatol Clin 1996;14:733–737.

Habif TP: Clinical Dermatology: A Color Guide to Diagnosis and Therapy, 3rd ed, pp 739–757. St. Louis, CV Mosby Company, 1996.

Hoffmann R, Happle R: Topical immunotherapy in alopecia areata: what, how, and why? Dermatol Clin 1996;14:739–744.

Rebora A: Telogen effluvium. Dermatology 1997;195:209–212.

Shapiro J, Price VH: Hair regrowth: therapeutic agents. Dermatol Clin 1998;16:341.

271 Atopic Dermatitis

Mitchell F. Finnie

Etiology

1. Cause is unknown.
2. Polygenic inherited tendency to dry, sensitive, pruritic skin with lowered itch threshold resulting in itch-scratch-rash cycle
3. Not an allergic condition, but possible immunologic basis

Symptoms

1. Pruritus is the sine qua non.
2. Infants demonstrate irritability, restlessness, poor sleep.
3. Seventy per cent of patients have family history of asthma, allergic rhinitis, or eczema.
4. Chronic condition of dry skin exacerbated by heat, dry air, and emotional stress

Key Symptoms

- Pruritus
- Family history of atopy
- Recurrent dry skin

Clinical Findings

1. Chronic, recurring dermatitis without unique lesions
   a. Distribution by age
      (1) Infants: face, cheeks, trunk, extensor surfaces
      (2) Children (2 to 12 years): Antecubital and popliteal fossae, neck, wrists, and ankles
      (3) Adults: Hands, face, genitalia, neck, flexural areas, and upper chest
   b. Morphology by age
      (1) Infants: scales, papulovesicules, oozing lesions
      (2) Children: inflammation, coalesced papules, lichenified areas
      (3) Adults: scales, erythema, lichenified areas

2. Secondary infections
   a. *Staphylococcus aureus*: weeping, crusted
   b. Herpes simplex (eczema herpeticum): can be life-threatening
   c. Molluscum contagiosum
   d. Dermatophytosis
3. Associated features
   a. Pigmentary changes, including pityriasis alba
   b. Extra infraorbital eyelid fold (Dennie-Morgan line)
   c. White dermatographism (white blanch after blunt stroke)
   d. Dry skin, xerosis, keratosis pilaris, ichthyosis vulgaris
   e. Facial erythema/pallor, conjunctivitis
   f. Cataracts (10 per cent), hyperlinear palms, hand dermatitis

Key Signs

- Dry skin and itching
- Erythema, inflammation
- Papules, crusting
- Typical distribution
- Scaling
- Lichenification

Laboratory Tests

1. No specific laboratory features to confirm diagnosis
2. Elevated serum immunoglobulin E and positive skin tests are common.

Differential Diagnosis

1. Consider any disorder manifested by dermatitis.
2. Differential depends on age-related presentation:
   a. Infants: irritant dermatitis, seborrhea, candidiasis
   b. Children: contact dermatitis, scabies, tinea, psoriasis, polymorphous light eruption, human immunodeficiency virus dermatitis
   c. Adults: psoriasis, lichen simplex chronicus, drug eruption, nummular eczema, contact dermatitis

3. Rare conditions of infancy
   a. Wiskott-Aldrich syndrome, ataxia-telangiectasia
   b. Phenylketonuria, acrodermatitis enteropathica
   c. Histiocytosis X (Letterer-Siwe, Hand-Schüller-Christian disease)

WARNING

Consider immunodeficiency and metabolic disorders if dermatitis appears before 2 months of age.

Treatment

1. Patients must understand natural history (chronicity) of disease.
2. Education is key to effective therapy.
   a. Avoid dry skin, irritants, and allergens.
   b. Eliminate inflammation and secondary infection.

Medication

1. Topical therapy
   a. Topical steroids for flares
      (1) Group V to VII for infants, face, skinfolds
         (a) Hydrocortisone (Hytone) 1% cream or ointment bid
         (b) Triamcinolone (Kenalog) 0.025% cream or ointment bid
      (2) Group I to IV for lichenified areas. May need occlusive therapy for 10 to 14 days.
         (a) Fluocinonide (Lidex) 0.05% cream or ointment
         (b) Mometasone (Elocon) 0.1% cream or ointment
      (3) Tar ointments (Fototar) are a safe but slow alternative.
   b. Moisturizers
      (1) Use frequently, chronically.
      (2) Petroleum jelly, Moisturel, Eucerin, Keri-Lotion
   c. Wet dressings for acute, weeping dermatitis (e.g., Burow's solution)
2. Systemic therapy
   a. Antibiotics for secondary infections
      (1) Erythromycin, 50 mg/kg/day or 250 to 500 mg qid
      (2) Dicloxacillin (Dynapen), 40 mg/kg/day or 250 to 500 mg qid
   b. Antihistamines (at bedtime) for pruritus

      (1) Hydroxyzine (Atarax), 0.5 to 1 mg/kg/dose of 10 mg/5 ml or 10 to 25 mg
      (2) Cetirizine (Zyrtec), ranitidine (Zantac)
   c. Consider phototherapy or psoralen and ultraviolet A (PUVA)
   d. Severe cases
      (1) Oral prednisone, 20 mg bid
      (2) Immunotherapy with cyclosporine or interferon

Diet
1. Dietary restrictions are controversial and usually not necessary.
2. In the rare food-sensitive child, avoid eggs, peanuts, milk, fish, soy, and wheat.

Activity
1. Avoid sweating, temperature extremes, low humidity, wool clothing.
2. Bathing: short, infrequent, tepid water; Cetaphil or mild soaps (Dove, Basis, Tone; *not* Ivory)

Patient Education
1. Control, not cure, is goal of therapy.
2. Keep skin well hydrated with moisturizers.
3. Not an allergy, but avoid known irritants and allergens, including cosmetics, detergents, fabric softeners, dust, animal dander, and tobacco smoke.
4. Not emotional disorder, but exacerbated by stress

Key Treatment

Drug of Choice	**Alternative Drugs**
• Topical steroids	• Antihistamines
Patient Education	• Antibiotics
• Skin hydration	
• Avoid drying, irritants.	
• Control environment and emotional stress.	

Follow-Up

1. Frequency of visits depends on severity of disease.
2. Maintenance therapy
   a. Mild soaps or soap substitute (Cetaphil)
   b. Moisturizer twice daily and after baths
   c. Antihistamines for itching as needed
   d. Topical steroid twice daily for 2 to 3 days for flares

3. Physician evaluation when maintenance therapy fails
4. Watch for complications and associated conditions.
   a. Asthma or hayfever will develop in 50 per cent.
   b. Secondary infections
   c. Steroid side effects, including striae and atrophy, with chronic use
5. Reassurance
   a. Infantile: Two thirds resolve by childhood.
   b. Childhood: Two thirds resolve by puberty.

Bibliography

Atopic dermatitis; eczema; non-infectious immunodeficiency disorders. In Arnold HL Jr, Odom RB, James WD (eds): Andrews' Diseases of the Skin, 8th ed, pp 68–74. Philadelphia, WB Saunders Company, 1990.

Habif TP: Clinical Dermatology: A Color Guide to Diagnosis and Therapy, 3rd ed, pp 100–121. St. Louis, CV Mosby Company, 1996.

Leung DYM, Rhodes AR, Geha RS: Atopic dermatitis. In Fitzpatrick TM, Eisen AZ, Wolff K, et al (eds): Dermatology in General Medicine, 4th ed, pp 1385–1408. New York, McGraw-Hill, 1993.

Rothe MJ, Grant-Kels JM: Atopic dermatitis: an update. J Am Acad Dermatol 1996;35:1–13.

Weston WL, Lane AT: Color Textbook of Pediatric Dermatology, pp 26–32. St. Louis, Mosby–Year Book, 1991.

272 Seborrheic Dermatitis

Gregory Bahtiarian

Etiology

1. Despite extensive investigation, the exact cause of seborrheic dermatitis (SD) is still unclear.

2. Although there are many theories as to the cause of SD, most have been thoroughly investigated without producing significant proof.

   a. Excessive sebum production

   b. Epidermal hyperproliferation

   c. Infectious

      (1) Bacterial

      (2) Yeast

3. Recently, attention has been placed on a lipophilic yeast, *Pityrosporum ovale*. The yeast seems to be more abundant in the areas affected by SD, and control of the yeast population appears to correlate with clinical improvement of the disease. More recent studies have demonstrated alterations of the cellular immune response to the *P. ovale* antigen, suggesting this as a mechanism for overcolonization.

4. There are multiple other variables that are associated with SD.

   a. Worse in the fall and winter and improves in the spring and summer

   b. Common in a variety of neurologic diseases, including Parkinson's disease, facial paralysis, and quadriplegia

   c. Appears to be worse in patients who are depressed and with increased emotional stress.

   d. Has a high frequency of occurrence in patients infected with human immunodeficiency virus, and the severity of symptoms seems to correlate with the clinical progression of acquired immunodeficiency syndrome.

   e. May be more common in alcoholics and in patients with diabetes mellitus.

   f. Appears to have a genetic predisposition.

Symptoms

1. Scaling of the involved areas is the predominant symptom.

2. Itching is usually present in varying degrees.

Key Symptoms

- Scaling lesions
- Itching

Clinical Findings

1. A common skin disorder with variable frequency and severity affecting adults and infants

   a. The average prevalence in the general population is about 2 per cent.

   b. Peak incidence is between 20 and 40 years of age.

   c. There is a male predilection.

   d. Clinical features vary with different age groups.

2. A chronic superficial inflammatory disease of the skin with recurrent exacerbations

3. Classic features include scaling lesions on an erythematous base.

   a. Lesions may be scales or crusts.

   b. White, gray-white, or yellow

   c. Dry or greasy

   d. A variety of sizes and thicknesses

   e. Initially somewhat adherent but become loose and flake with scratching

   f. Scales or crusts may coalesce to involve a large area or may be found in small patches.

4. Affects a variety of areas.

   a. Most commonly the scalp, face, and chest

   b. Affects the hair-bearing areas, including the scalp, hairline, eyebrows, beard and mustache areas, and parasternal area.

   c. Also affects the paranasal areas, nasolabial folds, glabella, eyelid margins, in and around the ears, and cheeks.

   d. Other areas are affected less frequently, including the central back, axilla, inframammary areas, umbilicus, groin, and gluteal cleft.

5. Individual areas are affected differently.

   a. SD of the scalp only causes scaling with minimal or no erythema.

b. The face, chest, and back are usually affected with scaling on an erythematous base.

c. The body creases are usually devoid of scales and just have erythema.

6. Pruritus is usually present and can be mild to moderate but may become worse with heat exposure and sweating.

7. Infantile SD is a common skin disorder of infancy.

   a. It usually occurs between 2 weeks and 4 months of life.

   b. Scales or crusts are usually greasy, thick, and yellow and may be on an erythematous base.

   c. The most commonly involved area is the scalp (cradle cap), but the forehead, eyebrows, eyelids, nasal folds, ears, neck, and intertriginous folds also may be involved.

   d. The disease may last for weeks to months but typically undergoes spontaneous remission by 1 year of age with a good prognosis.

   e. Rarely it can progress to a severe form called erythroderma desquamativum (Leiner's disease).

     (1) This is associated with diffuse inflammation of the skin with severe cracking and thickening.

     (2) The infant is usually severely ill with fever, diarrhea, and vomiting and has a poor prognosis.

8. The histopathology of SD is nondiagnositic, with nonspecific features that are similar to those of other low-grade inflammatory diseases such as psoriasis and atopic dermatitis.

Key Signs

- Loose, gray-white scales
- Erythematous base
- Involvement of the scalp, face, chest
- Pruritus

Laboratory Tests

No specific laboratory test is available or necessary.

1. Diagnosis is based on clinical features.

2. Biopsy is very rarely indicated, and would be nonspecific and therefore probably not helpful.

Differential Diagnosis

1. The differential diagnosis for SD is limited and varies depending on the extent of the disease; diagnosis made based on the distribution and type of skin lesions as compared with other skin disorders.

2. The most significant problem is to differentiate SD from psoriasis. However, certain elements unique to psoriasis usually distinguish it from SD.

3. Atopic dermatitis is also in the differential, especially with respect to infants. However, atopic dermatitis usually involves the arms and legs.

4. The malar rash commonly seen in lupus can resemble SD of the face.

5. The following skin diseases can all be included in a broad differential:

   a. Contact dermatitis

   b. Tinea versicolor

   c. Tinea corporis or capitis

   d. Pityriasis rosea

   e. Impetigo

Treatment

1. SD is a chronic disease without a cure. The treatment is directed toward reducing the exacerbations and limiting the severity.

2. A variety of treatments are available, mainly medicated shampoos and topical steroids.

3. The majority of treatments have one or more of the following activities:

   a. Cytostatic

   b. Antimycotic

   c. Anti-inflammatory

Medication

1. The mainstay of treatment involves the use of medicated shampoos that can be used on all affected areas (not just the scalp). The frequency of shampooing depends on the severity of the disease, but two times per week is the minimum. A number of shampoos are available and usually include one of the following active agents:

   a. Selenium sulfide (Selsun) 1% or 2.5% has a cytostatic as well as antimycotic effects and is a very effective treatment.

   b. Pyrithione zinc (Head & Shoulders) 1% or 2% also has cytostatic and antimycotic effects and is also very effective.

   c. Ketoconazole (Nizoral) 2% has antimycotic effects and is a newer treatment that has been shown to be very effective. Most studies show similar results when compared with selenium sulfide; however, a few studies suggest a lower relapse rate and better tolerance.

   d. Sulfur, salicylic acid, and tar derivatives are

other ingredients with differing modes of activity. Shampoos with these agents seem less effective.

2. Besides shampoos, a number of creams and lotions are available. They may be more useful in areas without hair but can be used to treat all affected areas. The most popular are the topical steroids, but ketoconazole cream is also effective.

   a. Topical steroids offer excellent treatment and can be found as creams, lotions, or solutions.

      (1) These can be applied to all affected areas one to three times per day.

      (2) The mainstay of the steroid preparations is hydrocortisone 1% cream or lotion.

      (3) The more potent steroids such as triamcinolone 0.1% or betamethasone 0.1% also can be used (except for the face) but should be reserved for more severe cases.

      (4) The risks of steroid use should always be explained to include steroid dermatitis, steroid atrophy, and steroid rebound, although these side effects are usually minimal, especially when using 1% hydrocortisone.

   b. Ketoconazole 2% cream is also very effective and can be applied two times per day to all affected areas. Topical ketoconazole is very safe with minimal side effects.

3. Treatment recommendations

   a. Selenium sulfide 2.5% shampoo two to three times per week

   b. Alternated with zinc pyrithione 2% two to three times per week

   c. Hydrocortisone 1% cream or lotion can be applied to all affected areas one to three times per day depending on the severity of the symptoms. Hydrocortisone 1% solution may be applied to the scalp one to two times per day if needed.

   d. If this regimen does not appear to be working after 1 month, then use ketoconazole 2% shampoo to be applied two times per week on all affected areas.

4. Infantile SD should be treated as follows:

   a. Remove crusts by shampooing with a mild baby shampoo two to three times per week (other medicated shampoos may be too irritating).

   b. Hydrocortisone 1% cream or lotion can be applied to the affected areas one to two times per day.

Diet and Activity

No special diet or restriction of activity

Patient Education

1. Patients need to be aware that SD is a chronic disease with exacerbations and remissions.

2. Patients should be instructed to apply shampoos to all affected areas. When treating the scalp, the shampoo needs to be left in for 3 to 5 minutes so that is can penetrate to the scalp.

3. Personal hygiene may have a small influence on SD.

   a. Patients should use a nondrying moisturizing soap.

   b. Women should avoid cosmetics.

   c. Men should shave regularly.

Key Treatment

Drugs of Choice	Alternative Drugs
• Selenium sulfide 2.5% shampoo	• Ketoconazole 2% shampoo
• Pyrithione zinc 2% shampoo	• Ketoconazole 2% cream
• Hydrocortisone 1% cream or lotion	• Other topical steroids

Follow-Up

1. Because SD is a chronic disease with recurrent exacerbations, follow-up initially should be frequent, every 1 to 2 months, to establish an individual treatment strategy. Once a therapeutic regimen is developed that is acceptable, less frequent follow-up is needed. More frequent follow-up can be arranged if severity or frequency worsen.

2. In more severe, refractory cases, consultation with a dermatologist may be necessary.

 Bibliography

Danby FW, Maddin WS, Margesson LJ, et al: A randomized, double-blind, placebo-controlled trial of ketoconazole 2% shampoo versus selenium sulfide 2.5% shampoo in the treatment of moderate to severe dandruff. J Am Acad Dermatol 1993;29:1008–1012.

Hay RJ, Graham-Brown RA: Dandruff and seborrheic dermatitis: causes and management. Clin Exp Dermatol 1997;22:3–6.

McGrath J, Murphy GM: The control of seborrheic dermatitis and dandruff by antipityrosporal drugs. Drugs 1991;41:178–184.

Rebora A, Rongioletti F: The red face: seborrheic dermatitis. Clin Dermatol 1993;11:235–242.

White JW: Localized eczematous disease. In Sams WM, Lynch PJ (eds): Principles and Practice of Dermatology, pp 403–407. New York, Churchill Livingstone, 1996.

273 Contact Dermatitis

Anne R. Lockett

Etiology

Contact dermatitis can be subdivided into allergic contact dermatitis (ACD) and irritant contact dermatitis (ICD).

1. ACD is a cell-mediated type IV delayed-type hypersensitivity reaction; therefore, sensitization is required.
    a. Antigenic substances penetrate the skin and bind to proteins in the epidermis.
    b. Langerhans' cells process the antigen and present it to T lymphocytes in regional lymph nodes.
    c. T lymphocytes start a cascade of events mediated by lymphokines, resulting in the observed inflammatory response.
    d. Common causes of ACD are
        (1) Plants (e.g., poison ivy and poison sumac)
        (2) Nickel (e.g., cheap pierced earrings and belt buckles)
        (3) Rubber (e.g., sterile gloves and shoes)
2. ICD is direct tissue damage after contact with an offending substance. No sensitization is required.
    a. The actual etiology is multifactorial, dependent on both the patient and the substance involved.
    b. Anything that alters the skin's ability to act as a barrier (e.g., age, sun damage, previous skin disease [especially atopic dermatitis], and chronic "super-hydration") makes a patient more susceptible.
    c. Concentration, duration of exposure, and temperature contribute to the "offensiveness" of a particular substance.
    d. Common causes of ICD are
        (1) "Wet work" (e.g., hairdressers and food handlers)
        (2) Strong alkalis (found in ready-mix cement)
        (3) Detergents and soaps

Symptoms

1. ACD
    a. Pruritis, stinging, burning, and pain
    b. Long latency period between exposure and eruption (24 to 48 hours)
2. ICD
    a. Minimal pruritis, burning, and pain
    b. Short latency period between exposure and eruption (minutes to hours)

Clinical Findings

1. For both ACD and ICD, clinical findings vary with the patient's susceptibility and the amount of offending substance contacting the skin.
2. Lesion is often in the shape of the object causing the reaction (e.g., necklace or shoe strap) or the distribution of the application of or exposure to the substance (e.g., lower face reacting to shaving lotion or hands reacting to a cleaning solution).
3. The cutaneous response in ICD is often indistinguishable from that of ACD:
    a. Acute lesions: erythema, edema, and vesicle formation
    b. Subacute lesions: erythema, edema, oozing, crusting, scaling
    c. Chronic lesions: thick plaques with accentuated skin lines and scaling
4. For other patients, ICD can appear as a more intense dermatitis with sharply demarcated erythema and even necrosis.

Key Signs

- Erythema
- Vesicles
- Bullae
- Scaling
- Thick plaques with accentuated skin lines
- Shape of lesion same as offending agent

Laboratory Tests

1. Standard patch testing
2. Controlled application of the suspected offending agent

Differential Diagnosis

1. Atopic dermatitis
   a. Tends to start in early childhood.
   b. Type I hypersensitivity reaction
   c. May be exacerbated by stress or change in temperature.
2. Lichen simplex chronicus
   a. Caused by repeated physical trauma, such as scratching
   b. Usually solid plaques with minimal scaling
   c. Characteristic distribution: nuchal area, scalp, lower extremity, and anogenital region
3. Nummular eczema
   a. Coin-shaped plaques comprising grouped small vesicles on an erythematous base
   b. Random distribution
4. Psoriasis
   a. May be accompanied by constitutional symptoms such as fever and arthritis.
   b. Characteristic plaques with scales. The adherent scale is silvery white and reveals bleeding points when removed (Auspitz's sign).
   c. Can have nail involvement resulting in pitting or onycholysis.
5. Seborrheic dermatitis
   a. Usually occurs in areas of high concentration of sebaceous glands (i.e., scalp, face, presternal area, and body folds).
   b. Lesions are typically white to yellowish, greasy, scaling macules and papules.
   c. Pruritis is variable.

Treatment

General Principles

1. Avoiding contact with the substance. (In the case of substance that may remain on the skin, copious irrigation to prevent further protein binding is important.)
2. If contact with the substance is unavoidable, may need protective clothing, gloves, or barrier creams.
3. Cool, wet compresses using plain water or Burow's solution

4. Steroids appropriate to severity of the reaction
   a. Topical steroids (e.g., triamcinolone cream [Aristocort] 0.1 or 0.5%) may be used for simple erythema, two to four times a day.
   b. Oral steroids such as prednisone, 20 mg bid for 6 days in widespread inflammation
   c. IM steroids (e.g., triamcinolone suspension [Kenalog], 40 mg/ml) may be used for severe, systemic reactions.
5. Symptomatic treatment may include
   a. Cool tub baths with colloidal oatmeal
   b. Oral antihistamines such as diphenhydramine (Benadryl), 25 to 50 mg orally every 4 hours as needed
6. Antibiotics for secondary infection

Specific Therapies

1. Acute
   a. Topical steroids (e.g., triamcinolone cream [Aristocort] 0.1 or 0.5%)
   b. Symptomatic treatment
2. Subacute
   a. No wet compresses because the lesions are dry
   b. Topical steroids under occlusion
   c. Lubrication with Lubriderm lotion, Nutraderm lotion, or Eucerin cream, 1 to 2 hours after application of the steroid three to four times a day
3. Chronic
   a. Potent topical steroids under occlusion for 1 to 3 weeks
   b. May consider intralesional steroid administration for resistant lesions.

Key Treatment

Treatment of Choice	Alternative Treatments
• Steroids	• Antihistamines
• Avoidance of substance	• Steroids
	• Symptomatic relief

Follow-Up

1. Lesions should be monitored for signs of secondary infection.
2. Patient should be encouraged to avoid the substance in the future.

Bibliography

Beltrani VP, Beltrani VS: Contact dermatitis. Ann Allergy Asthma Immunol 1997;78:160–173.

Goh CL: Nonoccupational contact dermatitis. Clin Dermatol 1998;16:119–127.

Leung DYM, Diaz LA, DeLeo V, et al: Allergic and immunological skin disorders. JAMA 1997;278:1914–1923.

Lushniak BD: The epidemiology of occupational contact dermatitis. Dermatol Clin 1995;13:671–680.

Shaw S: Managing contact dermatitis. Practitioner 1996; 240:16–24.

274 Miliaria

Gregory T. Soltner

Etiology

1. Miliaria is caused by blockage of sweat glands at the level of the epidermis or dermis.

2. Subtypes of miliaria are based on the depth at which the blockage occurs.

   a. *Miliaria crystallina* results from mild damage to the keratin layer of the epidermis. For example, a thermal injury such as sunburn causes keratin to slough off and clog sweat pores at the most superficial portion. When sweating occurs, the classic thin-walled vesicles are seen. Inflammation is minimal. In the newborn, miliaria crystallina may result from immature sweat glands or may be seen after phototherapy.

   b. *Miliaria rubra* (prickly heat) results from blockage in the mid to lower level of the epidermis. Sodium chloride from dried sweat and thermal injury have been implicated in the pathogenesis. It is very common in hot, humid areas and may also occur in hot, dry areas if pores are blocked by clothing. In addition, greasy topical agents may block sweat glands.

   c. *Miliaria profunda* is a rare disorder that results from a deeper blockage of sweat ducts in the lower epidermis or dermis. History will reveal prolonged heat exposure in tropical areas while performing heavy physical activity. Exhaustion and heat intolerance may be associated.

Symptoms

1. Miliaria crystallina is asymptomatic and very rarely causes clinical problems.

2. Patients with miliaria rubra have stinging, pruritic lesions mostly confined to the face, neck, and upper trunk. Symptoms are usually worse with the initiation of sweating.

3. Patients with miliaria profunda often describe lesions similar to miliaria rubra as the primary lesion. As heat exposure and physical activity continue, discrete vesicular lesions appear. There is decreased or absent sweating in the area of the lesions. Inability to sweat may lead to heat intolerance and exhaustion.

Key Symptoms

- Crystallina: none
- Rubra: stinging, itching
- Profunda: decreased sweating

Clinical Findings

1. Miliaria crystallina results in the formation of 2- to 3-mm thin-walled vesicles that are easily ruptured. Distribution is often over the face, neck, and upper trunk. The lesions have no associated erythema but may occur in areas of desquamating sunburn. It is often seen in newborn and bed-bound elderly patients.

2. Miliaria rubra is an erythematous papulovesicular rash that usually occurs over clothed (covered) skin. The lesions are pinhead-sized and spare the palms and soles.

3. When miliaria profunda does occur, it is often the result of progression from miliaria rubra. Discrete vesicular lesions occur with decreased sweating. Fever and exhaustion may occur.

Key Signs

- Crystallina: thin-walled vesicles, no erythema
- Rubra: papulovesicular lesion with surrounding erythema
- Profunda: vesicles in areas of decreased sweating, fever, fatigue (late)

Laboratory Tests

Laboratory tests are not useful in the diagnosis of the miliarias. Diagnosis is based on history and physical findings. A biopsy would demonstrate sweat gland obstruction.

Differential Diagnosis

1. Miliaria rubra can resemble folliculitis, papular urticaria, and erythema toxicum.

2. Miliaria rubra usually has less associated erythema than papular urticaria and erythema toxicum.

3. Miliaria rubra can be distinguished from folliculitis by its nonfollicular distribution.

Treatment

1. Treatment common to all forms of the miliarias includes moving to a cooler environment; application of cool compresses; wearing lightweight, loose-fitting clothing; and avoidance of greasy topical agents.
2. Afterward, natural desquamation will occur.

Medication

The stinging and itching of miliaria rubra may be relieved with the application of anhydrous lanolin or calamine lotion. Topical corticosteroids have demonstrated limited benefit.

Diet

Assess for signs of dehydration; ensure adequate hydration.

Activity

Rest, along with moving to a cooler environment, is important to decrease sweating.

Patient Education

The disorder is self-limiting once the provoking factors have been eliminated.

Key Treatment

- Cool environment
- Loose clothing
- Natural desquamation
- Anhydrous lanolin or calamine for stinging

Follow-Up

Follow up for re-evaluation if the expected resolution does not occur over several days.

Bibliography

Arnold HL Jr, Odom RB, James WD: Diseases of the Skin: Clinical Dermatology, 8th ed, pp 23–25. Philadelphia, WB Saunders Company, 1990.

Champion RH, Burton JL, Ebling FJ: Disorders of sweat glands: In Textbook of Dermatology, 5th ed, pp 1745–1762. Boston, Blackwell Scientific, 1992.

Freedberg IM, Eisen AZ, Wolff K, et al (eds): Fitzpatrick's Dermatology in General Medicine, 5th ed. New York, McGraw-Hill, 1999.

Hurwitz S: Clinical Pediatric Dermatology, 2nd ed, pp 156–159. Philadelphia, WB Saunders Company, 1993.

Kirk JF: Miliaria profunda. J Am Acad Dermatol 1996; 35:854–856.

Zitelli BJ, Davis HW: Atlas of Pediatric Physical Diagnosis, 3rd ed, St. Louis, Mosby-Wolfe, 1997.

275 Hyperhidrosis

Erik O. Gilbertson

Etiology

1. Unclear. Various hypotheses, including increased cholinergic tone, especially with respect to eccrine glands of acral skin.
2. Primary and secondary forms.
3. On occasion, strong family history.
4. Significant social, professional, and emotional consequences.

Symptoms

1. Excessive sweating, predominantly of the extremities (especially palms, soles, axillae)
2. With sudden, new and/or unilateral process, must consider an underlying central nervous system (CNS) tumor/endocrinopathy

Key Symptom

Excessive sweating

Clinical Findings

1. Copious clear sweating with or without malodor and with or without emotional stressors that trigger sweating of the palms, soles, and/or axillae.
2. Profuse sweating may also lead to maceration and subsequent secondary infection and osmidrosis.

Key Sign

Copious sweating with or without malodor

Laboratory Tests

Rule out underlying CNS process or endocrinopathy if spontaneous in appearance or unilateral.

Treatment

Essentially, directly affect sweat glands or modify their innervation.

1. Medication—topical
   a. Aluminum chloride 12% solution in anhydrous ethanol (Drysol)
      (1) Apply to completely dry skin at night; slowly increase hours of application, then use on a nightly basis (i.e., 6 to 8 hours) until acceptable control. Avoid eyes! Wash off in morning. Use twice a week as needed for maintenance.
      (2) If too irritating, may switch to the 6.25% solution or use a concomitant topical steroid initially. If lack of sufficient response after 2 to 3 weeks of nightly application, may try occlusion with sock or plastic wrap.
   b. Topical glycopyrrolate cream
2. Medication—oral
   a. Glycopyrrolate (Robinul) may work for some, but usually limiting anticholinergic side effects occur with doses required for adequate control of hyperhidrosis.
   b. Others have tried clonidine, anxiolytics, and β-blockers, especially if the sweating is situational.
3. Interventional/behavioral
   a. Iontophoresis: Special galvanic generator units for tap water immersion or direct-contact units for passage of low electrical current. Usually no prescription needed; available from Drionics Units—Underarms, Hands, and/or Feet, General Medical Company, Los Angeles, CA (phone: 1-800-432-5362).
   b. Botulinum toxin: New, limited information. Localized injections seem to block cholinergic nerve terminals with long duration of response.
   c. Behavioral/biofeedback, especially if situational/generalized anxiety or the like
4. Surgical
   a. Sympathetic blockade
   b. Excision of affected area (i.e., axillary area)
   c. Transthoracic endoscopic sympathectomy: Main risks are pneumothorax (as a result of the procedure) and compensatory hyperhidrosis. See an experienced neurosurgeon.

Key Treatment

- Aluminum chloride (Drysol)
- Glycopyrrolate (Robinul)
- Iontophoresis

Bibliography

Atkin SL, Brown PM: Treatment of diabetic gustatory sweating with topical glycopyrrolate cream. Diabetes Med 1996;13:493–494.

Berger TG: Hyperhidrosis. In Berger TG, Elias PM, Wintroub BU (eds): Manual of Therapy for Skin Diseases, pp 152–153. New York, Churchill Livingstone, 1990.

Drott C, Gothberg G, Claes G: Endoscopic thoracic sympathectomy: an efficient and safe method for the treatment of hyperhidrosis. J Am Acad Dermatol. 1995;33: 78–81.

Naumann M, Hofman U, Bergmann I, et al: Focal hyperhidrosis: effective treatment with intracutaneous botulinum toxin. Arch Dermatol 1998;134:301–304.

Shelley WB, Talanin NY, Shelley ED: Botulinum toxin therapy for palmar hyperhidrosis. J Am Acad Dermatol 1998;38(2 Pt 1):227–229.

276 Erysipelas

Joseph R. Masci

Etiology

1. Erysipelas is a specific type of superficial cellulitis accompanied by pronounced lymphedema.
2. Almost all cases are caused by group A β-hemolytic streptococci (*Streptococcus pyogenes*). Other organisms, including *Staphylococcus aureus*, other streptococci, or even gram-negative bacteria, are occasionally implicated.
3. Erysipelas is seen most commonly in young children and elderly adults. The following may be predisposing conditions:
   a. Pre-existing lymphedema secondary to lymphatic occlusion (e.g., malignancies or postoperative)
   b. Pre-existing breaks in the epidermis (e.g., xerosis, ichthyosis, fungal infections)
   c. Venous stasis

Symptoms

1. Pain and swelling in the involved area
2. Fever and chills are common.
3. Painful swelling in regional lymph nodes may be seen.

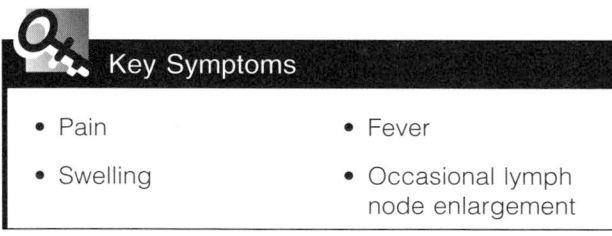

Key Symptoms

- Pain
- Swelling
- Fever
- Occasional lymph node enlargement

Clinical Findings

1. Most common sites of involvement are the face and the lower extremities.
2. Characteristic features include
   a. Erythema and lymphedema in the involved area
   b. Palpable advancing margin that may progress over hours to days. Formation of bullae may be seen. Multiple sites of involvement are unusual.
3. Systemic signs of infection are often present; these may include
   a. Fever

b. Peripheral leukocytosis
c. Lymphangitis and regional tender lymphadenopathy
d. Approximately 5 per cent of patients have positive blood cultures. Rarely, the sepsis syndrome may be seen with hypotension, systemic acidosis, and disseminated intravascular coagulation.

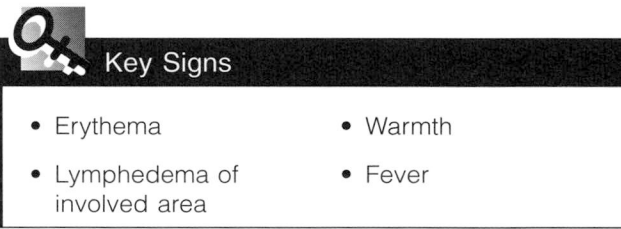

Key Signs

- Erythema
- Lymphedema of involved area
- Warmth
- Fever

Laboratory Tests

1. Culture and Gram's stain of aspirate from advancing margin of lesion if possible
2. The following blood tests should be considered in severe cases:
   a. Complete blood count
   b. Blood urea nitrogen, creatinine, electrolytes
   c. Blood cultures

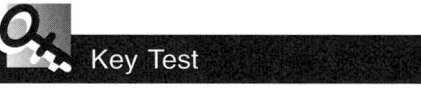

Key Test

Consider culture of aspirate of involved area in severe cases or when response to therapy is delayed.

Differential Diagnosis

1. Other bacterial soft tissue infections
2. A variety of other disorders may be confused with erysipelas; these include
   a. Seborrheic dermatitis
   b. Erythema chronicum migrans
   c. Early herpes zoster
   d. Contact dermatitis
3. Erysipelas usually may be distinguished from these disorders on the basis of the following criteria:
   a. Soft tissue infections caused by other bacte-

ria are less commonly associated with significant lymphedema and a palpable advancing margin.

  b. Other aids in diagnosis include

    (1) Fever rarely occurs in association with seborrheic dermatitis or contact dermatitis but is seen commonly with erysipelas.

    (2) Erythema chronicum migrans should be considered in persons who have recently traveled to areas endemic for Lyme disease.

    (3) Herpes zoster typically occurs in a dermatomal distribution. The appearance of grouped vesicles suggests the diagnosis of herpes zoster.

Treatment

1. Treatment consists of antibiotic therapy, which may be instituted on the basis of characteristic physical findings of erysipelas.
2. Local care and bed rest may be beneficial.

Medication

1. Penicillin is the antibiotic of choice. Oral therapy with phenoxymethyl penicillin (7.5 mg/kg four times daily for 7 to 10 days) may be sufficient for mild cases in healthy individuals. Hospitalization and parenteral therapy with penicillin G (1 to 2 million units every 4 hours) may be necessary for more severe cases or in elderly or debilitated hosts.
2. For patients allergic to penicillin, erythromycin (500 mg by mouth four times daily) is the drug of choice for oral therapy. Clindamycin (Cleocin), 600 mg intravenously every 8 hours, may be used if parenteral therapy is required.
3. Underlying skin disorders, if present, should be treated.
4. Antipyretics and cool and wet dressings as necessary for comfort

Diet

No modification in diet necessary.

Activity

1. Bed rest, elevation of involved area
2. Hospitalized patients should be placed on skin precautions.

Patient Education

1. Underlying skin disorders should be treated, if possible.
2. Recurrence of erysipelas may be seen in areas of recurrent breaks in the dermis or of lymphatic or venous occlusion.

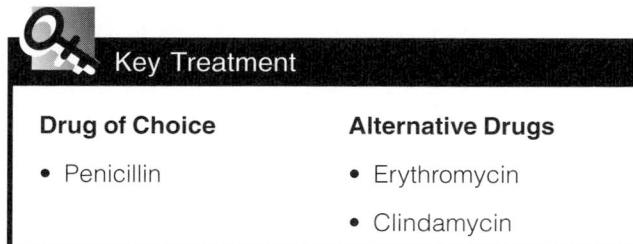

Key Treatment	
Drug of Choice	**Alternative Drugs**
• Penicillin	• Erythromycin
	• Clindamycin

Follow-Up

1. Response to therapy usually occurs within several days.
2. Patient should return if worsening or no improvement occurs within 48 hours.
3. Follow-up evaluation of underlying skin conditions, if present, including
  a. Xerosis, ichthyosis, fungal infections
  b. Venous stasis

 Bibliography

Dreizen S: The butterfly rash and the malar flush: what diseases do these signs reflect? Postgrad Med 1991;89: 225–228 and 233–234.

Eriksson B, Jorup-Tonstrom C, Karkkonen K, et al: Erysipelas: clinical and bacteriologic spectrum and serological aspects. Clin Infect Dis 1996;23:1091–1098.

Feingold DS, Hirschmann JV: Cellulitis. In Gorbach SL, Bartlett JG, Blacklow NR (eds): Infectious Diseases, pp 1072–1074. Philadelphia, WB Saunders Company, 1992.

Kahn RM, Goldstein EJ: Common bacterial skin infections: diagnostic clues and therapeutic options. Postgrad Med 1993;93:175–182.

Sjoblom AC, Bruchfeld J, Eriksson B, et al: Skin concentrations of phenoxymethylpenicillin in patients with erysipelas. Infection 1992;30:30–33.

277 Acne (Vulgaris)

Gary I. Levine

Etiology

1. Acne is an inflammatory disorder of the psilosebaceous unit.
2. Key etiologic factors
   a. Overproduction of androgens (dehydroepiandrosterone sulfate) and testosterone, generally at puberty
   b. Hyperresponsiveness of the psilosebaceous unit to androgens
   c. Hypersensitivity to the metabolic products of *Propionibacterium acnes*
3. Pathophysiology
   a. Androgens stimulate sebum production and follicle keratinocyte proliferation.
   b. Keratin plug obstructs the follicle opening, causing sebum to accumulate and distend the follicle.
   c. *Propionibacterium acnes* proliferates in the plugged follicle, metabolizes sebum into free fatty acids, produces chemotactic factors and proinflammatory mediators, and activates complement.
   d. Presence of inflammatory substances results in inflammation of the follicle and adjacent dermis.
4. Incidence/prevalence: Most commonly seen in adolescents—age 16, 80 to 90 per cent affected; age 25 to 34, 8 per cent affected; age 35 to 44, 3 per cent affected

Symptoms

1. Pain
2. Psychological distress: low self-esteem, social isolation, and depression

Key Symptoms

- Pain
- Psychological distress

Clinical Findings

1. Distribution of lesions: central forehead, nose, paranasal area and chin, upper back, and chest
2. Types of lesions

   a. Noninflammatory
      (1) Open comedones (blackheads)
      (2) Closed comedones (whiteheads)
   b. Inflammatory: papules, pustules, nodules, and cysts
   c. Excoriations (self-induced)
   d. Scars: "ice pick," atrophic, hypertrophic, and depressed

Key Signs

- Comedones
- Papules, pustules, nodules, and cysts
- Excoriations
- Scars

Laboratory Tests

1. There are no specific laboratory tests utilized in the diagnosis of acne.
2. Woman with late-onset acne (age >25) may benefit from investigation for androgen excess.
3. Females of reproductive age taking *isotretinoin* (Accutane) should have a negative pregnancy test, and all patients should have baseline lipid (triglyceride, cholesterol, high-density lipoprotein cholesterol) levels, complete blood count (CBC), and liver function tests (LFTs: aspartate transaminase, alanine transaminase) prior to beginning therapy with this agent. Pregnancy tests should ideally be done monthly; lipid levels, CBC, and LFTs every 1 to 2 weeks until stable, then every 4 to 8 weeks for the duration of therapy.

Key Tests

Closely monitor pregnancy test (females), lipids, CBC, and liver function tests in patients taking isotretinoin

Differential Diagnosis

1. Acne cosmetica
2. Acne rosacea

3. Chloracne
4. Folliculitis
5. Occupational exposure to tars, oils, and greases
6. Perioral dermatitis
7. Pseudo–folliculitis barbae
8. Steroid-induced acne

Treatment

Medication

1. Treatment regimens
   a. Comedonal (noninflammatory) acne: topical keratinolytic agent
   b. Mild inflammatory (papulopustular) acne: topical antibacterial agent
   c. Moderate inflammatory (papulopustular or nodulocystic) acne: topical retinoid once daily with a topical or systemic antibacterial agent
   d. Severe cystic acne: isotretinoin

2. Topical keratinolytics
   a. Tretinoin (Retin-A)—0.025%, 0.05%, 0.1% cream; 0.01%, 0.025% gel; 0.05% solution: Apply nightly after washing. Start with lowest concentration of cream and advance as tolerated. May cause an initial flare of lesions; side effects include erythema, dryness, scaling.
   b. Adapalene (Differin) 0.1% gel: Apply nightly after washing. Better tolerated than tretinoin and equally effective.
   c. Tazarotene (Tazorac) 0.05%, 0.1% gel: Apply nightly. Newer agent with side effects similar to those of tretinoin
   d. Azelaic acid (Azelex) 20% cream: Apply bid. Is keratinolytic, anti-inflammatory, and antibacterial.
   e. Salicylic acid: 0.5% to 2.0% hydroalcoholic

3. Topical antibacterials
   a. Benzoyl peroxide 0.25%, 5%, 10% lotion, cream, and gel: Apply thin film one to two times a day, preferably at bedtime.
   b. Benzoyl peroxide–erythromycin (Benzamycin) 5%/3% gel: Apply bid.
   c. Erythromycin (A/T/S, Emgel, Erycete, T-stat) 2% gel or solution: Apply bid.
   d. Clindamycin (Cleocin T, Dalacin T) 1% solution, lotion, gel: Apply bid.
   e. Tetracycline (Topicycline) 0.22% solution: Apply bid.

4. Systemic antibiotics
   a. Tetracycline, 500 to 1000 mg daily: Begin at high dose, and taper in 2 to 4 weeks if patient responds. Do not use in children less than 8 years old; may cause photosensitivity.
   b. Minocycline (Minocin), 50 to 200 mg daily: Most effective and expensive of tetracycline group. Less photosensitivity than tetracycline, side effects include vertigo, autoimmune hepatitis, and lupus-like syndrome.
   c. Doxycycline (Vibramycin), 50 to 200 mg daily: Can take with food, but higher incidence of photosensitivity.
   d. Erythromycin, 500 to 1000 mg daily
   e. Trimethoprim-sulfamethoxazole (Bactrim, Septra), 1 double-strength tablet once or twice daily: Used for gram-negative folliculitis or resistance to tetracycline

5. Systemic retinoids: Isotretinoin (Accutane), 0.5 to 1.0 mg/kg/day given bid
   a. Usually given for 12 to 20 weeks to a total dose around 120 mg/kg. Sixty to 90 per cent of patients achieve remission within 16 weeks; side effects include cheilitis, xerosis, arthralgias, myalgias, hyperlipidemia, and elevated liver enzymes.
   b. *Highly teratogenic*—absolutely contraindicated in pregnancy, and strict contraceptive precautions are absolutely necessary in women of childbearing age.

6. Oral contraceptives
   a. Triphasic formulation combining ethinyl estradiol with norgestimate (Tri-cyclen) is efficacious in women with acne.
   b. Norgestimate, desogestrel, and ethynodiol diacetate have low androgenic activity and are preferred progestational agents.

7. Intralesional injection of triamcinalone, 0.5 to 1.0 ml (Kenalog, 2 mg/ml) via 30-gauge needle: Used for large cystic lesions.

Diet

There is no evidence that ingesting foods such as chocolate, fatty or greasy foods, or nuts worsens acne, and there is no benefit to dietary restriction in the treatment of acne.

Activity

1. Activities that reduce stress may be beneficial.
2. Sun exposure is of questionable benefit in improving acne, and may be harmful in patients taking tetracycline derivatives.
3. Women taking isotretinoin should not engage in unprotected sex (two forms of effective contraception are recommended).

Patient Education

1. Acne is a common chronic illness of adolescents that can be controlled with medication in most

individuals. It is not caused by improper diet or inadequate hygiene.

2. Obsessive scrubbing of the face or picking pimples can be harmful.

Key Treatment

- Comedonal: topical retinoid

- Mild inflammatory: topical antibacterial

- Moderate inflammatory: topical retinoid + topical or oral antibacterial

- Severe cystic: isotretinoin

Follow-Up

1. Patients being treated with topical or systemic antibiotics should be seen regularly until stable improvement is noted; monthly visits would be reasonable.

2. Patients receiving isotretinoin should receive close clinical and laboratory monitoring by providers trained in the use of this agent.

Bibliography

Kaminer MS, Gilchrest BA: The many faces of acne. J Am Acad Dermatol 1995;32:S6–S14.

Landow K: Dispelling myths about acne. Postgrad Med 1997;102:94–111.

Leyden JJ: Therapy for acne vulgaris. N Engl J Med 1997;336:1156–1162.

Strasburger VC: Acne—what every pediatrician should know about treatment. Pediatr Clin North Am 1997; 44:1505–1523.

Usatine RP, Quan MA, Strick R: Acne vulgaris—a treatment update. Hosp Pract 1998;Feb:111–127.

278 Impetigo

Laeth S. Nasir

Etiology

1. *Staphylococcus aureus*: Coagulase-positive *Staphylococcus* has become the dominant microorganism in all forms of this superficial skin infection. *Staphylococcus* is considered to be the sole cause of bullous impetigo, a manifestation of localized infection with phage group II staphylococci. The severest form of this infection is known as "staphylococcal scalded skin syndrome." *Streptococcus*, *Staphylococcus*, or mixed strep-staph infection causes impetigo contagiosa. All forms of impetigo are highly contagious and spread by direct contact, insect vectors, and fomites.

2. *Streptococcus pyogenes* (group A β-hemolytic streptococci): The major consequence of infection with this organism is the nonsuppurative sequelae caused by infection with nephritogenic strains of *Streptococcus*. Scarlet fever and erythema multiforme also may occur. Antibiotic treatment of impetigo has not been demonstrated to reduce the incidence of poststreptococcal glomerulonephritis. Rheumatic fever is not a sequela of skin infection.

Symptoms

1. Impetigo contagiosa: May present with an itching, crusting, often indolent rash. Exposed or traumatized skin are the sites most commonly affected.

2. Bullous impetigo: often a dramatic presentation with rapidly growing blisters in localized areas; may become very large. This condition is most commonly seen in neonates.

Key Symptoms

- Itching
- Crusting
- Blisters

Clinical Findings

1. Impetigo contagiosa: Begins as tender papules, becoming vesicular and subsequently rupturing, leaving the classic "honey-colored crusts." Removal of this crust reveals superficial weeping erosions. Regional lymphadenopathy is seen in the majority of cases. Constitutional symptoms are absent.

2. Bullous impetigo: Begins as a small vesicle, rapidly enlarging to bullae filled with purulent fluid. Spontaneous rupture occurs, leaving red, tender erosive areas. Lymphadenopathy and constitutional symptoms are absent. Both bullous and nonbullous forms of impetigo heal without scarring.

Key Signs

- Red papules early
- Vesicles
- Pustules
- Bullae
- Honey-colored crusts
- Regional lymphadenopathy
- Absence of constitutional symptoms

Laboratory Tests

Diagnosis is clinical. Laboratory tests are not performed routinely. However, in special situations, the following tests may be considered:

1. Gram's stain
2. Culture and sensitivity
3. Tzanck's smear to rule out herpes simplex infection
4. Antihyaluronidase and antideoxyribonuclease B serum titers to rule out or confirm group A β-hemolytic streptococcal infections. Streptolysin O production (by streptococci) is inhibited by lipids in the skin; therefore, antistreptolysin O titer is not useful in diagnosis.

Differential Diagnosis

1. Ecthyma: considered a "deep" form of impetigo. Lesions often covered with a thicker and more adherent crust than observed in impetigo. Removal of the crust reveals purulent red ulcers with raised margins.

2. Folliculitis: Lesions localized to hair follicles with inflammation and central pustules.

3. Eczema: often seen around the nose and mouth in a distribution similar to that observed in impetigo. Additionally, these lesions may become secondarily impetiginized.
4. Herpes simplex: also susceptible to secondary impetigination. Tends to be more painful than impetigo.

Treatment

1. Topical antibiotic therapy. Treatment of localized, easily accessible lesions is best accomplished through topical antibiotic therapy and débridement of lesions as outlined under "Patient Education."
2. Systemic antibiotic therapy. Indications for systemic antibiotic therapy are
    a. Widely disseminated or inaccessible lesions
    b. Outbreaks of impetigo in multiple family members or others in close contact, such as day care
    c. Bullous impetigo
3. Duration of both systemic and topical forms of therapy is 7 to 10 days or until complete resolution occurs.

Medication

1. Drug of choice
    a. Topical therapy: mupirocin (Bactroban) ointment applied tid to affected areas
    b. Systemic therapy
        (1) Erythromycin: adult dose, 1 gm/day divided dose; pediatric dose (erythromycin estolate [Ilosone]), 40 mg/kg/day every 6 hours
        (2) Cephalexin (Keflex): adult dose, 250 to 500 mg qid; pediatric dose, 25 to 50 mg/kg/day every 6 hours
2. Alternative drugs
    a. Dicloxacillin (Dynapen): adult dose, 250 to 500 mg qid
    b. Azithromycin (Zithromax)
        (1) Adult dose: 500 mg on day 1, followed by 250 mg once daily on days 2 through 5
        (2) Pediatric dose: 10 mg/kg as a single dose (not to exceed 500 mg) on day 1, followed by 5 mg/kg/day (not to exceed 250 mg) on days 2 through 5
        (3) Azithromycin is administered 1 hour before or 2 hours after a meal.
    c. Clindamycin (Cleocin): adult dose, 300 mg every 8 hours; pediatric dose, 20 mg/kg/day every 6 hours

d. Ciprofloxacin (Cipro), 500 mg bid (adults only)

Patient Education

1. Débridement of crust with wet soaks for 20 minutes three times daily, followed by gentle scrubbing with a washcloth
2. Fingernails should be kept short and scratching discouraged to avoid spread of infection.
3. Impetigo is extremely contagious. Use of an antibacterial soap, as well as avoidance of towels and washcloths used by the affected individual, is crucial to avoiding spread of infection.
4. Children should be removed from day care until 24 hours after antibiotic treatment is initiated.

Key Treatment

Drugs of Choice	Alternative Drugs
• Mupirocin	• Dicloxacillin
• Erythromycin	• Azithromycin
• Cephalexin	• Clindamycin
	• Ciprofloxacin

Follow-Up

1. If lesions clear promptly (3 to 5 days), no further follow-up is necessary.
2. Failure to eradicate the lesions within 7 days or acute spread of lesions necessitates prompt reevaluation of the diagnosis and/or treatment.
3. If a nephritogenic strain of *Streptococcus* is strongly suspected as the causative organism, follow-up with a urinalysis in 2 weeks may be a reasonable precaution.

Bibliography

American Academy of Pediatrics: Children in out-of-home child care. In Peter G (ed): Red Book: Report of the Committee on Infectious Diseases, 24th ed, p 83. Elk Grove Village, IL, American Academy of Pediatrics, 1997.

Bass JW, Chan DS, Creamer KM, et al: Comparison of oral cephalexin, topical mupirocin and topical bacitracin for the treatment of impetigo. Pediatr Infect Dis J 1997;16:708–710.

Darmstadt GL, Lane A: Cutaneous bacterial infections. In Behrman RE, Kliegman RM, Arvin AM (ed): Nelson Textbook of Pediatrics, 15th ed, pp 1890–1891. Philadelphia, WB Saunders Company, 1996.

Parish LC, Witkowski JA: Systemic management of cutaneous bacterial infections. Am J Med 1991;91(6A):106–110.

Rice TD, Duggan AK, DeAngelis C: Cost effectiveness of erythromycin versus mupirocin for the treatment of impetigo in children. Pediatrics 1992;89:210–214.

279 Basal and Squamous Cell Carcinoma

Marsha DuPree

Etiology

1. Basal cell carcinoma (BCC) is the most common malignancy in the United States, and squamous cell carcinoma (SCC) is the second most common cutaneous malignancy. Approximately 750,000 new cases of nonmelanoma skin cancer occur yearly, and the incidence is increasing.

2. Definitions
   a. BCC is a malignant tumor arising from basal cell layer of epidermis.
   b. SCC is a malignant tumor arising from keratinizing cells of epidermis.

3. Risk factors
   a. Excessive cumulative sun exposure
   b. Light complexion, light hair, light eyes
   c. History of radiation treatment in area, trauma, or arsenic ingestion
   d. Immunosuppression (SCC seen most commonly)
   e. Genetic syndromes: xeroderma pigmentosa, albinism, and basal cell nevus syndrome

Symptoms

BCC and SCC are generally asymptomatic.

Clinical Findings

1. Basal cell carcinoma
   a. Average age of onset 64 years, more common in males
   b. Common sites
      (1) Face, especially nose
      (2) Neck, chest, and upper back
      (3) Very rare on mucous membranes, hands, and extremities
   c. Clinical presentation
      (1) Nodular BCC: white, translucent papule, telangiectasia, with or without ulcer
      (2) Superficial BCC: scaly, erythematous macule, telangiectasia, with or without crust
      (3) Pigmented BCC: nodular BCC with irregular pigmentation
      (4) Morpheaform or sclerosing (rare form, approximately 0.1 per cent): waxy, yellow "scar-like" plaque, telangiectasia

   (5) Metastasis very rare

2. Squamous cell carcinoma
   a. Average age of onset 66.2 years; 3:1 male/female ratio
   b. Common sites
      (1) Face
      (2) Dorsal hands, lower extremities (chronic ulcers, burns)
      (3) Mucous membranes (especially lower lip, glans penis)
   c. Clinical presentation
      (1) Early lesions (actinic keratosis, solar keratosis, SCC in situ) scaly, erythematous macule (<5 mm) with telangiectasia
      (2) Later lesions firm, scaly plaque or nodule with telangiectasia or ulceration
   d. Metastasis: Increased incidence of metastasis in SCC involving
      (1) Eyelid, external ear, scalp, dorsal hand, mucous membranes
      (2) Areas of burns, ulcers, and immunocompromised hosts
      (3) Recurrent lesions
      (4) Large lesions greater than 2 cm
      (5) Aggressive histologic pattern (see "Laboratory Tests")

Key Findings

BCC	SCC
• Translucent, white papule	• Scaly erythematous papule or plaque
• Scaly patch with crust	• Firm papule or plaque
• Telangiectasia	• Telangiectasia
• Ulceration centrally	• Central ulceration
• Face and upper back	• Face, dorsal hand, and lower lip

Laboratory Tests

1. The only laboratory procedure for confirming the diagnosis of BCC or SCC is biopsy (shave or punch). Biopsy before treatment because this

will help determine treatment. *Always do a punch biopsy if you suspect a skin cancer at the site of a scar.*

2. The histopathology of BCC and SCC is important in determining treatment.

   a. BCC (nodular or superficial): foci or lobules of basaloid cells extending from epidermis

   b. Aggressive variants of BCC

      (1) Morpheaform or sclerosing BCC

      (2) Infiltrating BCC

      (3) Metatypical or basosquamous cell carcinoma

      (4) Tumors with perineural invasion

   c. SCC

      (1) Irregular downward proliferation of atypical keratinocytes showing individual cell keratinization, atypical mitosis, and invasion into the dermis

      (2) Actinic keratosis shows these features confined to epidermis.

   d. Aggressive variants of SCC

      (1) Spindle cell SCC

      (2) Adenoid SCC

      (3) Verrucous carcinoma

 Key Test

Biopsy (shave or punch)

Differential Diagnosis

1. Clinical mimics easily diagnosed on histology.

   a. Pigmented BCC can mimic melanoma.

   b. Keratoacanthoma (rapidly growing, crater-like nodule) mimics SCC.

2. Genetic diseases (important in differential diagnosis of young people with skin cancers)

   a. Basal cell nevus syndrome (autosomal dominant) (see Habif, 1996): nevus-like lesions arising at puberty, associated with mutations of patched gene

   b. Albinism

   c. Xeroderma pigmentosa (see Habif, 1996)

Treatment

It is important to evaluate the *anatomic site* (area involved), the *histologic type*, whether the lesion is a *recurrence*, and the *age* of patient in choosing treatment. *Appropriate initial treatment offers the best cure rates and best cosmetic results.*

1. *Surgical excision* (recurrence rate approximately 10 per cent)

   a. Surgical margins for nonaggressive BCC less than 2 cm are 2 to 4 mm.

   b. Surgical margins for nonaggressive SCC less than 2 cm are 5 to 6 mm.

   c. If surgical margins are positive, then immediate re-excision or Mohs' surgery.

   d. *Contraindications*: medically unstable patient, histologically aggressive tumors

2. *Electrodesiccation and curettage* (recurrence rate approximately 7 per cent)

   a. Simple procedure in skilled hands

   b. Good for small (<2 cm) nodular and superficial BCC

   c. Good for tumors on firm surfaces (chest, forehead, temple, ears)

   d. *Contraindications*: recurrences, histologically aggressive tumors, scalp tumors

3. *Cryosurgery* (recurrence rate 7.5 per cent in experienced hands)

   a. Actinic keratosis, BCC, and nonaggressive SCC

   b. Can be used on larger tumors, patients on anticoagulants or with pacemakers, and on difficult anatomic sites (nasal ala, ears, eyelid)

   c. *Contraindications*: recurrences, lower leg tumors (delayed healing)

4. *Radiotherapy* (recurrence rate 8.7 per cent)

   a. BCC, SCC, recurrences, or residual tumors

   b. Facial areas (where cosmesis and function are important, such as the eyelid)

   c. Larger size (1 to 5 cm), patients on anticoagulants, or keloid formers

   d. Age 40 years or older, because treated areas deteriorate cosmetically with time

   e. *Contraindications*: recurrences treated initially with radiation, scalp tumors

5. *Mohs' micrographic surgery*: procedure where the tumor is excised and frozen sections of the entire cut surgical margin are evaluated until the margins are clear (usually same day).

   a. Best used in

      (1) Recurrent tumors

      (2) Tumor with aggressive pathology (see "Laboratory Tests")

      (3) Large tumors

      (4) Tumors where recurrence rate is high (see BCC and SCC recurrence)

   b. *Tissue-sparing* aspect of Mohs' is helpful in functionally and cosmetically difficult areas

   c. *Recurrence rates*: for primary, 1 per cent; for recurrent tumors, 5.6 per cent

d. Disadvantages: expensive and difficult for patients in poor health

6. *Chemotherapy*
   a. Topical 5-fluorouracil
      (1) Extensive actinic keratosis, keratoacanthoma, and superficial BCC
      (2) Patients are often noncompliant because of pain and erosions (temporarily cosmetically disfiguring).
   b. Intralesional interferon-α
      (1) Useful in superficial and nodular BCC; has shown an approximate 80 per cent cure
      (2) Side effects: some flu-like symptoms and pain in area
   c. Retinoid (oral)
      (1) Useful in patients with genetic syndromes (see "Differential Diagnosis")
      (2) Numerous severe side effects in long-term use

7. *Photodynamic therapy*: newer treatment combining laser and photoactive drugs

Prevention

1. Education on sunscreens
2. Avoiding exposure to midday sun and burning
3. A 3-inch brim on hats
4. Protect children: *Remember, it is cumulative ultraviolet radiation that causes skin cancer.*

Key Treatment

- Surgical excision
- Electrodesiccation, curettage
- Cryosurgery
- Radiotherapy
- Mohs' micrographic surgery
- Chemotherapy
- Photodynamic therapy

Follow-Up

1. First year: every 3 months for recurrence and new BCC or SCC
2. At least yearly for 5 years; some authors believe a lifetime, because more than 50 per cent of patients will develop a *new* BCC or SCC within 4 to 5 years.

Recurrence: BCC

- Areas of common recurrences: nose, ears, lips, periorbital, scalp
- Large size (>2 cm)
- Aggressive histologic variants
- Previously treated lesions

Recurrence: SCC

- Sites of common recurrences: lip, nose, ear, scalp, dorsum of hand
- Occurrence in scar site
- Large size (>2 cm)
- Previously treated lesions
- Immunocompromised host
- Aggressive histologic types

Bibliography

AAD Committee on Guidelines of Care (Lynn A. Drake, chairman): Guidelines of care for cutaneous squamous cell carcinomas. J Am Acad Dermatol 1993;28:628–631.

Arnold HL, Odom RB, James WD: Epidermal nevi, neoplasms, and cysts. In Andrews' Diseases of the Skin, 8th ed, pp 763–782. Philadelphia, WB Saunders Company, 1990.

Goldstein AM, Bale SJ, Peck GL, et al: Sun exposure and basal cell carcinoma in the nevoid basal cell carcinoma syndrome. J Am Acad Dermatol 1993;29:34–41.

Habif TP: Clinical Dermatology: A Color Guide to Diagnosis and Therapy, 3rd ed, pp 649–669. St. Louis, Mosby, 1996.

NIAMS Scientific Workshop Summary: Patient outcome in basal cell and squamous cell carcinoma, December 2–3, 1996.

Indications

1. Punch: Establish or confirm diagnosis of skin lesions.
2. Shave: Removal of benign dome-shaped papules such as intradermal nevus, skin tags, dermatofibroma, seborrheic keratosis

Contraindications

1. Punch: Lesions on eyelids, or directly over cartilaginous areas (tip of nose, ears), prominent veins, tendons, or joints

> **Note**
> Lesions suspected of being a malignant melanoma should be completely excised rather than punch or shave biopsied.

2. Shave: Nonelevated lesions or inflammatory conditions

Preparation

1. Consent: Include possibility of infection (cellulitis), minor bleeding; also discuss possible need for further treatment (i.e., complete excision), specialist referral (depending on histologic diagnosis).
2. Antiseptic (e.g., povidone-iodine, isopropyl alcohol): Cleanse immediate area (2 to 3 cm diameter around lesion).
3. Sterile draping is generally unnecessary.

Equipment

1. Shave
   a. No. 15 scalpel (or half a straight razor blade [or Derma Blade] for flexible blade shave biopsy)
   b. A 1- or 3-ml syringe
   c. A 30-gauge needle
   d. 1% lidocaine with or without epinephrine
   e. Smooth-tipped forceps (not toothed)
   f. Povidone-iodine swabs/pads, alcohol pads
   g. Electrocautery unit (e.g., Hyfrecator) or Monsel's solution (20% ferric subsulfate)
   h. Specimen bottle with fixative
   i. 4 × 4 gauze pads
2. Punch
   a. A 1- or 3-ml syringe
   b. A 30-gauge needle
   c. 1% lidocaine
   d. Povidone-iodine or alcohol pads
   e. Smooth-tipped (not toothed forceps)
   f. Scissors (to remove specimen)
   g. Disposable Baker-type punch; 2, 3, 4 mm most commonly used (2 mm for facial lesions).
   h. Optional: 4-0, 5-0, or 6-0 nylon suture (see "Technique")
   i. Specimen bottle with fixative
   j. 4 × 4 gauze pads

Anesthesia

1. Local anesthesia with 1% lidocaine with 1:100,000 epinephrine (except for fingertips, toes, tip of nose, pinna). Epinephrine prolongs the anesthetic effect of the lidocaine and helps to control bleeding. For intradermal and subcutaneous administration (vs. nerve block) anesthesia is immediate. The vasoconstrictive effect of epinephrine may take a few minutes.
2. For shave excision, intradermal infiltration (e.g., just like raising a wheal for administering a tuberculin skin test), to cover approximately 1 mm outside the lesion's boundary, is all that is necessary.
3. For punch biopsy, both intradermal and subcutaneous infiltration are required. If the punch defect is to be sutured (e.g., on the face), a wider area of anesthesia may be needed.
4. To reduce pain associated with anesthetic injection
   a. Use 30-gauge needle; inject slowly.
   b. Hold ice or cold pack to lesion for 30 to 60 seconds before injection.
   c. Add 1 ml 7.5% $NaHCO_3$ to 5 ml lidocaine.
   d. Hand-warm the solution before injecting.

Precautions

1. Allergic reactions to lidocaine are rare (most reactions are vasovagal). For true lidocaine-allergic patients, inject bacteriostatic saline (it contains benzyl alcohol, which has a weak anesthetic effect) in a volume two to three times the volume required for 1% lidocaine. The anesthetic effect is briefer than that of lidocaine.
2. Location of biopsy (see "Contraindications" above). For punch biopsies, use caution in areas over vessels, nerves, joints. It is possible to manually retract skin overlying such structures in a way that safely allows the biopsy (e.g., manually retract an upper eyelid lesion up over the supraorbital ridge).
3. Wound hemostasis

a. Monsel's solution (20% ferric subsulfate) leaves a pigmented stain, so do not use on the face.

b. Aluminum chloride solution is less effective for hemostasis but can be used on the face.

c. Silver nitrate sticks are caustic to tissues and stain black; therefore, these are not recommended at all in these procedures.

d. Light electrocautery (e.g., Hyfrecator low setting, 25 to 35 units; grounding of patient is unnecessary)

Technique

1. Prep and anesthesia
   a. Antiseptic prep of immediate area (1 to 2 cm surrounding the lesion). Sterile draping optional; use universal precautions.
   b. Anesthetic infiltration as described above

2. Shave
   a. Intradermal infiltration of anesthetic results in immediate anesthesia, so, unless there is a need to wait for the vasoconstrictive effect of epinephrine (i.e., for a vascular lesion), you may proceed immediately. For a vasoconstrictive effect wait 3 to 5 minutes.
   b. It is often helpful, using the tip of a No. 15 scalpel, to first "outline," with the blade parallel to the surrounding skin, the perimeter of the lesion to be excised, then "shave" the blade across the base of the lesion, flush with the surrounding skin (especially important for good cosmesis).

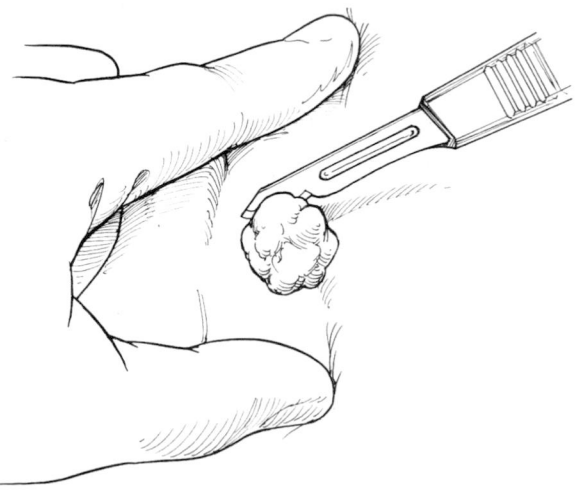

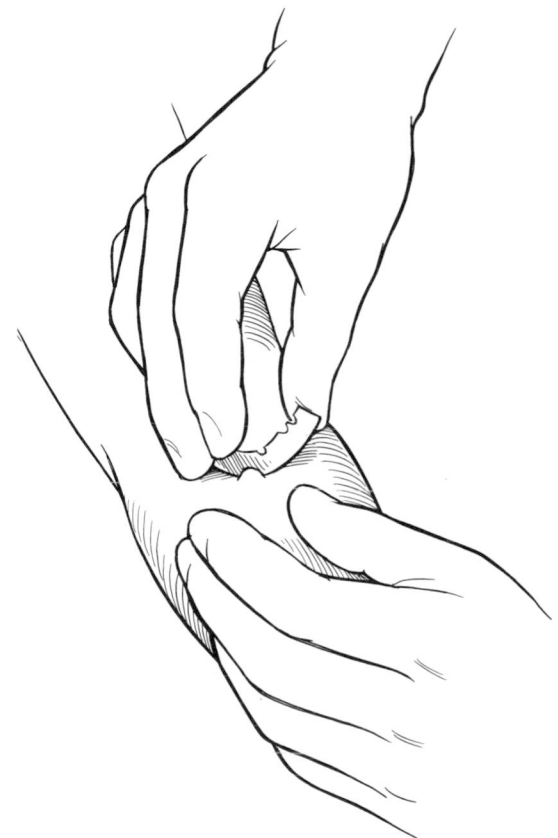

   c. Alternatively, a flexible blade (a longitudinal half of a straight-edged razor blade or Derma Blade) can be used to shave, with a side-to-side cutting motion while slowly moving the blade forward across the base of the lesion.

This tends to have a slight "scooping" effect that may be desirable in certain cases where a slightly deeper excision would be helpful symptomatically (e.g., dermatofibroma) or histologically (basal cell carcinoma—which, of course, would require further treatment).

   d. The resultant wound usually requires hemostasis either with direct pressure, light cautery, or chemical hemostasis as described above (see "Precautions").

3. Punch
   a. After intradermal and subcutaneous anesthesia, select the appropriate-size punch. Complete excision of lesions requiring larger than a 4-mm punch is better accomplished (with respect to wound healing and cosmesis) with elliptical excision. If sampling a larger lesion, orient the punch at the lesion's edge and, in fact, include a portion of the surrounding

normal skin. This is helpful for histologic interpretation.

b. Hold the skin surrounding the wound taut for stabilization, with tension directed perpendicular to normal skin lines. This will also give the resultant wound more of an oval shape, which makes wound closure (if done) easier and results in a less noticeable scar.

c. Using a rotary motion, back and forth, exert pressure downward so the cutting edge of the punch cuts down through the dermis to the subcutaneous tissue.

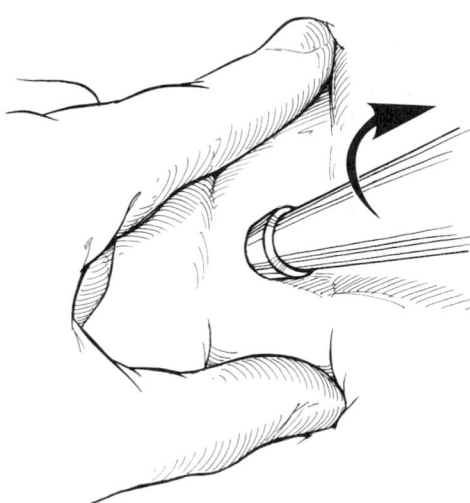

Depending on underlying structures, use caution when finishing the cut through the dermis. Be aware of differences in the thickness of the dermis (e.g., infraorbital area, 1 mm; periscapular area, 5 to 6 mm). After cutting through the dermis into the subcutaneous tissue, remove the punch. With a smooth-tipped (or at least not a single-toothed) forceps, carefully elevate the plug of tissue, using care not to crush the skin portion.

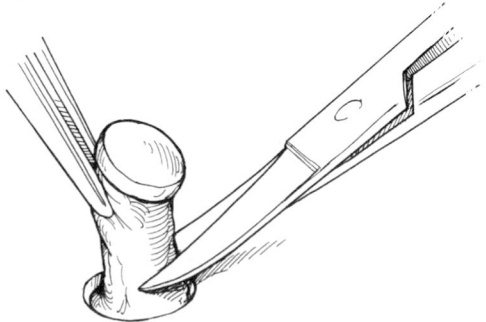

d. Another technique is to elevate the plug out of the wound using the needle from the anesthetic syringe. Remove the sample by cutting through the subcutaneous tissue and place it in the specimen bottle.

e. Once hemostasis is achieved, place one or two sutures to close the wound. Alternatively, place a small pressure dressing that can be removed after 12 hours. Facial punch biopsy wounds, even 2-mm wounds, should be sutured for optimal cosmesis.

Follow-Up

1. Depending upon the location on the body, sutures should be removed in 2 days (face) to 7 days (extremity). Results of histologic examination are reviewed with the patient at the time of follow-up and further therapeutic plans developed accordingly.

2. For malignant lesions, special follow-up is required. Acceptable tumor-free margins may be as little as 2 mm for certain basal cell carcinomas, between 4 and 6 mm for most squamous cell carcinomas, and up to 2 cm for malignant melanoma.

Note

If one is uncertain about proper definitive treatment for a specific dermatologic malignancy, referral should be made to the appropriate specialist for wide excision or other therapy as indicated.

Bibliography

Achar S: Principles of skin biopsies for the family physician. Am Fam Physician 1996;54:2411–2418.

Epstein E: A flexible scalpel for shave excision of skin lesions. J Am Acad Dermatol 1997;36(6 Pt 1):1030–1031.

Habif TP: Dermatologic surgical procedures. In: Clinical Dermatology: A Color Guide to Diagnosis and Therapy, 3rd ed, pp 808–816. St. Louis, Mosby, 1996.

Sams WM Jr: Diagnostic procedures. In Sams WM Jr, Lynch PJ (eds): Principles and Practice of Dermatology, 2nd ed, pp 45–51. New York, Churchill Livingstone, 1996.

280 Melanoma

Roger J. Zoorob

Melanoma is a skin disease that results from malignant proliferation of melanocytes. It is a cancer that is increasing in incidence and potentially fatal.

Etiology and Epidemiology

1. White collar workers, men and women equally, are mostly affected.
2. Fair complexion and the tendency to burn, rather than tan, are definite risk factors.
3. Exposure to ultraviolet rays early in life increases the incidence. Regular use of sunscreens may not help.
4. Ten per cent of patients have one family member with melanoma.
5. A very important risk factor is the number of melanocytic nevi.

Symptoms

Patient will present with a pigmented skin lesion that can be described as follows:

1. Asymptomatic
2. Increasing in size
3. Variegated color
4. Itchy
5. Bleeding
6. Irregular borders

Key Symptom

Ugly-looking mole

Clinical Findings

Melanoma is classified according to growth patterns:

1. *Superficial spreading* (75 per cent of melanomas): Tumor occurs on trunk and lower extremities. Grows horizontally for months or years, then develops a nodular component.
2. *Lentigo maligna* (5 per cent of melanomas): Mostly on the head and neck of patients over 60 years old. Lesion grows in a radial pattern.
3. *Nodular* (20 per cent of melanomas): Non—weight-bearing areas of the foot often affected but can occur anywhere. Nodule grows in a ver-

tical pattern and may invade deeper tissues early.

4. *Acral lentiginous* (<3 per cent of melanomas): Occurs in the palms and soles of middle-aged African Americans. Invades deeper tissues very early.
5. *Amelanotic*: A nonpigmented, usually pink nodule. Increased morbidity as a result of failure of recognition.

The acronym ABCDE is very important in the physical examination of a skin lesion suspected to be melanoma. Characteristics to be noted are: *a*symmetry, *b*order, *c*olor, *d*iameter, and *e*nlargement/*e*levation.

Key Signs

- Asymmetric lesion
- Border irregularity
- Color changes
- Diameter greater than 6 mm
- Enlargement/elevation

Laboratory Tests

1. Excisional biopsy with a 2-mm normal skin margin. Avoid a shave biopsy because it prevents assessment of the thickness of the lesion.
2. Incisional biopsy for large lesions that cannot be excised. Biopsy the thickest part of the lesion.
3. Complete blood count, liver function tests
4. Chest radiograph

Key Test

Excisional biopsy

WARNING

Shave biopsy inappropriate

Differential Diagnosis

1. Simple and halo nevus, compound nevus, junctional nevus, blue nevus, dysplastic nevus
2. Actinic and seborrheic keratosis, simple lentigo, pigmented basal cell carcinoma
3. Keratoacanthoma, dermatofibroma, Kaposi's sarcoma
4. Pyogenic granuloma, subungual hematoma, hemangioma

Treatment

Primary Lesion

Wide excision of the melanoma. Excision margin depends on thickness.

1. In situ melanoma: 0.5-cm margin
2. Less than 1 mm thick: 1-cm margin
3. One to 4 mm thick: 2-cm margin
4. More than 4 mm thick: at least 2- to 3-cm margin
5. Subungual melanoma: digital amputation

WARNING

Avoid Mohs' surgery in all melanomas.

Metastatic Disease

1. In-transit metastasis: local excision or carbon dioxide ablation. Recurrence around 100 per cent. Dinitrochlorobenzene (DNCB) injection in small dermal metastasis may be successful.
2. Remote nodal and soft tissue: Do better with complete resection.
3. Palliative but sometimes curative resection can be attempted in visceral metastasis. Best result with resection of solitary pulmonary metastasis.

Adjuvant Therapy

1. Interferon-alfa 2b (Intron A): Prolongs relapse-free survival by 11 per cent and overall 5-year survival by 9 per cent for nodal metastasis.
2. Radiotherapy as an adjunct to local node dissection results in around 85 per cent local control.

Patient Education

1. Avoid sunburn and sunbathing.
2. All patients with family history of melanoma should be examined periodically.
3. Check any mole appearing after puberty.
4. Check any mole that changes in color, size (especially >6 mm), or border.
5. Educate patient about self-examination, especially ABCDE.

Key Treatment

Excision with adequate margin

Follow-Up

1. Most recurrences are within 3 years after excision.
2. For thin melanomas, follow up every 6 months for 1 year, then yearly.
3. For thick lesions, follow up every 3 months for 2 years, then every 6 months for 5 years, then yearly.
4. Follow up with history and physical examination, as well as yearly chest radiograph and liver function tests.
5. Further testing depends on the above factors.
6. Educate patient and family about how to detect recurrence or a second melanoma (5 per cent risk).

Bibliography

Coit D, Wallack M, Balch C: Melanoma surgical practice guidelines. Oncology 1997;11:1317–1323.

Johnson TM, Yolanda AM, Chang AE, et al: Advances in melanoma therapy. J Am Acad Dermatol 1998;38:731–741.

Rossi CR, Foletto M, Vecchiato A, et al: Management of cutaneous melanoma: state of the art and trends. Eur J Cancer 1997;33:2302–2312.

Seykora J, Elder D: Dysplastic nevi and other markers of melanoma. Semin Oncol 1996;23:682–686.

Stadelmann WK, McMasters K, Polk HC: Diagnosis and treatment of cutaneous melanoma of the head and neck. J Ky Med Assoc 1998;96:47–55.

281 Kaposi's Sarcoma

Avra Goldman

Etiology

Kaposi's sarcoma (KS) is a proliferation of an atypical collection of cells that occurs in the presence of immunosuppression. It appears to spring from an infectious agent.

1. Major etiologic agents: Evidence indicates that these factors are necessary, but may not be sufficient for the development of KS.
   a. Human herpesvirus 8 (HHV8), also known as Kaposi's sarcoma herpesvirus (KSHV): a newly identified virus found in the KS cells, believed to pass most easily through male-to-male sexual contact.
   b. Immunosuppression
      (1) Human immunodeficiency virus (HIV) infection
      (2) Corticosteroids and other immunosuppressive drugs after organ transplantation
      (3) Malnutrition: in endemic KS in Africa
2. Likely potentiating factors
   a. Androgenic hormones: KS disproportionately affects men (96 per cent of KS in acquired immunodeficiency syndrome in gay men).
   b. HIV: an important cofactor apart from its immunosuppressive effects
   c. Cytokines: growth-promoting agents
   d. Genetic factors: Many patients are positive for human leukocyte antigen DR5.

Symptoms

The symptoms and manifestations of KS vary markedly depending on the location of the tumor. It can occur in any part of the body, with five areas most commonly involved.

1. Cutaneous system: skin and mucous membranes, particularly face and genitalia; pain secondary to infection and ulceration
2. Oral cavity
   a. Pain with chewing and swallowing
   b. Bleeding in the mouth
   c. Tooth loss
3. Lymphatic system: Swelling can cause limitation of function.

4. Gastrointestinal (GI) tract
   a. Abdominal pain, dyspepsia
   b. Nausea and vomiting
   c. Early satiety
   d. GI bleeding: Can be substantial.
   e. GI KS is often *asymptomatic*.
5. Respiratory tract
   a. Dyspnea
   b. Hemoptysis
   c. Chest pain

Key Symptoms

- Pain
- Hemorrhage
- Dyspnea

Clinical Findings

There can be a broad spectrum of involvement, ranging from a pinpoint nodule to a life-threatening mass.

1. Cutaneous system
   a. Raised red, purple, or brown, very vascular nodule, seen especially in sun-exposed areas and areas of trauma; does not blanch with compression.
   b. Ulceration
2. Oral cavity
   a. Discoloration of palate
   b. Nodule
3. Lymphatic system
   a. Lymphedema: Masses can cause obstruction to flow.
   b. Lymphadenopathy
4. GI tract: Can occur anywhere throughout system; abdominal distention and tenderness secondary to obstruction.
5. Respiratory tract: no distinctive signs on physical examination

Key Signs

- Raised, vascular, nonblanching nodules
- Lymphedema

Laboratory Tests

The definitive method of diagnosis for KS in any organ system is tissue biopsy.

1. Biopsy: Spindle cells are the hallmark of KS. Epithelial, inflammatory cells, macrophages full of hemosiderin.
2. Stool for occult blood: a good screening test of GI KS
3. Chest radiograph: May show dense bilateral lower lobe infiltrates, pleural effusions, loss of heart border; no distinctive sign to distinguish it from *Pneumocystis carinii* pneumonia, fungal, or viral lung infections

Key Tests

- Biopsy
- Stool for occult blood
- Chest radiograph

Differential Diagnosis

1. Common skin conditions
   a. Ecchymoses
   b. Nevi
   c. Congenital hemangiomata
2. Other malignancies
   a. Melanoma
   b. Lymphoma
3. Unusual infections
   a. Cutaneous mycobacterial infections
   b. Bacillary angiomatosis

Treatment

There are no clear guidelines for treatment, and many methods remain experimental. No treatment has been found to affect survival, and lesions typically recur after completion of treatment. Treatment should thus be aimed at palliation of symptoms.

1. Antiretroviral therapy: New evidence shows this may be the most effective strategy; with increased CD4 counts, KS has been seen to go into complete remission.
2. Intralesional therapy: for small, localized dis-

ease that is causing troublesome symptoms or is disfiguring
   a. Intralesional radiation: effective; can cause mucositis.
   b. Intralesional chemotherapy: Vinblastine quite effective.
   c. Cryotherapy
   d. Laser treatment: Effective but may increase viral spread.
3. Systemic therapy: for disseminated disease or problematic visceral involvement. The benefits of therapy must be weighed against the significant risk of opportunistic infections and neutropenia. Disease almost always recurs after cessation of treatment, which is invariably toxic.
   a. Vinblastine
   b. Interferon-alfa
   c. Combination therapy with vinblastine, bleomycin, and doxorubicin or daunomycin—very effective and very toxic
4. New treatment possibilities
   a. Cytokine inhibitors
   b. Antiviral agents (e.g., foscarnet, hydroxyurea)
   c. Numerous miscellaneous agents (e.g., apolipoprotein E, TNP-470, thalidomide)

Key Treatment

- Antiretroviral agents
- Intralesional radiation and chemotherapy
- Systemic chemotherapy

Follow-Up

No treatment reliably cures KS (except perhaps antiretroviral drugs that successfully suppress viral load). The physician must watch vigilantly for serious disease recurrence. It is also important to remember that opportunistic infections will likely coexist with KS.

 Bibliography

Dezube BJ: Clinical presentation and natural history of AIDS-related Kaposi's sarcoma. Hematol Oncol Clin North Am 1996;10:1023–1029.

Ganem D: KSHV and Kaposi's sarcoma: the end or the beginning? Cell 1997;91:157–160.

Morris AK, Valley AW: Overview of the management of AIDS-related Kaposi's sarcoma. Ann Pharmacother 1996;30:1150–1163.

Myskowski PL, Ahkami R: Advances in Kaposi's sarcoma. Dermatol Clin 1997;15:177–188.

Sung JC, Louis SG, Park SY: Kaposi's sarcoma: advances in tumor biology and pharmacotherapy. Pharmacotherapy 1997;17:670–683.

282 Psoriasis

Josiah Friedlander

Etiology

1. Psoriasis is a skin ailment characterized by localized areas of accelerated turnover of keratinocytes. This leads to epidermal thickening and increasing skin shedding.
2. It is lifelong and is characterized by exacerbations and remissions.
3. Exacerbations are often attributed to stress, changing weather, and certain medications, including lithium carbonate, β-blockers, and antimalarials.
4. Psoriasis has a prevalence of 1 to 3 per cent worldwide, occurs equally among men and women, and is genetically linked to human leukocyte antigen Cw6.
5. On a molecular basis, studies show that those with psoriasis have higher serum levels of interleukin (IL)-8 and lower levels of IL-10 than controls, and these levels trend toward normal with aggressive treatment of the disease.
6. Most commonly starts in third or fourth decade of life.

Symptoms

1. Pruritic, desquamative rash most commonly involving the extensor surfaces of the elbows, knees, and scalp
2. Rash usually spares palms, soles, and face. Scale is not usually visible in intertriginous areas.
3. Symptoms improve after exposure to sunlight.
4. Rash tends to wax and wane.
5. Nail pitting and onycholysis are not uncommon.
6. Rash can develop in areas of prior trauma (Koebner's phenomenon).
7. Pinpoint bleeding occurs when flakes are picked off (Auspitz's sign).
8. Ten per cent of patients develop arthritis.

Key Symptoms

- Pruritic, erythematous desquamative rash on extensor surfaces
- Pitting of nails
- Joint pain/swelling

Clinical Findings

1. Classic psoriasis
   a. Location: extensor surfaces, most commonly on the elbows and the knees
   b. Appearance: red, raised, clearly circumscribed with an obvious demarcation between normal-appearing and affected skin
   c. The skin desquamates easily and can break down and split when the lesions become sufficiently thick and friable.
   d. Auspitz's sign: punctate bleeding when scale is pulled away from a lesion
   e. Nail changes, including pitting or ridging
   f. Koebner's phenomenon: Frequently psoriasis will develop at the site of previously traumatized skin (e.g., lacerations or incision sites) in those with a history of psoriasis.
   g. Psoriatic arthritis
      (1) Five to ten per cent of those with psoriasis will also develop psoriatic arthritis, an asymmetric arthritis involving one or more small joints in the feet and hands.
      (2) Arthritis most commonly follows the development of skin lesions, but can antedate or occur simultaneously.
      (3) *Arthritis mutilans* (a rare variant) aggressively destroys small bones of the hands and feet.
      (4) Effective treatment of the skin lesions usually improves the arthritis.
2. Guttate psoriasis
   a. Sudden appearance 1 to 2 weeks after upper respiratory infection/strep throat of multiple pinpoint to 1-cm red, scaling papules
   b. Heralds onset of chronic psoriasis.
3. Generalized pustular psoriasis: Rare, sometimes life-threatening condition where small, sterile pustules coalesce into lakes of pus; responds well to etretinate.
4. Psoriasis inversus: primarily in skinfolds, such as axillae, groin, gluteal cleft, auricular fold
5. Human immunodeficiency virus (HIV)–induced psoriasis
   a. Often atypical, involving groin, axillae, palms, soles, scalp

b. Later onset, in thirties to forties; family history of psoriasis

c. CD4 cell count less than 300/mm^3 usually

d. Management directed at HIV with antiretroviral therapy.

Key Signs

- Raised erythematous plaques
- Desquamation
- Clear delineation between normal and abnormal skin
- Nail pitting
- Arthritis
- Koebner's phenomenon

Laboratory Tests

1. Skin biopsy may reveal an increase in mitoses.
2. Enlarged and tortuous capillaries adjacent to the skin surface explain the punctate bleeding associated with removal of scale and the erythema.

Key Test

Skin biopsy (only necessary if rash cannot be diagnosed clinically based on appearance and location)

Differential Diagnosis

1. Tinea corporis (ringworm): central clearing, KOH-positive for hyphae
2. Seborrheic dermatitis: red, greasy, scaly rash in areas with sebum glands (e.g., scalp, eyebrows, nasal folds, presternal)
3. Lichen planus: small, flat, violaceous, shiny, pruritic papules of the skin and mucous membranes
4. Pityriasis rosea: salmon/light brown plaques with central fine scale and peripheral looser scale
5. Secondary syphilis: symmetric polymorphic pink rash, nonpruritic, involving palms and soles

Treatment

Phototherapy

1. Ultraviolet B (UVB) exposure

a. Sunlight

b. Artificial source, narrow band UVB is preferable

c. Tanning booths are not effective (low potency UVA and UVB)

2. Psoralen and ultraviolet A (PUVA): photochemotherapy combining oral psoralen with UVA

a. UVA usually from a specially designed light box.

b. Safe and frequently effective in experienced hands

c. Increased risk of squamous cell cancer of the skin proportionate to the duration and intensity of treatment

d. Not effective for scalp lesions because the UVA fails to penetrate the hair.

WARNING

PUVA therapy can increase risk of squamous cell cancer.

Medication

1. Topical

a. Coal tar: available in over-the-counter preparations, including shampoo, as well as by prescription

b. Anthralin (Lasan, Anthra-Derm, Drithrocreme) 0.1% to 0.5% ointment, 0.1% to 1.0% cream: Apply once daily and rinse after 1 hour.

c. Corticosteroids

(1) Creams generally less potent but also less messy than ointments. Be careful using under occlusion, which also augments potency. Be careful using in skinfolds and near the face because thinning of the skin can occur easily in these areas.

(2) Very high potency: augmented betamethasone 0.05% qd or bid

(3) High potency: betamethasone dipropionate 0.05% qd or bid

(4) Medium potency: triamcinolone 0.1% or 0.5% qd or bid

WARNING

Chronic use of potent topical corticosteroids, particularly under occlusion, can cause acne, thinning of the skin, and even suppression of the hypothalamic-pituitary-adrenal axis.

---

d. Calcipotriene (vitamin D analogue) 0.005% ointment applied bid.
e. Combination therapy with corticosteroid and salicylic acid (e.g., 0.1% mometasone furoate and 5% salicylic acid ointment) or corticosteroid with calcipotriene
f. Scalp involvement
   (1) Scale can be removed using shampoo with tar and salicylic acid.
   (2) Underlying skin then treated with topical corticosteroid solution.
   (3) Some patients respond to ketoconazole shampoo or oral ketoconazole, 400 mg/day
2. Intralesional corticosteroids: Triamcinolone (Kenalog), 5 mg/ml
3. Systemic therapy
   a. Methotrexate, 5 mg q12h times three doses per week: *not in pregnant women!*

> **WARNING**
>
> **Methotrexate is an antimetabolite and is contraindicated in pregnancy. Its use will likely lead to spontaneous miscarriage.**

   b. Cyclosporine (Neoral), 5 mg/kg/day
   c. Etretinate (Tegison), 1 mg/kg/day divided bid: *not in pregnant women!* Has been used with excellent results for both skin and arthritis.

> **WARNING**
>
> **Etretinate is a teratogen and is contraindicated in pregnancy.**

   d. Systemic corticosteroids should be avoided because the disease worsens significantly beyond its presteroid state when the steroids are finally withdrawn.

Patient Education/Exacerbating Factors

1. Initiation or increase in the dosage of lithium will necessitate more aggressive psoriasis treatment
2. β-Blockers and antimalarials variably worsen psoriasis.

Key Treatment

First Line
- Topical corticosteroids
- Coal tar
- Calcipotriene
- Phototherapy

Second Line
- Methotrexate
- Etretinate
- Cyclosporine

Follow-Up

1. Watch carefully for toxicities of medications and of phototherapy.
2. Frequency of follow-up dependent on response to therapy and severity of disease.

Bibliography

Cuellar ML, Espinoza LR: Methotrexate use in psoriasis and psoriatic arthritis. Rheum Dis Clin North Am 1997;23:787–809.

Habif TP: Clinical Dermatology, 3rd ed, pp 143–161. St. Louis, CV Mosby Company, 1995.

Spuls PI, Witkamp L, Bossuyt PM, et al: A systematic review of five systemic treatments for severe psoriasis. Br Dermatol 1997;137:943–949.

Van der Kerkhof PC: The management of psoriasis. Neth J Med 1998;52:40–45.

283 Pityriasis Rosea

Stephen D. Saglio

Etiology

1. Unknown
   a. Most likely caused by an infectious agent
      (1) Discrete clinical course
      (2) Apparent lifelong immunity after illness
   b. Relatively noncontagious, uncommon case clusters
2. Moderately common
   a. Worldwide distribution
   b. All races affected
   c. Typical spring and autumn peaks in temperate zones
   d. Females affected slightly more than males
   e. Patients usually 10 to 43 years old
3. An increased incidence described with
   a. Atopy
   b. Seborrheic dermatitis
   c. Acne vulgaris
   d. Dandruff
4. Medications reported to cause rashes resembling pityriasis rosea (PR)
   a. Bismuth
   b. Barbiturates
   c. Captopril
   d. D-Penicillamine
   e. Gold
   f. Isotretinoin
   g. Metronidazole
   h. Sulfa drugs

Symptoms

1. Occasionally a mild prodromal syndrome
   a. Malaise
   b. Nausea
   c. Decreased appetite
   d. Fever
   e. Arthralgias
   f. Fatigue
   g. Headache
   h. Sore throat
2. Pruritus of the rash
   a. None: 25 per cent of cases
   b. Mild: 50 per cent of cases
   c. Severe: 25 per cent of cases

Key Symptoms

- Occasional mild "viral syndrome"–type prodrome
- Mild pruritus

Clinical Findings

1. A self-limited illness
2. The classic disease progression (80 per cent of cases) is pathognomonic.
3. Primary lesion (or "herald patch")
   a. Large, typically 2 to 6 cm in diameter
   b. Located on the torso
   c. Precedes the general rash by 2 to 21 days.
4. Secondary lesions
   a. Miniatures of the primary lesion
   b. Appear in crops.
   c. 0.5 to 1.5 cm in diameter
   d. Papulosquamous
   e. Erythematous
   f. Oval with central clearing
   g. The border is darker, thin, and scaly.
5. Lesions may continue to appear for 2 to 3 weeks.
6. Complete resolution of the rash by 6 to 8 weeks (may take up to 14 weeks)
7. The distribution of PR is mainly on the torso.
   a. Classic "Christmas tree" pattern
   b. May also affect the proximal extremities.
8. Recurrences occur in no more than 3 per cent of cases.
9. Involvement of internal organs is never seen.

Key Signs

- "Herald patch"
- "Christmas tree" pattern
- Papulosquamous
- Erythematous
- Central clearing
- Secondary rash in 2 to 21 days
- Truncal distribution
- Oval
- Discrete
- Thin, scaly border

Laboratory Tests

1. None are of diagnostic importance.
2. A syphilis test should be obtained.
3. On biopsy, the pathology is nonspecific.

Key Test

Syphilis serology recommended

Differential Diagnosis

1. Tinea versicolor
   a. The lesions are more brown.
   b. The borders are not as ovoid.
   c. KOH testing is usually positive for hyphae.
2. Drug eruptions
   a. Usually no "herald patch"
   b. History of exposure to suspicious medications
   c. Very resistant to therapy
   d. Protracted course and larger lesions
3. Secondary syphilis
   a. Not pruritic
   b. Often a history of prior genital lesions
   c. Positive serology
   d. More common on palms and soles
4. Psoriasis
   a. Found predominantly on the extremities and scalp
   b. Rash has a whitish, thicker scale.
   c. A more chronic course
5. Seborrheic dermatitis
   a. A chronic clinical course
   b. Irregular, greasy scales
   c. On the sternum and other hairy areas
   d. No "herald patch"
6. Lichen planus
   a. More papular and violaceous
   b. Involving mucosa of the mouth and lips

7. Kaposi's sarcoma
   a. Oval, violaceous plaques
   b. May have a "Christmas tree" pattern.
   c. No scaling
8. Nummular eczema
   a. Usually not confined to the trunk
   b. Round lesions
   c. More chronic than PR

Treatment

1. Keep as mild as possible to prevent complications. Avoid soap, wool, and sweating; minimize irritation.
2. Sunlight and ultraviolet (UV) therapy modestly helpful

Medications

1. Used mainly to control pruritus
   a. Oatmeal collodial bath, every day or every other day
   b. Calamine lotion
   c. Oral antihistamines
   d. Topical steroids in a hydrophilic cream base
2. Systemic steroids for severe pruritis
   a. Prednisone, 20 to 40 mg daily, taper over 1 to 2 weeks
   b. Triamcinolone acetonide, 40 mg intramuscularly

Patient Education

Very important to reassure patient that
1. PR is essentially noncontagious.
2. No other organs are involved.
3. The rash should resolve completely.
4. Recurrences are rare (3 per cent of cases).

Key Treatment

Primary	Alternative
• Exposure to sunlight	• UV therapy
• Oatmeal collodial baths	• Prednisone, 20 to 40 mg, taper over 1 to 2 weeks
• Calamine lotion	
• Oral antihistamines	
• Topical steroids in hydrophilic base	• Triamcinolone acetonide, 40 mg intramuscularly

Bibliography

Bjornberg A: Pityriasis rosea. In Fitzpatrick TB, Eisen AZ, Wolff K, et al (eds): Dermatology in General Medicine, 4th ed, pp 1117–1123. New York, McGraw-Hill, 1993.

Fitzpatrick TB, Johnson RA, Polano MK, et al: Pityriasis rosea. In Color Atlas and Synopsis of Clinical Dermatology: Common and Serious Diseases, 3rd ed, pp 104–107. New York, McGraw-Hill, 1997.

Gibson LE, Perry HO: Papulosquamous eruptions and exfoliative dermatitis. In Moscella SL, Hurley HJ (eds): Dermatology, 3rd ed, pp 622–625. Philadelphia, WB Saunders Company, 1992.

Sauer GC, Hall JC: Manual of Skin Diseases, 7th ed, pp 143–147. Philadelphia, Lippincott-Raven, 1996.

Vidimos AT, Camisa C: Tongue and cheek: oral lesions in pityriasis rosea. Cutis 1992;50:276–280.

284 Lichen Planus

Rajani Katta

Etiology
1. Cause unknown
2. Thought to be an autoimmune disease mediated by T cells

Symptoms
Most patients experience intense pruritus, although some may be asymptomatic.

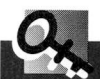

Key Symptom

Pruritic skin lesion

Clinical Findings
1. Cutaneous lichen planus (LP)
   a. The skin lesions exhibit a characteristic morphology.
      (1) Violaceous, polygonal, flat-topped papules and plaques
      (2) Surface may exhibit a thin reticulated pattern of white scale known as Wickham's striae.
      (3) Lesions often resolve with intense hyperpigmentation.
      (4) Lesions may occur in areas exposed to trauma, such as lacerations. This is known as an isomorphic response, or Koebner's phenomenon.
   b. Distribution: The flexor surfaces of the extremities are commonly involved. A very typical area of involvement is the flexor wrist.
   c. Although the most common form of cutaneous LP is the "classic" type described above, other variants exist:
      (1) Hypertrophic LP, most common on the anterior legs
      (2) Vesiculobullous LP displays blisters within plaques.
      (3) Actinic LP occurs within sun-exposed areas and is more common in Middle Eastern countries.
2. Oral, genital, nail, and scalp LP: Although LP often involves only cutaneous surfaces, it may involve other areas of the body alone or in conjunction with the cutaneous involvement.
   a. Oral
      (1) Classic morphology is a reticular lacy pattern. Other morphologies include papular lesions, atrophic lesions, or erosive areas.
      (2) Buccal and glossal mucosa are the most commonly involved.
   b. Genital
      (1) In men, the classic lesions are violaceous papules on the glans penis.
      (2) In women, atrophic plaques, leukoplakia, erythroplakia, or desquamative vaginitis may occur.
   c. Nails
      (1) LP may involve fingernails or toenails.
      (2) A pterygium is formed when the proximal nail fold extends distally onto the nail. This finding, when seen, is typical of nail LP.
      (3) Nail involvement may manifest in multiple ways that are not specific for LP.
   d. Scalp
      (1) Lichen planopilaris manifests as areas of hair loss with keratotic follicular papules.
      (2) The end stage manifests as scarring alopecia.

Key Signs

The 6 "P"s of Lichen Planus
- Pruritic
- Polygonal
- Planar (flat-topped)
- Purple
- Papules
- Plaques

Laboratory Tests

1. Punch biopsy of the skin should be obtained in order to examine the epidermis and dermis.
2. Histopathology of LP reveals characteristic findings, with a lichenoid lymphocytic infiltrate at the epidermal-dermal junction.
3. Multiple studies support a higher incidence of hepatitis C in patients with LP. These patients may be asymptomatic. Therefore, serum transaminases and anti–hepatitis C antibodies should be tested in all patients.

Key Tests

- Punch biopsy of lesion
- Anti–hepatitis C antibodies and serum transaminases

Differential Diagnosis

1. Cutaneous LP
   a. Lichenoid drug eruptions may be clinically indistinguishable from LP. Histopathology may not even be able to distinguish. Many medications may cause this eruption, including thiazide diuretics, angiotensin-converting enzyme inhibitors, β-blockers, gold, antimalarials, quinidine, and penicillamine, in addition to multiple others.
   b. Lupus, psoriasis, and secondary syphilis may all have morphology similar to LP.

> **WARNING**
>
> **Always consider a lichenoid drug eruption in the differential diagnosis of lichen planus, because clinically they may be indistinguishable.**

2. Oral LP
   a. In the white reticular or papular form, consider a benign bite line, leukoplakia, *Candida*, or secondary syphilis.
   b. In erosive LP, consider blistering diseases that involve the oral mucosa, including pemphigus and pemphigoid, or erythema multiforme.

Treatment

Medication

1. Topical steroids
   a. For localized cutaneous disease, topical steroids are the mainstay of therapy.
   b. High potency steroids are typically used.
   c. Topical steroids are the first-line therapy for oral lichen planus. Administer in an adhesive gel for use in the oral cavity (e.g., Orabase).
2. Intralesional steroids: For resistant or hyperkeratotic plaques, intralesional triamcinolone acetonide (Kenalog) may be used.
3. Systemic steroids
   a. Oral prednisone is the most commonly used treatment for generalized cutaneous lichen planus. Dosages of 30 to 60 mg/day are used, tapering over 6 weeks.
   b. Many think that treatment with systemic steroids reduces the duration of disease.
4. Retinoids: Controlled trials demonstrate the efficacy of acitretin (Soriatane), at a dose of 30 mg/day for 8 weeks in the treatment of cutaneous LP. This medication is highly teratogenic and requires careful monitoring.
5. Psoralen and ultraviolet (PUVA): Consider as an alternative treatment.

Diet

1. In cutaneous LP, no specific dietary restrictions are imposed except those indicated when taking certain medications.
2. In oral LP, if erosive lesions are present, patients should avoid acidic foods such as citrus fruits. If the erosive lesions are extensive, a soft diet may be indicated.

Activity

No restrictions on activity are necessary.

Patient Education

1. Advise that lesions often resolve with hyperpigmentation, which may take months to fade.
2. Reassurance that spontaneous remissions of cutaneous LP occur in the majority of cases after 1 year.

Key Treatment

- For localized cutaneous disease, topical steroids are the first-line treatment.
- For generalized cutaneous disease, oral prednisone is used. Alternatives include acitretin and PUVA.
- For oral LP, topical steroids in an adhesive vehicle are the first-line treatment.

Follow-Up

1. The frequency of physician visits depends on the severity of disease.
2. There is a higher incidence of squamous cell carcinoma in patients with oral LP, so monitor the oral mucosa. Any changes or suspicious areas should be biopsied.

WARNING

Patients with oral lichen planus have an increased risk of oral squamous cell carcinoma.

Bibliography

Boyd A, Nelder K: Lichen planus. J Am Acad Dermatol 1991;25:593–619.

Cribier B, Frances C, Chosidow O: Treatment of lichen planus. Arch Dermatol 1998;134:1521–1530.

Gadenne A, Bigby M, Camisa C: Lichen planus. In Arndt K, Leboit P, Robinson J, et al (eds): Cutaneous Medicine and Surgery, Vol. 1, pp 235–240. Philadelphia, WB Saunders Company, 1996.

Halevy S, Shai A: Lichenoid drug eruptions. J Am Acad Dermatol 1993;29:249–255.

Imhof M, Popal H, Lee J, et al: Prevalence of hepatitis C virus antibodies and evaluation of hepatitis C virus genotypes in patients with lichen planus. Dermatology 1997;195:1–5.

285 Vitiligo

Marc A. Darr

Etiology and Epidemiology

1. Etiology is uncertain. Vitiligo is thought to be autoimmune in nature, because it is often seen in conjunction with other autoimmune disorders (thyroid disease, diabetes mellitus, Addison's disease, and pernicious anemia).
2. Affects both sexes equally but more noticeable in dark-skinned persons.
3. Incidence is approximately 1 per cent.
4. Vitiligo is an acquired condition; congenital cases are extremely rare. Incidence peaks between 10 and 30 years.
5. Approximately 30 per cent of patients have a family member with the disease. Exact inheritance pattern is unclear.

Symptoms

1. White spots on skin
2. Patient may have a history of premature graying of hair.
3. Patient may have a history of alopecia.

Key Symptom

White spots on skin

Clinical Findings

1. Hypopigmented macule(s) ranging from 1 mm to several centimeters in diameter
   a. Usually white, but may be off-white or tan in color
   b. Tend to be circular or oval-shaped.
   c. Accentuated by viewing with Wood's lamp, especially in light-skinned patients
   d. Often have scalloped edges.
   e. May be focal, segmental, or generalized.
   f. Generalized vitiligo usually occurs in a very symmetric pattern.
   g. Common sites include extensor surfaces (knees, elbows, back of hands), body folds (axilla, genitalia), and skin around body orifices (mouth, eyes, nostrils, nipples, umbilicus).
   h. Macules also occur frequently at sites of skin trauma (elbows, collar, waistband) and previously sunburned areas. This is known as Koebner's phenomenon.
2. Other skin findings may include
   a. Leukotrichia
   b. Halo nevi
   c. Alopecia areata
3. Iritis is seen in 10 per cent of patients with vitiligo.
4. Patients may have associated signs of hyperthyroidism, diabetes, pernicious anemia, or Addison's disease.

Key Signs

- White, oval-shaped macules
- Symmetric pattern
- Lack of other skin changes
- Lesions accentuated by Wood's lamp
- Koebner's phenomenon

Laboratory Tests

1. Diagnosis is usually made by history and physical examination. Laboratory tests are rarely necessary.
2. If performed, skin biopsy reveals normal skin, except for an absence of melanocytes.
3. Once diagnosis of vitiligo is established, the clinician should consider screening for vitiligo-associated conditions:
   a. Thyroxine and thyroid-stimulating hormone for thyroid disease
   b. Complete blood count for pernicious anemia
   c. Fasting blood sugar for diabetes
   d. Na^+, K^+, and/or cortisol level for Addison's disease

Differential Diagnosis

1. Tinea versicolor
2. Tuberous sclerosis
3. Pityriasis alba
4. Postinflammatory hypopigmentation

5. Leprosy
6. Lupus erythematosus
7. Chemical leukoderma
8. Nevus anemicus

Treatment

1. The patient's need/desire for treatment must be determined.
   a. Vitiligo is primarily of cosmetic and social concern. The significance of vitiligo is much greater in darker-skinned individuals. In some cultures, the social stigmata attached to vitiligo can be devastating.
   b. Vitiligo tends to be stable initially and then slowly progresses over several years.
   c. Untreated vitiligo lesions usually remain for life, but some individuals develop spontaneous repigmentation.

Treatment Options

1. Education and reassurance often are all that is necessary in mild cases.
2. Sunscreens (skin protection factor [SPF] >30) should be used by all patients with vitiligo. Sunscreen will diminish tanning; tanning makes hypopigmented areas more noticeable. Sunscreen also decreases the risk of koebnerization and actinic damage.
3. Cosmetics: Makeups, skin dyes, and instant-tanning preparations may provide good results.
4. Repigmentation
   a. Topical steroids for isolated lesions
   b. Topical or oral psoralen and ultraviolet A (PUVA) photochemotherapy for more extensive disease
5. Depigmentation: useful for patients with extensive disease. This procedure involves "bleaching" the remaining normal skin with monobenzylether of hydroquinone (monobenzone [Benoquin]). This provides a permanent, uniform, and usually highly satisfactory result. Patients will, however, be at increased risk of sunburn after this procedure.

Medication

1. Topical steroids as noted above. Use hydrocortisone (1% or 2.5%) on the face and skinfolds, more potent steroids elsewhere. Interrupted schedule should be used if steroids are given for more than 6 to 8 weeks. Follow closely for evidence of steroid atrophy.
2. Topical psoralen (methoxsalen [Oxsoralen]) for isolated macules. Topical psoralen is highly phototoxic. Patients must avoid sunlight for 3 days after treatment.

3. Oral psoralen is effective treatment for widespread vitiligo.

WARNING

Oral psoralens should not be used in children under age 12.

---

4. Monobenzone as above for depigmentation

Diet
No special dietary measures.

Activity
Full

Patient Education

1. Benign nature of disease should be explained.
2. Patient should be instructed to use high-SPF sunscreens.
3. Avoid sun exposure at midday.
4. Risks and benefits of repigmentation and depigmentation should be explained to patients considering these therapies.

Key Treatment

- Drug of choice depends on severity of disease.
- Reassurance
- Sunscreen
- Cosmetics
- Repigmentation with steroids, PUVA
- Depigmentation with monobenzone

Follow-Up

1. Follow-up varies depending on the treatment plan.
2. Most patients with mild disease will require only periodic skin examinations as part of their overall health care maintenance.
3. Patients on repigmentation/depigmentation regimens will require multiple visits over several months to years.
4. All patients should have an eye examination by an ophthalmologist.

Bibliography

Arnold HL, Odom RB, James WD: Andrew's Diseases of the Skin: Clinical Dermatology, 8th ed, pp 1000–1003. Philadelphia, WB Saunders Company, 1990.

Fitzpatrick TB, Johnson RA, Polano MK, et al: Color Atlas and Synopsis of Clinical Dermatology: Common and Serious Diseases, 3rd ed, pp 287–295. New York, McGraw-Hill, 1997.

Habif TP: Clinical Dermatology: A Color Guide to Diagnosis and Therapy, 3rd ed, pp 616–620. St. Louis, CV Mosby Company, 1996.

Lavine N: Pigmentary disorders. In Rakel RE (ed): Conn's Current Therapy, pp 853–854. Philadelphia, WB Saunders Company, 1998.

Mosher DB, Fitzpatrick TB, et al: Disorders of pigmentation. In Fitzpatrick TB, Eisen AZ, Wolff K, et al (eds): Dermatology in General Medicine, 5th ed, vol 1, pp 949–960. New York, McGraw-Hill, 1999.

286 Herpes Simplex Infection

Arthur R. Slaughter

Etiology

1. Herpes simplex virus types 1 and 2 (HSV-1 and HSV-2) are herpes DNA viruses that cause either recognized or unrecognized primary infection, most often as herpes labialis or gingivostomatitis (HSV-1) or genital herpes (HSV-2). Each type can infect any site; digital and eye herpetic infections usually are caused by HSV-1.
2. Thereafter, either type may reactivate off and on throughout life to cause annoying and infectious skin disease.
3. HSV-1 does confer some partial immunity to HSV-2.
4. Disseminated simplex and simplex encephalitis may occur.

Symptoms

1. Primary infection begins with lesions 2 to 21 days after topical inoculation.
2. In addition to oral area sores and sore throat, herpes labialis often begins with fever, headache, myalgia, and cervical lymphadenopathy.
3. Primary genital herpes may present as painful urination; burning vulvar, scrotal, or penile pain; local swelling; erythema; fatigue; backache; or joint, abdominal, or suprapubic pain.
4. Reactivation of labial lesions may come at times of stress or excess sun exposure as extended painful lips for several days, with single or multiple lesions, often limited to an area involving the mucocutaneous borders of the lips.
5. Reactivation of genital herpes may be preceded by hours or days with genital pain, paresthesia, or numbness. The lesions tend to be unilateral. The degree of discomfort varies but is less than with primary infection.
6. Herpetic whitlow (HSV on finger), herpetic keratoconjunctivitis; and a pox-like eruption in atopic dermatitis (one cause of Kaposi's varicelliform eruption) are other ways primary or reactivated HSV may appear.

 Key Symptoms

- Local discomfort
- Grouped lesions

Clinical Findings

1. In HSV-1, clusters of small, clear vesicles on the lips, face, buccal mucosa, soft palate, floor of the mouth, and throat; within 1 to 3 days the vesicles break and leave painful ulcers that take 4 to 14 days to crust.
2. In HSV-2, typical grouped vesicles, pustules, and painful erosions or ulcers may then appear, sometimes with a vaginal discharge.

 Key Signs

- Clustered vesicles
- Painful erosions or ulcers
- Local swelling
- Regional lymphadenopathy

Laboratory Tests

1. Tzanck's smear (scrape base of a lesion, smear on a slide, and stain with Wright's or Giemsa's) can be done in the office; shows multinucleated giant cells often with inclusion bodies; does not distinguish between varicella-zoster virus and herpes simplex virus (HSV).
2. Viral culture taken by Dacron swab from scraped base of lesion into special media takes 2 to 14 days for results.
3. Antibody testing of sera is positive if fourfold or greater rise between acute and convalescent (at 2 weeks) samples.

 Key Tests

- Tzanck's smear
- HSV culture
- Antibody testing

Differential Diagnosis

1. Impetigo
2. Aphthous stomatitis
3. Herpangina

4. Syphilitic chancre
5. Stephens-Johnson syndrome
6. Varicella, coxsackievirus, or HSV may cause Kaposi's varicelliform eruption.

Treatment

1. May use topical Campho-Phenique for recurrent herpes labialis for local relief.
2. Occasionally children with severe gingivostomatitis may require intravenous hydration.
3. If patient is unable to void because of periurethral involvement, suggest sitting in warm bath or pouring cup of warm water over genitals to urinate.
4. Topical cool compresses with Burow's solution for 15 minutes four to five times daily may be soothing.
5. Women with a history of genital herpes or who have a sex partner with genital herpes should have HSV cultures obtained at delivery to aid in decisions for the newborn. Women with active genital lesions at the time of labor should have cesarean section; the neonate should be cultured and treated with intravenous acyclovir if cultures are positive or clinical disease develops.

Medication

1. Drugs of choice—see Table 286-1
2. IV acyclovir
   a. For severe initial genital HSV in normal host or any HSV in immunocompromised patient: 5 mg/kg (250 mg/m² for age <12 years) IV over 1 hour every 8 hours for 7 to 14 days
   b. For HSV encephalitis, neonatal HSV, or disseminated HSV: 10 mg/kg (500 mg/m² for age <12 years) IV over 1 hour every 8 hours for 14 to 21 days.

   c. Patients require adequate hydration during intravenous acyclovir administration.
   d. Adjust dosage for significant renal insufficiency.
   e. Because of safety concerns, reserve acyclovir use in pregnancy for IV treatment of severe or complicated HSV; notify the registry of the manufacturer and the Centers for Disease Control and Prevention (1-800-722-9292, ext. 58465).
3. HSV keratoconjuctivitis: Use trifluridine (Viroptic) 1% solution topically, 1 drop every 2 hours (up to 9 drops daily) for 10 days; care by ophthalmologist is recommended.
4. Alternative drugs
   a. Foscarnet (Foscavir), 40 mg/kg IV every 8 hours, for immunocompromised patients who develop episodic resistance to acyclovir, valacyclovir, and famciclovir.
   b. Cidofovir gel (Forvade) effective topically in acyclovir-resistant mucocutaneous herpes simplex in acquired immunodeficiency syndrome patients.

Diet

1. Normal diet usually
2. Nonacid solids or liquids for HSV gingivostomatitis

Patient Education

1. Avoid kissing or sexual intercourse until lesions are crusted.
2. Encourage use of condoms for all sexual intercourse that is not mutually monogamous, whether or not lesions are present.
3. Avoid contact with immunocompromised persons or neonates while lesions are active (not crusted).

TABLE 286-1.   ANTIVIRAL DRUGS OF CHOICE FOR HERPES SIMPLEX

DRUG	HERPES LABIALIS	PRIMARY GENITAL HERPES	RECURRENCE OF GENITAL HERPES	PROPHYLAXIS FOR GENITAL HERPES
Acyclovir* (Zovirax)		400 mg PO tid or 200 mg PO 5 times daily ×7-10 d	400 mg PO tid or 200 mg PO 5 times daily ×5 d	400 mg PO bid
Valacyclovir* (Valtrex)		1 gm PO bid ×10 d	500 mg PO bid ×5 d	500 mg PO qd for <10 episodes/yr; 1 gm PO qd for ≥10 episodes/yr
Famciclovir* (Famvir)		250 mg PO tid ×5-10 d†	125 mg PO bid ×5 d	250 mg PO bid
Penciclovir (Denavir) 1% cream	Topical q2h while awake for 4 days			

*Reduce dosages with significant renal insufficiency.
†Not approved by Food and Drug Administration for this indication.

4. Wash hands often both to prevent spread to others and to prevent autoinoculation of other sites.

5. Inform of widespread prevalence of HSV (>90 per cent of population) to put problem into perspective for the patient.

Key Treatment

- Topical compresses
- Penciclovir
- Acyclovir
- Valacyclovir
- Famciclovir

Follow-Up

1. Have patient return if complications are suspected (such as pneumonia) or if disease severity warrants more aggressive intervention.

2. For patients who take acyclovir, famciclovir, or valacyclovir chronically to suppress recurrences of genital HSV, monitor at least annually; try drug-free intervals and/or reduce the dose to least that remains effective in reducing recurrences.

Bibliography

Arbesfeld DM, Thomas I: Cutaneous herpes simplex infections. Am Fam Physician 1991;43:1655–1664.

Drugs for non-HIV viral infections. Med Lett 1997;39:69–76.

Dwyer DE, Cunningham AL: Herpes simplex virus infection in pregnancy. Ballieres Clin Obstet Gynecol 1993;7:75–105.

Glickman FS: Herpes simplex virus infection. Fam Pract Recertif 1993;15:21–32.

Vestry JP, Norval M: Mucocutaneous infections with herpes simplex virus and their management. Clin Exp Dermatol 1992;17:221–237.

287 Herpes Zoster Infection

Arthur R. Slaughter

Etiology

Varicella-zoster virus (VZV), a herpes DNA virus, causes a primary infection (*varicella*, or chickenpox), most often during childhood. After dormancy for months to years in the sensory ganglia, VZV then may cause *herpes zoster* (shingles) when reduction in cellular immunity allows the latent virus to spread along a dermatome, usually in adulthood.

Symptoms

1. Herpes zoster often has prodrome of burning, itching sensations in skin, or boring or sharp pains lasting hours to days before rash occurs.
2. Lesions appear along a specific dermatome, unilaterally.
3. These begin as red papules that become clustered vesicles, often with malaise, fatigue, or low-grade fever.
4. Vesicles become pustular or hemorrhagic by days 3 to 4.
5. Dry crusting occurs by 7 to 10 days and resolves by days 14 to 21, often leaving scars of varying pigmentation.
6. Pain usually resolves with the rash, but in about 15 per cent an irritating postherpetic neuralgia may persist for over 1 month after the rash, especially in persons over age 40 (in 50 per cent over age 60).
7. Herpetic neuralgia may occur without clinical evidence (zoster sine herpete).
8. Motor neuralgias occasionally occur with paralysis or paresis of the involved areas; these usually resolve within 1 year with minimal residua.
9. Immunocompromised persons may have lesions more diffusely and more severely.

Key Symptoms

- Painful prodrome
- Dermatome, unilateral
- Afebrile or low-grade fever

Clinical Findings

1. Zoster may present initially with no signs, with dysesthesia within a dermatome unilaterally, or with typical lesions.

2. Lesions start as small papules and then become vesicles, often in groups, all within a dermatome on one side.
3. Occasionally, one to three lesions may cross the midline or appear in remote sites.
4. By 3 to 4 days lesions are pustular or hemorrhagic; dry crusts form by 7 to 10 days and resolve by 2 to 3 weeks, often with scars of varying pigmentation.
5. Zoster ophthalmicus, involving the first division of the trigeminal nerve, requires ophthalmologic evaluation and therapy to optimally treat potential ocular involvement (in 50 per cent), especially if the nasociliary branch is involved (in 33 per cent), with lesions visible on the tip of the nose.

Key Signs

- Papules, vesicles, pustules
- Clear or cloudy appearance
- Umbilication, excoriation, crusting
- Dermatomal, unilateral
- Afebrile or low-grade fever

Laboratory Tests

1. Tzanck's smear from scraping of base of vesicle takes minutes and is positive in 75 per cent; a positive Tzanck's smear shows multinucleated giant cells but does not differentiate between varicella-zoster (VZV) and herpes simplex virus.
2. Viral culture from scraped base of lesion may require up to 2 weeks and is positive in 44 per cent.
3. Polymerase chain reaction technique, when clinically available, can be final in 24 hours and positive in 97 per cent; may be done on unstained slide made for Tzanck's smear.
4. Antibody testing, although useful for establishing cause, usually takes too long for clinical impact on contemporaneous diagnosis and treatment.

- Tzanck's smear

- Viral culture

- Antibody testing

Differential Diagnosis

1. Kaposi's varicelliform eruption
2. Dermatitis herpetiformis
3. Herpes gestationis (in pregnant patients)
4. Insect bites

Treatment

1. Soothing baths with baking soda added to water or topical compresses with Burow's solution applied 15 minutes four times daily may give symptomatic relief.
2. Non-narcotic analgesics such as acetaminophen may reduce pain of zoster.
3. For postzoster neuralgia, capsaicin cream (0.025%) applied three to five times daily may begin to decrease pain after 14 days.
4. Low-dose amitriptyline, begun at 10 to 25 mg daily, may reduce postzoster discomfort.

Medication

1. Drugs of choice
   a. Acyclovir, valacyclovir, or famciclovir may attenuate the duration and severity of zoster and may decrease the occurrence and duration of postherpetic neuralgia if given within 48 to 72 hours of onset of rash.

Key Drugs and Dosages for Herpes Zoster

- Acyclovir (Zovirax), 800 mg PO five times daily ×7 days

- Famciclovir (Famvir) 500 mg PO three times daily ×7 days

- Valacyclovir (Valtrex) 1000 mg PO three times daily × 7 days

- (Reduce all dosages in renal insufficiency.)

---

   b. Intravenous acyclovir, 10 mg/kg every 8 hours (500 mg/m² q8h in children) for 7 to 10 days, is indicated for patients with zoster who are severely immunocompromised.
2. Alternative drugs
   a. Foscarnet (Foscavir), may be considered for immunocompromised persons with zoster who do not respond to acyclovir.

   b. Vidarabine (Vira-A), 15 mg/kg/day over 12 hours IV for 7 days, occasionally is used in immunocompromised patients with zoster, but it is less efficacious and more toxic than acyclovir.
   c. Leukocyte interferon may decrease severity and number of days of new lesions but can also decrease granulocyte counts and cause fever and neurasthenia.
3. Universal childhood varicella vaccine
   a. Now recommended by the Advisory Committee on Immunization Practices, the American Academy of Pediatrics, and the American Academy of Family Physicians; may reduce the occurrence and severity of herpes zoster when compared to natural infection.
   b. For children ages 12 months through 12 years, a single 0.5-ml dose is given; for age 13 years and up, two doses at least 4 weeks apart.
   c. Early side effects include pain and redness at the injection site, a varicella-like rash at injection site (1 to 3 per cent; usually two to four lesions), and a mild varicella-like syndrome (1 to 4 per cent; afebrile with average of 42 lesions compared to febrile illness with average of 300 lesions with natural infection).
   d. In geriatric populations, the vaccine can bolster cell-mediated immunity.
   e. Controversy about universal varicella vaccination remains. Concerns include
      (1) The unknown duration of immunity
      (2) Decrease in the number of subclinical infections that currently help boost immunity
      (3) Whether future booster doses, if required, would actually be obtained by adults.
      (4) Whether more serious primary varicella may occur in an adult
      (5) Whether or not zoster will be prevented many years later.

Diet
No restrictions

Activity

1. Strict isolation is indicated for cases occurring in a hospital.
2. Health care workers who have no immunity and who have been exposed to an active case of varicella or active herpes zoster lesions should stay away from immunocompromised patients from days 10 to 21 after exposure

(days 10 to 28 if varicella immune globulin is given).

Patient Education

Warn patients to avoid exposure to all immuno-compromised individuals and pregnant women who are not immune to varicella-zoster virus.

Key Treatment

- Baths or compresses
- Antipruritics
- Avoid aspirin
- Analgesics: acetaminophen
- Acute medications: acyclovir, famciclovir, valacyclovir
- Postzoster neuralgia: capsaicin, amitriptyline

Follow-Up

Follow zoster patients until pain has resolved; on rare occasions of motor impairment, follow until improved significantly (usually by 1 year).

Bibliography

Brody MB, Moyer D: Varicella-zoster virus infection. Postgrad Med 1997;102:187–194.

Drugs for non-HIV viral infections. Med Lett 1997;39:69–76.

Levin MJ, Hayward AR: Prevention of herpes zoster. Infect Dis Clin North Am 1996;10:657–675.

Ljungman P: Herpes virus infections in immunocompromised patients: problems and therapeutic interventions. Ann Med 1993;25:329–333.

MacFarlane LL, Sanders ML, Carek PJ, et al: Concerns regarding universal varicella immunization. Arch Fam Med 1997;6:537–541.

288 Warts and Nevi

Virginia E. Robertson

Warts and nevi are generally benign skin lesions; however, certain subclasses of each are associated with premalignant conditions.

Warts

Etiology

1. All *verruca vulgaris* (warts) are caused by human papillomaviruses (HPVs).
2. Over 60 different types of HPV are known. Different types will be associated with different clinical manifestations, but there is overlap.
3. Some HPV types are found to have oncogenic potential.
   a. *Cervical intraepithelial neoplasia* is associated especially with HPV types 16 and 18, as well as types 31, 33, and 35.
   b. Benign HPV lesions may become associated with neoplasia in immunosuppressed hosts.
4. *Epidermodysplasia verruciformis* is a rare inherited disease that yields numerous HPV papules and macules.
   a. Degeneration into malignant lesions is common.
   b. It is believed to be autosomal recessive.

Symptoms

1. The cosmetic effect may be of most concern to the patient, depending on the size and location of the wart.
2. The patient will note a painless papule or a cluster of papules, generally asymptomatic, that are skin-toned.
3. *Plantar warts* may be painful or present as a foreign-body sensation in ambulatory patients.
4. Hoarseness may be prominent in patients with laryngeal warts.

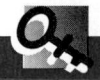
Key Symptom

Papular skin lesion

Clinical Findings

1. *Common warts* appear most often on the distal extremities and the face.
   a. Variably sized from 1 or 2 mm to 1 cm
   b. Firm, solid, nontender lesion
   c. Dome-shaped, sessile papule or nodule
   d. Hyperkeratotic, corrugated surface
   e. Skin-colored, with black punctae evident on close inspection, representing capillary loops
   f. Singular or clustered with satellite lesions from local spread. Clusters may become dense and matted.
2. *Flat warts* or *verruca plana* also may appear on the extremities and face, notably the eyelids, but may be less noticeable.
   a. Slightly raised, sessile lesions
   b. Smooth, flat-topped
   c. Skin-colored or slightly darker
3. *Plantar warts* occur on the sole of the foot, most often at high-pressure points such as the heel or metatarsal heads.
   a. Endophytic papule, partially or fully inverted (in nonmobile patients, may be more exophytic)
   b. Covered by thick callus
   c. Black punctae evident on close inspection (capillary loops) or after callus removed
   d. Tender with pressure
4. *Anogenital warts* or *condyloma acuminata* appear on the anogenital mucosal surfaces in women and men.
   a. A sexually transmitted disease (STD)
   b. Can resemble common warts in appearance or soft, pedunculated, moist lesions
   c. Single or clustered
   d. Skin-colored or hyperkeratotic (leukoplakia)
   e. On cervical epithelium, HPV can induce subclinical changes that may be noted only on Pap smear, colposcopy, or biopsy.
5. *Larnygeal warts* are most often found in infants and children and may cause obstruction, necessitating emergent care; hoarseness, stridor, and signs of respiratory distress.

Laboratory Tests

1. Diagnosis can usually be based on clinical findings.
2. Consider biopsy of suspect skin or mucosal lesions, including those resistant to therapy.
3. Pap smears can document HPV-associated cytology of the cervix.
4. Colposcopy with biopsy may be indicated when there are cervical cell changes (squamous intraepithelial lesions).

Differential Diagnosis

1. Simple plantar corns may be mistaken for plantar warts. Corns do not have black punctae and have a central translucency when the lesion is pared away.
2. Skin tags or seborrheic keratoses
3. Epidermal nevi and nevus sebaceus
4. Occasionally, premalignant and malignant lesions, including actinic keratoses and squamous cell carcinoma, may be mistaken for warts.

Treatment

A wide range of treatment options exists, all with side effects and none with a guaranteed cure. Treatment choice(s) depend on the type, location, size, responsiveness, cosmetic effect, and premalignant potential of the lesion and the side effects of the treatment.

1. *Watch and wait* may be acceptable for small common or flat warts, because a certain percentage of these will disappear without intervention over time.
2. *Chemical destruction* can be done in home or office:
   a. Presoak lesion in warm water for 5 minutes.
   b. Rub away loose wart with an emery board, pumice stone, or scalpel.
   c. Avoiding normal skin, apply agent to wart and cover with plaster or tape to improve penetrance.
   d. Repeat daily or bid for 2 to 3 months until response is adequate.
   e. Agents and side effects include
      (1) Topical salicyclic acid 15 to 40 per cent; local irritation may be relieved by temporary cessation of therapy.
      (2) Topical formalin, especially for plantar warts; drying and fissuring of skin with occasional allergic reaction
      (3) Weekly office application of caustic agents such as trichloroacetic acid 50%, washed off after 2 hours; occasional scarring of surrounding tissue
3. *Cryotherapy* by the clinician with liquid nitrogen or CO_2 can be used for any type of wart.
   a. Soak the lesion, then scrape excess keratin with scalpel blade.
   b. Using a cotton-tipped swab or spray attachment, apply agent directly and continuously to wart until a whitened halo of 1 to 2 mm appears around the base of the lesion.
   c. After the lesion has thawed, reapply a second time.
   d. Initially, the lesion will have an erythematous ring, then a blister may form with clear, cloudy, or hemorrhagic fluid. Patient may use a sterile needle to puncture the blister if painful or in an awkward location.
   e. The blister or wart will crust and fall off after 1 week; reapply cryotherapy if needed in 2- to 3-week cycles until adequate effect is achieved.
   f. Burning and throbbing, especially during the thaw phase, are uncomfortable but generally well tolerated by most patients.
   g. Side effects include occasional scarring, depigmentation or hyperpigmentation, and sensory loss depending on site.
4. *Pharmacologic agents* may be applied topically by clinician or patient or intralesionally by the clinician.
   a. Podophyllin, 25% resin solution, can be applied weekly by the clinician to plantar or anogenital warts. Systemic absorption can yield side effects when large surface areas are covered. Side effects include nausea and vomiting, seizures, peripheral neuropathy, and coma.
   b. Purified podophyllotoxin, 0.5% solution (Condylox), is available for home application by patients for anogenital warts. Side

effects are milder, generally only local erythema and irritation.

c. Cantharidin, 0.7% collodion solution (Cantharone) for common and plantar warts

(1) Application is followed by occlusion for 24 hours.

(2) A blister forms, which heals within a week.

(3) Major side effects are pain from the blister or formation of a ring wart (treatable).

d. Retinoic acid, 0.05% solution or 0.5% cream for flat warts

(1) Apply daily until desquamation occurs.

(2) Local irritation is the major side effect.

e. 5-Fluorouracil 5% for recalcitrant flat warts

f. Interferon intralesional injections

g. Bleomycin intralesional injections

5. *Surgery* is reserved for recalcitrant warts.

a. Electrosurgery

b. CO_2 laser

6. *Immunotherapy* also would be reserved for recalcitrant warts: dinitrochlorobenzene.

Patient Education

1. Careful counseling about treatment options, side effects, time course, and expected outcomes should occur before any therapy is begun.

2. For patients with anogenital warts, STD counseling is advisable, including recommendations for condom use, partner notification, and testing for other STDs as appropriate. Partners should be examined and treated.

Key Treatment

- Watch and wait
- Topical chemical agents
- Cryotherapy
- Topical podophyllin and other pharmacologic agents

Nevi

Etiology

Clustering of melanocytic nevus cells in the skin causes nevi or *moles*. Sun exposure is a key factor.

Symptoms

1. Generally asymptomatic, with patients noticing the presence or appearance of lesions in various locations. New nevi commonly form through middle age, especially in sun-exposed areas, but tend to regress in later years.

2. If itching or morphologic changes are noted, the clinician needs to consider whether malignant features are present.

Key Symptom

Presence of macule/papule

Clinical Findings

1. *Common acquired melanocytic nevi* are benign lesions that are subdivided into three classes, based on the location of the nevus cells in the skin. They have little potential for malignant degeneration.

a. Junctional nevi

(1) Pinpoint to few-millimeter macules

(2) Well-circumscribed

(3) Uniform in color; typically brown-black

(4) Widely distributed but especially in sun-exposed areas

b. Compound nevi

(1) Slightly elevated or dome-shaped

(2) Uniform in color; may have a hypopigmented "halo"

(3) Smooth surface but may become rough with age

c. Dermal nevi

(1) Dome-shaped, polypoid, pedunculated

(2) Skin-colored to black

(3) A variant is called a *blue nevus*, given its characteristic color

2. *Congenital nevi* may be premalignant lesions, especially giant congenital melanocytic nevi.

a. Present at birth; can be found on any skin surface.

b. Variably sized but may cover entire body parts

c. Medium-dark brown, variegated color across lesion

d. Rough or lobulated surface, increasingly so with age

e. Coarse hair growth

f. May involve leptomeninges if lesion occurs on head.

3. *Dysplastic nevi* can occur sporadically or following a familial, autosomal dominant pattern. These have premalignant potential.

a. Five- to 10-mm or larger macules or papules

b. Most often on trunks and limbs

c. Variegated in color within lesion: pink, tan, brown

d. Irregular border and surface

Key Signs

- Pigmented macule/papule

- Generally well circumscribed

- Other appearances, depending on type

Laboratory Tests

1. Clinical diagnosis of nevus/nevi is usually adequate.

2. Biopsy may be done for confirmation of initial diagnosis or for lesions with malignant characteristics.

Key Test

None or skin biopsy

Differential Diagnosis

1. Malignant melanoma

2. Squamous or basal cell carcinomas: Dermal nevi may be indistinguishable from basal cell carcinoma.

Treatment

Many nevi require no treatment. Those with malignant potential require careful monitoring for changes. Excision with adequate margins may be recommended for some nevi with high malignant potential, especially giant congenital melanocytic nevi.

Patient Education

1. Advise patient to look for possible indications of malignant changes.

a. Change in borders (e.g., less distinct, asymmetric, larger)

b. Change in pigmentation (e.g., more varied or stippled)

c. Crusting or bleeding, erosion

d. Pruritus, pain, tenderness

2. Adequate protection from sun exposure should be encouraged.

Key Treatment

- Monitor for changes

- Excision of some nevi

Follow-Up

Yearly complete skin examinations; more frequently (every 6 months or more) in patients with dysplastic nevi or other nevus conditions with high malignant potential

Bibliography

For general text and atlas, see
Fitzpatrick TB, Eisen AZ, Wolff K, et al: Dermatology in General Medicine, 4th ed. New York, McGraw-Hill, 1993.

For detailed review of wart treatments, see
Benton EC: Therapy of cutaneous warts. Clin Dermatol 1997;15:449–455.

For discussion of cervical HPV and dysplasia, see
Kitchener KC: The role of HPV in the genesis of cervical cancer. Cancer Treat Res 1994;70:29–41.

For review of research on HPV and skin carcinoma, see
Pfister H, Ter Schegget J: Role of HPV in cutaneous premalignant and malignant tumors. Clin Dermatol 1997; 15:335–347.

For discussion on atypical mole recognition and management, see
Williams ML, Sagebiel RW: Malanoma risk factors and atypical moles. West J Med 1994;160:343–350.

Cryosurgery

Indications

1. Treatment of warts and seborrheic and actinic keratoses
2. Treatment of epitheliomas should not be attempted without thermocouple temperature control apparatus and experience in this technique.

Contraindications

1. Melanocytes and neural tissue are more susceptible to cold injury than other anatomic structures.
2. Cryosurgery of skin lesions in African Americans and other darkly complected individuals can result in permanent depigmentation of the area.
3. Cryosurgery must be avoided over superficially situated motor nerves, including the ulnar nerve at the ulnar groove and the common peroneal nerve at the fibular condyle.
4. Cryosurgery over the digital nerves at the fingerwebs and lateral fingers usually results in temporary sensory deficit.

Preparation

1. Informed consent
2. Selection of appropriate lesions
3. Cleansing of the site. Not a sterile technique.

Equipment

1. Source of liquid nitrogen: Most dermatology offices have a tank of liquid nitrogen that is refilled when necessary by a supplier via tank truck.

2. Application apparatus
   a. Cotton swabs: Applicator stick with extra cotton, most commonly used with a styrofoam cup or metal-insulated flask with vented cap. If the metal (i.e., not disposable) flask is used each swab should be dipped in only once to avoid blood contamination. Glass-lined vacuum flasks should not be used because of danger of explosion.
   b. Spray apparatus (e.g., Cry-AC) is more efficient and eliminates danger of contamination of nitrogen.
3. Eye shields

Anesthesia

1. Anesthesia is usually not necessary.
2. EMLA cream somewhat helpful for brief freezing of, for example, flat warts
3. Local anesthesia may be administered (e.g., 1% plain lidocaine) to prevent pain.
4. Local anesthesia can be used to elevate a lesion, separating it from underlying nerves—for instance, over the lateral fingers.

Precautions

1. See "Contraindications."
2. Cryosurgery near the frontal and temporal hairlines can induce headaches.
3. Skin on penile shaft should be pouted to avoid freezing of corpora cavernosa, which is very painful.
4. Eyes must be protected, particularly from cryospray injury, with eyeshields or with cones to prevent spread of nitrogen. Cones can be purchased from manufacturers of the spray apparatus.

Technique

1. The swab is applied or the spray directed at the center of the lesion and the lesion frozen until a 1-mm halo of hard freeze is achieved.

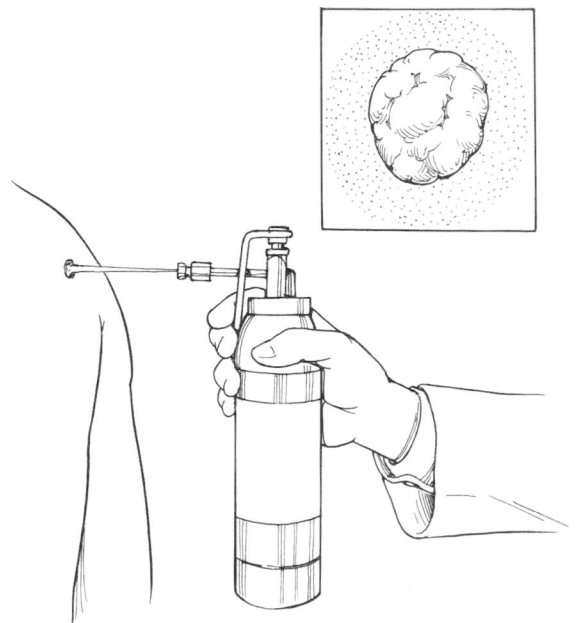

The **C** tip is useful for most applications. Tiny 1- to 2-mm lesions are most accurately treated with a pointed cotton swab.

2. The lesion is allowed to thaw and the procedure is repeated once. Thicker lesions require longer times to achieve complete freezing. Larger lesions require that the nitrogen be applied to more than one spot.

Follow-Up

1. A blister will ensue, frequently a hemorrhagic one.

2. Blister should be left intact in most instances and allowed to dry and slough in 10 to 14 days.

3. A very tense, painful bulla can be punctured in the office or at home with a sterilized needle.

4. Progressive spread of blisters, usually on the dorsal hand of elderly patients with atrophic skin, can be handled similarly to item 3.

5. If blister opens or is drained, lesion must be treated as an open wound with bacitracin, mupirocin, or povidone-iodine and dressing to prevent infection.

6. Analgesia usually not necessary, but pain may persist for up to a day, particularly on digits. Acetaminophen, aspirin, or ibuprofen can be used.

Electrosurgery

Indications

1. Destruction of benign skin lesions, including verrucae, benign keratoses, and skin tags

2. With curettage, destruction of appropriately selected small epitheliomas previously subjected to biopsy

3. Adjunctive after shave excision of benign melanocytic nevi for control of bleeding

Contraindications

1. Allergy to local anesthesia

2. Presence of a pacemaker or defibrillator

3. Suspicion of malignant melanoma

4. Large epithelioma

5. Epitheliomas not amenable to electrosurgical eradication (e.g., morpheaform basal cell carcinomas, many squamous cell carcinomas, tumors near tissue planes)

6. Lesions in areas where depressed scarring is likely (e.g., ala nasae) (a relative contraindication)

7. Lesions in areas where hypertrophic scarring is likely (a relative contraindication)

8. Surgery over nail matrix should be done with great caution to avoid injury.

9. Surgery near eyes should be done with caution to avoid ectropion, eye trauma.

Preparation

1. Informed consent

2. Selection of appropriate lesions

3. Cleansing of site; usually done in clean, not sterile, setting

Equipment

1. Gloves: Examination gloves adequate.

2. Mask with visor for eye protection or additional goggles.

3. Waterproof gown

4. Alcohol or povidone-iodine prep pads

5. Anesthesia in disposable syringe with disposable fine 27- to 30-gauge needle

6. No. 15 disposable scalpel blade for biopsy and biopsy container with formalin

7. 3 × 3 gauze pads or applicator sticks

8. Dermal curette, disposable or sterile

9. Appropriate electrosurgical instrument (e.g., Birtcher hyfrecator, Bovie with disposable tip or autoclaved tip and sleeve for working electrode)

Anesthesia

1. Use 1% or 2% lidocaine plain or with 1:100,000 epinephrine.
2. Isotonic saline can be used for brief procedures in the event of history of "Caine" allergy.
3. Epinephrine should be avoided in patients with arrhythmia, with significant hypertension, and those taking β-blockers.

Precautions

1. Patient should be in supine position.
2. Patient should not be in contact with ground (i.e., metal table parts).
3. See "Contraindications"; "Anesthesia."

Technique

1. Operative area is cleaned, lesion to be removed is anesthetized, and the area is draped if appropriate.
2. Eyes and mouth are protected where appropriate.
3. Shave biopsy or excision is performed when indicated (see "Indications").
4. Machine is set: a low setting appropriate for small lesions or those in close proximity to eyes; higher setting for larger lesions.
5. Electrode is brought in close proximity (fulguration) or in contact (desiccation) with the lesion or wound.

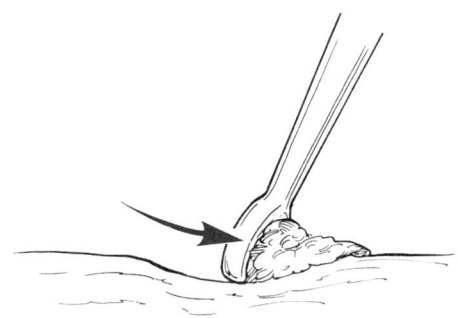

8. Desiccation/fulguration is again performed until homeostasis is complete. Electrosurgery instruments are ineffective in grossly bloody field. Wound can be kept from filling with blood by pressure with gauze pad or applicator stick, which is slowly withdrawn laterally as the wound or lesion is desiccated.

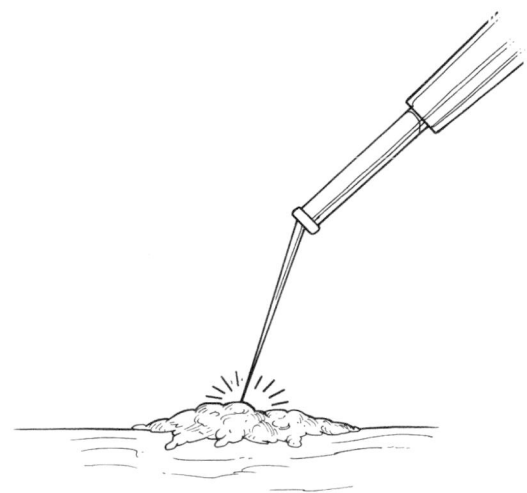

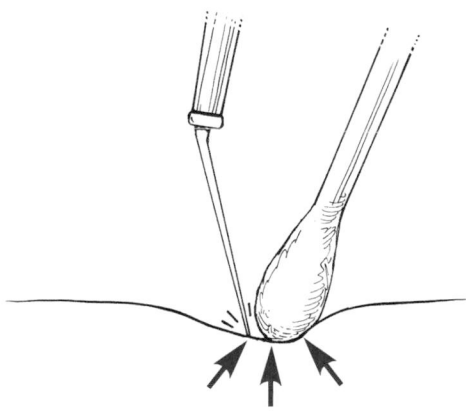

6. Foot or hand switch is depressed and held until lesion has been destroyed and bleeding stopped.
7. Curettage is performed on base of now dry wound until lesion removal is complete.

9. Procedure as outlined in items 7 and 8 is repeated at least three times or until curettage indicates complete removal of epithelioma.
10. Wound is dressed with gauze and bacitracin ointment or other suitable topical antiseptic or antibiotic.

Follow-Up

1. Wound care instructions: daily dressing change, application of bacitracin, mupirocin, povidone-iodine, or similar ointment and bandage

2. Occlusive dressings enhance comfort and speed re-epithelialization in wound healing studies.

3. Most facial wounds re-epithelialize in 10 to 14 days, trunk and extremity lesions in 14 to 21 days.

4. If biopsy is benign, no further follow-up is required.

5. Development of hypertrophic scars is possible in upper trunk electrosurgery, and patient should be so advised. Intralesional steroid injection is sometimes necessary.

Bibliography

Dawler RPR, Walker NPJ: Physical and surgical therapy. In Champion RH, Burton JL, Ebeling PJ (eds): Rook's Textbook of Dermatology, 5th ed, pp 3100–3111, 3113–3114. Boston, Blackwell, 1992.

Demetrius RW, Randle HW: High-risk nonmelanoma skin cancers. Dermatol Surg 1998;24:1272–1292.

Guidelines of American Academy of Dermatology on cryotherapy. Dermatol World 1993; August (Suppl).

Kuflik EG: Cryosurgery updated. J Am Acad Dermatol 1994;31:925–944.

Riordan AT, Gamete C, Fiasco SW: Electrosurgery and cardiac devices. J Am Acad Dermatol 1997;37:250–255.

289 Condyloma Acuminata

Anne Cather Cutlip

Etiology

1. Human papillomavirus (HPV) types 6 and 11 account for 90 per cent of the condyloma acuminata or genital warts (GW), the most prevalent viral sexually transmitted disease (STD) in the United States. It is believed that HPV gains access through microabrasions in the skin as may occur during sex. Condyloma may recur or persist after treatment, undergo malignant transformation, or regress spontaneously.

2. There are over 80 genotypes. More than one genotype can coexist in a patient. Types 6 and 11 are considered low risk, whereas types 16 and 18 are considered high risk for oncogenic potential. HPV is the strongest of the risk factors associated with cervical neoplasia.

3. Children may develop condylomata via infection during vaginal delivery or through sexual abuse. Manual contact or direct contact with fomites can be a possible etiology.

4. Risk factors for condyloma include
   a. Sex with an infected partner.
   b. Increased number of lifetime sexual partners.
   c. Increased number of years of sexual activity.
   d. History of STD (e.g., *Chlamydia trachomatis*)
   e. Cigarette smoking
   f. Lack of condom use

5. About two thirds of persons whose sexual partner has condylomata will themselves develop condylomata within an average of 3 months (range 1 to 9 months). A large percentage of persons develop subclinical infection. Autoinoculation is possible.

6. Areas of clinically apparent disease may represent a small amount of the actual infected area. If GW are seen in area of the anogenital tract, infection is likely elsewhere.

7. The greatest prevalence is between ages 17 and 33. Males more commonly have overt disease. Females have a higher prevalence of infection.

Symptoms

1. GW are usually asymptomatic except for obvious presence of palpable lesion.

2. Some patients complain of pruritis, burning, pain, or bleeding.

Clinical Findings

1. Pink to flesh-colored, papillomatous, pedunculated or sessile mass in the anogenital area or other moist areas. May be pigmented.

2. Single or multiple lesions. Initially small but may grow, become confluent, and form a cluster or "cauliflower" mass. Giant condylomata, flesh or brown colored, have uncertain malignant potential.

3. Males commonly develop condylomata on the distal half of penis. Uncircumcised men will more often have GW on inner aspect of foreskin. GW are less common on the scrotum, meatus, and anus.

4. Females commonly develop condylomata on the posterior introitus, fourchette, and labia minora. Can also be found on the clitoris, vagina, cervix, urethra, and anus.

Key Signs

- Papillomatous, pedunculated or sessile
- Pink or flesh colored
- Anogenital area
- Single or multiple
- Small (1 to 2 mm) to giant size

Laboratory Tests

1. Diagnosis is usually made clinically, based on typical appearance and location. Magnification or colposcopy allows for detection of clinically unapparent lesions. Anoscopy should be available. Application of 3% to 5% acetic acid typically produces an "acetowhitening" of the condyloma within several minutes. This is not diagnostic.

2. No culture methods are available. Testing for seroreactivity to several proteins of the oncogenic HPV types (types 16 and 18) is available.

3. Histology and cytology can confirm the diagnosis. Typical histologic features include koilocytes (large epithelial cells with small, dense nuclei and clear perinuclear areas) and hyperkeratosis, dyskeratosis, or acanthosis.

4. HPV DNA–detecting assays are not usually used to screen. Typing may be used to identify which lesions may be at greater risk for progressing to cancer. Current methods include Southern blot, dot blot, in situ hybridization, polymerase chain reaction (PCR), and solution hybridization. Of these, PCR is the most sensitive.

Differential Diagnosis

1. Common benign lesions: verruca vulgaris (common wart), seborrheic keratoses, nonpigmented nevi, pearly penile papules (1 to 2 mm papules on proximal edge of the glans), vulvar vestibular papillae (benign, bilateral papillae)

2. Sexually transmitted lesions: condyloma latum (moist, rounded, white papule of syphilis), molluscum contagiosum (smooth, round papule with central umbilication)

3. Neoplastic lesions: bowenoid papulosis (flat, multicentric, resembles warts; may regress, or progress to squamous cell carcinoma), Bowen's disease (flat, whitish plaque with well-defined borders; may be ulcerated), malignant melanoma

Treatment

1. Before treatment, biopsy is important to rule out malignancy in suspicious lesions: giant or rapidly growing condylomata; pigmented, friable, ulcerated, or confluent hyperkeratotic lesions, or rapid recurrence after treatment.

2. Examine entire anogenital tract because of widespread nature of HPV. Consider testing for other STDs because of frequent coexistence.

3. No single procedure is remarkably superior to any other. Treatment modality should be guided by patient preference and consideration of the number of office visits, expense, response, convenience, and potential for adverse effects.

4. No therapy effectively eliminates HPV infection and replication or prevents associated progression toward malignancy.

5. Recurrence rate for any treatment regimen is generally 30 per cent. Up to 70 per cent of HPV infections regress after 24 months. The factors associated with regression are undefined.

6. There are no studies determining if exophytic GW versus subclinical infections are more infectious, or whether removal of warts reduces transmission.

7. Treatment options: Pretreatment with lidocaine/prilocaine (EMLA) cream provides relief of pain for the procedures noted below.

   a. Physical treatments

   (1) Cryotherapy (liquid nitrogen or nitrous oxide): freeze until iceball extends several millimeters beyond the base of the lesion. Repeat every 1 to 2 weeks until clear. Usual treatment of choice because of few complications and safety in pregnancy. May need local anesthesia.

   (2) Local excision: simple excision, punch biopsy, or loop electrosurgical excisional procedure (LEEP). Easy and available in most offices. Safe in pregnancy. Use local anesthesia.

   (3) Electrocautery: not an initial treatment. Wear mask to avoid viral particles in the plume. Use local anesthesia. Expensive.

   (4) CO_2 laser vaporization: not an initial treatment. Wear mask to avoid viral particles in the plume. Requires expert skills. Use local or general anesthesia. Expensive.

   b. Chemical treatments

   (1) Trichloroacetic acid (TCA) or bichloroacetic acid (BCA): up to 80 per cent acid in 70% ethyl alcohol applied with cotton applicator (by physician or patient) once to twice a week until clear. Can be used on the vagina, cervix, or penis.

   (2) Podofilox (Condylox): 0.5% solution of purified podophyllotoxin applied to external warts twice a day for 3 consecutive days, withheld for 4 days, and then the cycle repeated weekly for total of 4 weeks. Side effects include burning, pain, inflammation, and erosion. Avoid use in perianal or mucous membrane areas. Patients may apply. No pregnancy use data available.

   (3) 5-Fluorouracil (5-FU) 5% cream: most often used for vaginal or periurethral warts or as prophylaxis after ablation. Typically one-third to one-half vaginal applicatorful once a week for 8 weeks. Recheck patient every 2 weeks. Can cause extensive erosions and scarring of vaginal and vulvar tissues and urethral strictures. Avoid in pregnancy. Newer studies of 5-FU/epinephrine gel administered as an injection show promising response rates.

   (4) Imiquimod: 5% cream applied three times a week at night and washed off 6 to 10 hours later. Side effects include erythema, erosion, and excoriation. Unknown safety during pregnancy. Food

and Drug Administration approved for patient application.

(5) Interferon-α group (alfa-2b [Intron A], alfa-n3 [Alferon N]): multiple intralesional injections several times a week. Use for refractory warts, not first-line therapy. Major side effect is flu-like symptoms. Expensive.

(6) Vaccines (prophylactic or therapeutic) are unlikely to be introduced in the near future.

Diet

No specific diet has been recognized to prevent, treat, or cause regression of condylomata.

Activity

Abstain from sexual activity during treatment; otherwise, activities as tolerated.

Patient Education

The key to prevention is education of those patients at risk about the nature of condylomata. Patients will continue to carry the virus and to have a potential for neoplasm. Encourage regular examinations and smoking cessation. Stress condom use and monogamy. Condoms are not 100 per cent effective. Many support groups are available.

Key Treatment

Physical	Chemical
• Cryotherapy	• TCA or BCA
• Local excision	• Podofilox
• Electrocautery	• 5-FU
• CO$_2$ laser vaporization	• Imiquimod
	• Interferon-α

Follow-Up

1. Treat until all condylomata are gone.
2. Infected patients should be thoroughly examined (including Pap smears) every 6 to 12 months initially. Some recommend a screening colposcopy at diagnosis.
3. Patients will be concerned about social stigma, pain, and spread of HPV. Counseling is important because patients may experience fear, shock, and disgust and develop feelings of decreased self-worth. Encourage partner notification. Suggest support groups.

Bibliography

Mayeaux EJ, Harper MB, Barksdale W, et al: Noncervical human papillomavirus genital infections. Am Fam Physician 1995;52:1137–1146.

Munk C, Savre EI, Poll P, et al: History of genital warts in 10,838 women 20 to 29 years of age from the general population: risk factors and association with Papanicolaou smear history. Sex Transm Dis 1997;24: 567–572.

Stone KM: Human papillomavirus infection and genital warts: update on epidemiology and treatment. Clin Infect Dis 1995;.20(Suppl 1):S91–S97.

Sykes NL: Condyloma acuminatum. Int J Dermatol 1995; 34:297–302.

Tyring S (ed): Perspectives on human papillomavirus infection. Am J Med 1997;102(5A):1–43.

290 Leukoplakia and Erythroplasia

John G. Spangler

Etiology

1. Cigarette or smokeless tobacco use
2. Repetitive oral trauma (malpositioned teeth, ill-fitting dentures, habitual cheek biting)
3. Long-term, excessive alcohol consumption
4. Oral infections; unproven roles of herpes simplex virus and human papillomavirus
5. Rarely, metabolic disturbances (e.g., avitaminosis A)
6. Betel nut chewing, lime-tobacco mixtures (Southeast Asia)
7. Large percentage of idiopathic cases

Symptoms

1. Usually asymptomatic (over 95 per cent of cases)
2. "Roughness" at site of lesion occasionally noticed.
3. Pain or ulceration rare but strongly associated with malignancy.

Key Symptoms

- Usually asymptomatic
- Roughness
- Pain (rare)

Clinical Findings

1. Leukoplakia: white surface mucosal lesions that do not wipe off
   a. Clinical appearance varies and may be
      (1) Thin, almost nonpalpable or thick, dense lesions
      (2) Faintly translucent white or speckled red and white or opaque gray colors
      (3) Single lesion (large or small) or scattered lesions with or without adjacent ulcerations
      (4) Associated with candidal superinfection (unfavorable sign but unknown if etiologic agent)
   b. Location
      (1) Fifty per cent of cases occur on tongue, mandibular alveolar ridge, and buccal mucosa; less frequently, palate, maxillary alveolar ridge, floor of mouth, retromolar regions
      (2) In smokeless tobacco or betel nut chewers, lesions usually occur at habitual site of quid placement.
      (3) Tongue and floor of mouth lesions have highest incidence of malignant transformation.
   c. Patient characteristics
      (1) Incidence unknown, but peak onset in fourth decade of life.
      (2) May occur in youths who use tobacco heavily (especially smokeless forms).
      (3) Male/female ratio greater than 2:1.
      (4) Leukoplakia in nonusers of tobacco has highest rate of malignant transformation (24 per cent).
   d. Histology ranges from hyperkeratosis to dysplasia to invasive carcinoma.
   e. Clinical course
      (1) One third regress with time, but may spontaneously recur.
      (2) Between 2 and 15 per cent (average 5 per cent) progress to carcinoma, especially if dysplasia found on biopsy.
      (3) Rest remain essentially unchanged.
   f. Malignant transformation more likely if
      (1) Tongue or floor of mouth location
      (2) Any redness to lesion (see below)
      (3) Papillomatous or verrucous appearance
      (4) Leukoplakia in tobacco nonuser
      (5) Continued exposure to irritants
      (6) Possible increased risk if there is overlying candidal infection.
2. Erythroplasia: bright red mucosal plaques or erosions
   a. Often associated with leukoplakia (erythroleukoplakia)
   b. Malignant potential greatly increased with any red component to leukoplakic lesion; 90 per cent of erythroleukoplakia is dysplastic or worse.

Key Signs

White Lesions	Increased Malignant Potential if
• Do not wipe off.	• Tongue, floor of mouth, or soft palate location
• Single or multiple lesions	• Any redness
• Nonpalpable or thick	• Papillomatous features
• Red component (erythroplakia)	• Nonuser of tobacco
	• Candidal superinfection

Laboratory Tests

1. Biopsy
   a. Necessary for definitive diagnosis
   b. Biopsy lesions at high risk for malignancy, such as lesions on tongue, lesions with overlying candidiasis, and verrucous or papillary lesions, and all red areas.
   c. Toluidine blue (tolonium chloride), a vital stain, helps direct biopsy to areas most likely to contain dysplasia or malignancy.
   d. If biopsy of small lesions suspected to be malignant will distort appearance, or if lesions are in areas difficult to access (e.g., base of tongue, piriform fossa), then physician who will perform definitive treatment should see lesion and preferably perform biopsy.
   e. Both incisional and punch biopsy techniques are acceptable.
   f. Large lesions may require multiple biopsies.
2. Cytologic smears
   a. Not a replacement for biopsy; helps to confirm clinical suspicion only, but cannot treat cancer on basis of cytologic smear alone.
   b. Analogous to Papanicolaou smears in collection and staining

Key Tests

- Biopsy for definitive diagnosis
- Toluidine blue to highlight dysplastic areas
- Cytologic smears (not a substitute for biopsy)

Differential Diagnosis

1. Lichen planus: frequently symptomatic, especially if erosive

2. Oral hairy leukoplakia: lingual manifestation of acquired immunodeficiency syndrome caused by Epstein-Barr virus
3. Systemic lupus erythematosus
4. White sponge nevus
5. Hereditary keratosis

Treatment

1. Remove or correct chronic irritants to allow inflammatory processes to heal. Treat *Candida* infection if KOH smear is positive for yeast; follow-up in 2 weeks.
2. Biopsy if high-risk lesions (see above) that persist at follow-up.
3. All lesions with histopathologic dysplasia must be totally excised.
   a. Carbon dioxide laser (most effective and frequently used)
   b. Electrodesiccation
   c. Cryotherapy
   d. Knife excision

Medication

Vitamin A derivatives and other antioxidants (e.g., vitamin C, vitamin E) show promise but as yet are not routinely recommended because of side effects or unknown long-term effects. Antifungal agents will not remove true leukoplakia.

Patient Education

1. Patients must understand 2 to 15 per cent potential for malignant transformation even of relatively benign-appearing lesions.
2. Importance of cessation of tobacco, alcohol, or other etiologic factors must be stressed, as well as follow-up.

Key Treatment

- Remove irritants.
- Treat *Candida* if present.
- Excise all dysplastic lesions:
  - CO_2 laser
  - Electrodesiccation
  - Cryotherapy
  - Knife excision
- Follow up regularly

Follow-Up

Regular follow-up is mandatory to detect appearance of dysplastic change or new lesions.

Bibliography

Axell T, Pindborg JJ, Smith CJ, et al: Oral white lesions with special reference to precancerous and tobacco-related lesions: conclusions of an international symposium held in Uppsala, Sweden, May 18–21, 1994. J Oral Pathol Med 1996;25:49–54.

Kaugars GE, Silverman S Jr, Lovas JG, et al: Use of antioxidant supplements in the treatment of human oral leukoplakia. Oral Surg Oral Med Oral Pathol 1996;81:5–14.

Lumerman H, Freedman P, Kerpal S: Oral epithelial dysplasia and the development of invasive squamous cell carcinoma. Oral Surg Oral Med Oral Pathol 1995;79:321–329.

Mashberg A, Samit A: Early diagnosis of asymptomatic oral and oropharyngeal squamous cancers. CA Cancer J Clin 1995;45:328–351.

Sciubba JJ: Oral leukoplakia. Crit Rev Oral Biol Med 1995;6:147–160.

Silverman S Jr: Oral Cancer, 4th ed. Hamilton, Ontario, BC Decker, Inc, 1998.

Silverman S Jr, Bhargava K, Mani NH, et al: Malignant transformation and natural history of oral leukoplakia in 57,518 industrial workers of Gujarat, India. Cancer 1976;38:1790.

291 Calluses and Corns

Janet L. Purkey

Calluses

Etiology

1. Hyperkeratotic lesions on the plantar surface of the foot caused by friction and pressure
   a. Natural protective barrier
   b. Becomes problematic when the underlying structures are irritated by hardened buildup.
2. Structural defects
   a. Excessive pronation causing abnormal pressure on the metatarsal heads
   b. Hammer toes, subluxation, and trauma
   c. Change in weight bearing, such as associated neuropathy
3. Improperly fitted footwear
   a. High heels, dancers (especially ballet), and athletes who wear poorly fitted shoes
   b. Proper footwear with abnormal weight bearing (see above)

Symptoms

1. Pain on weight bearing
2. Pruritus and burning

Clinical Findings

1. A circumscribed area of varying size of hypertrophied and keratinized skin on the plantar surface
2. Callus may form on any area exposed to abnormal pressure and friction.

WARNING

The diabetic patient needs special attention to the foot examination because ulceration and infection involving callus increase morbidity.

 Key Signs

- Circumscribed area of hypertrophied and keratinized skin on plantar surface primarily over metatarsophalangeal joints

- May be noted on any area of the forefoot

Laboratory Tests

None

Differential Diagnosis

1. Plantar keratosis is usually an inherited condition of hyperkeratosis.
2. Plantar wart caused by human papillomavirus is differentiated in that it is not histologically similar and usually does not occur over the metatarsophalangeal joints.

Treatment

1. Educating the patient concerning home care
   a. Weekly use of a pumice stone or emery board
   b. Care must be taken not to disrupt the healthy epithelium.
   c. Softening the callus in a 20-minute warm soak prior to exfoliation
   d. The diabetic patient must *not* damage healthy skin or cause the callus to bleed.
   e. A small amount of callus must be left to provide protection.
2. Office care for painful callus
   a. Immediate improvement obtained by débridement with a surgical blade.
   b. Paring the callus with small parallel strokes allows for safe débridement.
   c. May be needed as often as every 2 or 3 months.
3. Preventing calluses requires replacement of offending footwear.
   a. Educate the patient on proper footwear.
   b. An appropriate fit involves proper length, width, depth of "toe box," and placement of the seams.
   c. Low-heeled and soft-soled shoes provide benefit.
   d. Custom footwear is an investment in foot care.
   e. Diabetic patients should wear leather enclosed-toe footwear.
4. Padding around pressure points
   a. A comma-shaped pad or "cookie" placed proximal to the prominent metatarsal head reduces pressure.

b. Special insoles relieve pressure points.

c. Moleskin is easily shaped for added comfort.

5. Topical keratolytic therapy for the recalcitrant callus

   a. Dilute solution of salicylic acid (15% to 20%, up to 40%) applied under an occlusive dressing for 1 to 7 days followed by débridement.

   b. Other keratolytic agents

      (1) Whitfield's ointment

      (2) Lactic acid in propylene glycol

      (3) Glycolic acid 20% in petrolatum

   c. Diabetic patients should not use any keratolytic agent because it may damage adjacent healthy skin.

6. Referral to an orthopedist or podiatrist

   a. Surgical correction of structural defects

      (1) The malaligned metatarsal head can be corrected.

      (2) Other bony prominences may be reduced surgically.

      (3) Procedures that lessen or eliminate excessive pronation

   b. Referral to a foot specialist for nonsurgical treatment as well

      (1) Débridement of patients with diabetes mellitus, peripheral vascular disease, rheumatoid arthritis

      (2) These specialists provide many of the special metatarsal pads, insoles, and molds that enhance nonsurgical therapy.

Key Treatment

- Educating patient concerning home care
  –Weekly use of pumice stone or emery board
  –Soften callus in a warm soak

- Office care for painful callus
  –Débridement with surgical blades

- Topical keratolytic therapy

- Surgical correction of structural defects

Follow-Up

1. Patients must wear properly fitted shoes.

2. Patients should be encouraged to use the pumice stone at home on a regular basis.

3. If these measures fail to eliminate a painful callus, patients should be followed in the office often for débridement.

4. Referral to an orthopedist or podiatrist should be based on the response to conservative measures.

Corns

Etiology

1. "Corns," "clavi," or "helomas" refer to small, hard, conical hyperkeratoses over a bony prominence caused by pressure and friction.

2. Accumulation of several layers of epidermis with an underlying avascular translucent central core

3. Ill-fitting shoes are a primary cause of the epidermal buildup.

4. Structural deformities

   a. Hammer toes with exostosis

   b. Other abnormal bony prominences

Symptoms

1. Corns produce pain when the foot is squeezed and placed in a tightly fitted shoe.

2. Plantar corns produce pain when weight bearing.

Clinical Findings

1. Hard corns are keratotic lesions most commonly observed on the dorsum of the lesser toes and lateral aspect of the fifth toes.

2. Soft corns are found in the web space between the toes.

   a. Most commonly observed in the fourth web space.

   b. The pressure point lies between two adjacent phalanges.

   c. The maceration of the corn in the moist web space makes it "soft."

3. Plantar clavi or seed corns are conical-shaped hyperkeratotic epidermal lesions with a central portion extending toward sensitive subcutaneous tissue found on the plantar surface of the foot.

Key Signs

- Hard corns most commonly observed on lateral aspect of fifth toe.

- Soft corns most commonly observed in fourth web space.

- Plantar corns are conical-shaped and have a central portion extending toward sensitive subcutaneous tissue.

Laboratory Tests
None

Differential Diagnosis
1. Plantar warts look like hyperkeratosis; however, they are quite vascular compared with corns.
2. Foreign bodies with secondary keratosis
3. In diabetics, ulcerations and infection must be ruled out.

Treatment
1. Débriding the excessive buildup of epidermis is crucial to treatment (See "Calluses").
2. Enucleation of the apex or central portion of the plantar corn
3. Aperture or corn pads reduce pressure over bony prominences.
4. Moleskin, lamb's wool, silicone toe splints relieve pressure from the tender central core.
5. Footwear with adequate length, width, and depth in the "toe box."
6. Liquid nitrogen and keratolytics are useful in plantar corns that are recalcitrant to other therapy. (See "Keratolytic Agents" under callus "Treatment".)
7. Referral to an orthopedist or podiatrist when above measures fail

Key Treatment

- Débridement of excessive buildup of epidermis
- Enucleation of apex or central portion of plantar corn
- Corn pads reduce pressure over bony prominences.
- Adequate footwear
- Liquid nitrogen and salicylic acid

Follow-Up
Same as under "Calluses."

Bibliography

Brahms MA: Corns and deformities of the small toes. In Jahss MH (ed): Disorders of the Foot and Ankle, 2nd ed, pp 1175–1197. Philadelphia, WB Saunders Company, 1991.

Day RD: Evaluation and management of interdigital corn. Clin Podiatr Med Surg 1996;13:201–206.

Dishan S, Singh D, Bentley G, et al: Callosities, corns and calluses. BMJ 1996;312:1403–1406.

George DH: Management of hyperkeratotic lesions in the elderly patient. Clin Podiatr Med Surg 1993;10:69–77.

Gordon GM: Exercise and the aging foot. South Med J 1994;87:36–41.

Richards RN: Calluses, corns, and shoes. Semin Dermatol 1991;10:112–114.

292 Lipoma

Joseph W. Gravel, Jr.

Lipomas are the most common soft tissue tumors (48 per cent) and are composed of fat cells in a thin fibrous capsule. They are freely mobile, subcutaneous masses with a rubbery consistency, most often small (1 to 3 cm) and solitary. However, many patients have large (>15 cm) and/or multiple tumors. By far the most common sites are the trunk, neck, proximal extremities, and axillae. Lipomas occur in all age groups but usually become manifest in middle age.

Etiology

1. Fifty to 80 per cent of solitary lipomas arise from a definable chromosomal abnormality; many of the cytogenetically "normal" lipomas probably have subtle changes not demonstrable by current methods of analysis.

2. Chromosomes 12 (30 per cent), 13 (13 per cent), and 6 (8 per cent) are the most commonly affected. The chromosome 12 abnormality has been localized to activation of the *HMGI-C* gene.

3. Multiple lipomas are more often angiolipomas. These are small, usually numerous, develop in younger people, are composed of fat cells and blood vessels (mostly capillaries), and have normal karyotypes.

4. Lipomas can also arise secondary to trauma, possibly from local inflammation inducing adipocyte proliferation.

5. Familial multiple lipomatosis is a fairly common condition, transmitted via an autosomal dominant inheritance pattern that becomes clinically apparent in the third and fourth decades.

6. Lipomas can also be part of several rare syndromes, including adiposis dolorosa (Dercum's disease), benign symmetric lipomatosis (Madelung's disease), congenital lipomatosis, and proteus syndrome. These are all idiopathic.

7. Multiple endocrine neoplasia type I (MEN-I) gene mutation may play a role in both MEN-I–associated lipomas and sporadic lipomas.

Symptoms

1. Most lipomas present as a small, localized, subcutaneous fatty tumor, the most bothersome symptom being a change in the skin contour. Regardless of their size, lipomas frequently engender a great deal of concern in patients until the physician can provide reassurance.

2. Lipomas usually do not cause pain unless they compress nerves or blood vessels. They are normally nontender, compressible, and freely mobile.

3. Trauma to lipomas can disrupt blood supply, causing necrosis and possible subsequent tenderness, hemorrhage, fibrosis, and/or calcification.

 Key Symptoms

- Change in skin contour/"lump"
- Usually painless (but may become painful)

Clinical Findings

1. Most lipomas are small (1 to 3 cm) and asymptomatic.

2. On palpation, they are usually nontender, well-circumscribed, freely mobile subcutaneous masses with a rubbery consistency. They rarely extend into fascia or muscle.

3. Lipomas generally occur on the trunk, neck, proximal extremities, and axillae. However, lipomas can occur almost anywhere in the body, including the joints (lipoma arborescens), colon, mesentery, spermatic cord, lung, pancreas, nasopharynx, heart, middle ear, retroperitoneal space, and (in children) the spinal canal.

4. Solitary lipomas occur with nearly equal frequency in men and women. Multiple lipomas occur more frequently in men.

5. Larger lesions, especially on the neck and back, may extend deeper than is apparent. For these lesions, consider excision in an operating room and/or surgical referral.

 Key Signs

- Nontender, rubbery, freely mobile mass
- Look for *peau d'orange* sign with lateral compression

Laboratory Tests

1. Most common test done is histologic diagnosis following excision or core biopsy.
   a. Lipomas consist of sheets of normal adipocytes interspersed with thin strands of fibrous tissue.
   b. Histologic diagnosis distinguishes benign lipomas from malignant liposarcomas (relatively rare), although this can usually be done on the basis of history and clinical findings.
   c. Histologic diagnosis also identifies uncommon benign lipomatous variants: angiolipoma, spindle cell/pleomorphic lipoma, angiomyolipoma, myelolipoma, chondroid lipoma, atypical lipoma (also known as well-differentiated liposarcoma of subcutis), lipoblastomas (seen in infants and young children), and hibernoma (lipoma of brown fat).
2. Ultrasonography can be used to distinguish lipomas from cystic masses.
3. Magnetic resonance imaging (MRI) (fat-suppressed T_1-weighted images enhanced with Gd-DTPA) can distinguish lipoma (thin-walled septa that do not enhance) from liposarcoma (enhanced thick septa with muscle fibers).
4. Fine-needle aspiration to differentiate lipoma from liposarcoma is not recommended because of a high false-negative rate.

Key Tests

- Histologic diagnosis of tissue is definitive.
- Ultrasonography if suspect cyst, MRI if suspect liposarcoma

Differential Diagnosis

1. Sebaceous cyst, abscess, dermoid cyst, ganglion cyst, thyroglossal duct cyst, lymph node, metastatic cancer (especially from breast, colon, ovary, carcinoid, malignant melanoma), liposarcoma or other soft-tissue sarcomas, diabetic lipodystrophy, acute panniculitis (nodular fat necrosis)
2. Most sarcomas present as painless, hard masses. Liposarcomas are softer than other sarcomas but firmer, less mobile than lipomas.
3. Larger masses (>10 cm) should be further evaluated, as should lymph nodes that are greater than 2 cm in diameter.
4. Firm, irregular, fixed masses should be biopsied.
5. Some sarcomas present with pain, heat, and skin changes resembling an abscess. Consider sarcoma if infection does not clear with antibiotics or center has necrotic, cheesy material.

Treatment

1. Reassurance of the patient with monitoring for changes is the standard treatment of lipoma.
2. If removal is desired, this can be easily performed by open surgical excision under local anesthesia, usually in the office. Deep sutures are normally needed for optimal wound closure.
3. Laparoscopic excision is becoming used more frequently to minimize scarring, particularly in cosmetically important areas.
4. Liposuction can be used for large lipomas when the diagnosis is ensured, but should not be done without a prior biopsy.

Medication

Steroid injections have been tried but are not generally effective.

Diet

There is no known correlation between diet and either onset or growth of lipomas.

Activity

Other than trauma, activity has no effect on lipomas.

Patient Education

1. If confident of the diagnosis, reassure the patient by emphasizing that lipomas are benign with no possibility of malignant transformation.
2. No prophylaxis is known to prevent lipomas or affect their growth.
3. No treatment is required unless the lipoma becomes symptomatic or for cosmesis.
4. Excision is generally a simple office procedure requiring only local anesthesia.
5. Recurrence rate is extremely low unless excision is incomplete.
6. Explain to the patient the characteristics of a lipoma: rubbery, freely mobile, well-circumscribed, and so forth, versus a hard, fixed, irregular mass (which would indicate need for further evaluation).

Key Treatment

- Reassurance
- Excision
- Liposuction

Follow-Up

1. Routine postoperative wound care after excision: Monitor for infection, seroma, hematoma, and wound dehiscence.
2. After initial evaluation, follow-up is unnecessary in the absence of a change in the lipoma.

Bibliography

Anders KH, Ackerman AB: Neoplasms of the subcutaneous fat. In Fitzpatrick TB, Eisen AZ, Wolff K, et al (eds): Dermatology in General Medicine, 4th ed, vol 1, pp 1348–1353. New York, McGraw-Hill, 1993.

Hosono M, Kobayashi H, Fujimoto R, et al: Septum-like structures in lipoma and liposarcoma: MR imaging and pathologic correlation. Skeletal Radiol 1997;26:150–154.

Munk PL, Lee MJ, Janzen DL, et al: Lipoma and liposarcoma: evaluation using CT and MR imaging. AJR 1996;169:589–594.

Rubin BP, Fletcher CDM: The cytogenetics of lipomatous tumors. Histopathology 1997;30:507–511.

Weiss SW: Lipomatous tumors. Monogr Pathol 1996;38:207–239.

Indications

1. Unsightly or bothersome
2. Recurrent infections or inflammation
3. Increasing size
4. Foul-smelling discharge
5. Pain or tenderness

Contraindications

1. Acute inflammation (requires incision and drainage, if fluctuant, followed by excision after inflammation has resolved)
2. Bleeding disorder

Preparation

1. Obtain informed consent.
2. Assemble equipment.
3. Prepare container for pathology specimen.

Equipment

1. Small procedure tray
   a. 4 × 4 gauze sponges
   b. Small curved scissors (Metzenbaum or iris scissors)
   c. Scalpel handle and No. 15 blade
   d. Small curved hemostats (2)
   e. Needle holder
   f. Small-toothed (Adson) forceps
   g. Fenestrated sterile drape
2. Povidone-iodine swabs
3. Syringe (6 ml) and needles (20- and 27- or 30-gauge)
4. Sterile gloves

5. Surgical masks
6. Face shield or goggles (universal precautions for human immunodeficiency virus)
7. Lidocaine, 1% (with epinephrine unless contraindicated)
8. Suture, 3-0 or 4-0 absorbable (chromic, Dexon), 4-0 or 5-0 nylon
9. Single-tooth skin hooks (2)
10. Specimen bottle with formalin
11. Dressing materials (Telfa, 2 × 2 gauze sponges, tincture of benzoin, 1-inch tape)

Anesthesia

1. Lidocaine 1% (with epinephrine unless contraindicated)
2. Use lidocaine *without* epinephrine in "end circulation" areas such as fingers, toes, ears, nose, and penis.
3. Do not use more than 20 ml of 1% lidocaine.

Precautions

1. Patients should be asked about allergy to local anesthetics, iodine, and tape.
2. Be certain that adequate resuscitation equipment is available.

WARNING

A common error is to rupture the cyst in the mistaken belief that sebaceous cysts are *subcutaneous* structures. Sebaceous cysts are *intradermal* structures; thus the skin incision directly over the cyst must be very superficial.

Technique

1. Prepare the skin with povidone-iodine and apply a sterile fenestrated drape.
2. Inject 1% lidocaine (with epinephrine unless contraindicated) using a 27- or 30-gauge needle. Inject the anesthetic so that it dissects the cyst away from the surrounding tissue. Do not inject into the cyst itself.

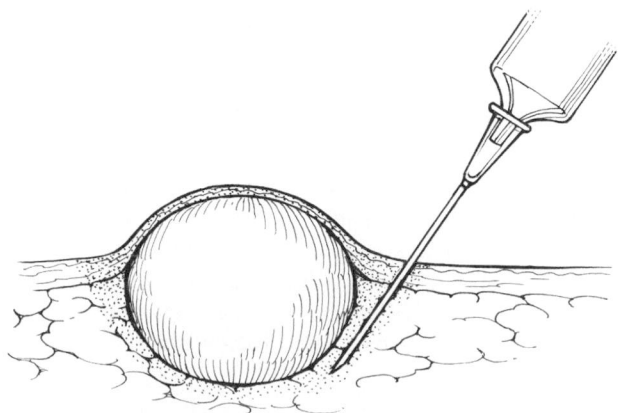

3. Make an elliptical incision that surrounds the central opening and is slightly longer than the diameter of the cyst.

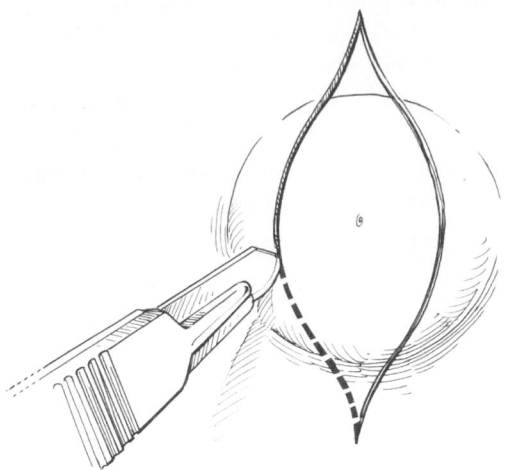

Make the incision parallel to the skin lines.

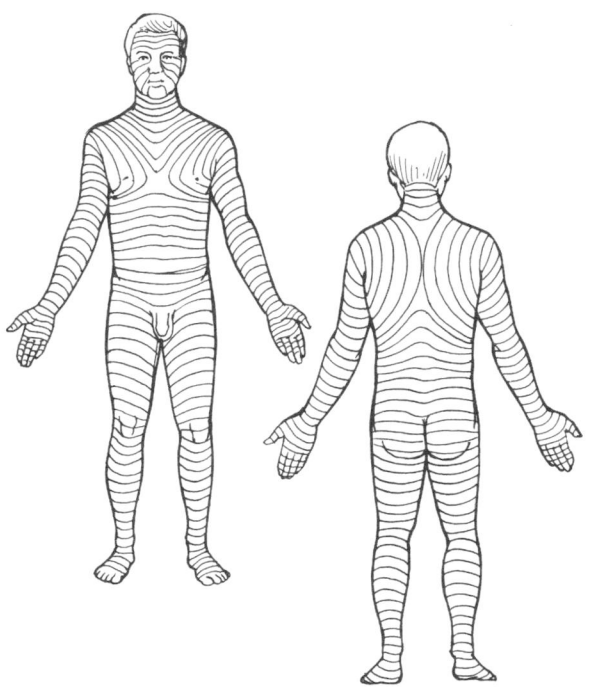

4. Incise the skin very superficially when directly over the cyst. The easiest way to avoid rupturing the cyst is to include, with the cyst, an ellipse of skin around the central opening where the skin is most adherent to the cyst wall.

5. Dissect into the subcutaneous tissue at the ends of the incision where the cyst is not as close to the surface. Grasp one corner of the skin that is to be removed with the cyst and apply upward traction. Use sharp and blunt dissection to carefully locate the fragile cyst wall.

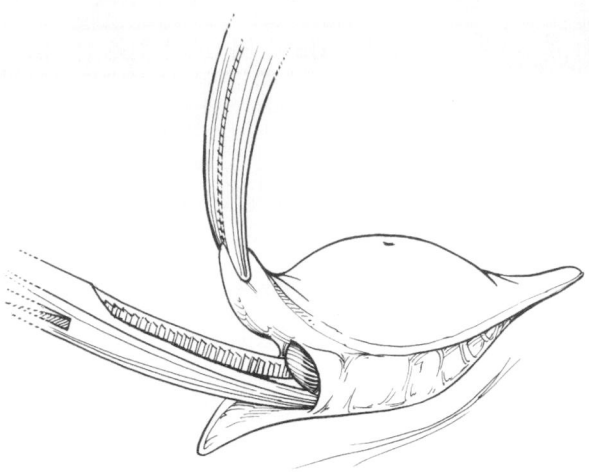

6. Develop a plane between the cyst wall and the surrounding tissue. This dissection is best accomplished by carefully spreading a hemostat or small curved scissors. Use the scissors to cut tissue adherent to the cyst wall.

7. If the cyst ruptures, remove as much keratinous material as possible. Then remove the entire cyst wall using a toothed forceps and scissors. If part of the wall remains, a new cyst may form.

8. Continue the dissection until the cyst is completely free of the underlying tissues, and send it for pathologic examination.

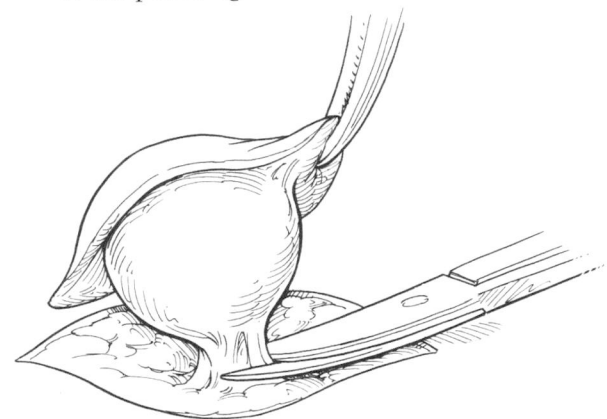

9. Obtain hemostasis with pressure, cautery, or suture ligation if necessary.

10. If the cyst was large, eliminate the dead space by approximating the subcutaneous tissue with absorbable sutures.

11. Close the skin with interrupted nylon sutures.

12. Apply a dressing.

Follow-Up

1. Instruct the patient to keep the wound covered and dry for at least 24 hours.

2. Explain the signs of wound infection to the patient.

3. Remove the sutures after 7 days. Sutures in the back or the extensor surface of joints should remain for 12 to 14 days with sterile adhesive strips applied after removal, because such wounds are prone to dehiscence.

Bibliography

English GM: Ear, nose, throat and sinuses. In Hill GJ (ed): Outpatient Surgery, 3rd ed, pp 169–230. Philadelphia, WB Saunders Company, 1988.

Goldstein BG, Goldstein AO: Practical Dermatology, 2nd ed. St. Louis, Mosby, 1997.

Goodnight JE: Tumors. In Wolcott MW (ed): Ambulatory Surgery and the Basics of Emergency Surgical Care, 2nd ed, pp 101–122. Philadelphia, JB Lippincott Company, 1988.

Habif TP: Clinical Dermatology, 3rd ed. St. Louis, Mosby, 1996.

McGowan GJ: Removing a skin cyst. In Driscoll CE, Rakel RE (eds): Patient Care: Procedures for Your Practice, 2nd ed, pp 287–289. Los Angeles, Practice Management Information Corporation, 1991.

Definition

Abscess: a collection of purulent material in a circumscribed closed cavity. The treatment objective is to create an open wound that will drain infected fluid, devitalized tissue, or foreign body and will heal by secondary intention.

Indications

1. An abscess that is not healing spontaneously or shows clinical worsening (enlargement, cellulitis, lymphangitis, systemic symptoms)
2. The timing is correct: a "ripe" abscess is one that is localized, fluctuant, tender, erythematous; the abscess needs to be ripe for best results.
3. The area is reachable percutaneously.
4. There is failure of conservative therapy (heat, antibiotics).

Contraindications

1. Absolute
   a. Location is such that specialist referral is indicated.
   b. Lack of patient consent
   c. Incorrect diagnosis (e.g., herpetic whitlow)
2. Relative
   a. Not yet "ripe," not localized
   b. Coagulopathy
   c. Immunosuppression
   d. Severe underlying medical problems requiring attention first

Preparation

1. Appropriate history and physical, including allergy
2. Informed consent items to mention should include allergic reaction to local anesthetic leading to death and scarring, bleeding, infection, poor results, no results, recurrence.

Equipment

1. A minor surgical tray
   a. Sterile drape
   b. Hemostat, plain forceps, surgical scissors
   c. Culturette, aerobic and anaerobic
   d. Iodoform gauze packing, 1/4 and 1/2 inch or plain
   e. Local anesthetic
   f. Dressings: 4 × 4 inch gauze and adhesive tape
   g. Irrigation solution; saline
   h. Needles: 18 gauge for aspiration and irrigation, 25 to 27 gauge for anesthesia
   i. Syringes: 6 ml injection, 25 ml for irrigation
   j. Scalpel blade: No. 11 pointed
   k. Antiseptic cleanser of skin: povidone-iodine (Betadine) solution, 70% ethyl alcohol, hexachlorophene (pHisoHex)
2. Sterile gloves; protective eye gear and clothing when appropriate

Anesthesia

1. Topical: Ethyl chloride spray—note that it is flammable and not to be used with cautery.
2. Local: Dosages should not exceed maximal allowable for size of patient.
   a. Lidocaine 1% with epinephrine (avoid epinephrine in fingers, toes, nose, penis, ears)
   b. Procaine (Novocaine) 1% for amide allergy
   c. Bupivacaine (Marcaine) 0.25% for longer duration of analgesia
   d. Add 8.4% sodium bicarbonate into same syringe as anesthetic in a 1:10 dilution to decrease pain of injection by increasing pH of anesthetic.
3. Oral: sodium pentobarbital, 100 mg, or diazepam, 5 to 10 mg, or meperidine hydrochloride, 100 mg, 1 hour before procedure
4. Intravenous and general anesthetic is generally not needed except for very large abscesses (perirectal), or very uncooperative patients (young children). Physicians must follow governmental regulations regarding conscious sedation.

Precautions

1. Use sterile technique to avoid contamination.
2. Avoid squeezing because it may rarely lead to bacteremia.
3. Make incision large enough so it will stay open and abscess does not recur.

Technique (Under Local Anesthesia)

1. Place patient in a comfortable position with area well exposed.
2. Clean area with antiseptic agent and allow to dry.
3. Drape as needed.
4. Infiltrate area subcutaneously with local anesthetic where incision is to be made.

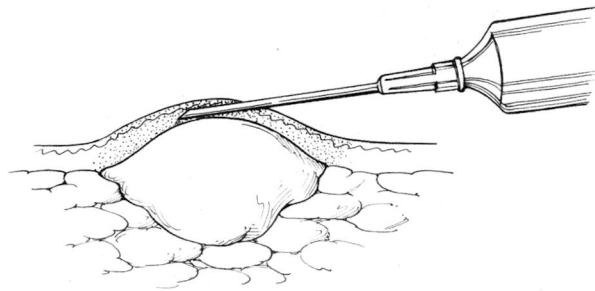

5. Following skin tension lines (see Procedure for Excision of a Sebaceous [Epidermal] Cyst), make stab incision and extend down to pus cavity.

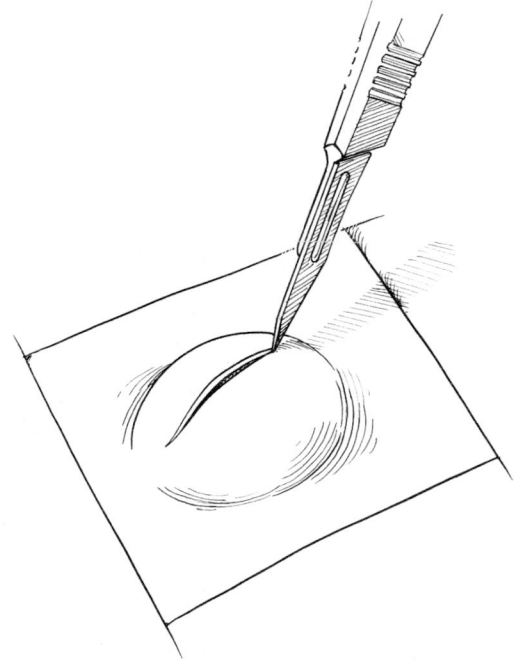

6. Extend incision enough to allow full drainage, widening as necessary.

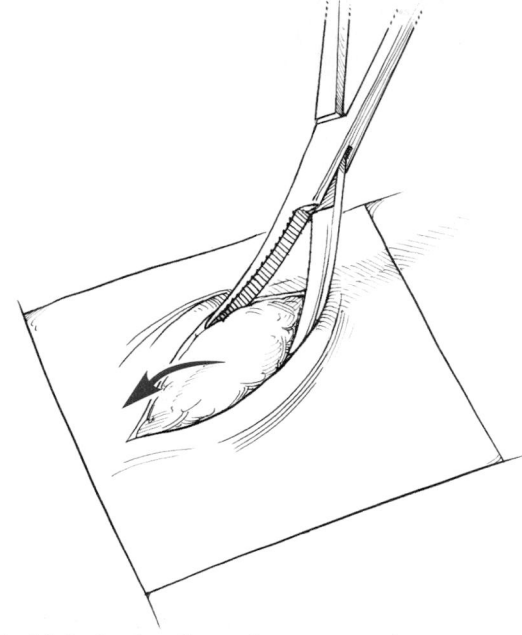

7. If desired, take culture (can also irrigate with saline and aspirate for culture).
8. Break adhesions/loculations within abscess cavity with gloved finger or blunt instrument.

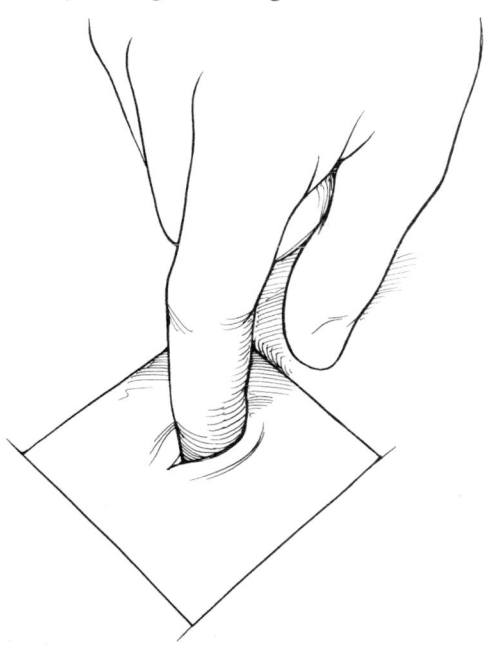

9. Irrigate cavity, especially if foreign material is present.
10. Hemostasis with packing or pressure; cautery is rarely necessary.
11. Insert iodoform gauze if indicated and pack lightly, leaving one end outside of skin acting as a wick.

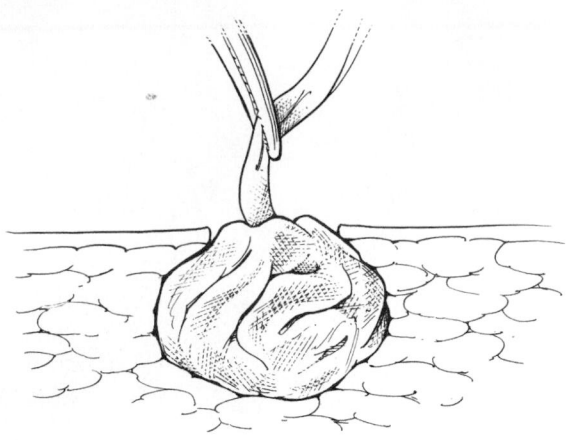

12. Apply sterile dressing.

Follow-Up

1. Elevate area if possible.
2. Apply heat: water soaks for 20 minutes four times daily for 5 to 7 days
3. Expect area to heal slowly by secondary intention over the next 5 to 7 days.

4. Antibiotics for surrounding cellulitis, lymphangitis, systemic symptoms
5. Follow-up visit can be in 1 to 3 days but sooner for problems.
6. If packing used, expect to change daily.

Bibliography

Derksen DJ: Incision and drainage of an abscess. In Pfenninger JL, Fowler CG (eds): Procedures for Primary Care Physicians, pp 50–53. St. Louis, Mosby, 1994.

Knudson RH: Incision and drainage of cutaneous abscess. In Driscoll CE, Rakel RE (eds): Patient Care: Procedures for Your Practice, 2nd ed, pp 307–311. Los Angeles, Practice Management Information Corporation, 1991.

Lawrence CM, Cox NH: Physical Signs in Dermatology: Color Atlas and Test, p 221. London, Mosby-Year Book Europe Limited, 1993.

Local Anesthetic Buffering Efficacy and Stability, Vol 81. Micromedex Inc, 1994.

Mayhew E, Rodgers A: Basic Procedures in Family Practice: An Illustrated Manual, pp 1–5. Bethany, CT, Fleschner Publishing Co., 1984.

293 Hair Disorders

Thomas B. Golemon

Telogen Effluvium

Etiology

1. Distinct physiologic stress causes a rapid, synchronous shift of hair follicles from the active (anagen) phase to the resting (telogen) phase. After 2 to 3 months, a diffuse, self-limited shedding occurs in large numbers (thus effluvium, or flood). Hair regrows in 6 to 12 months.
2. Most common example is parturition, but high fever, shock states, crash diets, severe psychiatric stress, and discontinuation of certain medications (long-term oral contraceptives, high-dose steroids) can trigger the process.
3. Because hair density may be reduced by 50 per cent before thinning is noticeable, the patient may or may not notice this.

Symptoms

Discrete onset of diffuse hair loss, with or without thinning; hair "clogs the drain."

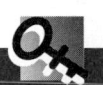
Key Symptom

Large-volume, diffuse hair loss, 2 to 3 months after physiologic trauma

Clinical Findings

1. Scalp is normal: no scaling, scarring, redness, or broken hairs.
2. Hair loss is diffuse; thinning may be unnoticeable (avoid blunder of stating the "hair looks normal" and "nothing is wrong"). No focal areas of baldness.

Key Signs

- Normal scalp examination
- Diffuse hair loss with minimal thinning

Laboratory Tests

1. None required with classic history and physical.
2. Hair pull test: 20 to 30 hairs grasped and pulled briskly between thumb and forefinger should yield no more than four to six normal club (telogen, light-colored bulb) hairs. False negatives possible depending on timing of evaluation.
3. Thyroid panel and complete blood count if diagnosis is uncertain

Differential Diagnosis

1. Endocrine disorders: hypo/hyperthyroidism, hypopituitarism, hypoparathyroidism
2. Deficiency states: protein-calorie, malabsorption (gluten enteropathy), iron, zinc, essential fatty acids (parenteral hyperalimentation)
3. Infectious: syphilis ("moth-eaten," scaly scalp), acquired immunodeficiency syndrome (diffuse loss, changes in texture and density of hair)

Treatment

1. Medication: None required.
2. Diet: no recommendations
3. Activity: no recommendations
4. Patient education
   a. Explanation of problem and self-limited nature
   b. Reassurance

Key Treatment

Education of the patient as to the self-limited nature of the problem

Follow-Up

Three months if hair loss has not slowed to normal

Alopecia Areata

Etiology

Unknown etiology (autoimmune, genetics, stress proposed)

Symptoms

1. One or more focal areas of baldness (alopecia areata) is most common and least severe of the three presentations. More severe: loss of all scalp hair (alopecia totalis) and loss of all body

hair (alopecia universalis). Peaks in 20 to 40-year-old range.

2. Rapid onset of oval lesions nearly devoid of hair, which may coalesce; occasionally see loss of all hair within a few days. Nonpigmented hair may be spared, thus patient's hair may seem to "turn white overnight."

3. Spontaneous remissions common, as are recurrences. Worse prognosis: onset in prepuberty, multiple episodes. Better prognosis: few, stable patches. In 50 per cent of cases, the duration of first episode is less than 1 year. Regrowth in 6 to 12 months, usually same color.

Key Symptom

Rapid-onset "bald spots" in younger patients

Clinical Findings

1. Sharply bordered 1 to 3 cm oval or circular patches of hair loss, leaving smooth, healthy-appearing scalp. Areas may coalesce with time to form larger lesions.

2. Pathognomonic stubby "exclamation point" hairs at periphery variably present.

3. Lesions may occur in eyebrows, beard, axillae.

4. Nail pitting (most common), ridging, splitting, and opacification may be seen, more often with alopecia totalis or universalis. Trachyonychia (rough nails) as descriptive term.

5. Alopecia areata has been reported in association with atopy, Down's syndrome, vitiligo, pernicious anemia, Addison's disease, and thyroid disease (especially in children).

Key Signs

- Sharply delineated bald spots on normal-appearing scalp

- Pathognomonic "exclamation point" hairs at periphery

Laboratory Tests

1. Biopsy of scalp (if necessary)
2. Syphilis serology; thyroid profile with autoantibodies (especially for children)

Differential Diagnosis

1. Trichotillomania: hairs broken rather than exclamation point; patches less discrete

2. Traction alopecia

3. Cicatricial alopecias (lichen planus, folliculitis decalvans, cutaneous lupus, linear scleroderma, sarcoidosis): scarring or inflammation notable; postinflammatory hyperpigmentation. Biopsy will prove.

4. Tinea capitis: erythema and scaling of scalp; examine for fungi.

5. Secondary syphilis: "moth-eaten" appearance to hair

Treatment

1. No curative treatment available, and all successes must be weighed against spontaneous cure rate.

2. Systemic steroids are not usually warranted (prompt recurrence at cessation, side effects) except for "follicle sparing" in rapid total losses. Topical steroids seem more effective in children and for small lesions. Intralesional triamcinolone and topical steroids used with greatest success; may result in significant atrophy, adrenal suppression.

3. Psoralen and ultraviolet A (PUVA) therapy of the scalp or entire body, and irritants such as anthralan or squaric acid, enjoy moderate success.

4. Topical minoxidil useful in some, and few side effects.

Medication

1. Intralesional triamcinolone acetonide, 3 to 10 mg/ml: very small aliquots deeply in dermis every 4 to 6 weeks; do not exceed 20 mg per session. Lessen pain by slow injection. Success rates of 71 per cent at 12 weeks for alopecia areata, 28 per cent for totalis.

2. Minoxidil (Rogaine) 2% solution, applied bid; improvement in up to 25 per cent but does not alter course of disease.

3. Anthralan cream 0.5% applied at bedtime and removed by shampooing in morning. Often combined with topical minoxidil for large areas or alopecia totalis, and especially good in children (85 per cent response). Referral to physician familiar with treatment recommended.

4. Topical betamethasone dipropionate cream (Diprosone) bid; requires at least 3 months for evaluation. Painless, and preferred starting point for children and some adults.

5. Finasteride (Propecia), a competitive inhibitor of type II 5α-reductase, reduces the conversion of testosterone to dihydrotestosterone (DHT) in the scalp and other areas. This has proven ef-

fective in producing hair growth in male pattern baldness, where the balding scalp contains miniaturized hair follicles and increased concentrations of DHT compared to the normal scalp. While helpful in about 66 per cent of patients with androgenic alopecia, there is no indication for its use with alopecia areata.

Diet

No recommendations

Activity

No recommendations

Patient Education

1. Emphasize no curative treatment, outline spontaneous remissions and possibility of recurrences. Side effects of treatment options must be covered.

2. Emotional support is critical in view of the chronicity and recurrences. Referral to the National Alopecia Areata Foundation, 714 C Street, Suite 216, San Rafael, CA 94901 (1-415-383-3444) may be beneficial.

Key Treatment

- Intralesional triamcinolone
- Topical minoxidil
- Topical steroids with or without anthralin in children

Follow-Up

Office visit every 4 to 6 weeks, depending on choice of treatment or referral

Bibliography

Fauci AS, Braunwald E, Isselbacher KJ, et al (eds): Harrison's Principles of Internal Medicine, 14th ed. New York, McGraw-Hill, 1998.

Fiedler VC: Alopecia areata: a review of therapy, efficacy, safety, and mechanism. Arch Dermatol 1992;128: 1519–1529.

Fitzpatrick TB, Eisen AZ, Wolff K, et al: Dermatology in General Medicine, 4th ed. New York, McGraw-Hill, 1993.

Headington JT: Telogen effluvium: new concepts and review. Arch Dermatol 1993;129:356–363.

Weitzner JM: Alopecia areata. Am Fam Physician 1990; 41:1197–1201.

294 Diseases of the Nails

Eckart Haneke

Nail diseases are almost as diverse as those of the skin. They may be unique to the nail or a symptom of another skin disease. Only a few of the most frequent and important disorders can be briefly mentioned.

Onychomycosis

Epidemiology

1. Fungal nail infections are the most frequent nail disorders, comprising 30 to 50 per cent of all nail diseases.
2. Their frequency steadily increases with age: very rare in children; seen in about 45 per cent of those over 70.
3. Toenails are about seven times more frequently infected than fingernails.

Etiology

1. The overwhelming majority of cases are due to dermatophyte infections (Table 294–1), with *Trichophyton rubrum* causing 80 to 85 per cent, *T. mentagrophytes* being responsible for approximately 10 per cent, molds isolated in less than 5 per cent, and yeasts, mainly *Candida albicans* and other *Candida* species, causing less than 10 per cent.
2. The pathogenic role of most molds is more and more disputed, with *Scytalidium dimidiatum* being the only one to be unanimously accepted as a primary nail pathogen.
3. *Candida albicans* is the primary pathogen in chronic mucocutaneous candidiasis and may secondarily invade a nail damaged by chronic recurrent paronychia, other nail pathogens, and trauma.
4. Almost all onychomycoses start with fungal infection of the surrounding skin.

Symptoms

Onychomycoses often go unnoticed by the patient. However, they may considerably interfere with daily activities such as walking and performing fine manual work, and the quality of life may be markedly impaired.

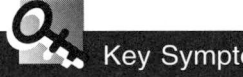

Key Symptom
None or pain

Clinical Findings

1. Proximal white subungual onychomycosis is characterized by whitish discoloration growing out from under the proximal nail fold, loss of transparency, detachment of the involved nail plate from the nail bed.
2. Superficial white onychomycosis is due, in temperate climates, to *T. mentagrophytes* growing on the surface and causing chalky white patches; molds such as *Fusarium* species and *Acremonium* species are rarely encountered in hot and humid climates.
3. Any type of fungal nail infection may eventually lead to total dystrophic onychomycosis. The nail plate is completely destroyed, keratotic remnants are grayish green, and there may be accompanying swelling of the nail folds.

TABLE 294–1. TYPES OF FUNGAL NAIL INFECTIONS

CLINICAL TYPE (METHOD OF FUNGAL INVASION)	MAIN PATHOGEN	FREQUENCY
Distal subungual onychomycosis	Dermatophytes	Most frequent
Proximal white subungual onychomycosis	Dermatophytes	Rare, but more frequent in acquired immunodeficiency syndrome
Superficial white onychomycosis	*T. mentagrophytes*	Relatively rare
Endonyx onychomycosis	*T. soudanense*	Very rare
Total dystrophic onychomycosis		
Primary form	*C. albicans*	Very rare
Secondary form	Dermatophytes	Relatively common

Tests

The key to correct diagnosis is the demonstration of fungal elements from the nail organ using a KOH preparation and their exact determination by culture.

Differential Diagnosis

1. The most important and most difficult differential diagnosis is nail psoriasis.
2. Nonspecific nail dystrophy in old age, arterial circulation disorders, venous insufficiency, and chronic trauma, as well as nail involvement in alopecia areata, lichen planus, and chronic allergic contact dermatitis, have to be considered.

Treatment

Therapy may be topical, systemic, surgical, and/or combined. However, surgical nail avulsion is no treatment per se and has to be considered as a serious trauma to the nail organ, increasing its susceptibility for fungal infection.

1. *Topical treatment* is only effective in mild cases and uses one of two approaches:
   a. Atraumatic nail avulsion with 40% urea paste or 50% potassium iodide ointment followed by topical application of an antifungal agent. This method should ideally remove all infected nail plate and subungual hyperkeratosis. The success rate is between 40 and 65 per cent when carried out consistently and correctly. However, treating several nails is time consuming, and matrix involvement usually cannot be cured.
   b. Nail lacquers containing 5% amorolfine or 8% ciclopirox offer cure rates of about 50 per cent provided there is no matrix involve-

ment. The drug is painted on the nail daily, then every other day, finally once or twice a week after filing the nail surface. Topical treatments have to be completed with therapy of the surrounding skin.

2. *Systemic therapy* allows treatment of the entire nail organ and surrounding skin.
   a. Itraconazole is the treatment of choice. Given as a pulse therapy at 200 mg bid daily for 1 week per month over two cycles for fingernail and three to four cycles for toenail infections, it provides cure rates of about 75 per cent. The clinical response continues to improve after cessation of treatment because the drug remains in the nail for 6 to 9 months in therapeutically relevant concentrations. Drug tolerance is excellent, although there are a number of drug interactions, particularly with those competing for cytochrome P-450.
   b. Griseofulvin is active against dermatophytes only. One gm/day over 6 to 8 months for fingernails and over 8 to 12 (up to 18) months for toenails offers cure rates of about 45 per cent. Griseofulvin is given with a meal rich in fat to increase its absorption.
   c. Ketoconazole (Nizoral), although more effective than griseofulvin, is no longer given for onychomycosis because of potential hepatotoxic side effects.
   d. Fluconazole (Diflucan) was recommended as a once-weekly treatment of 150 mg. Clinical trials are still ongoing; however, the duration of treatment is several months and the dose might not be sufficient for people weighing over 60 to 70 kg.
   e. Terbinafine (Lamisil) is the first systemically active fungicidal drug. It is given in a daily dose of 250 mg for 6 weeks in fingernail and 12 weeks in toenail infections. Cure rates are as high as 80 per cent. The drug is well tolerated, but some serious cutaneous and extracutaneous side effects have been reported.

3. *Surgical treatment* is very rarely indicated, usually only in total dystrophic onychomycosis to get rid of most of the infected material, which no drug can reach in sufficient concentrations. After nail avulsion, systemic or combined treatment must follow.

4. *Combined treatment* using a nail lacquer or atraumatic removal of the infected nail and a topical antifungal plus systemic treatment offers the best success and cuts the failure rate to about one half.

Patient Education

Patients should be educated that there is apparently an inherited susceptibility to develop onychomycosis, requiring lifelong prophylaxis against a relapse/reinfection. This is carried out with consistent hygiene, keeping the feet dry, and using antimycotic sprays for the feet and powder for the shoes. Other factors predisposing to onychomycosis have to be treated separately.

Key Treatment

- Itraconazole
- Terbinafine

Paronychia

Acute paronychia is usually due to bacteria or viruses, whereas chronic paronychia is mainly caused by *C. albicans*, foreign bodies, or contact allergy to foods.

1. Acute paronychia from herpes simplex virus (HSV)
   a. Characterized by marked pain, early lymphangitis, and then blisters that are first clear but then tend to become putrid
   b. The diagnosis is confirmed with a Tzanck's smear or viral culture.
   c. Differential diagnosis is mainly acute bacterial paronychia.
   d. Treatment may be expectant in case of less severe symptoms, or systemic acyclovir or famciclovir may be used. Surgical treatment as a felon is contraindicated. Relapse rate depends on the type of HSV, with HSV-2 causing considerably more relapses than HSV-1.
   e. Medical personnel and dentists must wear gloves when treating patients with herpes simplex infections.
2. Acute bacterial paronychia
   a. Mainly due to either *Staphylococcus aureus* or streptococci.
   b. The nail wall is swollen, erythematous, and painful.
   c. A swab should be taken to identify the pathogen and its antibiotic sensitivity.
   d. Treatment is by removing the blister roof or incising at the point of maximum pain on probing and systemic antibiotic treatment. Splinting of the lower arm is recommended in severe cases.
3. Chronic paronychia

   a. Mainly due to *C. albicans*
   b. This condition is chronic with recurrent (sub)acute flares, the latter causing some pain. The nail fold is swollen, the cuticle disappears, the proximal nail fold no longer adheres to the underlying nail so that foreign material may get under the nail fold, and the nail plate develops irregular transverse grooves and often a grayish-greenish discoloration from secondary infection with *Pseudomonas*, *Klebsiella*, or *Proteus* species.
   c. Treatment involves cleaning the space under the nail fold with a mouth douche, keeping the area dry, and applying anticandidal drugs topically and systemically. In cases of contact dermatitis, testing of foods is necessary and potent topical steroids are used.
   d. The patient must be educated that wet work and contact with carbohydrates and food predispose to chronic paronychia.

Ungual Psoriasis

Psoriasis is the dermatosis most frequently affecting the nail. Some 50 per cent of psoriatics present with nail changes, but about 90 per cent of patients develop nail involvement over their lifetimes.

Symptoms

Most patients just feel cosmetically embarrassed, but manual work may be considerably impaired.

1. Pits—small depressions of the surface of the nail—are the most frequent and characteristic alterations, representing matrix pathology.
2. Salmon spots and onycholysis represent nail bed psoriasis.
3. Nail destruction, leukonychia, splinter hemorrhages, nail thickening, brittleness, and subungual hyperkeratosis may develop.
4. Fingernails are much more frequently involved than toenails.

Laboratory Tests

Absence of fungal elements from nail specimens differentiates this condition from onychomycosis.

Differential Diagnosis

The most important differential diagnosis is onychomycosis (Table 294–2). Other diagnoses to be considered are lichen planus, alopecia areata, contact dermatitis, and nail dystrophy.

Treatment

1. Nail psoriasis is notoriously difficult to treat. However, any systemic therapy improving skin lesions usually also improves nail changes.

TABLE 294–2. DIFFERENTIAL DIAGNOSIS OF PSORIASIS AND ONYCHOMYCOSIS

SIGN OR SYMPTOM	PSORIASIS	ONYCHOMYCOSIS
Digits mainly involved	Fingers	Toes
Pits	Very frequent, regular	Rare, irregular in size and arrangement
Subungual hyperkeratosis	Frequent	Frequent
Nail discoloration	Frequent	Frequent
Onycholysis	Frequent	Frequent
Salmon spots	Frequent	Very rare
Nail destruction	Depends on matrix involvement	Depends on matrix involvement
Demonstration of fungal elements	Usually no, but onychomycosis may occur in psoriasis	Prerequisite for the diagnosis
Other skin lesions	Common: psoriasis	Common: tinea
Overall frequency	1–2% of Caucasian population	Up to 30% in population

a. Key treatments are potent topical steroids, calcipotriol, and 5-fluorouracil, as well as sublesional injections of triamcinolone acetonide crystal suspension; the latter have been shown to be effective, but they are painful and have to be repeated at regular intervals.

b. Systemic psoriasis treatment with cyclosporin A or methotrexate, or photochemotherapy with psoralen and ultraviolet A (PUVA), also improve nail changes.

2. The patient should be educated that trauma to the nail may initiate a Koebner's phenomenon with new lesions.

3. Psoriasis is due to an inherited predisposition. Recurrences may occur at any time.

Nail Lesions Caused by Other Skin Diseases

Other dermatoses may also affect the nail organ and cause alterations that give the experienced physician a hint as to the diagnosis. However, in isolated nail involvement, it is often difficult to make the correct diagnosis.

Skin Diseases with Nail Involvement

1. *Lichen planus* shows nail lesions in about 5 to 10 per cent of cases; isolated nail involvement may occur. The nails are longitudinally striated, rough, and lusterless and tend to split at the free margin (onychorrhexis). Chronic disease insidiously causes thinning, permanent nail dystrophy with pterygium formation, and eventually nail loss.

2. *Alopecia areata* may affect the nail; the more extensive the alopecia, the more likely are nail lesions. The nail develops multiple fine pits, loses its luster and transparency, looks like it has been sandpapered, and may become brittle, although the plate may appear thickened.

3. *Contact dermatitis*, either allergic or irritative, may be localized to the distal phalanx. The cu-

ticle slowly disappears, permitting various organisms, allergens, and irritants to wash under the nail fold, which in turn swells, detaching it even further from the plate. This sets up a vicious cycle of infection, irritation, and inflammation, ultimately distorting the nail plate by laterally positioned transverse ridges, discoloration, and loss of nail sheen.

4. *Twenty-nail dystrophy* is a term delineating rough nails of virtually all digits. It is not clear whether it is an entity or merely a presentation of isolated nail lichen planus, alopecia areata, or another hitherto unidentified spongiotic dermatitis of the matrix and nail bed.

Differential Diagnosis
The differential diagnosis of nail changes accompanying skin diseases is extensive (Table 294–3).

Treatment
Key treatments for these conditions are potent topical steroids, sublesional steroid injections in lichen planus, and avoidance of allergens and irritants in contact dermatitis.

Melanonychia

1. Brown to black nail pigmentation, particularly as a longitudinal streak, is extremely common in dark-skinned people. It is said to be more often malignant than benign when it occurs in an adult fair-skinned person or when a single brown streak in a dark-skinned person turns jet black and becomes wider. A diagnostic biopsy, preferably excisional, is mandatory in these cases.

2. It must be stressed that one quarter to one third of ungual melanomas are amelanotic, often mimicking granulation tissue, pyogenic granuloma, or ingrowing nail.

TABLE 294–3. DIFFERENTIAL DIAGNOSTIC LIST OF CHARACTERISTIC NAIL CHANGES

CLINICAL SIGN	MOST FREQUENT CAUSES
Onycholysis	Minor trauma (overzealous manicure), onychomycosis, psoriasis, circulatory disorders, photosensitivity, candidiasis (proximal onycholysis)
Thickening and subungual hyperkeratosis	Onychomycosis, psoriasis, onychogryposis, "eczema," pachyonychia congenita
Lamellar nail splitting	"Idiopathic," wet work, trauma
Longitudinal ridging	Old age, lichen planus, alopecia areata, dyskeratosis follicularis Darier, twenty-nail dystrophy, trauma
Single deep longitudinal groove	Myxoid pseudocyst, ungual fibrokeratoma
Transverse ridging	Reil-Beau's line from previous illness, trauma, chronic eczema, chronic relapsing paronychia, Raynaud's disease, carpal tunnel syndrome
Pain	Trauma, ingrowing nail, herpetic whitlow, paronychia, glomus tumor, keratoacanthoma, other rapidly growing tumors
Discoloration	
White	Leukonychia, liver disease, trauma, renal disease, psoriasis, dermatophyte infection
Yellow	Yellow nail syndrome, slow growth, *Candida* infection, some drugs, exogenous stains
Green	Infection with *Pseudomonas, Aspergillus, Candida*
Brown to black	Hematoma, nevi, melanoma, fungal infection (*S. dimidiatum, T. rubrum* var. *nigricans*), bacteria, exogenous stains (potassium permanganate, tobacco)

Clinical Findings

Signs raising suspicion of malignant melanoma of the nail unit are listed below.

Key Signs

- Acquired longitudinal brown streak in a fair-skinned Caucasian adult

- Brown streak wider than 5 to 6 mm

- Appearance of periungual pigmentation (Hutchinson's sign)

- Development of nail dystrophy with the pigmentation

- Nodular growth with or without pigmentation and with tendency to bleed

Differential Diagnosis

Main differential diagnoses are hematoma and microbial pigmentation, which rarely present as longitudinal pigmented bands.

Treatment

Early diagnosis and treatment are the keys to successful therapy of this highly malignant lesion. Key treatment is complete surgical excision of the lesion.

Bibliography

Baran R, Kechijian P: Longitudinal melanonychia (melanonychia striata): diagnosis and management. J Am Acad Dermatol 1989;21:1165–1175.

Daniel CR 3rd, Daniel MP, Daniel CM, et al: Chronic paronychia and onycholysis: a thirteen-year experience. Cutis 1996;58:397–401.

de Berker DA, Lawrence CM: A simplified protocol of steroid injection for psoriatic nail dystrophy. Br J Dermatol 1998;138:90–95.

Elewski BE: Onychomycosis: pathogenesis, diagnosis, and management. Clin Microbiol Rev 1998;11:415–429.

Haneke E: Fungal infections of the nail. Semin Dermatol 1991;10:41–53.

Tosti A, Peluso AM, Fanti PA, et al: Nail lichen planus: clinical and pathologic study of twenty-four patients. J Am Acad Dermatol 1993;28:724–730.

Indications

1. Repetitive trauma from short or tight-fitting shoes
2. Improper trimming of nails, leaving rough edges or spicules to abrade nail fold
3. Excessive curvature or wide nails
4. Fungal infections of the nail plate and nail bed
5. Excessive moisture
   a. Stage I: Erythema and swelling of lateral nail fold
   b. Stage II: Infection of nail fold with edema and purulent drainage
   c. Stage III: Formation of granulation tissue with hypertrophy of nail fold

Contraindications

No absolute contraindications

Preparations

1. Conservative management
   a. Culture and treat with appropriate antibiotics and/or systemic antifungals.
   b. Regular and correct trimming of nails
   c. Appropriate shoe fitting
   d. Hydrogen peroxide on cotton-tipped applicator applied between nail plate and nail fold
2. If conservative management fails, proceed to partial or total nail plate resection.

Equipment

1. Straight mosquito hemostatic forceps
2. 3/8-inch Penrose drain or thick, sterilized rubber band
3. 3 × 3 gauze sponges
4. Freer septum elevator
5. Straight hemostat
6. English anvil nail-splitter
7. Straight scissors
8. Dermal curette
9. Scalpel with No. 15 blade
10. Fine-toothed forceps
11. Cotton with toothpicks
12. Liquid phenol 88%
13. Needle holder
14. 4-0 to 5-0 Prolene suture
15. If desired, electrosurgical unit with insulated straight probe

Anesthesia

1. Lidocaine 1% to 2% without epinephrine, 2 to 3 ml, for field block
2. EMLA cream may be used topically preoperatively to reduce discomfort in anxious patients.
3. Bupivacaine, levobupivacaine, or ropivacaine 1%, 1 to 1.5 ml, as wing block for prolonged postoperative analgesia

Precautions

1. Rule out osteomyelitis, particularly in chronic or recurrent paronychia, by radiography of infected digits.
2. Evaluate for neuropathy, vasculopathy, and infection in
   a. Patients with diabetes mellitus
   b. Other immunocompromised patients
   c. Patients with circulatory disease
3. Evaluate for bleeding disorders.
4. Evaluate for potential for methemoglobinemia (if using ELMA cream).
5. Evaluate for allergy to medication, anesthetic agents.
6. Evaluate for prosthetic devices, artifical valves.

Technique

1. Optional: Apply EMLA cream, 2 gm/10 cm^2 of skin surface under occlusive dressing for at least 1 hour prior to beginning procedure (primarily for anxious and pediatric patients).
2. Apply field block of toe and wait 10+ minutes to ensure adequate anesthesia. Infected toenails take longer to achieve satisfactory anesthesia.

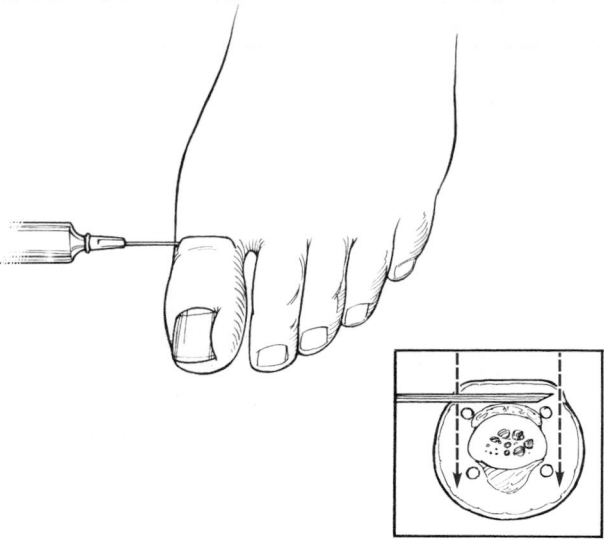

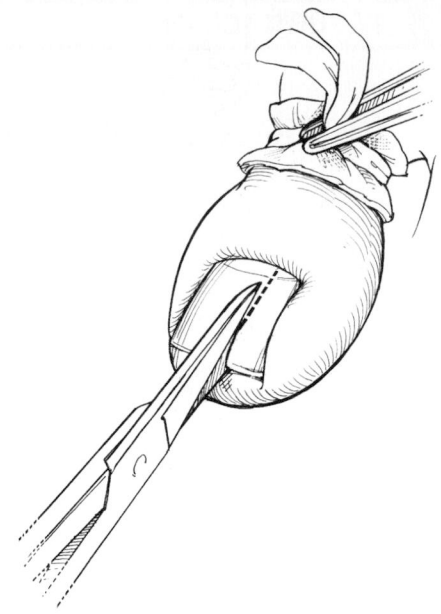

3. Prepare skin with antiseptic solutions, such as chlorhexidine or povidone-iodine.

4. Apply a few layers of gauze to base of toe to protect neurovascular bundles and then apply Penrose drain as tourniquet, held with forceps, to ensure bloodless field.

5. Free cuticle back to base of nail plate and then free portion of nail to be removed from the nail bed back to the base of the nail, using the Freer septum elevator or straight forceps.

7. Grasp the nail with a straight hemostat and rotate the portion to be removed in the direction of the healthy portion of the nail, to avulse it.

8. Curette the proximal nail matrix and any granulation tissue present.

9. *Phenol method*: Protect surrounding skin with antibiotic ointment. Apply fresh 88% liquid phenol to proximal matrix, using cotton-tipped toothpick, to cauterize any remaining matrix and assist in postoperative hemostasis. The tissue touched by the phenol will turn white. After three applications of phenol of 30 to 60 seconds each, irrigate the area with 70% isopropyl alcohol.

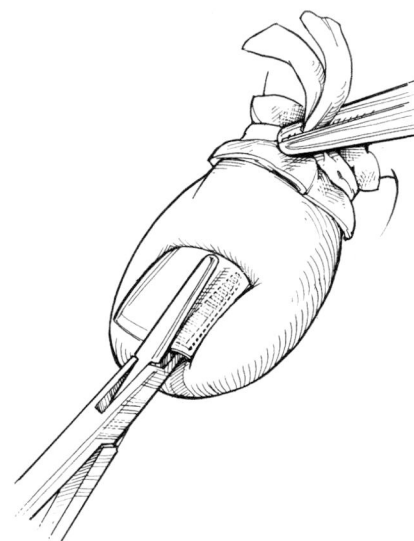

6. Separate the portion of the nail to be removed with straight scissors or anvil nail-splitter.

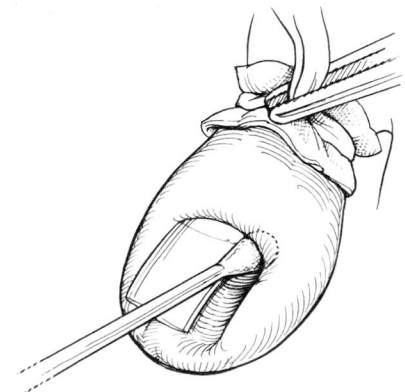

10. Electrocautery to the proximal matrix is also a successful procedure to prevent regrowth of the nail.

11. If hypertrophic nail fold is present, this may be excised in elliptical fashion and the free edge of the skin sutured to remaining nail plate.

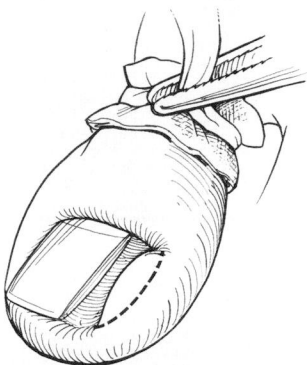

6. Healing is usually complete in 4 weeks.

Follow-Up

1. Remove tourniquet; apply antibiotic ointment to wound followed by a nonadherent, bulky pressure dressing.

2. Elevate the foot and apply ice initially to prevent bleeding and pain.

3. Prescribe acetaminophen with codeine for pain the first 2 to 3 days.

4. Dressings may need to be changed daily if oozing occurs, otherwise in 4 to 7 days. Reapply antibiotic ointment with each dressing change until healed.

5. Some serous drainage after phenol application is to be expected.

 Bibliography

Brewster NT, Howie CR: Excision of the germinal matrix: a modification. J R Coll Surg Edinb 1995;40:59.

Giacalone VF: Phenol matricectomy in patients with diabetes. J Foot Ankle Surg 1997;36:264–267; discussion 328.

Kinata Y, Uetake M, Tsukada S, et al: Follow-up study of patients treated for ingrown nails with the nail matrix phenolization method. Plast Reconstr Surg 1995; 95:719–724.

Salasche SJ: Nail unit surgery. In Robinson J, Arndt KA, LeBoit PE, et al (eds): Atlas of Cutaneous Surgery, pp 189–200. Philadelphia, WB Saunders Company, 1996.

Thompson GH: Bunions and deformities of the toes in children and adolescents. Instr Course Lect 1996;45: 355–367.

295 Venous Stasis Ulcer

David E. Trachtenbarg

Etiology

Underlying causes of stasis ulcers include venous insufficiency secondary to incompetence of the deep vein valves, and deep vein thrombosis.

Symptoms

1. Patients usually present with an ulcer on the lower leg that will not heal in the "gaiter area" between the knee and the foot.
2. The ulcer is usually not painful unless infected.
3. There is often associated aching and swelling of the lower leg aggravated by prolonged standing.
4. There may be a previous history of trauma or vascular surgery or a history of deep vein thrombosis, venous valvular incompetence, or varicosities.

Key Symptom

Painless ulceration of lower leg

Clinical Findings

1. Stage of ulcer: Staging cannot be confirmed unless the wound base is visible.
   a. Stage I: erythema not resolving within 30 minutes of pressure relief with intact epidermis
   b. Stage II: partial-thickness ulcer not extending through the dermis
   c. Stage III: full-thickness ulcer extending through the dermis
   d. Stage IV: ulcer extending through subcutaneous tissue to fascia, muscle, or bone
2. The ulcers typically have minimal pain or are painless. Exudate is usually serosanguineous.
3. The surrounding skin often has edema, brownish discoloration, or dermatitis. Varicosities are usually present.
4. Watch for signs of significant local or systemic infection, including marked surrounding erythema, copious purulent exudate, significant pain and fever. A fecal odor is a sign of secondary anaerobic infection.

Key Signs

- An ulcer in the "gaiter area" above the foot and below the knee
- Edema and brownish discoloration of surrounding skin

Laboratory Tests

1. Cultures usually show polymicrobial flora, and bacteria isolated do not correlate with clinical response.
   a. Perform a culture if a systemic infection or significant surrounding cellulitis is suspected.
   b. Cultures should be done following cleansing of the wound base.
2. Consider the possibility of underlying osteomyelitis for stage III and IV ulcers.
3. Venous Doppler testing is useful for selected patients, particularly if surgery is contemplated.

Key Tests

- Cultures are generally not helpful.
- Venous Doppler testing in selected patients

Differential Diagnosis

1. The diagnosis is usually straightforward.
2. Consider a mixed ulcer or an arterial ulcer if there is arterial peripheral vascular disease.

WARNING

Consider biopsy if the ulcer is not healing or there are other signs of disease to rule out carcinoma.

Treatment

1. Necrotic tissue must be removed to promote healing.
   a. Wet-to-dry dressings are often the most cost-effective way of doing this.

b. Other options include
  (1) Dressings that enhance leukocyte migration and cause autolysis for shallow wounds (Op-Site, Tegaderm, Comfeel, DuoDERM)
  (2) Enzymatic débridement (Travase, Elase, Santyl, Biozyme C)
  (3) Surgical débridement for wounds with a large amount of necrotic tissue
2. Maintain a moist environment. Options include the following:
  a. Saline dressings are cost-effective for many patients.
  b. Hydrocolloid dressings (Comfeel, Duo-DERM) and transparent dressings (Op-Site, Tegaderm) are useful for selected patients because they may be left in place for several days.
  c. Remove excess wound exudate by thorough cleansing at each dressing change.
    (1) The solution of choice is normal saline, which does not destroy tissue.
    (2) Betadine, hydrogen peroxide, Dakin's solution (potassium hypochlorite), and acetic acid can inhibit wound healing by destroying cells.
3. Eradicate clinical infection
  a. Use systemic antibiotics if cellulitis or systemic infection is present. Common organisms are *Staphylococcus aureus*, *Streptococcus pyogenes*, and *Pseudomonas aeruginosa*.
  b. Topical agents such as silver sulfadiazine (Silvadene) and polymyxin B–bacitracin-neomycin (Neosporin) also may be useful but have not consistently been shown to promote wound healing. Watch carefully for signs of sensitization, especially with polymyxin B–bacitracin-neomycin.
4. Eliminate edema (venous compression).
  a. Possible choices for venous compression include
    (1) Elastic stockings with at least 35 mm of compression
    (2) Zinc oxide bandages (Unna boot); change weekly.
    (3) Elastic wraps (Ace wrap, multilayer bandage)
    (4) Intermittent mechanical compression
  b. When using venous compression, monitor patient for circulatory compromise, including swelling, color changes, and temperature changes.
5. Give appropriate nutritional support to provide protein, calories, vitamins, and minerals essential for healing.
6. Maintain adequate circulation and oxygenation to the wound bed. Correct peripheral vascular disease when possible, or use an agent such as Trental to improve the circulation if arterial disease is present.
7. Surgery is indicated for selected patients who do not respond to nonsurgical therapy.
8. Using stockings with 30 to 40 mm of compression after ulcer healing will prevent many recurrences.

Patient Education
1. Keep legs elevated above the heart when lying down.
2. Avoid sitting with the legs crossed.
3. Avoid standing for prolonged periods.
4. Ambulate intermittently throughout the day.
5. Avoid constrictive clothing.
6. Use a moisturizer such as Eucerin or Alpha Keri to keep surrounding skin clean and pliable.
7. Avoid heating pads, hot water bottles, heat lamps, hot solutions, cold solutions, and ice packs to prevent thermal trauma.
8. Reportable symptoms
  a. Change in color
  b. Change in temperature
  c. Pain or other change in sensation
  d. Change in drainage or odor
9. Inspect feet and legs daily.

Key Treatment

- Venous compression to reduce venous stasis and edema
- Moist wound surface promotes wound healing.

Follow-Up
Stasis ulcers heal very slowly. Office visits more often than every 1 to 2 weeks are usually not necessary unless an acute infection is being treated.

Bibliography

Alguire PC, Mathes BM: Chronic venous insufficiency and venous ulceration. J Gen Intern Med 1997;12: 374–383.
Fletcher A, Cullum N, Sheldon TA: A systematic review of compression treatment for venous leg ulcers. BMJ 1997;315:576–580.

McGuckin M, Stineman M, Goin J, et al: Draft guideline: diagnosis and treatment of venous leg ulcers. Ostomy Wound Manage 1996;42(April):100, 102, 104.

McGuckin M, Stineman M, Goin J, et al: Draft guideline: diagnosis and treatment of venous leg ulcers. Ostomy Wound Manage 1996;42(May):48, 50–52, 54.

Samson RH, Showalter DP: Stockings and the prevention of recurrent venous ulcers. Dermatol Surg 1996;22:373–376.

University of Pennsylvania: Update: venous leg ulcer guideline. Ostomy Wound Manage 1997;43:80–82.

296 Decubitus Ulcer

David P. Losh

Etiology

1. Pressure over a bony prominence
2. Friction, such as pulling patient across a bed sheet
3. Shear forces, such as partial reclining position
4. Moisture, such as incontinence
5. Contributing factors
   a. Decreased mobility
   b. Decreased sensation
   c. Poor nutrition
   d. Dementia

Symptoms

1. Pain over a bony prominence in stage 1 or 2
2. Relatively pain free in stage 3 or 4

Key Symptom

Often unnoticed in early stages

Clinical Findings

1. Location: 95 per cent over lower extremities—ischial tuberosities, trochanters, sacrum, heels
2. Clinical staging
   a. Stage 1: nonblanching erythema lasting over 30 minutes after relief of pressure. Epidermis intact.
   b. Stage 2: partial-thickness skin loss. Extends into but not through the dermis.
   c. Stage 3: full-thickness through the dermis and into subcutaneous tissue; shallow crater that may include eschar, exudate, infection, necrotic tissue, undermining or sinus tracts
   d. Stage 4: deep penetration to fascia or bone

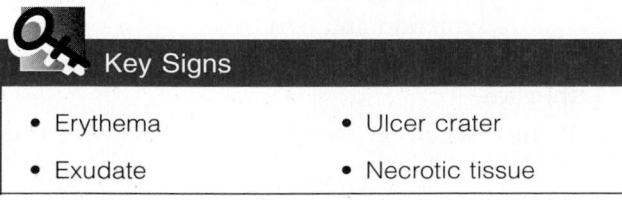

Key Signs

- Erythema
- Exudate
- Ulcer crater
- Necrotic tissue

Laboratory Tests

1. Cultures of ulcer indicated *only* if signs of sys-temic infection or deep lesions with purulent or foul smelling drainage.
2. Tests for malnutrition
   a. Serum albumin: 3.5 gm/dl or lower
   b. Complete blood count (CBC): hemoglobin less than 12 mg/dl in men, less than 10 mg/dl in women; lymphocytes below 1500/mm³
   c. Serum transferrin: less than 200 mg/dl
3. Screening tests for osteomyelitis
   a. White blood cells greater than 15,000/mm³
   b. Westergren sedimentation rate: greater than 100 mm/hour
   c. Plain radiograph: lytic lesions, reactive bone formation, periosteal elevation

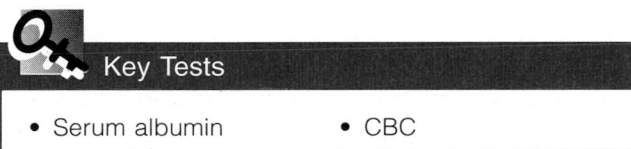

Key Tests

- Serum albumin
- CBC

Differential Diagnosis

1. Venous stasis ulcer: edema, hyperpigmentation, lower extremity
2. Diabetic ulcer: most on forefoot and toes, neurotrophic or ischemic origin
3. Ulceration from arterial insufficiency: resting pain, pale atrophic skin, hair loss, nail dystrophy
4. Ecthyma gangrenosum: *Pseudomonas* infection and neutropenia, gluteal or perineal ulcers
5. Skin cancer: basal cell, squamous cell, other
6. Pyoderma gangrenosum: underlying inflammatory or malignant disease, purple margin
7. Self-induced (factitial) ulcers: underlying psychosocial disorder; geometric straight margins, only on reachable skin

Treatment

Medications and Dressings

1. Débriding methods
   a. Wet-to-damp saline and gauze dressings: used for early débridement but may cause epithelial damage if allowed to dry
   b. Enzymatic ointments or creams (Travase, Elase, Santyl, Granulex, Panfil)

c. Whirlpool soaks

d. Irrigation, normal saline

e. Surgical débridement for thick eschars or deep necrotic tissue

2. Lotions, ointments, creams, and topical antibiotics

a. Emollients aid in good skin care (Eucerine lotion, KeriLotion, others).

b. Silver sulfadiazine or combination antibiotic ointment for superficial infections

c. Avoid antiseptic agents that are toxic to granulation tissue, such as chlorhexidine, povidone-iodine, acetic acid, and hydrogen peroxide.

3. Synthetic dressings: preferred treatment to maintain protected, moist wound environment

a. Semipermeable transparent film dressings (Op-Site, Tegaderm, Bioclusive, Blisterfilm): best for stage 1 to 3 without heavy exudate

b. Hydrocolloid and occlusive dressings (DuoDERM, Restore, Comfeel): best on low- to moderate-exudate wounds. May be difficult on areas of irregular contour.

c. Hydrogels (Vigalon, Geliperm, IntraSite): best on moist, granulating nonexudative, non–weight-bearing surfaces. Cooling effect helps with pain control. Require daily changes.

d. Calcium alginate (Kaltostat): for stage 2 to 3 exuding ulcers prior to re-epithelization. Ineffective in dry ulcers.

4. Antibiotics

a. If treating systemic infection or deep purulent lesions, use a broad spectrum β-lactam antibiotic, quinolone, or combination to cover aerobic and anaerobic organisms.

b. Specific therapy should be guided by culture results from soft tissue aspirate, blood culture, or bone biopsy.

c. *Pseudomonas aeruginosa* and *Providencia* are associated with worsening pressure ulcers.

Diet

1. Identify signs of malnutrition: nonvolitional weight loss, hypoalbuminemia

2. Begin nutritional support early. Set realistic treatment goal of at least 35 kcal/kg/day. Use team approach, including nutritionist.

3. Consider high-protein diet: 1.0 to 1.2 gm/kg/day.

4. Consider supplementation with multivitamin and mineral preparation in patients suspected of vitamin deficiency.

Activity

Encourage ambulation, frequent repositioning, physical therapy if appropriate.

Key Treatment

- Reduce pressure, moisture, shearing, friction.

- Use débridement method least damaging to tissue.

- Keep well humidified and protected with appropriate dressing.

Prevention

1. Identify high-risk patients

a. Elderly

b. Recent hospitalization

c. Immobile

d. Incontinence: moisture and fecal incontinence

e. Poor nutrition

f. Skin abnormalities

g. Quadriplegia or paraplegia

2. Reduce pressure

a. Reposition on side at 30-degree angle more frequently than every 2 hours.

b. Consider pressure relief devices and select on the basis of cost, ease of use, and severity of condition.

(1) Chair cushions, splints, heel protectors, cradle boots: Do not use donut-type devices.

(2) Special mattresses and overlays

(a) Static foam mattresses, sheepskin fleeces: least pressure reduction; results similar to alternating air pressure pads.

(b) Alternating air pressure pads: intermediate pressure reduction, increased mechanization and cost; results similar to static devices

(3) Air-fluidized beds: maximum pressure reduction and cost

3. Reduce friction: Use draw sheets for patient transfer.

4. Reduce shearing: Avoid partially reclining bed position.

5. Reduce moisture.

a. Regular toileting and incontinence treatment

b. Barrier ointments and absorptive products

Follow-Up

A preventative regimen and plan of therapeutic interventions should be based on the patient's and family's overall goals and should involve a team including the physician, nurses, nutritionist, and physical and/or occupational therapists.

Bibliography

Bergstrom N, Bennett M, Carlson C, et al: Pressure Ulcers in Adults: Prediction and Prevention. Guideline Report No. 3. (AHCPR Publication No. 93-0013). Rockville, MD, Agency for Health Care Policy and Research, 1992.

Bergstrom N, Bennett M, Carlson C, et al: Treatment of Pressure Ulcers. Clinical Practice Guideline No. 15. (AHCPR Publication No. 95-0652). Rockville, MD, Agency for Health Care Policy and Research, 1994.

Findlay D: Practical management of pressure ulcers. Am Fam Physician 1996;54:1519–1528.

Thomas D, Allman R (eds): Pressure Ulcers. Clin Geriatr Med 1997;13(3).

Thomas D: Pressure ulcers. In Cassel C, et al (eds): Geriatric Medicine, 3rd ed, pp 767–785. New York, Springer-Verlag, 1997.

297 Scabies

Peter S. P. Lee

Etiology

1. The arthropod itch mite *Sarcoptes scabiei* subspecies *hominis* causes the dermatitis scabies in humans. (The subspecies *canis*, responsible for sarcoptic mange in dogs, can neither burrow nor breed on human skin and so survives only a few weeks and produces milder and self-limited scabies.)

2. Transmission of the itch mite occurs between people either via skin-to-skin contact or indirectly via bedlinens or clothing. Infectivity is higher with prolonged and intimate contact and exposure to the rarer but more severe form known as Norwegian or crusted scabies, wherein an individual lesion harbors 10^4 to 10^6 organisms versus only about 10 in an ordinary scabies case.

3. Infestation of the skin by the itch mite begins when a pregnant female is incidentally deposited on the skin. Within 1 hour of arrival and then principally at nighttime, it feeds by burrowing into and then within the epidermis. During each day it defecates and lays two to four eggs in the burrow. About 4 days later the eggs hatch, and in 2 weeks mature into adults. They mate on the skin; the male soon dies, and the female completes a 30-day lifecycle. An obligate ectoparasite, the itch mite survives only 48 hours off its human host in good conditions and it is known to die within 2 hours at temperatures above 120° F (50° C).

4. Hypersensitivity to mite protein antigen and mite fecal irritants generate most of the skin manifestations. An individual having no prior mite infestation may have delay symptoms in 4 to 6 weeks, whereas prior sensitization precipitates a reaction in 1 to 4 days of infestation.

5. Prevalence of scabies is worldwide, but endemic in some countries. It involves all socioeconomic classes, and blacks are affected less frequently. Epidemics are thought to last 15 years and wane for 15 years, although there has been a worldwide pandemic since 1964. It involves especially those at institutional settings such as at day care centers, nursing homes, and mental health facilities.

Symptoms

1. Severe pruritus, especially during nighttime or after a hot shower.
2. Rash

Key Symptoms

- Intense pruritus, worse at night
- Rash

Clinical Findings

1. Burrows are the characteristic finding, but may not be discernible at an early stage or after trauma from scratching.
2. Erythematous papules, pustules
3. Reddish brown nodules 5 to 20 mm, develop in 7 to 10 per cent of scabies patients (*nodular scabies*).
4. Thick hyperkeratotic or crusted lesions (*Norwegian scabies*—typically in immunologically and neurologically impaired individuals)
5. Secondary changes: excoriation, eczematization, partial healing, secondary infection (especially *Streptococcus pyogenes* and *Staphylococcus aureus*)
6. Body part distribution predilection
   a. In adults and older children: interdigital web spaces > flexures of wrists/elbows > penis/genitalia > feet > anterior axillae/areolae > beltline/buttocks > other (rarely involves face)
   b. In children less than 2: also head and neck

Key Signs

- Burrows, although infrequently found
- Pleomorphic lesions: erythematous papules, pustules, nodules
- Distribution pattern: webs of fingers, flexures of wrists and elbows, genitalia, axillae

Laboratory Tests

1. History and skin examination alone may make the diagnosis.
2. Obtaining a positive test can be difficult.
3. Failures in correctly diagnosing scabies have earned it the nickname "the great imitator."
4. Naked-eye or magnified examination of a suspicious lesion in vivo may reveal a white- or black-appearing organism at one end of the burrow (body length <0.5 mm).
5. Skin shavings under microscope
   a. Select high-yield lesions: more mites tend to be located on unscathed primary burrows on hands.
   b. Moisten No. 15 scalpel blade or needle tip with mineral oil or water.
   c. Scrape, shave, or extract portion of suspected lesion onto slide.
   d. Examine under microscope at low power.
   e. Inspect for any multilegged, rounded creatures, unhatched or hatched eggs, or fecal pellets (scybala).
6. Burrow ink test
   a. Paint fountain pen ink onto lesion.
   b. After few minutes, remove surface ink with alcohol pad
   c. If burrow is present, ink within canaliculus will appear as dark zig-zag line.
   d. An alternative to ink is liquid tetracycline, which fluoresces yellow-green under a Wood's lamp.
7. Punch biopsy: often performed in diagnostic dilemmas, may reveal mite presence.
8. "Therapeutic test": If treatment is curative, may make presumptive diagnosis.

Key Tests

- Visual inspection
- Microscopy of skin shavings
- Burrow ink test

Differential Diagnosis

1. Insect bites
2. Atopic dermatitis: Scabies may also exacerbate.
3. Contact or irritant dermatitis
4. Dermatitis herpetiformis
5. Lichen planus
6. Secondary syphilis
7. Impetigo: Scabies may be the underlying disorder.
8. Urticaria (e.g., drug reaction)
9. Pruritic urticarial papules and plaques of pregnancy (PUPPP)
10. Pruritus caused by systemic disease (e.g., uremia)
11. Delusion of parasitosis

Treatment

Untreated scabies will last months to years, the origin of the saying "the seven year itch."

Medication

1. Scabecides
   a. Who should receive?
      (1) Index patient, sexual partners, household members, caregivers (babysitter, etc.)
      (2) Casual contacts usually not necessary. Notable exception is exposure to a patient with Norwegian scabies which has high mite count.
      (3) Simultaneous prophylactic treatment warranted even in asymptomatic close contacts because may be in incubation period (up to 4 to 6 weeks).
   b. Principles of topical application
      (1) Cut nails, apply subungually with toothbrush, reapply to hands after hand washing, and dispose of toothbrush.
      (2) Apply from chin to soles in adults and older children.
      (3) Include head/scalp for children less than 2 and refractory or severe cases.
      (4) Avoid body orifices, mucous membranes, conjunctivae (especially Lindane).
      (5) Absorption higher on "open" wounds or after bathing.
      (6) Avoid in pregnant and nursing mothers, infants less than 2 months (especially Lindane).
      (7) Overnight applications are usually more convenient.
   c. Permethrin (Elimite) 5% cream, 30 gm/dose for adult of average body surface area
      (1) Drug of choice: One dose generally curative, relatively safe, more expensive.
      (2) Apply, leave on 8 to 14 hours, wash off.
   d. Lindane (Scabene, G-well) 1% lotion, 30 ml/adult dose

(1) Apply, leave on 8 to 12 hours (6 to 8 hours in young children), wash off.

(2) May repeat in 1 week.

WARNING

There are many reports of adverse effects with Lindane use (seizures, aplastic anemia especially among children), but almost all are due to overuse and misuse (e.g., caution against licking).

---

e. Crotamiton (Eurax) 10% cream or lotion, 60 gm/two adult applications

(1) May have antipruritic properties.

(2) Even two applications associated with more treatment failures than Permethrin or Lindane.

(3) Apply, 24 hours later repeat, 48 hours later wash off.

f. Precipitated sulfur 6% to 10% in petrolatum or emollient

(1) Time-honored but messy, smelly, stains clothing, causes dry skin.

(2) Apply, repeat at 24 and 48 hours. Wash 24 hours after each application.

g. Ivermectin (Stromectol), 0.200 mg/kg orally: Not Food and Drug Administration–approved for scabies, but used in similar single dose for strongyloidiasis and onchocerciasis.

h. Regimens for Norwegian scabies include ivermectin, or several weeks of permethrin on day 1 and sulfur on days 2 through 7. Dosing and routes as above.

2. Symptomatic medications for pruritus

a. Sedating antihistamines (e.g., hydroxyzine [Atarax, Vistaril] or diphenhydramine [Benadryl]) 25 to 50 mg orally qhs (May also mitigate insomnia caused by pruritus.)

b. Emollients for dry skin (e.g., Eucerin, Lubriderm, Aveeno)

c. Corticosteroids: May alter disease, making it unrecognizable ("scabies incognito").

(1) Topical, medium or low potency (e.g., triamcinolone 0.1% or hydrocortisone 1% cream tid)

(2) Systemic (e.g., prednisone 14-day taper, first day 1 mg/kg)

(3) Intralesional injection (e.g., triamcinolone, 5 mg/ml into nodule)

3. Bacterial secondary infection: antibiotic (e.g., macrolide, first-generation cephalosporin, amoxicillin-clavulanate)

Environmental Control

1. Clothes/sheets/towels and the like used in past 48 hours: avoid human contact with for 3 days; or launder and dry cycle, or dry clean.

2. In institutions, to prevent outbreaks prior to treatment completion, consider fastidious use and discarding of disposable gloves/gowns for patient contact.

Patient Education

1. Need to notify and treat close contacts.

2. Once diagnosed, avoid overzealous attempts at hygiene (i.e., overbathing), which can cause excessive skin dryness and additional itchiness.

3. Once scabetic therapy completed, expect rapid decline of symptoms by 24 hours. Yet expect that mite remains/feces may cause itchiness for weeks until exfoliated. No further scabecide indicated.

4. Okay to return to school/work 24 hours after therapy completed. Meanwhile, maintain contact isolation.

 Key Treatment

Drug of Choice
- 5% Permethrin

Symptomatic (Pruritus)
- Antihistamines
- Topical or systemic steroids

Alternative Drugs
- 1% Lindane, 10% crotamiton

If Secondarily Infected
- Antibiotic

Treat Contacts and Environment

Follow-Up

1. See the patient in 1 to 4 weeks, depending on circumstances: generally sooner for uncertain diagnosis, for more likely anticipated treatment failure, or for more severe infestations requiring further intervention (e.g., antibiotic, oral steroids).

2. For treatment failures: reconsider diagnosis, inadequate medication application, medication resistance, contact or fomite transmission.

Bibliography

Habif TB: Infestations and bites. In Baxter S (ed): Clinical Dermatology: A Color Guide to Diagnosis and Therapy, 3rd ed, pp 445–453. St. Louis, Mosby, 1996.

Hurwitz S: Insect bites; Parasitic infestations. In Hurwitz S (ed): Clinical Pediatric Dermatology, 2nd ed, pp 405–413, 428–429. Philadelphia, WB Saunders Company, 1993.

Maunder JW: Lice and scabies: myths and realities. Dermatol Clin 1998;16:843–845.

Meinking TL, Taplin D, Hermida JL, et al: The treatment of scabies with ivermectin. N Engl J Med 1995;633:26–30.

Scabies. In Peter G (ed): Red Book: The Report of the Committee on Infectious Diseases, 24th ed, pp 468–470. Elk Grove Village, IL, American Academy of Pediatrics, 1997.

298 Pediculosis (Body and Head Lice)

Jean Forman

Etiology

Lice are blood-sucking ectoparasites transmitted by direct contact. The existence of lice and their interaction with man has been documented in the earliest writings. Several mentions are made in the Bible and in early Greek literature.

1. Two distinct species
   a. *Pediculus humanus*
   b. Head louse (*P. humanus capitis*)
   c. Body louse (*P. humanus corporis*): morphologically similar to the head louse, but larger
   d. *Pthirus pubis*: the pubic (crab) louse
2. Head lice
   a. Infest only the scalp.
   b. Do not transmit disease.
   c. Are highly contagious.
   d. Commonly found in schoolchildren—12 million are estimated to be infected annually.
   e. Cut across social class and level of personal cleanliness.
   f. Lower incidence in blacks in the United States: It is difficult for lice to grip curled hair shafts.
   g. Likelihood of infestation not affected by keeping hair short, brushing, or shampooing.
   h. Transmitted by direct contact: helmets, hats, combs, and brushes.
   i. Overcrowding is a factor.
3. Body lice
   a. Not found on the body.
   b. Cling to fibers in the seams of clothing, then feed on the body.
   c. Responsible for the spread of diseases such as
      (1) Typhus: caused by *Rickettsia prowazeki*
      (2) Louse-borne relapsing fever
      (3) Trench fever
   d. Seen primarily on the homeless and indigent.
   e. Transmitted by direct body contact or sharing of contaminated clothing or bedding.
4. Crab lice
   a. Spread by sexual contact.

b. Most often seen in adults 15 to 40 years of age.
   c. Highly contagious: Most cases (95 per cent) occur after only one exposure.
5. Immunosuppressed patients are at higher risk of infestation.

Symptoms

Head Lice
1. Most cases are asymptomatic.
2. Up to 38 per cent present with itching, excoriation, and crusting.

Body Lice
1. Severe pruritis with excoriation
2. Red papules on the body
3. Areas most affected: axillae, groin, and truncal areas

Pubic Lice
1. Pruritis of the genital and anal area
2. May be asymptomatic during a 30-day incubation period.

 Key Symptom

Pruritus

Clinical Findings

Head Lice
1. Adult lice or eggs (nits) found by careful inspection of the scalp.
   a. Adult: The life span of a female is about 40 days, during which time she produces 7 to 10 eggs a day. A nymph hatches after 8 to 10 days.
   b. Nits: white dots clinging to a hair shaft. Finding these is the most common means of diagnosis. Nits are attached at locations that ensure suitable incubation temperature; most likely found at the nape of the neck and behind the ears. Duration of the infestation can be estimated by the location on the hair shaft as a result of hair growth. Those within 3 to 4 mm of the scalp reflect active infestation.

2. Nits are firmly attached. This distinguishes them from normal hair scale.
3. Black dust (feces or molted skins of the lice) may be noticed on pillows or collars.
4. Erythematous papules usually on the occiput, nape of the neck, and postauricular region.
5. Regional adenopathy is rare but can be due to secondary bacterial infection.

Body Lice

1. Papules, urticaria, pyoderma, and postinflammatory hyperpigmentation are common.
2. Lice and/or nits in the seams of clothing

Pubic Lice

1. Erythematous papules and excoriations
2. Blue-gray macules (maculae ceruleae) may be seen on surrounding skin. Maculae ceruleae are caused by degradation of blood pigments by louse saliva. They are characteristic but not common. They are painless and disappear in a few days with no lasting effect.
3. Nits can be seen on pubic hair shafts and, infrequently, on the trunk, beard, eyelashes, and axillary areas.
4. Feces of crab lice often cause stains on underwear as reddish or black spots, produced by the feces becoming sticky when moistened by perspiration.

Key Signs

- Erythematous papules
- Excoriations
- Nits
- Maculae ceruleae

Laboratory Tests

Microscopic examination may reveal an adult louse or a nit.

1. An adult head louse is 2 to 4 mm and gray. Its legs (three pairs) are equipped with hook-like claws that enable it to grasp scalp hairs.
2. A nit is oval and has a lid (operculum) covering the free end.
3. The pubic louse is shorter and has widespread claws on the second and third pairs of legs.

Key Tests

Examination for nits

Differential Diagnosis

1. Head lice
   a. Seborrhea
   b. Psoriasis
   c. Tinea capitis
   d. Impetigo
   e. Artifacts (i.e., hair spray)
   f. Hair casts: moveable cylinders
   g. White piedra
   h. Trichonodosis
   i. Trichorrhexis nodosa
2. Body and pubic lice
   a. Scabies

Treatment

Head Lice

1. Permethrin (Nix): Destroys both lice and eggs.
   a. An over-the-counter synthetic pyrethroid, safe and effective; 95 per cent cure rate
   b. Apply to scalp after shampoo and rinse off after 10 minutes. One treatment is usually sufficient. Ovicidal activity is still detectable after 10 days.
   c. Side effects: 1 per cent experience mild dermatitis.
2. Lindane (Kwell, Scabene): Not recommended because of resistance.
   a. Less effective; less than 90 per cent cure rate
   b. Apply as a shampoo; massage into scalp and leave on 4 minutes before rinsing. Repeat after 7 days.
   c. Side effects: Neurotoxicity (resulting from percutaneous absorption) from misuse. Avoid use in infants, pregnant and nursing women, and anyone with a neurologic disorder.
3. Pyrethrin (R&C Shampoo, Rid, A-200, and Lice-Enz)
   a. Over-the-counter preparation, safer than Lindane; less than 90 per cent cure rate
   b. Naturally occurring insecticide extracted from chrysanthemum flowers.
   c. Apply to scalp, leave on for 10 minutes before rinsing.
   d. Not as ovicidal as permethrins.
4. Acetomicellar complex (SH-206TM, Pharmascience): a natural product; no published studies of effectiveness
5. Malathion (Ovide): 98 per cent cure rate in one study; not recommended because of unknown long-term side effects

Use all of the above per package instructions. *Do not use in infants less than 2 months of age.* Inspect every day after treatment. If live lice are seen 48 hours after treatment, resistance is a possibility. If this is the case, a different product should be used and repeated in 7 days. Pruritis may continue up to 10 days after successful treatment. Advise parents to repeat treatments only if lice or nits are seen.

Body Lice

1. Improved hygiene
2. Washing and drying clothing and bedding at high temperatures
3. Pediculicides are necessary only for epidemics.

Pubic Lice

1. Permethrin 1% creme rinse applied for 10 minutes
2. Lindane 1% shampoo applied for 4 minutes, then rinsed off
3. Treat sexual partners simultaneously.
4. Pediculicides should not be used around the eyes.
5. Eyelash infestations: Petroleum gel applied five times a day asphyxiates lice, or gentle removal with baby shampoo may help.
6. Clothing and bed linens washed and dried on a hot setting

Patient Education

1. It may be possible to eliminate head lice without medical treatment by daily combing of wet hair with a fine metal comb. The procedure must continue for up to 1 to 2 weeks until no further lice or nits are found. Even with the use of medication, metal combs are recommended to remove the nits from the hair shaft. Backcombing is helpful.
2. Close contacts, classmates, and family should be inspected and treated.

3. Can return to work or school after the first medical treatment. However, some schools and workplaces require hair to be free of nits before return.
   a. Wash clothes and linens in hot water and dry on hot settings if possible.
   b. Soak combs and brushes in hot water at least 10 minutes or wash in a pediculicide.
   c. Dry cleaning also kills lice and nits.
   d. Vacuum mattresses, carpets, and upholstery.
   e. Fumigation of the house is not necessary.
5. Careful follow-up by schools helps contain spread.
6. Reinfection is usually due to nonadherence to treatment plan.

Key Treatment

- Permethrin shampoo
- Lindane shampoo
- Pyrethrin
- Wash clothing and bed linen at high temperatures

Bibliography

Burgess IF: Human lice and their management. Adv Parasitol 1995;36:271–320.

Epstein SE, Orkin M: Pediculosis: clinical aspects. Part II: Cutaneous infestations: pediculosis. In Orkin M, Maibach HI (ed): Cutaneous Infestations and Insect Bites, vol 4, pp 159–237. New York, Marcel Dekker, 1985.

Forsman KE: Pediculosis and scabies. Postgrad Med 1995;98:89–100.

Parker J: Treatment of head lice [letter]. N Engl J Med 1997;336:734–735.

Public Health: the facts of lice. Can Med Assoc J 1997; 157:747.

Sander Stichele RH, Dezeure EM, Bogaert MG: Systematic review of clinical efficacy of topical treatments for head lice. BMJ 1995;311:604–608.

299 Fungus Infections of the Skin

David M. Adelson

Etiology

1. Fungal infections of the skin are usually caused by dermatophytes or fungi of the genus *Candida* or *Malassezia*.

2. Dermatophytes are of three genera: *Microsporum*, *Trichophyton*, and *Epidermophyton*. These aerobic organisms parasitize keratin of the skin, hair, and nail. Deeper penetration occurs with local or systemic immunosuppression.

   a. Geophylic dermatophytes normally are found in the soil but can infect humans or animals. Zoophilic dermatophytes are found on animals but can infect humans, and anthropophilic dermatophytes have humans as their only host.

   b. Certain species more commonly infect specific areas. *Microsporum* species generally invade the hair and glabrous skin. *Epidermophyton* infection usually involves the groin or feet. *Trichophyton* species infect the hair, skin, and nails.

   c. Transmission is from direct contact with infected persons, animals, or fomites.

3. *Candida albicans* is usually responsible for cutaneous candidiasis, but non-*albicans* candidal organisms can also cause infection. The mucosal epithelium or stratum corneum is invaded in areas of maceration or in patients with decreased cell-mediated immunity. Antibiotic therapy, diabetes, pregnancy, and the use of oral contraceptives can increase the risk of candidiasis.

4. *Malassezia furfur* causes tinea versicolor, a common superficial fungal infection and *Malassezia* (*Pityrosporum*) folliculitis. This organism can exist in two yeast forms called *P. ovale* and *P. orbiculare*.

Symptoms

1. Dermatophyte infections may be pruritic or asymptomatic. Occasionally there is tenderness and inflammation. Other symptoms depend on location.

   a. Scalp (tinea capitis): alopecia, scaling, occasionally swelling, occasionally purulent discharge

   b. Feet (tinea pedis): scaling, thickened soles, occasionally small blisters

   c. Nails (onychomycosis): thickening, brittleness, and subungual debris

2. Candidiasis: itching and burning, swelling, redness; scaly, creamy exudate

3. *Malassezia* infections

   a. Tinea versicolor: Usually asymptomatic but occasionally pruritic; often hypopigmented macules, especially in summer; mild scale with scratching

   b. *Malassezia* folliculitis: Asymptomatic or pruritic acne-like rash

Key Symptoms

- Itching
- Inflammation
- Scaling
- Tenderness
- Alopecia
- Blisters (rare)

Clinical Findings

Clinical findings depend on the organism and location of the infection.

1. Dermatophyte infections

   a. Scalp (tinea capitis)

      (1) Noninflammatory form: One or multiple scaly patches or plaques, and/or stubs (black dots); alopecia with minimal inflammation.

      (2) Inflammatory form: Papular or nodular erythematous plaque; alopecia. Can develop into a boggy, purulent nodule, often with a surface yellow crust (kerion).

   b. Body (tinea corporis): Erythematous plaque with central clearing and sharp margins. There is an advancing scale and an erythematous papular edge trailing this scaling. Occasionally intense inflammation with or without pustules.

   c. Groin (tinea cruris): Morphology similar to infections on the body. Papules, vesicles, or pustules may stud the border. The scrotum and penis are usually spared.

   d. Feet (tinea pedis): The most frequent form of

cutaneous fungal infection. There are three common forms of presentation.

   (1) Interdigital tinea pedis: macerated, red and scaly toe web space. Often associated fissuring. The fourth web space is most commonly involved.

   (2) Moccasin type: Dry, scaly, thick skin on soles and sides of feet. Soles are erythematous. May be seen on two feet and one hand or one foot and two hands.

   (3) Vesicular type: erythema, vesicles, and scaling, usually of the instep. The vesicles may coalesce into larger bullae.

   e. Nails (onychomycosis): Three clinical variants of dermatophyte nail infection exist:

   (1) Distal subungual onychomycosis: Thickening of the skin and collection of debris under the distal edge of the nail. The thickened nail becomes brittle and crumbles. The disease progresses from the distal edge proximally.

   (2) Proximal subungual onychomycosis: Thickening and crumbling of the nail begins at the proximal nail fold with disease progressing toward the tip.

   (3) Superficial white onychomycosis: White, chalky adherent plaques on the surface of the nail.

2. Candidal infections

   a. Intertrigo: Body folds such as the axillae, groin, gluteal folds, inframammary skin, interdigital spaces, corners of mouth, and retroauricular skin are involved. The area is intensely red, moist, and edematous. The edge is sharply marginated and there are usually surrounding satellite pustules or papules. With severe maceration, the pustules are usually absent and there is a cheesy exudate. In the groin the scrotum is often involved.

   b. Paronychia: erythema and edema around nailfold. The cuticle is lost. Subsequent dystrophic nail transverse ridging occurs that may progress to a thickened and brittle nail. Purulent exudate is often expressed from the proximal nail fold.

   c. Diaper candidiasis: maceration, intense erythema involving the skin folds and satellite pustules. Papular and nodular lesions can occur.

   d. Oral candidiasis: whitish patches loosely adherent to the mucosa; red beefy tongue at times; smooth patch with loss of papillae in central tongue

   e. Balanitis: red pinpoint pustules or papules on the glans and foreskin

3. *Malassezia* infections

   a. Tinea versicolor: small red, tan-brown, or hypopigmented macules with fine scale. Usually seen on the sternal skin, back, lateral chest, and sides of neck. Facial lesions can occur on infants and children.

   b. *Malassezia* folliculitis: pruritic acne-like papules and pustules on the chest or back

---

Key Signs

- Annular plaque
- Erythema and scale
- Dry, thickened soles
- Satellite pustules (*Candida*)
- Alopecia
- Broken hairs
- Thickened nails
- Cheesy exudate (*Candida*)

Laboratory Tests

1. Potassium hydroxide (KOH) preparation: Skin or nail scrapings or hair plucks from the edge of the involved sites are obtained. Samples are placed on a glass slide, 10% to 20% KOH is applied, followed by a cover slip, and the slide is gently heated. The slide is then viewed microscopically for fungus.

   a. Chlorozol black E is a stain that combines KOH and a fungal stain that stains fungus a blue-black color. It contains dimethylsulfoxide; therefore, heating is not necessary.

   b. Hyphae are seen in dermatophyte infections, pseudohyphae in candidal infections, and short, fat hyphae and/or yeast in diseases caused by *Malassezia*.

2. Wood's light (black light) shown on the affected area in a pitch-black room

   a. Yellow or green-yellow fluorescence of hair shafts suggests fungal infection.

   b. Coral-red fluorescence is seen in primary or secondary erythrasma (see "Differential Diagnosis").

3. Fungal culture: skin scrapings, nail clippings, or hair plucks from the involved area

   a. Sabouraud's dextrose agar: standard in mycology labs

   b. Dermatophyte test media (DTM) contains a pH color indicator. Dermatophyte growth raises the pH of the media, changing the color to red.

4. Skin biopsy: Rarely necessary; however, fungal infections can be diagnosed when not initially expected. Histologic fungal stains will show the organism.

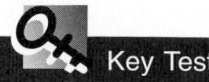
Differential Diagnosis

1. Dermatophyte infection
   a. Tinea capitis: psoriasis, seborrheic dermatitis, alopecia areata, trichotillomania, discoid lupus
   b. Tinea corporis: psoriasis, nummular eczema, pityriasis rosea, secondary syphilis
   c. Tinea cruris: psoriasis, seborrheic dermatitis, erythrasma, intertrigo, candidal intertrigo
   d. Tinea pedis
      (1) Interdigital type: erythrasma and mixed intertriginous infection caused by secondary bacterial infection
      (2) Moccasin type: psoriasis, irritant foot dermatitis, keratoderma, secondary syphilis
      (3) Vesicular type: dyshidrotic eczema, palmoplantar psoriasis
   e. Onychomycosis: nail psoriasis, traumatic nail dystrophy, lichen planus
2. Candidal infection
   a. Intertrigo: same as tinea cruris above
   b. Paronychia: bacterial paronychia, usually staphylococcal
   c. Diaper candidiasis: irritant diaper dermatitis, seborrheic dermatitis, psoriasis; rare: histiocytosis X, congenital syphilis, acrodermatitis enteropathica
   d. Oral candidiasis: lichen planus, leukoplakia, oral hairy leukoplakia
   e. Balanitis: herpes genitalis, lichen planus, psoriasis
3. *Malassezia* infections
   a. Tinea versicolor: pityriasis rosea, seborrheic dermatitis, secondary syphilis, vitiligo
   b. *Malassezia* folliculitis: bacterial folliculitis, acne vulgaris

Treatment

1. Keep infected area clean and dry.
2. When used as a single agent, topical antifungals are ineffective in treating fungal infections of the scalp, beard area, or nails.
3. An oral agent is also preferred if extensive body areas are infected.

Medication—Available Agents

1. Topical antifungals
   a. Imidazole compounds: effective in treating dermatophyte, *Candida*, and *Malassezia* infections. Low cost and wide spectrum make them the drug of choice for uncomplicated, limited disease. Included in this group are clotrimazole (Lotrimin), miconazole (Monistat), ketoconazole (Nizoral), econozole (Spectazole), sulconazole (Exelderm), oxiconazole (Oxistat), and terconazole (Terazol).
   b. Allylamines: include naftifine (Naftin) and terbinafine (Lamisil). Have a wide spectrum and are fungicidal for dermatophytes and fungistatic for *Candida*.
   c. Ciclopirox olamine (Loprox): effective broad-spectrum fungicidal agent
   d. Nystatin: a polyene antibiotic that is only effective in *Candida* infections
2. Oral antifungals
   a. Griseofulvin: effective in dermatophyte but ineffective in *Candida* or *Malassezia* infections. Some reports of resistant dermatophytes.
   b. Oral imidazoles: Broad spectrum of activity; include ketoconazole, fluconazole, and itraconazole.
   c. Oral allylamines: fungicidal against dermatophytes, not as active against yeasts.

Medication—Drug of Choice

Because medication dosages often change, please check all dosages prior to dispensing.

1. Dermatophyte infection
   a. Tinea capitis
      (1) Adult: griseofulvin (ultramicrosize), 250 to 375 mg/day; pediatric: griseofulvin (ultramicrosize), 5.5 to 7.3 mg/kg/day. Treat for 6 weeks.
      (2) Alternates: None of these alternatives are presently indicated by the Food and Drug Administration (FDA) for the treatment of tinea capitis.
         (a) Itraconazole (Sporanox), 100 mg/day (or 3 to 5 mg/kg/day) for 4 weeks
         (b) Fluconazole (Diflucan), 6 mg/kg/day for 3 to 6 weeks; not FDA approved for the treatment of dermatophyte infection
         (c) Terbinafine (Lamisil), 62.5 mg/day if less than 20 kg, 125 mg/day if 20 to 40 kg, 250 mg/day if greater than 40 kg, for 4 weeks

(3) Adjuvant therapy: Shampoo with selenium sulfide 2.5% or ketoconazole shampoo two times per week. Include close family contacts.

b. Tinea corporis
   (1) Limited: topical imidazole for 2 to 3 weeks. Medication should continue for at least 1 week after clinical cure.
   (2) Extensive or in beard area: griseofulvin (ultramicrosize), 250 to 375 mg/day. Treat for 4 weeks.
   (3) Alternates: itraconazole, 200 mg bid for 7 days; terbinafine, 250 mg/day for 2 weeks

c. Tinea cruris
   (1) Topical imidazole (DTIC-Dome) for 2 to 3 weeks. Medication should continue for at least 1 week after clinical cure.
   (2) Alternates: itraconazole, 200 mg bid for 7 days; terbinafine, 250 mg/day for 2 weeks

d. Tinea pedis
   (1) Topical imidazole for 4 weeks
   (2) Alternates: itraconazole, 200 mg bid for 7 days; terbinafine, 250 mg/day for 2 weeks

e. Onychomycosis
   (1) Itraconazole, 200 mg bid for 7 days, repeat monthly for 2 months (fingernails) or 3 months (toenails); or terbinafine, 250 mg/day for 6 weeks (fingernails) or 12 weeks (toenails)
   (2) Alternate: fluconazole, 150 mg/week for 12 months; Not FDA approved for the treatment of dermatophyte infection

2. Candidal infection
   a. Topical imidazole, nystatin, cyclopirox, or allylamine
   b. Alternates: If recalcitrant: oral ketoconazole, 200 mg/day; fluconazole, 100 mg/day; itraconazole, 100 mg/day

3. *Malassezia* infections
   a. Tinea versicolor
      (1) Limited: selenium sulfide 2.5% lathered on for 5 minutes, then rinsed, or topical imidazole. Alternate: 50% propylene glycol bid for 2 weeks.
      (2) Extensive: ketoconazole, 400 mg in a single dose, repeated in 1 week; or fluconazole 400-mg single dose

   b. *Malassezia* folliculitis: selenium sulfide 2.5% lathered on for 5 minutes, then rinsed

Diet

No restrictions

Activity

No restrictions

Patient Education

1. Reinfection is common, so avoid sharing personal hygienic tools, shoes, or clothing with others.
2. With tinea pedis, avoid occlusive footwear; wear shower shoes in shower shared with public (i.e., health club or hotel).
3. Others in the family should be evaluated for infection, particularly with tinea capitis.

 Key Treatment

Drugs of Choice	Alternative Drugs
• Topical imidazole (body)	• Topical allylamine
• Griseofulvin (scalp)	• Topical cyclopirox
• Terbinafine (nails)	• Oral itraconazole
• Itraconazole (nails)	• Oral fluconazole

Follow-Up

1. Persistent or recurrent infections should be reevaluated.
2. A post-therapy fungal culture should be obtained in patients with tinea capitis.

 Bibliography

Elgart ML, Warren NG: The superficial and subcutaneous mycoses. In Moschella SL, Hurley HJ (eds): Dermatology, 3rd ed, vol 1, pp 869–912. Philadelphia, WB Saunders Company, 1992.

Fallon-Friedlander S: Pediatric antifungal therapy. Dermatol Clin 1998;16:527–533.

Gupta AK, Sauder DN, Shear NH: Antifungal agents: an overview. Part I. J Am Acad Dermatol 1994;30:677–698.

Gupta AK, Sauder DN, Shear NH: Antifungal agents: an overview. Part II. J Am Acad Dermatol 1994;30:911–933.

Katz HI: Systemic antifungal agents used to treat onychomycosis. J Am Acad Dermatol 1998;38:S48–S51.

Odom RB: New therapies for onychomycosis. J Am Acad Dermatol 1996;35:S26–S30.

300 Burns

Augustine J. Sohn

Classification

Burns can be classified in many different ways.
1. According to the etiology of burns
   a. Scalding burn: exposure to hot liquid, most common cause
   b. Chemical burns: caused by either acid or alkali exposure
   c. Electrical burns: caused by exposure to electrical current
   d. Inhalation burn: usually caused by exposure to closed-space burns; have more serious problems in systems such as respiratory system.
2. According to the depth of burn injury
   a. First-degree burns: Usually involve epidermis; like sunburn; no blisters.
   b. Second-degree burns
      (1) Superficial: Involve papillary dermis and have blisters; painful.
      (2) Deep: Involve reticular dermis; have blisters; painful.
   c. Third-degree burns: Involve full-thickness dermis and subcutaneous tissue, usually pale in appearance and painless because the nerve endings were destroyed.
   d. Fourth-degree burns: Involve the muscles and bones.
3. According to the severity of burns
   a. Minor burns: less than 15 per cent of total body surface area in adult and less than 10 per cent of total body surface area in child; no third-degree burns
   b. Moderate burns: between 15 and 25 per cent of total body surface area in adult and 10 to 20 per cent of total body surface area in child; less than 10 per cent third-degree burns
   c. Severe burns: more than 25 per cent of total body surface in adult and more than 20 per cent of total body area in child; more than 10 per cent third-degree burns. Also includes serious burn to eyes, ears, face, hands, feet, perineum; inhalation injury; electrical burn; other trauma; and high-risk patient.
   d. Calculation of total body area of burn is based on "Rule of Nines."

Rule of Nines

The body can be divided into several areas of 9 per cent, with the head and each arm being 9 per cent each. The anterior trunk, posterior trunk, and each leg are each 18 per cent. This leaves 1 per cent for the genitalia and perineum. The size of the palm of the patient's hand is approximately 1 per cent of total body surface area.

Symptoms

1. First- and second-degree burns: pain with burn injury
2. Third-degree burn: no pain with burn injury

Key Symptom

The main difference between first- and second-degree burns and third-degree burns is the absence of pain in third-degree burns because of the death of nerve endings.

Clinical Findings

1. First-degree burn: erythema, no blister
2. Second-degree burn
   a. Superficial: blisters, erythema, capillary refills, intact pain sensation
   b. Deep: blisters, pale white or yellow color, no capillary refill, absent pain sensation
3. Third-degree burn: absence of blisters, pale and no sensation on touch because of nerve damage, no capillary refill
4. Fourth-degree burn: burn to the muscles and bones

Key Sign

Main difference between first-degree and second-degree burn is the absence of blisters in the first-degree burn. Sometimes it takes a few days to be able to differentiate between deep second-degree burns and third-degree burns.

Laboratory Tests

Usually laboratory tests are not necessary in minor and moderate burns. In major burns, an arterial blood sample for pH, blood gases, carboxyhemoglobin level, serum electrolytes, urea nitrogen, glucose, and hematocrit should be obtained.

WARNING

It should be remembered that tests for oxygen saturations and arterial blood gases will not reveal the extent of tissue hypoxia because oximeters do not detect carboxyhemoglobin in case of inhalation burn injury

---

WARNING

Differential diagnosis may not be difficult in diagnosing burn injury based on symptoms and clinical findings, but may need more thorough investigation in infants and children for evidence of lack of parental supervision (which might necessitate involvement of community services in further accident prevention) or the suspicion of child abuse or neglect (may necessitate department of child and family service involvement in case).

Treatment

The following burns require hospitalization:

1. All "major" burns
2. Burns with suspected inhalation injury
3. Deep burns of scalp; burns of eye, buttock, and/or perineum
4. Crushing burns, especially of the hands or feet
5. Circumferential burns of the chest, which might impair ventilation, or a limb, which might embarrass circulation
6. Severe electrical burn
7. Patients whose home circumstances make it impossible for them to be managed as outpatients

Management of Minor Burns at Outpatient Office

1. First aid: Immediately cooling the burned area is still the best way to control the pain and to limit the inflammatory damage by limiting thermal damage. Cooling can be achieved the best with 20° to 25°C cool water within 30 minutes of injury.
2. Pain control: May require opiates in severely painful cases such as superficial second-degree burns. Aspirin should be avoided because it can cause platelet dysfunction, thereby worsening the coagulation-anticoagulation phenomenon of the inflammatory cascade.

3. Débridement: Débride any bullae exceeding 2 cm in diameter, which may be vulnerable to rupture; small bullae if they are draining; and erosions that are necrotic or contain purulent material. The easiest way is to cut all the way around the blister using an iris scissors and forceps.
4. Infection control: Coat the wound with antibiotic ointment such as Bactroban (mupirocin) or Silvadene cream (silver sulfadiazine). Although burn wounds are initially sterile, hair follicles and sweat glands are a source of wound contamination. For gram-positive organism such as *Staphylococcus* and *Streptococcus pyogenes*, which are seen during the first week, mupirocin is effective. Silver sulfadiazine provides much broader coverage, including that against *Pseudomonas aeruginosa*, *Escherichia coli*, and other gram-negative infections that occur during the second week.
5. Wound cleansing: Clean gently with tap water and soap.
6. Dressings: Use nonstick occlusive topical dressings to avoid causing pain when the dressing is changed. Dressing change should be done every 3 days until epithelialization occurs.
7. Patient education: Patients should call if purulent or greenish drainage develops, edema or pain increases, or there are signs of systemic toxicity.

Management of Major Burns

1. Airway establishment is the first step, especially when there is an inhalation injury.
2. Fluid resuscitation:
   a. First day: Lactated Ringer's solution, 4 ml/kg of body weight multiplied by the percentage of body surface area burned for 24 hours; first half in 8 hours and second half in 16 hours.
   b. Second day: Half of first day's lactated Ringer's solution.
   c. Third day and after: Alter the rate of fluid administration using an hourly urine output in adults of 0.5 ml/kg; in children who weigh less than 25 kg, an output of 1.0 ml/kg is necessary.
3. Topical antimicrobial agents prolong the interval between injury and colonization and maintain low levels of the wound flora. Only three agents have proven efficacy in major burns: 8.5% mafenide acetate cream, 1% silver sulfadiazine cream, and 0.5% silver nitrate solution.
4. Surgical treatment of deep burns: skin graft if necessary

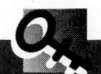

Key Treatment

- Except for first-degree burns, all burn wound patients need tetanus prophylaxis.

- Immediate cooling

- Débride large bullae

- Antibiotic ointment and nonstick dressings

- Lactated Ringer's solution in major burns

Bibliography

Greenhalgh D: Physical and chemical injuries: burns. In Rakel R (ed): Conn's Current Therapy, pp 1169–1174. Philadelphia, WB Saunders Company, 1997.

Herndon D: Physical and chemical injuries: burns. In Rakel R (ed): Conn's Current Therapy, pp 1155–1159. Philadelphia, WB Saunders Company, 1998.

Marsden AK: Minor burns. In Settle JAD (ed): Principles and Practice of Burn Management, pp 203–208. New York, Churchill Livingstone, 1996.

Monafo W: Initial management of burns. N Engl J Med 1996;335:1581–1585.

Pruitt BA Jr, Cood CG Jr, Pruitt SK: Burns including cold, chemical, and electric injuries. In Sabiston D (ed): Textbook of Surgery: The Biological Basis of Modern Surgical Practice, 15th ed, pp 221–252. Philadelphia, WB Saunders Company, 1997.

301 Rosacea

Elizabeth E. Brownell

Etiology

1. Rosacea is a chronic episodic skin disorder with onset between the ages of 30 and 50 years. It affects women three times more than men.
2. The cause of rosacea is unknown. There are many postulated causes, several of which include
   a. Genetic predisposition: Celtic origin
   b. Hypertension
   c. *Demodex folliculorum* mites
   d. Gastrointestinal disease
3. Known contributing factors to rosacea are
   a. Persons predisposed to flushing and blushing
      (1) Dietary and environmental precipitation
      (2) Menopause
      (3) Vasodilator drug therapy
   b. Exposure to sunlight and heat

Symptoms

1. Excessive flushing and blushing with persistence of facial heat and redness
2. Sensitive skin that may sting and burn after use of lotions, cosmetics, or astringents
3. Persistent painful papules and cysts unresponsive to antiacne therapy

Key Symptoms

- Facial heat and redness
- Sensitive skin
- Painful papules and cysts

Clinical Findings

1. Rosacea affects the central face, especially the forehead, cheeks, chin, nose, and glabella. The hallmarks of rosacea, after an episode of flushing, are erythema, telangiectasias, papules, and papulopustules. Comedones are classically *absent*.
2. Rosacea occurs as intermittent but progressively more severe episodes.
   a. Mild erythema lasting for hours to days and a few scattered telangiectasias
   b. Moderate erythema, more telangiectasias, papules, and pustules that may persist for weeks
   c. Bright erythema, networks of telangiectasias, papules, and pustules. Variable patches of edema affect primarily the cheeks and nose.
3. Characteristic of more severe rosacea are chronic inflammation, connective tissue hypertrophy with collagen deposition, and diffuse sebaceous gland hyperplasia.
   a. Disfiguring deformities resulting from these tissue changes are the "phymas." The most characteristic is rhinophyma, a gross deformity of the nose primarily affecting men.
   b. Ocular rosacea may develop and can cause blepharitis, conjunctivitis, and corneal ulcers.

Key Signs

- Erythema
- Telangiectasias
- Papules
- Papulopustules

Laboratory Tests

1. The diagnosis of rosacea is based on clinical findings. There are no definitive laboratory tests.
2. Histopathology is variable, and a combination of findings may support the diagnosis of rosacea, but biopsies are not routinely performed for diagnoses.

Differential Diagnosis

1. Acne vulgaris
2. Perioral dermatitis
3. Seborrheic dermatitis
4. Contact dermatitis
5. *Staphylococcus aureus* folliculitis
6. Lupus erythematosus
7. Carcinoid flush
8. Cutaneous tuberculosis

Treatment

1. Rosacea can be treated, but complete cure is usually not possible.

2. Treatment is based on the predominant clinical findings and severity of the disease. Options include topical therapy, systemic therapy, and dietary and environmental modifications.

Medication

1. Topical therapy
   a. Topical antibiotics can be effective against papulopustular rosacea: tetracycline, erythromycin, or clindamycin in a 0.5 to 2.0% concentration applied twice daily.
   b. Metronidazole (0.75% MetroGel) applied twice daily
      (1) Greatest effect on papules and pustules
      (2) Little effect on erythema and telangiectasias
   c. Drying lotions applied once or twice daily
      (1) Benzoyl peroxide
      (2) Sulfur-containing lotions
   d. Hydrocortisone cream 1% may be useful in decreasing the erythema and inflammation of rosacea. Fluorinated steroids should *not* be used. Although initially effective, prolonged use causes a rebound worsening of rosacea symptoms.
   e. Telangiectatic vessels may be treated by superficial electrodesiccation or laser surgery.
   f. Soft tissue hypertrophy in rhinophyma is most effectively treated with CO_2 laser surgery, dermabrasion, or electrosurgery.
   g. Ocular complications should be evaluated by an ophthalmologist.
2. Systemic therapy
   a. Systemic antibiotics are effective in treating the inflammatory lesions (papules and pustules) of rosacea.
      (1) Tetracycline, 250 mg orally four times daily, until symptoms diminish; then taper or discontinue the medication.
      (2) Erythromycin or minocycline, 50 to 100 mg twice daily, is an alternative if tetracycline is ineffective.
      (3) Metronidazole, 250 mg twice daily, may be as effective as tetracycline in a first-line approach or as an alternative if tetracycline is ineffective.
   b. Isotretinoin (13-*cis*-retinoic acid) (Accutane)
      (1) Isotretinoin may be effective in severe rosacea or rosacea unresponsive to other forms of therapy.
         (a) Standard dose: 0.5 to 1.0 mg/kg/day for 15 to 20 weeks. Used primarily in refractory rosacea. Adverse effects can limit course of treatment.

(b) Low dose: 0.1 to 0.2 mg/kg/day. Improvement may take longer than standard dose. Fewer adverse effects
(c) Minidose: 2.5 to 5 mg daily (*not* adjusted for body weight). Improvement may take up to 6 months. Adverse effects are minimal.
      (2) Adverse effects are dose-related.
         (a) Ocular
            (i) Blepharitis
            (ii) Dry eyes
         (b) Hepatotoxicity
         (c) Teratogen: contraindicated in pregnant women

Diet

Avoid any foods that might cause vasodilation of blood vessels and therefore facial flushing, including hot liquids, alcohol, tea, spicy foods, coffee, and tobacco.

Activity

Avoid extremes of weather: prolonged sun exposure, heat, wind, and cold.

Patient Education

1. See "Diet" above.
2. Sunscreens with a sun protection factor (SPF) of 15 or higher
3. Use a mild, nondrying soap.
4. Avoid local skin irritants: alcohol-based facial cleansers, peeling agents, abrasive facial cleansers, topical medications.
5. Stress management may be helpful.

Key Treatment

- Topical therapy
- Systemic therapy

Follow-Up

Determined by individual treatment and severity of disease.

Bibliography

Arndt AA: Rosacea and periorofacial (perioral) dermatitis. In Bernhardt MS (ed): Manual of Dermatologic Therapeutics, 5th ed, pp 160–163. Boston, Little, Brown, 1995.

Fitzpatrick TB, Johnson RA, Wolff K: Rosacea. In Wonsiewicz MJ, Englis MR, McCurdy PA (eds): Color Atlas and Synopsis of Clinical Dermatology: Common and

Serious Disease, 3rd ed, pp 12–15. New York, Mc-
Graw-Hill, 1997.

Habif TP: Acne, rosacea and related disorders. In Baxter
S (ed): Clinical Dermatology: A Color Guide to Diag-
nosis and Therapy, 3rd ed, pp 182–183. St Louis,
Mosby, 1996.

Moschella SL, Hurley HJ: Rosacea. In Fletcher J (ed):
Dermatology, 3rd ed, vol 2, pp 1487–1491. Philadelphia, WB Saunders Company, 1992.

Plewig G: Rosacea. In Fitspatrick TB, Eisen AZ, Wolff K,
et al. (eds): Dermatology in General Medicine, 4th ed,
vol 1, pp 727–735. New York, McGraw-Hill, 1993.

Wilken JK: Rosacea: pathophysiology and treatment.
Arch Dermatol 1994;130:359–362.

302 Tattoo Removal

Mark D. Wells

Human skin has served as a canvas for artistic expression for thousands of years. Tattoos result from exogenous material being implanted in the dermis, most often by tattoo artists, cosmetologists, or trauma. Modern puncture tattoos probably date back to 8000 BC. It is estimated that approximately 10 million people in the United States have decorative tattoos, with the ratio of males to females being approximately 10:1.

Etiology

1. Amateur tattoos: Self-inflicted tattooing is easily accomplished by dipping the point of a needle in ink and puncturing the skin repeatedly. These tattoos are characterized by variability in pigment depth, making removal more problematic.
2. Professional tattoos: These tattoos are performed under antiseptic conditions using a rapidly moving electric needle. A variety of pigments can be at a relatively constant depth within the papillary dermis.
3. Posttraumatic tattoos: Foreign bodies are embedded within the dermis following accidental abrasion of the skin. The epithelial elements regenerate, resulting in permanent entrapment of particulate matter within the dermis.
4. Medical and cosmetic tattoos
   a. Historically, tattooing was used medically in an attempt to camouflage vascular malformations of the skin. Generally, the results of this treatment were cosmetically unacceptable. More recently, tattooing has been used successfully to create the areola after mastectomy and breast reconstruction.
   b. Placement of tattoos is on the rise by cosmetologists. Application of permanent lip liner, eyeliner, and brow pigmentation has become very popular.

Histopathology

1. Initial reaction
   a. Wheal-and-flare reaction with edema
   b. Nonspecific inflammatory reaction
   c. Superficial crusting of the epidermis
   d. Some loss of pigment as it extrudes through the needle holes
2. Over months
   a. Unassimilated granules remain between collagen bundles within the dermis.
   b. Some of the pigment is transported to regional lymph nodes.
3. Over years
   a. Mild perivascular lymphocytic inflammation causes dermal fibrosis with loss of tattoo definition.
   b. Color of tattoo begins to fade.
   c. Fading process is accelerated by sun exposure.

Potential Complications

1. Pyogenic infections
   a. Superficial
      (1) Impetigo
      (2) Ecthyma
   b. Deep
      (1) Furunculosis
      (2) Erysipelas
      (3) Cellulitis
2. Nonpyogenic infections
   a. Syphilis
   b. Hepatitis B
   c. Tetanus
   d. Human immunodeficiency virus
   e. Molluscum contagiosum
   f. Tuberculosis cutis
   g. Leprosy
3. Cutaneous diseases that localize in tattoos
   a. Vaccinia
   b. Verruca vulgaris
   c. Herpes simplex and zoster
   d. Psoriasis
   e. Lichen planus
   f. Darier's disease
   g. Chronic discoid lupus
   h. Keratoacanthoma
4. Acquired tattoo pigment sensitivity
   a. Mercury (red)
   b. Chromium (green)
   c. Cadmium (yellow)
   d. Cobalt (blue)

5. Miscellaneous reactions
   a. Hypertrophic scarring
   b. Keloid
   c. Sarcoid granulomas
   d. Lymphadenopathy
   e. Localized scleroderma
   f. Erythema multiforme

Treatment

The disdain that society at large holds toward people with tattoos frequently motivates individuals with tattoos to have them removed. Tattoos that are often requested to be ablated include antisocial messages, obscene subjects, or the names of past acquaintances. Additionally, tattoos in highly visible regions such as the hands and face are more likely to require subsequent removal. Despite many practitioners' claims, there is no technique that can remove a tattoo without risk of scarring or pigmentary change.

1. Overtattooing: Tattoo artists are often asked to modify unacceptable tattoos. Their methods include overtattooing or retattooing with a lighter pigment in an attempt to mask a dark tattoo. Alternatively, older unacceptable tattoos can be incorporated into new ones, albeit at the cost of a larger tattoo.

2. Cauterization: Do-it-yourself methods of removing tattoos include cauterization with cigarettes and hot coat hangers. The third-degree burns caused by these methods may be associated with wound sepsis or unacceptable scarring. Cauterization is *not* recommended.

3. Salabrasion
   a. An irritating substance (bleach, salicylic acid, tannic acid) is applied to the tattoo for several days, after which table salt is rubbed into the tattoo site. The result is epidermal abrasion with underlying inflammation. Pigment is leached out during the healing phase.
   b. Often the processes must be repeated several times to be effective. Scarring, which is sometimes hypertrophic, is not uncommon.

4. Dermabrasion
   a. The tattoo is anesthetized and abraded with a high-speed mechanical wheel. Only the epidermis and part of the upper dermis is removed. The epidermis is allowed to regenerate from the residual adnexal structures.
   b. If the pigment is buried deep within the dermis, incomplete removal may occur. Additionally, there is a significant risk of unacceptable scarring with this method.

5. Chemical peel
   a. The tattoo is treated with topical phenol or trichloroacetic acid. These chemicals are allowed to react with the skin until they induce coagulative necrosis to the level of the papillary dermis. The epidermis is allowed to regenerate from the uninjured dermal elements.
   b. Incomplete pigment removal, scarring, hypopigmentation, and arrhythmias (phenol) are all possible complications with this method.

6. Cryosurgery: Freon, carbon dioxide, liquid oxygen, and liquid nitrogen have all been advocated. All result in necrosis of the epidermis and the papillary dermis with sloughing of a portion of the pigment. This technique has generally been abandoned because of poor results.

7. Acids: When caustic substances such as hydrochloric acid or nitric acid are used to remove tattoos, a third-degree burn often results, with healing by secondary intention. The risk of infection is high and the resultant scarring unacceptable.

8. Surgery
   a. Small tattoos may be amenable to surgical excision and direct closure. Larger tattoos however, are often more problematic.
      (1) Serial excision of a portion of the tattoo in two or three stages allows removal of a larger area than would otherwise be possible in one stage.
      (2) Tissue expansion also has been advocated. By progressively stretching the normal skin adjacent to a tattoo over several weeks with a mechanical device, it may be possible to excise the tattoo and resurface the region with a local advancement flap. This technique has the advantage of resurfacing the tattooed region with tissue of similar texture and quality. However, a major disadvantage is the time required for expansion and the need for two stages. Additionally, expander extrusion and infection are not uncommon, particularly in the extremities.
   b. Some professional tattoos may be amenable to tangential excision of pigment within the papillary dermis with a dermatome blade. The epithelial elements are allowed to regenerate over a period of 7 to 10 days depending on the depth of excision. Alternatively, if the excision extends into the subcutaneous fat, split- or full-thickness skin grafting can be performed to resurface the wound.

9. Laser

a. In the newest technique to remove tattoo pigment within the dermis, lasers are used to vaporize the pigment.

b. Early studies used the carbon dioxide and argon lasers. Both of these devices caused disruption of the epidermis and dermis with extrusion of the pigment. These lasers rely on the tattoo pigment being carried away in the posttreatment exudate as well as dermal sclerosis to obscure residual deeper pigment. Their use was associated with variable degrees of hypertrophic scarring and hypopigmentation.

c. More recently, Q-switched laser technology has been advocated.

   (1) The laser light is selectively absorbed by the targeted ink and preferably ignored by the surrounding chromophobes in the skin, such as melanin and hemoglobin. Exposure time is limited so that the heat generated is confined to the target pigment and not allowd to diffuse to the surrounding soft tissues.

   (2) Q-switched lasers have a pulse duration that can be measured in nanoseconds, wavelengths well absorbed by most tattoo inks, and high peak powers. These characteristics allow the laser to be used for selective photothermolysis of ink particles. Q-switched lasers fracture the large ink particles into smaller ones, so they can be more easily scavenged by resident macrophages.

d. The ability of a particular wavelength to remove colored ink particles can be predicted by the ink's absorption spectra.

   (1) Red-containing pigments are best treated with 510-nm wavelengths (pulsed dye green laser).

   (2) Green-containing pigments are best treated at 694-nm (Q-switched ruby laser) or 755-nm (Q-switched alexandrite laser) wavelengths.

   (3) Black ink responds well to red light and less so to green.

   (4) Short-wavelength lasers can often injure melanocytes, creating hypopigmentation, particularly in dark-skinned individuals. For darker individuals, the use of the 1064-nm wavelength (Q-switched neodymium: yttrium-aluminum-garnet laser) shows less interference with cutaneous melanin.

   (5) All these lasers can produce pigmentary changes (hypo- and hyperpigmentation) in susceptible individuals. Skin textural changes are usually minimal.

e. The need for multiple treatments and the expense of the equipment are major disadvantages of the laser procedure.

Key Treatment

- Overtattooing
- Cauterization
- Salabrasion
- Dermabrasion
- Chemical peel
- Cryosurgery
- Acids
- Surgery
- Lasers

Bibliography

Achauer BM: Lasers in plastic surgery. Plast Reconstr Surg 1997;99:1442–1450.

Bjarnesen JP, Wester JU, Sienssen SS, et al: External skin stretching for closure of skin defects in 22 patients. Acta Orthop Scand 1996;67:182–184.

Cronin ED, Harber JL: A new technique of dermabrasion for traumatic tattoos. Ann Plast Surg 1996;36:401–402.

Kilmer SL: Laser treatment of tattoos. Dermatol Clin 1997;3:409–417.

O'Donnell BP, Mulvaney MJ, James WD, et al: Thin tangential excision of tattoos. Dermatol Surg 1995;21:601–603.

Goals

1. Return tissue to as near preinjury state as possible (normally functioning, cosmetically pleasing with scar as small as possible).
2. Excise devitalized tissue.
3. Close primarily whenever possible.
4. Low or no tension. May require advancement or rhomboid flap closure (see Procedure on Wound Revision).

> **Note**
> See the next procedure, Wound Revision, for preparation and follow-up.

Equipment

1. Anesthetic and syringes
2. Sterile minor surgical tray (disposable or autoclaved)
   a. Instruments
      (1) Needle holder
      (2) Adson tissue forceps (with and without teeth)
      (3) Skin hooks—commercial or home-made (see below)
      (4) Iris scissors
      (5) Hemostats (2 or more)
      (6) No. 15 scalpel handle and blade (or disposable)
      (7) (Optional) Metzenbaum scissors
   b. Materials
      (1) Sterile 4 × 4 gauze pads
      (2) Sterile towels (cloth or paper)
      (3) Sterile saline
      (4) Sterile gloves
      (5) Additional sterile syringes/needles as needed
      (6) Appropriate sutures (or staples or glue)

Anesthesia

1. Generally local infiltration
   a. Materials
      (1) A 10-ml syringe
      (2) An 18- to 20-gauge needle to pull up anesthetic from vial
      (3) A 26- to 30-gauge needle for administration of anesthetic
      (4) 1% lidocaine, with or without epinephrine: Buffer with 1:10 $NaHCO_3$ to lidocaine.
      (5) Nonsterile gloves for anesthetic administration
      (6) Alcohol to cleanse skin at injection site (if necessary)
   b. Inject buffered anesthetic slowly through wound margins into subcuticular layer to minimize discomfort.
2. Field blocks as appropriate (intraoral or facial wounds).
3. Consider topical anesthetic, especially in children (e.g., tetracaine, adrenalin, and cocaine [TAC] or lidocaine, adrenalin, and tetracaine [LAT]).

Precautions

1. Be gentle with tissue.
   a. Never place a crushing clamp on any tissue (except for hemostasis) that will remain in the wound after repair is complete.
   b. Adson forceps can crush tissue. Skin hooks are much less traumatic.
   c. Sharply excise devitalized, severely injured, or contaminated tissue.
   d. Never put toxic materials (povidone-iodine, soap, etc.) into the wound. Irrigate copiously with saline.
2. Assess function of underlying nerves, tendons, and vessels before repair. *Sensation must be evaluated before anesthetic.*
3. Ensure hemostasis.
4. Close dead space.
5. Avoid skin tension: undermine; consider flaps (see Procedure on Wound Revision).
6. Prepare sharp vertical margins for closure.
7. Verify tetanus status.
8. Avoid epinephrine in sensitive areas: "fingers and toes, ears and nose," genitalia, and the like.

Technique

1. Inspect all wounds.
   a. Ensure function of deeper structures.
   b. Cleanse *skin* around wound with povidone-iodine or Hibiclens.

c. Anesthetize (local or topical).

d. Remove all foreign bodies and devitalized tissue.

e. Irrigate wound copiously with saline.

2. Ensure hemostasis.

a. Most bleeding stops spontaneously. Use hemostat if necessary (may be released after 1 to 2 minutes)

b. Use figure-of-eight sutures around hemostat.

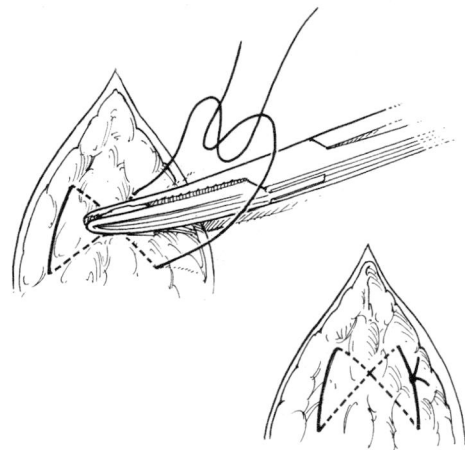

c. Electrocauterize if necessary: Tips can be sterilized and handle placed inside sterile glove to bring into sterile field.

3. Prepare wound margins.

a. Clean and square irregular or devitalized edges with scalpel or scissors. Divide all skin layers with a single cut. (Do not make "hesitation marks.")

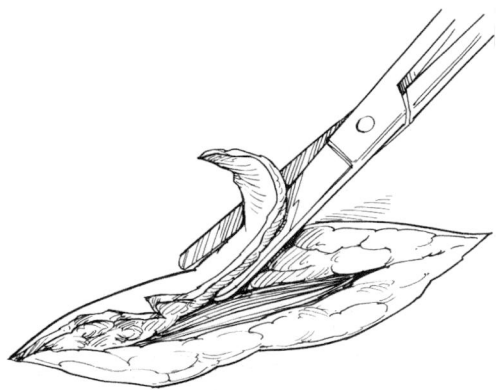

b. Tangenital wounds mound or pit when they heal and retract and make unsightly scars. Convert to vertical margins.

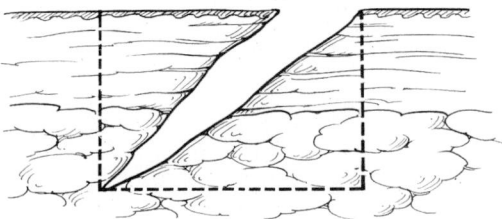

4. Facial wounds: Preserve as much tissue as feasible.

a. Reapproximate irregular margins like a jigsaw puzzle.

b. If too irregular or macerated, consider excising entire wound and converting into fusiform incision for closure.

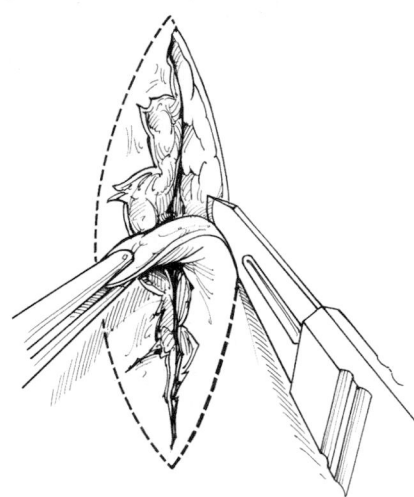

5. Undermine skin margins sufficiently to reduce tension, especially where natural tension exists (as in lower leg) or where tissue loss has occurred.

a. Use scalpel or scissors.

b. Optimal level for undermining is just below skin-fat junction—major vessels and nerves are usually deeper.

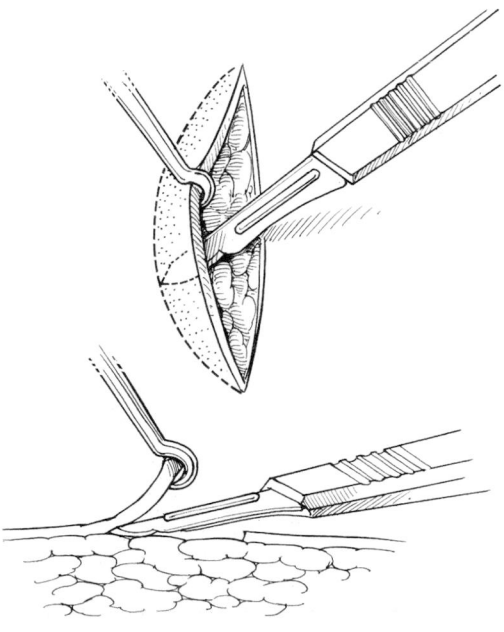

6. Constructing skin hooks

a. Start with a 22- to 26-gauge needle.

b. Grasp tip in needle holder and rotate needle holder to bend needle around it (180 to 270 degrees).

c. Grasp loop at base with needle holder and reverse bend at this point to customize hook

d. Completed skin hook should look something like this:

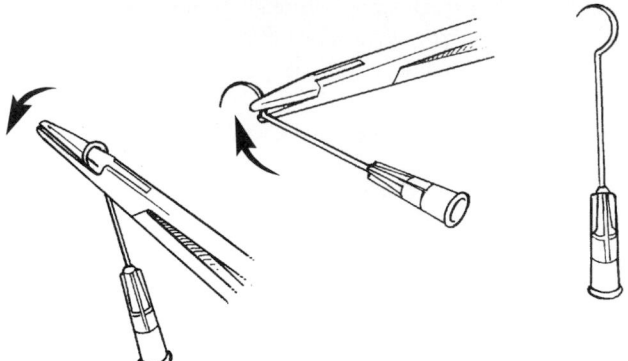

Attach to tuberculin or 2-ml syringe to use as handle.

e. Skin hooks make excellent retractors, move flaps and approximate margins well, and cause minimal trauma.

 Bibliography

Moy RL: Management of acute wounds. Dermatol Clin 1993;11:759–766.

Pfenninger JL: Procedures for Primary Care Physicians. St. Louis, Mosby–Year Book, 1994.

Rapport NH: Laceration repair. Am Fam Physician 1984; 30:115–123.

Reiter D: Methods and materials for wound closure. Otolaryngol Clin North Am 1995;28:1069–1080.

Zuber TJ, DeWitt DE: The fusiform excision. Am Fam Physician 1994;49:371–376.

Indications

Wounds that
1. Cross flexor creases
2. Require significant tension for closure
3. Are cosmetically unacceptable, either now (e.g., dog-ears, etc.) or later (e.g., trap doors, wounds oriented perpendicular to relaxed skin tension [RST] lines)

Contraindications

1. Infection or severe contamination
2. Complicated wounds: significant injury to deeper structures
3. Wounds beyond expertise of physician
4. Systemic process that delays healing (coagulopathy, long-term high dose steroids, etc.)
5. Uncooperative or noncompliant patient
6. Wound more than 12 to 24 hours old (relative contraindication)

Preparation

1. Cleanse skin with povidone-iodine or Hibiclens—keep these solutions out of wound.
2. Confirm function of tendons, nerves, and the like.
3. Anesthetize.
4. Irrigate wound copiously with saline.

> **Note**
> See preceding procedure, Wound Management, for equipment, anesthesia, and precautions.

Technique

1. RST lines usually coincide with age lines and generally run perpendicular to underlying muscles.
    a. Wounds parallel to RST lines heal with thinner, less noticeable scar.
    b. Whenever possible orient wounds along RST lines.

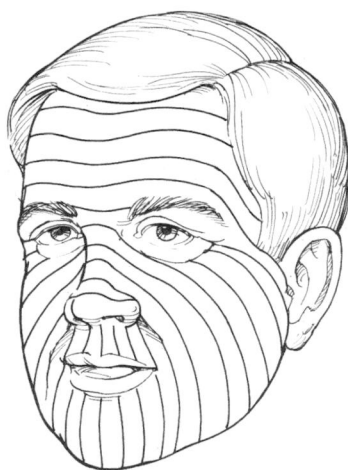

    c. Compare injured area to other side of body for clues to RST lines.
    d. Especially on the face, have patient grimace, smile, whistle, and so forth to verify RST lines.
    e. If you still cannot tell, undermine and wait 5 minutes. Wound will frequently orient itself along RST lines.

2. Properly repaired wounds should lie flat.
    a. Central wound tension, inequality of wound margins, or the tendency of wounds oblique to RST lines to slide (shear) may result in elevated tissue mounds at wound ends.
    b. These protruding corners are called "dog-ears."
3. Large dog-ear defects create unacceptable scars.
    a. Tendency to dog-ear can be minimized by placing end sutures carefully perpendicular to the wound margin. This tends to shift tissue (that would otherwise "bunch up" to create a dog-ear), allowing it to lie flat along scarline.
    b. For large dog-ears, excising the redundant tissue to create an elliptical continuation of the wound makes a simple repair.

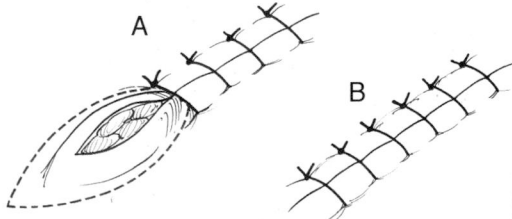

    c. The improved appearance more than compensates for the short extension of the scarline.
4. Wounds that cross flexion creases can result in limited joint function when scars contract; Z-plasty allows redirection of the scarline.

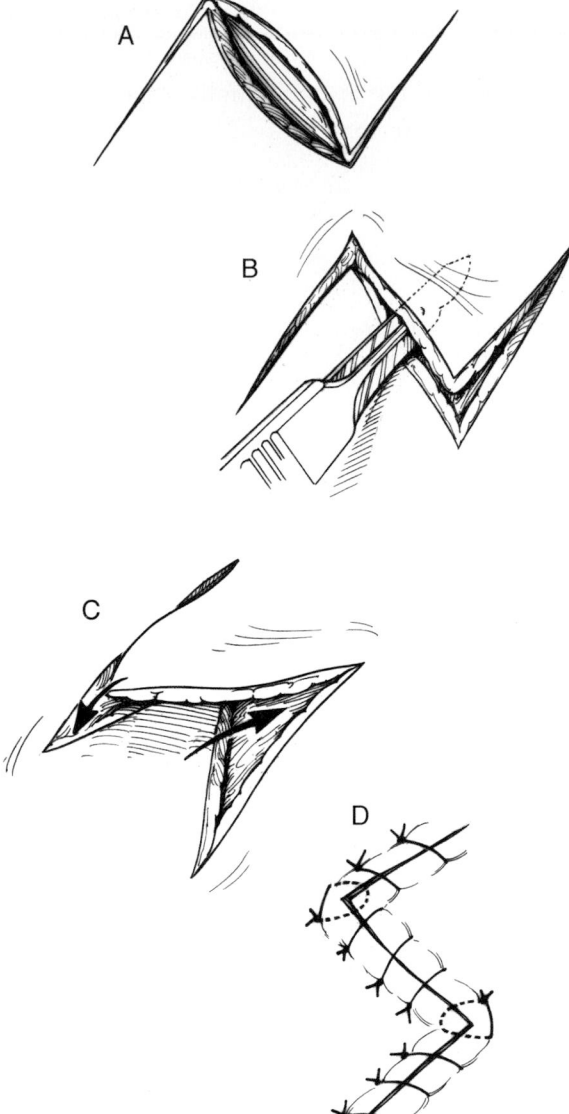

5. Large defects may require extensive mobilization of tissue to effect closure.
   a. Local tissue can be rearranged to close a defect.
   b. Creating a flap from nearby skin can facilitate closure of a defect.

> **Important**
> In general, a flap's length should *never* exceed twice its width at the base (that is where the blood supply comes from).

   c. Advancement flap: As the skin is advanced over the defect, dog-ears will develop unless triangles of tissue are excised from the *outside* skin edges at the far end of the flap.

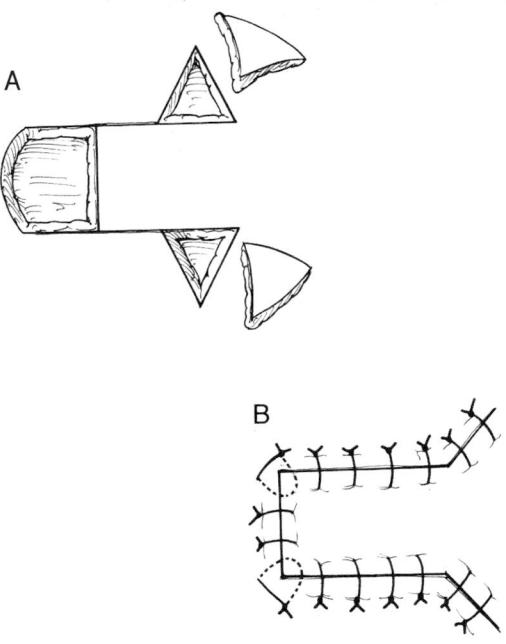

a. At each end of the wound, make incisions approximately the length of the wound directed at a 60-degree angle to the wound.
b. Make each incision on the opposite side of the wound (forming the letter **Z**) (see A above).
c. Undermine skin creating two triangular skin flaps (see B above).
d. Transpose the corners of the triangular flaps (see C above).
e. Suture the wound. The central portion of the wound now lies at 90 degrees to the original wound direction (see D above).
f. Because **Z**-plasty transfers some tissue from the transverse to the longitudinal axis, the circumference of a digit may shrink enough to compromise circulation.
g. If the wound is long, consider doing multiple **Z**-plasties.

Follow-Up
1. Apply direct pressure to surgical site for 2 to 24 hours after the procedure.
2. Apply antibiotic ointment daily until wound is healed.
3. Examine wounds promptly if signs of infection or hematoma develop.
4. Remove sutures after appropriate interval.

Bibliography

Borges AF: Dog-ear repair. Plastic Reconstr Surg 1982; 69:707–713.
Edgerton MT: The Art of Surgical Technique. Baltimore, Williams & Wilkins, 1988.
Gusman D: Wound closure and special suture techniques. J Am Podiatr Med Assoc 1995;85:2–10.
Hudson-Peacock MJ, Lawrence CM: Comparison of wound closure by means of dog-ear repair and elliptical excision. J Am Dermatol 1995;32:627–630.
Usatine RP, Moy RL, Tobinick EL, et al: Skin Surgery: A Practical Guide. St. Louis, Mosby, 1998.

Indications

1. Laceration
2. Incision/excision repair

Contraindication

1. Contaminated wound
2. Disrupted nerves or tendons (refer?)

Preparation

1. Copious irrigation (laceration) with saline or lactated Ringer's solution
2. Proper débridement as necessary to remove devitalized tissue
3. Povidone-iodine wash
4. Anesthetic
5. Draping
6. Inform patient of procedure, risks of scarring, infection, discomfort

Equipment

1. A 27-gauge, 1½-inch needle and syringe
2. Needle holders
3. Fine tissue scissors/skin hooks
4. Suture scissors
5. No. 15 blade and scalpel handle
6. Sterile gloves
7. Two sterile drapes (one fenestrated)
8. 4 × 4 sterile gauzes
9. 5-0 or 6-0 nylon or Prolene suture for face
10. 3-0 or 4-0 nylon or Prolene suture for trunk, extremities
11. 3-0 or 4-0 Vicryl or Dexon for buried suture
12. Possible Steri-Strips

Anesthesia

See Procedures on local and regional anesthesia (Chapters 46 and 211). If repairing a laceration, enter through the laceration.

Precautions

1. Use antistaphylococcal antibiotics for prophylaxis in dirty wounds, in immune-suppressed, diabetic, and elderly patients, and when there is vascular-compromised tissue.
2. Check tetanus status.
3. Before repairing a laceration, document intact neurovascular and tendon structures.
4. Do not use epinephrine with the lidocaine in "dirty wounds" or in the fingers, nose, penis, toes, or earlobes.
5. When holding tissue with pickups, do not close the pickups tightly. This traumatizes the tissue. Using skin hooks avoids this problem and facilitates repair.
6. Close all dead spaces in wound.
7. Approximate but do not strangulate wound edges.
8. Make deeply buried stitches support any wound tension so that skin margins are slightly tented up but without tension.

Technique

1. Simple interrupted

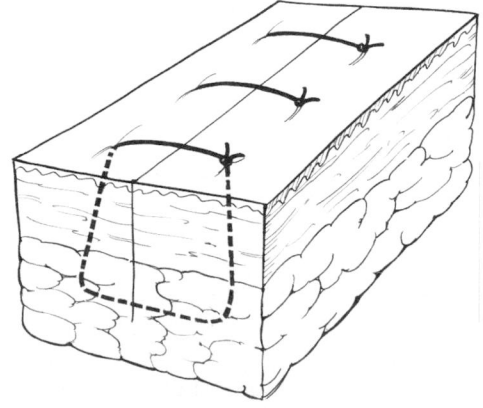

a. The shape of the path of the suture should look like an Erlenmeyer flask.
b. The closer the sutures, the less wound tension and thus less scarring. Sutures should be placed as far apart as they traverse across the wound.
c. The levels of tissue should be approximated to the same levels on the opposite side. This closure can be used for most wounds.

2. Running stitch

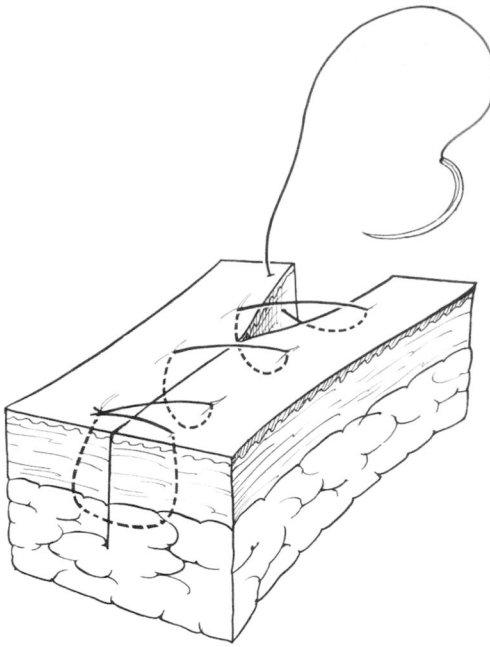

Advantages are that this closure is quick and provides some hemostasis. Use where scarring is not important (e.g., scalp).

3. Two-layered closure—deep inverted stitch

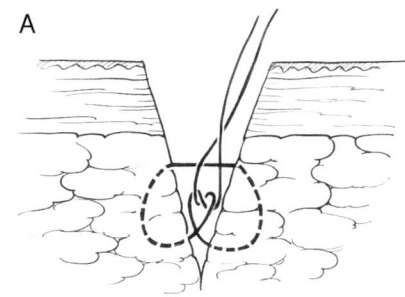

A

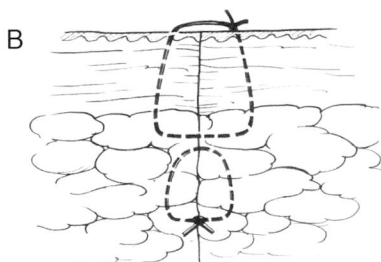

B

Use with deep wounds, in conjunction with undermining to close wounds under tension, or with a significant gap of wound margins. Remember "bottoms up" to obtain an inverted knot—start at the bottom of the wound, go up, across, and then down. The knot ends up at the bottom of the wound, where it will cause less inflammation.

4. Subcuticular closure

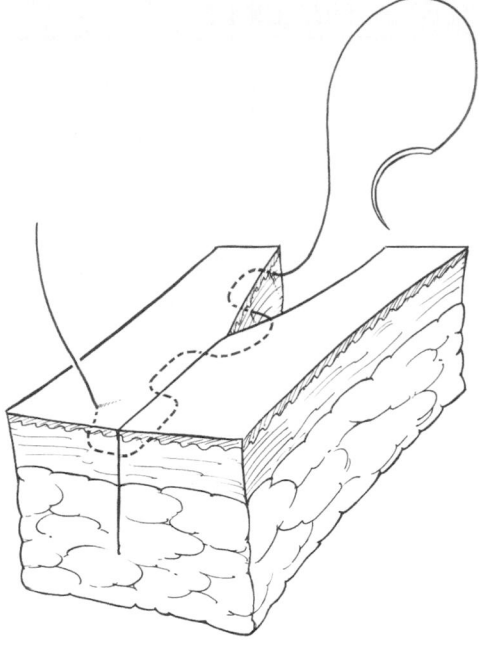

Use only if skin margins lie opposed without tension. Real advantage is minimal scarring. May be left in place 2 weeks or more. Use Prolene—it is more slippery and stronger than nylon.

5. Mattress sutures

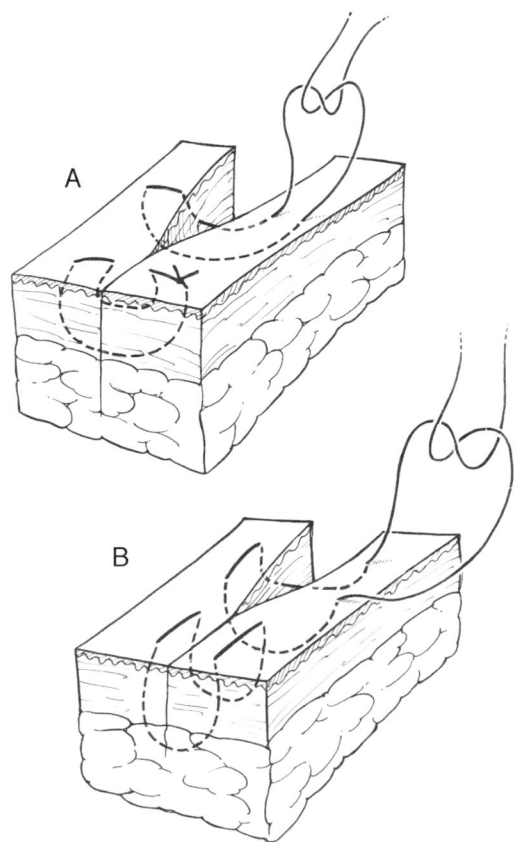

A

B

Use where there is significant wound tension or with very thin or very thick skin.

6. The corner stitch (half-buried mattress)

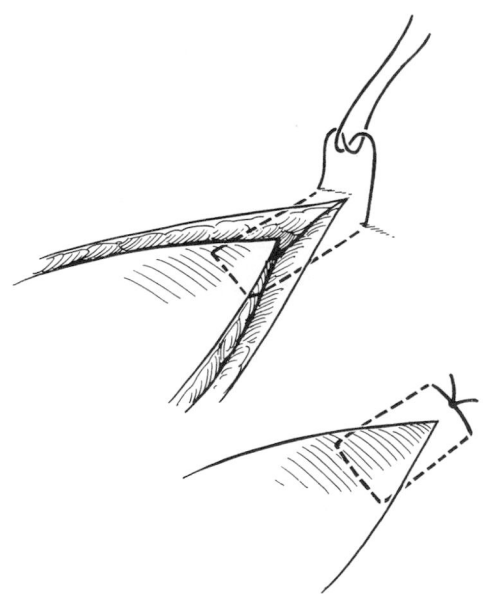

Important to use in all V- and T-shaped lacerations to avoid tip necrosis.

Follow-Up

1. Keep area dry for 24 hours, and then wash gently with mild soap and water three to four times a day. May cover with antibiotic ointment.

2. Report redness, drainage, or persistent pain (indications of infection).

3. Use acetaminophen or ibuprofen for pain.

4. Rest as appropriate; possible elevation and/or ice

5. Antibiotics as indicated

6. Suture removal according to the following:

   a. Face, 4 to 7 days

   b. Trunk, 10 to 12 days

   c. Extremities, 10 to 14 days

Method of Suture Removal

Cut near knot where suture enters skin.

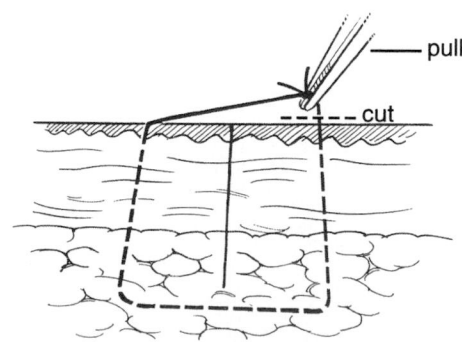

Pull suture across wound edge to avoid pulling "dirty" suture through the wound; pressure tends to pull wound edges together.

Use of Tissue Glues (Cyanoacrylate Tissue Adhesives)

Indications

1. Nonmucosal lesions
2. Facial, torso, extremity wounds
3. May be used after deep sutures placed if skin tension minimal.
4. Length of wound less than 8 cm
5. Low-tension wounds (gap < 0.5 cm)

Contraindications

1. Mucosal lesions
2. Significant wound margin tension
3. Noncompliant patients (must not pull at wound)
4. Pregnancy (?)
5. Soiled or heavily contaminated wounds needing débridement
6. Animal or human bites or scratch wounds
7. Puncture wounds
8. Stellate crush wounds
9. Hand and joint lacerations (with repetitive movement and washing, the adhesive will peel off with the top layer of epidermis in only a few days)

Advantages

1. Faster than sutures
2. Less painful
3. No anesthetic needed
4. As effective as suturing in properly selected individuals
5. The medically approved agents are more flexible, stronger.
6. No reports of toxic effects or carcinogenicity
7. May decrease wound infection when properly applied.
8. No need for follow-up visit for suture removal
9. Reduces risk of needle-stick injuries.
10. Low cost

Disadvantages

1. Wound strength on first day is significantly less (approximately 10 to 15 per cent) than with suture. Wound dehiscence most common complaint.

2. Inadvertent spillage can cause unwanted adherence of uninvolved tissues.

Material

Octylcyanoacrylate adhesive (Dermabond)

Technique

1. Approximate wound edges with fingers or forceps.

2. Paint tissue adhesive over manually opposed wound edges (not deep in wound) with applicator tip.

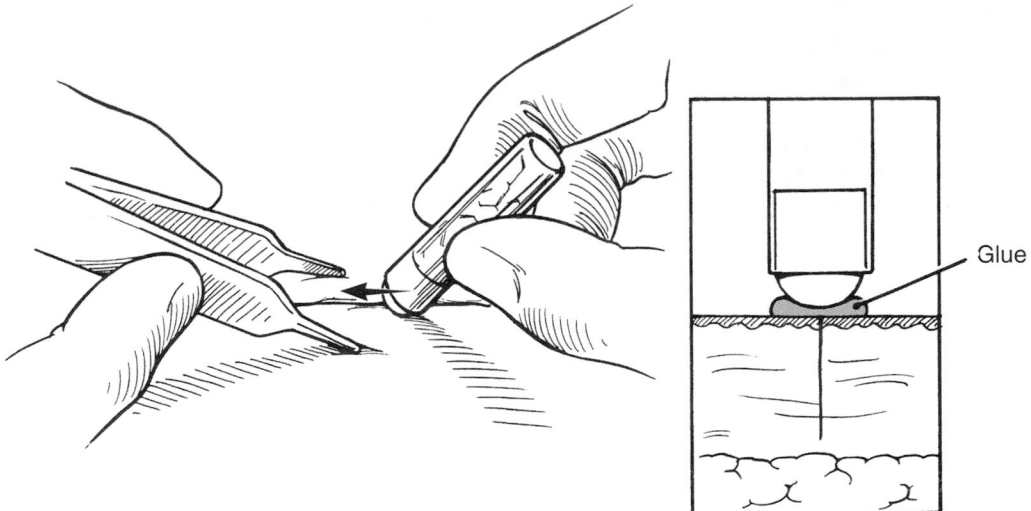

Glue

Deep application may impair wound healing and cause foreign body reaction.

3. Hold for 30 seconds.

Postoperative Care

1. No dressing required
2. Will slough after 7 to 14 days.
3. Patient may shower but should avoid washing or soaking area.

 ## Bibliography

Leversee J, McCall MW, Salascke SJ: Office excision of facial lesions. Patient Care 1990;Feb:26–41.

Moy RL, Lee A, Zalka A: Commonly used suturing techniques in skin surgery. Am Fam Physician 1991;44: 1625–1634, 2123–2128.

Quinn J, Wells G, Sutcliffe T, et al: A randomized trial comparing octylcyanoacrylate tissue adhesive and sutures in the management of lacerations. JAMA 1997; 277:1527–1530.

Pfenninger JL: The Reimbursement Manual for Office Procedures, 6th ed. Midland, MI, The National Procedures Institute, 1999.

Snell G: Laceration repair. In Pfenninger JL, Fowler GC (eds): Procedures for Primary Care Physicians. St. Louis, Mosby–Year Book, 1994.

Usatine RP, Moy RL, Tobinich EL, et al: Suturing Techniques. In: Skin Surgery: A Practical Guide, pp 88–100. St. Louis, Mosby, 1998.

Zuber TJ, DeWitt DE: The fusiform excision. Am Fam Physician 1994;49:371–378.

303 Common Neurologic Symptoms

1. Dizziness is an erroneous perception of self- or object motion or an unpleasant distortion of static gravitational orientation. It is caused by a mismatch between the three sensory systems: the vestibular, visual, and somatosensory systems. These systems are mutually interactive and redundant, in that simultaneous reafferent cues of all systems guide orientation and balance. Because the functional ranges of the three systems overlap, they are able to compensate in part for each other's deficiencies. Thus dizziness is not a well-defined disease entity, but rather a multisensory syndrome induced either by stimulation of the intact sensorimotor system by motion (e.g., as in motion sickness or height vertigo), or by pathologic dysfunction of any of the stabilizing sensory systems (e.g., as in vestibular neuritis).

2. Although in clinical practice dizziness is often a vague complaint encompassing many varying disease processes, four typical forms can serve as a guide for differential diagnosis. At first vertigo as an illusion of rotatory motion has to be differentiated. After that major factors to be considered are, first, the episodic nature, duration, frequency, and position eliciting vertigo, and, second, the associated ear or brain stem signs, headache, family history, and patient's age.

   a. Attacks of rotational vertigo
   b. Sustained rotational vertigo
   c. Positional vertigo
   d. Dizziness with postural imbalance

Differential Diagnosis and History

After this first rough classification, the differential diagnosis must differentiate between peripheral labyrinthine and central vestibular vertigo syndromes. Important manifestations include ear signs (Ménière's disease, perilymphatic fistula, neurovascular cross-compression) or brain stem signs (central positional vertigo, vertebrobasilar ischemia, basilar migraine,

paroxysmal ataxia/dysarthria); certain provoking factors such as head motion (benign paroxysmal positioning vertigo, central positional vertigo, neurovascular cross-compression, bilateral vestibulopathy); or family history (congenital vertigo). Furthermore, psychogenic dizziness must be considered, in particular in patients with anxiety, depression, and personality disorders and less frequently in those with psychosis.

1. Attacks of rotational vertigo
   a. In adults, recurrent vertigo attacks lasting for some seconds to minutes may occur as
      (1) A central vertigo syndrome secondary to transient vertebrobasilar ischemia, vestibular migraine, and paroxysmal central vertigo and ataxia in multiple sclerosis
      (2) A peripheral labyrinthine vertigo syndrome secondary to vestibular paroxysmia (neurovascular cross-compression of the eighth nerve) and perilymph fistulas
   b. Attacks lasting half an hour to a few hours (or even a few days) may be due to Ménière's disease (with associated hearing loss and tinnitus), or in rare cases familial periodic ataxia/vertigo.
   c. In children, short attacks are most likely due to benign paroxysmal vertigo of childhood, a migraine equivalent, or rarely to Ménière's disease.

2. Sustained rotational vertigo
   a. Over several hours or a few days, it occurs as a single episode
      (1) Either with acute unilateral peripheral loss of vestibular function (vestibular neuronitis, labyrinthitis, labyrinthine concussion), *or*
      (2) With pontomedullary brain stem or cerebellar vermis lesions near the vestibular nuclei. Etiology of the central lesion can be vascular, inflammatory, tumorous, or traumatic.

b. Chronic unilateral vestibular lesions, as in acoustic neurinoma, are mostly asymptomatic as a result of central compensation.

3. Positional (positioning) vertigo is due to

a. Cupulolithiasis, also called benign paroxysmal positioning vertigo (BPPV), a mechanical disorder of the inner ear

(1) A precipitating positioning of the head induces an abnormal stimulation, usually of the posterior semicircular canal of the undermost ear.

(2) Patients with this most common form of vertigo develop brief attacks of rotational vertigo and concomitant rotatory nystagmus that are precipitated by rapid head tilt toward the affected ear or by head extension. This typically occurs when turning over in bed, extending the neck to look up, or lifting the head after bending over.

(3) The clinician can induce the symptoms by rapid position changes (e.g., from a sitting to a head-hanging position— Hallpike's maneuver).

(4) Rotatory nystagmus starts after a few seconds of latency and beats with a crescendo-decrescendo rate.

(5) The most common causes are idiopathic (50 per cent), head injury (17 per cent), viral neurolabyrinthitis (15 per cent), and long bed confinement.

(6) In general, it is a disease of the elderly that has a peak of occurrence between the ages of 50 and 70.

b. Neurovascular cross-compression or vestibular paroxysmia, in which vertigo attacks depend on the particular head position (changes of position can modify the duration) and last for seconds to minutes

(1) Vertigo occurs in combination with hypoacusis or tinnitus.

(2) Auditory or vestibular deficits are measurable by neurophysiologic methods.

c. All central positional vertigo syndromes involve the region around the vestibular nuclei. Nystagmus is often vertical or diagonal, changing in direction, and of longer duration; it does not exhibit fatigability.

4. Dizziness and unsteadiness of gait

a. Nonspecific but frequently described symptoms

b. Differential diagnosis is difficult because it comprises central and peripheral vestibular disorders but also nonvestibular syndromes such as visual dizziness, presyncopal faintness or light-headedness (e.g., caused by hyperventilation, orthostatic hypotension, vasovagal attacks, decreased cardiac output, hypoglycemia, drug intoxication), and psycho-physiologic dizziness.

Clinical Findings

1. Clinical phenomena include postural, perceptual, oculomotor, and vegetative symptoms, which manifest with ataxia, nystagmus, vertigo, and nausea.

2. These four manifestations correlate with different aspects of vestibular function:

a. Postural imbalance and vestibular ataxia are due to an abnormal activation or dysfunction of vestibulospinal pathways.

b. Nystagmus is due to a direction-specific imbalance in the vestibulo-ocular reflex–activating brain stem neuronal circuitry.

c. Vertigo itself is due to a disturbance of cortical spatial orientation.

d. The unpleasant vegetative effects (nausea and vomiting) are due to an activation of the reticular formation, the vomiting center, in the medullary brain stem.

Tests

1. A thorough neurologic examination: brain stem signs, Hallpike's maneuver, stepping test; exclusion of sensory polyneuropathy

2. Otologic examination of cochlear function (audiometry)

3. Vestibular testing: electronystagmography with a rotational chair, testing of otolith function (measurements of visual vertical and objective rotational eye position), posturography

4. Magnetic resonance imaging of the eighth nerves, brain stem, and cerebellum

5. Cardiovascular examination with orthostatic blood pressure, electrocardiogram with monitoring (arrhythmia?), echocardiogram, ultrasound Doppler sonography of the arteries to the brain

6. Possibly an ophthalmologic examination because of visual vertigo (cataract, monocular diplopia)

Management

1. The underlying etiology determines the management. Because the central nervous system has a strong impulse to compensate for, or habituate to, a persisting sensory mismatch, all therapy for vertigo should avoid disturbing these naturally compensatory mechanisms, a

center of which is within the vestibular nuclei. It must be stressed that the central nervous system needs the stimulus of the sensory mismatch for habituation and compensation.

2. Adequate therapy for vertigo must consider that antivertiginous drugs will suppress such mechanisms, because most of these drugs are vestibular sedatives. Therefore, vestibular suppressants should only be applied when vertigo is accompanied by distressing nausea and vomiting—in acute peripheral vestibulopathy and acute brain stem and cerebellar lesions (near the vestibular nuclei), or to prevent motion sickness. These drugs are not indicated in patients suffering from chronic dizziness or positioning vertigo. If possible, specific therapies directed at the underlying cause should be chosen.

1. *Peripheral-Labyrinthine Vertigo Syndromes*
   a. BPPV: liberatory maneuvers, no pharmacologic therapy
   b. Acute peripheral vestibulopathy (vestibular neuronitis, trauma)
      (1) Vestibular sedatives on days 1 to 3, when nausea and vomiting are severe.
      (2) Treatment with steroids (methylprednisolone sodium succinate), because they may accelerate the process of central compensation as well as peripheral restoration
      (3) Physical therapy
   c. Bacterial labyrinthitis: antibiotics
   d. Vestibular paroxysmia: carbamazepine (phenytoin, gabapentin) before contemplating surgery
   e. Ménière's disease: see Ch. 323.

2. *Central Vestibular Vertigo Syndromes*
   a. Transient vertebrobasilar ischemia: antiplatelet agents or anticoagulants

   b. Basilar/vestibular migraine or benign paroxysmal vertigo of childhood
      (1) Pharmacologic management of the acute migraine attack is identical to that of other migraine attacks: ergotamines, sumatriptan, acetylsalicylic acid, paracetamol.
      (2) When the attacks occur at least twice a month or present with significant brain stem deficits: preventative medication with a β-blocker (metoprolol, propranolol) is indicated for a period of 9 to 12 months. Others: flunarizine and serotonin antagonists.
   c. Paroxysmal central vertigo/ataxia in multiple sclerosis: carbamazepine
   d. Familial periodic ataxia: Acetazolamide (Diamox), alprazolam, or the calcium-entry blocker flunarizine can also be tried.

3. *Psychogenic Vertigo Syndromes*: acrophobia or phobic postural vertigo
   a. Psychotherapy is dominated by behavioral approaches, which can be classified as either systematic or in vivo desensitization procedures.
   b. Drugs used for symptomatic relief from panic attacks are either tranquilizers or antidepressants, such as imipramine.

B Bibliography

Baloh RW: Neurootology. In Baillière's Clinical Neurology. London, Baillière Tindall, 1994.

Baloh RW, Halmagyi GM: Disorders of the Vestibular System. New York, Oxford University Press, 1996.

Brandt T: Vertigo: Its Multisensory Syndromes. London, Springer-Verlag, 1999.

Sharpe JA, Barber HO: The vestibulo-ocular reflex and vertigo. New York, Raven Press, 1993.

SYMPTOM TREMOR

Thomas R. Pellegrino

1. *Tremor* is defined as a rhythmic, oscillating, involuntary movement that may involve the extremities, the trunk, or the head and neck. Like other involuntary movements, it may be temporarily suppressed by the patient and is absent during sleep. Tremor is frequently worsened by anxiety or fatigue and by a wide variety of medications. Tremor may present as an isolated phenomenon or may be a symptom of some underlying disease.

2. Most individuals have experienced tremor at some time, usually when anxious or fatigued or following excess use of caffeine, alcohol, or over-the-counter medications; such tremors are self-limited and usually cause no impairment of function, so such persons rarely seek medical attention.

3. In some persons, tremor may be virtually constant and may cause significant embarrassment or annoyance; tremor also may cause serious impairment of function. Handwriting and other fine movements are often affected, but some patients may experience difficulty with speech, eating, or working.

Differential Diagnosis

Tremors traditionally are characterized as either resting or action tremors depending on when they are most evident, but this distinction is not absolute. In addition, more than one kind of tremor may be present in a given patient.

1. Action tremors: typically increased with muscle activity and reduced or absent at rest.

    a. Physiologic tremor: most evident in extremities held in fixed position against gravity. Usually of low amplitude, fast (6 to 12 Hz). Most evident in fingers and hands; little functional impairment.

    b. Essential tremor: most evident during active use of affected muscles. Low or moderate amplitude, fast (6 to 12 Hz). May involve extremities or head and neck. May cause significant functional impairment.

    c. Cerebellar tremor: classic "intention" tremor. Moderate or high amplitude, relatively slow (3 to 5 Hz). Often causes severe functional impairment.

2. Resting tremors: typically maximal when the involved extremities are at rest and relieved or absent during voluntary activity. Parkinsonian tremor may be associated with idiopathic Parkinson's disease or with parkinsonism of some other cause.

The most important diagnostic distinction is between parkinsonian tremor and essential tremor; note that *both* may be present in a given patient. Parkinsonian tremors, as noted, are typically most evident at rest; they may be asymmetric and involve the extremities, sparing the head and neck. The typical movement is alternation of pronation and supination of the forearm or "pill-rolling" movements of the fingers. Essential tremor, on the other hand, is most evident during activity; it is usually symmetric and may involve the head and neck as well as the extremities. The typical movement is flexion-extension.

> Refer to Ch. 316, Parkinson's Disease.

History: Key Questions to Ask

1. Is the tremor present primarily at rest or with activity?

2. Which parts of the body are affected? Does the tremor affect both sides of the body equally?

3. What makes the tremor better or worse? Ask about the effects of any drugs, caffeine, alcohol.

4. Does the patient use any regular drugs (with or without medical advice)? What about alcohol?

5. How does the tremor affect the patient? Is the effect only cosmetically limiting, or does the tremor impair specific activities?

6. Are there other symptoms of neurologic disease? Ask specifically about weakness, "stiffness" or slowness of movement, impaired gait or balance, slurred speech, and altered handwriting.

7. Is there any family history of tremor?

Clinical Findings

1. Is the tremor present primarily at rest or with activity? What parts of the body are affected?

2. Is the movement flexion-extension or pronation-supination? Is "pill-rolling" present?

3. Is muscle tone normal or increased? Is cogwheel rigidity present?

4. Is there any abnormality of speech, gait, or posture?

The clinical examination is helpful to clarify the details of the history and to look for other signs of neurologic disease that may not have been reported by the patient. In most patients presenting for evaluation of tremor, a fairly comprehensive neurologic examination will be necessary.

Tests

In most cases, the diagnosis of a specific tremor is based entirely on the history and clinical examination. There are no specific laboratory or imaging studies needed unless the clinical evaluation suggests some underlying disease.

Management

1. Physiologic tremor

    a. Reassure patient that no "disease" is present.

    b. Avoid caffeine and other stimulants.

    c. Anxiolytics for *occasional* use in specific stressful situations

    d. *Propranolol* in small doses (10 to 20 mg tid) is sometimes helpful.

2. Essential tremor

    a. Avoid caffeine and other stimulants.

    b. Alcohol in small amounts frequently is very helpful but should be recommended with *great caution*.

    c. Either *propranolol* or *primidone* may be helpful. If one drug is ineffective or not tolerated, try the other.

    (1) Propranolol, 20 mg tid to start; increase as needed and tolerated.

    (2) Primidone, 50 mg at bedtime to start; gradually increase to 250 to 300 mg/day in divided doses.

3. Cerebellar tremor: usually very difficult to treat unless underlying disease can be treated. In some patients, physical or occupational therapy can be helpful. No specific drug therapy available.

4. Parkinsonian tremor
   a. Stop or reduce any drugs that might exacerbate parkinsonism.
   b. In patients with Parkinson's disease, use standard treatment regimens.

Bibliography

Alexander GE: Parkinson's disease. In Johnson RT, Griffin JW (eds): Current Therapy in Neurologic Disease, 5th ed, pp 268–274. St. Louis, Mosby–Year Book, 1997.

Calne DB: Treatment of Parkinson's disease. N Engl J Med 1993;329:1021–1027.

Koller WC, Busenbark K, Miner K: The relationship of essential tremor to other movement disorders: a report on 678 patients. Ann Neurol 1994;35:717–723.

Weiner WJ, Lang AE: Movement Disorders: A Comprehensive Survey, pp 221–256. Mt. Kisco, NY, Futura, 1989.

Young RR: Essential-familial tremor. In Johnson RT, Griffin JW (eds): Current Therapy in Neurologic Disease, 5th ed, pp 294–296. St. Louis, Mosby–Year Book, 1997.

SYMPTOM PARESTHESIAS

James P. McKenna

1. *Paresthesias* are abnormal sensations arising spontaneously without an apparent stimulus. These sensations have been described variously as tingling, pins and needles, prickling, electric, burning, vibrating, buzzing, or crawling.

2. Paresthesias often arise from compression of peripheral nerves but also may result from ectopic foci in the peripheral or central nervous system.

3. Brief paresthesias occurring from resting on the sciatic, peroneal, or ulnar nerve may be experienced as the limb "falling asleep" and have no significance; however, persistent paresthesias warrant further evaluation.

Differential Diagnosis
1. Most common
   a. Entrapment neuropathies
      (1) Carpal tunnel syndrome: median nerve at the wrist
      (2) Cubital tunnel syndrome: ulnar nerve at the elbow
      (3) Peroneal neuropathy: peroneal nerve lateral at the head of the fibula
      (4) Meralgia paresthetica: lateral femoral cutantous nerve at the inguinal ligament
   b. Radiculopathy
      (1) Cervical—C5, C6, or C7
      (2) Lumbosacral—L5 or S1
   c. Restless legs syndrome
   d. Diabetic polyneuropathy
   e. Vitamin B$_{12}$ deficiency
   f. Alcoholic polyneuropathy
2. Less common
   a. Multiple sclerosis
   b. Guillain-Barré syndrome
   c. Medication (isoniazid, vincristine, diuretics, nonsteroidal anti-inflammatory drugs [NSAIDs])
   d. Hypocalcemia
   e. Carcinomatous neuropathy (breasts and lung cancer)
   f. Human immunodeficiency virus infection

Carpal tunnel syndrome, the most common compression mononeuropathy, is often bilateral, with the dominant hand more severely affected. Median nerve entrapment is usually idiopathic or occupational but may be secondary to pregnancy, hypothyroidism, rheumatoid arthritis, or injury, and rarely is due to amyloidosis, acromegaly, or multiple myeloma. Vitamin V$_{12}$ deficiency is most often due to pernicious anemia but may be secondary to gastric disease (gastrectomy, tumor) or small intestine malabsorption (Crohn's disease, celiac sprue, blind loop). Rare causes of paresthesias include leprosy, polycythemia vera, tumors of peripheral nerves, rabies, focal sensory seizures, and other causes of neuropathy, including less common entrapment neuropathies.

Refer to Ch. 174, Diabetes Mellitus, Type I; Ch. 175, Type II; Ch. 230, Carpal Tunnel Syndrome and Other Nerve Entrapments; Ch. 319, Multiple Sclerosis; and Ch. 324, Guillain-Barré Syndrome.

History: Key Questions to Ask
1. What is the distribution of the paresthesias?
2. How long have the sensations been present?
3. Does any position or activity alter those sensations?

4. Does pain, numbness, weakness, stiffness, or clumsiness exist?

5. Have there been any recent changes in medication?

Paresthesias that occur only in the distribution of single peripheral nerves are most often secondary to entrapment neuropathies. Pain, numbness, and weakness, if present, are confined to the distribution of the nerve and usually are of gradual onset. Pain from radiculopathy, usually caused by degenerative disk disease, is typically abrupt in onset, increased by twisting and bending, and exacerbated by heavy lifting or the Valsalva maneuver. The restless legs syndrome manifests as uncomfortable, crawling, dull, tingling sensations in the lower legs that occur at rest, especially at night, and produce an irresistible urge to move the legs. Distal sensory polyneuropathy is the most common diabetic neuropathy and occurs in about 40 per cent of diabetics whose illness has spanned 25 years. Symptoms may include paresthesias, numbness, and severe aching, deep pain. About 70 per cent of patients with neurologic symptoms from vitamin B_{12} deficiency experience paresthesias, typically in a glove-and-stocking distribution. Twenty per cent of patients with multiple sclerosis present with paresthesias. Paresthesias are the earliest symptom in most cases of Guillain-Barré syndrome, followed by rapidly progressing ascending weakness.

Clinical Findings

1. Tinel's sign (percussing an entrapped nerve heightens distal paresthesias) may be present in carpal tunnel and cubital tunnel syndromes.

2. Phalen's sign (flexion of the wrists enhancing median nerve paresthesias) may be present with carpal tunnel syndrome.

3. Sensory abnormalities in common entrapment syndromes
   a. Carpal tunnel syndrome: palmar surface of radial three and one-half fingers
   b. Cubital tunnel syndrome: ulnar side of the fourth finger and fifth finger
   c. Peroneal nerve: lateral aspect of the leg
   d. Meralgia paresthetica: anterolateral thigh

4. Radiculopathy may cause decreased strength, sensation, and reflexes in the corresponding affected nerve root.

5. Physical findings in restless legs syndrome occur only in cases secondary to iron or folate deficiency or uremia.

6. Diabetic polyneuropathy is predominantly sensory, with bilateral loss of sensation for pain, touch, temperature, and proprioception distally with minimal weakness.

7. Vitamin B_{12} deficiency may cause paresthesias only early in the course of the illness or may occur with anemia, glossitis, abnormal position and vibration sense, weakness, spasticity, decreased deep tendon reflexes, and a wide variety of psychiatric features ranging from mood and personality changes to psychosis and delirium. The Romberg's sign is often present.

8. Multiple sclerosis manifestations may be protean and depend on the locations of the plaques (see Ch. 319, Multiple Sclerosis).

9. Guillain-Barré syndrome is characterized by an ascending paralysis and hyporeflexia with much less significant or absent sensory disturbance.

10. Lhermitte's sign (flexion of the neck causing paresthesias radiating from the neck into the limbs) is classically present in cervical cord disease caused by multiple sclerosis but may be present with other cervical cord lesions.

11. Paresthesias may occur with no abnormal physical findings early in vitamin B_{12} deficiency, multiple sclerosis, Guillain-Barré syndrome, and entrapment neuropathies.

Tests

1. In most cases of paresthesias, a careful history and physical examination will reveal the cause of the paresthesias.

2. Electromyography and nerve conduction studies help identify the source of the abnormality.

3. Glucose and glycosylated hemoglobin levels demonstrate the degree of control in diabetes.

4. If a vitamin B_{12} deficiency exists, the levels are usually less than 200 pg/ml. Schilling's test locates the malabsorption site.

5. Polysomnography demonstrates periodic movements of sleep in restless legs syndrome but is rarely necessary.

6. Magnetic resonance imaging is the most reliable imaging study in multiple sclerosis.

7. Cerebrospinal fluid demonstrates rising serum protein in Guillain-Barré syndrome and oligocolonal banding in multiple sclerosis.

8. Normal values of ferritin, blood urea nitrogen, creatinine, bicarbonate, and folate exclude secondary causes of restless legs syndrome.

9. Normal serum calcium levels exclude hypocalcemia.

10. Elevated liver function tests (especially gammaglutamyl transferase) and an elevated mean corpuscular volume suggest alcohol abuse.

Management

1. Entrapment neuropathies

a. Carpal tunnel syndrome: wrist cock-up splint, anti-inflammatory medication, surgical decompression

b. Cubital tunnel syndrome: elbow splint to prevent elbow flexion, surgical decompression if necessary

c. Peroneal nerve: Avoid crossing legs.

d. Meralgia paresthetica: Avoid compression, weight loss, hydrocortisone injections.

2. Radiculopathy: Avoid activities that increase pain; physical therapy, nonsteroidal anti-inflammatory drugs, limited bed rest; surgery if unresponsive.

3. Diabetes: Improve diabetic control; amitriptyline (Elavil) or desipramine (Norpramin), from 10 to 25 mg at bedtime up to 125 to 150 mg, for painful neuropathy. Carbamazepine (Tegretol) or gabapentin (Neurontin) may also help.

4. Vitamin B_{12} deficiency: 1000 μg intramuscularly weekly for 1 month and then once a month for life

5. Guillain-Barré syndrome: Initiate plasmapheresis early.

6. Multiple sclerosis: Corticosteroids are the mainstay of therapy for acute multiple sclerosis relapses. Interferon beta-1a (Avonex) and -1b (Betaseron) and glatiramer acetate (Copaxone) are used to treat relapsing-remitting multiple sclerosis.

Follow-Up

Follow-up is essential to ensure that the causes of paresthesias have been appropriately evaluated.

PEARLS

- Transient paresthesias do not suggest a neurologic lesion.

- If paresthesias persist and no abnormality is found, re-examine the patient.

- Neurologic abnormalities may precede hematologic abnormalities in vitamin B_{12} deficiency.

B Bibliography

Diseases of the peripheral nerves. In Adams RD, Victor M (eds): Principles of Neurology, 6th ed, pp 1302–1369. New York, McGraw-Hill, 1997.

Griffin JW, Hsieh ST, McArthur JC, et al: Laboratory testing in peripheral nerve disease. Neurol Clin 1996; 14:119–134.

Poncelet AN: An algorithm for the evaluation of peripheral neuropathy. Am Fam Physician 1998;57:755–764.

Posner JB: Disorders of sensation. In Bennett JC, Plum F (eds): Cecil Textbook of Medicine, 20th ed, pp 2030–2038. Philadelphia, WB Saunders Company, 1996.

Rudick RA, Cohen JA, Weinstock Guttman B, et al: Management of multiple sclerosis. N Engl J Med 1997;337:1604–1611.

Thompson HG, Roland LT: Pain and paresthesias. In Roland LT (ed): Merritt's Textbook of Neurology, 9th ed, pp 27–30. Philadelphia, Lea & Febiger, 1995.

SYMPTOM **PERIPHERAL NEUROPATHY**

Steven K. Rothschild

Peripheral neuropathy is neither one symptom nor one disease. There are several types of peripheral nerves, and they may be damaged by more than 100 different diseases and toxins. To understand peripheral neuropathy, the physician must utilize history and physical examination to categorize the nerve damage into an anatomic-pathologic syndrome. Each syndrome, or pattern of nervous involvement, will have its own diagnostic considerations and unique approach to the diagnostic evaluation. Although physicians are often pessimistic about the work-up of peripheral neuropathy, using a systematic approach to evaluation will lead to diagnosis in as many as 80 per cent of cases, often with the identification of a treatable cause.

Etiology

1. The common process in all peripheral neuropathies is damage to peripheral nerves.

2. Three major patterns of nerve damage in neuropathies

   a. Damage to the cell body of the axon (neuronopathies)

   b. Demyelination

   c. Distal degeneration of the axon (axonopathies)

Symptoms

1. Symptoms depend upon which nerves are affected: motor, sensory, or autonomic.

   a. Motor: Weakness is the primary symptom, but this may present subtly:

      (1) Difficulty with daily activities (e.g., dressing, turning a key, carrying groceries, buttoning clothes) may be first thing patient notices.

      (2) Occasionally presents with cramping or fasciculations.

(3) Distal or small muscle groups are usually affected first, with proximal involvement later. Exceptions: inflammatory neuropathies, porphyria.

   b. Sensory: Numbness, tingling (paresthesias), or loss of feeling are primary symptoms. Other presentations include

     (1) Pain syndromes or a burning sensation (dysesthesias)

     (2) Unsteady feeling, especially in a dark room (loss of proprioception)

   c. Autonomic: often the most subtle; patients may not volunteer symptoms.

     (1) Postural hypotension, lightheaded upon arising

     (2) Abnormal sweating: excess or absent

     (3) Constipation, urinary retention

     (4) Impotence

2. Consider the distribution of the problem:

   a. Does the symptom represent an isolated nerve or plexus?

   b. Can it be explained by a radiculopathy?

   c. Are complaints more distal in nature or proximal?

   d. Is there no logical connection, or a patchy distribution?

3. Other key history

   a. Onset and time course: acute, subacute, chronic, or lifelong

   b. Age of onset

   c. Family history: A thorough genogram may be critical in unusual genetic causes.

   d. Are there relapses or spontaneous improvements?

   e. Other medical conditions associated with neuropathy.

   f. Alcohol, medications, toxins

Clinical Findings

1. Motor examination

   a. Distinguish proximal muscle groups (hips, shoulder girdle) from distal muscle groups

   b. Look for atrophy, loss of motor tone

   c. Deep tendon reflexes may be slowed or absent in demyelination of motor nerves

2. Sensory examination

   a. Include proprioception, vibration (128-Hz tuning fork), temperature

   b. Light touch: cotton wisp, 10-gm monofilament (for evaluation of feet)

3. Autonomic examination

   a. Orthostatic blood pressure measurements

   b. Postvoid residual

Laboratory Tests

> **Important**
> Do not order tests in a "shotgun" fashion: History and physical should guide classification, and classification should guide the work-up!

1. Electrodiagnostic studies: Nerve conduction studies (NCS) and electromyography (EMG) are of great help in identifying the clinical-anatomic distribution.

   a. Can also distinguish axonal degeneration from demyelination. (Demyelination is characterized by slowed nerve conduction.)

   b. May reveal patterns of nerve damage not detected on clinical examination.

   c. Caveats in using EMG and NCS

     (1) False negatives seen in pure small-fiber sensory neuropathies.

     (2) False positives, or clinically unimportant findings, may distract from actual diagnosis.

2. Additional laboratory testing to consider (based on neurologic syndrome)

   a. Blood tests: complete blood count (CBC), erythrocyte sedimentation rate (or C-reactive protein), fasting glucose, vitamin B_{12} (especially if macrocytosis noted on CBC), thyroid function testing, Venereal Disease Research Laboratory test, human immunodeficiency virus (HIV), antinuclear antigen

   b. Serum protein electrophoresis (SPEP): In motor neuropathies, when monoclonal gammopathy is a consideration, consider immunofixation electrophoresis to avoid false-negative SPEPs.

   c. Screening for heavy metals is rarely of benefit, unless there is known exposure.

   d. Lumbar puncture: Elevated cerebrospinal fluid protein level is suggestive of chronic inflammatory demyelinating polyradiculopathy (CIDP)

   e. Nerve biopsies (e.g., sural nerve biopsy) are not needed in most cases. Utilize when vasculitis, amyloidosis, leprosy, or sarcoidosis is suspected.

   f. Antibody assays are often used by neurologists, including anti-glycolipid antibodies, anti-Hu antibodies (present in occult malignancies in patients with subacute ataxia), and anti–calcium channel antibodies.

   g. Genetic testing is increasingly available to identify hereditary neuropathies.

Differential Diagnosis

Differential diagnoses are organized here by clinical syndrome; they are *not* listed in order of frequency.

1. Mononeuropathies, radiculopathies
   a. Direct compression or entrapment, such as by disk, tumor, carpal tunnel syndrome
   b. Diabetic neuropathy, vasculitis
2. Mononeuritis multiplex
   a. Diabetes mellitus
   b. Rheumatologic: systemic lupus erythematosus, vasculitis
   c. Malignancy
   d. Leprosy, sarcoid, Lyme disease
   e. Hereditary neuropathy with predisposition to pressure palsies (HNPP)
3. Motor neuropathy
   a. Guillain-Barré syndrome
   b. CIDP
   c. Paraproteinemic neuropathies (associated with monoclonal gammopathies)
   d. Hereditary causes: Charcot-Marie-Tooth disease, muscular dystrophies
   e. Amyotrophic lateral sclerosis (motor neuron disease)
   f. Acute porphyria
4. Sensory neuropathy
   a. Diabetes mellitus: most frequent peripheral neuropathy in industrialized nations
   b. Leprosy: most frequent worldwide cause of peripheral neuropathy
   c. Deficiencies of vitamin B_{12}, thiamine
   d. Malignancy
   e. Vasculitis
5. Pain syndromes
   a. Alcohol, nutritional deficiencies
   b. HIV infection
   c. Diabetes mellitus
   d. Cryoglobulinemia
   e. Malignancy (paraneoplastic syndrome)
   f. Arsenic or thallium poisoning
   g. Vasculitis
6. Acute-onset neuropathies
   a. Guillain-Barré syndrome
   b. Porphyria
   c. Toxic, such as arsenic

Treatment

1. Treatment will vary widely with the syndrome and etiology of the neuropathy; underlying pathology must be treated in the presence of nerve compression, paraneoplastic syndromes, vasculitis, or infection such as syphilis.
2. Nonspecific immunomodulating therapies: corticosteroids, intravenous immune globulin, plasmapheresis, and immune suppressants (such as cyclosporine, azothioprine, and cyclophosphamide)
3. Painful neuropathies, such as those seen in diabetics, may often respond to tricyclic antidepressants (amitriptyline or nortriptyline, in doses up to 100 mg/day) or anticonvulsants (such as carbamazepine, phenytoin, or gabapentin).
4. Activity and patient education must be determined by etiology. Consider
   a. Physical and occupational therapies
   b. Educating patients about risk reduction, especially in sensory neuropathies

Bibliography

Barohn RJ: Approach to peripheral neuropathy and neuronopathy. Semin Neurol 1998;18:7–18.

Bromberg MB: Peripheral neuropathy in the nondiabetic patient. Hosp Pract 1997;32:97–99, 103–104, 132–135.

Dyck PJ, Dyck PJB, Grant IA, et al: Ten steps in characterizing and diagnosing patients with peripheral neuropathy. Neurology 1996;47:10–17.

McLeod JG: Investigation of peripheral neuropathy. J Neurol Neurosurg Psychiatry 1995;58:274–283.

Ravitts J: Recent advances in the treatment of neuropathies. West J Med 1998;168:268–269.

304 Stroke

Douglas C. McCrory

Etiology

1. Ischemic strokes are the most common type (70 per cent of all strokes) and may occur as a result of
   a. Thrombus related to atherosclerosis of carotid or large intracranial arteries: 30 per cent
   b. Embolus from cardiac source (e.g., chronic atrial fibrillation): 20 percent. Note that secondary hemorrhage may follow embolic stroke.
   c. Lacunar (small vessel) stroke: 20 per cent
   d. Unknown, multiple, or uncommon causes: 30 per cent
2. Intracerebral hemorrhage: 15 per cent of all strokes
   a. Bleeding directly into brain parenchyma.
   b. Etiology: amyloid angiopathy in the elderly; hypertensive arterial disease; arteriovenous malformations (AVMs); or anticoagulant drugs or bleeding diatheses
3. Subarachnoid hemorrhage: 15 per cent of all strokes
   a. Bleeding around the brain.
   b. Caused by ruptured congenital ("berry") aneurysm; amyloid angiopathy in the elderly; or inflammatory or infectious processes or drug abuse

Symptoms

1. Focal symptoms
   a. Focal or multifocal neurologic deficit persisting for more than 24 hours
   b. Carotid (anterior circulation) system symptoms can involve the upper and/or lower extremity and/or face on the opposite side, the opposite visual field, or the eye on the same side.
      (1) Motor dysfunction: dysarthria, weakness, clumsiness
      (2) Sensory symptoms: numbness, paresthesia, loss of vision in either of two patterns: monocular blindness (same side eye) or homonymous hemianopia (opposite visual field)
      (3) Aphasia
      (4) Hemispatial neglect
   c. Vertebrobasilar (posterior circulation) system symptoms can involve any combination of upper and lower extremities and face, left and/or right sides.
      (1) Motor dysfunction, sensory symptoms, and aphasia as for carotid system
      (2) Loss of balance, ataxia, vertigo, diplopia, or dysphagia
2. Nonfocal symptoms: Suggest increased intracranial pressure and are common in subarachnoid hemorrhage, hypertensive cerebral hemorrhage, or major ischemic stroke with cerebral edema.
   a. Headache
   b. Vomiting
   c. Impaired level of consciousness (restlessness, drowsiness, coma)
   d. Cranial nerve palsies

Key Symptoms

Focal

- Aphasia
- Dysarthria
- Hemiparesis
- Monocular blindness

Nonfocal

- Headache
- Coma

Clinical Findings

1. Physical exam clues to etiology
   a. Carotid bruit: a systolic murmur heard over the mid- to upper neck; indicates the presence of stenosis of the carotid artery.
   b. Hollenhorst's plaque: atheromatous emboli visible in retinal arterioles on ocular fundus examination

2. Anatomic localization (see "Symptoms")
   a. Sidedness of neurologic deficits
   b. Pattern of neurologic deficits

Key Signs

- Carotid bruit
- Hollenhorst's plaque

Laboratory Tests

1. Computerized cranial tomography (CCT scan) can help to distinguish ischemic and hemorrhagic stroke, and guide choice of treatment.
2. Electrocardiography: Can identify atrial fibrillation or other dysrhythmias
3. Echocardiography: Identifies intracardiac thrombi and valvular heart disease, which may be sources of embolic stroke.
4. Carotid artery duplex Doppler ultrasonography: Useful in carotid territory symptoms to screen for carotid stenosis and identify potential candidates for carotid endarterectomy
5. Cerebral angiography
   a. Determines the degree and location of a known carotid stenosis before carotid endarterectomy.
   b. Identifies aneurysm or AVM suspected from CCT scan in hemorrhagic stroke.

Key Tests

- CCT scan
- Electrocardiogram
- Carotid artery duplex Doppler ultrasound
- Transthoracic echocardiography

Differential Diagnosis

1. Migraine prodrome
2. Subdural hematoma
3. Brain tumors
4. Seizure disorder
5. Arteritis
6. Multiple sclerosis
7. Central nervous system infection

Treatment

1. Acute-phase care
   a. Thrombolytic therapy: Recombinant tissue-type plasminogen activator (rt-PA, alteplase [Activase]) should be used for ischemic stroke if it can be given within 3 hours of symptom onset and cerebral hemorrhage and other bleeding risks have been ruled out.
   b. Monitor with serial neurologic examinations to recognize progressing stroke.
   c. Control excessively high systemic blood pressure; however, aggressive blood pressure control may be dangerous except in the setting of hypertensive encephalopathy or acute myocardial infarction.
   d. Avoid hypotonic fluids (e.g., 5% dextrose in water), which may exacerbate cerebral edema.
2. Prevention of acute-phase medical complications
   a. Deep vein thrombosis prophylaxis with heparin or enoxaparin in nonambulatory patients
   b. Avoid prolonged use of intravenous and indwelling urinary catheters to prevent infection.

Surgery

1. Carotid endarterectomy is useful for secondary prevention of ischemia in patients with anterior circulation nondisabling strokes and an ipsilateral carotid stenosis of more than 70 per cent.
2. Craniotomy may be useful for treatment of intracranial aneurysm or AVM.

Diet

1. Nothing by mouth for the first 24 hours
2. Clinically assess swallowing to exclude aspiration before initating diet.
3. Begin enteral nutrition (e.g., via nasoduodenal tube or gastrostomy tube) within a week if unable to take oral feeding.

Activity

1. Frequent turning and appropriate bedding for immobile patients to prevent bed sores
2. Range-of-motion exercises to avoid contracture
3. Early physical therapy to improve bed mobility, transfers, ambulation, and activities of daily living

Patient Education

1. Discuss expectations for recovery with patient and family.
2. Begin planning for postacute care in rehabilitation facility, nursing home, or home.

Key Treatment

Drugs of Choice	Alternative Drugs
• rt-PA for acute treatment of ischemic stroke • Aspirin to prevent recurrent ischemic stroke	• Clopidogrel (Plavix) or ticlopidine (Ticlid) (long term) to prevent recurrent ischemic stroke • Warfarin anticoagulation (long term) to prevent cardiogenic emboli

Follow-Up

1. General: Monitor for depression, which is common following stroke.
2. Prevent recurrent stroke
   a. Aspirin is useful for secondary prevention of ischemic stroke.
   b. Clopidogrel (Plavix) or ticlopidine (Ticlid) are alternatives to aspirin when it fails or if patients are aspirin intolerant.
   c. Long-term warfarin anticoagulation for secondary prevention of cardiogenic emboli in chronic atrial fibrillation
   d. Risk factor modification
      (1) Control chronic hypertension with diet or drug treatment.
      (2) Assess cigarette smoking status and encourage cessation in smokers.
      (3) Measure cholesterol and aggressively treat hypercholesterolemia.
      (4) Control blood glucose in patients with diabetes mellitus.
      (5) Assess alcohol use and encourage cessation in heavy drinkers.
3. Rehabilitation: speech, physical, or occupational rehabilitation at home or in specialized facility

 Bibliography

Alberts MJ: Hyperacute stroke therapy with tissue plasminogen activator. Am J Cardiol 1997;80(4C):29D–34D.

Goldstein LB, Matchar DB: Clinical assessment in the evaluation of stroke. JAMA 1994;271:1114–1120.

Gresham GE, Duncan PW, Stason WB, et al: Post-Stroke Rehabilitation. Clinical Practice Guideline No. 16. (AHCPR Publication No. 95-0662). Rockville, MD, Agency for Health Care Policy and Research, 1995.

Landis DM, Tarr RW, Selman WR: Thrombolysis for acute ischemic stroke. Neurosurg Clin North Am 1997; 8:219–226.

Matchar DB, McCrory DC, Barnett HJM, et al: Medical treatment for stroke prevention. Ann Intern Med 1994; 121:41–53.

305 Transient Ischemic Attack

Glen F. Aukerman

Etiology

Transient ischemic attack (TIA) is a transient episode of focal cerebral dysfunction causing sudden weakness, numbness, or difficulties with vision or speech. It has a rapid onset and a variable duration, lasting from a few minutes to 24 hours. Most TIAs have a duration of 2 to 15 minutes. Patients who experience TIAs are at increased risk for stroke.

1. Common causes
   a. Partial blockage in an artery in the brain, often caused by a small clot that has broken away from a blood vessel
   b. Atherosclerotic disease of the carotid and vertebral arteries
   c. Carotid or vertebrobasilar ischemia that is localized to the portion of the brain supplied by that vascular system
   d. Arteritis primarily caused by noninfectious necrotizing vasculitis
   e. Large stenosis of the carotid or vetebral arteries
   f. Ventricular thrombosis
   g. Thrombus formation caused by atrial fibrillation
   h. Embolic sources from valvular disease
   i. Carotid or vertebral dissection from trauma or injury

2. Less common causes include sympathomimetic drugs, which are associated with hypercoagulable states; aggregation; vasospasm; dysrhythmia; transient hypertension and hyperdynamic states; and vasculitis.

3. Risk factors
   a. Advanced age
   b. Smoking
   c. Diabetes
   d. Heart attack
   e. Hypertension
   f. History of stroke
   g. Cardiac disease
   h. Asymptomatic carotid stenosis
   i. Diet high in cholesterol
   j. Heavy alcohol use or binge drinking
   k. Sickle cell disease

Symptoms

Symptoms appear suddenly and usually disappear within 24 hours.

1. Loss of speech
2. Temporary weakness or numbness of the face, arm, leg, or one side of the body
3. Sudden loss of vision in one or both eyes or visual disturbance
4. Sudden severe headache
5. Confusion
6. Fainting or dizziness without loss of consciousness
7. Chest pain not relieved by resting or medication
8. Difficulty swallowing

Key Symptoms

- Transient weakness
- Numbness
- Difficulty with speech or vision

Clinical Findings

A complete physical examination, including a detailed neurologic examination, is required for a patient with a suspected TIA. When eliciting a history and chief complaint from the patient, family members, caregivers, or others close to the patient at the time of the event should also be involved to help document the symptoms during the episode. The physician should determine the onset, duration, and intensity of all symptoms. He or she should also ask follow-up questions to clarify symptoms as necessary, determining when symptoms first began, if patterns of symptoms emerge, and so forth. It is important to remember that a TIA is symptomatic of an underlying cerebrovascular problem that needs to be identified and treated.

1. Vital signs should include
   a. Blood pressure
   b. Respiratory rate
   c. Respiratory pattern
   d. Rectal temperature

e. Pulse oximetry

f. Rapid finger-stick glucose

2. General appearance should be evaluated, including
   a. Development
   b. Hydration
   c. Language
   d. Memory skills

3. Head and neck should be examined for signs of
   a. Vasculitis
   b. Meningitis
   c. Mastoiditis
   d. Sinusitis

4. Carotid arteries should be checked for
   a. Bruit
   b. Pulse upstroke
   c. Presence of carotid endarterectomy scars

5. Ophthalmoscopy should be conducted to check for
   a. Retinal plaques
   b. Retinal pigmentation
   c. Pupil reaction to light exposure

6. Chest examination should look for
   a. Surgical scars
   b. Signs of cardiac disorder
   c. Pacemaker

7. Cardiac assessment should be used to identify unusual rhythms, rates, murmurs, or rubs.

8. A thorough neurologic examination should assess the patient's
   a. Mental status (through a mini-mental status examination)
   b. Cerebellar system, looking for signs of past-pointing and dystaxia, hypotonia, overshooting, gait dystaxia, and nystagmus in ocular movement
   c. Gait
   d. Finger-to-nose and heel-to-toe

9. Cranial nerve function, looking for signs of dysfunction including
   a. Asymmetrical mouth retraction
   b. Loss of the nasolabial crease

10. Ocular dysmotility
    a. Forehead wrinkling asymmetry
    b. Incomplete eyelid closure, swallowing difficulty
    c. Weak shoulder shrugging
    d. Visual field deficit

11. Somatic motor skills
    a. Using the standard grading system of 0 to 4, test deep tendon reflexes of biceps, triceps, brachioradialis, patellar, and Achilles.
    b. Test strength of the upper extremity, shoulder girdle, abdominal muscle, and lower extremity.
    c. Test passive movement of major joints to check for spasticity, clonus, or rigidity.

Key Signs

- Transient neurologic symptoms, including weakness, numbness, difficulty with vision or speech without residual neurologic effect

- Patient alert and oriented

Laboratory Tests

1. Serum chemistry profile
2. Erythrocyte sedimentation rate
3. Glucose level
4. Renal, liver, and endocrine studies
5. Complete blood count
6. Cerebrospinal fluid
7. Syphilis serology
8. Hematocrit measurement
9. Coagulation studies
10. Platelet count
11. Antiphospholipid antibodies
12. Cardiac index
13. Possible other studies include
    a. Noncontrast computerized cranial tomography to rule out ischemia or infarction, locate a silent infarction from a previous stroke, or exclude other lesions that simulate a TIA. CT is preferred to rule out a solid lesion, MRI to rule out a vascular lesion or demyelination.
    b. Magnetic resonance imaging to rule out acute infarcts
    c. Cerebral arteriography to evaluate the carotid, vertebral, and basilar arteries and to define intracranial stenosis or occlusion
    d. Cerebral arterial imaging
    e. Twelve-lead electrocardiogram
    f. Lumbar puncture

- Serum chemistry profile
- Erythrocyte sedimentation rate
- Glucose level

Differential Diagnosis

1. Migraine
2. Seizures
3. Transient global amnesia
4. Ménière's disease
5. Hypoglycemia
6. Narcolepsy
7. Cataplexy
8. Periodic paralysis
9. Sensory phenomena associated with
   a. Hyperventilation
   b. Electrolyte imbalance
   c. Syncope or near-syncope caused by hypotension
   d. Cerebral infarction with transient symptoms

Treatment

The goal of therapy is to prevent a future stroke.

Medication

Pharmocologic treatments fall into two categories: antiplatelets and anticoagulants

1. Antiplatelet agents
   a. Aspirin, 325 mg/day (range 30 to 1300 mg/day)
   b. Dipyridamole (Persantine), 75 to 100 mg PO qid
   c. Ticlopidine (Ticlid), 250 mg twice a day
   d. Clopidogrel (Plavix), 75 mg PO daily
2. Anticoagulants
   a. Warfarin: dose based on raising the international normalized ratio (INR)
   b. Heparin: IV dose to raise the INR to 2.0 to 3.0

WARNING

Warfarin is contraindicated in pregnancy. Heparin is usually safe; however, the benefits must outweigh the risks. Safety of dipyridamole and ticlopidine during pregnancy has not been established.

Surgery

For patients with carotid stenosis of 70 per cent or greater, carotid endarterectomy is advised.

Diet

Well-balanced diet, low in fat, cholesterol, and salt, is recommended. Limit alcohol intake.

Activity

Refrain from strenuous activity until the nature of such an episode is determined.

Patient Education

1. Prevention
   a. Regular moderate exercise for cardiovascular fitness: 30 to 45 minutes three to four times a week
   b. Avoid smoking.
   c. Limit alcohol intake.
   d. Treat high blood pressure, diabetes, or other conditions if needed.
   e. Well-balanced diet low in fat, cholesterol, and salt
2. Patients should be told to return to the emergency department if symptoms return.

Key Treatment

Antiplatelet Agents

- Aspirin
- Dipyridamole
- Ticlopidine

Follow-Up

If the patient presents to an emergency room or acute care facility with symptoms of a TIA, it is important for the emergency room or urgent care physician to communicate the events to the patient's primary care physician so he or she may continue to monitor the patient's progress. Discussion should include coordination of tests and the need for additional inpatient or outpatient care and follow-up. It is also important to talk with family members to assess the safety and responsiveness of home and work environments for the patient. Follow-up should be with the primary care or personal physician.

Bibliography

Albers GW: Management of acute ischemic stroke: an update for primary care physicians. West J Med 1997; 166:253–262.

Broderick JP, Santilli JD: Prevention and Treatment of Ischemic Stroke (American Family Physician Monograph No. 3). Kansas City, MO, American Academy of Family Physicians, 1998.

Brown RD, Evans BA, Wiebers DO, et al: Transient ischemic attack and minor ischemic stroke: an algorithm for evaluation and treatment. Mayo Clin Proc 1994; 69:1027–1039.

Feinberg WM, Albers GW, Barnett HJM, et al: Guidelines for the management of transient ischemic attacks: from the Ad Hoc Committee on Guidelines for the Management of Transient Ischemic Attacks of the Stroke Council of the American Heart Association. AHA Medical/Scientific Statement 1994;89:2590–2965.

Sacco RL, Lipset CH: Stroke risk factors: identification and modification. In Fisher M (ed): Stroke Therapy, pp 1–28. Stoneham, MA, Butterworth Heinemann, 1995.

306 Falls in the Elderly

James T. Pacala

Falls and injurious sequelae of falls are increasingly common with age. About one third of community-dwelling individuals over age 75 fall at least once in a given year; half fall multiple times. Approximately 5 per cent of falls result in a fracture; 1 per cent cause a hip fracture.

Etiology

The cause of most falls is multifactorial. Risk factors for falls can be divided into intrinsic (i.e., characteristics of the faller) and extrinsic (i.e., characteristics of the faller's environment) factors.

1. Intrinsic factors (implicated in about 50 per cent of falls)
   a. Neurologic disorders arising from a number of conditions (e.g., Alzheimer's disease, stroke, Parkinson's disease)
      (1) Vestibular dysfunction
      (2) Proprioceptive dysfunction
      (3) Cognitive impairment
   b. Musculoskeletal disorders commonly caused by deconditioning, arthritis, or paralysis
      (1) Muscular weakness
      (2) Joint pain
      (3) Foot problems
   c. Sensory impairment
      (1) Visual disturbance
      (2) Hearing impairment
   d. Cardiovascular disorders
      (1) Postural hypotension
      (2) Cardiac arrhythmia
   e. Acute medical illness
   f. Medications (can adversely affect all the above)
   g. Risky behaviors
      (1) Hurrying or running (especially while carrying a heavy object)
      (2) High-risk activities (e.g., standing on a chair to reach a high object)
2. Extrinsic factors (implicated in about 50 per cent of falls)
   a. Environmental obstacles (e.g., uneven door thresholds)
   b. Slippery surfaces (e.g., throw rugs)
   c. Ill-fitting clothes and footwear
   d. Poor lighting
   e. Inappropriate furniture
   f. Unsafe stairs

Risk Assessment

1. Assess risk for falling by inquiring about conditions listed above as risk factors.
2. In those who have fallen, characterize the fall.
   a. Type: Did the patient fall because of
      (1) Stumbling over an object?
      (2) Slipping (what type of surface)?
      (3) Weakness ("legs gave out")?
      (4) Loss of balance?
      (5) Loss or near-loss of consciousness?
   b. Location: room in home, other building, outside
   c. Activity just before fall: walking, standing still, arising from bed or chair, climbing stairs, hurrying
   d. Level of consciousness: light-headedness, dizziness

Key Symptoms

- Light-headedness
- Loss of equilibrium
- Loss of consciousness (prior to fall)
- Slip
- Stumble or trip
- Weakness, especially in lower extremities

Clinical Findings

1. Abnormal balance
   a. Loses balance after nudge from behind
   b. Unsteady gait on
      (1) Flat surfaces: vestibular dysfunction
      (2) Uneven surfaces: proprioceptive dysfunction
      (3) Turning: proprioceptive, sensory, muscular problems
2. Abnormal gait: decreased step height, festination

3. Cognitive deficit on mental status testing

4. Muscle weakness: difficulty getting up from and sitting down in a chair; paralysis, weakness on examination

5. Foot problems: bunions, calluses

6. Vision problems: cataract, field cut, decreased acuity

7. Hearing problems: cerumen impaction, presbycusis

8. Postural hypotension

9. Contributing medications

   a. Antidepressants

   b. Barbiturates

   c. Benzodiazepines

   d. Nonthiazide diuretics

   e. Phenothiazines

10. Extrinsic hazards on home or institutional assessment, including poor lighting, throw rugs, deep-pile carpet, absence of grab bars in shower and toilet, electrical cords and loose items on the floor, poorly fitting shoes

Key Signs

- Abnormal balance
- Abnormal gait
- Muscle weakness
- Risky medical regimen
- Environmental hazards
- Postural hypotension

Laboratory Tests

1. Performance-based balance and gait testing is essential.

   a. The easiest test is to have the patient get up from a chair, walk down a hallway, turn, walk back, and sit down again.

   b. Other, more quantitative tests can be easily accomplished in the office setting, for example, the "get-up and go" test (see Mathias et al, 1986).

   c. Formal balance and gait testing can be performed at referral centers.

2. Other tests should be guided by history and physical examination. Examples:

   a. Electrocardiogram and Holter monitoring should be obtained if there was dizziness, light-headedness, or loss of consciousness before the fall.

   b. Vitamin B_{12} and glucose testing is indicated if peripheral neuropathy is present.

Key Test

Simple balance and gait assessment: Have patient rise from a chair, walk down a hall, turn, walk back, and sit again; evaluate step height, symmetry, path deviation, and balance.

Differential Diagnosis

1. Remember that most falls are caused by several factors.

2. The challenge for clinicians is figuring out which risk factors are implicated.

3. Although they are rare causes of falls (about 1 per cent of the time), arrhythmia and aortic stenosis should be excluded if there has been loss or near-loss of consciousness prior to the fall.

Treatment

Medications

1. *Reduction* or *discontinuation* of medicines that can contribute to falls is essential.

2. In cases of postural hypotension, fludrocortisone can be useful as part of the therapeutic regimen.

Diet

1. Adequate caloric intake to help prevent muscular weakness

2. Adequate hydration to minimize postural hypotension

Activity

1. Balance training

2. Gait training

3. Muscle strengthening

4. Correction of vision and hearing problems

5. Correction of foot problems

6. Treatment of acute medical illnesses

7. Elimination of environmental hazards

   a. Remove electrical cords, loose items from floors.

   b. Use shallow-pile carpet or nonskid wax floors.

   c. Grab bars in bathroom (toilet and shower)

   d. Properly fitting shoes

   e. Improve lighting, eliminate glare.

Patient Education

1. Instruction in risk factors on falls

2. Counsel regarding behavioral risk factors

3. Home safety checklist

Key Treatment

A multidisciplinary team approach (physician, physical therapist, podiatrist, home assessment nurse or physical therapist) works best to detect and treat all intrinsic and extrinsic risk factors.

Follow-Up

1. After a fall, patients should be seen monthly for 3 months and then quarterly to follow status of risk factors.

2. Many older adults underreport falls. Having them keep a falls diary can be of help.

Bibliography

Malmivaara A, Heliovaara M, Knedt P, et al: Risk factors for injurious falls leading to hospitalization or death in a cohort of 19,500 adults. Am J Epidemiol 1993;138: 384–394.

Mathias S, Nayak US, Isaacs B: Balance in elderly patients: the "get-up and go" test. Arch Phys Med Rehabil 1986;67:387–389.

Studenski S, Duncan PW, Chandler J, et al: Predicting falls: the role of mobility and nonphysical factors. J Am Geriatr Soc 1994;42:297–302.

Tinetti ME, Baker DI, McAvay G, et al: A multifactorial intervention to reduce the risk of falling among elderly people living in the community. N Engl J Med 1994; 330:1769–1775.

Tinetti ME, Speechley M: Prevention of falls among the elderly. N Engl J Med 1989;320:1055–1059.

307 Delirium

F. Allan Martin

Etiology

1. Often goes undiagnosed and is associated with a 20 to 30 per cent mortality rate
2. Predisposing factors
   a. Young age but more commonly advanced age
   b. Prior history of dementia or other primary degenerative brain disease
   c. Multiple coexistent medical problems
   d. Presence of polypharmacy, especially psychoactive drugs, but almost any drug or combination can be related to delirium in susceptible persons.
   e. Abuse of alcohol or other drugs
3. Frequently the heralding symptom of underlying major medical or surgical pathology
4. Multiple possible causes exist, and several causes may coexist in any individual patient with delirium (Table 307–1).

Symptoms

1. Multiple areas of possible dysfunction may be variably affected in delirium (Table 307–2).
2. Delirium seems to correlate best with the symptom complex of suddenness of onset and fluctuating course over time with prominent impairment in attention.

Clinical Findings

1. Evaluation of a patient's cognitive status is essential but may be difficult to obtain.
2. Key clinical signs usually can be elicited from an interview and thorough physical examination of the patient combined with data from the patient's family and nursing staff. Especially important is the record of all medication use, both prescribed and over the counter.
3. No single set of diagnostic criteria exists for all patients.
4. Physical findings usually correlate with the underlying disease processes that caused the delirium.
5. A few nonspecific physical findings may suggest the presence of delirium in an acutely confused patient:
   a. Autonomic dysfunction, such as tachycardia, bradycardia, flushing, pallor, hyper- or hypotension, impairment of pupillary or sweating function
   b. New onset of asterixis, tremor, or seizure

 Key Signs

Altered mental status with evidence of the following:

- Acute onset and fluctuating course over the day
- Inattention
- Disorganized thinking
- Altered level of consciousness

Presence of the first two plus either the third or the fourth strongly suggests delirium.

From Inouye SK, Van Dyck CH, Alessi CA, et al: Clarifying confusion: the confusion assessment method, a new method for detection of delirium. Ann Intern Med 1990;113:947, with permission.

TABLE 307–1.   FREQUENT CAUSES OF DELIRIUM

Drugs, dehydration
Electrolyte imbalances, environmental changes (e.g., location, extremes of temperature)
Liver disease (e.g., encephalopathy), lungs (hypoxia)
Infection (especially urinary tract infection and pneumonia), immune system dysfunction, intracranial lesions, inflammation (meningitis, encephalitis, vasculitis)
Retention (urinary or fecal)
Ischemia (cerebral or cardiac), intoxication, intestinal obstruction
Uremia
Myocardial disease (e.g., infarction, arrhythmia, congestive heart failure), metabolic abnormalities

Laboratory Tests

1. Should be directed by history and physical examination
2. Screening laboratory examinations
   a. Chemistry profile to include electrolytes, magnesium, calcium; liver, renal, and thyroid function tests; albumin, glucose, vitamin B_{12}, folate levels; creatine phosphokinase, and serum ammonia levels.
   b. Complete blood count and differential, clot-

TABLE 307-2. CLINICAL FEATURES OF DELIRIUM, DEMENTIA, AND ACUTE FUNCTIONAL PSYCHOSIS

	DELIRIUM	DEMENTIA	ACUTE FUNCTIONAL PSYCHOSIS
Onset	Sudden	Insidious	Sudden
Course over 24 hours	Fluctuating, with nocturnal exacerbation	Stable	Stable
Consciousness	Reduced	Clear	Clear
Attention	Globally disordered	Normal, except in severe cases	May be disordered
Cognition	Globally disordered	Globally impaired	May be selectively impaired
Hallucinations	Usually visual or visual and auditory	Often absent	Predominantly auditory
Delusions	Fleeting, poorly systematized	Often absent	Sustained, systematized
Orientation	Usually impaired, at least for a time	Often impaired	May be impaired
Psychomotor activity	Increased, reduced, or shifting unpredictably	Often normal	Varies from psychomotor retardation to severe hyperactivity, depending on the type of psychosis
Speech	Often incoherent, slow or rapid	Patient has difficulty finding words, perseveration	Normal, slow, or rapid
Involuntary movements	Often asterixis or coarse tremor	Often absent	Usually absent
Physical illness or drug toxicity	One or both are present	Often absent, especially in Alzheimer's disease	Usually absent

From Lipowski ZJ: Current concepts-geriatrics: delirium in the elderly patient. N Engl J Med 1989;320:578. Copyright 1989 Massachusetts Medical Society, with permission.

ting studies, arterial blood gases, or pulse oximetry

  c. Urinalysis with cultures of urine and blood

  d. Serum levels of ingested drugs, although even therapeutic levels may cause delirium

  e. Screen for illicit drugs and alcohol level as indicated.

  f. Chest radiograph and electrocardiogram

3. Tests possibly indicated if preceding not diagnostic:

  a. Electroencephalogram, looking for a diffuse slow-wave pattern, common in patients with reduced arousal, or low-voltage fast activity, seen in more agitated patients

  b. Computerized tomography or magnetic resonance imaging of head may be indicated, especially with history of head trauma or focal/abnormal neurologic examination.

  c. Lumbar puncture with cerebrospinal fluid evaluation if meningitis/encephalitis is suspected, especially if patient has potential for immunosuppression

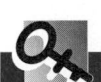 **Key Test**

No pathognomonic laboratory tests available.

Differential Diagnosis

1. Must first distinguish delirium from other neuropsychiatric disorders (see Table 307-2)

2. After delirium is recognized, then pursuit of likely medical/surgical cause can proceed.

Treatment

1. Specifically targeted at correction of medical disorder

2. Attempt nonpharmacologic therapy initially, such as well-lighted room, avoidance of over- or understimulating environment, gentle one-on-one interaction, attempt to reorient patient, and close communication with family.

3. Restraints may be used in the short term if patient's behavior compromises medical care or presents a significant threat to themselves or others.

4. Attempt to withdraw, reduce, or stop all nonessential medications.

Medication

1. Benzodiazepines have benefits of rapid onset of action with relatively few side effects during short-term use (Table 307-3).

2. Antipsychotics are particularly effective in patients with hallucinations, delusions, and paranoia (see Table 307-3).

Diet

1. Maintain adequate nutrition, either intravenously or orally.

2. Provide adequate vitamins and minerals as indicated, especially folate, thiamine, magnesium, multivitamins, and B$_{12}$.

TABLE 307–3. DRUGS USEFUL IN SYMPTOMATIC TREATMENT OF DELIRIUM

TARGETED SYMPTOMS	DRUG	DOSING*	MAXIMUM DAILY DOSE
Acute agitation with or without psychosis	Lorazepam (Ativan)[†]	0.5–1.0 mg q1–2 h IV, IM, PO	10 mg
Acute agitation with prominent psychosis	Haloperidol (Haldol)[‡]	2–5 mg q30–60 min IM, PO	100 mg
Alcohol withdrawal	Chlordiazepoxide (Librium)[†]	50–100 mg q2–4 h IV, PO	Titrated to sedation

*Should decrease dose to one quarter to one half of these doses in elderly or debilitated patients.
[†]Benzodiazepines may further impair attention.
[‡]Close monitoring for onset of extrapyramidal effects is indicated.

Activity

1. Very close observation until delirium clears
2. Resolution of delirium may take longer than improvement or resolution of precipitating metabolic abnormalities.

Patient Education

1. Avoidance of precipitating factors, such as alcohol and illicit drugs
2. Disease-specific information for patients and families to maximize self-care and recognition of recurrence

Key Treatment

- Supportive care

- Treat underlying precipitating illnesses

- Drug therapy as indicated

Follow-Up

1. Once delirium clears, follow-up can be tailored to the precipitating medical or surgical causes and the age of the patient.

2. Geriatric patients who survive an episode of delirium have a higher likelihood of institutionalization and mortality. They may therefore need more stringent aftercare.

3. In delirious patients, there probably exists a more fragile metabolic homeostasis and tenuous reserve capacity, with the onset of delirium merely a marker for such.

Bibliography

American Psychiatric Association: Diagnostic and Statistical Manual of Mental Disorders, 4th ed, pp 123–133. Washington, DC, American Psychiatric Press, 1994.

Inouye SK, Charpentier PA: Precipitating factors for delirium in hospitalized elderly persons. JAMA 1996; 275:852–857.

Inouye SK, van Dyck CH, Alessi CA, et al: Clarifying confusion: the confusion assessment method, a new method for detection of delirium. Ann Intern Med 1990;113:941–948.

Jacobson SA: Delirium in the elderly. Psychiatr Clin North Am 1997;20:91–110.

Lipowski ZJ: Delirium in the elderly patient. N Engl J Med 1989;320:578–582.

308 Headache

Glen D. Solomon

Headache is the most common pain complaint of humankind. It may represent a distinct syndrome without identified underlying pathology (primary or benign headache) or be a symptom of an underlying disease (secondary or organic headache). The number of different types of headache, and their associated causes, signs, symptoms, natural history, and treatments, often can make headache difficult to diagnose and treat. Most headaches can be treated effectively, however, once the diagnosis is made.

Primary Headache Disorders

- Migraine headache

- Cluster headache

- Tension-type headache

Epidemiology

1. Lifetime prevalence of headache is 96 per cent (women 99 per cent, men 93 per cent).

2. Lifetime prevalence of migraine is 16 per cent (women 25 per cent, men 8 per cent). Male/female ratio is 1:3.

3. Lifetime prevalence of tension-type headache is 78 per cent (women 88 per cent, men 69 per cent).

4. Chronic tension-type headache (tension-type headache occurring ≥180 days/year) is noted by 3 to 4 per cent of the population.

5. Cluster headache is seen in 1 male per 1000. The male/female ratio is about 5:1.

Differential Diagnosis

1. Migraine is a syndrome of intermittent, moderate- to severe-intensity headaches, lasting from 4 to 72 hours. The headaches are typically unilateral, throbbing, associated with nausea or vomiting, and aggravated by light and/or noise. Aura, usually scintillating scotomata or fortification spectra, precedes the headache in about 15 per cent of patients.

2. Tension-type headache is typically described as a bilateral headache having a pressing or tight-ening quality of mild to moderate severity. Unlike migraine, it is neither aggravated by physical activity nor associated with vomiting. Chronic tension-type headache is usually a daily or almost-daily headache.

3. Cluster headache is marked by cycles of headache lasting 1 to 4 months, separated by remissions of 6 to 24 months. The cluster headache attacks are always unilateral, and are located around the eye, temple, or upper jaw. Associated symptoms include reddening and tearing of the eye, drooping of the eyelid, nasal stuffiness, and rhinorrhea. The attacks generally last from 15 minutes to 2 hours, occur one to four times daily, and often awaken the patient from sleep. The pain is excruciating, and the patient commonly will pace the floor during an attack.

4. In medical practice, most headaches are not caused by underlying disease. It is important to recognize, however, that headache can be the presenting symptom of several diseases or be an adverse effect from medication.

Diseases That May Present With Headache

Rheumatologic	*Endocrine*
• Systemic lupus erythematosus	• Hyperthyroidism
• Vasculitis	• Hypothyroidism
• Giant cell arteritis	• Adrenal insufficiency
• Fibromyalgia	• Hyperparathyroidism/ hypercalcemia
	• Hyponatremia
	• Pheochromocytoma

Miscellaneous

• Fever/infection	• Depression
• Malignant hypertension	• Polycythemia/anemia
• Sleep apnea	• Hypoxemia
• Chronic renal failure	

The Headache History

1. Duration of headache disorder
   a. Sudden onset
      (1) Hemorrhage
      (2) Meningitis
   b. Chronic
      (1) Migraine
      (2) Tension-type
      (3) Cluster
2. Age at onset
   a. Childhood
      (1) Migraine
      (2) Tension-type
   b. Puberty: migraine
   c. Twenties
      (1) Migraine
      (2) Tension-type
      (3) Cluster
3. Temporal pattern
   a. Daily
      (1) Chronic tension-type
      (2) Analgesic rebound
      (3) Chronic cluster
   b. Constant: chronic tension-type
4. Quality of pain
   a. Throbbing: migraine
   b. Pressure/ache: tension-type
   c. Boring: cluster
   d. Shock-like: trigeminal neuralgia
5. Duration of attacks
   a. Seconds
      (1) Trigeminal neuraliga
      (2) Idiopathic stabbing
   b. Minutes: cluster/chronic primary headache
   c. Hours
      (1) Migraine
      (2) Episodic tension-type
6. Location of pain
   a. Unilateral
      (1) Cluster
      (2) Trigeminal neuralgia
      (3) Migraine (two thirds)
   b. Bilateral
      (1) Tension-type
      (2) Migraine (one third)
7. Trigger factors
   a. Migraine
      (1) Hormonal changes/menses
      (2) Changes in sleep
      (3) Poststress
      (4) Foods
      (5) Missing meals
      (6) Weather changes
   b. Cluster: alcohol
   c. Tension-type: stress

Key History

- Duration of headache disorder
- Age of onset
- Temporal pattern
- Quality of pain
- Location of pain
- Trigger factors

Symptoms

Associated Symptoms

1. Migraine
   a. Aura
   b. Premonitory symptoms
   c. Photo/phonophobia
   d. Anorexia/nausea/vomiting
   e. Exacerbation with exertion
2. Cluster: lacrimation/rhinorrhea/Horner's syndrome
3. Tension-type
   a. Dysthymia
   b. Depression

Symptoms Suggesting Organic Headaches

1. New, massive, or gradually increasing headache
2. Personality changes
3. Constant, worsening in horizontal position
4. Headaches in late nights or morning

Clinical Findings

1. Patients with benign headache disorders will

have a normal physical and neurologic examination.

2. The following signs strongly suggest headaches of organic cause:
   a. Tender temporal arteries
   b. Papilledema
   c. Fever plus rigidity of the neck
   d. Loss of local neurologic function, including loss of sight

Diagnostic Testing

1. Diagnostic tests for headache patient should be chosen on the basis of the results of the history and physical examination. In a patient with a typical headache history and a normal neurologic examination, no further evaluation may be needed.

2. All patients older than 60 with new-onset headache or a change in their headache pattern should have their sedimentation rate or C-reactive protein levels measured to evaluate for giant cell arteritis (sedimentation rate 50 to 120 mm per hour [usually >80 mm per hour]). If either measurement is elevated, a temporal artery biopsy should be obtained to confirm the diagnosis.

3. Most patients suffering from acute severe headaches should undergo imaging with computerized tomography or magnetic resonance imaging to rule out the organic causes.

Management

Migraine

1. Prophylactic therapy
   a. β-Blockers
   b. Calcium channel blockers
   c. NSAIDs
   d. Antidepressants
   e. Methysergide
   f. Cyproheptadine
   g. Valproic acid
2. Abortive therapy
   a. Serotonin agonists: triptans or ergots
   b. Isometheptene mucate combination
   c. NSAIDs
   d. Antiemetics
   e. Analgesics

Tension-Type Headache

1. Prophylactic therapy
   a. NSAIDs

   b. Antidepressants
   c. Muscle relaxants
2. Abortive therapy
   a. NSAIDs
   b. Muscle relaxants

Cluster Headache

1. Prophylactic therapy
   a. Verapamil
   b. Corticosteroids
   c. Methysergide
   d. Lithium
2. Abortive therapy
   a. Oxygen
   b. Sumatriptan: subcutaneous
   c. Ergotamine: sublingual or parenteral
   d. Lidocaine

Nonpharmacologic Therapy

Nonpharmacologic therapy is also important in the management of chronic headache syndromes.

1. Reducing trigger factors may reduce the frequency of attacks.
2. Biofeedback can help patients to change vasomotor tone and to relax tight muscles.
3. Physical therapy is used to train patients to strengthen neck muscles, improve mobility, and correct poor posture.
4. Guided imagery has been shown to reduce headache disability and improve quality of life.

Patient Education

Counseling the patient on the mechanisms of headache, trigger factors, and expected outcome of therapy ("control" of headaches and improvement in lifestyle without "cure" of disease) and reassurance of the absence of serious disease are key components of patient education. Further discussion on the wide varieties of therapies available to aid the headache sufferer should encourage the patient to continue care if the initial treatment is ineffective or poorly tolerated.

Follow-Up

The management of chronic headache disorders requires frequent follow-up to ensure that patient goals are met and therapy is successful with a minimum of adverse effects. The headache diagnosis should be re-evaluated at each visit because secondary headaches can develop in patients with a primary headache disorder.

Bibliography

Diamond M, Solomon GD (eds): Diamond and Dalessio's The Practicing Physician's Approach to Headache, 6th ed. Philadelphia, WB Saunders Company, 1998.

Olesen J, Tfelt-Hansen P, Welch KMA (eds): The Headaches. New York, Raven Press, 1993.
Solomon GD: Headache. In Rakel RE (ed): Conn's Current Therapy, pp 915–921. Philadelphia, WB Saunders Company, 1997.

Solomon GD, Lee TG, Solomon CS: Clinician's Manual on Migraine, 2nd ed. London, Science Press, Ltd, 1998.
Tollison CD, Kunkel RS (eds): Headache: Diagnosis and Treatment. Baltimore, Williams & Wilkins, 1993.

309 Migraine Headache

Michael B. Stevens

Etiology

1. Release of vasoactive substances from trigeminal nerve fibers causes a neurogenic "sterile inflammation" in the tissue surrounding various blood vessels in the brain, especially near the trigeminal nerve.

2. New antimigraine compounds are potent agonists to the specific serotonin receptor 5-hydroxytryptamine-1D ($5HT_{1D}$). Their possible mechanisms of action include carotid territory vasoconstriction and inhibitory effects on the pain-producing trigeminal nerve.

Symptoms

1. Specific symptoms often vary with the specific type of migraine headache. The "basic types" of migraine headaches as proposed by the Headache Classification Committee of the International Headache Society are listed in Table 309–1.

2. Before the onset of the actual headache, some patients may experience a prodrome, or "aura," of visual, sensory, motor, or affective manifestations. Visual auras and especially "scintillating scotoma" (shimmering vision and flashing lights) are the most common.

3. Following the aura (if present), the patient develops a deep, throbbing, and often debilitating headache. The pain may be unilateral or bilateral.

4. Associated symptoms may be nausea, photophobia, and phonophobia. Vomiting may occur.

TABLE 309–1. BASIC TYPES OF MIGRAINE HEADACHES

CLASSIFICATION NO.	NAME
1.1	Migraine without aura
1.2	Migraine with aura
1.3	Ophthalmoplegic migraine
1.4	Retinal migraine
1.5	Childhood periodic syndromes
1.6	Complications of migraine
1.7	Other migraine disorders

Source: Headache Classification Committee of the International Headache Society.

Key Symptoms

- Aura, usually visual (if present)
- Deep, throbbing headache on one or both sides
- Nausea, photophobia

Clinical Findings

1. Patients may have an ill appearance and pallor.

2. Physical examination, including funduscopic and neurologic examination, is unremarkable. Meningismus is absent.

Key Signs

Other than an ill appearance, the physical findings are *normal*.

Laboratory Tests

1. Given a medical history consistent with migraine and a normal physical examination, laboratory testing is not helpful or cost-effective.

2. Laboratory testing, especially brain imaging studies (computerized tomography or magnetic resonance imaging), is useful and necessary in patients who have historical details or physical markers (except meningismus) for serious pathology.

3. If meningismus is present, a lumbar puncture is indicated.

Key Tests

Laboratory and radiographic testing is useless, except for the exclusion of other disease.

Differential Diagnosis

1. Before making the diagnosis of migraine, other serious systemic illnesses must be considered and excluded. These are cerebral hemorrhage, cerebral infarction, encephalitis, intracranial mass, meningitis, and others.

2. During the history and physical examination, the physician should be watchful for any symptoms and signs of possible serious disease (see Warning box below). In their absence, the physician may safely make the diagnosis of migraine if supported by the patient's historical and physical findings.

WARNING: SYMPTOMS AND SIGNS OF POSSIBLE SERIOUS DISEASE

- **Patients whose frequent headaches begin after age 25**

- **Progressive headaches over days or weeks, localizing to one area, and increasing in severity**

- **Headaches associated with altered mental status, meningismus, neurologic deficits, papilledema, or seizure**

- **Headaches *caused* by exertion (bending over, coughing, exercise, sneezing, or orgasm)**

- **Headaches with an abrupt onset and intense severity**

- **Headaches that represent a radical change from a pre-existing headache pattern**

- **Headaches refractory to first-line treatment**

Treatment

Medication

1. The treatment of migraine headache is a three-faceted approach: *abortive* (at the *immediate* onset of the headache), *interval* (during the headache), and *prophylactic* (to prevent the headache).

2. Abortive therapy is *only* useful during the aura (if present) or start of the migraine headache. Abortive medications include the various oral ergot compounds (e.g., Cafergot), nasal dihydroergotamine (Migranal), and subcutaneous and nasal sumatriptan (Imitrex).

3. Interval therapy is directed at treating the migraine headache. These medications include analgesics and antiemetics to provide relief of symptoms and selective serotonin receptor ($5HT_{1D}$) agonists such as oral naratriptan (Amerge), subcutaneous/nasal/oral sumatriptan (Imitrex), nasal dihydroergotamine (Migranal), and oral zolmitriptan (Zomig) to resolve the migraine. Other medications such as tricyclic antidepressants and methysergide (Sansert) may act via $5HT_2$ receptors to prevent attacks.

4. Prophylactic therapy is used to prevent or reduce the frequency and/or severity of migraines. The commonly used medications are the β-blockers, calcium channel blockers, and antidepressants. The new selective serotonin-reuptake inhibitor antidepressants may have a theoretical yet unproven advantage over other antidepressants.

5. Medications may be administered by subcutaneous injection, intranasal application, or orally. Sumatriptan (Imitrex) by subcutaneous injection is the drug of choice because of its rapid onset of action. All selective serotonin receptor ($5HT_{1D}$) agonists are contraindicated in patients who are pregnant or at risk for coronary artery disease.

Diet

Numerous foods and food additives (Table 309–2) can precipitate a migraine headache in those susceptible.

Activity

1. Rest is an important mainstay of therapy.

2. The frequency and severity of migraine headaches may be reduced with regular exercise, sexual activity, and proper sleep habits.

3. Heat or cold applications, relaxation therapy, biofeedback, and hypnotherapy may be used as adjunctive therapies.

4. If stress or depression is a major co-factor of migraine headache, individual or family counseling may be helpful.

Patient Education

1. The best treatment for migraines is preventive.

2. Patients who are prone to migraine headaches should be encouraged to adopt a lifestyle that

---

TABLE 309–2.   FOOD/FOOD ADDITIVE PRECIPITANTS OF MIGRAINE

SUBSTANCE	MAJOR FOOD SOURCE
Nitrates/nitrites	Reddened (colored with additives) meats (e.g., hot dogs)
Phenylethylamines	Aged cheeses, red and blush wines, beer, champagne, chocolates, certain nuts, and beans
Monosodium glutamate (MSG)	Many prepared foods, Oriental foods
Caffeine (by withdrawal)	Coffee, tea, sodas, and cola beverages
Other	Fruits, cultured dairy products, shellfish

will help to eliminate or reduce migraine headaches by reducing inciting agents or activities. These lifestyle changes include avoiding known precipitants, exercising regularly, and maintaining good sleep habits.

Follow-Up

1. Patients with migraine headaches should be followed up according to their degree of frequency and severity: A more frequent or severe headache demands a more urgent follow-up.

2. Headache journals (records of the date and severity [e.g., 1 to 10 scale] of headaches) are useful to determine a baseline, to determine if therapy is working, and to discover precipitants (e.g., menses in women).

Bibliography

Headache Classification Committee of the International Headache Society: Classification and diagnostic criteria for headache disorders, cranial neuralgias and facial pain. Cephalalgia 1988;8(Suppl 7):19–28.

Lance JW: The pathophysiology of migraine. In Dalessio DJ, Silberstein SD (eds): Wolff's Headache and Other Head Pain, 6th ed, pp 59–95. New York, Oxford University Press, 1993.

Moore KL, Noble SL: Drug treatment of migraine. Part I. Acute therapy and drug-rebound headache. Am Fam Physician 1997;56:2039–2048.

Noble SL, Moore KL: Drug treatment of migraine. Part II. Preventive therapy. Am Fam Physician 1997;56: 2279–2286.

Silberstein SD, Saper JR: Migraine: diagnosis and treatment. In Dalessio DJ, Silberstein SD (eds): Wolff's Headache and Other Head Pain, 6th ed, pp 96–170. New York, Oxford University Press, 1993.

310 Seizure Disorder

Milton C. Chavez

Etiology

1. A seizure can be defined as the behavioral manifestation of abnormal neuronal activity. It is a self-limited but excessive and repetitive, hypersynchronous electrical discharging of the neurons in the cerebral cortex.

2. Epilepsy is a pattern of two or more recurrent seizures. It can occur at any time during a patient's life but, in general, has two peaks of incidence, in early childhood before age 1 and in later adulthood after the age of 65.

3. Up to 75 per cent of seizures are idiopathic. The remainder of cases, for which a cause can be identified (25 percent), fall under genetic, acquired, or environmentally induced seizures and are classified as symptomatic. A stimulus, if potent enough, may precipitate a seizure in an otherwise healthy person (see "Patient Education").

4. Seizures are classified under two general headings based on the origin of the focus:
   a. Partial seizures: The discharge begins as a single focus in one cerebral hemisphere. There are three subclassifications:
      (1) Simple (consciousness not impaired)
      (2) Complex (consciousness impaired)
      (3) Secondarily generalized (simple or complex seizures that generalize)
   b. Generalized seizures: Activity begins symmetrically (both hemispheres) and synchronously (simultaneously). Alteration of consciousness is a key feature of generalized seizures. There are two subclassifications:
      (1) Convulsive: tonic, clonic, tonic-clonic
      (2) Nonconvulsive: absence, atonic, myoclonic

Symptoms

Seizures present in a variety of ways depending on the origin of the epileptogenic focus.

1. Partial seizures may present with a prodrome and usually present with an aura.
   a. The prodrome is an emotional dysphoria that may begin several days before the seizure.
   b. The aura is a motor or sensory warning that begins immediately before the seizure and gives valuable clues to the origin of the seizure focus. Examples:
      (1) Motor symptoms: twitching of an extremity
      (2) Somatosensory or special sensory symptoms: paresthesias of one side of the face
      (3) Vegetative symptoms: nausea, sweating
      (4) Psychic symptoms: déjà vu

2. Secondarily generalized seizures initially present as partial seizures and continue on as generalized seizures, which are characterized by immediate altered consciousness with or without convulsions.

3. Most seizures end within 5 minutes of onset. As consciousness is regained, the confusional state that ensues is known as the postictal state.

Key Symptoms

- Prodrome
- Aura
- Other motor-sensory phenomena

Clinical Findings

1. The most important clinical findings are those that are witnessed.

2. Signs of epilepsy can be broadly classified into a limited number of categories: alteration of consciousness, behavior, posture, tone or motor activity, sensation, and autonomic function.

3. General physiologic changes are usually noted during or immediately after the epileptic seizure in the so-called postictal phase. Many of the findings relate to autonomic dysfunction, such as excessive salivation, urine and/or stool incontinence, and pilomotor phenomena. Other clinical findings relate to hypertension, hyperthermia, cardiac rhythm disturbances, hypoxemia, and respiratory changes.

4. The neurologic examination is usually normal after the occurrence of the seizure. A focal finding will localize the site of a cortical lesion.

5. Seizures arising secondary to other medical illnesses are treated by early introduction of antiepileptic drugs (AEDs) while attending to the underlying cause.

Key Signs

- Autonomic dysfunction
- Postictal confusion

Laboratory Tests

1. Ruling out other possible causes of a seizure helps make the diagnosis of epilepsy.

2. After a careful history and neurologic examination, the following tests should be ordered for an initial seizure: electroencephalogram (EEG), electrocardiogram (ECG), computerized tomography (CT) scan (with and without contrast), complete blood count (CBC), and blood and urine chemistries. AEDs can be started after these initial tests.

3. If seizures persist despite medication, magnetic resonance imaging (MRI) (with and without contrast) and surveillance with closed-circuit television (CCTV) are advisable. The MRI improves the diagnostic yield and can detect low-grade tumors, and CCTV helps distinguish between seizures and nonepileptic events.

4. EEGs should be repeated in a week and serially two to three times throughout the year. EEGs help diagnose epilepsy as well as help distinguish between generalized and partial seizures with secondary generalization. This distinction will guide therapeutic management.

Key Tests

- Serial EEGs
- CT scan (with and without contrast)
- ECG
- CBC
- Blood and urine chemistries

Differential Diagnosis

1. Seizures can be mimicked by several other conditions known as "spells" or nonepileptic events (NEEs).

   a. Seizures are paroxysmal and stereotypical. In other words, they "come out of the blue and are always the same." Spells are not paroxysmal and are rarely stereotypical.

   b. Seizures usually last less than 5 minutes and respond favorably to AEDs. NEEs usually last for greater than 5 minutes and do not generally respond to AEDs.

   c. NEEs that can be confused with seizures are usually paroxysmal and transient symptoms of either cardiopulmonary, cerebrovascular, metabolic, toxic, or psychiatric states.

2. The most common differential diagnoses

   a. Migraines
   b. Syncope
   c. Transient ischemic attacks
   d. Hyperventilation syndrome
   e. Cataplexy

Treatment

Treatment is aimed at finding the single best AED to control the seizure (Table 310–1). Doses must be tailored to patient responsiveness.

Activity

Patients with epilepsy can live a relatively normal life. Contraindications to certain activities should be tailored to the individual patient:

1. Absolute contraindications: swimming, scuba diving, football, boxing
2. Relative contraindications: driving, skiing, and other contact sports

Patient Education

Patients need to be counseled on certain exacerbating factors, which will often lower the seizure threshold and may induce a seizure.

1. Sleep deprivation
2. Alcohol
3. Trauma
4. Toxic or metabolic processes

TABLE 310–1. ANTIEPILEPTIC MEDICATIONS AND DOSAGES

	AED	INITIAL DAILY DOSE
Partial seizures	Carbamazepine (Tegretol)	400 mg per day (max 400–1200)
	Phenytoin (Dilantin)	4–7 mg/kg/day
Generalized seizures	Valproic acid (Depakene, Depakote)	15 mg/kg (max 60 mg/kg)
	Phenytoin	4–7 mg/kg/day

5. Fever or infection
6. Stress
7. Known convulsive drugs

Key Treatment

Partial Seizures

• First choice: carbamazepine (Tegretol)

• Second choice: phenytoin (Dilantin)

Generalized Seizures

• First choice: cabamazepine

• Second choice: valproic acid (Depakene)

Follow-Up

1. Self-management and adherence to the medication regimen is essential to obtain good outcomes. Significant lifestyle changes must include proper rest, diet, and stress management for the entire family. Patients must learn the side effects of their medication, as well as early seizure warning signs. Patients must also be aware of their prognosis and that they will never be "cured" of their seizures.

2. If a patient has been seizure free for a period of at least 2 years with a consistently normal EEG while on medication, then an attempt to taper and stop the AED over a period of 4 to 6 months is reasonable. If the seizures recur, restart the AED at the original dosage. The only exception is juvenile myoclonic epilepsy. These patients should be on medication for life.

3. Persistent seizures should alert the physician to the following possibilities: misdiagnosis, incorrect choice of AED, low drug levels, an occult brain tumor, or a nonadherent patient. Persistent seizures, pregnancy, and uncertainty in the diagnosis or management are the most important reasons for referring patients to a specialist.

Bibliography

Clancy RR: Valproate: an update—the challenge of modern pediatric seizure management. Probl Pediatr 1990; XX(4).

Giuffra ME: Seizure disorders. In Noble J (ed): Textbook of Primary care Medicine, 2nd ed, pp 1378–1385. St. Louis, Mosby, 1996.

Moore-Sledge C: Evaluation and management of first seizures in adults. Am Fam Physician 1997;56:1113–1120.

Pruitt A: Approach to the patient with a seizure. In Goroll A, May L, Mulley A Jr, et al (eds): Primary Care Medicine, 3rd ed, pp 851–858. Philadelphia, JB Lippincott Company, 1995.

Smith M, Buelow J: Epilepsy. Dis Mon 1996;42:725–828.

311 Reading Disabilities, Including Dyslexia

William G. Elder, Jr.

Etiology

1. Reading disability (RD) is a general term for a heterogeneous group of deficits that result in poor acquisition and use of reading. Most definitions require that reading achievement be significantly inferior to intellectual ability. Intrinsic central nervous system (CNS) dysfunction is assumed. Sensory deficit, mental retardation, low motivation, and educational deprivation do not cause RDs. RDs affect 4 to 8 per cent of children, with males and females equally affected.

2. RDs comprise a subset of learning disabilities (LDs). Spelling and mathematical disabilities are other LD types, depending on the area of academic achievement impacted. RDs account for 80 to 90 per cent of LDs and are the best researched. Common terms for RD are *dyslexia*, *congenital word blindness*, and *reading retardation*. The *Diagnostic and Statistical Manual of Mental Disorders* (DSM-IV) uses the terms "reading *disorder*" and "learning *disorder*" rather than reading disability and learning disability. Learning disabilities are conceptualized as intrinsic, whereas learning disorders may be acquired.

3. RDs are idiopathic. The following is generally agreed about their basis:

   a. RDs can be familial and heritable. Concordance rates are 60 and 35 per cent for monozygotic and first-degree relatives, respectively. Chromosomes 6 and 15 have been linked to specific RD subtypes.

   b. Phonologic processing deficits are the core problem in most cases.

   c. Left cerebral hemisphere anomalies have been frequently found:

      (1) Expected planum temporal asymmetries are absent (left ≯ right). *Note:* Typical, normal brains exhibit an enlarged left temporal lobe.

      (2) Cerebral blood flow differences that implicate left temporal and parietal lobes

      (3) Cell size differences in visual and auditory channels that may slow processing speeds

   d. Deficits exist on a severity continuum sug-

gesting that multiple brain factors are involved.

   e. Perinatal and postnatal factors associated with acquired learning disorders include prematurity, low birth weight, toxemia, hyperbilirubinemia, recurrent otitis, meningitis, encephalitis, and anemia.

Common Myths

1. Causal theories implicating allergies, spatial disorientation, and left-right confusion

2. Letter reversals (e.g., reading or writing "d" instead of "b"): common in early development and diagnostic only in the later elementary school years

3. Soft neurologic signs: May be associated findings but are not diagnostic with regard to RD.

Symptoms

1. The diagnosis of RD is based on reading achievement that is substantially below expectations for age, intelligence, and educational exposure. As a heuristic, reading performance should be 2 or more years less than grade level.

2. Symptoms include inaccurate word recognition, inaccurate and slow oral reading, and poor comprehension of written text

3. Early signs include delayed language development, word confusion, mispronunciations, hesitations, and word-finding difficulties.

Key Symptoms

- Reading level less than expected
- Word recognition errors
- School adjustment problems
- Low self-esteem

Course

1. The child patient typically presents with parental or teacher complaints of academic difficulties, usually when formal reading instruction begins in the first grade. Bright children able to compensate for deficits may be identified later,

perhaps in the fifth grade, when reading demands increase.

2. Findings differ as to ultimate educational and vocational impact. Reading difficulties tend to improve with age but residual difficulties are often apparent. Severity of the RD, strength of other intellectual abilities, success of intervention, and match between vocational demands and reading deficits are factors in adjustment.

3. The physician should be alert for adults with reading and other disabilities. For various reasons, adults may not divulge their disability and, because most adults with RD can read, detection may be difficult. However, residual reading difficulties can greatly impair understanding of medical information. Table 311–1 gives suggestions to enhance practice with adults with LD.

Clinical Findings

1. Deficient phonologic processing appears to be the core problem for most RD cases. Phonologic processing refers to the ability to decode words and includes segmenting sound sequences and accessing representations of word sounds.

2. Common findings include limited speech, limited vocabulary, word-finding problems, and poor use of pronouns. Semantics and syntax may or may not be normal.

TABLE 311–1. ENHANCING CARE OF ADULTS WITH LEARNING DISABILITIES

Awareness and recognition	Observe waiting-room behaviors
	Check ability to fill out forms
	Observe coherence or adequacy of history
	Monitor comprehension
Communication	Ask simply worded, direct questions
	Use simple vocabulary
	Avoid medical terminology
	Speak slowly
	Encourage questions
	Office staff may help with forms
Giving instructions	Review instructions
	Ask the patient to repeat instructions
	Explain graphic or pictorial information
	Involve other family members
	Limit amount of information given in each visit
Checking compliance	Ask in detail how medications are taken
	Use weekly medication dispenser with compartments
	Have staff telephone patients to remind of appointments
	Schedule follow-up appointment or telephone call

From Kelly MS, Gottesman RL: Adults with severe reading and learning difficulties. J Am Board Fam Pract 1997;10:199–205, with permission.

3. Other abilities, such as music reading or memory for nonsense words, should remain intact.

4. Individuals with mixed or other types of LDs may exhibit a wide range of cognitive problems, including visual-spatial deficits, time confusion, left-right disorientation, and poor planning, aprosody, and social interaction deficits.

WARNING

- Intellectual functioning, including bright or dull performance, is independent of RD.
- The Mini-Mental Status Exam and neurologic examinations are not sensitive to RD.
- Letter reversals are normal in early reading development.

---

5. The potentially devastating emotional consequences of RD are well known. Persons with RD may report a pervasive sense of inadequacy, shame, and worthlessness. Attitudes, self-esteem, goal striving, and peer and family relationships may suffer. Questions to understand children's perception of RD and its emotional consequences include

a. How is school going for you?

b. How important are good grades?

c. What do others say about your grades? How does that feel?

d. How have you been feeling about yourself lately?

e. What is your best (worst) feature?

f. What does having a LD mean to you? How do you feel about it?

 Key Signs

- No major neurologic or psychiatric disorder
- History of delayed language development

Laboratory Tests

An educational diagnostician (usually a psychologist) should evaluate RD.

1. Statistically significant discrepancy between intellectual abilities and reading achievement will be established using standardized tests such as the Wechsler Intelligence Scale for Children–III (WISC-III), the Wide Range Achievement Test–3 (WRAT-3), and the Woodcock-Johnson Psycho-Educational Battery–Revised.

2. Expect specialized tests of ability to sound words, nonwords, phonemes, and letters in text and in isolation.
3. Family, school, and other environmental/situational variables will be evaluated qualitatively.
4. Emotional functioning and co-morbid psychiatric conditions will be assessed using interview and standardized tests such as the Achenbach Child Behavior Checklist, the Personality Inventory for Children, and the Conners Behavior Rating Scale.
5. Ethical psychological assessment practice includes discussion of test results with the patient and/or parents at an appropriate level.

Evaluating the Evaluator

Request a copy of the evaluation. A parental release is required.

- Were parents and teachers interviewed?

- Was developmental history considered?

- Are tests standardized and relevant?

- How much discrepancy between academic achievement and intellectual ability was found?

- Are co-morbid conditions ruled out or weighted?

- Are environmental factors (teacher, family) adequately considered?

- Is there an over-reliance on psychological constructs and theories?

- Are the child's strengths noted and used in the individualized education program?

- Are recommendations practical and helpful?

Key Tests

- Intelligence test (e.g., WISC-III)

    comparison to

- Reading-specific test (e.g., WRAT-3)

Differential Diagnosis

1. The primary diagnostic task of the physician is to rule out any medical causes of academic difficulties, while the educational diagnostician will assess intellectual, academic, and psychosocial functioning to determine if a LD diagnosis is appropriate.
2. RD has a high degree of co-morbidity with psy-

---

chiatric disorders such as attention-deficit hyperactivity disorder (ADHD) (20 to 25 per cent), conduct disorder, and depression. Explanations for this association suggest that the psychiatric disorders may be

a. Emotional and/or behavioral expressions of CNS dysfunction
b. Emotional and/or behavioral sequelae to suffering RD, especially failure experiences
c. Secondary to poor processing, where social perception or communication is impacted.

All explanations have good support and should be considered in case formulation.

Causes of Academic Performance Problems

- Learning disabilities

- Neurologic disorders

- Chronic medical illnesses

- Medications affecting CNS functioning

- Speech, visual, or auditory impairment

- Mental retardation

- ADHD

- School refusal/phobia

- Depressive, anxiety, and other internalizing disorders

- Conduct (delinquency) and other externalizing disorders

- Poor family involvement or dysfunctional family

- Inadequate schooling (frequent changes or absences)

Note
A distinction is sometimes made between verbal and nonverbal LDs, largely depending on cerebral hemisphere and associated abilities believed to be affected. RD involving language areas usually localized to the left hemisphere is a verbal LD.

Treatment

Treatment for children is usually long term, addresses broad and systemic issues, and should include specific interventions.

1. The physician may coordinate care but, more commonly, may serve by contributing to an interdisciplinary team effort originating at the child's school. Public Law 94-142 (Education for All Handicapped Children Act) requires

states to provide free appropriate public education to all children with disabilities. All children receiving special services must have an individual education program (IEP) on file. Parent, teacher, administrator, diagnostician, and physician develop the IEP to provide the best and least restrictive educational experience for the child.

2. Some controversy exists as to whether bright children reading at the average level should receive treatment. Policies vary across school systems.

3. Take advantage of longitudinal exposure to the child and the family to preserve self-esteem. Encourage the child and the family to discuss their feelings about the disability. Monitor for changes in self-concept and emotional difficulties.

4. Pharmacotherapy for RD is experimental, but treatment for co-morbid conditions may be helpful. Medications with CNS side effects should be at lowest possible doses.

5. Work with the family. Children with disabilities often require extra family time and resources, especially in the presence of co-morbid conditions. Allow the family to discuss their experience. Be alert for parental reading or other cognitive difficulties and assist with problem solving.

6. Advise the family as to the genetic and biologic basis of RD to avoid a view of the child as lazy or oppositional.

7. Help the family to avoid useless treatments. Programs addressing visual-perceptual training, chiropractic, vestibular treatment, and dietary supplementation have little support.

8. Young children may benefit from remedial interventions, whereas older children and adults may benefit most from accommodations.

9. Remediation should address weaknesses or teach to strengths.

   a. Programs addressing phonologic processing weakness offer direct instruction in letter-sound associations. For example, Orton Gil-

lingham and DISTAR teach letter sounds and then syllables and words. "Analytic" approaches such as Merrill and the SRA Basic Reading program teach whole words and then have students deduce associations.

   b. Programs that teach to strengths avoid phonologic processes and use visual associations. For example, the Bridge Reading Program trains students in picture/symbol-word associations.

Patient Education

Resources for the patient and family

1. The National Center for Learning Disabilities
   381 Park Avenue South, Suite 140
   New York, NY 10016
   1-888-575-7373
   www.ncld.org

2. Learning Disabilities Association of America
   4156 Library Road
   Pittsburgh, PA 15234-1349
   1-412-341-1515
   www.ldanatl.org

 Key Treatment

- Individualized tutoring for remediation
- Counseling for emotional sequelae
- Supportive parents

 Bibliography

American Psychiatric Association: Diagnostic and Statistical Manual of Mental Disorders, 4th ed, Washington, DC, American Psychiatric Press, 1994.

Beitchman JH, Young AR: Learning disorders with a special emphasis on reading disorders: a review of the past 10 years. J Am Acad Child Adolesc Psychiatry 1997; 36:1020–1032.

Kelly MS, Gottesman RL: Adults with severe reading and learning difficulties. J Am Board Fam Pract 1997;10: 199–205.

Sattler JM: Clinical and Forensic Interviewing of Children and Families. San Diego, Sattler Publishing, 1998

Shaywitz SE: Clues to dyslexia in school-age children. N Engl J Med 1998;338:307–312.

312 Sleep Disorders

J. Steven Poceta

Narcolepsy

Etiology

Altered sleep and rapid eye movement (REM) sleep mechanisms underlie the symptoms of narcolepsy. For example, cataplexy has the appearance of REM-like atonia of skeletal muscle outside the context of a REM period. The sleepiness is probably due to dopaminergic and noradrenergic neural transmission. There is a strong linkage with human leukocyte antigen (HLA) alleles DR-2 and DQB1*0602, but not all cases are familial. The gene abnormality in canine narcolepsy has recently been described. Onset is usually in adolescence or young adulthood.

Symptoms

1. Sleepiness is the primary symptom, sometimes in the form of "sleep attacks." Although sleep and sleepiness occur at times outside the habitual sleep period (night), the total amount of sleep attained by narcoleptics in a 24-hour day is not increased compared with normal individuals. Daytime naps are usually refreshing. "Automatic behavior" refers to waking activity of which the patient may not be aware, such as driving home without memory of such or acting strangely. Presumably, automatic behavior is the result of microsleeps invading waking activities.

2. Cataplexy is pathognomonic for the classic narcolepsy syndrome and consists of partial or total loss of muscle tone without loss of consciousness, usually provoked by anticipatory emotion. Laughter, surprise, and their anticipation are the most common inciting emotions. Injury to the patient can occur, and this symptom can be disabling depending on the patient's occupation and goals. The most common muscles involved are proximal, especially the neck and jaw.

3. Sleep paralysis is the experience of being awake but unable to move, usually occurring near sleep onset or offset, and usually quite frightening. The attack usually lasts for seconds. Eye movements remain intact, and some patients use them to help abort the spell.

4. Hypnogogic hallucinations are vivid dream-like experiences that the patient cannot distinguish from reality. These may occur during daytime naps.

5. Disturbed nocturnal sleep is common in narcoleptics, especially older narcoleptics. This problem compounds the daytime sleepiness and contributes to disability.

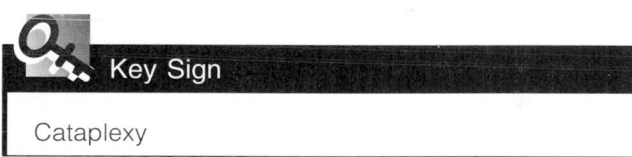

Key Symptoms

- Sleepiness
- Cataplexy
- Sleep paralysis
- Hypnogogic hallucinations
- Disturbed nocturnal sleep

Clinical Findings

1. The examination is normal, by definition, except perhaps for manifest sleepiness.

2. Cataplexy can be diagnosed by observing loss of deep tendon reflexes during an attack and the prompt resumption of reflexes after the attack.

Key Sign

Cataplexy

Laboratory Tests

1. The diagnosis is confirmed by an overnight sleep study followed by a multiple sleep latency test (MSLT). The MSLT is a series of daytime naps with measurement of electroencephalogram-defined sleep and will show a mean sleep latency of under 7 minutes with at least two sleep-onset REM periods. Normal patients would show a sleep latency of greater than 10 minutes and no REMs.

2. HLA typing is useful only in occasional cases that do not fit a standard pattern. The associated phenotypes are common in the general population, but their absence is evidence against classic narcolepsy with cataplexy.

Differential Diagnosis

1. Sleep apnea, even mild forms in which snoring disturbs sleep without frank apnea, can cause sleepiness. Nocturnal myoclonus also can present as sleepiness. These conditions are ruled out by the overnight polysomnogram

2. Idiopathic hypersomnolence is a related syndrome of sleepiness but without the REM-related symptoms of narcolepsy; its distinction from narcolepsy can be difficult.

3. Psychiatric conditions may cause complaints of sleepiness, fatigue, and altered sleep and dream content.

4. Antisocial personality disorders might manifest with periods of inactivity or withdrawal that can be confused with true sleepiness.

5. Medical conditions causing sleepiness, such as hypothyroidism or hydrocephalus, also must be ruled out.

6. Cataplexy must be distinguished from seizures and ischemic vertebrobasilar drop attacks.

Treatment

Treatment of the sleepiness consists primarily of stimulant medication. When cataplexy is mild, the stimulants can sometimes control it effectively. Cataplexy and the other REM-related symptoms are treatable with REM-suppressant agents such as the tricyclic antidepressants and selective serotonin-reuptake inhibitors (SSRIs).

Medication

1. A variety of stimulant agents can be used successfully, and individuals vary greatly in their responses and needs.
   a. Pemoline (Cylert), 37.5 to 150 mg daily in one or two divided doses
   b. Methylphenidate (Ritalin), 20 to 60 mg daily in two or three divided doses: available in regular and sustained-release forms
   c. Dextroamphetamine or methamphetamine, 20 to 60 mg daily in one or two divided doses; available in regular and sustained-release forms
   d. Modafinil (Provigil), 100 to 200 mg twice a day

2. REM-related symptoms such as cataplexy can be controlled with agents that increase central nervous system synaptic norepinephrine.
   a. Tricyclic agents, especially clomipramine (Anafranil), 25 to 75 mg daily, and protriptyline (Vivactil), 5 to 20 mg daily, are effective, although their use is sometimes limited by anticholinergic side effects.
   b. Fluoxetine (Prozac), 20 to 80 mg daily, is an alternative. Other SSRIs may be effective but are less well documented.

Patient Education

Planned naps after lunch and after work can be helpful. Often, a brief nap before a drive is as effective as a take-as-needed stimulant. Patients should avoid shifts in their sleep schedule. Patients must be warned to respect the dangers of their sleepiness when involved in activities such as driving.

Restless Legs Syndrome and Nocturnal Myoclonus

Etiology

1. Restless legs syndrome (RLS) is a condition in which patients experience an unpleasant and hard-to-describe feeling in the limbs when they are at rest, particularly in the evening. It often interferes with sleep.

2. Nocturnal myoclonus, also called periodic limb movement disorder (PLMD), is a related condition of repetitive, periodic, and stereotypical movements of the limbs, usually the legs, during quiet waking or non-REM sleep. About 85 per cent of patients with RLS have PLMD, but many patients with PLMD do not have restless legs and may present instead with insomnia or excessive daytime sleepiness.

3. Both conditions can be idiopathic or secondary. Causes of secondary RLS and PLMD include iron deficiency and peripheral neuropathy. There is speculation that circulatory insufficiency or lumbar disk disease predisposes to RLS. However, neurochemical deficiencies probably underlie RLS—especially the idiopathic form. Alterations in dopamine or perhaps endogenous opioid systems are postulated. It is not known what level of the nervous system

is abnormal, although electrophysiologic studies suggest an alteration in mechanisms at the pontine level or higher. RLS is usually idiopathic, and familial in about one half of cases. No genetic pattern or gene defect has yet been established. Certain medications, such as tricyclic antidepressants or lithium, can aggravate RLS.

Symptoms

1. RLS is diagnosed on the basis of the symptoms and history. The sensation should be bilateral, very disagreeable, but not painful. It is often described as a tingling, prickling, tense, or "creepy-crawly" feeling. As mentioned, it is most notable when the patient is at rest, particularly in the evening. The urge to rub or to move the affected limbs is irresistible. Dyskinetic movements, myoclonic jerking, and marching in place are not uncommon. Most patients with RLS also have PLMD, which emerges during sleep.

2. PLMD is diagnosed on the basis of sleep-related repetitive, periodic, and stereotypical movements of the limbs, usually the legs. These take a form similar to a triple-flexion response with Babinski's sign and have both jerky and sustained components, last 0.5 to 5 seconds, and occur every 20 to 40 seconds. They may be disruptive to sleep or to a bedpartner's sleep. The symptom produced is either insomnia or excessive daytime sleepiness, and this condition should be considered in any patient with these complaints. Many patients have PLMD that is asymptomatic and does not require treatment.

Key Symptoms

- Irresistible restless sensation of the limbs, especially the legs, interfering with sleep
- Repetitive and periodic leg movements during sleep causing insomnia or sleepiness

Clinical Findings

By definition, the examination is normal in idiopathic RLS with PLMD.

Laboratory Tests

Nocturnal polysomnography is capable of demonstrating PLMD. Certain specific variations of these sleep studies can sometimes quantitate RLS as well. Considering that the available treatments have potential risks, documentation of the condition is sometimes desirable.

Key Test

Nocturnal polysomnography

Differential Diagnosis

1. RLS and PLMD have been associated in small series with many medical conditions, including pregnancy, uremia, neuropathy, myelopathy, amyloidosis, and anemias. Studies show an increased prevalence in neuropathy and iron deficiency. Chronic obstructive pulmonary disease, Isaacs' syndrome, Huntington's disease, and leukemias also have been reported in patients with RLS or PLMD. These conditions should be considered when evaluating a patient.

2. RLS and PLMD should be distinguished from other sleep-related movements, such as hypnic jerks. Myoclonic epilepsy and partial seizures might be confused with the jerky motions of PLMD. RLS should be distinguished from neuropathic pain and from akathisia. Akathisia produces a similar restless sensation and is often caused by neuroleptic use or by dyskinetic movement disorders. REM behavior disorder and sleep apnea are significant conditions with an increased prevalence of PLMD and should be ruled out prior to treatment. For example, arousals from apneas may appear to be leg-induced arousals to a casual observer.

Treatment

Treatment is aimed at either reducing the dysesthesia of RLS or at improving sleep quality in PLMD to eliminate insomnia or daytime sleepiness.

Medication

1. Dopaminergic agents are effective in up to 70 per cent of patients with RLS, and the benefit can be sustained for several years. L-Dopa with carbidopa is most often used, but direct dopamine agonists also appear to be effective. Both the subjective dysesthesias and the number of leg movements in sleep are reduced. Carbidopa-levodopa (Sinemet) is usually given in doses of 25/100 mg or 50/200 mg at bedtime with a repeat dose in the middle of the night if needed. The continuous-release form is also useful because of the sustained action. Side effects have been minor, such as nausea or dizziness. Daytime rebound of the sensation occurs in about one third of patients, often leading to daytime use of L-dopa. Dopamine agonists such as pergolide (Permax) are also effective and might produce less rebound. A typical dose would be

pergolide, 0.10 to 0.50 mg in the evening. These agents are not FDA approved for this indication.

2. Benzodiazepines, particularly temazepam (Restoril) and clonazepam (Klonopin), have been shown to improve sleep quality and to aid sleep onset in patients with RLS and PLMD. Their effect on the number of leg movements is less than that of L-dopa, but the arousals associated with the movements are reduced. Clonazepam is usually used in doses of 0.5 to 2.0 mg at bedtime; temazepam in doses of 15 to 30 mg. Tolerance and escalation of effective doses are sometimes encountered, as well as morning sedation.

3. Opioids, particularly propoxyphene and oxycodone, have been shown to relieve RLS and to decrease the number of leg movements, but the effect is not as robust as with L-dopa. Nonetheless, these agents are useful in many patients, and long-term side effects are better defined. Propoxyphene (Darvon) is used in doses from 65 to 195 mg at bedtime.

Key Treatment

- Dopaminergic agents, such as L-dopa and pergolide
- Benzodiazepines, such as temazepam and clonazepam
- Opioids, such as propoxyphene and oxycodone

Bibliography

Fry JM (ed): Current issues in the diagnosis and management of narcolepsy. Neurology 1998;50(Suppl 1):1S–48S.

Mitler MM, Aldrich MS, Koob GF, Zarconc VP: Narcolepsy and its treatment with stimulants. Sleep 1994; 17:352–371.

Nishino S, Mignot E: Pharmacological aspects of human and canine narcolepsy. Prog Neurobiol 1997;52:27–78.

Poceta JS: Restless legs syndrome. In Poceta JS, Mitler MM (eds): Sleep Disorders: Diagnosis and Treatment, pp 75–93. Totowa, NJ, Humana Press, 1998.

Silber MH: Concise review for primary-care physicians. Mayo Clin Proc 1997;72:261–264.

313 Bell's Palsy

Charles B. Eaton

Bell's palsy is an acute, complete or partial paralysis of the peripheral facial nerve striking approximately 25 in 100,000 people annually. No consensus on the etiology or best treatment exists; therefore, each patient should be evaluated based upon the severity of the symptoms, age of the patient, and the patient's expectations.

Etiology

Controversy exists as to the etiology of Bell's palsy, with various proponents suggesting metabolic, genetic, autoimmune, vascular, entrapment, and infectious etiologies. New evidence using molecular biology techniques suggests that reactivated herpes simplex virus may be implicated in 70 per cent of cases, leading to a viral-induced neuritis.

1. Idiopathic: diagnosis of exclusion
2. Infectious
   a. Viral: herpes simplex, herpes zoster (Ramsey-Hunt syndrome), human immunodeficiency virus (HIV), mumps, adenovirus, coxsackievirus, influenza, Epstein-Barr, polio.
   b. Bacterial: otitis media, Lyme, syphilis, leprosy
3. Pregnancy
4. Inflammatory: sarcoidosis
5. Demyelinating disease: multiple sclerosis, post-infectious demyelination
6. Chronic diseases: Diabetes mellitus, hypothyroidism, and hypertension are risk factors, although probably not etiologic agents.

Symptoms

1. Acute or subacute onset of facial weakness of upper and lower facial musculature (usually unilateral)
2. Subjective facial numbness: Suggests sensory dysfunction of cranial nerve V.
3. Postauricular pain
4. Abnormal lacrimation
5. Hyperacusis: Stapedial nerve affected.
6. Dysgeusia: Lingual nerve affected.

Key Symptoms

- Unilateral, acute facial weakness of the lower motor neuron type
- Postauricular pain
- Unilateral lacrimation

Clinical Findings

1. Lower motor neuron–type facial weakness, suggested by smooth forehead (loss of wrinkle lines), flattened nasolabial fold, asymmetric smile, is present. Usually the paresis is unilateral, but bilateral involvement is present in 1 per cent of cases. The paresis is progressive for 7 to 10 days.
2. More than one branch of facial nerve is usually involved, including the motor branch to upper and lower facial musculature, the lingual branch of the chordi tympani (taste perversion on anterior two thirds of tongue), the stapedial branch (diminished stapedial reflex), and the greater superficial petrosal nerve (lacrimation). Isolated facial nerve branch involvement suggests other etiologies.
3. Eye examination may reveal a widened palpebral fissure, diminished corneal reflex, possibly increased or decreased tearing, weakness of orbicularis oris musculature associated with Bell's phenomenon.
4. Remainder of neurologic examination is normal, including normal visual acuity, ocular movements, balance, and deep tendon reflexes.
5. Normal skin examination (no evidence of herpes zoster vesicles, erythema migrans, or café-au-lait lesions), normal parotid gland examination, and a normal ear examination.

Key Signs

- Facial weakness, usually unilateral, of the upper and lower facial musculature
- The remainder of the neurologic examination is normal.

Laboratory Tests

With a careful history and physical examination, 90 per cent of cases of Bell's palsy can be diagnosed without costly diagnostic tests. Selected laboratory tests to consider based upon the history and physical examination include

1. Baseline complete blood count (CBC), sedimentation rate, thyroid-stimulating hormone (TSH), and electrolytes, blood urea nitrogen (BUN), and glucose are recommended.
2. Pure-tone audiometry with stapedial reflex testing is suggested on all patients.
3. Lyme titer if suspicious of Lyme disease: Antibiotic therapy should be started early, prior to diagnostic test results, if Lyme disease is suspected.
4. Serologic tests for syphilis, HIV may be indicated based upon the patient's history.
5. Herpes simplex, Epstein-Barr, and herpes zoster titers can be done for confirmation of clinical suspicion.
6. Cerebrospinal fluid analysis is indicated if central nervous system syphilis, sarcoidosis, or demyelinating disease is suspected.
7. Magnetic resonance imaging with gadolinium contrast is indicated if demyelinating disease, neurofibromatosis, parotid tumor, acoustic neuroma, or Burkitt's lymphoma is suspected.
8. Computerized tomography scan is indicated if temporal bone fracture, cholesteatoma, or mastoiditis is suspected.
9. Angiotensin-converting enzyme and chest radiograph are indicated if sarcoidosis is suspected.
10. Modified tear test can be performed to assess baseline and reflex-induced tearing if lacrimation is affected.
11. Electrodiagnostic testing is expensive and requires serial evaluation. Electrical testing must be correlated with clinical progression of the paralysis. Electrodiagnostic testing is indicated when there is evidence of early, complete paralysis and suspected complete denervation, which has a poorer prognosis.

Key Tests

- CBC, sedimentation rate, TSH, and electrolytes, BUN, and glucose are recommended.

- Pure-tone audiometry with stapedial reflex testing is suggested on all patients. An intact stapedial reflex suggests incomplete paralysis and therefore a good prognosis.

- Selected tests based upon the patient's presentation, appropriate differential diagnosis, and severity of paralysis and therefore prognosis for recovery.

Differential Diagnosis

Slow onset of paralysis (weeks), associated tics and spasm, paralysis of isolated branch of the facial nerve, loss of balance, or other neurologic symptoms are *not* typical presentation of Bell's palsy and should trigger review of the differential diagnoses listed below.

1. Cerebrovascular accident
2. Trauma: fracture of the temporal bone, especially in newborn infants
3. Otitis media, cholesteatoma, mastoiditis
4. Herpes zoster (Ramsey-Hunt syndrome)
5. Neurosyphilis
6. Lyme disease: Important to consider in endemic areas and when patient presents with bilateral paralysis
7. HIV disease
8. Neoplasms, including cerebellopontine angle tumors, schwannoma, parotid gland tumors, Burkitt's lymphoma, and metastatic tumors
9. Demyelinating disease such as multiple sclerosis
10. Guillain-Barré syndrome
11. Sarcoidosis

Treatment

Treatment should be individualized based upon the severity of patient's paralysis, risks and contraindications of treatment, and patient's expectations. The sooner treatment is initiated, the better the outcome.

1. Pharmacologic
   a. Corticosteroids: If not contraindicated, oral prednisone, 1 mg/kg/day (minimum of 30 mg bid) for 5 days and then taper over 5 days, has been shown to be effective in several clinical trials if started within 72 hours of the onset of symptoms.
   b. Acyclovir (Zovirax), 400 mg 5 times a day for 10 days, has been shown to be more effective in combination with prednisone compared to prednisone alone if started within 72 hours of the onset of symptoms. Other clinical trials using acyclovir 800 mg tid have not shown acyclovir by itself to be as effective as prednisone alone.
2. Supportive care
   a. Protection of the eye with artificial tears during the daytime, ocular lubricant and lid taping if evidence of exposure keratitis is sug-

gested. Rarely tarsorrhaphy is needed if keratitis persists despite lid taping and ocular lubricants.

b. Physiotherapy with electrical stimulation has *not* been shown to be effective, and some experimental evidence suggests it may inhibit nerve regeneration; therefore, it is not recommended.

3. Surgical: Surgical decompression is advocated by some experts for patients with severe nerve degeneration (>90 per cent within 2 weeks of symptoms), with an 85 per cent recovery rate compared to 50 per cent for those treated conservatively.

Patient Education

1. Inform the patient of the importance of reporting ocular dryness or pain and the need for prevention of exposure keratitis.

2. Inform patient that most patients recover within 6 to 12 weeks and that up to 10 per cent of patients may experience a recurrence.

 Key Treatment

Oral prednisone, 1 mg/kg/day for 5 days and then taper over 5 days, plus acyclovir, 400 mg 5 times a day for 10 days

Follow-Up

1. Because nerve degeneration takes 7 to 10 days to be complete, all patients should be evaluated 1 week after initial evaluation to assess efficacy of treatment and prognosis. Incomplete paralysis has the best prognosis. Complete paralysis of rapid onset (within 72 hours) is associated with severe denervation and has a worse prognosis.

2. Serial electrodiagnostic testing is useful in patients with complete, early paralysis suggestive of severe nerve degeneration, which has a poorer prognosis, and to assess the potential for surgical decompression.

3. Consider referral to ophthalmology, neurology, or otolaryngology specialist when

a. Patient has persistent eye pain or evidence of nonhealing exposure keratitis.

b. Patient has documented abnormalities on neurologic examination other than a peripheral facial weakness or has abnormal balance.

c. Rapid onset of complete paralysis suggestive of severe degeneration with a poor prognosis, hearing loss or other otologic symptoms, or the isolated involvement of a single branch of peripheral facial nerve suggestive of tumor

ACKNOWLEDGMENTS: The author gratefully acknowledges Daniel Lombardi for his assistance with this manuscript.

 Bibliography

Adour KK: Medical management of idiopathic (Bell's) palsy. Otolaryngol Clin North Am 1991;24:663–673.

Adour KK, Ruboyianes JM, Von Doersten PG, et al: Bell's palsy treatment with acyclovir and prednisone compared to prednisone alone: a double-blind, randomized controlled trial. Ann Otol Rhinol Laryngol 1996;105:371–378.

Bauer CA, Coker NJ: Update on facial nerve disorders. Otolaryngol Clin North Am 1996;29:446–454.

Bleicher JN, Hamiel S, Gengler JS, et al: A survey of facial paralysis: etiology and incidence. Ear Nose Throat J 1996;75:355–358.

DeDiego JI, Prim MP, De Sarria MJ, et al: Idiopathic facial paralysis: a randomized, prospective, and controlled study using single dose prednisone versus acyclovir three times daily. Laryngoscope 1998;108:573–575.

314 Trigeminal Neuralgia

Howard Tung

Etiology

1. The etiology of trigeminal neuralgia is thought to be related to compression of the trigeminal nerve at some point between the gasserian ganglion and the pons.

2. Frequently, a vascular loop at the level of the root entry zone where the trigeminal nerve enters the pons is found to be the etiologic factor for trigeminal neuralgia.

3. Other common causes of trigeminal nerve root compression include benign tumors (meningioma, epidermoid cyst, acoustic neuroma) or plaque formation in multiple sclerosis.

Symptoms

1. Trigeminal neuralgia, or tic douloureux, is a symptom characterized by paroxysms of intense, stabbing pain within the distribution of the trigeminal nerve. The pain is often described as lancinating or shock-like in quality, lasting a few seconds to a minute or two.

2. A patient may suffer from one or two attacks per day to as many as 10 or 20 attacks per hour. The pain is typically more pronounced during the day, with markedly fewer episodes experienced at night. Many times, "trigger points" such as touching of the face, wind blowing across the face, or hot or cold liquids may initiate the pain. The pain also may begin spontaneously or with innocuous facial movements such as speaking, chewing, or swallowing.

3. In general, the pain syndrome is usually unilateral, involving the second or third divisions of the trigeminal nerve and rarely involving the ophthalmic division.

4. The majority of patients are over age 50, with women affected more often than men.

Key Symptoms

- Paroxysms of stabbing pain on one side of the face

- Attacks last only seconds to a minute or two

Clinical Findings

1. Most often, examination of the sensory and motor components of the fifth cranial nerve is normal in idiopathic trigeminal neuralgia.

2. Association of the cranial nerve abnormalities suggests other pathology, such as a cerebellopontine angle mass.

Laboratory Tests

Neuroradiologic work-up, including magnetic resonance imaging (MRI) of the head, is usually normal but important in excluding tumors or substantiating other neurologic disease processes (e.g., multiple sclerosis) that may present with trigeminal neuralgia.

Key Tests

None (MRI to rule out tumor or diagnose multiple sclerosis)

Differential Diagnosis

The diagnosis of trigeminal neuralgia rests mainly on strict clinical criteria and is usually readily distinguishable from other craniofacial neuralgias or pain arising from the jaw, teeth, or sinuses. The differential diagnosis includes

1. Multiple sclerosis
2. Glossopharyngeal neuralgia
3. Postherpetic neuralgia
4. Raeder's paratrigeminal syndrome
5. Atypical facial neuralgia
6. Chronic cluster syndrome (Horton's cephalgia)
7. Cluster headaches
8. Post-traumatic facial neuralgia
9. Temporomandibular joint pain
10. Pain secondary to disease of dental, sinus, or orbital origin

Treatment

Medication

Medical therapy is the treatment of choice for idiopathic trigeminal neuralgia, and a number of medications have proven effective in the relief of pain.

1. Approximately 80 per cent of patients will ob-

tain pain relief with the anticonvulsant carbamazepine (Tegretol), whereas phenytoin (Dilantin) will improve up to 50 per cent of patients.

a. Begin the Tegretol dose gradually with an initial dose of 200 mg/day. The dose may then be increased slowly (e.g., 100 to 200 mg every 2 or 3 days) until pain relief is achieved or drug toxicity develops. A typical dose may be 600 to 800 mg/day in three divided doses, but doses as high as 1200 to 1800 mg/day may be required to achieve pain relief in some.

b. It is important for patients to have their complete blood count and liver function tests followed periodically because carbamazepine may cause hematosuppression or liver dysfunction.

2. Baclofen (Lioresal) and clonazepam (Klonopin) also have proven useful but overall are less effective than carbamazepine or phenytoin and are considered secondary forms of medical therapy.

3. Gabapentin (Neurontin) is being used with success in patients with trigeminal neuralgia. It should be started at a low dose (e.g., 300 mg PO once a day) and escalated over 1 to 2 weeks to 300 mg PO tid as tolerated. The most common side effect is cognitive slowing.

Surgery

Surgical therapy also has proven to be effective in the treatment of trigeminal neuralgia. Surgical treatment is reserved for patients refractory to medical treatment or for those who develop untoward side effects to medical therapy. In general, surgical treatment for trigeminal neuralgia is divided into percutaneous trigeminal neurolysis and microvascular decompression.

1. Percutaneous trigeminal neurolysis

a. Percutaneous approaches to the gasserian ganglion have proven excellent in obtaining relief for the pain of trigeminal neuralgia. These techniques utilize placement of a needle or electrode through the foramen ovale to the trigeminal cistern of Meckel's cave, with a subsequent procedure to destroy the gasserian ganglion and retrogasserian rootlets.

b. The major advantages of percutaneous procedures include avoidance of general anesthesia as compared with open microvascular decompression, short hospital stays (1 day), and the procedure may be repeated easily if necessary.

c. In our series of over 500 patients with glycerol injection, initial pain relief has been achieved in over 85 per cent. Reported recurrence rates are variable in the literature, but, generally, 20 to 25 per cent may experience recurrence of pain in 2 to 3 years, which is consistent with my experience.

d. Side effects include sensory numbness in many patients, but this is usually well tolerated. Rarely, corneal anesthesia (without keratitis) or hyperesthesia may occur, but I have found this to be transient.

e. Radiofrequency thermocoagulation lesions offer results similar to glycerol injections. Instead of chemical destruction of the gasserian ganglion and rootlets with glycerol, thermocoagulation of the ganglion is carried out with a temperature-monitoring electrode. I have found the side effects with radiofrequency lesions similar to those of glycerol injections, except that the sensory disturbances tend to be more severe, with severe dysesthesias and anesthesia dolorosa occurring rarely.

f. Neurolysis via balloon compression of the trigeminal ganglion may be performed through a needle in a manner similar to radiofrequency lesioning or glycerol injection. General anesthesia is required because compression of the trigeminal ganglion is extremely painful and may cause a severe vagal response. The results are about the same as for radiofrequency lesioning: in most series more than 90 per cent of patients get immediate pain relief, with a 21 per cent recurrence rate.

g. When surgical treatment has been successful, patients then are slowly tapered off their medication regimen.

2. Microvascular decompression

a. The frequent finding of vascular compression of the root entry zone of the trigeminal nerve in patients with trigeminal neuralgia was first commented on by Dandy in 1934. Clinical and anatomic studies of patients with trigeminal neuralgia have supported this finding. However, the fact that vascular compression is not the sole cause of trigeminal neuralgia is attested to by the observation that compression is not found in as many as 10 to 15 per cent of patients at surgery.

b. Microvascular decompression is suitable for patients with typical trigeminal neuralgia intractable to medical therapy and who are otherwise healthy and without excessive anesthesia risks.

c. Presently, I perform microvascular decompression through a small retromastoid craniectomy with mobilization of the offending vascular structure (usually the superior cerebellar artery) away from the root entry zone of the trigeminal nerve and subsequent placement of a Teflon pledget between the artery and nerve.

d. Advantages of microvascular decompression include treating the apparent cause of pain, which can be curative and usually affords longer pain-free periods compared with percutaneous procedures. The procedure is nondestructive, sparing the nerve, and generally carries fewer of the sensory disturbances noted with other procedures.

e. Risks of microvascular decompression include the need for general anesthesia and retromastoid craniectomy, with increased potential for serious complications (e.g., meningitis, hemorrhage, cerebrospinal fluid leak, cranial nerve deficit).

Therapeutic Approach to Patients With Trigeminal Neuralgia

1. When first evaluating a patient with trigeminal neuralgia, there is no substitute for an accurate and careful history and physical examination. If the patient appears to have typical trigeminal neuralgia, diagnostic studies (e.g., MRI with and without contrast) are indicated to rule out the possibility of a posterior fossa tumor or lesion. If these are negative, medical treatment is indicated with Tegretol. Dilantin is later used if maximal doses of Tegretol are unsuccessful. If medical therapy fails or untoward side effects occur, surgical treatment is considered.

2. In elderly, medically infirm patients, we recommend percutaneous trigeminal neurolysis procedures. In my hands, glycerol injections have proven highly effective in relieving trigeminal neuralgia pain with fewer side effects versus trigeminal radiofrequency rhizotomy. This procedure also has been attractive to patients for its short hospital stay, with patients often returning to work the next day with a high rate of success. In addition, I have found this procedure also useful for trigeminal neuralgia related to multiple sclerosis.

3. In younger patients, a careful discussion of microvascular decompression and percutaneous trigeminal neurolysis, with expected results and possible risks of each procedure, is undertaken and a choice made by the patient. Although surgery is curative in a majority of cases, if the condition recurs after microvascular decompression, it can then be treated by percutaneous technique or re-exploration with partial division of the trigeminal sensory root.

Key Treatment

- All patients should be given a therapeutic trial of carbamazepine (Tegretol), which provides at least partial relief in most cases.

- Patients who are good operative candidates should be considered for microvascular decompression.

Bibliography

Hamlyn PJ, King TT: Neurovascular compression in trigeminal neuralgia: a clinical and anatomical study. J Neurosurg 1992;76:948–954.

Jannetta PJ: Observations on the etiology of trigeminal neuralgia, hemifacial spasm, acoustic nerve dysfunction and glossopharyngeal neuralgia: definitive microsurgical treatment and results in 117 patients. Neurochirurgia 1977;20:145–154.

Lunsford LD, Apfelbaum RI: Choice of surgical therapeutic modalities for treatment of trigeminal neuralgia: microvascular decompression, percutaneous retrogasserian thermal or glycerol rhizotomy. Clin Neurosurg 1985;32:319.

Tenser RB: Trigeminal neuralgia: mechanisms of treatment. Neurology 1998;51:17–19.

Waltz TA, Dalessio DJ, Copeland B, Abbott G: Percutaneous injection of glycerol for the treatment of trigeminal neuralgia. Clin J Pain 1989;5:195–198.

315 | Reflex Sympathetic Dystrophy

Robert J. Schwartzman

Etiology

1. New definitions of what has been called reflex sympathetic dystrophy (RSD) are now in use.

   a. If no specific nerve injury is identified, the syndrome is called complex regional pain syndrome type I (CRPS I); analogous to RSD (old definition).

   b. If a specific nerve is injured and the symptoms of RSD occur, the syndrome is now known as complex regional pain syndrome type II (CRPS II); analogous to causalgia.

2. Epidemiology: All age groups are susceptible. Particular injuries that are associated with RSD are

   a. Brachial plexus traction injuries

   b. Carpal tunnel surgery

   c. Arthroscopic knee surgery

   d. Fractures with concomitant nerve injury

   e. Radiculopathy and soft tissue injury

3. Risk factors

   a. A few families have been reported with RSD. There appears to be no genetic predisposition.

   b. Fifty per cent of all patients with RSD have been casted. Most of these patients have had sprains, Colles' fractures, or trimalleolar ankle fractures.

   c. A completely severed nerve does not cause RSD.

   d. Damage to blood vessel walls and nerves from electrical injury, ergotamine toxicity, or vein stripping may incite the process.

Symptoms

1. All features of RSD may be present in the affected extremity, whereas the contralateral extremity demonstrates subtle subclinical signs and symptoms of specific components of the syndrome.

2. The process in its early stages is sympathetically maintained but with time becomes sympathetically independent. It may spread to the entire body surface and can involve the visceral autonomic nervous system and bone.

3. Pain

   a. *Hyperalgesia*: lower pain threshold with enhanced pain perception

   b. Mechanical and thermal *allodynia*: pain induced by innocuous mechanical or thermal stimuli

   c. *Hyperpathia*: increased pain threshold that, once exceeded, induces severe pain that reaches maximum intensity explosively and continues when the stimulus is withdrawn

4. Hypoesthesia: Some patients with RSD are hypoesthetic in the affected area. The pain spreads both proximally and distally and does not respect a nerve or dermatomal distribution. It frequently is more severe on extensor surfaces.

Key Symptoms

- Pain out of proportion to injury
- Burning pain
- Deep ache
- Allodynia
- Hyperalgesia

Clinical Findings

1. Edema: Edema is seen in both early and late stages of the illness at the site of injury, distal to it and at times over major areas of the body. The edematous skin has a brawny-reddened quality.

2. Autonomic dysfunction: Autonomic dysfunction is present in all stages of RSD.

   a. Early in the illness, the involved extremity may be warm, suffused, red, and dry but with time becomes pale, cool, hyperhidrotic, and cyanotic.

   b. Temperature changes from warm to cool may vary within a short period of time in stage I disease.

   c. Generalized capillary circulatory dysfunction occurs in all fingers and toes of the affected extremity rather than in a nerve or dermatomal distribution.

3. Movement disorder: All patients with RSD manifest some aspects of its concomitant movement disorder. These features are

    a. An inability to initiate movement rapidly

    b. Dystonia

    c. Weakness

    d. Spasm

    e. Hyperactive reflexes

    f. Tremor

4. Dystrophy and atrophy

    a. Early in the course of the illness, the nails become thickened, ridged, and brittle. Hair becomes darker and grows more rapidly. Edematous areas demonstrate brawny, reddened, thickened skin.

    b. In later stages, nails break, hair is lost in the affected area, and the skin becomes shiny and atrophic. There is profound muscle atrophy, bone demonstrates periarticular resorption, and there is tendon and cartilage degeneration.

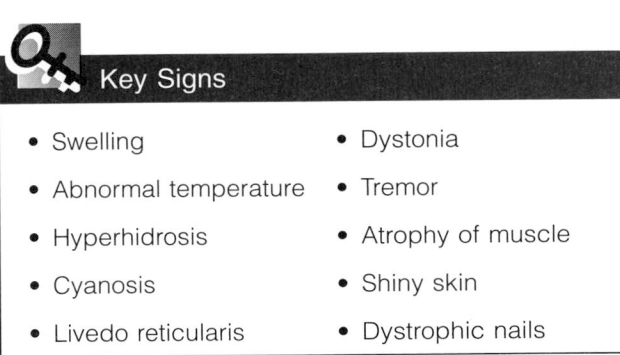

Key Signs

• Swelling	• Dystonia
• Abnormal temperature	• Tremor
• Hyperhidrosis	• Atrophy of muscle
• Cyanosis	• Shiny skin
• Livedo reticularis	• Dystrophic nails

Laboratory Tests

The underlying cause of the illness must be identified.

1. Thermography identifies small-fiber abnormalities (sympathetic and C-fiber in several dermatomes in the affected areas in a characteristic pattern).

2. A triple-phase bone scan may demonstrate abnormal pooling and increased periarticular uptake in 30 per cent of patients.

3. Sympathetic blockade of the affected area will afford dramatic relief of pain if the process is still sympathetically maintained. If the process is sympathetically independent, it will not relieve pain.

4. An intravenous phentolamine test (α_1-adrenergic antagonist) will be positive (pain relief) if the process is still sympathetically maintained.

5. Plain radiographs reveal clear periarticular and cystic bone changes in late-stage disease.

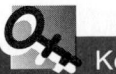

Key Tests

• Thermogram

• Triple-phase bone scan

• Response to sympathetic blockade

Differential Diagnosis

1. Autonomic dysfunction, edema, and pain from underlying soft tissue injury or fracture

2. Thrombophlebitis

3. Ergotism

4. Small-fiber neuropathy

Treatment

1. Diagnosis and treatment of the underlying injury

2. Sympathetic blockade

    a. Sympathetic blockade of the upper extremity: placement of an intrapleural block with continuous 0.05% bupivacaine for 3 days, followed by intensive physical therapy

    b. Sympathetic blockade of the lower extremity: placement of epidural catheter for a 3 to 5 day 0.05% bupivacaine block, followed by weight bearing, stretching and strengthening exercises

    c. Patients with generalized RSD (CRPS I/II): Intravenous lidocaine, 4 to 6 mg/minute, may be administered to decrease pain. If successful, mexiletine may be used in full cardiac dose.

3. Amitriptyline (Elavil) for sleep and diflunisal (Dolobid), 250 mg tid for pain in early stages

4. In sympathetic independent pain, a dorsal column stimulator is placed. In refractory single-extremity problems, a combination of nerve and dorsal column stimulation is utilized.

5. In generalized RSD that is refractory to all other forms of treatment, a morphine intrathecal pump is utilized. Approximately 35 mg/day relieves most patients.

6. Experimental new treatments

    a. Phenoxybenzamine (Dibenzyline)

    b. Nifedipine (Procardia, Adalat)

    c. SNX-III (voltage-gated calcium channel blocker)

Key Treatment

- Relieve underlying cause
- Sympathetic blockade
- Intense physical therapy
- Dorsal column stimulation
- Morphine pump

Bibliography

Benrath J, Eschenfelder C, Zimmerman M, et al: Calcitonin gene-related peptide, substance P and nitric oxide are involved in cutaneous inflammation following ultraviolet radiation. Eur J Pharmacol 1995;293:87–96.

Birklein F, Claus D, Riedl B, et al: Effects of cutaneous histamine application in patients with sympathetic reflex dystrophy. Muscle Nerve 1997;20:1389–1395.

Boas RA: Reflex sympathetic dystrophy. In Jänig W, Stanton-Hicks M (eds): Progress in Pain Research and Management, pp 79–92. Seattle, IASP Press, 1996.

Bowersox SS, Gadbois T, Singh T, et al: Selective N-type neuronal voltage-sensitive calcium channel blocker, SNX-111, produces spinal antinociception in rat models of acute, persistent and neuropathic pain. J Pharmacol Exp Ther 1996;279:1243–1249.

Cao YQ, Mantyh DW, Carlson EJ, et al: Primary afferent tachykinins are required to experience moderate to intense pain. Nature 1998;392:390–394.

316 Parkinson's Disease

John T. Slevin

Etiology

Anatomy, Biochemistry, Pathology

1. Parkinson's disease (PD) is an *idiopathic* condition resulting from neuronal degeneration and loss of pigmented brain stem nuclei.

2. Losses are prevalent in the zona compacta of the substantia nigra, a pigmented nucleus containing dopaminergic neurons projecting (via the *nigrostriatal pathway*) to the putamen and caudate nuclei. Functionally, this loss of inhibitory dopaminergic input is thought to account for much of the hypokinetic motor symptoms of PD.

3. The Lewy body, an eosinophilic intracytoplasmic neuronal inclusion, is considered the sine qua non of idiopathic PD but has been reported in several other neurologic diseases.

4. Recent evidence lends support to an *oxidant theory*: PD may result from either an extrinsic mechanism (oxidation of a protoxin, e.g., methylphenyltetrahydroperidine [MPTP]) or an intrinsic mechanism whereby free radicals are generated by dopamine metabolism among other mechanisms.

Biometric Data

1. The most common movement disorder in clinical practice—prevalence: 100 cases per 100,000 population; incidence: 20 cases per 100,000 population per year

2. Onset between ages 40 and 70 (peak onset in mid 50s)

3. No definite gender, ethnic, geographic, or socioeconomic predispositions are known.

4. Rare families may be predisposed to PD, with apparent autosomal dominant inheritance.

Symptoms

1. Slowness of movement: Leads to difficulties in grooming, dressing, feeding, and walking.

2. Stiffness: Affects both flexors and extensors of limbs and axial muscles, with patients complaining that they feel wooden or are moving against great resistance.

3. Tremor: Usually unilateral at onset, it can progress to involve the face and lower extremities. Exaggerated by anxiety; absent in sleep.

4. Posture/gait abnormalities: Patients assume a stooped posture and develop a disturbance of equilibrium leading to frequent falls.

5. Other: autonomic disturbances, including orthostatic hypotension, constipation, hyperhydrosis; muscle cramps and aching; micrographia; slurred, hypophonic, monotonous speech. Ultimately, dementia is seen in over half of patients.

Clinical Findings

1. Bradykinesia: Patient sits immobile on the examining table. Appearance of *masked facies*, or poker face, with decreased eyeblink.

2. Rigidity, usually *cogwheel rigidity*, wherein passive movement of a joint causes sequential catches as in turning a ratchet; resistance is uniform throughout range of motion. Often unilateral at disease onset, rigidity becomes increasingly prominent and generalized in later stages of the disease.

3. Gait disturbance: An initial lack of arm swing with walking evolves into a propulsive, or *festinating*, shuffling, small-stepped gait with en bloc, or whole-body, turning.

4. A resting, *pill-rolling* tremor of 3 to 6 Hz that diminishes with movement is an initial symptom in 70 per cent of patients. Tremor may be unilateral or generalized.

5. Exaggerated *glabellar reflex* (Myerson's sign): blinking that does not reduce or stop with repeated tapping on the forehead

6. Mild orthostatic hypotension, sialorrhea, moist greasy face with seborrheic dermatitis

Key Symptoms/Signs

Cardinal	Secondary
• Akinesia/bradykinesia	• Dysarthria
• Postural/gait abnormalities	• Micrographia
• Rigidity	• Seborrhea
• Tremor	• Sialorrhea

Laboratory Tests

1. PD is a clinical diagnosis with no definitive laboratory test(s).
2. Computerized tomography and magnetic resonance imaging either are normal or show nonspecific atrophy.
3. Electroencephalogram, blood, and cerebrospinal fluid studies are typically normal.

Differential Diagnosis

1. Isolated depression: When manifested as psychomotor retardation, major depression may be confused with PD, with which a reactive depression is not uncommon. There is evidence to suggest a primary depression in PD as a result of the diminution of biogenic amines.
2. Essential tremor: characterized by a postural and kinetic (not resting) tremor of the hands and head without bradykinesia and rigidity. It frequently decreases temporarily with ingestion of ethanol, and more than 50 per cent of patients respond to propranolol, primidone, or thalamic stimulation (see below). Frequently positive family history.
3. "Parkinson plus" syndromes: differentiated from idiopathic PD by the presence of various associated signs and symptoms.
   a. Parkinsonism + disturbances of ocular motility: progressive supranuclear palsy
   b. Parkinsonism + cerebellar signs and symptoms: olivopontocerebellar degenerations
   c. Parkinsonism + severe autonomic insufficiency: Shy-Drager syndrome
4. Secondary parkinsonism
   a. Head trauma (e.g., from professional boxing)
   b. Metabolic disorders, especially hypoparathyroidism
   c. Postviral encephalitis: rare, sporadic cases
   d. Toxins and industrial exposure (especially consider in the younger patient): carbon tetrachloride, carbon monoxide, carbon disulfide, cyanide, manganese, methanol, MPTP (the by-product of a street drug)
   e. Drugs: the most common cause of secondary parkinsonism, which itself is the most common drug-induced movement disorder
      (1) Neuroleptics, especially haloperidol, fluphenazine
      (2) Antiemetics, especially prochlorperazine, metoclopramide
      (3) Reserpine
      (4) α-Methyldopa (rarely)
      (5) Lithium carbonate (rarely)

Treatment

1. PD is relentlessly progressive; no treatment modalities have been shown to categorically slow disease progression. Treatment is palliative and directed at relieving symptoms.
2. Several surgical procedures are currently performed:
   a. Thalamic (deep brain) stimulation by means of an electrode connected to a battery usually implanted in the chest provides contralateral control of tremor.
   b. Unilateral pallidotomy is primarily effective in reducing contralateral dyskinesia and bradykinesia.
   c. Stimulation of either the subthalamic nucleus or globus pallidus, implantation of either human or porcine fetal nigral cells, and installation of trophic factors are all investigational procedures.
3. Choice of medication(s) depends on stage (see below) of illness; only oral preparations are available.

Medication

1. Dopaminergic agents
   a. All act by enhancing activity at central dopamine receptors and all have common side effects, including
      (1) Anorexia, vomiting, dizziness, orthostatic hypotension
      (2) Dyskinesia: usually choreiform movements; the effect is dose dependent and usually occurs after prolonged therapy.
      (3) Psychotic episodes, dementia, depression: Half of patients on chronic dopamine replacement therapy develop psychiatric side effects. Visual hallucinations and vivid nightmares are frequent early signs. Psychotic episodes usually take the form of paranoid delusions. Symptoms usually improve with reduction of dopaminergic agents.
   b. Precursor therapy: levodopa-carbidopa (Sinemet, Atamet); controlled release form (SinemetCR)
      (1) Levodopa crosses the blood-brain barrier (BBB) and is then converted to dopamine. Carbidopa, which cannot cross the BBB, blocks the peripheral decarboxylation of levodopa to dopamine, allowing more levodopa to reach the site of action in the brain.
      (2) Additional side effects
         (a) Cardiac arrhythmia: rare in preparations including carbidopa

(b) Orthostatic hypotension: usually transient, early in treatment, and resolves

(3) Dosing: Initial dose of carbidopa-levodopa, 25/100-mg tablet tid. As disease progresses, more frequent dosing is required to maintain relief. Extended-release preparations are helpful in patients who show excessive symptomatic fluctuations.

c. Direct receptor agonists: bromocriptine (Parlodel), pergolide (Permax), pramipexole (Mirapex), ropinirole (Requip)

(1) Permit use of lower dosages of levodopa with improvement in side effect profile (including dyskinesia) and fewer symptomatic fluctuations; can be used as monotherapy.

(2) Additional side effects

(a) Bromocriptine: exacerbation of peptic ulcer disease and *erythromelalgia*, a painful reddish skin discoloration.

(b) Ropinirole: somnolence

(c) An irresistable urge to sleep has been reported in patients who were taking pramipexole or ropinirole. All of the reported attacks occurred while driving, leading to motor vehicle accidents.

d. *Monoamine oxidase-B inhibitor*: selegiline (Eldepryl)

(1) Increases level of intrinsically/extrinsically derived dopamine by blocking catabolism. It has been suggested that drugs of this class may help slow the progression of PD; to date, studies have shown little significant effect in this regard.

(2) Additional side effects: insomnia; will potentiate side effects of levodopa.

e. *Catechol-O-methyltransferase (COMT) inhibitor*: tolcapone (Tasmar)

(1) Blocks peripheral catabolism of levodopa by COMT thereby enhancing the absorption and brain availability of exogenous levodopa.

(2) Helps smooth the course of fluctuating patients, in theory, by reducing pulsatile stimulation of dopamine receptors through its influence on levodopa pharmacokinetics.

(3) Should only be used in conjunction with levodopa.

(4) Tolcapone has been associated with severe, potentially fatal liver disease. At press time, FDA recommendations are to obtain liver function tests every two weeks for the first year of therapy. Changes in LFTs may not predict liver failure until damage has already occurred.

f. *Indirect agonist* (and an anti-A2 viral agent): amantidine (Symmetrel)

(1) Used in early PD; useful in treating tremor, can delay the need for levodopa.

(2) Additional side effects: congestive heart failure, urinary retention, livedo reticularis

2. Anticholinergic agents: trihexyphenidyl (Artane), benztropine (Cogentin), others

a. Blocking the relative excess cholinergic activity provides relief for some patients. First choice in treatment of patients with primarily tremor. No effect on hypokinesia or rigidity.

b. Side effects: Dry mouth, constipation, and blurred vision common; urinary retention in men; may cause confusion in older patients. Be alert to signs of closed-angle glaucoma.

Rational Treatment Strategy and Problems

1. At the onset of functional impairment, treat with selegiline and/or amantadine; use anticholinergics to treat tremor.

2. With deterioration in early disease, use a dopamine agonist or levodopa and be prepared to initiate combined therapy, rather than high-dose monotherapy, before the disease has reached its mid-course.

3. In later stages of PD, add a COMT inhibitor to modulate response fluctuations (see below) and consider surgery when control with medical therapy becomes unacceptable.

4. Treatment problems include

a. Dyskinesias: see side effects of dopaminergic agents above

b. On-off phenomena: marked, rapid fluctuations between a parkinsonian state and normal or dyskinetic state that do not directly correlate with time of dosing

c. Loss of efficacy: Patients lose response to medications as PD progresses, usually not before the fifth year of overt symptoms.

Diet

1. Patients should eat a balanced diet that contains sufficient fiber and fluid to prevent constipation and enough calcium to maintain existing bone structure.

2. Some patients will exhibit a significant delay or, occasionally, no response after levodopa dosing. Efficacy may be improved by dosing *before* meals or by reducing dietary protein (especially breakfast and lunch).

3. Patients who have more trouble with the peripheral side effects of levodopa (nausea and vomiting) often improve with dosing *after* meals.

Activity

Patients with PD, like everyone, should participate in a regular exercise program. They should focus on maintaining range of mobility and muscle strength. A physical therapist familiar with PD can often help individualize an exercise program.

Patient Education

1. Encourage participation in support groups that can offer psychological and social benefits to both patient and family and encourage membership in a national support group, most of which provide newsletters.

2. When appropriate, occupational counseling may help with adaptions to improve productivity and reduce stress in the workplace.

3. Expert advice in the form of legal/financial counseling from attorneys and estate planners who specialize in elder law may help patients cope with anxiety associated with concerns of increasing physical disability.

Key Treatment

- No treatment modality has categorically slowed disease.

- Treatment is palliative and aimed at relieving symptoms.

Follow-Up

1. One must know the interval between levodopa dosing and the clinical examination and whether the patient feels *off* or *on* when examined to determine if a change in therapy is necessary, usually at two to three yearly visits.

2. Of many rating scales used for PD, the Hoehn-Yahr Staging Scale has been in use for over 25 years.
   a. Stage 0: no signs of disease
   b. Stage I: unilateral disease
   c. Stage II: bilateral or midline involvement
   d. Stage III: stage II + impaired balance
   e. Stage IV: severe disability, able to walk
   f. Stage V: wheelchair bound/bedridden

Bibliography

Duvoisin RC: Parkinson's Disease: A Guide for Patient and Family, 4th ed. Philadelphia, Lippincott-Raven, 1996.

Jankovic J, Marsden CD: Therapeutic strategies in Parkinson's disease. In Jankovic J, Tolosa E (eds): Parkinson's Disease and Movement Disorders, 2nd ed, pp 115–144. Baltimore, Williams & Wilkins, 1993.

Olanow CW, Koller WC (eds): An algorithm (decision tree) for the management of Parkinson's disease: treatment guidelines. Neurology 1998;50(Suppl 3):S1–S57.

Paulson HL, Stern MB: Clinical manifestations of Parkinson's disease. In Watts RL, Koller WC (eds): Movement Disorders: Neurologic Principles and Practice, pp 183–199. New York, McGraw-Hill, 1997.

$\mathbf{317}$ Alzheimer's Disease

Robert J. Moss

Epidemiology

1. Major public health problem affecting over 4 million persons
2. Fourth leading cause of death, with 46,000 deaths per year
3. Costs may exceed $90 billion per year
4. Major risk factors
   a. Advanced age
   b. Family history
   c. Head trauma
   d. Educational background
   e. Apolipoprotein E4 genotype

Etiology

1. Histopathologic changes (frontal, temporal, and parietal lobes):
   a. Intracellular neurofibrillary tangles: abnormal filamentous accumulation in cytoplasm of neurons. Major ultrastructural unit is paired helical filament that contains protein tau.
   b. Extracellular neuritic plaques: abnormal nerve processes with central β-amyloid protein core. β-Amyloid is derived from amyloid precursor protein.
2. Cholinergic hypothesis
   a. Cholinergic neurons are selectively vulnerable to injury, with retrograde degeneration of the three subcortical nuclei.
   b. Choline acetyltransferase and acetylcholine, as well as other cholinergic markers, are decreased.
   c. Degree of cognitive impairment directly related to loss of cholinergic neurons and neurotransmitters.
3. Genetics
   a. Three causal or determinant genes have been identified for early-onset familial Alzheimer's disease.
      (1) Chromosome 21 has the amyloid precursor protein gene—20 families.
      (2) Chromosome 14 has the presenilin 1 gene—100 families.
      (3) Chromosome 1 has the presenilin 2 gene—few families.
   b. Two susceptibility genes have been identified for late-onset or sporadic Alzheimer's disease (majority of Alzheimer's disease).
      (1) Chromosome 19: Apolipoprotein E4 allele increases risk of disease before the age of 70 to 30 per cent.
      (2) Chromosome 12 recently reported to be involved.

Symptoms

1. Progressive memory loss (short and long term)
2. Impairment in at least one other area of cognitive function
   a. Abstract thinking
   b. Judgment
   c. Visual-spatial function
   d. Language
   e. Apraxia
   f. Agnosia
   g. Personality change
3. Impairment in social functioning (home, job, activities of daily living)
4. Consciousness not clouded (absence of delirium)

Key Symptoms

- Progressive memory loss
- Impairment in at least one other area of cognitive functioning
- Impaired social functioning
- Clear sensorium

Clinical Findings

1. Abnormal mental status screening examination (such as Folstein Mini-Mental State Examination)
2. Physical and neurologic examinations fail to identify other causes of dementia.

Laboratory Tests

1. Thyroid-stimulating hormone (TSH) to exclude hyper- or hypothyroidism
2. Erythrocyte sedimentation rate to exclude underlying inflammatory disease
3. Chemistry profile to exclude metabolic, renal, or hepatic disease
4. Urinalysis to exclude renal disease
5. Complete blood count (CBC) to exclude anemia
6. Folate and vitamin B_{12} to exclude nutritional deficiency
7. Fluorescent treponemal antibody absorption (FTA-Abs) test for syphilis to exclude tertiary syphilis
8. Human immunodeficiency virus (HIV) titer to exclude HIV infection for individuals at risk
9. Lumbar puncture to rule out slow viral or fungal disease if fever or nuchal rigidity present or to measure level of protein tau (not generally necessary to support diagnosis)
10. Neurodiagnostic testing: Yield is 3.5 per cent for pathogenic abnormalities.
    a. Electroencephalogram to rule out underlying seizure disorder, delirium, or Creutzfeldt-Jakob disease
    b. Computerized tomography (CT) brain scan to exclude tumor, subdural hematoma, stroke, normal-pressure hydrocephalus
    c. Magnetic resonance imaging (MRI): more sensitive to small-vessel disease, focal atrophy, and posterior fossa changes than CT brain scan
    d. Positron emission tomography (PET) scan determines functional abnormalities that predict cognitive changes with characteristic patterns for Alzheimer's disease.
    e. Single-photon emission computerized tomography (SPECT) scan used as PET scan, with characteristic pattern of decreased uptake in temporoparietal areas seen in Alzheimer's disease.
11. Genetic testing for susceptibility to disease not recommended. May be diagnostic in familial Alzheimer's disease and used as adjunctive test to support diagnosis in sporadic or late-onset disease. Genetic counseling recommended because of many potential psychosocial consequences of testing.
12. Brain biopsy is the only definitive test for diagnosis.

Differential Diagnosis

1. Delirium: acute onset with fluctuating levels of consciousness
2. Depression: fluctuating cognitive loss with depressed mood, "I don't know" answers and impaired concentration.
3. Other dementia syndromes
   a. Multiple infarct dementia: stepwise decline with multiple cardiovascular risk factors and focal neurologic signs
   b. Medications: sedatives, antihypertensives, antidepressants, neuroleptics, antihistamines, anticholinergic agents
   c. Alcohol
   d. Normal-pressure hydrocephalus: triad of urinary incontinence, dementia, and gait ataxia
   e. Toxic, metabolic, nutritional, infectious, and other neurologic causes
   f. Dementia with Lewy bodies: rapid course, visual hallucinations, extrapyramidal symptoms, very sensitive to neuroleptic medications.

Treatment

1. Acetylcholinesterase inhibitors
   a. Donepezil (Aricept)
      (1) Has shown modest cognitive and functional improvement 36 per cent of the time and may slow disease progression by 6 months.
      (2) A 5-mg tablet once a day; no liver function testing required; 10 per cent cholinergic side effect profile. Cautious use in persons with history of gastrointestinal bleeding, bradyarrhythmias, and chronic obstructive pulmonary disease or asthma.

(3) Two dose ranges: 5-mg and 10-mg tablet titrated after 1 month

b. Tetrahydroaminoacridine (tacrine HCl [Cognex])

(1) Similar benefits to donepezil

(2) Older drug; initial dose 10 mg four times a day with maximal dose of 160 mg daily; requires liver function testing every other week for the first 16 weeks. Thirty per cent of patients develop reversible increases in liver enzymes.

c. Other drugs under evaluation include metrifonate, which may also have benefits on behavioral symptoms and rivastigmine (Exelon) awaiting FDA approval.

2. Antioxidants

a. Vitamin E: May clinically impact rate of functional decline, although no impact on cognition; may interact adversely with warfarin (Coumadin).

b. Selegiline: Similar effect to vitamin E but no additive effect; has increased side effect profile and drug interactions.

c. *Ginkgo biloba*: May have positive impact on cognition and function. Many different preparations. Can inhibit platelets, and cases of hemorrhage have been reported.

3. Estrogen: Observational studies suggest a 29 per cent decrease in risk of developing a dementia in women who have taken postmenopausal estrogen. Its role in prevention and treatment not defined.

4. Nonsteroidal anti-inflammatory drugs: Cross-sectional studies suggest a decreased incidence of dementia. Their role in prevention and treatment not defined.

Behavioral Syndromes

1. Depression and anxiety occur in 30 per cent of patients. Consider structured activities-based program and treatment with short-acting anxiolytics or antidepressants with low anticholinergic side effects.

2. Delusions and hallucinations occur in 25 to 50 per cent of patients. Consider high-potency or novel neuroleptic medication with low anticholinergic side effects. Effective approximately 50 per cent of the time.

3. Agitation: Consider behavioral program, environmental manipulation, redirection. High-potency or novel neuroleptic medication, short-acting benzodiazepines, trazodone, β-blockers, buspirone, selective serotonin reuptake inhibitors, carbamazepine, and valproate are alternatives. Become familiar with side effect profile of each.

Diet

1. Weight loss commonly seen and can be a marker for inadequate self-care.

2. May need reminders to eat; meals often need to be prepared, and hand feedings or finger food offered.

3. Mechanical soft diet with thick liquids may become necessary to prevent aspiration.

4. Nutritional supplements are important.

5. Many ethical issues surrounding tube feedings should be discussed if necessary.

Patient Education

1. Explain diagnosis.

2. Caregiver support

a. Respite

b. Support groups, live-in help, adult day care

3. Financial planning

4. Anticipate home care and placement needs.

5. Review behavior syndromes (include falls, incontinence, sleep disturbance, and wandering).

6. Discuss advance directives, guardianship, and other ethical issues.

 Key Treatment

Drugs that augment acetylcholine, such as cholinesterase inhibitors

 Bibliography

American Psychiatric Association: Diagnostic and Statistical Manual of Mental Disorders, 4th ed. Washington, DC, American Psychiatric Press, 1994.

Post SG, Whitehouse PJ, Binstock RH, et al: The clinical introduction of genetic testing for Alzheimer's disease: an ethical perspective. JAMA 1997;277:832–836.

Rogers SL, Farlow MR, Doody RS, et al: A 24-week, double-blind, placebo-controlled trial of donepezil in patients with Alzheimer's disease. Neurology 1998;50: 136–145.

Sano M, Ernesto C, Thomas RG, et al: A controlled trial of selegiline, alpha-tocopherol, or both as treatment for Alzheimer's disease. N Engl J Med 1997;336:1216–1222.

Small GW, Rabins PV, Barry PP, et al: Diagnosis and treatment of Alzheimer disease and related disorders: consensus statement of the American Association for Geriatric Psychiatry, the Alzheimer's Association, and the American Geriatrics Society. JAMA 1997;278: 1363–1371.

Yaffe K, Sawaya G, Lieberburg I, et al: Estrogen therapy in postmenopausal women: effects on cognitive function and dementia. JAMA 1998;279:688–700.

318 Myasthenia Gravis

John J. Hart

Etiology

1. Myasthenia gravis (MG) is an autoimmune disease caused by antibody and T-cell attack on the nicotinic acetylcholine receptors (AChR) of the muscle endplate.

   a. Between 85 and 95 per cent of MG patients have antibodies to their AChRs.

   b. T-cell immunity is theorized to occur after sensitization in the thymus to a protein similar or identical to the embryonic AChR.

2. MG age classification and respective etiologies

   a. Adult MG: autoimmune etiology as described above

   b. Childhood MG

      (1) Transient neonatal MG: MG mothers passively transfer antibodies to 10 to 20 per cent of their children.

      (2) Congenital MG: caused by a variety of neuromuscular junction defects and *is not* autoimmune-mediated

      (3) Juvenile MG: etiology identical to adult MG, earlier onset

Symptoms

1. Voluntary muscle weakness and increased fatigability

2. Diplopia

3. Dysphagia

4. Jaw weakness while chewing

5. Choking

6. Fluid regurgitation through nose when swallowing

7. Difficulty maintaining volume of voice

8. Myasthenic crisis: respiratory failure

Key Symptoms

- Easily fatigued, weak muscles
- Diplopia

Clinical Findings

1. Muscle weakness initially is transitory.

2. Weakness is exacerbated with continuous use, warmer surroundings, at the end of the day, and with physiologic and psychosocial stress.

3. Order of muscle group involvement from most to least common: ocular, bulbar, neck, limb girdle, and distal extremity

4. Forty per cent of MG patients eventually develop bulbar muscle problems.

5. Ninety per cent of MG patients develop ocular findings (ptosis, acquired strabismus). Of those whose symptoms stay localized to the eyes for 1 year, 90 per cent will have ocular MG.

6. Clinical classification

   a. Ocular only

   b. Generalized

      (1) Mild: ocular with gradual progression to skeletal and bulbar muscles, no respiratory symptoms

      (2) Moderate: more rapid and involved progression, no respiratory symptoms

      (3) Severe

         (a) Acute fulminating

         (b) Late severe: severe symptoms after approximately 2 years

Key Signs

- Ptosis
- Muscle weakness
- Dysarthria

Laboratory Tests

1. AChR antibody assay: Antibody is elevated up to 95 per cent of the time in generalized MG but less with ocular MG. Overall assay is positive 74 per cent of the time.

2. Edrophonium (Tensilon) test: This anticholinesterase is administered intravenously and the patient is observed for improvement; 90 per cent true positive.

   a. Children heavier than 75 pounds and adults: 2 mg edrophonium is given intravenously over 15 to 30 seconds. The test is positive if muscular strength increases. If a positive response does not occur, an additional 8 mg of edrophonium is given and muscular strength is again evaluated. Decreased doses are used for infants and children less than 75 pounds.

b. False-negative results occur, especially with ocular MG. It is sometimes combined with other ocular tests to better diagnose ocular MG.

c. False-positive results have been reported in amyotrophic lateral sclerosis, Lambert-Eaton syndrome, brain tumors.

3. Electromyogram

a. A decremental response is seen with MG.

b. Repetitive nerve stimulation tests and stimulated single-fiber electromyography (SF-EMG)—the most sensitive

Key Tests

No single test is adequate for diagnosis; all three are used, that is:

- Acetylcholine antibody assay

- Edrophonium test

- Electromyogram

Differential Diagnosis

1. Lambert-Eaton syndrome
2. Muscular dystrophies
3. Brain tumors
4. Endocrine myopathies
5. Amyotrophic lateral sclerosis
6. D-Penicillamine administration (may induce AChR antibodies)
7. Chronic progressive external ophthalmoplegia
8. Polymyositis

Treatment

1. Thymectomy improves most MG; less so with ocular and mild MG. Best for moderate and severe MG.
2. Plasmapheresis gives short-term improvement and is useful in acute situations and before surgery.

Medication

1. Acetylcholinesterase inhibitors
   a. Pyridostigmine (Mestinon)
   b. Neostigmine bromide (Prostigmin)
2. Immunosuppressive medicines

a. Corticosteroids
b. Cyclophosphamide (Cytoxan)
c. Cyclosporine (Sandimmune)
d. Azathioprine (Imuran)
3. Intravenous human immune globulin

Diet

Monitor for metabolic abnormalities secondary to prednisone and correct, such as potassium supplementation, caloric restriction.

Activity

Overexertion may exacerbate MG.

Patient Education

1. Physiologic and emotional stress may exacerbate MG.
2. Many common medicines exacerbate MG.
   a. Antibiotics: aminoglycosides, polymyxins, tetracyclines
   b. Cardiac drugs: verapamil, β-blockers
   c. Others: phenytoin, chlorpromazine
3. Side effects of key medicines used to treat MG
   a. Pyridostigmine (Mestinon): diarrhea, bradycardia, sweating, salivation
   b. Prednisone: subclinical presentations of infections

Key Treatment

Drugs of Choice

- Pyridostigmine (Mestinon)

- Prednisone

Follow-Up

1. Progression of weakness
2. Thyroid function studies
3. Watch and screen for other autoimmune diseases.

Bibliography

Berrouschot J, Baumann I, Kalischewski P, et al: Therapy of myasthenic crisis. Crit Care Med 1997;25:1228–1235.

Busch C, Machens A, Pichlmeier U, et al: Long-term outcome and quality of life after thymectomy for myasthenia gravis. Ann Surg 1996;224:225–232.

Marx A, Wilisch A, Schultz A, et al: Pathogenesis of myasthenia gravis. Virchows Arch 1997;430:355–364.

Massey JM: Acquired myasthenia gravis. Neurol Clin 1997;15:557–595.

Wittbrodt ET: Drugs and myasthenia gravis—an update. Arch Intern Med 1997;157:399–408.

319 Multiple Sclerosis

Michael D. Kaufman

Etiology

1. Theories of pathogenesis of multiple sclerosis (MS)
   a. Autoimmune disease directed against myelin proteins, oligodendroglia cells, or other antigens
   b. Chronic viral (e.g., human herpesvirus-6) or bacterial (e.g., *Chlamydia pneumoniae*) infection of the central nervous system (CNS)
2. Increasingly prevalent in some locations, including areas of the United States and Europe
3. Environmental determinants
   a. More common as distance from the equator increases
   b. Outbreaks suggest transmission of an agent that induces disease.
   c. Susceptibility depends on childhood residence.
4. Genetic contributions: Multiple genes involved.
   a. High prevalence in whites (90 to 95 per cent of U.S. patients); some ethnic groups appear resistant to MS
   b. Increased incidence among family members (Table 319–1)
   c. Gender: three females to one male

Symptoms

1. Primarily affects young adults, usually starting unilaterally or focally but eventually becoming bilateral, disseminated, and progressive
2. Common: limb weakness, numbness and paresthesia, chronic aching pain, monocular impairment of vision, double vision, slurred speech, imbalance, vertigo, urgency, constipation, impotence, depression, fatigue, cool extremities, radiating paresthesias associated with neck flexion (Lhermitte's sign), heat intolerance, mild cognitive changes
3. Less common: radicular pains, facial weakness, hearing loss, trigeminal neuralgia, euphoria, confusion, oscillating vision, paroxysmal symptoms lasting seconds to minutes, dysesthesias, bilateral visual blurring
4. Uncommon: severe apraxias or aphasia, extrapyramidal movement disorders, seizures, perineal pains, hypersomnolence, hemianopsia, severe dementia
5. Symptoms may be vague and precede recognizable signs, falsely suggesting somatization or hysteria.
6. Course
   a. Benign: 10 to 30 per cent; never becomes progressive
   b. Relapsing-remitting/secondary progressive: more than 50 per cent; exacerbations without obvious progression at onset, then becomes progressive
   c. Primary progressive: 10 to 20 per cent; often affects spinal cord; no exacerbations
   d. Relapsing-progressive: 5 to 10 per cent progressive at onset but with superimposed exacerbations
   e. Less common patterns: optic neuritis and myelitis (Devic's disease), recurrent optic neuritis, acute MS, associated with diseases of known etiology

TABLE 319–1. MS RISK WHEN FAMILY MEMBER AFFECTED

RELATIONSHIP	LIFETIME MS RISK
General Caucasian population	<0.2%
Sibling or parent with MS	1–3%*
Dizygotic twin with MS	2–4%
Monozygotic twin with MS	17–40%

*May be as high as 25 per cent in women with more than one first-degree relative developing MS at a young age. Overall, brothers of siblings with MS have a 1 per cent risk while sisters have a 3 per cent risk of developing MS.

WARNING

Some patients report what appears to be a benign course for years, only then to experience rapid progression. Prediction of disease outcome for an individual is problematic.

Key Symptoms

- Neurologic symptoms lasting days to weeks in a young adult

- Symptoms involving distant parts of CNS often appearing together

- Monocular visual blurring or binocular diplopia

- Worsening symptoms with vigorous activity or heat

- Bowel, bladder, and sexual dysfunction

Clinical Findings

1. Common: asymmetric weakness, patchy sensory loss, pale optic disks, internuclear ophthalmoplegia, nystagmus, hyperreflexia, spastic gait, ataxia, diminished visual acuity, afferent pupillary defect

2. Less common: hyporeflexia, writhing facial muscles (myokymia), oscillating eye movement, deafness, atrophy of muscle, significant dementia

3. Uncommon (may suggest another diagnosis): homonomous hemianopsia, choreoathetosis, aphasia, apraxia, well-defined sensory level

Key Signs

- Brisk reflexes

- Weakness in an upper motor neuron pattern

- Ataxia or abnormal gait

- Internuclear ophthalmoplegia

- Unilateral diminished visual acuity

Laboratory Tests

1. No tests are pathognomonic.

2. Magnetic resonance imaging (MRI): relatively specific, but false-positive and false-negative results

   a. Ovoid high-intensity areas on T_2-weighted scan involving white matter of brain and spinal cord. Three characteristic lesions preferred. Enchancement suggests acute inflammation.

   b. Serial MRIs have shown that the majority of high-intensity areas (about 80 per cent) appear without clinical exacerbation.

   c. Newer techniques: fluid-attenuated inversion recovery (FLAIR), magnetization transfer and MRI spectroscopy

   d. Disability: related to T_1 changes, atrophy, and roughly to T_2 lesion load

3. Cerebrospinal fluid (CSF): Findings in MS are relatively specific.

   a. Cell count: usually less than 40 white blood cells, predominantly lymphocytes

   b. Protein: under 100 mg/dl; usually normal

   c. Oligoclonal immunoglobulin bands: positive in CSF, negative in serum

   d. Immunoglobulin G (IgG) index: above 0.70

   IgG index = CSF (IgG/albumin)/serum

   (IgG/albumin)

4. Evoked potentials: relatively nonspecific; includes visual, brain stem, somatosensory, cortical motor evoked potentials and blink reflex

   a. Can find subclinical areas of disease.

   b. If no history of optic neuritis visual evoked potentials can be relatively specific.

Key Tests

- MRI scans

- CSF oligoclonal immunoglobulin bands and IgG index

WARNING

MS is diagnosed only when physiologically consistent symptoms and signs and laboratory tests converge to suggest involvement of white matter projections from multiple areas within the CNS. Signs and symptoms fluctuate with time. No other pathology can exist to explain the complaints and findings.

Differential Diagnosis

1. Differential diagnosis varies with the patient's symptoms and with the duration of disease. Most difficult diagnostic problems arise with initial exacerbations, progressive myelopathies, and uncommon patterns.

2. MS can be mimicked by and can mimic conversion reactions.

3. Multiple small strokes, arteriovenous malformations, Arnold-Chiari malformation, sarcoidosis, CNS lymphoma, and some degenerative diseases may be confused with MS.

Treatment

1. Many disease-specific therapies now investigational: T-cell vaccination, interleukin-10, intravenous immune globulin, myelin basic protein–proteolipid protein (MBP-PLP) complexes, mitoxantrone, antibiotics
2. Symptomatic therapy often multidisciplinary; important to involve neurologist, physiatrist, social services, vocational rehabilitation for many patients.

Medication

1. Symptomatic treatment (Table 319–2)
2. Disease-specific
   a. Exacerbations: new or reappearance of previous symptom(s) evolving days or weeks (range minutes to months) not due to a metabolic disturbance and preceded by at least 30 days of stability
      (1) Methylprednisolone, 1 gm intravenously daily for 3 to 5 days; may speed recovery from and possibly delay further exacerbations. Follow with tapering, low dose of steroid.
      (2) Adrenocorticotropic hormone (ACTH), intravenously or intramuscularly
      (3) Antiadhesion molecule therapies under study.
   b. Relapsing-remitting/secondary progressive
      (1) Interferon beta-1b (Betaseron), interferon beta-1a (Avonex, Rebif)
      (2) Glatiramer acetate (Copaxone)
   c. Primary and secondary progressive (treatment not universally accepted)
      (1) Cyclophosphamide (Cytoxan): Controversial, but may be helpful in patients under age 40.
      (2) Low-dose azathioprine and methotrexate show a trend toward stability.
      (3) Boluses of methylprednisolone help some patients.
      (4) Interferon beta under study for secondary progressive disease.

Diet

1. No specific diet recommended.
2. Assess dysphagia with modified barium swallow.

Activity

1. Physical therapy: restorative and maintenance
2. Occupational therapy: energy conservation and adaptive devices
3. Aquatic therapy

Patient Education

1. Patients need to understand that treatment is palliative and the course is unpredictable.
2. Address social, insurance, and employment issues early.
3. Treatments that are expensive and potentially dangerous require extensive informed consent and patient cooperation.
4. National MS Society (1-800-FIGHT-MS) provides supplementary patient education.
5. Pharmaceutical houses have programs for patients:
   a. Berlex: 1-800-788-1467
   b. Biogen: 1-800-456-2255
   c. Teva Marion: 1-800-887-8100

Follow-Up

1. Neurologic or MS center consultation advised.
2. Interferon beta-1b may cause a depression of the white blood count and elevation of liver function tests. Follow monthly for 3 months and then periodically. Greater than fivefold persistent elevations of liver transaminase functions should prompt withdrawing treatment until liver tests are normal; then reinstitution at half the dose. Check thyroid function every 1 to 2 years. Subcutaneous injections may cause significant skin lesions. Interferon beta-1a has

TABLE 319–2. SYMPTOMATIC THERAPY

SYMPTOM	TREATMENT
Fatigue	Amantadine and stimulants; look for depression
Depression/demoralization	Antidepressants and counseling
Spasticity	Baclofen (PO and intrathecal), tizanidine, dantrolene, botulinium injections, phenol injections
Urgency/hesitancy	Anticholinergics if bladder spastic; intermittent catheterization if bladder will not empty, α-adrenergic inhibitors for hesitancy
Constipation	Fiber, softeners, suppositories, enemas, oral lactulose, cisapride
Neuralgic pain	Carbamazepine, antidepressants, gabapentin, phenothiazines
Chronic aching pains	Physical therapy and complementary therapies, antidepressants and phenothiazines
Dysmetria	High-dose isoniazid and clonazepam; hard to treat; odansetron
Postural tremor	Propranolol, primidone

similar profile but less severe. Interferon beta causes flu-like symptoms that can be managed with nonsteroidal anti-inflammatory drugs, steroids, pentoxifylline (Trental), and dose reduction.

3. Pseudoexacerbations caused by fever and infection should be treated appropriately, not with methylprednisolone or ACTH.

4. Glatiramer acetate (Copaxone), may cause systemic reaction in approximately 1 of 2500 injections: flushing, tachycardia, shortness of breath lasting 30 seconds to several minutes. Rarely lymphadenopathy may be seen.

Bibliography

Abramsky O, Ovadia H (eds): Frontiers in Multiple Sclerosis: Clinical Research and Therapy. St. Louis, Mosby, 1997.

Matthews WB (ed): McAlpine's Multiple Sclerosis, 2nd ed. New York, Churchill Livingstone, 1991.

Paty DW, Ebers GC: Multiple sclerosis. Contemp Neurol Series 1998;50.

Rudick RA, Cohen JA, Weinstock-Guttman B, et al: Management of multiple sclerosis. N Engl J Med 1997; 337:1604–1611.

Sadovnick AD, Yee IML, Ebers GC, et al: Effect of age at onset and parental disease status on sibling risks for MS. Neurology 1998;50:719–723.

320 Preferred Imaging Modalities in Common Specific Conditions

Sidney C. Ontai

General Principles

1. Ultrasound
   a. Most widely available, including outpatient clinics
   b. Low cost, medium resolution
   c. Cannot penetrate bone/air/tissue interfaces.
2. Computerized tomography (CT)
   a. Available in many hospitals
   b. Medium cost, high resolution; magnetic resonance imaging (MRI) better for soft tissue contrast.
   c. Spiral CT may replace some MRI functions.
   d. Avoid intravenous contrast in renal failure, hypovolemia, or iodine allergy
3. Nuclear scan
   a. Available in many hospitals, depending on frequency of use of test and half-life of specific isotope
   b. Medium to high cost, low resolution
   c. Measures tissue function.
4. MRI
   a. Limited availability
   b. High cost, highest resolution. CT better for bone contrast.
   c. Need patient history that rules out presence of internal ferrous material. Interferes with critical care monitors.

Preferred Imaging Modalities in Specific Conditions

1. Central nervous system, head
   a. Abscess: CT with contrast initially; MRI with contrast when stable
   b. Brain death: cerebral blood flow scan with technetium-99m-labeled hexamethyl-propyleneamine oxime (HMPAO)
   c. Dementia: MRI, cerebral blood flow scan
   d. Epilepsy: MRI
   e. Headache: CT with IV contrast
   f. Sinusitis: CT
   g. Movement disorders: MRI
   h. Neoplasm: MRI
   i. Stroke: CT initially; MRI for follow-up
   j. Transient ischemic attack: MRI, carotid duplex Doppler
2. Neck
   a. Goiter: iodine-123 scan. Scan differentiates "hot" (benign) from "cold" (malignant) thyroid nodules.
   b. Nasopharyngeal neoplasm: MRI
   c. Thyroid cancer: ultrasound. Localizes nodules for fine-needle aspiration.
3. Shoulder—rotator cuff tear, impingement syndrome: MRI
4. Chest
   a. Persistent pulmonary infiltrate or mass: CT
   b. Pulmonary embolism: perfusion lung scan
      (1) Pulmonary angiography still the gold standard; spiral CT emerging as useful for proximal emboli.
      (2) Doppler venous ultrasonography to correlate with deep venous thrombosis
   c. Trauma: CT (after chest radiography); transesophageal echocardiography for suspected cardiac trauma
5. Heart—coronary artery disease: thallium-201 stress test. Use more sensitive/specific thallium scan when electrocardiographic stress test equivocal.
6. Abdomen
   a. Abscess: CT. Ultrasound often used as initial modality, but CT has higher (92 vs. 87 per cent) sensitivity.
   b. Bleeding: labeled red cell scan
   c. Inflammatory bowel disease: indium-111– or gallium-67–labeled white blood cell (WBC) scan
   d. Meckel's diverticulum: technetium-99m pertechnetate scan
   e. Metastases: CT
   f. Peptic ulcer disease: carbon-14 urea breath test for *Helicobacter pylori*
   g. Right upper quadrant pain, obstructive jaundice, pancreatitis: ultrasound, CT
      (1) Magnetic resonance cholangiopancreatography (MRCP) may challenge endoscopic retrograde cholangiopancreatography (ERCP) as gold standard.

    (2) Hepatic ^{99m}Tc-iminodiacetic acid (HIDA) scan can be used to assess hepatobiliary function.

   h. Trauma: CT with contrast

7. Kidney—urinary obstruction: ultrasound; ^{99m}Tc-labeled mercaptoacetyltriglycine (MAG3) scan. Renal scan differentiates loss of glomerular function from anatomic dilatation of renal pelvis in ultrasound.

8. Pelvis

   a. Abnormal vaginal bleeding: transvaginal ultrasound

   b. Ectopic pregnancy: transvaginal ultrasound

   c. Metastases: CT

   d. Ovarian abscess/cyst: ultrasound

9. Testicle

   a. Torsion: Doppler ultrasound

   b. Tumor: ultrasound

10. Knee—cruciate tear, meniscal tear: MRI

11. General musculoskeletal

   a. Osteomyletis: ^{99m}Tc-labeled methylene diphosphonate scan; MRI. ^{99m}Tc scan is not specific. CT can also be used; not as sensitive as MRI.

   b. Osteoporosis: dual-energy x-ray absorptiometry (DEXA)

   c. Septic arthritis: CT or MRI. Detects joint effusion for aspiration.

   d. Aseptic necrosis of femoral head: MRI

12. Skin—soft tissue tumors: MRI. Lipomas, hemangiomas, and ganglion cysts can be differentiated with MRI.

13. Systemic—fever of unknown origin: CT of abdomen; gallium-67– or indium-111–labeled WBC scan

Bibliography

Frassica FJ, Thompson RC Jr: Evaluation, diagnosis, and classification of benign soft-tissue tumors. J Bone Joint Surg [Am] 1996;78:126–140.

Gilman S: Medical progress: imaging the brain (first of two parts). N Engl J Med 1998;338:812–820.

Herzog RJ: Magnetic resonance imaging of the shoulder. J Bone Joint Surg [Am] 1997;79:933–953.

Prvulovich EM, Bomanji JB: Fortnightly review: the role of nuclear medicine in clinical investigation. BMJ 1998; 316:1140–1146.

321 Meningitis

Dawn Schissel

Etiology

Aseptic

1. Viral
   a. Enteroviruses: coxsackievirus, echovirus
   b. Adenoviruses
   c. Mumps virus
   d. Epstein-Barr virus
   e. Herpes simplex virus
2. Fungal: found most commonly in immunocompromised patients
   a. *Candida albicans*
   b. *Coccidioides immitis*
   c. *Cryptococcus neoformans*
3. Tuberculosis: *Mycobacterium tuberculosis*
4. Syphilis

Bacterial (in Order of Prevalence)

1. Neonates
   a. Group B streptococcus
   b. *Escherichia coli*
   c. *Listeria monocytogenes*
2. Infants and toddlers: Highest incidence of meningitis in this age group (3 months to 2 years).
   a. *Haemophilus influenzae*
   b. *Neisseria meningitidis*
   c. *Streptococcus pneumoniae*
3. Older children and adolescents
   a. *Streptococcus pneumoniae*
   b. *Neisseria meningitidis*
   c. *Haemophilus influenzae*
4. Adults
   a. *Streptococcus pneumoniae*
   b. *Neisseria meningitidis*
   c. *Haemophilus influenzae*
   d. *Listeria monocytogenes*

Symptoms

1. Headache: sudden onset, severe, frontal
2. Fever: less than 40° C if aseptic; often greater than 40° C if bacterial
3. Photophobia
4. Stiff neck
5. Nausea and vomiting

6. Viral prodrome common in aseptic meningitis
7. Neonates present with decreased feeding, lethargy, increased irritability, and respiratory distress.

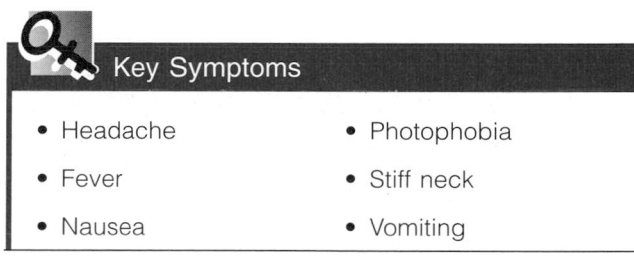

Key Symptoms

- Headache
- Fever
- Nausea
- Photophobia
- Stiff neck
- Vomiting

Clinical Findings

Meningeal signs

1. Nuchal rigidity
2. Kernig's sign: Patient lies supine, flexes knee and hip, and then extends knee. If pain occurs, positive sign.
3. Brudzinski's sign: Patient lies supine, bends neck forward. If knees flex spontaneously, positive sign.
4. Purpura or petechiae
5. Fever, tachycardia
6. Altered sensorium, ranges from confusion to coma
7. Increased white blood cell (WBC) count on complete blood count, with a predominance of neutrophils and immature cells

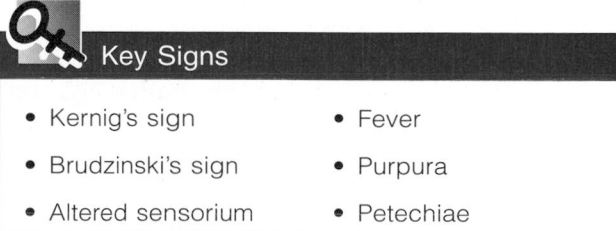

Key Signs

- Kernig's sign
- Brudzinski's sign
- Altered sensorium
- Fever
- Purpura
- Petechiae

Laboratory Tests

Aseptic

1. Cerebrospinal fluid (CSF) evaluation
   a. No growth on cultures
   b. Negative Gram's stain

c. Latex agglutinins negative

d. WBC count less than 1000/mm³, predominantly mononuclear cells

e. Protein: normal to slightly elevated

f. Glucose: normal to slightly decreased

2. Clinical evaluation

Bacterial

1. CSF evaluation

a. Increased opening pressure of more than 180 mm Hg

b. Decreased glucose: less than 40 mg/dl

c. Increased protein: greater than 50 mg/dl

d. WBC count greater than 1000/mm³, less than 10,000/mm³; primarily polymorphonuclear cells.

e. Gram's stain positive for organisms 70 to 90 per cent of the time.

f. Latex agglutinin studies for *S. pneumoniae, H. influenzae,* and *N. meningitidis* available.

2. Blood culture: Positive in 50 per cent of cases.

3. Clinical evaluation

Key Test

Lumbar puncture for CSF evaluation

Differential Diagnosis

1. Brain abscess: Abnormalities seen on CT scan, focal neurologic deficits.

2. Subarachnoid hemorrhage: Lumbar puncture is persistently bloody.

3. Epidural abscess: Neurologic deficits are generally focal.

Treatment

Aseptic

1. Uncomplicated, mild: symptomatic treatment with intravenous or oral fluids, pain relief, rest, acetaminophen

2. Severely ill: Treat empirically with intravenous antibiotics.

a. Ceftriaxone (Rocephin): adults, 1 gm every 24 hours; children, 50 mg/kg every 24 hours

b. Cefotaxime (Claforan): adults, 1 gm every 8 hours; children, 50 mg/kg/day in divided doses every 12 hours

c. May add a penicillin (e.g., ampicillin): adults, 2 gm every 6 hours; children, 100 mg/kg/day in divided doses every 6 hours

3. If unclear, hospitalize and observe for 24 hours. Consider repeat lumbar puncture and watch for WBC shift from polymorphonuclear cells to mononuclear cells.

Bacterial

1. Antibiotic treatment (intravenous) must be initiated emergently, and agent must cross the blood-brain barrier. Hospitalize patient.

2. Neonates

a. Ampicillin, 100 to 200 mg/kg/day in divided doses every 6 hours *plus*

b. Gentamicin, 7.5 mg/kg/day every 8 hours, or cefotaxime, 50 to 100 mg/kg/day in divided doses every 8 hours

3. Children and adolescents

a. Ampicillin, 100 to 200 mg/kg/day in divided doses every 6 hours *plus*

b. Third-generation cephalosporin

(1) Cefotaxime, 50 to 100 mg/kg/day in divided doses every 12 hours

(2) Ceftriaxone, 50 mg/kg every 24 hours

4. Adults

a. Ampicillin, 2 gm every 6 hours *plus*

b. Third-generation cephalosporin

(1) Cefotaxime, 1 gm every 8 hours

(2) Ceftriaxone, 1 gm every 24 hours

(3) If *Pseudomonas* is suspected, ceftazidime, 1.5 gm every 8 hours.

c. If penicillin-resistant *S. pneumoniae* is suspected, substitute vancomycin, 2 gm every 12 hours, for ampicillin until sensitivities are obtained.

5. Treatment consists of intravenous antibiotics for 10 to 14 days unless pathogen is a gram-negative bacillus; then intravenous therapy is 21 days in duration.

6. Repeat lumbar puncture is not necessary if patient is responding clinically to therapy.

7. Intravenous fluids should be limited in neonates and children to no more than two thirds maintenance to decrease risk of cerebral edema.

Tuberculosis

1. Isoniazid, 15 to 20 mg/kg/day (maximum 500 mg/day) in children and 8 to 10 mg/kg/day (maximum 300 mg/day) in once- or twice-daily doses

2. Rifampin, 15 to 20 mg/kg/day (maximum 600 mg/day) in adults or children in once- or twice-daily doses

Key Treatment

- Ampicillin
- Third-generation cephalosporin
- Acetaminophen

Follow-Up

1. Adults need no follow-up, because permanent neurologic sequelae are rare when meningitis is treated promptly.
2. Children should have hearing tested when treatment is complete and clinical picture has normalized.

Bibliography

Bradley JS: Meningitis. Hosp Pract 1993;28(Suppl 2):15–19.

Choi C: Bacterial meningitis. Clin Geriatr Med 1992;8:889–902.

Feigin R, McCracken G, Klein J: Diagnosis and management of meningitis. Pediatr Infect Dis J 1992;11:785–814.

Polito JM, Stollerman GH: Aseptic meningitis: a case for clinical experience. Hosp Pract 1992;27(May 30):27–39.

Tunkel AR, Scheld WM: Issues in the management of bacterial meningitis. Am Fam Physician 1997;56:1355–1362.

Indications

1. Central nervous system infection
   a. Bacterial meningitis (characterized by fever, headache, and stiff neck): Lumbar puncture (LP) is essential to diagnosis.
   b. Consider fungal, syphilitic, tuberculous, viral, and asceptic meningitis as diagnostic possibilities too.
   c. LP is less sensitive in detecting ventriculoperitoneal shunt infections.
2. Subarachnoid hemorrhage (SAH)
   a. LP is the most sensitive diagnostic tool to diagnose SAH.
   b. If feasible, do computed tomography (CT) first; LP not indicated if SAH is diagnosed on CT.
3. Carcinomatous meningitis: especially with lymphoma, leukemia, melanoma, and breast and lung cancer
4. Various inflammatory conditions: multiple sclerosis, Guillain-Barré syndrome
5. Miscellaneous conditions (the LP may be therapeutic as well as diagnostic): pseudotumor cerebri, normal-pressure hydrocephalus
6. Introduction of diagnostic and therapeutic substances: contrast media, antibiotics, anesthetics, chemotherapy, radionuclides

Contraindications

1. Evidence of increased intracranial pressure (ICP) from mass lesions such as neoplasm, abscess, or parenchymal hemorrhage. Consider raised ICP if
   a. Papilledema is present.
   b. Focal neurologic signs are detected.
   c. CT or magnetic resonance imaging (MRI) findings suggest raised ICP.
2. Infection in skin or other tissue overlying the anticipated LP site
3. Anticoagulated state
   a. Bleeding diathesis (e.g., prolonged prothrombin time)
   b. Thrombocytopenia (e.g., platelets less than $50,000/mm^3$)

Preparation

1. Explain procedure fully to patient and/or family.
2. Obtain signed informed consent.
3. Full-length examination table (preferred), firm flat bed, or stretcher; well-lighted room

Equipment

1. Antiseptic solutions, such as povidone-iodine, alcohol
2. Sterile drapes, gloves, gauze, Band-Aid
3. 20- to 22-gauge spinal needle with stylet
4. Manometer, three-way stopcock, four labeled collection tubes

Anesthesia

1. 3- to 5-ml syringe with 22- to 25-gauge long needle
2. 1- to 3-ml plain lidocaine, 1% to 2%

Precautions

1. CT or MRI before LP unless bacterial meningitis is strongly suspected, because delay in this diagnosis substantially increases morbidity and mortality.
2. Reverse anticoagulation at least 1 hour before LP.

Technique

1. Patient position
   a. Lateral recumbent position on a firm mattress or examination table is preferred.
      (1) Neck, trunk, hips, and knees are flexed, but avoid respiratory embarrassment.
      (2) Axis of spine is parallel to the floor, but hips and shoulders are perpendicular to the bed or table.
   b. Patient sitting curled forward initially may help locate landmarks in an obese patient or infant.
2. Select puncture site low enough to avoid puncturing spinal cord (cord ends as L1–L2).
   a. Palpate superior aspects of iliac crests; an imaginary line between these two points selects the appropriate lumbar interspace in adults (L3–L4, L4–L5).

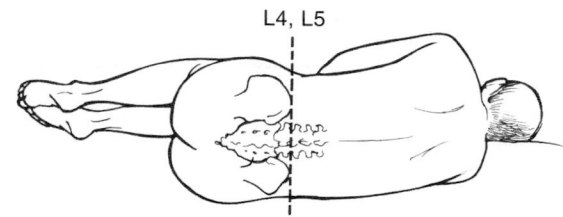

L4, L5

b. Use lower interspaces in infants because their spinal cords end at L3.

3. Prepare puncture site.

   a. Glove, cleanse area with povidone-iodine, wipe with alcohol, and then place sterile drapes.

   b. Reglove to avoid iodine contamination of LP needle.

4. Anesthetize interspace subcutaneously and into deeper tissues with lidocaine.

5. Needle insertion

   a. Insert the needle with stylet in place in midpoint of selected interspace.

   b. Direct needle 10 to 20 degrees cephalad, that is, toward umbilicus; bevel parallel to the long axis of the spine to separate, not transect, dural fibers and nerve roots.

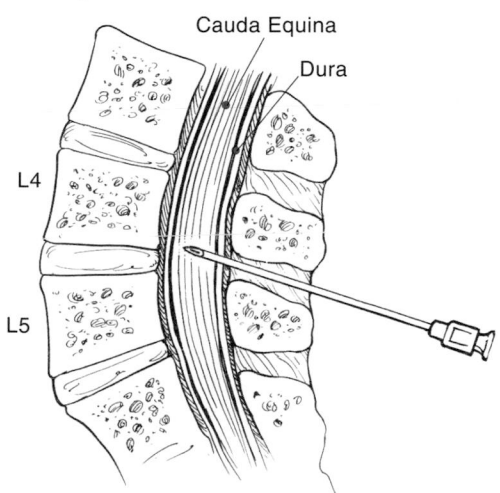

Cauda Equina

Dura

L4

L5

   c. Withdraw stylet after penetrating the dura, characterized by a pop. Check for spinal fluid.

      (1) If no pop is felt or needle has been advanced 3 to 6 cm without fluid, the stylet should be removed and replaced every 2 to 3 mm as the needle continues to slowly advance.

      (2) If the tap is dry, rotate needle 90 to 180 degrees.

      (3) If hard resistance is met, check to ensure midline interspace position. Withdraw needle with stylet and either redirect needle angle or restart procedure.

(4) Very obese or spondylotic patients may be done under fluoroscopy via paramedian approach by experienced clinicians only.

(5) Lateral C1 to C2 or cisterna magna puncture may be required if the LP is unsuccessful or the lumbar area is infected.

6. Cerebrospinal fluid (CSF) pressure measurement and sample collection

   a. Replace the stylet until the manometer or three-way stopcock is attached.

   b. Extend neck and legs, thereby preventing an artificially raised opening pressure.

   c. Open the stopcock to the manometer, and record the opening pressure (normal <200 mm H$_2$O).

   d. Close the stopcock to the manometer, and collect 1 to 2 ml of CSF in each of four labeled tubes.

7. Withdrawing LP needle

   a. Replace the stylet, and withdraw slowly to avoid aspiration of nerve roots.

   b. Apply a Band-Aid to the puncture site.

Follow-Up

1. Have the patient lie supine for 2 to 3 hours after procedure to avert a spinal headache.

2. Order CSF studies:

   a. Obtain a cell count (see Table 321–1) and differential (perform on first and fourth collection tubes if a traumatic tap is suspected), Gram's stain, bacterial cultures, and CSF and serum glucose.

   b. Other CSF tests are determined by diagnosis being considered: quantitative protein; protein electrophoresis; myelin basic protein; bacterial, viral, fungal antigens and cultures; mycobacterial and fungal stains; mycobacterial cultures; Venereal Disease Research Laboratory test; cytology; other tumor markers.

3. Complications and measures used to try to avoid them

   a. Headache occurs 10 to 20 per cent of the time: Hydrate, ensure bed rest supine, use small-gauge LP needle.

   b. Infection: Use aseptic technique, puncture in noninfected area.

   c. Bleeding: Check coagulation status, use atraumatic technique, delay post-LP anticoagulation.

   d. Backache: Minimize number of punctures, use atraumatic technique.

TABLE 321–1. TYPICAL CEREBRAL SPINAL FLUID (CSF) CHARACTERISTICS IN VARIOUS DIAGNOSES*

CONDITION	APPEARANCE	PRESSURE (mm H₂O)	GLUCOSE (mg/dl)	PROTEIN (mg/dl)	CELL COUNT (per mm³)
Normal	Clear, colorless	<200	60–70% of peripheral glucose	15–45	≤5 leukocytes (mononuclear)
Meningitis					
Bacterial	Cloudy	↑	↓	↑	↑ 500–10,000, neutrophils predominate
Tuberculous, fungal	Clear, maybe cloudy	↑	N or ↓	Slightly ↑	↑ 10–500, lymphocytes predominate
Viral/asceptic	Clear	N or ↑	N	N or ↑	>6, lymphocytes predominate
Other Conditions					
Meningeal carcinomatosis	Clear	↑	N or ↓	N or ↑	10–500, lymphocytes predominate
Subarachnoid hemorrhage	Bloody, does not clot, xanthochromic supernatant	↑	N	↑	1000–3.5 × 10⁶ RBCs, RBC:WBC ratio higher than ratio in peripheral blood
Traumatic tap	Blood clots, supernatant is not xanthochromic	N	N	↑	No. of RBC in CSF = no. of RBCs in peripheral blood; fewer RBCs in collection tube 4 than in tube 1
Multiple sclerosis	Clear	N	N	N or ↑	0–20 lymph
Guillain-Barré syndrome	Clear or xanthochromic	N or ↑	N	↑↑	N
Pseudotumor cerebri	Clear	↑	N	N	N

*↑, increase; ↓, decrease; N, normal; RBC, red blood cell; WBC, white blood cell.

e. Epidermoid transplant: Use stylet to avoid epidermal implantation in spinal canal.

f. Paresthesias: Use stylet, do not aspirate CSF or nerve roots.

g. Herniation: Avoid LP if mass lesion or acutely raised ICP is suspected.

WARNING

Herniation, which is usually fatal, can occur if LP is performed on patient with acutely increased ICP or if a mass lesion is present.

 Bibliography

Devinsky O, Weinreb HJ, Feldman E, et al: The resident's neurology book. Philadelphia, FA Davis, 1997.

Gilman S: Clinical examination of the nervous system. New York, McGraw-Hill, 1999.

Gilroy J: Infectious diseases. In Basic Neurology, 2nd ed, pp 251–254. New York, Pergamon Press, 1990.

Martin K, Gean A: Review: The spinal tap: a new look at an old test. Ann Intern Med 1986;104:840–848.

Quality Standards Sub-Committee of the American Academy of Neurology: Practice parameters, lumbar puncture. Neurology 1993;43:625–627.

Wood J: Cerebrospinal fluid: techniques of access and analytical interpretation. In Wilken R, Rengachary S (eds): Neurosurgery, pp 165–177. New York, McGraw-Hill, 1996.

322 Brain Tumor

Benjamin C. Warf

Etiology

1. *Primary brain tumors* arise from cells that are intrinsic to the brain or its coverings. These include
   a. Gliomas: astrocytoma, oligodendroglioma, glioblastoma
   b. Ependymoma
   c. Choroid plexus papilloma
   d. Primitive neuroectodermal tumors (e.g., medulloblastoma)
   e. Pineal tumors (e.g., pineocytoma, germinoma)
   f. Hemangioblastoma
   g. Primary central nervous system lymphoma
   h. Pituitary adenoma
   i. Meningioma
   j. Schwannoma (cranial nerve origin)
2. *Congenital intracranial tumors* are nonmalignant masses that arise during development, such as
   a. Craniopharyngioma
   b. Epidermoid
   c. Dermoid
   d. Colloid cyst
   e. Teratoma
   f. Chordoma
3. *Metastatic brain tumors* arise by seeding to the brain from primary tumors elsewhere. The more common tumors that metastasize to brain are
   a. Lung cancer (most common)
   b. Breast cancer
   c. Melanoma
   d. Renal cancer
   e. Lymphoma
4. Certain *genetic diseases* are known to predispose to the development of intracranial tumors, such as neurofibromatosis and tuberous sclerosis.
5. *Genetic anomalies* have been identified in a variety of brain tumor types, including chromosomal abnormalities, tumor suppressor gene mutations, and oncogene amplifications.

Symptoms

1. Neurologic symptoms
   a. Weakness or clumsiness
   b. Unsteady gait
   c. Cognitive or personality changes
   d. Language dysfunction
   e. Diminished level of consciousness
   f. Visual field deficit
   g. Seizures
2. Symptoms from elevated intracranial pressure
   a. Headache
   b. Nausea and vomiting
   c. Diplopia
   d. Declining vision or visual obscurations

Key Symptoms

- Headache
- Vomiting
- Diplopia
- Blurred vision
- Lateralized weakness
- Unsteady gait
- Seizures
- Mental status change

WARNING

Posterior fossa tumor with obstructive hydrocephalus is the most common presentation of brain tumor in children, the chief symptom of which initially may be chronic, intermittent vomiting.

Clinical Findings

1. *Neurologic deficit* depends on the location of the tumor and the degree of surrounding mass effect on other structures from edema or tumor mass.
   a. Mental status change: cerebral hemisphere
   b. Aphasia: dominant cerebral hemisphere
   c. Lateralized motor weakness: anywhere along corticospinal pathway from motor cortex to internal capsule to brain stem
   d. Cranial nerve abnormalities: brain stem or cranial nerve

e. Ataxia, dysmetria, or nystagmus: cerebellum

f. Visual field defect: chiasm, optic radiations, occipital lobe

g. Signs of brain stem compression from herniation

   (1) Depressed level of consciousness

   (2) Nonreactive or asymmetric pupils

   (3) Posturing movements

   (4) Abnormal breathing pattern

   (5) Hypertension and bradycardia

WARNING

Herniation is a neurologic emergency, and treatment must be instituted immediately!

---

2. *Papilledema* can result from prolonged increase in intracranial pressure and may be the only clinical sign of obstructive hydrocephalus.

3. *Endocrine and metabolic abnormalities* can occur with pituitary tumors and masses in the hypothalamic–third ventricle region.

4. *Signs of a primary cancer* may be evident in a patient presenting with a metastatic brain tumor, such as lung lesion on chest radiograph, breast mass, or skin lesion.

Key Signs

- Motor weakness
- Ataxia/dysmetria
- Visual field deficit
- Altered mental status
- Papilledema
- Cranial nerve deficits

Laboratory Tests

1. Computerized tomography (CT) or magnetic resonance imaging (MRI) of the head with and without contrast

2. *Metastasis work-up* if clinically indicated

Key Test

Brain imaging (CT, MRI)

WARNING

Do not perform a lumbar puncture unless an intracranial mass and obstructive hydrocephalus have been ruled out by CT or MRI.

Differential Diagnosis

1. Differential diagnosis of an intracranial mass lesion

   a. Tumor

      (1) Primary tumor

      (2) Metastatic tumor

   b. Infection

      (1) Brain abscess

      (2) Subdural empyema

      (3) Epidural abscess

      (4) Toxoplasmosis

      (5) Tuberculoma

      (6) Parasite

   c. Hemorrhage

      (1) Intracerebral hemorrhage

      (2) Chronic subdural hematoma

      (3) Acute subdural or epidural hematoma

   d. Other

      (1) Acute multiple sclerosis plaque

      (2) Acute infarction with swelling

      (3) Arachnoid cyst

      (4) Vascular malformation

      (5) Giant aneurysm

2. Other intracranial processes to consider with neurologic signs or symptoms in the absence of a mass lesion

   a. Infarct

   b. Primary seizure disorder

   c. Complicated migraine

   d. Toxic or metabolic encephalopathy

   e. Vasculitis

   f. Meningeal carcinomatosis

   g. Subarachnoid hemorrhage

   h. Hydrocephalus

   i. Multiple sclerosis

   j. Encephalitis

   k. Neurodegenerative disease (e.g., Alzheimer's disease)

Treatment

1. The discovery of an intracranial tumor necessitates neurosurgical consultation.

2. The appropriate treatment often will require biopsy or resection, in addition to possible adjuvant therapy.

3. Hydrocephalus may require urgent treatment with ventricular drainage.

4. Diet: nothing by mouth if neurosurgical intervention is imminent

5. Activity: no activity (e.g., driving) that presents potential harm to the patient or others

6. Patient education
   a. Risks and benefits of any procedures to be performed
   b. Prognosis depends on tumor pathology and location.

Key Treatment

- Biopsy or resection with possible adjuvant therapy
- Possible urgent ventricular drainage for hydrocephalus

Drug of Choice

- Initial management often includes the administration of *dexamethasone* to diminish brain edema.

Alternative Drugs

- *Mannitol*, in addition to intubation and hyperventilation, may be administered in critical cases of intracranial hypertension.
- *Anticonvulsants* are indicated for treatment of accompanying seizures (see Ch. 310, Seizure Disorder).

Follow-Up

This will be in conjunction with the neurosurgical consultant.

Bibliography

For more information on classification, diagnosis, and treatment of gliomas, see
Saleman M: Supratentorial gliomas: clinical features and surgical therapy. In Wilkins RH, Rengachary SS (eds): Neurosurgery, pp 777–788. New York, McGraw-Hill, 1996.

For more information on diagnosis and management of brain metastases, see
Sawaya R, Bindal RK: Metastatic brain tumors. In Kaye, AH, Laws ER (eds): Brain Tumors: An Encyclopedic Approach, pp 923–946. Edinburgh, Churchill Livingstone, 1995.

For more information on posterior fossa tumors in children, see
Albright L: Posterior fossa tumors. Neurosurg Clin North Am 1992;3:881–891.

For more information on intracranial hypertension and brain herniation, see
Cohen DS, Quest DO: Increased intracranial pressure, brain herniation, and their control. In Wilkins RH, Rengachary SS (eds): Neurosurgery, pp 345–356. New York, McGraw-Hill, 1996.

For more information on the intensive care management of the brain tumor patient, see
Morita M, Andrews BT, Gutin PH: The intensive care management of patients with brain tumors. In Andrews BT (ed): Neurosurgical Intensive Care, pp 375–389. New York, McGraw-Hill, 1993.

323 Ménière's Disease

Normandi Omar

Etiology

Ménière's disease is an idiopathic disease involving endolymphatic hydrops in the inner ear characterized by vertigo, tinnitus, hearing loss, and aural fullness. The incidence is equal in men and women, most common in adults between ages 20 and 60, but more frequent in the fifth decade of life. Both ears are affected with equal frequency; may be bilateral in 20 to 30 per cent of cases. Twenty per cent of patients have a family history of Ménière's disease.

1. Pathophysiologic theories in the etiology of Ménière's disease
   a. Metabolic
   b. Vascular
   c. Genetic
   d. Viral
   e. Immunologic
   f. Anatomic
   g. Psychological
2. Possible mechanisms
   a. Metabolic debris (immune complexes, viral debris) silting the vestibular duct, leading to increased endolymphatic pressure and dilatation of endolymph spaces and sac
   b. Chronic inflammation of anatomically narrow endolymphatic duct

Symptoms

1. Ménière's disease is defined using criteria based on the classical triad of hearing loss, vertigo, and tinnitus. These symptoms are fluctuant in nature and may or may not develop simultaneously; thus diagnosis may be difficult initially.
   a. Vertigo (episodic spinning or whirling) lasting minutes to hours, possibly accompanied by nausea and vomiting.
   b. Fluctuating, low frequency, sensorineural hearing loss
   c. Tinnitus described as roaring that may vary with hearing, may be present prior to or during attacks, or may be constant.
   d. Fullness in the ear that varies with hearing loss
   e. Persistent feelings of imbalance or disequilibrium that may last for days
2. The disease process may be divided into three

stages according to the progression of symptoms:
   a. Stage I: Vertigo predominates; presence of aural fullness and tinnitus. Duration is highly variable.
   b. Stage II: Absence of vertigo but hearing threshold deteriorates, is fluctuant, although not profound. May revert to stage I or progress to stage III.
   c. Stage III: No longer have acute vertigo episodes but may have constant disequilibrium. Hearing loss no longer fluctuates and is profound. Usually develops 5 to 10 years after onset, with 20 to 30 per cent involvement of the contralateral ear.

Key Symptoms

- Vertigo
- Hearing loss
- Tinnitus

Clinical Findings

Ménière's disease can be diagnosed on clinical assessment and audiometry. Evaluation should include a thorough history, head and neck examination, and neuro-otologic examination. Findings include

1. Peripheral vertigo without a positional component on Hallpike-Dix maneuvers
2. Nystagmus
3. Tinnitus
4. Sensorineural hearing loss in low frequencies, with higher frequencies being affected later in the disease course

WARNING

Because of the fluctuant nature of the disease and its variable presentation, it may be difficult to diagnose on clinical grounds alone initially.

Laboratory Tests

Ménière's disease is classified as idiopathic, and diagnosis is that of exclusion of other diseases with similar presentations.

1. Tests to exclude other disease states
   a. Serum electrolytes
   b. Serologic test for syphilis
   c. Thyroid function tests
   d. Gadolinium-enhanced magnetic resonance imaging (MRI) to rule out central nervous system (CNS) pathology, mainly acoustic neuroma when indicated
2. Tests to establish the diagnosis
   a. Electrocochleography: An increased ratio of summating potential to action potential is the chief finding.
   b. Glycerol dehydration test: improved audiometric response in low-frequency hearing scores after administration of oral glycerol. This change is not observed with other conditions.
   c. Caloric testing
   d. Audiometry

Differential Diagnosis

Dizziness is a common presentation of many conditions. Diseases that mimic Ménière's disease may be central, peripheral, or metabolic.

1. Central conditions
   a. Acoustic neuroma: Unilateral, nonfluctuating, high-frequency hearing loss helps distinguish this from Ménière's disease.
   b. Multiple sclerosis: fluctuating hearing loss and vertigo. Diagnostic testing includes MRI looking for intramural plaques and a lumbar puncture looking for multiple sclerosis-related changes.
   c. Vascular loop compression syndrome: anatomic situation in which a wrapped vessel compresses the eighth nerve complex. Magnetic resonance (MR) angiography helps delineate vascular anatomy.
   d. Vertebrobasilar vascular insufficiency and atherosclerosis: MR angiography aids in diagnosis.
   e. Cerebellar infarcts: Computerized tomography or MRI aids in diagnosis.
   f. Aneurysms of the cerebellum and brain stem: MR angiography aids in diagnosis.
   g. Tumors of cerebellum (meningiomas, glioblastomas): MRI aids in diagnosis.
2. Peripheral conditions
   a. Benign paroxysmal positional vertigo: positional symptoms that last seconds without hearing loss
   b. Vestibular neuronitis: usually preceded by upper respiratory infection; possibly viral; may last for 8 months but not recurrent and there is no hearing loss.
   c. Labyrinthitis: Mimics neuronitis but hearing loss may occur, although only in the high-frequency range.
   d. Migraine-induced vertigo: characterized by headaches before or after vertigo spells
   e. Presbycusis (degeneration of vestibular system that occurs with aging): May or may not be accompanied by hearing loss in the high-frequency range.
3. Metabolic conditions
   a. Hyperthyroidism or hypothyroidism
   b. Diabetes and hypoglycemia
   c. Anemia
   d. Infections: syphilis, chronic otitis media, Lyme disease
   e. Autoimmune disorders
   f. Cardiogenic disorders
   g. Leukemia

Treatment

1. Nonsurgical treatment of Ménière's disease is effective in controlling symptoms in 80 per cent of patients and forms the primary mode of therapy. However, no treatment has prospectively modified the disease course or prevented the progressive hearing loss.
2. Pharmacologic interventions include vestibular suppressants, antiemetics, and diuretics.

Medication

1. Vestibular suppressants
    a. Diazepam (Valium), 5 mg orally every 3 hours. Lorazepam (Ativan) may also be used.
    b. Meclizine (Antivert, Bonine), 25 to 100 mg orally daily
    c. Dimenhydrinate (Dramamine), 50 to 100 mg orally tid
    d. Diphenhydramine (Benadryl), 50 mg orally every 4 to 6 hours
2. Antiemetics
    a. Phenothiazines, including promethazine (Phenergan), 12.5 to 25 mg orally or suppository every 4 to 6 hours, and prochlorperazine (Compazine), 10 mg orally or IM every 4 to 6 hours.
    b. Because of the fluctuant nature of the disease, long-term treatment is not recommended unless to prevent frequent acute attacks.
3. Diuretics are used for maintenance therapy to control or arrest the disease process.
    a. Hydrochlorothiazide (HCTZ), 50 mg orally qd
    b. HCTZ and triamterene (Dyazide), one orally qd
    c. Furosemide (Lasix), 10 to 80 mg orally daily
4. Tricyclics can be tried in resistant cases. After 3 months of therapy, treatment failures are unlikely to improve and surgical options should be considered.

WARNING

- Phenothiazines may cause extrapyramidal reactions, hypotension, and abnormal cardiac conduction.

- HCTZ may cause hypokalemia: potassium supplement or substituting a potassium-sparing diuretic may be necessary.

Surgical Interventions

Although controversial, surgical therapy should be considered in patients with refractory Ménière's disease.

1. Ablative procedures have the highest rates of success. The objective of these procedures is to destroy all remaining vestibular function in the involved ear.
    a. Ablative procedures that preserve hearing
        (1) Vestibular nerve section
        (2) Aminoglycoside (streptomycin or gentamicin) perfusion of the labyrinth or instillation into the middle ear
    b. Ablative procedures that destroy hearing: labyrinthectomy and translabyrinthine vestibular nerve dissection
2. Nonablative options include decompression techniques such as endolymphatic sac–subarachnoid shunts, endolymphatic-mastoid shunts, and wide bony decompression of the endolymphatic sac. These techniques produce very variable success results, suggesting a strong placebo effect.

Diet

Dietary modifications include sodium restriction (<1 gm/day) and avoidance of caffeine, alcohol, and nicotine.

Activity

Bed rest is recommended initially for severe cases. As the vestibular loss stabilizes, vestibular exercises may be effective in management of symptoms. Patients with active, fluctuant disease are not good candidates for vestibular rehabilitation.

WARNING

The status of the contralateral ear with respect to vestibular function needs to be assessed because Ménière's disease is bilateral in 20 to 30 per cent of cases. If vestibular function is poor in the contralateral ear, the patient may not compensate well from an ablative procedure and may experience oscillopsia.

Patient Education

Patients affected by Ménière's disease should be informed that

1. The disorder is mild and clears up spontaneously.
2. The frequency may vary from every few weeks to every few years.
3. In long-lasting cases, the attacks become less severe but hearing loss and tinnitus may continue between attacks.
4. Severe attacks may return and may lead to serious or total hearing loss in at least one ear.
5. The cause of Ménière's disease is unknown, and therefore there is nothing the patient can do to prevent the disorder. However, the following instructions could aid in reducing severity and frequency of symptoms.
    a. Lying down and resting during an attack
    b. Following a diet low in salt and caffeine

c. Restricting fluid intake

d. Stopping smoking

Key Treatment

- Diazepam initially

- Meclizine if refractory to diazepam

- HCTZ with potassium supplement or Dyazide for maintenance therapy

Follow-Up

The fluctuant nature of the disease makes it difficult to conduct well-established placebo-controlled trials to assess the effectiveness of medical and surgical treatment. Most studies indicate that 80 per cent of patients with Ménière's disease respond to medical therapy alone.

1. Patients asymptomatic after a 3-month course of vestibular suppressants and dietary modifications

    a. Continue to follow dietary modification.

    b. Discontinue medications and follow up immediately if symptoms reoccur.

2. Patients remaining symptomatic after 3 months of therapy or who do not respond to vestibular suppressants

    a. Add a second vestibular suppressant of a different class.

    b. Add a diuretic.

    c. Investigate other etiologies, including MRI for CNS pathology.

3. Ménière's disease refractory to all medical therapy

    a. Decompression techniques: control of vertigo in 65 to 80 per cent of cases with little difference in hearing

    b. Ablative procedures

       (1) Vestibular neurectomy if decompression techniques fail. Procedure of choice in patients who can tolerate it because it relieves vertigo in 90 to 95 per cent of all cases by totally eliminating vestibular input from the operative ear without compromising existing serviceable hearing in that ear in 20 to 60 per cent of patients.

       (2) Labyrinthectomy with translabyrinthine nerve section in patients who are elderly or with compromised health who may not tolerate a vestibular neurectomy, or in those with no serviceable hearing in the affected ear. This procedure is 90 to 95 per cent effective but causes deafness in the operative ear.

       (3) Streptomycin and gentamicin perfusion thru fenestration of semicircular canal are some other techniques gaining favor. Similar results to decompression techniques but may be ototoxic and therefore may diminish hearing.

    c. Cochlear implantation: End-stage bilateral Ménière's disease indication for this procedure.

> **WARNING**
>
> For all the above ablative procedures, the status of the contralateral ear must be considered because if its labyrinthine function is poor, compensation for the surgical ear will not occur and oscillopsia may develop.

Bibliography

Knox G, McPherson A: Ménière's disease: differential diagnosis and treatment. Am Fam Physician 1997;55: 1185–1194.

La Rouere M: Surgical treatment of Ménière's disease. Otolaryngol Clin North Am 1996;29:311–322.

Saeed S: Diagnosis and treatment of Ménière's disease. BMJ 1998;316:368–372.

Slattery WH, Fayed JN: Medical treatment of Ménière's disease. Otolaryngol Clin North Am 1997;30:1027–1037.

Weber P, Adkins WY: The differential diagnosis of Ménière's disease. Otolaryngol Clin North Am 1997;30: 977–986.

324 Guillain-Barré Syndrome

Andrew H. Zalski

Etiology

Guillain-Barré syndrome (GBS) is an acute demyelinating polyneuropathy that occurs at a rate of 1 case per 1 million population per month. In about two thirds of the cases there is an antecedent febrile illness reported by patients days or weeks prior to the development of the ascending paralysis that is the hallmark of the syndrome.

1. Antecedent events

   a. Upper respiratory infection

   b. Diarrheal illness

   c. Herpesvirus infection

   d. Cytomegalovirus infection

   e. *Campylobacter jejuni* gastroenteritis

   f. Vaccinations: strong association with the swine flu vaccination in 1975

2. Reported associations

   a. Viral hepatitis

   b. Hodgkin's lymphoma

   c. Human immunodeficiency virus (HIV) disease

   d. Systemic lupus

   e. Mycoplasma

   f. Lyme disease

   g. Sarcoidosis

   h. Surgery

Symptoms

The symptoms in GBS generally appear 1 to 2 weeks after the resolution of an upper respiratory or gastrointestinal illness.

1. Ascending paralysis: initial involvement of the legs followed within a few days by the arms

2. Difficulty walking, getting up out of chairs, climbing stairs

3. Gait instability

4. Difficulty swallowing

5. Urinary retention

6. Respiratory depression

7. Paresthesias

Key Symptoms

- Ascending paralysis
- Difficulty walking
- Paresthesias

Clinical Findings

For most patients (70 to 80 per cent), the weakness is progressive over a 1- to 3-week course. Rare patients present with a fulminant, rapidly progressive course that proceeds to maximal paralysis within 1 or 2 days.

1. Weakness in proximal as well as distal muscles

2. Symmetric limb weakness

3. Progressive symmetric loss of deep tendon reflexes

4. Hypotonia

5. Blood pressure and heart rate fluctuations

6. Bulbar involvement in about 50 per cent of patients presenting with oropharyngeal weakness and/or facial palsy.

Key Signs

- Symmetric limb weakness
- Progressive and symmetric loss of deep tendon reflexes

Laboratory Tests

Symptoms and clinical presentation generally determine diagnosis of GBS. Examination of cerebrospinal fluid (CSF) and electromyography (EMG) may support the diagnosis of GBS.

1. Examination of CSF

   a. Elevation of CSF protein without pleocytosis. Serial CSF studies may be necessary to demonstrate CSF protein elevation because it may take up to 3 weeks before CSF protein elevation develops.

   b. If pleocytosis is present in the CSF, consider HIV disease, Lyme disease, or sarcoidosis.

2. EMG and nerve conduction studies
   a. Presence of a demyelinating peripheral neuropathy
   b. Slowed nerve conduction velocities
   c. F-wave prolongation
3. Magnetic resonance imaging should be considered in patients with symptoms suggesting a spinal cord lesion.

Key Tests

- CSF with elevated protein without increased cellularity
- EMG with F-wave slowing

Differential Diagnosis

The differential diagnosis includes the diseases causing acute or subacute paralysis.

1. Peripheral neuropathies of other causes
   a. Heavy metal poisoning
   b. Toxins such as organophosphates and hexacarbons
   c. Other disease states, such as diabetes, systemic lupus, rheumatoid arthritis, amyloidosis, lymphoma, multiple myeloma, polyarteritis nodosa, polio, uremia, myasthenia gravis, botulism
   d. Drugs, including dapsone, nitrofurantoin, chloroquine, gold, isoniazid, hydralizine, disulfiram, metronidazole
2. Spinal cord pathology
   a. Transverse myelitis
   b. Spinal cord compression
   c. Spinal cord tumors
   d. Spinal cord infarction
3. Hereditary causes of polyneuropathy
   a. Charcot-Marie-Tooth disease
   b. Roussy-Lévy disease
   c. Anderson-Fabry disease
   d. Krabbe's disease

Treatment

Cornerstone of treatment is hospitalization, careful medical support, and anticipatory management of respiratory insufficiency or failure.

1. General medical support
   a. Arterial blood gas measurement and vital capacity. Vital capacity less than 1000 ml and pO_2 less than 70 may indicate need for mechanical ventilation.
   b. Management of blood pressure and cardiac arrhythmias
   c. Expectant management of complications, including pneumonia, pulmonary embolus, bladder dysfunction, syndrome of inappropriate antidiuretic hormone secretion
   d. Adequate pain control
   e. Physical therapy to prevent contractures and for rehabilitation
2. Plasmapheresis
   a. May decrease the time on mechanical ventilation and shorten the time for the patient to be able to ambulate.
   b. Most effective when started within 2 weeks of onset of symptoms
3. Intravenous immune globulin (IVIG)
   a. Efficacy of IVIG is similar to plasmapheresis, although IVIG may have fewer complications.
   b. Generally mild side effects include headache, fever, nausea, and myalgias.

Key Treatment

- Plasmapheresis
- IVIG

Follow-Up

Recovery is generally slow. About 85 per cent of patients are ambulatory by 6 months. There is a recurrence rate of about 3 per cent. Fifteen per cent of patients with GBS have residual motor weakness at 1 year and about 5 per cent remain severely disabled.

1. Extended physical therapy and rehabilitation are needed to improve and restore physical functioning.
2. Patients may need psychological support and therapy to deal with the disability and reduction of functioning caused by GBS.
3. Support groups are valuable and may be located by contacting the:
   Guillain-Barré Foundation International
   P.O. Box 262
   Wynnewood, PA 19096
   1-610-667-0131
4. Further information is available on the Internet, including support groups and new therapies. The National Institutes of Health has a web site at: *www.ninds.nih.gov/healinfo/disorder/guillain/guillain.htm.*

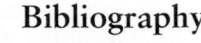

Bibliography

Bouget J, Chevret S, Chastang C, et al: Plasma exchange morbidity in Guillain-Barré syndrome: results from the French prospective, double-blind, randomized, multicenter study. Crit Care Med 1993;21:651–658.

Bril V, Ilse WK, Pearce R, et al: Pilot trial of immunoglobulin versus plasma exchange in patients with Guillain-Barré syndrome. Neurology 1993;43:1034–1036.

Hartung HP, Pollard JD, Harvey GK, et al: Immunopathogenesis and treatment of the Guillain-Barré syndrome: Part I. Muscle Nerve 1995;18:137–153.

Hartung HP, Pollard JD, Harvey GK, et al: Immunopathogenesis and treatment of the Guillain-Barré syndrome: Part II. Muscle Nerve 1995;18:154–164.

Pascuzzi RM, Fleck JD: Acute peripheral neuropathy in adults: Guillain-Barré syndrome and related disorders. Neurol Clin 1997;15:529–547.

325 Head Injuries in Sports

Aaron Rubin

Etiology

Most commonly caused by a forceful blow to the head.

1. Head injuries are common injuries in contact sports such as football, hockey, rugby, soccer, boxing, and wrestling, as well as "noncontact" sports such as basketball, baseball, cycling, auto racing, motocross, and gymnastics. Head injuries include minor head injuries (concussions), severe head injuries, and second-impact syndrome (SIS).

   a. It has been estimated that up to 20 per cent of high school football players (over 250,000) suffer a concussion in a given year.

   b. Severe head injuries include cerebral contusion, intracranial hemorrhage, epidural hematoma, and subdural hematoma. These are fortunately rare in sports. Most severe head injuries are readily recognizable by immediate and prolonged (greater than 5 minutes) loss of consciousness (LOC).

   c. SIS is rapid development of diffuse brain swelling and herniation following a second head injury. These may be seemingly minor injuries but with devastating consequences. The National Center for Catastrophic Sports Injury Research in Chapel Hill, North Carolina, identified 51 cases of head injury death between 1980 and 1991. Of these, 29 appear to be due to SIS.

2. Biomechanical forces and mechanism of head injury

   a. Blow to resting movable head usually produces maximal injury beneath the point of impact (coup injury).

   b. Moving head contacting a nonmobile object results in maximal injury to opposite side of brain injury (contrecoup injury).

   c. Epidural hematoma commonly occurs with a temporal skull fracture tearing the middle meningeal artery. The patient may have a lucid interval after the injury until the hematoma expands, leading to mass effect and eventual brain herniation. The underlying brain is generally not significantly injured, and rapid evaluation and treatment have good results.

   d. Acute subdural hematoma is often associated with a higher degree of brain damage and swelling and a poor prognosis, even with rapid evaluation and treatment.

   e. Intracerebral hematoma is associated with severe acceleration injury with prolonged LOC. Mortality varies depending on the location of the lesion and level of consciousness at the time of presentation.

   f. Subarachnoid hemorrhage results from rupture of a congenital vascular lesion like an aneurysm or arteriovenous malformation that may occur in conjunction with trauma.

   g. SIS is probably due to lack of autoregulation of the brain leading to vascular engorgement and edema of the brain with herniation and coma. *This is a major reason for careful evaluation of the head-injured athlete and caution with return to play.*

   h. Minor head injuries (concussions) are by far the most common of head injuries. There are various grading systems for concussions (Table 325–1). Concussion has been defined by

TABLE 325–1. GRADING SYSTEMS FOR CONCUSSION

GRADE	CANTU (1986)	COLORADO (1991)	AAN (1997)*
1	No LOC	No LOC	No LOC
	Dazed, HA, PTA <30 min	Confusion without amnesia	Symptoms <15 min
2	LOC <5 min or	No LOC	No LOC
	PTA >30 min	Dazed confusion with amnesia	Symptoms >15 min
3	LOC > 5 min or	LOC (any length)	LOC (any length)
	PTA >24 hr		

Abbreviations: HA, headache; LOC, loss of consciousness; PTA, post-traumatic amnesia.
*AAN, American Academy of Neurology (see Kelly and Rosenberg, 1997).

the Congress of Neurological Surgeons as "an immediate and transient impairment of neural function such as alteration of consciousness, disturbance of vision, equilibrium, and other similar symptoms."

Symptoms

1. LOC and alteration of mental status are the primary signs of head injury. Serious head injury is usually associated with LOC.

2. Symptoms include headache, dizziness, difficulty concentrating, amnesia (post-traumatic as well as retrograde), irritability, confusion, hyperexcitability, and LOC.

3. Concussion may have mild symptoms and at times may only be noted with careful neuropsychiatric testing. Even mild concussion may impair attention and information processing.

4. Postconcussion syndrome may follow mild head injury.

    a. Common symptoms (reported in greater than 20 per cent): headache (muscle contraction, migraine, cluster), dizziness, fatigue, nonspecific psychological symptoms (irritability, anxiety, depression), mild memory loss, difficulty concentrating

    b. Less common (1 to 20 per cent): positional vertigo, hearing loss, anosmia, photophobia, sleep disturbance, hyperacusis

    c. Rare problems (less than 1 per cent): delayed subdural and epidural hematoma, seizure disorder, transient global amnesia, movement disorder, Parkinson's disease, torticollis.

Key Symptoms

- LOC
- Headache
- Amnesia
- Difficulty concentrating
- Dizziness
- Irritability
- Confusion

Clinical Findings

1. Evaluation of airway, breathing, and circulation (ABCs) and the cervical spine is performed initially.

2. Initial evaluation should include an estimate of the Glasgow coma scale (Table 325–2) or the AVPU system (*a*lert, responds to *v*erbal, responds to *p*ain, *u*nresponsive)

3. History of mechanism of injury; complaints of headache, tinnitus, blurred vision, nausea, or unsteadiness; problems concentrating; or emotional lability should be obtained, as well as history of previous head injury.

4. Neurologic examination should be performed, including pupillary response, Romberg's test, heel-to-toe gait, finger to nose, extraocular motion, concentration (digits repeated backward, months in reverse order), memory (details of injury, previous games, president, governor).

5. History and examination should be repeated 5, 10, and 20 minutes after injury. Before return to play, examination should be repeated with provocative maneuvers such as a short sprint, push-ups, and sit-ups. Symptoms or neurologic findings should prevent return to play.

Key Signs

- Memory loss
- Inability to concentrate
- Gait disturbance
- Abnormal Glasgow score
- Abnormal pupillary response

Laboratory Tests

1. Radiographs are generally not considered helpful in mild head injuries. They do not predict intracranial trauma. They should be used in suspected cases of skull fracture.

2. Computerized tomography (CT) is helpful in diagnosing intracranial pathology. This should generally be reserved for patients with Glasgow

TABLE 325–2. GLASGOW COMA SCALE*

I. BEST MOTOR RESPONSE		II. VERBAL RESPONSE		III. EYE OPENING	
Obeys	6	Oriented	5	Spontaneous	4
Localizes	5	Confused conversation	4	To speech	3
Withdraws from pain (flexion)	4	Inappropriate words	3	To pain	2
Abnormal flexion	3	Incomprehensible sounds	2	None	1
Abnormal extension (decerebrate posturing)	2	None	1		
None	1				

*I + II + III = coma score: 13 to 15, minor; 9 to 13, moderate; less than 8, coma; 5 to 8, severe.

coma scale score less than 15, abnormal mental status, or focal neurologic deficits.

3. Magnetic resonance imaging (MRI) is more sensitive than CT but is more expensive and less available, and has not been found to affect clinical outcome. MRI is better than CT at finding contusions, providing some information on diffuse axonal injury, and possibly predicting delayed traumatic intracerebral hematoma, but not in influencing surgical intervention.

4. Electroencephalography has limited sensitivity and specificity in minor head injuries but may be helpful when a post-traumatic seizure disorder is suspected.

5. Auditory brain stem response may be abnormal after mild head injury. Again, the clinical usefulness is uncertain.

6. Neuropsychiatric testing is helpful in evaluating and following individuals with head injury.

Key Tests

- CT scan
- MRI

Differential Diagnosis

1. In the comatose individual: subdural hematoma, epidural hematoma, subarachnoid bleed, intracerebral hematoma, drug or alcohol overdose, and metabolic disease

2. Minor head injuries and postconcussion syndrome: migraines, psychiatric disorder, drug and alcohol abuse, and underlying learning disorders

Treatment

1. Planning for the evaluation and care of the seriously head-injured athlete should occur prior to the event. An emergency plan should be in place for all athletic practices and games.

   a. Initial assessment of the head-injured athlete should be performed by a certified athletic trainer or the team physician. All coaches and other supervisors should be made aware of the seriousness of head injury for events when the athletic trainer or physician is not available.

   b. Cervical (C) spine injury should be assumed in any unconscious athlete.

      (1) Initial assessment should be performed without moving the athlete. As always, *airway, breathing, and circulation* (ABCs) should be addressed.

      (2) The athlete should be carefully moved to his or her back with control of the cervical spine only by appropriately trained persons. Removing a football helmet is not recommended because of unnecessary movement of the C-spine and problems managing the C-spine in a player with shoulder pads. Face mask should be removed by cutting the attachments with an instrument designed to do such. This should be practiced by all appropriate personnel.

      (3) Airway should be maintained by jaw thrust and oxygen given to all comatose individuals.

      (4) The athlete should be placed on a spine board and the C-spine stabilized for transport to the nearest neurosurgical emergency facility.

   c. Intubation should be considered in the comatose athlete with hyperventilation to decrease the partial pressure of CO_2. Blood pressure should be maintained near normal. Hypotonic intravenous fluids should be avoided. There have not been satisfactory studies to support the routine use of corticosteroids in management of closed head injury.

   d. Evaluation of the C-spine and further evaluation of coma should be carried out at the neurosurgical facility.

2. Sideline management of minor head injury also should be planned.

   a. The athlete who is conscious and without neck pain or tenderness may be removed from the playing field for evaluation on the sidelines or in the locker room. Worsening symptoms or examination may require initiation of the emergency action plan.

   b. The athlete should remain under observation with repeat examinations at regular intervals every 5 to 10 minutes.

   c. If the athlete is agitated, he or she should be moved to a quiet place with rapid access to the medical team. If any concern about the degree of injury is present, the athlete should be transported to the emergency room for further observation.

   d. If the player does remain on the sideline, care should be taken to prevent his or her premature return to the contest. This may occur as a result of the athlete's denial about the potential seriousness of the injury, confusion resulting from the injury, or the "heat of the battle."

TABLE 325–3. RETURN TO PLAY BASED ON COMMON GRADING SYSTEMS

GRADE	CANTU (1986)	COLORADO (1991)	AAN (1997)
1	Asymptomatic for 1 wk 2nd: may return in 2 wk if asymptomatic for 1 wk 3rd: terminate season	May return after 20 min if asymptomatic; CT/MRI* 2nd in same contest: remove 3rd: terminate season (at least 3 mo off)	May return after 15 min if asymptomatic 2nd in same contest: remove 4th: terminate season
2	Asymptomatic for 1 wk 2nd: minimum of 1 mo; may return if asymptomatic for 1 wk; consider terminating season 3rd: terminate season	Asymptomatic for 1 wk: CT/MRI* 2nd: 1 mo off 3rd: terminate season	Asymptomatic for 1 wk, CT/MRI* 2nd: 2 wk and asymptomatic 3rd: terminate season
3	Minimum of 1 mo; may return if asymptomatic for 1 wk 2nd: terminate season	Minimum of 1 mo; may return if asymptomatic for at least 2 wk; conditioning drills may resume if asymptomatic after 2 wk, CT/MRI	Brief (seconds) LOC: may return when asymptomatic for 1 wk Prolonged (minutes) LOC: may return after asymptomatic for 2 wk 2nd: withhold until asymptomatic for 1 mo

*CT or MRI if symptoms persist longer than 1 week or based on clinical judgment of physician.

 e. If the athlete is allowed to return home, a responsible adult should be instructed in the care of the athlete, with written instructions.

3. Treatment of postconcussion syndrome is often in the realm of family physicians (see Ch. 326, Postconcussion Syndrome).

 a. Recognition of the preceding symptoms is the first step. Patients with symptoms of fatigue, headache, tinnitus, problems concentrating, and the like should be questioned about previous head injuries.

 b. Postconcussion headaches have been treated with amitriptyline, nonsteroidal anti-inflammatory drugs, muscle relaxants, propranolol, and calcium channel blockers, as well as transcutaneous electrical nerve stimulation (TENS) and biofeedback.

 c. Teachers should be made aware of possible learning difficulties, problems with concentration and focus, and emotional lability that may occur after a minor head injury.

 d. Family should be counseled about the problem and its treatment and prognosis.

Key Treatment

- Basic life support with cervical spine precautions
- Oxygen
- Intubation with hyperventilation
- Transport to neurosurgical emergency hospital

Follow-Up

1. Follow-up should continue until symptoms have resolved. Do not forget about postconcussion syndrome and the potentially long course it may take.

2. Return-to-play issues are difficult. Three guidelines are provided (Table 325–3). These are only guidelines, and all have limitations. Many athletes with mild head injury have limited or no symptoms. The goal of limiting return to play is to avoid the disaster of the second-impact syndrome and morbidity resulting from repeated head injury.

Bibliography

Cantu RC: Cerebral concussion in sport. Sports Med 1992;14:64–74.

Colorado Medical Society: Guidelines for the Management of Concussion in Sports. 1990 (revised 1991). (P.O. Box 17550, Denver, CO 80217-0550; phone: 1-303-779-5455)

Evans RW: The postconcussion syndrome and the sequelae of mild head injury. Neurol Clin 1992;10:815–845.

Henderson JM, Browning DG: Head trauma in young athletes. Med Clin North Am 1994;78:289–303.

Kelly JP, Rosenberg JH: The diagnosis and management of concussion in sports. Neurology 1997;48:575–580.

326 Postconcussion Syndrome

Randolph W. Evans

Etiology

1. Definition: a constellation of symptoms and signs that may occur alone or in combination following usually mild head injury. Loss of consciousness does not have to occur for the postconcussion syndrome to develop. Mild head injury is defined as an injury resulting in an initial Glasgow Coma Scale score of 13 to 15.

2. Epidemiology
   a. The annual incidence of mild head injury per 100,000 population is about 150.
   b. Mild head injury accounts for about 75 per cent of all head trauma.
   c. Estimates of the relative causes of head trauma in the United States are as follows: motor vehicle accidents, 45 per cent; falls, 30 per cent; occupational accidents, 10 per cent; recreational accidents, 10 per cent; and assaults, 5 per cent.
   d. Perhaps 50 per cent of patients with mild head injury will develop the postconcussion syndrome.

3. Neuropathology
   a. Damage to the scalp, skull, and meninges can lead to scalp lacerations, skull fractures, and subdural and epidural hematomas.
   b. Damage to brain parenchyma by coup and contrecoup injuries can lead to brain contusions, lacerations, and hemorrhages.
   c. Diffuse axonal injury may account for many aspects of the postconcussion syndrome.
   d. A neurochemical substrate of mild head injury may consist of release of excitatory neurotransmitters such as acetylcholine and glutamate.

Symptoms

1. A multitude of symptoms and signs can follow mild head injury (Table 326–1).
2. Headaches have been variably reported as occurring in 30 to 90 per cent of patients who are symptomatic. The most common type is muscle-contraction headaches often associated with greater occipital neuralgia. This headache type also can be due to neck and temporomandibular joint injuries. Much less often, migraine and, rarely, cluster-type headaches may develop after mild head injury.
3. Dizziness is reported by 53 per cent of patients within 1 week of the injury. The different causes include labyrinthine concussion, benign positional vertigo, and rarely a perilymph fistula.

TABLE 326–1. KEY SYMPTOMS: SEQUELAE OF MILD HEAD INJURY

Headaches
Muscle contraction type
Migraine
Cluster
Greater occipital neuralgia
Supraorbital and infraorbital neuralgia
Secondary to neck injury
Secondary to temporomandibular joint syndrome
Caused by scalp laceration or local trauma
Mixed

Cranial Nerve Symptoms and Signs
Dizziness
Vertigo
Tinnitus
Hearing loss
Blurred vision
Diplopia
Convergence insufficiency
Light and noise sensitivity
Diminished smell and taste

Psychological and Somatic Complaints
Irritability
Anxiety
Depression
Personality change
Fatigue
Sleep disturbance
Decreased libido
Decreased appetite

Cognitive Impairment
Memory impairment
Impaired concentration and attention
Slowing of reaction time
Slowing of information processing speed

Rare Sequelae
Subdural and epidural hematomas
Seizures
Transient global amnesia
Tremor
Dystonia

From Evans RW: Postconcussion syndrome. In Evans RW, Baskin DS, Yatsu FM (eds): Prognosis of Neurological Disorders, p. 98. New York, Oxford University Press, 1992, with permission.

Occasionally, sensorineural hearing loss and tinnitus can result.

4. Fourteen per cent of patients report blurred vision, most often due to convergence insufficiency. Occasionally, third, fourth, and sixth cranial nerve palsies occur, resulting in diplopia.

5. About 5 per cent of patients report decreased smell and taste. The olfactory filaments can be damaged by mild head injury. About 10 per cent report light and noise sensitivity.

6. Over 50 per cent report nonspecific psychological symptoms, including irritability, personality change, anxiety, and depression. Fatigue and sleep disturbance are less commonly reported. A post-traumatic stress disorder also can develop following mild head injury.

7. Four weeks after the injury, about 20 per cent of patients complain of memory problems and difficulty with concentration. Deficits in cognitive functioning that may occur include a reduction in speed of information processing and attention, prolonged reaction time, and decreased memory for new information.

Clinical Findings

1. There may be no physical findings on examination.

2. In cases of greater occipital neuralgia, the symptoms are reproduced with palpation over the greater occipital nerve, which is located approximately midway between the inion and posterior mastoid just below the occipital crest.

3. Rotatory nystagmus may be present in patients with vertigo as a result of peripheral vestibular dysfunction.

Laboratory Tests

1. Skull radiographs are usually not necessary to evaluate patients with mild closed head injury.

2. A computerized tomographic (CT) scan, when indicated, is the preferred imaging modality for evaluation of acute head trauma. In patients who have had a mild head injury and have a normal neurologic examination, the yield of CT scans is quite small. After mild head injury, the incidence of neurosurgical complications such as subdural and epidural hematoma is between 1 and 3 per cent.

3. Magnetic resonance imaging (MRI) is more sensitive than CT scan in evaluating extra-axial and intra-axial lesions in the acute and chronic stages following head injury but rarely affects outcome.

4. Electroencephalogram (EEG) studies are usually not indicated for evaluating mild head injury because of limited sensitivity and specificity. However, an EEG is helpful when a post-traumatic seizure disorder is suspected. Brain mapping and auditory brain stem response studies are not indicated for the evaluation of mild head injury.

5. Electronystagmography (ENG) studies may be helpful in evaluating dizziness. Audiograms are indicated in patients with hearing complaints.

6. In patients with prominent visual complaints, formal visual field testing is part of the evaluation.

7. In patients with significant cognitive complaints, neuropsychological testing is often worthwhile

Key Tests

When indicated:

- CT scan or MRI of the head
- EEG
- ENG
- Audiogram
- Visual fields
- Neuropsychological testing

Differential Diagnosis

1. In patients with progressive clinical symptoms or an abnormal neurologic examination, consider a delayed or chronic subdural or epidural hematoma.

2. With time, postconcussion syndrome will generally not worsen. In cases where structural pathology has been excluded, consider possibilities such as depression, anxiety, hysteria, somatiform disorder, compensation neurosis, and malingering.

Treatment

1. Treatment is individualized after each of the problems is properly diagnosed.

2. Muscle contraction–type headaches may respond to simple analgesics, barbiturate-narcotics (with caution), nonsteroidal anti-inflammatory drugs, antidepressants (particularly tricyclics), and muscle relaxants. For greater occipital neuralgia, a nerve block may be helpful. Biofeedback, physical therapy, and transcutaneous electrical nerve stimulation (TENS) may help intractable headaches.

3. Migraines may respond to the usual prophylactic and symptomatic medications.

4. The treating physician or, if indicated, a psychologist or psychiatrist should provide the pa-

tient with psychological support. When psychological symptoms are prominent, psychotropic medications may be used.

Activity

1. Patients usually can return to normal activities within a few weeks. Some patients have prolonged disability.
2. Return to contact sports is discussed in Ch. 325, Head Injuries in Sports.

Patient Education

1. Education of the patient and family members is essential and in many cases is the most important part of treatment.
2. The general public may be midled by the "Hollywood head injury myth" into believing that mild head injuries should not cause persistent symptoms. Head injuries are presented in two contexts in the movies or on television. In the first, in action, detective, martial arts, western, and boxing films, the injuries may appear serious but do not result in significant sequelae. The public is led to overestimate how much head injury a person can withstand. In the second context, in slapstick and cartoons, head trauma not only is not serious but can be very funny. Counterexamples such as knockouts and the "punch drunk" state in boxers may be helpful in patient education.

Key Treatment

- Individualize for each symptom
- A number of treatments are available for each headache type.
- Psychological support and education of the patient are crucial.

Follow-Up

1. Prevention: Encourage patients to use helmets for activities such as bicycle or motorcycle riding.

2. Monitoring: periodic follow-up visits for patients with persistent symptoms even if only for psychological support

3. Prognosis
   a. Symptoms persist more often in patients who are women, over age 40, or with a prior history of head injury.
   b. Although headaches resolve in about 50 per cent of patients by 3 months, some 20 per cent may still complain of headaches 3 years after the injury.
   c. Cognitive impairment usually resolves within 3 to 6 months after the injury. A small percentage of patients have deficits that may persist indefinitely.
   d. Some physicians believe that patients who sustain injuries resulting in litigation have persistent symptoms caused by compensation neurosis or malingering. Although this is true for a small number, most plaintiffs still symptomatic at the time of litigation are not cured by a verdict. Litigants have similar symptoms, improving with time, and similar cognitive test results to nonlitigants.

Bibliography

Alves W, Macciocchi SN, Barth JT: Postconcussive symptoms after uncomplicated mild head injury. J Head Trauma Rehabil 1993;8:48–59.

Duus BR, Lind B, Christensen H, et al: The role of neuroimaging in the initial management of patients with minor head injury. Ann Emerg Med 1994;23:1279–1283.

Evans RW: The postconcussion syndrome and the sequelae of mild head injury. In Evans RW (ed): Neurology and Trauma, pp 91–116. Philadelphia, WB Saunders Company, 1996.

Evans RW: The postconcussion syndrome. In Evans RW, Baskin DS, Yatsu FM (eds): Prognosis of Neurological Disorders, 2nd ed. New York, Oxford University Press, 2000.

Fisher JM, Williams AD: Neuropsychologic investigation of mild head injury: ensuring diagnostic accuracy in the assessment process. Semin Neurol 1994;14:53–59.

McAllister TW: Neuropsychiatric sequelae of head injuries. Psychiatr Clin 1992;15:395–413.

327 Subdural Hematoma

Erol Taşdemiroğlu

Definitions

1. Subdural hematoma or hemorrhage is characterized by a collection of blood between the dura mater and the arachnoid membranes of the central nervous system.
2. Depending on the rapidity of bleeding and the size of the blood vessel that is torn, subdural hematomas are classified as acute, subacute, or chronic. Acute and subacute hematomas are associated with contusion and laceration of the cerebral parenchyma and are sometimes called "complicated subdural hematomas."
3. Infantile subdural effusions are considered a separate entity. The source of bleeding may be arterial or venous.
4. If a rupture of the arachnoid membrane accompanies the formation of a hematoma, the condition is called a "complex subdural hygroma."
5. Subdural hematomas can be located in the supratentorial region (convexity, interhemispheric, subtemporal, or suboccipital hematomas), the infratentorial region (posterior fossa subdural hematomas), or the spine.

Etiology

1. Trauma: birth trauma, physical child abuse
2. Coagulopathy: secondary to cancer chemotherapy, hepatic and hematologic diseases, hemophilia, anticoagulant therapy, vitamins C or K, hypovitaminosis
3. Arteriovenous malformation or rupture of an aneurysm into the subdural space
4. Ventricular shunting procedures or lumbar puncture
5. Neoplasms: primary neoplasms or metastases to the subdural space
6. Other: alcoholism, hypertension, hemodialysis, infusion of osmotic diuretics, intracranial operations, infections

Symptoms

1. Acute subdural hematomas: Symptoms occur within the first 24 hours of injury. Acute subdural hematomas generally extend over large portions of the brain. Two types of traumatic acute subdural hematomas have been described:
   a. Bleeding is associated with cortical and parenchymal lacerations. Usually the underlying primary brain injury is severe. The size of the hematoma is insignificant. Often there is no lucid interval.
   b. Hematoma characterized by massive hemorrhage caused by a tear in large bridging veins or the dural sinuses. Primary brain damage is less severe, and a lucid interval may occur. Acute subdural hematomas are occasionally caused by birth trauma.
2. Subacute subdural hematomas: Clinical symptoms occur within an interval of 3 to 21 days after injury. Signs and symptoms are usually similar to those of chronic subdural hematomas.
3. Chronic subdural hematomas: Symptoms start at least 3 weeks after head injury. Symptoms can mimic transient ischemic attacks and may show fluctuations. Bilateral chronic subdural hematomas are seen in 15 to 20 per cent of patients.

Key Signs and Symptoms: Subacute and Chronic Subdural Hematomas

- Dull headaches, seizures
- Changes in personality and mental status
- Hemiparesis, dysphasia, hemisensory changes
- Papilledema, retinal hemorrhage, photophobia

4. Subdural hematoma in infants and children
   a. Chronic subdural hematomas or subdural effusions are seldom seen in patients more than 2 years of age unless a shunt procedure was carried out; they rarely occur in adolescents less than age 20. Chronic infantile subdural collections are usually bilateral and frequently communicate under the falx.
   b. Calcified chronic subdural hematomas are usually bilateral and may remain asymptomatic for years. Calcification and/or ossification of chronic subdural hematoma can appear after approximately 3 years. They

only manifest themselves when seizure activity or mental retardation becomes apparent.

Key Signs and Symptoms: Subdural Hematomas in Infants and Children

- Increased intracranial pressure (abnormal width and tension of the fontanelle, palpable separation of the cranial sutures, "cracked-pot" percussion sound of the skull, irritability and vomiting)—in 60 per cent

- Seizures (local or generalized)—in 40 per cent

- Macrocrania (characterized by biparietal enlargement and distention of superficial scalp veins)

- Retinal or subhyaloid hemorrhage

- Anemia

- Generalized hypertonicity of the extremities

- Lateralizing or focal motor deficits

5. Spinal subdural hematomas: Spinal subdural hematomas can complicate lumbar puncture (therapeutic or diagnostic), can follow spinal surgery (e.g., lumbar disk surgery), or may occur spontaneously. This type of hematoma is most commonly located in the lower thoracic or thoracolumbar regions. Clinical symptoms often include sphincter dysfunction, paralysis of the lower extremities, and back pain.

6. Posterior fossa subdural hematomas: Posterior fossa subdural hematomas constitute fewer than 1 per cent of all subdural hematomas. These hematomas are usually acute in nature and characterized by bleeding from torn bridging veins or posterior fossa dural sinuses.

7. Subdural hygroma: Subdural hygromas appearing during the post-traumatic period are characteristically subdural fluid collections that are crystal clear or mildly xanthochromic. Subdural hygromas are called "simple" if they occur alone or "complex" when they are associated with parenchymal injuries. These hygromas are also seen after monitoring and vigorous treatment of increased intracranial pressure in patients with Reye's syndrome. The clinical manifestations are similar to those of subdural hematomas.

Diagnosis

1. Skull radiographs may reveal skull fracture line, shift of physiologic midline calcifications (falx cerebri and pineal gland), and calcified subdural hematoma membrane.

2. Subdural tap is another procedure used to diagnose infantile chronic subdural effusions. In newborns, the results of taps of the subdural space through the fontanelle or the coronal suture may be misleading, because the hematoma is usually coagulated and solid.

3. Cerebral angiography is characterized by biconvex avascular extracerebral mass.

4. Electroencephalogram may be abnormal; diffuse reduction of voltage and/or unilateral suppression of alpha rhythm on the side where the hematoma is located.

5. Radioisotope brain scan shows increased activity over the cortex on the side where the hematoma is located.

6. B-mode ultrasonography is a relatively easy, harmless, noninvasive, and economical way to diagnose and follow chronic infantile subdural hematomas.

7. Computerized tomographic (CT) scan (Table 327–1): Cerebral edema is frequently seen. Acute subdural hematomas are hyperintense on CT scans (Fig. 327–1) and are usually localized over the convexity. Acute subdural hematomas are sometimes isointense to brain when patients

TABLE 327–1. SUBDURAL HEMATOMA DENSITY CHANGES ON CT AND MRI WITH TIME

STAGE	CT SCAN	MRI Hemoglobin	MRI T_1-Weighted	MRI T_2-Weighted
Hyperacute (<24 hr)	Hyperdense Intracellular iron	Oxyhemoglobin	Hypointense to brain parenchyma	Hyperintense (CSF density) to brain parenchyma
Acute (1–3 d)	Hyperdense Intracellular iron	Deoxyhemoglobin	Isointense to brain parenchyma	Hypointense to brain
Early subacute (3–7 d)	Isodense Intracellular iron	Methemoglobin	Hyperintense to brain (+)	Hypointense to brain
Late subacute (>7 d)	Isodense Extracellular iron	Methemoglobin	Hyperintense to brain (++)	Hyperintense to brain
Chronic (>3 wk)	Hypodense Extracellular iron	Methemoglobin	Hyperintense to brain (+)	

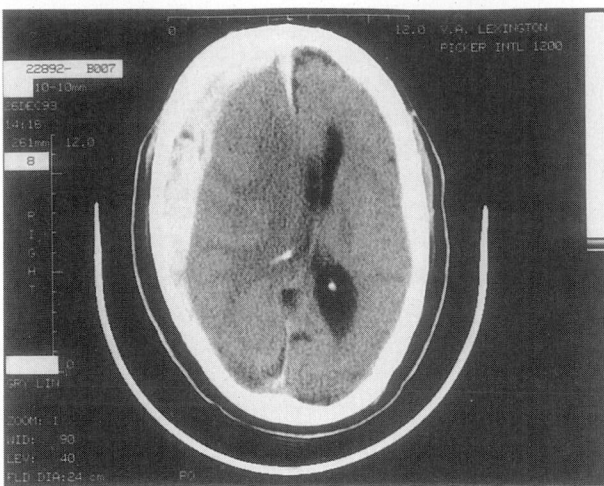

Figure 327–1 Axial CT scan of the head without contrast enhancement shows supratentorial large hyperdense acute subdural hematoma and cerebral edema with mass effect resulting in midline shift.

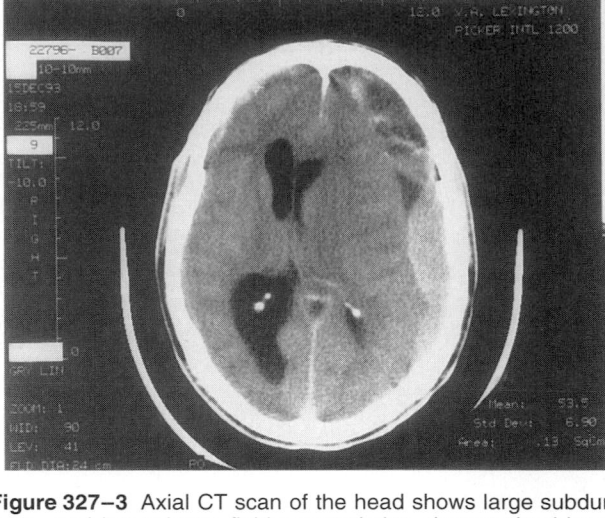

Figure 327–3 Axial CT scan of the head shows large subdural hypo- and hyperdense fluid accumulation characterized by rehemorrhage into the subdural space.

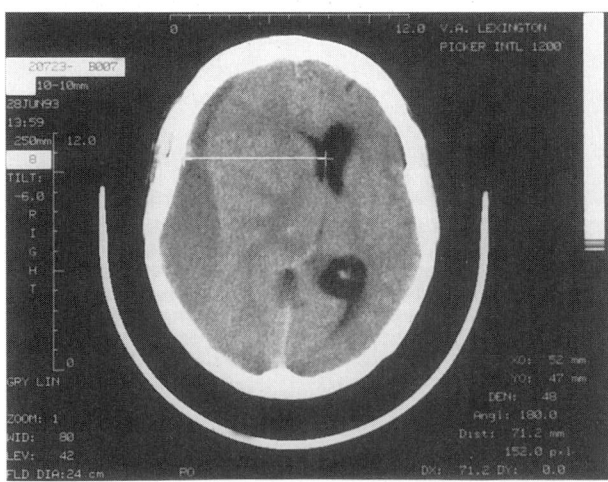

Figure 327–2 Axial CT scan of the head without contrast enhancement shows large hypodense fluid collection over the right hemisphere with significant midline shift.

have low hemoglobin levels or when cerebrospinal fluid from torn arachnoid dilutes the extravasated blood. Whereas subacute subdural hematomas are 70 per cent isointense on axial CT scan, chronic subdural hematomas are 76 per cent hypointense (Fig. 327–2) and 16 per cent isointense on axial CT scans. However, layering phenomena and repeated episodes of hemorrhage may produce hematomas of variable attenuation and size (Fig. 327–3).

8. Magnetic resonance imaging (MRI) (Table 327–1): The MRI appearance of subdural hematoma shows an evolving pattern of variable signal intensity. When recurrent bleeding occurs in a subdural hematoma, the different events may be distinguishable by the variable signal intensities on MRI (Fig. 327–4).

Treatment

Surgery

1. Acute and subacute subdural hematomas: If the collection of blood in a symptomatic hematoma is thicker than 1 cm at its thickest point, rapid surgical evacuation should be considered. Hematomas characterized by massive hemorrhage should be evacuated rapidly. The primary treatment of subacute subdural hematomas is also surgical drainage.

2. Chronic subdural hematoma: Surgical evacuation of the hematoma is indicated for symptomatic lesions with maximum thickness greater than about 1 cm. If a significant re-collection is demonstrated, a short course of dexamethasone, 2 to 4 mg four times daily for a period ranging from 7 to 14 days, is instituted. Only when this regimen fails to improve the situation is reoperation considered. Residual subdural collections after treatment are common and may require up to 6 months for complete resolution. Persistent fluid collections, especially those evident on CT scan during the first 20 postoperative days, should not be re-evacuated unless they increase in size, as demonstrated by CT scan, or the patient shows no signs of recovery or deteriorates neurologically.

3. Subdural hematoma in infants and children: Although many authors recommend observation for patients with no symptoms or with only enlarging head and development delay, at least

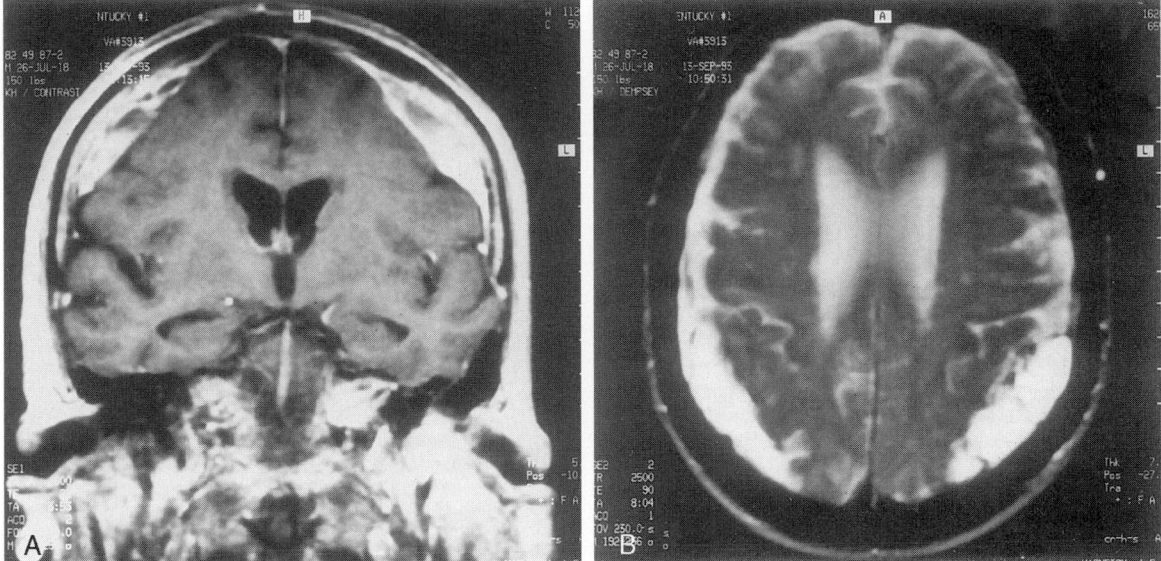

Figure 327–4 Gadolinium-enhanced coronal T₁-weighted (*A*) and axial T₂-weighted (*B*) MRI images show inhomogeneous subdural fluid collection that represents different ages of the blood products within.

one percutaneous subdural tap should be performed to rule out infection. Treatment options for symptomatic cases include serial percutaneous subdural taps, burr-hole drainage, and extremely low-pressure subdural-peritoneal shunt placement. The subdural-peritoneal shunt is usually removed after 2 to 3 months of drainage because, as a result of foreign body reaction, mineralization of the dura and arachnoid membranes increases the seizure activity.

4. Calcified subdural hematoma: Calcified subdural hematoma is not responsible for seizures or mental retardation. The surgical indications for treating such a lesion are progressive mental retardation, an increase in the number of seizures, or other progressive neurologic deficit.

5. Spinal subdural hematoma: A laminectomy should be performed as soon as possible after the diagnosis is made so that the amount of neurologic damage can be held to a minimum.

6. Subdural hygroma: Surgical evacuation is unnecessary for patients who are clinically improving or stable.

Medication

1. Because the development of chronic subdural hematoma is an inflammatory process, inhibition of inflammatory reaction would be beneficial.

   a. Glucocorticoids have been shown to inhibit neomembrane formation and neovascularization in experimental subdural hematomas.

   b. Intravenous hyperosmolar agents such as mannitol with or without steroids are the cornerstone of medical treatment.

   c. Small and mildly symptomatic chronic subdural hematomas could be treated with steroids.

2. Seizure prophylaxis is considered.

Prognosis and Outcome

1. The overall mortality rate associated with acute subdural hematomas is 66 per cent, and functional recovery is 19 per cent. Postoperative seizures occur in 9 per cent and do not correlate with outcome, but these rates are higher for aged patients (82 per cent) and for patients who use anticoagulants (90 per cent). Subacute subdural hematomas carry a much better prognosis than acute subdural hematomas. However, in posterior fossa, subdural hematoma prognosis is related to the patient's neurologic condition and the severity of the head injury.

2. The mortality rates after treatment of a chronic subdural hematoma are reported at less than 10 per cent in large series, and approximately 75 per cent of patients are able to resume normal functioning. The mortality rate drops to 5 per cent in patients who are alert or drowsy (grades 0 to 2; see Table 327–2).

3. After treatment of chronic subdural effusions, although approximately 75 per cent of infants show normal development, 5 per cent show some degree of psychomotor retardation.

327 Subdural Hematoma • 1409

TABLE 327–2. GRADING OF CHRONIC SUBDURAL HEMATOMA

GROUP	DESCRIPTION
0	Neurologically normal
1	Alert and oriented; mild symptoms, including headache, reflex asymmetry, seizure
2	Lethargic or disoriented with variable neurologic deficits such as hemiparesis
3	Stuporous but responds appropriately to noxious stimuli; severe focal signs such as hemiplegia
4	Comatose; decerebrate or decorticate posturing

From Markwalder TM, Steinsiepe KF, Rohner M, et al: The course of chronic subdural hematomas after burr-hole craniostomy and closed-system drainage. J Neurosurg 1981;55:390–396, with permission.

Bibliography

Becker DP, Gade GF, Young HF, Feuerman TF: Diagnosis and treatment of head injury in adults. In Youmans JR (ed): Neurological Surgery: A Comprehensive Guide to the Diagnosis and Management of Neurosurgical Problems, 3d ed, vol 3, pp 2017–2148. Philadelphia, WB Saunders Company, 1990.

Bradley WG Jr: Hemorrhage and brain iron. In Stark DD, Bradley WG Jr (eds): Magnetic Resonance Imaging, 2d ed, vol 1, pp 721–769. St Louis, Mosby–Year Book, 1992.

Drapkin AJ: Chronic subdural hematoma: pathophysiological basis for treatment. Br J Neurosurg 1991;5:467–473.

Greenberg MS: Handbook of Neurosurgery, 4th ed. Lakeland, FL, Greenberg Graphics, 1997.

Hamilton MG, Frizzell JB, Tranmer BI: Chronic subdural hematoma: the role of craniotomy re-evaluated. Neurosurgery 1993;33:67–72.

328 Common Behavioral Symptoms

Syed M. Ahmed

1. Insomnia reflects the perception by a person of nonrestful or inadequate sleep resulting from problems with sleep initiation, sleep maintenance, and/or nonrestorative sleep. If insomnia does not cause daytime problems (e.g., fatigue, irritability, somnolence, distractibility), it is not clinically significant. Approximately 30 per cent of the population complain of insomnia, making it one of the most common complaints of patients. Because insomnia may be symptomatic of a variety of diseases, a careful history and physical examination is needed to come to an appropriate diagnosis.

2. Insomnia is classified on the basis of duration of symptoms as
   a. Transient insomnia: up to several days
   b. Short-term insomnia: up to 3 weeks
   c. Chronic insomnia: more than 3 weeks

3. Transient insomnia is usually precipitated by life stress, excitement, grief, jet lag, or withdrawal from a drug. Chronic insomnia can result from maladaptive coping strategies or inadequate treatment of transient insomnia. It is most common in individuals with a predisposition, such as a predilection for anxiety.

Differential Diagnosis

1. Primary insomnias: In primary insomnias, no identifiable medical or psychiatric cause can be established. These chronic sleep disorders are usually diagnosed in a sleep laboratory by nocturnal polysomnography. Ten to 20 per cent of insomnias are primary sleep disorders.
   a. Obstructive sleep apnea syndrome. About 5 to 15 per cent of adults suffer from sleep apnea. Overweight, middle-aged men more commonly suffer from this problem. Loud snoring is typical. Recurrent periods of apnea associated with desaturation and arousal from sleep lead to excessive daytime drowsiness and fatigue.
   b. Restless legs syndrome: This disorder is caused by unpleasant sensations in the calves and a persistent urge to move the legs.
   c. Periodic limb movement disorder: Repeated muscle contractions of the legs (and occasionally arms) cause frequent awakenings.
   d. Circadian rhythm sleep disorders: Jet lag and work shift changes can cause transient insomnia. In older people, advanced sleep-phase disturbances are characterized by falling asleep early in the evening and waking early in the morning. In young adults, falling asleep early in the morning and waking late in the day are characteristics of delayed sleep-phase disturbances.
   e. Psychophysiologic insomnia: Negative conditioning usually causes difficulty in initiating and maintaining sleep. Insomnia needs to be present for more than a month to have a diagnosis of psychophysiologic insomnia.

2. Secondary insomnias: Insomnias caused by psychological, medical, or other factors are noted in Table 328–1. About 50 per cent of all insomnias are related to psychiatric causes. Major depression is classically associated with early morning awakening, but can also be manifested by initial or middle insomnia.

History

Physicians should attempt to identify the underlying cause of insomnia rather than simply prescribe a medication to treat it. History taking should be thorough and include exploring medical and psychiatric history. Physicians need to evaluate sleep pattern, duration, and frequency of insomnia. Talking to the sleeping partner can provide valuable insights. Table 328–2 identifies a number of domains to be investigated when taking a history.

Clinical Findings

1. Patients with insomnia usually present with a complaint of inadequate sleep (Table 328–3).
2. Depending on the underlying causes, patients

TABLE 328–1. CAUSES OF SECONDARY INSOMNIA

Psychiatric Causes
Major depression
Generalized anxiety disorder
Manic-depressive disorder
Obsessive-compulsive disorder
Psychosis
Pain disorder
Somatoform pain disorders

Medical/Surgical Causes
Hyperthyroidism/hypothyroidism
Arthritis
Fibromyalgia
Gastroesophageal reflux disease
Asthma/chronic obstructive pulmonary disease
Congestive heart failure
Angina
Urinary tract infection
Benign prostatic hypertrophy
Hyperglycemia
Gallbladder disease
Delirium
Dementia
Pain of any origin

Prescription Drugs
Diuretics
Steroids
Theophylline
Phenytoin
Levodopa

Nonprescription Drugs
Cough preparations
Decongestants
Diet aids

Other
Alcohol
Cigarettes
Coffee
Tea
Cola
Chocolate

Tests

1. Sleep diary: Physicians should ask a patient to keep a daily sleep diary for 2 weeks. This sleep log documents bedtimes, time on arising, estimates of time needed to fall asleep, number of nocturnal awakenings, total amount of sleep each night, timing and quantity of meals, use of alcohol, exercise, smoking, and medications. This information can provide valuable clues to underlying causes of insomnia and help tailor treatment for each patient.

2. Polysomnography: In a sleep laboratory, polysomnography is used to evaluate complicated chronic insomnias or sleep apnea syndrome. In polysomnography, a continuous all-night recording of a patient's respirations, eye movement, muscle tone, electroencephalogram, blood oxygen saturation, and electrocardiogram is made.

Management

Physicians should explore a causative foundation of insomnia because this can lead to a specific treatment strategy. Physicians need to provide both nonpharmacologic and pharmacologic treatment as deemed appropriate.

1. Nonpharmacologic therapy

   a. Sleep hygiene: The physician needs to review

may show other clinical findings. In obstructive sleep apnea, obesity, short thick neck, long uvula, or somnolence may be noted. In patients with congestive heart failure or chronic obstructive pulmonary disease, dyspnea may be seen.

TABLE 328–2. MISCELLANEOUS DOMAINS TO SURVEY FOR INSOMNIA HISTORY

DOMAIN	QUESTIONS FOR CONSIDERATION
Onset	Precipitating events?
	Age at onset?
Frequency	Every night, intermittent, or only on specific nights?
	In response to particular circumstances?
Severity of daytime consequences	Lethargy, sleepiness, napping, dozing?
	Deficits in cognition, performance, and mood (e.g., mild depression and irritability)?
Response to treatment	Was the treatment trial adequate, efficacious?
What improves sleep?	Sleeping away from home?
	Sleeping the night before a day off?
What worsens sleep?	Clock watching at night?
	Sleeping with a bed partner?
	Are Sunday nights worse?
Medical status	Pain, discomfort?
	Disorders that produce daytime sedation or increase arousal?
Drugs	Pharmacotherapy: arousing drugs?
	Tolerance to sedating drugs?
	Drugs that induce daytime sleep?
	Side effects?
	Illicit drugs: alerting and sedating substances interfering with sleep?
Alcohol	Disrupting continuity and depth of sleep?
Psychiatric disorders	Depression, anxiety, personality or other disorders?
Work	Demands, coping capacity, work schedule?
Family	Staying up late? (e.g., consistent with family's sleep habits, waiting up for family members to come home)

Adapted from Spielman AJ, Nunes J, Glovinsky PB: Insomnia. Neurol Clin 1996;14:513–543, with permission.

TABLE 328-3. INSOMNIA COMPLAINTS

Not enough sleep
Trouble falling asleep
Difficulty staying asleep
Early morning awakening
Light or unrefreshing sleep
Needs sleeping pills to fall asleep
Unpredictable sleep
Unable to sleep when work schedule permits (e.g., shift work)

Adapted from Spielman AJ, Nunes J, Glovinsky PB: Insomnia. Neurol Clin 1996;14:513–543, with permission.

TABLE 328-5. STIMULUS CONTROL INSTRUCTIONS

1. Lie down to sleep only when you are sleepy.
2. Use your bed only for sleep or sexual activity.
3. If you are unable to fall asleep after 10 minutes, get up and leave the bedroom.
4. Repeat Step 3 as often as necessary.
5. Get up at the same time each morning.
6. Do not nap during the day.

From Bootzin RR, Perlis ML: Nonpharmacologic treatments of insomnia. J Clin Psychiatry 1992;53(Suppl):37–45, with permission. Copyright 1992, Physicians Postgraduate Press.

appropriate sleep hygiene with the patient. Using sleep diary, physicians can evaluate problem areas and advise on healthier sleep habits (Table 328–4).

b. Stimulus control: Some behavior modification strategies can help implement coping activities that can reduce episodes of insomnia (Table 328–5).

c. Relaxation techniques: Physicians may recommend relaxation techniques, including meditation, biofeedback, deep muscle relaxation, self-hypnosis, or yoga, as nonpharmacologic modalities to treat insomniacs.

d. Cognitive therapy: Cognitive therapy can be helpful in insomniacs with anxiety or affective disorder. It can help an insomniac to recognize and balance exaggerated negative

cognitions and overcome the vicious cycle of insomnia.

e. Sleep restriction therapy: The basic premise in sleep restriction therapy is the recognition that exposure to sleep deprivation significantly increases the need for sleep. In this technique, the patient and therapist decide on an initial period of time that the patient will spend in bed. For example, the patient goes to bed at 12:00 PM and gets up at 5:00 AM. Although he had only a maximum of 5 hours of sleep, he is not allowed any napping during the day. Once the patient has been successful on initial sleep pattern, sleep interval is gradually increased.

2. Pharmacologic therapy (Table 328–6): All sedative-hypnotics are indicated for short-term or intermittent use. The lowest effective dose should be used. In the elderly or in patients with

TABLE 328-4. SLEEP HYGIENE MEASURES

1. Sleep as much as needed to feel alert during the day, but not more. Curtailing the time in bed seems to solidify sleep; excessive time spent in bed seems to fragment sleep.
2. Establish a regular awakening time in the morning that you can adhere to every day, including weekends and vacations. Such regularity strengthens circadian cycling.
3. Exercise performed regularly (but not too close to bedtime) probably deepens sleep.
4. Excessive noise may disturb sleep; insulate your room against loud noises.
5. Excessive warmth disturbs sleep. Keep the room temperature at a comfortable level.
6. A light snack prior to bedtime may improve sleep, although a large meal and excessive fluids close to bedtime may have the opposite effect.
7. Caffeinated beverages disturb sleep, even though you may be aware of their effect.
8. Alcoholic beverages, which may assist in falling asleep, can significantly fragment sleep.
9. If you feel angry and frustrated because you cannot fall asleep, do not try harder to fall asleep. Instead, leave the bedroom and do something not very stimulating, like reading a boring book.
10. The chronic use of tobacco disturbs sleep.

Adapted from Doghramji K: The evaluation and management of sleep disorders. In Stoudemire A (ed): Clinical Psychiatry for Medical Students, 2nd ed, p 636. Philadelphia, JB Lippincott Company, 1994, with permission.

TABLE 328-6. DRUGS FOR INSOMNIA: DOSAGES AND DURATION OF ACTION

MEDICATION (TRADE NAME)	USUAL DAILY DOSAGE* (mg)
Benzodiazepines	
Short acting	
Triazolam (Halcion)	0.125–0.25
Zolpidem (Ambien)†	5–10
Zaleplon (Sonata)	5–10
Intermediate acting	
Temazepam (Restoril)	15–30
Estazolam (Prosom)	1–2
Long acting	
Flurazepam (Dalmane)	15–30
Quazepam (Doral)	7.5–15
Antidepressants	
Amitryptyline (Elavil)	10–25
Nortriptyline (Pamelor)	25–50
Trazodone (Desyrel)	50–100
Antihistamine	
Diphenhydramine	25–50

*For elderly patients, initial dose at one half the minimal dose may suffice.
†Chemically unrelated to benzodiazepines but binds the same receptors.

renal or hepatic disease, dose should be reduced. Most of these drugs can cause habituation, withdrawal, and rebound insomnia upon abrupt cessation.

a. Benzodiazepines

   (1) Benzodiazepines, nonselective agonists of γ-aminobutyric acid (GABA) receptors, are the most commonly used drugs in the treatment of insomnia. The choice of a drug for a specific patient is based on the duration of action of the drug, age of the patient, and whether the beginning, middle, or end of the night is affected. A shorter acting agent may be helpful for the patient with difficulty initiating sleep. A longer acting compound may help a patient with early morning awakening and daytime anxiety.

   (2) In general, most benzodiazepines have relatively benign side effect profiles. Daytime sedation and ataxia are the most commonly reported side effects. Benzodiazepines should be avoided in patients with obstructive sleep apnea because of their potential to suppress respiration. For elderly patients, long-acting drugs should be avoided because of the higher occurrences of falls and injuries. Memory impairment and rebound insomnia are the side effects to watch for while using benzodiazepines.

b. Nonbenzodiazepine GABA receptor agonists: Zolpidem, an imidazopyridine hypnotic agent, binds selectively to benzodiazepine or omega brain receptor. It has rapid onset of action and a short half-life, and lacks significant potential for drug addiction. Zaleplon (Sonata) is a pyrazolopyrimidine derivative that binds selectively to the benzodiazepine BZ_1 receptor subtype. It is less potent than zolpidem and has a shorter half-life. It offers an alternative to zolpidem and the benzodiazepines (especially triazolam) in the treatment of insomnia.

c. Tricyclic antidepressants: Amitryptyline (10 to 25 mg), nortriptyline (25 to 50 mg), and trazodone (50 to 150 mg) are commonly used agents for insomnia. Trazodone does not have significant anticholinergic effects, but it can precipitate orthostatic hypotension secondary to its α-adrenolytic properties.

d. Antihistamines: Diphenhydramine (25 to 50 mg) is used as an over-the-counter sedative agent. It has marked anticholinergic side effects.

e. Other drugs

   (1) Melatonin: Exogenous melatonin has been demonstrated to have positive effects on human sleep. One study noted that 5 mg of melatonin significantly increased sleep propensity. Endogenous sleep-promoting substances, such as polypeptides (interleukins, interferons) and prostaglandins, are currently the subject of research.

   (2) Chloral hydrate: Chloral hydrate (500 to 2000 mg) is useful for stress-related transient insomnia (e.g., as a sedative the night before surgery). Its effect lasts less than 2 weeks because of rapid development of tolerance.

PEARLS

- Physicians should look for underlying cause(s) of insomnia.

- There are patients who are natural "short sleepers." They may sleep less than 7 hours and do well.

- By adequately managing sleep disturbances, the physician is in a position to prevent a chronic insomnia from developing.

- Although a patient wishes an immediate solution, a physician should educate a patient that insomnia may take weeks or months to improve.

- Sedative-hypnotic drugs are best used for a limited time and in conjunction with nonpharmacologic therapy.

- All insomniacs should be encouraged to maintain sleep hygiene.

- Forty to 50 per cent of patients presenting with insomnia have major depression.

Bibliography

Kupfer DJ, Reynolds CF III: Management of insomnia. N Engl J Med 1997;336:341–346.

Pary R, Tobias CR, Webb WK, et al: Treatment of insomnia. Postgrad Med 1996;100:195–210.

Perlis ML, Giles DE, Mendelson WB, et al: Psychophysiological insomnia: the behavioral model and a neurocognitive perspective. J Sleep Res 1997;6:179–188.

Spielman AJ, Nunes J, Glovinsky PB: Insomnia. Neurol Clin 1996;14:513–543.

Winokur A: Insomnia. In Rakel RE (ed): Conn's Current Therapy, 50th ed, pp 31–35. Philadelphia, WB Saunders Company, 1998.

Fatigue, also called "tiredness" or "lassitude," may be a primary complaint or may accompany other symptoms. It is a nonspecific, subjective sensation of ill-being that reflects emotional, social, or physical dysfunction. For the patient, fatigue interferes with quality of life and productivity. For the primary care physician, fatigue is a challenge requiring a broad approach, sound clinical reasoning, negotiation, and interpersonal skills.

Differential Diagnosis

1. Mood disorder, especially depression
2. Stress, whether social or physical
3. Infection, including hepatitis, human immunodeficiency virus (HIV), and mononucleosis
4. Endocrine or metabolic disorder, including thyroid disease, diabetes, menopause, adrenal dysfunction, and electrolyte imbalance
5. Hematologic disorder, including anemias and leukemia
6. Medication side effect or other toxic exposure, including carbon monoxide, gasoline or organic solvents, and substance abuse
7. Cardiovascular disease
8. Collagen-vascular disease
9. Lifestyle, including sleep, diet, exercise, work, and substance use habits
10. Malignancy

Etiology

Most complaints of fatigue will have a nonorganic cause. Fifty to 60 per cent will be functional or psychological in origin and 40 to 50 per cent will be physical; depression is the most common diagnosis and occurs in 20 to 30 per cent of cases. The role of stress and lifestyle factors is unknown but likely large. More exhaustive lists of physical diagnoses can be found in the Bibliography.

History

1. Patient concerns, expectations, and theory of disease (illness explanatory model)
2. Duration of symptoms: Less than 4 weeks more likely to be physical while more than 4 months more likely to be psychosocial.
3. Character of symptoms
   a. Progressive instead of fluctuating suggests physical.
   b. Worse in morning suggests psychosocial.
   c. Nonspecific and multiple symptoms suggest psychosocial.

4. Symptoms suggesting alternate diagnostic algorithms
   a. Fever
   b. Organ- or system-specific symptoms (e.g., dyspnea on exertion, polyuria/polydipsia/polyphagia, arthritis)
   c. Menstrual abnormality (i.e., pregnancy, menopause, dysfunctional bleeding)
5. Demographics or habits placing patient in a high-risk category for underlying illness such as hepatitis, HIV, lupus, anemia, heart disease, or malignancy
6. Symptoms of depression (mood, sleep, appetite, social activity, etc.) and other psychiatric disorders
7. Social context
   a. Stressors and supports (family, economic/financial, school/work)
   b. Family transitions (birth, marriage, divorce, death, illness)
   c. BATHE questions (see Procedure on The BATHE Technique)
8. Medications
9. Lifestyle
   a. Sleep, diet, activity, work, and sexual habits
   b. Substance use and habits; consider CAGE questions (see Table 344–3).

Duration and character of symptoms may help differentiate physical from psychosocial causes. Because of their high incidence, depression and psychosocial causes must be screened for. Using a problem-solving approach, the presence of certain symptoms such as fever, weakness, or arthritis would suggest alternate diagnostic algorithms; a history of risk factors would prompt additional evaluation. Establishing patient concerns, expectations, and illness explanatory model allows the physician and patient to negotiate the extent and pace of evaluation and treatment.

Clinical Findings

1. General appearance: Ill suggests physical, whereas anxious or depressed suggests psychosocial.
2. Weakness suggests physical.
3. Mental status examination may be abnormal.

There are no specific signs for tiredness, but the above may suggest the cause. A complete physical examination may reveal clues to a physical diagnosis.

Tests

1. Complete blood count
2. Glucose
3. Thyroxine and thyroid-stimulating hormone
4. Electrolytes
5. Erythrocyte sedimentation rate
6. Other tests based on risk factors (e.g., hepatitis B surface antigen, hepatic panel, antinuclear antigen, follicle-stimulating hormone, HIV)
7. Appropriate routine cancer screening (e.g., Pap smear, fecal occult blood)
8. Consider psychological screening tests (e.g., Beck, Zung).
9. Consider screening tests for support and stress (e.g., genogram, Duke Social Support and Stress Scale [DUSOCS], Family APGAR, Family Circle).

Cost-effectiveness evaluations of laboratory testing have markedly reduced the number of tests recommended in the absence of an obvious physical diagnosis. Abnormal tests occur no more than 25 per cent (and often less than 10 per cent) of the time, and frequently do not influence the diagnosis. The high frequency of psychosocial causes places the emphasis on psychological and social screening.

Management

1. Treat underlying medical illness, if present.
2. Establish therapeutic relationship: listen, reassure, and provide empathy.
3. Initiate brief counseling or refer for cognitive-behavioral psychotherapy, if indicated.
4. Formulate plan to reduce or manage stressors.

Medication

1. Withdraw any suspected medications.
2. Begin appropriate therapy if underlying disease is found.
3. Consider an empirical trial of antidepressants (tricyclics and monoamine oxidase inhibitors may be more effective).

Diet

Encourage a balanced, low-fat, high-fiber diet and regular meals.

Activity

1. Prescribe moderate aerobic exercise.
2. Consider a diary of symptoms.

Patient Education

1. Provide disease-specific education if an underlying disease is found.
2. Explain the interaction of psychosocial and somatic functioning (mind-body connection).

3. Provide guidance and support appropriate for life stage.
4. Teach or recommend resources for stress and personal management skills.

Follow-Up

1. Schedule a complete physical examination in follow-up of brief initial examination.
2. Review interval history for evolution of symptoms that may make the cause more apparent ("test of time").
3. Review compliance with exercise, diet, stress reduction, and other interventions.
4. If a physical problem was present, monitor appropriate parameters.
5. At each visit, negotiate the extent and pace of evaluation and treatment based on patient concerns and expectations.
6. Continue to build on therapeutic relationship.
7. Periodically revisit psychosocial issues, especially those that patient may be hesitant to reveal.
8. Schedule frequent, regular visits for those with multiple somatic complaints or many concerns.
9. Avoid excessive tests or procedures.

PEARLS

- Fatigue is a nonspecific symptom, not a diagnosis.

- The majority of cases will have a nonorganic cause; depression is the most common diagnosis.

- Diagnosis is mostly based on history and an understanding of the epidemiology; routine laboratory testing should be minimized.

- Duration of symptoms less than 4 weeks and a progressive deterioration suggest a physical cause.

- Duration of symptoms more than 4 months, peak symptomatology in the morning, and nonspecific and multiple symptoms suggest a psychosocial cause.

- Physician-patient negotiation, a therapeutic relationship, and a broad approach are cornerstones of successful management.

Bibliography

Llewelyn MB: Assessing the fatigued patient. Br J Hosp Med 1996;55:125–129.

McGee SR: Fatigue. In Fihn SD, McGee SR (eds): Outpatient Medicine, pp 72–74. Philadelphia, WB Saunders Company, 1992.

Sharpe M, Chalder T, Palmer I, et al: Chronic fatigue syndrome: a practical guide to assessment and management. Gen Hosp Psychiatry 1997;19:185–199.

Solberg LI: Lassitude: a primary care evaluation. JAMA 1984;251:3272–3276.

Valdini AF: Fatigue of unknown aetiology—a review. Fam Pract 1985;2:48–53.

SYMPTOM IRRITABILITY

Linda F. Pessar

Irritability may be viewed as the opposite of equanimity. It refers to a lowered threshold for feeling frustrated and reacting negatively. It is often a person's response to physical or psychological stressors. Its nonspecific nature and the absence of characteristic physical findings require that the physician take a careful history to determine if treatment is necessary. Although often a response to the inconveniences and indignities of daily life, irritability may also reflect underlying psychiatric, medical, or neurologic disorders. Whenever possible, the underlying etiology should be identified.

Differential Diagnosis

1. Psychiatric conditions
   a. Mood disorders: depression, dysthymic disorder, bipolar disorder
   b. Anxiety disorders
   c. Personality disorders: antisocial, borderline, narcissistic, paranoid
   d. Conduct disorder
   e. Attention-deficit hyperactivity disorder
2. Substance use and withdrawal syndromes
   a. Substance use: amphetamine, cocaine, and phencyclidine
   b. Withdrawal from alcohol, opiates, nicotine, benzodiazepines, barbiturates
3. Medication side effects: sympathomimetics, glucocorticoids
4. Endocrine and metabolic disorders
   a. Hyperthroidism
   b. Hypothyroidism
   c. Premenstrual syndrome
   d. Menopausal dysphoria
   e. Hepatic disease
   f. Uremia
   g. Electrolyte disturbances
   h. Vitamin B deficiencies
5. Neurologic disorders
   a. Dementia
   b. Disinhibiting frontal lobe syndromes
   c. Post-traumatic brain syndrome
6. Disruption to homeostasis
   a. Disrupted sleep
   b. Disordered eating
   c. Chronic pain
   d. Fatigue
   e. Psychosocial stressors

History: Key Questions to Ask

1. What is the patient's age?
2. What is the course of irritability: acute or gradual onset; intermittent or pervasive; diurnal variation; known triggers?
3. Is the patient taking medications?
4. Is the patient using alcohol or substances?
5. Is irritability associated with other symptoms?
6. What are the stressors in the patient's life? Is there a temporal association between the stressors and irritability? Is there conflict in the patient's family?
7. Investigate issues that the patient may be ashamed to raise: Has the patient been involved in domestic violence or sexual abuse? Is the patient newly sexually active? Might the patient be pregnant?
8. Has the patient's irritability affected ability to function and quality of relationships?
9. What relieves or diminishes the symptom?
10. Does the patient have psychiatric, neurologic, or medical illnesses?

Clinical Findings

1. Abnormal mental status findings may be present in many disorders.
2. Vital signs may reflect autonomic disturbance in substance use and withdrawal syndromes and endocrine disorders.
3. Many of the conditions that cause irritability will not produce findings on physical examination.

Tests

1. Because irritability is a nonspecific symptom, history and clinical findings will guide the choice of tests. Underlying illness is suggested by abrupt onset without identifiable psychosocial stressors, or irritability severe enough to

disrupt the patient's activities and relationships. Patient or family report of "a change in personality" should also alert the physician to an underlying disorder or illness.

2. It is helpful to have the patient keep a diary that records frequency, severity, and circumstances of irritability.

3. Interview with family members may be useful in shedding light on family tensions and patient behavior.

4. If the symptom is worrisome and history and clinical examination are not revealing, a screening battery of tests would include

   a. Electrolytes, glucose, blood urea nitrogen, liver function tests

   b. Complete blood count with indices

   c. Thyroid screening tests

   d. Pregnancy test

   e. Vitamin B_{12} level

   f. Toxicology screen

Management

The treatment for irritability will be determined by the etiology of the symptom. When no single cause can be determined, general measures to re-establish equilibrium should be found. The patient should be encouraged to regulate sleep and eating. Relaxation and other behavioral techniques should be taught to reduce the patient's baseline tension. Educational materials appropriate to the patient's diagnosis should be provided. Family counseling or referral for psychotherapy should be offered to patients with substantial psychosocial stressors. Although the patient may request anxiolytic medication, this should be avoided unless the cause for the irritability is known and is time-limited. Psychiatric consultation should be sought when there is no apparent medical etiology and general management strategies have failed to alleviate the symptom.

PEARLS

- Irritability is a nonspecific symptom.

- Abrupt onset or disruption of function or relationships should raise the possibility of underlying disorder.

- Mood disorders, anxiety disorders, and substance and alcohol use are common causes.

Bibliography

American Psychiatric Association: Diagnostic and Statistical Manual of Mental Disorders, 4th ed. Washington, DC, American Psychiatric Press, 1994.

Leigh H, Kramer SI: The psychiatric manifestations of endocrine disease. Adv Intern Med 1984;29:413–445.

Lishman WA: Organic Psychiatry: The Psychological Consequences of Cerebral Disorder, 2nd ed. Oxford, Blackwell Scientific Publications, 1987.

O'Connor PG, Schottenfeld RS: Alcohol problems. N Engl J Med 1998;338:592–602.

Pearlstein TB: Hormones and depression: what are the facts about premenstrual syndrome, menopause and hormone replacement therapy? Am J Obstet Gynecol 1995;173:646–653.

329 Marital Discord

Judith Z. Clark

Etiology

1. The roots of marital conflict are complex and may lie in arrested intrapersonal development, personality disorder, isolated or repetitive behavior, external stressors, miscommunication, or misunderstanding. Individual problems or pathology afflicting one partner may color interactions to the degree that marital conflict ensues.

2. Marital discord can represent a chronic condition in an ongoing marriage, or may lead to the disintegration of marriage. The U.S. divorce rate has been estimated to be between 50 and 67 per cent for first marriages, and up to 10 per cent higher for subsequent marriages.

Symptoms

1. Negative interactions are the distinguishing feature of discordant marriages; negativity tends to be the pervasive tone overall. Negative interactions can range from verbal or physical attacks to emotional or sexual withdrawal. Research suggests that negative nonverbal behavior is a particularly good indicator of discord, because couples asked to "fake good" or "fake bad" nonverbal behavior were unable to fool their partners.

2. Couples in distressed marriages tend to engage in negative trait attribution ("you always," "you never"), and to attribute negative motivation to even neutral and benign communications.

3. The ultimate negative outcome of marital discord, divorce, has been correlated with shortened life span, greater risk for a variety of illnesses, and elevated rates of suicide and substance abuse.

4. Individuals in discordant marriages often suffer from concomitant depression.

Clinical Findings

1. Studies by different researchers have resulted in fairly consistent observations concerning negativity in discordant marriages.

   a. Results of studies suggest discordant couples reciprocate verbal and nonverbal negative behavior with negative behavior, whereas nondistressed couples do not demonstrate negative reciprocity to any reportable degree. Although both groups evidence positive reciprocity, the distressed couples are more consistent in this pattern.

   b. It has been suggested the reason may be greater rigidity and more highly structured interactions among distressed couples. In troubled marriages, a negative interaction tends to suppress positive spousal responses. In nontroubled marriages no significant tendency for a partner to suppress positive responses after a negative spousal interaction has been noted.

2. Discordant couples do not tend to have more problem-focused interactions; however, the manner in which they discuss problems is different.

   a. Distressed couples tend to respond with negativity to both negative and positive interactions in problem discussions. The discussions are more emotional overall than problem discussions by nondistressed couples.

   b. Nondistressed couples engage in more validation (positive reaction to problem descriptions), and more positive reciprocity (positive following positive). Research suggests distressed couples engage in more devaluation (negative following positive), lengthier continuation of negative sequences (fighting on), and negative start-up sequences ("yes-butting," another form of negative following positive).

   c. Nondistressed couples are more likely to not react to a negative statement, and distressed couples are more likely to not react to a positive statement; nondistressed couples are more likely to respond positively to a problem discussion, and distressed couples are more likely to respond negatively to a problem discussion.

   d. Efforts to repair a negative interaction tend to occur in the middle of the sequence for both types of couples. Generally, a verbalization aimed at repair ("Don't interrupt me") will be delivered with unpleasant affect. In distressed marriages the negative affect is the focus of the partner ("I wouldn't interrupt if you ever gave me a chance to speak"), whereas in nondistressed marriages the repair attempt tends to be the partner's focus ("I'm sorry; finish what you were saying"). It has been suggested that the inability to repair conflict correlates with an inability to soothe the self and the partner.

3. In discordant marriages couples tend to engage in negative attribution, or negative sentiment override. In happy marriages a spouse's behavior perceived as negative is likely to be attributed to a momentary condition ("He was just tired"). In discordant marriages a negative attribution tends to be assigned to positively perceived behaviors ("He's just in a good mood because he had a big week at work," or "He's just buttering me up so he can . . . "). Pervasive negative sentiment toward the spouse and the marriage cause couples to mentally override behaviors that seem inconsistent with overall negative perceptions.

4. Behaviors that tend to recur in discordant marriages are criticism, defensiveness, and contempt.

    a. A specific sequence of negative behavior called the wife demand–husband withdraw or wife pursuer–husband distancer pattern has been repeatedly researched. Psychophysiologic studies have suggested males trying to persuade their wives show a significant increase in systolic blood pressure before and during discussion, which is accompanied by increased anger. It has been hypothesized that the discomfort of these physiologic effects combined with the influence of socialization may account for the tendency of males to withdraw in spousal arguments.

    b. According to studies, females experience more disruption of endocrine and immune functions in discordant marriages.

Key Signs and Symptoms

- Pervasive negativity
- Negative reciprocity
- Distress-maintaining attributions
- Wife demand–husband withdraw pattern
- Recurring behaviors: criticism, defensiveness, and contempt

Tests

1. Temperament differences may lead to discord, particularly when one partner believes his or her temperament style is "right" and the partner's style is "wrong." Therapists may use temperament assessment instruments such as the Meyers-Briggs Type Indicator or the Taylor-Johnson Temperament Analysis Profile to interpret differences to the couple.

2. If one or both partners appears to be suffering from personality pathology, an instrument such as the Minnesota Multiphasic Personality Inventory-2 or the Millon Clinical Multiaxial Inventory-2 may be employed diagnostically.

3. Therapists also use instruments aimed at assessing couple behavior, such as the Marital Interaction Coding System or Olson's PAIR.

Key Tests

- Temperament tests
- Personality instruments
- Marital behavior inventories

Treatment

Research findings in the area of marital therapy suggest positive treatment outcomes across different types of treatment. There is also some evidence in the literature that there may be considerable overlap in actual treatment practices across orientations. Studies suggest there tends to be a short-term decrease in marital distress with therapy, and that more studies need to be conducted to determine the long-term efficacy of marital therapy.

1. Several of the more common treatments include behavioral marital therapy, cognitive-oriented marital therapy, emotion-focused marital therapy, psychodynamic treatment models, and structured systemic therapies. Each of the different orientations is based upon specific assumptions about how negative behavior becomes entrenched and about how people learn. Therapists across different orientations tend to focus on communication and problem solving in the context of their particular orientation.

    a. A behavioral marital therapist might use exercises to change a discordant marital dynamic, such as a specific communication strategy, contingency contracting, or prescribing shared positive experiences. An example of a behavioral marital therapy communication exercise might be to have one partner state a problem or explain an emotional wound and to have the other partner repeat what was said in his or her own words. This process would continue until the wounded partner felt the other partner truly heard and understood his or her distress. Then the roles would be reversed.

b. Cognitive therapists focus on perceptions such as negative attribution, and on underlying assumptions, called "core beliefs," of which the individual is often not consciously aware. In cognitive-oriented marital therapy, couples are taught to look beneath what is expressed in their negative communications. For example, bullying behavior may arise from the belief that the individual is actually weak and likely to be overwhelmed in interpersonal relationships. When the bullying partner uncovers and acknowledges this vulnerability, more adaptive ways of feeling strong and effective can be adopted in the relationship.

c. Emotion-focused couples therapy trains couples to identify and communicate about the emotions underlying problematic behavior. The different marriage encounter–type programs fall in this category. Couples learn to identify feelings underlying behaviors and communicate in a pattern, "I feel __ because __."

d. Some couples therapies are based on psychodynamic models. Insight-oriented marital therapy involves working with conflicted emotional processes in one or both of the partners, between the two partners, and in the larger family system. Some psychodynamic couple's therapies are based on developmental models of marriage that mirror developmental stages of the individual. Bader and Pearson have a model based on Mahler's early stages of development. Their therapy approach involves facilitating intrapersonal development while maintaining the integrity of the bond through the challenges of growth and change.

e. Family systems and structural therapies made seminal contributions to work with couples and families. The focus of treatment in these methods is on the family system and how the dysfunctional structure of the marriage is being maintained in the service of some need of the couple or family unit.

2. Research suggests that concurrent individual therapy or concurrent sex therapy does not interfere with successful outcomes in couples' therapy. Before making a referral to sex therapy, it is important to rule out the possibility that the sexual dysfunction is the symptom of a narcissistic vulnerable alliance. In the narcissistic vulnerable marriage, secondary sexual problems tend to ameliorate when emotional wounds are healed. This healing process can take place with as simple an intervention as one partner expressing sincere understanding of the other's hurt and apologizing.

Key Treatment Modalities

- Behavioral marital therapy
- Cognitive-oriented marital therapy
- Emotion-focused marital therapy
- Psychodynamic treatment models
- Structured systemic therapies

Follow-Up

Scheduling a follow-up session for a "tune-up" is recommended because of the lack of definitive research on long-term treatment results of marital therapy. One theory suggests that couples who have difficulty soothing themselves and each other may derive this soothing function from the therapist during treatment rather than solidly developing the skills themselves. Although not all couples will agree to return several months to a year after initial treatment has ended, it is an advisable practice to recommend.

Bibliography

Bader E, Pearson PT: In Quest of the Mythical Mate: A Developmental Approach to Diagnosis and Treatment in Couples Therapy. New York, Bruner/Mazel Publishers, 1988.

Gottman JM: Psychology and the study of marital processes. Annu Rev Psychol 1998;49:169–197.

Lebow JL: Research assessing couple and family therapy. Annu Rev Psychol 1995;46:27–57.

Smueli A, Clulow C: Marital therapy: definition and development. Curr Opin Psychiatry 1997;10:247–250.

Wallerstein JS: The Good Marriages: How and Why Love Lasts. Boston, Houghton Mifflin Company, 1995.

330 Domestic Violence

Howard A. Holtz

Etiology

1. Power imbalance in intimate adult relationships often reflects historical and present-day gender bias. Subjugation of women or misogyny in society can be reflected in interpersonal relationships; that is, the private may mirror the public.

2. Male moral development and socialization are marked by absolute principles (right and wrong), taking control, and action, while women typically develop more contextual ethics and collaborative and emotional processing skills. These differences may help explain why women are so often the recipients and men the perpetrators of domestic violence.

3. Despite these important sex differences, female-to-male and homosexual domestic violence does occur. However, male-to-female domestic violence is the major public health problem.

4. Observing violence in one's family or community or in repeated cultural exposures may model behavior or even teach that violence often works to achieve one's goals.

5. Alcohol and other drugs may be a permissive factor and are commonly associated with episodes of domestic violence, but are not thought to be causal.

Symptoms

1. The main risk factor is being a woman; females most frequently experience the effects of domestic violence perpetrated by men. Because domestic violence is so common (3 to 4 million adult women battered every year in the United States) and the symptoms so varied, all women should be asked about physical, emotional, and sexual abuse in the social history. Women who state they are not currently in a relationship are not protected from domestic violence. In fact, being single, separated, or divorced is associated with a higher risk.

2. The response to domestic violence may manifest as chronic pain, headaches, functional gastrointestinal (GI) or gynecologic symptoms (irritable bowel, pelvic pain), or musculoskeletal complaints. These somatic presentations are thought to occur more commonly in battered women because of the stress of living in violent relationships. Sensorineural hearing loss, bruises, soft-tissue swelling, fractures, and "spontaneous" abortions may result directly from physical abuse. Before *any* psychiatric diagnosis is given to a woman, especially panic disorder, post-traumatic stress disorder, depression, personality disorder, dysthymia, generalized anxiety disorder, or somatization disorder, one must ask about a history of domestic violence. The diagnosis often changes from "major depression" to "major depression secondary to domestic violence."

Key Symptoms

- Chronic pain
- Headache
- Functional GI, gynecologic, musculoskeletal complaints

Clinical Findings

There are no pathognomonic physical signs. Most injuries are non–life-threatening soft-tissue injuries. The lack of findings to support an organic disease process should prompt the physician to ask about domestic violence as an underlying social cause of the patient's complaints.

Key Sign

None or repeated soft-tissue injuries

Laboratory Tests

1. Occasionally, occult trauma can be detected radiographically (i.e., healed fractures, bony fragments, or calcification from previous internal bleeding); however, the most useful diagnostic tests are questions in the history.

2. Screening questions: Does your partner ever lose his temper? What happens when he does? Have you ever been slapped, hit, or kicked by your partner? Are you ever afraid to speak your mind with your partner? Have you ever been forced to engage in sexual activity? Have you

ever had to call the police or obtain a restraining order against your partner?

3. Case-finding questions: I see many women who have problems similar to yours who have been humiliated or beaten at home; has this ever happened to you? Did someone do this to you?

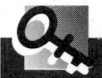

Key Test

Radiograph (or none)

Differential Diagnosis

1. Accidental trauma
2. Migraine or tension headache
3. Fibromyalgia
4. Irritable bowel syndrome, functional dyspepsia
5. Affective and anxiety disorders
6. Somatoform disorders, personality disorders
7. Dyspareunia, pelvic pain, endometriosis
8. Disorders associated with recurrent "spontaneous" abortion
9. Substance abuse (may be associated problem in abuser or victim)

Treatment

Medication

Do not overprescribe psychotropic drugs if domestic violence is the primary problem; occasionally, temporary symptom control with anxiety-reducing drugs or antidepressants is required. Make it clear in the medical record that the *primary* problem is domestic violence and not psychiatric.

Patient Education: ABCDES

1. *A* stands for *alone*. Acknowledge the loneliness and isolation your patient has most likely experienced. Tell her how common a problem violence against women is and how commonly you identify it in your practice. Validate the anguish that she and other women in abusive relationships endure in facing the problem alone.
2. *B* stands for *belief*. This is your belief that the violence is wrong, that it is a crime inside as well as outside the home. Articulate your conviction that violence is the responsibility of the batterer. Regardless of specific problems in a relationship, violence is not an acceptable solution. If her self-esteem has been seriously eroded by the abuser, this statement of belief correctly defines the problem. It categorizes the violence as a problem of the abuser and begins the process of empowering the woman.

3. *C* stands for *confidentiality*. Adult domestic violence is not child abuse, where the legal and developmental incompetence of the victim requires providers to report to public protective agencies. Unless your state has a specific domestic violence mandatory reporting statute, let the patient know that it is important to document the findings regarding domestic violence in the chart but that the information will not be released or disclosed without her permission. Explain that as a "medicolegal" document, her medical record can be very helpful in child custody and divorce proceedings, in obtaining restraining orders, or in criminal prosecutions, if pursued in the future.

4. *D* stands for *documentation*. As noted above, the medical record can be pivotal in future court decisions. Even when women are unable to admit that they have been battered, it is appropriate to make an assessment of battering if this is the most likely diagnosis:

"The pattern and frequency of injuries, as well as the anxiety demonstrated by the patient when discussing her husband, are characteristic of battered women syndrome."

Avoid pejorative negative descriptors and psychiatric labels, such as "hysterical" or "borderline." The emotional reaction of being out of control is a logical reflection of what the woman experienced. Women may more accurately be described as frightened, trembling, angry, anxious, crying, or re-experiencing a traumatic event, but, most important, the reaction must be described as secondary to the domestic violence.

5. *E* stands for *education*.

a. It is imperative that women be given referrals to community resources. Battered women's shelters often provide much more than emergency shelter. They often provide 24-hour hotline numbers, non-resident counseling and support groups, programs for children who have witnessed their mother's abuse, and programs for batterers. Some provide legal advocacy for victims and community education for professionals and their staffs. Women's organizations, coalitions for battered women, hospital-based programs, and government-sponsored victim's assistance programs also may provide these and other services.

b. Referrals to private mental health providers must be based on their expertise and appreciation of the dynamics of domestic violence.

The consultants' professional group (social worker, counselor, psychologist, psychiatrist) is less important than their knowledge of domestic violence. Couples counseling is generally inappropriate and a potentially dangerous therapy in relationships characterized by power imbalance. If a shelter or coalition cannot recommend a counselor/therapist, it is important to question potential consultants about their approach to domestic violence victims. Do they express a strong *belief*, as noted above, or do they tend to practice a form of victim blaming by exploring the victim's personality to look for provocative or facilitating traits?

   c. Legal options, such as the availability of temporary restraining orders, also can be discussed. Excellent patient education pamphlets are available and can be displayed in waiting rooms, bathrooms, and examining areas.

6. *S* stands for *safety*.

   a. A safety plan is an essential aspect of the patient encounter. A quick escape plan should be rehearsed, similar to a fire drill. If it is feasible, advise the woman to hide important documents, money, an extra set of car keys, clothes, and meaningful items for the children for quick getaways. Risk increases when there is concomitant sexual abuse, threats of death, a pattern of escalating violence, or when weapons are available. However, it is the woman who can best assess the potential for serious injury or death. If she tells you her husband will not respect a temporary restraining order and may attack her on the courthouse steps, believe her. Too many women have died because professionals have underestimated how an abuser will react to a changing domestic situation or legal restraints.

   b. If emergency shelter is not available, you can admit a patient to the hospital. The ICD diagnosis and code are Adult Physical Abuse: 995.81. The following safeguards should be in place to protect a victim admitted to the hospital: visitor restriction, patient information blackout, notification of hospital security, and contacting local police.

Follow-Up

Women often cannot extricate themselves from violent relationships because abusers continue to stalk them or threaten worse abuse if they leave; other reasons include financial or emotional barriers. Do not become angry and judgmental if a woman does not leave a violent relationship on your time schedule. Include domestic violence as a chronic problem and ask about it on follow-up visits; leave your door open as an informed advocate who can help her when she is ready to make changes.

Bibliography

Flitcraft AH, Hadley SM, Hendriks-Matthews MK, et al: Diagnostic and Treatment Guidelines on Domestic Violence. Chicago, American Medical Association, 1992.

Holtz HA, Esposito CN, Podhorin R: A domestic violence primer for clinicians. NJ Med 1994;91:848–850 (part 1), 853–854 (part 2).

McCauley J, Kern DE, Kolodner K, et al: The "battering syndrome": prevalence and clinical characteristics of domestic violence in primary care internal medicine practices. Ann Intern Med 1995;123:737–746.

McCauley J, Yurk RA, Jenckes MV, et al: Inside "Pandora's Box": Abused women's experiences with clinicians and health services. J Gen Intern Med 1998;13:549–555.

Rodriguez MA, Bauer HM, McLoughlin E, et al: Screening and intervention for intimate partner abuse: practices and attitudes of primary care physicians. JAMA 1999;282:468–474.

Sullivan CM, Bybee DI: Reducing violence using community-based advocacy for women with abusive partners. J Consult Clin Psychol 1999;67:43–53.

331 Sexual Assault

Harold J. May

Incidence

1. Sexual assault represents the most rapidly growing violent crime in the United States. Each year, over 700,000 women are sexually assaulted, yet only 50 per cent of rapes are reported.

2. Whereas 20 per cent of sexual assaults occurred by assailants unknown to the victim, the vast majority of assaults are committed by friends, acquaintances, or family members. Date rape has become increasingly common among adolescents, with 61 per cent of victims under age 18. Male victims represent five per cent of reported sexual assaults.

3. At least 20 per cent of adult women, 15 per cent of college women, and 12 per cent of adolescent women have experienced some form of sexual abuse or assault during their lifetimes. Sexual assault is also reported by 33 to 46 per cent of women who experience domestic violence by their husbands.

The Physician's Role

The role of the physician is not to determine if assault has occurred. Rape is a legal, not medical, term. The physician's responsibilities are

1. History documentation
2. Careful physical examination
3. Treatment of physical injuries
4. Collection of legal evidence
5. Prevention of sexually transmitted diseases (STDs)
6. Prevention of pregnancy
7. Psychological support
8. Arrangement for follow-up counseling

Any sexual assault should be considered a medical and psychological emergency, and physicians should become familiar with the rape kit available in their community and the accepted procedure for evidence collection. Obtain written formal consent or document any inability to provide consent, such as age, intoxication, or trauma.

Key Points—Safe Environment

- Place patient in quiet and private area
- Speak and move slowly
- Do not leave patient alone
- Ask permission to call a friend, family member, or victim advocate

Pertinent History

1. Identifying information of victim and assailant(s): age, race, stature
2. Circumstances of assault: date, time, place, number of assailants
3. Type of physical and sexual abuse; use of weapons, threats, restraints
4. Use of drugs or alcohol by victim or assailant
5. Type of intercourse or sexual act; ejaculation or urination
6. Activities since assault: bathing, douching, urination, defecation, clothing change
7. Sexual history: date of last voluntary coitus, infections
8. For males: homosexual, bisexual, and heterosexual experience
9. For females: last menstrual period, pregnancy history, contraception use, gynecologic surgery

Clinical Findings

1. Fewer than one third of assault victims seek medical care, yet 8 to 45 per cent of victims show external trauma. The most common sites of trauma are the mouth, throat, wrists, breasts, and thighs. Male victims may present with greater injury.

2. Even if the victim is uncertain about prosecution, physical evidence should still be collected. Evidence not collected within 48 to 72 hours is often invalid or inadmissible.

3. Items for collection on physical examination

   a. Each item of clothing placed in a separate paper bag

   b. Blood samples dictated by protocol, using equipment in the kit

c. Perform oral examination and collect saliva for secretor status

d. Collect fingernail scrapings from under all nails.

e. Document all physical injuries.

f. Use a Wood's light to inspect the patient.

g. Perform pelvic and rectal examination slowly and gently.

h. Record any flashbacks of the attack that may occur during the examination.

i. Collect samples of body, head, and pubic hair.

j. Collect pubic hair and other combings.

k. Vaginal (and anal) swab or aspirate: Use sterile cotton-tipped applicators; send for sperm detection, acid phosphatase, and other semen marker (p30 and MHS-5) analysis.

l. Ask the patient to supply a urine sample.

Sexually Transmitted Diseases

1. Counseling about and prophylaxis for STDs is crucial for the assault victim. Decisions about STD testing should be made based on the patient's medical and sexual history, sites of penetration and visual examination.

2. Although acquiring a STD is estimated to occur in 5 to 10 per cent of cases following an assault, approximately half of victims do not return for follow-up cultures or care. Therefore, the decision to test for STDs becomes a public health, legal, forensic, and medical issue. Rule out preexisting STDs if legal charges are being considered.

3. In some states, human immunodeficiency virus testing is mandated as part of the protocol.

STD Prophylaxis—Key Points

- The Centers for Disease Control and Prevention recommends antimicrobial therapy for chlamydia, gonorrhea, trichomoniasis, and bacterial vaginosis.

- Immunize against hepatitis B and give postexposure prophylaxis using hepatitis B immune globulin.

Pregnancy

1. Female patients should be counseled about options for pregnancy prevention. Should the physician have moral reservations, he or she is responsible for having someone else provide information concerning risks and interventions to prevent contraception.

2. Although pregnancy occurs at less than a 5 per cent rate in fertile victims, pregnancy testing is recommended for all women. The physician should document the woman's decision concerning postcoital contraception medication.

3. Common prophylaxis regimens include

a. Low-dose ethinyl estradiol–norgestrel, 4 tablets PO, followed by 4 tablets in 12 hours

b. Ethinyl estradiol–norgestrel, 2 tablets PO, followed by 2 tablets in 12 hours

c. Conjugated estrogens, 50 mg/day IV ×2 days or 30 mg/day PO ×5 days

Psychological Care of the Victim

1. Emotional sequelae following assault can be significant and long-lasting.

a. One third of victims report they have not recovered 4 to 6 years after the assault.

b. Hypervigilance, recurrent fears, and self-blame can lead to chronic anxiety or depression. Twenty-four per cent of victims meet *Diagnostic and Statistical Manual of Mental Disorders, Fourth Edition* (DSM-IV) criteria for major depression in the first few months following assault.

c. Suicide attempts or drug and alcohol abuse is present in 22 per cent of victims, with adolescents especially at risk.

d. Sexual dysfunction is reported in 25 to 40 per cent of victims 1 to 6 years postassault.

Common Emotional Sequelae

- Depression
- Post-traumatic stress disorder
- Somatization
- Sexual dysfunction
- Anxiety, panic, or phobic disorders

2. The rape trauma syndrome is a post-traumatic stress disorder.

a. The physician should discuss the normal psychological consequences of assault with the patient, partner, and family to ensure that the patient is involved in follow-up counseling.

b. The most important factor in recovery is social support.

c. Providing early treatment in a caring fashion, with attention to both the medical and psychological aspects of assault, can positively affect recovery.

Rape Trauma Syndrome

- Acute phase (few days to weeks): shock, disbelief, numbness, lability, feelings of violation

- Reorganization phase (months to years): adjustment, integration, recovery

Bibliography

American Academy of Pediatrics, Committee on Adolescence: sexual assault and the adolescent. Pediatrics 1994;94:761–765.

American Medical Association: Strategies for the Treatment and Prevention of Sexual Assault. Chicago, American Medical Association, 1995.

Braaten LS: Sexual dysfunction in sexually traumatized women. The Health Psychologist 1996;18:6–19.

Gostin LO, Lazzarini Z, Alexander D, et al: HIV testing, counseling and prophylaxis after sexual assault. JAMA 1994;271:1436–1444.

Young WW, Bracken AC, Goddard MA, et al: Sexual assault: review of a national model protocol for forensic and medical evaluation. Obstet Gynecol 1992;80:878–883.

332 Personality Disorders

Ruth Levine

Borderline Personality Disorder

Etiology

1. Biological theories
   a. Genetic basis: Borderline personality disorder (BPD) patients have more relatives with mood disorders than controls.
   b. Impulsivity and aggression have been associated with decreased serotonergic function.
   c. Affective instability has been tentatively linked to alterations in the cholinergic and noradrenergic systems.
2. Psychological/psychodynamic theories
   a. Impaired parenting
      (1) Impaired early attachment
      (2) Mismanagement of 2- to 3-year-old child's efforts at autonomy
      (3) Inattention to child's emotions and attitudes
      (4) Exaggerated maternal frustration that aggravates the child's anger
   b. Early trauma or neglect
      (1) Physical and/or sexual abuse
      (2) Traumatic early abandonment

Symptoms

1. Frantic efforts to avoid real or imagined abandonment
2. A pattern of unstable and intense interpersonal relationships characterized by alternating between extremes of idealization and devaluation
3. Identity disturbance: markedly and persistently unstable self-image or sense of self
4. Impulsivity in at least two areas that are potentially self-damaging (e.g., spending, sex, substance abuse, reckless driving, binge eating)
5. Recurrent suicidal behavior, gestures, or threats or self-mutilating behavior
6. Affective instability as a result of a marked reactivity of mood (e.g., intense episodic dysphoria, irritability, or anxiety usually lasting a few hours and only rarely more than a few days)
7. Chronic feelings of emptiness

8. Inappropriate, intense anger or difficulty controlling anger (e.g., frequent displays of temper, constant anger, recurrent physical fights)
9. Transient, stress-related paranoid ideation or severe dissociative symptoms

Differential Diagnosis

1. Axis I disorders
   a. Mood disorders: BPD has symptoms similar to those of major depression and bipolar disorder.
   b. Schizophrenia: BPD patients lack prolonged psychotic episodes and thought disorder.
2. Axis II disorders
   a. Schizotypal personality disorder: These patients show peculiar thinking, strange ideation, and ideas of reference, and lack the affective instability of BPD.
   b. Paranoid personality disorder: Patients can show anger and suspiciousness but lack the impulsivity, self-destructiveness, and abandonment concerns of BPD.
   c. Narcissistic personality disorder: patients have a stable and idealized self-image, whereas BPD patients have unstable identities and feelings of being evil or bad.
   d. Antisocial personality disorder: These patients display impulsivity and aggression for the purpose of obtaining materialistic gains, whereas the behavior of BPD patients is interpersonally oriented and for the purpose of gaining support.
   e. Histrionic personality disorder: These patients are dramatic, manipulative, and seductive, but lack the affective instability and behavioral dyscontrol of BPD.

Treatment

1. Psychotherapies
   a. Individual psychotherapy: Dynamic and supportive approaches emphasize developing a stable, trusting relationship with a therapist who does not retaliate to patient's anger and disruptive behaviors. Basic therapeutic principles

(1) Identify and treat co-morbid problems such as substance abuse or major depression.

(2) Differentiate nonlethal self-harm intentions from true suicidal ideation.

(3) Stress that the therapy is collaborative.

(4) Management of countertransference is essential.

(5) Have a low threshold for seeking consultation.

b. Cognitive-behavioral therapies

(1) Cognitive therapies target disturbed cognitions that develop early, have maladaptive consequences, and are self-perpetuating.

(2) Linehan's "dialectical behavior therapy" combines individual and group approaches to teach coping skills and attack self-destructive behaviors.

c. Family therapy

(1) Focuses on families in which there is either overinvolvement or neglect.

(2) Utilizes supportive and psychoeducational approaches.

(3) Therapist can help facilitate independence, communication, confrontation (when necessary), and reconciliation.

d. Group therapy: helpful in identifying maladaptive interpersonal behavior patterns, providing support, and enhancing coping skills and overall social functioning

e. Social skills training

(1) Focus is on improvement of interpersonal behavior.

(2) Helps patients see how their actions affect others.

2. Pharmacotherapy: useful for specific features of the disorder

a. Antidepressants

(1) Serotonin reuptake inhibitors: a first-line choice for impulsive aggression, depressed mood, and affective lability

(2) Monoamine oxidase inhibitors: effective but limited by side effects

(3) Tricyclic antidepressants: not recommended because of low efficacy and danger in overdose

b. Benzodiazepines: May help with anxiety but can be abused and cause disinhibition so should be used with extreme caution.

c. Mood stabilizers (lithium, carbamazepine, and valproic acid): May help with affective lability and impulsivity.

d. Antipsychotics: May be helpful in low dosages for psychotic-like symptoms, anger, hostility, labile mood, and anxiety.

Follow-Up

1. Most psychotherapies take 3 to 5 years.

2. Pharmacotherapy should be closely monitored and tailored to specific symptoms.

Dependent Personality Disorder

Etiology

1. Psychological theories

a. Classic psychoanalytic theory: oral fixation

b. Object relations: Disruptions in infant-caregiver relationship lead to interference in the childhood task of separation-individuation.

c. Ethologic theory: Poor early bonding and subsequent doubt of an attachment figure's availability leads to anxious and dependent attachments.

2. Social learning models

a. Dependency of infancy and childhood is reinforced while independence is discouraged

b. Distortion of information processing so that individuals view themselves as powerless, helpless, and ineffective

c. Parental overprotectiveness and authoritarianism

Symptoms

1. Difficulty making everyday decisions without an excessive amount of advice and reassurance from others

2. Needs others to assume responsibility for most major areas of his or her life.

3. Difficulty expressing disagreement with others because of fear of loss of support or approval

4. Difficulty initiating projects or doing things on his or her own because of a lack of self-confidence in judgment or abilities rather than because of a lack of motivation or energy

5. Goes to excessive lengths to obtain nurturance and support from others, to the point of volunteering to do things that are unpleasant.

6. Feels uncomfortable or helpless when alone, because of exaggerated fears of being unable to care for himself or herself.

7. Urgently seeks another relationship as a source of care and support when a close relationship ends.

8. Unrealistic preoccupation with fears of being left to take care of himself or herself

Differential Diagnosis

1. Axis I disorders
   a. Anxiety disorders: Panic disorder or agoraphobic patients may become highly dependent. There are higher degrees of anxiety than found in dependent personality disorder (DPD) patients.
   b. Major depression: Patients may be very dependent during the course of their illness.
2. Axis II disorders
   a. Histrionic personality disorder: Relationships are superficial and for the purpose of obtaining attention. DPD relationships are more deep and longstanding.
   b. Borderline personality disorder: Both types of patients fear abandonment, but BPD relationships are more unstable, intense, and manipulative.
   c. Avoidant personality disorder (APD): Both types of patients lack self-confidence in social situations, but APD patients withdraw from relationships to avoid rejection.

Treatment

1. Psychotherapy: general issues
   a. DPD patients are more likely to seek and stay in treatment, leading to better prognosis than other patients with personality disorders.
   b. Transference and countertransference problems
      (1) Demands for direct help can lead therapist either to be too directive or to emotionally withdraw.
      (2) Attempts to have therapist take on responsibility can reinforce dependency and interfere with development of independent coping skills.
      (3) Patients may linger in therapy to maintain attachment to the therapist.
      (4) If a therapist pushes the patient to change a problem relationship, this may lead to panic or early termination of the therapy.
2. Individual dynamic psychotherapy
   a. A dependent transference is encouraged to promote emotional growth.
   b. Therapist promotes assertiveness and independent decision making.
3. Cognitive-behavioral therapy
   a. Promotion of accurate self-appraisal
   b. Emphasis on independence in problem solving and general behavior
4. Time-limited dynamic psychotherapy
   a. Useful in light of patients' reluctance to terminate
   b. Forces confrontation of anxieties regarding loss and independence.
5. Pharmacotherapy: recommended when there is a concurrent axis I disorder

Follow-Up

Therapist should remain available after active therapy is over.

 ## Bibliography

American Psychiatric Association: The Diagnostic and Statistical Manual of Mental Disorders, 4th ed. Washington, DC, American Psychiatric Press, 1994.

Bornstein RF: The dependent personality: developmental, social, and clinical perspectives. Psychol Bull 1992;112: 3–23.

Gunderson JG, Links P: Borderline personality disorder. In Gabbard GO (ed): Treatment of Psychiatric Disorders II, pp 2291–2309. Washington, DC, American Psychiatric Press, 1995.

Hirschfeld RMA, Shea MT, Weise R: Dependent personality disorder. J Pers Disord 1991;5:135–149.

Kaplan HI, Sadock BJ (eds): Synopsis of Psychiatry, 8th ed. Baltimore, Williams & Wilkins, 1998.

Perry JC: Dependent personality disorder. In Gabbard GO (ed): Treatment of Psychiatric Disorders II, pp 2355–2366. Washington, DC, American Psychiatric Press, 1995.

Phillips KA, Gunderson JG: Personality disorders. In Hales RE, Yudofsky SC, Talbott JA (eds): The American Psychiatric Press Textbook of Psychiatry, 2nd ed, pp 795–823. Washington, DC, American Psychiatric Press, 1997.

Trestman RL, DeVegvar M, Siever LJ: Treatment of personality disorders. In Schazberg AF, Nemeroff CB (eds): The American Psychiatric Textbook of Psychopharmacology, pp 753–768. Washington, DC, American Psychiatric Press, 1995.

333 Childhood Behavioral Problems

Laeth S. Nasir

Thumbsucking

1. About 50 per cent of normal children suck their thumbs persistently for some period of time. In most children, the behavior extinguishes itself as the child ages.
2. Most authorities recommend ignoring thumbsucking until the child is 5 or 6 years old. After that time, teasing by other children and problems with malocclusion of the teeth may cause problems.
3. Conditions such as herpetic whitlow, eczema, and chronic paronychia may necessitate intervention.

Treatment

1. Ignore behavior and reinforce the child for times that the thumb is out of the mouth. "Sticker charts" to monitor progress and provide positive reinforcement are recommended.
2. Aversive conditioning by applying bad-tasting substances on the thumb (e.g., "Thumzit") to remind the child not to suck his or her thumb
3. Occasionally the behavior is a "combination" habit (e.g., holding a blanket or twirling hair while sucking the thumb). Hiding the blanket or cutting hair short may extinguish the thumbsucking as well.
4. Rarely, dental or digital appliances are used to prevent thumbsucking.

Patient Education

1. Reassure the parents that this behavior is not associated with "mental problems" and has no prognostic significance for the future. As a rule, once the behavior is extinguished, "replacement" behaviors do not occur.
2. Encourage the caregivers to monitor the child's environment to ascertain whether situations such as boredom or frustration are contributing to the problem.

Key Treatment

- Reinforce child for times that the thumb is out of the mouth.
- Aversive conditioning
- Rarely, the use of appliances to prevent thumbsucking

Breath Holding

Etiology

Dysregulation of the autonomic nervous system is thought to be the etiology of breath-holding spells. However, some authors have noted the frequent coexistence of these spells with disturbed family dynamics. A familial predisposition has been proposed, and an association with iron deficiency anemia has been noted. Virtually all patients are younger than 24 months at the onset of this disorder.

Symptoms

1. Breath holding is seen after an episode that provokes or frightens a child between the neonatal period and 5 or 6 years of age.
2. Typically, the episode is heralded by a shrill cry, then breathlessness, followed by onset of pallor ("pallid spell" that corresponds to vasodepressor syncope) or cyanosis ("cyanotic spell"). The child may lose consciousness, followed by hypotonia and occasionally brief myoclonic jerks.
3. Urinary incontinence may occur.

Key Signs

- Cyanosis or pallor that follows a provoking stimulus
- May or may not progress to loss of consciousness and hypotonia.
- Loss of consciousness may be followed by myoclonic jerks.
- Todd's paralysis is absent, but child may appear drowsy for several minutes after episode.

Clinical Findings

1. Physical examination is normal.
2. Reproduction of episode in 25 per cent of cyanotic spells and 60 to 78 per cent of pallid spells with gentle bilateral ocular compression for 10 seconds.

History

1. Precise description of the episode: Are "spells" always preceded by emotional upset?
2. Family history of breath-holding spells
3. History of anemia
4. Inquiry into parent-child and sibling interactions

Laboratory Tests

None required with typical history and normal physical examination.

Differential Diagnosis

1. Seizures: no history of emotional stimulus preceding episode. Loss of consciousness and tone occur first, followed by cyanosis.
2. Arrhythmias: Can usually be detected by history and physical examination. Electrocardiogram can detect long Q-T syndrome.
3. Brain stem lesions (e.g., such as tumor, Arnold-Chiari malformation, Rett's syndrome): These rare causes are usually detectable on history and physical examination.

Treatment

1. Placing the child in a safe place and avoiding positive interactions with the child for a specified period after the episode
2. Treatment of iron deficiency anemia, if present
3. In refractory cases of "pallid spells" (vasodepressor syncope), oral atropine sulfate 0.01 mg/kg/dose every 6 hours
4. Piracetam (an orphan drug) has been reported to be effective in the treatment of cyanotic spells.

Patient Education

1. Reassure parents that the episodes are not dangerous and do not represent seizures.
2. Avoid reinforcing behavior by "giving in" to the child's demands inappropriately to avoid "spells."
3. Fifty per cent of cases resolve by 4 years of age, and 90 per cent by 6 years of age.

Key Treatment

- Reassurance
- Avoid inadvertent reinforcement of episodes.
- Treatment of associated iron deficiency anemia
- Atropine sulfate for refractory vasodepressor syncope

Sleep Problems

Twenty-five to 50 per cent of children between the ages of 6 and 12 months suffer from sleep disturbances. Although night waking and difficult bedtime "settling" are most common, other sleep disorders, such as night terrors and somnambulism (sleep walking), are frequently seen in older children.

Sleep Refusal

Symptoms

1. Refusal to go to bed (or stay in bed)
2. Repeated requests for snacks or trips to the bathroom after bedtime
3. Excessive anxiety at bedtime, often expressed by reports of monsters or strange noises

Key Symptoms

- Refusal to stay in bed
- Excessive anxiety at bedtime
- Bedtime tantrums

Differential Diagnosis

1. Separation anxiety
2. Delayed sleep phase
3. Part of a pattern of oppositional behavior

Treatment

1. For all patients: the establishment of good sleep hygiene, by avoiding frightening, vigorous, or exciting activities prior to bedtime, establishing regular sleep and wake times, consistent nap schedules, and bedtime routines.
2. Children should be put to bed while awake. The bedroom environment should be conducive to sleep.
3. Sleep-phase disorder: Allow child to fall asleep when he or she becomes drowsy, then gradually "push back" the child's bedtime by 5 or 10

minutes a night until the desired bedtime is reached.

4. Separation anxiety: Leaving the bedroom door open or using a nightlight may be useful. In some cases, it may be necessary for the parent to sit quietly in the child's room until the child sleeps.

5. Oppositional behavior: Firmly return the child to bed without engaging in argument or expressing anger toward the child.

Key Treatment

- Good sleep hygiene
- Avoiding positive reinforcement of undesired behavior

Night Waking

Most children begin sleeping through the night at around 6 months of age. About 25 per cent may have persistent problems with nighttime awakening and inability to spontaneously resume sleep through the first year of life. Night waking usually comes to the physician's attention as a problem when parental expectations and the child's need for sleep are discordant.

Key Symptom

Inability to resume sleep after a spontaneous nighttime awakening

Differential Diagnosis

1. Acute medical illness (e.g., otitis media)
2. Hunger
3. Family stress

Treatment

1. Institute sleep hygiene measures (as above).
2. Encouraging the parents not to respond immediately to crying, and to check briefly to make sure the child is safe. The parent should avoid picking up or interacting with the child. Further crying should be ignored, or brief checking on the child may continue, with increasing intervals between each check.

Key Treatment

- Good sleep hygiene
- Avoiding positive reinforcement of crying

Bibliography

Blum NJ, Carey WB: Sleep problems among infants and young children. Pediatr Rev 1996;17:87–92.

DiMario FJ: Breath holding spells in childhood. Am J Dis Child 1992;146:125–131.

Peterson J, Schneider P: Oral habits: a behavioral approach. Pediatr Clin North Am 1991;44:1724–1728.

Rosenberg MD: Thumbsucking. Pediatr Rev 1995;16:73–74.

334 Attention-Deficit Hyperactivity Disorder

Esther Entin

Attention-deficit hyperactivity disorder (ADHD) is a neuropsychological syndrome that, although most commonly identified in school-age children, is found in preschool children, adolescents, and adults. Neurobiologic dysfunctions, both anatomic and biochemical, are thought to play significant roles in its etiology and manifestations.

Symptoms and Signs

1. Diagnostic criteria for childhood ADHD are specified in the *Diagnostic and Statistical Manual of Mental Disorders, Fourth Edition* (DSM-IV). (Diagnostic criteria for ADHD diagnosed in adulthood: Wender Utah Rating Scale; see Bibliography)

   a. Either inattention or hyperactivity-impulsivity must be present.

   (1) *Inattention*: Six (or more) of the following symptoms have persisted for at least 6 months to a degree that is maladaptive and inconsistent with developmental level.

   (a) Often fails to give close attention to details or makes careless mistakes in schoolwork, work, or other activities.

   (b) Often has difficulty sustaining attention in tasks or play activities.

   (c) Often does not seem to listen when spoken to directly.

   (d) Often does not follow through on instructions and fails to finish schoolwork, chores, or duties in the workplace (not caused by oppositional behavior or failure to understand instructions).

   (e) Often has difficulty organizing tasks and activities.

   (f) Often avoids, dislikes, or is reluctant to engage in tasks that require sustained mental effort (such as schoolwork or homework).

   (g) Often loses things necessary for tasks or activities (e.g., toys, school assignments, pencils, books, or tools).

   (h) Is often easily distracted by extraneous stimuli.

   (i) Is often forgetful in daily activities.

   (2) *Hyperactivity-impulsivity*: Six (or more) of the following symptoms have persisted for at least 6 months to a degree that is maladaptive and inconsistent with developmental level.

   (a) Hyperactivity

   (i) Often fidgets with hands or feet or squirms in seat.

   (ii) Often leaves seat in classroom or in other situations in which remaining seated is expected.

   (iii) Often runs about or climbs excessively in situations in which it is inappropriate (in adolescents or adults, may be limited to subjective feelings of restlessness).

   (iv) Often has difficulty playing or engaging in leisure activities quietly.

   (v) Is often "on the go" or often acts as if "driven by a motor."

   (vi) Often talks excessively.

   (b) Impulsivity

   (i) Often blurts out answers before questions have been completed.

   (ii) Often has difficulty awaiting turn.

   (iii) Often interrupts or intrudes on others (e.g., butts into conversations or games).

   b. Some hyperactive-impulsive or inattentive symptoms that caused impairment were present before age 7 years.

   c. Some impairment from the symptoms is present in two or more settings (e.g., at school or work and at home).

   d. There must be clear evidence of clinically significant impairment in social, academic, or occupational functioning. The symptoms do not occur exclusively during the course of a pervasive developmental disorder, schizophrenia, or other psychotic disorder and are not better accounted for by another mental disorder (e.g., mood disorder, anxiety disorder, dissociative disorder, or personality disorder).

2. Classification depends on predominant symptoms:
   a. Attention-Deficit/Hyperactivity Disorder, Combined type
   b. Attention-Deficit/Hyperactivity Disorder, Predominantly Inattentive Type
   c. Attention-Deficit/Hyperactivity Disorder, Predominantly Hyperactive-Impulsive Type

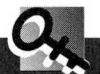

Key Symptoms

- Inattention
- Impulsivity
- Overactivity

Clinical Presentations

1. Vary with environment, age, and developmental stage; change through the life cycle.
2. Are described in DSM IV diagnostic criteria.
3. Other manifestations: cognitive impulsivity, impersistence, mental fatigue, absence of quality control, behavioral unpredictability, affective lability, insensitivity to feedback, diminished reinforceability, insatiability, egocentricity

Differential Diagnosis

Includes many conditions that can be primary diagnoses that mimic ADHD, that develop secondary to ADHD, or that are co-morbid with ADHD.

1. Medical, including
   a. Neurologic conditions (e.g., post-traumatic encephalopathy, seizures)
   b. Endocrine abnormalities (e.g., thyroid conditions)
   c. Congenital or acquired syndromes (e.g., fragile X syndrome, fetal alcohol syndrome, Tourette's syndrome)
   d. Toxic ingestions (e.g., lead)
2. Developmental abnormalities, including
   a. Learning disabilities/processing disorders
   b. Developmental delay/mental retardation
   c. Autism/pervasive developmental delay
   d. Sensory impairment: hearing/vision
3. Emotional/psychiatric, including
   a. Conduct disorder
   b. Oppositional defiant disorder
   c. Depression
   d. Anxiety
   e. Substance abuse
   f. Temperament
4. Environmental, including
   a. Chaotic/disruptive/dysfunctional family
   b. Inappropriate school placement (e.g., bored gifted child)

Tests

Evaluation must be multifaceted and must explore co-morbid and secondary conditions.

1. Physical/neurologic/extended neurologic examination (e.g., stressed gaits, timed motor output tasks, looking for "soft signs" of neuromaturational delay)
2. Hearing/vision screening
3. Developmental assessment
4. Complete patient and family history, including family history of ADHD and learning disabilities
5. Psychological assessment: screen for anxiety, depression, poor self-esteem
6. Psychosocial assessment: parent and family functioning, peer relationships, impact of ADHD behaviors on patient and family
7. Psychoeducational assessment: cognitive ability, achievement, language processing—neuropsychological testing
8. School assessment: classroom environment
9. Rating scales: Used by teachers, parents, and patients; provide objective measurements of symptoms for diagnosis and for monitoring therapy. Examples:
   a. Psychosocial functioning/ADHD behaviors: Achenback Child Behavior Check List, Conners Scales for teachers and parents, AN-SER, Yale Children's inventory, DSM IV questionnaire
   b. Anxiety: Children's Manifest Anxiety Scale
   c. Depression: Children's Depression Inventory
   d. Home and school behavior: Home/School Situations Questionnaire

Treatment

Treatment must be multimodal and tailored to the needs of the child and family and should address ADHD behaviors, co-morbid and secondary conditions, and psychosocial impact of ADHD.

1. Education and demystification of parents, family members, teachers/coaches, patient
   a. Reading/reference material

b. Support groups

c. Office visits

2. Psychosocial/behavioral interventions

a. Individual counseling for ADHD patients

(1) To help with low self-esteem

(2) If complicated by depression/anxiety

(3) To develop problem-solving skills, self-management, and stress reduction strategies

(4) Social skills training to improve peer relationships

b. Family counseling

(1) If family dysfunction is contributing to ADHD symptoms

(2) If ADHD has caused significant family disruption

3. School-based interventions

a. Academic support/tutoring

b. Accommodations based on Section 504 of the Rehabilitation Act of 1973

(1) Allows for free appropriate education: an education comparable to the education provided to nonhandicapped students.

(2) Does not require "special education" designation to qualify; a formal individualized education program (IEP) is not required.

(3) Allows for reasonable accommodations, including modifications to regular programs and provision of different programs, such as shorter assignments, taped textbooks, changes in test-taking requirements, seating adjustments, aides or readers.

c. Management of co-morbid learning disabilities

d. Facilitation of medication dosing during school hours

e. Ongoing surveillance of progress via teacher rating scales and conferences

4. Home-based interventions

a. Modification of environments and routines

b. Behavioral management techniques

5. Medication (Table 334–1)

a. General considerations

(1) Should be used in conjunction with other interventions.

(2) Should be used to modify target behaviors and administered when such behaviors are likely to significantly interfere with functioning.

(3) Should be started on a short-term trial basis.

(4) Should be monitored for efficacy and side effects.

(5) Should be periodically reassessed via objective measures such as rating scales.

(6) Selection based on primary diagnosis, co-morbid conditions, and contraindications.

b. Stimulant medications (methylphenidate, dexedrine, pemoline) most commonly used.

(1) Decrease distractibility and impulsivity and disinhibition, enhance ability to focus.

(2) Common side effects: appetite suppression, insomnia, rebound irritability, emotional lability, tics

(3) Preparations

(i) Methylphenidate (Ritalin): rapid onset, short acting but also available in long-acting, sustained release preparations

(ii) Dexedrine and Adderal (dexedrine and three amphetamines combined): longer half life than methylphenidate and requires less frequent dosing. Dexedrine is the only stimulant approved for children 3 to 6 years of age.

(iii) Pemoline (Cylert): Concern about liver function has decreased the popularity; requires regular blood tests to check for liver abnormalities.

c. α-Adrenergic agents: clonidine (Catapres) and guanfacine (Tenex)

(1) Especially effective with hyperactivity, impulsivity, co-morbid tic disorders or Tourette's syndrome, conduct disorder, or obsessive compulsive disorder.

(2) Decrease hyperarousal; may not be as effective in improving distractibility.

(3) May be first-line treatment or used in conjunction with methylphenidate.

(4) May cause somnolence, headache, dizziness, lightheadedness; may enhance central nervous system depression secondary to alcohol, barbiturates, and the like.

(5) Must be increased slowly up to desired dose and must be tapered when medication is withdrawn to avoid possible rebound phenomena.

(6) Contraindications: significant cardiovas-

TABLE 334–1. COMMONLY USED MEDICATIONS FOR ADHD

MEDICATION	DOSAGE RANGE	SIDE EFFECTS/REMEDY	EFFECTIVENESS
Methylphenidate (Ritalin) 5, 10, 20 mg	0.3–0.6 mg/kg per dose; short-acting	Loss of appetite (brief) Rebound; adjust dose. Sleep difficulty; adjust dose. Overfocused state, tics (rarely); lower dose.	67–96%
20 mg sustained release	Long-acting; 0.6–1.2 mg/kg/dose	Same as above; more complaints of stomach upset.	Not as effective sometimes (return to short-acting). Advantage: no dose in school, therefore better compliance.
Dextroamphetamine Dexedrine: 5 mg Spansules: 5, 10, 15 mg Dextrostat: 5 mg	0.15–0.3 mg/kg/dose	More loss of appetite. More overfocused.	Similar to methylphenidate, more side effects. Longer acting, may need only AM dose (even short-acting preparations). Less expensive; short-acting.
Pemoline (Cylert) (Not recommended)		Same as above. Some data suggest may trigger more tics. Liver function abnormalities.	Similar to methylphenidate.
Desipramine* (Norpramin)	25–100 mg	Cardiac in prepubertal, can cause prolonged Q-T; get baseline electrocardiogram and at intervals in all patients.	Can be effective; may be drug of choice for some adolescents.
Clonidine* (Catapres)	0.1–0.4 mg, usual 0.1–0.3 mg	Sleepiness or sleep disturbance, hypotension, dizziness.	Can be helpful adjunct, especially for impulsivity, tics.
Guanfacine* (Tenex)	0.1–0.4 mg	Similar to clonidine; sleep said to be less of a problem.	Similar to clonidine, longer half-life.
Dextroamphetamine saccharate and sulfate; amphetamine aspartate and sulfate (Adderall)	0.15–0.3 mg/kg/dose	Similar to Dexedrine	See Dexedrine

Adapted from Kiessling LS: Attention deficit hyperactivity disorder (ADHD). In: Rakel RE (ed): Conn's Current Therapy, p 915. Philadelphia, WB Saunders Company, 1999, with permission.
*Not approved by the Food and Drug Administration for this indication.

cular disease and known allergic reactions, depressive symptomatology or history of depression in patient or family

(7) Not approved by Food and Drug Administration for this indication

(8) Guanfacine has a longer plasma half-life than clonidine and is less sedating.

d. Tricyclic antidepressants: imipramine, desipramine, nortriptylene

(1) Can be used as second-line drug for ADHD or first line in patients with co-morbid depression or anxiety disorder.

(2) Contraindications: known hypersensitivity to tricyclic antidepressants, children or adolescents with cardiac conduction abnormalities, simultaneous administration or recent withdrawal (less than 2 weeks) of a monoamine oxidase inhibitor

(3) Cautions: May lower seizure threshold

and may activate psychotic process in schizophrenic patients.

(4) Must monitor electrocardiogram and drug levels.

(5) Several reported cases of sudden death in prepubertal patients taking desipramine. No consensus on this issue.

e. Newer antidepressants (bupropion, buspirone, paroxetine) can be useful in children with co-morbid anxiety and depression.

Key Treatment

- Education—patient, teacher, family
- Psychosocial intervention, behavioral management
- Stimulant medications
- Management of co-morbid conditions

Follow-Up

1. Should include monitoring of
   a. School performance (academic and behavioral) via teaching rating scales, report cards, parent and child reports, school visits
   b. Psychosocial functioning, including peer and family relationships, via parent and child interviews/rating scales
   c. Co-morbid conditions: medical/psychological/psychoeducational
   d. Medication side effects: Adjust dosing or change medications as necessary.
2. Re-evaluate periodically for emergence of new manifestations of ADHD or co-morbid conditions.

Bibliography

American Psychiatric Association: Diagnostic and Statistical Manual of Mental Disorders, 4th ed. Washington, DC, American Psychiatric Press, 1994.

Culbert T, Banez G, Reiff M: Children who have attention disorders: interventions. Pediatr Rev 1994;15:5–14.

Kelly D, Aylward G: Attention deficit in school-aged children and adolescents. Pediatr Clin North Am 1992;39:487–509.

Levine MD, Carey WB, Crocker AC: Developmental-Behavioral Pediatrics, 2nd ed. Philadelphia, WB Saunders Company, 1992.

Wender P: Attention Deficit Hyperactivity Disorder in Adults. New York, Oxford University Press, 1995.

335 Autism

Susan Hart-Hester

Etiology

1. Occurs once in every 1000 births (including pervasive developmental disorders and Asperger's syndrome).
2. Higher ratio of males diagnosed autistic (4:1).
3. No known cause for the disorder has been identified.
4. Several theories are offered for causation:
   a. Imbalance of serotonin that adversely affects β and α receptors
   b. Administration of antibiotics early in development
   c. Exposure to toxic chemicals
   d. Leaky-gut syndrome
   e. Genetic conditions

Symptoms

Behaviors associated with autism can be categorized into four areas of dysfunction:

1. *Language and communication problems*: little or no speech, delayed speech, normal development of speech then regression; echolalic; high-pitched, sing-song, or monotone voice; uses gestures to communicate.
2. *Socialization problems*: does not understand social cues, body language, facial expressions; treats people like objects; many lack affection or are affectionate on own terms.
3. *Sensory problems*: hyposensitive or hypersensitive to tactile and/or auditory stimulation; may engage in self-injurious behaviors and/or self-stimulatory behaviors.
4. *Other characteristics*: problems in sequencing and generalizing events and skills, may have strong ability in one area of development, poor discrimination between important and irrelevant information, difficulty making transitions, perseverates on objects/people/ideas.

Key Symptoms/Behaviors

- Inappropriate laughing/giggling
- Insensitivity to pain
- Little or no eye contact
- Spinning objects/self
- Ritualistic behaviors
- Inappropriate attachments
- Hyposensitive or hypersensitive
- Socially isolated
- Self-injurious behaviors
- Delayed speech or no speech

Clinical Findings

1. Classified within the *Diagnostic and Statistical Manual of Mental Disorders, Fourth Edition* (DSM-IV) category of pervasive developmental disorders.
2. Usually occurs within the first 3 years of life.
3. Is a syndrome of behaviors that exist along a continuum from mild to severe.

Key Signs

- Onset prior to age 3
- Social dysfunction
- Delayed speech or no speech development
- Stereotypic behaviors

Screening Tests

1. Behavior Observation Scale
2. Autism Screening Instrument for Education Planning
3. Autism Checklist
4. Childhood Autism Rating Scale (CARS)
5. Useful in describing and measuring movement abnormalities
   a. Abnormal Involuntary Movement Scale (AIMS)
   b. Abbreviated Dyskinesia Rating Scale (ADRS)

- Childhood Autism Rating Scale
- Parental observations
- Teacher observations

Differential Diagnosis

Accurate diagnosis requires a developmental history assessing specific autistic behaviors concomitant with cognitive abilities.

1. *Rett's disorder*: only in females; after age 4— head growth deceleration; awkward gait; limited social interactions early in development

2. *Childhood disintegrative disorder*: later onset following normal development; deterioration of acquired abilities

3. *Asperger's syndrome*: pronounced deficit in social skills; normal language development; often called high-functioning autism.

4. *Landau Kleffner's syndrome*: higher cognitive functioning; identified electroencephalographic pattern

5. *Childhood schizophrenia*: impaired thought patterns; manifests after normal developmental period.

6. *Elective mutism*: selective speech in identified settings (home/school); use of gestures

Treatment

Most successful approaches begin with early identification. A number of approaches have proven successful:

1. *Behavioral intervention*: Focuses on modifying specific behaviors.

2. *Sensory integration therapy*: Incorporates activities that involve each of the sensory receptor areas, enabling the autistic child to develop appropriate responses to his or her environment.

3. *Auditory integration therapy (AIT)*: Utilizes the auditory tract to desensitize the autistic child to environmental stimuli. This approach has proven to enhance social interactions and increase attention span, as well as improve gross and fine motor skills.

4. *Pressure therapy*: Utilizes deep pressure against the body or specific areas of the body to reduce anxiety, tension, and self-stimulating behaviors. Studies have documented the calming effects of deep pressure therapy for persons with autism.

5. *Psychopharmacologic therapies*: four categories of commonly used drugs
   a. *Dopaminergic drugs*: Initially autism was

thought to be a form of childhood schizophrenia; therefore, the antipsychotic drugs or dopamine antagonists were used.
   (1) Typical: Effective but have limited long-term use because of adverse effects (i.e., extrapyramidal symptoms [EPS] and tardive dyskinesia)
   (2) Atypical: May yield effective results in decreasing agitation and hyperactivity with fewer risks of EPS adverse effects. Long-term use should be routinely evaluated.

   b. *Serotonergic drugs*: Studies have shown that between 40 and 70 per cent of autistic individuals have hyperserotonemia. Serotonin reuptake inhibitors are effective in lessening repetitive, perseverative, and aggressive behaviors.

   c. *Opiate antagonists*: Varied results in the treatment of self-injurious behaviors. The safety and efficacy with long-term administration of opiate antagonists are not yet known.

   d. *Noradrenergic drugs*: Research has suggested the efficacy of using β-blockers to decrease aggressiveness and self-injury in autistic individuals.
   (1) Clonidine and propranolol: May have limited mediating effect on hyperactivity and irritability in autistic persons; however, further study is needed.
   (2) Methylphenidate (Ritalin): Can reduce target symptoms of inattention, impulsivity, and overactivity in higher functioning autistics and adolescents with autistic disorder; however, its use may worsen stereotypies, impair cognition, and increase irritability.

Because of the complexity of the autism syndrome and the tremendous variance in severity and intensity of behaviors across settings, treatments should be tailored to the individual.

6. *Other biomedical interventions*: Alternative approaches have been investigated:
   (1) *Antifungal agents*: effective when the autistic disorder is yeast-related (*Candida albicans*)
   (2) *Vitamins*: Ascorbic acid (vitamin C), niacinamide, pantothenic acid, and pyridoxone (B_6) have been studied. (*Note*: High-dose pyridoxone therapy can deplete magnesium and other B-complex vitamins.)
   (3) *Food allergies*: Avoidance of foods that

cause allergy response has shown varied success.

Patient Education

1. Crucial to the successful management of the autistic child is parental education.
2. Successful treatment involves consistent implementation of therapies at home and at school.
3. Generally, treatment involves combination therapies: behavior management, integration training, and pyschopharmacologic medicines.

Key Treatment

- Behavior therapy
- Psychopharmacology
- Sensory integration therapy
- Patient education

Follow-Up

Autism is a lifelong developmental disability; therefore, continued monitoring of patient progress is encouraged.

Bibliography

American Psychiatric Association: Diagnostic and Statistical Manual of Mental Disorders, 4th ed, pp 65–78. Washington, DC, American Psychiatric Press, 1994.

Autism Society of America: Fact sheet. Bethesda, MD, Autism Society of America, 1977.

Edelson S, Edelson M, Kerr D, et al: Behavioral and physiological effects of deep pressure on children with autism: A pilot study evaluating the efficacy of Grandin's Hug Machine. Am J Occup Ther 1999;53:145–152.

Gilman J, Tuchman R: Autism and associated behavioral disorders: pharmacotherapeutic intervention. Ann Pharmacother 1995;29:47–56.

Potenza M, McDougle C: New findings on the causes and treatment of autism. Medscape Mental Health 1997; 2(8).

Rapin I: Autism. N Engl J Med 1997;337:97–104.

336 Somatoform Disorders

Dale A. Matthews

Etiology

1. Predisposing factors
   a. Frequent or severe illness during childhood
   b. Overprotective parents and family
   c. Personal or family histories of psychiatric illness, alcoholism, and drug addiction, physical and sexual abuse, divorce, and antisocial behavior
   d. Lower educational attainment and socioeconomic class
2. Precipitating factors
   a. Stressful life events (e.g., bereavement, acute physical illness or injury)
   b. Overwork or strenuous activity prior to the illness (i.e., "burnout")
3. Perpetuating factors
   a. Development and maintenance of the "sick role"
   b. Poor self-esteem, impaired social and occupational skills, ongoing disability claims (and other forms of "secondary gain")
   c. Physicians' somatization through excessive diagnostic testing or an unwillingness to explore psychosocial concerns

Symptoms

Recurrent somatic symptoms occur in multiple organ systems that are unexplained by medical illness or known pathophysiologic mechanisms; or, if disease is present, the symptoms are in excess of what would be expected.

Key Symptoms

- Chest pain
- Abdominal pain
- Back pain
- Headaches
- Dysmenorrhea
- Fatigue
- Weakness
- Paralysis
- Dizziness
- Palpitations
- Nausea
- Vomiting
- Anorexia
- Food intolerance
- Sexual indifference

Clinical Findings

1. Multiple, diffuse, or vague complaints; fear and conviction of serious illness; and preoccupation with, or exaggeration of bodily symptoms.
2. Usually seen in general medical or surgical settings: patients generally eschew psychiatrists. Extensive use of medical care system. Patients seek care assiduously, yet are often highly dissatisfied with their care. Many doctors are consulted (often concurrently) and patients undergo many types of diagnostic tests and treatments (including multiple medications and surgeries) to little avail. Iatrogenic illness (e.g., surgical complications and increased side effects from medications) is common.
3. Often, a histrionic personality style is found with dramatic, emotional, seductive and/or shallow affect and vague, inconsistent, and/or contradictory history of presenting illness.
4. A low pain threshold, heightened sensitivity to stimuli, excessive fear of illness, aging, and death, and overconcern about appearance may be found. Self-esteem is low. Many are overly self-conscious, vulnerable to stress, and prone to excessive self-criticism and feelings of shame and guilt, and may believe that they deserve punishment. They tend to be anxious, depressed, hostile, and dependent.
5. The illness or symptom may have a symbolic meaning (e.g., deafness after "hearing bad news"), thereby serving as a means of communicating distress. Alexithymia (inability to express emotion in verbal terms) may be present. Patients may vigorously deny the role of psychological factors in the development of symptoms and disparage clinicians who propose a psychogenic etiology for their symptoms.

Key Signs

- Abnormal affect
- Nondermatomal pain
- Multiple tender points
- Voluntary weakness

Laboratory Tests

1. No laboratory findings are pathognomonic, although extensive testing is commonly per-

formed. If minor abnormalities are found, symptoms may be in excess of the usual clinical findings associated with that laboratory value. If significant abnormalities are found, organic illness must be considered.

2. Diagnostic restraint is advisable: tests should be done only when classic presentations of illness or objective signs of disease are found.

Key Tests

- Complete blood count with differential
- Sedimentation rate
- Chemistry panel
- Thyroid function tests
- Antinuclear antibodies
- Rheumatoid factor
- A 24-hour urine for coproporphyrins and porphobilinogen

Differential Diagnosis

1. The somatoform disorders include:
   a. Body dysmorphic disorder: preoccupation with some perceived defect in appearance
   b. Conversion disorder: loss or impairment of functioning suggestive of a physical disorder that is, instead, an expression of a psychological conflict or need
   c. Hypochondriasis: preoccupation with fear of having a serious disease
   d. Somatization disorder: a longstanding history of recurrent and multiple somatic complaints or belief that one is sickly
   e. Somatoform pain disorder: preoccupation with pain in the absence of adequate physical findings to account for the pain or its intensity
   f. Undifferentiated somatoform disorder: one or more physical complaints (e.g., fatigue) causing significant distress or impairment without sufficient medical explanation; or the complaints are greatly in excess of what would be expected for that medical condition

2. Other psychiatric illnesses to consider: mood and anxiety disorders (particularly major depression and panic disorder), substance abuse, personality disorders (e.g., histrionic, borderline, passive-dependent, narcissistic), schizophrenia, prolonged grief reactions, and couvade.

3. Medical illnesses to consider: myasthenia gravis, multiple sclerosis, systemic lupus erythematosis, acute intermittent porphyria, and endocrine disorders (hypo/hyperthyroidism, hypo/hypercortisolism, and hyperparathyroidism).

4. Overlapping syndromes in which somatization may be present: chronic fatigue syndrome, fibromyalgia, mitral valve prolapse, "reactive" hypoglycemia, irritable bowel syndrome, multiple chemical sensitivity, Gulf War syndrome, systemic candidiasis

Treatment

1. Listen patiently to the "organ recital" of complaints. Take each symptom seriously, negotiating and prioritizing which symptoms to evaluate during the visit. Perform a brief, focused physical examination at each visit.

2. Accept and acknowledge the symptoms as genuine expressions of suffering, thereby giving "permission" to the patient to receive the care he or she desperately needs. Do not dispute the reality of the complaint, but do not promise quick relief or cure. The goal is to minimize disability and maximize functional capacity and the patient's sense of control over the symptom.

3. Gently, gradually begin to encourage (by selective attention and reinforcement) verbal expression of problems and feelings in lieu of new somatic symptoms. Recognize and reward any incipient personal insights and growth, healthy behaviors, and coping mechanisms.

4. Do not just "rule out" organic illness, but "rule in" treatable psychiatric illness, using standard psychiatric criteria. However, do not prematurely assume that the complaint reflects psychologic stress and not treatable organic illness.

5. Use a multimodal approach, incorporating fitness training, relaxation, and other stress management approaches. Inquire about and consider use of alternative and complementary approaches.

6. Find something to admire and respect in the patient (e.g., ability to endure despite prolonged and severe discomfort). Empathize and try to understand his or her point of view. Discover the patient's model of illness and expectations regarding care and negotiate together an acceptable explanation of the illness and treatment plan. Address conflicts explicitly.

7. Validate and legitimize the need for continued medical attention and ensure long-term continuity and availability. Focus on establishing a long-term, trusting relationship. Use referral sparingly. Collaborate with a psychiatrist adept in the medicine-psychiatry interface. Encourage group therapy and individual cognitive-behavioral therapy, although patients are often

reluctant to undergo psychotherapy. Discourage "doctor shopping."

8. Be realistic about the goals of treatment, which should focus on containing symptoms and reducing disability and unneeded health care expenditures: care, not cure. Set appropriate personal and professional limits. Obtain support from colleagues to avoid building frustration and resentment.

Medication

Treat depression, anxiety, or other concomitant psychiatric disorders as needed; otherwise try to avoid medicines. Smaller than customary doses of psychotropic medicines may be effective. Troubling side effects are, however, common.

Diet

1. No specific diet is necessary, but a healthy, well-balanced diet tailored to individual needs is a useful adjunct.

2. In a desperate search to get well, some try a great variety of dietary regimens or other self-help methods with little success. Unusual, "fad" diets with extravagant claims (and price tags) should be discouraged.

Activity

General conditioning and aerobic exercise is a useful general aid to health by building self-esteem and confidence.

Patient Education

Patients should be notified whenever tests and examinations do not reveal evidence of significant medical illness. They should always be told that their symptoms and their suffering are real (i.e., not "all in their head") and that they have increased sensitivity to painful stimuli, but that no serious or life-threatening illness is present. They should also be informed that continued careful observation is advisable.

Key Treatment

- Establish long-term relationship of trust and mutual respect.

- Validate symptoms and need for ongoing treatment.

- Use psychotropic medicine for symptoms of depression and anxiety.

Follow-Up

1. To ensure careful follow-up and to prevent the patient from feeling rejected or abandoned, follow-up appointments should always be scheduled on a regular basis (e.g., every 1 to 4 weeks at the beginning) and not made contingent upon the development of new symptoms.

2. The appointments can be brief (15 to 20 minutes) and should always include a brief physical examination tailored to the patient's presenting complaints.

Bibliography

For details of classification of somatoform disorders, see
American Psychiatric Association: Diagnostic and Statistical Manual of Mental Disorders, 4th ed. Washington, DC, American Psychiatric Press, 1994.

For comprehensive reviews of the subject from a psychiatric perspective, see
Kellner R: Diagnosis and treatment of hypochondriacal syndromes. Psychosomatics 1992;33:278–289.
Kellner R: Somatization: theories and research. J Nerv Ment Dis 1990;178:150–160.

For comprehensive reviews of the subject from a primary care perspective, see
Kaplan C, Lipkin M, Gordon G: Somatization in primary care: patients with unexplained and vexing medical complaints. J Gen Intern Med 1988;13:177–190.
Kroenke K, Spitzer RL, deGruy FV, et al: Multisomatoform disorder. Arch Gen Psychiatry 1997;54:352–358.
Smith RC: Somatization disorder: defining its role in clinical medicine. J Gen Intern Med 1991;6:168–175.

For studies demonstrating the cost-effectiveness of training physicians in diagnosing and treating somatoform disorders, see
Kashner TM, Rost K, Cohen B, et al: Enhancing the health of somatization disorder patients: effectiveness of short-term group therapy. Psychosomatics 1995;36:462–470.
Smith GR, Rost K, Kashner M: A trial of the effect of a standardized psychiatric consultation on health outcomes and costs in somatizing patients. Arch Gen Psychiatry 1995;52:238–243.

For techniques on how to care for patients with somatization, see
Bass C, Benjamin S: The management of chronic somatisation. Br J Psychiatry 1993;162:472–480.
Creed F, Guthrie E: Techniques for interviewing the somatising patient. Br J Psychiatry 1993;162:467–471.
Morrison J: Managing somatization disorder. Dis Mon 1990;36:537–591.

The BATHE technique is a verbal procedure consisting of a series of four questions followed by an empathic response.

> **B**ackground: What is going on in your life?
>
> **A**ffect: How do you feel about that?
>
> **T**rouble: What troubles you about that?
>
> **H**andling: How are you handling that?
>
> **E**mpathy: That must be very difficult.

Indications

1. To answer the question, "Why is the patient here now" as part of constructing a medical history
2. To establish personal rapport with patients
3. To serve as a rough screening test for anxiety, depression, or situational stress disorders
4. To probe for possible psychosocial precipitants related to somatic complaints
5. To operationalize the biopsychosocial model by establishing the context of the patient's illness
6. To help patients connect their physical symptoms to their emotional responses and the circumstances of their lives
7. To explore a patient's reaction to a diagnosis
8. To handle an unexpected psychosocial revelation at the end of an interview
9. To explore lack of compliance, requests for inappropriate referrals, or other difficult situations in the doctor-patient relationship
10. As a structure for a brief counseling session or a family interview

Contraindications

1. Patients in severe pain or life-threatening circumstances
2. Resistance on the part of the patient, expressed as suspiciousness or hostility
3. Active psychosis

4. Modifications may need to be made for patients with developmental disorders, physical handicaps, of different cultural backgrounds or when language is a barrier.
5. Strict limits must be set when used for patients with severe personality disorders.
6. Not sufficient in itself for suicidal patients, battered spouses, sexual abuse victims, or substance abusers

Preparation

The BATHE technique needs little preparation. In the routine patient interview, it follows the exploration of the reason for the visit and history of the present illness. Patients can be BATHE'd repeatedly during a visit as relevant material emerges.

Equipment

None required. The physician should sit, make eye contact, listen attentively, and refrain from taking notes, reading the chart, or otherwise distracting the patient.

Precautions

1. Try to say nothing except the BATHE questions.
2. Do not allow patients to elaborate at length on the circumstances or details of their situations. Do summarize briefly and ask the next question.
3. Do not analyze or interpret patients' responses.
4. Avoid giving advice.
5. When patients fail to answer the "affect" question and provide more background information, intervene quickly by repeating, "Yes, but how do you *feel* about that?", "How does it make you feel?", or "How does it affect *you*?" until you get a response.
6. When patients express positive feelings, do not assume that there is nothing "troubling" them. Modify the "T" question appropriately such as: "Is there anything about it that troubles you?"
7. Recognize that it is not your job to fix the patient's problems, only to empower them and provide support or clarification.

Technique

1. **B** (background: "What is going on in your life?") ascertains the context of the visit. If the patient has already discussed this, go directly to affect.

2. **A** (affect: "How do you feel about that?") elicits the patient's emotional response. It is therapeutic for the patient to label the feeling(s).

3. **T** (trouble: "What troubles you the most about this?") gets at the symbolic meaning for the patient.

4. **H** (handling: "How are you handling that?") helps to assess their resources and response to the situation.

5. **E** (empathy: "That must be very difficult for you") acknowledges reasonable coping responses. Ideally you would

    a. State the feeling of the patient (i.e., "You are really angry . . .").

    b. Paraphrase your understanding of the circumstances (i.e., "your wife decided . . .").

    c. Then state that you *can* understand that this must be difficult. Anyone would be upset by this situation. This normalizes the patient's reaction.

6. In a family conference, each member in turn is BATHE'd. This provides information and opens communications.

Follow-Up

1. When a psychosocial problem is uncovered, the patient is asked to return to discuss the situation further.

2. At the return visit, the opening BATHE question becomes "Tell me what's been happening since I saw you."

3. For further information and additional techniques, see *The Fifteen Minute Hour*.

 Bibliography

Bloom BL: Stuart and Lieberman's "fifteen minute hour." In Planned Short-Term Psychotherapy: A Clinical Handbook, pp 273–277. Boston, Allyn & Bacon, 1992.

Lieberman JA III, Stuart MR: Practicing biopsychosocial medicine. In RE Rakel (ed): Textbook of Family Medicine, 5th ed, pp 55–61. Philadelphia, WB Saunders Company, 1995.

Lieberman JA III, Stuart MR: Principles of office counseling. In R Taylor (ed): Manual of Family Practice, pp 193–195. Boston, Little, Brown, 1996.

Stuart MR, Lieberman JA III: Current Concepts in Psychotherapy: Applied Psychotherapy for the Primary Care Physician [monograph]. Blue Bell, PA, Aetna–US Healthcare, 1997.

Stuart MR, Lieberman JA III: The Fifteen Minute Hour: Applied Psychotherapy for the Primary Care Physician, 2nd ed. Westport, CT, Praeger, 1993.

337 Depression

Robert E. Rakel

Etiology

1. Epidemiology: Depression will affect one third of adults in the United States at some time during their lives, with a female-male ratio of 3:1.
2. Genetic: Although a responsible gene has not been identified, sites on chromosomes 18 and 21 have been suggested.
3. Familial predisposition: The risk of depression is two to three times higher if a first-degree relative has been affected. The incidence of depression in both monozygotic twins is 65 per cent but is only 14 per cent in dizygotic twins.
4. Neurochemical: Depression is associated with a deficiency of norepinephrine and serotonin in the central nervous system. Suicide victims have depleted amounts of serotonin in the cerebrospinal fluid, and postmortem studies show a compensatory increase in the number of certain norepinephrine receptors.
5. Co-morbidity: Approximately 60 per cent of depressed patients have another medical illness; most common are cardiac, neurologic, metabolic, and endocrine (e.g. coronary artery disease, stroke, cancer, Parkinson's disease, and diabetes mellitus). Almost half of post–myocardial infarction patients will have some depression within 10 days, with an increased risk of sudden death.
6. Medication (e.g., reserpine, β-adrenergic blockers, benzodiazepines, oral contraceptives, steroids, codeine, and sedative-hypnotics).

Symptoms

1. Depressed mood most of the day nearly every day, or loss of interest or pleasure in previously enjoyed activities (anhedonia), and at least four of the following:
   a. Insomnia or hypersomnia
   b. Fatigue or loss of energy
   c. Decrease or increase in appetite
   d. Difficulty concentrating
   e. Restlessness, anxiety, or slowed actions
   f. Feelings of worthlessness or inappropriate guilt
   g. Recurrent thoughts of death or suicidal ideation

2. Anxiety: Mixed anxiety and depression is common.
   a. Sixty per cent of depressed patients have anxiety.
   b. Panic disorder is common and may be a depressive disorder because the treatment is an antidepressant.
   c. Patients with mixed anxiety and depression are more refractory to treatment and have a more prolonged illness.

3. Somatic complaints
   a. Rule out depression in a patient with multiple recurring physical complaints, especially when there is no medical explanation or the complaints involve a variety of body systems.
   b. Half of patients with more than five physical complaints are probably depressed or have mixed anxiety and depression.
   c. Pain is one of the most frequent complaints, often associated with the gastrointestinal or musculoskeletal systems.

Key Symptoms

- Little interest or pleasure in usual activities
- Feeling down, depressed, or hopeless
- Insomnia, especially early morning awakening
- Appetite change
- Multiple somatic symptoms, usually including pain

Clinical Findings

1. A sad or easy-to-cry patient who moves slowly and appears excessively concerned or preoccupied with physical symptoms.
2. No medical cause of physical symptoms can be found.
3. Patients may be irritable, angry, agitated, or worry excessively.

Tests

1. Specific laboratory tests are not available. The dexamethasone suppression test is not reliable.
2. Thyroid function studies, complete blood count, and blood chemistry panel, including liver and renal function tests, plus electrolytes to rule out medical causes
3. Beck Depression Inventory
4. Zung Self-Rating Depression Scale
5. Carroll Depression Self-Rating Scale
6. Center for Epidemiologic Studies/Depressed Mood Scale
7. Primary Care Evaluation of Mental Disorders (PRIME-MD)

Differential Diagnosis

1. Bipolar disorder
2. Dementia
3. Anxiety disorder
4. Somatoform disorder
5. Substance abuse disorder
6. Schizophrenia and schizoaffective disorder
7. Attention-deficit hyperactivity disorder
8. General medical disorder (e.g., thyroid or other endocrine problem)

Treatment

1. *Assess the potential for suicide.* Inquire about thoughts or plans of suicide. Suicidal patients usually communicate their intent to others, and most have seen a physician within the previous month. At greatest risk are depressed alcoholics who have attempted suicide in the past and white elderly unmarried men who live alone.

2. *Electroconvulsive therapy*: Usually reserved for patients who are suicidal or who do not respond to medication. Effective in more than 90 per cent of patients within 1 or 2 weeks. Treatments are usually given three times a week until improvement occurs.

3. *Psychotherapy*: Supportive psychotherapy, including active ongoing encouragement, is essential whether or not medication is used. Specific techniques include interpersonal, cognitive-behavioral, and psychodynamic. Marital therapy and group psychotherapy may also be helpful.

4. *Bright light therapy*: Effective for patients with seasonal affective disorder. Given in the morning hours; works best if used in combination with pharmacotherapy.

5. *Exercise*: About as effective as psychotherapy in treating mild to moderate depression. The added cardiovascular benefit should make this a standard recommendation for patients who are receptive.

Medication

1. Effectiveness
   a. All antidepressants are equally effective, so choice is usually made on the basis of minimal risk and side effects. Tables 337–1 and 337–2 list the antidepressants currently available and their side effects.
   b. Most primary care physicians prefer to use a drug that is safe if taken in overdose. The lethal dose of a tricyclic is 1.5 gm, or about 10 times the daily therapeutic dose.

2. *Selective serotonin reuptake inhibitors* (SSRIs)
   a. Drugs of first choice because of their excellent patient acceptance. Side effects include nausea, agitation, and sexual dysfunction.
   b. If the patient's primary complaint is tiredness, an activating SSRI may be preferred, whereas if anxiety is a major component, a more sedating drug such as nefazodone may work best.
   c. Patients should be seen weekly, effectiveness of the medication assessed, and dose gradually increased to maximum if necessary.

3. *Monoamine oxidase inhibitors* (MAOIs)
   a. Do not mix an MAOI with another antidepressant.
   b. MAOIs are rarely used in primary care because of their severe side effects, the most serious of which is potentially fatal hypertensive crisis if taken with certain drugs or with foods containing tyramine.

4. *Augmentation therapy*

TABLE 337–1. ANTIDEPRESSANT FORMS AND DOSAGES

Drug	Dosage Forms* (mg)	Initial Dose† (mg/d)	Range (mg/d)	Frequency	Half-Life	Safe in Overdose
Selective Serotonin Reuptake Inhibitors						
Fluoxetine (Prozac)	10, 20 Pulvules; 20/5 ml liquid	20	20–60	qd (AM)	2–9 d	Yes
Sertraline (Zoloft)	25, 50, 100 ST	50	50–200	qd	1–4 d	Yes
Paroxetine (Paxil)	10, 20, 30, 40 CT	20	20–50	qd	10–24 hr	Yes
Fluvoxamine (Luvox)	50, 100 ST	50	50–300	qd (hs)	15 hr	Yes
Citalopram (Celexa)	20, 40 ST	20	20–60	qd	35 hr	Yes
Miscellaneous						
Venlafaxine (Effexor)	25, 37.5, 50, 75, 100 ST	75	75–275	bid	5–11 hr	Yes
	37.5, 75, 150 XR	37.5	75–375	qd (hs)	5–11 hr	Yes
Nefazodone (Serzone)	50, 100, 150, 200, 250 ST	200	200–600	bid	2–4 hr	Yes
Trazodone (Desyrel)	50, 100, 150, 300 ST	150	150–600	bid	4–9 hr	Yes
Bupropion (Wellbutrin)	75, 100 tablets;	200	200–450	tid‡	8–24 hr	Yes
	100, 150 SR	150	200–450	bid	8–24 hr	Yes
Tricyclics						
Amitriptyline (Elavil)	10, 25, 50, 75, 100, 150 CT	50–75	50–300	qd (hs)	31–46 hr	No
Clomipramine (Anafranil)	25, 50, 75 tablets	25	25–250	qd (hs)	19–37 hr	No
Doxepin (Sinequan)	10, 25, 50, 75, 100, 150 capsules; 10/ml solution	50–75	25–300	qd (hs)	81–24 hr	No
Imipramine (Tofranil)	10, 25, 50 CT	50–75	30–300	qd (hs)	11–25 hr	No
Trimipramine (Surmontil)	25, 50, 100 capsules	50–75	50–300	qd (hs)	7–30 hr	No
Desipramine (Norpramin)	10, 25, 50, 75, 100, 150 CT	50–75	25–300	qd (hs)	12–24 hr	No
Nortriptyline (Pamelor)	10, 25, 50, 75 capsules; 10/5 ml solution	25–50	30–100	qd§	18–44 hr	No
Protriptyline (Vivactil)	5, 10 CT	10–15	15–60	tid	67–89 hr	No
Amoxapine (Asendin)	25, 50, 100, 150 ST	100–150	50–600	qd§	8 hr	Yes
Tetracyclics						
Maprotiline (Ludiomil)	25, 50, 75 ST	50–75	50–225	qd (hs)	21–25 hr	No
Mirtazapine (Remeron)	15, 30 ST	15	15–60	qd (hs)	20–40 hr	Yes?
Monoamine Oxidase Inhibitors						
Phenelzine (Nardil)	15 CT	45	45–90	tid	2–4 hr	No
Tranylcypromine (Parnate)	10 CT	30	30–60	tid	2.4–2.8 hr	No

*CT, coated tablets; SR, sustained-release tablets, ST, scored tablets; XR, extended-release tablets.
†Initial daily adult dose. Elderly persons should receive half the starting dose.
‡Initial dose 100 mg bid for 3 days, then 100 mg tid.
§Start in divided doses (tid); maintenance may be once daily at bedtime [qd (hs)].

a. If the selected drug is only partially effective, add a second agent from another class (except an MAOI). If the combination is still ineffective, lithium, buspirone, or thyroid hormone can be a potentiating agent.

b. If an SSRI does not achieve the anticipated effect, add a drug from the miscellaneous group or a tricyclic or switch to another SSRI, because failure to respond to one does not predict poor response to another.

c. Venlafaxine, although it has side effects similar to the SSRIs and can cause hypertension at doses greater than 225 mg/day, can be useful in patients who do not respond to other agents.

Patient Education

1. Patient and family: Emphasizing the biomedical nature of depression will help relieve the stigma that many attach to mental illness.

2. Insight regarding probable side effects will help the patient remain on the medication until the side effects have passed. Emphasize the importance of daily dosing and not stopping the drug without physician supervision.

3. Educate the patient to be alert to any recurrence of symptoms.

TABLE 337–2. ANTIDEPRESSANT SIDE EFFECTS

DRUG	ANTICHOLINERGIA	SEDATION	INSOMNIA/AGITATION	ORTHOSTATIC HYPOTENSION	ARRHYTHMIA	NAUSEA	WEIGHT GAIN*	SEXUAL DYSFUNCTION
Amitriptyline (Elavil)	++++	++++	0	++++	+++	0	++++	++
Desipramine (Norpramin)	+	+	+	+++	++	0	+	++
Doxepin (Sinequan)	+++	++++	0	+++	++	0	+++	++
Imipramine (Tofranil)	+++	+++	+	++++	+++	+	+++	++
Nortriptyline (Pamelor)	++	+	0	+++	++	0	+	++
Protriptyline (Vivactil)	+	+	0	+++	++	0	0	++
Trimipramine (Surmontil)	+	++++	0	+++	+++	0	+++	++
Amoxapine (Asendin)	++	++	++	++	+	0	++	0
Maprotiline (Ludiomil)	++	++	0	++	+	0	++	0
Mirtazapine (Remeron)	+	++	0	+	0	0	+++	0
Trazodone (Desyrel)	0	++++	0	++	+	+	+	0
Nefazodone (Serzone)	0	+++	0	0	+	+	0	0
Bupropion (Wellbutrin)	0	0	++	0	0	+	0	0
Venlafaxine (Effexor)	0	0	++	0	0	++	0	+
Fluoxetine (Prozac)	0	0	++++	+	0	+++	0	++
Paroxetine (Paxil)	0	0	++	0	0	+++	0	++
Sertraline (Zoloft)	0	0	+++	0	0	+++	0	++
Fluvoxamine (Luvox)	0	0	+++	0	0	+++	0	++
Citalopram (Celexa)	0	0	++	0	0	+++	0	+

Key: 0, none; +, minimal; ++, mild; +++, moderate; ++++, strong.
*Over 13 pounds.
Adapted from: Depression Guideline Panel: Depression in Primary Care: Detection, Diagnosis, and Treatment (Quick Reference Guide for Clinicians, No. 5). Rockville, MD, U.S. Department of Health and Human Services, Agency for Health Care Policy and Research, 1993.

Key Treatment

Drugs of Choice

- Fluoxetine
- Paroxetine
- Sertraline
- Citalopram

Follow-Up

1. Weekly or bi-weekly visits until improved and optimal dosage identified, then every 2 to 4 weeks *for a minimum of 6 months* after asymptomatic. Many patients should be maintained on medication for 1 to 2 years.

2. When withdrawal is indicated, taper slowly and observe for recurrence of symptoms.

3. If the patient has had two or more episodes of depression, long-term therapy may be of benefit to prevent recurrences.

Bibliography

Brody DS, Hahn SR, Spitzer RL, et al: Identifying patients with depression in the primary care setting: a more efficient method. Arch Intern Med 1998;158:2469–2475.

DeWester JN: Recognizing and treating the patient with somatic manifestations of depression. J Fam Pract 1996;43(Suppl):3–15.

Greden JF, Schwenk TL: Major mood disorders. In Knesper DJ, Riba MB, Schwenk TI (eds): Primary Care Psychiatry, pp 107–131. Philadelphia, WB Saunders Company, 1997.

Richelson ER: Mood disorders. In Rakel RJ (ed): Conn's Current Therapy, pp 1135–1145. Philadelphia, WB Saunders Company, 1999.

Rosenbaum JF, Fava M: Approach to the patient with depression. In Stern TA, Herman JB, Slavin PL (eds): The MGH Guide to Psychiatry in Primary Care, pp 1–14. New York, McGraw-Hill, 1998.

338 Suicide Assessment

Sherry L. Robbins

1. In the United States each year approximately 30,000 people commit suicide. This number may be conservative, because one must maintain a high index of suspicion for motor vehicle accidents, drug overdoses, and gunshot wounds as being possibly intentional rather than accidental. Social stigma, survivor denial, and concerns over insurance coverage may lead to underreporting.

2. Although commonly assumed, suicidality is not *necessarily* synonymous with depression. It may be a feature of a personality disorder (borderline) or a well-considered plan to end physical suffering or ensure a death with dignity. It may also be the result of attention-seeking or manipulative behavior.

3. Numbers of suicidal threats/attempts far outweigh the number of those who complete the suicide, but it is difficult to identify those who will succeed.

Symptoms

1. A feeling of hopelessness—the most universal finding among suicide victims.

2. Suicidal ideation: Any expression of suicidal thoughts should be taken seriously.

3. Plan for suicide: If the patient can verbalize the precise method by which he or she intends to take his or her life, the risk should be considered to be imminent.

4. Previous attempt of suicide: Increases the risk.

5. Positive family history of suicide: Increases the risk.

6. Precipitating acute life events: Anniversary reactions, holidays, loss, or acute stressors

7. Presence of command hallucinations: Although these are extremely dangerous in psychotic patients, their absence should not give false reassurance.

8. Giving away valued possessions: Especially important in children.

9. Precipitating recent media events: There is an increased rate of suicide attempts by adolescents after publicity of adolescent suicide.

Key Symptoms

- Feelings of hopelessness
- Previous suicide attempts
- Suicidal ideation
- Acute life events/ unemployment
- Isolation
- Symptoms of depression
- Positive family history of suicide
- Plan for suicide
- Giving away possessions
- Presence of command hallucinations

Clinical Findings

In addition to the presence of some of the increased risk factors in the history, a suicidal patient may present with positive findings on mental status examination. He or she may display a disturbance of affect and/or mood. Suicidal ideation may be revealed either by the patient or by significant others. Disorders of speech, thought, or sensorium may be evident, depending upon the presence of a psychiatric disorder or drug effects.

1. Suicidal ideation on mental status examination

2. Co-morbid factors have been found in 70 to 80 per cent of completed suicides.

   a. Depression (unipolar or bipolar): Lifetime risk of suicide is 15 and 19 per cent, respectively.

   b. Schizophrenia: Greatest risk within the first 10 years of illness, but is increased lifelong.

   c. Panic disorder: It is unclear as to whether this relationship is direct or indirect.

   d. Personality disorder: Primarily, borderline personality disorder

   e. Debilitating or terminal disease: cancer, human immunodeficiency virus/acquired immunodeficiency syndrome, Huntington's disease, amyotrophic lateral sclerosis, multiple sclerosis, and the like

3. Substance use/abuse: Patients who commit suicide often have alcohol or illicit drugs in their systems at the time an attempt is made. "CAGE" questions may be helpful (see Ch. 344, Alcoholism).

4. Presence of demographic factors that may represent increased suicide risk
   a. Male sex: more likely to use methods of greater lethality and to complete the suicide
   b. Age: Suicide is more likely to be completed in the elderly (more co-morbidity, fewer physical reserves, less likely to be found, less likely to give warning, and use of more lethal means).

tween decreased levels and suicide. However, the clinical significance of this finding is currently limited.
   b. Depression inventory tests (Beck or Zung) and/or anxiety scales (Hamilton) may be helpful in determining whether an underlying affective disorder is present. These tests are particularly helpful in terminally ill patients who request physician-assisted suicide.

Key Signs

- Abnormal affect
- Male sex
- Elderly
- Co-morbid factors (depression, schizophrenia, panic disorder, borderline personality disorder, or debilitating/terminal disease)
- Depressed mood
- Marital status (divorced/widowed)
- Current substance use (alcohol/drugs)

WARNING

Despite the value of demographic information, it may fail to be predictive of the outcome for the individual patient being evaluated. Each situation must be assessed and a determination made as to the degree of risk by a gestalt approach, rather than by a tabulation of risk factors alone.

Laboratory Tests

1. The assessment of an attempted suicide necessitates a complete physical examination and appropriate diagnostic testing to ascertain the effects of the method used.
   a. In general, urine and serum drug screens, complete blood count (CBC), electrolyte panel, and cardiac monitoring represent the minimum evaluation for most overdosages.
   b. A thyroid-stimulating hormone (TSH) level should be performed in the work-up of patients suspected of having a psychiatric disorder.
2. No specific diagnostic test can definitively determine suicidal risk; however, various instruments have attempted to do so. None at this point has been established as a standard of care.
   a. Studies of levels of serotonin in cerebrospinal fluid have demonstrated a correlation be-

---

Key Tests

May be helpful before a suicide attempt is made or if physician-assisted suicide is being considered:

- Depression inventory tests
- Anxiety rating scales
- TSH

May be helpful immediately following a suicide attempt:

- Drug screens, alcohol level
- CBC, metabolic panel, telemetry
- Other tests specific to the method used (electrocardiogram, chest radiograph, arterial blood gases, drug levels, etc) (See Ch. 351, Poisonings.)

Differential Diagnosis

The differential diagnosis of a suicide attempt includes accidents, effects of drugs and/or alcohol, and attention-seeking or manipulative behavior without actual intent to harm oneself. It also includes a possible attempt to end suffering by a patient with a debilitating or terminal illness. For patients who request physician-assisted suicide, an unrecognized or untreated psychiatric disorder must be excluded.

Treatment

1. Medication
   a. Selective serotonin reuptake inhibitors (SSRIs): drugs of choice in suicidal patients with depression, because they are less lethal than monoamine oxidase inhibitors or tricyclics. For patients who fail to respond, check for therapeutic dosing, consider following drug levels, and consider electroconvulsive therapy.
   b. Pain medication to adequately treat pain in terminally ill patients
   c. Appropriate medical treatment of other co-morbid disorders

d. Avoid dispensing large amounts of potentially lethal medications for patients at risk.

e. For acute overdosage, syrup of ipecac, activated charcoal, and specific antidotes may be indicated. (See Ch. 351, Poisonings.)

2. Activity
a. Emergency commitment for patients believed to be at imminent risk; they should be accompanied by a capable person (emergency medical services personnel, police, or medical personnel) until commitment is achieved.

b. Ask the family to remove from home any means by which the patient could kill himself or herself.

c. Avoid alcohol and illicit drugs.

d. Refer the patient for counseling.

3. Patient education
a. Foster community/school suicide awareness groups.

b. Encourage less isolation among the elderly.

c. Patients/family members should contact physician if suicidal thoughts or high-risk behaviors occur.

d. Encourage a change in perspective from *hopelessness* to *hopefulness*; focusing upon reasons that prevent the patient from acting upon suicidal ideation is helpful.

Key Treatment

- Prevention should be the main focus of treatment of suicidality, including adequate and appropriate treatment of depression. Query all depressed patients about suicidal thoughts and modify risk factors.

- SSRIs are the drugs of choice for depressed patients at risk of suicide.

Follow-Up

1. For patients with suicidal ideation who are not thought to be at imminent risk, close follow-up is essential. Because the threshold for suicide may be met over the course of time, it may be necessary to see or contact these patients every few days to weeks. Suicide contracts, in which a patient promises to not harm himself or herself, have been used frequently. It is important to realize that these contracts are *therapeutic* and may not be legally binding.

2. Depressed patients should have close follow-up after antidepressant treatment is initiated, because patients may commit suicide after showing some initial improvement. This phenomenon is thought to be due to an increase in energy and motivation, preceding improvement in the depressed mood.

3. Following a completed suicide, it is important to have follow-up with the family. The effects on survivors can be far-reaching and devastating, and counseling is usually required.

Bibliography

Besseghini VH: Depression and suicide in children and adolescents. Ann N Y Acad Sci 1997;816:94–98.

Hirschfeld RMA, Russell JM: Assessment and treatment of suicidal patients. N Engl J Med 1997;337:910–915.

Hughes DH: Suicide and violence assessment in psychiatry. Gen Hosp Psychiatry 1996;18:416–421.

Mann JJ: Suicide. Psychiatr Clin North Am 1997;20:499–690.

Oquendo MA, Malone KM, Mann JJ: Suicide: risk factors and prevention in refractory major depression. Depression Anxiety 1977;5:202–211.

339 Panic Disorder

Mark A. Zamorski

Etiology

We all have the capacity to panic, and the panic response is constructive to the extent that the physical and psychological changes prepare for defensive or evasive action. In panic disorder, such panic attacks occur "out of the blue," without any trigger, and are associated with significant anxiety and disability. Numerous pieces of evidence, including its strong familial tendency, suggest that panic disorder has a neurobiologic basis.

Symptoms

Panic attacks occur in panic disorder as well as in other psychiatric diagnoses. Patients will have a number of the symptoms noted in Table 339–1. Symptoms of attacks begin abruptly and peak within about 10 minutes; attacks last for a few minutes to an hour or more.

Key Symptoms

- Chest pains: Approximately one half of primary care patients with this complaint meet criteria for panic disorder
- Dizzy spells
- Palpitations

Clinical Findings

During an acute panic attack, patients appear agitated and fearful, having tachycardia, hypertension, tachypnea, diaphoresis, and other signs of adrenergic excess.

TABLE 339–1. SYMPTOMS OF PANIC ATTACKS

Somatic	Psychological
Chest pain	Fear of dying
Palpitations	Fear of losing control or going crazy
Dyspnea	Derealization or depersonalization
Choking	
Chills or hot flushes	
Diaphoresis	
Paresthesias	
Dizziness	
Tremor	
Nausea	

Laboratory Tests

Laboratory studies are unremarkable in patients with panic disorder. Electrocardiography and Holter monitoring may show sinus tachycardia and increased ectopic beats.

Differential Diagnosis

The key to diagnosing panic disorder is to strongly suspect it when young patients present with recurrent, fearful spells. Most such patients will prove to have panic disorder, but medical, substance-related, and other psychiatric diagnoses should be considered.

1. The most serious *medical disorders* that can mimic panic disorder include
   a. Coronary ischemia: The most useful distinguishing feature is that panic disorder has an average age of onset of 25 years and is more common in women than men; onset after age 40 is rare.
   b. Pulmonary embolism: Heightened suspicion is appropriate in patients with recognized risk factors for venous thromboembolism.
   c. Temporal lobe seizures: These are typically briefer than panic attacks, lasting a few seconds to a minute or two. Features suggestive of seizures include loss of awareness during attacks, amnesia for attacks, and odd, psychomotor behaviors during attacks.
2. Other medical diagnoses to consider include
   a. Ménière's disease should be considered in patients with vertiginous attacks, fluctuating hearing loss, and tinnitus. Other vestibular disorders are also a consideration, but panic disorder should be suspected when there is disproportionate anxiety about attacks or any phobic avoidance.
   b. Patients diagnosed with mitral valve prolapse, "hypoglycemia," and esophageal spasm often actually have panic disorder, and respond well to antipanic treatments.
   c. Hyperthyroidism and pheochromocytoma do not cause typical panic attacks.
   d. Asthma may cause dyspneic episodes, but they are almost always preceded by familiar triggers, and coughing and/or wheezing are present at some time in almost all patients.

e. About one half of patients with irritable bowel syndrome also meet criteria for panic disorder.

3. Panic attacks may be *substance-related*, caused by intoxication with hallucinogens or stimulants (including caffeine), or withdrawal from sedatives.

4. *Psychiatric disorders* in which panic attacks are seen include

   a. Panic disorder, in which recurrent attacks occur, at least initially, "out of the blue," associated with one or more of the following:

      (1) Concern about having future attacks

      (2) Worry about the implications or consequences of the attacks

      (3) A significant change in behavior related to the attacks

   b. Panic attacks can occur within the context of the specific fears seen in phobias, obsessive compulsive disorder, post-traumatic stress disorder, and psychotic disorders. If the panic attacks are fully accounted for by another disorder (e.g., attacks only occur during public speaking in social phobia), the additional diagnosis of panic disorder is not warranted.

5. *Normal individuals* may have rare spontaneous or stress-induced panic attacks.

6. The most important psychiatric co-morbidities of panic disorder are

   a. Agoraphobia, the fear or avoidance of places in which escape might be difficult or help unavailable in the event of a panic attack. Agoraphobia is present in about one half of patients with panic disorder, and it often causes substantial disability.

   b. Depression, which will be present at some point in two thirds of patients with panic disorder.

   c. Substance abuse, which precludes the use of benzodiazepines in patients with this co-morbidity.

Treatment

Patients with panic disorder require specific treatment to prevent panic attacks and their related disability. The two main choices for therapy are medications and cognitive-behavioral therapy.

1. Medication

   a. The selective serotonin reuptake inhibitors (SSRIs) are the first choice for the drug treatment of panic disorder. Both paroxetine and sertraline have well-documented efficacy. Patients with anxiety disorders are especially sensitive to the temporary activating effects of SSRIs. For this reason, start with half of the normal starting dose for depression, and increase the dose weekly or as tolerated. Patients with panic disorder appear to require, on the average, higher doses of SSRIs than do depressed patients.

   b. The tricyclic antidepressants (TCAs) are an inexpensive alternative to the SSRIs. Activation is less of a problem with the TCAs, although low starting doses (e.g., 10 to 25 mg/day of imipramine) are recommended. The target dose is the full antidepressant dosage for most patients.

   c. The high-potency benzodiazepines (lorazepam, alprazolam, and clonazepam) are effective at preventing panic attacks if given at high doses (e.g., 2 to 6 mg/day of alprazolam). Lower doses improve anticipatory and generalized anxiety but do not prevent attacks. Because of their abuse potential, sedative side effects, lack of convincing efficacy for treatment of co-morbid depression, and propensity to cause physiologic dependence, the benzodiazepines should be reserved as third-line agents for panic disorder. Some patients benefit from short-term, regularly administered, low-dose benzodiazepine therapy while other antipanic agents are being initiated.

   d. Ineffective agents include buspirone, bupropion, and β-adrenergic blockers.

2. A specific, relatively unfamiliar type of short-term psychotherapy called cognitive-behavioral therapy (CBT) is highly effective for panic disorder (and co-morbid agoraphobia). Agoraphobia usually responds better to CBT than to medications. Unfortunately, quality CBT is often not available in smaller communities, and insurance issues, time pressures, and lack of acceptability make CBT less appealing to most patients. Nevertheless, if available, CBT is an excellent choice for patients who prefer to avoid medications.

3. All patients benefit from patient education handouts (see Bibliography), which serve to legitimatize the diagnosis. Self-help and support groups are helpful for some patients.

Key Treatment

- An SSRI, TCA, or cognitive-behavioral therapy

- Short-term benzodiazepines if needed; avoid long-term benzodiazepines.

Follow-Up

1. Frequent (every week or two) follow-up is required during the first month or two after diagnosis as medications are adjusted; weeks are required before medications are effective for preventing panic attacks.
2. Like depression, panic disorder is a chronic, relapsing condition. Treatment should continue for at least 12 to 24 months (and often lifelong) depending on the degree of disability, comorbidities (e.g., chronic depression), number of previous exacerbations, and patient tolerance and preferences

B Bibliography

Ballenger JC, Davidson JR, Lecrubier Y, et al: Consensus statement on panic disorder from the International Consensus Group on Depression and Anxiety. J Clin Psychiatry 1998;59(Suppl 8):47–54.

Katon W: Panic Disorder in the Medical Setting (NIH Publication No. 94-3482). Bethesda, MD, National Institutes of Health, 1994.

Nesse R, Zamorski MA: Anxiety disorders in primary care. In Knesper DJ, Riba MB, Schwenk TL (eds): Primary Care Psychiatry, pp 132–162. Philadelphia, WB Saunders Company, 1997.

Sources for patient education materials: The National Institute of Mental Health Information Line (1-800-647-2642) or *http://www.nimh.nih.gov/publicat/anxiety.htm.*

340 Generalized Anxiety Disorder

Thomas L. Leaman

Etiology

1. May result from unresolved adjustment disorder with anxious mood
2. In 50 per cent of cases a precipitating emotional stressor can be identified.
3. In the other 50 per cent no stressor can be identified; a disturbance of the neurotransmitters is presumed to be the cause.

Symptoms

1. Worry and anxiousness over multiple real or projected problems. The worry is out of proportion to the situation and out of control.
2. At least three of the following symptoms:
   a. Restlessness
   b. Fatigue
   c. Trouble concentrating
   d. Irritability
   e. Sleep disturbance
   f. Muscle tension
3. Frequently characterized by episodes of severe autonomic symptoms
   a. Cardiac: chest pain, palpitations, tachycardia, tachypnea
   b. Pulmonary: hyperventilation, smothering sensations, dyspnea
   c. Gastrointestinal: globus hystericus, indigestion, abdominal pains, flatulence, diarrhea, constipation
   d. Genitourinary: frequency, menstrual irregularities, sexual dysfunction
   e. Dermatologic: paresthesias, sweating, hot flushes, chills, pruritus

Key Symptoms

- Worry
- Fatigue
- Chest pain, palpitations
- Smothering sensation
- Indigestion

Clinical Findings

Consider in any patient with the underlying symptoms described above, especially if accompanied by episodes of autonomic symptom clusters.

Key Signs

- Agitation
- Sweating, tremor
- Scattered mentation
- Hyperventilation

Tests

Instruments useful in helping to confirm or refute the diagnosis:

1. Sheehan Patient Rated Anxiety Scale: Self-administered, 35 questions; useful both for diagnosis and monitoring response to treatment. Scores may be tabulated directly by patient.
2. Hopkins Symptom Checklist (SCL90): Lengthy questionnaire, requires training in interpretation.
3. Hamilton Anxiety and Depression Scales: Both are physician administered but require some training.
   a. HAM-A (anxiety) consists of 14-item checklist of anxiety symptoms.
   b. HAM-D (depression) is a 17-item, interview-based scale.
4. Zung Anxiety Self-Assessment Scale: Self-administered scale; interpretation requires physician analysis.
5. Covi Anxiety and Raskin Depression Scales: Three items on each scale; interpreted by physician; useful in differentiating between anxiety and depression.

Key Tests

- Hamilton Anxiety and Depression Scales
- Covi Anxiety and Raskin Depression Scales

Differential Diagnosis

1. Somatic diseases
   a. None of the symptoms of generalized anxiety disorder is pathognomonic, and all may be caused by a wide variety of other diseases. Among the most prominent are endocrine disorders (especially hyperthyroidism), cardiac diseases (especially coronary artery dis-

ease), and pulmonary disorders (especially chronic obstructive pulmonary disease).

b. It is not necessary, or even possible, to rule out every conceivable disease that could be responsible for the symptoms exhibited. Rather, it is important to rule out those that are most dangerous or most likely.

c. The diagnosis should be suspected on the basis of the pattern of symptoms over time. The somatic symptoms tend to occur in clusters, usually subsiding within a few weeks. They tend to recur in a variable period of time, involving the same organ system again or an entirely different system or even multiple systems.

2. Mental diseases: The diagnosis is not made if the patient has a psychosis or bipolar disease or is under the effects of drugs (abuse or medication).

3. Other anxiety disease: The diagnosis is not made if the patient has another anxiety disease.

4. Depression: Most people with generalized anxiety disorder (GAD) have symptoms of depression at some stage in their disease. It is usually possible to determine which is the primary disease on the basis of a careful history.

a. Symptoms common to both anxiety and depression
(1) Fatigue
(2) Tearfulness
(3) Eating disturbances
(4) Irritability
(5) Excessive worry
(6) Difficulty concentrating

b. Symptoms especially characteristic of anxiety
(1) Difficulty falling asleep or staying asleep
(2) Pain syndromes: Pain tends to be acute, sharp.
(3) Patients often complain of nervousness, want help.
(4) Mood may be elevated.
(5) Autonomic symptoms prominent

c. Symptoms especially characteristic of depression
(1) Early morning awakening
(2) Pain syndromes: Pain tends to be chronic, dull.
(3) Patients often unaware of their illness, want to be left alone
(4) Mood may be depressed.
(5) Anhedonia
(6) Suicidal thoughts

Treatment

There are three treatment modalities: psychotherapy, pharmacotherapy, and patient education. Most people with GAD require both of the first two; all need the last.

1. Psychotherapy
a. In many patients with GAD there is an identifiable stress factor in the cause of the disease. Any such stressors should be sought and the patient's coping mechanisms explored. In anyone who has GAD, particularly if it has gone undiagnosed or misdiagnosed for a prolonged period of time, the disease itself may serve as a perpetuating stressor.

b. Supportive counseling, cognitive therapy, psychodynamic psychotherapy, family therapy, or various behavior therapies are most frequently used in GAD.

c. Other techniques that may be helpful adjuncts, but not necessarily of proven value, include exercise, meditation, progressive relaxation, biofeedback, yoga, and t'ai chi.

2. Pharmacotherapy. Three groups of drugs have proven useful in the management of GAD.
a. Azipirones: Currently, there is only one approved drug in this group, buspirone (BuSpar). It can be useful in the management of acute anxiety, provided that patients are properly prepared to expect some delay before significant improvement. Buspirone is especially indicated in the long-term therapy often needed in GAD.
(1) Advantages: well tolerated, does not interact with alcohol or benzodiazepines, and does not cause drug dependency.
(2) Disadvantages: very slow to work (2 to 4 weeks), not always effective, and in some people can cause the side effects of dizziness, drowsiness, nausea, and headache.

b. Benzodiazepines (BZDs): BZDs are usually grouped according to their duration of action; the long-acting (up to 100 hours), the intermediate, and the short-acting (5 to 15 hours). Short-acting BZDs are sometimes considered the drugs of choice in acute anxiety because of their effectiveness and prompt action. They are especially favored if there is a history of panic attack or adrenergic symptoms are most prominent. If longer therapy is needed (beyond 3 to 6 weeks), it is recommended that patients gradually be switched to buspirone or an antidepressant. Either of these can be used concomitantly with the BZD as it is being withdrawn.

(1) Advantages: effectiveness, prompt action, side effects tend to diminish with time, rarely addictive

(2) Disadvantages: May cause drug dependency; symptoms of withdrawal may mimic anxiety symptoms; abrupt withdrawal of the short-acting BZDs after prolonged high dosage may cause convulsions; slow, tapered withdrawal essential.

(3) Possible side effects: sedation, dizziness, and ataxia

c. The antidepressant most frequently studied and shown to be effective in the treatment of GAD is imipramine. Antidepressants may be used in therapy of acute anxiety, so long as patients are aware of a probable delay before significant improvement. The antidepressants, especially imipramine, are especially useful in long-term management.

(1) Advantages: well tolerated, no drug dependency, high rate of effectiveness, side effects tend to diminish with time.

(2) Disadvantages: slow to work (3 to 5 weeks), sedation, orthostatic hypotension, and anticholinergic effects.

Patient Education

Crucial in the management of anxiety diseases

1. Anxiety disorders are "closet" diseases, often not openly discussed.

2. Patients tend to blame themselves.

3. Anxiety patients have trouble concentrating, remembering.

Key Treatment

- Counseling, supportive psychotherapy
- BuSpar, BZDs, tricyclic antidepressants
- Patient education

Follow-Up

GAD is a chronic disease with many somatic manifestations. Patients should be encouraged to remain under continuous monitoring.

Bibliography

Leaman TL: Healing the Anxiety Diseases. New York, Plenum Press, 1992.

McGlynn TJ, Metcalf HL: Diagnosis and Treatment of Anxiety Disorders: A Physician's Handbook, 2nd ed. Washington, DC, American Psychiatric Press, 1992.

Schweitzer E, Rickels K: The long-term management of generalized anxiety disorder: issues and dilemmas. J Clin Psychiatry 1996;57(Suppl 7):9–12.

Schweitzer E, Rickels K: Strategies for treatment of generalized anxiety disorder in the primary care setting. J Clin Psychiatry 1997;58(Suppl 3):27–31.

Walley EJ, Beebe DK, Clark JL: Management of common anxiety disorders. Am Fam Physician 1994;50:1745–1752.

Indications

1. Maladaptive levels of stress, anxiety, anger, and hostility
2. Important component in treatment of generalized anxiety disorder, panic disorder, simple phobia, speech anxiety, and test anxiety
3. Anxiety and maladaptive arousal as causative factors in onset or exacerbation of stress-related physical disorders: essential hypertension, migraine headache, tension headache, low back pain, bruxism, temporomandibular joint syndrome, Raynaud's disease
4. Component in preparation of patients for stressful medical procedures and distress following surgery
5. For prevention and treatment of anticipatory nausea and vomiting as side effects of cancer chemotherapy
6. Component in treatment of acute pain and chronic pain syndromes
7. Primary insomnia

Contraindications

1. Intervention is generally very safe with rare side effects; when they occur, side effects tend to be mild and generally present early in the process.
2. Avoid use with psychotic patients because they may precipitate psychotic episode.
3. Beware of underlying organic problems that may mimic anxiety (such as hyperthyroidism, pheochromocytoma, withdrawal reactions) or cause physical symptoms (such as headache caused by brain tumor), which if left medically untreated could endanger health of patient.
4. Side effects (≤1 per cent of time) include anxious feelings, depersonalization, elicitation of repressed thoughts, and tension headache.

Preparation

1. Rule out organic causes for patient's symptoms.
2. Conduct biopsychosocial formulation of presenting problem based on interview, observation, past history, self-report measures, and physiologic measures; pinpoint how maladaptive arousal or anxiety is implicated in problem manifested.
3. Determine need for alternative pharmacologic and/or psychosocial intervention instead of, or in conjunction with, deep muscle relaxation.
4. Present problem formulation to patient, and educate patient about causative role of stress, anxiety, or arousal in problem.

5. Provide treatment rationale for deep muscle relaxation—why it would be expected to help—without overstating case.
6. Foster positive expectation for change, and nurture and bolster motivation.
7. Explore and address fears, concerns, myths, and anticipations about relaxation therapy.
8. Identify prior experiences, if any, with relaxation-based techniques: type, duration, and outcome.
9. Present relaxation as skill to be acquired through practice.
10. Present it as an active coping strategy for patient to use in the future.
11. Outline the specific muscle groups, and explain concept of tension-relaxation cycle.
12. Demonstrate a tension-relaxation cycle for each muscle group, and emphasize need to relax only one group at a time.
13. Screen for present or past injuries to muscle groups that may interfere with tension-relaxation cycles.
14. Teach patient use of self-monitoring chart to track symptoms during baseline, treatment, and follow-up as a measure of efficacy.
15. Provide patient with relaxation chart to facilitate reminder for practice and promote adherence.

Equipment

1. Physical environment free of distractions and interruptions and conducive to relaxation
2. A comfortable chair able to provide full support of body (e.g., recliner)
3. Dimmed lighting to create relaxing atmosphere

Precautions

1. Although rare, watch for precipitation of "relaxation-induced anxiety" in patients who fear the following: loss of control, the physical feelings accompanying the relaxed state, feelings possibly associated with prior traumas, feelings of floating, and the "letting go" experience.
2. With patients prone to excessive cognitive worriment, consider use of relaxing imagery.
3. Overcontrolled perfectionistic patients with obsessive-compulsive tendencies who "try hard" to relax
4. Hypervigilant patients excessively focused on physical sensations

TABLE 340–1. OUTLINE FOR ADMINISTERING DEEP MUSCLE RELAXATION

MUSCLE	INSTRUCTIONS FOR TENSING	INSTRUCTIONS FOR FOCUSING ON SENSATIONS (8–10 s)	INSTRUCTIONS FOR RELAXING (RELEASING TENSION)	INSTRUCTIONS FOR FOCUSING ON RELAXATION AND THE CONTRAST
Right hand	Make a fist as tightly as you can . . . tighter and tighter.	Hold the tension and concentrate on tension in your fist.	Let go of the tension. Allow your hand to relax, letting your fingers go loose. Actively relax the tension away.	Focus on relaxing sensations in your hand and examine the contrast between tension and relaxation.
Left hand	Make a fist as tightly as you can . . . tighter and tighter.	Hold the tension and concentrate on tension in your fist.	Let go of the tension. Allow your hand to relax, letting your fingers go loose. Actively relax the tension away.	Focus on relaxing sensations in your hand and examine the contrast between tension and relaxation.
Right/left forearms	Press arms downward on the arm of the recliner. (Alternative: Lift arms and place them straight out in front of you away from your body, making them straighter and straighter, as straight as possible.)	Hold the tension and concentrate on the tension in your forearms.	Let your arms relax and rest comfortably on your lap.	Focus on the relaxing sensations in your forearms, noticing the difference between tension and relaxation.
Right/left arms	Bring your arms toward your shoulders, bending at the elbow.	Hold the tension and focus on the tension in your arms.	Allow your arms to relax and rest comfortably.	Focus on the relaxing feelings in your arms, once again noticing the difference.
Toes	Curl your toes as tightly as you can.	Hold the tension in your toes and examine it.	Let go of the tension in your toes and let your toes rest comfortably.	Concentrate on the relaxing sensations and examine the difference.
Calves	Lift both feet slightly off the ground and point your toes away from you.	Hold the tension there and examine the feelings of tension in your calves.	Let your legs rest comfortably now and feel the relaxing sensations.	Focus on the relaxing sensations in your calves and take notice of the difference between tension and relaxation.
Thighs	Tighten your thigh muscles by pressing the heels of your feet into the floor as hard as you can.	Hold the tension there and pay attention to the sensations of tension in your thighs.	Now, just let the tension go.	Focus on those relaxed feelings and focus on the difference.
Abdomen	Tighten your abdominal muscles tighter and tighter.	Hold the tension there.	Gradually release the tension in your abdomen by letting go.	Concentrate on the relaxing sensations and the difference.
Chest	Take a deep breath and fill up your lungs as much as you can.	Hold your breath and concentrate on the sensations of tension in your chest.	Gradually exhale while saying the word "relax" to yourself.	As you are exhaling, focus on the relaxing sensations that accompany letting go. Now, focus on the difference between tension and relaxation.
Neck	Bend your head forward and let your chin touch your chest.	Keep your head forward and hold the tension in your neck.	Bring your neck back to its normal position.	Just focus on the relaxed feelings in your neck and note the difference.
Jaw	Clench your jaw as tightly as you can . . . tighter and tighter.	Hold the tension there and concentrate on the tension there.	Now, just let your jaw relax comfortably.	Focus on the relaxing feelings in your jaw and focus on the difference.
Lips	Press your lips together as tightly as possible, tighter.	Hold your lips pressed together.	Let your lips relax.	Concentrate on the relaxing sensations in your lips and notice the difference.
Eyes	With eyes closed, close your eyes tighter and tighter.	Hold the tension around your eyes and focus on the tension.	Now, just let your eyes relax.	Concentrate on the relaxation and study the difference.
Forehead	Wrinkle your forehead by raising your eyebrows as high as you can.	Keep your forehead wrinkled and concentrate on the tension there.	Now, relax your forehead by smoothing it out as much as you can . . . smoother and smoother.	Notice the difference between tension and relaxation.

Adapted from material in Barlow and Cerney (1988), Clum (1990), Masters et al (1987), and Poppen (1998).

5. Patients with unrealistic expectations about relaxation
6. Patients with past or present physical injuries where tensing muscles may cause discomfort
7. Patients who suffer from paranoia, dissociative states, and thyroid problems
8. Relaxation may enhance effects of sedatives and insulin; may also create tiredness and temporary hypotension and hypoglycemia.

Technique

1. Instruct patient to settle back into the recliner and close eyes.
2. Follow outline provided in Table 340–1 and conduct two tension-relaxation cycles for each muscle group.
3. Repeatedly focus the patient's attention to slowing breathing rate during the exercise.
4. Provide explicit instruction and suggestions to enhance the relaxation and active "letting go" of tension by patient.
5. Teach patient to associate the relaxed state with the cue word "relax" by repeatedly pairing the word "relax" with exhalation and relaxed sensations throughout.
6. At conclusion of the total tension-relaxation exercise, instruct patient to follow path of relaxation through each muscle group from toes to forehead as in the accompanying table, with added suggestions of sensations of relaxation, warmth, and heaviness.
7. Finally, at end of entire exercise, instruct patient, when ready, to count backward from 5 to 1; open eyes at count of 1 with suggestion to feel relaxed, alert, and refreshed.
8. The entire exercise is administered by physician, who observes patient for signs of increased relaxation.
9. Formal sessions are conducted once a week until patient is proficient at inducing relaxed state on own.
10. Clinician may audiotape a relaxation session for home use by patient.
11. Patient is encouraged to practice technique once or twice daily.

Follow-Up

1. Track improvements in patient's symptoms through patient and physician monitoring.
2. Provide continued reinforcement for practice of relaxation.
3. Incorporate and plan relapse-prevention strategies designed to prevent tension from reaching maladaptive levels.
4. Gradually increase intervals between sessions to foster practice and generalization.
5. Remind patient to use tension as a cue to relax.
6. Plan periodic booster sessions to foster maintenance of gains.

Bibliography

Barlow DH, Cerney JA: Psychological Treatment of Panic, pp 96–119. New York, Guilford Press, 1988.
Carlson CR, Bernstein DA: Relaxation skills training: abbreviated progressive relaxation. In O'Donohue W, Krasner L (eds): Handbook of Psychological Skills Training: Clinical Techniques and Applications, pp 20–35. Boston, Allyn & Bacon, 1995.
Clum GA: Coping with Panic: A Drug-Free Approach to Dealing With Panic Attacks, pp 69–91. Pacific Grove, CA, Brooks/Cole Publishing, 1990.
Everly GS: A Clinical Guide To The Treatment of the Human Stress Response, pp 166–169. New York, Plenum Press, 1989.
Masters JC, Burish TG, Hollon SD, et al: Behavior Therapy Techniques and Empirical Findings, 3rd ed, pp 36–77. Fort Worth, Harcourt Brace Jovanovich, 1987.
Poppen R: Behavioral Relaxation Training and Assessment, 2nd ed. New York, Pergamon Press, 1998.

341 Hyperventilation Syndrome

Randolph W. Evans

Etiology

1. Definition: a syndrome characterized by a variety of somatic symptoms induced by physiologically inappropriate hyperventilation and usually reproduced in whole or in part by voluntary hyperventilation
   a. Acute hyperventilation with obvious rapid breathing accounts for only 1 per cent of all cases.
   b. Chronic hyperventilation without obvious rapid breathing is responsible for 99 per cent of cases. May occur with a small imperceptible increase in tidal volume or a mild increase in resting respiratory rate or both. Once established, an occasional deep breath will keep the partial pressure of oxygen (pCO_2) low.
2. Epidemiology
   a. Occurs in about 6 to 11 per cent of the general patient population.
   b. Occurs two to seven times more frequently in females.
   c. Most patients range in age between 15 and 55 years, but can occur in childhood and in the elderly.
3. Pathophysiology
   a. Hyperventilation produces a reduction in arterial pCO_2, resulting in alkalosis.
   b. Respiratory alkalosis produces the Bohr effect, a left shift of the oxygen dissociation curve with increased binding of oxygen to hemoglobin and reduced oxygen delivery to tissues.
   c. Alkalosis also causes a reduction in plasma Ca^{2+} concentration. Hypophosphatemia may occur as a result of intracellular shifts of phosphorus caused by altered glucose metabolism. In chronic hyperventilation, bicarbonate and potassium levels may be decreased as a result of increased renal excretion.
   d. Stress can trigger a hyperadrenergic state that may trigger hyperventilation caused by β-adrenergic stimulation.
   e. Cerebral blood flow can be reduced by 30 to 40 per cent by low pCO_2–induced cerebral vasoconstriction. Coronary vasoconstriction can occur in patients with occlusive disease or Prinzmetal's angina.
4. Mechanisms of symptom production
   a. Chest pain may arise from the intercostal or anterior chest muscles, occasionally from angina.
   b. Shortness of breath or difficulty getting a good breath may be due to overinflation of the chest.
   c. Dry mouth, bloating, belching, flatulence, and epigastric fullness may be due to aerophagia.
   d. Dizziness, headache, visual disturbance, tinnitus, ataxia, syncope, and various psychological symptoms may be produced by diminished cerebral blood flow.
   e. The cause of paresthesias is not certain. Possibilities include decreased cerebral perfusion and increased peripheral nerve axonal excitability.
   f. Muscle spasms and tetany may be due to respiratory alkalosis and hypocalcemia.
   g. In chronic hyperventilation, hypophosphatemia may result in tiredness, dizziness, poor concentration, disorientation, and paresthesias. Hypokalemia can cause muscle weakness and lethargy.
   h. A hyperadrenergic state with anxiety may result in tremor, tachycardia, anxiety, and sweating.
5. Pathogenesis
   a. Acute hyperventilation may be triggered by acute stress, anxiety, or emotional upset.
   b. Chronic hyperventilation may be a bad habit of exaggerated thoracic breathing with episodes triggered by any physical or emotional disturbance that produces increased ventilation.

Symptoms

1. The symptoms and signs are protean and can occur alone or in various combinations. Dizziness, dyspnea, chest pain, and paresthesias are the most frequent.
2. Include general, cardiovascular, gastrointestinal, neurologic, psychological, and respiratory manifestations

3. Paresthesias may be symmetric, involving one or various combinations of sites including the face, especially periorally, and the extremities, especially the hands and feet. Unilateral paresthesias also can occur affecting the left side of the face and body more often than the right.

4. Unusual psychological complaints may be reported, such as feelings of unreality and hallucinations.

Key Symptoms

- General: fatigability, exhaustion, weakness, sleep disturbance, nausea, sweating

- Cardiovascular: chest pain, palpitations, tachycardia, Raynaud's phenomenon

- Gastrointestinal: aerophagia, dry mouth, pressure in throat, dysphagia, globus hystericus, epigastric fullness or pain, belching, flatulence

- Neurologic
  - Headache, pressure in the head, fullness in the head, head warmth
  - Blurred vision, tunnel vision, momentary flashing lights, diplopia
  - Dizziness, faintness, vertigo, giddiness, unsteadiness
  - Tinnitus
  - Numbness, tingling, coldness of face, extremities, trunk
  - Muscle spasms, muscle stiffness, carpopedal spasm, generalized tetany, tremor
  - Ataxia, weakness
  - Syncope and seizures

- Psychological
  - Impairment of concentration and memory
  - Feelings of unreality, disorientation, confused or dream-like feeling, déjà vu
  - Hallucinations
  - Anxiety, apprehension, nervousness, tension, fits of crying, agoraphobia, neuroses, phobic, panic

- Respiratory: shortness of breath, suffocating feeling, smothering spell, unable to get a good breath or breathe deeply enough, frequent sighing, yawning

From Evans RW: Neurologic aspects of hyperventilation syndrome. Semin Neurol 1995;15:115–125, with permission. Copyright Thieme Medical Publishers, Inc.

Clinical Findings
1. With acute hyperventilation, tachypnea is present; with chronic, there may be no obvious signs.
2. Tetany and carpopedal spasm occur rarely.

Key Signs

- Tachypnea in acute hyperventilation
- Rarely tetany or carpopedal spasm

Laboratory Tests
1. The diagnosis depends on reproducing some or all of the symptoms with the hyperventilation test and excluding other possible causes by either clinical reasoning or laboratory testing when indicated.

2. The hyperventilation test can be performed with either an increased ventilation rate of up to 60 breaths per minute or simply deep breathing for 3 minutes.

   a. The hyperventilation test should *not* be performed in patients with ischemic heart disease, cerebrovascular disease, pulmonary insufficiency, hyperviscosity states, significant anemia, sickle cell disease, and uncontrolled hypertension.

   b. Dizziness, unsteadiness, and blurred vision commonly develop within 20 to 30 seconds, especially with the patient in the standing position; paresthesias usually start later. Chest pain is reported by 50 per cent of patients after 3 minutes of hyperventilation and by all by 20 minutes.

   c. For clinical purposes, measurement of arterial or end-tidal volume pCO_2 is not necessary. There is no clear correlation between arterial pCO_2 and neurologic manifestations.

   d. For some patients with hyperventilation syndrome, symptoms cannot be reliably reproduced during the hyperventilation test. The provocation test lacks test-retest reliability. Antecedent anxiety and stress may need to be present to reproduce symptoms.

3. Hyperventilation can produce electrocardiogram changes, including T-wave inversion, ST segment depression, and ST segment elevation in patients without coronary artery disease.

Key Test

Hyperventilation provocation test

Differential Diagnosis
1. Salicylism, caffeinism, and other drug effects
2. Cirrhosis and hepatic coma, acute pain such as with a myocardial infarction, splenic flexure

syndrome, cholecystitis, fever and sepsis, dissecting aortic aneurysm, respiratory dyskinesia, pulmonary embolism, pneumothorax, interstitial lung disease, asthma, heat and altitude acclimatization, and a variety of neurologic conditions including brain stem strokes and intracranial hypertension.

3. Similar transient neurologic and psychological symptoms may occur in migraine aura, partial and partial complex seizures, multiple sclerosis, transient ischemic attacks, and panic attacks.

Treatment

1. There is a lack of well-controlled treatment trials for the various approaches available.

2. Patient education and breathing instructions for attacks are the most important and often only treatment necessary.

3. Medications may be helpful in selected cases.

4. Breathing exercises and diaphragmatic retraining may be helpful for some patients.

5. Biofeedback and hypnosis may help patients who do not respond to usual treatments.

6. Psychological and psychiatric referral may be necessary in patients with significant anxiety, depression, or panic disorder.

Medication

1. β-Blockers may reduce palpitations, tremor, and anxiety.

2. Benzodiazepines may be helpful for anxious patients when prescribed for a short period of time.

3. Antidepressant medications may be helpful in patients with underlying depression or panic disorder.

Patient Education

1. An explanation of the difference between acute and chronic hyperventilation should be provided. Many patients with the chronic form will protest that they do not breathe rapidly as in the hyperventilation test. Explain how breathing a little too fast or too deeply can cause a drop in pCO_2. Then explain briefly how the symptoms may be produced by physiologic changes.

2. Reassuring patients that they do not have a serious condition is crucial. If the diagnosis is clear-cut, avoid laboratory testing.

3. Explain how anxiety and various emotional states might trigger symptoms. Alternatively, if a patient chronically hyperventilates because of stress or out of habit, explain this connection.

4. Once the patient understands the pathophysiology, then treatment of an acute episode by elevating the pCO_2 makes sense. Suggest that if the patient has additional episodes, he or she should try a breathing treatment. Options include holding the breath and counting to 10, followed by breathing every 6 seconds for a minute or so or breathing into a small paper bag placed over the nose and mouth for up to several minutes.

Key Treatment

Treatment of Choice	Alternative Treatment
• Patient education	• Medications
• Instruction in "breathing treatment"	

Follow-Up

1. Monitoring

   a. Have the patient check in by telephone a week or so after the initial visit.

   b. If the symptoms persist, a follow-up visit and discussion of additional treatment may be necessary.

2. Prognosis: For most patients, education, reassurance, and instruction in "breathing treatment" will lead to resolution of episodes.

 ## Bibliography

Evans RW: Neurologic aspects of hyperventilation syndrome. Semin Neurol 1995;15:115–125.

Gardner WN: Hyperventilation syndromes. Respir Med 1992;86:273–275.

Lum LC: Hyperventilation syndromes in medicine and psychiatry: a review. J R Soc Med 1987;80:229–231.

Magarian GJ: Hyperventilation syndromes: infrequently recognized common expressions of anxiety and stress. Medicine 1982;61:219–236.

Saisch SGN, Wessely S, Garnder WN: Patients with acute hyperventilation presenting to an inner-city emergency department. Chest 1996;110:952–957.

342 Phobias

Jeanne Parr Lemkau

1. Phobias are acute anxiety and avoidance reactions in response to specific feared objects or situations. Phobic individuals generally recognize that their anxiety responses are out of proportion to realistic threat.

2. Phobias are common across the lifespan. Treatment is indicated when symptoms restrict life and interfere with functioning, contribute to avoidance of necessary medical or dental care, or cause the individual to experience significant distress or secondary complications, such as substance abuse or depression.

3. Three types of phobic disorder are recognized within current psychiatric nosology:

   a. *Simple phobias* are of various types, including phobias of animals, elements of the natural environment (heights, water, etc.), blood-injection-injury, or situations (bridges, airplanes, elevators).

   b. *Social phobias* are characterized by fear of scrutiny by others in social/performance situations.

   c. *Agoraphobia* is characterized by fear of places or situation from which escape might not be possible or where help might not be available should panic/anxiety occur. Agoraphobia usually develops secondary to the onset of panic attacks.

4. Once well-established in adult patients, phobias are highly persistent and rarely remit without treatment.

Etiology

Theories abound as to the general etiology of phobias, although the source(s) in the individual case are often elusive and not necessary to identify in order for treatment to be successful. Etiological theories variously emphasize

1. *Classical conditioning* and stimulus generalization from negative experiences (a child who develops a "white coat" phobia after a noxious medical procedure)

2. *Psychodynamic processes* emphasizing psychological defenses (a marital conflict is symbolically expressed as a fear of leaving home).

3. *Genetic predispositions* toward anxiety disorders and/or the misfiring of innate protective mechanisms related to adaptive fears (a blood phobia).

Symptoms

1. *Marked persistent fear* of an object or situation out of proportion to realistic threat

2. Acute *anxiety or panic upon exposure* to the feared object or situation. Panic attacks are common among agoraphobic individuals and those who seek help in medical settings for anxiety disorders.

3. *Avoidance* of the feared object or situation or intense distress upon exposure

Key Symptoms

- Dry mouth, trembling, palpitations, shortness of breath, and/or other symptoms of anxiety in response to specific stimulus

- Avoidance of feared situation or stimulus

Clinical Findings

The diagnosis of a phobic disorder is made on the basis of history and clinical presentation.

1. *Signs of anxiety* described or observed may include palpitations, trembling, sweating, blushing, fainting, muscular tension, fears of going crazy, and other manifestations of autonomic nervous system arousal.

2. The anxiety reaction is *in direct response to a specific object or situation.*

3. *Other behavior described or observed* may include secondary attempts to manage anxiety (substance abuse) and/or co-morbid conditions (depression).

4. *Panic attacks* may or may not be present. When present, their onset typically precedes the onset of phobic avoidance.

Key Signs

- Physiologic signs of anxiety when confronted with feared object or situation, such as
  - Palpitations
  - Dry mouth
  - Fainting or dizziness
  - Hyperventilation

Laboratory Tests

Although not routinely indicated, laboratory tests may be helpful to rule out medical illness or substance abuse in individual cases.

Differential Diagnosis

Numerous nonphobic disorders may present with symptoms of anxiety for which different treatments are indicated. Differential diagnosis of phobias includes generalized anxiety disorder, obsessive compulsive disorder, post-traumatic stress disorder (PTSD), separation anxiety, avoidant personality disorder, paranoid and psychotic states, depression, and organic anxiety disorder.

1. In *generalized anxiety disorder*, excessive anxiety and worry is not restricted to a specific object or situation.

2. In *obsessive compulsive disorder*, fear is cued by obsessions about contamination.

3. In *PTSD*, symptoms represent the re-experience of trauma and/or avoidance of stimuli associated with the trauma.

4. In *separation anxiety*, onset is usually in childhood and anxiety is specific to anticipated or actual separation from attachment figures.

5. In *avoidant personality disorder*, the dominant fear is of social rejection rather than the embarrassment feared by the social phobic.

6. *Paranoid and psychotic states and schizophrenia* are distinguished from social phobia or agoraphobia by broader symptomatology and impaired reality testing.

7. *Depression* with social withdrawal is distinguished from social phobia by the presence of vegetative signs and depressed mood. Depression is a frequent co-morbid condition with agoraphobia.

8. *Organic disorders* that may generate symptoms of anxiety, fear, avoidance, and physiological arousal include cerebrovascular accident, brain tumor, and substance abuse.

Note

When alcohol or drug problems develop secondary to social phobia, treatment of phobia is indicated in addition to substance abuse treatment.

Treatment

Exposure-based behavioral treatment by a behaviorally oriented psychologist or psychiatrist is the treatment of choice for phobic disorders. The efficacy of such treatment has been well supported by empirical research. Exposure-based treatments are typically carried out over several weeks or months. Cognitive approaches that integrate patient education and address maladaptive thought patterns that underlie anxiety symptoms, and stress management techniques that address physiologic arousal, are often integrated with behavioral techniques. Depending on the individual situation, adjunctive treatment may include marital therapy with agoraphobic individuals, social skills training with social phobics, relaxation training, and bibliotherapy.

1. Patient education should include basic information on phobia, panic, and treatment as appropriate to the patient. Patients should be advised to limit caffeine intake, which can exacerbate anxiety and panic in sensitive individuals.

2. Exposure-based behavioral treatments that have received strong empirical support for their efficacy include

   a. *Graduated in vivo exposure*: The patient is supported to practice exposure to the feared stimulus in progressive steps, often in conjunction with relaxation training.

   b. *Systematic desensitization*: Imaginal confrontation of the feared stimulus is visualized in progressive steps, often in conjunction with relaxation training and in vivo exposure.

   c. *Imaginal flooding*: The patient is supported to confront and maintain exposure to the feared stimulus in fantasy until extinction of learned anxiety responses has occurred.

   d. *Participant modeling and reinforced practice*: The patient watches others engage in feared behavior and is rewarded for progressive practice.

3. Medication may be needed to supplement behavioral treatment or to treat co-morbid conditions; its use should be evaluated on a case-by-case basis.

   a. Medication is more helpful in cases of *generalized anxiety* than in cases of *specific pho-*

bias. Empirical support for treating simple phobia with medication is weak.

b. For *panic disorder* that often underlies agoraphobia, antidepressants, anxiolytics, and β-blockers may be helpful.

c. Care should be taken to *avoid iatrogenic complications* of prescribing anxiolytic drugs to social phobics, for whom substance abuse is a frequent complication.

4. Use other treatment approaches as appropriate to dominant symptoms of patient (i.e., social skills training for socially inept individuals, progressive relaxation for those with prominent physiological arousal, etc.).

Key Treatment

- Patient education

- Referral for exposure-based behavioral treatment

- Medication for panic or co-morbid conditions

- Other therapies as indicated

Follow-Up

Occasional "booster" sessions of cognitive-behavioral treatment are sometimes required to maintain gains achieved through comprehensive treatment.

Bibliography

American Psychiatric Association: Diagnostic and Statistical Manual of Mental Disorders, 4th ed. Washington, DC, American Psychiatric Press, 1994.

Fones CS, Manfro GG, Pollack MH: Social phobia: an update. Harvard Rev Psychiatry 1998;5:247–259.

Knapp S, VandeCreek L: Anxiety Disorders: A Scientific Approach for Selecting the Most Effective Treatment. Sarasota, FL, Professional Resource Press, 1994.

Rachman S: Anxiety. East Sussex, UK, Psychology Press Ltd, 1998.

Stein MM, McQuaid JR, Laffaye C, et al: Social phobia in the primary care medical setting. J Fam Pract 1999; 48:514–519.

343 Wernicke-Korsakoff Syndrome

Randy K. Ward

Etiology

1. Wernicke's encephalopathy and Korsakoff's amnestic syndrome can be viewed as two facets of the same pathophysiologic process. This process is a nutritional deficiency disorder secondary to lack of thiamine. The deficiency results in an alteration in central nervous system (CNS) carbohydrate metabolism that leads to neuronal dysfunction and damage. The primary areas affected are in the brain stem, diencephalon, and cerebellum.

2. In the western world the main cause is chronic alcohol dependence in the context of malnutrition.

3. Other more rare causes are starvation, persistent vomiting, malignancies, and inadequate parenteral nutrition.

Symptoms

1. Wernicke's encephalopathy presents as an acute onset of symptoms.
   a. Confusion, visual disturbances, and gait problems compose the classic triad.
   b. Many patients will not recognize the symptoms because of their confusion and concurrent alcohol use.
   c. The symptoms may begin as isolated difficulties of vision or gait and progress to an acute confusional state.

2. Korsakoff's amnestic syndrome may develop after one or more episodes of Wernicke's encephalopathy.
   a. Patients develop severe anterograde and retrograde amnesia (inability to form new memories or recall distant memories).
   b. Confusion and lack of insight are present secondary to the memory deficits.

Key Symptoms

Wernicke's Encephalopathy

- Confusion
- Visual disturbances
- Gait problems

Korsakoff's Amnestic Syndrome

- Anterograde and retrograde amnesia
- Confusion

Clinical Findings

1. The diagnosis of Wernicke's encephalopathy requires opthalmic signs and at least one other clinical sign of the triad. It usually occurs in patients with chronic alcoholism and malnutrition.
   a. The most common opthalmic sign is horizontal or vertical nystagmus.
      (1) Lateral rectus weakness or palsy is also common.
      (2) Other oculomotor weakness or palsy may be present.
   b. Stance is wide based and gait is slow and uncertain.
   c. Mental status examination shows a global confusional state.
      (1) Apathy, indifference, inattentiveness
      (2) Disorientation, misidentification, poor judgment and insight
      (3) Stupor and coma are rare.

2. Korsakoff's amnestic syndrome occurs after one or more episodes of Wernicke's encephalopathy and results in anterograde and retrograde amnesia.
   a. Short-term memory is markedly impaired. Patients cannot commit new information to memory.
   b. Remote memory loss is severe and may cover a period of many years.
   c. These deficits result in confusion and difficulties in intellectual functioning.

Key Signs

Wernicke's Encephalopathy

- Ophthalmoplegia and nystagmus
- Wide-based, ataxic gait
- Confusion with a clear sensorium

Korsakoff's Amnestic Syndrome

- Severe anterograde and retrograde amnesia
- Confusion and lack of insight

Laboratory Tests

Wernicke-Korsakoff syndrome is a clinical diagnosis.

1. Magnetic resonance imaging (MRI) can help confirm characteristic CNS structural damage.
2. Neuropsychological testing can confirm and clarify memory deficits.

Key Test

MRI

Differential Diagnosis

1. Wernicke's encephalopathy
   a. Delirium
   b. Intoxication
   c. Seizure
   d. Trauma
   e. CNS vascular or mass lesion
2. Korsakoff's amnestic syndrome
   a. Dementia
   b. Anoxia
   c. Trauma
   d. Herpes encephalitis
   e. CNS vascular or mass lesion

WARNING

Any patient suspected of being alcohol dependent or malnourished should receive parenteral thiamine prior to administration of glucose or any form of nutrition, in order to prevent Wernicke-Korsakoff syndrome.

Treatment

1. Wernicke's encephalopathy
   a. This is a medical emergency, and requires immediate treatment with parenteral thiamine. The usual dose is 100 mg IV or IM.
   b. The resolution of confusion may be rapid but is variable. Ocular manifestations usually begin to recover within hours, and ataxia within days.
   c. Supportive fluids and nutrition should be given after administration of thiamine.
   d. Continued treatment with oral or parenteral thiamine, vitamin supplementation, and an appropriate diet is required.
   e. The patient should be evaluated for alcohol withdrawal and other sequelae of chronic alcoholism and malnutrition.
2. Korsakoff's amnestic syndrome
   a. Proper nutrition and abstinence from alcohol are crucial in recovery.
   b. There is no specific pharmacotherapy for the cognitive deficits. There have been trials with clonidine and selective serotonin reuptake inhibitors.
   c. Patients may require pharmacologic management of anxiety and agitation secondary to their cognitive deficits.

Key Treatment

- Thiamine
- Avoidance of alcohol

Follow-Up

1. Wernicke's encephalopathy
   a. Continued monitoring is necessary to evaluate the resolution of the patient's symptoms. Residual nystagmus and gait problems may remain.
   b. The patient may go on to develop Korsakoff's amnestic syndrome.
2. Korsakoff's amnestic syndrome
   a. Approximately 20 per cent of patients will eventually fully recover, 25 per cent will show no improvement, and the remainder show partial recovery over time.
   b. Patients may require behavioral management, pharmacotherapy of anxiety and aggression, or placement in supervised living settings depending on the severity of their deficits.

Bibliography

Adams RD, Victor M, Ropper AH: Principles of Neurology, 5th ed, pp 1139–1145. New York, McGraw-Hill, 1997.

Gastfriend DR, Renner JA, Hackett TP: Alcoholic patients—acute and chronic. In Cassem NH (ed): Massachusetts General Hospital Handbook of General Hospital Psychiatry, 4th ed, pp 211–230. St. Louis, Mosby–Year Book, 1997.

Guido ME, Brady W, DeBehnke D: Reversible neurological deficits in a chronic alcohol abuser: a case report of Wernicke's encephalopathy. Am J Emerg Med 1994; 12:238–240.

Lishman WA: Organic Psychiatry: The Psychological Consequences of Cerebral Disorder, 3rd ed, pp 575–585. Oxford, Blackwell Scientific Publications, 1998.

Messing R: Nutritional disorders of the nervous system. In Bennett JC, Plum F (eds): Cecil Textbook of Medicine, 20th ed, pp 2039–2041. Philadelphia, WB Saunders Company, 1994.

344 Alcoholism

Warren G. Thompson

Etiology

1. Genetic: Sons of alcoholics are four times as likely to be alcoholic as sons of nonalcoholics whether they are raised by biologic or adoptive parents. Adoptions studies on daughters of alcoholics are less clear, but a recent twin study in women found higher concordance in monozygotic twins, suggesting that heredity is also important in women. Studies of genetic markers and of a specific gene for alcoholism are inconclusive.

2. Ethnicity and culture: Rates among American Indians are very high, whereas rates among Asian Americans appear to be lower than the general population. France has a much higher prevalence of alcoholism than Italy even though the per capita alcohol consumption in Italy is slightly higher.

3. Occupations: bartenders, painters, and physicians

4. Social influences: Legal restrictions and increased price decrease rates of alcoholism.

5. Sex: Rates are much higher in men than in women. Women living with a substance-abusing male are at high risk.

6. Tolerance: Sons of male alcoholics and possibly other men who have increased tolerance for alcohol are at increased risk.

Natural History

1. The majority of heavy young male drinkers reduce drinking to nonproblem drinking as they get older without intervention. Inner city men begin problem drinking about 10 years earlier (ages 25 to 30) than college graduates. Surprisingly, inner city men are more likely to be abstinent at long-term follow-up (30 vs. 10 per cent), but they are also more likely to die (30 vs. 15 per cent). Mortality in both groups is greatly increased by smoking. Continued abstinence can only be reliably predicted by 5 years of not drinking; 40 per cent of men abstinent for 2 years or longer relapse.

2. The typical onset of problem drinking in females occurs later than in males (after age 25). However, progression is more rapid and females usually enter treatment earlier. Women

are more likely to abuse prescription drugs with alcohol.

3. The spontaneous remission rate of alcoholism is 10 to 30 per cent.

4. In one study only 31 per cent of men with a self-defined drinking problem sought help from a physician. These men often did not reveal they had a problem with drinking, and only 50 per cent of those who sought help were asked about their alcohol intake. Only 25 per cent of the problem drinkers were either encouraged to reduce their intake or warned about the health hazards of drinking, and only 3 per cent of these heavy drinkers were referred to a treatment program by their physician. Physicians need to learn to screen effectively for alcoholism (Table 344-1).

Diagnosis

Medical symptoms, clinical findings, and laboratory tests are not sufficiently sensitive to be useful in the diagnosis of alcoholism. Screening and diagnosis require an assessment of the consequences of alcoholism in several domains (see below).

Symptoms

1. Patients with alcoholism may complain of abdominal pain, diarrhea, weight loss, palpitations, sexual dysfunction, memory loss, depression, blackouts, or seizure or give a history of gastrointestinal bleeding.

2. The patient may present with symptoms of the consequences of alcoholism (holiday heart syn-

TABLE 344-1. WHY SCREEN FOR ALCOHOLISM?

- The problem is common (between 10 and 20 per cent in general medical outpatient populations).
- Effective screening tests are available.
- If one does not screen, the diagnosis is likely to be missed (50–90 per cent of alcohol problems are missed in the office).
- Effective treatments are available (especially if diagnosis is made early).
- Early identification can prevent physical and psychosocial problems from developing in the patient, family, and society.

Adapted from Cyr MG, Sherman SE: Screening, assessment, making the diagnosis. In Bigby JA (ed): Substance Abuse Education in General Internal Medicine: A Manual for Faculty, p 3. Washington, DC, Society of General Internal Medicine, 1993, with permission.

344 Alcoholism • 1473

drome, cirrhosis, alcoholic hepatitis, Wernicke's encephalopathy).

Key Symptoms

- Abdominal pain
- Diarrhea
- Weight loss
- Palpitations
- Sexual dysfunction
- Memory loss
- Depression
- Blackouts

Clinical Findings

1. Patients with alcoholism may present with gynecomastia, testicular atrophy, spider angiomas, hepatomegaly, abdominal tenderness, evidence of cerebellar dysfunction, or hypertension.
2. Alcohol odor on breath
3. Bilateral parotid gland enlargement
4. Unexplained tremulousness

Key Signs

- Alcohol odor on breath
- Bilateral parotid gland enlargement
- Unexplained tremulousness

Laboratory Tests

1. γ-Glutamyltransferase (GGT) and mean corpuscular volume are the most sensitive (about 50 per cent) laboratory tests.
2. Other liver function tests, creatinine kinase, amylase and lipase, magnesium, phosphorus, uric acid, and triglycerides may also provide clues to the diagnosis.

Key Test

Blood alcohol level (Table 344–2) is the most specific and most underutilized test for diagnosis of alcoholism.

TABLE 344–2. BLOOD ALCOHOL LEVELS DIAGNOSTIC OF ALCOHOLISM

Blood alcohol level >300 at any time
Blood alcohol level >150 if not obviously intoxicated
Blood alcohol level >100 on a routine office visit

Screening

1. The most practical screening tool is the CAGE questionnaire (Table 344–3).
2. The Alcohol Use Disorders Identification Test (AUDIT), which has 10 questions, has been shown to be superior to the CAGE because it is better at detecting binge drinkers and people who drink too much but are not alcohol dependent. These questions should be asked after the CAGE questions.
3. Table 344–3 contains a set of questions (including some questions from AUDIT) that are practical for office use and will pick up most patients presenting with alcoholism. In addi-

TABLE 344–3. SCREENING FOR ALCOHOLISM

General Population*
1. Do you drink alcohol at all?
   If yes: go to questions 2–5
   If no: Have you ever had a drinking problem?
         Has anyone in your family had a drinking problem?
2. CAGE questionnaire: follow up on positive questions with questions about the circumstances and the reasons
   –Have you ever felt the need to Cut down on your drinking?
   –Have people Annoyed you by criticizing your drinking?
   –Have you ever felt bad or Guilty about your drinking?
   –Have you ever had a drink first thing in the morning to steady your nerves or get rid of a hangover? (Eye-opener)
3. How often do you have a drink containing alcohol?
4. How many drinks containing alcohol do you have on a typical day when you are drinking?
5. Other questions that are often useful
   –How often do you have 6 or more drinks on one occasion?
   –How often during the past year have you found that you were not able to stop drinking once you had started?
   –Do you ever have an irresistible craving for alcohol?
   –Have you had blackouts or memory loss after drinking?
   –Is your drinking different now than 5 years ago?
   –Have you ever been arrested for drinking, such as for driving under the influence?
   –Have you ever gotten in trouble at work because of drinking?
   –Have you neglected your family, work, or obligations for 2 or more days in a row because you were drinking?
   –Have you ever been to an AA meeting?

Geriatric Population†
1. Did you find your drinking increased after someone close to you died?
2. Does alcohol make you sleepy so that you often fall asleep in your chair?

Adolescent Population‡
1. Do you drink alone?
2. Do you ever miss school to go drinking or because you have a hangover?

*Adapted from Cyr MG, Sherman SE: Screening, assessment, making the diagnosis. In Bigby JA (ed): Substance Abuse Education in General Internal Medicine: A Manual for Faculty, pp 3–14. Washington, DC, Society of General Internal Medicine, 1993, with permission.
†Adapted from AMA Council on Scientific Affairs: Alcoholism in the elderly. JAMA 1996;275:797–801, with permission.
‡Adapted from Elster AB, Kuznets NJ: AMA guidelines for adolescent preventive services, p 125. Baltimore, Williams & Wilkins, 1994, with permission.

tion, these questions provide the main tools needed to make the diagnosis of alcoholism.

Formal Diagnosis

1. The *Diagnostic and Statistical Manual of Mental Disorders, Fourth Edition* (DSM-IV) defines alcohol abuse as continued use despite familial or occupational consequences or recurrent use in hazardous situations (driving while intoxicated) over a 12-month period; the patient does not meet the criteria for physical dependence.

2. The diagnosis of alcohol dependence requires three or more of the following eight symptoms:
   a. Continued drinking despite physical or psychological consequences caused or exacerbated by alcohol
   b. Neglect of other activities
   c. Inordinate time spent drinking and recovering
   d. Drinking more or over a longer period than intended
   e. Inability to control drinking
   f. Tolerance (increased amounts needed for effect)
   g. Withdrawal symptoms on cessation of drinking
   h. Drinking to relieve or avoid withdrawal symptoms

Treatment

1. Naltrexone (ReVia), 50 mg once daily, blocks opiate receptors in the brain and reduces craving for alcohol. In two 12-week trials abstinence increased from 33 to 54 per cent. Liver function tests should be less than three times normal, and the drug should not be used until patients are off alcohol (and opiates) for at least 1 week. The cost is about $4.50 a day.

2. Acamprosate, which affects γ-aminobutyric acid receptors, has been shown to be effective as well but is available only in Europe.

3. The largest trial of disulfiram (Antabuse) showed very little benefit.

Patient Education

1. Brief physician advice reduces alcohol intake, lowers GGT levels, and reduces hospital days.

2. A trial period of controlled drinking with careful follow-up may be appropriate for a diagnosis of alcohol abuse. Complete abstinence is the only treatment for alcohol dependence.

3. The physician should present the diagnosis in a nonjudgmental fashion that emphasizes the consequences of alcohol on that patient's life and the need for complete abstinence. The word "alcoholic" should be avoided. Indicate that responsibility for change is up to the patient. If the patient does not believe there is a problem, suggest a 2-week trial of abstinence and suggest bringing a family member to the next appointment.

4. Alcoholics Anonymous (AA) should be strongly recommended.
   a. Physicians should have literature about AA available to patients. The address is AA General Service, P.O. Box 459, Grand Central Station, New York, NY 10163.
   b. One does not have to be religious to go to AA. Patients should attend at least five different meetings in order to find a compatible meeting (an inner city resident may be uncomfortable at a suburban meeting and vice versa). Women may do better at meetings open only to women.
   c. Hospitalized patients should be encouraged to call from the hospital (AA will send someone to talk to them if the patient makes the contact).
   d. Patients need to attend meetings regularly (daily at first) and for a sufficient length of time (usually 2 years or more) because recovery is a difficult and lengthy process.

5. In the beginning, patients should remove alcohol from their home and avoid bars and other establishments where there is strong pressure to drink.

6. If the patient has an antisocial personality (severe problems with family, peers, school, and police before age 15 and before the onset of alcohol problems), recovery is unlikely. If the patient has a primary depression (depression that antedates problems with alcohol or is a significant problem during long periods of sobriety), this problem should be addressed.

7. Family members of alcoholics should be strongly encouraged to contact Al-Anon and Alateen. The address is Al-Anon Family Group Headquarters, P.O. Box 182, Madison Square Garden Station, New York, NY 10159-0182.

Key Treatment

- Naltrexone
- Patient education

Follow-Up

1. Frequent follow-up is essential to support the patient in recovery. Patients should be asked

TABLE 344–4. STRATEGIES IN RELAPSE PREVENTION

1. Learning to say no to drinking in social situations
2. Handling heavy-drinking friends who will try to undermine the patient's sobriety
3. Handling stress (do not ignore symptoms of anxiety)
4. Avoiding boredom (patients have previously been spending a great deal of time drinking and recovering and now they have time on their hands)
5. Learning to get along again with family and close friends (family problems often increase when drinking stops)
6. Identifying other situations that can lead to drinking again and develop ways to cope with these situations

Adapted from Schuckit MA: Treatment of alcoholism in office and outpatient settings. In Mendelson JH, Mello NK (eds): Medical Diagnosis and Treatment of Alcoholism, p 381. New York, McGraw-Hill, 1992, with permission.

about attendance at AA meetings and about their relationship with their sponsor.

2. The key step for the patient is to realize that treatment does not end with sobriety. Recovery means that patients can handle the stresses of everyday life without alcohol. Therefore, the patient must develop and rehearse strategies to cope with high-risk situations (Table 344–4).

Attending to these situations is essential for both treatment and follow-up.

Bibliography

For more information on diagnosis, see
American Psychiatric Association: Diagnostic and Statistical Manual of Mental Disorders, 4th ed. Washington, DC, American Psychiatric Press, 1994.

For more information on improving skills in diagnosis and treatment and on teaching about alcoholism, see
Bigby JA (ed): Substance Abuse Education in General Internal Medicine: A Manual for Faculty. Washington, DC, Society of General Internal Medicine, 1993.

For more information on diagnosis and treatment of alcoholism, see
O'Connor PG, Schottenfeld RS: Patients with alcohol problems. N Engl J Med 1998;338:592–602.

For comparison of the CAGE questionnaire and the AUDIT, see
Steinbauer JR, Cantor SB, Holzer CE, et al: Ethnic and sex bias in primary care screening tests for alcohol use disorders. Ann Intern Med 1998;129:353–362.

For documentation of the importance of early recognition and physician advice to stop drinking, see
Fleming MF, Barry KL, Manwell LB, et al: Brief physician advice for problem alcohol drinkers: a randomized controlled trial in community-based primary care practices. JAMA 1997;277:1039–1045.

345 Fetal Alcohol Syndrome

Esther Entin

1. Fetal alcohol syndrome (FAS) is a physical and neurodevelopmental syndrome with a characteristic triad of craniofacial dysmorphology, growth deficiencies, and central nervous system dysfunction. It results from exposure of the developing fetus to alcohol and causes lifelong morbidity. Quantity of alcohol, gestational timing of exposure, and genetic background influence the severity of the manifestations. The most devastating impact is on cognitive development, and the degree of intellectual impairment parallels the severity of the craniofacial abnormalities.

2. The designation fetal alcohol effect (FAE) may be used for a patient who has been exposed to alcohol in utero and manifests characteristic neurodevelopmental/behavioral/cognitive features, but lacks growth retardation or full phenotypic facial features.

Etiology

1. Maternal alcohol consumption during pregnancy
   a. Critical period: from conception through the first 2 months of pregnancy.
   b. Dose-related effect
      (1) Mild FAS can be induced by as little as 1 ounce of absolute alcohol daily.
      (2) Complete syndrome seen with consumption of four to five drinks (60 to 75 ml absolute alcohol) per day.
      (3) No absolutely safe level of ethanol consumption during pregnancy has yet been established.

2. Paternal alcohol consumption
   a. Heavy alcohol intake by the father prior to conception has been suspected of producing FAS.
   b. Conclusive evidence lacking but American Medical Association states that growth retardation and some adverse aspects of fetal development may be due to paternal influence.

Clinical Findings

The diagnosis of FAS requires that items 1, 2, and 3 below be present (Fig. 345–1).

1. Craniofacial dysmorphology
   a. Typical facies: short palpebral fissures, hypoplastic upper lip with thinned vermillion, diminished to absent philtrum, midfacial and mandibular growth deficiency
   b. Other findings
      (1) Eyes: ptosis, strabismus, epicanthal folds, myopia, microphthalmia, blepharophimosis
      (2) Ears: poorly formed concha, posterior rotation, eustachian tube dysfunction
      (3) Nose: short upturned
      (4) Mouth: prominent lateral palatine ridges, retrognathia in infancy, micrognathia or relative prognathia in adolescence, cleft lip or palate, small teeth with faulty enamel, malocclusion, poor dental alignment
      (5) Maxilla: hypoplastic

2. Central nervous system: most debilitating symptom
   a. Microcephaly
   b. Cognitive deficits: mild to moderate retardation (extent parallels degree of craniofacial abnormality), specific arithmetic deficiency, difficulty with abstraction and concept of cause and effect, poor generalization, inattention, poor concentration, memory deficit, impaired judgment, low adaptive functioning

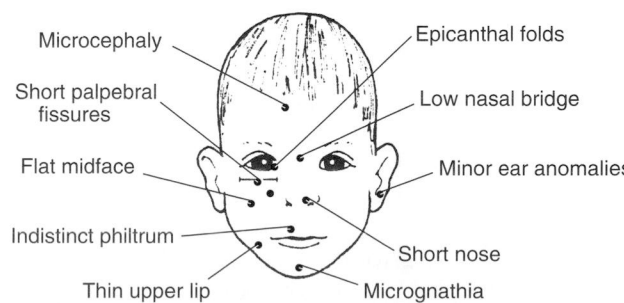

Figure 345–1 Facies in fetal alcohol syndrome. Modified from Streissguth AP, LaDue RA, Randels SP: A manual on adolescents and adults with fetal alcohol syndrome with special reference to American Indians. Indian Health Service, Public Health Service, U.S. Dept. of Health and Human Services, 1988, p 7.

c. Motor deficits:
   (1) Fine motor dysfunction: weak grasp, poor eye-hand coordination, and/or tremulousness
   (2) Hypotonia
d. Behavioral characteristics
   (1) Infancy and newborns: irritable and tremulous, poor suck and hyperacusis for weeks to months
   (2) Attention-deficit hyperactivity disorder in childhood
   (3) Adult: maladaptive behaviors, poor social skills
3. Growth
   a. Prenatal growth deficiency in length and weight: small-for-gestational-age infants
   b. Postnatal deficiency in length, weight, and head circumference, usually remain more than two standard deviations below the mean for height and weight; decreased adipose tissue
4. Other major and minor malformations, variably present
   a. Cardiac murmurs, atrial septal defect, ventricular septal defect, great vessel anomalies, tetralogy of Fallot
   b. Renogenital anomalies, labial hypoplasia, hypospadias
   c. Cutaneous: hemangiomas, hirsutism in infancy
   d. Skeletal: abnormal palmar creases, pectus excavatum, restriction of joint movement, nail hypoplasia, radioulnar synostosis, pectus carinatum, bifid xiphoid, Klippel-Feil anomaly, scoliosis
   e. Muscular hernias of diaphragm, umbilicus or groin; diastasis recti

Key Signs

- Craniofacial dysmorphology
- Developmental, behavioral, neurologic abnormalities
- Growth deficiencies

Differential Diagnosis
Shares some phenotypic symptoms with other syndromes:
a. Fetal hydantoin
b. Cornelia de Lange's syndrome
c. Noonan's syndrome

d. Williams' syndrome
e. Trisomy 18

Outcome/Course
1. Craniofacial
   a. Facial anomalies become more subtle in adolescents and adults.
   b. Dental malalignments, malocclusions secondary to maxillary hypoplasia
   c. Eustachian tube dysfunction leads to chronic serous otitis.
2. Growth abnormalities
   a. Often present with failure to thrive in infancy and childhood.
   b. May have some improvement in growth and weight-to-height proportion.
   c. Persistent short stature
   d. Persistent microcephaly
3. Central nervous system developmental outcome
   a. Developmental and cognitive handicaps persist.
   b. Most FAS individuals fail to achieve independent housing and income.
   c. Low-average academic functioning; fourth grade often highest educational level
   d. Social: poor judgment, distractibility, difficulty recognizing social cues

Medical Intervention
1. Identification of syndrome from characteristic stigmata
2. Referral for specific treatments based on individual needs (e.g., craniofacial surgery, ear-nose-throat surgery)
3. Behavioral management
4. Educational interventions
5. Anticipation of needs through the life cycle
6. Treatment of associated malformations as indicated

Prevention
1. Preconception and prenatal counseling regarding alcohol intake
2. Treatment of alcohol abuse
3. Awareness of unrecognized sources of alcohol (e.g., medications)

Bibliography

Astley SJ, Clarren SK: A case definition and photographic screening tool for the facial phenotype of fetal alcohol syndrome. J Pediatr 1996;129:33–41.

Briggs G, Freeman R, Yaffe S: Drugs in Pregnancy and Lactation, 4th ed. Baltimore, Williams & Wilkins, 1994.

Clarren SK, Smith, DW: The fetal alcohol syndrome. N Engl J Med 1978;298:1063–1067.

Spohr HL, Willms J, Steinhausen HC: Prenatal alcohol exposure and long term developmental consequences. Lancet 1993;341:907–910.

Streissguth AP, Aase JM, Clarren SK, et al: Fetal alcohol syndrome in adolescents and adults. JAMA 1991;265: 1961–1967.

Weinberg NZ: Cognitive and behavioral deficits associated with parental alcohol use. J Am Acad Child Adolesc Psychiatry 1997;36:1177–1186.

346 Substance Abuse

Ernest Frugé

Etiology

1. There are a number of competing theories of etiology (e.g., biological, psychodynamic, sociopolitical).
2. Substance abuse is best conceptualized as a biopsychosocial disease resulting from an interplay of physical, psychological, and social factors unique to each patient.
3. It is most important to determine for each patient what factors may maintain drug use, motivate quitting, and precipitate relapse following treatment.

Definition of Key Terms

1. *Substance abuse*: the use of a substance in a way that is not medically or socially (e.g., legally) sanctioned and/or causes harm to self or others
2. *Addiction*: repeated use despite negative physical, psychological, or social consequences
3. *Tolerance*: diminishing effect of a drug with regular use; significant increase over time in amount of drugs needed to produce the desired results
4. *Dependence*: physical adaptation so that rapid removal of the drug causes a withdrawal syndrome
5. *Withdrawal*: reduction in amount of substance taken in. Depending on the rate of reduction and class of drug, a drug-specific withdrawal syndrome can occur, ranging from mild flu-like symptoms to severe reactions (e.g., seizures, cardiovascular collapse).
6. *Overdose*: toxic or lethal amount of substance
7. *Detoxification*: management of withdrawal symptoms by administering declining doses of the substances or of a cross-tolerant drug
8. *Relapse*: return to substance abuse after a period of abstinence

Epidemiology

1. About 35 to 40 per cent of the U.S. population will use illicit drugs at some time in their lives, and 6 to 8 per cent will meet the formal criteria for dependence. These percentages do not include the abuse of alcohol or prescription drugs. The U.S. Department of Health and Human Services has estimated that 20 to 40 per cent of hospitalized patients are there because of complications of drug and alcohol use.
2. It is likely that an individual will abuse more than one substance simultaneously.
3. Particular populations present greater risks for substance abuse. Keeping substance abuse in mind when dealing with these populations is important.
   a. Adolescents and young adults: Children are experimenting with drugs at earlier ages. Between 40 and 50 per cent of high school seniors admit some use of illicit drugs. Use of alcohol and smoking cigarettes are correlated with the use of illicit drugs. Drugs are frequently involved in crimes, high-risk sexual behavior, and accidents and injuries (including homicide and suicide), the leading causes of death in this age range.
   b. Neonates: Drug use during pregnancy is correlated with birth complications and defects. Exposure can be particularly damaging if it occurs within the first trimester. Infants born to addicted mothers also may display signs of withdrawal.
   c. Elderly: This group is at risk for self-overmedication or poly-pharmacy because of lack of coordination between multiple physicians involved in their care. Symptoms of substance abuse may be hidden by family members, misdiagnosed as other medical conditions, or mistakenly viewed as simply a by-product of "aging" (e.g., problems in attention).
   d. Disadvantaged populations: This includes ethnic and racial minorities, homeless individuals, and the disabled.

Symptoms and Clinical Findings

1. Arylcyclohexylamines
   a. Examples: phencyclidine (PCP), ketamine
   b. Effects
      (1) Desired effects include altered sensory perceptions and reduced inhibition.
      (2) Tolerance develops in high-dose users.
      (3) Dependence and withdrawal have not been conclusively documented.
   c. Signs of overdose: disorientation, coma, cat-

atonia, nystagmus, hypertension, and seizures

2. Hallucinogens
   a. Examples: lysergic acid diethylamide (LSD), mescaline, methylene dioxyamphetamine (MDA), methylene dioxymethamphetamine (MDMA), 1-(2,5-dimethoxy-4-methylphenyl)-2-aminopropane (DOM/STP), trimethoxyamphetamine (TMA), *N,N*-dimethyltryptamine (DMT), *N,N*-diethyltryptamine (DET), psilocybin
   b. Effects
      (1) Desired effects include altered sensory perception and stimulation.
      (2) Tolerance develops rapidly.
      (3) Dependence and withdrawal do not occur.
   c. Signs of overdose: disorientation, dilated pupils, nausea, rambling speech, perceptual distortions, seizures (severe cases)

3. Cannabis (marijuana)
   a. Examples: hashish, tetrahydrocannabinol (THC)
   b. Effects
      (1) Desired effects include euphoria, central nervous system (CNS) depression.
      (2) Tolerance and dependence develop with high-dose use.
      (3) Withdrawal is mild and does not appear for 8 to 10 days because of long half-life. Symptoms may include anxiety, insomnia, and nausea.

4. Opiates
   a. Examples: heroin, morphine, methadone, codeine, pentazocine, butorphanol, meperidine, buprenorphine, hydromorphone, propoxyphene
   b. Effects
      (1) Desired effects include euphoria, CNS depression, analgesia.
      (2) Tolerance develops rapidly to euphoria and CNS depression, less rapidly to analgesia.
      (3) Dependence develops rapidly to short-acting drugs (morphine, heroin, and methadone) and less rapidly to long-acting drugs (codeine and partial agonist drugs).
      (4) Withdrawal symptoms are uncomfortable but not life threatening and vary with the amounts and lengths of time opiates are used. Common symptoms include craving, irritability, agitation, tachycar-

dia, hypertension, headache, perspiration, abdominal cramps, nausea, anorexia, anxiety, broken sleep, dysphoria, muscle aches, fatigue, and rhinorrhea.
   c. Signs of overdose: decreased respiration, miotic pupils, bradycardia, hypotension, pulmonary edema, coma

5. Sedative-hypnotics
   a. Examples: barbiturates, benzodiazepines, sleeping pills, muscle relaxants, "minor tranquilizers"
   b. Effects
      (1) Desired effects include euphoria and CNS depression.
      (2) Tolerance develops more rapidly to desired effects than to therapeutic effects and more rapidly to therapeutic effects than to lethality, except for benzodiazepines, where lethal doses are rare. Cross-tolerance exists for all sedative-hypnotics.
      (3) Dependency develops more rapidly to short-latency, short-acting drugs and less rapidly to the long-acting drugs.
      (4) Withdrawal may be life-threatening.
   c. Signs of overdose: respiratory depression, nystagmus, depressed deep tendon reflexes, hypotension, dysarthria, coma

6. Solvents (inhalants)
   a. Examples: gasoline, halogenated hydrocarbons (Freon), nitrous oxide, toluene, carbon tetrachloride, airplane glue, amyl nitrite, butyl nitrite
   b. Effects
      (1) Desired effects include euphoria, CNS depression, "rush" of blood pressure, and respiration changes.
      (2) Tolerance may develop with prolonged use.
      (3) Dependence and withdrawal not well-documented.
   c. Signs of overdose: disorientation, odor of solvent, arrhythmia, hypoxia

7. Stimulants
   a. Examples: amphetamines, prescription diet pills, methylphenidate, cocaine, caffeine
   b. Effects
      (1) Desired effects include stimulation of the CNS, euphoria, and appetite control.
      (2) Tolerance develops rapidly, particularly the anorexiant effect.
      (3) Dependence is now thought to develop;

however, withdrawal symptoms are relatively mild.

   c. Signs of overdose

     (1) Acute signs include hyperactivity, diaphoresis, dilated pupils, tremor, tachycardia, hypertension, hyperpyrexia, stereotypical behavior, seizures, and paranoia.

     (2) Within 24 to 36 hours, patient may experience hypersomnolence, hyperphagia, and electroencephalographic changes. After several weeks, insomnia and depression

8. Anabolic steroids

   a. Examples

     (1) Oral: ethylestrenol (Maxibolin), fluoxymesterone (Halotestin), methyltestosterone (Android-5, Virilon)

     (2) Injectable: nandrolone decanoate (Deca-Durabolin), testosterone cypionate (Depo-Testosterone), testosterone enanthate (Testaval 90/4)

   b. Effects

     (1) Desired effects include increased muscle mass, strength, and fighting ability. Desired effects also include decreased healing time following injury and decreased recovery time following weight training.

     (2) Adverse effects include psychiatric disorders such as depression, mania, psychosis, and marked aggressiveness.

     (3) Unclear evidence for physical dependence and withdrawal, but psychological dependence develops, compounded by the social reinforcement linked with enhanced appearance and performance.

   c. Signs of overuse

     (1) Short-term signs include rapid increase in musculature, behavioral and mood alterations (particularly increased aggressiveness), and excessive acne.

     (2) Chronic signs of overuse include hypercalcemia, diabetes, testicular atrophy, impotence, virilization and voice changes in females, arthritis, hyperlipidemia, liver tumors, hepatic cholestasis, jaundice, and hepatocellular carcinoma.

Diagnosis

1. General considerations in diagnosis

   a. Early detection and intervention are associated with better treatment outcomes.

   b. Scanning for drug use should be incorporated into routine history taking and should focus on problems that are often associated with substance abuse.

   c. Early indicators are typically behavioral, psychological, and social.

   d. Medical complications are usually associated with chronic abuse and overdose.

   e. Other psychiatric disorders (e.g., anxiety, depression, personality disorders) often coincide with substance abuse.

2. Leading psychosocial indicators

   a. Psychological/behavioral: anxiety, depression, distractibility, mood swings, irritability, violence, poor judgment, memory loss, psychosis (e.g., hallucinations, delusions)

   b. Work/school: declining and/or disrupted performance, frequent absences or tardiness, frequent job changes

   c. Family and social relations: spouse or child abuse, emotional and behavioral disorders in patient's children, loss of friends (or development of antisocial friends in children and adolescents), neglect of children's welfare

   d. Legal and financial: crime (including delinquency); arrests for driving while under the influence, theft, public intoxication or disturbing the peace; financial mismanagement (e.g., defaulted loans); selling possessions

3. Medical complications potentially associated with substance abuse

   a. Cardiovascular: arrhythmias, arteritis, cardiomyopathy, cor pulmonale, endocarditis, hypertension, myocardial infarction, myocarditis, thrombophlebitis, vasculitis

   b. Pulmonary: abscess, cellulitis, hemorrhage, edema, pneumothorax, reduced pulmonary function, respiratory depression, foreign-body reactions

   c. Gastrointestinal: abdominal cramping and diarrhea, anorexia, cirrhosis, chronic constipation

   d. Neurologic: ataxia, delirium, ischemia, peripheral nerve lesions, seizures, stroke, coma

   e. Reproductive: impaired sperm production, complications in pregnancy (intrauterine growth retardation), congenital abnormalities, infertility, irregular menses, neonatal distress, sexually transmitted disease, testicular enlargement or atrophy

   f. Septicemia and infections: fungal ophthalmitis, hepatitis, renal disease, human immunodeficiency virus infection, tetanus

   g. Other physical examination findings: conjunctivitis, hepatomegaly, increased sweating, jaundice, malnutrition, miosis, muscle weakness or wasting, mydriasis, nystagmus, poor hygiene, repeated injuries, rhinorrhea, scleral icterus

h. Seeking to obtain psychoactive drugs from the physician without clear medical indications

Laboratory Tests and Detection

1. Toxicology screens with combining procedures such as immunoassays and chromatographic assays are useful in determining which drugs are involved in emergency situations.

2. Drug testing is of limited use in general practice because of the limited span of time reflected in the tests.

Differential Diagnosis

1. Primary mental disorder (e.g., mental disorders resulting from a general medical condition, dementia, psychosis, mood disorders, anxiety disorders)

2. Nonpathologic substance use (e.g., medical or recreational purposes)

3. Dual psychiatric diagnosis (e.g., anxiety, depression)

Treatment

1. General considerations

a. Selection of treatment strategies is determined by the severity of the problem and cooperation of the patient.

b. It is crucial that the physician maintain confidentiality and a supportive, nonjudgmental stance, focusing on the physical health and well-being of the patient.

c. Patients often deny or distort their drug-use pattern.

(1) If substance abuse is suspected, generally assume that patients are underestimating or denying substance use unless proved otherwise.

(2) Use collateral sources of information (e.g., spouses, parents) whenever possible and appropriate.

(3) Some patients, however, may exaggerate use (e.g., adolescents attempting to shock their parents).

d. Moving from physical findings to implications for health and competence (e.g., sexual difficulties) may be a doorway to increase motivation.

e. Early identification, education, and brief interventions can have very positive effects. Once substance abuse is discovered, it is important to determine the following:

(1) Range and patterns of substances used over time and currently (e.g., types, duration, frequency, routes of administration)

(2) Concurrent high-risk behavior (unprotected sex)

(3) Current (and predicted future) negative consequences of continued use/abuse

(4) Incentives for continued use/abuse and incentives for quitting

(5) Personal vulnerabilities, sources of support, resources and strengths

f. A frank discussion of use patterns and the short- and long-term negative consequences along with suggestions on how to modify habits may promote change or set the stage for future treatment efforts.

g. In severe cases the physician may be asked to coordinate or participate in a meeting of significant others in the patient's social network (e.g., spouse, children, employer, friends).

(1) The aim of this type of meeting (sometimes referred to as an "intervention") is to overcome a patient's denial of substance abuse or dependency and secure an agreement by the patient to pursue treatment.

(2) The participants rehearse in advance and then present specific evidence of the negative consequences of the problem both present and future (e.g., a spouse may announce the intention to divorce). Such presentations should be done in a compassionate, matter-of-fact manner, not judgmental, guilt-inducing, or threatening.

2. General rules for treatment of withdrawal and overdose

a. Withdrawal

(1) Withdrawal (detoxification) often can be managed on an outpatient basis but requires clear commitment to abstinence by the patient, a reliable caregiver, and daily monitoring by the physician.

(2) Inpatient detoxification is indicated for sedatives (and alcohol), when there are serious medical complications (e.g., sepsis, history of seizures), or when the conditions for patient compliance and daily physician monitoring are not present.

(3) Use long-acting drugs showing cross-dependence with the drug of abuse.

(4) Withdraw drugs in blind fashion using fixed-volume dosages.

(5) All drugs that produce dependence lead to a protracted abstinence syndrome that lasts for months.

b. Overdose

(1) Ensure adequate airway and respiration.

(2) Maintain the cardiovascular system.

(3) Assess the patient's level of consciousness.

(4) Draw appropriate blood studies before starting an intravenous line.

(5) Administer a 50% glucose solution and naloxone, 2 mg.

c. Drugs taken orally

(1) Determine the amount of time since the drug was taken.

(2) If the patient is fully conscious, administer an emetic and activated charcoal.

(3) In comatose patients, perform a gastric lavage with an endotracheal tube in place to prevent aspiration. Then administer activated charcoal through a nasogastric tube.

3. Treatment programs

a. Formats for treatment can range from outpatient programs to partial hospitalization (day or evening), inpatient programs, and residential programs (e.g., "therapeutic communities").

b. At this time, there is no evidence that one format of treatment for substance abuse (e.g., inpatient versus outpatient) is generally better than any other.

c. Referral to more expensive, restrictive inpatient programs should be determined by factors such as the following:

(1) Repeated failure of prior outpatient or partial hospital treatment efforts

(2) Serious medical or psychiatric concurrent conditions (e.g., high suicidal risk)

(3) Lack of (or seriously disturbed) social support system

d. Choice of treatment modalities is often limited by the patient's ability to pay.

e. Physicians should become familiar with the local range of programs available in both the public and private sectors, refer based on the best estimate of fit with patient characteristics, and evaluate program effectiveness over time.

f. Physicians can begin to evaluate programs by asking program representatives the following questions:

(1) What is the program's theoretical model, basic structure, and staffing?

(2) How does the program evaluate outcome?

(3) What is the cost of treatment?

(4) What is the scope and content of the assessment and treatment plan?

(5) Does the program include detoxification?

(6) What is the nature and cost of the relapse-prevention strategies and aftercare programs (postdischarge components)?

(7) What is the relationship between the program and referring physician?

4. Self-help groups

a. Twelve-step programs

(1) There are a number of nonprofit programs derived from the fundamental model of Alcoholics Anonymous that focus on other substances of abuse (e.g., Narcotics Anonymous, Cocaine Anonymous).

(2) These programs offer the addicted patient an opportunity to overcome the denial and develop new principles for life without drugs in an atmosphere of mutual support and anonymity.

(3) The groups emphasize the spiritual aspects of recovery yet are not religious organizations.

(4) The 12-step programs designed to help the families of addicted patients (e.g., Al-Anon) can be of substantial help to both loved ones and the patient.

b. Other resources

(1) Additional self-help programs may be available in the patient's area.

(2) Most local and state governments have offices dealing with drug abuse and can provide additional information.

Follow-Up

1. General

a. Recovery is a long-term process requiring extensive personal changes and often involving several relapses.

b. Continuity of compassionate care by the primary care physician for both the identified patient and his or her family can be a crucial element in maintaining the process of recovery.

2. Primary prevention
   a. Physicians can have positive effects through education of their child and adolescent patients and involvement in the community as well (e.g., school-based programs on the health risks of drugs and alcohol).
   b. Substance abuse cuts across all socioeconomic, racial, and ethnic groups. There are additional factors that can create vulnerability to substance abuse, including poverty, family disruption, negative peer influence, and parents with a history of substance abuse.
   c. The National Clearinghouse for Alcohol and Drug Abuse Information has validated the Problem Oriented Screening Instrument for Teenagers (POSIT) as a method for screening for substance abuse and developmental risk factors.

Bibliography

American Academy of Family Physicians: Diagnosis and Treatment of Drug Abuse in Family Practice (American Family Physician Monograph). Kansas City, MO, American Academy of Family Physicians, 1994.

Augenstein WL (ed): Emergency aspects of drug abuse. Emerg Med Clin North Am 1990;8:467–730.

Blondell RD (ed): Clinics in office practice: substance abuse. Primary Care 1993;20:1–276.

Lange WR, White N, Robinson N: Medical complications of substance abuse. Postgrad Med 1992;92:205–214.

Lowinson JH, Ruiz P, Millman RB (eds): Substance abuse: a comprehensive textbook. Baltimore, Lippincott, Williams & Wilkins, 1997.

347 Nicotine Dependence

Jack L. Cox

Epidemiology

1. In 1995, approximately 47 million U.S. adults were current cigarette smokers and, in 1991, 5.3 million adults were smokeless tobacco users (Table 347–1).
2. Adult cigarette use
   a. A total of 24.7 per cent of U.S. adults were current smokers in 1995; 44.3 million adults were former smokers. This rate has been flat for the last 5 years.
   b. Among current smokers, 32 million (68.2 per cent) wanted to quit and 17.3 million (45.8 per cent) had stopped smoking for at least 1 day during the preceding year.
3. Adult smokeless tobacco use
   a. In 1991, 2.9 per cent of U.S. adults were current smokeless tobacco users; 7.9 million adults were former smokeless tobacco users.
   b. The rate of smokeless tobacco use has tripled from 1972 to 1991.
4. High school student tobacco use
   a. An estimated 80 per cent of tobacco use occurs for the first time among individuals under 18 years old.
   b. Approximately 3000 adolescents begin smoking each day; 750 of these will die from tobacco-related diseases.
   c. In 1997, 42.7 per cent of high school students used cigarettes, smokeless tobacco, or cigars within 30 days prior to a Centers for Disease Control and Prevention survey. The number of current cigarette smokers increased from 27.5 per cent in 1991 to 36.4 per cent in 1997, a 32 per cent increase (Table 347–2).

Morbidity and Mortality

1. In 1990, 419,000 deaths were directly attributable to smoking. One out of every five deaths in the United States is directly related to smoking.
   a. Smoking kills more U.S. adults each year than all deaths caused by alcohol, illicit drugs, homicide, suicide, car accidents, fires, and acquired immunodeficiency syndrome combined. Most deaths from smoking are cardiovascular-related, neoplasm-related, or respiratory-related (Table 347–3).
   b. Average life expectancy for a 30-year-old man who smokes 1 pack per day is 64.8 years; for a 30-year-old man who never smoked it is 82.7 years.
   c. An individual who quits smoking at any time in his or her life increases the quality and quantity of life. For example, an individual who quits smoking before 50 years of age decreases overall mortality by 50 per cent over the next 15 years.
   d. Cigarette smoking is related to increased risk for complications in pregnancy (low birth weight, ectopic pregnancy frequency, spontaneous abortion, premature birth, placenta abruption), osteoporosis in women, cataract formation, and respiratory infections.
2. Environmental tobacco smoke (ETS) accounts for approximately 53,000 deaths annually: 37,000 from cardiovascular disease, 3700 from lung cancer, and 12,000 from other neoplasms.
   a. ETS has been labeled a class A carcinogen by the Environmental Protection Agency.
   b. ETS has been associated with an increased frequency of sudden infant death syndrome;

TABLE 347–1. ADULT TOBACCO USE PREVALENCE

	CIGARETTES (% OF POPULATIONS, 1995)	SMOKELESS TOBACCO (% OF POPULATIONS, 1991)
Men	27.0 (24.5 million)	5.6 (4.8 million)
Women	22.6 (22.5 million)	0.6 (533,000)
White	25.6	3.1
Black	25.8	2.3
<12 years education	29.5	4.6
≥16 years of education	14.0	1.4

TABLE 347-2. HIGH SCHOOL STUDENT CURRENT TOBACCO USE PREVALENCE (1997)

	CIGARETTE	SMOKELESS TOBACCO	CIGARS	ANY CURRENT TOBACCO USE
Male	37.7	15.8	31.2	48.2
Female	34.7	1.5	10.8	36.0
White	39.7	12.2	22.5	46.8
Black	22.7	2.2	19.4	29.4
Hispanic	34.0	5.1	20.3	36.8
Total	36.4	9.3	22.0	42.7

Adapted from Tobacco use among high school students–United States, 1997. MMWR Morb Mortal Wkly Rep 1998;47:229–232.

an increased incidence of pneumonia, asthma, and upper respiratory symptoms in childhood; and increased respiratory symptoms in adults.

3. Smokeless tobacco users are at an increased risk of oropharnygeal cancer, teeth/gum disease, coronary artery disease, and peptic ulcers.

Why People Use Tobacco

Addiction

1. Nicotine in tobacco products is at least as addictive as cocaine or heroin and is the reason most people use tobacco.
   a. Eighty per cent of smokers attempting to quit "cold turkey" undergo physiologic withdrawal symptoms. These symptoms usually peak in 48 to 72 hours and last for up to 4 to 6 weeks (Table 347–4).
   b. Nicotine withdrawal is the primary reason for relapse to smoking early on in attempted cessation.

TABLE 347-3. SMOKING-RELATED DEATHS

Cardiovascular Ischemic heart disease (myocardial infarct) Cerebrovascular disease (stroke) Hypertension Atherosclerosis	180,000 deaths
Neoplasms Cervix uteri Esophagus Kidney Larynx Lip, oral cavity, pharynx Lung Pancreas Urinary bladder	150,000 deaths
Respiratory Disease Pneumonia/influenza Emphysema/chronic bronchitis	84,000 deaths

2. Nicotine dependence is high if a smoker smokes within 30 minutes of awakening, smokes more than 20 cigarettes per day, or has had significant withdrawal symptoms with a previous quit attempt.

Psychosocial

1. Most smokers start smoking in response to peer, sibling, or parental smoking.
2. Smokers use tobacco for stress reduction, relaxation, and/or reward. Stress is the most common reason for late relapse in quit attempts. Coping mechanisms must be addressed for the quitting smoker in order to prevent relapse.
3. There is a higher incidence of underlying depression in smokers versus nonsmokers.

Habit

1. There are many cues that may precipitate craving for tobacco. These include the smell of coffee or cigarette smoke, seeing someone smoke, after meals, and with alcohol use.
2. These cues can be used to help a smoker quit by recognizing which cues are important and formulating plans for avoiding or handling them.

Treatment

Pharmacologic

1. Current pharmacologic therapies shown to be consistently helpful in smoking cessation include nicotine polacrilex (gum), nicotine transdermal patches, nicotine nasal spray, nicotine

TABLE 347-4. WITHDRAWAL SYMPTOMS

Anxiety/irritability	Nicotine craving
Headaches	Restlessness
Impaired concentrating	Sleep disturbance
Increased hunger	Somnolence

TABLE 347–5.   AVAILABLE PHARMACOLOGIC THERAPIES FOR SMOKING CESSATION

Nicotine polacrilex (OTC)	Nicorene (2 mg; gum), SmithKlein Beecham Pharmaceuticals
	Nicorette DS (4 mg; gum), SmithKlein Beecham Pharmaceuticals
Nicotine transdermal patches (OTC)	Nicoderm CQ (21, 14, 7 mg; 24-hour patch), SmithKlein Beecham Pharmaceuticals
	Habitrol (21, 14, 7 mg; 24-hour patch), Novartis
	Prostep (22, 11 mg; 24-hour patch), Lederle
	Nictrol (15 mg; 16-hour patch), McNeil
Nicotine nasal spray	Nicotrol NS (0.5 mg/spray), McNeil
Nicotine inhaler	Nicotrol Inhaler, McNeil
Bupropion HCl	Zyban (150-mg tablets), Glaxo Wellcome

inhaler, and bupropion (Table 347–5). There are not enough studies as of now on pharmacologic therapies in smokeless tobacco cessation.

2. Clonidine, Inderal, benzodiazepines, silver acetate, and lobeline have not been shown to consistently improve 1-year smoking cessation rates versus placebo.

3. The more intensive the behavioral intervention, the more successful abstinence; pharmacologic therapy doubles 1-year success rates of any behavioral intervention.

Behavioral Approaches

(Adapted from Smoking Cessation (Clinical Practice Guidelines No. 18. Bethesda, MD, Agency for Health Care Policy and Research, 1996.)

1. Ask about each patient's smoking status at every opportunity: former, current, never, or passive smoke exposure.
   a. About 70 per cent of smokers visit a physician's office at least once per year, yet 54 per cent of smokers in one study reported not being asked if they smoked or told to quit.
   b. Simply asking a patient if he or she smokes and telling him or her to quit increases chances for abstinence.

2. Advise all smokers to quit in a supportive, caring, nonjudgmental way, and let them know that, if they have problems quitting, you will help them. Cutting down is a step in the right direction, but complete abstinence should be the goal.

3. Assess motivation to quit (J. O. Prochaska's model for behavioral change):
   a. Precontemplators are individuals not currently interested in quitting.
   b. Contemplators are thinking of quitting within the next 6 months.
   c. Smokers in preparation are considering quitting within the next month and actively looking at strategies to quit.
   d. Smokers in the action phase are involved in changing their behavior and environment to quit.
   e. Patients in the maintenance phase have quit for over 6 months and are addressing ways to prevent relapse.

4. Assist smokers in quitting with a quit plan.
   a. Precontemplators need clear information on the hazards of smoking and the benefits of quitting.
   b. Contemplators need advice on strategies to help them quit: setting a quit date, offering pharmacologic therapy, skills training, and educational material.
   c. Individuals in the preparation and action phases need reassurance in their ability to quit and stay quit. Most smokers have made three to seven attempts at quitting before being successful. Setting a quit date greatly increases long-term success.
   d. Individuals in the maintenance phase benefit from positive feedback and advice on relapse prevention.
   e. All smokers should be offered pharmacologic therapy.

5. Arrange follow-up for all smokers attempting to quit, preferably at 1 week, 1 month, and 3 months after the quit date, or individualize. If a smoker relapses, identify the reason, and encourage another attempt to quit or continued abstinence.

 ## Bibliography

For a more in-depth discussion on smoking and smoking cessation, including the risk and benefits, see

Cigarette smoking among adults–United States, 1995. MMWR Morb Mortal Wkly Rep 1997;46:1217–1220.

Fiore M (ed): Cigarette smoking. Med Clin North Am 1992;76:289–539.

The Agency for Health Care Policy and Research smoking cessation clinical practice guideline. JAMA 1996; 275:1270–1280.

Tobacco use among high school students–United States, 1997. MMWR Morb Mortal Wkly Rep 1998;47:229–233.

For more information on stages of quitting, see
Prochaska JO, DiClemente CL, Norcross JC: In search of how people change: application to addictive behaviors. Am Psychol 1992;47:1102–1114.

For more information on the AHCPR Guideline No 18, contact
AHCPR Publications Clearinghouse; PO Box 8547; Silver Spring, MD 20907, or *http://www.ahcpr.gov/guide/*.

348 Schizophrenia

Linda B. Andrews

Etiology

1. One per cent lifetime prevalence; men and women equally affected; average age of onset, late teens to early adulthood; similar prevalence worldwide

2. Specific etiology not known.

3. Neurodevelopmental model: Central nervous system abnormalities, occurring probably as early as second trimester, alter normal neurotransmitter and subsequent limbic and cortical development. Symptoms appear when complicated neurobehavioral tasks are required in late adolescence/early adulthood.

4. Dopamine hypothesis: Hypoactive dorsolateral prefrontal cortex (DLPFC) dopamine neurons (secondary to problems in migration of neural tissue in early development) cause hyperactive limbic system dopamine neurons. Adolescence triggers the need to use one's DLPFC as higher cognitive functions develop.

5. Genetics: The closer the genetic relationship to the proband, the higher the risk of developing schizophrenia (i.e., monozygotic twins, 47 per cent; dizygotic twins, 12 per cent; general population, 1 per cent). Similar incidence in twins separated at birth and reared in different environments

6. Stress-diathesis model: Both neurophysiologic and psychosocial factors appear to be important. An individual has specific vulnerability or genetic predisposition that when acted on by stressors, allows the development of symptoms of schizophrenia.

Symptoms

1. Psychotic symptoms (active phase) for at least *1 month* (a, b, or c)

   a. Prominent hallucinations (hallucination is a perception of an external stimulus when no external stimulus is present)

   b. Bizarre delusions (delusion is a false belief not shared by others who have the same knowledge, experience, or cultural background that is firmly maintained even though it is contraindicated by social reality)

   c. Two of the following: less prominent hallucinations or delusions, disorganized speech (frequent loosening of associations [LOA] or incoherence), grossly disorganized or catatonic behavior, or negative symptoms (flat affect, poverty of speech, lack of initiative).

   These are sometimes called the "positive symptoms of schizophrenia" and may be related to the hyperactive limbic system dopamine neurons.

2. Some symptoms (chronic phase) for at least 6 *months*: isolation, withdrawal, decreased work performance, peculiar behavior, poor hygiene, flat affect, speech changes, odd beliefs, unusual perceptions, lack of initiative, interest, or energy. These are sometimes called the "negative symptoms of schizophrenia" and may be related to the hypoactive DLPFC dopamine neurons.

3. Decreased level of functioning (work, social, self-care)

4. No prominent mood symptoms (i.e., no prominent symptoms of depression or mania)

5. No "organic" (general medical) cause for symptoms

6. Subtypes of schizophrenia

   a. Paranoid: prominent paranoid ideations, best prognosis and generally later onset

   b. Catatonic: significant psychomotor changes, including stupor, negativism, rigidity, excitement, or posturing

   c. Disorganized: LOA, disinhibition, and grossly disorganized behavior

   d. Undifferentiated: not clearly one of the preceding three subtypes

   e. Residual: no active-phase symptoms but has two or more of the chronic-phase symptoms

Key Symptoms

- Hallucinations

- Delusions

- Decreased level of functioning

- Not attributable to another medical or psychiatric condition

Clinical Findings

1. Premorbid history: often a history of being a quiet, passive, withdrawn child, few friends, introverted, loner, daydreamer
2. Often positive family history of schizophrenia
3. Chronic deteriorating course of exacerbations and remissions
4. Positive symptoms: hallucinations, delusions, LOA. Negative symptoms: isolation, withdrawal, poor hygiene, flat affect, lack of initiative, interest, or energy
5. Fifty per cent attempt suicide; 10 per cent succeed.
6. Mental status examination
   a. Orientation: usually alert and oriented with clear sensorium and no fluctuation in level of consciousness
   b. Motor activity: May fluctuate between agitation and psychomotor retardation.
   c. Affect and mood: The most common affective presentations are either blunted emotional responsiveness or overly labile/inappropriate emotions. The blunted affect can represent symptoms of the illness, parkinsonian side effects of medications used to treat the illness, or a superimposed depression.
   d. Thought process/content: when psychotic, often illogical, not goal-directed, may include LOA, flight of ideas, thought blocking, or delusions (persecutory, grandiose, religious, somatic or thought-control, thought-broadcasting, thought-withdrawal)
   e. Perception: when psychotic, often prominent hallucinations (usually auditory)
   f. Insight: often poor
   g. Judgment: when psychotic, poor; when not psychotic, adequate
   h. Memory and abstraction: often impaired
7. Physical examination findings: Frequently soft neurologic symptoms, abnormal eye movements (increased rate of blinking, abnormal rapid eye movements, and decreased ability to follow an object through space with smooth eye pursuit), tics, stereotypes, grimacing, impaired fine motor skills, abnormal motor tone; no physical findings are diagnostic or pathognomonic.
8. Computerized tomography (CT) scan: Static ventricular enlargement, indicative of decreased cortical mass, is present at onset of illness in 10 to 50 per cent of patients (not diagnostic). Positron emission tomography scan: decreased frontal lobe metabolism, especially during psychological tests that stress this area of the brain
9. Electroencephalogram (EEG) findings: Significant number of patients have abnormal records with some tendency toward left-sided abnormalities (not diagnostic).
10. Psychological testing: When psychotic, projective tests (Rorschach) abnormal.

Key Signs

- Hallucinations
- Delusions
- Positive family history of schizophrenia
- Chronic deteriorating course

Laboratory Tests

1. There are no laboratory tests that definitively diagnose schizophrenia.
2. The work-up to evaluate schizophrenia should include tests necessary to exclude other medical conditions that can present with psychotic symptoms (toxicology screens, complete blood count, rapid plasma reagin, CHEM-20, thyroid function tests, CT scan, EEG).
3. Mental status examination

Key Test

Mental status examination

Differential Diagnosis

1. Medical disorders or substance abuse (intoxication or withdrawal) that present with psychotic symptoms
2. Schizophreniform disorder: diagnosed if the patient has had symptoms for less than 6 months
3. Brief psychotic disorder: diagnosed if the symptoms have been present at least 1 day but less than 1 month
4. Schizoaffective disorder: diagnosed if depressive or manic symptoms are at least as prominent as the psychotic symptoms
5. Mood disorders with psychotic symptoms: diagnosed if the psychotic symptoms are brief relative to the mood symptoms. Cross-sectionally, mania can mimic schizophrenia.
6. Delusional disorder: diagnosed if the patient has nonbizarre delusions for at least 6 months

and does not have any of the other symptoms of schizophrenia

7. Personality disorders: Patients with borderline, paranoid, schizoid, and schizotypal personality disorders all may have brief periods of psychotic symptoms.

Treatment

First assess whether or not the patient needs to be hospitalized for diagnostic purposes, stabilization on medications, patient's safety (i.e., suicidal ideations), or patient's lack of ability for self-care.

Medication

1. General guidelines
   a. Define target symptoms to be treated.
   b. Choose an antipsychotic medication that has worked for the patient or family member in the past, if tolerated.
   c. Give patient an adequate trial (4 to 6 weeks on medication) at adequate doses.
   d. If patient does not respond, try medications from different chemical classes.
   e. Monitor for compliance.
2. Antipsychotic medications (previously called "neuroleptics" or "major tranquilizers") are the medications of choice for schizophrenia.
   a. Newer atypical antipsychotics such as clozapine (Clozaril), risperidone (Risperdal), or olanzapine (Zyprexa) may be more effective, especially for negative symptoms. Clozapine does have a serious potential side effect of agranulocytosis.
   b. All traditional (typical) antipsychotics are equally efficacious. Traditional antipsychotics can generally be grouped based on high or low affinity for blocking dopamine$_2$ receptors.
      (1) High-potency
          (a) Haloperidol (Haldol)
          (b) Fluphenazine (Prolixin)
          (c) Trifluoperazine (Stelazine)
      (2) Low-potency
          (a) Chlorpromazine (Thorazine)
          (b) Thioridazine (Mellaril)
   c. Acute episodes of psychotic symptoms generally respond to 5 to 30 mg of high-potency antipsychotics or 300 to 1000 mg of low-potency antipsychotics.
   d. Side effects for high-potency antipsychotics include extrapyramidal symptoms (acute dystonic reactions, akathisia-restlessness, induced parkinsonism) and neuroleptic malignant syndrome (fever, rigidity, autonomic instability, altered mental status), a life-threatening side effect that occurs in 0.5 to 1 per cent of patients treated with these medications. Anticholinergic medications (diphenhydramine [Benadryl], benztropine [Cogentin]) can be used to treat acute dystonic reactions.
   e. Side effects for low-potency antipsychotics include anticholinergic side effects (dry mouth, blurred vision, urinary retention, constipation), postural hypotension, and sedation.
   f. Most antipsychotics also can cause weight gain and impotence.
   g. A long-term and usually irreversible side effect of all typical antipsychotics is tardive dyskinesia. Tardive dyskinesia occurs in 15 to 20 per cent of patients treated with typical antipsychotics.
   h. Atypical antipsychotics combine dopamine and serotonin blockade and may cause less extrapyramidal symptoms, including less risk for tardive dyskinesia.

Patient Education

1. Patient and family education about schizophrenia is crucial for compliance (Alliance for the Mentally Ill is a national referral resource: 1-800-950-NAMI).
2. Supportive group therapy also may be useful to reduce social isolation and improve reality testing.

Key Treatment

Treatment of Choice	Other Treatment
• Antipsychotic medications	• Patient/family education
	• Supportive group therapy

Follow-Up

1. Decisions to maintain patients on antipsychotics are based on the severity of the illness as well as the availability of family and community support.
2. Greater than two thirds of patients relapse within the first 6 months following the discontinuation of antipsychotic medication. Therefore, the patient must be instructed that he or she may need this medication indefinitely. Once stabilized, the patient can be followed as an outpatient as frequently as weekly or as infre-

quently as every 3 to 6 months depending on symptom stability.

Bibliography

Andreasen NC: Schizophrenia: From Mind to Molecule. Washington, DC, American Psychiatric Press, 1994.

Bymaster FP, Rasmussen K, Calligaro DO, et al: In vitro and in vivo biochemistry of olanzapine: a novel, atypical antipsychotic drug. J Clin Psychiatry 1997; 58(Suppl 10):28–36.

Davis KL, Kahn RS, Ko G, et al: Dopamine and schizophrenia: a review and reconceptualization. Am J Psychiatry 1991;148:1474–1486.

Kapur S, Remington G: Serotonin-dopamine interaction and its relevance to schizophrenia. Am J Psychiatry 1996;153:466–476.

Weinberger DR: Implications of normal brain development for the pathogenesis of schizophrenia. Arch Gen Psychiatry 1987;44:660–669.

349 Obsessive Compulsive Disorder

Norman H. Rasmussen

Obsessive compulsive disorder (OCD) is characterized by recurrent and intrusive thoughts, ideas, impulses, or images (*obsessions*) and/or by the presence of stereotyped repetitive behaviors (*compulsions*). Obsessive compulsive disorder is a generally chronic and often disabling condition with a lifetime prevalence of 2 to 3 per cent based on epidemiologic studies. Recent epidemiologic studies indicate that OCD is slightly more common in females. Approximately one third of adult cases are of childhood onset.

Etiology

1. The specific cause of OCD is unknown.
2. Genetic evidence
   a. Recent twin studies indicate a concordance rate in the 50 to 90 per cent range for monozygotic twins as compared with the 40 per cent range for dizygotic twin pairs.
   b. In family studies of OCD probands, up to 25 per cent of the fathers and 9 per cent of the mothers have OCD. When subclinical OCD is included, approximately 35 per cent of all first-degree relatives are affected.
3. Neurobiologic basis for OCD
   a. Neuroimaging studies (positron emission tomography [PET], single-photon emission computed tomography, magnetic resonance imaging) of nontreated and treated OCD patients have revealed neurophysiologic abnormalities in primarily three brain areas: orbital frontal cortex, cingulate cortex, and head of the caudate.
   b. Although there are no published postmortem studies in OCD, the morphology of the brain in living patients, as evidenced primarily on computerized tomography (CT) findings, reveals no consistent evidence of structural pathology.
   c. The prevailing neurophysiologic model of OCD implicates a dysfunction in central serotonin neurotransmission, that is, an abnormal decrease of serotonergic (inhibitory) activity in the brain.
4. Psychosocial causes
   a. Freudian psychodynamic factors based primarily on the ego-defense mechanisms of reaction formation, isolation, and undoing
   b. Learning theory views obsessions as a conditioned stimulus to anxiety and compulsions as an anxiety reduction response.
5. To summarize, the cause of OCD is poorly understood, but the extant research suggests multiple determinants, including neurophysiologic abnormalities, heredity, and learning history. Overall, it appears that genetic and neurobiologic factors constitute the primary etiologic roles, with psychosocial determinants exacerbating the OCD disorder.

Symptoms

1. The essential sign is either recurrent obsessions or compulsions.
   a. Obsessions
      (1) Recurrent and persistent thoughts, ideas, images, or impulses viewed as intrusive and senseless
      (2) Attempts are made to suppress, ignore, or neutralize the obsession with some other thought or an action.
   b. Compulsions
      (1) Intentional and repetitive behavior performed in response to an obsession or in a stereotyped ritualistic manner according to certain rules
      (2) Compulsions can either be overt behaviors (e.g., hand washing, ordering, checking) or covert mental acts (e.g., silently counting or praying).
      (3) The purpose is to neutralize or prevent anticipated distress or a dreaded event, but the compulsive act is not connected in a realistic way to what it is designed to prevent or neutralize.
   c. There are patients who are purely obsessional or purely ritualizers, but the most common pattern (approximately 75 per cent) is a combination of the two essential features.
2. Obsessions and compulsions share several common features:
   a. The thought or impulse to act persistently invades the person's conscious awareness.
   b. The thought or impulse to act is ego-dystonic or ego-alien.

c. The thought or impulse to act is recognized as irrational, but the person is unable to prevent it.

d. There is a strong desire to resist the idea or impulse.

e. The obsessions and compulsions are time-consuming and lead to fatigue.

3. The obsessions and compulsions significantly interfere with the patient's normal routine, work performance, or social functioning because of the marked distress and/or excessive time (i.e., take more than 1 hour per day) involved.

4. Onset of symptoms

   a. Mean age of onset is 16 years in the United States.

   b. Over 50 per cent experience the onset of symptoms before age 24 and 80 per cent by age 35.

   c. Approximately one third of cases in adults have their onset in childhood.

5. Associated features frequently include depression, anxiety, and personality disorders.

Key Symptoms

- Obsession of contamination followed by washing compulsion

- Obsession of doubt followed by a compulsion of checking

- Obsessional slowness or taking excessive time to carry out activities of daily living

Clinical Findings

1. The OCD patient is frequently embarrassed or ashamed of his or her symptoms and therefore will not confide in the physician during a regular office visit. Thus the physician must be alert to recognize associated physical and/or psychological signs.

   a. Possible physical indicators

      (1) Chapped or eczematoid-appearing hands from frequent washings

      (2) Gum lesions from excessive teeth brushing

   b. Possible psychological indicators

      (1) Depressed mood

      (2) Insistent concerns or firm belief that she or he has an infectious disease (e.g., acquired immune deficiency syndrome)

2. Brief office-based screening index

   a. If the physician is suspicious of possible OCD based on physical and/or psychological indicators, ask the following brief questions:

      (1) Do you overly worry about contamination from dirt or other environmental substances?

      (2) Do you have to wash your hands repeatedly?

      (3) Do you have the need to repeatedly check locks or switches?

   b. If the patient answers yes to any of the screening questions, there is a strong possibility of OCD.

   c. Patients with anxiety disorders consult their family doctor, rather than a mental health professional, up to 80 per cent of the time. A high index of suspicion for OCD is necessary because approximately one third of patients with OCD see their family physician without ever mentioning the psychiatric symptoms.

Key Signs

- Acknowledgment or observation of excessive handwashing or other cleaning rituals

- Acknowledgment or observation of repeating rituals, such as going in and out of a door

- Acknowledgment or observation of checking rituals, such as locked doors, appliances, or car brakes

Laboratory Tests

1. Neuroimaging studies such as CT are not yet routinely indicated because the findings do not clearly lead to a differential treatment plan.

2. Formal personality testing on instruments such as the Minnesota Multiphasic Personality Inventory (MMPI) and the Millon Clinical Multiaxial Inventory (MCMI-II) is indicated for several reasons.

   a. The high prevalence (i.e., 60 to 70 per cent) of concomitant personality disorders in OCD patients

   b. There are relationships between the personality subtype and treatment participation, compliance, and outcome; for example, patients with no evident personality pathology and those with dependent qualities demonstrate the best outcome, whereas schizotypal personality disorder consistently predicts a poorer outcome.

3. Formal clinician-rated testing on the Yale-Brown Obsessive Compulsive Scale (Y-BOCS) is important for making treatment decisions and assessing treatment progress related to
   a. Content and severity of specific OCD symptoms
   b. Degree of self-control over specific OCD symptoms

Key Tests

- Minnesota Multiphasic Personality Inventory (MMPI)
- Millon Clinical Multiaxial Inventory (MCMI-II)
- Yale-Brown Obsessive Compulsive Scale (Y-BOCS)

Differential Diagnosis

1. Major neurologic disorders to consider in the differential diagnosis
   a. Tourette's disorder
   b. Chronic motor or vocal tic disorder
   c. Transient tic disorder
   d. Temporal lobe epilepsy
2. Primary psychiatric disorders that need to be differentiated from OCD
   a. Schizophrenia
      (1) In schizophrenia, the symptoms are generally more bizarre.
      (2) The OCD patient has more insight into his or her disorder as compared with the schizophrenic.
   b. Depression
      (1) The obsessing in depression is milder and of the brooding and ruminative type as compared with the severe, persistent, and intrusive ego-dystonic obsessional thinking in OCD.
      (2) The presence or absence of other symptoms (e.g., recurrent thoughts of death) indicative of major depression can help to make this differentiation.
   c. Phobias
      (1) In the phobias, the avoidance behavior is generally of a more circumscribed nature.
      (2) OCD patients tend to be less successful in avoiding the feared object than are phobic patients.

   d. Obsessive compulsive personality disorder
      (1) There are no true obsessions or compulsions in obsessive compulsive personality disorder.
      (2) The degree of social and occupational impairment is significantly greater in OCD.
3. Other medical conditions
   a. Postpartum onset
   b. Sydenham's chorea

Treatment

1. Interdisciplinary treatment, including both behavioral therapy and psychopharmacology, is indispensable for several reasons.
   a. Each treatment has differential therapeutic effects on symptoms and types of patients.
   b. Some patients who obtain no therapeutic benefit with behavior therapy improve on medication, and vice versa.
   c. Patients who refuse one of the treatments may use the other as an alternative.
   d. Patients who are noncompliant with one may adhere to the other.
2. Behavior therapy
   a. Between 65 and 75 per cent of OCD patients improve on behavioral therapy.
   b. Appears to be the most beneficial on the compulsive rituals with a secondary effect on the associated obsessions.
   c. There are neurophysiologic changes (e.g., decreased cerebral glucose metabolism in the right caudate region) on PET similar to that produced by fluoxetine (Prozac) treatment.
   d. The behavioral treatment of choice is exposure and response prevention (ERP).
      (1) Exposure: deliberately facing the feared and avoided thought, situation, place, or object
      (2) Response prevention: delaying, diminishing, or preventing the anxiety-reducing compulsive rituals
      (3) The rationale for ERP: The obsession creates a high level of discomfort and a parallel urge to engage in a compulsive ritual or to avoid the feared stimulus; avoidance and/or compulsive rituals are self-reinforcing because they produce a partial anxiety reduction; exposure and response prevention break this self-reinforcing chain and chronic pattern because the anxiety is gradually diminished (habituation) when the patient refrains from performing the compulsive ritual in

response to the anxiety-evoking stimulus; the urge to perform the compulsive ritual or avoidance behavior is progressively decreased.

e. Behavioral group therapy and individual behavioral therapy are equally effective, although individually based treatment usually results in more rapid reductions in OCD symptom severity.

3. Pharmacotherapy
   a. Medications generally produce a 30 to 90 per cent reduction in OCD symptoms.
   b. Pharmacologic treatment for OCD should begin with an orally administered SRI (serotonin reuptake inhibitor). The usual average daily dose and range (initial to maximum) and for a minimum trial duration of 10 to 12 weeks are
      (1) Clomipramine (Anafranil), 200 mg/day (25 to 250 mg)
      (2) Fluoxetine (Prozac), 50 mg/day (20 to 80 mg)
      (3) Fluvoxamine (Luvox), 200 mg/day (50 to 300 mg)
      (4) Paroxetine (Paxil), 50 mg/day (20 to 60 mg)
      (5) Sertraline (Zoloft), 150 mg/day (50 to 200 mg)
   c. If the patient does not respond to the average dose of an SRI, gradually increase the dose to its maximum within 4 to 8 weeks from the start of treatment. When a patient partially responds to an average dose of an SRI, gradually increase the dose to its maximum within 5 to 9 weeks from the start of treatment. Experts recommend switching to another SRI if there is no response after 4 to 6 weeks at the maximum dose.
   d. If treatment response to a single orally administered SRI is partial but inadequate, the concurrent administration of another agent is indicated. Usual initial and maximum dosages of augmenting agents for treatment-resistant OCD for a recommended trial duration of 4 to 8 weeks are:
      (1) Buspirone (BuSpar), 15 to 60 mg/day
      (2) Clonazepam (Klonopin), 0.5 to 6 mg/day
      (3) Fenfluramine (Pondimin), 20 to 60 mg/day
      (4) Haloperidol (Haldol), 1 to 5 mg/day
      (5) Olanzapine (Zyprexa), 5 to 20 mg/day
      (6) Risperidone (Risperdal), 2 to 10 mg/day
   e. Haloperidol has demonstrated efficacy as an augmentation of an SRI in patients with co-morbid tic disorders.
   f. Intravenous administration of clomipramine appears to be a viable treatment for some OCD patients who do not adequately respond to orally administered SRIs.

4. Psychodynamic psychotherapy has not been demonstrated to be an effective treatment.

5. Neurosurgery should be considered only if the patient, despite adequate pharmacologic and behavioral treatment trials, remains severely disabled. Current neurosurgical procedures target tracts within the cingulate gyrus (cingulotomy) the subcaudate area (subcaudate tractotomy), their combination (limbic leucotomy), and the anterior limb of the internal capsule (anterior capsulotomy).

6. Most effective treatment: ERP behavior therapy combined with SRIs.

Key Treatment

- Exposure and response prevention (ERP) behavior therapy
- Serotonergic reuptake inhibitors (SRIs)

Follow-Up

1. Most patients treated with a combination of behavioral therapy and medication can expect significant long-term symptom improvement but not complete remission.

2. Common reasons for treatment failure
   a. Misdiagnosis, such as schizophrenia
   b. Inadequate treatment, such as medication trial too short or medication dosage too low
   c. Treatment noncompliance, such as patient refuses medication because of a fear of long-term effects or inability to tolerate the initial increased anxiety associated with behavioral therapy.

3. Preliminary evidence indicates a relapse rate of over 90 per cent soon after medication-only treatment.

4. Family counseling is useful in preventing the avoidant behavior that is a serious complication of OCD.

Bibliography

For a comprehensive and detailed treatise on the diagnosis and treatment of OCD, see
Jenike MA, Baer L, Minichiello WE (eds): Obsessive-Compulsive Disorders: Theory and Management, 2nd ed. Chicago, Year Book Medical Publishers, 1990.

For patient education, see
Foa E, Wilson R: Stop Obsessing! How to Overcome Your Obsessions and Compulsions. New York, Bantam, 1991.

For more information on treatment-resistant patients, see
Goodman WK, McDougle CJ, Barr LC, et al: Biological approaches to treatment-resistant obsessive compulsive disorder. J Clin Psychiatry 1993;54(Suppl)6:16–26.

For an overview of OCD for the family physician, see
Levine N: Selections from current literature: obsessive compulsive disorder. Fam Pract 1997;14:258–261.

For more information on the pharmacologic treatment of OCD, see
Osterheld JR, Osser DN: Drug interactions in augmentation strategies for pharmacotherapy of obsessive-compulsive disorder. J Prac Psych Behav Health 1999; 5:179–183.

For Expert Consensus Guidelines for the treatment of OCD, see
Frances A, Docherty JP, Kahn DA: Treatment of obsessive-compulsive disorder. J Clin Psychiatry 1997; 58(Suppl 4):5–72.

350   Common Poisoning Symptoms

Abdominal pain can result from a vast array of underlying medical and psychological problems. In the context of poisoning and environmental problems, however, one must consider the wide range of possible ingestions and exposures and then narrow the field using the more probable ones.

Differential Diagnosis

1. Food poisoning
   a. Bacterial toxins: Cases of food poisoning present with abdominal pain, nausea, vomiting, and diarrhea and are often associated with outbreaks. Patients are usually afebrile.
      (1) Staphylococcal poisoning results from improperly prepared and stored protein-containing foods.
      (2) *Clostridium* toxin can be found in cooked meats.
      (3) *Bacillus cereus* toxin is often associated with fried rice.
      (4) Scombroid fish poisoning occurs with ingestion of tuna or mackerel.
      (5) Paralysis may occur in neurotoxic seafood poisoning (NSP) and botulism.
   b. Mushrooms and plants
      (1) Poisonous mushrooms, especially those of the genus *Amanita*
      (2) Toxalbumin-producing plants, such as jequirty bean and rosary bean
2. Drug and household chemical ingestion: A great number of pharmaceutical products can cause symptoms of abdominal pain when excessive dosages are ingested.
   a. Common drugs
      (1) Digoxin
      (2) Theophylline
      (3) Iron (Fe) supplements
      (4) Erythromycin can cause abdominal pain in therapeutic doses.

   b. Other medications: Abdominal pain often occurs in eosinophilia-myalgia syndrome (EMS) caused by contaminated L-tryptophan supplements. Intake of iodine-containing topical solutions also may cause abdominal pain.
   c. Household chemicals: The ingestion of household chemicals and cleaning products can be a common problem, especially with young children.
      (1) Caustics (e.g., acids, alkalis, bleach) cause abdominal pain through direct irritant effect.
      (2) Halogenated hydrocarbons found in solvents, floor waxes, and adhesive cements
      (3) Pesticides
      (4) Arsenic (As)–containing products, such as insecticides, rodenticides, and wood preservatives
3. Occupational and environmental exposures
   a. Occupational exposures: Exposures to hazardous materials from manufacturing and industry can cause abdominal pain in employees working directly in these settings and in people living and working nearby. Agricultural chemicals can affect farm laborers and may contaminate groundwater supplies.
      (1) Heavy metals such as lead (Pb), arsenic, mercury (Hg), and thallium (Tl)
      (2) Other exposures include benzene, formaldehyde, pesticides (e.g., fluoride salts, organophosphates [OP], pentachlorophenol [PCP], phosphorus), and polychlorinated biphenyls (PCBs).
   b. Environmental exposures: Other environmental exposures resulting in abdominal pain include
      (1) Carbon monoxide
      (2) Agent Orange (AO) and phenoxy herbicides

(3) Lead

(4) Chemical warfare agents (similar in action to organophosphate pesticides)

4. Effects of the physical environment: Decreased partial pressures of oxygen and increased 2,3-diphosphoglycerate at high altitudes can promote sickling of erythrocytes in people with sickle cell anemia, resulting in abdominal pain. In rare cases, abdominal angina can occur at high elevations as a result of lowered oxygen tensions, especially in the postprandial setting. These patients usually have underlying atherosclerosis or vasculitis.

> Refer to Ch. 85, Appendicitis; and Ch. 351, Poisonings

History

1. Possible exposures

   a. Foods: Ask about recent picnics, dining out, recent seafood consumption, and home canning.

   b. Medications: What medications are available to the patient in his or her household?

   c. Occupational exposures: Ask about exposure to heavy metals, pesticide production, agricultural practices, and ventilation.

   d. Travel: Ask about recent travel to areas where water may be contaminated, pesticides used, or exotic plants available.

   e. Household exposures: What cleaning products and insecticides are used? Where are they kept? Is there peeling or cracking paint on the walls? What is the age of the dwelling?

2. Duration of abdominal pain

   a. Acute pain: Effects are seen almost immediately with caustics and usually occur within 1 to 24 hours after ingestions of contaminated foods, poisonous plants, and mushrooms.

   b. Chronic pain: Chronic pain is more common with medical therapy (e.g., digoxin or theophylline toxicity) and household or occupational exposures to heavy metals, PCBs, and carbon monoxide.

3. Associated symptoms: Symptoms (Table 350–1) can help narrow the field of possible exposures.

4. Concomitant medical problems: Include in the past medical history information on atherosclerosis, hepatic and renal dysfunction, pulmonary disease, sickle cell disease, and multiple transfusions.

Clinical Findings

1. General (Table 350–2)

   a. Hyperpyrexia with possible pesticide exposure suggests PCP poisoning.

   b. Dehydration is commonly found in food poisoning and also with arsenic toxicity.

TABLE 350–1. SYMPTOMS COMMONLY ASSOCIATED WITH POISONINGS THAT CAUSE ABDOMINAL PAIN

Symptom	Food Poisoning	Medications	Caustics and Hydrocarbons	Pesticides	Heavy Metals	PCBs and Agent Orange
Nausea and vomiting	+	+		+	Fe, As, Hg	AO
Diarrhea	+	+		+	Tl, Fe, As, Hg	AO
Constipation					Pb	
Anorexia		Digoxin			As	AO
Oral irritation	Plants		+			
Stomatitis					As	
Metallic taste					Hg	
Salivation				OP	Hg	
Breath odor				Phosphorus	As	
Skin rash	Scombroid				As	+
Hair loss					As, Tl	
Sweating				OP		
Wheezing				OP		
Visual changes		Digoxin				
Peripheral neuropathy					Pb, As	
Incontinence				OP		
Tremors/fasciculations		Theophylline		Fluorides, OP		
Paralysis	Bot., NSP				Tl	AO
Cognitive changes			Hydrocarbons		Pb	AO, PCB
Headache					Pb	AO, PCB
Anxiety		Theophylline				

Symptoms related to a general category are indicated by "+." Specific agents are identified by name or symbol.
See text for explanation of abbreviations.

TABLE 350–2. CLINICAL PRESENTATIONS AND SIGNS COMMONLY FOUND IN POISONINGS THAT CAUSE ABDOMINAL PAIN

CLINICAL SIGNS	FOOD POISONING	MEDICATIONS	CAUSTICS AND HYDROCARBONS	PESTICIDES	HEAVY METALS	PCBs AND AGENT ORANGE
General						
Dehydration	+				As	
Hypotension	+	+			Fe, As, Tl	
Hyperpyrexia				PCP		
Mental status changes			Hydrocarbons		Pb	+
Cardiovascular						
Tachycardia	Mushrooms	Theophylline				
Bradycardia		Digoxin		OP		
Respiratory						
Wheezing				OP		
Pulmonary edema				PCP, OP		
Skin						
Rash	Scombroid					
Follicular dermatitis					As	
Chloracne						+
Neurologic						
Miosis				OP		
Extensor weakness					Pb	
Fasciculations		Theophylline		OP, Fluorides		
Paralysis	Bot., NSP			Fluorides		
Musculoskeletal						
Myalgias		EMS				
Renal						
Acute tubular necrosis					Hg	

Signs occurring in general categories are indicated by "+." Specific agents are identified by name or symbol.
See text for explanation of abbreviations.

c. Hypotension can result from dehydration or bradycardia or effects of iron, thallium, and arsenic.

d. Mental status changes are associated with hydrocarbon, carbon monoxide, and lead toxicity.

2. Cardiovascular

a. Bradycardia may be found in digitalis toxicity and OP poisoning.

b. Tachycardia is associated with theophylline toxicity and mushroom poisoning.

3. Respiratory

a. Bronchorrhea and wheezing are commonly found in OP poisoning.

b. Pulmonary edema can be found in OP or PCP poisoning.

4. Skin

a. A rash associated with recent seafood ingestion may indicate scombroid.

b. Follicular or eczematous dermatitis can be found in chronic arsenic poisoning.

c. Chloracne, characterized by cysts filled with straw-colored liquid, is highly suggestive of PCBs.

5. Neurologic signs

a. Miosis occurs with OP poisoning as a result of cholinergic stimulation.

b. Extensor muscle weakness may occur with lead toxicity.

c. Fasciculations suggest theophylline toxicity or poisoning with OPs or fluoride salts.

d. Paralysis occurs in botulism, NSP, and poisoning from fluoride salts and thallium.

6. Musculoskeletal: Incapacitating myalgias are the hallmark of EMS.

7. Renal: Acute tubular necrosis may occur in mercury poisoning.

Tests

1. Food poisoning

a. Food contamination: Culture food, vomitus, or stool. Bioassay of food and serum for toxin if botulism or NSP is suspected.

b. Mushroom poisoning: Follow renal and hepatic function tests and prothrombin times.

2. Medications
   a. Digitalis toxicity: electrocardiogram (ECG), electrolytes (especially potassium), and serum digoxin level
   b. Theophylline: ECG, serum theophylline level, serum glucose, and consider serum pH
   c. EMS: Obtain complete blood count (CBC) with differential if EMS is suspected.
3. Caustics and hydrocarbons
   a. Caustics: Consider upper gastrointestinal (GI) endoscopy to define extent of tissue damage for all ingestions of caustic material, including acids, alkalis, and formalin. Obtain chemistry survey and blood gases to assess possible hypocalcemia, hyperkalemia, and metabolic acidosis.
   b. Hydrocarbons: Follow liver function tests.
4. Pesticides: Assess plasma and erythrocyte cholinesterase activity levels. These will be lowered to less than 50 per cent of normal levels in OP poisoning. Follow calcium levels if fluoride salt poisoning.
5. Heavy metals: Consider abdominal radiographs if ingestion of iron tablets or elemental lead is suspected.
   a. Iron: Obtain serum iron, total iron-binding capacity, and ferritin levels. Also, consider serum glucose and pH.
   b. Lead: Obtain levels of serum lead, blood urea nitrogen, creatinine, and free erythrocyte protoporphyrin. Also obtain CBC with differential (microcytic anemia with basophilic stippling).
   c. Arsenic: 24-hour urine for arsenic. Check CBC for signs of anemia.
   d. Mercury: serum and urine Hg level. Look for active urine sediment.
6. Carbon monoxide: Obtain carboxyhemoglobin level. Consider ECG.

Management
1. Basic life support
2. Discontinuation or limitation of exposure
   a. Ingestions
      (1) Dilute caustics and carefully lavage (consider early endoscopy before lavage).
      (2) Eliminate others using *emesis, lavage, activated charcoal,* and *cathartics* (ELACC).
   b. Topical absorption of OP pesticides: Health care providers should be gowned and gloved. Remove patient's clothing, shampoo hair, and clean all skin surfaces.

   c. Inhalations: Remove from place of exposure. Displace carbon monoxide using 100 per cent oxygen. Assisted ventilation may be necessary. Also consider use of hyperbaric chamber.
3. Specific interventions

   a. Food poisoning
      (1) Food poisoning is usually self-limited. Public health department should be notified of outbreak.
      (2) Paralysis (e.g., botulism, NSP) may require hospitalization and mechanical ventilation.
      (3) Treat mushroom poisoning as above (ELACC). Institute vigorous intravenous fluid rehydration with forced diuresis (>300 ml/hour of urine output). Penicillin, silymarin, and cimetidine may be useful. With severe hepatic toxicity, liver transplantation is a final option.
   b. Medications: Decrease absorption as above.
      (1) Digoxin: Symptomatic bradycardia may be treated with atropine (0.5 to 2.0 mg intravenously). Lidocaine may be used for other dysrhythmias. Digoxin antibody may be given in extreme cases.
      (2) Theophylline: Intravenous esmolol (25 to 50 μg/kg/min) or propranolol (0.5 to 1.0 mg) may be given for symptomatic tachycardia.
      (3) EMS: Glucocorticoids may be of some benefit.
   c. Caustics
      (1) Acids and formalin: Dilute with water or milk. *Do not induce emesis.* Consider early upper GI endoscopy. Provide supportive care with correction of metabolic acidosis.
      (2) Halogenated hydrocarbons: Emesis and lavage are controversial because of risk

of aspiration pneumonitis. Consider possible hemodialysis.

(3) Others: Follow management for ingestions above.

d. Pesticides

(1) OPs: Support respiration and follow management above. Use atropine (0.02 to 0.05 mg/kg intravenously every 15 minutes) until some effects are manifested. Administer pralidoxime (20 to 50 mg/kg intravenously every 2 to 12 hours).

(2) Fluoride salts and phosphorus: Dilute with milk or calcium gluconate. Follow management for ingestions above. Then administer intravenous solution of 10% calcium gluconate to maintain serum calcium. Supportive care.

(3) PCP: Avoid atropine. *Lower body temperature.* Supportive care.

e. Heavy metals: If acute ingestion, follow management for ingestions above.

(1) Iron: Administer deferoxamine (10 to 15 mg/kg/hour intramuscularly or intravenously) until serum iron less than 250 $\mu g/dl$.

(2) Lead: Chelation with calcium EDTA (50 mg/kg/day intravenous infusion for 5 days)

(3) Arsenic: Administer dimercaprol (BAL) (2.5 to 3.0 mg/kg intramuscularly as 10% solution in oil, then 2 to 3 mg/kg intramuscularly every 4 hours for 2 days). Then administer oral penicillamine (25 mg/kg/day every 6 hours for 7 days, maximum 2 gm/day).

(4) Mercury: Dimercaprol as above. Maintain appropriate urine output.

(5) Thallium: Administer potassium chloride and Prussian blue (potassium ferrichexacyanoferrate). Consider hemodialysis.

PEARLS

- The telephone numbers of the 51 regional poison control centers certified by the American Association of Poison Control Centers are listed in the back of the *Physicians' Desk Reference.* The trained personnel at these centers are available 24 hours per day and are invaluable sources of information in the management of poisoning and overdose.

- The federal Hazardous Substances Act requires content labeling of hazardous household products.

- POISINDEX is a detailed toxicology data base available on CD-ROM with information on 750,000 substances (Micromedix Inc., 6200 South Syracuse Way, Suite 300, Englewood, CO 80111).

B Bibliography

For more information on treatment of drug overdose, see
Olson KR (ed): Poisoning & Drug Overdose, 2nd ed. Norwalk, CT, Appleton & Lange, 1994.

For overview of poisoning and drug overdose, see
Linden CH, Lovejoy FH: Poisoning and drug overdose. In Fauci AS, Braunwald E, Isselbacher KJ, et al (eds): Harrison's Principles of Internal Medicine, 14th ed, vol 2, pp 2523–2544. New York, McGraw-Hill, 1998.

For more information on occupational chemical exposures, see
National Institute for Occupational Safety and Health: Pocket Guide to Chemical Hazards (DHSS [NIOSH] Publication No. 91-116). Bethesda, MD, National Institute of Occupational Safety and Health, 1994.

For more information on wide spectrum of poisoning, see
Ellenhorn MJ: Ellenhorn's Medical Toxicology: Diagnosis and Treatment of Human Poisoning, 2nd ed. Baltimore, Williams & Wilkins, 1997.

For more information on occupational and environmental exposures, including heavy metals, see
Rom WN (ed): Environmental and Occupational Medicine, 3rd ed. Philadelphia, Lippincott Raven, 1998.

SYMPTOM NAUSEA AND VOMITING
Thomas Masciangelo

Nausea, an impending urge to expel upper gastrointestinal (GI) contents, usually precedes the forceful ejection of gastric contents through the upper oral cavity: the act of vomiting. Toxic exposures and ingestion of either excessive doses of prescribed drugs or poisonous compounds can evoke rapid onset of upper GI myoelectric and muscular phenomena (vomiting mechanism). Two medullary centers, the chemoreceptor trigger zone (CTZ) and the vomiting center (VC), are responsible for inducing vomiting. Diverse drugs and toxins directly influence the former (CTZ), which reacts to secrete neurotransmitters such as dopamine that in turn catalyze a series of reactions in the VC. Multiple efferent tracts diverge from the VC to numerous end-organ targets to coordinate the actual act of emesis. The VC receives afferent signals from several sources; however, it is particularly sensitive to those propagated from visual or olfactory centers, among others (cortical center, labyrinthine apparatus, and CTZ).

Determining the etiology of the intoxication is mandatory. Assistance by local poison control centers can prove beneficial.

Differential Diagnosis

1. *Medications* are among the most common causes.
   a. Chemotherapeutic agents such as cyclophosphamide, cisplatin, daunorubicin, BCNU
   b. GI irritants: aspirin, nonsteroidal anti-inflammatory agents, sulfasalazine
   c. Cardiovascular drugs: digitalis, calcium channel blockers, β-blockers, and antiarrhythmics
   d. Antibiotics: erythromycin, sulfonamides, antituberculosis medications, acyclovir
   e. Central nervous system agents that treat Parkinson's disease; anticonvulsants, benzodiazepines, tricyclic antidepressants
   f. Respiratory modifiers such as theophylline
2. *Inhalation* poisoning most commonly occurs in carbon monoxide exposure, in which at least 30 to 40 per cent saturation of carboxyhemoglobin induces nausea, vomiting.
3. *Infections*, particularly gram-negative bacteria such as enterotoxigenic *Escherichia coli*, *Campylobacter*, *Salmonella*, *Shigella*, *Vibrio*, *Clostridium*, and viral hepatitis
4. Narcotic drugs (opiates, cocaine) and alcohol intoxication
5. Heavy metal ingestion: Includes iron, mercury, lead, arsenic, gold.
6. Occupational exposures from organophosphates, petroleum and its derivatives, and ethylene glycol

History: Key Questions to Ask

1. Time, route, and duration of exposure when appropriate. Time of presentation relative to time of exposure
2. Drug name or classification, quantity ingested, or exposure concentration
3. Symptom nature, onset, severity, and if there are associated findings relevant to diagnosis
4. Medical and psychiatric history (look for suicide note on patient or among belongings, as well as prematurely empty prescription bottles)
5. Medication history
6. Have first aid measures or antidotes been administered?

7. Number of episodes and quantity of emesis
8. Concomitant diarrhea, fever, or hematochezia

Clinical Evaluation

1. Evaluate mental status and the presence of an adequate airway with a reasonable respiratory rate.
2. Skin color, cyanosis, warmth, turgor, ulcerative lesions; look for puncture marks that indicate use of needles.
3. Blood pressure and pulse to provide sufficient organ perfusion. Body temperature, diaphoresis
4. Abdominal distention or rigidity, bowel sounds, organomegaly
5. Determine if drug-containing packets or containers are present in any orifices.
6. Is patient excited, depressed, discordant, or normal? Have convulsions been observed?

Tests

1. Anion gap indicates metabolic acidosis, and implicates methanol, ethylene glycol, or salicylate intoxication.
2. Serum lactate level rises in hypoxia, hypoperfusion, organ failure, and seizure activity.
3. Elevated serum magnesium or calcium suggests intoxication with ethanol, propylene glycol, lithium, iodine, or nitrates.
4. Osmolal gap becomes elevated with high concentration of low-molecular-weight solutes like alcohol, and with high serum ketone or glucose levels as seen in diabetic ketoacidosis or lactic acidosis.
5. Blood glucose levels are higher in acetone ingestion, β-agonist or calcium channel antagonist overdose, and theophylline intoxication. Hypoglycemia, in contrast, occurs in excessive β-blocker, salicylate, and oral hypoglycemia ingestion.
6. Hypokalemia is seen in overdose of β-agonists, diuretics, theophylline, and barium intake. Hyperkalemia occurs in digitalis, β-blocker, and fluoride toxicity.
7. Chest radiograph is useful to evaluate pulmonary edema, infiltrative opacities as seen with inhalation of toxic fumes, gases, vapors, or dusts (carbon monoxide, cyanide, paraquat, ammonia, metal oxides, mercury, or aspiration of gastric contents).
8. Abdominal radiograph may show radiopaque areas caused by ingestion of heavy metals, calcium salts, or psychotherapeutic agents.
9. Electrocardiogram is helpful for assessment of bradycardia, atrioventricular block, and QRS complex or QT interval prolongation.

10. Urinalysis and serum drug screens to identify drugs and metabolites
11. Liver function tests to check hepatic toxicity and involvement of poison on liver integrity

Management

1. Supportive care is of primary significance.
   a. Maintain a patent airway that provides adequate ventilation and oxygenation.
   b. Prevent hypotension and hypoperfusion by fluid resuscitation and replacement of intravascular volume.
   c. Treat arrhythmias aggressively to maintain adequate cardiac output. Ventricular tachyarrhythmias may require intravenous lidocaine or phenytoin.
   d. Seizures must be controlled by anticonvulsants specifically aimed at the toxin ingested.
2. For slow poison absorption
   a. Activated charcoal can be suspended in water and administered orally by straw, cup, or nasogastric tube. The recommended dose is 1 to 2 gm/kg body weight. Sorbital may be added plus a cathartic for faster evacuation from the bowel.
   b. Serum of ipecac can be used if the ingestion has not already provoked vomiting, and if charcoal is not available. Doses range from 30 ml for adults to 15 ml for children (age 1 to 12 years) and 10 ml for infants (age 6 to 12 months). Onset of action is about 20 to 25 minutes after ingestion.
   c. Whole GI washout is achieved with an agent high in electrolytes and polyethylene glycol (GoLYTELY, Colyte). The high quantity needed may make it necessary to insert a nasogastric tube.
   d. Extracorporeal elimination can be accomplished by peritoneal dialysis, hemodialysis, hemofiltration, plasmapheresis, or exchange transfusion. Low-molecular-weight toxins that are water soluble and have minimal protein binding and small volumes of distribution are good candidates for removal by dialysis. Such compounds include barbiturates, bromide, ethylene glycol, alcohol, lithium, methanol, procainamide, theophylline, and salicylate.

3. Antidotes may be given to neutralize the toxin, either by chemical binding or inactivation by an antibody-antigen complex. Care must be taken in administering these medications because they also can be potentially toxic; therefore, accurate diagnosis and identification of the toxin is mandatory.

Prevention

1. The most effective and permanent preventive measure is education of patients regarding the toxic effects of prescribed medications or over-the-counter drugs.
2. Education of family members or caregivers concerning the daily dose and frequency of medications if the patient is confused or incapable of proper self-administration
3. Child-proofing all containers, cabinets, receptacles where medication or poisonous substances are located is an absolute necessity. Access to medication or toxic compounds should be restricted not only for children and infants, but also if the adult patient is mentally incapable of discerning safety of ingested substances.
4. Patients who have proven to be noncompliant with daily intake should be prescribed a limited quantity and few refills to enable the strict monitoring of intake, response, and compliance.

Bibliography

Block JB: The Signs and Symptoms of Chemical Exposure. Springfield, IL, Charles C Thomas, 1980.
Ellenhorn MJ, Barceloux DG: Medical Toxicology: Diagnosis and Treatment of Human Poisoning. New York, Elsevier, 1988.
Haddad LM: Acute poisoning. In Bennett JC, Plum F, Gill GN, et al (eds): Cecil Textbook of Medicine, 20th ed, pp 503–510. Philadelphia, WB Saunders Company, 1996.
Hasler WL: Approach to the patient with nausea and vomiting. In Kelley WN, DuPont HL, Glick JH, et al (eds): Textbook of Internal Medicine, pp 608–617. Philadelphia, Lippincott-Raven, 1997.
Klaasen CD, Amdur MO, Doull J (eds): Casarett and Doull's Toxicology: The Basic Science of Poisons, 5th ed. New York, McGraw-Hill, 1996.
Linden CH, Lovejoy FH Jr: Poisoning and drug overdosage. In Fauci AS, Braunwald E, Isselbacher KJ, et al (eds): Harrison's Principles of Internal Medicine, 14th ed, pp 2523–2544. New York, McGraw-Hill, 1998.

351 Poisonings

Lars C. Larsen

Etiology

More than 2 million human poison exposure cases were reported by U.S. poison control centers in 1995. Ingestions accounted for over 1.5 million cases and represented 73.6 per cent of all poison exposures.

1. Ingestions of analgesics, antidepressants, stimulants and street drugs, and cardiovascular drugs caused the largest number of deaths.

2. The risk of fatality was greatest in patients who ingested stimulants and street drugs, cardiovascular drugs, and antidepressants.

3. Children less than 6 years of age accounted for 53 per cent of all poison exposures, but less than 3 per cent of the fatalities.

4. Patients over 19 years of age accounted for over 90 per cent of drug-related fatalities, primarily because their poisonings are more commonly intentional.

5. Although most oral poisonings occur acutely, a significant percentage may be caused by chronic ingestion of near-therapeutic amounts of medications.

Symptoms

Symptoms may not be present initially, depending upon the toxicity of the ingested substance(s), the amount ingested, and the time since ingestion. Also, poisonings (acute or chronic) in the presence of concurrent medical conditions can produce confusing clinical findings.

1. Patients with acute poisonings often present with neurologic symptoms, gastrointestinal symptoms, or respiratory depression.

2. Chronic ingestions may produce less specific symptoms, including tiredness, malaise, anorexia, and vague gastrointestinal complaints.

3. Information obtained from family, friends, other health care professionals (e.g., clinicians, pharmacists), medication remnants, and medication labels is often more useful than information obtained from the patient, especially in intentional poisonings.

4. Symptoms may present as characteristic "toxidromes" (see "Clinical Findings").

Clinical Findings

A brief initial physical assessment should be performed on all patients to determine the effects of the ingestants and the presence of concurrent conditions such as head trauma, penetrating body injuries, and chronic medical conditions. Focal neurologic signs or other findings not consistent with poisoning should alert the clinician to the presence of other conditions. Clinical findings may rapidly change (e.g., cyclic antidepressant poisoning) and patients must be closely monitored until stable.

1. The skin should be examined for needle tracks, chemical injuries, and other signs of trauma.

2. Odors and medication remnants (e.g., pill fragments) may aid in identification of the poison.

3. Clinical syndromes ("toxidromes") may be present and allow early identification and management of specific poisonings:

   a. *Physiologic stimulants* (cocaine, amphetamines, caffeine, theophylline, antihistamines, early tricyclic antidepressant poisoning, and hallucinogens): Often produce tremor, tachycardia, mydriasis (dilated pupils), irritability, diaphoresis, mania, convulsions, and tachyarrhythmias.

   b. *Physiologic depressants* (alcohol, benzodiazepines, barbiturates, muscle relaxants, chloral hydrate): Often produce lethargy, decreased responsiveness to verbal and physical stimulation, miosis (constricted pupils), hypothermia, and coma.

   c. *Cyclic antidepressants*: central nervous system (CNS) excitability, confusion, fever, mydriasis, dry mouth, blurred vision, tachycardia, arrhythmias, hypotension, respiratory depression, coma, seizures

   d. *Acetaminophen*: malaise, nausea, vomiting, right upper quadrant abdominal pain, confusion, jaundice, somnolence, coma in severe poisonings

e. *Salicylates*: nausea, vomiting, fever, hyperpnea, tinnitus, coma, lethargy, seizures, abdominal pain, diaphoresis, disorientation

f. *Benzodiazepines*: lethargy, drowsiness, ataxia, dysarthria, hypotension, hypothermia, coma, respiratory depression with large overdoses

g. *Cocaine*: headache, euphoria, anxiety, confusion, chest pain, tachycardia, tachypnea, fever, twitching, vomiting, mydriasis, abdominal cramps, hallucinations, seizures, cardiopulmonary arrest, hypertension, hypotension, dysrhythmias, diaphoresis

h. *Narcotics*: drowsiness, respiratory depression, cyanosis, nausea, vomiting, miosis, coma, seizures, noncardiac pulmonary edema

Key Signs

- Needle marks
- Focal neurologic signs
- Respiratory depression
- Mental status changes
- Head or penetrating body trauma
- Miosis or mydriasis

Laboratory Tests

Laboratory evaluation is indicated if the ingestion was intentional, if the poison has significant potential toxicity, when the ingestants are unknown, and if patients are symptomatic.

1. Tests to obtain with most poisonings include a complete blood count, serum electrolytes (with calculation of the anion gap), serum glucose, renal function tests (blood urea nitrogen and creatinine), hepatic function tests (aspartate transaminase, alanine transaminase, bilirubin, alkaline phosphatase, lactate dehydrogenase, prothrombin time), calcium, and urinalysis.

2. If poisoning with ethylene glycol, isopropanol, or methanol is suspected, measurement of the serum osmolarity and calculation of the osmolar gap may be helpful in confirming the diagnosis.

3. Although toxicology screening has limited value, it has become the standard of care in most communities. *Qualitative screening* can be helpful when the poison is unknown, when multiple toxic substances are taken, and when the physical findings are not compatible with the suspected ingestant. *Quantitative screening* is indicated when knowledge of serum drug lev-

els may affect the management of patients. Examples include ingestion of salicylates, acetaminophen, digoxin, iron, lithium, theophylline, anticonvulsants, ethanol, ethylene glycol, methanol, and isopropyl alcohol.

4. An electrocardiogram should be obtained in patients with arrhythmias or suspected ingestions of cardiotoxic drugs.

5. Chest radiographs are indicated in comatose patients, patients with suspected aspiration, and when ingestion of medications that cause noncardiogenic pulmonary edema (sedative-hypnotics, narcotics, salicylates, paraquat) is suspected.

6. Abdominal radiographs may reveal ingestions of drug packets, calcium salts, heavy metals (e.g., iron tablets), salicylates, or foreign bodies.

Key Tests

- Serum electrolytes
- Renal and hepatic function tests
- Serum glucose
- Electrocardiogram

Treatment

1. Patients with suspected overdoses must initially be resuscitated and stabilized with attention to the "ABCs" (*a*irway, *b*reathing, *c*irculation). Patients with altered mental status may respond to naloxone or dextrose and thiamine.

a. Patients with suspected hypoglycemia should have rapid reagent testing and, if the value is less than 80 mg/dl, should receive intravenous dextrose (neonates, 5 ml/kg of 10% dextrose; children, 4 ml/kg of 25% dextrose; adults, 50 ml of 50% dextrose). If rapid reagent testing is not available, dextrose may be given empirically. If intravenous access is difficult, 1 mg of glucagon IM may be given pending placement of the intravenous line. To prevent Wernicke's encephalopathy, all patients treated with dextrose should receive intravenous thiamine (children, 10 to 25 mg; adults, 100 mg).

b. Naloxone (Narcan) may be given to patients with respiratory and/or CNS depression caused by suspected narcotic overdoses, and may be administered intramuscularly, intravenously, endotracheally, subcutaneously, or intralingually. Doses:

(1) Adults, for respiratory depression: 2 mg initially, repeated every 2 minutes as needed up to a total of 10 mg

(2) Adults without respiratory depression or suspected narcotic-dependent patients; 0.1 mg initially, doubled every 2 minutes up to a total of 10 mg

(3) Children older than 5 years or over 20 kg: 2 mg initially for respiratory depression or 0.1 to 0.8 mg if respiratory depression is not present

(4) Neonates and young children: 0.1 mg/kg initial dose

2. Following resuscitation and stabilization, gastrointestinal decontamination should be considered:

a. Gastric lavage is the preferred method to empty the stomach.

(1) Emptying the stomach beyond 4 hours after the ingestion is not useful except in massive ingestions or when concretions may occur.

(2) Indications for lavage include ingestion of highly toxic substances; ingestion of iron, lead, lithium, or methanol (substances not well absorbed by activated charcoal); and patients with jeopardized airways. Lavage is contraindicated following ingestion of most hydrocarbons and corrosives.

(3) A No. 36 to 40 French tube is appropriate for adults; a No. 28 to 36 French tube may be used for children. Normal saline or tap water is used until the lavage return is clear (in children, 15 ml/kg until clear; in adults, 300-ml aliquots until clear, up to 10 to 20 L if needed).

b. Syrup of ipecac may be useful for the telephone management of patients unable to be seen at a health care facility within 1 hour of the ingestion. It should not be used in children less than 6 months of age, in patients with decreased responsiveness or gag reflexes, or in patients who may have rapid changes in sensorium from their poisonings. Also, it should not be given to patients who have ingested corrosives, sharp objects, most hydrocarbons, and if activated charcoal will be given within 60 to 90 minutes. Dosages:

(1) Adolescents and adults, 30 ml followed by 8 to 16 oz of water

(2) Children 1 to 12 years of age, 15 ml followed by 4 to 8 oz of water

(3) Children 6 to 12 months of age, 10 ml followed by 5 to 15 ml/kg of water.

c. *Activated charcoal is the preferred method of gastrointestinal decontamination* and is effective without gastric emptying in most poisonings.

(1) It is *not* effective for ingestions of corrosives, alcohols, heavy metals (e.g., iron, arsenic), and lithium.

(2) The dose for children and adults is 1 to 2 gm/kg, usually given in a single dose combined with a cathartic. Multiple doses, 1 gm/kg every 2 to 6 hours, is effective following ingestions of salicylates, digitalis, theophylline, phenobarbital, phenytoin, carbamazepine, and dapsone.

(3) Cathartics should be combined with the activated charcoal only for the first dose and *not* with subsequent doses.

d. Whole-bowel irrigation may be useful following ingestions of toxins that are not adsorbed by activated charcoal or not amenable to lavage. Examples include packets containing cocaine; lithium; iron; and slow-release potassium. Isosmotic cathartic solutions (Colyte, Golytely) are administered orally or via nasogastric tube at 2 L/hour in adults and 0.5 L/hour (or 25 to 40 ml/kg/hour) in children until the rectal effluent is clear. Abdominal radiographs may be useful to document passage of drug packets and iron tablets.

3. Antidotes to specific toxins (Table 351–1) should be considered after the patient has been resuscitated and stabilized, and evaluated for gastric decontamination. The duration of action of the toxin is often longer than the effect of the antidote, and monitoring in a specialized hospital unit is usually indicated following the use of an antidote. Clinicians not experienced in using an antidote should contact a poison

TABLE 351–1. COMMONLY USED ANTIDOTES

TOXINS	ANTIDOTES*
Acetaminophen	N-acetylcysteine (Mucomyst)
Cyclic antidepressants	Bicarbonate
Opiates	Naloxone (Narcan)
Benzodiazepines	Flumazenil (Romazicon)
Digoxin	Digoxin immune Fab (Digibind)
Calcium channel blockers	Calcium
β-blockers	Glucagon
Anticholinergic agents	Physostigmine (Antilirium)
Methanol, ethylene glycol	Ethanol
Iron	Deferoxamine (Desferal)

*If not familiar with the indications, dosage, and potential complications from use of an antidote, consultation with a poison control center is recommended.

control center for management assistance and suggestions.

4. Hemodialysis is indicated for patients with methanol and ethylene glycol poisonings, and severe poisonings with lithium or salicylates. Hemoperfusion may be useful in selected cases of theophylline or barbiturate poisoning. Consultation with a poison control center is generally indicated when these methods are being considered.

Key Treatment

- Resuscitation and stabilization
- Antidote if indicated
- Activated charcoal
- Supportive care

Follow-Up

1. Most patients require only supportive care, and many can be safely sent home from the health care facility following evaluation and limited treatment. Patients with intentional poisonings require psychological assessment before discharge.

2. All patients admitted to the hospital should be placed in hospital units with sufficient staff and resources to manage potential complications, especially patients who have received antidotes.

3. Consultation with a certified poison control center is indicated for unanswered questions about management of poisoning victims.

Bibliography

Herrington AM, Clifton GD: Toxicology and management of acute drug ingestions in adults. Pharmacotherapy 1995;15:182–200.

Litovitz TL, Smilkstein M, Felberg L, et al: 1996 Annual report of the American Association of Poison Control Centers Toxic Exposure Surveillance System. Am J Emerg Med 1997;15:447–500.

Phillips S, Gomez H, Brent J: Pediatric gastrointestinal decontamination in acute toxin ingestion. J Clin Pharmacol 1993;33:497–507.

Shannon MW, Haddad LM: The emergency management of poisoning. In Haddad LM, Shannon MW, Winchester JF (eds): Clinical Management of Poisoning and Drug Overdose, 3rd ed, pp 2–31. Philadelphia, WB Saunders Company, 1998.

Vernon DD, Gleich MC: Poisoning and drug overdose. Crit Care Clin 1997;13:647–667.

352 Food Poisoning

Katherine R. Schlaerth

Significant recent changes in lifestyle, including dual-career families, ubiquitous fast food outlets, and the creation by the food industry of packaged and frozen meals to replace the traditional food prepared from basic ingredients in the home have added to the risk of food poisoning already increased by worldwide shipment of foodstuffs and mass production of pooled meat and other products. Food preparation errors that formerly put a small number of people at risk now threaten large numbers who are exposed to tainted food on a much larger scale. A knowledge of the ways food poisoning can present and a high level of suspicion serve the clinician well in uncovering cases that might otherwise be attributed to different agents.

Etiology

Bacterial food poisoning refers to the illnesses produced by consumption of food contaminated with bacteria or their toxic products. Generally not included are illnesses that could be but are not necessarily caused by the ingestion of contaminated food, unless causative bacteria can be associated through laboratory identification of outbreaks as being responsible for similar disease in two or more individuals ingesting a contaminated food. Certain species of *Vibrio*, *Shigella*, toxigenic *Escherichia coli*, *Campylobacter*, *Yersinia*, *Listeria*, and *Aeromonas*, many of which cause either lower gastrointestinal (GI) tract symptoms or disseminated disease, fall under the latter definition.

PEARL

- Diseases caused by the ingestion of fish contaminated with toxin produced by a marine dinoflagellate give different symptoms from those commonly ascribed to traditional food poisoning.
  —Ciguatera poisoning, after the ingestion of large fish like barracuda, red snapper, amberjack, and grouper, causes nausea, vomiting, diarrhea, and abdominal pain within a few hours of ingestion, followed by perioral and extremity paresthesias with hot-cold reversal.
  —Scomboid poisoning after mahi-mahi ingestion does not cause GI symptoms. Rather, flushing, oral blisters, and

---

erythema develop within minutes of ingestion, although abdominal pain, diarrhea, and bronchospasm may sometimes be seen too.

Differential Diagnosis:

1. The agents most commonly associated with food poisoning in the United States include *Salmonella*, *Staphylococcus aureus*, *Clostridium perfringens*, and *Bacillus cereus*.

   a. *Staphylococcus aureus* produces an enterotoxin that is ingested preformed in food, especially foods with a high salt content (ham, canned meats) or high sugar content (cream or custard pastries). Symptoms appear within 1 to 6 hours of ingestion, usually consisting of nausea, vomiting, and diarrhea, that resolve within 4 hours or so.

   b. *Bacillus cereus* produces two toxins.

      (1) One, preformed, is associated with fried rice and causes vomiting and abdominal cramps generally within 2 hours of ingestion. Diarrhea is present in only one third of cases, and symptoms resolve within 8 to 10 hours.

      (2) The other toxin, not preformed, causes diarrhea, cramps, and vomiting after an incubation period of 6 to 14 hours, and the duration of illness is much longer—20 to 36 hours. Many foods can harbor the organism, including cream, dried milk and potatoes, and various spices and sauces; food contamination occurs prior to cooking.

   c. *Clostridium perfringens* type A is associated with bulk-prepared meat whose internal cooking temperature is insufficient to kill the spores. Cooling allows the spores to germinate, and, within 8 to 22 hours of ingestion, watery diarrhea and severe crampy abdominal pain supervene, lasting no longer than 24 to 36 hours.

   d. *Salmonella*, found ubiquitously in nature but usually associated with the ingestion of eggs, meat, or poultry, requires a large inoculum to produce disease. The incubation period is 24 to 36 hours and clinical manifestations include fever, vomiting, abdominal cramps, and diarrhea (occasionally bloody), generally lasting 2 to 3 days.

   e. *Vibrio parahaemolyticus* outbreaks, common in the summer and associated with the ingestion of toxin in improperly refrigerated seafood, are characterized by explosive watery diarrhea, vomiting, moderately severe abdominal cramps, chills, and low-grade fever.

2. Symptoms similar to those of food poisoning can be associated with many other infectious and noninfectious diseases, including rotavirus, enteroviruses, Norwalk agent, other bacterial pathogens as delineated above, and such noninfectious causes as appendicitis and pyelonephritis in young children, an acute abdomen, central nervous system disease, and even drug side effects. The history and physical examination become critical in sorting out the many illnesses that can present with vomiting and/or diarrhea in different age groups.

Key Symptoms:

- Clustering of cases

- Vomiting, diarrhea, abdominal discomfort

- Occasionally low-grade fever and/or dehydration

History: Key Questions to Ask

1. What foods were ingested in the past 48 hours? Has anyone else ingesting the same foods developed similar symptoms?

2. Are there underlying conditions such as achlorhydria, immunodeficiencies, or chronic use of narcotics that could facilitate the colonization of the GI tract with offending organisms?

3. Has there been any history of travel, ingestion of foods from other areas of the world, or ingestion of raw, improperly cooked, or reheated foods (especially if prepared institutionally)?

4. Are symptoms or signs present that might point to other organ systems rather than the GI tract as being the source of symptoms? (For example, severe headache and nuchal rigidity with meningitis; dysurea or malodorous urine in the young child with pyelonephritis and parenteral diarrhea).

Clinical Findings

Food poisoning is usually self-limited, but can be more severe in those with underlying illnesses, and in the very young and very old. In addition to a brief physical examination to rule out similarly presenting illnesses, with attention paid to the presence of neurologic signs and flank tenderness, the work-up should include evaluation for

1. Dehydration: tachypnea, tachycardia, orthostatic hypotension, dry mucous membranes, lack of tears or urine, lethargy; in the infant, sunken fontanelle or shock; in the older adult, confusion and headache

2. Abdominal signs and symptoms: distention, organomegaly, guarding or rebound, heel-strike, bowel sounds, others

3. Mental status, especially in the infant and the elderly.

Key Findings

- Dehydration evidenced by tachycardia, tachypnea, drop in blood pressure greater than 20 mm Hg on standing, dry mucous membranes, decreased tearing and urine output in moderate food poisoning

- Rarely, shock and altered mental status in severe episodes

Diagnostic Tests

1. General tests to access the acuity of the illness

   a. Complete blood count (CBC)

   b. Electrolytes and blood urea nitrogen (BUN), creatinine if dehydration is evident on physical examination

   c. Other tests to rule out similarly presenting diseases, which may include amylase, urinalysis and culture, and liver function tests

Key Tests

- For dehydration:
  - BUN, creatinine, electrolytes
  - CBC and differential

- For identification of pathogen:
  - Isolation of bacteria on select media
  - Toxin identification

2. Specific identification of pathogens: See Table 352–1.

Management

Medication

1. Antiemetics and antimotility agents are contra-

TABLE 352–1. TESTS FOR IDENTIFICATION OF PATHOGENS IN FOOD POISONING

ORGANISM	SAMPLE SOURCE	ASSAY OR CULTURE
Bacillus cereus	Vomitus, stool, food	Culture on special agar, with stool control and serotyping
Clostridium perfringins	Stool, rectal swab, food or contaminated surfaces	Special agar with typing
Vibrio parahaemolyticus	Stool, rectal swab, food, surfaces, seawater	Special agar, serotyping
Staphylococcus aureus	Stool, vomitus, any lesions on the body of food preparer, contaminated surfaces	Special agar with tests for enterotoxin
Salmonella	Stool or rectal swab from food preparer or patient, food if available	SS agar with phage typing
Other GI organisms	Stool, food, surfaces	Alert lab as to what organisms offer concern so appropriate isolation media can be used

indicated in toxin-induced and bacterial food poisoning.

2. Antibiotics can prolong the carrier state in salmonella infections, and are used in salmonellosis only under specific conditions, as in immunocompromised hosts, neonates at risk of sepsis, and with certain hemoglobinopathies.

3. In dehydration, appropriate fluid and electrolyte management, through either oral or intravenous access, is mandatory.

Diet

1. Most food poisoning is self-limited.

2. Oral hydration with an appropriate electrolyte solution (such as the World Health Organization rehydration packets or various commercial solutions) can be given in small quantities with increased frequency of intake.

3. Some sports drinks need to be diluted because their large glucose content can cause an osmotic diarrhea.

4. Solids low in fat and acid content can be introduced initially after the food poisoning has resolved, with appropriate advancement to a normal diet.

Activity

As tolerated, avoiding dehydrating activities or environments

Patient Education

1. Proper preparation and storage of food cannot be emphasized enough.

2. Food purchased at fast food outlets should be thoroughly cooked.

3. Hygiene should be carefully maintained in cooking areas, with appropriate cleaning of counters, washing of hands, and use of disposable gloves for group food preparation.

4. Cooking utensils should be washed before each usage.

5. Individuals traveling to other countries should ingest only foods thoroughly cooked or those that can be peeled.

PEARL

The ice cubes used in beverages can spread organisms in countries where the water is contaminated.

Follow-Up

All instances of commercial and other clusters of food poisoning should be reported to the local health department for investigation and prevention of recurrences.

Bibliography

Northrup RS, Flanigan TP: Gastroenteritis. Pediatr Rev 1994;15:461–471.

Reeves-Darby VG, Mathias JR: Toxigenic Diarrheas. In Snape WJ Jr (ed): Consultations in Gastroenterology, pp 372–380. Philadelphia, WB Saunders Company, 1996.

Section IV: Topics Involving Multiple Organs. In Feldman M, Scharschmidt BF, Sleisenger MH (eds): Sleisenger & Fordtran's Gastrointestinal and Liver Disease, 6th ed, vol 1, pp 301–450. Philadelphia, WB Saunders Company, 1998.

Section X: Small and large intestines. In Feldman M, Scharschmidt BF, Sleisenger MH (eds): Sleisenger & Fordtran's Gastrointestinal and Liver Disease, 6th ed, vol 1, pp 1624–1627. Philadelphia, WB Saunders Company, 1998.

Tamkin GW: An approach to diarrhea. Emerg Med 1998; June:16–36.

353 Lead Poisoning

Thomas F. Heston

Etiology

1. Lead poisoning is a major public health problem in industrialized countries. In terms of the threat to human health, lead is listed second only to arsenic by the Centers for Disease Control and Prevention's list of the top 275 hazardous substances. Lead poisoning is largely determined by proximity to environmental sources and age.

2. The blood lead level (BLL) is usually highest between 9 and 18 months of age. Children are at increased risk for lead poisoning because of
   a. Repeated hand-to-mouth activity
   b. Higher gastrointestinal absorption of lead
   c. Pica (ingestion of nonfood products)
   d. Incompletely developed blood-brain barrier

3. The major environmental source of lead is paint in old housing. Leaded gasoline (used prior to 1995 in the United States) has contaminated the soil of congested urban areas. Major sources of lead exposure are
   a. Pre-1977 housing with lead-based interior paint
   b. Contaminated soil from smelters, hazardous waste, or gasoline
   c. Lead-soldered pipes contaminating drinking water
   d. Occupational exposure (mining, metal smelters, radiator and battery shops)
   e. Hobbies (ceramics, stained glass)
   f. Folk remedies, cosmetics, food, and retained bullets

Symptoms

1. Most lead poisoning is asymptomatic. Symptomatic lead poisoning is considered a medical emergency. The major organ systems affected are the gastrointestinal tract, central nervous system, and renal system.

2. Chronic low-level toxicity (BLL 10 to 35 μg/dl or possibly less) may have lifelong effects:
   a. Attention-deficit hyperactivity disorder
   b. Decreased intelligence
   c. Poor social adjustment
   d. Hypertension
   e. Osteoporosis

3. Mild toxicity (BLL 35 to 50 μg/dl in children): nonspecific abdominal discomfort, mild fatigue, myalgias, paresthesias, and irritability

4. Moderate toxicity (BLL 50 to 70 μg/dl): headache, tremor, lethargy, difficulty concentrating, emesis, constipation, and weight loss

5. Severe toxicity (BLL >70 μg/dl): paresis or paralysis, encephalopathy (seizures, altered level of consciousness), blue-black lead line on the gingiva, colic

Key Symptoms

- Usually asymptomatic
- Abdominal pain
- Myalgias
- Cognitive deficits
- Lethargy
- Irritability
- Seizures
- Encephalopathy

Clinical Findings

1. Physical examination is generally not helpful in diagnosing lead poisoning.

2. Affected children may
   a. Be pale from anemia
   b. Be irritable
   c. Show cognitive deficits
   d. Have decreased hearing
   e. Have congenital abnormalities with severe prenatal exposure

3. Children should routinely be screened for lead poisoning.
   a. Universal BLL screening in areas with 27 per cent or more of housing built before 1950, or where the percentage of 1- and 2-year-olds with elevated BLLs is 12 or higher
   b. Targeted BLL screening recommended for all others based on risk factors.

4. Risk factors for lead poisoning include
   a. Children living in or regularly visiting a house with peeling or chipping paint built before 1978
   b. Having a sibling or playmate with lead poisoning
   c. Living with an adult who works with lead

d. Living near a point source of lead (e.g., a smelter)

e. Living and playing in urban areas near congested motor vehicle traffic

Laboratory Tests

1. Measurement of the venous BLL is the most accurate test for diagnosis. A level greater than 9 μg/dl is considered positive. Capillary lead levels must be confirmed by venous samples. The erythrocyte protoporphyrin level is rarely used for screening because of its poor sensitivity below 30 μg/dl.

2. Other tests to be considered:

   a. Radiographs of the abdomen for accidental ingestions

   b. Complete blood count with peripheral smear

   c. Blood urea nitrogen and creatinine level

   d. Urinalysis

 Key Test

Venous BLL is the preferred test.

Differential Diagnosis

Because the presenting signs and symptoms are nonspecific, lead poisoning may be confused with other causes of

1. Neurologic diseases and seizures

2. Developmental delay and behavioral problems

3. Anemia

4. Gastrointestinal disorders

5. Porphyria

WARNING

- **All U.S. children are at risk for lead poisoning and should be screened routinely.**

- **Public health efforts are targeted to the primary prevention of lead poisoning.**

Treatment

1. Because lead poisoning has lifelong effects, the best cure is prevention. The source of lead exposure is identified and removed. Public health authorities are notified. All symptomatic cases receive immediate chelation therapy.

2. Management of asymptomatic children depends on the BLL:

   a. BLL less than 10 μg/dl: routine screening only

   b. BLL 10 to 14 μg/dl: Parental counseling, recheck in 4 months. If 12 per cent or more of children screened are in this category, community-wide prevention activities and universal BLL screening is triggered.

   c. BLL 15 to 19 μg/dl: in addition, environmental evaluation

   d. BLL 20 to 44 μg/dl: medical and environmental evaluation and intervention. Consider chelation.

   e. BLL 45 to 69 μg/dl: outpatient chelation therapy

   f. BLL greater than 70 μg/dl: Hospitalize for intensive chelation therapy.

Medication

Chelating agents reduce the total body burden of lead. Chelation is done only in consultation with a toxicology specialist. Chelating agents include

1. Edetate calcium disodium (calcium EDTA), intravenous: Dosage in children is 50 mg/kg/day divided tid; in adults, 1 gm bid. Give for 3 to 5 days with BAL in oil.

2. Dimercaprol (BAL in oil), intramuscular: Avoid in glucose-6-phosphate dehydrogenase deficiency, hepatic or renal failure. Dosage is 3 to 4 mg/kg every 4 hours for 3 to 5 days. Used with calcium EDTA.

3. Penicillamine (Cuprimine), oral: Cross-sensitivity may occur with penicillin-allergic patients. Used as adjunctive treatment, or as solo therapy in mild toxicity (not approved by Food and Drug Administration). The usual dose is 250 mg qid in adults, or 30 mg/kg/day divided qid in children.

4. Succimer (DMSA), oral: Used for outpatient chelation. Pediatric dose is 10 mg/kg tid for 5 days followed by 10 mg/kg bid for 14 days.

Diet

The diet of children with lead poisoning should have adequate amounts of iron, calcium, zinc, and protein. A low-fat diet can decrease absorption.

Activity

1. Minimize pica.

2. Hand washing, especially before bedtime, reduces inadvertant ingestion.

3. Parents exposed to lead at work can shower and change clothes before coming home.

4. Cigarette smoke and dirt from animals are kept outside.

Patient Education

1. Educate parents about potential sources of lead poisoning.

2. Review probable symptoms of lead poisoning and potential complications.

3. Parents should be aware of ways to decrease the risk of exposure (e.g., renovation and remodeling techniques, wet mopping, and food storage).

4. Household members of affected individuals should be screened.

Key Treatment

- Primary prevention
- Remove lead sources
- Reduce exposure
- Educate parents
- Chelating agents

Follow-Up

1. Make sure the source of lead exposure has been identified and abated. This is done in collaboration with public health agencies. Abatement is completed before children are allowed to return to their environment.

2. BLL of children treated with chelating agents is rechecked 2 weeks after therapy to evaluate for rebound effects and to guide further treatment.

 ## Bibliography

Agency for Toxic Substances and Disease Registry: The 1997 Comprehensive Environmental Response, Compensation, and Liability Act Priority List of Hazardous Substances. Atlanta, Centers for Disease Control and Prevention, 1997. (Contact Division of Toxicology, 1600 Clifton Road, E29, Atlanta, GA 30333, or *http://atsdr1.atsdr.cdc.gov:8080/97list.html*)

American Academy of Pediatrics, Committee on Environmental Health: Screening for elevated blood lead levels. Pediatrics 1998;101:1072–1078.

Environmental Protection Agency, Office of Pollution Prevention and Toxics, 401 M Street SW, Washington, DC 20460 (*http://www.epa.gov/lead/index.html*)

Mendelsohn AL, Dreyer BP, Fierman AH, et al: Low-level lead exposure and behavior in early childhood. Pediatrics 1998;101:E10.

Silbergeld EK: Preventing lead poisoning in children. Annu Rev Public Health 1997;18:187–210.

Update: blood lead levels—United States, 1991–1994. MMWR Morb Mortal Wkly Rep 1997;46(7):141–146. (Published erratum appears in MMWR Morb Mortal Wkly Rep 1997;46:607.)

White RF, Diamond R, Proctor S, et al: Residual cognitive deficits 50 years after lead poisoning during childhood. Br J Ind Med 1993;50:613–622.

354 Animal Bites

James R. Blackman

Etiology

1. Between 1 and 3 million mammalian bites to humans occur annually in the United States; 1 million seek medical attention (1 to 2 per cent of emergency department visits). Most occur indoors.

2. Dog bites represent 70 to 90 per cent of all bites. The dog frequently belongs to family or a close neighbor. More than half of victims are children, a result of poorly supervised animal-child interaction.

3. Cat bites represent 5 to 20 per cent of mammalian bites, have a higher incidence of infection (deep puncture wounds), and are more common in women.

4. Human and rodent bites make up most of the remainder of mammalian bites.

5. Predisposing factors include
   a. Youth
   b. Disturbing a sleeping, feeding, injured, or unfamiliar animal
   c. Teasing, kissing, or playing recklessly with an animal
   d. Separating fighting animals
   e. Chasing wild animals
   f. Fist-fighting (human)
   g. Occupations such as animal control, police work, postal work, veterinary medicine, farming, and hunting
   h. Unprovoked attacks from feral (wild) dogs and cats, and sick or injured wild animals such as skunks, squirrels, or bats; some may have rabies.

Symptoms

The following information should be recorded in any animal bite history:

1. Concerning the animal
   a. Type of animal (including breed if known)
   b. Relationship of the animal to the victim
   c. Circumstances of the bite (provoked or unprovoked)
   d. Time and location of the incident
   e. Vaccination and health status of the animal (if known)
   f. Current location of animal (if known)

2. Concerning the victim
   a. First aid measures given
   b. Tetanus immunization status
   c. Past history of diseases of immunologic compromise
   d. Symptoms of musculoskeletal, neurologic, or vascular compromise

Clinical Findings

1. The extremities are involved in 75 per cent of cases when victims handle or attempt to avoid the animal. Head and neck injuries are the next most common.

2. Serious problems may result from
   a. Skull penetration following a bite to the cranium in a small child
   b. Bites over a joint
   c. Puncture wounds
   d. Lip and face bites in children

3. Wounds (abrasions, crush injuries, lacerations, and punctures) should be described as to size, location, and type. Include diagrams. If infected, describe adenopathy and diagram extent of cellulitis.

4. Wounds should be classified as high risk or low risk, facilitating management as regards suturing and empiric antibiotic therapy.
   a. High-risk wounds include all human and cat bites, hand and foot wounds (including closed fist injuries); wounds surgically débrided; puncture wounds; wounds involving joints, ligaments, tendons, and bones; bites with treatment delay exceeding 12 hours; and bites in immunocompromised individuals (primary immunologic disorder, human immunodeficiency virus [HIV], chronic alcoholism, asplenia, diabetes mellitus, presence of prosthetic valves or joints, immunosuppressive therapy).
   b. Low-risk wounds include lacerations involving the extremities, face, and body.

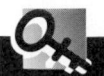

Key Signs

- Large hematoma
- Motor weakness
- Decreased capillary refill
- Decreased sensation
- Loss of function

Laboratory Tests

For most mammalian bites, laboratory tests and radiographs are unnecessary.

1. If significant blood loss is expected, hematocrit may be indicated, followed by type and cross match.
2. Cultures of wounds are necessary only in those cases in which an immunocompromised patient is infected, when there is evidence of sepsis, or when empiric antibiotic therapy fails. Organisms come from animal oral flora and human skin and include aerobes and anaerobes.

Key Organisms

Human Bites	Animal Bites
• Staphylococcal species	• Staphylococcal species
• Streptococcal species	• Streptococcal species
• *Eikenella*	• *Pasteurella multocida*
	• *Capnocytophaga*
	• Variety of aerobic and anaerobic bacteria

3. Gram's stains and cultures on fresh, uninfected wounds correlate poorly with subsequent infections and waste financial resources.
4. Radiographs are indicated when bony penetration is suspected: hands, wrists, feet, head (skull films or cranial computerized tomography).

Key Complications

- Neurovascular damage
- Bony or joint penetration with infection
- Compartment syndrome
- Cellulitis
- Septic shock
- Musculotendinous injury
- Severe crush injury
- Meningitis and cerebral abscess
- Prosthetic valve and joint infection
- Scarring and disfiguration

Treatment

1. Control airway, breathing, and circulation, and inspect for major crush injury or penetrating trauma.
2. Provide meticulous wound care.
   a. Inspect carefully for depth and extent of injury and neurovascular and musculoskeletal integrity. Bite wounds may be more severe than they appear.
   b. Débride and irrigate wound.
      (1) Provide mechanical cleansing and careful excision of devitalized tissues; crushed, devitalized tissue is particularly common with dog bites (do not soak).
      (2) Keep débridement to a minimum for facial lacerations.
      (3) Leave enough tissue to close the wound and preserve function.
      (4) Irrigate with 18- or 19-gauge needle on a 15- or 20-ml syringe using normal saline or, preferably, 1% povidone-iodine solution. If high risk of rabies transmission, use 20% soap and water or ethyl alcohol for at least 10 minutes followed by 1% benzalkonium chloride. More potent antiseptics devitalize tissue. Finish irrigation with normal saline to remove antiseptic.
   c. Repair.
      (1) Meticulous irrigation and débridement may allow wound closure.
      (2) Low-risk wounds may be sutured primarily.
      (3) High-risk wounds should be closed secondarily.
      (4) Wounds of questionable risk may be managed with delayed primary closure (some hand wounds).
3. Empiric antibiotic therapy is indicated for all high-risk wounds. Regimens are based on the most likely offending organisms. Give one parenteral dose prior to emergency room care.
4. Treat established wound infections aggressively.
   a. Provide adequate surgical débridement and drainage.
   b. Perform Gram's stain and culture.
   c. Hospitalize patients with severe blood loss, sepsis, open fracture, osteomyelitis, severe hand injury, and deep tissue injury; provide parenteral antibiotics covering gram-positive and gram-negative aerobes and anaerobes.
   d. Follow up bite wounds frequently in office to evaluate for infection and wound healing (24 and 48 hours).

5. Provide tetanus prophylaxis in standard manner (Table 354–1).
6. Review rabies postexposure prophylaxis guidelines. Exposure is defined as an open bite or wound in contact with body fluids.
    a. Wild animals
        (1) Provide prophylaxis for bites from rabies-endemic species (bats anywhere in the United States; raccoons, skunks, foxes, based on local public health recommendations).
        (2) Provide prophylaxis for bites from wild carnivores (e.g., coyotes, bobcats) and groundhogs living in a rabies-endemic area.
        (3) No treatment is necessary for provoked exposure from animals where rabies is not endemic in the species involved or in other animals in the area (e.g., rodents, rabbits, and many wild animals).
    b. Domestic animals
        (1) No treatment is indicated if animal is immunized or healthy and available for 10 days of observation.
        (2) Treatment indicated
            (a) Dogs in most developing countries and in the United States along Mexican border
            (b) Animal rabid or suspected rabid
    c. If health or immunization status is unknown at time of exposure, consult public health officials for current recommendations.
    d. Consult state or local health departments for any questions.

7. Specific treatment recommendations
    a. In previously vaccinated individuals with documented antibody response, give two doses of human diploid cell vaccine (HDCV), rabies vaccine adsorbed (RVA), or purified chick embryo cell culture (PCEG) vaccine, 1.0 ml intramuscularly (deltoid), one each on days 0 and 3. Rabies immune globulin (RIG) should not be given.
    b. In unvaccinated individuals give RIG, 20 IU/kg, as much as possible infiltrated into wound and remainder intramuscularly (gluteal); then five doses of HDCV or RVA, 1.0 ml intramuscularly (deltoid), one each on days 0, 3, 7, 14, and 28 (day 0 indicates the first day of treatment).
8. Review for possibility of hepatitis B or C transmission in human bites and provide immunoprophylaxis for hepatitis B if indicated (administer hepatitis B immune globulin, 0.06 ml/kg intramuscularly, immediately and repeat in 30 days).
9. Precautions should be taken if human bite is by a known HIV carrier.

Patient Education

1. Animals are territorial and will not attack unless territory is entered.
2. Virtually all animals give some kind of warning sign.
3. Children should never be left alone with an animal.
4. Wild animals are never safe, and pet ferrets are particularly dangerous.
5. Foster attitudes of animal love and respect.

TABLE 354–1. TETANUS PROPHYLAXIS

NEED FOR TETANUS TOXOID AND TETANUS IMMUNE GLOBULIN BASED ON HISTORY OF IMMUNIZATIONS	LOW RISK*		HIGH RISK[†]	
	Toxoid[‡]	TIG[§]	Toxoid	TIG
Not known	Yes	No	Yes	Yes
Zero	Yes	No	Yes	Yes[‖]
One	Yes	No	Yes	Yes[‖]
Two	Yes	No	Yes	Yes
Three or more				
Last booster <5 yr	No	No	No	No
Last booster <10 yr	No	No	Yes	Yes
Last booster >10 yr	Yes	No	Yes	Yes

*Low risk: Clean, little devitalized tissue, easily débrided (and irrigate).
[†]High risk: Dirty, deep, much devitalized tissue, difficult to débride (and irrigate).
[‡]Toxoid: Adult, 0.5 ml dT IM
        Child <5, 0.5 ml DPT IM
        Child >5, 0.5 ml DT IM
[§]TIG (tetanus immune globulin): 250–500 U IM in limb opposite of toxoid.
[‖]Plus completion of immunization (three injections) with booster doses, at 30 and 60 days after initial injection.

6. Provide obedience training in companion animals
7. Keep animals under control.
8. Do not run if confronted by a threatening dog.

Key Treatment

Human Bites

- Amoxicillin–clavulanic acid (Augmentin), followed by dicloxacillin plus penicillin

- If penicillin-allergic, tetracycline (but not in children and during pregnancy)

Cat Bites

- Amoxicillin–clavulanic acid followed by dicloxacillin or penicillin G followed by penicillin V

- If penicillin-allergic, erythromycin

Dog Bites

- Amoxicillin–clavulanic acid followed by dicloxacillin or cefazolin followed by cephalexin

- If penicillin-allergic, erythromycin

Bibliography

Blackman JR: Man's best friend? J Am Board Fam Pract 1998;11:167–169.
Callanan ML, French SP: Bites and injuries inflicted by mammals. In Auerbach PS (ed): Management of Wilderness and Environmental Emergencies, 3rd ed, pp 927–993. St. Louis, Mosby–Year Book, 1995.
Groleau G: Rabies. Emerg Med Clin North Am 1992;10: 361–368.
Kelleher AT, Gordon SM: Management of bite wounds and infection in primary care. Cleveland Clin J Med 1997;64:137–141.
Tisovec RW, Kakaiya R: Dog bites: hidden danger of fulminant sepsis. J Am Board Fam Pract 1998;11:152–153.

355 Insects and Spiders

Thomas C. Michels

Etiology

1. Bites: insects (fleas, bed bugs, flies, mosquitoes) and others (spiders, ticks, chiggers)
2. Stings: Hymenoptera (honeybee, wasp, yellow jacket, hornet, fire ant) and scorpions

Symptoms (see also Table 355–1)

1. Local minor reactions
   a. Normal reaction following any sting or bite
      (1) Immediate local pain with swelling; subsides in 1 to 2 hours.
      (2) Early pruritis that may persist for several days
      (3) Ticks usually cause itching and local wheal, but can transmit diseases such as tick bite fever, tick paralysis, Rocky Mountain spotted fever, and Lyme disease.
   b. Large local reaction
      (1) Swelling extending from sting site over a large area, such as entire extremity
      (2) Peaks at 48 hours, may last up to a week.
2. Local major (dermonecrotic) reactions
   a. Prototype is bite of brown recluse spider (*Loxosceles reclusa*): cutaneous loxoscelism.
   b. Bite may go unnoticed or victim may feel mild stinging or burning.
   c. May note a sore at the site with pain and tenderness 2 to 72 hours later.
   d. Necrotic ulcer later develops (in 20 per cent of those seeking care) and may take weeks to heal.
3. Anaphylaxis
   a. Most commonly with hymenoptera envenomation, can occur with other bites or stings.
   b. Same symptoms as with anaphylaxis from any cause
4. Systemic toxic reactions: most commonly caused by neurotoxins in arthropod venom
   a. Systemic loxoscelism
      (1) Symptoms start 6 to 72 hours after bite of brown recluse spider.
      (2) Fever, malaise, rash, arthralgias, nausea, and vomiting; may progress to collapse.
   b. Latrodectism: bite of the black widow spider (*Latrodectus mactans*) or its relatives
      (1) Bite often unnoticed, but victim may feel a pinprick sensation.
      (2) In 20 to 30 minutes, limb and lymph node pain, local swelling, itching, or hives develops.
      (3) May progress to crampy pain in thighs, abdomen, chest, with sialorrhea, nausea, and vomiting.
   c. Scorpion stings
      (1) Most bites in United States are due to the bark scorpion (*Centruroides sculpturatus*); endemic to Southwest, but can be transported anywhere.
      (2) Shortly after bite, local itching, regional paresthesias; then diaphoresis, dyspnea, sialorrhea, lacrimation, muscle pain, nausea, vomiting may begin.

Key Symptoms

- Stinging, burning
- Extremity pain or paresthesias

If severe:

- Abdominal pain
- Sialorrhea
- Nausea and vomiting

Clinical Findings

1. Local minor reactions
   a. Normal reaction has small papule or wheal, with or without evidence of excoriation.
   b. Papular urticaria described after flea bites and others.
   c. Painful wheals, then vesicles and pustules typical for fire ant bite in Southeastern United States.
   d. Large local reaction has wheal at bite site; may have regional edema and erythema.
2. Local major (dermonecrotic) reactions
   a. Early: red, edematous, or blanched area sur-

TABLE 355–1. SUMMARY OF SELECTED FEATURES OF MAJOR CLINICAL SYNDROMES

SYNDROME	ETIOLOGY	SYMPTOMS	SIGNS	DIFFERENTIAL DIAGNOSIS	TREATMENT	FOLLOW-UP
Local minor reaction	Any arthropod bite or sting	Local pain, swelling, pruritis	Papule or wheal; possibly vesicles, regional edema	Atopic or contact dermatitis; viral or drug eruption	Cool compresses; topical lotions; antihistamines	Usually none; watch for secondary infection; general protective measures
Local major (dermonecrotic) reaction	Brown recluse spider	Mild local stinging, then a sore at site	Sinking blue macule with surrounding erythema; later blister and purpura; occasionally necrotic ulcer	Vasculitis, trauma, septic embolus, purpura, pyoderma	Immobilization, cleanse wound, tetanus prophylaxis, expectant management, rarely surgery	To determine extent of necrosis, necessity of surgery; general protective measures
Anaphylaxis	Hymenoptera (multiple causes)	Pruritis, throat irritation, dyspnea, nausea, faintness	Hypotension, tachycardia, stridor, syncope, urticaria	Acute cardiovascular or respiratory event	Epinephrine, antihistamines, steroids	Allergy testing and immunotherapy; general protective measures
Systemic toxic reaction	Black widow spider, brown recluse spider, scorpions (less common)	Regional pain, swelling, nausea, vomiting, malaise, rash	Hypotension, tachycardia, muscle spasms and rigidity; flushing, diaphoresis	Acute renal failure, disseminated intravascular coagulation, acute abdomen from any cause	ABCs, general supportive measures: intravenous fluids, oxygen; tetanus prophylaxis; muscle relaxants	Follow for resolution of symptoms; general protective measures

rounding bite; classically a sinking blue macule with halo of erythema

   b. Later: hemorrhagic blister surrounded by irregular purpura

   c. Eschar forms days later; necrotic ulcer that may take months to heal; more extensive in areas with more subcutaneous fat (thighs, abdomen, buttocks).

3. Anaphylaxis: same as anaphylxis from any cause

4. Systemic toxic reactions

   a. Systemic loxoscelism: fever, hypotension, shock, self-limited hemolysis; rarely scarlatiniform rash, splenomegaly

   b. Latrodectism

     (1) Hypertensive, restless patient, flushed, sweating face, contorted with spasm or pain

     (2) Prominent muscle rigidity, including abdominal muscles

   c. Scorpion stings

     (1) Initially tachycardia, hypotension; can progress to shock.

     (2) Involuntary motor activity; can progress to seizures; cranial nerve dysfunction.

Key Signs

- Erythematous papules
- Central punctum
- Hemorrhagic blister

If severe:

- Hypertension or hypotension
- Muscle rigidity
- Involuntary movement

Laboratory Tests

1. Few specific diagnostic tests: venom-specific immunoglobulin E in serum of patient with anaphylaxis indicates specific allergy.

2. Tests search for complications or monitor supportive care.

3. Leukocytosis and hyperglycemia usual in stress reactions.

4. Severe reactions: elevated creatine phosphokinase or renal failure; loxoscelism may show hemolysis or evidence of disseminated intravascular coagulation (DIC) (see Ch. 171, Disseminated Intravascular Coagulation).

Key Tests

None (glucose, white blood cell count, blood urea nitrogen, creatinine, urinalysis, coagulation studies useful in severe cases)

Differential Diagnosis

1. History of exposure and bite; have patient bring the offending organism in for identification.

2. Local minor reactions: Many "bug bites" have similar presentation.

   a. Ask for history of travel, exposure to outdoor or unhygienic environments, pets, or others with same condition.

   b. Papules grouped on exposed surfaces or snug spots in clothing suggest infestation or flea bites.

   c. Examination should look for urticarial papules with a central punctum.

   d. Chigger (harvest mite) bites (Southern United States): discrete, bright-red papules of legs and waist with hemorrhagic puncta and intense pruritis

   e. Differential includes atopic dermatitis, allergic or irritant contact dermatitis, and viral or drug eruption.

3. Dermonecrotic reactions: Early differential includes vasculitis, trauma, septic embolus, or purpura; later: pyoderma.

4. Anaphylaxis: same as anaphylaxis from any cause

5. Systemic toxic reactions

   a. Systemic loxoscelism: Severe reactions can present as acute renal failure or DIC from any cause.

   b. Latrodectism

     (1) Severe reactions can present as acute abdomen; history of bite, abrupt onset, tender muscles, and patient writhing in pain help distinguish.

     (2) Differential includes tabic crisis, acute psychosis, meningitis, or acute renal failure.

   c. Scorpion stings: Severe reactions may present as insecticide poisoning.

Treatment

1. Minor local reactions: cool compresses; topical lotions such as calamine, camphor-menthol

   a. Secondary infection requires antibiotic treatment as with cellulitis.

b. Large local reactions: antihistamines (e.g., chlorpheniramine, 4 to 8 mg, or diphenhydramine, 50 mg every 6 hours) or steroids (e.g., prednisone, 40 mg daily for 2 to 3 days)

2. Dermonecrotic reactions
   a. Initial management: Immobilize limb, apply cold compresses.
   b. Hospital care: Carefully cleanse wound; tetanus prophylaxis; avoid local injections into wound and steroids; antibiotics only for secondary infection.
   c. Although dapsone, steroids, colchicine, and hyperbaric oxygen are all advocated by some, none have been shown better than conservative expectant management; each has its own risks.
   d. Corrective surgery rarely required; graftings should be delayed for 8 weeks to allow for adequate tissue demarcation of necrosis.

3. Anaphylaxis: same as anaphylaxis from any cause

4. Systemic toxic reactions
   a. Identification of biting or stinging arthropod critical if specific antivenom to be considered.
   b. General supportive measures important: airway, breathing, and circulation (ABCs) of resuscitation; intravenous volume expansion; monitoring; oxygen.
   c. Systemic loxoscelism: general supportive measures; treat acute renal failure or DIC if present.
   d. Latrodectism
      (1) Cool compresses to bite site
      (2) General supportive measures
      (3) Muscle relaxants provide symptomatic relief.
         (a) Diazepam: 5 to 10 mg IM or IV, may repeat in 3 to 4 hours; in children 1 month to 5 years, 1 to 2 mg per dose; larger doses may be required for severe spasm.
         (b) Methocarbamol: 15 mg/kg slowly IV; followed by oral therapy
         (c) Calcium gluconate 10% solution, 1 to 2 ml/kg up to 10 ml per dose; often affords more striking relief, although transient.
      (4) Tetanus prophylaxis
      (5) Antivenom of equine origin available from Merck Sharpe & Dohme: for severely affected patients; experts with most experience rarely advocate its use.

e. Scorpion stings
   (1) General supportive measures
   (2) Local compresses, analgesics
   (3) Tetanus prophylaxis
   (4) Treat hypertension, tachycardia with β-blockers.
   (5) Specific antivenom available for severe cases from Arizona State University.

Patient Education

1. Patients with hymenoptera sensitivity
   a. Minimize exposure: no bare feet outdoors; wear long pants, gloves when gardening; avoid perfumes, hair sprays, pastel or white clothing.
   b. Self-administration of epinephrine; commercially available kits (ANA-Kit, EpiPen)

2. Avoidance measures for all patients with outdoor exposure
   a. Wear work gloves when cleaning up debris.
   b. Consider use of pesticides in heavily infested areas.
   c. Brush off, do not swat, if something crawling on body.
   d. Check outdoor clothing, shoes before putting them on.
   e. Insect repellents useful against many insects and ticks.

Key Treatment

- Cool compresses
- Antihistamines
- Tetanus prophylaxis
- Muscle relaxants
- Specific antivenin (rarely, in severe cases)

Follow-Up

1. Most patients with sting or bite reactions have self-limited course.
2. Ongoing desensitization therapy for hymenoptera sensitivity
3. Follow-up to determine if débridement or excision necessary in dermonecrotic reaction.
4. Follow-up for those with systemic toxic reactions determined by specific clinical syndrome.

Bibliography

For an overview of common bites and stings with differential features, see
Paller A: Insect bites and infestations. In Dershewitz RA (ed): Ambulatory Pediatric Care, 2nd ed, pp 275–279. Philadelphia, JB Lippincott Company, 1993.

For details on hymenoptera sensitivity and other reactions, see
Reisman RE: Stinging insect allergy. Med Clin North Am 1992;76:883–894.

For a detailed review of spider and scorpion envenomation, including photographs of these arthropods, see
Allen C: Arachnid envenomations. Emerg Med Clin North Am 1992;10:269–288.

For a broad overview briefly covering many insects and arachnids, see
Stawiski MA: Insect bites and stings. Emerg Med Clin North Am 1985;3:785–808.

For a practical review by an experienced clinician, see
Anderson PC: Spider bites in the U.S. Dermatol Clin North Am 1997;15:307–311.

For a review of brown recluse spider bites, see
Cacy J, Mold JW: The clinical characteristics of brown recluse spider bites treated by family physicians: an OKPRN study. J Fam Pract 1999;48:536–542.

356 Snakebite

Gregory Juckett

Etiology

1. There are about 8000 venomous snakebites per year in the United States, most of which occur between April and October; however, only 10 to 15 of these at most result in death.

2. Pit vipers of the family Crotalidae include rattlesnakes, cottonmouths (water moccasins), and copperheads. These are responsible for the vast majority (99 per cent) of U.S. venomous native snakebites. Pit vipers are named after a small, heat-sensitive pit located between the eye and the nostril. They have broad heads, vertical pupils, and a single row of subcaudal scales below the anal plate.

   a. Rattlesnakes (*Crotalus* or *Sistrurus*) are responsible for most fatalities because they are present through most of the continental United States excepting Maine, Delaware, and Rhode Island. Multiple species exist (timber, canebrake, prairie, Pacific, sidewinder, massasauga, Mojave, pygmy, and eastern and western diamondbacks), of which the latter two are the largest and most dangerous. Contrary to popular belief, rattlesnakes do not always rattle to warn of an impending strike.

   b. Cottonmouths or water moccasins (*Agkistrodon piscivorus*) are aggressive semiaquatic snakes most common in the southeast. Their venom is intermediate in toxicity between rattlesnake and copperhead venom.

   c. Copperheads (*Agkistrodon contortrix*) are common pit vipers of the eastern United States but have the least toxic venom. Their bite is usually not fatal in adults, but supportive treatment is necessary to prevent complications.

3. Coral snakes of the family Elapidae are small, nonaggressive, colorful snakes of the deep south, with subspecies in the eastern United States, Texas, and Arizona. The bite of the eastern coral snake (*Micrurus*) is much more serious than that of the Arizona type (*Micruroides*). Coral snakes seldom bite but, when they do, they introduce venom by chewing instead of injection. Their distinctive pattern of red, yellow, and black bands can be distinguished from nonvenomous mimics because the red and yellow bands are adjacent ("red on yellow, kill a fellow; red on black, fear may lack"). This rule is applicable only in the United States and northern Mexico, however, becoming unreliable south of Mexico City.

4. Exotic venomous snakes: Increasing numbers of snakebites now occur from captive exotic species such as cobras, all too often kept as pets by individuals. The availability of exotic antivenins can be determined at any time by calling the Arizona Poison Control Center at 1-520-626-6016. Consultation with snakebite experts is also available there.

Symptoms

1. Pit viper envenomation

   a. With the exception of some Mojave rattler bites, painful in 5 minutes, with local swelling and ecchymosis soon developing

   b. Other symptoms may include fasciculations, unusual taste, oral paresthesias, vomiting, confusion, seizures, and hemorrhage possibly leading to hypovolemic shock and death.

   c. Anxiety symptoms are common and must be distinguished from those of envenomation.

   d. The venom consists of a stable mixture of toxic proteins and enzymes that results in tissue necrosis and hemolysis. Mojave venom is an exception because it blocks neuromuscular transmission and may induce paralysis.

   e. Unless a vein is entered, pit viper bites are not immediately fatal.

2. Coral snake envenomation usually lacks local pain, although numbness is common. The venom is neurotoxic, however, and cranial nerve palsies, respiratory paralysis, and death can quickly develop. Systemic symptoms are difficult to reverse once they begin.

Key Symptoms

- Local pain and swelling (numbness if coral snake)

- Vomiting, cramps, abnormal taste, confusion, bleeding

Clinical Findings

1. Pit viper bites classically appear as two fang punctures with local swelling and tissue necrosis. Occasionally, only one or (rarely) three fang marks are visible. Extremity bites can be complicated by infection, gangrene, and occasionally compartment syndromes. Systemic reactions may involve disseminated intravascular coagulation, acute renal failure, hypovolemic shock, and death.

2. Coral snake bites are easy to miss, consisting of multiple tiny fang punctures with no other visible change. Local sensation may be diminished. Systemic signs include weakness, ptosis, diplopia, dysphagia, salivation, diaphoresis, loss of tendon reflexes, and most seriously, respiratory depression and paralysis.

Key Signs

- Fang marks, edema, tissue necrosis, ecchymoses, bullae

- Hemorrhage, hematuria, renal failure, hypotension

- Numbness, weakness, ptosis and cranial nerve signs, respiratory depression (coral snake, occasionally Mojave rattlesnake)

Laboratory Tests

1. Routine laboratory tests for suspected snakebite envenomation should usually include the following.

    a. Complete blood cell (CBC) count with platelets and differential

    b. Coagulation studies: prothrombin time (PT), partial thromboplastin time (PTT), fibrinogen, fibrin degradation products. Repeat studies within 12 hours.

    c. Type and cross match

    d. Blood chemistries: electrolytes, glucose, blood urea nitrogen (BUN), creatinine, liver transaminases, bilirubin, creatinine kinase (CK)

    e. Urinalysis

    f. Arterial blood gases (ABGs)

    g. Stool hemoccult

    h. Electrocardiogram (ECG)

2. Laboratory abnormalities in severe envenomation may include leukocytosis, hemolytic anemia, thrombocytopenia, prolonged PT/PTT, hypofibrinogenemia, hematuria, proteinuria, elevated BUN and creatinine and CK.

Key Tests

- CBC
- Urinalysis
- ABGs
- PT/PTT/fibrinogen
- BUN/creatinine
- ECG
- Electrolytes, liver function tests, glucose
- CK
- Type and cross match

Treatment

1. First aid measures for snakebite have been radically revised in recent years because tourniquets and wound incisions often exacerbated rather than helped the patient's condition. The following measures are currently recommended:

    a. Calm patient and immobilize the extremity. Remove jewelry. Avoid exertion.

    b. A wide constriction band may be applied proximal to the bite to block lymphatic drainage but not blood flow. It should be easy to insert one finger beneath this band without difficulty. Splint upper extremities at heart level.

    c. Do not incise fang marks. If available within 3 minutes of being bitten, a Sawyer extractor applied over the site and left on for 30 minutes may help.

    d. Transport as quickly as possible to the nearest equipped medical facility.

    e. Things *not* to do: *Do not apply ice or a tourniquet*, and do not use electric shock. Do not try to kill or capture snake (this can result in another bite), but try to identify it from a safe distance. If the snake is already dead, do not pick it up with hands because it may still bite by reflex action. Do not consider antivenin administration in the field. Do not cut the site or suck it out with the mouth.

2. Determine if envenomation has occurred. At least 25 per cent of venomous snakebites are "dry" and no reaction occurs. Asymptomatic pit viper bites should be observed for at least 6 hours before discharge. Measure affected limb circumference frequently. Coral snake and other elapid bites should always be admitted for 24 hours' observation. Although dry coral snake bites are common, any suspected envenomation by eastern coral snakes should be treated with antivenin immediately. Do not wait for symptoms because it is diffi-

cult to reverse them with antivenin once they appear.

3. Resuscitation measures as needed: oxygen, monitors, two large-bore intravenous lines, intravascular volume expansion with crystalloids; draw lab specimens, including type and cross match.

4. Clean wound and consider tetanus toxoid or tetanus immune globulin if not immunized.

5. Consider antivenin for moderate to severe pit viper envenomations, remembering that antivenin administration can be almost as dangerous as the snakebite.

   a. *Antivenin (Crotalidae) polyvalent* is suitable for rattlesnake, cottonmouth, and copperhead bites, whereas the eastern coral snake requires *Micrurus fulvius antivenin.*

   b. Exotic species have specific antivenins the location of which is available from the Arizona Poison Control Center.

   c. Antivenin is best administered within 4 hours but is effective for at least the first 24 hours (possibly up to 72 hours for coagulopathy). It should only be given intravenously using a strict protocol with the physician in attendance and epinephrine and antihistamines available at the bedside.

   d. A safer sheep-derived (ovine) antivenin is currently under consideration by the Food and Drug Administration.

6. Once antivenin is deemed necessary, skin testing should be performed with the test kit dose of horse serum according to the package insert (unless the patient is in extremis). If the patient does react to skin testing, antivenin should only be administered if there is a true threat to life or limb, with careful monitoring, hydration, and premedication.

7. Pit viper antivenin dose is usually based on clinical grading of envenomation:

   a. Grade 0: no envenomation, no local or systemic findings—avoid antivenin.

   b. Grade 1: minimal envenomation with local pain and edema—consider 5 vials; however, antivenin may be unnecessary (e.g., most copperhead bites). Smaller doses of pit viper antivenin are not indicated. Dose not reduced for children.

   c. Grade 2: moderate envenomation, local with mild systemic and/or lab findings—5 to 15 vials.

   d. Grade 3: severe envenomation, severe local, systemic and lab abnormalities—15 to 20+ vials. Remember, grades can change over time.

8. Antivenin administration: reconstitute by injecting supplied 10-ml sterile water diluent into each vial and swirling without shaking to mix. Reconstituted antivenin is then diluted in 500 ml of normal saline or 5% dextrose in water and a trial dose of 5 to 10 ml is administered intravenously over 5 minutes. If no reaction occurs, adjust the rate to give up to 10 vials in the first hour. Additional infusions should be given every 2 hours until signs and symptoms are resolving.

9. Fasciotomy is rarely indicated and should not be done prophylactically. However, monitoring for compartment syndromes is still necessary for many pit viper bites.

10. Eastern coral snake antivenin should be given immediately for any suspected envenomation rather than waiting for neurologic symptoms to develop. Local symptoms are often absent. Antivenin is not available for Arizona coral snake (*Micruroides*), which is not associated with human fatality.

   a. Give 3 to 5 vials *Micrurus* antivenin if envenomation suspected but no signs or symptoms present.

   b. Give 6 to 10+ vials if systemic symptoms exist.

11. If bite infection occurs, treat with broad-spectrum antibiotic.

12. Complications from antivenin therapy are common, including hypersensitivity reactions (including anaphylaxis) and, after 1 to 4 weeks, serum sickness. Serum sickness develops in a majority of antivenin patients and presents with itching, urticarial rash, fever, and arthralgias. It responds well to oral prednisone therapy.

Key Treatment

- Supportive first aid with rapid transport to hospital
- Treatment is determined by degree of envenomation.
- Antivenin is the only specific treatment but poses significant risks.

Prevention

1. Wear protective clothing and boots when walking where snakes may occur.

2. Take a friend with you on wilderness excursions and avoid drugs and alcohol.

3. Watch where you step and place your hands. Avoid tall grass and underbrush.

4. Leave snakes alone—many bites are provoked by attempting to kill, handle, or tease.

5. Do not keep venomous snakes as pets.

6. Do not walk after dark; if you do, carry a flashlight.

Bibliography

Gold BS, Wingert WA: Snake venom poisoning in the U.S.—a review of therapeutic practice. South Med J 1994;87:579–589.

Lichtenhan JB: Emergency management of poisonous snakebites. Physician Sports Med 1995;23:73–88.

Newman JG: Bites and stings. In Howell JM (ed): Emergency Medicine, vol 2, pp 1585–1597. Philadelphia, WB Saunders Company, 1998.

Norris RL: Snake venom poisoning in the U.S.—assessment and management. Emerg Med Rep 1995;16:87–93.

Sullivan JB Jr, Wingert WA, Norris RL Jr: North American venomous reptile bites. In Auerbach PS (ed): Wilderness Medicine, 3rd ed, pp 680–709. St. Louis, Mosby–Year Book, 1995.

357 Heat-Related Illness

Michael L. O'Dell

Etiology

1. Definition: Heat-related illnesses include heat cramps, heat syncope, heat exhaustion, and heat stroke. These syndromes occur during prolonged exposure to high environmental temperatures, especially if the affected individual is engaged in heavy exertion or is elderly.

   a. Heat cramps are muscle cramps during or immediately following exercising in excessive heat conditions. The muscle cramps usually involve the exercised muscle group.

   b. Dizziness, weakness, and fatigue following exposure to excessive heat conditions define heat exhaustion.

   c. Heat syncope involves loss of consciousness by a person who has been exposed to high ambient temperatures. Heat exhaustion generally precedes loss of consciousness.

   d. Heat stroke is characterized by rapidly progressive elevation of core body temperature to greater than 105° F following exposure to high ambient heat conditions. Classic heat stroke occurs primarily in older or chronically ill individuals during heat waves and is often not related to exertion. Exertional heat stroke generally occurs in younger persons vigorously exerting themselves in high ambient heat conditions.

2. Epidemiology

   a. Heat load is subject to several factors, including metabolic heat production, air temperature, humidity, radiant heat, and air movement. The last four of these are measured by the "heat index." The incidence of heat-related illness climbs dramatically when the 24-hour average temperature exceeds 90° F, particularly when elevated temperature occurs suddenly, not allowing for acclimatization.

   b. Metabolic heat production can be increased through vigorous exercise. Other modifiers include febrile illness, hyperthyroidism, and use of certain drugs, such as cocaine.

   c. Heat index factors can be modified voluntarily by clothing and through seeking cooler surroundings, such as an air-conditioned room.

3. Predisposing factors: Factors that contribute to heat-related illness include social, behavioral, and medical factors.

   a. Social factors: Air conditioning is a potent modifier of heat-related illness. Air conditioning markedly lessens the risk of heat-related illness. Fans contribute to convective heat load at temperatures greater than 90° F, and worsen heat stress. Social isolation (few friends, family, or pets) is a predictor of heat-related illness.

   b. Behavioral factors: Heavy exercise in high heat raises the risk of heat-related illness. Over 2 weeks, healthy and fit individuals can increase their tolerance to heat through acclimatization. Limiting work and exercise to periods of the day when the temperature is lower reduces the risk of heat-related illness. Consuming alcohol or engaging in illicit drug abuse, such as cocaine use, increases the risk of heat-related illness.

   c. Medical factors: Numerous medical factors contribute to heat-related illness, including illness that results in being confined to bed or otherwise unable to care for self; mental illness; heart disease; pulmonary disease; and obesity.

Symptoms

1. Heat cramps: muscle cramps during or following exercise in heat stressed conditions, especially if fluid intake has not been adequate

2. Heat exhaustion: Heat exhaustion is the most common syndrome seen by clinicians. Weakness, confusion, and lightheadedness are common. Symptoms are likely related to poor perfusion as a result of peripheral pooling and poor hydration. Nausea, headache, anxiousness, and an urge to defecate are also common symptoms.

3. Heat syncope: Heat syncope involves loss of consciousness during high heat conditions.

4. Heat stroke: Heat stroke is divided into two categories, exertional and classical.

   a. Exertional heat stroke occurs in healthy, young individuals engaging in heavy exertion in high ambient heat conditions. Loss of consciousness may be the first symptom, although preceding symptoms of heat exhaustion have often been present. Headache, vertigo, faintness, abdominal distress, confusion, and delirium are other common symptoms.

b. Classical heat stroke occurs primarily in older or chronically ill individuals during heat waves. Loss of consciousness may be the first symptom. Headache, vertigo, faintness, abdominal distress, confusion, and delirium are other common symptoms

Key Symptoms

- Cramping of muscle groups following exertion
- Confusion or altered mental status

Clinical Findings

1. Heat cramps: Body temperature is normal. Sweating is normal or excessive.
2. Heat exhaustion: Skin is often ashen-gray in color. The skin is cool and clammy. Body temperature is normal or subnormal. Sweating is normal or excessive. Hyperventilation and tachycardia are often present, and blood pressure may be low. Pupils are often dilated.
3. Heat syncope: Signs are those of heat exhaustion in an unconscious patient.
4. Heat stroke: In both syndromes rectal temperature is elevated, often greater than 105° F.
   a. Exertional heat stroke: The patient continues to sweat. The patient is confused, unconscious, or delirious.
   b. Classic heat stroke: The skin is hot and dry, and sweating is not present. Blood pressure is low and shock is common. Muscle tone is flaccid with decreased deep tendon reflexes.

Key Signs

- In heat cramps, heat exhaustion, and heat syncope, body temperature is normal or subnormal. In heat stroke, core body temperature is elevated, often above 105° F.
- In classical heat stroke, the skin is hot and dry. However, in exertional heat stroke, sweatiness may still be present.

Laboratory Tests

1. Heat cramps, heat exhaustion, and heat syncope: Normal laboratory findings are the rule.

2. Heat stroke
   a. Exertional heat stroke: Hemoconcentration, hyponatremia, hypocalcemia, abnormal liver and muscle enzymes, and hypophosphatemia are often present. Coagulation studies often reveal disseminated intravascular coagulation (DIC). Acute renal failure may be present, and lactic acidosis is common.
   b. Classical heat stroke: Initial laboratory studies may be normal, but liver and muscle enzyme abnormalities are common. Hypocalcemia and hypophosphatemia are often present. DIC and coagulopathy may be present. Respiratory alkalosis followed by metabolic acidosis is often present. Leukocytosis, proteinuria, and elevation of blood urea nitrogen (BUN) are common. Electrocardiograms may show tachycardia, flattened or inverted T waves, and depression of ST segments.

Key Tests

- Laboratory studies are generally normal in heat cramps, heat exhaustion, and heat syncope.
- Liver and muscle enzymes, calcium, phosphate, BUN are often abnormal in heat stroke.
- Leukocytosis and DIC are often present in heat stroke.

Differential Diagnosis

1. Heat cramps: Consider electrolyte disturbance, exposure to toxins, and tetanus.
2. Heat exhaustion: Consider dehydration, dysrhythmias, or other causes of hypotension.
3. Heat syncope: Differential that of heat exhaustion. Also consider common causes of unconsciousness, including trauma, infection, and metabolic disorders.
4. Heat stroke: Findings may be confused with overwhelming sepsis or thyroid storm.

Treatment

1. Prevention of heat illness should be a priority. Exercise should be moderate and early in the day until acclimatized. Heavy exertion should not be scheduled during high ambient heat conditions. Adequate intake of fluid is necessary for the prevention of heat-related illness. Elderly, chronically ill, or isolated persons should have access to air conditioning during high heat conditions.

2. All heat-related illnesses require removal from high ambient heat to cooler spaces.

3. Heat cramps, heat exhaustion, and heat syncope all respond well to rehydration and cooling. World Health Organization oral rehydration formula or similar fluids are particularly suitable for rehydration, although copious amounts of water are satisfactory. Affected individuals should be assumed to be at least 10 per cent dehydrated. Unconscious or confused patients may require parenteral administration of fluids.

4. Heat stroke is a medical emergency. Cooling blankets or ice to lateral torso should be accompanied by vigorous massage to aid in decreasing peripheral vasoconstriction. Immersion in ice water bath renders the patient less accessible and is no more effective than massage and ice. Hydration should be monitored via Swan-Ganz catheterization and urinary output. Airway management is critical, particularly in comatose or seizing patients.

Key Treatment

- Prevention, through acclimatization, hydration, and careful scheduling of activities, is important for all heat-related illnesses.

- Removal from the heat-stressed environment is necessary for all patients with heat-related illness.

- Hydration is a critical issue in all patients with heat stress.

- Prompt cooling is critical for patients with heat stroke.

Follow-Up

1. Heat cramps, heat exhaustion, and heat syncope: Patients should be counseled regarding appropriate fluid intake, acclimatization, and appropriate times of day to exercise.

2. Heat stroke

   a. Young and previously healthy patients are more likely to survive heat stroke. All patients surviving heat stroke should be instructed to avoid high heat conditions in the future. Surviving patients should be educated in fluid intake and assessing heat conditions.

   b. Prompt recovery is a favorable prognostic sign, although 21 per cent of patients initially surviving succumb in 2 to 3 weeks.

   c. Continued disability and excessive deaths occur several months beyond the initial heat stroke. Of surviving patients, one study found 28 per cent mortality at 1-year follow-up. Close ongoing follow-up must occur.

Bibliography

Dematt J, O'Mara K, Buescher J, et al: Near fatal heat stroke during the 1995 heat wave in Chicago. Ann Intern Med 1998;129:173–181.

Heat related mortality—United States, 1997. MMWR Morb Mortal Wkly Rep 1998;47(23).

Kilbourne E, Choi K, Jones S, et al: Risk factors for heat stroke—a case control study. JAMA 1982;24:3332–3336.

Marzuk P, Tardiff M, Leon A, et al: Ambient temperature and mortality from unintentional cocaine overdose. JAMA 1998;279:1795–1800.

Semenza J, Rubin C, Falter K, et al: Heat related deaths during the July 1995 heat wave in Chicago. N Engl J Med 1996;35:84–90.

358 Frostbite

Frank S. Celestino

Etiology

1. Tissue injury and destruction are due to freezing. Extracellular ice crystals increase the extracellular osmotic gradient, leading to cell death. Progressive vascular ischemic thrombosis and occlusion occur via red cell sludging, platelet aggregation, endothelial injury, and the local generation of prostaglandins and thromboxanes, causing vasoconstriction.

2. Risk factors
   a. Prolonged exposure to cold climate
   b. Previous frostbite injury
   c. Inappropriate or wet clothing
   d. Immobility
   e. Impaired cognition
   f. Extremes of age
   g. Malnutrition
   h. Smoking
   i. Psychiatric illness
   j. Sedative and alcohol use
   k. Hypothyroidism
   l. Pre-existing cardiac or vascular disease
   m. Lack of acclimatization
   n. Skin damage
   o. Extremes of temperature and wind chill factor
   p. Cold exposure at high altitude
   q. Homelessness

Symptoms

1. Superficial injury: partial to complete skin involvement only
   a. Paresthesias, tingling, and moderate numbness
   b. Burning, throbbing, or aching discomfort
   c. Prickly or itchy sensations
   d. Painful dysesthesias and burning on rewarming
2. Deep injury: skin plus varying involvement of subcutaneous tissue, muscle, bone
   a. Profound numbness/anesthesia
   b. Stiffness and immobility
   c. Heaviness and "block of wood" feeling
   d. Joint pains/arthralgias
   e. Burning, throbbing, tingling, aching, or shooting pains on rewarming

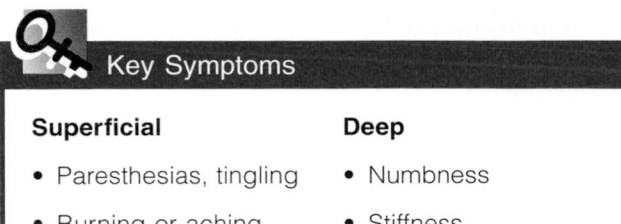

Key Symptoms

Superficial	Deep
• Paresthesias, tingling	• Numbness
• Burning or aching	• Stiffness

Clinical Findings

1. Most injuries (90 per cent) involve fingers or toes; less commonly nose, ears, cheeks, and penis.
2. Superficial injury
   a. Cold, frozen, white, nonblanchable, and waxy-appearing skin
   b. Soft, pliable, and resilient subcutaneous tissue before thawing
   c. Erythema, mild to moderate edema, bleb formation with clear fluid, and occasional desquamation on thawing
   d. No permanent tissue loss occurs.
3. Deep injury
   a. Icy, hard, and wooden skin
   b. Nonresilient and hard subcutaneous tissue
   c. Intense hyperemia, marked edema, cyanosis, hemorrhagic blisters, skin necrosis, gangrene, and even mummification after thawing
   d. Permanent tissue loss occurs.

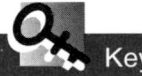

Key Signs

Superficial Injury

• Nonblanchable, waxy-appearing skin

• Soft, resilient subcutaneous tissue before thawing

Deep Injury

• Icy, hard, and wooden skin/limb

• Hard, nonresilient subcutaneous tissue before thawing

Laboratory Tests

1. Complete blood count
2. Serial radionuclide angiography and/or triple-phase bone scans have traditionally been used in deep frostbite injuries to help with the identification and débridement of nonviable tissue. These studies are unreliable in the first 2 to 4 days after injury because of effects of persistent vascular spasm and instability. More recently, magnetic resonance (MR) imaging and MR angiography have been shown to be superior to bone scanning for tissue demarcation.
3. Wound and blood cultures if superimposed infection is suspected
4. Other laboratory tests and radiographs are needed only to detect and manage multisystem complications of any concomitant systemic hypothermia.

Key Tests

Serial radionuclide angiography and/or bone scanning for deep injuries

Differential Diagnosis

1. Frostnip: transient, localized, very superficial skin cooling without sequelae
2. Chilblain (pernio): nondestructive, cold-induced, chronic hypersensitivity (vasculitic) skin reaction causing itching, burning, violaceous discoloration, mild edema
3. Immersion foot (trench foot): nonfreezing pedal tissue injury caused by prolonged exposure to wet and cold conditions
4. Systemic hypothermia: cold-induced decrease from average homeothermic core body temperature (37° C) to less than 35° C because of environmental exposure or immersion

Treatment

1. Protect involved part from mechanical trauma; no rubbing or massaging.
2. Avoid rewarming if there is *any* risk of refreezing, even if this means walking on frozen feet.
3. Admit to the hospital all patients except those with the most superficial and localized injuries.
4. Initiate treatment for any associated systemic hypothermia.
5. Begin rapid but controlled rewarming by immersing the frozen body part in circulating warm water bath heated precisely to 40° to 42° C (*not any warmer*). A flushed appearance of the involved part, usually occurring after 20 to 30 minutes, signals reperfusion and the need to cease rewarming.
6. Early (within 36 to 72 hours) regional sympathectomy is controversial.
7. Subsequent supportive measures include protection of the limb from infection and trauma, twice-daily hydrotherapy in a warm (37° to 40° C) water/disinfectant (hexachlorophene) bath for 30 to 60 minutes, nicotine avoidance, limb elevation, and use of sterile dressings.

Medication

1. Narcotics are given as needed for pain, especially during rewarming.
2. Unless contraindicated, give ibuprofen (minimum of 12 mg/kg orally per day) for 1 week to combat prostaglandin-mediated ischemia and inflammation.
3. Tetanus prophylaxis as indicated
4. Prophylactic antibiotics are controversial. In one nonrandomized trial using 500,000 units of penicillin every 6 hours intramuscularly, treated patients had less tissue loss and a lower amputation rate. Subsequent antibiotics are based on culture results.
5. Débride blisters and cover with aloe vera gel (a potent antiprostaglandin agent) every 6 hours.
6. Thrombolytic therapy is experimental. A very small recent trial using recombinant tissue plasminogen activator infused directly into the involved limb showed promising results.
7. Possibly helpful, but unproven, adjuvant medications include nifedipine, pentoxifylline, superoxide dismutase, prostaglandin E analogs, and hyperbaric oxygen. Anticoagulants and corticosteroids have no usefulness.

Diet

As tolerated

Activity

1. Protect injured body part.
2. Initiate physical therapy once edema significantly lessens.

Patient Education

1. Regarding risk factors for frostbite and early signs and symptoms
2. Establishment of buddy system during wilderness exploration
3. Concerning possible sequelae
   a. Hypersensitivity with painful dysesthesias, especially on re-exposure to cold
   b. Hyperhidrosis
   c. Skin discoloration

d. Joint pain

e. Growth plate abnormalities in children

f. Vasomotor instability

g. Muscle atrophy

h. Gangrene and tissue loss

Key Treatment

- Do not rewarm if there is *any* risk of refreezing.

- Admit almost all patients to the hospital.

- Rapid controlled rewarming in warm water bath (40° to 42° C) for 20 minutes.

- Subsequent elevation, protection, daily hydrotherapy, surveillance for infection.

Follow-Up

1. Escharotomy may be necessary if impaired circulation or movement. Fasciotomy occasionally needed to alleviate a compartment syndrome resulting from extensive tissue edema.

2. Because early prediction of the extent of nonviable tissue is difficult in frostbite, amputation should not be considered until it is definitively established that tissues are dead. Aphorisms such as "frostbite in January, amputate in July" illustrate this principle. Autoamputation of digits involved in deep frostbite may avoid surgical intervention and help limit the amount of tissue that would have been removed.

3. Only indication for early débridement is uncontrolled infection. Otherwise, delay débridement for 1 to 3 months until the level of gangrene is demarcated.

4. Researchers are exploring the use of serial radionuclide scintigraphy and MR imaging to allow earlier assessment of ultimate tissue viability and the need for débridement/amputation.

Bibliography

Britt DL, Dascombe WH, Radriguez A: New horizons in the management of hypothermia and frostbite injury. Surg Clin North Am 1991;71:345–370.

McAdams TR: Frostbite: a review and orthopedic perspective. Am J Orthop 1999;28:21–26.

McCauley RL, Smith DJ, Robson MC, et al: Frostbite and other cold-induced injuries. In Auerbach PS (ed): Wilderness Medicine, 3rd ed, pp 315–346. St. Louis, Mosby–Year Book, 1995.

Mills WJ Jr, O'Malley J, Kappes B: Cold and freezing: a historical chronology of laboratory investigation and clinical experience. Alaska Med 1993;35:89–116.

Pulla RJ, Pickard LJ, Carnett TS: Frostbite: an overview with case presentations. J Foot Ankle Surg 1994;33:53–63.

Reamy BV: Frostbite: review and current concepts. J Am Board Fam Pract 1998;11:34–40.

359 Altitude Sickness

Paul J. Hughes

Etiology

1. Acute exposure to altitudes above 8000 feet (2438 m) can result in a constellation of symptoms referred to as altitude sickness (AS). Although these symptoms may be similar to many other illnesses, a history of high-altitude exposure separates this entity from other items in the differential diagnosis. Entities included in AS are acute mountain sickness (AMS), high-altitude cerebral edema (HACE), and high-altitude pulmonary edema (HAPE).

2. The principal physiologic insult from high-altitude exposure is hypoxia. The partial pressure of oxygen decreases with increasing altitude. The primary response to hypoxia is an increase in minute ventilation. This increase in ventilatory rate causes a drop in the partial pressure of carbon dioxide in the alveoli, resulting in a respiratory alkalosis.

3. Other physiologic responses to high-altitude exposure include a decrease in plasma volume, an increase in erythropoietin, and a bicarbonate diuresis. There is also an increase in sympathetic activity, causing an increased heart rate, pulmonary vasoconstriction, and increased cerebral blood flow.

4. Physical conditioning does not appear to affect the occurrence of AMS. The limiting factor in exercise at altitude is lung function.

Signs and Symptoms

1. Acute mountain sickness
   a. History of rapid ascent to an altitude greater than 8000 feet
   b. Shortness of breath
   c. Headache
   d. Anorexia
   e. Dizziness
   f. Nausea
   g. Insomnia, disturbed sleep
   h. Lassitude, difficulty concentrating
2. High-altitude pulmonary edema
   a. Most often occurs on the second night at altitude
   b. Early signs and symptoms
      (1) Dyspnea
      (2) Dry cough
      (3) Decreased exercise tolerance
      (4) Confusion
   c. Late signs and symptoms
      (1) Dyspnea at rest
      (2) Cyanosis
      (3) Rales
      (4) Pink frothy sputum
      (5) Tachycardia
      (6) Tachypnea
3. High-altitude cerebral edema
   a. Uncommon below 12,000 feet
   b. Early signs and symptoms essentially the same as AMS
   c. Late signs and symptoms
      (1) Increasing confusion
      (2) Ataxia
      (3) Seizures

Key Symptoms	
• Headache	• Nausea
• Insomnia	• Confusion
• Dyspnea	

Clinical Findings

1. Early in the development of AMS, HAPE, and HACE, the findings are nonspecific and therefore not diagnostic. In advanced HACE and HAPE, signs and symptoms of central nervous system involvement and pulmonary congestion manifest themselves.

2. The emergence of symptoms in the proper setting and a high index of suspicion are the most important diagnostic factors.

Laboratory Tests

1. There are no useful laboratory studies for the evaluation of AMS, HAPE, or HACE. Therefore, diagnostic information comes from the history and physical examination, which dem-

onstrate signs and symptoms of AS in the appropriate clinical setting.

2. In HAPE the chest radiograph may show pulmonary congestion and/or patchy, fluffy infiltrates. However, patients with no symptoms may have a similar radiographic picture.

Treatment

1. At altitude
   a. Early recognition is paramount.
   b. The primary therapy for all the forms of altitude sickness is to "GO DOWN."
   c. A descent of at least 2000 feet, preferably to an altitude of less than 10,000 feet, is imperative. Descend early while the patient is able to assist in the descent.
   d. Supplemental oxygen is useful in relieving hypoxia-related symptoms. This is especially helpful with sleep-aggravated hypoxia. Oxygen bottles are cumbersome, however, and therefore, are not usually carried on many treks.
   e. A Gamow Bag can be used to temporarily increase the ambient pressure. This portable hyperbaric chamber can simulate descent and, together with supplemental oxygen, is useful in buying time until a descent is possible.
   f. Nifedipine (Procardia, Adalat) may be effective in HAPE. It reduces pulmonary artery pressure and improves oxygenation. It is dosed 10 mg sublingually (open or pierced capsule) and 20 mg q6–8h, until a descent is possible.
   g. Dexamethasone, 4 mg q6h for two doses, given at altitude may reduce the symptoms in HACE. This should be followed by an immediate descent.

2. In hospital
   a. Primary hospital care consists of high-flow, continuous oxygen and bed rest.
   b. Diuretics are not indicated.
   c. Assisted ventilation is not indicated and in some cases may slow improvement.
   d. A decrease in tachycardia, tachypnea, and dyspnea, and an improvement in mental status are indications of resolution.

Key Treatment

- Descent
- Supplemental oxygen

Prevention

1. Fitness: Good physical conditioning improves exercise tolerance, although this may not prevent altitude-related illness. An improved hemodynamic response to exercise may be of some benefit in preventing HAPE and HACE.
2. Good health: Poorly controlled hypertension, diabetes, or other chronic diseases may have a negative effect.
3. Control the rate of ascent.
4. Begin below 8000 feet. Travel by automobile rather than air, if possible. This provides time to acclimate.
5. Rest the first day.
6. Ascend about 1000 feet per day. If symptoms start, descend.
7. Climb high, sleep low.
8. Avoid alcohol.
9. Keep well hydrated.
10. Acetazolamide (Diamox), 125 to 1250 mg/day starting 12 to 24 hours before arrival and continuing for 3 to 4 days, can significantly reduce the severity of AMS symptoms. This drug should not be used in patients with allergies to sulfa.
11. Dexamethasone, 4 mg bid starting with the first day of ascent and continuing for a few days. Because of its side-effect profile, dexamethasone should be reserved for those patients who are unable to tolerate acetazolamide.

Bibliography

Curtis R: Outdoor Action Guide to High Altitude: Acclimatization and Illnesses. *www.princeton.edu/~oa/altitude.html*, downloaded April 1998.

Dietz TE: Altitude Illness Clinical Guide for Physicians. *www.gorge.net/hamg/AMS-medical.html*, January 1998, downloaded April 1998.

McMurray SJ: High altitude medicine for family physicians. Can Fam Physician 1994;40:711–718.

Sutton JR: Mountain sickness. Neurol Clin 1992;10: 1015–1030.

Tom PA, Garmel GM, Auerbach PS, et al: Environment dependant sports emergencies. Med Clin North Am 1994;78:305–325.

360 Aquatic Injuries

Bruce Flareau

Jellyfish Stings

Etiology

The tentacles of the jellyfish contain thousands of venom-containing stinging cells known as nematocysts. These remain active for several days after the creature's death such that injuries may result from brushing against live or dead tentacle fragments.

Symptoms

Abrupt development of painful erythematous eruptions in linear welts or patches.

Differential Diagnosis

1. Cousins of the jellyfish, the Portuguese man-of-war and the blue bottle, are found off the coasts of Florida and Hawaii, respectively. Symptoms are similar to those produced by jellyfish, but more severe, with fever, wheezing, vomiting, or even paralysis. These lesions may require steroids and supportive care.
2. Sea anemones also possess nematocysts that may cause mild stings if brushed against.

Treatment

1. Immediate application of vinegar to deactivate any remaining undischarged nematocysts.
2. After 3 to 5 minutes, the tentacles may be scraped off.
3. Jellyfish stings should not be rinsed in fresh water because this may cause the nematocyst to discharge.
4. In the Chesapeake Bay area, the most common jellyfish is the sea nettle, which has unique vinegar-resistant nematocysts. In these waters, a paste of saltwater and baking soda should be applied.
5. Cold packs may ease skin pain.
6. Topical steroids may help mild itching.
7. Systemic steroids should be used for severe cases of delayed hypersensitivity.

Stingray Lacerations

Etiology

Stingrays are usually found burrowed in the sand in shallow water and will hurl their barbed "tail" upward in a defensive response to being stepped on or disturbed. The resulting wound may be both a laceration and a venomous puncture.

Symptoms

1. The victim usually presents with disproportionally painful lesions.
2. The sharp, shooting pain of a stingray laceration usually peaks in a few hours and, if untreated, resolves within a few days.
3. These lesions may cause nausea, weakness, and even respiratory distress.

Tests

Marine puncture wounds should be routinely radiographed for retained fragments.

Differential Diagnosis

Like the stingray, bony fish (i.e., lion, weaver, scorpion, cat, and stone fish) can inject venom using their spines. The toxin remains potent for 24 to 48 hours such that one can sustain injuries after the death of the animal, even with refrigeration.

Treatment

1. Stingray and bony fish lesions should be soaked in water as hot as can be tolerated (115° to 120° F) for 60 to 90 minutes in order to inactivate the heat-labile toxins. The wound should be thoroughly cleansed and débrided. Retained fragments should be removed when possible, and surgical removal may be necessary.
2. As with any puncture wound, tetanus prophylaxis is recommended. Antibiotics are optional depending on the physician's level of suspicion for infection (see "Marine Infections" below).

Marine Infections (Cutaneous)

Etiology

1. Streptococci and staphylococci are the common infecting organisms.
2. Of concern, however, are the marine-specific bacteria such as *Erysipelothrix, Mycobacterium marinum, Pseudomonas* species, and the halophilic (salt-loving) *Vibrio* species. Of these, *Vibrio* appears to be the most prevalent.

Symptoms

Patients typically complain of pain, swelling, tenderness, or loss of function.

Clinical Findings

Patients may present with nonhealing abrasions, granulomas, painful red swollen lesions of acute cellulitis, or a more maculopapular, nonvesiculating infection of the hands.

Laboratory Tests

Wound cultures may be performed with attention to halophilic bacteria and atypical *Mycobacterium* culture media.

Differential Diagnosis

1. Fish handlers' disease is caused by infection with *Erysipelothrix* bacteria. It is a rash-like infection of the palmar surfaces of the hands most commonly seen in those who handle or prepare fish.
2. Wound granulomas may be caused by infection with *M. marinum*; however, coral cuts and other retained foreign matter such as sea urchin spines or sponge spicules may present as granulomas. Empiric antibiotic therapy, cultures, and occasionally wound biopsies may be necessary to arrive at a diagnosis.

Treatment

1. Cleanse the wound to remove foreign debris and reduce the possibility of granuloma formation.
2. Tetanus prophylaxis should be administered as with any tetanus-prone wound.
3. Antibiotic selection
   a. Resistant to penicillins and cephalosporins, the *Vibrio* species require quinolones, sulfa agents, or tetracycline for adequate treatment. Because of photosensitivity, the tetracyclines are poorly tolerated in the Sunbelt; for this reason, the quinolones (Cipro or Floxin) or trimethoprim-sulfamethoxazole (Bactrim or Septra) are often the selected agents. Any marine infection not responding to a penicillin derivative should be given a trial with one of these agents. Remember that quinolone antibiotics are poor coverage for streptococcal infections and thus may not be the best first-line treatment.
   b. Fish handlers' disease should be treated with penicillin, erythromycin, or a cephalosporin, or based on culture sensitivity results.
   c. *Mycobacterium marinum* infection is a difficult infection to eradicate and may require surgical excision for definitive therapy. Antibiotic selection may include minocycline, trimethoprim-sulfamethoxazole, or rifampin plus ethambutol.

Marine Ingestions

Etiology

Ingestion of marine life may result in a variety of food poisonings. Causes range from endogenous poisons within the fish itself to animal-ingested toxins and bacterial decomposition. Focus is on the latter two in this discussion of scombroid and ciguatera poisoning.

Scombroid

Scombroid poisoning is the result of decaying fish being ingested. The amino acid histidine is converted to histamine by bacteria, and the individual has a massive histamine exposure that presents much like anaphylaxis.

Symptoms

Flushing, headaches, dizziness, nausea, diarrhea, and vomiting may begin within minutes to hours of the ingestion.

Clinical Findings

May include bronchospasm, respiratory distress, palpitations, supraventricular tachycardia, and mild hypotension.

Laboratory Tests

None commercially available

Differential Diagnosis

Any disorder presenting with gastrointestinal symptoms, including gastroenteritis, hepatitis

Treatment

Cardiovascular support and antihistamine (H_1 and H_2) therapy. Symptoms usually resolve within 12 to 24 hours.

Ciguatera

Ciguatera is acquired by ingesting fish that themselves have ingested the offending dinoflagellate. Thought to be a type of reef flora, it concentrates up the food chain until a critical mass is ingested by the patient. The majority of implicated fish are grouper, snapper, jack, and barracuda, although almost any fish can be involved. The offending agent, known as ciguatoxin, is tasteless and unaffected by refrigeration or cooking.

Symptoms

1. Within 6 hours of ingestion the victim may experience gastrointestinal and neurologic symptoms.
2. Initially, gastrointestinal symptoms predominate with abdominal cramps, nausea, vomiting, and diarrhea. These usually resolve within 24 to 48 hours and may be followed by neurologic symptoms on the third to fifth day.
3. The hallmark of this illness is the reversal of hot-cold sensation, which may last for months.
4. Severe cases may be complicated by bradycardia, shock, respiratory failure and rarely death.

Treatment

Treatment is supportive but may involve diphenhydramine for concomitant pruritus and mannitol for neurologic symptoms. Mannitol doses of up to 1 gm/kg at a rate of 500 mg/hour have been used with success in small studies. Fortunately, the disease is usually self-limited, and treatment other than prevention unnecessary.

Prevention

Recurrent episodes tend to have increased severity, and thus victims should eliminate fish and fish derivatives from their diet. Other foods such as nuts and alcohol may precipitate recurrence and should be avoided for at least 6 months.

Bibliography

For more information on jellyfish stings, see
Fenner PJ, Williamson JA: Worldwide deaths and severe envenomation from jellyfish stings. Med J Aust 1996; 165:658–661.

For more information on marine infections, see
Czachor JS: Unusual aspects of bacterial water-borne illnesses. Am Fam Physician, 1992;46:797–804.

For more information on ciguatera toxicity, see
Levine DZ: Ciguatera: current concepts. 1995;95:193–198.

For more information on marine injuries, see
Flareau B: Hazardous marine animals. In Rakel RE (ed): Conn's Current Therapy, pp 1082–1086. Philadelphia, WB Saunders Company, 1995.
Frey C: Marine injuries—prevention and treatment. Orthop Rev 1994;23:645–649.
Schwartz S, Meinking T: Venomous marine animals of Florida: morphology, behavior, health hazards. J Florida Med Assoc 1997;84:433–440.

Reference Intervals for the Interpretation of Laboratory Tests

William Z. Borer

Most of the tests performed in a clinical laboratory are quantitative in nature. That is, the amount of a substance present in blood or serum is measured and reported in terms of concentration, activity (e.g., enzyme activity), or counts (e.g., blood cell counts). The laboratory must provide reference intervals to assist the clinician in the interpretation of laboratory results. These reference intervals comprise the physiologic quantities of substance (concentrations, activities, or counts) to be expected in healthy individuals. Deviation above or below the reference range may be associated with a disease process, and the severity of the disease process may be associated with the magnitude of the deviation. Unfortunately a sharp demarcation rarely exists to distinguish between physiologic and pathologic values, and the time of transition between the two is often gradual as the disease process progresses.

The terms *normal* and *abnormal* have been used to describe the laboratory values that fall inside or outside of the reference range, respectively. Use of these terms is inappropriate, because no good definition of normality exists in the clinical sense and because the term *normal* may be confused with the statistical term *Gaussian*. Reference ranges are established from statistical studies in groups of healthy volunteers. These study subjects must be free of disease, but they may have lifestyles or habits that result in variations in their laboratory values. Examples of these variables include diet, body mass, exercise, and geographic location. Age and gender may also affect reference values.

When the data from a large cohort of healthy subjects fits a Gaussian distribution, the usual statistical approach is to define the reference limits as two standard deviations above and below the mean. By definition, the reference range excludes the 2.5 per cent of the population with the lowest values and the 2.5 per cent with the highest values. Non-Gaussian distributions are handled by different statistical methods, but the result is similar in that the reference range is defined by the central 95 per cent of the population. In other words, the probability is 1 in 20 that a healthy individual will have a laboratory result that falls outside the reference range. If 12 laboratory tests are performed, the probability increases to about 50 per cent that at least one of the results will be outside the reference range. This means that all healthy individuals are likely to have a few laboratory results that are unexpected. The clinician must then integrate these data with other clinical information such as the history and physical examination to arrive at an appropriate clinical decision. The reference intervals for many tests (especially enzyme and immunochemical measurements) varies with the method used. Accordingly each laboratory must establish reference intervals that are appropriate for the methods used.

SI Units

During the 1980s a concerted effort was made to introduce SI units (le Système International d'Unités). The rationale for conversion to SI units is sound. Laboratory data are scientifically more informative when the units are based on molar concentration rather than mass concentration. For example, the conversion of glucose to lactate and pyruvate or the binding of a drug to albumin is more easily understood in units of molar concentration. Another example is illustrated as follows:

Conventional Units

1.0 gm of hemoglobin
  —Combines with 1.37 ml of oxygen
  —Contains 3.4 mg of iron
  —Forms 34.9 mg of bilirubin

SI Units

4.0 mmol of hemoglobin
  —Combines with 4.0 mmol of oxygen
  —Contains 4.0 mmol of iron
  —Forms 4.0 mmol of bilirubin

The use of SI units would also enhance the standardization of nomenclature to facilitate global communication of medical and scientific information. The units, symbols, and prefixes employed in the International System are shown in Tables 1, 2, and 3.

Unfortunately, problems have arisen with the im-

TABLE 1. BASE SI UNITS

PROPERTY	BASE UNIT	SYMBOL
Length	meter	m
Mass	kilogram	kg
Amount of substance	mole	mol
Time	second	S
Thermodynamic temperature	kelvin	K
Electric current	ampere	A
Luminous intensity	candela	cd
Catalytic amount	katal	kat

TABLE 2. DERIVED SI UNITS AND NON-SI UNITS RETAINED FOR USE WITH THE SI

PROPERTY	UNIT	SYMBOL
Area	square meter	m^2
Volume	cubic meter	m^3
	liter	L
Mass concentration	kilogram/cubic meter	kg/m^3
	gram/liter	g/L
Substance concentration	mole/cubic meter	mol/m^3
	mole/liter	mol/L
Temperature	degree Celsius	C (=K − 273.15)

TABLE 3. STANDARD PREFIXES

PREFIX	MULTIPLICATION FACTOR	SYMBOL
yocto	10^{-24}	y
zepto	10^{-21}	z
atto	10^{-18}	a
femto	10^{-15}	f
pico	10^{-12}	p
nano	10^{-9}	n
micro	10^{-6}	u
milli	10^{-3}	m
centi	10^{-2}	c
deci	10^{-1}	d
deca	10^{1}	da
hecto	10^{2}	h
kilo	10^{3}	k
mega	10^{6}	M
giga	10^{9}	G
tera	10^{12}	T

plementation of SI units in the United States. Their introduction in 1987 prompted many medical journals to report laboratory values in both SI and conventional units in anticipation of complete conversion to SI units in the early 1990s. The lack of a coordinated effort toward this goal has forced a retrenchment on the issue. Physicians continue to think and practice using laboratory results expressed in conventional units, and few if any American hospitals or clinical laboratories exclusively use SI units. Complete conversion to SI units is not likely to occur in the foreseeable future, yet most medical journals will probably continue to publish both sets of units. For this reason, the tables of reference ranges in this appendix (Tables 4 through 12) are given in both conventional units and SI units.

TABLE 4. REFERENCE INTERVALS FOR HEMATOLOGY

TEST	CONVENTIONAL UNITS	SI UNITS
Acid hemolysis (Ham test)	No hemolysis	No hemolysis
Alkaline phosphatase, leukocyte	Total score 14–100	Total score 14–100
Cell counts		
Erythrocytes		
Males	4.6–6.2 million/mm^3	4.6–6.2 × 10^{12}/L
Females	4.2–5.4 million/mm^3	4.2–5.4 × 10^{12}/L
Children (varies with age)	4.5–5.1 million/mm^3	4.5–5.1 × 10^{12}/L
Leukocytes, total	4500–11,000/mm^3	4.5–11.0 × 10^9/L
Leukocytes, differential counts*		
Myelocytes	0%	0/L
Band neutrophils	3–5%	150–400 × 10^6/L
Segmented neutrophils	54–62%	3000–5800 × 10^6/L
Lymphocytes	25–33%	1500–3000 × 10^6/L
Monocytes	3–7%	300–500 × 10^6/L
Eosinophils	1–3%	50–250 × 10^6/L
Basophils	0–1%	15–50 × 10^6/L
Platelets	150,000–400,000/mm^3	150–400 × 10^9/L
Reticulocytes	25,000–75,000/mm^3 (0.5–1.5% of erythrocytes)	25–75 × 10^9/L
Coagulation tests		
Bleeding time (template)	2.75–8.0 min	2.75–8.0 min
Coagulation time (glass tube)	5–15 min	5–15 min
D-dimer	<0.5 μg/ml	<0.5 mg/L
Factor VIII and other coagulation factors	50–150% of normal	0.5–1.5 of normal
Fibrin split products (Thrombo-Welco test)	<10 μg/ml	<10 mg/L
Fibrinogen	200–400 mg/dl	2.0–4.0 g/L
Partial thromboplastin time (PTT)	20–35 s	20–35 s
Prothrombin time (PT)	12.0–14.0 s	12.0–14.0 s
Coombs' test		
Direct	Negative	Negative
Indirect	Negative	Negative
Corpuscular values of erythrocytes		
Mean corpuscular hemoglobin (MCH)	26–34 pg/cell	26–34 pg/cell
Mean corpuscular volume (MCV)	80–96 μm^3	80–96 fL
Mean corpuscular hemoglobin concentration (MCHC)	32–36 g/dl	320–360 g/L
Haptoglobin	20–165 mg/dl	0.20–1.65 g/L
Hematocrit		
Males	40–54 ml/dl	0.40–0.54
Females	37–47 ml/dl	0.37–0.47
Newborns	49–54 ml/dl	0.49–0.54
Children (varies with age)	35–49 ml/dl	0.35–0.49
Hemoglobin		
Males	13.0–18.0 g/dl	8.1–11.2 mmol/L
Females	12.0–16.0 g/dl	7.4–9.9 mmol/L
Newborn	16.5–19.5 g/dl	10.2–12.1 mmol/L
Children (varies with age)	11.2–16.5 g/dl	7.0–10.2 mmol/L
Hemoglobin, fetal	<1.0% of total	<0.01 of total
Hemoglobin A$_{1C}$	3–5% of total	0.03–0.05 of total
Hemoglobin A$_2$	1.5–3.0% of total	0.015–0.03 of total
Hemoglobin, plasma	0.0–5.0 mg/dl	0.0–3.2 μmol/L
Methemoglobin	30–130 mg/dl	19–80 μmol/L
Sedimentation rate (ESR)		
Wintrobe		
Males	0–5 mm/hr	0–5 mm/hr
Females	0–15 mm/hr	0–15 mm/hr
Westergren		
Males	0–15 mm/hr	0–15 mm/hr
Females	0–20 mm/hr	0–20 mm/hr

*Conventional units are percentages; SI units are absolute cell counts.

TABLE 5. REFERENCE INTERVALS* FOR CLINICAL CHEMISTRY (BLOOD, SERUM, AND PLASMA)

ANALYTE	CONVENTIONAL UNITS	SI UNITS
Acetoacetate plus acetone		
Qualitative	Negative	Negative
Quantitative	0.3–2.0 mg/dl	30–200 μmol/L
Acid phosphatase, serum (thymolphthalein monophosphate substrate)	0.1–0.6 U/L	0.1–0.6 U/L
ACTH (see Corticotropin)		
Alanine aminotransferase (ALT, SGPT), serum	1–45 U/L	1–45 U/L
Albumin, serum	3.3–5.2 g/dl	33–52 g/L
Aldolase, serum	0.0–7.0 U/L	0.0–7.0 U/L
Aldosterone, plasma		
Standing	5–30 ng/dl	140–830 pmol/L
Recumbent	3–10 ng/dl	80–275 pmol/L
Alkaline phosphatase (ALP), serum		
Adult	35–150 U/L	35–150 U/L
Adolescent	100–500 U/L	100–500 U/L
Child	100–350 U/L	100–350 U/L
Ammonia nitrogen, plasma	10–50 μmol/L	10–50 μmol/L
Amylase, serum	25–125 U/L	25–125 U/L
Anion gap, serum, calculated	8–16 mEq/L	8–16 mmol/L
Ascorbic acid, blood	0.4–1.5 mg/dl	23–85 μmol/L
Aspartate aminotransferase (AST, SGOT), serum	1–36 U/L	1–36 U/L
Base excess, arterial blood, calculated	0 ± 2 mEq/L	0 ± 2 mmol/L
Bicarbonate		
Venous plasma	23–29 mEq/L	23–29 mmol/L
Arterial blood	21–27 mEq/L	21–27 mmol/L
Bile acids, serum	0.3–3.0 mg/dl	0.8–7.6 μmol/L
Bilirubin, serum		
Conjugated	0.1–0.4 mg/dl	1.7–6.8 μmol/L
Total	0.3–1.1 mg/dl	5.1–19.0 μmol/L
Calcium, serum	8.4–10.6 mg/dl	2.10–2.65 mmol/L
Calcium, ionized, serum	4.25–5.25 mg/dl	1.05–1.30 mmol/L
Carbon dioxide, total, serum or plasma	24–31 mEq/L	24–31 mmol/L
Carbon dioxide tension (pCO$_2$), blood	35–45 mm Hg	35–45 mm Hg
β-Carotene, serum	60–260 μg/dl	1.1–8.6 μmol/L
Ceruloplasmin, serum	23–44 mg/dl	230–440 mg/L
Chloride, serum or plasma	96–106 mEq/L	96–106 mmol/L
Cholesterol, serum or EDTA plasma		
Desirable range	<200 mg/dl	<5.20 mmol/L
LDL cholesterol	60–180 mg/dl	1.55–4.65 mmol/L
HDL cholesterol	30–80 mg/dl	0.80–2.05 mmol/L
Copper	70–140 μg/dl	11–22 μmol/L
Corticotropin (ACTH), plasma, 8 AM	10–80 pg/ml	2–18 pmol/L
Cortisol, plasma		
8:00 AM	6–23 μg/dl	170–630 nmol/L
4:00 PM	3–15 μg/dl	80–410 nmol/L
10:00 PM	<50% of 8:00 AM value	<50% of 8:00 AM value
Creatine, serum		
Males	0.2–0.5 mg/dl	15–40 μmol/L
Females	0.3–0.9 mg/dl	25–70 μmol/L
Creatine kinase (CK), serum		
Males	55–170 U/L	55–170 U/L
Females	30–135 U/L	30–135 U/L
Creatine kinase MB isoenzyme, serum	<5% of total CK activity	<5% of total CK activity
	<5% ng/ml by immunoassay	<5% ng/ml by immunoassay
Creatinine, serum	0.6–1.2 mg/dl	50–110 μmol/L
Estradiol-17β, adult		
Males	10–65 pg/ml	35–240 pmol/L
Females		
Follicular	30–100 pg/ml	110–370 pmol/L
Ovulatory	200–400 pg/ml	730–1470 pmol/L
Luteal	50–140 pg/ml	180–510 pmol/L
Ferritin, serum	20–200 ng/ml	20–200 μg/L
Fibrinogen, plasma	200–400 mg/dl	2.0–4.0 g/L
Folate		
Serum	3–18 ng/ml	6.8–41 nmol/L
Erythrocytes	145–540 ng/ml	330–1220 nmol/L
Follicle-stimulating hormone (FSH), plasma		
Males	4–25 mU/ml	4–25 U/L
Females, premenopausal	4–30 mU/ml	4–30 U/L
Females, postmenopausal	40–250 mU/ml	40–250 U/L
Gamma-glutamyltransferase (GGT), serum	5–40 U/L	5–40 U/L
Gastrin, fasting, serum	0–100 pg/ml	0–100 mg/L
Glucose, fasting, plasma or serum	70–115 mg/dl	3.9–6.4 nmol/L
Growth hormone (hGH), plasma, adult, fasting	0–6 ng/ml	0–6 μg/L

Table continued on following page

TABLE 5. REFERENCE INTERVALS* FOR CLINICAL CHEMISTRY (BLOOD, SERUM, AND PLASMA) (*Continued*)

ANALYTE	CONVENTIONAL UNITS	SI UNITS
Haptoglobin, serum	20–165 mg/dl	0.20–1.65 g/L
Immunoglobulins, serum (see Table 11)		
Iron, serum	75–175 µg/dl	13–31 µmol/L
Iron-binding capacity, serum		
Total	250–410 µg/dl	45–73 µmol/L
Saturation	20–55%	0.20–0.55
Lactate		
Venous whole blood	5.0–20.0 mg/dl	0.6–2.2 mmol/L
Arterial whole blood	5.0–15.0 mg/dl	0.6–1.7 mmol/L
Lactate dehydrogenase (LD), serum	110–220 U/L	110–220 U/L
Lipase, serum	10–140 U/L	10–140 U/L
Lutropin (LH), serum		
Males	1–9 U/L	1–9 U/L
Females		
Follicular phase	2–10 U/L	2–10 U/L
Midcycle peak	15–65 U/L	15–65 U/L
Luteal phase	1–12 U/L	1–12 U/L
Postmenopausal	12–65 U/L	12–65 U/L
Magnesium, serum	1.3–2.1 mg/dl	0.65–1.05 mmol/L
Osmolality	275–295 mOsm/kg water	275–295 mOsm/kg water
Oxygen, blood, arterial, room air		
Partial pressure (p_aO_2)	80–100 mm Hg	80–100 mm Hg
Saturation (S_aO_2)	95–98%	95–98%
pH, arterial blood	7.35–7.45	7.35–7.45
Phosphate, inorganic, serum		
Adult	3.0–4.5 mg/dl	1.0–1.5 mmol/L
Child	4.0–7.0 mg/dl	1.3–2.3 mmol/L
Potassium		
Serum	3.5–5.0 mEq/L	3.5–5.0 mmol/L
Plasma	3.5–4.5 mEq/L	3.5–4.5 mmol/L
Progesterone, serum, adult		
Males	0.0–0.4 ng/ml	0.0–1.3 mmol/L
Females		
Follicular phase	0.1–1.5 ng/ml	0.3–4.8 mmol/L
Luteal phase	2.5–28.0 ng/ml	8.0–89.0 mmol/L
Prolactin, serum		
Males	1.0–15.0 ng/ml	1.0–15.0 µg/L
Females	1.0–20.0 ng/ml	1.0–20.0 µg/L
Protein, serum, electrophoresis		
Total	6.0–8.0 g/dl	60–80 g/L
Albumin	3.5–5.5 g/dl	35–55 g/L
Globulins		
$Alpha_1$	0.2–0.4 g/dl	2.0–4.0 g/L
$Alpha_2$	0.5–0.9 g/dl	5.0–9.0 g/L
Beta	0.6–1.1 g/dl	6.0–11.0 g/L
Gamma	0.7–1.7 g/dl	7.0–17.0 g/L
Pyruvate, blood	0.3–0.9 mg/dl	0.03–0.10 mmol/L
Rheumatoid factor	0.0–30.0 IU/ml	0.0–30.0 kIU/L
Sodium, serum or plasma	135–145 mEq/L	135–145 mmol/L
Testosterone, plasma		
Males, adult	300–1200 ng/dl	10.4–41.6 nmol/L
Females, adult	20–75 ng/dl	0.7–2.6 nmol/L
Pregnant females	40–200 ng/dl	1.4–6.9 nmol/L
Thyroglobulin	3–42 ng/ml	3–42 µg/L
Thyrotropin (hTSH), serum	0.4–4.8 µIU/ml	0.4–4.8 mIU/L
Thyrotropin-releasing hormone (TRH)	5–60 pg/ml	5–60 ng/L
Thyroxine, free (FT_4), serum	0.9–2.1 ng/dl	12–27 pmol/L
Thyroxine (T_4), serum	4.5–12.0 µg/dl	58–154 nmol/L
Thyroxine-binding globulinn (TBG)	15.0–34.0 µg/ml	15.0–34.0 mg/L
Transferrin	250–430 mg/dl	2.5–4.3 g/L
Triglycerides, serum, after 12-hr fast	40–150 mg/dl	0.4–1.5 g/L
Triiodothyronine (T_3), serum	70–190 ng/dl	1.1–2.9 nmol/L
Triiodothyronine uptake, resin (T_3RU)	25–38%	0.25–0.38
Urate		
Males	2.5–8.0 mg/dl	150–480 µmol/L
Females	2.2–7.0 mg/dl	130–420 µmol/L
Urea, serum or plasma	24–49 mg/dl	4.0–8.2 nmol/L
Urea nitrogen, serum or plasma	11–23 mg/dl	8.0–16.4 nmol/L
Viscosity, serum	1.4–1.8 × water	1.4–1.8 × water
Vitamin A, serum	20–80 µg/dl	0.70–2.80 µmol/L
Vitamin B_{12}, serum	180–900 pg/ml	133–664 pmol/L

*Reference values may vary depending upon the method and sample source used.

TABLE 6. REFERENCE INTERVALS FOR THERAPEUTIC DRUG MONITORING (SERUM)

ANALYTE	THERAPEUTIC RANGE	TOXIC CONCENTRATIONS	PROPRIETARY NAMES
Analgesics			
Acetaminophen	10–20 μg/ml	>250 μg/ml	Tylenol, Datril
Salicylate	100–250 μg/ml	>300 μg/ml	Aspirin, Bufferin
Antibiotics			
Amikacin	25–30 μg/ml	Peak >35 μg/ml	Amikin
		Trough >10 μg/ml	
Gentamicin	5–10 μg/ml	Peak >10 μg/ml	Garamycin
		Trough >2 μg/ml	
Tobramycin	5–10 μg/ml	Peak >10 μg/ml	Nebcin
		Trough >2 μg/ml	
Vancomycin	5–35 μg/ml	Peak >40 μg/ml	Vancocin
		Trough >10 μg/ml	
Anticonvulsants			
Carbamazepine	5–12 μg/ml	>15 μg/ml	Tegretol
Ethosuxamide	40–100 μg/ml	>150 μg/ml	Zarontin
Phenobarbital	15–40 μg/ml	40–100 ng/ml (varies widely)	Luminal
Phenytoin	10–20 μg/ml	>20 μg/ml	Dilantin
Primidone	5–12 μg/ml	>15 μg/ml	Mysoline
Valproic acid	50–100 μg/ml	>100 μg/ml	Depakene
Antineoplastics and Immunosuppressives			
Cyclosporine	50–400 ng/ml	>400 ng/ml	Sandimmune
Methotrexate, high dose, 48 hr	Variable	>1 μmol/L 48 hr after dose	
Tacrolimus (FK-506), whole blood	3–10 μg/ml	>15 μg/ml	Prograf
Bronchodialators and Respiratory Stimulants			
Caffeine	3–15 ng/ml	>30 ng/ml	
Theophylline (aminophylline)	10–20 μg/ml	>20 μg/ml	Elixophyllin, Quibron
Cardiovascular Drugs			
Amiodarone*	1.0–2.0 μg/ml	>2.0 μg/ml	Cordarone
Digitoxin[†]	15–25 ng/ml	>35 ng/ml	Crystodigin
Digoxin[‡]	0.8–2.0 ng/ml	>2.4 ng/ml	Lanoxin
Disopyramide	2–5 μg/ml	>7 μg/ml	Norpace
Flecainide	0.2–1.0 ng/ml	>1 ng/ml	Tambocor
Lidocaine	1.5–5.0 μg/ml	>6 μg/ml	Xylocaine
Mexiletine	0.7–2.0 μg/ml	>2 μg/ml	Mexitil
Procainamide	4–10 μg/ml	>12 μg/ml	Pronestyl
Procainamide plus NAPA	8–30 μg/ml	>30 μg/ml	
Propranolol	50–100 ng/ml	Variable	Inderal
Quinidine	2–5 μg/ml	>6 μg/ml	Cardioquin, Quinaglute
Tocainide	4–10 ng/ml	>10 ng/ml	Tonocard
Psychopharmacologic Drugs			
Amitriptyline	120–150 ng/ml	>500 ng/ml	Elavil, Triavil
Bupropion	25–100 ng/ml	Not applicable	Wellbutrin
Desipramine	150–300 ng/ml	>500 ng/ml	Norpramin, Pertofrane
Imipramine	125–250 ng/ml	>400 ng/ml	Tofranil, Janimine
Lithium[§]	0.6–1.5 mEq/L	>1.5 mEq/L	Lithobid
Nortriptyline	50–150 ng/ml	>500 ng/ml	Aventyl, Pamelor

*Obtain specimen more than 8 hours after last dose.
[†]Obtain specimen 12 to 24 hours after last dose.
[‡]Obtain specimen more than 6 hours after last dose.
[§]Obtain specimen 12 hours after last dose.

TABLE 7. REFERENCE INTERVALS FOR CLINICAL CHEMISTRY (URINE)*

ANALYTE	CONVENTIONAL UNITS	SI UNITS
Acetone and acetoacetate, qualitative	Negative	Negative
Albumin		
Qualitative	Negative	Negative
Quantitative	10–100 mg/24 hr	0.15–1.5 μmol/day
Aldosterone	3–20 μg/24 hr	8.3–55 nmol/day
δ-Aminolevulinic acid (δ-ALA)	1.3–7.0 mg/24 hr	10–53 μmol/day
Amylase	<17 U/hr	<17 U/hr
Amylase/creatinine clearance ratio	0.01–0.04	0.01–0.04
Bilirubin, qualitative	Negative	Negative
Calcium (regular diet)	<250 mg/24 hr	<6.3 nmol/day
Catecholamines		
Epinephrine	<10 μg/24 hr	<55 nmol/day
Norepinephrine	<100 μg/24 hr	<590 nmol/day
Total free catecholamines	4–126 μg/24 hr	24–745 nmol/day
Total metanephrines	0.1–1.6 mg/24 hr	0.5–8.1 μmol/day
Chloride (varies with intake)	110–250 mEq/24 hr	110–250 mmol/day
Copper	0–50 μg/24 hr	0.0–0.80 μmol/day
Cortisol, free	10–100 μg/24 hr	27.6–276 nmol/day
Creatine		
Males	0–40 mg/24 hr	0.0–0.30 mmol/day
Females	0–80 mg/24 hr	0.0–0.60 mmol/day
Creatinine	15–25 mg/kg/24 hr	0.13–0.22 mmol/kg/day
Creatinine clearance (endogenous)		
Males	110–150 ml/min/1.73 m²	110–150 ml/min/1.73 m²
Females	105–132 ml/min/1.73 m²	105–132 ml/min/1.73 m²
Cystine (or cysteine)	Negative	Negative
Dehydroepiandrosterone		
Males	0.2–2.0 mg/24 hr	0.7–6.9 μmol/day
Females	0.2–1.8 mg/24 hr	0.7–6.2 μmol/day
Estrogens, total		
Males	4–25 μg/24 hr	14–90 nmol/day
Females	5–100 μg/24 hr	18–360 nmol/day
Glucose (as reducing substance)	<250 mg/24 hr	<250 mg/day
Hemoglobin and myoglobin, qualitative	Negative	Negative
Homogentisic acid, qualitative	Negative	Negative
17-Hydroxycorticosteroids		
Males	3–9 mg/24 hr	8.3–25 μmol/day
Females	2–8 mg/24 hr	5.5–22 μmol/day
5-Hydroxyindoleacetic acid		
Qualitative	Negative	Negative
Quantitative	2–6 mg/24 hr	10–31 μmol/day
17-Ketogenic steroids		
Males	5–23 mg/24 hr	17–80 μmol/day
Females	3–15 mg/24 hr	10–52 μmol/day
17-Ketosteroids		
Males	8–22 mg/24 hr	28–76 μmol/day
Females	6–15 mg/24 hr	21–52 μmol/day
Magnesium	6–10 mEq/24 hr	3–5 mmol/day
Metanephrines	0.05–1.2 ng/mg creatinine	0.03–0.70 mmol/mmol creatinine
Osmolality	38–1400 mOsm/kg water	38–1400 mOsm/kg water
pH	4.6–8.0	4.6–8.0
Phenylpyruvic acid, qualitative	Negative	Negative
Phosphate	0.4–1.3 g/24 hr	13–42 mmol/day
Porphobilinogen		
Qualitative	Negative	Negative
Quantitative	<2 mg/24 hr	<9 μmol/day
Porphyrins		
Coproporphyrin	50–250 μg/24 hr	77–380 nmol/day
Uroporphyrin	10–30 μg/24 hr	12–36 nmol/day
Potassium	25–125 mEq/24 hr	25–125 mmol/day
Pregnanediol		
Males	0.0–1.9 mg/24 hr	0.0–6.0 μmol/day
Females		
Proliferative phase	0.0–2.6 mg/24 hr	0.0–8.0 μmol/day
Luteal phase	2.6–10.6 mg/24 hr	8–33 μmol/day
Postmenopausal	0.2–1.0 mg/24 hr	0.6–3.1 μmol/day
Pregnanetriol	0.0–2.5 mg/24 hr	0.0–7.4 μmol/day
Protein, total		
Qualitative	Negative	Negative
Quantitative	10–150 mg/24 hr	10–150 mg/day
Protein/creatinine ratio	<0.2	<0.2
Sodium (regular diet)	60–260 mEq/24 hr	60–260 mmol/day
Specific gravity		
Random specimen	1.003–1.030	1.003–1.030
24-hour collection	1.015–1.025	1.015–1.025
Urate (regular diet)	250–750 mg/24 hr	1.5–4.4 mmol/day
Urobilinogen	0.5–4.0 mg/24 hr	0.6–6.8 μmol/day
Vanillylmandelic acid (VMA)	1.0–8.0 mg/24 hr	5–40 μmol/day

*Values may vary depending upon the method used.

TABLE 8.   REFERENCE INTERVALS FOR TOXIC SUBSTANCES

ANALYTE	CONVENTIONAL UNITS	SI UNITS
Arsenic, urine	<130 μg/24 hr	<1.7 μmol/day
Bromides, serum, inorganic	<100 mg/dl	<10 mmol/L
Toxic symptoms	140–1000 mg/dl	14–100 mmol/L
Carboxyhemoglobin, blood	*% Saturation*	*Saturation*
Urban environment	<5%	<0.05
Smokers	<12%	<0.12
Headache	>15%	>0.15
Nausea and vomiting	>25%	>0.25
Potentially lethal	>50%	>0.50
Ethanol, blood	<0.05 mg/dl <0.005%	<1.0 mmol/L
Intoxication	>100 mg/dl >0.1%	>22 mmol/L
Marked intoxication	300–400 mg/dl 0.3–0.4%	65–87 mmol/L
Alcoholic stupor	400–500 mg/dl 0.4–0.5%	87–109 mmol/L
Coma	>500 mg/dl >0.5%	>109 mmol/L
Lead, blood		
Adults	<25 μg/dl	<1.2 μmol/L
Children	<15 μg/dl	<0.7 μmol/L
Lead, urine	<80 μg/24 hr	<0.4 μmol/day
Mercury, urine	<30 μg/24 hr	<150 nmol/day

TABLE 9.   REFERENCE INTERVALS FOR TESTS PERFORMED ON CEREBROSPINAL FLUID (CSF)

TEST	CONVENTIONAL UNITS	SI UNITS
Cells	<5/mm^3; all mononuclear	<5 × 10^6/L, all mononuclear
Protein electrophoresis	Albumin predominant	Albumin predominant
Glucose	50–75 mg/dl (20 mg/dl less than in serum)	2.8–4.2 mmol/L (1.1 mmol less than in serum)
Immunoglobulin G (IgG)		
Children under 14	<8% of total protein	<0.08 of total protein
Adults	<14% of total protein	<0.14 of total protein
IgG index: $\left(\dfrac{\text{CSF/serum IgG ratio}}{\text{CSF/serum albumin ratio}}\right)$	0.3–0.6	0.3–0.6
Oligoclonal banding on electrophoresis	Absent	Absent
Pressure, opening	70–180 mm H$_2$O	70–180 mm H$_2$O
Protein, total	15–45 mg/dl	150–450 mg/L

TABLE 10. REFERENCE INTERVALS FOR TESTS OF GASTROINTESTINAL FUNCTION

TEST	CONVENTIONAL UNITS
Bentiromide	6-hour urinary arylamine excretion greater than 57%; excludes pancreatic insufficiency
β-Carotene, serum	60–250 ng/dl
Fecal fat estimation	
Qualitative	No fat globules seen by high-power microscope
Quantitative	<6 g/24 hr (>95% coefficient of fat absorption)
Gastric acid output	
Basal	
Males	0.0–10.5 mmol/hr
Females	0.0–5.6 mmol/hr
Maximum (after histamine or pentagastrin)	
Males	9.0–48.0 mmol/hr
Females	6.0–31.0 mmol/hr
Ratio: basal/maximum	
Males	0.0–0.31
Females	0.0–0.29
Secretin test, pancreatic fluid	
Volume	>1.8 ml/kg/hr
Bicarbonate	>80 mEq/L
D-Xylose absorption test, urine	>20% of ingested dose excreted in 5 hours

TABLE 11. REFERENCE INTERVALS FOR TESTS OF IMMUNOLOGIC FUNCTION

TEST	CONVENTIONAL UNITS	SI UNITS
Complement, serum		
C3	85–175 mg/dl	0.85–1.75 g/L
C4	15–45 mg/dl	150–450 mg/L
Total hemolytic (CH$_{50}$)	150–250 U/ml	150–250 U/ml
Immunoglobulins, serum, adult		
IgG	640–1350 mg/dl	6.4–13.5 g/L
IgA	70–310 mg/dl	0.70–3.1 g/L
IgM	90–350 mg/dl	0.90–3.5 g/L
IgD	0.0–6.0 mg/dl	0.0–60 mg/L
IgE	0.0–430 ng/dl	0.0–430 μg/L

Lymphocyte subsets, whole blood, heparinized

ANTIGEN	CELL TYPE	PERCENTAGE	ABSOLUTE CELL COUNT
CD3	Total T cells	56–77	860–1880
CD19	Total B cells	7–17	140–370
CD3 and CD4	Helper-inducer cells	32–54	550–1190
CD3 and CD8	Suppressor-cytotoxic cells	24–37	430–1060
CD3 and DR	Activated T cells	5–14	70–310
CD2	E rosette T cells	73–87	1040–2160
CD16 and CD56	Natural killer (NK) cells	8–22	130–500

Helper/suppressor ratio: 0.8–1.8

TABLE 12. REFERENCE INTERVALS FOR SEMEN ANALYSIS

TEST	CONVENTIONAL UNITS	SI UNITS
Volume	2–5 ml	2–5 mL
Liquefaction	Complete in 15 min	Complete in 15 min
pH	7.2–8.0	7.2–8.0
Leukocytes	Occasional or absent	Occasional or absent
Spermatozoa		
Count	$60–150 \times 10^6$/ml	$60–150 \times 10^6$/ml
Motility	>80% motile	>0.80 motile
Morphology	80–90% normal forms	>0.80–0.90 normal forms
Fructose	>150 mg/dl	>8.33 mmol/L

Bibliography

American Medical Association: Drug Evaluations Annual. Chicago, American Medical Association, 1994.

Bick RL (ed): Hematology: Clinical and Laboratory Practice. St. Louis, Mosby–Year Book, 1993.

Borer WZ: Selection and use of laboratory tests. In Tietz NW, Conn RB, Pruden EL (eds): Applied Laboratory Medicine, pp 1–5. Philadelphia, WB Saunders Company, 1992.

Campion EW: A retreat from SI units. N Engl J Med 1992;327:49.

Friedman RB, Young DS: Effects of Disease on Clinical Laboratory Tests, 3rd ed. Washington, DC, AACC Press, 1997.

Henry JB: Clinical Diagnosis and Management by Laboratory Methods, 19th ed. Philadelphia, WB Saunders Company, 1996.

Hicks JM, Young DS: DORA '97–99: Directory of Rare Analyses. Washington, DC, AACC Press, 1997.

Jacobs DS, Demott WR, Grady HJ, et al: Laboratory Test Handbook, 4th ed. Baltimore, Williams & Wilkins, 1996.

Kaplan LA, Pesce AJ: Clinical Chemistry: Theory, Analysis, and Correlation, 3rd ed. St. Louis, CV Mosby Company, 1996.

Kjeldsberg CR, Knight JA: Body Fluids: Laboratory Examination of Amniotic, Cerebrospinal, Seminal, Serous and Synovial Fluids, 3rd ed. Chicago, ASCP Press, 1993.

Laposata M: SI Unit Conversion Guide. Boston, NEJM Books, 1992.

Scully RE, McNeely WF, Mark EJ, et al: Normal reference laboratory values. N Engl J Med 1992;327:718–724.

Speicher CE: The Right Test: A Physician's Guide to Laboratory Medicine, 2nd ed. Philadelphia, WB Saunders Company, 1993.

Tietz NW (ed): Clinical Guide to Laboratory Tests, 3rd ed. Philadelphia, WB Saunders Company, 1995.

Wallach J: Interpretation of Diagnostic Tests: A synopsis of Laboratory Medicine, 6th ed. Boston, Little, Brown and Company, 1996.

Young DS: Determination and validation of reference intervals. Arch Pathol Lab Med 1992;116:704–709.

Young DS: Implementation of SI units for clinical laboratory data. Ann Intern Med 1987;106:114–129.

Young DS: Effects of Drugs on Clinical Laboratory Tests, 4th ed. Washington, DC, AACC Press, 1995.

Young DS: Effects of Preanalytical Variables on Clinical Laboratory Tests, 2nd ed. Washington, DC, AACC Press, 1997.

Tables of Reference Intervals

Some of the values included in Tables 4 through 12 have been established by the Clinical Laboratories at Thomas Jefferson University Hospital, Philadelphia, PA, and have not been published elsewhere. Other values have been complied from the sources cited in the Bibliography. These tables are provided for information and educational purposes only. Laboratory values must always be interpreted in the context of clinical data derived from other sources, including the medical history and physical examination. Users must exercise individual judgment when employing the information provided in this appendix.

Index

Note: Page numbers in *italics* refer to illustrations; page numbers followed by t refer to tables.

Bezold-Jarisch reflex, in shock, 292
Bicarbonate. See *Sodium bicarbonate.*
Biceps tendinitis, 966, 971
Biceps test, for shoulder pain, 967
Bicuspid valve, congenital, 349
Bile acid sequestrants, for hyperlipidemia, 303
Biliary cirrhosis, diagnosis of, 485
Biliary colic, 499, 500t
Biliary tract. See also *Gallbladder.*
  dyskinesia of, 499, 500t
  nuclear scanning of, 501
  obstruction of, diagnosis of, 485
  symptoms of diseases of, 475–486. See also individual symptoms.
  ultrasonography of, 486
Bilious vomitus, 393
Bilirubin, excess of. See *Hyperbilirubinemia; Jaundice.*
  in ascitic fluid, 484
  in hemolytic anemia, 774
  measurement of, 476, 500t
  production and elimination of, 493–494
Bioelectromagnetic applications, 47
Biofeedback, 47
Biopsies. See also specific organs.
  for fever, 1109–1110
Bird fancier's lung, 200
Bisacodyl, 412t
Bismuth subsalicylate, for diarrhea, 41, 407, 408, 1123, 1126, 1126t
  for *Helicobacter pylori* infection, 427, 427t
  for peptic ulcers, 429
Bisphosphonates, for hypercalcemia, 244
  for osteoporosis, 930
  for Paget's disease, 933
Bites, animal, 1516–1519
  cat, 1516–1519
  dog, 1516–1519
  insect and spider, 1520–1523, 1521t
  snake, 1525–1528
Bitot's spots, 1140
Black cohosh, pharmacology of, 51t
Black widow spider, 1520, 1521t, 1522, 1523
Blackouts, alcoholic, 1474
Bladder cancer, 748–750
  hematuria from, 688
  staging of, 749t
Bladder irritability, from cancer, 748
Bladder obstruction, renal failure from, 713
Bladder tap, 732, 732–733, 733
Blastomycosis, 1111–1113
  adrenal insufficiency from, 863
  clinical findings in, 1112
  laboratory tests for, 1112
  laryngitis from, 83, 161
  symptoms of, 1111
  treatment of, 1112–1113
Bleeding. See *Hemorrhage.*
Bleeding disorders, 808–810. See also specific disorder.
  acquired, 808
  congenital, 808
  etiology of, 808
  laboratory tests for, 809, 809t
  treatment of, 810
Bleeding time, for epistaxis, 78
Bleomycin, for warts, 1249
  scleroderma from, 1037
Blepharitis, 56
  corneal ulceration from, 110
  management of, 57
Blindness, glaucoma and, 99
  in HIV disease, 947

Blood cultures, for *Borrelia burgdorferi,* 1152
  for endometritis, 592
  for fever, 1106
  for neutropenia, 785
  for orbital cellulitis, 143
  for pyelonephritis, 722
  for shock, 293
  for toxic shock, 1119
  for typhoid fever, 1160
Blood pressure. See also *Hypertension; Hypotension.*
  measurement of, 299
Blood products. See also *Transfusions.*
  anaphylaxis from, 959
Blood tests, for anemia, 764t
  hemolytic, 774
  megaloblastic, 771
  for back pain, 977
  for cardiomyopathy, 341
  for chest pain, 274
  for constipation, 411
  for diarrhea, 407, 409
  for GI bleeding, 401
  for heart failure, 327
  for hemoptysis, 156
  for leukemia, 792
  for neutropenia, 785
  for peripheral neuropathies, 1326
  for *Plasmodium,* 1157
  for sickle cell disease, 777
  for snakebites, 1526
  for thrombocytopenia, 789
  for vaginal bleeding, 517
  of sugar, for diabetes, 830
    for ketoacidosis, 837
  reference intervals for, 1543t–1544t
Blood transfusions. See *Transfusions.*
Blood typing, for first trimester bleeding, 656
  for pregnancy, 637
Blood urea nitrogen (BUN), in food poisoning, 1511
  in glomerulonephritis, 720
  in ketoacidosis, 838
  in prostatic hyperplasia, 739
  in renal failure, 713, 714, 716
Blood urea nitrogen/creatinine ratio, for oliguria, 697
Blood vomitus, 393
Bloom's syndrome, leukemia and, 791
"Blue bloater," 184
Blue dot sign, 525
Blue nevus, 1249
  differential diagnosis of, 1226
Blue toe syndrome, 389
Body composition analysis, 908
Body dysmorphic disorder, 1443
Body lice, 1294–1296
Body mass index, 903, 911, 911t
  calculations for, 915
Body temperature, measurement of, 1104
Body weight, excess. See *Obesity.*
  ideal, 908, 910t, 911
  loss of. See *Weight loss.*
  malnutrition and, 916
  measurement of, 908, 910t
Boeerhave's syndrome, 393
Bone biopsy, for Paget's disease, 933
Bone diseases, 926–936. See also *Musculoskeletal disorders; Osteo* entries.
  from blastomycosis, 263
  Paget's, 932–934
  symptoms of, 926–927
Bone marrow, aspiration and biopsy of, 794–796
  contraindications for, 794

Bone marrow (*Continued*)
  for Hodgkin's disease, 806
  for iron deficiency anemia, 767–768
  for leukemia, 792
  for lymphadenopathy, 800
  for lymphoma, 802
  for megaloblastic anemia, 770–771
  for neutropenia, 785
  for thrombocytopenia, 789
  indications for, 794
  technique for, 795, 795–796
  failure of, differential diagnosis of, 792–793
  transplantation of, for sickle cell disease, 779
  for thalassemia, 783
Bone marrow stain, for histoplasmosis, 260, 260t
Bone metastasis, hypercalcemia and, 244
Bone mineral density, 929
  classification of, 928t
  measurement of, 929, 929t
Bone pain, 926–927
  differential diagnosis of, 315
  from leukemia, 791
  from osteomyelitis, 935
  from Paget's disease, 932
  from polycythemia, 797
  tests for, 926–927
  treatment of, 927
Bone radiographs. See *Radiography.*
Bone scans, for ankle fractures, 1094
  for ankle pain, 989
  for back pain, 977
  for hand and wrist disorders, 975
  for knee pain, 987
  for leukemia, 792
  for neck pain, 963
  for pain and swelling, 926
  for reflex sympathetic dystrophy, 1366
  for tendinitis, 1001
Bone swelling, 926–927
BOOP (bronchiolitis obliterans with organizing pneumonia), 179, 183
Borderline personality disorder, 1428–1429
  differential diagnosis of, 1428, 1430, 1443
Bordetella parapertussis, bronchitis from, 178
Bordetella pertussis, bronchiectasis from, 182
  bronchitis from, 178
Borrelia burgdorferi, 1151–1153. See also *Lyme disease.*
  vaccine for, 11
Botanical medicine, 47
Botulinum toxin, for hyperhidrosis, 1210
Bouchard's nodules, 1010
Boutonnière deformity, 1091
Bowel cancer, diarrhea from, 408
Bowel sounds, abnormal, from diverticulitis, 462
Bowenoid papulosis, differential diagnosis of, 1256
Bowen's disease, differential diagnosis of, 1256
Boxer's fracture, 973
Brachial artery, arterial access via, 191, *191*
Brachial plexus traction injuries, 1365
Bradyarrhythmias, shock and, 292
  syncope and, 275
Bradycardia, in shock, 292
Bradykinesia, in Parkinson's disease, 1368
Brain abscess, differential diagnosis of, 1384
  from animal bites, 1517
  imaging of, 1381

Brain death, imaging of, 1381
Brain scan, for subdural hematoma, 1407
Brain stem aneurysms, differential diagnosis of, 1393
Brain stem auditory evoked responses, 69
Brain stem lesions, differential diagnosis of, in children, 1432
Brain tumor, 1389–1391
  clinical findings in, 1389–1390
  differential diagnosis of, 1376, 1390
  etiology of, 1389
  treatment of, 1390–1391
Branchial cleft cyst, 851
Brazelton Neonatal Behavioral Assessment Scale, 21
BRCA genes, 36
  breast cancer and, 530
  ovarian cancer and, 564, 565
Breast, abscess of, 649
  atypical hyperplasia of, 530
  cancer of, 241t, 530–532
    diagnosis of, 242
    differential diagnosis of, 528, 529
    estrogen replacement and, 598
    male, gynecomastia and, 825
    ovarian cancer and, 564
    screening for, 36
  duct atresia of, 509–510
  enlargement of, in pregnancy, 636
  pain of, 649
  fibrocystic disease of, 528–529
  fine-needle aspiration of, 531, *534, 534–535, 535*
  lumpectomy of, 531
  nipple discharges in, 509–510. See also *Nipple.*
  self-examination of, 36, 531
  stereotactic biopsy of, 531
Breast-feeding, 648–650
  hyperprolactinemia in, 870
  jaundice from, 475, 476, 477, 493, 494
  otitis media prevention and, 123
  pain and, 649
  physician promotion of, 648
  physician support of, 648–649
  postpartum depression and, 668
Breath holding, 1431–1432
Breath odor, abdominal pain and, from poisoning, 1500t
Breath test, for diarrhea, 409
Breathing, in CPR, 279–281, *280*
Breathlessness, from hyperventilation, 1464
Bretylium, for cardiac arrest, 319
Bright light therapy, for depression, 1448
Brodie-Trendelenburg test, for varicose veins, 376
Bromocriptine, for amenorrhea, 515
  for hyperprolactinemia, 871
  for Parkinson's disease, 1370
  for restless leg syndrome, 1032
Bronchial atresia, atelectasis from, 203
Bronchiectasis, 182–183
  pneumothorax and, 221
  treatment of, 183
Bronchiocephalic vein, displaced or dilated, 204–205
Bronchiolitis, 159, 167–168
  treatment of, 167–168
Bronchiolitis obliterans with organizing pneumonia (BOOP), 179, 183
Bronchitis, 178–180
  acute exacerbation of chronic, 179–180
    treatment of, 179–180, 180t
  acute infectious, 178–179
  chronic, 184–186

Bronchitis (*Continued*)
  atelectasis from, 202
  hemoptysis from, 155
Bronchoalveolar lavage, for interstitial lung disease, 197–198
  for sarcoidosis, 267
Bronchodilators, for asthma, 174t
  for bronchiectasis, 183
  for COPD, 185
  therapeutic range for, 1545t
Bronchogenic carcinoma, 205, 237–238. See also *Lung(s), cancer of.*
Broncholithiasis, atelectasis from, 202
Bronchopulmonary dysplasia, fetal lung immaturity and, 169
Bronchoscopy, for atelectasis, 203
    therapeutic, 205
  for cough, 149
  for hemoptysis, 156
  for interstitial lung disease, 197
  for lung cancer, 238
  for pleural effusion, 227
Bronze skin coloring, from hemochromatosis, 820
Brow block, 146, *146*
Brown-Marie syndrome, optic neuritis in, 115
Brown recluse spider, 1520, 1521t, 1522
Brucellosis, epididymitis from, 678
Brudzinski's sign, 1383
Bruit(s), arterial, from claudication, 290
  in peripheral disease, 384
  carotid, 1328
    TIAs and, 1332
  from temporal arteritis, 1044
Bruton agammaglobulinemia, 938, 939t
Budd-Chiari syndrome, ascites and, 480
  cirrhosis from, 496
Budesonide, for asthma, 175t
  for nasal polyps, 134
Buerger's disease, 384
  claudication from, 289
Bulimia nervosa, 919–921
  laboratory tests for, 920, 920t
  parotid gland enlargement in, 65
Bulk-forming laxatives, 412, 412t
Bullous impetigo, 1217
Bullous myringitis, 64
BUN. See *Blood urea nitrogen (BUN).*
Bundle-branch block, ECG of, *364*
  myocardial infarction and, 316
Bunion, 990
Buphthalmos, 99
Bupivacaine, for head and neck procedures, 145
  for reflex sympathetic dystrophy, 1366
Buprenorphine, abuse of, 1481
  for pain, 45t
Bupropion, for depression, 1449t, 1450t
  for nicotine withdrawal, 1488t
  therapeutic range for, 1545t
Burkitt's lymphoma, tumor lysis syndrome and, 246
Burns, 1301–1303
  classification of, 1301
  prevention of, 15
  Rule of Nines on, 1302
  treatment of, 1302
Burrow ink test, for scabies, 1291
Bursae, types of, 995
Bursectomy, 997
Bursitis, 966, 995–997
  differential diagnosis of, 997, 1043
  etiology of, 995
  iliopectineal or iliopsoas, 981
  ischial, 982

Bursitis (*Continued*)
  of heel, 989
  pes anserine, 986
  pes anserinus, 1048
  sites of, 996
  subacromial, injection for, 1017, *1017*
  symptoms of, 995
  tendinosis and, 998
  treatment of, 997
  trochanteric, 982
Buspirone, for obsessive compulsive disorder, 1497
Busulfan, for leukemia, 793
Butoconazole, for candidal vulvovaginitis, 569
Butorphanol, 1481
  for upper GI endoscopy, 432
Butyropenones, for nausea/vomiting, 394
Byssinosis, 200

C

C1 esterase inhibitor deficiency, 1188
CA 19-9 levels, in pancreatic cancer, 507
CA-125 levels, in ovarian cancer, 565
Cabergoline, for hyperprolactinemia, 871
Caffeine, abuse of, 1481
  headache and, 1346t
  palpitations and, 285
CAGE questions, 1415, 1474, 1474t
Calamine, for pruritus, 1187
Calcaneal apophysitis (Sever's disease), 989, 1000, 1000t
Calcaneal bursitis, 996
Calcaneal fracture, 989, 1073
Calcaneal spur, posterior, 1073
Calcifications, from hypercalcemia, 876
Calcinosis, subcutaneous, in scleroderma, 1037
Calcipotriene, for psoriasis, 1231
Calcitonin, assay of, for goiter, 828
  for hypercalcemia, 245, 877
  for osteoporosis, 930
  for Paget's disease, 933
Calcitriol, for hypocalcemia, 881
Calcium, deficiency of, 879–881
  excess of, 876–878
  for hypertension in pregnancy, 674
  for hypocalcemia, 880–881
  for menopause, 598
  for osteoporosis, 930
  measurement of, in hypercalcemia, 877
    in hypocalcemia, 880
  sequestration of, hypocalcemia from, 879
Calcium channel blockers, adverse effects of, 300
  antidote to, 1508t
  for cardiomyopathy, 341
  for coronary artery disease, 310
  for heart failure, 328
  for hypertension, 300
    in pregnancy, 674
  for myocardial infarction, 315
  for pulmonary edema, 325
  for Raynaud's phenomenon, 389
  for scleroderma, 1037
  for urinary incontinence, 702t
Calcium chloride, for sinus bradycardia, 363
Calcium gluconate, for latrodectism, 1523
Calcium oxalate crystals, 697, 709t, 710t
Calcium pyrophosphate deposition disease, differential diagnosis of, 1011, 1020
Calcium stones, renal, 708, 709t, 710t
  treatment of, 711

Closed-chest compression, in CPR, 281–282
Clostridial infections. See also specific species.
    anemia from, 773
Clostridium difficile, diarrhea from, 406, 1121, 1123, 1125
    in HIV disease, 948
    management of, 1125
    gastritis from, 425
    pseudomembranous colitis and, 1125
    treatment of, 407
Clostridium perfringens, abdominal pain from, 1499, 1500t
    diarrhea from, 406, 1121
    food poisoning from, 1510, 1512t
Clotrimazole, for candidiasis, in HIV disease, 949
    vulvovaginal, 520, 520t, 569
    for cutaneous mycoses, 1299
    for *Trichomonas vaginalis* infection, 569
Clozapine, for schizophrenia, 1492
Clubbing, from lung cancer, 238
    in interstitial lung disease, 197
Cluster headache, 1341, 1342, 1343
    differential diagnosis of, 1341, 1342, 1362
CMV. See *Cytomegalovirus (CMV)*.
Coagulation disorders, 808–810
    purpura from, 1193
    tendinitis and, 1001
Coagulation tests, for hemorrhoids, 466
    for leukemia, 792
    for snakebites, 1526
Coagulopathies, postpartum hemorrhage from, 663, 665
    subdural hematoma from, 1406
    transfusions for, 811–812
    vaginal bleeding in, 517
Coal tar, for psoriasis, 1230
Coal-miner's knee, 996
Cobalamin deficiency, 762, 770–772
    differential diagnosis of, 771
    treatment of, 771
Cocaine, abuse of, 1481
    for head and neck procedures, 145
    orbital cellulitis from, 142
    poisoning from, 1507
Coccidioidin skin test, 258
Coccidioidomycosis, 257–259, 1111–1113
    adrenal insufficiency from, 863
    clinical findings in, 258, 1112
    diagnosis of, 947
    disseminated, 258–259
    hypercalcemia in, 876
    in HIV disease, 257, 947
        treatment of, 949
    laboratory tests for, 1112
    laryngitis from, 83
    meningitis from, 1383
    pulmonary, 258
    symptoms of, 1111
    treatment of, 259, 1113
Cochlear implantation, for Ménière's disease, 1395
Codeine, 1481
    for common cold, 159
    for pain, 45t
    for restless leg syndrome, 1032
Cognitive-behavioral therapy, for personality disorders, 1429, 1430
Cognitive disorders, from fetal alcohol syndrome, 1477
    postconcussion, 1403t
Cognitive marital therapy, 1421

Cogwheel rigidity, in Parkinson's disease, 1368
Coitus interruptus, 609
Colchicine, for gout, 1020–1021
    for purpura, 1194
    for stomatitis, 95
Cold-induced urticaria, 1189
Cold intolerance, from anorexia, 919
    in hypothyroidism, 841
Cold-reactive antibodies, anemia and, 773
Cold-related disorders, 1532–1534
"Cold sores," 93, 94, 421–422
Colitis, amebic, 1174, 1175, 1175t, 1176
    diarrhea from, 408
    differential diagnosis of, 453, 457
    infectious, 457
    ischemic, 457
    pseudomembranous, 1125
    rectal bleeding from, 416
    ulcerative, 456–458. See also *Ulcerative colitis*.
Collagen vascular disease. See also individual diseases.
    aortic regurgitation and, 350
    cardiomyopathy in, 339
    pulmonary, 196
    stomatitis from, 93, 421
    tendinitis and, 1001
Collar, soft, for cervical spine injuries, 965
Colles' fracture, 973, 1087
    pediatric, 1087, 1088
    reduction of, 1088
    reverse, 1087
Colloid cyst, brain, 1389
Colon, alpha loops of, 444
    ascending, 444
    Crohn's disease of, 452
    descending, 444
    examination of, 444
    transverse, 444
Colonic transit studies, for constipation, 411
Colonoscopy, 442–445, *443, 444*
    for abdominal pain, 391
    for colorectal cancer, 439, 440, 441
    for Crohn's disease, 453
    for diarrhea, 1123
    for pelvic pain, 521
    for rectal bleeding, 418
    for ulcerative colitis, 457
    patient preparation for, 442
Colorectal cancer, 438–441, *439*
    differential diagnosis of, 457, 463, 473
    etiology of, 438–439
    genetics and, 438–439, *439*
    staging of, 440, 441t
    tests for, 440
        screening, 37, 439–440, 458
    treatment of, 440–441, 441t
        with estrogen, 596
Colorectal diseases. See also specific diseases.
    rectal bleeding from, 416
Colposcopy, 541–543, *541–543*
    contraindications for, 540, 541
    for cervical cancer, 548
    for vulvar pruritus, 523
    indications for, 539, 541
    technique for, *540–542, 542–543*
Comedones, 1214
Commissurotomy, for mitral stenosis, 347
Common cold, 158–160
    treatment of, 159
Common variable immunodeficiency disease, 938, 939t
Common warts, 1247

Compartment syndrome, elbow, 971
    from animal bites, 1517
    rhabdomyolysis and, 1029
    tendinitis and, 1000
Complement disorders, 939–940
Complement fixation test, for histoplasmosis, 261
Complement tests, for glomerulonephritis, 720
    for proteinuria, 692
Complete blood count (CBC), for abdominal pain, 391
    for abruptio placentae, 660
    for appendicitis, 436
    for ascariasis, 1183
    for ascites, 481
    for asthma, 173
    for bleeding disorders, 809, 809t
    for cheilitis, 97
    for costochondritis, 1023
    for decubitus ulcers, 1287
    for diverticulitis, 463
    for endometritis, 592
    for epistaxis, 78
    for fatigue, 1416
    for first trimester bleeding, 656
    for food poisoning, 1511
    for glomerulonephritis, 720
    for hematuria, 689
    for hip pain, 982
    for HIV disease, 943
    for Hodgkin's disease, 806
    for hookworms, 1184
    for hypernatremia, 893
    for hypertension, pregnancy-induced, 673
    for iron deficiency anemia, 767
    for ketoacidosis, 838
    for leukemia, 792
    for lymphoma, 802
    for malaria, 1157
    for neutropenia, 785
    for pelvic pain, 521
    for peripheral neuropathies, 1326
    for placenta previa, 659
    for poisonings, 1507
    for polycythemia, 798
    for polymyalgia rheumatica, 1042
    for postpartum hemorrhage, 664
    for pregnancy, 637
    for preterm labor, 653
    for rectal bleeding, 418
    for renal failure, 714
    for seizures, 1349
    for shock, 293
    for sickle cell disease, 777
    for Sjögren's syndrome, 104
    for snakebites, 1526
    for thrombocytopenia, 789
    preoperative, 30
Complex regional pain syndrome, 1365
    of ankle, 988, 989
Compression stockings, for leg edema, 289
    for stasis, 1285
    for varicose veins, 375
Compulsions, 1494. See also *Obsessive compulsive disorder*.
Computed tomography (CT), for abdominal pain, 391
    for Alzheimer's disease, 1373
    for amenorrhea, 515
    for ankle fractures, 1094
    for ankle pain, 989
    for aortic dissection, 353
    for appendicitis, 436
    for ascites, 481
    for atelectasis, 203

Cystitis, bladder cancer and, 748
  candidal, 1112
  from *Chlamydia trachomatis,* 577
  interstitial, dysuria from, 694
    treatment of, 695
  menopause and, 595
  pyelonephritis and, 722
  treatment of, 726t
Cystoid macular edema, 116
Cystoscopy, for bladder cancer, 749
  for hematuria, 690
  for penile discharge, 699
Cystourethrogram, voiding, in children, 730
Cystourethroscopy, for pelvic pain, 521
Cytarabine (ara-C), for leukemia, 793
Cytogenetics, for cancer, 241t
Cytokines, hypercalcemia of cancer and, 244
Cytomegalovirus (CMV), adrenal insufficiency from, 863
  aphthous stomatitis from, 93
  fever from, 1108
  from transfusions, 815
  hyperbilirubinemia from, 494
  in HIV disease, diagnosis of, 948
    treatment of, 950
  infectious mononucleosis from, 1142
  jaundice from, 479
  parotitis from, 65
  prevention of, in transfusions, 812
  pulmonary, 200
  stomatitis from, 421
  treatment of, 950
Cytosine arabinoside, hypocalcemia from, 879
Cytotoxic therapy. See also individual agents.
  for hemolytic anemia, 775
  for interstitial lung disease, 198
  leukemia from, 791
  neutropenia from, 784

D

Dacryoadenitis, 59
Dacryocystitis, 59, 143
Danazol, adverse effects of, 589
  for contraception, 609
  for endometriosis, 518, 589
  for purpura, 1194
Dapsone, for *Pneumocystis carinii* infection, 944, 949
    in HIV disease, 950
  for purpura, 1194
  for toxoplasmosis, 945
Daunorubicin, for Kaposi's sarcoma, 950
  for leukemia, 793
  nausea and vomiting from, 1504
de Musset's sign, 350
de Quervain's tenosynovitis, 973, 975
de Quervain's thyroiditis, 844, 845, 853t, 857–858
Deafness. See *Hearing loss.*
Débridement, of animal bite wounds, 1517
  of burns, 1302
  of frostbite wounds, 1533
Decision-making capacity, 30, 34
Decongestants, for rhinitis, 131
  for sinusitis, 141
Decubitus ulcers, 1287–1289
  prevention of, 1288–1289
  treatment of, 1287–1288
Deep muscle relaxation exercises, 1461–1463

Deep venous thrombosis (DVT), 379–383
  cellulitis and, 1128
  clinical findings in, 379
  differential diagnosis of, 380, *381*
  etiology of, 379
  laboratory findings in, 380
  treatment of, 381–383, 381t, 382t
DEET, 41
Deferiprone, for hemochromatosis, 821
Deferoxamine, 1503
  for hemochromatosis, 821
Defibrillation, 282, 320, 321–323
  for heart failure, 329
  indications for, 321
  technique for, 321–323, *322, 323*
Dehydration, from food poisoning, 1511
  from poisoning, 1501t
  shock and, 291
Dehydroepiandrosterone, hirsutism from, 823
  measurement of, 823
Delavirdine, 944, 949
Delirium, 1338–1340
  causes of, 1338, 1338t
  clinical findings in, 1338, 1339t
  differential diagnosis of, 1373
  treatment of, 1339–1340, 1340t
Delta agent, 491
Delusional disorder, 1491–1492
Delusions, 1339t
  in Alzheimer's disease, 1374
  in schizophrenia, 1490
Dementia, Alzheimer's, 1372–1374
  differential diagnosis of, 1339t
  drug-induced, 1373
  imaging of, 1381
  multiple infarct, 1373
  with Lewy bodies, 1373
Demodex folliculorum, rosacea and, 1304
Dennie-Morgan line, 1199
Dental health, assessment of, 14t, 15
Dental procedures, anesthesia for, 145–147
Dental sinusitis, nasal polyps and, 133
Denture stomatitis, 96
Denver Developmental Screening Test II (DDST II), 21, 26, 27–28
Deoxycoformycin, for leukemia, 793
Dependence. See also *Alcoholism; Substance abuse.*
  definition of, 1480
Dependent personality disorder, 1429–1430
Depigmentation, for vitiligo, 1239
Depot medroxyprogesterone acetate (Depo-Provera), 606–607
  adverse effects of, 607
Depression, 1447–1451
  alcoholism and, 1474
  Alzheimer's disease and, 1374
  anxiety and, 1459
  appetite loss from, 902, 903t
  assessment of, 12
  differential diagnosis of, 1369, 1373, 1430, 1443, 1448, 1459, 1496
  etiology of, 1447
  hyperprolactinemia and, 870
  medications for, 1448–1449, 1449t, 1450t
    dosages of, 1449t
    side effects of, 1450t
  panic attacks and, 1456
  phobia and, 1468
  postpartum, 667–669
  suicide and, 1452
  tests for, 1448
  treatment of, 1448–1449
Dercum's disease, 1264

Dermabrasion, for tattoo removal, 1308
Dermatitis, 1199–1206
  atopic, 1199–1201, 1206
    differential diagnosis of, 1290
  contact, 1205–1206
    differential diagnosis of, 1206, 1212, 1213, 1290, 1304
    nails and, 1279
  drug-induced, 953
  herpetiformis, 1245
    differential diagnosis of, 1290
  malnutrition and, 908
  periorbital, differential diagnosis of, 1304
  pruritus from, 1186
  seborrheic, 1202–1204
    differential diagnosis of, 1203, 1206, 1213, 1230, 1233, 1304
    vulvar pruritus in, 523
  vaginal, 518
Dermatofibroma, 1226
Dermatographism, 1189
  atopic dermatitis and, 1199
Dermatology. See *Skin; Skin diseases.*
Dermatomyositis, 1039–1041
  interstitial lung disease in, 196
  treatment of, 1040
Dermatophyte infections, 1297–1300
  dermatitis from, 1199
  of nails, 1276, 1276t
Dermoid tumors, brain, 1389
  orbital, 59
Dermonecrotic lesions, from spider bites, 1520, 1521t, 1522
  treatment of, 1523
Desensitization, for drug allergy, 954
  for phobia, 1468
Desipramine, for attention deficit hyperactivity disorder, 1436, 1437t
  for depression, 1449t, 1450t
  therapeutic range for, 1545t
Desmopressin, for enuresis, 704
  for hemophilia, 810
  for uterine bleeding, 556
Detoxification, from alcohol, 1475
  from drugs, 1480, 1483–1484
Development, accident and injury prevention by stages of, 12, 14t, 15
  charts on, *22–24*
  delays in, 25
    epidemiology of, 25
    etiology of, 25
    prevention of, 29
    risk factors for, 25
    screening for, 26–29
  disorders of. See also *Growth, abnormal.*
    attention deficit and, 1435
    bronchiectasis in, 182
    guidelines on, 18–24
    screening for, 21, 25
    surveillance of, 25–29
Devic's disease, 1377
Dexamethasone, for adrenal insufficiency, 865
  for croup, 165
  for fetal lung immaturity, 171
  for hirsutism, 824
  for nasal polyps, 134
  for pain, 45t
  for preterm labor, 654
  for purpura, 1194
  for spinal cord compression, 246
  for stomatitis, 94
  suppression test with, for Cushing's syndrome, 861
Dexedrine, for attention deficit hyperactivity disorder, 1436, 1437t

Elderly, appetite loss in, 902, 903t
  falls of, 1335–1337
  fecal impaction in, 472
  fever in, 1106
  osteoporosis in, 930
  stomatitis in, 96
  substance abuse in, 1480
  urinary tract infections in, 725
Electrocardiography (ECG), defibrillation
    and, 321
  for aortic regurgitation, 350
  for aortic stenosis, 349
  for atrioventricular blocks, 372, 372,
    373, 373
  for cardiac arrest, 318
  for cardiomyopathy, 340
  for chest pain, 274
  for coronary artery disease, 309
  for costochondritis, 1023
  for GI bleeding, 401
  for heart failure, 327
  for hyperkalemia, 887, 887
  for hypokalemia, 890
  for ketoacidosis, 838
  for mitral regurgitation, 343
  for mitral stenosis, 346
  for myocardial infarction, 314
  for nausea and vomiting, 1504
  for obesity, 912
  for palpitations, 285–286
  for pericarditis, 361
  for pneumothorax, 222
  for poisonings, 1507
  for pulmonary edema, 324
  for sarcoidosis, 267
  for sepsis, 1115
  for shock, 293
  for sinus rhythms and ectopic beats, 363–
    366, 363–366, 363t
  for stress testing, 311, 311–312, 312
  for stroke, 1329
  for supraventricular tachyarrhythmias,
    367–369, 367–369
  for syncope, 276
  preoperative, 30
  stress, for coronary artery disease, 309
Electrocautery, for anogenital warts, 1256
  for skin diseases, 1252–1254, 1253
Electrocochleography, for Ménière's disease,
    1393
Electroconvulsive therapy, for depression,
    1448
Electrodessication and curettage, for basal
    and squamous cell carcinoma, 1220
Electroencephalography (EEG), for Alzhei-
    mer's disease, 1373
  for delirium, 1339
  for head trauma, 1401
  for postconcussion syndrome, 1404
  for schizophrenia, 1491
  for seizures, 1349
  for subdural hematoma, 1407
Electrolytes, disorders of, cardiac arrest
    from, 318
    delirium and, 1338
    food poisoning and, 1511
    hypovolemia and, 899t
    palpitations and, 285
  in parenteral nutrition, 924
  measurement of, for fatigue, 1416
    for glomerulonephritis, 720
    for leukemia, 792
    for snakebites, 1526
Electromyography (EMG), for back pain, 977
  for elbow pain, 972
  for Guillain-Barré syndrome, 1397

Electromyography (Continued)
  for hand and wrist disorders, 975
  for myasthenia gravis, 1376
  for neck pain, 963
  for paresthesias, 1324
  for peripheral neuropathies, 1326
  for polymyositis, 1040
  for shoulder pain, 967
Electron microscopy, in cancer, 241t
Electronystagmography, for postconcussion
    syndrome, 1404
Electrophoresis, for polycythemia, 797t
Electrophysiologic studies, for heart failure,
    328
  for syncope, 276
ELISA. See Enzyme-linked immunosorbent
    assay (ELISA).
Elliot's sclerocorneal trephine, for glaucoma,
    100
Elliptocyes, 774
Elliptocytosis, hereditary, 763, 773
  spherocytic, 773
  stomatocytic, 773
Embolism. See also Thromboembolism.
  air, from transfusions, 815
  claudication from, 289
  pulmonary, 206–207. See also Pulmonary
    embolism.
EMG. See Electromyography (EMG).
EMLA cream, for circumcision, 751
  for head and neck procedures, 145
Emollients, for atopic dermatitis, 1200
  for dry skin, 1191–1192
  for pruritus, 1187
Emotion-focused couple therapy, 1420,
    1421
Emotional status, assessment of, 12, 13t
Emphysema, 184–186
Emphysematous gastritis, 425
Empyema, tube thoracostomy for, 224–225
Enalapril, for heart failure, 328
  for pulmonary edema, 325
Enalaprilat, for hypertension, 300
Encephalitis, from herpes simplex virus,
    1242
  from Lyme disease, 1151
  optic neuritis in, 115
Encephalomyelitis, acute disseminated, optic
    neuritis in, 115
Encephalopathy, from toxic shock, 1118
  Wernicke's, 1470–1471
Endobronchial obstruction, atelectasis from,
    202
  bronchiectasis from, 182
Endobronchial tumors, atelectasis from, 202
  hemoptysis from, 155
Endocarditis, 355–359
  aortic regurgitation and, 350
  etiology of, 355, 355t
  fever from, 1108
  from aspergillosis, 1112
  glomerulonephritis and, 719, 720
  immune status and, 937
  in IV drug abusers, 355, 355t, 358
  native valve, 355, 355t
  prophylaxis for, 357t, 358t, 359
    in mitral valve prolapse, 345
  prosthetic valve, 355, 355t, 358
  tests for, 356
  treatment of, 356–357, 357t
Endocrine disorders. See also specific disor-
    ders.
  amenorrhea and, 514
  common symptoms of, 823–829
  eating disorders and, 921
  from brain tumor, 1390

Endocrine disorders (Continued)
  from exercise, 306
  hypertension from, 300
  irritability from, 1417
  leg edema and, 287, 288
  male sexual dysfunction from, 628
  management of, in preoperative setting, 31
  myofascial syndromes and, 1025
  myopathies from, 1376
  nausea/vomiting in, 393
  obesity from, 911, 912
  osteoporosis from, 930t
  pruritus from, 1186
  undescended testicle and, 686
  vaginal bleeding in, 516
Endocrine effects, of exercise, 305
Endocrinopathies, anemia from, 762
Endometrial biopsy, for vaginal bleeding,
    517
Endometriosis, 588–590
  differential diagnosis of, 512, 565
  dysmenorrhea and, 510, 511
  infertility and, 625
  pelvic inflammatory disease and, 573
  pelvic pain in, 521
  vulvar, 585
Endometritis, 591–594
  differential diagnosis of, 592
  etiology of, 591
  from Chlamydia trachomatis, 577
  laboratory findings in, 592
  risk factors for, 592
  treatment of, 592–593
Endometrium, biopsy of, 551, 552, 558–
    560, 559
    for abnormal uterine bleeding, 555
    for infertility workup, 627t
    uterine dilatation and curettage after,
      561–563
  cancer of, 551–553, 551t, 552t
    biopsy for, 558–560
    estrogen replacement and, 598
    laboratory findings in, 551–552
    risk factors for, 551t
    screening for, 37
    staging of, 552t
  cultures of, for endometritis, 592
  dilatation and curettage of, 551–552,
    561–563
  hyperplasia of, 552
    biopsy for, 558–560
  inflammation of, 591–594. See also En-
    dometritis.
  polyps of, vaginal bleeding in, 517
  thickening of, uterine bleeding and, 554
Endophthalmitis, candidal, 1112
Endoscopic papillotomy, for pancreatitis,
    504
Endoscopic retrograde cholangiopancreatog-
    raphy, 486, 495, 501, 504, 507,
    1381
Endoscopy, for amebiasis, 1176
  for colorectal cancer, 440
  for constipation, 411
  for diverticulitis, 463
  for gastritis, 426
  for gastroesophageal reflux, 423
  for GI bleeding, 401–402
  for heartburn, 398
  for intestinal obstruction, 447
  for peptic ulcer diagnosis, 429
  for variceal bleeding, 402
  intraoperative, for rectal bleeding, 419
  upper gastrointestinal, 432–434, 433, 434
Endotoxins, 1114
  atelectasis from, 203

Hereditary nonpolyposis colorectal cancer, 438
Hernia, disk, 964
  hiatal, pain of, 397
    reflux esophagitis and, 423
  incarcerated, 525
  inguinal, 525
  small bowel, 446
  undescended testicle and, 685
Heroin, 1481. See also *Opioids.*
Herpangina, differential diagnosis of, 1241
  sore throat and, 151
Herpes gestationis, 1245
Herpes labialis, 93, 94, 421–422, 1241, 1242
  treatment of, 1242, 1242t
Herpes simplex virus (HSV), 1241–1243
  Bell's palsy and, 1359
  cervicitis from, 571–572, 1241
  conjunctivitis from, 106, 108, 1241, 1242
  dermatitis from, 1199
  differential diagnosis of, 582, 583, 1241–1242
  fever from, 1108
  genital, 1241
    treatment of, 1242, 1242t
  in HIV disease, 947
    prophylaxis for, 949
  laboratory tests for, 1241
  meningitis from, 1383
  of nails, 1278
  oral, 1241, 1242
  Pap smear and, 538
  screening for, in pregnancy, 637
  skin lesions from, 1241–1243
    differential diagnosis of, 1218
  sore throat and, 151, 1241
  stomatitis from, 93, 94, 96, 421–422, 1241
  symptoms of, 1241
  treatment of, 1242, 1242t
  urethritis from, 699, 734
  vaginal, 518
Herpes zoster, 1131, 1133–1134, 1244–1246. See also *Varicella-zoster virus (VZV).*
  differential diagnosis of, 1023, 1212, 1213
  in HIV disease, 1133
  ophthalmicus, 59, 1244
Herpetic gingivostomatitis, 93, 94, 96, 1241
  acute primary, 421
Herpetic whitlow, 1241
Hiatal hernia, pain of, 397
  reflux esophagitis and, 423
Hiccups, 90–92
  causes of, 90, 90t
  management of, 91–92, 91t
High-altitude disorders, 41–42, 1535–1536
High-frequency ventilation, 214–215
Hill-Sachs lesion, 1075
Hill's sign, 350
Hip, fracture of, 981
  osteoporosis and, 928
  pain in, 981–983
    differential diagnosis of, 981–982
    management of, 983
    rheumatoid arthritis in, 1013
Hip flexor stretching, 980
Hip joint aspiration, 983
Hirsutism, 823–824, 1196
  in Cushing's syndrome, 860
  management of, 824
Histamine 1 blockers, for anaphylaxis, 961

Histamine 2 blockers, for anaphylaxis, 961
  for gastroesophageal reflux, 424
  for heartburn, 399
  for peptic ulcers, 429
  for scleroderma, 1037
  for urticaria, 1190
Histiocytosis X, dermatitis in, 1200
Histoplasma antigen assay, 260, 260t
Histoplasmosis, 260–262, 1111–1113
  adrenal insufficiency from, 863
  atelectasis from, 202
  clinical findings in, 1112
  differential diagnosis of, 268, 806
  disseminated, 260
  fever from, 1108
  gastritis from, 425
  hypercalcemia in, 876
  in HIV disease, diagnosis of, 948
    treatment of, 950
  laboratory tests for, 1112
  laryngitis from, 83, 161
  pulmonary, 199, 260
  symptoms of, 1111
  treatment of, 261–262, 261t, 950, 1113
Histrionic personality disorder, 1428, 1430
HIV. See *Human immunodeficiency virus (HIV).*
Hives. See *Urticaria.*
HLA types, narcolepsy and, 1355
  scleroderma and, 1036
  Sjögren's syndrome and, 103
  temporal arteritis and, 1044
HMG CoA reductase inhibitors, for hyperlipidemia, 303, 304t
HMGI-C gene, 1264
Hoarseness, 83–85
  acute, 83–84
  chronic, 84
  from laryngitis, 161
  from lung cancer, 238
  management of, 84–85
  rhinolaryngoscopy for, 86
Hodgkin's disease, 240, 805–807
  laboratory tests for, 805–806
  lymphadenopathy in, 801t, 805
  staging of, 806
  symptoms of, 805
  treatment of, 806
Holotranscobalamin II, 771
Holter monitoring, for palpitations, 286
  for syncope, 276
Homan's sign, 379
Home Screening Questionnaire, 28
Homeopathy, 46–47
Homeostatic disorders, irritability from, 1417
Homocystinuria, claudication from, 289
Homosexuals, diarrhea in, 406
  hepatitis in, 478
  HIV disease in, 941
  lymphogranuloma venereum in, 579
Honeybee stings, 1520–1523
Hookworm infections, 1166, 1167, 1184–1185
Hopkins Symptom Checklist, 1458
Hordeolum, 59
Hormonal tests, for ectopic pregnancy, 600
  for hair loss, 1197
Hormonal therapy. See also specific hormones.
  breast cancer and, 530, 532
  for endometriosis, 589
  for male sexual dysfunction, 629
  for uterine bleeding, 556
  for vaginal bleeding, 517
Horner's syndrome, from lung cancer, 238

Hornet stings, 1520–1523
Horse chestnut, pharmacology of, 53t
Horton's cephalalgia, 1362
Hot flashes, menopause and, 595
Household chemical ingestions, abdominal pain from, 1499
Housemaid's knee, 996
HPV. See *Human papillomavirus (HPV).*
HSV. See *Herpes simplex virus (HSV).*
Human bites, 1516
Human herpesvirus 8, Kaposi's sarcoma and, 1227
Human immunodeficiency virus (HIV), 941, 943
  diagnosis of, 941, 943–944
  from transfusions, 815
  screening for, in pregnancy, 637
Human immunodeficiency virus (HIV) disease, 941–950
  adrenal insufficiency in, 863
  anemia in, 762
  asymptomatic, 941–942
  Bell's palsy and, 1359
  CD4 cell counts in, 941, 942, 943, 944, 945, 947, 949
  cervical cancer and, 36
  coccidioidomycosis in, 257, 947, 949
  cryptococcosis in, 948, 949–950
  cytomegalovirus in, 948, 950
  diarrhea in, 407, 410
    diagnosis of, 1123
  differential diagnosis of, 941, 944
  early symptomatic, 943–946
  etiology of, 941
  fever in, 1108
  hair disorders in, 1273
  herpes zoster in, 1133
  histoplasmosis in, 948, 950
  Hodgkin's disease and, 805
  immunizations in, 942, 945
  infectious mononucleosis in, 1142
  influenza vaccine and, 1149
  Kaposi's sarcoma in, 948, 1227–1228
  laboratory tests for, in asymptomatic phase, 941
    in early symptomatic phase, 943–944
  late symptomatic, 947–950
  lymphadenopathy in, 801t
  lymphoma and, 802
  Mycobacterium avium-complex in, 947, 948, 949, 950
  neutropenia in, 784
  opportunistic infections in, diagnosis of, 944, 947–948
    prophylaxis against, 942, 944–945, 949
    treatment of, 945, 949–950
  optic neuritis from, 115
  paresthesias in, 1323
  parotitis in, 65
  protozoal/helminthic infections and, 1166
  psoriasis in, 1229–1230
  sexual abuse and, 1426
  stomatitis and, 93, 94, 95, 96, 421
  syphilis and, 584, 944
  thrombocytopenia and, 787
  toxoplasmosis in, 944, 948, 950
  treatment of, in asymptomatic stage, 941–942
    in early symptomatic phase, 944–945
    in late symptomatic phase, 949–950
  tuberculosis and, 248, 948, 949, 950
  vulvovaginal pruritus in, 523
Human leukocyte antigen types. See *HLA types.*

Preterm labor, 651–655, 654t
  laboratory findings in, 653
  prevention of, 654–655
  treatment of, 653–654
Priapism, from sickle cell disease, 777
PRICE(M) mnemonic, for ankle sprains, 993
  for bursitis, 997
  for hand and wrist injuries, 975
  for tendinitis, 1001
Prickly heat, 1208
Primaquine, for malaria, 41
Primidone, therapeutic range for, 1545t
Prinzmetal's angina, pain from, 273
  shock and, 292
Probenecid, for gout, 1021
Probucol, for hyperlipidemia, 303
Procainamide, therapeutic range for, 1545t
Procarbazine, for Hodgkin's disease, 806
Prochlorperazine, for Ménière's disease, 1394
Proctitis, from ulcerative colitis, 456, 457
  penile discharge and, 699
  treatment of, 457
  ulcerative, management of, 410
Proctocolitis, from lymphogranuloma venereum, 579
Proctosigmoidoscopy, for rectal bleeding, 418
Progesterone, for menopause, 597, 597t
  for premenstrual syndrome, 603
  test of, for ectopic pregnancy, 600
  for infertility workup, 627t
Progestin, challenge test of, 515
  contraception with, 608, 609. See also *Oral contraceptives.*
  adverse effects of, 608
  cycle of, amenorrhea and, 515
  replacement of, in menopause, 597, 597t
  uterine bleeding and, 554, 556
Projectile vomiting, 393
Prokinetic agents, for gastroesophageal reflux, 424
  for heartburn, 399
  for irritable bowel syndrome, 460
Prolactin, assay of, 515
  excess of, 870–872
Prolactinomas, 514
  hyperprolactinemia from, 870
Prolymphocytic leukemia, 791
Promethazine, for Ménière's disease, 1394
Pronator teres syndrome, 971
Propamidine isethionate, for corneal ulceration, 111
Propantheline, for urinary incontinence, 702t
Propionibacterium, acne from, 1214
  otitis externa from, 127
Propofol, for endotracheal intubation, 211
Propoxyphene, abuse of, 1481
  for pain, 45t
  for restless leg syndrome, 1032, 1358
Propranolol, for aortic dissection, 354
  for autism, 1440
  for esophageal varices, 497
  for hyperthyroidism, 846
  hypoglycemia from, 882
  therapeutic range for, 1545t
Propylthiouracil, for goiter, 829
  for hyperthyroidism, 846
Prostacyclins, for Raynaud's phenomenon, 389
Prostaglandin(s), E₁, for male sexual dysfunction, 629
  for Raynaud's phenomenon, 389
  F₂ₐ, for postpartum hemorrhage, 666

Prostaglandin(s) (*Continued*)
  for induction of labor, 671
  for peptic ulcers, 430
  septic shock and, 1114
Prostate, cancer of, 241t, 242, 742–744
  diagnosis of, 242, 743
  differential diagnosis of, 740, 933
  hematuria from, 688
  screening for, 38
  staging of, 742t
  treatment of, 743–744, 743t
  examination of, 738
  fine-needle aspiration of, 743
  hyperplasia of, benign, 739–741
    hematuria from, 688
    oliguria from, 696
  transurethral resection of, for cancer, 742, 743
    for hyperplasia, 740
Prostate-specific antigen (PSA), 739, 742, 743
Prostatectomy, for cancer, 743
  for hyperplasia, 740
Prostatitis, 737–738
  bacterial, 737
  differential diagnosis of, 738, 740
  dysuria from, 693
  epididymitis and, 678
  immune status and, 937
  nonbacterial, 737
  penile discharge and, 698
  treatment of, 695, 738
Prostatocystitis, dysuria from, 693
Prostatodynia, 737
Prostatosis, 737
Protease inhibitors, 942, 944, 949
Protein, determination of requirements for, 910, 917
  in parenteral nutrition, 924
  in ascitic fluid, 484
  measurement of body, 909, 910t
  in malnutrition, 917
Protein C deficiency, deep venous thrombosis and, 379
Protein S deficiency, deep venous thrombosis and, 379
Protein-energy malnutrition, 497, 908, 916, 923
  corneal ulceration from, 110
  hair disorders in, 1273
Proteinuria, 690–693
  glomerular, 690
  in children, 728–729
  orthostatic, 693
  overflow, 691, 692
  pregnancy-related hypertension and, 672, 673t
  transient, 691, 692, 693
  tubular, 691, 692
Proteus, Bartholin's gland abscess from, 586
  endometritis from, 591
  epididymitis from, 678
  gastritis from, 425
  pneumonia from, 199
  pyelonephritis from, 722
  urinary tract infections from, in children, 728
Proteus syndrome, 1264
Prothrombin time, in bleeding disorders, 809, 809t
  in cirrhosis, 497
  in DIC, 818
  in epistaxis, 78
  in hematuria, 689
Proton pump inhibitors, for gastroesophageal reflux, 424
  for heartburn, 399

Proton pump inhibitors (*Continued*)
  for peptic ulcers, 429, 430
  for scleroderma, 1037
Protozoal infections, 1166–1168, 1174–1176. See also individual species and diseases.
  diarrhea from, 406
  geographic distribution of, 1166t
  symptoms of, 1166–1169
Protriptyline, for depression, 1449t, 1450t
  for narcolepsy, 1356
  for sleep apnea, 272
Proximal interphalangeal joint, dislocation of, 1081–1082
Pruritic urticarial papules and plaques of pregnancy, 1186, 1291
Pruritus, 1186–1188
  anal, from pinworms, 1170
  etiology of, 1186
  from atopic dermatitis, 1199
  from food allergy, 956
  from Hodgkin's disease, 805
  from pityriasis rosea, 1233
  from polycythemia, 797
  from renal failure, 716
  from seborrheic dermatitis, 1203
  from varicella, 1132
  jaundice and, 478, 479
  management of, 1187–1188
  tests for, 1187
  vulvar, 523–524
PSA (prostate-specific antigen), 739, 742, 743
Pseudoephedrine, for common cold, 159
  for rhinitis, 131
  for sinusitis, 141
Pseudogout, differential diagnosis of, 1011, 1014, 1020
Pseudohyperkalemia, 885
Pseudohypoglycemia, 884
Pseudokidney sign, in intussusception, 450
Pseudomembranous colitis, 1125
Pseudomonas, from aquatic injuries, 1537–1538
  from transfusions, 816
  otitis externa from, 127
  septic shock from, 1114, 1116
  urinary tract infections from, in children, 728
Pseudoprolactinomas, 871
Pseudotumor cerebri, CSF characteristics in, 1388t
Psilocybin, 1481
Psittacosis, pulmonary, 200
Psoas sign, 435–436
Psoralen, for alopecia, 1198
  for psoriasis, 1230
  for vitiligo, 1239
Psoriasis, 1229–1231
  differential diagnosis of, 583, 1203, 1206, 1233, 1236
  guttate, 1229, 1230
  in HIV disease, 1229–1230
  inversus, 1229
  of nails, 1229, 1278–1279, 1279t
Psoriatic arthritis, 1229, 1230
  differential diagnosis of, 1014
Psychiatric disorders, 1411–1498. See also *Behavioral disorders.*
  alcoholism and, 1473–1476
  chest pain from, 273
  depression and, 1447–1451
  diarrhea in, 408
  eating disorders and, 921
  generalized anxiety and, 1458–1460
  hyperventilation and, 1464–1466

ISBN 0-7216-8002-X

90071